Cardiovascular Pharmacotherapeutics

SECOND EDITION

NOTICE

Medicine is an ever-changing science. As new research and clinical experience broaden our knowledge, changes in treatment and drug therapy are required. The editors and the publisher of this work have checked with sources believed to be reliable in their efforts to provide information that is complete and generally in accord with the standards accepted at the time of publication. However, in view of the possibility of human error or changes in medical sciences, neither the editors nor the publisher nor any other party who has been involved in the preparation or publication of this work warrants that the information contained herein is in every respect accurate or complete, and they disclaim all responsibility for any errors or omissions or for the results obtained from use of the information contained in this work. Readers are encouraged to confirm the information contained herein with other sources. For example and in particular, readers are advised to check the product information sheet included in the package of each drug they plan to administer to be certain that the information contained in this work is accurate and that changes have not been made in the recommended dose or in the contraindications for administration. This recommendation is of particular importance in connection with new or infrequently used drugs.

Cardiovascular Pharmacotherapeutics

SECOND EDITION

EDITED BY:

William H. Frishman, M.D., M.A.C.P.
The Barbara and William Rosenthal
Professor and Chairman
Department of Medicine
Professor of Pharmacology
New York Medical College
Director of Medicine
Westchester Medical Center
Valhalla, New York

Edmund H. Sonnenblick, M.D.
Edmond J. Safra Distinguished Professor of Medicine
Chief Emeritus, Division of Cardiology
Albert Einstein College of Medicine
Bronx, New York

Domenic A. Sica, M.D.
Professor of Medicine and Pharmacology
Chairman, Section of Clinical Pharmacology
Division of Nephrology
Medical College of Virginia
Virginia Commonwealth University
Richmond, Virginia

McGRAW-HILL
MEDICAL PUBLISHING DIVISION

New York   Chicago   San Francisco   Lisbon   London
Madrid   Mexico City   Milan   New Delhi   San Juan
Seoul   Singapore   Sydney   Toronto

Cardiovascular Pharmacotherapeutics, Second Edition

Copyright © 2003, 1997 by The **McGraw-Hill Companies**, Inc. All rights reserved. Printed in the United States of America. Except as permitted under the United States Copyright Act of 1976, no part of this publication may be reproduced or distributed in any form or by any means, or stored in a database or retrieval system, without the prior written permission of the publisher.

1 2 3 4 5 6 7 8 9 0 KGP/KGP 0 9 8 7 6 5 4 3 2

ISBN 0-07-136981-3

This book was set in Times Roman by TechBooks.
The editors were Darlene Cooke and Nicky Panton.
The production supervisor was Catherine Saggese.
The cover designer was Janice Bielawa.
The index was prepared by Jerry Ralya.
Quebecor/Kingsport was the printer and binder.

This book is printed on acid-free paper.

Library of Congress Cataloging-in-Publication Data

Cardiovascular pharmacotherapeutics / [editors] William H. Frishman, Edmund
   Sonnenblick, Domenic Sica.
        p.   cm.
     Includes bibliographical references and index.
     ISBN 0-07-136981-3
     1. Cardiovascular agents.   I. Sonnenblick, Edmund H., 1932–   II. Frishman, William H.,
1946–   III. Sica, Domenic A.

RM345 .F75   2002
616.1′061—dc21   2002017298

*To our patients and students who
have made our careers in medicine worthwhile.*

*To our wives, children, and grandchildren
who have made our lives worthwhile.*

Contents

Contributors

Jonathan Abrams, M.D.   [14]
Department of Medicine
Division of Cardiology
University of New Mexico School of Medicine
Albuquerque, New Mexico

Naveen Acharya, M.D.   [35]
Department of Internal Medicine
Cleveland Clinic Foundation
Cleveland, Ohio

Yogesh K. Agarwal, M.D.   [25]
Department of Medicine
Division of Cardiology
New York Medical College
Westchester Medical Center
Valhalla, New York

Brian A. Ahangar, M.D.   [43]
Department of Medicine
New York Medical College
Westchester Medical Center
Valhalla, New York

Piero Anversa, M.D.   [37, 42]
Cardiovascular Institute
Department of Medicine
New York Medical College
Valhalla, New York

Masoud Azizad, M.D.   [25]
Department of Medicine
USC School of Medicine
Santa Barbara Cottage Hospital
Santa Barbara, California

Michael Balazy, Ph.D.   [45]
Department of Pharmacology
New York Medical College
Valhalla, New York

Steven R. Bergmann, M.D., Ph.D.   [4]
Departments of Medicine & Radiology
Columbia University College of Physicians & Surgeons
New York, New York

Laura Bienenfeld, M.D.   [2]
Department of Medicine
Mt. Sinai Medical Center
New York, New York

D. Craig Brater, M.D.   [Foreword]
Office of the Dean
Indiana University School of Medicine
Indianapolis, Indiana

Mary Welna Brown, R.N., M.S.   [3]
University of Rochester School of Medicine
Rochester, New York

Peter M. Buttrick, M.D.   [41]
Departments of Medicine & Physiology
Division of Cardiology
University of Illinois School of Medicine
Chicago, Illinois

Erdal Cavusoglu, M.D.   [12]
Department of Medicine
Division of Cardiology
Mt. Sinai School of Medicine and
Bronx VA Medical Center
New York, New York

Pamela Charney, M.D.   [Appendices]
Department of Medicine
Norwalk Hospital
Norwalk, Connecticut
and
Obstetrics & Gynecology and Women's Health
Albert Einstein College of Medicine
Bronx, New York

Judy W.M. Cheng, Pharm.D.   [27]
Department of Pharmacy
Mt. Sinai Medical Center
New York, New York
and
Arnold & Marie Schwartz College of Pharmacy
    & Health Sciences of Long Island University
Brooklyn, New York

Angela Cheng-Lai, Pharm.D.   [Appendices]
Department of Pharmacy
Montefiore Medical Center
Bronx, New York

Peter Chien, M.D.   [2]
Department of Medicine
Division of General Internal Medicine
New York Medical College
Westchester Medical Center
Valhalla, New York

Youngsoo Cho, M.D.   [27]
Department of Medicine
Brown University School of Medicine
Rhode Island Hospital
Providence, Rhode Island

Andrew Y. Choi, M.D.   [46]
Department of Radiology
Winthrop University Hospital
Mineola, New York
and
SUNY Health Sciences Center at Stony Brook
Stony Brook, New York

Jay D. Coffman, M.D.   [50]
Department of Medicine
Boston University School of Medicine
Boston Medical Center
Boston, Massachusetts

Piyush K. Dhanuka, M.D.   [3]
Department of Medicine
Division of General Internal Medicine
New York Medical College
Westchester Medical Center
Valhalla, New York

Robert T. Eberhardt, M.D.   [50]
Department of Medicine
Division of Cardiology
Boston University School of Medicine
Boston Medical Center
Boston, Massachusetts

William J. Elliott, M.D., Ph.D.   [29]
Departments of Preventive Medicine
Internal Medicine and Pharmacology
Rush Medical College of Rush University-
    Presbyterian-St. Luke's Medical Center
Chicago, Illinois

Mariana Fernandez, M.D.   [39]
Department of Medicine
Cornell University Medical College
St. Barnabas Hospital Center
Bronx, New York

Robert Forman, M.D.   [19]
Department of Medicine
Division of Cardiology
Albert Einstein College of Medicine
Montefiore Medical Center
Bronx, New York

Ruth Freeman, M.D.   [36]
Departments of Medicine & Obstetrics-Gynecology
Albert Einstein College of Medicine
Montefiore Medical Center
Bronx, New York

William H. Frishman, M.D.   [1–3, 7–14, 18–40, 42–44, 46, 47, 49, appendices]
Departments of Medicine & Pharmacology
New York Medical College
Westchester Medical Center
Valhalla, New York

W. Bruce Fye, M.D.   [6]
Department of Medicine
Division of Cardiology
Mayo Clinic & Medical School
Rochester, Minnesota
and
President
American College of Cardiology
Bethesda, Maryland

Isaac Galandauer, M.D.   [28]
Department of Medicine
New York Medical College
Westchester Medical Center
Valhalla, New York

Amanda Ganem, M.D.   [37, 38]
Department of Medicine
Long Island Jewish Medical Center
Albert Einstein College of Medicine
New Hyde Park, New York

Todd W.B. Gehr, M.D.   [10, 11]
Department of Medicine
Division of Nephrology
Medical College of Virginia of
    Virginia Commonwealth University
Richmond, Virginia

Michael Gewitz, M.D.   [49]
Department of Pediatrics
Division of Pediatric Cardiology
New York Medical College
Children's Hospital at Westchester Medical Center
Valhalla, New York

Eugenia Gianos, M.D.   [32]
Department of Medicine
Long Island Jewish Medical Center
Albert Einstein College of Medicine
New Hyde Park, New York

Stephen P. Glasser, M.D.   [2]
Department of Epidemiology & Graduate Studies in Clinical Research
University of Minnesota School of Public Health
Minneapolis, Minnesota

Renée J. Goldberg Arnold, Pharm.D.   [5]
Pharmacon International Inc.
New York, New York;
Arnold & Marie Schwartz College of Pharmacy & Health
    Sciences of Long Island
Brooklyn, New York
and
Rutgers University College of Pharmacy
Piscataway, New Jersey

Mardi Gomberg-Maitland, M.D.   [36]
Department of Medicine
Division of Cardiology
Mt. Sinai School of Medicine & Medical Center
New York, New York

Alice Guh, M.D.   [46]
Department of Medicine
Georgetown University School of Medicine & Hospital Center
Washington, DC

Nils Guttenplan, M.D. [42]
Department of Medicine
New York Medical College
St. Vincent's Catholic Medical Center
New York, New York

Richard M. Hays, M.D. [33]
Division of Nephrology
Albert Einstein College of Medicine
Montefiore Medical Center
Bronx, New York

Armin Helisch, M.D. [33]
Max-Planck Institute for Physiological & Clinical Research
Bad Nauheim, Germany

Hilary Hotchkiss, M.D. [26]
Department of Pediatrics
Division of Pediatric Nephrology
Mt. Sinai School of Medicine & Hospital Center
New York, New York

Jamal Hussain, M.D. [23]
Department of Medicine
Division of Cardiology
Wayne State University School of Medicine
Detroit Medical Center
Detroit, Michigan

Anjum Ismail, M.D. [22]
Heart Institute of Nevada
Las Vegas, Nevada

Andre Scott Jung, M.D. [39]
Department of Medicine
UC-San Diego School of Medicine & Medical Center
San Diego, California

Daniel W. Kang, M.D. [25]
Department of Medicine
University of Hawaii
Tripler Army Medical Center
Honolulu, Hawaii

Diana J. Kaniecki, Pharm.D. [5]
Pharmacon International Inc.
New York, New York
and
Rutgers University College of Pharmacy
Piscataway, New Jersey

Sukhdeep Kaur, M.D. [31]
Department of Medicine
Division of General Internal Medicine
New York Medical College
Westchester Medical Center
Valhalla, New York

David Khaski M.D. [37]
Department of Internal Medicine
Beth Israel Medical Center
Albert Einstein College of Medicine
New York, New York

Marc Klapholz, M.D. [35]
Department of Medicine
Division of Cardiology
New York Medical College
St. Vincent's Catholic Medical Center
New York, New York

Michael D. Klein, M.D. [18]
Department of Medicine
Division of Cardiology
Boston University Medical School
Boston Medical Center
Boston, Massachusetts

Peter R. Kowey, M.D. [17]
Department of Medicine
Division of Cardiology
Jefferson Medical College
Philadelphia, Pennsylvania
and
Lankenau Hospital & Main Line Health System
Wynnewood, Pennsylvania

Lawrence R. Krakoff, M.D. [15, 16]
Department of Medicine
Mt. Sinai School of Medicine
New York, New York
and
Englewood Hospital Center
Englewood, New Jersey

Nathan A. Kruger, M.D. [23, 24]
Department of Medicine
Yale University School of Medicine
Yale-New Haven Hospital
New Haven, Connecticut

Tom Ky, M.D. [22]
Department of Internal Medicine
University of California-Irvine School of Medicine &
    Medical Center
Orange, California

Brian R. Landzberg, M.D. [40]
Department of Medicine
New York Hospital
Cornell Medical Center
New York, New York

Michal Laniado-Schwartzman, Ph.D. [45]
Department of Pharmacology
New York Medical College
Valhalla, New York

Eliot J. Lazar, M.D. [4]
Department of Clinical Medicine
Weill Medical College of Cornell University
New York, New York
and
Department of Medicine
Division of Cardiology
Columbia Presbyterian Medical Center
New York, New York

Benjamin Y. Lee, M.D.   [28]
Department of Medicine
UCLA School of Medicine
Cedars Sinai Medical Center
Los Angeles, California

Jay Lee, M.D.   [32]
Department of Medicine
Greenwich Hospital
Greenwich, Connecticut

Wei-Nchih Lee, M.D., MPH   [2, 3]
Department of Medicine
Division of General Internal Medicine
New York Medical College
Westchester Medical Center
Valhalla, New York

Christine Leehealey, M.D.   [42]
Department of Internal Medicine
University California-Irvine Medical Center
Orange, California

Thierry H. LeJemtel, M.D.   [13]
Department of Medicine
Division of Cardiology
Albert Einstein College of Medicine
Montefiore Medical Center
Bronx, New York

Robert G. Lerner, M.D.   [18]
Department of Medicine
Division of Hematology
New York Medical College
Westchester Medical Center
Valhalla, New York

Walter G. Levine, Ph.D.   [1]
Department of Molecular Pharmacology
Albert Einstein College of Medicine
Bronx, New York

Cherry Lin, M.D.   [34]
Department of Medicine
Kaiser Permanente
Pleasonton, California

George Lin, M.D.   [47]
Colima Medical Group
Hacienda Heights, California

Jason Lyons, M.D.   [33]
Department of Medicine
University of Rochester School of Medicine
Strong Memorial Hospital
Rochester, New York

Adam B. Mayerson, M.D.   [35]
Department of Medicine
Yale School of Medicine
Yale-New Haven Hospital
New Haven, Connecticut

John C. McGiff, M.D.   [45]
Department of Pharmacology
New York Medical College
Valhalla, New York

Jeffrey A. Medin, M.D.   [41]
Department of Medicine
Division of Hematology & Oncology
University of Illinois School of Medicine
Chicago, Illinois

B. Robert Meyer, M.D.   [8]
Department of Medicine
Weill Medical College of Cornell University
New York, New York
and
New York Presbyterian Medical Center
New York, New York

Eric L. Michelson, M.D.   [17]
Astra Zeneca LP
Wayne, Pennsylvania
and
Jefferson Medical College
Philadelphia, Pennsylvania

John Misailidis, M.D.   [37]
Departments of Medicine & Pediatrics
University of Hawaii School of Medicine
Honolulu, Hawaii

Daniel Mobati, M.D., DDS   [39]
Department of Medicine
New York Medical College
Valhalla, New York

Rajesh Mohandas, M.D.   [37]
Department of Medicine
Division of Geriatrics
New York Medical College
Westchester Medical Center
Valhalla, New York

Nauman Naseer, M.D.   [33]
Department of Medicine
New York Medical College
Westchester Medical Center
Valhalla, New York

James Nawarskas, Pharm.D.   [44]
University of New Mexico
College of Pharmacy
Albuquerque, New Mexico

Devraj U. Nayak, M.D.   [24]
Department of Medicine
Division of Cardiology
New York Medical College
Westchester Medical Center
Valhalla, New York

Michael A. Nelson, M.D.   [38]
Department of Medicine
Yale University School of Medicine
Yale-New Haven Hospital Center
New Haven, Connecticut

Joel M. Neutel, M.D. [21]
University of California-Irvine School of Medicine
Integrated Research
Orange, California

Lionel H. Opie, M.D. [48]
Cape Heart Centre Medical School
Cape Town, South Africa

Donald Orlic, Ph.D. [37]
National Human Genome Research Institute
National Institutes of Health
Bethesda, Maryland

Sameet A. Palkhiwala, M.D. [30, 39]
Department of Medicine
Columbia University College of Physicians & Surgeons
St. Lukes-Roosevelt Hospital Center
New York, New York

Denise Park, M.D. [36]
Department of Medicine
New York Medical College
Westchester Medical Center
Valhalla, New York

Jonathan Passeri, M.D. [38]
Department of Medicine
Harvard University School of Medicine
Massachusetts General Hospital
Boston, Massachusetts

Stephen J. Peterson, M.D. [2, 3, 47]
Departments of Medicine & Pharmacology
Division of General Internal Medicine
New York Medical College
Westchester Medical Center
Valhalla, New York

Alex Huanphong Phan, M.D. [28]
Department of Medicine
Santa Barbara Cottage Hospital
Santa Barbara, California

Shadi Qasqas, M.D. [39]
Department of Medicine
Washington University School of Medicine
Barnes-Jewish Hospital
St. Louis, Missouri

Atif Qureshi, M.D. [36]
Department of Medicine
SUNY Buffalo School of Medicine & Biomedical Sciences
Buffalo General Hospital
Buffalo, New York

Vikram Rajan, M.D. [44]
Department of Medicine
UCLA School of Medicine
Cedars Sinai Medical Center
Los Angeles, California

Avi Retter, M.D. [37, 39]
Department of Medicine
Temple University School of Medicine & Hospital Center
Philadelphia, Pennsylvania

Fay Rim, M.D. [30, 39]
Department of Medicine
New York Medical College
Westchester Medical Center
Valhalla, New York

Mira Roganovic, M.D. [18]
Department of Medicine
Cornell University Medical College
St. Barnabas Hospital Center
Bronx, New York

James A. Schoenberger, M.D. [50]
Department of Preventive Medicine
Rush Medical College of Rush University-
Presbyterian-St. Luke's Medical Center
Chicago, Illinois

Jessica Sekhon, M.D. [37]
Department of Pediatrics
George Washington University School of Medicine &
  Health Sciences
Children's National Medical Center
Washington, DC

Neil S. Shachter, M.D. [20]
Department of Medicine
Columbia University College of Physicians & Surgeons
New York Presbyterian Medical Center
New York, New York

Michael H. Shanik, M.D. [34]
Department of Medicine
Long Island Jewish Medical Center
New Hyde Park, New York

Farooq Sheikh, BS [37]
National Human Genome Research Institute
National Institutes of Health
Bethesda, Maryland
and
New York Medical College
Valhalla, New York

Domenic A. Sica, M.D. [9–12, 27, 44, 45, 51]
Department of Medicine
Divisions of Nephrology & Clinical Pharmacology
Medical College of Virginia
  of Virginia Commonwealth University
Richmond, Virginia

Stephen T. Sinatra, M.D. [47]
Department of Medicine
Division of Cardiology
University of Connecticut School of Medicine &
  Eastern Connecticut Health Network
Farmington, Connecticut

Inderpal Singh, M.D. [31]
Department of Medicine
Division of Cardiology
New York Medical College
Westchester Medical Center
Valhalla, New York

Sanjai Sinha, M.D. [43]
Department of General Medicine
Mt. Sinai School of Medicine
Bronx VA Medical Center
New York, New York

Tatjana N. Sljapic, M.D. [17]
Department of Medicine
Division of Cardiology
Lankenau Hospital
Wynnewood, Pennsylvania

Bradley G. Somer, M.D. [27, 32]
Department of Medicine
University of Pennsylvania School of Medicine
Hospital of the University of Pennsylvania
Philadelphia, Pennsylvania

Edmund H. Sonnenblick, M.D. [13, 42]
Department of Medicine
Division of Cardiology
Albert Einstein College of Medicine
Montefiore Medical Center
Bronx, New York

Adam Spiegel, BS [Appendices]
New York College of Osteopathic Medicine
Westbury, New York

Praveen Tamirisa, M.D. [31]
Northwest Ohio Cardiology Consultants
Toledo, Ohio

Babak A. Vakili, M.D. [24]
Department of Medicine
Division of Cardiology
Albert Einstein College of Medicine
Montefiore Medical Center
Bronx, New York

Christos Vavasis, M.D. [39]
Department of Medicine
New York University School of Medicine
North Shore University Hospital
Manhasset, New York

Michael A. Weber, M.D. [21]
Office of the Dean & Department of Medicine
SUNY Health Science Center-Brooklyn
Brooklyn, New York

Melvin Weiss, M.D. [40]
Department of Medicine
Division of Cardiology
New York Medical College
Westchester Medical Center
Valhalla, New York

Paul Woolf, M.D. [49]
Department of Pediatrics
Division of Pediatric Cardiology
New York Medical College
Children's Hospital at Westchester
  Medical Center
Valhalla, New York

Joyce Wu, M.D. [49]
Department of Pediatrics
University of Washington School of Medicine
Children's Hospital Regional Medical Center
Seattle, Washington

Austin Yu, M.D. [30]
Department of Medicine
UCLA/Veterans Affairs Medical Center
Greater LA Health Care Systems
Los Angeles, California

Peter Zimetbaum, MD [20]
Department of Medicine
Division of Cardiology
Harvard Medical School
Beth Israel Deaconess Hospital
Boston, Massachusetts

Foreword

We have been and will continue to be immersed in a flood of new medical information. Arguably, the biggest wave of this informational assault is in the area of therapeutics; namely, devices and drugs. Practicing physicians will increasingly face a daunting challenge of keeping up with new therapeutic information and deciding how to apply it in their practices for the betterment of patients.

Despite this increase in therapeutic knowledge, most texts are oriented toward specific diseases or organ systems. Therein, efficiently finding answers to questions about drugs is often a challenge. This second edition of *Cardiovascular Pharmacotherapeutics* solves the problem. The text is co-edited and co-authored by three distinguished physician-scientists with a long record of research accomplishments in cardiovascular pharmacology and pathophysiology, and includes contributions from many of the leading investigators in cardiovascular drug development. The book is primarily oriented toward specific drugs and drug classes. Of particular relevance is the section on "New Drug Classes in Development (Part III)," which aims to keep readers abreast of this rapidly evolving therapeutic area. Moreover, an added feature is the section on "Special Topics (Part IV)" which provides additional information on drug-drug interactions, complementary medicine, the use of cardiovascular drugs in children, the treatment of peripheral vascular disease, and quality of life issues. The concluding appendices present practical information on drug utilization in clinical practice.

What all this means is that *Cardiovascular Pharmacotherapeutics* is not just another text. Indeed, it fills a niche that benefits a broad spectrum of health care professions.

Craig D. Brater, M.D.
Dean
Indiana University School of Medicine
Indianapolis, Indiana

Preface

The objectives of this book have not changed since the publication of the 1st edition six years ago. It is a formidable challenge even for the cardiovascular specialist to keep up with the rapid pace of drug discovery and the introduction of new therapeutic agents. *Cardiovascular Pharmacotherapeutics* is designed to provide a compendium of updated information for the clinician using drug therapy to manage patients with cardiovascular disease, which also includes preventative strategies. The scientific basis behind every pharmacotherapy advance is also included.

The editors have almost one hundred years of experience in both basic science investigations and the clinical research of cardiovascular drugs. The editors have also authored or co-authored almost all the book chapters while carefully editing the chapters of other noted contributors to bring a consistency to the entire text.

Similar to the previous edition, the textbook is organized into five main sections. The introductory section includes chapters related to relevant clinical pharmacology, patient compliance issues, new drug development, the placebo effect, pharmacoeconomics, and concludes with a history of cardiac drug development by W. Bruce Frye, the current President of The American College of Cardiology.

In the next section, the available cardiovascular drugs are reviewed, with each drug class organized into separate chapters. Included in these chapters are detailed discussions on how to utilize the drugs for the treatment of various cardiovascular disorders and for the prevention of disease. Compared to the first edition, there are hundreds of new reference citations included with discussions of recently approved drugs and drug indications that were only considered pharmacologic concepts in the previous edition.

Part III is unique among textbooks of pharmacology and medicine for its detailed discussions of drugs in development and potential drug targets for innovative drug discovery that have been outgrowths of advances in our knowledge of receptor and ion channel biology, cell growth, neurohumoral control, biochemistry and pathophysiology. Many drugs that were only investigational in the previous edition are now approved for clinical use and include bosentan, an endothelin receptor antagonist for primary pulmonary hypertension; fenoldopam, a selective dopamine agonist for hypertensive emergencies; and nesiritide, a natriuretic peptide for acute heart failure. New chapters in this section discuss innovative pharmacologic targets that include matrix metalloproteinases, ecosanoids, angiogenesis, growth factors in cell therapy, and unique inhibitors of cholesterol synthesis and absorption.

The fourth section deals with special topics relevant to cardiovascular pharmacotherapy and includes chapters on complementary medicine, drug-drug interactions, cardiovascular drug use in children, drug therapy of peripheral vascular disease, and drug therapy and quality of life. As a complementary volume to other standard textbooks of cardiovascular medicine, this section of the book has been shortened from the first edition and no longer includes chapters on specific disease treatments, which are best addressed in the current editions of *Harrison's Principles of Internal Medicine* and *Hurst's The Heart*.

The book concludes with an eight-part appendix section. The first addresses relevant pharmacokinetic information on all the available cardiovascular drugs, the second practical drug prescribing information, and the remaining six appendices are guides on how to use cardiovascular drugs in specific patient populations.

This newest edition of *Cardiovascular Pharmacotherapeutics* encompasses the major advances in drug development over the last 30 years and points to new directions for expanding our therapeutic armamentarium in the years to come.

The editors are indebted to the many contributors to the book and to our trainees and colleagues who serve as research collaborators, critics, and constant sources of intellectual stimulation. A special acknowledgment must be given to Joanne Cioffi-Pryor who has been the editorial assistant for both editions of *Cardiovascular Pharmacotherapeutics,* as well as other textbooks and medical journals we have published over a 20-year period. Her meticulous attention to detail and organizational skills have contributed to the successful completion of this text.

We wish to acknowledge our editor, Darlene Cooke and the production staff at McGraw-Hill, especially Susan Noujaim and Nicky Panton for their efforts in guiding the book through the publishing process.

Finally, our most important contributors are our families who provide the support and love that have enabled our academic careers to flourish.

We feel privileged to have been part of a research enterprise that has advanced to the forefront of medical therapeutics and patient management. We hope that this new edition of *Cardiovascular Pharmacotherapeutics* will continue to energize current and future investigators to pursue ongoing scholarly activities in the important pursuit of new drug development.

William H. Frishman, M.D.
Edmund H. Sonnenblick, M.D.
Domenic A. Sica, M.D.
November 2002

Cardiovascular
Pharmacotherapeutics

SECOND EDITION

PART I

Introductory Chapters

Basic Principles of Clinical Pharmacology Relevant to Cardiology

Walter G. Levine

William H. Frishman

This chapter focuses on some of the basic pharmacologic principles that influence the manner by which cardiovascular drugs manifest their pharmacodynamic and pharmacokinetic actions. A discussion of drug receptor pharmacology is followed by a review of drug disposition, drug metabolism, excretion, and effects of disease states on pharmacokinetics.

RECEPTORS

For nearly 100 years, it has been recognized that, in order to elicit a response, a drug must interact with a receptor, the interface between drug and body, and principal determinant of drug selectivity. The receptor (1) recognizes and binds the drug, (2) undergoes changes in conformation and charge distribution, and (3) transduces information inherent in the drug structure (extracellular signal) into intracellular messages, resulting in a change in cellular function. A receptor may be any functional macromolecule and is often a receptor for endogenous regulatory substances, such as hormones or neurotransmitters.

Nature of Receptors

Receptors typically are proteins, lipoproteins, or glycoproteins including (1) regulatory proteins that mediate the action of endogenous substances such as neurotransmitters, hormones, etc.; (2) enzymes, which typically are inhibited by drugs; (3) transport proteins such as Na^+,K^+-ATPase; and (4) structural proteins such as tubulin.

1. Gated channels involve synaptic transmitters (e.g., acetylcholine, norepinephrine) and drugs mimicking their action. These receptors regulate ion flow through membranes, altering transmembrane potentials. The well-characterized nicotinic acetylcholine receptor is a protein consisting of five subunits, two of which selectively bind acetylcholine, opening the Na^+ channel through conformational alterations. In the absence of agonist, the channel remains closed. Other drugs—e.g., certain anxiolytics—act similarly at GABA-regulated Cl^- channels. The time sequence is extremely fast (milliseconds).
2. G proteins (which interact with guanine nucleotides) diffuse within the cell membrane, interacting with more than one receptor. They regulate enzymes, such as adenyl cyclase, or ion channels. Their large number and great diversity may account for drug selectivity in some cases. A prominent example is the role of a specific G protein in the regulation of muscarinic receptors in cardiac muscle. Activation enhances potassium permeability, causing hyperpolarization and depressed electrical activity.
3. Transmembrane enzymes—e.g., protein tyrosine kinases—recognize ligands such as insulin and several growth factors. These bind to an extracellular domain of the receptor and allosterically activate the enzyme site at the cytoplasmic domain, enabling phosphorylation of receptor tyrosines. The signaling process proceeds to phosphorylation of other intracellular proteins, involving serine and threonine as well. Downregulation of these receptors is frequently seen, limiting the intensity and duration of action of the ligand (drug).
4. Intracellular receptors. Here the lipophilic drug (agonist) penetrates the plasma membrane and binds selectively to an intracellular macromolecule. The drug-receptor complex subsequently binds to DNA-modifying gene expression. Response time is slow (up to several hours) and duration of hours or days after disappearance of the drug due to turnover time of the proteins expressed by the affected gene.

The four major classes of receptors are depicted in Fig. 1-1. Transmembrane signal transduction also involves a number of second messenger systems that respond to receptor activation. These systems include (1) cyclic AMP, which is formed by the action of ligand-activated adenyl cyclase on ATP and, through activation of selective protein kinases, mediates numerous hormonal and drug responses. (2) Phosphatidyl inositol, which, through hydrolysis by phospholipase C within the cell membrane, yields water-soluble inositol triphosphate, which enters the cell and releases bound Ca^{2+}, and lipid-soluble diacylglycerol, which remains in the membrane, where it activates protein kinase C.

Kinetics of Drug-Receptor Interactions

Drug or agonist interacts with its receptor as follows:

$$A + R \underset{k_2}{\overset{k_1}{\rightleftarrows}} AR$$

where R = unoccupied receptor
AR = drug-receptor complex

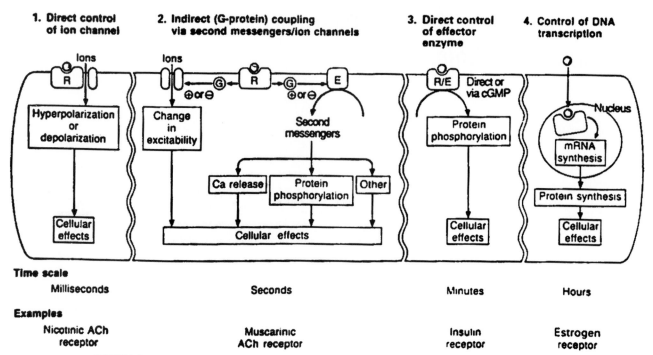

FIGURE 1-1. Scheme for the four major types of drug receptors and linkage to their cellular effects. E = enzyme; G = G protein; R = receptor molecule.

According to the law of mass action, the forward reaction rate is given by $k_1[A][R]$ and the reverse reaction rate by $k_2[AR]$.

$$\text{The dissociation constant (K}d) = \frac{[A][R]}{[AR]} \text{ relates to } \frac{k_2}{k_1}$$

$$\text{The binding (affinity) constant (K}a) = \frac{1}{\text{K}d} \text{ relates to } \frac{k_1}{k_2}$$

Each constant is characteristic of a drug and its receptor.

Drug-receptor interaction may involve any type of bond: van der Waals, ionic, hydrogen, covalent. The interaction is usually of the weaker, reversible type, since covalent binding would effectively destroy receptor function (which may be desirable in the case of an irreversible inhibitor such as the cholinesterase inhibitors, echothiophate, and parathion). Affinity for receptors varies considerably in a teleologically satisfactory manner. Postsynaptic receptors have low affinity for endogenous neurotransmitters released in high concentrations into the synaptic cleft. In contrast, intracellular steroid receptors have high affinity for hormones, which are found in the circulation in very low concentration.

Quantitative Considerations

If one measures an effect at varying drug doses (concentrations) and plots the drug response versus the dose, a rectangular hyperbola is obtained (Fig. 1-2A). Since quantitative comparisons among drugs and types of receptors are best described in terms of ED_{50} (the dose eliciting 50% maximal response), it is necessary to plot the response versus the log dose. In this way, the ED_{50} can be more accurately determined (Fig. 1-2B), since it is found in a relatively linear part of the curve. This relationship is valid when a graded response is discernible.

The log dose–response curve can also be used to distinguish competitive and noncompetitive inhibition, characteristic of many commonly used drugs. Competitive inhibition implies that the agonist and antagonist compete for binding at the active site of the receptor (e.g., beta-adrenergic-receptor blocking drugs are competitive inhibitors at beta-adrenergic receptor sites). Binding of the antagonist to the active site induces no biological response but causes a shift to the right of the log dose–response curve, indicating that more agonist is required to attain a maximal response (Fig. 1-3A). A noncompetitive inhibitor, on the other hand, binds at other than the active site, preventing the agonist from inducing a maximal response at any dose (Fig. 1-3B). There may also be blockade of an action distal to the active site of the receptor. For example, verapamil and nifedipine are calcium channel blockers and prevent influx of calcium ions, nonspecifically blocking smooth muscle contraction.

A partial agonist induces a response qualitatively similar to that of the true agonist but far less than the maximal response. Of critical importance is the lack of full response to the agonist in the presence of the partial agonist, the latter thereby acting as an inhibitor. The nonselective beta-blocker pindolol exhibits prominent partial agonist activity. The original hope that such a drug would be valuable in cardiac patients with asthma or other lung diseases has not been fulfilled.

Two fundamental properties of drugs, efficacy (intrinsic activity) and potency, must be distinguished (Fig. 1-4A). A partial agonist, unable to elicit a full response, has lower efficacy than does the true agonist. *Efficacy* is actually a property of the drug-receptor complex, since the efficacy of a drug may change from one receptor system to another. *Potency* refers to the concentration or dose of drug required to elicit a standard response. Figure 1-4B shows that a series of drugs acting on the same receptor and differing in potency, may possess similar efficacy; with increasing dose, each can induce the same maximal response. In Fig. 1-4C are log dose–response curves for several agonists with similar potencies but with varying efficacies. Potency is often considered to be a function of the drug-receptor binding constant. Clinically, a drug that undergoes

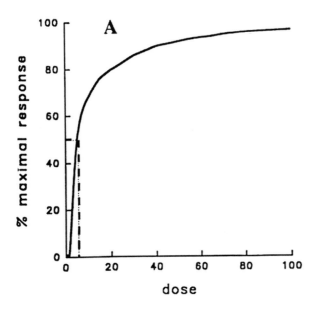

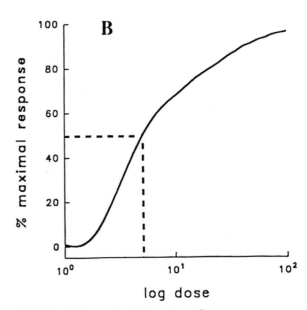

FIGURE 1-2. Theoretical dose (concentration)–response curves. (*A*) Arithmetic dose scale. (*B*) Log dose scale. Dashed lines = determination of 50% effect.

extensive first-pass metabolism, is rapidly inactivated, or has other impediments to accessing its receptor, and may actually require a high dose despite demonstration of high receptor affinity in vitro. High potency in itself is not a therapeutic advantage for a drug. The therapeutic index must always be considered. A twofold increase in potency may be accompanied by a similar increase in toxicity, yielding no advantage.

A fundamental tenet in receptor theory is that a receptor must be "occupied" by an agonist to elicit a biological response and that the biological response is proportional to the number of receptors occupied. However, the ultimate response—e.g., change in blood pressure, renal function, secretion, etc—may not exhibit a simple proportional relationship owing to the complexity of postreceptor events. The spare-receptor theory states that a maximal response may be attained prior to occupancy of all receptors at a particular site. This is strictly a quantitative concept since the spare (unoccupied) receptors do not differ qualitatively from other receptors at the same site. Spare receptors may represent 10 to 99% of the total and may allow agonists of low affinity to exert a maximal effect.

Modulation of receptor function is frequently seen. Downregulation is the decrease in the number of receptors upon chronic exposure to an agonist, resulting in lower sensitivity to the agonist. The receptor number may later normalize. For example, administration of a dobutamine infusion to patients with cardiac failure often leads to loss of efficacy of the drug due to downregulation of myocardial beta adrenoceptors. Upregulation was first illustrated by

denervation supersensitivity. Sympathetic denervation reduces the amount of neurotransmitter (norepinephrine) to which the postsynaptic adrenoceptor is exposed. Over a period of time, the receptor population increases, resulting in a heightened sensitivity to small doses of agonist. Drug-induced depletion of sympathetic neurotransmitter (reserpine, guanethidine) elicits a similar response. The increase in cardiac beta receptors during hyperthyroidism increases the sensitivity of the heart to catecholamines. Thus, thyrotoxicosis is accompanied by tachycardia, which responds to propranolol.

DRUG DISPOSITION AND PHARMACOKINETICS

Although binding of a drug to its receptor is required for most drug effects, the amount bound is a small fraction of the total within the body. The mechanisms controlling the movement, metabolism, and excretion of total drug within the body are critical. Upon them depend the dose, route of administration, onset and duration, intensity of effect, frequency of administration, and, often, toxic side effects.

Passage of Drugs Across Cell Membranes

Movement of nearly all drugs within the body requires transport across cell membranes by filtration (kidney glomeruli), active transport (renal tubules), passive transport, and facilitated diffusion. Most drugs cross most membranes under most conditions by simple

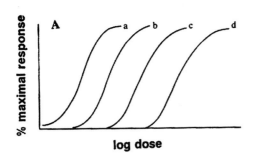

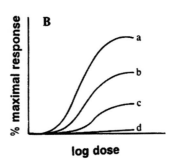

FIGURE 1-3. Log dose – response curves illustrating competitive (*A*) and noncompetitive (*B*) antagonism. In (*A*), a is the curve for agonist alone; b, c, and d are curves obtained in the presence of increasing concentration of a competitive inhibitor. In (*B*), a is the curve for agonist alone; b, c, and d are the curves obtained in the presence of increasing concentrations of a noncompetitive inhibitor.

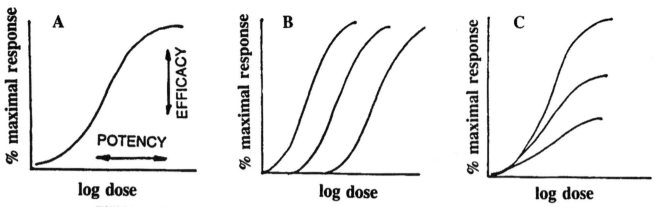

FIGURE 1-4. (*A*) Log dose–response curves distinguishing potency from efficacy (intrinsic activity). (*B*) Response to three drugs with similar efficacies but differing in potency. (*C*) Response to three drugs with similar potencies but differing in efficacy. In each case the receptor system is the same.

diffusion. Passive flux of molecules down a concentration gradient is given by Fick's law.

$$\text{Flux (molecules per unit time)}$$

$$= C_1 - C_2 \frac{(\text{area} \times \text{permeability coefficient})}{\text{thickness}}$$

where C_1 and C_2 = the higher and lower concentrations, respectively
area = area of diffusion
permeability coefficient = mobility of molecules within the diffusion pathway
thickness = that of the diffusion path

Therefore, rate and direction of passage depend on (1) concentration gradient across the membrane of unbound drug and (2) lipid solubility of drug. Most drugs, being weak organic bases or acids, will be ionized or un-ionized depending on their pK and the pH of their environment. The *un-ionized* form, being more lipid-soluble, readily diffuses across the membrane, whereas the *ionized* form is mainly excluded from the membrane. This principle is adhered to most rigidly in the brain, where the tight gap junctions in cerebral capillaries prevent intercellular diffusion of hydrophilic drugs, creating the so-called blood–brain barrier. Drugs having a charge at physiologic pH—e.g., terfenadine (Seldane) and neostigmine—are generally excluded from the brain. By contrast, in the liver, blood passes through sinusoids that are highly fenestrated, allowing plasma constituents, including charged and noncharged drugs, to pass readily into the interstitial space and have direct contact with the liver cells, where selectivity for drug transport is far less.

Absorption

Absorption of drugs from sites of administration follows the general principles described above. Other factors include solubility, rate of dissolution, concentration at site of absorption, circulation to site of absorption, and area of the absorbing surface.

Routes of Drug Administration

Sublingual

Sublingual administration avoids destruction due to the acidic environment of the stomach and bypasses the intestine and liver,

avoiding loss through absorption and enzymatic destruction (first-pass effect). It is used for nitroglycerin (angina pectoris), ergotamine (migraine), and certain testosterone preparations (avoids prominent first-pass effects).

Oral Route

In addition to the convenience of this route, the structure, surface area, and movement of the intestines are conducive to absorption, which takes place throughout the GI tract. Rules for passive transport are applicable; pH gradient along the tract influences absorption of drugs with varying pK. Aqueous and lipid solubility of drug may be competing factors—i.e., a drug may be lipid-soluble, favoring absorption, but so insoluble in water that absorption is very poor or erratic. Rate of absorption is partially regulated by intestinal blood flow, which serves to remove drug from the absorption site, thus maintaining a high GI tract–blood concentration gradient and gastric emptying time (most drugs are mainly absorbed in the intestine). Absorption varies with pH, presence and nature of food, mental state, GI and other diseases, endocrine status, and drugs that influence GI function.

Drugs may be extensively (high extraction) or minimally (low extraction) cleared from both the portal and systemic circulation by the liver. The extent of removal is referred to as the *extraction ratio*. It follows that the rate of plasma clearance of high-extraction drugs is very sensitive to hepatic blood flow. An increase or decrease in hepatic blood flow will enhance or depress, respectively, drug clearance from the plasma. Conversely, variations in hepatic blood flow have minimal influence on removal of low-extraction drugs, since so little is removed per unit time. Diminished hepatic extraction capacity, as seen in severe liver disease and aging, can significantly decrease the first-pass effect and plasma disappearances of high-extraction drugs.

Rectal Route

This route is reserved mainly for infants, cases of persistent vomiting, and the unconscious patient. Absorption follows rules for passive transport but is often less efficient than in other parts of the GI tract. Since blood flow in the lower part of the rectum connects directly with the systemic circulation, portions of rectally administered drugs bypass the first-pass effect.

Pulmonary Route

The pulmonary route is used primarily for gaseous and volatile drugs as well as nicotine and other drugs of abuse, such as crack cocaine. These are rapidly absorbed due to their high-lipid solubility and small molecular size and the vast alveolar surface area (approximately 200 M^2).

Transdermal Route

This route has come into vogue for the administration of certain cardiac, central nervous system (CNS), and endocrine drugs for a slow, sustained effect. The large surface area (2 M^2) and blood supply of the skin (30%) are conducive to absorption. Advantages include more stable blood levels, avoidance of first-pass effect, better compliance—since frequency of administration is greatly diminished, no injection risks, and elimination of variability in oral absorption. The drug must be relatively potent—i.e., effective in low dose—sufficiently lipid, and water-soluble to penetrate the several layers of the skin; it must also be nonirritant and stable for several days. Inflammation, by increasing cutaneous blood flow, enhances drug absorption. Drugs administered by the transdermal route include scopolamine, nitrate, clonidine, and estradiol.

Injection

This route avoids the first-pass effect. The *intravenous* route allows rapidity of access to the systemic circulation and a degree of accuracy for dosage not possible with other routes. *Intramuscular* and *subcutaneous* routes require absorption into the systemic circulation at rates dependent upon the lipid-solubility of the drug and circulation to the injected area. Epinephrine may be added to subcutaneous injection to constrict blood vessels and thus retard absorption. Drugs can also be administered into regional circulations through *indwelling catheters* (e.g., vascular growth factors) and injected directly into the vascular endothelium and myocardium (e.g., gene therapy).

Bioavailability

There are two aspects of this concept: (1) Absolute bioavailability, or the proportion of administered drug gaining access to the systemic circulation after oral as opposed to IV administration, reflecting the first-pass effect. (2) Relative bioavailability of different preparations of the same drug.

By plotting plasma concentration versus time, one can calculate the area under the curve (AUC), a measure of bioavailability (Fig. 1-5). The curve also indicates peak plasma levels and time to attain peak levels. Bioequivalent preparation should be identical in each of these parameters. However, considerable variation may be seen among different preparations, reflecting extent and rate of drug release from its dosage form (pill, capsule, etc.) within the GI tract. Factors that may affect bioavailability include conditions within the GI tract, pH, food, disease, other drugs, metabolism, and/or binding within the intestinal wall and liver. Ideally, preparations should be tested for bioavailability under identical conditions in the same subject. The narrower the therapeutic index of a drug, the greater the concern for variation in bioavailability. Examples of varying bioavailabilities are given in Table 1-1.

Distribution to Tissues

Vascularity and plasma concentration of drug are the main determinants of tissue distribution. Organs receiving a high blood supply—e.g., kidney, brain, and thyroid—are rapidly exposed to drugs, whereas bone and adipose tissue receive only a minor fraction of the dose. High plasma concentrations of drugs result in high tissue levels due to mass action and passive diffusion across cell

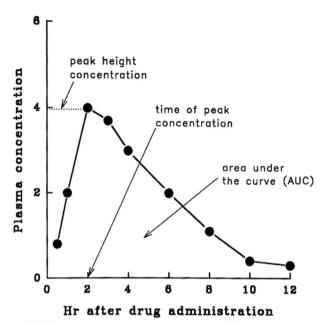

FIGURE 1-5. Theoretical plasma levels of drug as a function of time. The curve is used to determine bioavailability, since it illustrates peak concentration, time of peak concentration, and area under the curve (AUC).

membranes. Lipid-soluble drugs readily pass the placenta, enabling distribution to and possible action on the developing fetus. Therefore, the use of any drug is not recommended during pregnancy; thiazide diuretics and warfarin, among others, are particularly discouraged. Redistribution of drugs can influence pharmacologic response. For example, it is well established that the actions of benzodiazepines and thiopental are terminated not by metabolism or excretion but by redistribution of the drugs away from the brain.

Site-specific drug delivery would enhance therapeutic effectiveness and limit side and toxic effects. This has been achieved for very few drugs, since normal body mechanisms are generally conducive to wide distribution to sites unrelated to the desired drug receptors. A type of organ targeting is seen with prodrugs such as L-dopa, which is converted to the active form, dopamine, in the CNS, and sulfasalazine, which is converted to the active salicylate by gut bacteria within the lower bowel.

Binding to Plasma Proteins

Most drugs are bound to plasma proteins to some extent. Albumin binds a wide spectrum of drugs, particularly those with acidic and

TABLE 1-1. Varying Drug Bioavailability (%)

Amiodarone (46)	Morphine (24)
Atropine (50)	Nifedipine (50)
Bretylium (20)	Phenytoin (90)
Caffeine (100)	Procainamide (83)
Digoxin (60–75)	Propranolol (26)
Diltiazem (40–90)	Quinidine (80)
Disopyramide (80)	Theophylline (96)
Flecainide (95)	Tocainide (89)
Lidocaine (35)	Verapamil (22)
Meperidine (52)	Warfarin (93)
Metoprolol (38)	

Source: Adapted from Levine WG: Basic principles of clinical pharmacology relevant to cardiology. In: Frishman WH, Sonnenblick EH, eds. *Cardiovascular Pharmacotherapeutics.* New York: McGraw Hill, 1997:9.

neutral characteristics. Binding is usually nonspecific, although some selective sites are known. Basic drugs may also bind to albumin, but mainly to alpha$_1$-acid glycoprotein, an acute-phase reactant protein. Lipoproteins also bind some lipophilic and basic compounds. A number of highly specific proteins exist that bind thyroxine, retinol, transcortin, etc., but these are of little consequence for drugs and other xenobiotics.

Binding to plasma proteins is always reversible, and the half-time of binding and release is exceedingly short (measured in milliseconds). Thus, even in the case of extensive (tight) binding, it is rapidly reversible under physiologic conditions. Since concentration gradients, which determine the rate of passive transport across membranes, are based solely on free drug, it follows that binding to plasma proteins slows the rate of removal of drug from plasma by diminishing the concentration gradient across capillary cell membranes. Thus, access to all extravascular sites, receptors, metabolism, storage, and excretion are to a great extent regulated by plasma protein binding. It follows that the half-lives of many drugs correlate with the extent of binding. On the other hand, active transport, as in the proximal tubule, is unaffected by plasma protein binding. For example, nifedipine, which is 96% bound to plasma proteins, has a half-life of only 1.8 h. In this case, the protein bound portion of the drug serves as a readily accessible reservoir due to rapid reversibility of binding.

Hepatic extraction is sensitive to plasma protein binding. For low-extraction drugs, binding is of considerable importance, whereas hepatic uptake of high extraction drugs is little influenced by binding.

Displacement of drugs from binding sites increases the proportion of free drug in the plasma and thus the effective concentration of the drug in extravascular compartments. Similarly, increasing the dose of a drug beyond binding capacity disproportionately increases the unbound fraction within the plasma and may lead to undesired pharmacologic effects. Plasma-binding proteins may be decreased in concentration or effectiveness under the following conditions:

Albumin: Burns, nephrosis, cystic fibrosis, cirrhosis, inflammation, sepsis, malnutrition, neoplasia, aging, pregnancy, stress, heart failure. Uremia causes decreased binding of acidic but not basic drugs.
Alpha$_1$-acid glycoprotein: Aging, oral contraceptives, pregnancy.

The possibility of altered drug disposition should be considered in each case.

Volume of Distribution

Under ideal conditions, drugs are considered to be distributed in one or more of the body fluid compartments. The apparent volume of distribution (Vd) is the body fluid volume that appears to contain the drug.

$$Vd = \frac{dose}{plasma\ concentration\ (after\ equilibration)}$$

For example, Vd = plasma volume (e.g., heparin) implies extensive binding of the drug to plasma proteins, with the bulk of the drug remaining in the plasma. Vd = total body water (e.g., phenytoin, diazepam) implies that the drug is evenly distributed throughout the body. However, one should avoid associating Vd values with a specific anatomic compartment, since binding at extravascular sites

(e.g., procainamide, verapamil, and metoprolol) may significantly affect Vd determinations. Their importance lies in the fact that Vd can vary with age, gender, disease, etc. Thus, changes in plasma protein synthesis, skeletal muscle mass, adipose tissue mass, adipose/muscle ratio, and body hydration will be reflected in Vd and may markedly alter the therapeutic as well as the toxic response to a drug. Values of Vd, if used intelligently, can provide information on body distribution of a drug, changes in body water compartments, implications for intensity of effect, and rate of elimination.

Half-Life and Clearance

The half-life (T$_{1/2}$) of a drug is the time for the plasma concentration to be decreased by one-half. It is usually independent of route of administration and dose. Assuming equilibration among all body fluid compartments, it theoretically is a true reflection of the T$_{1/2}$ within the total body and correlates closely with duration of action. T$_{1/2}$ is derived from a first-order reaction calculated from a semilog plot of the plasma concentration versus time during the elimination phase, which reflects metabolism and excretion of the drug (Fig. 1-6). Linearity of this phase reflects exponential kinetics (first order), in which plasma concentrations of drug do not saturate the rate-limiting step in elimination. The process may be expressed as a rate constant, k, the fractional change per unit time. T$_{1/2}$ and k are related by the following equation:

$$T_{1/2} \times k = 0.693 \ (\ln 0.5)$$

or

$$T_{1/2} = 0.693/k$$

After oral administration, the initial period is called the *absorption phase*. Here too, T$_{1/2}$ is calculated from the elimination phase. In a few cases (alcohol, phenytoin, high-dose aspirin), the rate-limiting step is saturated and plasma disappearance rate is zero order. For

FIGURE 1-6. Theoretical plasma disappearance curve for a drug after IV or oral administration. During the elimination phase, the straight line obtained from a semilog plot reflects first-order kinetics.

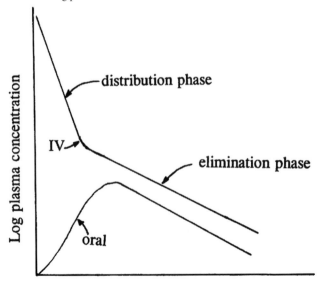

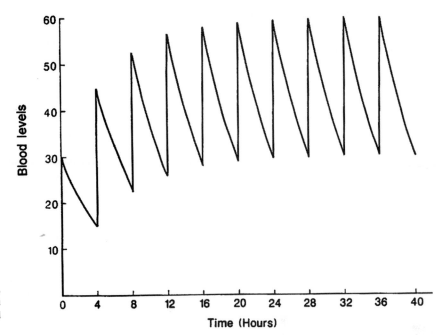

FIGURE 1-7. Blood level–time profile for a drug, half-life = 4 h, administered every 4 h. The plateau effect determines that 95% of the final mean blood level is attained in four to five half-lives.

phenytoin, this may lead to difficulty in controlling blood levels to maintain efficacy while avoiding toxicity.

Total body clearance (Cl_T) is an expression of the fluid Vd cleared per unit time. It is calculated as the product of the elimination rate constant and the Vd.

$$Cl_T = k\,Vd$$

It follows that

$$T_{1/2} = \frac{0.693\,Vd}{Cl}$$

This concept assumes clearance from a single body fluid compartment and is the sum of renal and hepatic clearances. Disease states, aging, and other conditions where Vd may be altered would change clearance. Clearance can be used to determine correct dosage when the desired plasma concentration has been predetermined but changes in physiologic parameters governing drug disposition occur, thus altering clearance.

$$Dosage = Cl \times C_{ss}$$

where Cl = clearance
C_{ss} = steady-state plasma drug concentration

Dosage therefore is a replacement of cleared drug.

Caution   Since clearance is calculated from Vd, a theoretical rather than a physiologic term, the number derived may itself not be truly physiologic. In therapeutics, it is the change of clearance that is a marker for altered drug disposition.

Steady-State Kinetics

During chronic oral administration of a drug, its steady-state plasma level is not a set concentration but a fluctuating concentration, reflecting periodic absorption and continual removal. When drug administration is begun, in accord with first-order kinetics, the elimination rate gradually increases with increasing plasma levels and, eventually, a steady state is attained where input equals output. This is the plateau effect (Fig. 1-7). It can be shown that

50% of steady state is attained after one half-life
75% of steady state is attained after two half lives
87.5% of steady state is attained after three half lives
93.75% of steady state is attained after four half lives

The rule of thumb is that steady state is attained in four to five half-lives. After drug withdrawal, the converse of the plateau effect is seen—i.e., plasma levels are reduced by

50% in one half-life
75% in two half-lives
87.5% in three half-lives
93.75% in four half-lives

When a long half-life—e.g., 14 h—and therapeutic demands preclude waiting four to five half-lives to attain desired plasma concentration of drug, a loading dose is used, calculated as follows:

$$LD = (Vd \times C)/F$$

where Vd = apparent volume of distribution
C = desired plasma concentration
F = fraction of oral dose that reaches the systemic circulation (first pass effect)

This is based on the need to fill the entire Vd to the desired concentration as rapidly as possible. The dose is limited by toxicity, distribution rate, and other variables.

For a drug given by intravenous infusion,

$$LD = \text{infusion rate} \times T_{1/2}$$

DRUG METABOLISM (BIOTRANSFORMATION)

Mechanisms and Pathways

Most drugs and other xenobiotics are metabolized prior to excretion. Although most drugs are ultimately converted to inactive products, many are transformed to pharmacologically active metabolites. In some instances, a drug is metabolized via several pathways, some of which represent inactivation, while others involve activation to toxic product(s).

For many drugs, the first step (phase I) is catalyzed by the cytochrome P450 (mixed-function oxidase) system of the endoplasmic reticulum (microsomal fraction). Cytochrome P450 is actually a large family of isozymes, members of which vary with species, gender, and age. Each has its own spectrum of substrates and can be independently influenced by induction and inhibition. Selective forms of cytochrome P450 (CYP) are shown in Table 1-2. Among the implications of this table is that patients lacking CYP2D6 will obtain little or no pain relief from codeine, since CYP2D6 converts codeine to morphine, the active analgesic metabolite of codeine.

The mixed-function oxidase system exists mainly in the liver but has been detected in nonhepatic tissue as well, particularly at other sites of xenobiotic entry—e.g., lung, skin, etc. Total metabolism in these tissues is a fraction of that of the liver. Nevertheless, since environmental chemicals often enter the body through the lungs and skin, these tissues are of considerable importance in their metabolism.

Major phase I pathways, microsomal and nonmicrosomal, include (1) aliphatic and aromatic hydroxylation, (2) *N*-dealkylation, (3) *O*-dealkylation, (4) sulfoxidation, (5) *N*-hydroxylation (commonly associated with toxic activation of aromatic amines, including a number of chemical carcinogens), (6) azo and nitro reduction, (7) *O*-methylation, and (8) hydrolysis by plasma esterase.

Conjugation (synthetic) pathways (phase II) often but not always follow phase I. They include (1) acylation, a common pathway for aliphatic and aromatic primary amines; (2) glucuronide formation; (3) sulfate formation; and (4) glutathione conjugate formation. Phase II reactions increase drug polarity and charge and thus promote renal excretion (see below).

Glutathione conjugation is a major inactivation mechanism for toxic metabolic intermediates of numerous drugs. For example, in normal dosage, a toxic metabolite of acetaminophen is effectively removed as a glutathione conjugate. In extreme overdose (10–15 g), the demand for glutathione exceeds its rate of hepatic biosynthesis and the accumulation of toxic intermediate leads to liver toxicity and, in rare cases, necrosis and death. Toxicity is treated with acetylcysteine, which serves to restore liver glutathione.

TABLE 1-2. Selective Forms of Cytochrome P450

CYP1A2*	CYP2D6[†]
CYP2C9	CYP2E1[‡]
CYP1C19	CYP3A4[§]

* Induced by smoking and charcoal-broiled foods.

[†] Polymorphism seen in 5 to 10% of the population.

[‡] Induced by alcohol.

[§] Metabolizes a high percentage of drugs; induced by phenobarbital, rifampin, glucocorticoids.

Factors Affecting Drug Metabolism

Species

A major problem in drug development and research.

Age

Few drugs are studied in young children prior to their approval by the U.S. Food and Drug Administration (FDA), presenting a considerable challenge in the treatment of this population. In the *neonate,* factors affecting drug disposition include prolonged gastric emptying time, fluctuating gastric pH, smaller muscle mass, greater cutaneous absorption of toxic substances (e.g., hexachlorophene), changing body water/fat ratio, less effective plasma protein binding, poor hepatic drug metabolism and low renal blood flow. Drugs that pass the placenta present problems of disposition to the fetus. The newborn often exhibits a deficiency in glucuronyl transferase, which catalyzes the essential step in bilirubin excretion. If this deficiency is unattended, kernicterus may ensue. The postneonatal period is also a time of rapid structural and physiologic changes, including the capacity to metabolize drugs. Therefore calculation of dosage based solely on body weight or surface area may not always be appropriate. In the elderly, one sees diminished renal plasma flow and glomerular filtration rate, decreased hepatic phase I, but not phase II drug metabolism, diminished Vd due to loss of body water compartment, decreased muscle mass, decreased or increased adipose tissue, and decreased first-pass effect.

Genetic Factors

Marked differences in rates of drug metabolism are often attributable to genetic factors. Approximately half the male population in the United States acetylates aromatic amines such as isoniazid rapidly and the other half acetylates slowly (Fig. 1-8). The slow-acetylator phenotype is inherited as an autosomal recessive trait. Neither slow nor fast acetylation is an advantage, since the toxicity of both isoniazid (peripheral neuropathies, preventable by pyridoxine administration) and its acetylated metabolite (hepatic damage) is known. Other affected drugs include procainamide, hydralazine, and sulfasalazine.

A small percentage (< 1%) of the population has an abnormal form of plasma pseudoesterase and is unable to hydrolyze succinylcholine at the normal rapid rate, leading to an exaggerated duration of action. Three forms of cytochrome P450 (CYP2D6, CYP2C19, and CYP2C9) exhibit polymorphism. The phenotypes are slow and rapid metabolizers of many drugs: CYP2D6—debrisoquin, tricyclic

FIGURE 1-8. Bimodal distribution of patients into rapid and slow acetylators of isoniazid. Slow acetylators are homozygous for an autosomal recessive gene.

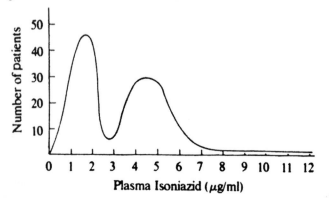

antidepressants, phenformin, dextromethorphan, and several beta blockers; CYP2C19—mephenytoin; CYP2C9—warfarin. Some 3 to 10% of the population has the slow trait, inherited in an autosomal recessive fashion.

Nutritional Deficiency

Multiple manifestations of malnutrition may significantly affect drug disposition. These include changes in GI and renal function, body composition (fluids, electrolytes, fat, protein, etc.), hepatic drug metabolism, endocrine function, and immune response. This is most likely among economically depressed populations and in diseases such as cancer, which are often accompanied by malnutrition. Obviously, hepatic or renal disease can have major consequences for drug disposition. Half-lives for many drugs increase in cirrhosis, hepatitis, obstructive jaundice, nephritis, and other types of kidney failure. Liver disease may result in altered hepatic blood flow, decreased extraction, or depressed metabolizing enzymes. Kidney disease may be manifest as altered renal blood flow and depressed glomerular filtration, active transport, or passive reabsorption. In cardiac failure, the decreased blood supply to most organs means delayed and incomplete absorption of drugs. On the other hand, decreased Vd may mean higher plasma drug levels and consequently exaggerated responses to drug.

Induction

Chronic exposure to any of a large number of drugs and other environmental chemicals induces the synthesis of specific forms of cytochrome P450 (Table 1-3); conjugation with glucuronic acid and glutathione may also be affected. The duration of action of some drugs is thereby shortened, their blood levels are lowered, and their potency is diminished. The half-lives of drugs with low hepatic extraction are mainly affected, whereas drugs not metabolized by these enzymes are not affected. Examples of well-known inducing agents are (1) lipid-soluble drugs such as phenobarbital, phenytoin, rifampin, and ethanol; (2) glucocorticoids; and (3) environmental pollutants such as benzo(a)pyrene and other polycyclic hydrocarbons formed in cigarette smoke, polychlorinated biphenyls, and dioxin. The effect of smoking on plasma drug levels is shown in Fig. 1-9.

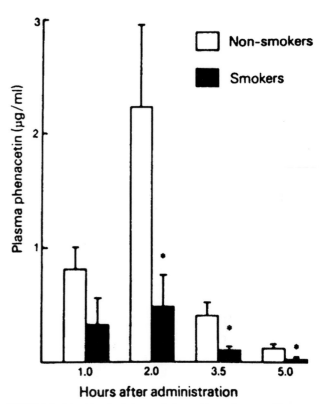

FIGURE 1-9. Blood levels of phenacetin in smoking and non-smoking populations, reflecting the inducing effect of components of cigarette smoke on drug metabolizing enzymes.

Inhibition

Inhibition of drug metabolism will have the opposite effect (Table 1-3), leading to a prolonged half-life and an exaggerated pharmacologic response. Drugs well known for their inhibitory effects include chloramphenicol, cimetidine, allopurinol, and monoamine oxidase inhibitors. Alcohol acutely depresses certain drug metabolism pathways (although chronically it induces them) and may lead to enhanced and prolonged effects of other drugs. Erythromycin and ketoconazole block the conversion of

TABLE 1-3. Major Inhibitors and Substrates of Different Cytochrome P450 (CYP450) Enzymes

CYP450 Enzymes	Inhibitors	Inducers
CYP1A2	Cimetidine, ciprofloxacin, clarithromycin, erythromycin, fluvoxamine, grapefruit juice, isoniazid, ketoconazole, levofloxacin, paroxetine	Phenobarbital, phenytoin, rifampin, ritonavir, smoking
CYP2C9	Amiodarone, chloramphenicol, cimetidine, fluvoxamine, omeprazole, zafirlukast	Carbamazepine, phenobarbital, phenytoin, rifampin
CYP2D6	Amiodarone, cimetidine, desipramine, fluoxetine, fluphenazine, haloperidol, paroxetine, propafenone, quinidine, ritonavir, sertraline	Carbamazepine, phenobarbital, phenytoin, rifampin, ritonavir
CYP3A4	Amiodarone, clarithromycin, erythromycin, fluconazole, fluoxetine, fluvoxamine, grapefruit juice, indinavir, itraconazole, ketoconazole, metronidazole, nefazodone, ritonavir, saquinavir, sertraline, zafirlukast	Carbamazepine, dexamethasone, ethosuximide, phenobarbital, phenytoin, rifabutin, rifampin, troglitazone

Source: From Cheng JWM: Cytochrome P450–mediated cardiovascular drug interactions. *Heart Disease* 2:254–258, 2000.

terfenadine (Seldane), a prodrug, to its active metabolite. Since the parent compound is arrhythmogenic, serious cardiac toxicity may be seen with such drug combinations. For this reason, terfenadine was banned, although its active metabolite is marketed as fexofenadine (Allegra), which lacks cardiotoxicity and CNS effects. It is suspected that there are many more such inhibitory drugs, but it is difficult to predict a priori when inhibition will occur.

Metabolism by Intestinal Microorganisms

The abundant flora of the lower gut includes many organisms capable of metabolizing drugs as well as their metabolic derivatives. Since the microflora consist mainly of obligate anaerobes and the gut environment is anaerobic, only pathways not requiring oxygen are seen. These bacteria make a significant contribution to drug metabolism, and suppression of the gut flora by oral antibiotics or other drugs will appreciably alter the fate and thus the effects of many other drugs. The various pathways include hydrolysis of glucuronides, sulfates, and amides; dehydroxylation; deamination; and azo and nitro reduction.

Enterohepatic Circulation

Many conjugated drugs are transported into the bile and pass into the intestine. Here, intestinal microorganisms hydrolyze the conjugate (glucuronides in particular), yielding the original, less polar compound, which can then be reabsorbed. This cycle tends to repeat itself and makes a major contribution to maintenance of drugs and certain endogenous compounds within the body. For example, bile salts are 90% recirculated through this mechanism. Suppression of gut bacteria by oral antibiotics will appreciably affect the half-lives and thus the plasma levels of compounds that undergo extensive enterohepatic circulation.

EXCRETION

All drugs are ultimately eliminated from the body via one route or another. Elimination rate, as reflected in plasma disappearance rate for most drugs, is generally proportional to the total amount in the body, following first-order kinetics.

1. The *kidney* is the major organ of excretion for most drugs and associated metabolites. Its large blood supply (25% of cardiac output) is conducive to efficient excretion. Drugs not bound to plasma proteins are filtered in the glomeruli with nearly 100% efficiency. Reabsorption within the tubule is mainly by passive diffusion. Thus, highly charged drugs (or metabolites) will be poorly reabsorbed and readily excreted. Changes in tubular pH alter excretion rates by influencing the net charge on the compound. Appropriate manipulation of urinary pH is helpful in facilitating excretion in cases of drug overdose. For example, raising the pH increases excretion of phenobarbital, an organic acid, while lowering the pH increases excretion of amphetamine, an organic base. Active transport of organic anions and cations takes place in the tubules. Penicillin, a weak organic acid, is actively pumped into the tubule's lumen by the tubular anion transport system, an action readily suppressed by probenecid, an inhibitor of the anion pump. Renal failure presents a major therapeutic problem due to accumulation of drug as well as toxic metabolites. Hemodialysis filters out unbound drugs from the plasma, thus assisting clearance. Drugs bound in extravascular areas are less affected by dialysis.

2. *Biliary* excretion is usually reserved for highly polar compounds with a molecular weight greater than 500. Bile empties into the duodenum, and drugs passing via this route are frequently reabsorbed in the intestinal tract (see "Enterohepatic Circulation," above). Unlike the mechanisms involving urine, those of bile formation and biliary excretion are poorly understood. Biliary secretion is greatly but not entirely dependent on bile salt transport. Bile salts may facilitate or inhibit biliary excretion of drugs, depending on the drug and the concentration of bile salts.

3. *Lungs* are the excretion route for many general anesthetics and other volatile substances. A clever utilization of the lungs as a route of excretion is the "aminopyrine breath test." Aminopyrine that has been labeled with radioactive carbon in its methyl moiety is administered. It is demethylated by the liver's P450 system, ultimately forming radioactive carbon dioxide, which is then collected from the expired air and counted. The amount of radioactivity is a reflection of hepatic drug metabolism and has been used as a noninvasive assessment of liver function in, for example, liver cirrhosis. In recent years erythromycin has been used as the test substance.

4. *Milk.* Considerable concern has been raised regarding drugs in breast milk in view of the increase in the past two decades in the number of nursing mothers. Drug entry into plasma is affected by pK of drug, pH of milk and plasma, binding to plasma and milk proteins, and fat composition of milk. Drugs enter the milk by passive diffusion. The pH of milk (6.5–7.0), its varying volume, and its high content of fat globules and unique proteins influence drug secretion, especially for lipid-soluble compounds. Drugs known to be secreted into milk include cardiovascular drugs (hydralazine, digoxin), CNS drugs (caffeine, amitriptyline, primidone, ethosuximide), drugs of abuse (nicotine, narcotics, cocaine), and others (metronidazole, medroxyprogesterone, nor-testosterone). This does not necessarily imply an incompatibility between nursing and taking any of these drugs. However, drugs contraindicated or to be used with caution during lactation include alcohol, amiodarone, atropine, chlorpromazine, cimetidine, cocaine, cyclosporine, doxorubicin, lithium, morphine, nitrofurantoin, phenytoin, phenindione, salicylates, tetracyclines, and tinidazole. At present, drugs must be evaluated individually when deciding on the safety of nursing infants. Similar considerations are valid for cow's milk, since these animals may be given drugs to increase milk production.

Another route of excretion being developed for noninvasive assessment of blood levels of drugs is saliva. For some drugs, a known equilibrium exists between the plasma and saliva. Although the work is only in its infancy, one can foresee the day when, if plasma levels are required, a patient will simply spit for the doctor rather than being stuck with a needle five or six times.

SUPPLEMENTAL READING

Berndt WO, Stitzel RE: Excretion of drugs. In: Craig CR, Stitzel RE, eds. *Modern Pharmacology,* 4th ed. Boston: Little Brown, 1994:47–53.

Bourne HR, Roberts JM: Drug receptors and pharmacodynamics. In: Katzung BG, ed. *Basic and Clinical Pharmacology,* 8th ed. Norwalk, CT: Appleton & Lange, 2001:9–33.

Cheng JWM: Cytochrome P450-mediated cardiovascular drug interactions. *Heart Disease* 2:254, 2000.

Correia MA: Drug biotransformation. In: Katzung BG, ed. *Basic and Clinical Pharmacology,* 8th ed. Norwalk, CT: Appleton & Lange, 2001:51–63.

Fleming WW: Mechanisms of drug action. In: Craig CR, Stitzel RE, eds. *Modern Pharmacology,* 4th ed. Boston: Little Brown, 1994:9–18.

Godin DV: Pharmacokinetics: disposition and metabolism of drugs. In: Munson PL, Mueller RA, Breese GR, eds. *Principles of Pharmacology: Basic Concepts and Clinical Applications.* New York: Chapman & Hall, 1995:39–84.

Gram TE: Drug absorption and distribution. In: Craig CR, Stitzel RE, eds. *Modern Pharmacology,* 4th ed. Boston: Little Brown, 1994:19–32.

Gram TE: Metabolism of drugs. In: Craig CR, Stitzel RE, eds. *Modern Pharmacology,* 4th ed. Boston: Little, Brown, 1994:33–46.

Gwilt PR: Pharmacokinetics. In: Craig CR, Stitzel RE, eds. *Modern Pharmacology,* 4th ed. Boston: Little Brown, 1994:55–64.

Holford NHG, Benet LZ: Pharmacokinetics and pharmacodynamics: Rational dose selection and the time course of drug action. In:

Katzung BG, ed. *Basic and Clinical Pharmacology,* 8th ed. Norwalk, CT: Appleton & Lange, 2001:35–50.

Hollenberg MD, Severson DL: Pharmacodynamics: drug receptors and receptors/mechanisms. In: Munson PL, Mueller RA, Breese GR, eds. *Principles of Pharmacology: Basic Concepts and Clinical Applications.* New York: Chapman & Hall, 1995:7–37.

Levine WG: Basic principles of clinical pharmacology relevant to cardiology. In: Frishman WH, Sonnenblick EH, eds. *Cardiovascular Pharmacotherapeutics.* New York: McGraw-Hill, 1997:3–15.

Nierenberg DW, Melmon KL: Introduction to clinical pharmacology and rational therapeutics. In: Carruthers SG, Hoffman BB, Melmon KL, Nierenberg DW, eds. *Melmon & Morrelli's Clinical Pharmacology,* 4th ed. New York: McGraw Hill, 2000:3.

Opie LH, Frishman WH: Drug interactions. In: Fuster V, Alexander RW, O'Rourke RA, et al., eds. *Hurst's The Heart,* 10th ed. New York: McGraw Hill, 2000:2251.

Rang HP, Dale MM, Ritter HM, Gardner P: *Pharmacology.* New York, Churchill Livingstone, 1995.

Sokol SI, Cheng-Lai A, Frishman WH, Kaza CS: Cardiovascular drug therapy in patients with hepatic diseases and patients with congestive heart failure. *J Clin Pharmacol* 40:11, 2000.

CHAPTER 2

The Placebo Effect in Cardiovascular Disease

William H. Frishman

Wei-Nchih Lee

Stephen P. Glasser

Laura Bienenfeld

Peter Chien

Stephen J. Peterson

There are three general reasons for clinical improvement in a patient's condition: (1) natural history and regression to the mean; (2) the specific effects of the treatment; and (3) the nonspecific effects of the treatment attributable to factors other than the specific active components (this latter effect being included under the heading of "placebo effect").[1] Each time a physician recommends a diagnostic or therapeutic intervention for a patient, there is built into this clinical decision the possibility of a placebo effect being involved, a clinical effect unrelated to the intervention itself.[2–4] Simple diagnostic procedures such as phlebotomy, or more invasive procedures such as cardiac catheterization, have been shown to have important placebo effects associated with them.[5,6] Indeed, Chalmers has stated that one only has to review the graveyard of therapies to realize how many patients would have benefited by being assigned to a placebo control group.[7] In fact, what might represent the first known clinical trial and one in which the absence of a placebo control group led to erroneous conclusions is a summary attributed to Galen in 150 BC, where he stated that "some patients that have taken this herb have recovered, while some have died; thus, it is obvious that this medicament fails only in incurable diseases."

Placebo effects are commonly observed in patients with cardiac disease who also receive drug and surgical therapies as treatments (Fig. 2-1). In this chapter, the placebo effect in cardiovascular disease is reviewed and the implication of this clinical phenomenon to the study of new treatments are discussed.

DEFINITION

Stedman's Medical Dictionary gives two meanings for the word *placebo*, which originates from a Latin verb meaning "I shall please": (1) an inert substance prescribed for its suggestive value and (2) an inert substance identical in appearance with the compound being tested in experimental research, which may or may not be known by the physician and/or the patient; and which is given to distinguish between a compound's action and the suggestive effect of the compound under study.[8]

Currently, there is some disagreement as to the exact definition of a placebo.[9,10] Many recent articles on the subject include a broader definition, as described by Shapiro in 1961[11]:

> ... any therapeutic procedure (or that component of any therapeutic procedure) which is given deliberately to have an effect or unknowingly has an effect on a patient, symptom, syndrome, or disease, but which is objectively without specific activity for the condition being treated. The therapeutic procedure may be given with or without conscious knowledge that the procedure is a placebo, may be an active (non-inert) or nonactive (inert) procedure, and includes, therefore, all medical procedures no matter how specific—oral and parenteral medication, topical preparations, inhalants, and mechanical, surgical and psychotherapeutic procedures. The placebo must be differentiated from the placebo effect which may or may not occur and which may be favorable or unfavorable. The placebo effect is defined as the changes produced by placebos. The placebo is also used to describe an adequate control in research.

A further refinement of the definition was proposed by Byerly in 1975[12]: "... any change in a patient's symptoms that is the result of the therapeutic intent and not the specific physiochemical nature of a medical procedure."

THE PLACEBO EFFECT IN CLINICAL TRIALS

Placebo controls in medical research date back to 1753, when Dr. James Lind advocated their use when he evaluated the effects of lime juice on scurvy.[13] After World War II, research protocols designed to assess the efficacy and safety of new pharmacologic therapies began to include the recognition of the placebo effect. Recognition of placebos and their role in controlled clinical trials occurred in 1946, when the Cornell Conference on therapy devoted a session to placebos and double-blind methodology. At that time, placebos were associated with increased heart rate, altered respiration patterns, dilated pupils, and increased blood pressure.[10] In 1951, Hill[14] concluded that for a specific treatment to be attributable to a

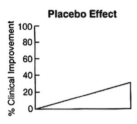
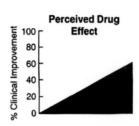
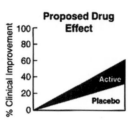

FIGURE 2-1. Any perceived total drug effect is likely to be composed of an active drug effect component and a placebo effect component. (*Reproduced with permission from Archer TP, Leier CV.*[41])

change for better or worse in a patient, this result must be repeatable a significant number of times in similar patients. Otherwise, the result was merely due to the natural history of the disease or simply the passage of time. He also proposed the inclusion of a control group that received identical treatment except for the inclusion of an "active ingredient." Thus, the active ingredient was separated from the situation within which it was used. This control group, also known as a placebo group, would help in the investigations of new and promising pharmacologic therapies.[14]

Beecher was among the first investigators to promote the inclusion of placebo controls in clinical trials.[15] He emphasized the importance of ensuring that neither the patient nor the physician know what treatment the experimental subject was receiving and referred to this as the "double unknown technique." Today, this is called the "double-blind trial" and ensures that the expectations and beliefs of the patient and physician are excluded from evaluation of new therapies. In 1955, Beecher reviewed 15 studies that included 1082 patients and found that an average of 35% of these patients benefited from placebo therapy.[15] He also concluded that placebos can relieve pain from conditions where either physiologic or psychologic etiologies were present. He described many diverse objective changes from placebo therapy. Some medical conditions improved, including severe postoperative wound pain, cough, drug-induced mood changes, pain from angina pectoris, headache, seasickness, anxiety, tension, and the common cold.

CHARACTERISTICS OF THE PLACEBO EFFECT

There appears to be an inverse relationship between the number of placebo doses that need to be administered and treatment outcomes. In a study of patients with postoperative wound pain, 53% of the subjects responded to one placebo dose, 40% to two or three doses, and 15% to four doses.[15]

In analyzing the demographics of placebo responders and nonresponders, Beecher and his associates could find no differences in gender ratios or intelligence quotients between the two groups.[16] They did find significant differences in attitudes, habits, educational backgrounds, and personality structure between consistent responders and nonresponders.[15] In attempting to understand the reproducibility of the placebo effect, they observed that there was no relationship between an initial placebo response and subsequent responses with repeated placebo doses of saline.[16] Beecher concluded that placebos are most effective when stress, such as anxiety and pain, is greatest.[15]

Placebos can produce both desirable and adverse reactions. Beecher and his associates described over 35 different adverse reactions from placebo; the most common ones are described in Table 2-1.[16a,b] These reactions were recorded without the patient's or physician's knowledge that a placebo had been administered. In one study where lactose tablets were given as a placebo, major adverse reactions occurred in three patients.[17] The first patient

experienced overwhelming weakness, palpitation, and nausea after taking placebo. The second patient experienced a diffuse rash that disappeared after discontinuing placebo administration. The third patient experienced epigastric pain followed by watery diarrhea, urticaria, and angioneurotic edema of the lips after receiving placebo.[17] Indeed, due to the substantial evidence of placebo "efficacy" and placebo "side effects," some have wittingly suggested that if placebo were submitted to the U.S. Food and Drug Administration (FDA) for approval, the agency, although impressed with the efficacy data, would probably recommend disapproval based on the high incidence of side effects. Some have questioned whether placebos are truly inert. Davis points out that "part of the problem with the placebo paradox is our failure to separate the use of an inert medication (if there is such a substance) from the phenomenon referred to as the placebo effect.[18] It might help us if we could rename the placebo effect the 'obscure therapeutic effect.'" That is, in lactase deficiency, could the amount of lactose in placebo tablets actually cause true side effects? Due to the small amount of lactose, this seems unlikely, but it is perhaps more likely that allergies to some of the so-called inert ingredients in placebos could cause reactions in predisposed individuals (although in the latter case it would seem unlikely that this could explain more than a small percentage of placebo side effects).

The most recent validation of the placebo effect occurred in 1962, when the United States enacted the Harris-Kefauver Amendments to the Food, Drug, and Cosmetic Act. These amendments require proof of efficacy as well as documentation of relative safety, in terms of the risk-to-benefit ratio for the disease to be treated, before an experimental agent can be approved for general use.[19] In 1970, the FDA published rules for "Adequate and Well-Controlled Clinical Evaluations." The federal regulations identified five types of controls (i.e., placebo, dose-comparison, active, historical, and no treatment) and identified utilization of the placebo control as an indispensable tool to achieve the standard.[20] However, it should be pointed out that the FDA does not mandate placebo controls, and in fact has stated that placebo groups are "...desirable, but need not be interpreted as a strict requirement... the speed with which blind comparisons with placebo and/or positive controls can be fruitfully

TABLE 2-1. Most Common Adverse Reactions from Placebo Therapy

Dry mouth	9%
Nausea	10%
Sensation of heaviness	18%
Headache	25%
Difficulty concentrating	15%
Drowsiness	50%
Warm glow	8%
Relaxation	9%
Fatigue	18%
Sleep disturbance	10%

undertaken varies with the nature of the compound."[21] In the FDA publication regarding "General Considerations for the Clinical Evaluation of Drugs," it further states that "it should be recognized that there are other methods of adequately controlling studies. In some studies, and in some diseases, the use of an active control drug rather than a placebo is desirable, primarily for ethical reasons."[21]

An important statistical concept and one that may mimic a placebo response is regression to the mean. Regression to the mean addresses the fact that in biologic systems, most variables increase and decrease around a mean (one might envision a sine wave to conceptualize this). Thus, it is likely that any value measured at a specific point in time will, by chance, either be above or below the mean, and that a second measurement will be at a different point around the mean and therefore different from the first measurement. This change between measurements could then represent an improvement or worsening and thereby mimic a placebo response. The presumption is that this variability about the mean will be the same in the placebo group as the active treatment group (assuming adequate sample size and randomization), so that differences between the two groups relative to regression to the mean will "cancel out."

A recent meta-analysis of randomized clinical trials with three arms—a treatment arm, a placebo arm, and a non-treatment arm—demonstrated a clear placebo effect when comparing continuous variable outcomes among subjects in the placebo arm with subjects in the nontreatment arm.[22] The beneficial effect, however, decreased with increasing sample size. The authors suggest that although placebo should continue to play a role in future clinical trials, it should not be used as an actual treatment.

Placebo in Ischemic Heart Disease and Chronic, Stable Exertional Angina Pectoris

The rate of improvement in the frequency of symptoms in patients with chronic, stable, exertional angina pectoris with placebo therapy

TABLE 2-2. Symptomatic Placebo Effects in Cardiovascular Disease

	Placebo Effect
Chronic, stable angina pectoris improvement	30–80%[23]
Heart failure improvement	25–35%[39]

has been assessed to be from 30 to 80%.[23] A summary of subjective and objective placebo effects in cardiovascular disease is provided in Tables 2-2 and 2-3. Due to the magnitude of the placebo effect, studies of new antianginal therapies had generally been performed with a placebo control.[23a] However, the safety of this practice came under scrutiny in the late 1980s due to the concern that patients with coronary artery disease would have periods of no drug treatment. As a result of this, Glasser et al. explored the safety of exposing patients with chronic, stable exertional angina to placebos during short-term drug trials with an average double-blind period of 10 weeks.[24] The study samples were taken from new drug applications (NDAs) submitted to the FDA. The results of these drug trials were submitted, whether favorable or not, and all adverse events were reported. Qualifying studies used symptom-limited exercise tolerance testing as an end point. No antianginal medication except sublingual nitroglycerin was taken after a placebo or drug-free washout period. The placebo-controlled samples consisted of 12 studies, 6 studies using beta-adrenergic blockers and 6 studies using calcium antagonists.[24] A total of 3161 patients entered the studies and 197 withdrew due to adverse cardiovascular events. Beta-blocker therapy was not significantly different when compared to placebo therapy. Conversely, calcium antagonist therapy had a significantly higher cardiovascular event rate compared to placebo therapy, leading to withdrawal from the trials. However, this significantly higher cardiovascular event rate was due to one calcium antagonist study reporting a disproportionately higher number of adverse events than the other five studies.

TABLE 2-3. Objective Placebo Effects in Cardiovascular Disease

	Placebo Effect
Heart failure	
Exercise tolerance testing	
with 1–2 baseline measurements	90–120 s[39]
with 3–10 baseline measurements	10–30 s[39]
Increase in ejection fraction of 5%	20–30% of patients[39]
Hypertension	
Measured by noninvasive, automatic, ambulatory 24-h monitoring	0%[55]
Arrhythmias based on comparison of one control 24-h monitoring period to one 24-h treatment period (variability is so great that it may be inadvisable to pool individual patient data to detect trends in ectopic frequency in evaluating new potential antiarrhythmic agents in groups of patients).	
Mean hourly frequency of ventricular tachycardia	<65%[66]
Mean hourly frequency of couplets	<75%[66]
All ventricular ectopics, without regard for complexity	<83%[66]
When differentiating proarrhythmia in patients with mixed cardiac disease and chronic ventricular arrhythmias from spontaneous variability, with a false-positive rate of only 1%.	
When baseline ventricular premature complexes (VPCs), >100/h	<3 times baseline[67]
When baseline VPCs <100/h	<10 times baseline[67]
Silent ischemic coronary disease	
Reduction in the frequency of ischemic events	44%[28]
Reduction of ST-segment integral	50%[28]
Reduction in duration of ST-segment depression	50%[28]
Reduction of total peak ST-segment depression	7%[28]
Other	
Compliance with treatment at a rate ≥75%	<3 times baseline[70,72]

This study found evidence supporting the safety of a placebo group in short-term drug trials for chronic, stable exertional angina.[24]

The safety of using placebo in longer-term drug trials for chronic, stable exertional angina has not been established. A placebo-controlled trial by a European group in 1986 enrolled 35 patients and followed them while administering placebo and short-acting nitroglycerin for 6 months.[25] This study of the long-term effects of placebo treatment in patients with moderately severe, stable angina pectoris found a shift toward the highest dosage during the titration period. Seven patients were kept on the lowest dosage. The average ending dosage was 65% more than the initial dose. The compliance, when determined by pill count, for 27 patients was >80%. During the first $2\frac{1}{2}$ months of the trial, all the patients who were noncompliant or could not physically continue the study were determined. No patients died or had a myocardial infarction.[25]

There is a paucity of data regarding any gender differences in placebo response. Female patients represented 43% of the population in the aforementioned European study[25] and were more likely to have angina despite normal coronary arteries. Since the placebo effect may be more pronounced in patients with normal coronary arteries, data from male patients were analyzed separately to be compared with the overall results. However, the data from male patients were very similar to the overall results. In fact, the functional status of males showed more improvement due to placebo (61%) than overall (48%) at 8 weeks. The results of this study showed no adverse effects of long-term placebo therapy with 65% of patients reporting subjective clinical improvement and 27% of patients reporting objective, clinical improvement on exercise performance.[25] Of note, improvement in exercise performance can occur when patients are repeatedly exposed to testing.[26]

The use and lack of use of placebo controls in most studies of antianginal drug therapy is evident. One problem inherent in all of the modern day antianginal trials relates to the fact that since anginal patterns vary and, with modern day treatments, attacks of angina are rather infrequent, a surrogate measure of antianginal effect has been adopted by the FDA and relates to treadmill walking time to the point of moderate angina. Also, just as there is a placebo effect on anginal frequency, a patient's treadmill walking time frequently (50–75%) improves with placebo therapy. There are other potential mechanisms that partially explain the improvement unrelated to a treatment effect in exercise walking time in antianginal studies: the so-called learning phenomenon, and the training effect. Patients frequently show an improvement in exercise walking time between the first and second treadmill test in the absence of any treatment. The presumption is that the first test is associated with anxiety and unfamiliarity, which are reduced during the second test. Of greater importance is the training effect, where the frequency of treadmill testing might result in a true improvement of exercise performance irrespective of treatment. The effect of placebo on exercise tolerance in patients with angina was demonstrated in the Transdermal Nitrate Therapy Study, which compared various doses of nitroglycerin administered for 24-h durations from transcutaneous patch formulations to placebo patch treatment.[27] This study was particularly important because it was the first large study to address the issue of nitrate tolerance with transcutaneous patch drug delivery in outpatient, ambulatory subjects. The net result of the study was the demonstration of tolerance in all treated groups in that the treated groups performed no better than placebo at study end. However, there was a striking improvement of 80 to 90 s in the placebo and active treatment groups in the primary efficacy end point of exercise walking time on a treadmill. This improvement in placebo could have masked any active treatment effect, but it also demonstrated the importance of placebo control, since without such a control one could have deduced a significant improvement due to active therapy.

Myocardial ischemia was assessed via 48-h ambulatory electrocardiographic (ECG) monitoring for ST-segment analyses in 250 males with stable angina pectoris and coronary artery disease based on at least 70% stenosis of one major coronary artery, previous myocardial infarction at least 2 months prior to screening, coronary artery bypass surgery, angioplasty, or a positive exercise tolerance test within the last 12 months prior to screening.[28] These participants were reassessed after 7 weeks of therapy with amlodipine or placebo by repeating the 48-h ambulatory ECG monitoring. The monitoring showed the well-known circadian pattern of ischemic activity with peaks in the morning and afternoon. Amlodipine significantly reduced ischemia compared to placebo. However, transient silent myocardial ischemia was less frequent in all groups, including the placebo group.

It was once thought that internal mammary artery ligation improved angina pectoris, until studies showed similar benefit in patients where a sham operation was performed—that is, skin incision with no ligation. Beecher tried to analyze the effect of doctors' personalities on clinical outcomes by comparing the results of the same placebo procedure performed by one of two groups, the "enthusiasts" or the "skeptics."[29] His analysis indicated that the enthusiasts achieved nearly four times more "complete relief" for patients than the skeptics, in spite of the fact that the procedure has no known specific effects.[29] Five patients receiving the sham operation emphatically described marked improvement.[30,31] Objectively, a patient undergoing the sham operation had an increase in work tolerance from 4 to 10 min with no inversion of T waves on ECG and no pain. This procedure was utilized in the United States for 2 years before it was discontinued, when it was disproven by three small, well-planned, double-blind studies.[32] Carver and Samuels also have addressed the issue of sham therapy in the treatment of coronary artery disease.[33] They point out that although the pathophysiology of coronary artery disease is well known, the awareness of many of the expressions of myocardial ischemia are subjective, rendering the placebo effect more important. This has resulted in a number of treatments that are based upon "testimonials" rather than hard scientific evidence and have been touted as "miracle cures" and "breakthroughs," etc. Among therapies cited by these authors are chelation therapy, various vitamin therapies, and mineral supplements. Chelation therapy is probably one of the most instructive examples of a sham and is briefly discussed here. It has been estimated that 500,000 patients per year are treated by this technique in the United States alone. Prior to 1995, the data to support claims regarding the effectiveness of chelation therapy were uncontrolled open-label studies. In 1994, van Rij and associates performed a double-blind, randomized, placebo-controlled study in patients with intermittent claudication and demonstrated no benefits of chelation over placebo.[34] A number of variables were evaluated, including both objective and subjective measures, with improvement in many of the measures of both therapies. Again, without the use of a placebo control, the results could have been interpreted as improvements related to chelation treatment.

At this time the National Institutes of Health has started a large multicenter, placebo-controlled trial to definitively assess whether chelation is of any clinical benefit in patients with coronary artery disease.

The Placebo Effect in Heart Failure

Until recently, the importance of the placebo effect in patients with congestive heart failure (CHF) had not been recognized. In the 1970s and early 1980s, vasodilator therapy was administered to patients in clinical trials without placebo control. Investigators believed that the cause of heart failure was predictable, so placebo-controlled trials were unnecessary. Another view of the unfavorable course of heart failure concluded that withholding a promising new agent was unethical. The ethical issues regarding placebo use in cardiovascular disease are discussed further on in this chapter.[35–38]

Upon inclusion of placebo controls in clinical trials, a 25 to 35% improvement in patients' symptoms was documented. This placebo response occurred in patients with mild to severe symptoms and did not depend on the size of the study. The assessment of left ventricular (LV) function can be determined by several methods, including noninvasive echocardiography, radionuclide ventriculography, or invasive pulmonary artery balloon-floatation catheterization. These methods measure the patient's response to therapy or the natural progression of the patient's heart failure.[39]

Noninvasive measurements of LV ejection fraction vary, especially when the ventricular function is poor and the time interval between tests is 3 to 6 months. Packer found that when a 5% increase in ejection fraction is used to determine a beneficial response to a new drug, 20 to 30% of patients show improvement while receiving placebo therapy. Overall, changes in noninvasive measures of LV function have not been shown to correlate closely with observed changes in clinical status of patients with CHF. Most vasodilator and inotropic drugs can produce clinical benefit without a change in LV ejection fraction. Conversely, LV ejection fraction may increase significantly in heart failure patients with worsening clinical status.[39]

In using invasive catheterization to evaluate the efficacy of a new drug, interpretation must be done carefully, since there may be spontaneous fluctuations in hemodynamic variables in the absence of drug therapy. To avoid recognition of spontaneous variability attributable to drug therapy, postdrug effects should be assessed at fixed times and threshold values should eliminate changes due to spontaneous variability. Another factor that can mimic a beneficial drug response by favorably affecting hemodynamic measurements is measurement performed immediately after catheterization of the right side of the heart or after ingestion of a meal. Following intravascular instrumentation, systemic vasoconstriction occurs and resolves after 12 to 24 h. When predrug measurements are done during the postcatheterization period, any subsequent measurements will show beneficial effects, since the original measurements were done during the vasoconstricted state. Thus, comparative data must be acquired after the postcatheterization vasoconstricted state has resolved.[39]

The most common test to evaluate drug efficacy for heart failure is the exercise tolerance test (ETT). An increased duration of ET represents a beneficial therapy. However, this increased duration is also recorded during placebo therapy, possibly due to the familiarity of the patient with the test and the increased willingness of the physician to encourage the patient to exercise to exhaustion. Placebo response to repeated ETT can be an increase in duration of 90 to 120 s when only one or two baseline measurements are done. This response can be reduced to 10 to 30 s when 3 to 10 baseline measurements are performed. The placebo response cannot be explained by changes in gas-exchange measurements during the ETT; presumably, it relates to an improvement in the subjects' mechanical efficiency of walking during the ETT.[39,40]

Since all methods used to measure efficacy of a treatment for heart failure include placebo effects, studies must include placebo controls in order to prove efficacy of a new drug therapy. Statistical analysis of placebo-controlled studies must compare between groups for statistical significance. "Between groups" refers to comparison of the change in one group, such as a new drug therapy, with the change in another group, such as a placebo.[39]

In 1992, Archer and Leier reported on placebo therapy for 8 weeks in 15 patients with CHF,[41] which resulted in a mean improvement in exercise duration of 81 s or 30% above baseline. This result was statistically significant compared to the 12-s improvement by the 9 patients in the nonplacebo control group. Using between-group statistical analysis, there were no statistically significant differences between the placebo and nonplacebo groups at baseline or at week 8 of treatment. Echocardiography studies showed no significant improvement in either group and no significant differences between the two groups at baseline or during the treatment period. To prove the existence of the therapeutic power of placebo treatment in CHF and to quantitate it, all studies were performed by the same principal investigator with identical study methods and conditions, and all patients were similarly familiarized with the treadmill testing procedure prior to baseline measurements. Also, the study used a well-matched, nonplacebo control group and illustrated the spontaneous variability of congestive heart failure.[41]

The Placebo Effect in Hypertension

Some studies of placebo response in hypertensive patients have shown a lowering of blood pressure[42–47] and others have not.[47–51] In the Medical Research Council study, no treatment compared to placebo therapy in patients with mild hypertension for several months found similar results in both groups, an initial fall in blood pressure followed by stabilization.[51] Of historical note is a study by Goldring and associates published in 1956.[52] These authors fabricated an "electron gun" designed to be as "dramatic as possible, but without any known physiologic action other than a psychogenic one." Initial exposure to "the gun" was for 1 to 3 min and was increased to 5 min three times daily. The investigators noticed a substantially lower pressure during therapy compared with pretherapy. In 6 of 9 hospitalized patients, there was a blood pressure reduction of 39/28 mm Hg.

An important factor to consider is the method used to measure blood pressure. In using standard sphygmomanometry, blood pressure falls initially. During placebo therapy, intraarterial pressures and circadian curves measured over 24 h did not show a decline in blood pressure or heart rate. Intraarterial blood pressure was lower at home compared to measurements at the hospital. The circadian curves from intraarterial ambulatory blood pressure monitoring were reproducible on separate days several weeks apart.[45,53]

Like 24-h invasive intraarterial monitoring, 24-h noninvasive automatic monitoring of ambulatory blood pressure also has been reported to be devoid of a placebo effect. Upon the initial application of the blood pressure device, a small reduction of ambulatory blood pressure values in the first 8 h occurred with placebo therapy. This effect, however, did not change the mean 24-h value. The home monitoring values were lower than the office measurements. Heart rate was also measured, with no variance in either setting. The office measurement of blood pressure but not the 24-h blood pressure was lower after 4 weeks of placebo therapy.[54] This study confirms the absence of a placebo effect in 24-h noninvasive ambulatory blood pressure monitoring suggested by several specific studies on large numbers of patients.[55–58] The 24-h monitoring was measured by the noninvasive automatic Spacelabs 5300 device (Spacelabs Inc., Redmond, Washington).[59] Another important factor in 24-h noninvasive monitoring is that the intervals of measurement were <60 min.[60]

In a study on the influence of observer's expectation on the placebo effect in blood pressure, 100 patients were followed for a 2-week single-blind period and for a 2-week double-blind period.[61] During this time, the patients' blood pressures were measured by two methods: a 30-min recording with an automatic oscillometric device and a standard sphygmomanometric measurement performed by a physician. All patients were seen in the same examining room, monitored by the same automatic oscillometric device, and seen by the same physician. The results during the single-blind period showed a slight but statistically significant decline in diastolic blood pressure detected by the automatic oscillometric device and no decline measured by the physician. During the double-blind period, there was no additional decline in diastolic blood pressure measured by the oscillometric device, but the physician measured significant decreases in both systolic and diastolic blood pressures. Overall, the blood pressures measured by the automatic oscillometric device in the absence of the physician were lower than those measured by the physician. However, there was significant correlation of the two methods. The investigators concluded that in correcting for the placebo effect in clinical trials in hypertension, the use of ambulatory monitoring should adhere to the same design standards as those in using conventional sphygmomanometry.[62]

Although there was a placebo effect in the measurement of blood pressure using auscultatory technique in the Systolic Hypertension in the Elderly Program (SHEP), this was not as significant as the reduction of blood pressure produced by active therapy in patients 60 years of age and older with isolated systolic hypertension.[63,64] In a subsequent study of patients with isolated systolic hypertension, it was observed that a substantial portion of the long-term blood pressure change observed during active treatment could be attributed to a placebo effect. Twenty-four-hour blood pressure monitoring was no more reliable than conventional sphygmomanometry in correcting for the actions of placebo.

The Placebo Effect in Arrhythmia

Spontaneous variability in the natural history of disease or in its signs and/or symptoms is another reason that placebo controls are necessary. In a study of ventricular arrhythmias, Michelson and Morganroth found marked spontaneous variability of complex ventricular arrhythmias such as ventricular tachycardia and couplets.[65] Their study followed 20 patients for 4-day periods of continuous ECG monitoring. They recommended that, in evaluating therapeutic agents, a comparison of one 24-h control period to four 24-h test periods must show a 41% reduction in the mean hourly frequency of ventricular tachycardia and a 50% reduction in the mean hourly frequency of couplets to demonstrate statistically significant therapeutic efficacy. They also suggested that individual patient data not be pooled to detect trends because the individual variability is so great.

A study by Morganroth et al. provides an algorithm to differentiate spontaneous variability from proarrhythmia in patients with benign or potentially lethal ventricular arrhythmias.[66] A total of 495 patients were evaluated with two or more Holter tracings during placebo therapy. The algorithm defines proarrhythmia as an increase of more than three times when the hourly frequency of baseline ven-

tricular premature complexes (VPCs) is >100 and >10 times when it is <100. The false-positive rate is 1% with this algorithm.

The Cardiac Arrhythmia Suppression Trial (CAST) evaluated the effect of antiarrhythmic therapy in patients with asymptomatic or mildly symptomatic ventricular arrhythmia.[67,68] Response to drug therapy was determined by an ≥80% reduction of ventricular premature depolarizations or a ≥90% reduction of runs of unsustained ventricular tachycardia as measured by 24-h Holter monitoring 4 to 10 days after the initiation of pharmacologic treatment—this response having previously been considered an important surrogate measure of antiarrhythmic drug efficacy. Ambulatory ECG (Holter) recording screened for arrhythmias. The CAST Data and Safety Monitoring Board recommended that encainide and flecainide therapy be discontinued based on the increased number of deaths from arrhythmia, cardiac arrest, or any cause compared to the placebo group (1455 patient were assigned to drug regimens). The CAST investigators' conclusion emphasized the need for more placebo-controlled clinical trials of antiarrhythmic drugs with a mortality end point.[67]

The Relationship of Treatment Adherence to Survival in Patients with and without History of Myocardial Infarction

One important consideration in determining study results is adherence to therapy and the presumption that any differences in adherence rates would be equal in the active versus the placebo treament groups. The Coronary Drug Project planned to evaluate the efficacy and safety of several lipid-influencing drugs in the long-term treatment of coronary heart disease.[69] This randomized double-blind placebo-controlled multicenter clinical trial found no significant difference in the 5-year mortality of 1103 men treated with the fibric acid derivative clofibrate compared to 2789 men given placebo. However, good adherers, patients taking ≥80% of the protocol drug, had lower mortality than poor adherers in both the clofibrate and placebo groups.[69]

A similar association between adherence and mortality was found in patients after myocardial infarction in the Beta-Blocker Heart Attack Trial (BHAT) data.[70] This same phenomenon was extended to women after myocardial infarction. On analysis of the BHAT data for 505 women randomized to both beta-blocker therapy and placebo therapy, there was a $2\frac{1}{2}$- to 3-fold increased mortality within the first 2 years in patients taking <75% of their prescribed medication. Adherence among men and women was similar at about 90%. However, the cause of the increased survival resulting from good adherence is not known. There is speculation about good adherence reflecting a favorable psychological profile—an individual's ability to make lifestyle adjustments that limit disease progression. Alternatively, adherence may be associated with other advantageous health practices or social circumstances not measured. Another possible explanation is that improved health status may facilitate good adherence.[71]

The Lipid Research Clinics Coronary Primary Prevention Trial did not find a correlation between compliance and mortality.[64] They randomized 3806 asymptomatic hypercholesterolemic men to cholestyramine or placebo. Over 7 years, the main effects of the drug compared to placebo on cholesterol and death or nonfatal myocardial infarction were shown. In the active drug group, a relationship between compliance and outcome existed, mediated by lowering cholesterol. However, no effect of compliance on cholesterol or outcome was observed in the placebo group.[72,73]

The Physicians' Health Study randomized 22,000 U.S. male physicians between the ages of 40 and 84 years who were free of myocardial infarction and cerebral vascular disease.[74] This study analyzed the benefit of differing frequencies of aspirin consumption on the prevention of myocardial infarction. Additionally, the study identified factors associated with adherence and analyzed the relationship of adherence with cardiovascular outcomes in the placebo group. In this study, an average compliance of 80% in the aspirin and placebo groups over the 60 months of follow-up was observed.[74] Adherence during the trial was associated with several baseline characteristics in the aspirin and placebo groups. Trial participants with poor adherence (<50% compliance with pill consumption) were more likely to be younger than 50 years at randomization, to smoke cigarettes, to be overweight, to not exercise regularly, to have a parental history of myocardial infarction, and to have angina relative to those with good adherence. These associations were statistically significant. In a multivariant logistic regression model, cigarette smoking, being overweight, and angina remained significant predictors of poor compliance. The strongest predictor of adherence during the trial was adherence during the run-in period. Baseline characteristics with little relationship to adherence included regular alcohol consumption and a history of diabetes and hypertension.[74]

Using an intention-to-treat analysis, the aspirin group had a 41% lower risk of myocardial infarction compared to the placebo group. On subgroup analysis, participants reporting excellent (≥95%) adherence in the aspirin group had a significant (51%) reduction in risk of first myocardial infarction relative to those with similar adherence in the placebo group. Lower adherence in the aspirin group did not produce a statistically significant reduction of first myocardial infarction compared to the placebo group with excellent adherence. Excellent adherence in the aspirin group was associated with a 41% lower relative risk of myocardial infarction than in those with lower adherence in the aspirin group. Excellent adherence in the placebo group did not show a reduction of relative risk.

The rate of stroke was different from myocardial infarction. Using an intention-to-treat analysis, the aspirin group had a nonsignificant (22%) increased rate of stroke than the placebo group. Excellent adherence in the placebo group produced a lower rate of strokes than among participants in the aspirin and placebo groups with poor (<50%) adherence. Excellent adherence in the placebo group was associated with a 29% lower risk of stroke than among those with excellent adherence in the aspirin group.

The overall relationship of adherence to aspirin therapy with cardiovascular risk considered a combined end point of all important cardiovascular events—including first fatal or nonfatal myocardial infarction or stroke or death from cardiovascular disease with no prior myocardial infarction or stroke. Using an intention-to-treat analysis, there was an 18% decrease in risk of all important cardiovascular events in the aspirin group compared to the placebo group. Participants with excellent adherence in the aspirin group had a 26% reduction of risk of a first major cardiovascular event compared to those with excellent adherence in the placebo group. However, those participants in the aspirin group with poor compliance had a 31% increased risk of a first cardiovascular event compared to those in the placebo group with excellent adherence. Within the placebo group, there was no association between level of adherence and risk of first cardiovascular event.

In analysis of death from any cause with no prior nonfatal myocardial infarction or stroke, poor adherence in both the aspirin and placebo groups was associated with a fourfold increase in the risk of death. In analysis of the 91 deaths due to cardiovascular causes,

similar risks were found to be associated with poor adherence in both the aspirin and placebo groups relative to excellent adherence in the placebo group.

The Physicians' Health Study found similar results to the Coronary Drug Project when all-cause mortality and cardiovascular mortality were considered.[69,74] These relationships remained strong when adjusted for potential confounding variables at baseline. The strong trend for higher death rates among participants with poor adherence in both the aspirin and placebo groups may be due to the tendency for individuals to lessen or discontinue study participation as individuals' health declines with serious illness. Acute events such as myocardial infarction did not accompany an increased risk associated with poor adherence in the placebo group. Thus, placebo effects seem to vary depending on the outcome considered.

CLINICAL TRIALS AND THE ETHICS OF USING PLACEBO CONTROLS

Since the 1962 amendments to the Food, Drug and Cosmetic Act, the FDA has had to rely on the results of "adequate and well-controlled" clinical trials to determine the efficacy of new pharmacologic therapies. Regulations governing pharmacologic testing recognize several types of controls that may be used in clinical trials to assess the efficacy of new pharmacologic therapies. These include (1) placebo concurrent control, (2) dose-comparison concurrent control, (3) no-treatment concurrent control, (4) active-treatment concurrent control, and (5) historical control. However, regulations do not specify the circumstances for the use of these controls because there are various study designs that may be adequate in a given set of circumstances.[75,76]

There is an ongoing debate concerning the ethics of using placebo controls in clinical trials of cardiac medications.[35,36,77] The issue revolves around the administration of placebo in lieu of a proven therapy. Two articles illustrate the debate.[20,37]

Rothman and Michels[37] state that patients in clinical trials often receive placebo therapy instead of a proven therapy for the patient's medical condition and assert that this practice is in direct violation of the Nuremberg Code and the World Medical Association's adaptation of this code in the Helsinki Declaration. The Nuremberg Code, a 10-point ethical code for experimentation in human beings, was formulated in response to the human experimentation atrocities that were recorded during the post–World War II trial of Nazi physicians in Nuremberg, Germany. According to Rothman and Michels,[37] violation occurs because the use of placebo as control denies the patient the best proven therapeutic treatment. It occurs despite the establishment of regulatory agencies and institutional review boards, although these authors seem to ignore the fact that informed consent is part of the current practice, as certainly was not the case with the Nazi atrocities.

One reason why placebo-controlled trials are approved by institutional review boards is that this type of trial is part of the FDA's general recommendation for demonstrating therapeutic efficacy before an investigational drug can be approved. When the investigational drug is found to be more beneficial than placebo, therapeutic efficacy is proven.[78] As more drugs are found to be more effective than placebo in treating disease, the inclusion of a placebo group is often questioned. However, this question ignores that, in many cases, drug efficacy had been established by surrogate measures and—as new and better measures of efficacy become available— additional study becomes warranted. For instance, the suppression of ventricular arrhythmia by antiarrhythmic therapy was later proven to be unrelated to survival; in fact, results with this therapy were worse than with placebo. Likewise, in studies of inotropic therapy for heart failure, exercise performance rather than survival was used as the measure of efficacy, and in fact a presumed efficacious therapy performed worse than placebo. In the use of immediate short-acting dihydropyridine calcium antagonist therapy for the relief of symptoms of chronic stable angina pectoris, again, a subject might have fared better had he or she been randomly assigned to placebo therapy.

Also important in the concept that established beneficial therapy should not necessarily prohibit the use of placebo in the evaluation of new therapies is that the natural history of a disease may change, and the effectiveness of the so-called established therapy (e.g., antibiotic agent for treatment of infection) may diminish. In deciding on the use of an investigational drug in a clinical trial, the prevailing standard is that there should be enough confidence to risk exposure to a new drug but also enough doubt about the drug to risk exposure to placebo. Thus, in this situation, the use of a placebo control becomes warranted, particularly as long as other life-saving therapy is not discontinued.

The use of placebo-controlled trials may be advocated on the basis of a scientific argument. When pharmacologic therapy has been shown to be effective in previous placebo-controlled clinical trials, conclusions drawn from trials without placebo controls may be misleading because the previous placebo-controlled trial becomes a historical control. These historical controls are the least reliable for demonstrating efficacy.[75] In active-controlled clinical trials, there is an assumption that the active control treatment is as effective under the new experimental conditions as it was in the previous placebo-controlled trial. This assumption can result in misleading conclusions when results with an experimental therapy are found to be equivalent to those with active, proven therapy. This conclusion of equivalence can be magnified by conservative statistical methods, such as the use of "intent to treat" approach, an analysis of all randomized patients regardless of protocol deviations, and an attempt to minimize the potential for introduction of bias into the study. Concurrent placebo controls account for factors other than drug-effect differences between study groups. When, instead of a placebo-control group, an untreated control group is used, blinding is lost and treatment-related bias may occur.[20,75,79–81]

Clark and Leaverton[20] and Rothman and Michel[37] agree that the use of placebo controls is ethical when there is no existing treatment to affect morbidity and mortality or survival favorably. Furthermore, there are chronic diseases for which treatment exists but does not favorably alter morbidity and mortality or survival. For example, no clinical trial has found the treatment of angina to increase a patient's survival. In contrast, treatment after a myocardial infarction with beta-blocking agents has been convincingly proven to increase a patient's survival.[20]

However, Clark and Leaverton[20] disagree with Rothman and Michels[37] in asserting that, for chronic disease, a placebo-controlled clinical trial of short duration is ethical because there is usually no alteration in long-term outcome for the patient. The short duration of the trial represents a small segment of the life-time management of a chronic disease. For instance, the treatment of chronic symptomatic CHF and a low ejection fraction (<40%) with enalapril was shown to decrease mortality by 16%. This decrease in mortality was most marked in the first 24 months of follow up, with an average follow-up period of 40 months. Therefore, only long-term compliance with pharmacologic therapy resulted in some decrease in mortality. Another example of a chronic medical condition that requires long-term

treatment and in which short-term placebo is probably not harmful is hypertension.[82] In some studies, men and women with a history of myocardial infarction and with a ≥80% compliance with treatment, including placebo therapy, had an increased survival. This increased survival was also described in patients in a 5-year study of the effect of lipid-influencing drugs on coronary heart disease.[71,83,84]

Therefore, Rothman and Michels[37] and Clark and Leaverton[20] agree that a placebo should not be included in a trial when there is a proven therapy that favorably affects morbidity and mortality, but they disagree with regard to chronic cardiovascular diseases and short-term trials. Brief interruption of effective therapy has not been found to alter long-term outcome when the effective treatment is a long-term therapy. The claim that the use of placebos in clinical trials violates the Nuremberg Code and the Helsinki Declaration if a proven therapy exists does not account for all of the information currently available. The proven therapies for chronic congestive heart failure and hypertension are long-term therapies. The belief that patients receiving placebo are being harmed is not accurate because there is no adverse effect on morbidity and mortality or survival when proven, long-term therapy is withheld for a short time.

A different argument for the ethical basis of using placebo controls relies on the informed consent process. Before a patient's participation in a clinical trial, the patient is asked to participate in the trial. The informed consent process includes a description of the use of placebo and other aspects of the trial. In this written agreement the patient is responsible for notifying the physician of any medical problems and is informed of his or her right to withdraw from the study at any time, as described in the Nuremberg Code and Helsinki Declaration. During this disclosure, patients are presented with some new concepts and with risks and benefits to understand. On the basis of this information, a patient voluntarily decides whether to participate, knowing that he or she may receive a placebo or investigational medication.

However, despite physicians' efforts to inform the patient of research methods and the risk and benefits of trial participation, some patients agree to participate simply because of their trust in their physician. This situation may produce conflict between the physician-patient relationship and the physician's role as investigator. A partial resolution of this conflict is the double-blind technique, in which neither the patient nor the investigator knows which therapy a patient is receiving. This technique allows the doctor and patient to make medical decisions on the basis of clinical signs and symptoms. In addition, because of the requirement for informed consent, the decision about participation in a clinical trial is shifted to the patient rather than left solely with the physician. However, the patient's physician evaluates the suitability of the patient for a particular trial before asking the patient to participate.

For every pharmacologic therapy, an assumption is made about patient compliance with the regimen. In clinical trials, investigators try to keep track of compliance by having patients bring their pill bottles to their appointments and counting the pills. Ultimately, the patient decides whether the beneficial effects of therapy outweigh the adverse effects. If a medication produces annoying and adverse side effects, then the patient may not continue to take the medication. Other factors affecting compliance are the number of pills taken per day or the frequency of dosing. For instance, it is easier to take a medication once a day rather than three times a day. Furthermore, studies of patient compliance have found increased survival in patients with at least an 80% rate of compliance with therapy, including placebo therapy.[71,83,84]

All parties should be responsible for their research and accountable for the ethical conduct of their research. Clinical trials failing to comply with the Nuremberg Code and the Helsinki Declaration should not be conducted and should not be accepted for publication. Yet there is disagreement in determining which research methods are in compliance with the Nuremberg Code and Helsinki Declaration. Scientific needs should not take precedence over ethical needs. Clinical trials need to be carefully designed to produce a high quality of trial performance. In addition, in experimentation involving human subjects, the Nuremberg Code and Helsinki Declaration must be used as universal standards.

Until the mechanism of the placebo action is understood and can be controlled, a clinical trial that does not include a placebo group provides data that should be interpreted with caution. The absence of a placebo group makes it difficult to assess efficacy of a therapy. It is easy to attribute clinical improvement to a drug therapy if there is no control group. As was found with heart failure, chronic diseases have variable courses. Until the variability in chronic diseases is understood, placebo controls are needed to help explain it. In addition, because each clinical trial has a different setting and different study design within the context of the physician-patient relationship, a placebo group helps the investigator differentiate true drug effects from placebo effects.

More important than the inclusion of a placebo group is a careful study design that includes frequent review by a data and safety monitoring board of each patient's medical condition and trends affecting the patients' mortality, morbidity, and survival. This monitoring is crucial to protect the study participants. To protect the participants, trials must include provisions that require a patient to be removed from a trial when the patient or doctor believe that removal is in the best interest of the patient. The patient can then be treated with currently approved therapies.

Patients receiving placebo may report subjective, clinical improvements and show objective, clinical improvements, for instance, on ETT or Holter monitoring of ischemic events. Findings such as these dispel the implication that placebo therapy is the same as no therapy and may occur because many factors are involved in the physician-patient relationship, such as the psychological state of the patient, the patient's expectations and conviction regarding the efficacy of the method of treatment, and the physician's biases, attitudes, expectations, and methods of communication.[85] An explanation of improvement in patients participating in trials is the close attention received by patients from the investigators. Baseline laboratory values are checked to ensure the safety of the patient and compliance with the study protocol. This beneficial response by the patient is called a positive placebo effect when found in control groups of patients receiving placebo therapy.[23,26,29,30,32,39,86,87]

Conversely, the condition of patients receiving placebos has also, in some cases, worsened in response to placebo therapy. Every drug has side effects. These side effects are also found with placebo therapy and can be so great that they preclude the patient's continuation with the therapy. This phenomenon is reported by patients in clinical trials receiving placebo.[17,25,39,86,88,89] Finally, placebos can act synergistically and antagonistically with other specific and nonspecific therapies. Therefore much is still to be discovered about the effect of placebo in cardiovascular medicine.

CONCLUSION

The effect of placebo on the clinical course of systolic hypertension, angina pectoris, silent myocardial ischemia, CHF, and ventricular tachyarrhythmias is well described, and continues to be the focus of much investigative interests.[71] In the prevention of myocardial infarction there appears to be a direct relation between compliance with placebo treatment and favorable clinical outcomes. The safety of short-term placebo-controlled trials has now been well documented in studies of drug treatment of angina pectoris. The ethical basis of performing placebo-controlled trials continues to be challenged in the evaluation of drugs for treating cardiovascular diseases[35,37]; however, as long as life-saving treatment is not being denied, the performance of placebo-controlled studies remains a prudent approach for obtaining reliable scientific information regarding the efficacy and safety of a new treatment.

REFERENCES

1. Turner JA, Deyo RA, Loeser JD, et al: The importance of placebo effects in pain treatment and research. *JAMA* 271:1609, 1994.
2. Benson H, Epstein MD: The placebo effect, a neglected asset in the care of patients. *JAMA* 232:1225, 1975.
3. Talbot M: The placebo prescription. *New York Times Magazine* January 9, 2000.
4. Weiner M, Weiner GJ: The kinetics and dynamics of responses to placebo. *Clin Pharmacol Ther* 60:247, 1996.
5. Packer M, Medina N, Yushak M: Hemodynamic changes mimicking a vasodilator drug response in the absence of drug therapy after right heart catheterization in patients with chronic heart failure. *Circulation* 71:76l, 1985.
6. Melmon K, Morrelli HF, Hoffman B, Nierenberg D, eds. *Melmon and Morrelli's Clinical Pharmacology: Basic Principles in Therapeutics,* 3rd ed. New York: McGraw-Hill, 1992.
7. Chalmers TC: Prophylactic treatment of Wilson's disease. *N Engl J Med* 278:910, 1968.
8. *Stedman's Medical Dictionary,* 25th ed. Baltimore: Williams & Wilkins, 1990.
9. Spiro HM: *Doctors, Patients and Placebos.* New Haven, CT: Yale University Press, 1986.
10. White L, Tursky B, Schwartz G, eds. *Placebo: Theory, Research, and Mechanisms.* New York: Guilford Press, 1985.
11. Shapiro AK: Factors contributing to the placebo effect: Their implications for psychotherapy. *Am J Psychother* 18:73, 1961.
12. Byerly H: Explaining and exploiting placebo effects. *Pers Biol Med* 19:423, 1976.
13. Lind JA: *A Treatise of the Scurvy.* Edinburgh: Scotland, 1753.
14. Hill AB: The clinical trial. *Br Med Bull* 7:278, 1951.
15. Beecher HK: The powerful placebo. *JAMA* 159:1602, 1955.
16. Lasagna L, Masteller F, von Felsinger JM, Beecher HK: A study of the placebo response. *Am J Med* 16:770, 1954.
16a. Barsky AJ, Saintfort R, Rogers MP, Borus JF: Nonspecific medication side effects and the nocebo phenomenon. *JAMA* 287:622, 2002.
16b. Feinstein AR: The placebo effect. In: *Education of Health Professionals in Complementary/Alternative Medicine.* Conference sponsored by Josiah Macy Jr. Foundation, Phoenix, AZ, Nov 2–5, 2000. Published by Josiah Macy Jr. Foundation, New York: New York, 2001.
17. Wolf S, Pinsky RH: Effects of placebo administration and occurrence of toxic reactions. *JAMA* 155:339, 1954.
18. Davis JM: Don't let placebos fool you. *Postgrad Med* 88:21, 1990.
19. Nies AS, Spielberg SP: Principles of therapeutics. In: Hardman JG, Limbird LE, eds. *Goodman and Gilman's the Pharmacological Basis of Therapeutics,* 9th ed. New York: McGraw Hill, 1996:55.
20. Clark PI, Leaverton PE: Scientific and ethical issues in the use of placebo controls in clinical trials. *Annu Rev Public Health* 15:19, 1994.
21. FDA Draft: Guidelines for the Clinical Evaluation of Anti-anginal Drugs. January 10, 1989.
22. Hrobjartsson A, Gotzsche PC: Is the placebo powerless? An analysis of clinical trials comparing placebo with no treatment. *N Engl J Med* 344:1594, 2001.
23. Amsterdam EA, Wolfson S, Gorlin R: New aspects of the placebo response in angina pectoris. *Am J Cardiol* 24:305, 1969.
23a. Kim MC, Kini A, Sharma SK: Refractory angina pectoris: Mechanism and therapeutic options. *J Am Coll Cardiol* 39:923, 2002.
24. Glasser SP, Clark PI, Lipicky RJ, et al: Exposing patients with chronic, stable, exertional angina to placebo periods in drug trials. *JAMA* 265:1550, 1991.

25. Boissel JP, Philippon AM, Gauthier E, et al: Time course of long-term placebo therapy effects in angina pectoris. *Eur Heart J* 7:1030, 1986.

26. McGraw BF, Hemberger JA, Smith AL, Schroeder JS: Variability of exercise performance during long-term placebo treatment. *Clin Pharmacol Ther* 30:321, 1981.

27. Transdermal Nitroglycerin Cooperative Study Group: Acute and chronic antianginal efficacy and continuous 24 hour application of transdermal nitroglycerin. *Am J Cardiol* 68:1263, 1991.

28. Deanfield JE, Detry JRG, Lichen PR, et al for the CAPE Study Group: Amlodipine reduces transient myocardial ischemia in patients with coronary artery disease: double-blind circadian anti-ischemia program in Europe (CAPE Trial). *J Am Coll Cardiol* 24:1460, 1994.

29. Beecher HK: Surgery as a placebo: A quantitative study in bias. *JAMA* 176:1102,1961.

30. Dimond EG, Kittle CF, Crockett JE: Evaluation of internal mammary artery ligation and sham procedures in angina pectoris. *Circulation* 18:712, 1958.

31. Dimond EG, Kittle CF, Crockett JE: Comparison of internal mammary artery ligation and sham operation for angina pectoris. *Am J Cardiol* 5:484, 1960.

32. Cobb LA: Evaluation of internal mammary artery ligation by double-blind technic. *N Engl J Med* 260:1115, 1959.

33. Carver JR, Samuels F: Sham therapy in coronary artery disease and atherosclerosis. *Pract Cardiol* 14:81, 1988.

34. van Rij AM, Solomon C, Packer SGK, Hopkins WG: Chelation therapy for intermittent claudication. *Circulation* 90:1194, 1994.

35. Martin Enserink: Are placebo-controlled drug trials ethical? *Science* 288:416, 2000.

36. Halpern SD, Karlawish JHT: Placebo-controlled trials are unethical in clinical hypertension research. *Arch Intern Med* 160:3167, 2000.

37. Rothman KJ, Michels KB: The continuing unethical use of placebo controls. *N Engl J Med* 331:394, 1994.

38. Bienenfeld L, Frishman W, Glasser SP: The placebo effect in cardiovascular disease. *Am Heart J* 132:1207, 1996.

39. Packer M: The placebo effect in heart failure. *Am Heart J* 120:1579, 1990.

40. Russel SD, McNeer FR, Beere PA, et al: Improvement in the mechanical efficiency of walking: An explanation for the "placebo effect" seen during repeated exercise testing of patients with heart failure. *Am Heart J* 135:107, 1998.

41. Archer TP, Leier CV: Placebo treatment in congestive heart failure. *Cardiology* 81:125, 1992.

42. Myers MG, Lewis GRJ, Steiner J, Dollery CT: Atenolol in essential hypertension. *Clin Pharmacol Ther* 19:502, 1976.

43. Pugsley DJ, Nassim M, Armstrong BK, Beilin L: A controlled trial of labetalol (Trandate), propranolol and placebo in the management of mild to moderate hypertension. *Br J Clin Pharmacol* 7:63, 1979.

44. Martin MA, Phillips CA, Smith AJ: Acebutolol in hypertension—a double-blind trial against placebo. *Br J Clin Pharmacol* 6: 351, 1978.

45. Report of Medical Research Council Working Party on Mild to Moderate Hypertension: Randomized controlled trial of treatment for mild hypertension: design and pilot trial. *Br Med J* 1:1437, 1977.

46. Gould BA, Mann SM, Davies AB, et al: Does placebo lower blood pressure? *Lancet* 2:1377, 1981.

47. Preston RA, Materson BJ, Reda DJ, et al: Placebo-associated blood pressure response and adverse effects in the treatment of hypertension: Observations from a Department of Veteran Affairs Cooperative Study. *Arch Intern Med* 160:1449, 2000.

48. Wilkinson PR, Raftery EB: A comparative trial of clonidine, propranolol and placebo in the treatment of moderate hypertension. *Br J Clin Pharmacol* 4:289, 1977.

49. Hanson L, Aberg H, Karlberg E, Westerlund A: Controlled study of atenolol in treatment of hypertension. *Br Med J* 2:367, 1975.

50. Veterans Administration Cooperative Study Group on Antihypertensive Agents: Effects of treatment on morbidity in hypertension: Results in patients with diastolic blood pressures averaging 115 through 119 mm Hg. *JAMA* 202:116, 1967.

51. Veterans Administration Cooperative Study Group on Antihypertensive Agents: Effects of treatment on morbidity in hypertension: Results in patients with diastolic blood pressures averaging 90 through 114 mm Hg. *JAMA* 213:1143, 1970.

52. Goldring W, Chasis H, Schreiner GE, Smith HW: Reassurance in the management of benign hypertensive disease. *Circulation* 14:260, 1956.

53. Raftery EB, Gould BA: The effect of placebo on indirect and direct blood pressure measurements. *J Hypertens* 8(Suppl 6):S93, 1990.

54. Mutti E, Trazzi S, Omboni S, et al: Effect of placebo on 24-h non-invasive ambulatory blood pressure. *J Hypertens* 9:361, 1991.

55. O'Brien E, Cox GP, O'Malley K: Ambulatory blood pressure measurements in the evaluation of blood pressure lowering drugs. *J Hypertens* 7:243, 1989.

56. Dupont AG, Van der Nieppen P, Six RO: Placebo does not lower ambulatory blood pressure. *Br J Clin Pharmacol* 24:106, 1987.

57. Coats AJS, Conway J, Sommers VK, et al: Ambulatory blood pressure monitoring in the assessment of antihypertensive therapy. *Cardiovasc Drugs Ther* 3:303, 1989.

58. Parati G, Pomidossi G, Casadei R, et al: Evaluation of the antihypertensive effect of celiprolol by ambulatory blood pressure monitoring. *Am J Cardiol* 61:27C, 1988.

59. Casadei R, Parati G, Pomidossi G, et al: Twenty-four hour blood pressure monitoring: Evaluation of Spacelabs 5300 monitor by comparison with intra-arterial blood pressure recording in ambulant subjects. *J Hypertens* 6:797, 1988.

60. Portaluppi F, Strozzi C, Uberti ED, et al: Does placebo lower blood pressure in hypertensive patients? A noninvasive chronobiological study. *Jpn Heart J* 29: 189, 1988.

61. Sassano P, Chatellier G, Corvol P, Menard J: Influence of observer's expectation on the placebo effect in blood pressure trials. *Curr Ther Res* 41:304, 1987.

62. Staessen JA, Thijs L, Bieniaszewski L, et al: On behalf of the Systolic Hypertension in Europe (SYST-EUR) Trial Investigators: Ambulatory monitoring uncorrected for placebo overestimates long-term antihypertensive action. *Hypertension* 27(Part 1):414, 1996.

63. SHEP Cooperative Research Group: Prevention of stroke by antihypertensive drug treatment in older persons with isolated systolic hypertension. Final results of the Systolic Hypertension in the Elderly Program (SHEP). *JAMA* 265:3255, 1991.

64. Davis BR, Wittes J, Pressel S, et al: Statistical considerations in monitoring the Systolic Hypertension in the Elderly Program (SHEP). *Control Clin Trials* 14:350, 1993.

65. Michelson EL, Morganroth J: Spontaneous variability of complex ventricular arrhythmias detected by long-term electrocardiographic recording. *Circulation* 61:690, 1980.

66. Morganroth J, Borland M, Chao G: Application of a frequency definition of ventricular proarrhythmia. *Am J Cardiol* 59:97, 1987.

67. The CAST Investigators: Preliminary report: Effect of encainide and flecainide on mortality in a randomized trial of arrhythmia suppression after myocardial infarction. *N Engl J Med* 321:406, 1989.

68. Capone RJ, Pawitan Y, El-Sherif N, et al and the CAST Investigators: Events in the Cardiac Arrhythmia Suppression Trial: Baseline predictors of mortality in placebo-treated patients. *J Am Coll Cardiol* 18: 1434, 1991.

69. The Coronary Drug Project Research Group: Influence of adherence to treatment and response to cholesterol on mortality in the Coronary Drug Project. *N Engl J Med* 303:1038, 1980.

70. Horwitz RI, Viscoli CM, Berkman L, et al: Treatment adherence and risk of death after a myocardial infarction. *Lancet* 336:542, 1990.

71. Gallagher EJ, Viscoli CM, Horwitz RI: The relationship of treatment adherence to the risk of death after myocardial infarction in women. *JAMA* 270:742, 1993.

72. Lipid Research Clinics Program: The Lipid Research Clinics Coronary Primary Prevention Trial Results: II. The relationship of reduction in incidence of coronary heart disease to cholesterol lowering. *JAMA* 251:365, 1984.

73. Sackett DL, Haynes RB, Gibson ES, Johnson A: The problem of compliance with antihypertensive therapy. *Pract Cardiol* 2:35, 1976.

74. Glynn RJ, Buring JE, Manson JE, et al: Adherence to aspirin in the prevention of myocardial infarction. *Arch Intern Med* 154: 2649, 1994.

75. Makuch RW, Johnson MF: Dilemmas in the use of active control groups in clinical research. *IRB Rev Hum Subj Res* 11:1, 1989.

76. Cleophas TJM: Clinical trials: Design flaws associated with use of a placebo. *Am J Ther* 3:529, 1996.

77. Fisher LD, Gent M, Büller HR: Active control trials: How would a new agent compare with placebo? A method illustrated with clopidogrel, aspirin, and placebo. *Am Heart J* 141:26, 2001.

78. Schechter C, Cagliano S, Traversa G, et al: Use of placebo controls (correspondence). *N Engl J Med* 332:60, 1995.

79. AI-Khatib SM, Califf RM, Hasselblad V, et al: Placebo-controls in short-term clinical trials of hypertension. *Science* 292:2013, 2001.

80. Moerman DE, Jonas WB: Deconstructing the placebo effect and finding the meaning response. *Ann Intern Med* 136:471, 2002.

81. Kaptchuk TJ: The placebo effect in alternative medicine: Can the performance of a healing ritual have clinical significance? *Ann Intern Med* 136:817, 2002.

82. Alderman MH: Blood pressure management: Individualized treatment based on absolute risk and the potential for benefit. *Ann Intern Med* 119:329, 1993

83. The Coronary Drug Project Research Group: Influence of adherence to treatment and response to cholesterol on mortality in the Coronary Drug Project. *N Engl J Med* 303:1038, 1980.

84. Horwitz RI, Viscoli CM, Berkman L, et al: Treatment adherence and risk of death after a myocardial infarction. *Lancet* 336:542, 1990.

85. Benson H, Epstein MD: The placebo effect, a neglected asset in the care of patients. *JAMA* 232:1225, 1975.

86. Sassano P, Chatellier G, Corvol P, Menard J: Influence of observer's expectation on the placebo effect in blood pressure trials. *Curr Ther Res* 41:304, 1987.

87. Morganroth J, Borland M, Chao G: Application of frequency definition of ventricular proarrhythmia. *Am J Cardiol* 59:97, 1987.

88. Roberts AH: The powerful placebo revisited: Magnitude of nonspecific effects. *Mind/Body Med* 1:35, 1995.

89. Drici MD, Raybaud F, DeLunardo C, et al: Influence of the behavior pattern on the nocebo response of healthy volunteers. *Br J Clin Pharmacol* 39:204, 1995.

CHAPTER 3

Compliance with Cardiovascular Drug Treatment

Piyush K. Dhanuka

Mary Welna Brown

Wei-Nchih Lee

Stephen J. Peterson

William H. Frishman

A key component of a successful plan for the management of cardiovascular disease is compliance with a prescribed medication regimen. However, patient compliance with a prescribed regimen is often difficult and frustrating to achieve. Reports in the cardiovascular literature denote that an average of 50% of patients do not follow prescribed medication instructions by not filling the prescription, not taking the correct medication dosage, not taking the medication at the correct time, and/or taking the medication with contraindicated compounds including certain food products, alternative medications, or over-the-counter medications.

Noncompliance is a costly and preventable problem that affects the patient, the health care industry, and society. Noncompliance usually results in suboptimal control of the patient's treated disease process and potentially serious sequelae. Noncompliance with prescribed medication regimens directly augments health care costs by increasing hospital or emergency room admissions, nursing home admissions, premature deaths, and the number of treatments and procedures that result from the problems of uncontrolled potential and existing disease processes or medication interactions. Indirect costs to overall society include work absences, employee turnover due to death or disability, and lost earnings of patients due to illness caused by noncompliance. The issue of cardiovascular medication compliance requires serious attention by health care providers.

DEFINITION OF COMPLIANCE

The general definition of *compliance* is "the extent to which a person's behavior (in terms of taking medications, following diets, or executing other lifestyle changes) coincides with the clinical prescription."[1] However, there is no universal definition of "good" or "bad" compliance in the published literature, and the varying quality of the compliance literature science makes it hard to draw concrete conclusions. This problem not only makes it difficult to conduct a comparative assessment of compliance literature statistics across studies but also to clearly define the difference between a compliant and noncompliant patient.[2] Compliance research studies have recently shifted away from looking at patient characteristics and other situational factors and placed more emphasis on the provider-patient relationship. Therefore, the definition of medication compliance in

this chapter is one of taking a prescribed cardiovascular medication regimen to achieve a desired therapeutic goal jointly determined by the provider and the patient.

As discussed above, variations in patients' medication-taking behavior can occur at various levels, and the provider needs to focus on the overall medication-taking behavior as well as its specific components—e.g., prescription filling, dose, frequency, dosing interval and timing of medication. Below we describe methods of assessment of cardiovascular medication compliance, characteristics that influence medication compliance, and strategies that the provider can utilize to improve medication compliance.

METHODS OF ASSESSMENT OF MEDICATION COMPLIANCE

It is extremely important that a health care provider assess whether the patient is therapeutically responding to a medication regimen. Reasons for poor therapeutic response may be noncompliance with the regimen or an ineffective medication regimen. It is important to distinguish the reasons for poor therapeutic response so as to utilize these methods of assessment of medication compliance appropriately.

There are indirect and direct methods of assessing medication compliance. Direct methods are based on tests that cannot be modified by the patient, and indirect methods rely on patient reporting or modifiable data. Since none of these methods is foolproof, it is usually best for the provider to use a combination of direct and indirect methods to most accurately assess compliance in patients whom a provider suspects as noncompliant.

Direct Methods

Direct methods of assessing medication compliance primarily include biologic measurements of blood or urine drug metabolites or serum drug concentration. It is possible to do measurements of metabolite and drug concentration in sweat, breath, or saliva samples. However, if a medication has a long half-life, a drug or metabolite concentration may not be a good indication that the patient took the medication in the few days prior to the sample date. Conversely, if a medication has a short half-life, the patient may have taken the medication in the few days or only on the day prior to the sample date. Therefore the presence of a metabolite or drug does not necessarily indicate that the patient took a medication on a regular basis and/or over a long time period.

Indirect Methods

There are numerous indirect methods of assessing medication compliance. Preprescription assessment methods include questioning patients whether they are willing to comply with a prescribed drug regimen and evaluating patients' medication compliance history. Following medication prescription, other indirect ways of evaluating patients' compliance include checking clinic attendance, asking patients to bring a prescription bottle to the clinic to assess that the amount taken is appropriate since the medication was prescribed or refilled, providing a diary or drug dispenser to patients to help them self-monitor medication intake, and measuring physiologic measures such as blood pressure or heart rate. However, the therapeutic response to a prescribed regimen varies among individual patients and may vary as often as daily in some individuals. The provider should remind patients that this fluctuation is normal, especially if patients are monitoring their own basic physiologic parameters, so discouragement does not ensue concerning the therapeutic value of a prescribed medication.

The utilization of specific questions such as "Are you taking your medications?" or "Describe what your routine is for taking your medications to me" is another method commonly utilized for compliance assessment. However, patients do not tend to report their own noncompliant behavior, and health care providers unfortunately overestimate patient compliance[3] even with increased experience and extensive contact with a given patient.[4–6] Often patients are not even aware that they were noncompliant, such as forgetting to take a dose at the appropriate time.

Electronic counters are a relatively new indirect method of measuring compliance that should become more widely commercially available in the near future. These counters are special medication caps containing a computer chip that records precisely when a bottle is opened. The chip can be interrogated using special computer software that providers can install on their office computers. This method is more costly, and the patient can unintentionally modify the system by opening a bottle without taking the recommended dose, transferring the dose to another container, or not taking the dose when the bottle is opened.[7,8] Patients may also open the bottle to show the device to others or to check that the bottle has been closed well. Therefore the information obtained by this method needs careful interpretation and should be combined with other methods of compliance assessment.[9] This method is becoming the new "gold standard" for compliance assessment and has many positive attributes.[8] One of the features of an electronic counting system is that it enables a practitioner to provide direct rapid feedback to the patient regarding the medication dosing pattern generated on a computer printout following chip interrogation. Computerized telephone feedback systems incorporated into electronic counting systems are currently in the research and development process. These systems automatically inform the health care provider when the patient does not take a prescribed medication dose within a specified period of time. These systems can also be designed to notify the patient within a preset time if a dose is omitted. Cramer[8] concluded that these systems are well worth the cost and will considerably reduce the economic consequences of medication noncompliance to the health care system and society.

CHARACTERISTICS THAT INFLUENCE MEDICATION COMPLIANCE

Multiple characteristics influence medication compliance in the cardiac patient. The distinct characteristics related to compliance have been traditionally divided into the following classification[10]:

1. Patient's sociodemographic characteristics
2. Characteristics of the health care provider
3. Medication characteristics
4. Disease characteristics

There are extensive conflicting data in the literature regarding the level of influence the preceding characteristics exert on compliance. Haynes came to this conclusion during his review of the compliance literature from 1979.[11] He clearly indicates that there are insufficient studies and conflicting data concerning identification of specific features that distinctively predict the level of medication compliance in the patient. Kjellgren and colleagues[12] substantiated those conclusions in 1995. No concrete universal agreement exists concerning single or multiple groups of characteristics that may contribute to medication noncompliance. Therefore it is impossible to identify the patient as compliant or noncompliant based on the presence of one or more of these characteristics. These characteristics and their significance to compliance vary among individual patients. This may account for the fact that the research studies have resulted in inconsistent findings. Since these characteristics influence each individual patient differently, the provider must specifically evaluate them in each patient. Table 3-1 presents these characteristics for consideration by the health care provider when assessing whether the patient will be compliant or not. A brief review follows that highlights the characteristics within each classification that publications commonly cite as having a significant influence on medication compliance in patients with cardiac disease.

Patient's Sociodemographic Characteristics

A review of the literature indicates there are several patient sociodemographic characteristics commonly related to cardiovascular medication compliance. Noncompliance with antihypertensive medications is found in both younger[13,14] and older patients.[15] According to Salzman,[16] the causes of noncompliance in elderly patients differ from those in young age groups. Salzman cites reasons for noncompliance in the elderly as increasing forgetfulness, leading to the use of too much or too little medication; confusion about dosage and reason for medication; increased frequency of side effects; and increased medication cost. In a study of prophylactic aspirin compliance in the elderly diagnosed with coronary artery disease, Carney et al.[17] found that major depression occurs more often in the elderly and leads to medication noncompliance. Patients who are poor,[14] African American,[18,19] less educated,[14] or cognitively impaired comply less well following a diagnosis of hypertension. Patients who have a high locus of control,[20] have a strong social support mechanism,[21] and perceive treatment to be beneficial[21,22] and lifelong[18] tend to comply better with hypertensive medications. Haynes[11] cited family instability and a history of previous noncompliance with other regimens as factors associated with

TABLE 3-1. Characteristics That Influence Medication Compliance

Patient's sociodemographic characteristics:

Age
Gender
Educational level
Socioeconomic status
Occupational status
Living status (alone vs. not alone)
Family stability and level of support
Mental stability
Race and ethnicity
Religious beliefs
Level of forgetfulness
State of knowledge of disease process or consequences and medication regimen
Strength of belief in treatment value
General attitude toward health care
Appropriateness of health beliefs
Expectations of prescribed regimen
Previous history of compliance
Appointment attendance

Characteristics of health care provider:

Length of time between start of problem and referral of patient to provider
Patient level of satisfaction with initial contact with provider
Interviewing and listening ability of provider
Ability level of provider to assess patient compliance and potential barriers to compliance
Length of time between contacts between provider and patient
Length of waiting time for provider services
Provider's ability to keep appointments
Length of time provider spends with patient
Continuity of care with provider
Level of support, empathy, and feedback that provider gives to the patient
Degree and ease of access that provider has to the patient
Quality of instruction given for taking prescribed regimen

Medication characteristics:

Type of medication
Complexity of dosing schedule
Degree of lifestyle changes required to adhere to prescribed medication regimen
Duration of therapy
Number of prescribed medications
Medication packaging
Side effects
Cost

Disease characteristics:

Symptomatology
Severity of illness
Duration of illness
Previous history of disease
Previous hospitalization
Level of disability caused by disease process

noncompliance. Increased patient knowledge of the disease process in congestive heart failure[23] and of prescribed hypertensive medications[22] has a positive effect on compliance. In their health belief model, Becker and Maiman[24] found that patients are more compliant if they believe that their disease is serious, think that their disease susceptibility is high, maintain faith that their disease treatment will be efficacious and beneficial, and perceive minimal adverse effects physical and psychological resulting from their treatment.

Characteristics of the Health Care Provider

All the characteristics listed under the "health care provider" classification point to one theme—how well health care providers render their services to patients, resulting in patient satisfaction with their health care and treatment plan. Patients want to choose their own competent health care provider. Patients want to maintain control over their health care by choosing providers who know their medical history, current medical problems, life outside the treatment setting, and family support systems. This enables the provider to implement the best treatment plan tailored to the patient's individual lifestyle. These personal aspects of health care delivery have become somewhat lost as health care providers become more reliant on tests and procedures for a diagnosis. The provider might prescribe a "cookbook" treatment plan to the patient in the last minutes of an office visit, usually immediately following the diagnosis. There is usually minimal individualized discussion of details and alternatives to these treatment plans and how they might affect the patient's lifestyle, thereby paving the way to potential noncompliance. Numerous research publications[25-27] in the academic arena as well as documented consumer surveys[28] demonstrate the desire for more personal communication between the health care provider and patient. Logistic issues such as waiting time, maintaining appointments, seeing the same provider at each visit, having appointments at a convenient location and time, and ongoing contact increase compliance, according to a review of multiple publications by Haynes.[11] The areas that increase medication compliance and require the most attention by the health care provider are providing time for support, empathy, and feedback from patients regarding their disease status; discussing options for treatment and choice of treatment tailored to patients' lifestyle[29]; providing clear instructions for adhering to prescribed therapeutic regimens; and identifying the treatment outcome and potential side effects that patients can expect from their treatment. Weintraub[30] noted in his 1975 publication that direct interpersonal contact between the health care provider and the patient results in increased knowledge about the specifics of the medication treatment plan and therefore increased compliance. However, Haynes[11] indicated that there is some controversy regarding whether it was truly the increased knowledge or the interpersonal attention that increased compliance. He concluded that the motivation resulting from the interpersonal provider-patient communication coupled with the increased knowledge leads to increased patient compliance.

Medication Characteristics

Several characteristics within this classification have a strong effect on medication compliance. Haynes[11] identified increased complexity of the regimen, extensive degree of behavioral changes required to maintain a specific medication regimen, and long duration of treatment as confirmed characteristics associated with noncompliance. Other studies identified a longer treatment period,[13] more drug side effects,[13] and an increased number of prescribed drugs as contributing to noncompliance.[14,31,31a] Fear of future health problems or disruption of routine life activities due to adverse events from hypertensive medications may lead to noncompliance.[20] However, one study contradicted the idea that increased side effects reduced compliance.[31]

New formulations that offer once-daily dosing options—such as transdermal and long-acting slow-release oral drugs—have been shown to increase compliance.[32,33,33a] However, the provider should determine whether treatment complexity may be the reason for

TABLE 3-2. Innovative Strategies for Improving Patient Compliance

Electronic monitoring devices
Pill containers with daily compartment for medication
Phone call refill reminders from pharmacies
Augmented medication counseling by pharmacists at time prescription is filled
Computerized lay-language medication instructions written by manufacturer for distribution at local pharmacies
Computerized dosage-schedule charts from pharmacies incorporating medication interactions of a prescribed
    regimen in over-the-counter medications and food products
Contact with pharmaceutical companies to provide medications for economically needy patients
Contact with pharmaceutical companies who offer compliance reminder programs
Community-based programs for patients by health care providers at schools and community centers
Compliance programs educating patients to be resourceful health care consumers
Compliance teams within health care facilities to educate and monitor patient compliance
Continuing education programs for health care providers on ways to increase patient compliance

noncompliance before prescribing these new formulations to increase patient compliance.[32] One study concluded that missing several doses of a once-daily medication may predispose the patient to an excessively low therapeutic level as opposed to the patient who may miss one dose of a medication that is taken two or three times per day.[34,35] Other medication characteristics also affect compliance. Medication packaging can be a deterrent to patient compliance if elderly or handicapped patients are unable to open the packaging. Cost of medication can be a factor if the patient has a limited source of income for purchasing some or all of the drug in a prescribed regimen and/or if this increased cost disrupts his or her lifestyle.[20] Patients will be less compliant if the process of taking the medication and its sequelae prove to be more troublesome to them than the problems resulting from the disease.

Disease Characteristics

An extensive review of the literature[31] indicates that disease characteristics have little influence on compliance with the following exceptions: psychiatric patients tend to be low compliers with treatment; increasing symptoms may be accompanied by decreasing compliance because the patient perceives that the medication regimen is ineffective; and disability resulting from the disease process may possibly increase compliance because of increased medical supervision for the disability. Asymptomatic disease contributes to noncompliance.[19,35a,35b] This is especially applicable to patients with hypertension, who may initially perceive themselves as acutely ill and symptomatic. As symptoms disappear, hypertensive patients may feel cured and stop medication because they do not perceive hypertension as having serious sequelae if it is not accompanied by symptoms.[21] This concept is clearly related not only to disease symptomatology but also to the patient's health beliefs, mentioned in a prior section of this chapter.

PRACTICAL AND INNOVATIVE STRATEGIES TO IMPROVE MEDICATION COMPLIANCE

Strategies to improve medication compliance include those that are practical and innovative. The research in the field of compliance interventions has been very sparse. In a review in 1996, Haynes and coauthors[36] found only six rigorous trials analyzing the efficacy of interventions to improve compliance with hypertension medications. Newell et al.[37] concluded in 1999 that strong recommendations were not possible because of suboptimal methodology of the located trials. These authors found only 20 randomized

trials of good or fair quality and made tentative recommendations for some strategies, such as providing written educational material to the patients, sending reminders, and supplying medications in compliance-enhancing packaging.

A plan for implementation of practical strategies to increase compliance is presented below. It has been shown that the best results are obtained when comprehensive interventions are used that combine educational, behavioral and affective strategies.[38,38a] The provider should use the innovative strategies identified in Table 3-2 to supplement the practical strategies. We acknowledge that pressure to control health care expenditures limits most providers' time for initiating the practical strategies to improve compliance. However, provider cooperation with a process to increase compliance is vital to helping the patient increase medication compliance and avoiding the multiple problems that result from noncompliance.[39] Much of the information presented previously in this chapter indicates that the evolution of a proactive, cooperative relationship between the health care provider and the patient is a key concept to improvement of compliance. This concept plays a major role in the implementation of the practical strategies. Both the patient and the provider must communicate to form a partnership to develop an individualized medication regimen that meets the therapeutic goals agreed on by the provider and patient. The "one size fits all" treatment plan does not work to increase medication compliance, and the provider must design a plan that allows patient participation to reflect the patient's individual needs, preferences, lifestyle patterns, and habits.[40] It is important for the provider to implement the partnership process in a caring and empathetic way.[41] The provider should also take into account the patient's sociodemographic, disease, and environmental characteristics, identified in the previous section, in implementing the practical strategies process described below. The steps of this process are described in the following sections.[34,40]

Assess, Inform, and Educate the Patient

The health care provider is responsible for ascertaining the required information from the patient to make a correct diagnosis. The provider should educate the patient on the details of the diagnosis—including cause, symptoms, time to expected improvement, potential sequelae, possible complications, prevention of recurrence, and how the disease process may impact the patients' health in general, especially in light of any significant medical history or coexisting disease processes.[34] The provider should request that a significant other be present so that there is someone who understands the patient's situation and is able to participate as a supportive partner to assist the patient to comply with the prescribed therapeutic regimen.[11]

At this time the provider should also consider whether any of the characteristics identified in the previous section of this chapter could influence the patient's compliance.

Empower Patients to Take Charge of Their Health Care and Set Therapeutic Goals

Motivating and empowering the patient encompasses the largest degree of change in the traditional authoritarian patient-provider relationship. The provider should recognize the patient as the major component in the treatment compliance process. The provider should make the patient an active participant in the choices of therapeutic goals and treatment plans. Self-monitoring by the patient of various end points—like blood pressure, body weight, and a symptom diary—can be effective in achieving this goal. Home monitoring of the blood pressure has been shown to improve compliance with hypertension treatment.[42,43]

Tailor a Medication Regimen That Is Workable by the Patient

The provider should present a medication regimen to the patient that is tailored to the patient's diagnosis, therapeutic goals, and lifestyle. The provider should give the patient some flexibility with formulations and dosing schedules and explain the rationale behind the chosen plan. The provider should tell the patient the significant potential adverse effects, cost, length of therapy needed to reach the agreed therapeutic goal, need for physiologic monitoring such as International Normalized Ratio (INR) or frequent blood pressure and pulse checks,[3,43] and lifestyle changes required by the various treatment plans.

Educate Patients on Implementation of the Medication Treatment Plan

The provider should ask patients why they believe the selected treatment plan would work best for themselves and whether patients will be compliant with the plan.[26] This information will give the provider insight into patients' understanding of the disease process, therapeutic goals, knowledge of some of the specifics of the medication regimen, and likelihood of compliance. Time should be allowed for patients to ask questions. At this point, the provider may want to assess whether to incorporate one of the innovative strategies identified in Table 3-2 into the treatment plan, such as providing patients with divided pillboxes or sources of financial assistance. Disabled patients should have medication packaging that is accessible and readable. If a significant other is present, the provider should ask this person how he or she might help the patient comply with the treatment plan. A written therapeutic plan should follow an oral teaching session, as reinforcement of the new knowledge that the patient has learned.[44] This written plan should include name, purpose, and dosing schedule. It should include whether the patient should take the prescribed medications with food, possible interactions with other medications, benefits, side effects, action to take if side effects occur, and other precautions such as not operating mechanical equipment. Sometimes a written provider-patient contract identifying the responsibilities of the provider and responsibilities of the patient is helpful for difficult patients. It is important that patients believe that the benefits of treatment are far more desirable than the disease or its sequelae. Last, the provider should present a medication dosage reminder chart to the patient tailored to the patient's lifestyle and incorporating the prescribed medications.[45,46] The patient should be asked to initiate a creative reminder system to take medications, such as notes or cues in frequented home areas. Reminders such as utilizing alarm clocks or incorporating self-medication administration into daily bathroom, bedtime, or meal rituals are also useful for some patients.[39,40] The provider should examine memory problems, especially in elderly patients, who often suffer from dementia or depression, and problem solve with these patients.

Evaluate Patient Compliance via Phone Contact and Repeat Visits

The provider should use a combination of the compliance assessment methods described in a previous section of this chapter following implementation of the medication treatment regimen. The provider should phone the newly diagnosed patient and/or see the patient in follow-up to check if there are questions, provide additional support, and assess compliance. The provider should increase the frequency of these contacts for patients requiring additional support. Appointment reminders, such as calls or reminder cards, should be sent to patients, and contact should be made with patients if an appointment is missed. The provider should make the purpose of the office appointment clear to the patient and stress that he or she wants to see the patient even if the patient is feeling better. This is especially important for the patient with more asymptomatic diseases such as hypertension, because the patient may not return to the provider when there are no overt symptoms. Achievable short-term therapeutic goals can be set for subsequent appointments so the patient has more motivation to be compliant to achieve the goal by the next appointment. The provider should minimize waiting time, make appointments at times that are convenient for the patient, and arrange transportation or parking reimbursement as needed. Communication via electronic mail can be extremely useful and time saving for monitoring patient compliance. E-mail reminders can be scheduled in such a way that they are automatically sent to patients at a predetermined time. However, the use of e-mail as a communication method requires careful attention to related ethical and legal issues. A detailed description of ethicolegal issues is beyond the scope of this chapter, but the reader can refer to the position paper by American Medical Informatics Association.[47] Website construction and hosting is becoming increasingly easy and more affordable, and many health care providers are using personal websites for interaction with their patients. Telemedicine is also being studied as a tool to monitor compliance and therapeutic goals. A recent study looked at the transmission of blood pressure data, using home monitoring devices, over telephone lines to health care providers.[48] Compared to controls who received usual care, the study group had significant improvement in blood pressure levels. While the results may in part be due to more frequent medication adjustments in the study group, they may also stem from improved compliance with prescription medications and lifestyle modifications. This is suggested by the authors' observation that even for those subjects in the study group who did not receive medication adjustments, blood pressure improved significantly.

Change the Prescribed Medication Regimen as Necessary

The provider should make modifications to the patient's medication regimen as needed. The provider should make the patient aware that it is possible to make changes in the regimen to accommodate his or her lifestyle or improve therapeutic response due to pharmacokinetic differences among drugs and/or delivery systems. The provider should be careful not to blame patients and make the them feel discouraged if a plan does not work. The provider should give patients positive feedback and discuss the plan with them, as indicated above, to encourage their participation. Sometimes a patient requires only extra counseling and encouragement to follow the initial regimen plan.

Refer the Patient for Extra Help as Needed

The provider should refer the patient for extra help as needed to increase compliance. This type of help can include cardiac rehabilitation programs, diet programs, support groups,[3,41] and/or extra individual counseling for psychiatric problems.

CONCLUSION

Improved compliance with cardiovascular medication regimens significantly decreases health care costs and helps prevent both occurrence and progression of cardiac disease. The key to increasing patient compliance is provider implementation of medication treatment strategies that enable the patient to participate as a health care partner by incorporating the therapeutic goals of the patient and individual patient attributes that influence compliance. Implementation of strategies to increase cardiovascular medication compliance requires investment and commitment on the part of patients, providers, and third-party payers. This investment of time and money into measures proven to increase cardiovascular medication compliance is well worth the positive long-term benefits to the patient, the health care industry, and society.

REFERENCES

1. Haynes RB: Introduction. In: Haynes RB, Taylor DW, Sackett DL, eds. *Compliance in Health Care.* Baltimore: Johns Hopkins, 1979:1–7.
2. Rand CS: Issue in the measurement of adherence. In: Shumaker SA, Schron EB, Okene JK, eds. *The Handbook of Health Behavior Change.* New York: Springer, 1990:102–110.
3. Haynes RB, Sackett DL, Gibson DW, et al: Improvement of medication compliance in uncontrolled hypertension. *Lancet* 1:1265, 1976.
4. Roth HP, Caron HS: Accuracy of doctors' estimates and patients' statements on adherence to a drug regimen. *Clin Pharm Ther* 23:361, 1978.
5. Mushlin AI, Appell FA: Diagnosing potential noncompliance: Physicians' ability in a behavioral dimension of medical care. *Arch Intern Med* 137:318, 1977.
6. Gilbert JR, Evans CE, Haynes RB, Tugwell P: Predicting compliance with a regimen of digoxin therapy in family practice. *Can Med Assoc J* 123:119, 1980.
7. Spilker B: Methods of assessing and improving patient compliance in clinical trials. In: *Patient Compliance in Medical Practice and Clinical Trials.* New York: Raven, 1991:37–56.
8. Cramer J: Microelectronic systems for monitoring and enhancing patient compliance with medication regimens. *Drugs* 49(3):321, 1995.
9. Arnet I, Haefeli WE: Overconsumption detected by electronic drug monitoring requires subtle interpretation. *Clin Pharmacol Ther* 67:44, 2000.
10. Blackwell B: Drug therapy? Patient compliance. *N Engl J Med* 289:249, 1973.
11. Haynes RB: A critical review of the "determinants" of patient compliance with therapeutic regimens. In: Taylor DW, Sackett DL, Haynes RB, eds. *Compliance in Health Care.* Baltimore: Johns Hopkins, 1979: 26–39.
12. Kjellgren KI, Ahlner J, Saljo R: Taking antihypertensive medication—controlling or cooperating with patients? *Int J Cardiol* 47:257, 1995.
13. Richardson MA, Simon-Morton B, Annegers JF: Effect of perceived barriers on compliance with antihypertensive medication. *Health Ed Q* 20:489, 1993.
14. Caldwell JR, Cobb S, Dowling MD, de Jongh D: The dropout problem in antihypertensive treatment. *J Chronic Dis* 22:579, 1970.
15. Evans L, Spelman M: The problem of noncompliance with drug therapy. *Drugs* 25:63, 1983.
16. Salzman C: Medication compliance in the elderly. *J Clin Psychol* 56:18, 1995.
17. Carney RM, Freedland KE, Eisen SA, et al: Major depression and medication adherence in elderly patients with coronary artery disease. *Health Psychol* 14:88, 1995.
18. Sharkness CM, Snow DA: The patient's view of hypertension and compliance. *Am J Prev Med* 8:141, 1992.
19. Cummings KM, Kirscht JP, Binder LR, Godley AJ: Determinants of drug treatment maintenance among hypertensive patients in inner city Detroit. *Public Health Rep* 97:99, 1986.
20. Stanton AL: Determinants of adherence to medical regimens by hypertensive patients. *J Behav Med* 10:377, 1987.
21. Meyer D, Leventhal H, Gutmann M: Common-sense models of illness: The example of hypertension. *Health Psychol* 4:115, 1985.
22. Given CW, Given BA, Simoni LE: The association of knowledge and perception of medications with compliance and health states among hypertensive patients: A prospective study. *Res Nurs Health* 1:76, 1978.
23. Fujita LY, Dungan J: High risk for ineffective management of therapeutic regimen: A protocol study. *Rehab Nurs* 19:75, 1994.
24. Becker MH, Maiman LA: Sociobehavioral determinants of compliance with health and medical care recommendations. *Med Care* 13:10, 1975.
25. Inui TS, Yourtee EL, Williamson JW: Improved outcome in hypertension after physician tutorials: A controlled trial. *Ann Intern Med* 84:646, 1976.
26. Eraker SA, Kirscht JP, Becker MH: Understanding and improving patient compliance. *Ann Intern Med* 100:258, 1984.
27. Roter D, Hall J: *Doctors Talking with Patients/Patients Talking with Doctors.* Westport, CT: Auburn House, 1992.
28. How is your doctor treating you? *Consumer Reports* February:81, 1995.
29. Conrad P: The meaning of medications: Another look at compliance. *Soc Sci Med* 20:29, 1985.
30. Weintraub M: Promoting patient compliance. *NYS J Med* 75:2263, 1975.
31. Haynes RB: Determinants of compliance: The disease and mechanics of treatment. In: Haynes RB, Taylor DW, Sackett DL, eds. *Compliance in Health Care.* Baltimore: Johns Hopkins, 1979:49–62.
31a. Sica DA: Rationale for fixed-dose combinations in the treatment of hypertension: The cycle repeats. *Drugs* 62:443, 2002.
32. Dwyer MS, Levy RA, Menander KB: Improving medication compliance through the use of modern dosage forms. *J Mod Pharm Tech* 2:166, 1986.
33. Lofdahl P: Compliance as a factor in the development of nitrate tolerance: A patient investigation. *J Intern Med Res* 21:51, 1993.
33a. Iskedjian M, Einarson TR, MacKeigan LD, et al: Relationship between daily dose frequency and adherence to antihypertensive pharmacotherapy: Evidence from a meta analysis. *Clin Ther* 24:302, 2002.
34. Keen PJ: What is the best dosage schedule for patients? *J R Soc Med* 84:640, 1991.
35. Elliott HL, Meredith PA: Nifedipine GITS. *Lancet* 341:306, 1993.
35a. Andrade SE, Walker AM, Gottlieb LK, et al: Discontinuation and antihyperlipidemic drugs—do rates reported in clinical trials reflect rates in primary care settings? *N Engl J Med* 332:1125, 1995.
35b. Simons LA, Levis G, Simons J: Apparent discontinuation rates in patients prescribed lipid-lowering drugs. *Med J Aust* 164:208, 1996.
36. Haynes RB, McKibbon KA, Kanani R: Systematic review of randomized trials of interventions to assist patients to follow prescriptions for medications. *Lancet* 348:383, 1996.
37. Newell SA, Bowman JA, Cockburn JD: A critical review of interventions to increase compliance with medication-taking, obtaining medication refills, and appointment-keeping in the treatment of cardiovascular disease. *Prev Med* 29:535, 1999.
38. Roter DL, Hall JA, Merisca R, et al: Effectiveness of interventions to improve patient compliance: a meta-analysis. *Med Care* 36:1138, 1998.

38a. Ockene IS, Hayman LL, Pasternak RC, et al: Task force #4: Adherance issues and behavior changes: Achieving a long-term solution. *J Am Coll Cardiol* 40:579, 2002.

39. Donavan JL, Blake DR: Patient noncompliance: Deviance or reasoned decision making? *Soc Sci Med* 34:507, 1992.

40. Rudd P: Clinicians and patients with hypertension: Unsettled issues about compliance. *Am Heart J* 130:572, 1995.

41. Squier RW: A model of empathetic understanding and adherence to treatment regimens in practitioner-patient relationships. *Soc Sci Med* 30:325, 1990.

42. Freis ED: Improving treatment effectiveness in hypertension. *Arch Intern Med* 159:2517, 1999.

43. Nessman DG, Carnahan JE, Nugent CA: Increasing compliance: Patient operated hypertension groups. *Arch Intern Med* 140:1427, 1980.

44. Cramer JA: Optimizing long-term patient compliance. *Neurology* 45:S25, 1995.

45. Gabriel M, Gagnon JP, Bryan CK: Improved patient compliance through use of a daily drug reminder chart. *Am J Public Health* 67:968, 1977.

46. Farmer KC, Jacobs EW, Phillips CR: Long-term patient compliance with prescribed regimens of calcium channel blockers. *Clin Ther* 16:316, 1994.

47. Kane B, Sands DJ: Guidelines for the clinical use of electronic mail with patients. *J Am Med Info Assoc* 5:104, 1998. [http://www.amia.org/positio2.htm]

48. Rogers MAM, Small D, Buchan DA, et al: Home monitoring service improves mean arterial pressure in patients with essential hypertension. *Ann Intern Med* 134:1024, 2001.

New Drug Development and FDA Approval

Eliot J. Lazar

Steven R. Bergmann

Recent advances in cardiovascular pharmacotherapeutics have radically altered the current practice of cardiology compared with that of just a few years ago. Cardiovascular specialists from the 1960s through the millennium have witnessed the development of entire new classes of agents, including the beta-adrenergic blockers, calcium blockers, thrombolytics, angiotensin converting enzyme (ACE) inhibitors, statins, and angiotensin receptor blockers (ARBs). Antiarrhythmics have come and gone, with few surviving the test of time. Reliable standbys such as digoxin, aspirin, and warfarin have undergone peaks and troughs in enthusiasm for their clinical use. Perhaps only in the area of infectious diseases are clinicians deluged by as many new products and indications.

When a pharmaceutical representative speaks about a new product or when an advertisement is viewed in a journal, physicians are seeing the culmination of many years and millions of dollars spent on drug research and development.[1] The process by which a new drug is initially developed, studied in terms of safety and efficacy, proven to be as good as or better than existing therapy, and finally released for use by the public is an arduous one, intimately tied to the regulatory process as governed by the U.S. Food and Drug Administration (FDA). It is important for clinicians to understand the rigorous testing which a product must undergo prior to FDA approval, but it is equally important to understand the limitations of this process. In this chapter, the process of drug development and approval is discussed, with particular attention given to clinical trials, special populations, and postmarketing surveillance.

HISTORICAL PERSPECTIVES

In the United States, the regulation of pharmaceutical products is governed by the FDA, administratively residing at present within the Department of Health and Human Services. The legislative history of FDA regulatory authority, though spanning most of the twentieth century, involves four major pieces of legislation.

The Pure Food and Drugs Act of 1906 provided a first step in the path to direct regulation of food and drug products. Although focusing on adulteration or misbranding, the 1906 act did not prohibit the existence of these products but rather their commercial transfer across state lines.[2] Although Congress mandated direct regulation of blood and blood products as early as 1902, it was not until the Food Drug and Cosmetic Act (FDCA) of 1938 that direct regulation of pharmaceutical company operations came under FDA purview.[2] The political climate of the New Deal shaped much of the course of this early regulation of food and drugs, but acceptance of federal

oversight was, nonetheless, a tough battle. An absorbing account of the political and legislative wrangling over these issues can be found in *Food and Drug Law*, published by the Food and Drug Law Institute based in Washington, D.C.[3] Regulation under the FDCA of 1938 operated through the denial of permission to market a given product rather than by approval of its release. It was not until the Kefauver-Harris amendments of 1962 that the role of the FDA and its drug approval process substantively changed to the current system of elaborate scientific, technical, and administrative requirements demanded by the agency before a new product can be marketed. Moreover, to obtain FDA approval, both the efficacy and safety of a new drug had to be demonstrated.[3] The Drug Price Competition and Patent Term Restoration Act of 1984 was the fourth of the major legislative initiatives. The principal purpose of this law was to establish an abbreviated new drug application (NDA) policy and set criteria as to when abbreviated NDAs may be submitted for approval of generic drugs. Such a policy was seen as essential to the marketing of less expensive generic drugs while still encouraging pharmaceutical companies to continue their research and development of new products. Additional legislative initiatives in the 1990s, particularly the FDA Modernization Act of 1997,[4] have contributed to speeding the approval process, modified the assessment of user fees, and addressed pharmaceutical testing in special populations.

CLINICAL TRIALS

The process by which a new chemical entity is tested and ultimately comes to market is both lengthy and costly. Recent estimates have indicated that the total cost to a pharmaceutical company to develop a single new drug averages more than $300 million.[1] The entire process of drug development from preclinical investigation to NDA submission and review by the FDA typically takes upward of 7 years (Fig. 4-1). Although a considerable portion of this time is spent by the developer performing basic and clinical research, the FDA approval process can be quite lengthy[5]; however, there is considerable variation in approval times across the industry.[6]

Recent initiatives by the agency have sought to decrease the review and approval time, particularly in conditions such as cancer and acquired immunodeficiency syndrome (AIDS). The process begins with development of a new chemical entity (NCE).

Various approaches are used by researchers to develop these compounds. Often, an NCE is synthesized to exhibit specific biochemical properties designed to produce a particular physiologic effect. As expected, there is considerable trial and error in these early

Testing in Humans				
	Number of Patients	Length	Purpose	Percent of Drugs Successfully Tested
Phase 1	20–100	Several months	Mainly safety	70 percent
Phase 2	Up to several hundred	Several months to 2 years	Some short term safety, but mainly effectiveness	33 percent
Phase 3	Several hundred to several thousand	1–4 years	Safety, effectiveness, dosage	25–30 percent

FIGURE 4-1. Of 100 drugs for which investigational new drug applications are submitted to the FDA, about 70% will successfully complete phase 1 and go onto phase 2; about 33% of the original 100 will complete phase 2 and go to phase 3; and 25 to 30% of the original 100 will clear phase 3 (and on average about 20 of the original 100 will ultimately be approved for marketing). *(Reproduced from FDA.[5])*

investigations. Currently, computer models with a focus on chemical receptors have been used. Advances in molecular biology are likely to alter drug development in the future, with agents prepared to specific molecular or genetic targets. In other instances, a beneficial property of an NCE has been fortuitously discovered, often when studying it for an unrelated use. Once an NCE with potential for therapeutic value is discovered, trials are begun in laboratory animals to establish toxicity data. Even though these studies do not require FDA permission, their results are used later by the FDA to determine whether to grant permission for human trials. The vast majority of NCEs never reach the phase of clinical investigation in humans. Data from the pharmaceutical industry suggest that only 1 in 1000 compounds that undergo preclinical testing are ultimately studied in humans. Of these, only 20% are ultimately approved for human use.[1,7]

Once a new entity has undergone animal trials, the company must apply for an investigational new drug (IND), more formally known as a Notice of Claimed Investigational Exemption for a New Drug.[2] This essentially grants the sponsor an exemption from the federal law that requires an approved marketing application prior to the transportation or distribution of a drug across state lines.[8] As outlined by FDA's Center for Drug Evaluation and Research, there are several types of INDs, including Investigator, Emergency Use, and Treatment.[8]

In determining whether the IND is to be granted, thus allowing human trials to begin, FDA staff review the preclinical data to assess safety, manufacturing specifications, and information on initial protocols and researchers.[8] The agency has 30 days from the time of submission to object to the initiation of human trials; otherwise the sponsor may begin human studies of the product.[2] The first human trials are known as phase I studies and involve a small number of usually healthy subjects. The purpose of these studies is to provide safety and toxicity data for human subjects. Phase I data generally do not address whether the new agent is effective for a specific medical use, only whether the drug can be safely tolerated. They essentially provide a green light to begin wider testing in humans. Phase I trials may also evaluate a potential drug's metabolism and mode of elimination. These studies generally last for several months, and 1 to 2 years may elapse between the beginning of phase I and the initiation

of phase II trials. Phase II trials involve a greater number of subjects and are designed to determine efficacy for the particular disease state being studied. A major difference between phase I and phase II trials is that the latter are performed in patients afflicted with the condition the drug is intended to treat. Dose-ranging studies and additional data on the drug's metabolism may also be obtained during phase II investigations. These studies may include several hundred subjects and last as long as 2 years.[5]

Phase III trials involve considerably larger numbers of patients and may last for several years. They focus on efficacy and determination of proper dosage in anticipation of submission to the FDA for approval. Phase IV studies are postmarketing studies that increasingly have been required by the FDA as part of the contingent approval of certain agents. These studies may provide additional data for original approved indications or may focus on use of an approved drug for new indications. They may also be used to obtain additional data on side effects with a longer duration of treatment.

Once data from the first three phases of clinical trials are analyzed, the sponsor submits an NDA, which includes a detailed compilation of product data, often after meeting with FDA staff.[2] NDAs received by the FDA are classified by their therapeutic potential[9]— e.g., standard or priority—the former representing minor improvement over existing products, while the latter represent a significant advance over current alternatives. From the time of submission, NDAs undergo extensive FDA review under prescribed time schedules, which gives the agency considerable time flexibility in completing these reviews.[2,10] If a product receives FDA approval, marketing can commence, but the pharmaceutical company must still maintain detailed records about the drug. As described later, all is not known about a given agent at the time of its approval.

For every 100 drugs submitted for IND approval for clinical testing, 20% are ultimately marketed for clinical use in humans.[5]

CLINICAL STUDY DESIGN

To approve a new drug, the FDA requires data from randomized, well-controlled clinical trials. Traditionally, this has been interpreted as a requirement for placebo-controlled studies. Typically, patients entered into studies of this type are randomized to one of two or more arms in a double-blind fashion; that is, neither the patient nor the investigator knows who is receiving which therapy. In a placebo-controlled trial, one of the arms involves administration of placebo therapy. Obviously, this becomes extremely difficult in conditions where therapy is thought to be lifesaving or to have a significant impact on morbidity or mortality. As more and more diseases, particularly in cardiovascular medicine, have established therapies of some efficacy, the concept of placebo control has become increasingly difficult to put into practice, owing to the ethical dilemma of withholding proven treatment for the sake of science (see Chap. 2).[11,12] Recent studies have been designed creatively to add a new agent—or placebo—to existing therapy; for example, digoxin versus placebo added to ACE inhibitors and diuretics. Regardless of the arm to which a patient is assigned, there is often an initial placebo run-in phase, so that all groups start from essentially the same baseline. After the run-in phase, patients receive either active drug or placebo in parallel. Predetermined parameters are measured at intervals depending on the nature of the drug and the disease under study, and target endpoints are assessed.[12a] In trials of cardiovascular agents, many of these end points have objective measurements such as blood pressure, anginal episodes, or arrhythmias detected by Holter monitoring. Often, interim analyses of the results are performed, which may lead to early cessation of the trial. This may be due to unexpectedly positive results, which ethically require the trial to be discontinued and the results made available for general clinical use. Negative results that demonstrate harm to the experimental population may also necessitate cessation of the study.[13]

Numerous variations on the basic theme of randomized, double-blind, placebo-controlled trials exist. A crossover study may be used in trials in which a small number of patients are enrolled. In this type of study, each patient receives both treatment options. During the first portion of the study, one-half the study population receives drug A, the other half drug B. After a specified time interval on active therapy, there is a placebo washout phase. Patients then enter a second active therapy phase and are switched to the opposite agent. Thus each patient serves as his or her own control. Variability between the groups, which is a more significant problem with smaller populations, is minimized. Newer studies are focusing not just on specific clinical end points but also on quality-of-life-improvement, measured by surveys or questionnaires.

PROTECTION OF HUMAN SUBJECTS

In 1962, the Kefauver-Harris amendments added informed consent to the FDCA of 1938[14]; however, the concept of an executed form, signed by the patient, became FDA policy as recently as 1967. In 1966, the U.S. Public Health Service delineated the fact that patients had a right to be informed about the benefits, risks, and objectives of research in which they might participate.[14]

In addition to approval by the FDA, studies in humans must also be approved by institutional review boards (IRBs) before any trials can be initiated. As the name implies, IRBs are review boards at hospitals or research facilities whose primary purpose is to protect human subjects. Since trials of pharmaceutical products are usually conducted by researchers or physician-investigators affiliated with institutions where the studies will be conducted and where human subjects will be recruited, the facility's IRB has evolved as

an appropriate entity to provide review.[15,16] In situations where investigations are to be conducted in the community at private offices or private clinics, noninstitutional review boards (NRBs) have been formed with similar responsibilities.

In little more than 30 years, IRBs have become familiar fixtures at health care institutions involved in any form of clinical research, serving as gatekeepers in the protection of human subjects. Indeed, FDA rules and regulations specifically call for IRB review of clinical investigations for the purpose of protecting the rights and welfare of human subjects involved in such investigations.[15] The function of an IRB or NRB is to determine in advance whether clinical research protocols satisfy certain criteria. In reviewing an experimental protocol, the review board must therefore consider whether the research design is sound, the balance between risks and benefits is reasonable, the selection of subjects is equitable, the informed consent is satisfactory, the monitoring of collected data is adequate, the privacy of individuals and the confidentiality of data are protected, and additional safeguards are in place when dealing with the vulnerable—i.e., populations comprising individuals who may be unable to give informed consent. These may include children, handicapped, or mentally disabled persons, economically or educationally disadvantaged individuals, and prisoners. There are additional safeguards for pregnant women.[15,16]

Even though all the components reviewed by the IRB are important, particular attention is usually given to the informed consent process. Every protocol includes an informed consent that must be signed by all subjects before they can be enrolled in the trial. The content of the informed consent is carefully examined by the committee. The form must contain all the information necessary to make an informed decision and must be written in language that a lay person can understand. In addition, every study subject must be made aware of other treatment options and their concomitant advantages and disadvantages, whether compensation or treatment is available for any unexpected event, and that participation is voluntary and the patient may withdraw from the trial at any time. A good informed consent form, however, is only a part of the process. The investigator must give the potential subject the opportunity to ask questions and discuss the protocol, ultimately being satisfied that the subject knows enough to make an informed decision regarding participation in the study.[11,17]

This highly regulated process reflects concern over past violations in human subject research, which culminated in the 1979 recommendations of the National Commission for the Protection of Human Subjects of Biomedical and Behavioral Research widely known as The Belmont Report.[16,18] The commission set ethical standards for the conduct of research involving human beings. The three basic ethical principles—respect for persons, beneficence, and justice—have thus become the essential guideposts in human subject research.[16,19,20] Yet as regulated as the process of drug approval appears, IRB members do have ample latitude in determining what is acceptable to them—conditions that may vary from protocol to protocol or in different clinical situations. For example, the balance of risks and benefits may be very different for drug trials in AIDS or certain malignancies than that for the treatment of diseases for which there are reasonable alternative treatment options, a concept of particular importance to incarcerated inmates.[21] Once a protocol receives IRB approval, the investigator may begin the trial. However, it should be noted that IRB involvement does not end with initial approval. Each phase of a trial and each change or amendment must be submitted for IRB consideration. In addition, approval may be granted for a period of no more than 2 years and is usually reviewed on an annual basis.[15,16] Adverse events must always be reported to the IRB.

TREATMENT WITH INVESTIGATIONAL NEW DRUGS

Historically, physicians have always been faced with clinical situations for which there is no established therapy. A new drug or product may show promise for a previously untreatable disease or condition but remain unproven pending controlled clinical trials. All too often patients would run out of time pending good data. In 1987 the FDA issued regulations permitting use of INDs as therapeutic options in selected circumstances.[8,22] The designation "treatment IND" indicates that a drug is being administered not just to determine safety and efficacy data but also to obtain a therapeutic response in a particular patient.[22] It is important to note that the regulations require informed consent of the patient, as in all trials, prior to institution of a treatment IND.

SPECIAL POPULATIONS

Traditionally, women and children as well as minorities have been excluded from clinical research. The FDA itself in 1977 issued guidelines that prohibited inclusion of women of childbearing age in early clinical trials.[23,24] This policy was due to concerns about the teratogenic effects of experimental drugs.[25] It had wide-ranging effects beyond the specific restrictions it enumerated. Examination of NDA databases as recently as 1994 revealed a distinct paucity of women subjects, even though there were no specific exclusion criteria in the protocols.[23] Some clinical researchers wished simply to avoid the entire issue and did not include women, even in circumstances such as life-threatening illnesses in which their inclusion was specifically permitted by the FDA.[23,24] The FDA has since rescinded this policy and issued new guidelines[23,25] stating that participation of both sexes, taking into account the prevalence of the disease in each sex, is expected and that this is part of a general FDA expectation that drugs will be evaluated in a reasonable sample of the people who will receive them.[23] In addition, the FDA has emphasized the importance of drug evaluation in children of various ages, preferring to no longer simply view children as "small adults" in the application of information obtained from adult studies.[26]

Concurrent with the FDA's policy change regarding inclusion of women in clinical trials, a legislative initiative was passed designed to improve representation of women and minorities in clinical trials. The NIH Revitalization Act of 1993 mandated the National Institutes of Health to develop specific policies for the inclusion of women and minorities in clinical research,[27,28] published in the *Federal Register* as follows:

- Ensure that women and members of minorities and their subpopulations are included in all human subject research.
- For phase III clinical trials, ensure that women and minorities and their subpopulations must be included such that valid analyses of differences in intervention effect can be accomplished.
- Not allow cost as an acceptable reason for excluding these groups.

- Initiate programs and support for outreach efforts to recruit these groups into clinical studies.

The 1993 act has received mixed reviews from the medical and scientific community.[29] Some believe that trying to generate data specific to subpopulations further dilutes the aggregate power of the results in terms of a specific disease entity. Others argue that subgrouping can go on ad infinitum with the inevitable conclusion that no result is really applicable to a more and more specific population. Over the last several years, the agency has been requiring sponsors to "analyze safety and effectiveness data for important demographic subgroups, including gender and racial subgroups."[5]

MedWatch: Adverse Drug Event Reporting

As excellent as the processes of drug development and FDA premarketing approval are, the full scope of clinical and side effects is often not known when a drug becomes available for widespread use. There are several reasons for this, some of which have been enumerated by FDA personnel and are included in the following list[30]:

1. *Short duration of clinical trials.* Side effects or complications with either long latency or delayed onset are often not detectable.
2. *Study population.* Clinical trials rarely represent all populations.
3. *Complicating factors.* Clinical trials often exclude patients with concurrent diseases so that the potential for interactions of the study drug and other agents is limited. Additionally, the size of most trials does not ensure a high likelihood that as wide a range of drugs that the general population will be concomitantly taking will be represented in the study population.
4. *Indications.* These evolve over time so that a drug with what appears to be a favorable profile may not actually be as safe when used in patients with a different disease.
5. *Small size of study population.* This certainly cannot address a significant number of potential drug interactions that can have an adverse effect.

The FDA has maintained several mechanisms for reporting adverse events related to a wide range of medical products for some years. In the early 1990s, FDA Commissioner David Kessler initiated a review of the reporting mechanisms for the various products regulated by the FDA, including drugs, medical devices, and biologics, with the intent of streamlining the process and making it more user friendly. A task force was formed to review the process, resulting in the development of MEDWATCH, the FDA Medical Products Reporting Program.

MEDWATCH was specifically designed to facilitate the reporting by health professionals of serious adverse events and product problems for all medical products, including drugs, biologics, medical devices, and special nutritional products. Serious adverse drug events (ADEs) are defined by the FDA as resulting in (1) death, (2) life-threatening event, (3) hospitalization (initial or prolonged), (4) disability, (5) congenital anomaly, or (6) medical or surgical intervention was required to prevent permanent damage.[30]

A sentinel example in the field of cardiovascular medicine, highlighting the importance of such postmarketing surveillance, is the interaction of terfenadine with ketoconazole. A young patient presented in 1989 with torsades de pointes after taking both drugs, and it

MEDWATCH
THE FDA MEDICAL PRODUCTS REPORTING PROGRAM

For **VOLUNTARY** reporting
by health professionals of adverse
events and product problems

Page ____ of ____

Form Approved: OMB No. 0910-0291 Expires:12/31/94
See OMB statement on reverse

FDA Use Only
Triage unit
sequence #

A. Patient information

1. Patient identifier

In confidence

2. Age at time of event:
or _____
Date of birth:

3. Sex
☐ female
☐ male

4. Weight
____ lbs
or
____ kgs

B. Adverse event or product problem

1. ☐ Adverse event   and/or   ☐ Product problem (e.g., defects/malfunctions)

2. Outcomes attributed to adverse event (check all that apply)
☐ death _____ (mo/day/yr)
☐ life-threatening
☐ hospitalization – initial or prolonged

☐ disability
☐ congenital anomaly
☐ required intervention to prevent permanent impairment/damage
☐ other: _____

3. Date of event (mo/day/yr)

4. Date of this report (mo/day/yr)

5. Describe event or problem

6. Relevant tests/laboratory data, including dates

7. Other relevant history, including preexisting medical conditions (e.g., allergies, race, pregnancy, smoking and alcohol use, hepatic/renal dysfunction, etc.)

C. Suspect medication(s)

1. Name (give labeled strength & mfr/labeler, if known)
#1
#2

2. Dose, frequency & route used
#1
#2

3. Therapy dates (if unknown, give duration) from/to (or best estimate)
#1
#2

4. Diagnosis for use (indication)
#1
#2

5. Event abated after use stopped or dose reduced
#1 ☐ yes ☐ no ☐ doesn't apply
#2 ☐ yes ☐ no ☐ doesn't apply

6. Lot # (if known)
#1
#2

7. Exp. date (if known)
#1
#2

8. Event reappeared after reintroduction
#1 ☐ yes ☐ no ☐ doesn't apply
#2 ☐ yes ☐ no ☐ doesn't apply

9. NDC # (for product problems only)
― ―

10. Concomitant medical products and therapy dates (exclude treatment of event)

D. Suspect medical device

1. Brand name

2. Type of device

3. Manufacturer name & address

4. Operator of device
☐ health professional
☐ lay user/patient
☐ other:
_____

5. Expiration date (mo/day/yr)

6.
model # _____
catalog # _____
serial # _____
lot # _____
other #

7. If implanted, give date (mo/day/yr)

8. If explanted, give date (mo/day/yr)

9. Device available for evaluation? (Do not send to FDA)
☐ yes ☐ no ☐ returned to manufacturer on _____ (mo/day/yr)

10. Concomitant medical products and therapy dates (exclude treatment of event)

E. Reporter (see confidentiality section on back)

1. Name, address & phone #

2. Health professional?
☐ yes ☐ no

3. Occupation

4. Also reported to
☐ manufacturer
☐ user facility
☐ distributor

5. If you do NOT want your identity disclosed to the manufacturer, place an " X " in this box. ☐

FDA

Mail to: **MEDWATCH**
5600 Fishers Lane
Rockville, MD 20852-9787

or FAX to:
1-800-FDA-0178

FDA Form 3500 (6/93)   Submission of a report does not constitute an admission that medical personnel or the product caused or contributed to the event.

FIGURE 4-2. MEDWATCH reporting form.

ADVICE ABOUT VOLUNTARY REPORTING

Report experiences with:

- medications (drugs or biologics)
- medical devices (including in-vitro diagnostics)
- special nutritional products (dietary supplements, medical foods, infant formulas)
- other products regulated by FDA

Report SERIOUS adverse events. An event is serious when the patient outcome is:

- death
- life-threatening (real risk of dying)
- hospitalization (initial or prolonged)
- disability (significant, persistent or permanent)
- congenital anomaly
- required intervention to prevent permanent impairment or damage

Report even if:

- you're not certain the product caused the event
- you don't have all the details

Report product problems – quality, performance or safety concerns such as:

- suspected contamination
- questionable stability
- defective components
- poor packaging or labeling

How to report:

- just fill in the sections that apply to your report
- use section C for all products except medical devices
- attach additional blank pages if needed
- use a separate form for each patient
- report either to FDA or the manufacturer (or both)

Important numbers:

- 1-800-FDA-0178   to FAX report
- 1-800-FDA-7737   to report by modem
- 1-800-FDA-1088   for more information or to report quality problems
- 1-800-822-7967   for a VAERS form for vaccines

If your report involves a serious adverse event with a device and it occurred in a facility outside a doctor's office, that facility may be legally required to report to FDA and/or the manufacturer. Please notify the person in that facility who would handle such reporting.

Confidentiality: The patient's identity is held in strict confidence by FDA and protected to the fullest extent of the law. The reporter's identity may be shared with the manufacturer unless requested otherwise. However, FDA will not disclose the reporter's identity in response to a request from the public, pursuant to the Freedom of Information Act.

The public reporting burden for this collection of information has been estimated to average 30 minutes per response, including the time for reviewing instructions, searching existing data sources, gathering and maintaining the data needed, and completing and reviewing the collection of information. Send your comments regarding this burden estimate or any other aspect of this collection of information, including suggestions for reducing this burden to:

Reports Clearance Officer, PHS
Hubert H. Humphrey Building,
Room 721-B
200 Independence Avenue, S.W.
Washington, DC 20201
ATTN: PRA

and to:
Office of Management and Budget
Paperwork Reduction Project
(0910-0230)
Washington, DC 20503

Please do NOT return this form to either of these addresses.

FDA Form 3500-back   **Please Use Address Provided Below – Just Fold In Thirds, Tape and Mail**

Department of Health and Human Services

Public Health Service
Food and Drug Administration
Rockville, MD 20857

Official Business
Penalty for Private Use $300

NO POSTAGE
NECESSARY
IF MAILED
IN THE
UNITED STATES
OR APO/FPO

BUSINESS REPLY MAIL
FIRST CLASS MAIL   PERMIT NO. 946   ROCKVILLE, MD

POSTAGE WILL BE PAID BY FOOD AND DRUG ADMINISTRATION

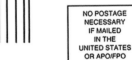

The FDA Medical Products Reporting Program
Food and Drug Administration
5600 Fishers Lane
Rockville, MD 20852-9787

FIGURE 4-2. *(Continued)*

was subsequently determined that ketoconazole interfered with the metabolism of terfenadine, resulting in accumulation of toxic levels of the latter. This effect on the levels of terfenadine when the drug is taken concomitantly with ketoconazole had not been previously observed. Based on the investigation that followed this incident, the labeling of terfenadine was modified to include a warning about this potentially serious side effect when the drug is used concomitantly with certain other pharmaceuticals.[28]

It is clear that ADEs are a significant cause of morbidity and mortality. Studies have reported that as many as 11% of acute care hospital admissions can be attributed to ADEs.[29] The MEDWATCH program facilitates reporting to the FDA, not only of serious adverse drug events but also of medical product problems, such as contaminants and defects. Dissemination of the safety measures resulting from the MEDWATCH information, an important component of this program, is now being done through journal articles, letters, and the *FDA Medical Bulletin*. It should be noted that there are also mandatory reporting requirements for certain categories of products regulated by the FDA. (At the time of this writing, the FDA telephone number for the MEDWATCH program is 1-800-FDA-1088.) The agency has also developed a universal form (Fig. 4-2) for voluntary reporting by health professionals.

CONCLUSION

The process of drug development in the United States today is an amalgam of scientific research, industry commitment, and legislated FDA oversight, all with the intended purpose of speeding safe and effective treatment to patients. It is a process with a rich evolution over the last century. It remains a lengthy and costly process spanning many years and requiring hundreds of millions of dollars. Practitioners of cardiovascular medicine and their patients have especially benefited from innovations in pharmacotherapy. The last 30 years have marked a renaissance in the pharmacologic treatment of cardiovascular disease. Dozens of new drugs and development of entire new classes of agents has resulted in explosive growth of pharmacotherapeutic options since 1960. If the next 30 years resemble the past, physicians and patients can eagerly anticipate major breakthroughs in the treatment of heart failure, arrhythmias, and atherosclerosis. Although targets for these agents may be the chromosome rather than the cell membrane receptor and although they may be more biologic than pharmacologic, a thorough understanding of the basic principles of clinical trials, informed consent, and postmarketing surveillance will still be essential for the cardiovascular practitioner who wishes to remain at the cutting edge.

REFERENCES

 1. Cohn J: The beginnings: Laboratory and animal studies: New drug development in the United States. *FDA Consumer* 2:2, 1995.
 2. Kleinfeld, Kaplan, Becker: Human drug regulation: Comprehensiveness breeds complexity. In: Cooper RM, ed. *Food and Drug Law.* Washington, DC: Food and Drug Law Institute, 1991:243–302.
 3. Hoffman J: The food and drug administrations administrative procedures. In: Cooper RM, ed. *Food and Drug Law.* Washington, DC: Food and Drug Law Institute, 1991:1–60.
 4. FDA: Benefit vs risk: How CDER approves new drugs. In: *From Test Tube to Patient: Improving Health Through Human Drugs.* Special Report. Washington, DC: US Food and Drug Administration, Sept 1999: 33–40.
 5. FDA: Testing drugs in people. In: *From Test Tube to Patient: Improving Health Through Human Drugs.* Special Report. Washington, DC: US Food and Drug Administration, Sept 1999:18–23.
 6. Feuerstein A: FDA not solely to blame for drug approval delays. http://aol.thestreet.com/stocks/biotech/10001581.html
 7. FDA: The beginnings: laboratory and animal studies. In: *From Test Tube to Patient: Improving Health Through Human Drugs.* Special Report. Washington, DC: US Food and Drug Administration, , Sept 1999:14–17.
 8. IND application process, Feb 26, 2001:1. www.fda.gov/cder/ regulatory/applications/ ind_pge_1.htm.
 9. FDA: FDA finds new ways to speed treatments to patients, in *From Test Tube to Patient: Improving Health Through Human Drugs.* Special Report. Washington, DC: US Food and Drug Administration, Sept 1999: 29–32.
10. Moore DL, Bernard S: Clinical trials in women's health research: Part I. The drug discovery and development process. *J Womens Health* 5:103, 1996.
11. Flieger K: Testing drugs in people. *FDA Consumer* 2:6, 1995.
12. Rothman KJ, Michels KB: The continuing unethical use of placebo controls. *N Engl J Med* 331:394, 1994.
12a. Lesko LJ, Atkinson AJ Jr: Use of biomarkers and surrogate end points in drug development and regulatory design making: Criteria, validation, strategies. *Ann Rev Pharmacol Toxicol* 41:347, 2001.
13. Sica D: Lessons learned from prematurely terminated clinical trials. *Curr Hypertens Rep* 3:360, 2001.
14. FDA: Protecting human subjects. In: *From Test Tube to Patient: Improving Health Through Human Drugs.* Special Report. Washington, DC: US Food and Drug Administration, Sept 1999:24–29.
15. Code of Federal Regulations, Part 56.101–56.124.
16. McGuire Dunn C, Chadwick G: *Protecting Study Volunteers in Research.* Boston: Center Watch, 1999.
17. Thompson RC: Protecting human guinea pigs. *FDA Consumer* 2:14, 1995.
18. Belmont Report: Ethical Principles and Guidelines for the Protection of Human Subjects of Research. *Federal Register* 79:1206s, 1979.
19. Faden RR: Beauchamp TL: *A History and Theory of Informed Consent.* London: Oxford University Press, 1986:213–218.
20. Levine RJ: *Ethics and Regulation of Clinical Research,* 2d ed. New Haven, CT: Yale University Press, 1986:11–18.
21. DeGroot AS, Bick J, Thomas D, Stubblefield E: HIV clinical trials in correctional settings: Right or retrogression? *AIO Read* 11:34, 2001.
22. Flieger K: FDA finds new ways to speed treatments to patients. *FDA Consumer* 2:19, 1995.
23. Sherman LA, Temple R, Merkatz RB: Women in clinical trials: A FDA perspective. *Science* 269:793, 1995.
24. Department of Health Education & Welfare, Food and Drug Administration: *General Considerations for the Clinical Evaluation of Drugs.* HEW Publication (FDA) 77-3040. Washington, DC: HEW, 1977.
25. Merkatz RB, Temple R, Sobel S, et al: Women in clinical trials of new drugs: A change in Food and Drug Administration policy. *N Engl J Med* 329:292, 1993.
26. Tauer CA: Testing drugs in pediatric populations: The FDA mandate. *Account Res* 7:37, 1999.
27. NIH Revitalization Act of 1993, 42 U.S.C. Sec. 289a–2.
28. NIH guidelines on the inclusion of women and minorities as subjects in clinical research. *Federal Register* 59:14508–14513, 1994.
29. Meinert CL: The inclusion of women in clinical trials. *Science* 269: 795, 1995.
30. Henkel J: MedWatch: FDA's "Heads Up" on Medical Product Safety. *FDA Consumer* 32(6):1998. http://www.FDA.gov/fdac/features/1998/ 698_med.html.
31. Seldane package insert. *Physicians' Desk Reference.* Montvale, NJ: Medical Economics, 1996:1536–1540.
32. Beard K: Adverse reactions as a cause of hospital admissions in the aged. *Drugs Aging* 2:356, 1992.

CHAPTER 5

Health Economic Considerations in Cardiovascular Drug Utilization

Renée J. Goldberg Arnold

Diana J. Kaniecki

INTRODUCTION

With limited health care dollars, an increasing burden is being placed on health care professionals to provide the best possible care while consuming the fewest possible resources. This is particularly the case when high-technology but costly interventions are a potential option, as in the treatment of patients with cardiovascular disease. Cardiovascular disease is the leading cause of complications and death in the United States, affecting nearly 60 million Americans in 1998 and costing an estimated $274.2 billion.[1]

Of particular interest, then, is the incremental benefit associated with the additional cost of a new therapeutic option. For example, tissue plasminogen activator (t-PA) has been demonstrated to reduce post–myocardial infarction (MI) mortality by 1.1% over streptokinase, but at an additional cost of approximately $2,800 per patient.[2] Another example is the up-front cost associated with angiotensin converting enzyme (ACE) inhibitor therapy as a treatment for heart failure, which may be associated with lower "downstream" hospitalization costs.[3] Often therapies with improved efficacy and/or safety profiles are more expensive, and it is not always clear whether the incremental benefit from the more expensive therapy is worth the additional cost.[2] The science of health economics (HE) allows one to determine whether this trade-off of efficacy for cost is worthwhile.

Cost-effectiveness analyses first became of interest in the 1970s and have assumed greater importance through the development of more sophisticated analytic techniques.[4] Because of the increasing prominence of these analyses in worldwide drug registration, formulary decision making, therapeutic guideline determination,[5] and individual patient decisions, it is incumbent upon the practicing cardiologist to understand the basic tenets of HE analyses and how these may be applicable to daily practice. Indeed, several comprehensive reviews of the cost-effectiveness of heart disease treatments have been published; these have been primarily in the U.S. literature.[6–9] The science of HE is more far-reaching than the question of which therapeutic options should be available within a particular setting. In fact, they are currently being conducted in some institutions to help determine which health professionals should initially be treating patients (e.g., generalist versus specialist[10–14]) and even which setting should be recommended.[13,15] Many influential groups, including the American Heart Association, support the tenet that cost-effectiveness, in addition to clinical effectiveness, must be determined to allow for appropriate treatment while maximizing allocation of scarce medical resources.[16]

FEATURES OF HEALTH ECONOMIC ANALYSES

Cost-Effectiveness

An effective HE or cost-effectiveness analysis is designed to answer certain questions, such as: Is the treatment effective? What will it cost? How do the gains compare with the costs? By combining answers to all of these questions, the technique helps decision makers to weigh the factors, compare alternative treatments, and decide which treatments are most appropriate for specific situations. Typically, one chooses the option with the least cost per unit of measure gained; the results are represented by the ratio of cost to effectiveness (C:E). With this type of analysis, called a cost-effectiveness analysis (CEA), various disease end points that are affected by therapy (risk markers, disease severity, death) can be assessed by corresponding indexes of therapeutic outcome (degree of blood pressure reduction, number of hospitalizations averted, and life-years saved, respectively).

"Average" cost-effectiveness is the result of dividing mean total costs by outcomes. Although this type of analysis allows one to view the actual numbers involved in the computation, average cost-effectiveness does not illustrate differences between competing strategies.[17,18] Thus, many researchers discuss the merits of an "incremental" cost-effectiveness ratio, i.e., additional cost for additional benefit, which may be calculated as follows:

$$\frac{\Delta C}{\Delta E} = \frac{\text{cost}_1 - \text{cost}_2}{\text{effectiveness}_1 - \text{effectiveness}_2}$$

where effectiveness$_1$ is greater than effectiveness$_2$.

The term *incremental* is commonly used interchangeably with the term *marginal* to denote the additional cost and outcome of an intervention.[18] As an example, consider the analysis by Eckman and colleagues[19] of the comparative cost-utility of aspirin, anticoagulation, and no anticoagulation in atrial fibrillation. Over a lifetime, providing anticoagulation therapy for a patient costs on average $2,200 more than aspirin therapy (i.e., cost$_1$−cost$_2$) and results in an average gain of 0.12 quality-adjusted life-years (QALYs) (i.e., effectiveness$_1$−effectiveness$_2$), concluding in a marginal

TABLE 5-1. Cost-Effectiveness Analysis

Strategies	Cost ($)	Effectiveness (QALYs*)	Marginal Cost ($) (Δ cost)	Marginal Effectiveness (Δ QALYs)	Marginal Cost-Effectiveness Ratio ($ per additional QALY)
Aspirin (ASA)	$8,544	6.74	—	—	—
Do not anticoagulate	$9,889	6.37	$1,345	−0.37 (vs. ASA)	Dominated
Anticoagulate with warfarin	$10,728	6.86	$2,184	0.12 (vs. ASA)	$18,200

*Quality-adjusted life-years.

Source: Adapted with permission from Eckman et al.[19]

cost-effectiveness ratio of $2,184/0.12 or $18,200 per QALY (Table 5-1). This type of analysis is useful in the following two instances: (1) where the new strategy is more costly but expected to be more effective or (2) where the new strategy is less costly but less effective.

In cases where these conditions do not apply, a negative cost-effectiveness ratio occurs—i.e., when the competing strategy produces cost savings without reducing effectiveness or when the comparator results in a net increase in costs and reduction in health. Such a strategy is said to be dominated by the more effective strategy. The cost-effectiveness ratio for a dominated strategy is, therefore, negative. Logically, no one would choose a treatment that costs more and is less effective; this results in a negative cost-effectiveness ratio and results are uninterpretable.[17,20]

As an example, again consider the analysis by Eckman and colleagues.[19] Since the cost-effectiveness ratio of "do not anticoagulate" is negative, i.e., less effective than either comparative strategy, only the aspirin and "anticoagulate with warfarin" strategies are evaluated.

An efficiency envelope illustrates the concept of incremental effectiveness versus cost. The curve of the outermost points forms the envelope or frontier and represents the most efficient options. Points within the envelope are dominated by at least one point along the envelope.[21] Relatively steep slopes from one strategy to another indicate a substantial increase in effectiveness for a modest increase in cost. As an example, once more consider the analysis by Eckman and colleagues (Fig. 5-1).[19] Here, aspirin and anticoagulation correspond to two points along the envelope where incremental cost-effectiveness is calculated; do not anticoagulate corresponds to the inside of the envelope.

The concepts that are of importance in understanding a HE analysis include its type, perspective, method used, data source(s),

ultimate use, time frame, patient subgroups, and robustness. Each of these is discussed in detail below and examples of cardiovascular analyses in the literature given.

Types of Analyses

Analyses may characterize differences between therapies and/or procedures used for treatment of disease. They can also be used to determine the cost-effectiveness of preventive measures. Several types of economic analyses have been developed to facilitate choices among therapies competing for the same health care dollars. HE analyses are generally categorized according to the type of analysis to be performed (Table 5-2).[22–24] Cost-minimization analysis (CMA) is most appropriately used when therapies are equally effective and only costs need be compared: the least expensive drug is preferred. Cost-benefit analysis (CBA) uses monetary terms to measure effectiveness; because it is difficult to place a monetary value on life and health, this approach has limited utility.

When a single dimension of effectiveness characterizes the relevant outcome for all therapies and alternative treatments do not have the same clinical effectiveness, CEA may be the most appropriate method of evaluation. It assesses the incremental gain in therapeutic benefits derived from additional costs and measures effectiveness in terms of health outcomes, such as life-years saved, cases of disease prevented, or complication-free therapy-months. Cost-utility analysis (CUA), which may be considered a type of CEA, evaluates the impact of a certain therapy on quality of life and measures effectiveness in terms of quality-adjusted units, such as the QALY. All of these methodologies may be carried out using either a retrospective or prospective approach, although the reliability of a CUA may be questionable when such a study is conducted retrospectively.

For example, prevention of primary and secondary MI and stroke via use of lysine acetylsalicylate was shown to be a cost-effective strategy in patients at high risk of cardiovascular and cerebrovascular events in a French model that used the social security perspective. Cost-effectiveness ratios varied according to underlying disease and dose of acetylsalicylate (see Table 5-3).[25] Likewise, Augustovski and colleagues[26] designed a Markov model to evaluate the utility of aspirin for primary prevention of cardiovascular events on expected length and quality of life for a hypothetical cohort over 10 years. Risk factors that were considered included gender, age, cholesterol levels, systolic blood pressure, smoking status, diabetes, and presence of left ventricular hypertrophy. Outcomes were MI, stroke, gastrointestinal bleed, ulcer, and death. The model indicated that those patients with the highest risk would garner the greatest benefit (gain of 11.3 quality-adjusted life-days), while those with the lowest risk would actually lose benefit (loss of 1.8 quality-adjusted

FIGURE 5-1. Aspirin and anticoagulation correspond to two points along the efficiency envelope where incremental cost-effectiveness is calculated; "do not anticoagulate" corresponds to the area inside of the envelope. (*Reproduced with permission from Eckman et al.[19]*)

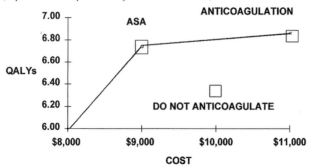

TABLE 5-2. Types of Economic Analysis

Type of Economic Analysis	Appropriate Uses	Limitations
Cost-consequence, cost-identification or component enumeration.	Costs and/or consequences of each therapy are presented in disaggregated form.	No combination analysis is attempted; difficult to ascertain total comparative costs.
Cost-minimization analysis (CMA) Identifies least costly selection among equally effective therapies.	Selecting among equally effective therapies (e.g., generic substitutions).	Difficult to establish identical clinical effectiveness in same/similar patient(s).
Cost-benefit analysis (CBA) Expresses effectiveness in monetary terms; monetary value placed on health-related outcomes as well as costs.	Choosing drugs or other therapy with highest net benefit or greatest cost-benefit ratio; comparing therapeutic regimens with different objectives.	Difficult to place monetary value on life or health.
Cost-effectiveness analysis (CEA) Assesses incremental gain in therapeutic benefits derived from additional costs; measures effectiveness in terms of health outcomes; compares regimens that measure effectiveness in terms of health outcomes and computes cost-effectiveness ratio for comparison.	Selecting among alternative treatments that do not have the same clinical effectiveness. Used when single dimension of effectiveness (e.g., cost/YLS*) characterizes outcome of all therapies.	Cannot compare different types of treatments; treatment strategies compared only for specific disease rather than across diseases.
Cost-utility analysis (CUA) Evaluates impact of certain therapy on quality of life and measures effectiveness in terms of quality-adjusted units.	Simultaneously synthesizing or summarizing several outcomes into single measure (e.g., impact of drugs on both pain and physical functioning).	Difficult to compare therapeutic impact across individuals. Preference for health state may differ according to current condition.

* Years of life saved.

Source: Adapted with permission from Goldberg et al,[22] CCOHTA guidelines,[23] and Eisenberg et al.[24]

life-days). The decision was extremely sensitive to variations in patient preference for taking aspirin and to aspirin's effects on cardiovascular mortality.

Perspective

The perspective of the analysis is typically that of the primary decision maker. Perspective dictates whether charges or actual costs to the payer should be recorded and employed in the evaluation. Examples of perspective include those of the patient, the third-party payer (e.g., Medicare, insurance companies), the institution (e.g., hospital or managed care organization), the provider, or society at large. The societal perspective frequently includes indirect costs, such as loss of productivity, home health care, and caregiver loss of wages, as well as direct costs of therapy, whereas the institutional perspective does not take these into consideration. Although

studies done in countries with a primarily socialized healthcare system frequently take the societal viewpoint,[27,28] U.S.-based studies rarely do, especially since indirect costs are frequently difficult to measure. Approaching the analysis from the appropriate perspective helps to ensure that the results will be useful. Importantly, different perspectives may be driving the issue, such as the individual physician's desire to hospitalize the patient and the managed care organization's (MCO's) desire to maximize profit margin.

RESOURCE AND COST COMPONENTS

The frequency and cost of resources that are typically incorporated into the cost component (numerator) of this ratio include outpatient visits, hospital days, emergency or urgent care visits, laboratory studies, treatment of adverse events, concomitant medications,

TABLE 5-3. Prevention of Primary and Secondary Myocardial Infarction (MI) and Stroke via Use of Acetylsalicylate

History	Follow-Up	C/E Metric	CE Ratio*
Unstable angina	1 year	Cost per avoided MI	$5,703 to $5,761 (1996 prices)
Prior MI	2 years	Cost per avoided MI	$15 (300-mg dose) to $494 (75-mg dose) (5% discount rate);
		Cost per avoided stroke	$37 to $1170
Ischemic stroke	3 years	Cost per avoided MI	$610 to $2,082
		Cost per avoided stroke	$176 to $599
Stable angina	4 years	Cost per avoided MI	$4,375 to $3,608

* In U.S. dollars.

CE = cost effectiveness.

monitoring for therapeutic effect and adverse events, generalist and specialist visits, primary drug therapy, and devices.

Costs may be recorded as charges or actual costs to the payer, depending on the perspective of the analysis. If costs are desired and only charges are available (as with patient bills), charges may be multiplied by cost-to-charge ratios (which may be available through accounting departments at institutions) to convert charges to costs. Care must be taken in this endeavor, however, since different cost centers may have a variety of cost-to-charge ratios. In addition, interpretation of results may be obscured by cost-shifting, i.e., shifting costs of procedures away from less profitable cost centers.[29] Several national sources of charges include the Medicare databases [e.g., Medicare Provider Analysis and Review (MEDPAR) available through the Centers for Medicare and Medicaid Services (formerly the U.S. Health Care Financing Administration)] and the resource-based relative value scale (RBRVS) of charges for physician-initiated procedures.[30] Costs may be collected, for example, via institutional examination [e.g., cost-accounting systems[31] in hospitals and health maintenance organizations (HMOs)], wholesale drug prices (e.g., *Red Book*[32]), and time and motion studies.

Resources may be broadly grouped as direct or indirect. Direct resources are those that are consumed in the immediate care of the patient, such as outpatient visits, while indirect resources are incurred as a consequence of the treatment or illness and are not directly consumed in carrying out the treatment strategy; indirect resources are those that may impact the patient or society at large, such as loss of income or leisure time.[17] On occasion, known costs may be used as proxies for unknown costs of items if these are felt to be comparable. For example, as a proxy for an adverse event cost, Podrid et al.[31] used the cost of a typical inpatient stay for a primary diagnosis of this event in a study of three antiarrhythmic agents. Sometimes, a cost-of-illness or burden-of-illness evaluation is undertaken. Such an analysis takes into consideration direct and indirect costs of illness[33] and may be useful in determining the potential impact of the intervention on the total cost of treating the disease.

TIME FRAME (DISCOUNTING AND TIME HORIZON)

Future costs and effects are discounted to reflect the fact that, in general, individuals and society have a positive rate of time preference.[34–36] That is, in general, they prefer desirable consequences to occur earlier and undesirable consequences to occur later. Thus, future benefits are discounted to reflect the fact that they are worth less simply because they occur in the future rather than now. Similarly, future costs are discounted to reflect the fact that we prefer them to occur in the future rather than the present.[4] Although the appropriate discount rate is controversial, 3 or 5% are currently the most accepted figures, since they are based on the real rate of return on long-term government bonds.[37] However, sensitivity analyses (see below) should encompass rates from 0% (i.e., no discounting) to 7%.

Time horizon, that is, the length of time into the future considered in the analysis over which costs and outcomes are projected, is also very important.[18] For example, if a clinical trial or the published literature report only short-term results for a chronic condition, the study outcome may come into question. This is where decision-analytic models may come into play, allowing one to project study results to clinically realistic time frames. In addition, these models can help in projecting thresholds (see "Robustness," below).[38]

EFFICACY VERSUS EFFECTIVENESS

Efficacy is typically considered as the measurement of therapeutic effect in clinical trials. Thus, it is a determination of the optimal benefit in an ideal setting, which may or may not be seen in routine clinical practice. In contrast, effectiveness is the therapeutic effect in a "real world" setting and is generally less favorable than efficacy because it includes effects such as noncompliance and less than ideal care. Effectiveness, rather than efficacy, is used in HE analyses because it is more representative of what clinicians experience in routine clinical practice.

Life expectancy is a frequently used effectiveness criterion.[39–44] Edelson et al. published a long-term cost-effectiveness study that compared propranolol, hydrochlorothiazide, nifedipine, prazosin, and captopril as monotherapy for mild-to-moderate hypertension.[42] These authors used the Coronary Heart Disease Policy Model (a computer simulation model) to calculate the cost per years of life saved (YLS) over 20 years of simulated therapy. Probabilities for cardiovascular events were determined from the Framingham Heart Study. The effects of the five agents on blood pressure and cholesterol were obtained via meta analysis of 153 reports. The cost per YLS (1987 dollars discounted at 5% annually) varied from $10,900 for propranolol to $72,100 for captopril. The analysis included savings due to avoided cardiovascular events but did not consider reduction in the risk of stroke.

In addition, compliance with these regimens was not considered. In fact, the Treatment of Mild Hypertension Study (TOMHS) examined this issue and demonstrated that after 4 years, 67.5% of patients remained on chlorthalidone, 77.8% on acebutolol, and 82.5% on amlodipine.[45] Similarly, discontinuation rates of antihyperlipidemic drugs in clinical trials were demonstrated in a study by Andrade et al.[46] not to be reflective of (higher than those of) managed care patients—e.g., 41 versus 31% for bile acid sequestrants, 46 versus 4% for niacin and 37 versus 15% for gemfibrozil in the managed care and clinical trials, respectively. Moreover, as demonstrated in Table 5-4, Kozma and coworkers showed that, regardless of initial diastolic BP, full compliance with the medication regimen would result in a cost per QALY that was about half that associated with partial compliance.[47]

A similar finding of reduced total costs among compliant patients was noted in a retrospective review of administrative claims data for congestive heart failure patients.[48] Clearly, these issues must be considered in long-term cost-effectiveness models.

If the therapies being evaluated are not necessarily lifesaving, if the time frame of the analysis does not lend itself to YLS, or if this measure is not clinically relevant to the question being studied, other measures may be employed to define the effectiveness component. Examples of these include complication-free therapy months[49]; coronary heart disease (CHD) events potentially avoided[50–52] or saved[53]; percent reduction in total cholesterol, LDL, HDL, and LDL/HDL[54]; degree of stenosis found[55];

TABLE 5-4. Influence of Compliance with Medication on Cost-Effectiveness

Diastolic Blood Pressure	Full Compliance ($/QALY)*	Partial Compliance ($/QALY)
≥105 mm Hg	$4,850	$10,500
95–104 mm Hg	$9,880	$20,400

*Quality-adjusted life-year.

blood pressure control[56]; surgical cure[57]; and thromboembolism averted.[58]

UTILITY ASSESSMENT AND QUALITY OF LIFE

CUA have gained increasing popularity since they incorporate a patient-oriented measure or subjective component, namely, patient preferences, into the effectiveness portion of the equation. In this regard, YLS may be "qualified" by the decrement in quality of life (QOL) during this time span, giving an effectiveness criterion such as QALYs.[4,19,50,59,60] Quality adjustment is important in that a treatment may not change life expectancy but may change QOL dramatically, so the net effect of a strategy will be completely missed if one does not consider QOL. For example, drugs to treat angina may not improve survival but may increase QOL. There are also strategies that may increase survival but reduce QOL, such as a pacemaker, where the patient is continually concerned about premature electrical discharge. For the remainder of the patient's life, his or her lifestyle will be dominated by this negative component of the therapy.

Quality adjustment is usually performed by polling a representative population (depending on the perspective of the analysis) to elicit their preferences for being in a particular state of health. These results, called "utilities," are typically expressed as numbers between "0" (death) and "1" (perfect health), which are then multiplied by the number of years in that health state. For example, 2 years with angina might be worth 1.6 years (2 years × 0.8 utilities or quality-adjustment factor) of perfect health. A number of methods, such as the standard gamble and time trade-off, have been developed to allow one to measure health-state utilities.[61–66] Although time trade-off has been generally considered easier to use than standard gamble, the latter may be more consistent or reliable.[8,37] Debates in this area have focused on potential states worse than death and on the definition of the utility of "1" (i.e., whose idea of perfect health?).[37,67] That is, while "0" is meant to represent the worst state of health, some believe that death is not always the worst health state.

Nonetheless, the importance of taking effectiveness and QOL into consideration may be illustrated as:

Treatment	Cost	QALYs	Cost per QALY
A	$10,000.00	10	$1,000.00
B	$ 8,000.00	6	$1,333.00

At face value, treatment B would be preferred because it is less expensive. However, if one takes into consideration the number of years lived and QOL during this time period for the average patient, treatment A is the preferred strategy.

METHOD USED

A variety of methods have been utilized to structure HE evaluations to assure inclusion of all applicable parameters. Some of these include decision trees (decision-analytic models), mathematical spreadsheets (e.g., using Microsoft Excel or Lotus), simulation models, and cost enumeration, among others.

Decision-Analytic Models

Decision-analytic models are structured methods of incorporating probabilities and costs of likely events for expected therapeutic pathways. These models use a tree structure and principles of expected utility to calculate both cost and effectiveness. Numerous evaluations have utilized this method for determining the most cost-effective strategy.[31,68–70] An example of this type of analysis was that undertaken by Danford and colleagues,[68] in which echocardiography followed by referral to the cardiologist was found more costly than initial evaluation by a cardiologist for evaluation of a pediatric heart murmur.

An example of a decision-analytic model that illustrates the need to target specific patient subgroups is the economic analysis carried out by Barrett and researchers to estimate the incremental cost per QALY of low (LOCM)- vs high (HOCM)-osmolality contrast media for cardiac angiography.[70] The decision-analytic model (Fig. 5-2) shows the three strategies that were examined—unrestricted use of LOCM or HOCM and selective use of LOCM in patients at high risk for contrast-media-related adverse events (e.g., those with unstable angina, recent MI, severe valvular disease, etc.). Nonfatal adverse events were characterized as severe (MI and stroke), moderate (ischemic, hemodynamic, electrophysiologic, and symptomatic events, including ventricular fibrillation and moderate-

FIGURE 5-2. The decision-analytic model shows the three strategies that were examined by Barrett and researchers to estimate the incremental cost per QALY of low- (LOCM) versus high (HOCM)-osmolality contrast media for cardiac angiography. These strategies include unrestricted use of LOCM or HOCM and selective use of LOCM in patients at high risk for contrast medium–related adverse events. (*Reproduced with permission from Barrett et al.*[70])

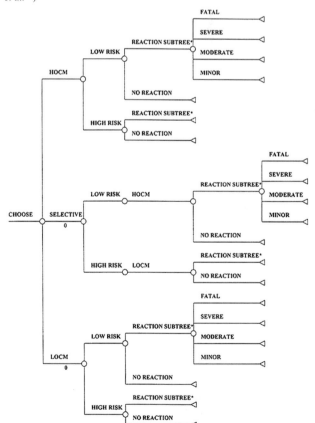

to-severe angina), and minor (nausea, mild angina). Data sources included clinical trial results and review of a large registry of cardiac catheterization complications. Incremental cost per QALY gained was dramatically different, depending on the study perspective and subgroup assessed—$649 to $17,264 in high-risk and $35,509 to $47,874 in low-risk patients, depending on the perspective taken. The results showed that only selective use of LOCM—i.e., in high-risk patients—would give a favorable cost-effectiveness ratio. Similarly, Steinberg and colleagues examined this issue and determined that there would be a 3.5-fold increase in incremental cost of each moderate adverse event avoided if LOCM were given to all rather than just high-risk patients.[60]

There are also special types of decision-analytic models, such as Markov models,[71] that can account for issues of time-sensitivity. That is, continuous risk and uncertain timing of events may depend on when events occur. For example, Eckman and colleagues[19] employed a Markov model in atrial fibrillation to discern the comparative cost-utility (using QALY as the effectiveness parameter) of anticoagulation versus no anticoagulation. Patients go on to develop three potential types of events—thromboembolic events, major bleeding events, or death from age-, gender-, race- and comorbidity-related causes. Using results from five nonvalvular atrial fibrillation trials, aspirin was shown to be both more effective and less costly than "do not anticoagulate"; thus, aspirin was the dominant strategy (see Table 5-1).

Likewise, a Markov model was used to evaluate the benefits and costs of nine diagnostic strategies—transthoracic echocardiography (TTE), transesophageal echocardiography (TEE), sequential approaches, selective imaging, and no imaging—to identify potential cardiovascular sources of emboli in patients who have had strokes.[72] Values for event rates, anticoagulation effects, utilities, and costs were obtained from the literature and Medicare data. Once again, it was more cost-effective to selectively perform diagnostic procedures ($9,000 per QALY versus $13,000 per QALY for TEE in patients with and without previous cardiac history, respectively). Cost savings and decreased morbidity and mortality rates associated with reduction in preventable recurrent strokes substantially offset examination costs and risks of anticoagulation. Since the major advantage of a computerized decision-analytic model is the ability to alter values for key variables and reevaluate the options (i.e., perform a sensitivity analysis) or to project long-term effectiveness when only short-term data are available, several "what-if" scenarios were undertaken. These sensitivity analyses demonstrated that the study results were moderately sensitive to efficacy of anticoagulation and incidence of intracranial bleeding during anticoagulation and were mildly sensitive to prevalence of left atrial thrombus, rate of recurrent stroke in patients with thrombus, QOL after stroke, cost of TEE and specificity of TEE. TTE, alone or in sequence with TEE, was not cost-effective compared with TEE.

Mathematical Spreadsheets

These models calculate the cost and cost-effectiveness of therapeutic strategies by multiplying the probability of an event by its cost. An example of this type of methodology is an Excel spreadsheet model developed by Arnold and colleagues to assess coronary heart disease (CHD) events potentially avoided (CEPA) in patients at risk for CHD.[52] In the base case, four HMG-CoA reductase inhibitors—lovastatin (L), pravastatin (P), simvastatin (S), and fluvastatin (F)—were evaluated. A multivariate regression equation used the following data to estimate the costs associated with CEPA: World Health Organization definition of CHD,[73] Framingham Heart Study coefficients for CHD based on relative risk,[74,75] National Cholesterol Education Program II Guidelines for initiation of treatment,[76,77] National Health and Nutrition Examination Survey II for distribution of low-density-lipoprotein cholesterol (LDL-C) in the U.S. population,[78] HCFA's MEDPAR CHD treatment costs, and *Red Book* (1994) for daily drug cost. Efficacy (LDL-C reduction) and drug monitoring and CHD treatment costs were analyzed. The average annual cost of CHD events per 1000 patients was $561,300 (F), $1,035,000 (P), $1,038,650 (S) and $1,108,000 (L) for the majority of patients. Compared to F, the marginal cost per CEPA was $473,700 (P), $477,350 (S), and $546,700 (L). To improve relevance to cost- and budget-conscious managed care clinicians, a matrix of the two population segments was developed to assess the drug budget impact.

Another example is an analysis performed by Najib and coauthors[79] to examine costs associated with managing patients with congestive heart failure in a managed care organization (MCO). Computerized administrative, clinical chart, and claims data from seven individual health care plans affiliated with the MCO were obtained. Medical records and claims data for 275 subjects (128 carvedilol and 147 control) were evaluated. The carvedilol patients were initially identified through the pharmacy and medical claims databases. Patients in the case group were health plan members with a pharmacy benefit chosen for this study. They also met all of the following criteria: (1) at least one carvedilol prescription, (2) a valid diagnosis of congestive heart failure (CHF) defined as a minimum of two claims with ICD-9-CM codes (428.x) at least 30 days apart between 5/1/1997 and 3/31/1999 in the outpatient setting, (3) between 18 and 64 years old as of the date of their first claim with a CHF diagnosis, (4) continuous carvedilol treatment for at least 4 months (continuous treatment was defined by having a prescription gap less than 90 days), (5) at least one of the concomitant drugs (diuretic, ACE inhibitor, or digoxin) taken within the 10-month period starting at the carvedilol index prescription date (the evaluation period), and (6) the latest start with the carvedilol index prescription date occurring before April 1, 1998. Control patients were included in the study if they met criteria two and three listed above but were not receiving carvedilol or any other beta blocker. Case patients were matched in approximately a one-to-one ratio with "noncarvedilol" control patients.

Using the claims data, the facility, professional services, and medication costs to the health plan during the 10 months following the index date for each patient were calculated. Charges submitted by providers to the health plan for their services were used to evaluate the costs associated with health care utilization. Costs were further divided into two groups, those for services with a corresponding CHF ICD-9-CM code plus carvedilol (carvedilol-related costs), and those services with a CHF ICD-9-CM code with no beta-blocker medication (non-carvedilol-related costs). All costs were adjusted to 1999 dollars using the medical care component of the Consumer Price Index. In addition to costs, the rates of facility and professional service utilization were calculated.

Even though no statistically significant differences were detected between treatment groups in terms of facility expenditures, the overall facility expenditures were lower for patients in the carvedilol group than for patients in the control group (Table 5-5*A* and *B*). The difference detected was approximately $9,000 in favor of carvedilol. This is consistent with the findings from the 1996 clinical trial conducted by Packer et al.,[80] which showed carvedilol

TABLE 5-5*A*. Comparison of Payer Costs by Type of Medical Service between Carvedilol (case) and Non-Carvedilol (control) Patients

	Total (*n* = 211) Mean (SD) [median]		Cases (*n* = 105) Mean (SD) [median]		Controls (*n* = 106) Mean (SD) [median]		*P* Value*
Type of Service Facility							
Inpatient	$12,426 ($34,075)	[$0]	$9,157 ($22,585)	[$0]	$15,664 ($42,376)	[$0]	.165
Outpatient hospital	$3,225 ($11,323)	[$339]	$2,186 ($5,411)	[$151]	$4,254 ($15,009)	[$464]	.185
Emergency room	$338 ($868)	[$0]	$368 ($873)	[$0]	$309 ($780)	[$0]	.605
Total facility expenses	$16,454 ($40,829)	[$2,880]	$11,987 ($25,620)	[$1,410]	$20,878 ($51,421)	[$4,771]	.113
Professional							
Cardiologist	$1,735 ($2,347)	[$903]	$1,886 ($2,456)	[$930]	$1,585 ($2,236)	[$864]	.353
Internist	$436 ($1,181)	[$0]	$445 ($1,502)	[$0]	$428 ($745)	[$116]	.914
Family practitioner	$343 ($751)	[$39]	$287 ($733)	[$0]	$399 ($769)	[$136]	.281
Other medical specialty	$2,812 ($4,814)	[$756]	$2,444 ($4,690)	[$510]	$3,176 ($4,929)	[$936]	.270
Total professional service expenses	$6,831 ($8,981)	[$3,616]	$6,559 ($9,050)	[$3,509]	$7,101 ($8,947)	[$3,696]	.662

*Statistical tests compare carvedilol (cases) to non-carvedilol (controls) using one-way analysis of variance with *T*-test.

to have a significant influence on reducing hospitalization-related expenditures. Indeed, in the current study, the mean cost of inpatient stay was approximately $6,500 greater in the control group than in the carvedilol group. The economic evaluation performed on the 6-month data from the clinical trial showed a difference of approximately $9,400 in favor of carvedilol,[81] which is also consistent with findings from the current study.

In another study,[82] Murdock and colleagues compared the clinical effectiveness and cost to convert recent-onset atrial fibrillation or flutter to sinus rhythm with intravenous ibutilide after 3 to 4 weeks of anticoagulation with direct-current (DC) cardioversion. Physician cost consisted of the summation of Medicare charges (CPT codes) submitted by cardiology and anesthesiology departments; hospital costs were obtained from charge data adjusted by cost-to-charge ratios appropriate for each cost center at the authors' hospital; and average wholesale price was used as a proxy for pharmaceutical costs. The low success rate with ibutilide made DC cardioversion the more clinical and cost-effective method to restore sinus rhythm. As noted by the authors, this is in contrast to a study by Zarkin and colleagues,[83] where ibutilide was shown to be more cost-effective as first-line therapy followed by DC cardioversion for patients who failed to convert versus proceeding directly to DC cardioversion. This discrepancy may have resulted from a number of confounding factors: Zarkin used published literature efficacy rates (and primarily for arrhythmia of recent onset) and assumed resource utilization and a lower cost for ibutilide, while Murdock et al. used actual efficacy rates in their hospital (although with an admittedly small

sample size of 30) and included patients with arrhythmia of duration up to 90 days (although mean duration of arrhythmia in each group was not noted); a preponderance of atrial fibrillation (versus atrial flutter) patients, both of which would be expected to reduce the efficacy of ibutilide; and average wholesale price (which is typically quite a bit greater than the price negotiated by institutions).

DATA SOURCE(S)

Prospective

The randomized prospective clinical trial may be a good source of clinical data; however, one must take care not to include costs of resource use required by protocols (so-called protocol-driven resource use), as these are artificially derived and may not be experienced in routine clinical care.[29] Perhaps a more reliable way to examine health care resource utilization is the prospective economic trial (PET),[84] in which patients are randomized to technologies to be evaluated and data on resource use are collected. However, this procedure may be lengthy and expensive. Moreover, there is no guarantee of external validity—that is, the ability to transfer resource use from one country or situation to another.[29] Califf and Eisenstein[3] attempted to account for this potential of nongeneralizability by prospectively enrolling typical patients undergoing percutaneous intervention (PCI) in examining the cost-effectiveness of abciximab versus placebo (EPIC trial),[85,86] then versus a lower

TABLE 5-5*B*. Comparison of Payer Costs by Type of Medical Service between Carvedilol (case) and Non-Carvedilol (control) Patients (*Continued*)

Medication	Mean (SD) [median]		Total (*n* = 211) Mean (SD) [median]		Cases (*n* = 105) Mean (SD) [median]		Controls (*n* = 106) *P* Value*
Carvedilol	$508 ($594)	[$0]	$1,020 ($428)	[$1,009]	$0 ($0)	[$0]	.0001
ACE inhibitors	$361 ($359)	[$310]	$449 ($403)	[$364]	$273 ($284)	[$239]	.0003
Diuretics	$89 ($207)	[$25]	$119 ($264)	[$28]	$59 ($121)	[$22]	.0347
Digoxin	$29 ($26)	[$27]	$33 ($26)	[$35]	$24 ($26)	[$14]	.0144
Other medications	$2,149 ($2,291)	[$1,589]	$2,182 ($1,929)	[$1,876]	$2,116 ($2,609)	[$1,313]	.8351
Total medication expenses	$3,135 ($2,552)	[$2,593]	$3,804 ($2,200)	[$3,329]	$2,472 ($2,709)	[$1,740]	.0001

*Statistical tests compare carvedilol (cases) to non-carvedilol (controls) using one-way analysis of variance with *T*-test.

ACE = angiotensin converting enzyme.

dose of heparin (EPILOG trial),[87] and then versus or in combination with stenting (EPISTENT trial).[88] Although these researchers demonstrated very favorable cost-effectiveness ratios of $6,213 per YLS for stents plus abciximab in comparison with stenting alone and $5,291 per YLS compared with abciximab alone, the use of glycoprotein IIb/IIIa agents in patients undergoing PCI remains at approximately 50% for PCI procedures.

Another method of using prospective, or clinical trial, data to project future events was undertaken by Caro and colleagues to estimate the cost-effectiveness of primary prevention with pravastatin compared to diet alone.[89] Using a generalized model of cardiovascular disease prevention, these researchers quantified the effect in terms of the avoidance of cardiovascular disease based on treatment-specific risks derived from West of Scotland Coronary Prevention Study (WOSCOPS) data. Country-specific costs were accounted for by expressing these in terms of the ratio of monthly treatment to that of managing a MI. Over multiple sensitivity analyses, cost-effectiveness ratios were consistently below $25,000 per life-year gained, with patients at higher baseline risk being the most cost-effective to treat.

Retrospective

A number of pharmacoeconomic researchers advocate retrospective analyses and modeling as alternatives to prospective trials. Sources for retrospective studies include patient charts,[49,69] individual or meta analyses of clinical trials in the literature, [31,40,44,52,70] medical and pharmacy claims data,[41,90] and Medicare databases,[91] among others. Claims or administrative databases have, in particular, recently gained favor as they are frequently computerized and reflect actual charges and payments for specific plans and populations. The disadvantages of these databases are as follows[92,93]:

- Diagnosis and procedure codes may reflect reimbursement strategies instead of clinically accurate diagnoses
- Limited information on important covariates
- Sparse outcomes data
- Lack of representativeness
- Lack of structure for research purposes

Indeed, in two comparisons of clinical and insurance claims databases in patients with ischemic heart disease, claims data failed to identify more than one half of patients with prognostically important conditions, including mitral insufficiency, CHF, peripheral vascular disease, old MI, hyperlipidemia, angina, and unstable angina.[94,95] Similar inconsistencies were noted in a study of coronary artery bypass surgery in which miscoding of diagnoses could be linked with the lack of specificity for an ICD-9-CM grouping and lack of reporting of coexisting conditions on discharge abstracts and claims.[94,95] Given the current state of these types of analyses, collection of original data for a representative percentage of the patient population should be undertaken to validate the clinical information contained therein.

Expert Opinion

Expert opinion is a source, frequently elicited by survey, used to obtain information where no or little data are available. For example, in our experience with a multicountry evaluation of health care resource utilization in atrial fibrillation, very little country-specific published information was available on this subject. Thus, the decision-analytic model is being supplemented with data from a physician expert panel survey to determine the following:

- Initial management approach: rate control versus cardioversion
- First-, second-, and third-line agents
- Doses and durations of therapy
- Type and frequency of studies that would be performed to initiate and monitor therapy
- Type and frequency of adverse events by body system and the resources used to manage them
- Place of treatment
- Adverse consequences of lack of atrial fibrillation control and cost of these consequences, e.g., stroke, CHF

This method may also be used in testing the robustness of the analysis.[31]

ULTIMATE USE

Economic evaluations are used in a variety of settings; they serve, among other things, as decision aids and for assisting in reimbursement strategies for national formularies. In fact, Australia and Canada have implemented guidelines for economic technology assessment. Although these and other countries do not yet require HE studies for drug registration, many countries in the European Union strongly suggest that these be undertaken. They are useful for policy makers who are concerned with health care resource allocation on a statewide or individual institutional level.[96] End users may include insurance companies, pharmaceutical manufacturers (who are interested in demonstrating the comparative cost-effectiveness of their agents to gold standards and/or to the most commonly used therapeutic options), government agencies (for establishing levels of reimbursement), MCO executives (to aid in establishing therapeutic guidelines), employers (who use these analyses as an aid in benchmarking the MCOs they are evaluating for their employees' health plans), and pharmacy benefits managers (PBMs) (who also wish to demonstrate that they have evaluated managed care plans to offer the most cost-effective one to employers). Similarly, individual clinicians are becoming increasingly interested in documenting that they have systematically identified the most cost-effective therapeutic options for their patients.

APPLICATION TO PATIENT SUBGROUPS (TARGETING)

Age, Gender, and Pretreatment Lipid Levels

Some therapies are cost-effective only in certain patient subgroups, and a number of patient-specific factors may influence economic outcomes.[8,18] This observation may be illustrated by cost-effectiveness analyses of the drug treatment of hypercholesterolemia. In general, these analyses have shown that the cost to produce health benefits of increased longevity and improved quality of life are lowest in groups with the highest near-term risk for CHD.[40,41,51,97] In a study designed to investigate the cost-effectiveness of lipid-lowering therapy in the primary prevention of CHD, Oster and Epstein examined the effects of cholestyramine therapy on men between 35 and 74 years of age with elevated levels of total plasma cholesterol.[40] The researchers found a wide range of values of cost-effectiveness of treatment, ranging from $36,000 to over $1 million per YLS. Cost-effectiveness was greatest for younger patients, for those with additional coronary risk factors such as smoking or hypertension, and for those whose course of treatment was of less than lifelong duration. These therapies were less cost-effective in older patients, for those with no additional coronary risk factors, and for patients who were treated for a lifetime. The investigators concluded that pharmacologic therapy may not be cost-effective for all patients with elevated cholesterol levels, especially those over 65 years of age.

To determine the cost-effectiveness of HMG-CoA reductase inhibitors for the primary and secondary prevention of CHD, Goldman et al. conducted an analysis based on the Coronary Heart Disease Policy Model.[43] This computer-simulation model estimates the risk factor–specific annual incidence of CHD and the risk of recurrent coronary events in persons with prevalent CHD. Primary prevention with HMG-CoA reductase inhibitors had favorable cost-effectiveness ratios only in selected subgroups based on cholesterol levels and other established risk factors. When used for secondary prevention, 20 mg of lovastatin was estimated to save lives and save costs in younger men with cholesterol levels above 250 mg/dL and to have a favorable cost-effectiveness ratio regardless of the cholesterol level. The only exception cited was in younger women with cholesterol levels below 250 mg/dL. Lovastatin doses of 40 mg daily had a favorable incremental cost-effectiveness ratio in men with cholesterol levels above 250 mg/dL.

Similarly, Grover and colleagues[98] performed simulations using the Cardiovascular Life Expectancy Model to estimate the long-term costs and benefits of treatment with simvastatin in diabetics with varying pretreatment LDL cholesterol values. Treatment with simvastatin for patients with cardiovascular disease was found to be cost-effective for both men and women with or without diabetes. Among diabetic individuals without cardiovascular disease, the benefits of primary prevention were also substantial and the cost-effectiveness ratios attractive across a wide range of assumptions (approximately $4,000 to $40,000 per YLS). In the absence of diabetes, cost-effectiveness ratios associated with primary prevention were substantially higher, ranging from $28,000 to $51,000 per YLS for men and $65,000 to $16,000 per YLS for women. The presence of diabetes was found to substantially increase the absolute risk of cardiovascular events and thereby to lower the cost-effectiveness of treating even modest levels of hyperlipidemia. These conclusions were robust even among diabetics with lower baseline LDL values and smaller LDL reductions.

Likewise, Weinstein and Stason used the regression coefficients from the Framingham Study to calculate the expected changes in the numbers of strokes and MIs resulting from treatment. The benefit of this treatment was found to vary by patient age and duration of therapy, being less for MI than stroke and ranging from about 40% in younger subjects to around 10% in 60-year-olds.[99] Gender was also an important influence, such that, as in the previously described study, cost-effectiveness improved as women aged but declined as men aged (Table 5-6).[99] This may reflect the propensity for women to develop cardiovascular disease later in life and the improved expected therapeutic effectiveness as a result. Low (good) cost-effectiveness ratios were also found in the Swedish Trial in Old Patients with Hypertension (STOP-Hypertension) study of men and women aged 70 and above, especially with beta blockers and diuretics.[100] In general, it appears cost-effective to treat

TABLE 5-6. Effect of Age and Gender on CEA (cost/QALY*)

Gender	Initial Diastolic Blood Pressure (mm Hg)	Age (years)		
		20	40	60
Male	100	$5,500	$8,700	$50,100
	110	$3,300	$5,700	$16,300
Female	100	$14,700	$10,000	$8,000
	110	$8,500	$6,100	$5,000

*Quality-adjusted life-year.

CEA = cost effective analysis.

patients 45 years of age and older with a diastolic blood pressure of ≥90 mm Hg.[101] The presence of other risk factors improves the cost-effectiveness of treatment, since these would be sicker patients, more likely to manifest hypertensive end-organ disease.

In contrast to Edelson,[42] Kawachi and Malcolm[102] reported a range of the cost-effectiveness of antihypertensive therapy from £11,058 to £63,760 per QALY gained in men and from £22,060 to £194,989 per QALY gained in women (costs and benefit discounted at 5%). Diuretic therapy produced the best (lowest) cost-effectiveness ratios, using as an example a 60-year-old woman with a DBP of 90 mmHg (£17,980 per QALY). For this woman, the cost per QALY was £67,678 on beta-blocker therapy and £111,230 per QALY on ACE inhibitors.

Pre-Treatment Blood Pressure

In addition to age and duration of therapy, the benefit (e.g., primary prevention of MI, prevention of CHD, QALYs, YLS) and cost-effectiveness of antihypertensive treatments vary according to pretreatment blood pressure.[103,104] These and other influences on the cost-effectiveness of antihypertensive treatment are summarized in Table 5-7. For example, evaluating data from the Hypertension Optimal Treatment (HOT) trial, researchers noted that the cost-effectiveness ratios, expressed as cost per year of life gained, were most favorable for the ≤90 mm Hg treatment target group ($4262) and for added aspirin treatment ($12,710). For moderately aggressive treatment (blood pressure ≤85 mm Hg), the cost-effectiveness ratio escalated incrementally to $86,360 and with intensive treatment to $658,370 per year of life gained. Thus, treatment to a target of 90 mm Hg and coadministration of aspirin were considered highly cost-effective, whereas treatments to lower the blood pressure further to 85 mm Hg were marginally cost-effective; intensive blood pressure lowering down to 80 mm Hg was not cost-effective.[104]

Comorbid Conditions

However, in patients with comorbid conditions that may accelerate the development of hypertensive sequelae, such as in those with type

TABLE 5-7. Influences on Cost-Effectiveness of Cardiovascular Treatment

Patient age
Comorbidities
Duration of therapy
Pretreatment goal (e.g., blood pressure)
Benefit sought (e.g., YLS, CHD event prevention, QALYs)
Medication compliance

CHD = coronary heart disease; QALYs = quality-adjusted life-years; YLS = years of life saved.

2 diabetes, tight control of blood pressure has been shown to substantially reduce the cost of complications, increase the interval without complications and survival, and have a cost-effectiveness ratio that compares favorably with many accepted health care programs. Indeed, the incremental cost per extra year free from diabetes-related end points amounted to £1,049 (costs and effects discounted at 6% per year) for patients randomized to tight control of blood pressure ($n = 758$) and £434 for patients in the less tight control group ($n = 390$)(costs discounted at 6% per year and effects not discounted). The incremental cost per life year gained was £720 (costs and effects discounted at 6% per year) and £291 (costs discounted at 6% per year and effects not discounted) for the two groups, respectively.[105]

These studies have demonstrated that HE analyses can aid decision making in the prevention of hypertensive complications. Indeed, HE analyses can clarify the value of alternative strategies for CHD prevention in specific populations, thereby helping to choose among them, given limited health care resources. Modification of major cardiovascular risk factors (blood cholesterol, high blood pressure, and smoking) is very cost-effective but needs to be better targeted if potential health gain is to be realized.[106] For example, the most cost-effective ratios in the treatment of hypertension are typically found in men of late middle age with the most severe hypertension and in those with multiple risk factors.[99,102,107–110] Population screening, stratified according to these cost-effectiveness criteria, can help identify patients in whom aggressive intervention via these disease management techniques is most desirable and in whom the best value is derived from treatment of hypertension. The utility of pharmacoeconomics in assisting in these decisions depends to a great extent upon the assumptions made and the quality of the data used for the analyses (e.g., the degree to which the data are evidence-based).[107]

ROBUSTNESS

In all analyses, there is uncertainty about the accuracy of the results that may be dealt with via sensitivity analyses.[4,21] In these analyses, one essentially asks the question "What if?" These allow one to vary key values over clinically feasible ranges to determine whether the

decision remains the same—that is, if the strategy initially found to be cost-effective remains the dominant strategy. Sensitivity analyses also allow one to determine threshold values for the key parameters at which the decision would change. For example, amiodarone was found to be a preferred strategy over implantable cardioverter-defibrillators (ICDs) when quality of life (utility) on amiodarone decreased to 40% lower than that with an ICD.[90] By performing sensitivity analyses, one can increase the level of confidence in the conclusions. Indeed, varying the effectiveness of a new therapy in reducing death, nonfatal MI, and revascularization (assuming all components contributed equally to the reduction in death) from 0.25 to 7.0% demonstrated a broad range of very cost-effective results (Fig. 5-3).[111]

CONCLUSION

HE analyses of cardiovascular therapies is a timely topic, especially in light of the fact that a number of governmental regulatory agencies are attempting to set reimbursement guidelines based upon these data. At this time, numerous studies have been completed for a variety of therapeutic options. However, there are no standardized guidelines for these studies; inclusion of resource use (e.g., direct, indirect), effectiveness criteria (e.g., CHD event avoided, QALYs), centralized cost sources, perspective, and incorporation of sensitivity analyses into the evaluation are quite variable. This underlies clinicians' concerns about premature efforts by regulatory agencies to dictate therapeutic options based upon an incomplete understanding of the true costs to payers and society and the benefits to the patient. Moreover, in addition to the societal and governmental perspectives regarding these analyses, there is inadequate information for the individual clinician attempting to treat an individual patient in terms of cost, general estimates of life expectancy, and overall likelihood of success of one particular treatment regimen versus another.

Furthermore, as newer and potentially more expensive therapies become readily available, decisions based on state-of-the-art analyses will be required to determine their place in therapy. Indeed, Eisenstein and colleagues[111] developed a decision model to evaluate the potential "economic attractiveness" of new therapies in patients with non-ST elevation acute coronary syndrome. Event probabilities at 30 days and 6 months were estimated from U.S. patients in the Global Use of Strategies to Open Occluded Coronary Arteries in Acute Coronary Syndromes (GUSTO) IIb trial and cost estimates were derived from patients enrolled in the Economics and Quality of Life substudy of this trial. Study results found that new therapies costing up to $2,000 per episode that reduce 6-month mortality by 0.5%, death and nonfatal MI by 1%, or a composite end point of death, nonfatal MI and revascularization by 3% may be cost-effective by current standards. New therapies costing up to $1,000 per episode reduce the absolute rate of death, nonfatal MI, and revascularization at 6 months by 6.5% or more and may be cost-saving.

Especially since the psychological component of many of these therapies—such as pacing, surgery and implantable devices—has not yet been sufficiently addressed, any future PETs should probably incorporate quality-of-life assessments. Such assessments of patients' desires, anticipated quality of life with a variety of interventions, and evaluators' perceptions about the representative nature of the study population from which the original cost estimates were derived will hopefully allow modulation of these and future HE

FIGURE 5-3. Cost-effectiveness of new therapies that reduce death, myocardial infarction (MI), and revascularization. YOLS = years of life saved. * Indicates that the therapy becomes dominant. (*Reproduced with permission from Eisenstein et al.*[111])

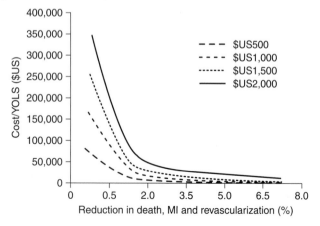

analyses. It is likely that these decisions will become increasingly common as health care reforms—such as capitation, initiated by organized health care delivery systems—become more evident.[10,29,67]

Although HE analyses will have an increasingly important role in resource allocation and even in individual health care decisions, there are some limitations to these assessments.[9] As mentioned throughout this chapter, although decision-analytic technique is an objective and well-established methodology, many other questions persist regarding basic issues such as uncertainty about costs and benefits, attribution of resources (e.g., if an adverse event requires a therapeutic switch, should future costs be attributed to the initial agent or to the switch agent), perspective, appropriateness of retrospective (e.g., claims) databases, appropriate time horizon and projection to clinically relevant time frames, QOL utility measurements (e.g., health states worse than death), and discount rate (e.g., if same for benefits as for costs, which value should be used), among others.

Despite these limitations, sensitivity analyses and ongoing updated evaluations will allow health care policy analysts to make the most informed decisions about the allocation of limited monetary resources to best treat the population with cardiovascular illnesses. Podrid and colleagues[84] (adapted from Wong [112]) and Kupersmith and coworkers[6–8] have published tables of comparative values or dollar cost (US$) per year or per QALY for cardiovascular therapies. These may be of use in performing comparative evaluations of available therapeutic options. HE analysis will also help guide the individual physician in making cost-effective decisions for individual patients. These decisions will also be guided by political forces and health care system requirements.

REFERENCES

1. Becker ER, Culler SD, Shaw LJ, et al: Economic aspects of transesophageal echocardiography and atrial fibrillation. *Echocardiography* 17:407–418, 2000.
2. Mark DB, Hlatky MA, Califf RM, et al: Cost effectiveness of thrombolytic therapy with tissue plasminogen activator as compared with streptokinase for acute myocardial infarction. *N Engl J Med* 332:1418–1424, 1995.
3. Califf RM, Eisenstein EL: Critical concepts in cost-effectiveness for cardiovascular specialists. *Am Heart J* 140:S143–147, 2000.
4. Weinstein MC, Stason WB: Foundations of cost-effectiveness analysis for health and medical practices. *N Engl J Med* 296:716–721, 1977.
5. Pare DS, Freed MD: Clinical practice guidelines for quality patient outcomes. *Nurs Clin North Am* 30:183–196, 1995.
6. Kupersmith J, Holmes-Rovner M, Hogan A, et al: Cost-effectiveness analysis in heart disease: Part III. Ischemia, congestive heart failure, and arrhythmias. *Prog Cardiovasc Dis* 37:307–346, 1995.
7. Kupersmith J, Holmes-Rovner M, Hogan A, et al: Cost-effectiveness analysis in heart disease: Part II. Preventive therapies. *Prog Cardiovasc Dis* 37:243–271, 1995.
8. Kupersmith J, Holmes-Rovner M, Hogan A, et al: Cost-effectiveness analysis in heart disease: Part I. General principles. *Prog Cardiovasc Dis* 37:161–184, 1994.
9. Weinstein MC, Stason WB: Cost-effectiveness of interventions to prevent or treat coronary heart disease. *Annu Rev Public Health* 6:41–63, 1985.
10. Mills PS, Michnich ME: Managed care and cardiac pacing and electrophysiology. *Pacing Clin Electrophysiol* 16:1746–1750, 1993.
11. Jaussi A: Continuing importance of the clinical approach. Observations on a regional collaboration between general practitioners, internists and cardiologists. *Schweiz Med Wochenschr* 124:2049–2052, 1994.
12. Goldstein S, Pearson TA, Colwill JM, et al: Task Force 4: The relationship between cardiovascular specialists and generalists. *J Am Coll Cardiol* 24:304–312, 1994.
13. Greenfield S, Nelson EC, Zubkoff M, et al: Variations in resource utilization among medical specialties and systems of care. Results from the medical outcomes study. *JAMA* 267:1624–1630, 1992.
14. Winslow R: Study compares role of doctors in cardiac cases. *Wall Street J* 1995.
15. Tarlov AR, Ware JE Jr, Greenfield S, et al: The Medical Outcomes Study. An application of methods for monitoring the results of medical care. *JAMA* 262:925–930, 1989.
16. Dustan HP, Francis CW, Allen HD, et al: Principles of access to health care. Access to Health Care Task Force, American Heart Association. *Circulation* 87:657–658, 1993.
17. Weinstein MC, Fineberg HV, Elstein AS, et al: Clinical decisions and limited resources. In: Weinstein MC, ed. *Clinical Decision Analysis.* Philadelphia: Saunders, 1980:228–265.
18. Detsky AS, Naglie IG: A clinician's guide to cost-effectiveness analysis. *Ann Intern Med* 113:147–154, 1990.
19. Eckman MH, Levine HJ, Pauker SG: Making decisions about antithrombotic therapy in heart disease. Decision analytic and cost-effectiveness issues. *Chest* 108:457S–470S, 1995.
20. US Congress, Office of Technology Assessment: *Effectiveness and Costs of Osteoporosis Screening and Hormone Replacement Therapy,* Vol I: *Cost-Effectiveness Analysis.* OTA-BP-H-160, August, 1995.
21. Eisenberg JM: Clinical economics. A guide to the economic analysis of clinical practices. *JAMA* 262:2879–2886, 1989.
22. Goldberg Arnold RJ, Kaniecki DJ, Frishman WH: Cost-effectiveness of antihypertensive agents in patients with reduced left ventricular function. *Pharmacotherapy* 14:178–184, 1994.
23. Canadian Coordinating Office for Health Technology Assessment. *Guidelines for economic evaluation of pharmaceuticals: Canada.* Ottawa: CCOHTA, 1994.
24. Eisenberg JM, Glick H, Koffer H: Pharmacoeconomics: Economic evaluation of pharmaceuticals. In: Strom BL, eds. *Pharmacoepidemiology.* West Sussex, UK: Wiley, 1994:338.
25. Marissal JP, Selke B, Lebrun T: Economic assessment of the secondary prevention of ischaemic events with lysine acetylsalicylate. *Pharmacoeconomics* 18:185–200, 2000.
26. Augustovski FA, Cantor SB, Thach CT, et al: Aspirin for primary prevention of cardiovascular events. *J Gen Intern Med* 13:824–835, 1998.
27. Freund DA, Dittus RS: Principles of pharmacoeconomic analysis of drug therapy. *Pharmacoeconomics* 1:20–32, 1992.
28. Drummond M, Stoddart G, Labelle R, et al: Health economics: An introduction for clinicians. *Ann Intern Med* 107:88–92, 1987.
29. Baker AM, Goldberg Arnold RJ, Kaniecki DJ: Considerations in measuring resource use in clinical trials. *Drug Inf J* 29:1421–1428, 1995.
30. Smith SL, Gallagher PE, eds: *Medicare RBRVS: The Physician's Guide 1995.* Chicago: American Medical Association, 1995.
31. Podrid PJ, Kowey PR, Frishman WH, et al: Comparative cost-effectiveness analysis of quinidine, procainamide and mexiletine. *Am J Cardiol* 68:1662–1667, 1991.
32. *1995 Drug Topics Red Book.* Oradell, NJ: Medical Economics, 1995.
33. Rice DP, Hodgson TA, Kopstein AN: The economic costs of illness: A replication and update. *Health Care Financ Rev* 7:61–80, 1985.
34. Gafni A, Torrance GW: Risk attitude and time preference in health. *Management Science* 30:440–451, 1984.
35. Lipscomb J: Time preference for health in cost-effectiveness analysis. *Med Care* 27:S233–S253, 1989.
36. Krahn M, Gafni A: Discounting in the economic evaluation of health care interventions. *Med Care* 31:403–418, 1993.
37. Mini-symposium: Cost-effectiveness in Health and Medicine. 17th Annual Meeting of the Society for Medical Decision Making, Tempe, AZ, 1995.
38. Beck JR, Salem DN, Estes NA, Pauker SG: A computer-based Markov decision analysis of the management of symptomatic bifascicular block: The threshold probability for pacing. *J Am Coll Cardiol* 9:920–935, 1987.
39. Kinosian BP, Eisenberg JM: Cutting into cholesterol. Cost-effective alternatives for treating hypercholesterolemia. *JAMA* 259:2249–2254, 1988.
40. Oster G, Epstein AM: Cost-effectiveness of antihyperlipemic therapy in the prevention of coronary heart disease. The case of cholestyramine. *JAMA* 258:2381–2387, 1987.

41. Goldman L, Weinstein MC, Goldman PA, et al: Cost-effectiveness of HMG-CoA reductase inhibition for primary and secondary prevention of coronary heart disease. *JAMA* 265:1145–1151, 1991.

42. Edelson JT, Weinstein MC, Tosteson AN, et al: Long-term cost-effectiveness of various initial monotherapies for mild to moderate hypertension. *JAMA* 263:407–413, 1990.

43. Goldman L, Sia ST, Cook EF, et al: Costs and effectiveness of routine therapy with long-term beta-adrenergic antagonists after acute myocardial infarction. *N Engl J Med* 319:152–157, 1988.

44. Krumholz HM, Pasternak RC, Weinstein MC, et al: Cost effectiveness of thrombolytic therapy with streptokinase in elderly patients with suspected acute myocardial infarction. *N Engl J Med* 327:7–13, 1992.

45. Liebson PR, Grandits GA, Dianzumba S, et al: Comparison of five antihypertensive monotherapies and placebo for change in left ventricular mass in patients receiving nutritional-hygienic therapy in the Treatment of Mild Hypertension Study (TOMHS). *Circulation* 91:698–706, 1995.

46. Andrade SE, Walker AM, Gottlieb LK, et al: Discontinuation of anti-hyperlipidemic drugs—do rates reported in clinical trials reflect rates in primary care settings? *N Engl J Med* 332:1125–1131, 1995.

47. Kozma CM, Reeder CE, Schulz RM: Economic, clinical and humanistic outcome: A planning model for pharmacoeconomic research. *Clin Ther* 15:1121–1132, 1993.

48. McGuigan KA, Sokol M, Yao J, et al: The value of compliance: Evidence from two patient cohorts (abstr). *Value in Health* 4:55, 2001.

49. Arnold RJ, Kaniecki DJ, Frishman WH: Cost-effectiveness of antihypertensive agents in patients with reduced left ventricular function. *Pharmacotherapy* 14:178–184, 1994.

50. Hatziandreu EI, Koplan JP, Weinstein MC, et al: A cost-effectiveness analysis of exercise as a health promotion activity. *Am J Public Health* 78:1417–1421, 1988.

51. Kinlay S, OConnell D, Evans D, et al: A new method of estimating cost-effectiveness of cholesterol reduction therapy for prevention of heart disease. *Pharmacoeconomics* 5:238–248, 1994.

52. Goldberg Arnold RJ, Kaniecki DJ, Tak Piech C, et al: An economic evaluation of HMG-CoA reductase inhibitors for cholesterol reduction in the primary prevention of coronary heart disease. Presented at the 11th International Conference on Pharmacoepidemiology. Montreal, 1995.

53. Himmelstein DU, Woolhandler S: Free care, cholestyramine, and health policy. *N Engl J Med* 311:1511–1514, 1984.

54. Schulman KA, Kinosian B, Jacobson TA, et al: Reducing high blood cholesterol level with drugs. Cost-effectiveness of pharmacologic management. *JAMA* 264:3025–3033, 1990.

55. England WL, Grim CE, Weinberger MH, et al: Cost effectiveness in the detection of renal artery stenosis. *J Gen Intern Med* 3:344–350, 1988.

56. Cantor JC, Morisky DE, Green LW, et al: Cost-effectiveness of educational interventions to improve patient outcomes in blood pressure control. *Prev Med* 14:782–800, 1985.

57. McNeil BJ, Varady PD, Burrows BA, et al: Measures of clinical efficacy. Cost-effectiveness calculations in the diagnosis and treatment of hypertensive renovascular disease. *N Engl J Med* 293:216–221, 1975.

58. Eckman MH, Beshansky JR, Durand-Zaleski I, et al: Anticoagulation for noncardiac procedures in patients with prosthetic heart valves. Does low risk mean high cost? *JAMA* 263:1513–1521, 1990.

59. Wong JB, Sonnenberg FA, Salem DN, et al: Myocardial revascularization for chronic stable angina. Analysis of the role of percutaneous transluminal coronary angioplasty based on data available in 1989. *Ann Intern Med* 113:852–871, 1990.

60. Steinberg EP, Moore RD, Powe NR, et al: Safety and cost effectiveness of high-osmolality as compared with low-osmolality contrast material in patients undergoing cardiac angiography. *N Engl J Med* 326:425–430, 1992.

61. Torrance GW: Measurement of health state utilities for economic appraisal: A review. *J Health Econ* 5:1–30, 1986.

62. Froberg DG, Kane RL: Methodology for measuring health-state preferences: II. Scaling methods. *J Clin Epidemiol* 42:459–471, 1989.

63. Guyatt GH, Veldhuyzen Van Zanten SJ, Feeny DH, et al: Measuring quality of life in clinical trials: A taxonomy and review. *Can Med Assoc J* 140:1441–1448, 1989.

64. Mehrez A, Gafni A: Quality-adjusted life years, utility theory, and healthy-years equivalents. *Med Decis Making* 9:142–149, 1989.

65. Weinstein MC: Challenges for cost-effectiveness research. *Med Decis Making* 6:194–198, 1986.

66. Tsevat J, Goldman L, Soukup JR, et al: Stability of time-tradeoff utilities in survivors of myocardial infarction. *Med Decis Making* 13:161–165, 1993.

67. Garson A, Jr: Health care reform and belt tightening: How can we become more cost effective? Commentary. *Curr Opin Cardiol* 10:29–32, 1995.

68. Danford DA, Nasir A, Gumbiner C: Cost assessment of the evaluation of heart murmurs in children. *Pediatrics* 91:365–368, 1993.

69. Jubran A, Gross N, Ramsdell J, et al: Comparative cost-effectiveness analysis of theophylline and ipratropium bromide in chronic obstructive pulmonary disease. A three-center study. *Chest* 103:678–684, 1993.

70. Barrett BJ, Parfrey PS, Foley RN, et al: An economic analysis of strategies for the use of contrast media for diagnostic cardiac catheterization. *Med Decis Making* 14:325–335, 1994.

71. Beck JR, Pauker SG: The Markov process in medical prognosis. *Med Decis Making* 3:419–458, 1983.

72. McNamara RL, Lima JA, Whelton PK et al: Echocardiographic identification of cardiovascular sources of emboli to guide clinical management of stroke: A cost-effectiveness analysis. *Ann Intern Med* 127:775–787, 1997.

73. Nomenclature and criteria for diagnosis of ischemic heart disease. Report of the Joint International Society and Federation of Cardiology/World Health Organization task force on standardization of clinical nomenclature. *Circulation* 59:607–609, 1979.

74. The Framingham Study: An Epidemiological Investigation of Cardiovascular Disease. In: US Department of Health and Human Services. The probability of developing certain cardiovascular diseases in eight years at specified values of some characteristics. Section 37: 1987.

75. Kannel WB, Dawber TR, Kagan A, et al: Factors of risk in the development of coronary heart disease—six year follow-up experience. The Framingham Study. *Ann Intern Med* 55:33–50, 1961.

76. Report of the National Cholesterol Education Program Expert Panel on Detection, Evaluation, and Treatment of High Blood Cholesterol in Adults. The Expert Panel. *Arch Intern Med* 148:36–69, 1988.

77. Summary of the second report of the National Cholesterol Education Program (NCEP) Expert Panel on Detection, Evaluation, and Treatment of High Blood Cholesterol in Adults (Adult Treatment Panel II). *JAMA* 269:3015–3023, 1993.

78. Carroll M, Sempos C, Briefel R, et al: *Vital and Health Statistics: Serum Lipids of Adults 20–74 Years: United States, 1976–1980.* Atlanta: U.S. Department of Health & Human Services, Public Health Service, 1993.

79. Najib MM, Arnold RJG, Kaniecki DJ, et al: Medical resource use and costs of congestive heart failure following use of carvedilol. *Heart Disease* 4:70, 2002.

80. Packer M, Bristow MR, Cohn JN, et al: The effect of carvedilol on morbidity and mortality in patients with chronic heart failure. *N Engl J Med* 334:349–1355, 1996.

81. Data on file, GlaxoSmithKline PLC.

82. Murdock DK, Schumock GT, Kaliebe J, et al: Clinical and cost comparison of ibutilide and direct-current cardioversion for atrial fibrillation and flutter. *Am J Cardiol* 85:503–506, 2000.

83. Zarkin GA, Bala MV, Calingaert B, et al: The cost-effectiveness of ibutilide versus electrical cardioversion in the conversion of atrial fibrillation and flutter to normal rhythm. *Am J Managed Care* 3:1387–1394,1997.

84. Podrid PJ, Arnold RJG, Kaniecki DJ: Pharmacoeconomic considerations in antiarrhythmic therapy. *Pharmacoeconomics* 2: 456–467, 1992.

85. The EPIC Investigators: Use of a monoclonal antibody directed against the platelet glycoprotein IIb/IIIa receptor in high-risk coronary angioplasty. *N Engl J Med* 330:956–61,1994.

86. Topol EJ, Ferguson JJ, Weisman HF, et al: Long-term protection from myocardial ischemic events in a randomized trial of brief integrin beta blockade with percutaneous coronary intervention. *JAMA* 278:479–484,1997.

87. The EPILOG Investigators: Platelet glycoprotein IIb/IIIa receptor blockade and low-dose heparin during percutaneous coronary revascularization. *N Engl J Med* 336:1689–1696,1997.

88. The EPISTENT Investigators: Randomised placebo-controlled and balloon-angioplasty-controlled trial to assess safety of coronary stenting with use of platelet glycoprotein-IIb/IIIa blockade. *Lancet* 352:87–92,1998.

89. Caro J, Klittich W, McGuire A, et al: International economic analysis of primary prevention of cardiovascular disease with pravastatin in WOSCOPS. West of Scotland Coronary Prevention Study. *Eur Heart J* 20:263–268, 1999.

90. Larsen GC, Manolis AS, Sonnenberg FA, et al: Cost-effectiveness of the implantable cardioverter-defibrillator: Effect of improved battery life and comparison with amiodarone therapy. *J Am Coll Cardiol* 19:1323–1334, 1992.

91. Altman DG, Flora JA, Fortmann SP, et al: The cost-effectiveness of three smoking cessation programs. *Am J Public Health* 77:162–165, 1987.

92. Adapted from *Using Administrative Data for Clinical (Disease) Management.* Tutorial on disease management methodologies. Philadelphia: Drug Information Association, 1995.

93. Lewis NJW, Patwell JT, Briesacher BA: The role of insurance claims databases in drug therapy outcomes research. *Pharmacoeconomics* 4:323–330, 1993.

94. Jollis JG, Ancukiewicz M, DeLong ER, et al: Discordance of databases designed for claims payment versus clinical information systems. Implications for outcomes research. *Ann Intern Med* 119:844–850, 1993.

95. Romano PS, Roos LL, Luft HS, et al: A comparison of administrative versus clinical data: Coronary artery bypass surgery as an example. Ischemic Heart Disease Patient Outcomes Research Team. *J Clin Epidemiol* 47:249–260, 1994.

96. Goldberg Arnold RJ, Kaniecki DJ, et al: Cost containment strategies in the United States: Role of cost-effectiveness research. *Drug Inf J* 30:609–619, 1996.

97. Hay JW, Wittels EH, Gotto AM Jr: An economic evaluation of lovastatin for cholesterol lowering and coronary artery disease reduction. *Am J Cardiol* 67: 789–796, 1991.

98. Grover SA, Coupal L, Zowall H, et al: Cost-effectiveness of treating hyperlipidemia in the presence of diabetes: Who should be treated? *Circulation* 102:722–727, 2000.

99. Weinstein MD, Stason WB: *Hypertension: A Policy Perspective.* Cambridge, MA: Harvard University Press, 1976.

100. Stason WB, Weinstein MC: Public-health rounds at the Harvard School of Public Health. Allocation of resources to manage hypertension. *N Engl J Med* 296:732–739, 1977.

101. Jonsson BG: Cost-benefit of treating hypertension. *J Hypertens* 12(Suppl):S65–S70, 1994.

102. Kawachi I, Malcolm LA: The cost-effectiveness of treating mild-to-moderate hypertension: A reappraisal. *J Hypertens* 9:199–208, 1991.

103. Whitworth J, Lang D, Henry D: Cost-effectiveness analysis in the treatment of hypertension: A medical view. *Clin Exp Hypertens* 21:999–1008, 1999.

104. Cost effectiveness of intensive treatment of hypertension. Based on presentations by Donald S. Shepard, PhD; and Dominic Hodgkin, PhD. *Am J Manag Care* 4:S765–S770, 1998.

105. Cost effectiveness analysis of improved blood pressure control in hypertensive patients with type 2 diabetes: UKPDS 40. UK Prospective Diabetes Study Group. *BMJ* 317:720–726, 1998.

106. Ebrahim S: Cost-effectiveness of stroke prevention. *Br Med Bull.* 56:557–570, 2000.

107. Fletcher AE, Bulpitt CJ: Pharmacoeconomic evaluation of risk factors for cardiovascular disease: An epidemiological perspective. *Pharmacoeconomics* 1:33–44, 1992.

108. Rorive G, Delporte JP: Pharmaco-economie du traitement de l'hypertension arterielle: Donnees et controverses. *Bull Mem Acad R Med Belg* 153:317–21,322–324, 1998.

109. Menard J: Cost-effectiveness of hypertension treatment. *Clin Exp Hypertens* 18:399–413, 1996.

110. Johannesson M: The cost effectiveness of hypertension treatment in Sweden. *Pharmacoeconomics* 7:242–250, 1995.

111. Eisenstein EL, Peterson ED, Jollis JG, et al: Evaluating the potential "economic attractiveness" of new therapies in patients with non-ST elevation acute coronary syndrome. *Pharmacoeconomics* 17:263–272, 2000.

112. Wong JB: *Cost-Effectiveness Analysis: Clinical Decision Analysis.* Advanced syllabus. San Diego: 1992, pp 132–133.

CHAPTER 6

Cardiovascular Pharmacology: A Historical Perspective

W. Bruce Fye

The processes of drug discovery, development, and distribution have changed dramatically during the past two centuries.[1-3] To illustrate this transformation, the introduction of digitalis, nitroglycerin, and thrombolytics into clinical practice is reviewed. Although most of the medicines used today to treat cardiovascular diseases were developed after World War II, there are two notable exceptions. Digitalis was first advocated as a cure for dropsy (the pathologic accumulation of fluid in various tissues or body cavities) in 1785 by William Withering, and nitroglycerin was first recommended for the treatment of angina pectoris in 1879 by William Murrell. Thrombolytic agents were first widely used to treat acute myocardial infarction in 1980. The circumstances surrounding the discovery of these drugs and their entry into the pharmacopeia provide valuable perspective on the history of cardiovascular pharmacology.

DIGITALIS

When digitalis was introduced into medical practice during the late eighteenth century, most medical discoveries and innovations in therapy came from doctors working alone. Only the activities of those few practitioners who published their observations, interpretations, and speculations are known. William Withering, the doctor who first recognized the therapeutic value of digitalis, was such a person. Born in Wellington, England, in 1741, Withering was the son of a successful apothecary.[4] He was one of the best-educated doctors of his era, having trained in Edinburgh, then a world center of medical education.[5] After receiving his medical degree in 1766 and touring several continental hospitals, Withering went into practice in the village of Stafford, near his hometown. There he became increasingly interested in botany; the countryside provided a wide variety of plants and flowers for study.

Withering recorded how he first recognized the therapeutic potential of the purple foxglove, *Digitalis purpurea:* "In the year 1775, my opinion was asked concerning a family receipt for the cure of the dropsy. I was told that it had long been kept a secret by an old woman in Shropshire, who had sometimes made cures after the more regular practitioners had failed." The physician-botanist explained that the woman's "medicine was composed of twenty or more different herbs; but it was not very difficult for one conversant in these subjects, to perceive that the active herb could be none other than the foxglove." Withering does not elaborate. Whereas other doctors had recognized that digitalis "produced violent vomiting and purging," he concluded that its "diuretic effects seemed to have been overlooked."[6]

Clinical experience gained by administering digitalis to several patients convinced Withering that it was an effective remedy for hydrothorax, ascites, and anasarca. Next, he encouraged several other physicians he knew to prescribe the drug for their patients with these conditions. Withering and his friends decided to use digitalis in a specific case mainly on the basis of the patient's symptoms, general appearance, and characteristics of the patient's pulse. A history of dyspnea and orthopnea or the presence of edema or ascites also suggested that digitalis might be beneficial. In Withering's time, doctors made therapeutic decisions without the clues that newer physical diagnosis and laboratory techniques would eventually provide.[7]

Physical examination of the chest was largely undeveloped in the eighteenth century; only rarely would a doctor palpate the precordium or apply an ear to the chest wall. Although Viennese physician Leopold Auenbrugger had invented percussion in 1761, very few doctors used the technique before French clinician Jean Nicholas Corvisart popularized it half a century later.[8] In 1819, René Theophile Hyacinthe Laennec reported his invention of the stethoscope, a tool that greatly facilitated diagnosis of diseases of the lungs and heart.[9] Even then, treatment was problematic because doctors had little understanding of the pathophysiology of the disorders they encountered or the mechanism of action of the remedies they prescribed.

In 1785, after using foxglove for a decade, Withering published his experience with the drug in 160 patients with a variety of medical problems.[6] Although many of his patients improved after they received digitalis, several experienced side effects as he tried to find the appropriate dose of the powerful (and poisonous) drug. Part of the problem was that it was impossible to accurately predict the potency of a given dose of digitalis. Withering prepared the plant in different ways in an attempt to address this problem. He initially prescribed a "decoction," made by boiling leaves of the foxglove plant, but he eventually used a powder made from dried leaves.[10]

As Withering varied the dose of digitalis, he carefully recorded the beneficial and harmful effects of the drug. He cautioned readers, "The foxglove when given in very large and quickly-repeated doses, occasions sickness, vomiting, purging, giddiness, confused vision, objects appearing green or yellow; increased secretion of urine... slow pulse, even as low as 35 in a minute, cold sweats, convulsions, syncope, death."[6]

Withering's book announced to the medical world that a powerful but potentially deadly remedy had been discovered. Within 6 months of its publication, Hall Jackson, a prominent New Hampshire doctor, asked Withering to send him seeds so he could introduce the plant—and the drug derived from it—into the United States.[11] As one of the few medicines shown to cause significant symptomatic improvement in some patients, many doctors were prescribing digitalis for dropsy by 1800. Many of them also used it in a variety of noncardiac conditions such as tuberculosis and pleurisy, however.

British physician John Ferriar was impressed with the effectiveness of digitalis in treating dropsy and credited Withering with teaching physicians how to use it "with safety and success." Writing in 1799, Ferriar reminded doctors that more experience was necessary to prove that digitalis was helpful in ailments other than dropsy. He warned, "Conclusions of so much moment to the welfare of mankind, cannot be formed from the events of a few weeks or months. They must depend on an estimate of the greater number of results, from many cases, under circumstances nearly similar. This is the foundation of experience with every rational man, not only in medicine, but in all reasoning concerning probable evidence. The mischief of precipitate conclusions is nowhere more sensibly felt, than in medical practice."[12] Ferriar and Withering would have been surprised to learn that the efficacy of digitalis in congestive heart failure was still being debated two centuries after it was introduced,[13] although a recent placebo-controlled study in patients with heart failure did conclude that digoxin reduced the rate of heart failure deaths or related hospitalizations with no apparent effect on overall survival.

NITROGLYCERIN

During the nineteenth century, laboratory experimentation gradually replaced empiric observation and clinicopathologic correlation as the chief research method in medicine as physiology, physiologic chemistry, and pharmacology emerged as distinct disciplines.[14,15] By midcentury, several European (especially German) universities had developed ambitious state-funded research programs that provided aspiring medical scientists with the time necessary to invent and use new tools and techniques to study the various functions of intact animals and isolated organs experimentally.[16] During the second half of the century, a few scientists used vivisection, new chemical techniques, and other innovative approaches to create the field of experimental pharmacology.[17]

But the nineteenth century was also a time when alternative systems of medicine such as homeopathy, botanic therapy, and hydrotherapy flourished.[18,19] The practitioners who used these and other nontraditional healing methods were outside the research tradition that was emerging in Europe. Their treatment regimens were not grounded in science; they were based on arcane principles articulated by the founder and promoters of each healing system. Nitroglycerin therapy can be traced to homeopathy, one of the most successful medical sects.

Nitroglycerin, still a mainstay of treatment for angina pectoris, is one of very few medications discovered before the twentieth century that is still in the pharmacopeia. It is also one of the few drugs that regular physicians adopted from homeopaths.[20] Nitroglycerin was identified as a useful medicine for anginal attacks because of the unlikely union of an irrational therapeutic system (homeopathy), a series of empiric observations, and sophisticated physiologic research.

Italian chemist Ascanio Sobrero synthesized nitroglycerin in 1847 by combining nitric and sulfuric acids with glycerin as part of a systematic search for new explosives after Christian Schönbein discovered guncotton 1 year earlier. Sobrero was impressed that he got a severe headache each time he touched his lips if there was any nitroglycerin on his hands. Understandably, he warned others about this unpleasant consequence of working with the new and powerful explosive.

Constantine Hering, a pioneer of American homeopathy, was intrigued by Sobrero's observations. His interest in nitroglycerin can be understood only in terms of one of homeopathy's fundamental principles: *similia similibus curantur* (like cures like). This curious notion led Hering to claim that nitroglycerin would cure headaches—because it predictably caused them. Before a medicine could be added to the homeopathic pharmacopeia, however, it had to be tested on volunteers using an approach devised by homeopathy's founder, German physician Samuel Hahnemann.[21]

To identify substances with therapeutic potential, Hahnemann elaborated a complex method of human experimentation, which he termed *Prüfung* (proving). In a proving, healthy individuals (provers) ingested small amounts of various substances and carefully recorded any bodily sensations that ensued, however slight. If the initial dose failed to produce any sensations, more was ingested. The dose and time of onset of any side effects were carefully recorded and compared among the participants who included healthy persons of various ages and both sexes. However irrational, Hahnemann's provings represented an innovation in therapeutics; they were a primitive precursor to present day approaches used to screen compounds for toxic and potential therapeutic effects.

Hering began to investigate nitroglycerin's therapeutic potential shortly after Sobrero synthesized the explosive. On the basis of a year of provings and in light of the doctrine of *similia similibus curantur,* he concluded that nitroglycerin was useful in headaches and a variety of other complaints. Hering and his homeopathic colleagues did not prescribe nitroglycerin for angina, however.[22]

In 1858 Alfred Field, a British regular physician, published a study of the side effects and potential therapeutic uses of nitroglycerin. He became interested in the substance after placing a small amount of it on his tongue at the urging of a homeopath. Field reported the dramatic side effects he experienced, including headache, a sense of fullness in his neck, and persistent nausea. Two London physicians, Henry Fuller of St. George's Hospital and George Harley of University College Hospital, repeated Field's experiments a few weeks later, but they were unimpressed. Fuller attributed the tachycardia associated with nitroglycerin ingestion to some unidentified contaminant.

A few other regular physicians and medical scientists, more impressed with the dramatic side effects of the nitrates, began to study them physiologically. High "arterial tension" was thought to be responsible for several diseases at the time, and they hoped to find drugs that would correct this problem by dilating the blood vessels. Johann Albers of Bonn published a sophisticated study of the physiologic effects of nitroglycerin in 1864. He concluded that its dramatic effects on the circulation were real and proposed that the drug acted through the central nervous system rather than on the heart directly.[23] Although a few regular practitioners began prescribing nitroglycerin for headache and neuralgia, it would be 15 years before anyone suggested that the drug might be useful in the treatment of angina.

Amyl nitrite, synthesized in 1844 by French chemist Antoine Balard, was the link between the homeopath's indiscriminate use of nitroglycerin and the modern use of vasodilators for the treatment of angina and heart failure.[24] London physician and part-time physiologist Benjamin Ward Richardson concluded that amyl nitrite was a vasodilator from research he performed in the mid-1860s. Working at the University of Edinburgh, Arthur Gamgee extended Richardson's experiments on amyl nitrite and stimulated medical student Thomas Lauder Brunton to further investigate the physiologic effects of the substance.

Brunton was a house physician at the Edinburgh Royal Infirmary in 1866 when he postulated that amyl nitrite might be useful for treating angina pectoris. Therapeutic bleeding with leeches and lancets had declined dramatically during the middle of the nineteenth century, but Brunton thought some patients with angina seemed to improve with bloodletting. He speculated that amyl nitrite, by reducing arterial tension, might have the same beneficial effect, without causing anemia. In the course of his research, Brunton used a new physiologic instrument, the sphygmograph, to prove that amyl nitrite reduced the arterial tension. Soon after he reported in *The Lancet,* in 1867, that amyl nitrite relieved angina, many doctors began prescribing the remedy.[25]

Twelve years later, British physician and part-time pharmacologist William Murrell reported that nitroglycerin was also an effective remedy for angina.[26] Murrell had recently completed his medical studies at University College, London, where he worked with physiologist John Burdon-Sanderson and part-time pharmacologist Sydney Ringer.[27] Aware of the earlier controversy as to whether nitroglycerin had any reproducible physiologic effects, Murrell decided to test the substance on himself. After touching the moistened cork stopper of a vial of nitroglycerin to his tongue, he developed a "violent pulsation" in his head, tachycardia, and a sense of forceful heart action.

This dramatic experience stimulated Murrell's interest in nitroglycerin. In addition to taking it several more times himself, he administered nitroglycerin to almost three dozen friends and patients. Each person experienced side effects similar to those that had so impressed Murrell. Familiar with Brunton's work on amyl nitrite, Murrell used a sphygmograph to record pulse tracings before, during, and after the administration of nitroglycerin. He noted a similarity between the pulse tracings recorded following the administration of amyl nitrite and nitroglycerin, although the effects of nitroglycerin came on more slowly and lasted longer. By analogy, Murrell concluded that nitroglycerin, like amyl nitrite, would be useful for the treatment of angina.[28]

Murrell began giving nitroglycerin to patients with angina in the summer of 1878. His first patient was a 64-year-old man, a heavy smoker, with typical angina. After taking a 1% solution of nitroglycerin three times a day for a week, the man's anginal attacks decreased in frequency and severity. If he took an additional dose at the onset of an attack, it would invariably shorten the episode. Murrell and his patient were impressed. Nitroglycerin's value in the treatment of angina was confirmed rapidly by other physicians. Shortly after Murrell published his report, a British doctor informed the editor of *The Lancet,* "I always found relief if I took the dose when I felt the first threatening of an attack, and the paroxysmal was staved off.... It is a great boon to have a remedy in which you can have perfect confidence that the painful attacks can be controlled."[29]

Nitroglycerin and amyl nitrite were not only effective in relieving a most distressing symptom, they demonstrated the value of physiologic research. One writer declared in 1882, "The applications of nitro-glycerine to the treatment of disease are directly deducible from the physiological study—another proof, if more were needed, of the value of the physiological method."[30]

THROMBOLYTIC THERAPY

In the late eighteenth century, William Withering discovered the therapeutic value of digitalis on his own—without any sophisticated laboratory apparatus or formal institutional base. A century later, Brunton and Murrell combined empiric observations and new experimental techniques to demonstrate the circulatory responses to vasodilators. These examples show how the process of drug discovery was gradually becoming more rigorous. The quantity and quality of medical and pharmacologic research continued to increase during the late nineteenth and early twentieth centuries as more scientists and clinical investigators had time and money to design and perform experiments.

Attracted by opportunities that did not exist in the United States, thousands of ambitious American physicians and aspiring scientists traveled to Europe during this time for clinical and laboratory training.[31] By World War I, a coalition of medical scientists, academic physicians, educational reformers, and philanthropists—impressed by the flood of new knowledge coming from European laboratories and clinics—succeeded in reinventing American medical education.[32] Their efforts culminated in the creation of the full-time faculty system and the adoption of the so-called research ethic by the nation's leading medical schools.[33,34]

Philanthropic and government financial support fueled the growth of academic medicine in the United States and elsewhere during the twentieth century.[35] Meanwhile, market forces stimulated the growth of the pharmaceutical industry. To enhance their research and development programs, many of these companies began to collaborate with investigators in universities and academic medical centers.[36,37] The combination of government-sponsored research and private initiatives set the stage for an explosion of new knowledge that, in turn, resulted in many clinically relevant advances.[38] It was in this context that the notion of antithrombotic therapy for acute myocardial infarction arose.

The clinical syndrome of acute myocardial infarction was first described just before World War I. This may seem strange when it is recalled that the original description of angina pectoris was published more than 200 years ago. Elsewhere, I have identified several factors that contributed to the long delay in recognizing acute myocardial infarction as a distinct syndrome.[39] During the second half of the nineteenth century, a series of observations and discoveries led to a clearer understanding of the pathologic sequelae of coronary artery disease and of sudden coronary occlusion.[40] Although some pathologists suggested that a causal relationship existed between thrombotic coronary occlusion and myocardial necrosis and scarring, clinicians were generally unaware of, or unimpressed by, their conclusions.[41]

In 1872, the German pathologist Georg Rindfleisch attributed fatty degeneration of the heart muscle, a condition now termed myocardial scarring, to "atheromatous degeneration of the coronary arteries with plugging of one of their larger branches by a thrombus ... in every instance."[42] Meanwhile, some physicians and medical scientists began to dispute the belief that coronary occlusion was invariably fatal. Researchers and astute clinicians were beginning to frame a new disease—acute myocardial infarction.[43] Although patients certainly had heart attacks before the twentieth century, their doctors did not recognize the symptoms and signs of that event as a discrete syndrome.

Russian physicians W. P. Obrastzow and N. D. Straschesko published the first paper describing the typical clinical features of acute myocardial infarction in 1910. Speculating that certain signs and symptoms accompanied acute coronary thrombosis, they emphasized two main findings: prolonged chest discomfort (status anginosus) and persistent dyspnea (status dyspnoeticus). After presenting case summaries with autopsy correlations, Obrastzow and Straschesko concluded that "the differential diagnosis of coronary thrombosis from angina pectoris is made by the presence of status anginosus with coronary thrombosis and its absence with isolated attacks of angina pectoris." They also stressed that the signs and symptoms of cardiac failure resolved promptly after a simple anginal attack but persisted following coronary thrombosis. Their paper, published in a German journal of clinical medicine, attracted little attention, however.[44,45]

Chicago physician James Herrick was familiar with Obrastzow and Straschesko's report. He deserves credit for convincing the English-speaking medical community that coronary thrombosis was not always fatal and could be recognized during life. Herrick's 1912 paper, "Certain Clinical Features of Sudden Obstruction of the Coronary Arteries," is a milestone in the understanding of the pathophysiology of coronary artery disease, angina pectoris, and acute myocardial infarction. Herrick provided a detailed explanation for the spectrum of signs and symptoms that he attributed to acute coronary thrombosis: "The clinical manifestations of coronary obstruction will evidently vary greatly, depending on the size, location and number of vessels occluded. The symptoms and end-results must also be influenced by blood pressure, by the condition of the myocardium not immediately affected by the obstruction, and by the ability of the remaining vessels properly to carry on their work, as determined by their health or disease. No simple picture of the condition can, therefore, be drawn."[46]

By 1920, it was generally accepted that sudden thrombotic occlusion of a diseased coronary artery caused acute myocardial infarction. During the next two decades, researchers in Europe and the United States made important observations on the new clinical syndrome and the value of electrocardiography in diagnosing it.[47] Other workers turned their attention to the treatment of the life-threatening condition. Shortly after the anticoagulants heparin and bishydroxycoumarin (dicumarol) were first used clinically (in 1937 and 1941, respectively), some clinical investigators thought these drugs might be useful in the treatment of heart attacks.

By 1946, anecdotal experience had convinced several clinicians and researchers that dicumarol significantly reduced mortality and embolic events following acute myocardial infarction.[48] Based on a multi-institutional study of 800 heart attack patients published 2 years later, academic internist Irving Wright and his colleagues concluded that those treated with anticoagulants had a lower incidence of death and thromboembolic events during the first 6 weeks following the index event than those who did not receive these agents. As a result, they advocated anticoagulating all patients following a "coronary thrombosis" unless there was a definite contraindication.[49] Enthusiasm for anticoagulant therapy following acute myocardial infarction gradually diminished, however, as other researchers criticized the design of Wright's and other studies and as the risks of chronic anticoagulation were recognized.[50] One reviewer explained that, by the 1970s, "the anticoagulant era, which had begun with such high hopes, ended with a whimper."[51]

Meanwhile, a few researchers had begun to study whether recently discovered fibrinolytic (thrombolytic) agents might be useful in the treatment of a variety of conditions, including acute myocardial infarction.[52] In 1933, William Tillett, a medical scientist trained at Johns Hopkins and the Rockefeller Institute Hospital, discovered that β-hemolytic streptococci produced a fibrinolytic substance that he termed *fibrinolysin* (later named *streptokinase*—the term used in this chapter for the sake of consistency).[53] Tillett continued his studies on thrombolytic agents at the New York University School of Medicine after he joined the faculty in 1937.

Sol Sherry, one of Tillett's long-time collaborators, recalled recently, "The time was right for Tillett to start the clinical investigation of streptokinase."[54] This statement reflects the fact that the federal government inaugurated an ambitious campaign of research funding after World War II that energized academic medicine in the United States.[55] The result was a steady stream of discoveries and inventions that transformed medicine in general and cardiology in particular.[56] The pace of discovery and the practical application of new knowledge accelerated dramatically as Washington pumped hundreds of millions of dollars into academic medicine and biomedical research.[57]

Streptokinase was first administered to humans in 1947 in an attempt to dissolve chronic empyemas. Five years later, Tillett's group reported that an intravenous infusion of streptokinase lysed blood clots they had induced in the ear veins of rabbits. On the basis of their experiments, they concluded that intravenous streptokinase created an "active lytic system."[58] In 1955, Tillett published the results of a clinical trial in which he and his associates administered streptokinase intravenously to 11 patients to assess its side effects. The most prominent adverse effects were fever and hypotension.[59]

Three years later, Anthony Fletcher, Sol Sherry, and their associates reported the results of a trial of "massive and prolonged" administration of intravenous streptokinase in 24 patients with acute myocardial infarction. Impressed with their findings, they speculated, "The rapid dissolution of a coronary thrombus by enzymatic means could result in reduction of the final area of muscle infarction, reduction of the degree of electrical instability present during the early critical phase of infarction and prevent the appearance of or lyse mural thrombi."[60] The following year (1959), they concluded that streptokinase was "a highly effective activator of human plasminogen."[61]

Concern about the pyrogenicity and antigenicity of streptokinase delayed its clinical application in thromboembolic disorders. But there was also a growing debate about the pathophysiology of acute myocardial infarction. For a quarter of a century after Herrick's 1912 paper, it was generally accepted that acute myocardial infarction was caused by abrupt thrombotic occlusion of an epicardial coronary artery. In 1939, New York cardiologist Charles Friedberg questioned this theory on the basis of a postmortem study of 1000 heart attack patients. Because 31% of the subjects did not have evidence of recent coronary thrombosis at autopsy, Friedberg concluded that acute myocardial infarction was not invariably caused by a blood clot forming in the diseased coronary artery. He thought the syndrome might "also be due solely to progressive coronary narrowing of extreme degree."[62]

During the 1950s and 1960s some pathologists and clinicians speculated that coronary thrombosis might *result from* rather than *cause* acute myocardial infarction.[63] Cardiac pathologist William Roberts of the National Institutes of Health agreed with this premise. In 1972, he claimed that a variety of postmortem findings "suggest that coronary thrombi are consequences rather than causes of acute myocardial infarction."[64] Other pathologists challenged this view. Michael Davies of England protested, in 1976, that it was "hardly credible that there should be continuing debate about what is ostensibly so simple a morphological problem, the relation of coronary thrombosis to acute myocardial infarction."[65]

While pathologists debated the role of coronary thrombosis in acute myocardial infarction, researchers in Europe and America continued to explore the therapeutic value of anticoagulants and thrombolytic agents. The European Working Party reported the results of their multicenter controlled trial of streptokinase in acute myocardial infarction in 1971. After reviewing the results of this trial in which 764 patients were randomized prospectively to treatment with intravenous streptokinase or heparin, they concluded that streptokinase was superior to heparin in reducing early mortality and reinfarction in the first 6 weeks following infarction. But because their study revealed only a "limited reduction in mortality," they advocated "further extensive trials."[66]

In 1976, E. I. Chazov and colleagues from Russia reported on two patients in whom they had performed coronary angiograms before and after the intracoronary administration of streptokinase and heparin during acute myocardial infarction. Reperfusion was successful in the patient who received thrombolytic therapy 4 hours after the onset of symptoms; it was unsuccessful in the patient who was treated 10 hours after the onset of symptoms.[67] This paper, published in Russian with a brief English summary, was unknown to most Europeans and Americans working in the area of thrombolytic therapy.[68]

The modern era of thrombolytic therapy for acute myocardial infarction can be traced to a 1979 paper by Peter Rentrop and his associates in Göttingen, Germany, in which they described the intracoronary administration of streptokinase in five patients. Rentrop accepted the "classical pathologic theory" that acute myocardial infarction was usually caused by "coronary thrombosis superimposed upon high-degree atherosclerotic lesions." Using selective coronary angiography before and after infusing streptokinase, he documented that the drug improved blood flow in the infarct-related artery in four of the five patients.[69]

Almost simultaneously, the European Cooperative Study Group for Streptokinase Treatment in Acute Myocardial Infarction reported the results of a randomized controlled trial of a 24-hour intravenous infusion of streptokinase. The mortality rate of patients treated with streptokinase was significantly lower at 6 months than of those who received placebo.[70] The ongoing debate about the causative role of thrombus in acute myocardial infarction was settled when Spokane cardiologist Marcus DeWood published a report on the prevalence of total coronary occlusion in the immediate postinfarction period. He performed coronary arteriograms in these patients and found that 87% of those studied within 4 hours of the onset of symptoms had occlusion of the infarctrelated artery.[71]

The papers by Rentrop and DeWood resulted in the rapid diffusion of intracoronary streptokinase therapy for acute myocardial infarction into clinical practice and greatly stimulated research on thrombolytic agents. Several European and American groups published studies in 1983 and 1984 demonstrating the efficacy of intravenous streptokinase.[72,73] This finding was especially relevant because most patients with acute myocardial infarction did not present initially to hospitals with cardiac catheterization laboratories. Intravenous thrombolytic therapy rapidly became a mainstay in the treatment of patients with heart attacks.

Meanwhile, another European group was interested in a different thrombolytic agent, tissue plasminogen activator (tPA),

discovered in 1947 by Danish biologists Tage Astrup and Per Permin.[74] In 1981, W. Weimar, Désiré Collen, and their associates in Belgium and the Netherlands reported that they had lysed a renal and iliofemoral thrombus in a renal transplant recipient with intravenous tPA. The authors were optimistic about the clinical potential of this agent because animal studies suggested that it caused thrombolysis without systemic fibrinolytic activation. The main problem they envisioned was the limited supply of tPA, which could then be obtained only from a specific malignant melanoma cell line. They speculated that a genetically engineered tPA was a distinct possibility, however.[75] Pharmacologic research now depended not only on the techniques of chemistry and experimental physiology, but it also drew upon many other disciplines, such as the rapidly expanding field of molecular biology.

Because tPA appeared to be clot-specific and had a short half-life, it was assumed that it would cause less systemic lytic activity and less bleeding than streptokinase or urokinase, the agents then approved for clinical use. Shortly after Collen began collaborating with Steven Bergmann, Burton Sobel, and other investigators at Washington University in St. Louis, they reported that tPA caused thrombolysis when it was administered to dogs in which an intracoronary thrombus had been induced experimentally. They claimed that once recombinant DNA technology made it possible to produce tPA in larger quantities the drug held "particular promise for widely applicable, prompt, safe dissolution of coronary thrombi accompanied by restitution of metabolism in jeopardized myocardium in patients."[76]

In 1983, Collen and several scientists at Genentech, Inc., a biotechnology company formed in San Francisco 7 years earlier, reported a method for producing human tPA using recombinant DNA technology. The successful cloning and expression of the human tPA gene meant that sufficient quantities of the substance could be produced for clinical research and commercial marketing if it proved to be effective and safe.[77]

Collen's group in Belgium and the investigators at Washington University reported the first clinical trial of intravenous and intracoronary tPA for acute myocardial infarction in 1984.[78] Later that year, they collaborated with researchers at Johns Hopkins and the Massachusetts General Hospital in a prospective, placebo-controlled clinical trial sponsored by Genentech. The authors concluded that intravenous or intracoronary tPA caused coronary thrombolysis without triggering clinically significant fibrinolysis in patients with evolving myocardial infarction.[79]

The many clinical trials of thrombolytic therapy during the 1980s and 1990s are beyond the scope of this historical review. They reflect the fact that today physicians, clinical investigators, and the Federal Drug Administration expect *proof* that new pharmaceutical products are both safe and effective before they are marketed. Withering, Brunton, and Murrell did not confront these expectations and regulations. As the cardiologic community was inundated with clever acronyms like GISSI (Gruppo Italiano per lo Studio della Supravivenza nell'Infarto Miocardico), ISIS (International Study of Infarct Survival), GUSTO (Global Utilization of Streptokinase and tPA for Occluded Coronary Arteries), and LATE (Late Assessment of Thrombolytic Efficacy), it became obvious that prompt thrombolytic therapy using either streptokinase or tPA saved lives.[80] The recent flood of publications on thrombolytic therapy is, in part, a manifestation of the magnitude of today's biomedical research effort.

Whereas Withering worked alone on digitalis and Brunton and Murrell had only a few colleagues who shared their interest in vasodilators, researchers in the area of thrombolytic therapy were part of a massive team of basic scientists, clinical investigators, and industry representatives. Last year, American pharmaceutical companies spent approximately $30 billion on research and development.[81] A significant portion of this impressive effort is devoted to developing drugs for the prevention and treatment of cardiovascular diseases—still the leading cause of morbidity and mortality in developed countries. It is easy to understand why so many new cardiovascular drugs have been introduced in recent years. The size and scope of this book is a palpable demonstration of the vitality of the intellectual enterprise.

REFERENCES

1. Weatherall M: *In Search of a Cure: A History of Pharmaceutical Discovery.* Oxford: Oxford University Press, 1990.
2. Leake CD: *An Historical Account of Pharmacology to the Twentieth Century.* Springfield, IL: Charles C Thomas, 1975.
3. Ackerknecht EH: *Therapeutics from the Primitives to the 20th Century.* New York: Hafner Press, 1973.
4. Peck TW, Wilkinson KD: *William Withering of Birmingham, M.D., F.R.S., F.L.S.* Bristol: John Wright & Sons, 1950.
5. Risse GB: *Hospital Life in Enlightenment Scotland: Care and Teaching at the Royal Infirmary of Edinburgh.* Cambridge: Cambridge University Press, 1986.
6. Withering W: *An Account of the Foxglove, and Some of Its Medical Uses.* Birmingham, England: GGJ & J Robinson, 1785.
7. Galdston I: Diagnosis in historical perspective. *Bull Hist Med* 9:367–384, 1941.
8. Faber K: *Nosography: The Evolution of Clinical Medicine in Modern Time.* 2d ed. New York: Paul B Hoeber, 1930.
9. Duffin JM: The cardiology of R.T.H. Laennec. *Med Hist* 33:42–71, 1989.
10. Aronson JK: *An Account of the Foxglove and its Medical Uses, 1785–1985.* London: Oxford University Press, 1985.
11. Estes JW: *Hall Jackson and the Purple Foxglove: Medical Practice and Research in Revolutionary America, 1760–1820.* Hanover, NH: University Press of New England, 1979.
12. Ferriar J: *An Essay on the Medical Properties of the Digitalis Purpurea, or Foxglove.* Manchester: Cadell & Davies, 1799.
13. Uretsky BF, Young JB, Shahidi FE, et al: Randomized study assessing the effect of digoxin withdrawal in patients with mild to moderate chronic congestive heart failure: Results of the PROVED trial. *J Am Coll Cardiol* 22:955–962, 1993.
14. Lesch JE: *Science and Medicine in France: The Emergence of Experimental Physiology, 1790–1855.* Cambridge, MA: Harvard University Press, 1984.
15. Kohler RE: *From Medical Chemistry to Biochemistry: The Making of a Biomedical Discipline.* New York: Cambridge University Press, 1982.
16. Coleman W, Holmes FL, eds: *The Investigative Enterprise: Experimental Physiology in Nineteenth-Century Medicine.* Berkeley: University of California Press, 1988.
17. Parascandola J: *The Development of American Pharmacology: John J. Abel and the Shaping of a Discipline.* Baltimore: Johns Hopkins University Press, 1992.
18. Gevitz N, ed: *Other Healers: Unorthodox Medicine in America.* Baltimore: Johns Hopkins University Press, 1988.
19. Warner JH: *The Therapeutic Perspective: Medical Practice, Knowledge, and Identity in America, 1820–1885.* Cambridge, MA: Harvard University Press, 1986.
20. Fye WB: Nitroglycerin: a homeopathic remedy. *Circulation* 73:21–29, 1986.
21. Kaufman M: *Homeopathy in America: The Rise and Fall of a Medical Heresy.* Baltimore: Johns Hopkins Press, 1971.
22. Hering C: Glonoin or nitro glycerine [Americanische Arzneiprüfungen], translated with additions. History as proved and applied by C. Hering, Philadelphia, 1847–1851. *New Engl Med Gaz* 9:9, 255–256, 337–352, 385–402, 433–448, 481–496, 529–544, 1874; 10:1–26, 1875.
23. Albers JFH: Die physiologische und therapeutische Wirkung des Nitroglycerins. *Deutsche Klin* 42:405–408, 1864.
24. Fye WB: Vasodilator therapy for angina pectoris: The intersection of homeopathy and scientific medicine. *J Hist Med Allied Sci* 45:317–340, 1990.
25. Brunton TL: On the use of nitrite of amyl in angina pectoris. *Lancet* 2:97–98, 1867.
26. Smith E, Hart FD: William Murrell, physician and practical therapist. *Br Med J* 3:632–633, 1971.
27. Fye WB: Sydney Ringer and the role of calcium in myocardial function. *Circulation* 69:849–853, 1984.
28. Murrell W: Nitro-glycerine as a remedy for angina pectoris. *Lancet* 1:80–81, 113–115, 151–152, 225–227, 1879.
29. Jameson G: Nitro-glycerine in angina pectoris. *Lancet* 1:578, 1879.
30. Nitro-gylcerine. *Med News* 40:408–409, 1882.
31. Bonner TN: *American Doctors and German Universities: A Chapter in International Intellectual Relations, 1870–1914.* Lincoln, NE: University of Nebraska Press, 1963.
32. Ludmerer KM: *Learning to Heal: The Development of American Medical Education.* New York: Basic Books, 1985.
33. Fye WB: *The Development of American Physiology: Scientific Medicine in the Nineteenth Century.* Baltimore: Johns Hopkins University Press, 1987.
34. Fye WB: The origin of the full-time faculty system: Implications for clinical research. *JAMA* 265:1555–1562, 1991.
35. Harvey AM: *Science at the Bedside: Clinical Research in American Medicine, 1905–1945.* Baltimore: Johns Hopkins University Press, 1981.
36. Swann JP: *Academic Scientists and the Pharmaceutical Industry.* Baltimore: Johns Hopkins University Press, 1988.
37. Liebenau J: *Medical Science and Medical Industry: The Formation of the American Pharmaceutical Industry.* Baltimore: Johns Hopkins University Press, 1987.
38. Comroe JH Jr, Dripps RD: *The Top Ten Clinical Advances in Cardiovascular-Pulmonary Medicine and Surgery 1945–1975.* Washington, DC: US Government Printing Office, 1978.
39. Fye WB: Acute myocardial infarction: a historical summary. In: Gersh BJ, Rahimtoola SH, eds. *Acute Myocardial Infarction.* New York: Elsevier Science Publishing, 1991:3–13.
40. Fye WB, ed: *Classic Papers on Coronary Thrombosis and Myocardial Infarction.* Birmingham, AL: Classics of Cardiology Library, 1991.
41. Leibowitz JO: *The History of Coronary Heart Disease.* London: Wellcome Institute of the History of Medicine, 1970.
42. Rindfleisch E: *A Manual of Pathological History to Serve as an Introduction to the Study of Morbid Anatomy* (transl EB Baxter). London: New Sydenham Society, 1872.
43. Rosenberg CF, Golden J, eds: *Framing Disease: Studies in Cultural History.* New Brunswick, NJ: Rutgers University Press, 1992.
44. Obrastzow WP, Straschesko ND: Zur Kenntnis der Thrombose der Koronararterien des Herzens. *Z Klin Med* 71:116–132, 1910.
45. Muller JE: Diagnosis of myocardial infarction: historical notes from the Soviet Union and the United States. *Am J Cardiol* 40:269–271, 1977.
46. Herrick JB: Certain clinical features of sudden obstruction of the coronary arteries. *JAMA* 59:2015–2020, 1912.
47. Fye WB: A history of the origin, evolution, and impact of electrocardiography. *Am J Cardiol* 73:937–949, 1994.
48. Wright IS: The discovery and early development of anticoagulants: a historical symposium. *Circulation* 19:73–134, 1959.
49. Wright IS, Marple CD, Beck DF: Report of the committee for the evaluation of anticoagulants in the treatment of coronary thrombosis with myocardial infarction. *Am Heart J* 36:801–815, 1948.
50. Gifford RH, Feinstein AR: A critique of methodology in studies of anticoagulant therapy for acute myocardial infarction. *N Engl J Med* 280:351–357, 1969.
51. Mitchell JRA: Anticoagulants in coronary heart disease—retrospect and prospect. *Lancet* 1:257–262, 1981.
52. Mueller RL, Scheidt S: History of drugs for thrombotic disease: Discovery, development, and directions for the future. *Circulation* 89:432–449, 1994.
53. Tillett WS, Garner RL: The fibrinolytic activity of hemolytic streptococci. *J Exp Med* 58:485–502, 1933.
54. Sherry S: *Reflections and Reminiscences of an Academic Physician.* Philadelphia: Lea & Febiger, 1993.
55. Strickland SP: *Politics, Science, and Dreaded Disease: A Short History of United States Medical Research Policy.* Cambridge, MA: Harvard University Press, 1972.

56. Fye WB: *American Cardiology: The History of a Specialty and Its College.* Baltimore: Johns Hopkins University Press, 1996.

57. Ginzberg E, Dutka AB: *The Financing of Biomedical Research.* Baltimore: Johns Hopkins University Press, 1989.

58. Johnson AJ, Tillett WS: The lysis in rabbits of intravascular blood clots by the streptococcal fibrinolytic system (streptokinase). *J Exp Med* 95:449–463, 1952.

59. Tillett WS, Johnson AJ, McCarty WR: The intravenous infusion of the streptococcal fibrinolytic principles (streptokinase) into patients. *J Clin Invest* 34:169–185, 1955.

60. Fletcher AP, Alkjaersig N, Smyrniotis F, Sherry S: The treatment of patients suffering from early myocardial infarction with massive and prolonged streptokinase therapy. *Trans Assoc Am Physicians* 71:287–296, 1958.

61. Fletcher AP, Alkjaersig N, Sherry S: The maintenance of a sustained thrombolytic state in man: I. Induction and effects. *J Clin Invest* 38:1096–1110, 1959.

62. Friedberg CK, Horn H: Acute myocardial infarction not due to coronary artery occlusion. *JAMA* 112:1675–1679, 1939.

63. Friedman M, Van den Bovenkamp GJ: The pathogenesis of a coronary thrombus. *Am J Pathol* 48:19–44, 1966.

64. Roberts WC, Buja LM: The frequency and significance of coronary arterial thrombi and other observations in fatal acute myocardial infarction: A study of 107 necropsy patients. *Am J Med* 52:425–443, 1972.

65. Davies MJ, Woolf N, Robertson WB: Pathology of acute myocardial infarction with particular reference to occlusive coronary thrombi. *Br Heart J* 38:659–664, 1976.

66. European Working Party. Streptokinase in recent myocardial infarction: A controlled multicentre trial. *Br Med J* 3:325–331, 1971.

67. Chazov EI, Matveeva LS, Mazaev AV, et al: Intracoronary administration of fibrinolysin in acute myocardial infarction. *Terapevticheskii Arkhiv* 48:8–19, 1976.

68. Braunwald E: The path to myocardial salvage by thrombolytic therapy. *Circulation* 76(Suppl II):3, (Suppl II):7, 1987.

69. Rentrop KP, Blanke H, Karsch KR, et al: Acute myocardial infarction: Intracoronary application of nitroglycerin and streptokinase. *Clin Cardiol* 2:354–363, 1979.

70. Streptokinase in acute myocardial infarction: European Cooperative Study Group for Streptokinase Treatment in Acute Myocardial Infarction. *N Engl J Med* 301:797–802, 1979.

71. DeWood MA, Spores J, Notske R, et al: Prevalence of total coronary occlusion during the early hours of transmural myocardial infarction. *N Engl J Med* 303:897–902, 1980.

72. Schröder R, Biamino G, Lettner E, et al: Intravenous shortterm infusion of streptokinase in acute myocardial infarction. *Circulation* 67:536–548, 1983.

73. Taylor GJ, Mikell FL, Moses HW, et al: Intravenous versus intracoronary streptokinase therapy for acute myocardial infarction in community hospitals. *Am J Cardiol* 54:256–260, 1984.

74. Astrup T, Permin PM: Fibrinolysis in the animal organism. *Nature* 159:681–682, 1947.

75. Weimar W, Stubbe J, Van Seyen AJ, et al: Specific lysis of an iliofemoral thrombus by administration of extrinsic (tissue-type) plasminogen activator. *Lancet* 2:1018–1020, 1981.

76. Bergmann SR, Fox KA, Ter-Pogossian MM, Sobel BE: Clot-selective coronary thrombolysis with tissue-type plasminogen activator. *Science* 220:1181–1183, 1983.

77. Pennica D, Holmes WE, Kohr WJ, et al: Cloning and expression of human tissue-type plasminogen activator cDNA in *E. coli. Nature* 301:214–221, 1983.

78. Van de Werf F, Ludbrook PA, Bergmann SR, et al: Coronary thrombolysis with tissue-type plasminogen activator in patients with evolving myocardial infarction. *N Engl J Med* 310:609–613, 1984.

79. Collen D, Topol EJ, Tiefenbrunn AJ, et al: Coronary thrombolysis with recombinant human tissue-type plasminogen activator: A prospective, randomized, placebo-controlled trial. *Circulation* 70:1012–1017, 1984.

80. Yusuf S, Colins R, Peto R, et al: Intravenous and intracoronary fibrinolytic therapy in acute myocardial infarction: Overview of results of mortality, reinfarction and side-effects from 33 randomized controlled trials. *Eur Heart J* 6:556–585, 1985.

81. Pharmaceutical Research and Manufacturers of America. http://www.phrma.org/publications/documents/backgrounders//2002-03-06.333.phtml.

PART II

Drug Classes

CHAPTER 7

Alpha- and Beta-Adrenergic Blocking Drugs

William H. Frishman

Catecholamines are neurohumoral substances that mediate a variety of physiologic and metabolic activities in humans. The effects of the catecholamines ultimately depend on their chemical interactions with receptors, which are discrete macromolecular structures located on the plasma membrane. Differences in the ability of the various catecholamines to stimulate a number of physiologic processes were the criteria used by Ahlquist in 1948 to separate these receptors into distinct types: alpha and beta-adrenergic.[1] Subsequent studies have revealed that beta-adrenergic receptors exist as three discrete subtypes called beta$_1$, beta$_2$, and beta$_3$ (Table 7-1).[2,3] It is now appreciated that there are two subtypes of alpha receptors, designated alpha$_1$ and alpha$_2$ (see Table 7-1).[4] At least three subtypes of both alpha$_1$- and alpha$_2$-adrenergic receptors are known,[5] but distinctions in their mechanisms of action and tissue location have not been defined.

This chapter examines the adrenergic receptors and the drugs that can inhibit their function. The rationale for use and clinical experience with alpha- and beta-adrenergic drugs in the treatment of various cardiovascular disorders is also discussed.

ADRENERGIC RECEPTORS: HORMONAL AND DRUG RECEPTORS

The effects of an endogenous hormone or exogenous drug depend ultimately on physiochemical interactions with macromolecular structures of cells called receptors. Agonists interact with a receptor and elicit a response; antagonists interact with receptors and prevent the action of agonists.

In the case of catecholamine action, the circulating hormone or drug ("first messenger") interacts with its specific receptor on the external surface of the target cells. The drug hormone-receptor complex, mediated by a G protein called Gs, activates the enzyme adenyl cyclase on the internal surface of the plasma membrane of the target cell, which accelerates the intracellular formation of cyclic adenosine monophosphate (cAMP). cAMP-dependent protein kinase ("second messenger") then stimulates or inhibits various metabolic or physiologic processes.[6-9] Catecholamine-induced increases in intracellular cAMP are usually associated with stimulation of beta-adrenergic receptors, whereas the stimulation of alpha-adrenergic receptors is mediated by a G protein known as Gi and is associated with lower concentrations of cAMP[7,10] and possibly increased amounts of guanosine-3'5'-monophosphate in the cell. These changes may result in the production of opposite physiologic effects from those of catecholamines, depending on what adrenergic receptor system is activated.

Until recently, most research on receptor action bypassed the initial binding step and the intermediate steps and examined either the accumulation of cAMP or the end step, the physiologic effect. Currently, radioactive agonists or antagonists (radioligands) that attach to and label the receptors have been used to study binding and hormone action.[7-11] The cloning of adrenergic receptors has also revealed important clues about receptor function.[7]

ALPHA-ADRENERGIC BLOCKERS

Clinical Pharmacology

When an adrenergic nerve is stimulated, catecholamines are released from their storage granules in the adrenergic neuron, enter the synaptic cleft, and bind to alpha receptors on the effector cell.[12] A feedback loop exists by which the amount of neurotransmitter released can be regulated: accumulation of catecholamines in the synaptic cleft leads to stimulation of alpha receptors in the neuronal surface and inhibition of further catecholamine release. Catecholamines from the systemic circulation can also enter the synaptic cleft and bind to presynaptic or postsynaptic receptors.

Initially it was believed that alpha$_1$ receptors were limited to postsynaptic sites, where they mediated vasoconstriction, whereas the alpha$_2$ receptors existed only at the prejunctional nerve terminals and mediated the negative feedback control of norepinephrine release. The availability of compounds with high specificity for either alpha$_1$ or alpha$_2$ receptors demonstrated that while presynaptic alpha receptors are almost exclusively of the alpha$_2$ subtype, the postsynaptic receptors are made up of comparable numbers of alpha$_1$ and alpha$_2$ receptors.[12] Stimulation of the postsynaptic alpha$_2$ receptors causes vasoconstriction. A functional difference does, however, exist between the two types of postsynaptic receptors. The alpha$_1$ receptors appear to exist primarily within the region of the synapse and respond preferentially to neuronally released catecholamine, whereas alpha$_2$ receptors are located extrasynaptically and respond preferentially to circulating catecholamines in the plasma.

Drugs having alpha-adrenergic blocking properties are of several types (Fig. 7-1)[12-18]:

1. Nonselective alpha blockers having prominent effects on both the alpha$_1$ and alpha$_2$ receptors (e.g., the older drugs such as phenoxybenzamine and phentolamine). Although virtually all of the clinical effects of phenoxybenzamine are explicable in terms of alpha blockade, this is not the case with phentolamine, which also possesses several other properties,

TABLE 7-1. Characteristics of Subtypes of Adrenergic Receptors*

Receptor	Tissue	Response
α_1[†]	Vascular smooth muscle, genitourinary smooth muscle	Contraction
	Liver[‡]	Glycogenolysis; gluconeogenesis
	Heart	Increased contractile force; arrhythmias
α_2[†]	Pancreatic islets (β cells)	Decreased insulin secretion
	Platelets	Aggregation
	Nerve terminals	Decreased release of norepinephrine
	Vascular smooth muscle	Contraction
β_1	Heart	Increased force and rate of contraction and AV-nodal conduction velocity
	Juxtaglomerular cells	Increased renin secretion
β_2	Smooth muscle (vascular, bronchial, GI and genitourinary)	Relaxation
	Skeletal muscle	Glycogenolysis; uptake of K+
	Liver[‡]	Glycogenolysis; gluconeogensis
β_3[§]	Adipose tissue	Lipolysis, thermogenesis

*This table provides examples of drugs that act on adrenergic receptors and of the location of subtypes of adrenergic receptors.

[†]At least three subtypes of each α_1- and α_2-adrenergic receptor are known, but their mechanisms of action and tissue locations have not been clearly defined.

[‡]In some species (e.g., rat), metabolic responses in the liver are mediated by α_1-adrenergic receptors, whereas in others (e.g., dog), β_2-adrenergic receptors are predominantly involved. Both types of receptors appear to contribute to responses in human beings.

[§]Metabolic responses in adipocytes and certain other tissues with atypical pharmacologic characteristics may be mediated by this subtype of receptor. Most β-adrenergic-receptor antagonists (including propranolol) do not block these responses.

Source: Adapted with permission from Hoffman and Taylor.[10]

including a direct vasodilator action and sympathomimetic and parasympathomimetic effects.

2. Selective alpha$_1$ blockers having little affinity for alpha$_2$ receptors (e.g., prazosin, terazosin, doxazosin, and other quinazoline derivatives). It is now clear that these drugs, originally introduced as direct-acting vasodilators, exert their major effect by reversible blockade of postsynaptic alpha$_1$ receptors.

Other selective alpha$_1$ blockers include indoramin, trimazosin, and urapadil (Table 7-2). Urapadil is of interest because of its other actions, which include stimulation of presynaptic alpha$_2$-adrenergic receptors and a central effect.

3. Selective alpha$_2$ blockers (e.g., yohimbine). The primary use of these drugs has been as tools in experimental pharmacology. Yohimbine is now marketed in the United States as an oral

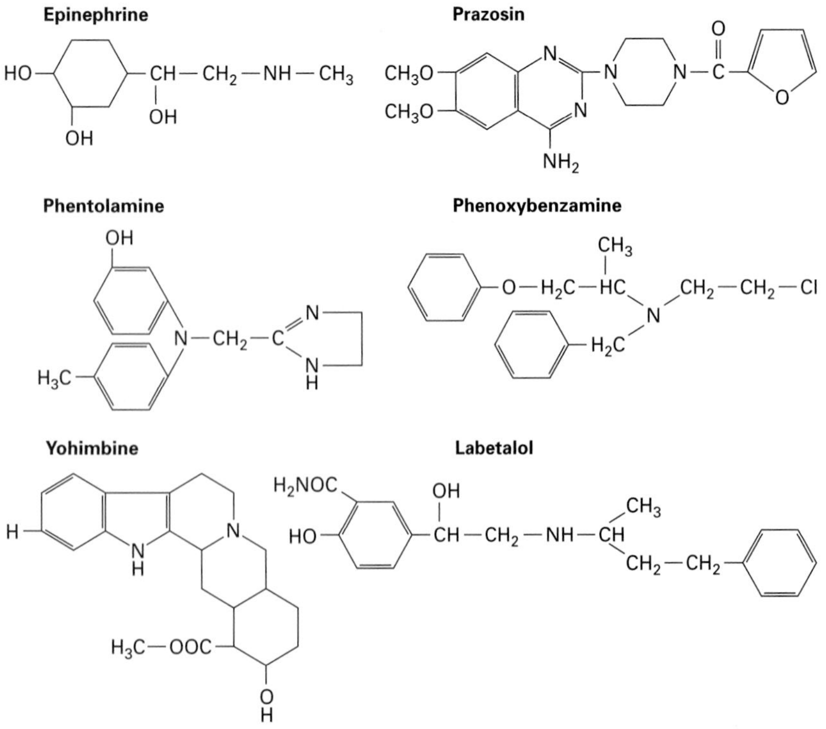

FIGURE 7-1. Molecular structure of the alpha-adrenergic agonist epinephrine and some alpha blockers.

TABLE 7-2. Pharmacokinetics of Selective α_1-Adrenergic Blocking Drugs

Selective α_1 Blocker	Daily Dose (mg)	Frequency per Day	Bioavailability (% of oral dose)	Plasma Half-Life (h)	Urinary Excretion (% of oral dose)
Doxazosin	1–16	1	65	10–12	NA
Indoramin*	50–125	2–3	NA	5	11
Prazosin	2–20	2–3	44–69	2.5–4	10
Terazosin	1–20	1	90	12	39
Trimazosin*	100–500	2–3	61	2.7	NA

*Investigational drug; NA = not available.

Source: Adapted with permission from Luther.[13]

sympatholytic and mydriatic agent. Male patients with impotence of vascular, diabetic, or psychogenic origin have been treated successfully with yohimbine.

4. Blockers that inhibit both alpha- and beta-adrenergic receptors (e.g., carvedilol, labetalol). Carvedilol and labetalol are selective alpha$_1$ blockers. Since these agents are much more potent as beta blockers than alpha blockers, they are discussed in greater detail in the section on beta blockers.

5. Agents having alpha-adrenergic blocking properties but whose major clinical use appears unrelated to these properties (e.g., chlorpromazine, haloperidol, quinidine, bromocriptine, amiodarone and ketanserin, a selective blocking agent of serotonin$_2$ receptors). It has been demonstrated that verapamil, a calcium-channel blocker, also has alpha-adrenergic blocking properties. Whether this is a particular property of verapamil and its analogues or is common to all calcium-channel blockers is not clear.[19] Also to be clarified is whether verapamil-induced alpha blockade occurs at physiologic plasma levels and helps to mediate the vasodilator properties of the drug.

All the alpha blockers in clinical use inhibit the postsynaptic alpha$_1$ receptor and result in relaxation of vascular smooth muscle and vasodilation. However, the nonselective alpha blockers also antagonize the presynaptic alpha$_2$ receptors, allowing for increased release of neuronal norepinephrine. This results in attenuation of the desired postsynaptic blockade and spillover stimulation of the beta receptors and, consequently, in troublesome side effects such as tachycardia and tremulousness and increased renin release. The alpha$_1$-selective agents that preserve the alpha$_2$-mediated presynaptic feedback loop prevent excessive norepinephrine release and thus avoid these adverse cardiac and systemic effects.

Because of these potent peripheral vasodilatory properties, one would anticipate, however, that even the selective alpha$_1$ blockers would induce reflex stimulation of the sympathetic and renin-angiotensin system similar to that seen with other vasodilators such as hydralazine and minoxidil. The explanation for the relative lack of tachycardia and renin release observed after prazosin, terazosin, and doxazosin may in part be due to the drugs' combined action of reducing vascular tone in both resistance (arteries) and capacitance (veins) beds. Such a dual action may prevent the marked increases in venous return and cardiac output observed with agents that act more selectively to reduce vascular tone only in the resistance vessels. The lack of tachycardia with prazosin, terazosin, and doxazosin use has also been attributed by some investigators to a significant negative chronotropic action of the drugs independent of their peripheral vascular effects.[20]

Use in Cardiovascular Disorders

Hypertension

Increased peripheral vascular resistance is present in the majority of patients with long-standing hypertension. Since dilation of constricted arterioles should result in lowering of elevated blood pressure, interest has focused on the use of alpha-adrenergic blockers in the medical treatment of systemic hypertension. Except for pheochromocytoma, the experience with nonselective alpha blockers in the treatment of hypertension was disappointing because of accompanying reflex stimulation of the sympathetic and renin-angiotensin system, resulting in frequent side effects and limited long-term antihypertensive efficacy. However, the selective alpha$_1$ blockers prazosin, doxazosin, and terazosin have been shown to be effective antihypertensive agents.[12,13,18,21]

Prazosin, doxazosin, and terazosin decrease blood pressure in both the standing and supine positions, although blood pressure decrements tends to be somewhat greater in the upright position. Because their antihypertensive effect is accompanied by little or no increase in heart rate, plasma renin activity, or circulating catecholamines, prazosin, doxazosin, and terazosin have been found useful as first-step agents in hypertension. Monotherapy with these agents, however, promotes sodium and water retention in some patients, although it is less pronounced than with other vasodilators. The concomitant use of a diuretic prevents fluid retention and in many cases markedly enhances the antihypertensive effect of the drugs. In clinical practice, prazosin, doxazosin, and terazosin have their widest application as adjuncts to one or more established antihypertensive drugs in treating moderate-to-severe hypertension. Their effects are additive to those of diuretics, beta blockers, alpha methyldopa, and the direct-acting vasodilators. The drugs cause little change in glomerular filtration rate or renal plasma flow, and can be used safely in patients with severe renal hypertension. There is no evidence for attenuation of the antihypertensive effect of prazosin, doxazosin, or terazosin during chronic therapy.

In large comparative clinical trials, the efficacy and safety of alpha$_1$ blockers have been well documented. In the TOMHS (Treatment of Mild Hypertension Study), doxazosin 2 mg/day given over 4 years reduced blood pressure as much as agents from other drugs classes.[22] In a large Veterans Administration Study where patients with severe hypertension were studied, prazosin 20 mg daily given over 1 year had a treatment effect that was significantly greater than placebo.[23] Doxazosin 2 to 8 mg daily was one of the drugs used in the ALLHAT (Antihypertensive and Lipid Lowering Treatment to Prevent Heart Attack Trial), which was designed to compare various antihypertensive agents and their effect on coronary morbidity and mortality in high-risk antihypertensives aged 55 years and older.[24] Doxazosin was withdrawn from this trial after an interim analysis showed a 25% greater rate of a secondary end point, combined cardiovascular disease, in patients on doxazosin than in those on chlorthalidone, largely driven by congestive heart failure.[25–26a] Based on this study, alpha$_1$ blockers should not be considered as first-line monotherapy treatment for hypertension but as part of a combination regimen to provide maximal blood pressure control.[27,28]

Selective alpha blockers appear to have neutral or even favorable effects on plasma lipids and lipoproteins when administered to hypertensive patients. Investigators have reported mild reductions in levels of total cholesterol, low-density lipoprotein (LDL) and very-low-density lipoprotein (VLDL) cholesterol, and triglycerides and elevations in levels of high-density lipoprotein (HDL) cholesterol and insulin sensitivity with prazosin, doxazosin, and terazosin.[29–34] With long-term use, selective alpha$_1$ blockers also appear to decrease left ventricular mass in patients with hypertension and left ventricular hypertrophy.[35]

A number of prazosin, doxazosin, and terazosin analogues have been developed (e.g., trimazosin) that in preliminary clinical trials have also shown promise as antihypertensive agents.[15,16,36] Doxazosin and terazosin have a longer duration of action than prazosin and have been shown to produce sustained blood pressure reductions with single daily administration. Indoramin, also a selective alpha$_1$ blocker, has been found to be effective in the treatment of systemic hypertension, but it produces many unwanted effects, such as lethargy and impotence, which may limit its clinical value. In contrast to prazosin, the drug appears to have little dilatory effect on the venous circulation. Prazosin, doxazosin, and terazosin are available for clinical use in the United States.

Congestive Heart Failure

Alpha-adrenergic blocking drugs appear particularly attractive for use in the treatment of heart failure because they hold the possibility of reproducing balanced reductions in resistance and capacitance beds. In fact, phentolamine was one of the earlier vasodilators shown to be effective in the treatment of heart failure.[37,38] The drug was infused into normotensive patients with persistent left ventricular dysfunction after a myocardial infarction and found to induce a significant fall in systemic vascular resistance accompanied by considerable elevation in cardiac output and a reduction in pulmonary artery pressure.[38] Because of its high cost and the frequent side effects that it produces, especially tachycardia, phentolamine is no longer used in the treatment of heart failure. Oral phenoxybenzamine has also been used as vasodilator therapy in heart failure; like phentolamine, it has been replaced by newer vasodilator agents.

Studies evaluating the acute hemodynamic effects of prazosin in patients with congestive heart failure consistently find significant reductions in systemic and pulmonary vascular resistances and left ventricular filling pressures associated with increases in stroke volume.[20,39] In most studies, there is no change or a decrease in heart rate. The response pattern seen with prazosin is similar to that observed with nitroprusside with the exception that the heart rate tends to be higher with the use of nitroprusside; therefore the observed increases in cardiac output are also higher with the latter agent.

Controversy still exists as to whether the initial clinical and hemodynamic improvements seen with prazosin are sustained during long-term therapy.[40] Whereas some studies have demonstrated continued efficacy of prazosin therapy after chronic use, others have found little hemodynamic difference between prazosin- and placebo-treated patients. Some investigators believe that whatever

tolerance to the drug does develop is most likely secondary to activation of counterposing neurohumoral forces; if the dose is raised and the tendency toward sodium and water retention is countered by appropriate increases in diuretic dose, prazosin is likely to remain effective. Others argue that sustained increases in plasma renin activity or plasma catecholamines are not seen during long-term therapy and that tolerance is not prevented or reversed by a diuretic. Some clinical studies suggest that patients with initially high plasma renin activity experience attenuation of beneficial hemodynamic effects more frequently. What appears clear is the need to evaluate patients individually as to the continued efficacy of their prazosin therapy. Whether there are subgroups of patients with heart failure (e.g., those with highly activated sympathetic nervous systems) who are more likely to respond to prazosin or other alpha blockers remains to be determined.

A multicenter study from the Veterans Administration hospitals has shown that prazosin, when compared with placebo therapy, did not reduce mortality with long-term use in patients with advanced forms of congestive heart failure.[41] In the same study, a favorable effect on mortality was seen with an isosorbide dinitrate–hydralazine combination.[41]

Doxazosin and metoprolol were combined and compared to metoprolol alone in the treatment of patients with chronic heart failure.[42] After 3 months of continuous therapy, both treatment groups showed similar and significant reductions in systemic vascular resistance and heart rate, with significant increases in cardiac index, ejection fraction, and exercise capacity. It was concluded that the combination of doxazosin and metoprolol was no better than metoprolol used alone.

There is increasing evidence that alpha$_1$-adrenergic receptors, different from those of other tissues, also exist in the myocardium and that an increase in the force of contraction may be produced by stimulation of these sites.[43,44] The mechanism of alpha-adrenergic positive inotropic response is unknown. What the biologic significance of alpha-adrenergic receptors in cardiac muscle is, and whether these receptors play a role in the response to alpha-blocker therapy in congestive heart failure, also remain to be determined.

Angina Pectoris

Alpha-adrenergic receptors help mediate coronary vasoconstriction.[45] It has been suggested that a pathologic alteration of the alpha-adrenergic system may be the mechanism of coronary spasm in some patients with variant angina.[46] In uncontrolled studies, the administration of alpha-adrenergic blockers, both acutely and chronically, has been shown effective in reversing and preventing coronary spasm. However, in a long-term, randomized, double-blind trial, prazosin was found to exert no obvious beneficial effect in patients with variant angina.[47] The demonstration of an important role for the postsynaptic alpha$_2$-receptors in determining coronary vascular tone may help explain prazosin's lack of efficacy. Further study in this area is anticipated.

Arrhythmias

It has been postulated that enhanced alpha-adrenergic responsiveness occurs during myocardial ischemia and that it is a primary mediator of the electrophysiologic derangements and resulting malignant arrhythmias induced by catecholamines during myocardial ischemia and reperfusion.[48] In humans, there have been favorable reports of the use of an alpha blocker in the treatment of supraventricular and ventricular ectopy. Whether there is a significant role for alpha-adrenergic blockers in the treatment of cardiac arrhythmias will be determined through further clinical study.

Use in Other Disorders

Pheochromocytoma

Alpha blockers have been used in the treatment of pheochromocytoma to control the peripheral effects of the excess catecholamines.[49] In fact, intravenous phentolamine was used as a test for this disorder, but the test is now rarely done because of reported cases of cardiovascular collapse and death in patients who exhibited exaggerated sensitivity to the drug. It is still rarely used in cases of pheochromocytoma-related hypertensive crisis. However, for long-term therapy, oral phenoxybenzamine is the preferred agent. Beta-blocking agents may also be needed in pheochromocytoma for control of tachycardia and arrhythmias. A beta blocker of any kind, but primarily the nonselective agents, should not be initiated prior to adequate alpha blockade, since severe hypertension may occur as a result of the unopposed alpha-stimulating activity of the circulating catecholamines.

Shock

In shock, hyperactivity of the sympathetic nervous system occurs as a compensatory reflex response to reduced blood pressure. Use of alpha blockers in shock has been advocated as a means of lowering peripheral vascular resistance and increasing vascular capacitance while not antagonizing the cardiotonic effects of the sympathomimetic amines. Although investigated for many years for the treatment of shock, alpha-adrenergic blockers are still not approved for this purpose.[50] A prime concern of the use of alpha blockers in shock is that the rapid drug-induced increase in vascular capacitance may lead to inadequate cardiac filling and profound hypotension, especially in the hypovolemic patient. Adequate amounts of fluid replacement prior to use of an alpha blocker can minimize this concern.

Pulmonary Disease

Pulmonary Hypertension

The part played by endogenous circulating catecholamines in the maintenance of pulmonary vascular tone appears to be minimal. Studies evaluating the effects of norepinephrine administration on pulmonary vascular resistance have found the drug to have little or no effect. The beneficial effects on the pulmonary circulation that phentolamine and other alpha blockers have demonstrated in some studies is most likely primarily due to their direct vasodilatory actions rather than to alpha blockade.[51] Like other vasodilators, in patients with pulmonary hypertension due to fixed anatomic changes, alpha blockers can produce hemodynamic deterioration secondary to their systemic vasodilatory properties.[52]

Bronchospasm

Bronchoconstriction is mediated in part through catecholamine stimulation of alpha receptors in the lung. It has been suggested that in patients with allergic asthma, a deficient beta-adrenergic system or enhanced alpha-adrenergic responsiveness could result in alpha-adrenergic activity being the main mechanism of bronchoconstriction.[53] Several studies have shown bronchodilation or inhibition of histamine and allergen- or exercise-induced bronchospasm with a variety of alpha blockers.[54] Additional studies are needed to define more fully the role of alpha blockers for use as bronchodilators.

Arterioconstriction

Oral alpha-adrenergic blockers can produce subjective and clinical improvement in patients experiencing episodic arterioconstriction (Raynaud's phenomenon). Alpha blockers may also be of value in the treatment of severe peripheral ischemia caused by an alpha agonist (e.g., norepinephrine) or ergotamine overdose. In cases of inadvertent infiltration of a norepinephrine infusion, phentolamine can be given intradermally to avoid tissue sloughing.

Benign Prostatic Obstruction

Alpha-adrenergic receptors have been identified in the bladder neck and prostatic capsule of male patients. In clinical studies, use of alpha blockers in patients with benign prostatic obstruction has resulted in increased urinary flow rates and reductions in residual volume and obstructive symptoms.[55] The drugs prazosin, terazosin, and doxazosin are approved as medical therapies for benign prostatic hypertrophy. Also available is tamsulosin, a long-acting partially selective blocker of the alpha$_1$ subtype that mediates prostatic smooth muscle tone and appears to be as effective as other alpha$_1$ blockers in the treatment of prostatism, but with little effect on blood pressure.[56]

Clinical Use and Adverse Effects

Oral phenoxybenzamine has a rapid onset of action, with the maximal effect from a single dose seen in 1 to 2 h.[57–59] The gastrointestinal absorption is incomplete, and only 20 to 30% of an oral dose reaches the systemic circulation in active form. The half-life of the drug is 24 h, with the usual dose varying between 20 and 200 mg daily in one or two doses. Intravenous phentolamine is initially started at 0.1 mg/min and is then increased at increments of 0.1 mg/min every 5 to 10 min until the desired hemodynamic effect is reached. The drug has a short duration of action of 3 to 10 min. Little is known about the pharmacokinetics of long-term oral use of phentolamine. The main side effects of the drug include postural hypotension, tachycardia, gastrointestinal disturbances, and sexual dysfunction. Intravenous infusion of norepinephrine can be used to combat severe hypotensive reactions. Oral phenoxybenzamine is approved for use in pheochromocytoma.

Prazosin is almost completely absorbed following oral administration, with peak plasma levels achieved at 2 to 3 h. The drug is 90% protein-bound. Prazosin is extensively metabolized by the liver. The usual half-life of the drug is $2\frac{1}{2}$ to 4 h; in patients with heart failure, the half-life increases to the range of 5 to 7 h.

The major side effect of prazosin is the first-dose phenomenon—severe postural hypotension occasionally associated with syncope, seen after the initial dose or after a rapid dose increment.[12,13] The reason for this phenomenon has not been clearly established but may involve the rapid induction of venous and arteriolar dilatation by a drug that elicits little reflex sympathetic stimulation. It is reported more often when the drug is administered as a tablet rather than a capsule, possibly related to the variable bioavailability or rates of absorption of the two formulations.[12] (In the United States, the drug is available in capsule form.) The postural hypotension can be minimized if the initial dose of prazosin is not higher than 1 mg and if it is given at bedtime. In treating hypertension, a dose of 2 to 3 mg/day should be maintained for 1 to 2 weeks, followed by a gradual increase in dosage titrated to achieve the desired reductions in pressures, usually up to 20 to 30 mg/day, given in two or three doses. In treating heart failure, larger doses (2–7 mg) may be used to initiate therapy in recumbent patients, but the maintenance dose is also usually not more than 30 mg. Higher doses do not seem to produce additional clinical improvement.

Other side effects of prazosin include dizziness, headache, and drowsiness. The drug produces no deleterious effects on the clinical course of diabetes mellitus, chronic obstructive pulmonary disease, renal failure, or gout. It does not adversely affect the lipid profile.

Terazosin, which has been approved for once-daily use in hypertension, may be associated with a lesser incidence of first-dose postural hypotension than prazosin.[18] The usual recommended dose range is 1 to 5 mg administered once a day; some patients may benefit from doses as high as 20 mg daily or from divided doses.

Doxazosin is also approved as a once-daily therapy for systemic hypertension. The initial dosage of doxazosin is 1 mg once daily. Depending on the patient's standing blood pressure response, the dosage may then be increased to 2 mg and, if necessary, to 4, 8, or 16 mg to achieve the desired reduction in blood pressure. Doses beyond 4 mg increase the likelihood of excessive postural effects including syncope, postural dizziness/vertigo, and postural hypotension.

The alpha$_2$ blocker yohimbine, 5.4 mg orally, is used four times daily to treat male impotence. Urologists have used yohimbine for the diagnostic classification of certain cases of male erectile dysfunction. Increases in heart rate and blood pressure, piloerection, and rhinorrhea are the most common adverse reactions. Yohimbine should not be used with antidepressant drugs.

BETA-ADRENERGIC BLOCKING DRUGS

Beta-adrenergic blocking drugs, which constitute a major pharmacotherapeutic advance, were conceived initially for the treatment of patients with angina pectoris and arrhythmias; however, they also have therapeutic effects in many other clinical disorders including systemic hypertension, hypertrophic cardiomyopathy, mitral valve prolapse, silent myocardial ischemia, migraine, glaucoma, essential tremor, and thyrotoxicosis.[60–62] Beta blockers have been effective in treating unstable angina and for reducing the risk of cardiovascular mortality and nonfatal reinfarction in patients who have survived an acute myocardial infarction.[63,64] Beta blockade is a potential treatment modality, with or without thrombolytic therapy, for reducing the extent of myocardial injury and mortality during the hyperacute phase of myocardial infarction.[65–68]

Recently, various beta blockers were approved for use in patients with New York Heart Association class II to IV heart failure who are receiving angiotensin converting enzyme inhibitors, diuretics, and digoxin, to reduce the progression of disease and mortality.[69–72]

Beta-Adrenergic Receptor

Radioligand labeling techniques have greatly aided the investigation of adrenoreceptors,[7–11] and molecular pharmacologic techniques have positively delineated the beta-adrenoceptor structure as a polypeptide with a molecular weight of 67,000.[8]

In contrast to the older concept of adrenoreceptors as static entities in cells that simply serve to initiate the chain of events, newer theories hold that the adrenoceptors are subject to a wide variety of controlling influences resulting in dynamic regulation of adrenoceptor sites and/or their sensitivity to catecholamines. Changes in tissue concentration of receptor sites are probably involved in mediating important fluctuations in tissue sensitivity to drug action.[9,11,73] These principles may have significant clinical

and therapeutic implications. For example, an apparent increase in the number of beta adrenoceptors, and thus a supersensitivity to agonists, may be induced by chronic exposure to antagonists.[9,73] With prolonged adrenoceptor-blocker therapy, receptor occupancy by catecholamines can be diminished and the number of available receptors can be increased.[73] When the beta-adrenoceptor blocker is withdrawn suddenly, an increased pool of sensitive receptors will be open to endogenous catecholamine stimulation. The resultant adrenergic stimulation could precipitate unstable angina pectoris and/or a myocardial infarction.[74] The concentration of beta adrenoceptors in the membrane of mononuclear cells decreases significantly with age.[7]

Using radioligand techniques, a decrease in beta-adrenoceptor sites in the myocardium has been demonstrated in patients with chronic congestive heart failure.[75,76] An apparent reduction in beta adrenoceptors and/or beta-adrenoceptor function has also been associated with the development of refractoriness or desensitization to endogenous and exogenous catecholamines,[77] a phenomenon probably caused by the prolonged exposure of these adrenoceptors to high levels of catecholamines.[78] This desensitization phenomenon is caused not by a change in receptor formation or degradation but rather by catecholamine-induced changes in the conformation of the receptor sites, thus rendering them ineffective.[79] More recently it has been determined that one of the most important mechanisms for explaining the rapid regulation of beta-adrenergic receptor function is agonist stimulation of receptor phosphorylation, which leads to decreased sensitivity to further catecholamine stimulation. When the receptors are phosphorylated by protein kinases, the end result is a decreased coupling to Gs and decreased stimulation of adenyl cyclase. A receptor-directed protein kinase, known as beta-adrenergic receptor kinase (BARK), phosphorylates the receptors only when they are occupied by an agonist.[80,81] It was subsequently discovered that BARK is a member of at least six protein-regulated receptor kinases that can phosphorylate an regulate a wide variety of G protein–coupled receptors.[10] Phosphorylation of the receptor is not sufficient to fully desensitize receptor function. A second reaction must occur, which involves an "arresting protein" known as arrestin.[82–84,84a] Agonists also produce reversible sequestration (internalization) of receptors. Beta-adrenoceptor blocking drugs do not induce desensitization or changes in the conformation of receptors but do block the ability of catecholamines to desensitize receptors.[79]

Basic Pharmacologic Differences among Beta-Adrenoceptor Blocking Drugs

More than 100 beta-adrenoceptor blockers have been synthesized during the past 35 years and over 30 are available worldwide for clinical use.[85] Selectivity for two subgroups of the beta-adrenoceptor population has also been taken advantage of: beta$_1$ receptors in the heart and beta$_2$ receptors in the peripheral circulation and bronchi.[60,86] More controversial has been the introduction of beta-blocking drugs with alpha-adrenergic blocking actions, varying amounts of selective and nonselective intrinsic sympathomimetic activity (partial agonist activity), calcium-channel blocker activity, antioxidant actions, effects on nitric oxide production, and nonspecific membrane stabilizing effects.[62,87–89] There are also pharmacokinetic differences between beta-blocking drugs that may be of clinical importance.[60,86]

Sixteen beta-adrenoceptor blockers are now marketed in the United States for cardiovascular disorders: propranolol for angina

TABLE 7-3. Pharmacodynamic Properties of β-Adrenergic Blocking Drugs

	β_1 Blockade Potency Ratio (propranolol = 1.0)	Relative β_1 Selectivity	Intrinsic Sympathomimetic Activity	Membrane Stabilizing Activity
Acebutolol	0.3	+	+	+
Atenolol	1.0	++	0	0
Betaxolol	1.0	++	0	+
Bisoprolol*	10.0	++	0	0
Carteolol	10.0	0	+	0
Carvedilol†	10.0	0	0	++
Esmolol	0.02	++	0	0
Labetalol‡	0.3	0	+	0
Metoprolol	1.0	++	0	0
Nadolol	1.0	0	0	0
Nebivolol§	10.0	++	0	0
Oxprenolol	0.5–1.0	0	+	+
Penbutolol	1.0	0	+	0
Pindolol	6.0	0	++	+
Propranolol	1.0	0	0	++
Sotalol¶	0.3	0	0	0
Timolol	6.0	0	0	0
Isomer-D-propranolol	—	—	—	++

++ = strong effect; + = modest effect; 0 = absent effect.

*Bisoprolol is also approved as a first-line antihypertensive therapy in combination with a very low dose diuretic.

†Carvedilol has peripheral vasodilating activity and additional α_1-adrenergic blocking activity.

‡Labetalol has additional α_1-adrenergic blocking activity and direct vasodilatory activity.

§Nebivolol can augment vascular nitric oxide release.

¶Sotalol has an additional type of antiarrhythmic activity.

Source: Adapted with permission from Frishman.[61]

pectoris, arrhythmias, systemic hypertension, migraine prophylaxis, essential tremor, and hypertrophic cardiomyopathy and for reducing the risk of cardiovascular mortality in survivors of an acute myocardial infarction; nadolol for hypertension and angina pectoris; timolol for hypertension and for reducing the risk of cardiovascular mortality and nonfatal reinfarction in survivors of myocardial infarction and in topical form for glaucoma; atenolol hypertension and angina and in intravenous and oral formulations for reducing the risk of cardiovascular mortality in survivors of myocardial infarction; metoprolol for hypertension, angina pectoris, moderate congestive heart failure, and in intravenous and oral formulations for reducing the risk of cardiovascular mortality in survivors of acute myocardial infarction; penbutolol, bisoprolol, and pindolol for treating hypertension; betaxolol and carteolol for hypertension and in a topical form for glaucoma; acebutolol for hypertension and ventricular arrhythmias; intravenous esmolol for supraventricular arrhythmias; sotalol for ventricular and atrial arrhythmias; labetalol for hypertension and in intravenous form for hypertensive emergencies; and carvedilol for hypertension and moderate-to-severe congestive heart failure.[60,62,69,90–97] In addition, oxprenolol has been approved for use in hypertension but is not marketed in the United States. Currently under investigation are two ultra-short-acting beta blockers for use in patients with arrhythmia, landiolol and ONO-1011,[98–99] and nebivolol for hypertension.[100]

Despite the extensive experience with beta blockers in clinical practice, there have been no studies suggesting that any of these agents have major advantages or disadvantages in relation to the others for treatment of many cardiovascular diseases. When any available blocker is titrated properly, it can be effective in patients with arrhythmia, hypertension, or angina pectoris.[60,62,86–97] However, one agent may be more effective than other agents in

reducing adverse reactions in some patients and for managing specific situations.[96]

Potency

Beta-adrenergic-receptor blocking drugs are competitive inhibitors of catecholamine binding at beta-adrenergic-receptor sites. The dose–response curve of the catecholamine is shifted to the right; that is, a given tissue response requires a higher concentration of agonist in the presence of beta-blocking drugs.[61] Beta$_1$-blocking potency can be assessed by the inhibition of tachycardia produced by isoproterenol or exercise (the more reliable method in the intact organism); the potency varies from compound to compound (Table 7-3).[61] These differences in potency are of no therapeutic relevance; however they do explain the different drug doses needed to achieve effective beta-adrenergic blockade in initiating therapy in patients or in switching from one agent to another.[60,79,101]

Structure-Activity Relationships

The chemical structures of most beta-adrenergic blockers have several features in common with the agonist isoproterenol (Fig. 7-2), an aromatic ring with a substituted ethanolamine side chain linked to it by an -OCH$_2$ group.[60,62,102] The beta blocker timolol has a catecholamine-mimicking side chain but a more complex ring.

Most beta-blocking drugs exist as pairs of optical isomers and are marketed as racemic mixtures. Almost all the beta-blocking activity is found in the negative (−) levorotatory stereoisomer. The two stereoisomers of beta-adrenergic blockers are useful for differentiating between the pharmacologic effects of beta blockade and membrane-stabilizing activity (possessed by both optical forms). The positive (+) dextrorotatory stereoisomers of beta-blocking agents have no apparent clinical value[60,101,102] except for

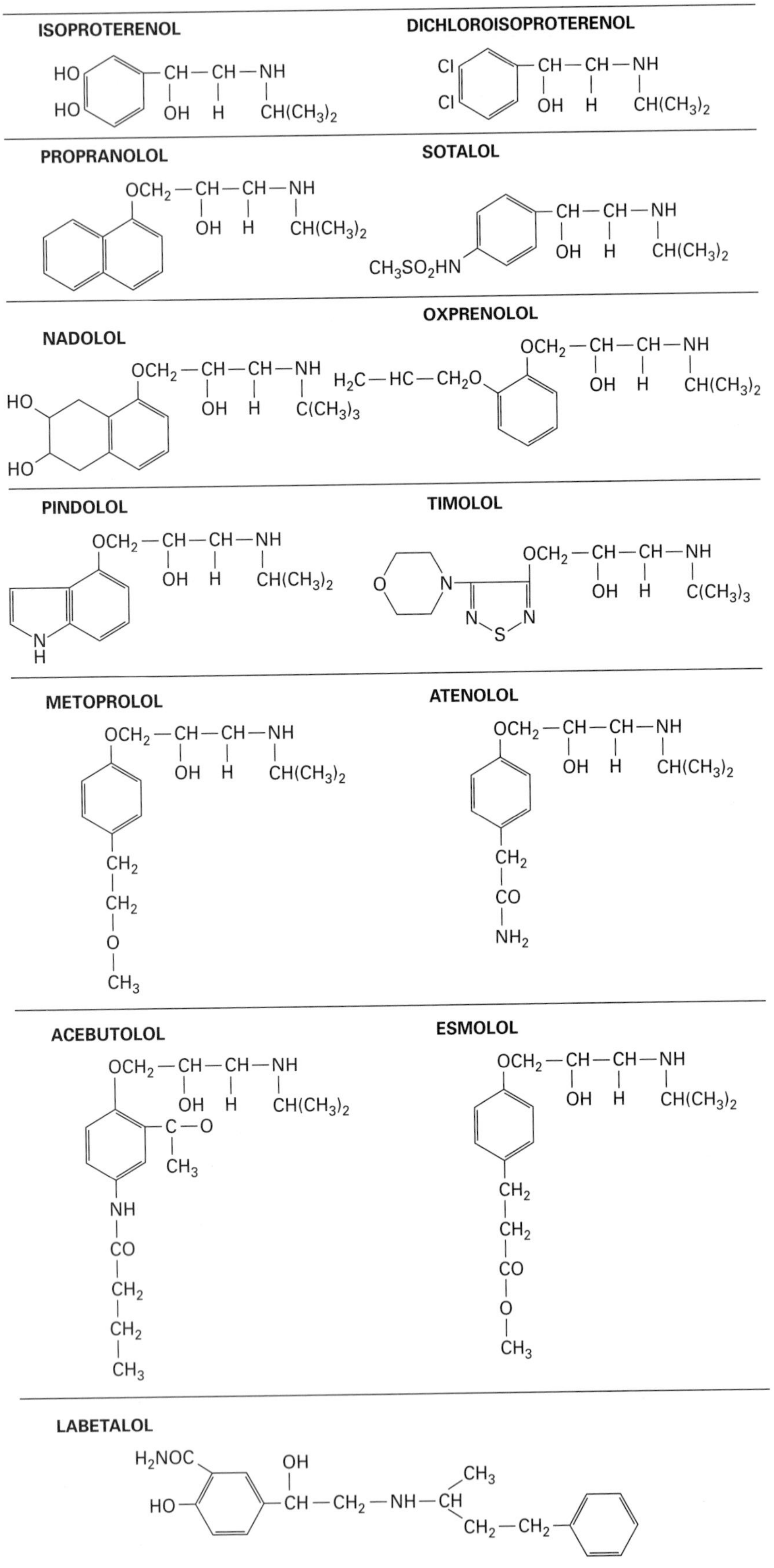

FIGURE 7-2. Molecular structure of the beta-adrenergic agonist isoproterenol and some beta-adrenergic blocking drugs.

FIGURE 7-3. Physiologic effects of beta-adrenergic blocking drugs with and without partial agonist activity in the presence of circulating catecholamines. When circulating catecholamines (●) combine with beta-adrenergic receptors, they produce a full physiologic response. When these receptors are occupied by a beta blocker lacking partial agonist activity (○), no physiologic effects from catecholamine stimulation can occur. A beta-blocking drug with partial agonist activity (⊕) also blocks the binding of catecholamines to beta-adrenergic receptors, but, in addition, the drug causes a relatively weak stimulation of the receptor. (*Reproduced with permission from Frishman.[93]*)

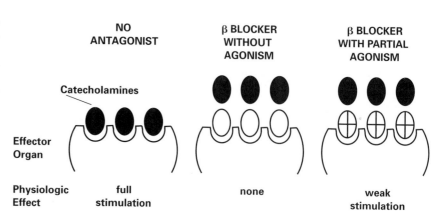

d-nebivolol, which has beta-blocking activity, and d-sotalol, which appears to have type III antiarrhythmic properties.[103] Penbutolol and timolol are marketed only in the l-form. As a result of asymmetric carbon atoms, labetalol and nebivolol have four stereoisomers and carvedilol has two.[104] With carvedilol, beta-blocking effects are seen in the (−) levorotatory stereoisomer and α blocking effects in both the (−) levorotatory and (+) dextrorotatory stereoisomers.

Membrane Stabilizing Activity

At concentrations well above therapeutic levels, certain beta blockers have a quinidine-like or local anesthetic membrane-stabilizing effect on the cardiac action potential. This property is exhibited equally by the two stereoisomers of the drug and is unrelated to beta-adrenergic blockade and major therapeutic antiarrhythmic actions. There is no evidence that membrane-stabilizing activity is responsible for any direct negative inotropic effect of the beta blockers, since drugs with and without this property equally depress left ventricular function.[105] However, membrane-stabilizing activity can manifest itself clinically with massive beta-blocker intoxications.[61,106,107]

Beta₁ Selectivity

Beta-adrenoceptor blockers may be classified as selective or nonselective, according to their relative abilities to antagonize the actions of sympathomimetic amines in some tissues at lower doses than those required in other tissues.[60,90] When used in low doses, beta₁-selective blocking agents such as acebutolol, betaxolol, bisoprolol, esmolol, atenolol, and metoprolol inhibit cardiac beta₂ receptors but have less influence on bronchial and vascular beta adrenoceptors (beta₂). In higher doses, however, beta₁-selective blocking agents also block beta₂ receptors. Accordingly, beta₁-selective agents may be safer than nonselective ones in patients with obstructive pulmonary disease, since beta₂ receptors remain available to mediate adrenergic bronchodilatation. Even selective beta blockers may aggravate bronchospasm in certain patients, so these drugs should generally not be used in patients with bronchospastic disease.

A second theoretical advantage is that unlike nonselective beta blockers, beta₁-selective blockers in low doses may not block the beta₂ receptors that mediate dilatation of arterioles. During infusion of epinephrine, nonselective beta blockers can cause a pressor response by blocking beta₂-receptor–mediated vasodilatation, since alpha-adrenergic vasoconstrictor receptors are still operative. Selective beta₁ antagonists may not induce this pressor effect in the presence of epinephrine and may lessen the impairment of peripheral blood flow. It is possible that leaving the beta₂-receptors

unblocked and responsive to epinephrine may be functionally important in some patients with asthma, hypoglycemia, hypertension, or peripheral vascular disease treated with beta-adrenergic blocking drugs.[60,62,90]

Intrinsic Sympathomimetic Activity (Partial Agonist Activity)

Certain beta-adrenoceptor blockers possess intrinsic sympathomimetic activity (ISA, partial agonist activity) at beta₁-adrenoceptor receptors sites, beta₂-adrenoceptor receptors sites, or both.[108] In a beta blocker, this property is identified as a slight cardiac stimulation that can be blocked by propranolol.[60,62,93,94,96] The beta blockers with this property slightly activate the beta receptor in addition to preventing the access of natural or synthetic catecholamines to the receptor (Fig. 7-3). Dichloroisoprenaline, the first beta-adrenoceptor blocking drug synthesized, exerted such marked partial agonist activity that it was unsuitable for clinical use.[96] However, compounds with less partial agonist activity are effective beta-blocking drugs. The partial agonist effects of beta-adrenoceptor blocking drugs such as pindolol differ from those of the agonist epinephrine and isoproterenol in that the maximum pharmacologic response that can be obtained is low, although the affinity for the receptor is high. In the treatment of patients with arrhythmias, angina pectoris of effort, and hypertension, drugs with mild-to-moderate partial agonist activity appear to be as efficacious as are beta blockers lacking this property. It is still debated whether the presence of partial agonist activity in a beta blocker constitutes an overall advantage or disadvantage in cardiac therapy.[93] Drugs with partial agonist activity cause less slowing of the heart rate at rest than do propranolol and metoprolol, although the increments in heart rate with exercise are similarly blunted. These beta-blocking agents reduce peripheral vascular resistance and may also cause less depression or atrioventricular conduction than drugs lacking these properties.[93,109] Some investigators claim that partial agonist activity in a beta blocker protects against myocardial depression, adverse lipid changes, bronchial asthma, and peripheral vascular complications, as caused by propranolol.[93,109,110] The evidence to support these claims is not conclusive, and more definitive clinical trials will be necessary to resolve these issues.

Alpha-Adrenergic Activity

Labetalol is a beta blocker with antagonistic properties at both alpha and beta adrenoceptors, and it has direct vasodilator activity.[61,62,111] Labetalol has been shown to be 6 to 10 times less potent than phentolamine at alpha-adrenergic receptors and 1.5 to 4 times less potent than propranolol at beta-adrenergic

TABLE 7-4. Pharmacokinetic Properties of Various Beta-Adrenoceptor Blocking Drugs

Drug	Extent of Absorption % of Dose	Extent of Bioavailability % of Dose	Dose-Dependent Bioavailability (major first-pass hepatic metabolism)	Interpatient Variations in Plasma Levels	β-Blocking Plasma Concentrations	Protein Binding (%)	Lipid Solubility*
Acebutolol	>90	≈40	Yes	7-fold	0.2–2.0 μg/mL	25	Low
Atenolol	≈50	≈40	No	4-fold	0.2–5.0 μg/mL	<5	Low
Betaxolol	>90	≈80	No	2-fold	0.005–0.05 μg/mL	50	Low
Bisoprolol	≈90	≈88	No	—	0.005–0.02 μg/mL	≈33	Low
Carteolol	≈90	≈90	No	2-fold	40–160 ng/mL	23–30	Low
Carvedilol	>90	≈30	Yes	5- to 10-fold	10–100 ng/mL	98	Moderate
Celiprolol	≈30	≈30	No	3-fold	—	22–24	Low
Esmolol†	NA	NA	NA	5-fold	0.15–1.0 μg/mL	55	Low
Labetalol	>90	≈33	Yes	10-fold	0.7–3.0 μg/mL	≈50	Moderate
Metoprolol	>90	≈50	Yes	10-fold	50–100 ng/mL	12	Moderate
Metoprolol LA	>90	65–70	Yes	10-fold	35–323 ng/mL	12	Moderate
Nadolol	≈30	≈30	No	7-fold	50–100 ng/mL	≈30	Low
Nebivolol	>90	12–96	Yes	7-fold	1.5 ng/mL	98	High
Oxprenolol	≈90	19–74	Yes	5-fold	80–100 ng/mL	80	Moderate
Penbutolol	>90	≈100	No	4-fold	5–15 ng/mL	80–98	High
Pindolol	>90	≈ 90	No	4-fold	50–100 ng/mL	57	Moderate
Propranolol	>90	30–70	Yes	20-fold	50–100 ng/mL	93	High
Propranolol LA	>90	30–40	Yes	20- to 30-fold	20–100 ng/mL	93	High
Sotalol	≈70	≈ 90	No	4-fold	1–3.2 μg/mL	0	Low
Timolol	>90	≈ 75	Yes	7-fold	5–10 ng/mL	≈10	Low-moderate

NA = not applicable or no data; LA = long-acting.

*Determined by the distribution ratio between octanol and water.

†Ultra-short-acting β blocker available only in intravenous form.

Source: Adapted with permission from Frishman.[61]

receptors; it is itself 4 to 16 times less potent at alpha than at beta adrenoceptors.[61,62,111] Like other beta blockers, it is useful in the treatment of hypertension and angina pectoris.[61,112,113] Unlike most beta blockers, however, the additional alpha-adrenergic blocking actions of labetalol lead to a reduction in peripheral vascular resistance that may maintain cardiac output.[61,111] Whether concomitant alpha-adrenergic blocking activity is actually advantageous in a beta blocker remains to be determined.[114,115]

Carvedilol is another beta blocker having additional alpha-blocking activity. Compared to labetalol, carvedilol has a ratio of alpha$_1$ to beta blockade of 1:10. On a milligram-to-milligram basis, carvedilol is about two to four times more potent than propranolol as a beta blocker.[116] In addition, carvedilol has antioxidant and antiproliferative activities.[117] Carvedilol has been used for the treatment of hypertension and angina pectoris and has been shown to be effective as a treatment for patients having symptomatic heart failure.[118]

Direct Vasodilator Activity

Bucindolol is a nonselective beta blocker which, in addition, has direct peripheral vasodilatory activity. It has undergone clinical evaluation as a treatment for symptomatic congestive heart failure,[118,119] with less success than the benefit observed with other beta blockers used for this indication.[120]

Nebivolol is a beta$_1$-selective adrenergic-receptor antagonist with a unique ability to increase vascular nitric oxide production,[121–125] and the drug is currently being evaluated as a treatment for hypertension.

Pharmacokinetics

Although the beta-adrenergic blocking drugs as a group have similar therapeutic effects, their pharmacokinetic properties are markedly different (Table 7-4).[61,101,105,126–128] Their varied aromatic ring structures lead to differences in completeness or gastrointestinal absorption, amount of first-pass hepatic metabolism, lipid-solubility, protein binding, extent of distribution in the body, penetration into the brain, concentration in the heart, rate of hepatic biotransformation, pharmacologic activity of metabolites, and renal clearance of a drug and its metabolites, which may influence the clinical usefulness of these drugs in some patients.[60,62,101,105,127] The desirable pharmacokinetic characteristics in this group of compounds are a lack of major individual differences in bioavailability and in metabolic clearance of the drug and a rate of removal from active tissue sites that is slow enough to allow longer dosing intervals.[60,62,129]

The beta blockers can be divided by their pharmacokinetic properties into two broad categories: those eliminated by hepatic metabolism, which tend to have relatively short plasma half-lives, and those eliminated unchanged by the kidney, which tend to have longer half-lives.[60] Propranolol and metoprolol are both lipid-soluble, are almost completely absorbed by the small intestine, and are largely metabolized by the liver. They tend to have highly variable bioavailability and relatively short plasma half-lives.[62,90,101,127] A lack of correlation between the duration of clinical pharmacologic effect and plasma half-life may allow these drugs to be administered once or twice daily.[60]

In contrast, agents such as atenolol and nadolol are more water-soluble, are incompletely absorbed through the gut, and are eliminated unchanged by the kidney.[91,92] In addition to longer half-lives, they tend to have less variable bioavailability in patients with normal renal function, allowing one dose a day.[91,92] The longer half-lives may be useful in patients who find compliance with frequent beta-blocker dosing a problem.[91]

Long-acting sustained-release preparations of propranolol and metoprolol are available (see Table 7-4).[129] A delayed-release long-acting propranolol formulation is now in clinical development. Studies have shown that long-acting propranolol and metoprolol can provide a much smoother curve of daily plasma levels than do comparable divided doses of conventional immediate-release formulations.[129–132]

Ultra-short-acting beta blockers are now available and may be useful where a short duration of action is desired (e.g., in patients with questionable congestive heart failure).[98,99] One of these compounds, esmolol, a beta$_1$-selective drug (see Tables 7-3 and 7-4) has been shown to be useful in the treatment of perioperative hypertension and supraventricular tachycardias.[133] The short half-life (approximately 15 min) relates to the rapid metabolism of the drug by blood and hepatic esterases. Metabolism does not seem to be altered by disease states.[134] A propranolol nasal spray that can provide immediate beta blockade has been tested in clinical trials,[135] as has a new sublingual immediate-release formulation (esprolol).[136] A delayed-release sustained-release chrono-therapeutic formulation of propranolol will soon be available for clinical use.

The specific pharmacokinetic properties of individual beta-adrenergic blockers (first-pass metabolism, active metabolites, lipid solubility, and protein binding) may be clinically important.[62,78,125] When drugs with extensive first-pass metabolism are taken by mouth, they undergo so much hepatic biotransformation that relatively little drug reaches the systemic circulation.[60,62,101,124] Depending on the extent of first-pass effect, an oral dose of beta blocker must be larger than an intravenous dose to produce the same clinical effects.[90,101,124] Some beta-adrenergic blockers are transformed into pharmacologically active compounds (acebutolol, nebivolol) rather than inactive metabolites.[137] The total pharmacologic effect therefore depends on the amount of the drug administered and its active metabolites.[125,126] Characteristics of lipid solubility in a beta blocker have been associated with the ability of the drug to concentrate in the brain,[60,62] and many side effects of these drugs, which have not been clearly related to beta blockade, may result from their actions on the central nervous system (CNS) (lethargy, mental depression, and hallucinations).[60,92] It is still not certain, however, whether drugs that are less lipid-soluble cause fewer of these adverse reactions.[78,91,92,138–140]

There are genetic polymorphisms that can influence the metabolism of various beta-blocking drugs, which include propranolol, metoprolol, timolol, and carvedilol.[141–143] A single codon difference of CYP2D6 may explain a significant proportion of interindividual variation of propranolol's pharmacokinetics in Chinese subjects.[142] There is no effect of exercise on propranolol's pharmacokinetics.[144]

Relationships between Dose, Plasma Level, and Efficacy

Attempts have been made to establish a relation between the oral dose, the plasma level measured by gas chromatography, and the pharmacologic effect of each beta-blocking drug.[125] After administration of a certain oral dose, beta-blocking drugs that are largely metabolized in the liver show large interindividual variation in circulating plasma levels.[60,62] Many explanations have been proposed to explain wide individual differences in the relation between plasma concentrations of beta blockers and any associated therapeutic effect. First, patients may have different levels of "sympathetic tone" (circulating catecholamines and active beta-adrenoceptor binding sites) and may thus require different drug concentrations to achieve adequate beta blockade.[101] Second, many beta blockers have flat

plasma–drug level response curves.[125] Third, active drug isomers and active metabolites are not specifically measured in many plasma assays. Fourth, the clinical effect of a drug may last longer than the period suggested by the drug's half-life in plasma,[101] since recycling of the beta blocker between receptor site and neuronal nerve endings may occur. Despite the lack of correlation between plasma levels and therapeutic effect, there is some evidence that a relation does exist between the logarithm of the plasma level and the beta-blocking effect (blockade of exercise- or isoproterenol-induced tachycardia).[90,101,125] Plasma levels have little to offer as therapeutic guides except for ensuring compliance and diagnosis of overdose. Pharmacodynamic characteristics and clinical response should be used as guides in determining efficacy.

Clinical Effects and Therapeutic Applications

The therapeutic efficacy and safety of beta-adrenoceptor blocking drugs has been well established in patients with angina pectoris, cardiac arrhythmias, congestive cardiomyopathy, hypertension, and for reducing the risk of mortality and possibly nonfatal reinfarction in survivors of acute myocardial infarction.[60,62,66] These drugs may be useful as a primary protection against cardiovascular morbidity and mortality in hypertensive patients.[145] The drugs are also used for a multitude of other cardiac (Table 7-5)[61,62,66,146–153] and noncardiac (Table 7-6)[61,62,78,154–160] uses.

Cardiovascular Effects

Effects on Elevated Systemic Blood Pressure

Beta-adrenergic blockers are effective in reducing the blood pressure of many patients with systemic hypertension (Tables 7-7 and 7-8), including elderly patients with isolated systolic hypertension,[59,161–163] and have been cited as a first-line treatment by the Fifth and Sixth Reports of the Joint National Committee on Prevention, Detection, Evaluation and Treatment of High Blood Pressure (JNC-V and VI).[164,165] However, in a recent meta analysis it was shown that the beneficial effects on clinical outcomes with diuretic treatment used as monotherapy in the elderly were more favorable

TABLE 7-5. Reported Cardiovascular Indications for β-Adrenoceptor Blocking Drugs

Hypertension* (systolic and diastolic)
Isolated systolic hypertension in the elderly
Angina pectoris*
"Silent" myocardial ischemia
Supraventricular arrhythmias*
Ventricular arrhythmias*
Reducing the risk of mortality and reinfarction in survivors of acute myocardial infarction*
Reducing the risk of mortality following percutaneous coronary revascularization
Hyperacute phase of myocardial infarction*
Dissection of aorta
Hypertrophic cardiomyopathy*
Reversing left ventricular hypertrophy
Digitalis intoxication (tachyarrhythmias)*
Mitral valve prolapse
QT interval prolongation syndrome
Tetralogy of Fallot
Mitral stenosis
Congestive cardiomyopathy*
Fetal tachycardia
Neurocirculatory asthenia

*Indications formally approved by the U.S. FDA.

TABLE 7-6. Some Reported Noncardiovascular Indications for β-Adrenoceptor Blocking Drugs

Neuropsychiatric
   Migraine prophylaxis*
   Essential tremor*
   Situational anxiety
   Alcohol withdrawal (delirium tremens)
Endocrine
   Thyrotoxicosis*
   Hyperparathyroidism
   Pheochromocytoma (after α blockers)*
Other
   Glaucoma*
   Portal hypertension and gastrointestinal bleeding
   Severe burns

*Indications formally approved by the U.S. FDA.

than those observed with beta blockers.[166] Most recently it was shown that losartan had a more favorable effect than atorolol on cardiovascular morbidity and mortality and a similar reduction in blood pressure in hypertensive patients with left ventricular hypertrophy.[166a] In a prospective cohort study, it was found that antihypertensive therapy with beta blockers was associated with a greater incidence of type II diabetes than treatment with ACE inhibitors, diuretics, and calcium blockers.[167] However, this increased risk of diabetes must be weighed against the proven benefit of beta blockers in reducing the risk of cardiovascular events.[168]

There is no consensus as to the mechanism(s) by which these drugs lower blood pressure. It is probable that some or all of the following proposed mechanisms play a part. Beta blockers without vasodilatory activity appear to be more efficacious in white patients and younger patients than they are in the elderly and in black patients.[169]

Negative Chronotropic and Inotropic Effects

Slowing of the heart rate and some decrease in myocardial contractility with beta blockers lead to a decrease in cardiac output, which in both the short and long term may lead to a reduction in blood pressure.[60] It might be expected that these factors would be of particular importance in the treatment of hypertension related to high cardiac output[170] and increased sympathetic tone.

Differences in Effects on Plasma Renin

The relation between the hypotensive action of beta-blocking drugs and their ability to reduce plasma renin activity remains controversial. Some beta-blocking drugs can antagonize sympathetically mediated renin release,[171] although adrenergic activity is not the only mechanism by which renin release is mediated.

TABLE 7-7. Proposed Mechanisms to Explain the Antihypertensive Actions of β Blockers

Reduction in cardiac output
Inhibition of renin
CNS effects
Effects on prejunctional β receptors: reductions in norepinephrine release
Reduction in peripheral vascular resistance
Improvement in vascular compliance
Reduction in vasomotor tone
Reduction in plasma volume
Resetting of baroreceptor levels
Attenuation of pressor response to catecholamines with exercise and stress

Source: Reproduced with permission from Frishman.[62]

Other major determinants are sodium balance, posture, and renal perfusion pressure.

The important question remains whether there is a clinical correlation between the beta blocker's effect on the plasma renin activity and the lowering of blood pressure. Investigators[171] have found that "high renin" patients do not respond or may even show a rise in blood pressure, and that "normal renin" patients have less predictable responses. In high-renin hypertensive patients, it has been suggested that renin may not be the only factor maintaining the high blood pressure state. At present, the exact role of renin reduction in blood pressure control is not well defined.

Central Nervous System Effect

There is now good clinical and experimental evidence to suggest that beta blockers cross the blood–brain barrier and enter the CNS.[172] Although there is little doubt that beta blockers with high lipophilicity (e.g., metoprolol, propranolol) enter the CNS in high concentrations, a direct antihypertensive effect mediated by their presence has not been well defined. Also, beta blockers that are less lipid-soluble and less likely to concentrate in the brain appear to be as effective in lowering blood pressure as propranolol.[91,92]

Peripheral Resistance

Nonselective beta blockers have no primary action in lowering peripheral resistance and indeed may cause it to rise by leaving the alpha-stimulatory mechanisms unopposed.[173] The vasodilating effect of catecholamines on skeletal muscle blood vessels is beta$_2$-mediated, suggesting possible therapeutic advantages in using beta$_1$-selective blockers, agents with partial agonist activity, and drugs with alpha-blocking activity. Since beta$_1$-selectivity diminishes as the drug dosage is raised, and since hypertensive patients generally have to be given far larger doses than are required simply to block the beta$_1$-receptors alone, beta$_1$-selectivity[174] offers the clinician little if any real specific advantage in the treatment of hypertension.[90,174]

Effects on Prejunctional Receptors

Apart from their effects on postjunctional tissue beta receptors, it is believed that blockade of prejunctional beta receptors may be involved in the hemodynamic actions of beta-blocking drugs. The stimulation of prejunctional alpha$_2$ receptors leads to a reduction in the quantity of norepinephrine released by the postganglionic sympathetic fibers.[175,176] Conversely, stimulation of prejunctional beta receptors is followed by an increase in the quantity of norepinephrine released by the postganglionic sympathetic fibers.[177–179] Blockade of prejunctional beta receptors should therefore diminish the amount of norepinephrine released, leading to a weaker stimulation of postjunctional alpha receptors—an effect that would produce less vasoconstriction. Opinions differ, however, on the contributions of presynaptic beta blockade to both a reduction in the peripheral vascular resistance and the antihypertensive effects on beta-blocking drugs.

Other Proposed Mechanisms

Less well documented effects of beta blockers that may contribute to their antihypertensive actions include favorable effects on arterial compliance,[180] venous tone and plasma volume,[60] membrane-stabilizing activity,[181,182] and resetting of baroreceptors.[182a]

Genetic polymorphisms of the beta$_1$ and beta$_2$ receptor and other genetic markers have been implicated as a cause for systemic hypertension and the responsiveness of patients to treatment with beta blockers.[183–186]

TABLE 7-8. Pharmacodynamic Properties and Cardiac Effects of β-Adrenoceptor Blockers

	Relative β_1-Selectivity	ISA	MSA	HR Rest/Exer	MC Rest	BP Rest/Exer	AV Conduction Rest	Antiarrhythmic Effect
Acebutolol	+	+	+	↓↔/↓	↓	↓/↓	↓	+
Atenolol	++	0	0	↓/↓	↓	↓/↓	↓	+
Betaxolol	++	0	+	↓/↓	↓	↓/↓	↓	+
Bisoprolol	++	0	0	↓/↓	↓	↓/↓	↓	+
Carteolol	0	+	0	↓↔/↓	↓↔	↓	↓	+
Carvedilol†	0	0	++	↓↔/↓	↓↔/	↓/↓	↓↔	+
Esmolol	++	0	0	↓/↓	↓	↓/↓	↓	+
Labetalol‡	0	+	0	↓↔/↓	↓↔	↓/↓↓	↓↔	+
Metoprolol	++	0	0	↓/↓	↓	↓/↓	↓	+
Nadolol	0	0	0	↓/↓	↓	↓/↓	↓	+
Nebivolol§	++	0	0	↓/↓	↓↔	↓/↓	↓↔	+
Oxprenolol	0	+	+	↓↔/↓	↓↔	↓/↓	↓↔	+
Penbutolol	0	+	0	↓↔/↓	↓↔	↓/↓	↓↔	+
Pindolol	0	++	+	↓↔/↓	↓↔	↓/↓	↓↔	+
Propranolol	0	0	++	↓/↓	↓	↓/↓	↓	+
Sotalol	0	0	0	↓/↓	↓	↓/↓	↓	+
Timolol	0	0	0	↓/↓	↓	↓/↓	↓	+
Isomer-D-propranolol	0	0	++	↔/↔	↔↓ ¶	↔/↔	↔↓ ¶	+ ¶

ISA = intrinsic sympathomimetic activity; MSA = membrane stabilizing activity; HR = heart rate; MC = myocardial contractility; BP = blood pressure; AV = atrioventricular; rest/exer = resting and exercise; ++ = strong effect; + = modest effect; 0 = absent effect; ↑ = elevation; ↓ = reduction; ↔ = no change.

*β_1 selectivity is seen only with low therapeutic drug concentrations. With higher concentrations, β_1 selectivity is not seen.

†Carvedilol has peripheral vasodilating activity and additional α_1-adrenergic blocking activity.

‡Labetalol has additional α_1-adrenergic blocking activity and direct β_2 vasodilatory activity.

§Nebivolol can augment vascular nitric oxide release.

¶Effects of D-propranolol with doses in human beings well above the therapeutic level. The isomer also lacks β blocking activity.

Source: Adapted from Refs. 2, 3, and 21, with permission.

Effects in Angina Pectoris

Ahlquist[1] demonstrated that sympathetic innervation of the heart causes the release of norepinephrine, activating beta adrenoreceptors in myocardial cells (Table 7-8). This adrenergic stimulation causes an increment in heart rate, isometric contractile force, and maximal velocity of muscle fiber shortening, all of which lead to an increase in cardiac work and myocardial oxygen consumption.[187] The decrease in intraventricular pressure and volume caused by the sympathetic-mediated enhancement of cardiac contractility tends, on the other hand, to reduce myocardial oxygen consumption by reducing myocardial wall tension (LaPlace's law).[188] Although there is a net increase in myocardial oxygen demand, this is normally balanced by an increase in coronary blood flow. Angina pectoris is believed to occur when oxygen demand exceeds supply, i.e., when coronary blood flow is restricted by coronary atherosclerosis. Since the conditions that precipitate anginal attacks (exercise, emotional stress, food, etc.) cause an increase in cardiac sympathetic activity, it might be expected that blockade of cardiac beta adrenoreceptors would relieve the anginal symptoms. It is on this basis that the early clinical studies with beta-blocking drugs in patients with angina pectoris were initiated.[189]

Three main factors—heart rate, ventricular systolic pressure, and the size of the left ventricle—contribute to the myocardial oxygen requirements of the left ventricle. Of these, heart rate and systolic pressure appear to be important (the product of heart rate multiplied by the systolic blood pressure is a reliable index to predict the precipitation of angina in a given patient).[190,191] However, myocardial contractility may be even more important.[192]

The reduction in heart rate effected by beta blockade has two favorable consequences: (1) a decrease in blood pressure, thus reducing myocardial oxygen needs, and (2) a longer diastolic filling time

associated with a slower heart rate, allowing for increased coronary perfusion.[193] Beta blockade also reduces exercise-induced blood pressure increments, the velocity of cardiac contraction, and oxygen consumption at any patient workload.[190,191] Pretreatment heart rate variability or low exercise tolerance may predict which patients will respond best to treatment with beta blockade.[192,194] Despite the favorable effects on heart rate, the blunting of myocardial contractility with β blockers may also be the primary mechanism of their antianginal benefit.[192,195]

Studies in dogs have shown that propranolol causes a decrease in coronary blood flow.[196] However, subsequent experimental animal studies have demonstrated that beta-blocking–induced shunting occurs in the coronary circulation, thus maintaining blood flow to ischemic areas, especially in the subendocardial region.[197] In human beings, concomitantly with the decrease in myocardial oxygen consumption, beta blockers can cause a reduction in coronary blood flow and a rise in coronary vascular resistance.[198] On the basis of coronary autoregulation, the overall reduction in myocardial oxygen needs with β-blockers may be sufficient cause for this decrease in coronary blood flow.[190,191]

Virtually all beta blockers—whether or not they have partial agonist activity, alpha-blocking effects, membrane-stabilizing activity, and general or selective beta-blocking properties—produce some degree of increased work capacity without pain in patients with angina pectoris. Therefore it must be concluded that this results from their common property: blockade of cardiac beta receptors.[190] Both D- and L-propranolol have membrane-stabilizing activity, but only L-propranolol has significant beta-blocking activity. The racemic mixture (D- and L-propranolol) causes a decrease in both heart rate and force of contraction in dogs, while the D-isomer has hardly any effect.[199] In human beings, D-propranolol, which has "membrane" activity but no beta-blocking properties, has been found to be ineffective in relieving angina pectoris even at very high doses.[200]

Beta blockers are recommended as the initial therapy for long-term management of angina pectoris.[201–206]

Although exercise tolerance improves with beta blockade, the increments in heart rate and blood pressure with exercise are blunted, and the rate-pressure product (systolic blood pressure × heart rate) achieved when pain occurs is lower than that reached during a control run.[207,208] The depressed pressure-rate product at the onset of pain (about 20% reduction from control) is reported to occur with various beta-blocking drugs, probably related to decreased cardiac output. Thus, although there is increased exercise tolerance with beta blockade, patients exercise less than might be expected. This may also relate to the action of beta blockers in increasing left ventricular size, causing increased left ventricular wall tension and an increase in oxygen consumption at a given blood pressure.[209]

Combined Use of Beta Blockers with Other Antianginal Therapies in Angina Pectoris

Nitrates

Combined therapy with nitrates and beta blockers may be more efficacious for the treatment of angina pectoris than the use of either drug alone.[190,201,206,210] The primary effects of beta blockers are to cause a reduction in both resting heart rate and the response of heart rate to exercise. Since nitrates produce a reflex increase in heart rate and contractility owing to a reduction in arterial pressure, concomitant beta-blocker therapy is extremely effective because it blocks this reflex increment in the heart rate. Similarly, the preservation of diastolic coronary flow with a reduced heart rate will also be beneficial.[190] In patients with a propensity for myocardial failure who may have a slight increase in heart size with the beta blockers, the nitrates will counteract this tendency by reducing heart size as a result of its peripheral venodilator effects. During the administration of nitrates, the reflex increase in contractility that is mediated through the sympathetic nervous system will be checked by the presence of beta blockers. Similarly, the increase in coronary resistance associated with beta-blocker administration can be ameliorated by the administration of nitrates.[190]

Calcium-Entry Blocker

Calcium-entry blockers are a group of drugs that block transmembrane calcium currents in vascular smooth muscle to cause arterial vasodilatation (see Chap. 9). Some calcium-entry blockers (diltiazem, mibefradil, verapamil) also slow the heart rate and reduce atrioventricular (AV) conduction. Combined therapy with beta-adrenergic and calcium-entry blockers can provide clinical benefits for patients with angina pectoris who still remain symptomatic with either agent used alone.[201,206,211–213] Because adverse cardiovascular effects can occur, however, patients being considered for such treatment must be carefully selected and observed.[211,212]

Angina at Rest and Vasospastic Angina

Angina pectoris can be caused by multiple mechanisms, including coronary vasospasm, myocardial bridging, and thrombosis, which appear to be responsible for ischemia in a significant proportion of patients with unstable angina and angina at rest.[214,214a] Therefore, beta blockers that primarily reduce myocardial oxygen

consumption but fail to exert vasodilating effects on coronary vasculature may not be totally effective in patients in whom angina is caused or increased by dynamic alterations in coronary luminal diameter.[190,212] Despite potential dangers in rest and vasospastic angina, beta blockers have been used successfully both as monotherapy and in combination with vasodilating agents in many patients.[13,215] The drugs have also been shown to favorably affect C-reactive protein concentrations in the blood, an important disease marker for active coronary artery disease.[215a]

Electrophysiologic and Antiarrhythmic Effects

Adrenoceptor-blocking drugs have two main effects on the electrophysiologic properties of specialized cardiac tissue (Table 7-9).[216] The first effect results from specific blockade of adrenergic stimulation of cardiac pacemaker potentials. In concentrations causing significant inhibition of adrenergic receptors, beta blockers produce little change in the transmembrane potentials of cardiac muscle. By competitively inhibiting adrenergic stimulation, however, beta blockers decrease the slope of phase 4 depolarization and the spontaneous firing rate of sinus or ectopic pacemakers and thus decrease automaticity. Arrhythmias occurring in the setting of enhanced automaticity—as seen in myocardial infarction, digitalis toxicity, hyperthyroidism, and pheochromocytoma—would therefore be expected to respond well to beta blockade.[61,216–218]

The second electrophysiologic effect of beta blockers involves membrane-stabilizing action, also known as "quinidine-like" or "local anesthetic" action, which is observed only at very high dose levels. This property is unrelated to inhibition of catecholamine action and is possessed equally by both the D- and L-isomers of the drugs (D-isomers have almost no beta-blocking activity).[216] Characteristic of this effect is a reduction in the rate of rise of the intracardiac action potential without an effect on the spike duration of the resting potential.[216] Associated features include an elevated electrical threshold of excitability, a delay in conduction velocity, and a significant increase in the effective refractory period. This effect and its attendant changes have been explained by inhibition of the depolarizing inward sodium current.[216] There is a greater antifibrillatory effect when beta blockers are combined with some other antiarrhythmics.[219]

Sotalol is unique among the beta blockers in that it possesses class III antiarrhythmic properties, causing prolongation of the action potential period and thus delaying repolarization.[220] Clinical studies have verified the efficacy of sotalol in the control and prevention of both atrial and ventricular arrhythmias,[221–232] but additional investigation will be required to determine whether its class III antiarrhythmic properties contribute significantly to its efficacy as an antiarrhythmic agent. A clinical study demonstrated an

TABLE 7-9. Antiarrhythmic Properties of β Blockers

β Blockade
  Electrophysiology: depress excitability and conduction
  Prevention of ischemia: decreased automaticity, inhibit reentrant
    mechanisms
Membrane-stabilizing effects
  Local anesthetic "quinidine-like" properties: depress excitability,
    prolong refractory period, delay conduction
  Clinically: probably not significant
Special pharmacologic properties
  β1-selectivity, intrinsic sympathomimetic activity (do not appear to
    contribute to antiarrhythmic effectiveness)

Source: Reproduced with permission from Frishman.[61]

increased mortality risk with d-sotalol, the stereoisomer with type III antiarrhythmic activity and no beta-blocking effect.[233,234]

There is a quantitative gender difference between men and women in response to d,l sotalol, which may explain the greater propensity of women to drug-induced torsades de pointes.[235] To ensure patient safety with sotalol use, it has been suggested that patients be admitted to the hospital for initiation of treatment.[236,237]

The most important mechanism underlying the antiarrhythmic effect of beta blockers, with the possible exclusion of sotalol, is believed to be beta blockade with resultant inhibition of pacemaker potentials. The contribution of membrane-stabilizing action does not appear to be clinically significant. In vitro experiments with human ventricular muscle have shown that the concentration of propranolol required for membrane stabilizing is 50 to 100 times the concentration that is usually associated with inhibition of exercise-induced tachycardia and at which only beta-blocking effects occur.[200] Moreover, D-propranolol, which possesses membrane-stabilizing properties but no beta-blocking action, is a weak antiarrhythmic even at high doses, while beta blockers devoid of membrane stabilizing action (atenolol, esmolol, metoprolol, nadolol, pindolol, etc.) have been shown to be effective antiarrhythmic drugs.[61,62,133] Differences in the overall clinical usefulness of beta blockers for arrhythmia are related to their other associated pharmacologic properties.[61,62]

Therapeutic Uses in Cardiac Arrhythmias

Beta-adrenergic blocking drugs have become an important treatment modality for various cardiac arrhythmias (Table 7-10), used alone and in combination with other antiarrhythmic drugs.[61,62,216,238–242] While it has long been believed that beta blockers are more effective in treating supraventricular arrhythmias than ventricular arrhythmias, this may not be the case.[243–246] These agents can be quite useful in the treatment of ventricular tachyarrhythmias in the setting of myocardial ischemia, mitral valve prolapse, and for other cardiovascular conditions (see Chap. 17).[246–253] A high prevalence of antibodies against beta$_1$ and beta$_2$ adrenoceptors has been observed in patients with atrial arrhythmias, ventricular arrhythmias, and conduction disturbances.[254,255]

TABLE 7-10. Effects of β Blockers in Various Arrhythmias

Supraventricular

Sinus tachycardia: treat underlying disorder; excellent response to β blocker if need to control rate (e.g., ischemia).

Atrial fibrillation: β blockers reduce rate, rarely restore sinus rhythm, may be useful in combination with digoxin.

Atrial flutter: β blockers reduce rate, sometimes restore sinus rhythm.

Atrial tachycardia: effective in slowing ventricular rate, may restore sinus rhythm; useful in prophylaxis.

Maintain patients in normal sinus rhythm after electrocardioversion of atrial and ventricular arrhythmias.

Ventricular

Premature ventricular contractions: good response to β blockers, especially digitalis-induced, exercise (ischemia-induced, mitral valve prolapse, or hypertrophic cardiomyopathy.

Ventricular tachycardia: effective as quinidine, most effective in digitalis toxicity or exercise (ischemia)-induced.

Ventricular fibrillation: electrical defibrillation is treatment of choice. β Blockers can be used to prevent recurrence in cases of excess digitalis or sympathomimetic amines; appear to be effective in reducing the incidence of ventricular fibrillation and sudden death post–myocardial infarction.

Source: Reproduced with permission from Frishman.[61]

TABLE 7-11. Possible Mechanisms by Which β Blockers Protect the Ischemic Myocardium

Reduction in myocardial consumption, heart rate, blood pressure, and myocardial contractility.

Augmentation of coronary blood flow; increase in diastolic perfusion time by reducing heart rate, augmentation of collateral blood flow, and coronary flow reserve, and redistribution of blood flow to ischemic areas.

Prevention of attenuation of atherosclerotic plaque, rupture, and subsequent coronary thrombosis.

Alterations in myocardial substrate utilization.

Decrease in microvascular damage.

Stabilization of cell and lysosomal membranes.

Shift of oxyhemoglobin dissociation curve to the right.

Inhibition of platelet aggregation.

Inhibition of myocardial apoptosis, allowing natural cell regeneration to occur.

Effects in Survivors of Acute Myocardial Infarction

Beta-adrenergic blockers have beneficial effects on many determinants of myocardial ischemia (Table 7-11).[61,191,256,257] The results of placebo-controlled, long-term treatment trials with some beta-adrenergic blocking drugs in survivors of acute myocardial infarction have demonstrated a favorable effect on total mortality; cardiovascular mortality, including sudden and nonsudden cardiac deaths; and the incidence of nonfatal reinfarction.[66,258,259] These beneficial results with beta-blocker therapy can be explained by both the antiarrhythmic (see Table 7-11) and the anti-ischemic effects of these drugs.[191,247,260–266a] It has also been proposed that beta-adrenergic blockers could reduce the risk of atherosclerotic plaque fissure and subsequent thrombosis.[267,268] Two nonselective beta blockers, propranolol and timolol, have been approved for reducing the risk of mortality in infarct survivors when started 5 to 28 days after an infarction. Metoprolol and atenolol, two beta$_1$-selective blockers, are approved for the same indication and can both be used intravenously in the hyperacute phase of a myocardial infarction. Beta blockers have also been suggested as a treatment for reducing the extent of myocardial injury[66,269,270] and mortality during the hyperacute phase of myocardial infarction,[67,271] but their exact role in this situation remains unclear.[272] Intravenous and oral atenolol has been shown to be effective in causing a modest reduction in early mortality when given during the hyperacute phase of acute myocardial infarction.[67] Atenolol and metoprolol reduce early infarct mortality by 15%,[67,271] an effect that may be improved upon when beta-adrenergic blockade is combined with acute thrombolytic therapy.[273] Metoprolol and atenolol combined with acute thrombolysis has been evaluated in the TIMI-II and GUSTO studies.[68,273a] Immediate beta-blocker therapy given to patients with acute myocardial infarction who have received tissue transminogen activator (t-PA) is associated with a significant reduction in the frequency of intracranial hemorrhage.[273a] Despite all the evidence showing that beta blockers are beneficial in patients surviving myocardial infarction,[274–278] they are considerably underused in clinical practice.

Recent studies have shown the cost-effectiveness of using beta blockers in a larger percentage of the postinfarction population,[279] including the elderly, diabetics, and patients with mild-to-moderate chronic obstructive pulmonary disease.[280–288] Beta blockers have also been shown to be effective in patients following coronary revascularization and in those with diminished ejection fraction post–myocardial infarction,[289,290] Attempts should be made to increase beta-blocker use in clinical practice.[291–293] Treatment with lower

TABLE 7-12. Results of β-Blocker Therapy in Recent Randomized Clinical Trials in Heart Failure

	Placebo (% of events)	β-Blocker Therapy (% of events)	Risk Reduction (%)	p Value
U.S. Carvedilol HF Program	(334)			
All-cause mortality	7.5	2.6	65	0.0001
Sudden death	3.8	1.7		
Death due to HF	3.3	0.7		
Hospitalization for cardiovascular causes	19.6	14.1	27	0.036
CIBIS-II[71]				
All cause mortality	17.3	11.8	34	<0.0001
Cardiovascular mortality	12	9	29	0.0049
Sudden death	6.3	3.6	44	0.0011
All cause hospital admission	39	33	20	0.0006
MERIT-HF[340]				
All cause mortality	11	7.2	34	0.0062
Cardiovascular mortality	6.4	10.1	38	0.0063
Sudden death	3.9	6.6	41	0.0002
Death due to worsening HF	1.5	2.9	49	0.0023
COPERNICUS[72]				
All cause mortality	16.8	11.2	3.5	0.001

CIBIS-II = Cardiac Insufficiency Bisoprolol Study II; MERIT-HF = Metoprolol CR/XL Randomized Intervention Trial in Congestive Heart Failure; COPERNICUS = Carvedilol Prospective Randomized Cumulative Survival Trial.

Source: Adapted with permission from Ambrosioni E, Bacchelli S, Esposti DD, Borghi C: β blockade in hypertension and congestive heart failure. *J Cardiovasc Pharmacol* 38(Suppl 3):S25, 2001.

doses of beta blockers than those used in large clinical trials is associated with at least as great a reduction in mortality as treatment with higher doses. In patients surviving a myocardial infarction in whom larger doses of beta blockers might be contraindicated, the use of smaller doses should be encouraged.[294] Studies have examined the use of beta-blockade by paramedics, before hospital admission, with some benefit observed.[295]

"Silent" Myocardial Ischemia

In recent years, investigators have observed that not all myocardial ischemic episodes detected by electrocardiography (ECG) are associated with detectable symptoms.[296] Positron emission tomography imaging techniques have validated the theory that these silent ischemic episodes are indicative of true myocardial ischemia.[297] Compared to symptomatic ischemia, the prognostic importance of silent myocardial ischemia occurring at rest and/or during exercise has not been determined. Beta blockers are as successful in reducing the frequency of silent ischemic episodes detected by ambulatory ECG monitoring as they are in reducing the frequency of painful ischemic events.[296–302]

Congestive Cardiomyopathy

The ability of intravenous sympathomimetic amines to affect an acute increase in myocardial contractility through stimulation of the beta-adrenergic receptor had prompted the hope that the use of oral catecholamine analogues could provide long-term benefit for patients with severe heart failure. However, recent observations concerning the regulation of the myocardial adrenergic receptor and abnormalities of beta-receptor–mediated stimulation of the failing myocardium have caused a critical reappraisal of the scientific validity of sustained beta-adrenergic-receptor stimulation.[7,303–305] Evidence suggests that beta-receptor blockade may, when tolerated, have a favorable effect on the underlying cardiomyopathic process,[306,307] perhaps by upregulation and preserving beta-receptor signaling.[308]

Recently it has been shown that excess catecholamine stimulation of beta receptors can result in receptor desensitization by the phosphorylation of inhibitory beta-adrenergic-receptor kinases with beta-receptor uncoupling from Gs due to beta-arrestin activity.[309,310] In addition, agonist anti-beta$_1$-adrenergic-receptor autoantibodies have been described in patients with heart failure, which can also cause receptor desensitization.[311]

Enhanced sympathetic activation is seen consistently in patients with CHF and is associated with decreased exercise tolerance,[312] hemodynamic abnormalities,[313] and increased mortality.[314] Increases in sympathetic tone can potentiate the patient's renin-angiotensin system, leading to increased salt and water retention, arterial and venous constriction, and increments in ventricular preload and afterload.[306] Catecholamines in excess can increase heart rate and cause coronary vasoconstriction.[315] They can adversely influence myocardial contractility on the cellular level,[316–318] while causing myocyte hypertrophy[317,319] and vascular remodeling. Catecholamines can stimulate growth and provoke oxidative stress in terminally differentiated cardiac cells; these two factors can trigger the process of programmed cell death known as apoptosis[320,321] Finally, they can increase the risk of sudden death in patients with CHF by adversely influencing the electrophysiologic properties of the failing heart.[322,323]

Controlled trials over the last 25 years with several different beta blockers in patients with both ischemic and nonischemic cardiomyopathy have shown that these drugs can improve symptoms, ventricular function, and functional capacity while reducing the need for hospitalization (Table 7-12).[324–333] A series of placebo-controlled clinical trials with the alpha-beta blocker carvedilol[69,72,334–337] showed a morbidity and mortality benefit in patients with New York Heart Association class II to IV heart failure when the drug was used in addition to diuretics, ACE inhibitors, and digoxin. Carvedilol has also been studied in symptomatic patients with low ejection fraction after an acute myocardial infarction, with a benefit shown on all-cause and cardiovascular mortality and recurrent nonfatal

TABLE 7-13. Possible Mechanisms by Which β-Adrenergic Blockers Improve Ventricular Function in Chronic Congestive Heart Failure

Upregulation of β receptors
Direct myocardial protective action against catecholamine toxicity
Improved ability of noradrenergic sympathetic nerves to synthesize norepinephrine
Decreased release of norepinephrine from sympathetic nerve endings
Decreased stimulation of other vasoconstrictive systems including renin-angiotensin-aldosterone, vasopressin, and endothelin
Potentiation of kallikrein-kinin system and natural vasodilatation (increase in bradykinin)
Antiarrhythmic effects raising ventricular fibrillation threshold
Protection against catecholamine-induced hypokalemia
Increase in coronary blood flow by reducing heart rate and improving diastolic perfusion time; possible coronary dilation with vasodilator–β blocker
Restoration of abnormal baroreflex function
Prevention of ventricular muscle hypertrophy and vascular remodeling
Antioxidant effects (carvedilol?)
Shift from free fatty acid to carbohydrate metabolism (improved metabolic efficiency)
Vasodilation (e.g., carvedilol)
Antiapoptosis effect, allowing myocardial cell regeneration to occur
Improved left atrial contribution to left ventricular filling
Modulation of postreceptor inhibitory G proteins
Normalization of myocyte Ca^{2+} regulatory proteins and improved Ca^{2+} handling
Increasing natriuretic peptide production
Attenuation of inflammatory cytokines
Restoring cardiac calcium release channel (ryanodine receptor)

myocardial infarction[290] It has been shown that patients treated with inotropic therapy (milrinone) can be titrated on carvedilol after reaching a stable state, with subsequent weaning of the inotrope.[338]

Placebo-controlled studies have also been done showing the benefit of using the beta$_1$-selective blockers, metoprolol (sustained-release) and bisoprolol, in patients with class II to III heart failure.[70,71,339,340,340a,340b] Sustained-release metoprolol was recently approved as a once-daily treatment for patients with congestive cardiomyopathy. A trial with the beta blocker-vasodilator bucindolol showed less benefit than with other beta blockers used to treatment congestive heart failure,[120] demonstrating that all beta blockers may not be interchangeable for this indication. A study is in progress comparing the alpha-beta blocker carvedilol to metoprolol in heart failure patients, which will also define whether the additional pharmacologic actions of carvedilol (beta$_2$ blockade, alpha blockade, antioxidant properties) provide any advantage over metoprolol.

The mechanisms of benefit with beta-blocker use are not known as yet. Possible mechanisms for beta-blocker benefit in chronic heart failure are listed in Table 7-13 and include the upregulation of impaired beta-receptor expression in the heart,[341,342] alteration of myocardial gene expression,[342a] augmentation of the cardiac natriuretic peptides,[343] and improvement in impaired baroreceptor functioning, which can inhibit excess sympathetic outflow.[344] It has been suggested that long-term therapy with beta blockers improves the left atrial contribution to left ventricular filling[345] and normalizes the abundance of myocyte Ca^{2+} regulatory proteins with improved Ca^{2+} handling.[346,346a,346b]

Other Cardiovascular Applications

Although beta blockers have been studied extensively in patients with angina pectoris, arrhythmias, and hypertension, they have also been shown to be safe and effective in diabetic patients[347] and for other cardiovascular conditions (see Table 7-5), some of which are described below.

Hypertrophic Cardiomyopathy

Beta adrenergic-receptor blocking drugs have been proven effective in therapy for patients with hypertrophic cardiomyopathy and idiopathic hypertrophic subaortic stenosis (IHSS).[146,348] These drugs are useful in controlling the symptoms of dyspnea, angina, and syncope.[61,62] Beta blockers have also been shown to lower the intraventricular pressure gradient both at rest and with exercise.

The outflow pressure gradient is not the only abnormality in hypertrophic cardiomyopathy; more important is the loss of ventricular compliance, which impedes normal left ventricular function. It has been shown by invasive and noninvasive methods that propranolol can improve left ventricular function in this condition.[349] The drug also produces favorable changes in ventricular compliance while it relieves symptoms. Propranolol has been approved for this condition and may be combined with the calcium-entry blocker verapamil in patients who do not respond to the beta blocker alone.

The salutary hemodynamic and symptomatic effects produced by propranolol derive from its inhibition of sympathetic stimulation of the heart.[350] There is no evidence that the drug alters the primary cardiomyopathic process; many patients remain in or return to their severely symptomatic state, and some die despite its administration.[146,348]

Mitral Valve Prolapse

This auscultatory complex, characterized by a nonejection systolic click, a late systolic murmur, or a midsystolic click followed by a late systolic murmur, has been studied extensively over the past 15 years.[351] Atypical chest pain, malignant arrhythmias, and nonspecific ST- and T-wave abnormalities have been observed with this condition. By decreasing sympathetic tone, beta-adrenergic blockers have been shown to be useful for relieving the chest pains and palpitations that many of these patients experience and for reducing the incidence of life-threatening arrhythmias and other ECG abnormalities.[148]

Dissecting Aneurysms

Beta-adrenergic blockade plays a major role in the treatment of patients with acute aortic dissection. During the hyperacute phase, beta-blocking agents reduce the force and velocity of myocardial contraction (dP/dt) and hence the progression of the dissecting hematoma.[352] Moreover, such administration must be initiated simultaneously with the institution of other antihypertensive therapy, which may cause reflex tachycardia and increases in cardiac output, factors that can aggravate the dissection process. Initially, propranolol is administered intravenously to reduce the heart rate to below 60 beats per minute. Once a patient is stabilized and long-term medical management is contemplated, the patient should be maintained on oral beta-blocker therapy to prevent recurrence.[352]

It has been demonstrated that long-term beta-blocker therapy may also reduce the risk of dissection in patients prone to this complication (e.g., Marfan's syndrome).[353,354] Systolic time intervals are used to assess the adequacy of beta blockade in children with Marfan's syndrome.[150]

Tetralogy of Fallot

By reducing the effects of increased adrenergic tone on the right ventricular infundibulum in tetralogy of Fallot, beta blockers have been shown to be useful for the treatment of severe hypoxic spells and hypercyanotic attacks.[150] With chronic use, these drugs have also been shown to prevent prolonged hypoxic spells. These drugs should be looked upon as palliative only, as definitive surgical repair of this condition is usually required.

QT Interval–Prolongation Syndrome

The syndrome of ECG QT-interval prolongation is usually a congenital condition associated with deafness, syncope, and sudden death.[149] Abnormalities in sympathetic nervous system functioning in the heart have been proposed as explanations for the electrophysiologic aberrations seen in these patients.[149,355] Propranolol and other beta blockers appear to be the most effective drugs for the treatment of this syndrome.[356] They reduce the frequency of syncopal episodes in most patients and may prevent sudden death. These drugs will reduce the ECG QT interval. Patients not responding to beta blockers should be candidates for implantable defibrillators.[357]

Regression of Left Ventricular Hypertrophy

Left ventricular hypertrophy induced by systemic hypertension is an independent risk factor for cardiovascular mortality and morbidity.[35] Regression of left ventricular hypertrophy with drug therapy is feasible and may improve patient outcome.[35] Beta-adrenergic blockers can cause regression of left ventricular hypertrophy, as determined by echocardiography, with or without an associated reduction in blood pressure.[35]

Atherogenesis

Beta blockers may have a direct antiatherosclerotic effect at a dose well below commonly prescribed regimens.[358] The mechanisms underlying this beta-blocker benefit is not known. An effect on reactive oxygen species has been proposed.[359] Recently it was shown that chronic propranolol treatment did not favorably influence the course of patients having abdominal aortic aneurysms.

Syncope

Vasovagal syncope is the most common form of syncope observed. Upright tilt-table testing with isoproterenol can help differentiate vasovagal syncope from other forms.[360] Beta blockers, including those with partial agonism, have been shown to be useful for both relieving symptoms and normalizing abnormal tilt-table tests in patients with syncope, with some studies showing no benefit.[360–362] The mechanism for benefit with beta blockers may be an interruption of the Bezold-Jarisch reflex or an enhancement of peripheral vasoconstriction by blockade of beta$_2$-adrenergic receptors.[363]

Myocardial Protection during Surgery

Beta blockers can protect patients at high risk for myocardial ischemia during and after major surgery.[364–366,366a,366b,366c] Prior beta-blocker therapy has also been shown to have a cardioprotective effect in limiting CK-MB release after percutaneous coronary interventions, associated with a lower mortality at intermediate-term follow up.[367,368,368a] However, a recent observational study did not support the contention that beta blockade can favorably influence CK-MB rise during angioplasty.[368b]

Noncardiovascular Applications

Beta-adrenergic receptors are ubiquitous in the human body, and their blockade affects a variety of organ and metabolic systems (Table 7-14).[61,62,78] Some noncardiovascular uses of beta blockers (glaucoma, migraine headache prophylaxis, essential tremor) have been approved by the U.S. Food and Drug Administration (FDA).[60,369–371] The combination of nitrates and beta blockers has been shown to be effective in preventing bleeding from esophageal varices.[372,373]

Adverse Effects of Beta Blockers

Evaluation of adverse effects is complex because of the use of different definitions of side effects, the kinds of patients studied, study design features, and different methods of ascertaining and reporting adverse side effects from study to study.[374–376] Overall, the types and frequencies of adverse effects attributed to various beta-blocker compounds appear similar.[375,376] The side-effect profiles resemble those seen with concurrent placebo treatments, attesting to the remarkable safety margin of the beta blockers.[374]

Adverse effects fall in two categories: (1) those from known pharmacologic consequences of beta-adrenoceptor blockade and (2) other reactions apart from beta-adrenoceptor blockade.

The first type includes asthma, heart failure, hypoglycemia, bradycardia and heart block, intermittent claudication, and Raynaud's phenomenon. The incidence of these adverse effects varies with the beta blocker used.[61,375,376]

Side effects of the second category are rare. They include an unusual oculomucocutaneous reaction and the possibility of carcinogenesis.[61,375,376]

Adverse Cardiac Effects Related to Beta-Adrenoceptor Blockade

Congestive Heart Failure

Despite benefit in many patients with congestive cardiomyopathy, blockade of beta receptors may cause congestive heart failure in an enlarged heart with impaired myocardial function where excessive sympathetic drive is essential to maintain the myocardium on a compensated Starling curve and where left ventricular stroke volume is restricted and tachycardia is needed to maintain cardiac output.

Thus, any beta-blocking drug may be associated with the development of heart failure. Furthermore, heart failure may also be augmented by increases in peripheral vascular resistance produced

TABLE 7-14. Pharmacodynamic Properties and Noncardiac Effects of β-Adrenoceptor Blockers

	Relative β_1 Selectivity	ISA	MSA	Bronchial Tone	Platelet Aggregability	PRA	PVR	RBF	GFR	HDL-C	LDL-C	VLDL-Tri
Acebutolol	+	+	+	↑↔↓		↓↔	↑↔	↓↔	↓↔	↔	↔	↔
Atenolol	++	0	0	↑↔↓		↓↔	↑↔	↓↔	↓↔	↔	↔	↔
Betaxolol	++	0	+	↑↔↓		↓↔	↑↔	↓↔	↔	↔	↔	↔
Bisoprolol	++	0	0	↑↔↓		↓↔	↑↔	↓↔	↓↔	↔	↔	↔
Carteolol	0	+	0	↑↔↓	↓	↓↔	↓↔↑	↓↔	↓↔	↔	↔	↔
Carvedilol*	0	0	++	↑↔↓	↓	↓↔	↓	↔↑	↔	↔	↔	↔
Esmolol	++	0	0	↑↔↓		↓↔	↑↔	?	?	?	?	?
Labetalol*	0	+	0	↑↔↓	↔	↓↔	↓	↔↑	↔	↔	↔	↔
Metoprolol	++	0	0	↑↔↓		↓↔	↑↔	↓↔	↓↔	↔↓	↔	↑↔
Nadolol	0	0	0	↔↓		↓↔	↑	↑	↑↔	?	?	?
Nebivolol†	++	0	0	↑↔↓	↓	↓	↓	↔	↓	↔	↔	↔
Oxprenolol	0	+	+	↑↔↓	↓	↓↔	↑↔	↓↔	↓	↔	↔	↔
Penbutolol	0	+	0	↑↔↓		↓↔	↓↔	?	?	?	?	?
Pindolol	0	++	+	↑↔↓	↓	↓↔↑	↔↓	↓↔	↓↔	↔	↔	↔
Propranolol	0	0	++	↔↓	↓	↓	↑	↓	↓	↓	↔	↑
Sotalol	0	0	0	↔↓		↓	↑	↓	↓	?	?	?
Timolol	0	0	0	↔↓	↓	↓	↑	↓	↓	?	?	?
Isomer-D-propranolol	0	0	++	↔	↓	↔	↔	↔	↔	?	?	?

ISA = intrinsic sympathomimetic activity; MSA = membrane stabilizing activity; PRA = plasma renin activity; PVR = peripheral vascular resistance; RBF = renal blood flow; GFR = glomerular filtration rate; HDL-C = high-density lipoprotein cholesterol; LDL-C = low-density lipoprotein cholesterol; VLDL-Tri = very low density lipoprotein triglycerides; ↑ = elevation; ↓ = reduction; ↔ = no change.

β_1 selectivity is seen only with low therapeutic drug concentrations. With higher concentrations, β_1 selectivity is not seen.

*Labetalol and carvedilol have additional α_1-adrenergic blocking activity and direct β_2 vasodilatory activity.

†Nebivolol can augment vascular nitric oxide release.

Source: Adapted with permission from Frishman.[61]

by nonselective agents (e.g., propranolol, timolol, sotalol).[376] It has been claimed that beta blockers with intrinsic sympathomimetic activity and alpha-blocking activity are better in preserving left ventricular function and less likely to precipitate heart failure.[377]

In patients with impaired myocardial function who require beta-blocking agents, digitalis, ACE inhibitors, and diuretics can be used.

Sinus Node Dysfunction and Atrioventricular Conduction Delay

Slowing of the resting heart rate is a normal response to treatment with beta-blocking drugs with and without intrinsic sympathomimetic activity. Healthy persons can sustain a heart rate of 40 to 50 beats per minute without disability unless there is clinical evidence of heart failure.[102] Drugs with intrinsic sympathomimetic activity do not lower the resting heart rate to the same degree as propranolol,[378] but all beta-blocking drugs are contraindicated (unless an artificial pacemaker is present) in patients with sick sinus syndrome.[376]

If there is a partial or complete AV conduction defect, the use of a beta-blocking drug may lead to a serious bradyarrhythmia.[376] The risk of AV impairment may be less with beta blockers that have intrinsic sympathomimetic activity.[379]

Overdosage

Suicide attempts and accidental overdosing with beta blockers are being described with increasing frequency. Since beta-adrenergic blockers are competitive pharmacologic antagonists, their life-threatening effects (bradycardia, myocardial and ventilatory failure) can be overcome with an immediate infusion of beta-agonist agents such as isoproterenol and dobutamine.[106] In situations where catecholamines are not effective, intravenous glucagon, amrinone, or milrinone have been used.[106]

Close monitoring of cardiorespiratory function is necessary for at least 24 h after the patient responds to therapy. Patients who recover usually have no long-term sequelae; however, they should be observed for the cardiac signs of sudden beta-blocker withdrawal.[106]

Beta-Adrenoceptor Blocker Withdrawal

After abrupt cessation of chronic beta-blocker therapy, exacerbation of angina pectoris and, in some cases, acute myocardial infarction and death have been reported.[74,380] Observations made in multiple double-blind randomized trials have confirmed the reality of a propranolol withdrawal reaction.[74,381] The mechanism for this reaction is unclear. There is some evidence that the withdrawal phenomenon may be due to the generation of additional beta adrenoceptors during the period of beta-adrenoceptor blockade. When the beta-adrenoceptor blocker is then withdrawn, the increased beta-receptor population readily results in excessive beta-receptor stimulation, which is clinically important when the delivery and use of oxygen are finely balanced, as occurs in ischemic heart disease. Other suggested mechanisms for the withdrawal reaction include heightened platelet aggregability, an elevation in thyroid hormone activity, and an increase in circulating catecholamines.[74] A beta-blocker withdrawal phenomenon with an increased risk for death has also been described in patients with heart failure who are withdrawn from beta blockers.[382]

Adverse Noncardiac Side Effects Related to Beta-Adrenoceptor Blockade

Effect on Ventilatory Function

The bronchodilatory effects of catecholamines on the bronchial beta$_2$-adrenoceptors are inhibited by nonselective beta blockers (e.g., propranolol, nadolol).[376] Beta-blocking compounds with partial agonist activity,[93,109] beta$_1$-selectivity,[6,91] and alpha-adrenergic blocking actions[383] are less likely to increase airways resistance in asthmatics. Beta$_1$-selectivity, however, is not absolute and may be lost with high therapeutic doses, as shown with atenolol and metoprolol. It is possible in treating asthma to use a beta$_2$-selective agonist (such as albuterol) in certain patients with concomitant low-dose beta$_1$-selective blocker treatment.[384] In general, all beta blockers should be avoided in patients with bronchospastic disease.

Peripheral Vascular Effects (Raynaud's Phenomenon)

Cold extremities and absent pulses have been reported more frequently in patients receiving beta blockers for hypertension than in those receiving methyldopa.[124] Among the beta blockers, the incidence was highest with propranolol and lower with drugs having beta$_1$-selectivity or intrinsic sympathomimetic activity. In some instances, vascular compromise has been severe enough to cause cyanosis and impending gangrene.[385] This is probably due to the reduction in cardiac output and blockade of beta$_2$-adrenoceptor-mediated skeletal muscle vasodilatation, resulting in unopposed beta-adrenoceptor vasoconstriction.[386] Beta-blocking drugs with beta$_1$-selectivity or partial agonist activity will not affect peripheral vessels to the same degree as does propranolol.

Raynaud's phenomenon is one of the more common side effects of propranolol treatment.[387] It is more troublesome with propranolol than with metoprolol, atenolol, or pindolol, probably because of the beta$_2$-blocking properties of propranolol.

Patients with peripheral vascular disease who suffer from intermittent claudication occasionally report worsening of the claudication when treated with beta-blocking drugs.[388,389] Whether drugs with beta$_1$-selectivity or partial agonist activity can protect against this adverse reaction has not been determined.[390]

Hypoglycemia and Hyperglycemia

Several authors have described severe hypoglycemic reactions during therapy with beta-adrenergic blocking drugs.[391] Some of the patients affected were insulin-dependent diabetics while others were nondiabetic. Studies of resting normal volunteers have demonstrated that propranolol produces no alteration in blood glucose values,[392] although the hyperglycemic response to exercise is blunted. Beta blockers can increase the incidence of type II diabetes.[167] Weight gain (average 1.2 kg) and insulin resistance have been reported with chronic beta-blocker use.[393]

The enhancement of insulin-induced hypoglycemia and its hemodynamic consequences may be less with beta$_1$-selective agents (where there is no blocking effect on beta$_2$ receptors) and agents with intrinsic sympathomimetic activity (which may stimulate beta$_2$ receptors).[394]

There is also marked diminution in the clinical manifestations of the catecholamine discharge induced by hypoglycemia (tachycardia).[395] These findings suggest that beta blockers interfere with compensatory responses to hypoglycemia and can mask certain "warning signs" of this condition. Other hypoglycemic reactions, such as diaphoresis, are not affected by beta-adrenergic blockade.

Hyperlipidemia

Nonselective beta-blocking agents can raise triglycerides and reduce HDL cholesterol.[396] This effect may not be seen with agents having partial agonism or alpha-blocking activity.[397]

Central Nervous System Effects

Dreams, hallucinations, insomnia, and depression can occur during therapy with beta blockers.[78,156] These symptoms provide evidence of drug entry into the CNS and may be more common with the highly lipid-soluble beta blockers (propranolol, metoprolol), which presumably penetrate the CNS better. It has been claimed that beta blockers with less lipid-solubility (atenolol, nadolol) cause fewer CNS side effects.[91,92] This claim is intriguing, but its validity has not been corroborated by other extensive clinical experiences.[138,139,398]

Miscellaneous Side Effects

Diarrhea, nausea, gastric pain, constipation, and flatulence have been noted occasionally with all beta blockers (2–11% of patients).[399] Hematologic reactions are rare. Rare cases of purpura[400] and agranulocytosis[401] have been described with propranolol. Beta blocker use early in pregnancy has been associated with fetal growth retardation (see Appendix 3).[402]

A devastating blood pressure rebound effect has been described in patients who discontinued clonidine while being treated with nonselective beta-blocking agents. The mechanism for this may be related to an increase in circulating catecholamines and an increase in peripheral vascular resistance.[403] Whether beta$_1$-selective or partial agonist beta blockers have similar effects following clonidine withdrawal has not been determined. This has not been a problem with labetalol.[404]

Adverse Effects Unrelated to Beta-Adrenoceptor Blockade

Oculomucocutaneous Syndrome

A characteristic immune reaction, the oculomucocutaneous syndrome—affecting one or both eyes, mucous and serous membranes, and the skin, often in association with a positive antinuclear factor—has been reported in patients treated with practolol, and has led to the curtailment of its clinical use.[376,405] Close attention has been focused on this syndrome because of fears that other beta-adrenoceptor blocking drugs may be associated with this syndrome.

Drug-Drug Interactions

Beta blockers are commonly employed, and the list of commonly used drugs with which they can interact is extensive (Table 7-15, see Chap. 48).[406,407] The majority of the reported interactions have been associated with propranolol, the best studied beta blocker, and may not necessarily apply to other drugs in this class.

How to Choose a Beta Blocker

The various beta-blocking compounds given in adequate dosage appear to have comparable antihypertensive, antiarrhythmic, and antianginal effects. Therefore, the beta-blocking drug of choice in an individual patient is determined by the pharmacodynamic and pharmacokinetic differences between the drugs, in conjunction with the patient's other medical conditions (Table 7-16).[61,62,93]

TABLE 7-15. Drug Interactions That May Occur with β-Adrenoceptor Blocking Drugs

Drug	Pharmacokinetic Interactions	Pharmacodynamic Interactions	Precautions
Alcohol	Enhanced first-pass hepatic degradation	None	May need increased doses of lipid soluble agents.
α-Adrenergic blockers		Increased risk for first-dose hypotension	Use with caution.
Aluminum hydroxide gel	Decreased β-blocker absorption	None	Clinical efficacy rarely altered.
Amiodarone	None	Enhanced negative chronotropic activity	Monitor response.
Aminophylline	Mutual inhibition		Observe patient's response.
Ampicillin	Impaired GI absorption leading to decreased β-blocker bioavailability		May need to increase β-blocker dose.
Angiotensin II–receptor blockers (losartan)	None	Enhanced blood pressure effects and bronchospasm	Monitor response.
Antidiabetics	Both enhanced and blunted responses seen	None	Monitor for altered diabetic response.
ACE inhibitors	None	Enhanced blood pressure effects and bronchospasm	Monitor response.
Calcium	Decreases β-blocker absorption		May need to increase β-blocker dose.
Calcium-channel blockers	Decreased hepatic clearance of lipid soluble and water soluble β blockers; decreased clearance of calcium blockers	Potentiation of AV nodal negative inotropic and hypotensive responses	Avoid use if possible, although few patients show ill effects.
Cimetidine	Decreased hepatic clearance of lipid soluble β blockers	None	Combination should be used with caution
Clonidine	None	Nonselective agents exacerbate clonidine withdrawal phenomenon	Use only β_1-selective agents or labetalol.
Diazepam	Diazepam metabolism reduced reduced		Observe patient's response.
Digitalis glycosides	None	Potentiation of bradycardic and AV blocks	Observe patient's response; interactions may benefit angina patients with abnormal ventricular function.
Epinephrine	None	Severe hypertension and bradycardia	Administer epinephrine cautiously; cardioselective β blocker may be safer.
Ergot alkaloids	None	Severe hypertension and peripheral artery hyperperfusion have been seen, though β blockers are commonly coadministered	Observe patient's response; few patients show ill effects.
Fluvoxamine	Decreased hepatic clearance of propranolol		Use with caution.
Glucagon	Enhanced clearance of lipid-soluble β blockers	None	Monitor for reduced response.
Halofenate			Observe for impaired response to β blockade.
Hydralazine	Decreased hepatic clearance of lipid-soluble β blockers	Enhanced hypotensive response	Cautious coadministration.
Indomethacin and Ibuprofen	None	Reduced efficacy in treatment of hypertension	Observe patient's response.
Isoproterenol	None	Cancels pharmacologic effect	Avoid concurrent use or choose selective β_1 blocker.
Levodopa		Antagonism of hypotensive and positive inotropic effects of levodopa	Monitor for altered response; interaction may have favorable results.
Lidocaine	Decreased hepatic clearance of lidocaine by lipid soluble β blockers	Enhanced lidocaine toxicity	Combination should be used with caution; use lower doses of lidocaine.
Methyldopa		Hypertension during stress	Monitor for hypertensive episodes.

(continued)

TABLE 7-15. (*Continued*)

Drug	Pharmacokinetic Interactions	Pharmacodynamic Interactions	Precautions
Monoamine oxidase inhibitors	Uncertain	Enhanced hypotension	Manufacturer of propranolol considers concurrent use contraindicated.
Nitrates	None	Enhanced hypotension	Monitor response.
Omeprazole	None	None	None.
Phenobarbital	Increased hepatic metabolism of β blockers		May need to increase lipid soluble β-blocker dose.
Phenothiazines	Increased phenothiazine and β-blocker blood levels	Additive hypotensive response	Monitor for altered response; especially with high doses of phenothiazine.
Phenylpropanolamine		Severe hypertensive reaction	Avoid use, especially in hypertension controlled by both methyldopa and β blockers.
Phenytoin		Additive ventricular depressive effects	Use with caution.
Reserpine		Depression, possible enhanced sensitivity to β-adrenergic blockade	Monitor closely.
Ranitidine	Not marked	None	Observe response.
Smoking	Enhanced first-pass metabolism	None	May need to increase dose of lipid-soluble β blockers.
Sulindac and naproxen	None	None	
Tricyclic antidepressants		Inhibits negative inotropic and chronotropic effects; enhanced hypotension	Use with caution with sotalol because of additive effects on ECG QT interval on ECG QT interval.
Tubucuraine		Enhanced neuromuscular blockade	Observe response in surgical patients, especially after high doses of propranolol.
Type I antiarrhythmics	Propafenone and quinidine decrease clearance of lipid soluble β blockers	Disopyramide is a potent negative inotropic and chronotropic agent	Cautious coprescription; use with sotalol can be dangerous because of additive effects on ECG QT interval.
Warfarin	Decreased clearance of warfarin	None	Monitor response.

TABLE 7-16. Clinical Situations That Would Influence the Choice of a β-Blocking Drug

Condition	Choice of β Blocker
Asthma, chronic bronchitis with bronchospasm	Avoid all β blockers if possible, but small doses of $β_1$-selective blockers can be used; $β_1$ selectivity is lost with higher doses; drugs with partial agonist activity and labetalol with α-adrenergic blocking properties can also be used.
Congestive heart failure	Drugs with partial agonist activity and vasodilatory activity (carvedilol, labetalol) may have an advantage, although all β blockers should be used with caution.
Angina	In patients with angina at low heart rates, drugs with partial agonist activity are probably contraindicated; patients who have angina at high heart rates but who have resting bradycardia may benefit from a drug with partial agonist activity; in vasospastic angina, labetalol may be useful; other β blockers should be used with caution.
AV conduction defects	β blockers are generally contraindicated, but drugs with partial agonist activity and labetalol can be tried with caution.
Bradycardia	β blockers with partial agonist activity and labetalol have less of a pulse-slowing effect and are preferable.
Raynaud's phenomenon, intermittent claudication, cold extremities	$β_1$-selective blocking agents, labetalol, and agents with partial agonist activity may have an advantage.
Depression	Avoid propranolol; substitute a β blocker with partial agonist activity.
Diabetes mellitus	$β_1$-selective blocking agents and partial agonist drugs are preferable.
Thyrotoxicosis	All agents will control symptoms, but agents without partial agonist activity are preferred.
Pheochromocytoma	Avoid all β blockers unless an α blocker is given first; labetalol may be used as a treatment of choice.
Renal failure	Use reduced doses of compounds largely eliminated by renal mechanisms (nadolol, sotalol, atenolol) and drugs whose bioavailability is increased in uremia (propranolol); also consider possible accumulation of active metabolites (propranolol, nebivolol).
Insulin and sulfonylurea use	There is a danger of hypoglycemia; possibly less using drugs with $β_1$ selectivity.
Clonidine	Avoid nonselective β blockers; there is a severe rebound effect with clonidine withdrawal.
Oculomucocutaneous syndrome	Stop drug; substitute with any β blocker.
Hyperlipidemia	Avoid nonselective β blockers; use agents with partial agonism, $β_1$ selectivity or α-blocking activity.

Source: Reproduced with permission from Frishman.[61]

REFERENCES

1. Ahlquist RP: Study of the adrenotropic receptors. *Am J Physiol* 153:486, 1948.
2. Lands AM, Luduena FP, Buzzo HJ: Differentiation of receptor systems responsive to isoproterenol. *Life Sci* 6:2241, 1967.
3. Emorine LJ, Marullo S, Briend-Sutren M-M, et al: Molecular characterization of the human β_2-adrenergic receptor. *Science* 245:1118, 1989.
4. Berthelsen S, Pettinger WA: A functional basis for classification of alpha-adrenergic receptors. *Life Sci* 21:596, 1977.
5. Minneman KP, Ebenshade TA: α-Adrenergic receptor subtypes. *Annu Rev Pharmacol Toxicol* 34:117, 1994.
6. Sutherland EW, Robinson GA, Butcher RW: Some aspects of the biological role of adenosine $3'5'$-monophosphate (cyclic AMP). *Circulation* 37:279–306, 1968.
7. Insel PA: Adrenergic receptors: evolving concepts and clinical implications. *N Engl J Med* 334:580, 1996.
8. Lefkowitz RJ, Caron MG: Adrenergic receptors: models for the study of receptors coupled to guanine nucleotide regulatory proteins. *J Biol Chem* 263:4993–4996, 1988.
9. Benovic JL, Bouvier M, Caron MG, Lefkowitz RJ: Regulation of adenyl cyclase-coupled beta-adrenergic receptors. *Annu Rev Cell Biol* 4:405–428, 1988.
10. Hoffman BB, Taylor P: Neurotransmission: the autonomic and somatic motor nervous systems. In: Hardman JG, Limbird LE, eds. *Goodman & Gilman's The Pharmacological Basis of Therapeutics,* 10th ed. New York: McGraw-Hill, 2001:115.
11. Watanabe AM: Recent advances in knowledge about beta-adrenergic receptors: application to clinical cardiology. *J Am Coll Cardiol* 1:82–89, 1983.
12. Frishman WH, Charlap S: α-Adrenergic blockers. *Med Clin North Am* 72:427, 1988.
13. Luther RR: New perspectives on selective α_1-blockade. *Am J Hypertens* 2:729, 1989.
14. Van Zwieten PA: Pharmacology profile of urapidil. *Am J Cardiol* 64:1D, 1989.
15. Elliott HL, Meredith PA, Vincent J, et al: Clinical pharmacological studies with doxazosin. *Br J Clin Pharmacol* 21:27S, 1986.
16. Reid JL, Meredith PA, Elliot HL: Pharmacokinetics and pharmacodynamics of trimazosin in man. *Am Heart J* 106:1222, 1983.
17. Archibald JL: Recent developments in the pharmacology and pharmacokinetics of indoramin. *J Cardiovasc Pharmacol* 8(Suppl 2):S16, 1986.
18. Frishman WH, Eisen G, Lapsker J: Terazosin: a new long-acting α_1-adrenergic antagonist for hypertension. *Med Clin North Am* 72:441, 1988.
19. Katz AM, Hager WD, Mesineo FC, et al: Cellular actions and pharmacology of the calcium channel blocking drugs. *Am J Med* 77:2, 1984.
20. Ribner HS, Bresnahan D, Hsieh AM: Acute hemodynamic responses to vasodilation therapy in congestive heart failure. *Prog Cardiovasc Dis* 25:1, 1982.
21. Grimm RH, Flack JM, Schoenberger JA, et al: α Blockade and thiazide treatment of hypertension. *Am J Hypertens* 9:445, 1996.
22. Neaton JD, Grimm RH, Prineas RI, et al for the Treatment of Mild Hypertension Study Research Group: treatment of mild hypertension study: final results. *JAMA* 270:713, 1993.
23. Materson BJ, Reda DJ, Cushman WC, et al: Single-drug therapy for hypertension in men. A comparison of six antihypertensives with placebo. *N Engl J Med* 328:914, 1994.
24. Davis BR, Cutler JA, Gordon DJ, et al, for the ALLHAT Research Group: Rationale and design for the Antihypertensive and Lipid Lowering Treatment to Prevent Heart Attack Trial (ALLHAT). *Am J Hypertens* 9:342, 1996.
25. The ALLHAT Officers and Coordinators for the ALLHAT Collaborative Research Group: Major cardiovascular events in hypertensive patients randomized to doxazosin vs chlorthalidone. The Antihypertensive and Lipid-Lowering Treatment to Prevent Heart Attack Trial (ALLHAT). *JAMA* 283:1967, 2000.
26. Frishman WH: Update in cardiology. *Ann Intern Med* 135:439, 2001.
26a. Davis BR, Cutler JA, Furberg CD, et al: Relationship of antihypertensive treatment regimens and change in blood pressure to risk for heart failure in hypertensive patients randomly assigned to doxazosin or chlorthalidone: Further analyses from the antihypertensive and lipid-lowering treatment to prevent Heart Attack Trial. *Ann Intern Med* 137:313, 2002.
27. Messerli FH: Doxazosin and congestive heart failure. *J Am Coll Card* 38:1295, 2001.
28. Black HR, Sollins JS, Garofalo JL: The addition of doxazosin to the therapeutic regimen of hypertensive patients inadequately controlled with other antihypertensive medications: a randomized, placebo-controlled study. *Am J Hypertens* 13:468, 2000.
29. Frishman WH, Patel K: Lipid-lowering drugs. In: Frishman WH, Sonnenblick EH, eds. *Cardiovascular Pharmacotherapeutics.* New York: McGraw-Hill, 1997:399.
30. Levy D, Walmsley P, Levenstein M for the Hypetension and Lipid Trial Study Group: Principal results of the Hypertension and Lipid Trial (HALT): a multicenter study of doxazosin in patients with hypertension. *Am Heart J* 131:966, 1996.
31. Andersson P-E, Lithell H: Metabolic effects of doxazosin and enalapril in hypertriglyceridemic, hypertensive men. *Am J Hypertens* 9:323, 1996.
32. Kinoshita M, Simazu N, Fujita M, et al: Doxazosin, an α_1-adrenergic antihypertensive agent, decreases serum oxidized LDL. *Am J Hypertens* 14:267, 2001.
33. Fajardo N, Deshaies Y: Long-term α_1 adrenergic blockade attenuates diet-induced dyslipidemia and hyperinsulinemia in the rat. *J Cardiovasc Pharmacol* 21:913, 1998.
34. Andersen P, Seljeflot I, Herzog A, et al: Effects of doxazosin and atenolol on atherothrombogenic risk profile in hypertensive middle-aged men. *J Cardiovasc Pharmacol* 31:677, 1998.
35. Hachamovitch R, Strom JA, Sonnenblick EH, Frishman WH: Left ventricular hypertrophy in hypertension and the effects of antihypertensive drug therapy. *Curr Probl Cardiol* 13:371, 1988.
36. Yasuda G, Umemura S, Ishii M: Characterization of bunazosin-sensitive α_1 adrenoceptors in human renal medulla. *J Cardiovasc Pharmacol* 30:163, 1997.
37. Gould L, Reddy CVR: Phentolamine. *Am Heart J* 92:392, 1976.
38. Majid PA, Sharma B, Taylor SH: Phentolamine for vasodilator treatment of severe heart failure. *Lancet* 2:719, 1971.
39. Gregorini L, Marco J, Palombo C, et al: Postischemic left ventricular dysfunction is abolished by alpha-adrenergic blocking agents. *J Am Coll Cardiol* 31:992, 1998.
40. Packer M: Vasodilator and inotropic therapy for severe chronic heart failure: passion and skepticism. *J Am Coll Cardiol* 2:841, 1983.
41. Cohn JN, Archibald DG, Ziesche S, et al: Effect of vasodilator therapy on mortality in chronic congestive heart failure: results of a Veterans Administration Cooperative Study (V-Heft). *N Engl J Med* 314:1547, 1986.
42. Kukin ML, Kalman J, Mannino M, et al: Combined alpha-beta blockade (doxazosin plus metoprolol) compared with beta blockade alone in chronic congestive heart failure. *Am J Cardiol* 77:486, 1996.
43. Scholz H: Inotropic drugs and their mechanism of action. *J Am Coll Cardiol* 4:389, 1984.
44. Kern MJ: Appreciating α adrenergic receptors and their role in ischemic left ventricular dysfunction. *Circulation* 99:468, 1999.
45. Baumgart D, Haude M, Gorge G, et al: Augmented α adrenergic constriction of atherosclerotic human coronary arteries. *Circulation* 99:2090, 1999.
46. Orlick AE, Ricci DR, Cipriano PR, et al: The contribution of alpha-adrenergic tone to resting coronary vascular resistance in man. *J Clin Invest* 62:459, 1978.
47. Winniford MD, Flipchuk N, Hillis DL: Alpha-adrenergic blockade for variant angina: a long-term double-blind randomized trial. *Circulation* 67:1185, 1983.
48. Corr PB, Shayman JA, Kramer JB, et al: Increased α-adrenergic receptors in ischemic cat myocardium: a potential mediator of electrophysiologic derangements. *J Clin Invest* 67:1232, 1981.
49. Manger WM, Gifford RW: *Pheochromocytoma.* New York: Springer-Verlag, 1977:304.
50. Honston MC, Thompson WL, Robertson D: Shock. *Arch Intern Med* 144:1433, 1984.
51. Fein SA, Frishman WH: The pathophysiology and management of pulmonary hypertension. *Cardiol Clin* 5:563, 1987.

52. Cohen ML, Kronzon I: Adverse hemodynamic effects of phentolamine in primary pulmonary hypertension. *Ann Intern Med* 95:591, 1981.

53. Henderson WR, Shelhamer JH, Reingold DB, et al: Alpha-adrenergic hyperresponsiveness in asthma. *N Engl J Med* 300:642, 1979.

54. Barnes PJ, Wilson NM, Vickers H: Prazosin, an alpha₁-adrenoceptor antagonist, partially inhibits exercise-induced asthma. *J Allergy Clin Immunol* 68:411, 1981.

55. Hedlund H, Andersson KE, Ek A: Effects of prazosin in patients with benign prostatic obstruction. *J Urol* 130:275, 1983.

56. Narayan P, Lowe FC: The effects of tamsulosin on vital signs in two multicenter, placebo-controlled studies. *Cardiovasc Rev Rep* September, 21:494, 2000.

57. van Zwieten PA: Alpha-adrenoceptor blocking agents in the treatment of hypertension. In: Laragh JH, Brenner BM, eds. *Hypertension: Pathophysiology, Diagnosis and Management*, Vol 2. New York: Raven Press, 1995:2917.

58. Pool JL: α-Adrenoceptor blockers. In: Oparil S, Weber MA, eds. *Hypertension. A Companion to Brenner & Rector's The Kidney.* Philadelphia: Saunders, 2000:595.

59. Frishman WH: Beta-adrenergic blockers. In: Izzo JL Jr, Black HR, eds. *Hypertension Primer*, 3rd ed. Dallas: American Heart Association, 2002, in press.

60. Frishman WH: β-Adrenoceptor antagonists: new drugs and new indications. *N Engl J Med* 305:500–506, 1981.

61. Frishman WH: *Clinical Pharmacology of the β-Adrenoceptor Blocking Drugs,* 2nd ed. Norwalk, CT: Appleton-Century-Crofts, 1984.

62. Frishman WH: β-Adrenergic blockers. *Med Clin North Am* 72:37–81, 1988.

63. The Norwegian Multicenter Study Group: Timolol induced reduction in mortality and reinfarction in patients surviving acute myocardial infarction. *N Engl J Med* 304:801–807, 1981.

64. Beta-Blocker Heart Attack Trial Research Group: A randomized trial of propranolol in patients with acute myocardial infarction. I. Mortality results. *JAMA* 247:1707–1714, 1982.

65. Braunwald E: Treatment of the patient after myocardial infarction. *N Engl J Med* 302:290–293, 1980.

66. Frishman WH, Furberg CD, Friedewald WT: β-Adrenergic blockade for survivors of acute myocardial infarction. *N Engl J Med* 310:30–837, 1984.

67. ISIS-I Collaborative Group: Randomized trial of intravenous atenolol among 16,027 cases of suspected acute myocardial infarction: ISIS-I. *Lancet* 2:57–66, 1986.

68. TIMI Study Group: Comparison of invasive and conservative strategies after treatment with intravenous tissue-type plasminogen activator in acute myocardial infarction: results of the thrombolysis in myocardial infarction (TIMI) trial phase II. *N Engl J Med* 320: 618–627, 1989.

69. Frishman WH: Carvedilol. *N Engl J Med* 339:1759, 1998.

70. MERIT-HF Study Group: Effect of metoprolol CR/XL in chronic heart failure: Metoprolol CR/XL Randomised Intervention Trial in Congestive Heart Failure (MERIT-HF). *Lancet* 353:2001, 1999.

71. CIBIS-II Investigators and Committee: The Cardiac Insufficiency Bisoprolol Study II (CIBIS-II): a randomised trial. *Lancet* 353:9, 1999.

72. Packer M, Coats AJS, Fowler MB, et al: for the Carvedilol Prospective Randomized Cumulative Survival Study Group: effect of carvedilol on survival in severe chronic heart failure. *N Engl J Med* 344:1651, 2001.

73. Glaubiger G, Lefkowitz RJ: Elevated beta-receptor number after chronic propranolol treatment. *Biochem Biophys Res Commun* 78:720–725, 1977.

74. Frishman WH: Beta-adrenergic blocker withdrawal. *Am J Cardiol* 59(13):26F–32F, 1987.

75. Bristow MR, Port JD, Sandoval A, et al: β-Adrenergic receptor pathways in the failing human heart. *Heart Failure* 5:77–90,1989.

76. Gilbert EM, Olsen SL, Renlund DG, Bristow MR: Beta-adrenergic receptor regulation and left ventricular function in idiopathic dilated cardiomyopathy. *Am J Cardiol* 71:23C, 1993.

77. Dishy V, Sofowora GG, Xie H-G, et al: The effect of common polymorphisms of the β₂-adrenergic receptor on agonist-mediated vascular desensitization. *N Engl J Med* 345:1030, 2001.

78. Hausdorff WP, Caron MG, Lefkowitz RJ: Turning off the signal desensitization of beta-adrenergic receptor function. *FASEB J* 41:2881, 1990.

79. Lefkowitz RJ, Caron MG, Stile GL: Mechanisms of membrane-receptor regulation. Biochemical, physiological and clinical insights derived from studies of the adrenergic receptors. *N Engl J Med* 310:1570–1579, 1984.

80. Benovic JL, Strasser RH, Caron MG, Lefkowitz RJ: β-Adrenergic receptor kinase: identification of a novel protein kinase that phosphorylates the agonist-occupied form of the receptor. *Proc Natl Acad Sci USA* 83:2797, 1986.

81. Akhter SA, Eckhart AD, Rockman HA, et al: In vivo inhibition of elevated myocardial β-adrenergic receptor kinase activity in hybrid transgenic mice restores normal β-adrenergic signaling and function. *Circulation* 100:648, 1999.

82. Lefkowitz RJ: G protein-coupled receptors. III. New roles for receptor kinases and beta-arrestins in receptor signaling and desensitization. *J Biol Chem* 273:18677, 1998.

83. Luttrell LM, Ferguson SSG, Daaka Y, et al: β-arrestin-dependent formation of β₂ adrenergic receptor–Src protein kinase complexes. *Science* 283:655, 1999.

84. McDonald PH, Chow C-W, Miller WE, et al: β-arrestin 2: a receptor-regulated MAPK scaffold for the activation of JNK3. *Science* 290:1574, 2000.

84a. Shenoy SK, McDonald P, Kohout TA, Lefkowitz RJ: Regulation of receptor fate by ubiquitination of activated β₂-adrenergic receptor and β-arrestin. *Science* 294:1307, 2001.

85. Cruickshank JM, Prichard BNC: *Beta-Blockers in Clinical Practice,* 2nd ed. Edinburgh: Churchill Livingstone, 1994:1055.

86. Frishman WH: The beta-adrenoceptor blocking drugs. *Int J Cardiol* 2:165–178, 1982.

87. Yamamoto N, Numura M, Okubo K, et al: Pharmacologic characterization of FR 172516: a new combined calcium channel-blocking and β-adrenoceptor-blocking agents. *J Cardiovasc Pharmacol* 33:587, 1999.

88. Yeh J-L, Liou S-F, Liang J-C, et al: Vanidipinedilol: a vanilloid-based β-adrenoceptor blocker displaying calcium entry blocking and vasorelaxant activities. *J Cardiovasc Pharmacol* 35:51, 2000.

89. Moser M, Frishman W: Results of therapy with carvedilol; a β-blocker vasodilator with antioxidant properties, in hypertensive patients. *Am J Hypertens* 11(1 Pt 2):15S, 1998.

90. Koch-Weser J: Metoprolol. *N Engl J Med* 301:698-703, 1979.

91. Frishman WH: Atenolol and timolol, two new systemic adrenoceptor antagonists. *N Engl J Med* 306:1456–1462, 1982.

92. Frishman WH: Nadolol: A new β-adrenoceptor antagonist. *N Engl J Med* 305:678–684, 1981.

93. Frishman WH: Pindolol: A new β-adrenoceptor antagonist with partial agonist activity. *N Engl J Med* 308:940–944, 1983.

94. Frishman WH, Covey S: Penbutolol and carteolol: two new beta-adrenergic blockers with partial agonism. *J Clin Pharmacol* 30:412–421, 1990.

95. Frishman WH, Tepper D, Lazar E, Behrmann D: Betaxolol: a new long-acting β₁-selective adrenergic blocker. *J Clin Pharmacol* 30:699–703, 1990.

96. Frishman W, Silverman R: Clinical pharmacology of the new beta-adrenergic blocking drugs. Part III: Comparative clinical experience and new therapeutic applications. *Am Heart J* 98:119–131, 1979.

97. Frishman WH, Cheng-Lai A, Chen J, eds. *Current Cardiovascular Drugs,* 3rd ed. Philadelphia: Current Medicine, 2000:120.

98. Sugiyama A, Takahara A, Hashimoto K: Electrophysiologic, cardiohemodynamic and β blocking actions of a new ultra-short-acting β blocker, ONO-1101, assessed by the in vivo canine model in comparison with esmolol. *J Cardiovasc Pharmacol* 34:70, 1999.

99. Atarashi H, Kuruma A, Yashima M-a, et al: Pharmacokinetics of landiolol hydrochloride, a new ultra-short-acting β blocker, in patients with cardiac arrhythmias. *Clin Pharmacol Ther* 68:143, 2000.

100. McNeely W, Goa KL: Nebivolol in the management of essential hypertension. *Drugs* 57:633, 1999.

101. Frishman W: Clinical pharmacology of the new beta-adrenergic blocking drugs. Part I: Pharmacokinetic and pharmacodynamic properties. *Am Heart J* 97:663–670, 1979.

102. Conolly ME, Kersting F, Dollery CT: The clinical pharmacology of beta-adrenoceptor blocking drugs. *Prog Cardiovasc Dis* 19:203–234, 1976.

103. Singh BN, Deedwania P, Nademanee K, et al: Sotalol: a review of its pharmacodynamic and pharmacokinetic properties and therapeutic use. *Drugs* 34:311–349, 1987.

104. Morgan T: Clinical pharmacokinetics and pharmacodynamics of carvedilol. *Clin Pharmacokinet* 26:335, 1994.
105. Opie LH, Yusuf S: Beta-blocking agents. In: Opie LH, Gersh BJ, eds. *Drugs for the Heart*, 5th ed. Philadelphia: Saunders, 2001:1.
106. Frishman W, Jacob H, Eisenberg E, Ribner H: Clinical pharmacology of the new beta-adrenergic blocking drugs. Part VIII: Self-poisoning with beta-adrenoceptor blocking drugs: recognition and management. *Am Heart J* 98:798–811, 1979.
107. Henry JA, Cassidy SL: Membrane stabilizing activity: a major cause of fatal poisoning. *Lancet* 1:1414–1417, 1986.
108. Huang Y-C, Wu B-N, Lin Y-T: Eugenodilol: A third-generation β-adrenoceptor blocker, derived from eugenol, a α-adrenoceptor blocking and β_2-adrenoceptor agonist-associated vasorelaxant activities. *J Cardiovasc Pharmacol* 34:10, 1999.
109. Frishman WH: Clinical perspective on celiprolol. *Am Heart J* 121:724–729, 1991.
110. Taylor SH, Silke B, Lee PS: Intravenous beta-blockade in coronary heart disease: is cardioselectivity or intrinsic sympathomimetic activity hemodynamically useful? *N Engl J Med* 306:631–635, 1982.
111. Frishman W, Halprin S: Clinical pharmacology of the new beta-adrenergic blocking drugs. Part VII: New horizons in beta-adrenoceptor blocking therapy: labetalol. *Am Heart J* 98:660–665, 1979.
112. Frishman WH, Strom J, Kirschner M, et al: Labetalol therapy in patients with systemic hypertension and angina pectoris: effects of combined alpha- and beta-adrenergic blockade. *Am J Cardiol* 48:97–928, 1981.
113. Frishman WH: Properties of labetalol, a combined β- and α-adrenergic blocking agents relevant to the treatment of myocardial ischemia. *Cardiovasc Drug Ther* 2:343–353, 1988.
114. Van Zwieten A: Pharmacology of antihypertensive agents with multiple actions. *Eur J Clin Pharmacol* 38:577–581, 1990.
115. Gilbert EM, Anderson JL, Deitchman D, et al: Long-term β-blocker vasodilator therapy improves cardiac function in idiopathic dilated cardiomyopathy: a double-blind randomized study of bucindolol versus placebo. *Am J Med* 88:223–229, 1990.
116. Ruffolo RR, Gallai M, Heible JP, Willette RN: Hemodynamic differences between carvedilol and labetalol in the cutaneous circulation. *Eur J Pharmacol* 38:S112, 1990.
117. Yue TL, Lysko PG, Barone FC, et al: Carvedilol, a new antihypertensive with unique antioxidant activity: potential role in cerebroprotection. *Ann NY Acad Sci* 738:230, 1994.
118. Foody JM, Farrell MH, Krumholz HM: β-Blocker therapy in heart failure. *Scientific Review JAMA* 287:883, 2002.
119. Ruffolo RR Jr, Boyle DA, Brooks DP, et al: Carvedilol: a novel cardiovascular drug with multiple actions. *Cardiovasc Drug Rev* 10:127, 1992.
120. The Beta Blocker Evaluation of Survival Trial Investigators: a trial of the beta-blocker bucindolol in patients with advanced chronic heart failure. *N Engl J Med* 344:1659, 2001.
121. Broeders MAW, Doevendans PA, Bekkers BCAM, et al: Nebivolol: a third-generation β blocker that augments vascular nitric oxide release. Endothelial β_2-adrenergic receptor-mediated nitric oxide production. *Circulation* 102:677, 2000.
122. Atlwegg LA, d'Uscio LV, Barandier C, et al: Nebivolol induces NO-mediated relaxations of rat small mesenteric but not large elastic arteries. *J Cardiovasc Pharmacol* 36:316, 2000.
123. Kubli S, Feihl F, Waeber B: Beta-blockade with nebivolol enhances the acetylcholine-induced cutaneous vasodilation. *Clin Pharmacol Ther* 69:238, 2001.
124. Tzemos N, Lim PO, MacDonald TM: Nebivolol reverses endothelial dysfunction in essential hypertension. A randomized, double-blind, crossover study. *Circulation* 104:511, 2001.
125. Reid JL: Nebivolol: the role of nitric oxide in hypertension—concluding remarks. *J Cardiovasc Pharmacol* 38(Suppl 3):S37, 2001.
126. Waal Manning HJ: Hypertension: which beta-blocker? *Drugs* 12:412–421, 1976.
127. Frishman WH, Lazar EJ, Gorodokin G: Pharmacokinetic optimization of therapy with beta-adrenergic blocking agents. *Clin Pharmacokinet* 20:311–318, 1991.
128. Frishman WH, Alwarshetty M: Beta-adrenergic blockers in systemic hypertension: pharmacokinetic considerations related to the JNC-VI and WHO-ISH guidelines. *Clin Pharmacokinet* 2002 (in press).
129. Frishman WH, Teicher M: Long-acting propranolol. *Cardiovasc Rev Rep* 4:100–1102, 1983.
130. Halkin H, Vered I, Saginer A, Rabinowitz B: Once-daily administration of sustained release propranolol capsules in the treatment of angina pectoris. *Eur J Clin Pharmacol* 16:387–391, 1979.
131. Abrahamsson B, Lucker P, Olofsson, et al: The relationship between metoprolol plasma concentration and beta$_1$-blockade in healthy subjects: a study on conventional metoprolol and metoprolol CR/ZOK formulations. *J Clin Pharmacol* 30:S46, 1990.
132. Sandberg A, Blomqvist I, Jonsson UE, Lundborg P: Pharmacokinetic and pharmacodynamic properties of a new controlled-release formulation of metoprolol: a comparison with conventional tablets. *Eur J Clin Pharmacol* 33(Suppl):S9, 1988.
133. Frishman WH, Murthy VS, Strom JA: Ultra-short acting β-adrenergic blockers. *Med Clin North Am* 72:359–372, 1988.
134. Murthy VF, Frishman WH: Controlled beta-receptor blockade with esmolol and flestolol. *Pharmacotherapy* 8:168–182, 1988.
135. Parker JO, Porter A, Parker JD: Propranolol in angina pectoris: comparison of long-acting and standard formulation propranolol. *Circulation* 65:1351–1355, 1982.
136. Matier WL, Patil G: Esprolol hydrochloride. A new beta adrenergic antagonist with a rapid onset of effect. *Heart Dis* 2:146, 2000.
137. Frishman WH: Acebutolol. *Cardiovasc Rev Rep* 6:979–983, 1985.
138. Wurzelmann J, Frishman W, Aronson M, et al: Neuropsychiatric effects of antihypertensive drugs in the old old. *Cardiol Clin* 5:689–699, 1987.
139. Carney RM, Rich MW, te Velde AJE, et al: Prevalence of major depressive disorders in patients receiving β-blocker therapy versus other medications. *Am J Med* 83:223–226, 1987.
140. Kostis JB, Rosen RC: Central nervous system effects of β-adrenergic blocking drugs: the role of ancillary properties. *Circulation* 75:204–212, 1987.
141. Cruickshank JM, Prichard BNC: *Beta-blockers in Clinical Practice*, 2nd ed. Edinburgh: Churchill Livingstone, 1994:277.
142. Ward SA, Walle T, Walle UK, et al: Propranolol's metabolism is determined by both mephenytoin and debrisoquin hydroxylase activities. *Clin Pharmacol Ther* 45:72, 1989.
143. Fujimaki M: Oxidation of the R(+) and S(−) carvedilol by rat liver microsome. Evidence for stereoselective oxidation and characterization of the cytochrome P450 isozymes involved. *Drug Metab Dispos* 22:700, 1994.
144. Panton LB, Guillen GJ, Williams L, et al: The lack of effect of aerobic exercise training on propranolol pharmacokinetics in young and elderly adults. *J Clin Pharmacol* 35:885, 1995.
145. Cohn JN: Nitroprusside and dissecting aneurysm of aorta (correspondence). *N Engl J Med* 295:567, 1976.
146. Cohen LS, Braunwald E: Amelioration of angina pectoris in idiopathic hypertrophic subaortic stenosis with beta-adrenergic blockade. *Circulation* 35:847–851, 1967.
147. Turner JRB: Propranolol in the treatment of digitalis-induced and digitalis-resistant tachycardia. *Am J Cardiol* 18:450–457, 1966.
148. Winkle RA, Lopes MG, Goodman DS, et al: Propranolol for patients with mitral valve prolapse. *Am Heart J* 93:422–427, 1970.
149. Krahn AD, Yee R, Chauhan V, et al: Beta blockers normalize QT hysteresis in long QT syndrome. *Am Heart J* 143:528, 2002.
150. Kornbluth A, Frishman WH, Ackerman M: Beta-adrenergic blockade in children. *Cardiol Clin* 5:629–649, 1987.
151. Meister SG, Engel TR, Feitosa GS, et al: Propranolol in mitral stenosis during sinus rhythm. *Am Heart J* 94:685–688, 1977.
152. Svedberg K, Hjalmarson A, Waagstein F, Wallentin I: Beneficial effects of long-term beta-blockade in congestive cardiomyopathy. *Br Heart J* 44:117–133, 1980.
153. Sullebarger JT, Liang C-s: Beta-adrenergic receptor stimulation and inhibition in chronic congestive heart failure. *Heart Failure* 7:154–160, 1991.
154. Kraus ML, Gottlieb LD, Horwitz RI, Anscher M: Randomized clinical trial of atenolol in patients with alcohol withdrawal. *N Engl J Med* 313:905–909, 1985.
155. Weber RB, Reinmuth OM: The treatment of migraine with propranolol. *Neurology (NY)* 22:366–369, 1972.
155a. Young RR, Growdon JH, Shahani BT: Beta-adrenergic mechanisms in action tremor. *N Engl J Med* 293:950–953, 1975.
156. Frishman WH, Razin A, Swencionis C, Sonnenblick EH: Beta-adrenoceptor blockade in anxiety states: a new approach to therapy. Update. *Cardiovasc Rev Rep* (Classics of the Decade Series) 13(2):8–13, 1992.

157. Ingbar SH: The role of antiadrenergic agents in the management of thyrotoxicosis. *Cardiovasc Rev Rep* 2:683–689, 1981.

158. Caro JF, Castro JH, Glennon JA: Effect of long-term propranolol administration on parathyroid hormone and calcium concentration in primary hyperparathyroidism. *Ann Intern Med* 91:740–741, 1979.

159. Lebrec D, Poynard T, Hillon P, Benhamou J-P: Propranolol for prevention of recurrent gastrointestinal bleeding in patients with cirrhosis. *N Engl J Med* 305:1371–1374, 1981.

160. Herndon DN, Hart DW, Wolf SE, et al: Reversal of catabolism by beta-blockade after severe burns. *N Engl J Med* 345:1223, 2001.

161. SHEP Cooperative Research Group: Prevention of stroke by antihypertensive drug treatment in older persons with isolated systolic hypertension: final results of Systolic Hypertension in the Elderly Program (SHEP). *JAMA* 265:3255, 1991.

162. Kostis JB, Berge KG, Davis BR, et al: Effect of atenolol and resperine on selected events in the Systolic Hypertension in the Elderly Program (SHEP). *Am J Hypertens* 8:1147, 1995.

163. Dahlof B, Lindholm LH, Hansson L, et al: Morbidity and mortality in the Swedish Trial in Old Patients with Hypertension (STOP Hypertension). *Lancet* 338:1281, 1991.

164. The Fifth Report of the Joint National Committee on Detection, Evaluation and Treatment of High Blood Pressure (JNC V). *Arch Intern Med* 153:154, 1993.

165. The Sixth Report of the Joint National Committtee on Prevention, Detection, Evaluation and Treatment of High Blood Pressure (JNC VI). *Arch Intern Med* 157:2413, 1997.

166. Messerli FH, Grossman E, Goldbourt U: Are β blockers efficacious as first-line therapy for hypertension in the elderly? *JAMA* 279:1903, 1998.

166a. Lindholm LH, Ibsen H, Devereux RB, et al: Cardiovascular morbidity and mortality in patients with diabetes in the Losartan Intervention for Endpoint reduction in hypertension study (LIFE), a randomised trial against atenolol. *Lancet* 359:1004, 2002.

167. Gress TW, Nieto J, Shahar E, et al for the Atherosclerosis Risk in Communities Study: Hypertension and antihypertensive therapy as risk factors for type 2 diabetes mellitus. *N Engl J Med* 342:905, 2000.

168. Sowers JR, Bakris GL: Antihypertensive therapy and the risk of type 2 diabetes mellitus (editorial). *N Engl J Med* 342:969, 2000.

169. Saunders E, Weir MR, Kong BW, et al: A comparison of the efficacy and safety of a β-blocker, a calcium channel blocker, and a converting enzyme inhibitor in hypertensive blacks. *Arch Intern Med* 150:1707, 1990.

170. Frohlich ED: Hyperdynamic circulation and hypertension. *Postgrad Med* 52:68–74, 1972.

171. Blumenfeld ID, Sealey JE, Manner SJ, et al: β-Adrenergic receptor blockade as a therapeutic approach for suppressing the renin-angiotensin-aldosterone system in normotensive and hypertensive subjects. *Am J Hypertens* 12:451, 1999.

172. Myers MG, Lewis PJ, Reid JL, Dollery CT: Brain concentration of propranolol in relation to hypotension effects in the rabbit with observations on brain propranolol levels in man. *J Pharmacol Exp Ther* 192:327–335, 1975.

173. Prichard BNC: Propranolol as an antihypertensive agent. *Am Heart J* 79:128–133, 1979.

174. Imhof PR: Characterization of beta-blockers as antihypertensive agents in the light of human pharmacology studies, In: Schweizer W, ed. *Beta-Blockers—Present Status and Future Prospects.* Bern: Huber, 1974:40–50.

175. Langer SZ: Presynaptic receptors and their role in the regulation of transmitter release. *Br J Pharmacol* 60:481–497, 1977.

176. Berthelsen S, Pettinger WA: A functional basis for classification of β-adrenergic receptors. *Life Sci* 21:595–606, 1977.

177. Yamaguchi N, de Champlain J, Nadeau RL: Regulation of norepinephrine release from cardiac sympathetic fibers in the dog by presynaptic α- and β-receptors. *Circ Res* 41:108–117, 1976.

178. Stjarne L, Brundin J: β-Adrenoceptors facilitate noradrenaline secretion from human vasoconstrictor nerves. *Acta Physiol Scand* 97:88–93, 1976.

179. Majewski HJ, McCulloch MW, Rand MJ, Story DF: Adrenaline activation of prejunctional β-adrenoceptors in guinea pig atria. *Br J Pharmacol* 71:435–444, 1980.

180. Savolainen A, Keto P, Poutanen V-P, et al: Effects of angiotensin converting enzyme inhibition versus β-adrenergic blockade on aortic stiffness in essential hypertension. *J Cardiovasc Pharmacol* 27:99, 1996.

181. Waal HJ: Hypotensive action of propranolol. *Clin Pharmacol Ther* 7:588–598, 1966.

182. Rahn KH, Hawlina A, Kersting F, Peanz G: Studies on the antihypertensive action of the optical isomers of propranolol in man. *Naunyn Schmiedebergs Arch Pharmacol* 286:319–323, 1974.

182a. Pickering TG, Gribbin B, Petersen ES, et al: Effects of autonomic blockade on the baroreflex in man at rest and during exercise. *Circ Res* 30:177–185, 1972.

183. Kato N, Sugiyama T, Morita H, et al: Association analysis of β_2-adrenergic receptor polymorphisms with hypertension in Japanese. *Hypertension* 37:286, 2001.

184. Bray MS, Krushkal J, Li L, et al: Positional genomic analysis identifies the β_2-adrenergic receptor gene as a susceptibility locus for human hypertension. *Circulation* 101:2877, 2000.

185. Bengtsson K, Melander O, Orho-Melander M, et al: Polymorphism in the β_1-adrenergic receptor gene and hypertension. *Circulation* 104:187, 2001.

186. Jia H, Hingorani AD, Sharma P, et al: Association of the $G_s\alpha$ gene with essential hypertension and response to β blockade. *Hypertension* 34:8, 1999.

187. Sonnenblick EH, Ross J Jr, Braunwald E: Oxygen consumption of the heart: newer concepts of its multifactorial determination. *Am J Cardiol* 22:328–336, 1968.

188. Sonnenblick EH, Skelton CL: Myocardial energetics: basic principles and clinical implications. *N Engl J Med* 285:668–675, 1971.

189. Black JW, Stephenson JS: Pharmacology of a new adrenergic beta-receptor blocking compound (Nethalide). *Lancet* 2:311–314, 1962.

190. Frishman WH: Beta-adrenergic blockade in the treatment of coronary artery disease. In: Hurst JW, ed. *Clinical Essays on the Heart,* Vol 2. New York: McGraw-Hill, l983:25.

191. Billinger M, Seiler C, Fleisch M, et al: Do beta-adrenergic blocking agents increase coronary flow reserve? *J Am Coll Cardiol* 38:1866, 2001.

192. Frishman WH, Gabor R, Pepine C, Cavusoglu E: Heart rate reduction in the treatment of chronic stable angina pectoris: experience with a sinus node inhibitor. *Am Heart J* 131:204, 1996.

193. Brouwer J, Viersma JW, van Veldhuisen DJ, et al: Usefulness of heart rate variability in predicting drug efficacy (metoprolol vs diltiazem) in patients with stable angina pectoris. *Am J Cardiol* 76:759, 1995.

194. Ardissino D, Savonitto S, Egstrup K, et al: Selection of medical treatment in stable angina pectoris: results of the International Multicenter Angina Exercise (IMAGE) study. *J Am Coll Cardiol* 25:1516, 1995.

195. Frishman W, Pepine CJ, Weiss R, Baiker WM for the Zatebradine Study Group: Addition of zatebradine, a direct sinus node inhibitor, provides no greater exercise tolerance benefit in patients with angina pectoris taking extended-release nifedipine: results of a multicenter, randomized, double-blind, placebo-controlled, parallel group study. *J Am Coll Cardiol* 26:305, 1995.

196. Parratt JR, Grayson J: Myocardial vascular reactivity after β-adrenergic blockade. *Lancet* 1:338–340, 1966.

197. Becker LC, Fortuin NJ, Pitt B: Effects of ischemia and anti-anginal drugs on the distribution of radioactive microspheres in the canine left ventricle. *Circ Res* 28:263–269, 1971.

198. Wolfson S, Gorlin R: Cardiovascular pharmacology of propranolol in man. *Circulation* 40:501–511, 1969.

199. Barrett AM: A comparison of the effect of (+) propranolol and (+) propranolol in anesthetized dogs: β-receptor blocking and hemodynamic action. *J Pharm Pharmacol* 21:241–247, 1969.

200. Bjorntorp P: Treatment of angina pectoris with beta-adrenergic blockade: mode of action. *Acta Med Scand* 184:259–262, 1968.

201. Fihn SD, Williams SV, Daley J, Gibbons RJ: Guidelines for the management of patients with chronic stable angina: treatment. *Ann Intern Med* 135:616, 2001.

202. Haim M, Shotan A, Boyko V, et al for the Bezafibrate Infarction Prevention (BIP) Study Group: effect of beta blocker therapy in patients with coronary artery disease in New York Heart Association classes II and III. *Am J Cardiol* 81:1455, 1998.

203. Heidenreich PA, McDonald KM, Hastie T, et al: Meta-analysis of trials comparing β blockers, calcium antagonists, and nitrates for stable angina. *JAMA* 281:1927, 1999.

204. Marie PY, Danchin N, Branly F, et al: Effects of medical therapy on outcome assessment using exercise thallium-201 single photon emission computer tomography imaging. Evidence from a protective effect of beta-blocking antianginal medications. *J Am Coll Cardiol* 34:113, 1999.

205. Task Force of the European Society of Cardiology: management of stable angina pectoris. Recommendations of the Task Force of the European Society of Cardiology. *Eur Heart J* 18:394, 1997.

206. Gibbons RJ, Chatterjee K, Daley J, et al: ACC/AHA/ACP-ASIM guidelines for the management of patients with chronic stable angina: Executive summary and recommendations. A report of the American College of Cardiology/American Heart Association Task Force on Practice Guidelines (Committee on Management of Patients with Chronic Stable Angina). *Circulation* 99:2829, 1999.

207. Frishman WH, Smithen C, Befler B, et al: Non-invasive assessment of clinical response to oral propranolol. *Am J Cardiol* 35:635–644, 1975.

208. Gauri AJ, Raxwal VK, Roux L, et al: Effects of chronotropic incompetence and β blocker use on the exercise treadmill test in men. *Am Heart J* 142:136, 2001.

209. Robinson BF: The mode of action of beta-antagonists in angina pectoris. *Postgrad Med J* 47:4l–43, 1971.

210. Packer M: Combined beta-adrenergic and calcium-entry blockade in angina pectoris. *N Engl J Med* 320:709, 1989.

211. Weiner DA, Klein MD: Calcium antagonists for the treatment of angina pectoris. In: Weiner DA, Frishman WH, eds. *Therapy of Angina Pectoris*. New York: Marcel Dekker, 1986:45–204.

212. Weiner DA: Calcium channel blockers. *Med Clin North Am* 72:83–115, 1988.

213. Frishman WH, Charlap S, Farham J, et al: Combination propranolol and bepridil therapy in stable angina pectoris. *Am J Cardiol* 55:43C–49C, 1985.

214. Schwarz ER, Klues HG, vom Dahl J, et al: Functional, angiographic and intracoronary Doppler flow characteristics in symptomatic patients with myocardial bridging: effect of short-term intravenous beta-blocker medication. *J Am Coll Cardiol* 27:1637, 1996.

214a. ACC/AHA 2002 Guidelines Update for the Management of Patients with Unstable Angina and Non-ST-Segment Elevation Myocardial Infarction. www.acc.org/clinical/guidelines/unstable.pdf 2002.

215. Doo Y-C, Kim D-M, Oh D-J, et al: Effect of beta blockers on expression of interleukin-6 and C-reactive protein in patients with unstable angina pectoris. *Am J Cardiol* 88:422, 2001.

215a. Jenkins NP, Keevil BG, Hutchinson IV, Brooks NH: Beta-blockers are associated with lower C-reactive protein concentrations in patients with coronary artery disease. *Am J Med* 112:269, 2002.

216. Miura D, Frishman WH, Dangman KH: Class II drugs. In: Dangman KH, Miura D, eds. *Basic and Clinical Electrophysiology and Pharmacology of the Heart*. New York: Marcel Dekker, 1991:665–676.

217. Nademanee K, Taylor R, Bailey WE, et al: Treating electrical storm. Sympathetic blockade versus advanced cardiac life support-guided therapy. *Circulation* 102:742, 2000.

218. Xu X, Zhang M, Kyker K, et al: Ischemic inactivation of G protein-coupled receptor kinase and altered desensitization of canine cardiac β-adrenergic receptors. *Circulation* 102:2535, 2000.

219. Tisdale JE, Sun H, Zhao H, et al: Antifibrillatory effect of esmolol alone and in combination with lidocaine. *J Cardiovasc Pharmacol* 27:376, 1996.

220. Cavusoglu E, Frishman WH: Sotalol: a new β-adrenergic blocker for ventricular arrhythmias. *Prog Cardiovasc Dis* 37:423, 1995.

221. Anderson JL, Prystowsky EN: Sotalol: an important new antiarrhythmic. *Am Heart J* 137:388, 1999.

222. Kühlkamp V, Mewis C, Mermi J, et al: Suppression of sustained ventricular tachyarrhythmias: a comparison of d,l-sotalol with no antiarrhythmic drug treatment. *J Am Coll Cardiol* 33:46, 1999.

223. Pacifico A, Hohnloser SH, Williams JH, et al for the d,l-Sotalol Implantable Cardioverter-Defibrillator Study Group: prevention of implantable defibrillator shocks by treatment with sotalol. *N Engl J Med* 340:1855, 1999.

224. Mewis C, Kühlkamp V, Mermi J, et al: Long-term reproducibility of electrophysiologically guided therapy with sotalol in patients with ventricular tachyarrhythmias. *J Am Coll Cardiol* 33:1989, 1999.

225. Lai L-P, Lin J-L, Lien W-P, et al: Intravenous sotalol decreases transthoracic cardioversion energy requirement for chronic atrial fibrillation in humans: assessment of the electrophysiological effects by biatrial basket electrodes. *J Am Coll Cardiol* 35:1434, 2000.

226. Southworth MR, Zarembski D, Viana M, Bauman J: Comparison of sotalol versus quinidine for maintenance of normal sinus rhythm in patients with chronic atrial fibrillation. *Am J Cardiol* 83:1629, 1999.

227. Tse H-F, Lau C-P, Ayers GM: Incidence and modes of onset of early reinitiation of atrial fibrillation after successful internal cardioversion, and its prevention by intravenous sotalol. *Heart* 82:319, 1999.

228. Gomes JA, Ip J, Santoni-Rugiu F, et al: Oral d,l sotalol reduces the incidence of postoperative atrial fibrillation in coronary artery bypass surgery patients: a randomized, double-bind, placebo-controlled study. *J Am Coll Cardiol* 34:334, 1999.

229. Benditt DG, Williams JH, Deering TF, et al for the d,l Sotalol Atrial Fibrillation/Flutter Study Group: Maintenance of sinus rhythm with oral d,l sotalol therapy in patients with symptomatic atrial fibrillation and/or atrial flutter. *Am J Cardiol* 84:270, 1999.

230. Bellandi F, Simonetti I, Leoncini M, et al: Long-term efficacy and safety of propafenone and sotalol for the maintenance of sinus rhythm after conversion of recurrent symptomatic atrial fibrillation. *Am J Cardiol* 88:640, 2001.

231. Amato Vincenzo de Paola A, Horta Veloso H, for the SOCESP Investigators: efficacy and safety of sotalol versus quinidine for the maintenance of sinus rhythm after conversion of atrial fibrillation. *Am J Cardiol* 84:1033, 1999.

232. Kochiadakis GE, Igoumenidis NE, Marketous ME, et al: Low dose amiodarone and sotalol in the treatment of recurrent, symptomatic atrial fibrillation: a comparative, placebo controlled study. *Heart* 84:251, 2000.

233. Waldo AL, Camm AJ, deRuyter H, et al for the SWORD Investigators: effect of d-sotalol on mortality in patients with left ventricular dysfunction after recent and remote myocardial infarction. *Lancet* 348:7, 1996.

234. Pratt CM, Camm AJ, Cooper W, et al for the SWORD Investigators: mortality in the Survival with Oral D-Sotalol (SWORD) Trial: Why did patients die? *Am J Cardiol* 81:869, 1998.

235. Lehmann MH, Hardy S, Archibald D, MacNeil DJ: JTc prolongation with d,l sotalol in women versus men. *Am J Cardiol* 83:354, 1999.

236. Chung MK, Schweikert RA, Wilkoff BL, et al: Is hospital admission for initiation of anti-arrhythmic therapy with sotalol for atrial arrhythmias required? Yield of in-hospital monitoring and prediction of risk for significant arrhythmia complications. *J Am Coll Cardiol* 32:169, 1998.

237. Barbey JT, Sale ME, Woosley RL, et al: Pharmacokinetic, pharmacodynamic, and safety evaluation of an accelerated dose titration regimen of sotalol in healthy middle-aged subjects. *Clin Pharmacol Ther* 66:91, 1999.

238. Kühlkamp V, Schirdewan A, Stangl K, et al: Use of metoprolol CR/XL to maintain sinus rhythm after conversion from persistent atrial fibrillation: a randomized, double-blind, placebo-controlled study. *J Am Coll Cardiol* 36:139, 2000.

239. Page RL: Beta blockers for atrial fibrillation: must we consider asymptomatic arrhythmias? *J Am Coll Cardiol* 36:147, 2000.

240. Farshi R, Kistner D, Sarma JSM, et al: Ventricular rate control in chronic atrial fibrillation during daily activity and programmed exercise: a crossover open-label study of five drug regimens. *J Am Coll Cardiol* 33:304, 1999.

241. Sager PT: Modulation of antiarrhythmic drug effects by beta-adrenergic sympathetic stimulation. *Am J Cardiol* 82:20I, 1998.

242. Boutitie F, Boissel J-P, Connolly SJ, et al and the EMIAT and CAMIAT Investigators: Amiodarone interaction with β blockers. Analysis of the merged EMIAT (European Myocardial Infarct Amiodarone Trial) and CAMIAT (Canadian Amiodarone Myocardial Infarction Trial) databases. *Circulation* 99:2268, 1999.

243. Antz M, Cappato R, Kuck K-H: Metoprolol versus sotalol in the treatment of sustained ventricular tachycardia. *J Cardiovasc Pharmacol* 26:627, 1995.

244. Pitzalia MV, Mastropasqua F, Massari F, et al: Holter-guided identification of premature ventricular contractions susceptible to suppression by β blockers. *Am Heart J* 131:508, 1996.

245. Reiter MJ, Reiffel JA: Importance of beta blockade in the therapy of serious ventricular arrhythmias. *Am J Cardiol* 82:9I, 1998.

246. Exner DV, Reiffel JA, Epstein AE, et al and the AVID Investigators: beta blocker use and survival in patients with ventricular fibrillation or symptomatic ventricular tachycardia: the Antiarrhythmics versus Implantable Defibrillators (AVID) trial. *J Am Coll Cardiol* 34:325, 1999.

247. Frishman WH, Cavusoglu E: β-Adrenergic blockers and their role in the therapy of arrhythmias. In: Podrid PJ, Kowey PR, eds. *Cardiac Arrhythmias: Mechanisms, Diagnosis and Management*. Baltimore: Williams & Wilkins, 1995:421–433.

248. Ryden L, Ariniego R, Arnman K, et al: A double-blind trial of meto-prolol in acute myocardial infarction: effects on ventricular tach-yarrhythmias. *N Engl J Med* 308:614–618, 1983.

249. Lichstein E, Morganroth J, Harrist R, et al for the BHAT Study Group: Effect of propranolol on ventricular arrhythmia—the Beta Blocker Heart Attack Trial Experience. *Circulation* 67:I5, 1983.

250. Szabo BM, Crijn HJGM, Wiesfeld ACP, et al: Predictors of mortal-ity in patients with sustained ventricular tachycardias or ventricular fibrillation and depressed left ventricular function: importance of β blockade. *Am Heart J* 130:281, 1995.

251. Mason JW for the Electrophysiologic Study Versus Electrocardio-graphic Monitoring (ESVEM): a comparison of seven antiarrhythmic drugs in patients with ventricular tachyarrhythmias. *N Engl J Med* 329:452, 1993.

252. Kennedy HL, Brooks MM, Barker AH, et al: Beta blocker therapy in the Cardiac Arrhythmia Suppression Trial. *Am J Cardiol* 74:674, 1994.

253. Steinbeck G, Andresen D, Bach P, et al: A comparison of electrophys-iologically guided antiarrhythmic drug therapy with beta blocker ther-apy in patients with symptomatic, sustained ventricular tachyarrhyth-mias. *N Engl J Med* 327:987, 1992.

254. Chiale PA, Rosenbaum MB, Elizari MV, et al: High prevalence of antibodies against beta$_1$- and beta$_2$-adrenoceptors in patients with primary electrical cardiac abnormalities. *J Am Coll Cardiol* 26:864, 1995.

255. Iwata M, Yoshikawa T, Baba A, et al: Autoantibodies against the sec-ond extracellular loop of beta$_1$-adrenergic receptors predict ventric-ular tachycardia and sudden death in patients with idiopathic dilated cardiomyopathy. *J Am Coll Cardiol* 37:418, 2001.

256. Braunwald E, Muller JE, Kloner RA, Maroko P: Role of beta-adrenergic blockade in the therapy of patients with myocardial in-farction. *Am J Med* 74:113–123, 1983.

257. Abrams J, Frishman W, Weitz J, Opie L: Pharmacologic options for treatment of ischemic disease. In: Antman E, ed. *Cardiovascu-lar Therapeutics. A Companion to Braunwald's Heart Disease*, 2nd ed. Philadelphia: Saunders, 2002:97.

258. Boissel-J-P, Leizorovicz A, Picolet H, et al for the APSI Investigators: secondary prevention after high risk myocardial infarction with low-dose acebutolol. *Am J Cardiol* 66:251, 1990.

259. Parks KC, Forman DE, Wei JY: Utility of beta-blockade treat-ment for older postinfarction patients. *J Am Geriatr Soc* 43:751, 1995.

259a. Freemantle N, Cleland J, Young P, et al: β blockade after myocar-dial infarction: systematic review and meta regression analysis. *BMJ* 318:1730, 1999.

260. Furberg CD, Hawkins CM, Lichstein E: Effect of propranolol in post-infarction patients with mechanical or electrical complications. *Circulation* 69:761–765, 1984.

261. Frishman WH: Role of β-adrenergic blockade. In: Fuster V, Ross R, Topol EJ, eds. *Atherosclerosis and Coronary Artery Disease*. New York: Lippincott, 1996:1205.

262. Frishman WH: Secondary prevention of myocardial infarction: the roles of β-adrenergic blockers, calcium-channel blockers, angiotensin converting enzyme inhibitors, and aspirin. In: Willich SN, Muller JE, eds. *Triggering of Acute Coronary Syndromes*. The Netherlands: Kluwer, 1996:367.

263. Frishman WH, Skolnick AE, Miller KP: Secondary prevention post infarction: The role of beta-adrenergic blockers, calcium-channel blockers, and aspirin. In: Gersh B, Rahimtoola S, eds. *Acute My-ocardial Infarction*, 2nd ed. New York: Chapman & Hall, 1996: 766.

264. Kendall MJ, Lynch KP, Hjalmarson A, Kjekshus J: β-Blockers and sudden cardiac death. *Ann Intern Med* 123:358, 1995.

265. Tuininga YS, Crijns HJGM, Brouwer J, et al: Evaluation of im-portance of central effects of atenolol and metoprolol measured by heart rate variability during mental performance tasks, physical exer-cise, and daily life in stable postinfarct patients. *Circulation* 92:3415, 1995.

266. Gottlieb SS, McCarter RJ: Comparative effects of three beta block-ers (atenolol, metoprolol, and propranolol) on survival after acute myocardial infarction. *Am J Cardiol* 87:823, 2001.

266a. β Blockers are best antiarrhythmics for reducing post-MI mortality. *Drugs Ther Perspect* 17:5, 2001.

267. Frishman WH, Lazar EJ: Reduction of mortality, sudden death and non-fatal reinfarction with beta-adrenergic blockers in survivors of

acute myocardial infarction: a new hypothesis regarding the cardio-protective action of beta-adrenergic blockade. *Am J Cardiol* 66:66G–70G, 1990.

268. Williams MJA, Low CJS, Wilkins GT, Stewart RAH: Randomised comparison of the effects of nicardipine and esmolol on coronary artery wall stress: implications for the risk of plaque rupture. *Heart* 84:377, 2000.

269. International Collaborative Study Group: Reduction of infarct size with the early use of timolol in acute myocardial infarction. *N Engl J Med* 310:9–15, 1984.

270. Hjalmarson A, Elmfeldt D, Herlitz J, et al: Effect of mortality of meto-prolol in acute myocardial infarction. A double-blind randomised trial. *Lancet* 2:823–827, 1981.

271. MIAMI Trial Research Group: Metoprolol in acute myocardial infarc-tion (MIAMI): a randomized placebo-controlled international trial. *Eur Heart J* 6:199–226, 1985.

272. Muller J, Roberts R, Stone P, et al: Failure of propranolol administra-tion to limit infarct size in patients with acute myocardial infarction (abstr). *Circulation* 68 (Suppl. III):III294, 1983.

273. Barron HV, Rundle AC, Gore JM, et al for the Participants in the Na-tional Registry of Myocardial Infarction-2. Intracranial hemorrhage rates and effect of immediate beta-blocker use in patients with acute myocardial infarction treated with tissue plasminogen activators. *Am J Cardiol* 85:294, 2000.

273a. Pfisterer M, Cox JL, Granger CB, et al for the GUSTO-I Investiga-tors: atenolol use and clinical outcomes after thrombolysis for acute myocardial infarction: the GUSTO-I experience. *J Am Coll Cardiol* 32:634, 1998.

274. Phillips BG, Yim JM, Brown EJ Jr, et al: Pharmacologic profile of survivors of acute myocardial infarction at United States academic hospitals. *Am Heart J* 131:872, 1996.

275. Ayanian JZ, Hauptman PJ, Guadagnoli E, et al: Knowledge and prac-tices of generalist and specialist physicians regarding drug therapy for acute myocardial infarction. *N Engl J Med* 331:1136, 1994.

276. Soumerai SB, McLaughlin TJ, Spiegelman D, et al: Adverse outcomes of underuse of beta blockers in elderly survivors of acute myocardial infarction. *JAMA* 277:115, 1997.

277. Gheorghiade M, Goldstein S: β-Blockers in the post-myocardial in-farction patient. *Circulation* 106:394, 2002.

278. Grand DA, Newcomer LN, Frieburger A, Tian H: Cardiologist's prac-tice compared with practice guidelines: use of beta blockade after acute myocardial infarction. *J Am Coll Cardiol* 26:1432, 1995.

279. Phillips KA, Shlipak MG, Coxson P, et al: Health and economic bene-fits of increased β blocker use following myocardial infarction. *JAMA* 284:2748, 2000.

280. Chen J, Radford MJ, Wang Y, et al: Effectiveness of beta blocker ther-apy after acute myocardial infarction in elderly patients with chronic obstructive pulmonary disease or asthma. *J Am Coll Cardiol* 37:1950, 2001.

281. Aronow WS, Ahn C: Effect of beta blockers on incidence of new coronary events in older persons with prior myocardial infarction and diabetes mellitus. *Am J Cardiol* 87:780, 2001.

282. Rochon PA, Tu JV, Anderson GM, et al: Rate of heart failure and 1-year survival for older people receiving low-dose β blocker therapy after myocardial infarction. *Lancet* 356:639, 2000.

283. Barron HV, Viskin S: Dispelling the myths surrounding the use of beta blockers in patients after acute myocardial infarction. *Prev Cardiol* 3:13, 1998.

284. Krumholz HM, Radford MJ, Wang Y, et al: National use and effec-tiveness of β blockers for the treatment of elderly patients after acute myocardial infarction. National Cooperative Cardiovascular Project. *JAMA* 280:623, 1998.

285. Krumholz HM, Radford MJ, Wang Y, et al: Early β blocker therapy for acute myocardial infarction in elderly patients. *Ann Intern Med* 131:648, 1999.

286. Chen J, Marciniak TA, Radford MJ, et al: Beta blocker therapy for secondary prevention of myocardial infarction in elderly diabetic pa-tients. *J Am Coll Cardiol* 34:1388, 1999.

287. Gottlieb SS, McCarter RJ, Vogel RA: Effect of beta blockade on mortality among high-risk and low-risk patients after myocardial in-farction. *N Engl J Med* 339:489, 1998.

288. Heller DA, Ahern FM, Kozak M: Changes in rates of β blocker use between 1994 and 1997 among elderly survivors of acute myocardial infarction. *Am Heart J* 140:663, 2000.

289. Chen J, Radford MJ, Wang Y, et al: Are β blockers effective in elderly patients who undergo coronary revascularization after acute myocardial infarction? *Arch Intern Med* 160:947, 2000.

290. The CAPRICORN Investigators: Effect of carvedilol on outcome after myocardial infarction in patients with left ventricular dysfunction: the CAPRICORN randomised trial. *Lancet* 357:1385, 2001.

291. Bradley EH, Holmboe ES, Matterna JA, et al: A qualitative study of increasing β blocker use after myocardial infarction. Why do some hospitals succeed? *JAMA* 285:2604, 2001.

292. Soumerai SB, McLaughlin TJ, Gurwitz JH, et al: Effect of local medical opinion leaders on quality of care for acute myocardial infarction: a randomized controlled trial. *JAMA* 279:1358, 1998.

293. Sarasin FP, Maschiangelo M-L, Schaller M-D, et al: Successful implementation of guidelines for encouraging the use of beta blockers in patients after acute myocardial infarction. *Am J Med* 106:499, 1999.

294. Barron HV, Viskin S, Lumdstrom RJ, et al: β Blocker dosages and mortality after myocardial infarction. Data from a large health maintenance organization. *Arch Intern Med* 158:449, 1998.

295. Gardtman M, Dellborg M, Brunnhage C, et al: Effect of intravenous metoprolol before hospital admission on chest pain in suspected acute myocardial infarction. *Am Heart J* 137:821, 1999.

296. Frishman WH, Teicher M: Antianginal drug therapy for silent myocardial ischemia. *Med Clin North Am* 72:185–196, 1988.

297. Andrews TC, Fenton T, Toyosaki N, et al for the Angina and Silent Ischemia Study Group (ASIS): subsets of ambulatory myocardial ischemia based on heart rate activity. Circadian distribution and response to anti-ischemic medication. *Circulation* 88:92, 1993.

298. Rogers WJ, Bourassa MG, Andrews TC, et al: Asymptomatic Cardiac Ischemia Pilot (ACIP) Study: Outcome at 1 year for patients with asymptomatic cardiac ischemia randomized to medical therapy or revascularization. *J Am Coll Cardiol* 26:594, 1995.

299. Pepine CJ, Cohn PF, Deedwania PC, et al for the ASIST (Atenolol/Silent Ischemia Study) Study Group: effects of treatment on outcome in mildly symptomatic patients with ischemia during daily life. *Circulation* 90:762, 1994.

300. Portegies MCM, Sijbring P, Gobel EJA, et al: Efficacy of metoprolol and diltiazem in treating silent myocardial ischemia. *Am J Cardiol* 74:1095, 1994.

301. von Arnim T for the TIBBS Investigators: prognostic significance of transient ischemic episodes: response to treatment shows improves prognosis. *J Am Coll Cardiol* 28:20, 1996.

302. Madjlessi-Simon T, Mary-Krause M, Fillette F, et al: Persistent transient myocardial ischemia despite beta-adrenergic blockade predicts a higher risk of adverse cardiac events in patients with coronary artery disease. *J Am Coll Cardiol* 27:1586, 1996.

303. Engelhardt S, Bohm M, Erdmann E, Lohse MJ: Analysis of beta-adrenergic receptor mRNA levels in human ventricular biopsy specimens by quantitative polymerase chain reactions: progressive reduction of $beta_1$-adrenergic receptor mRNA in heart failure. *J Am Coll Cardiol* 27:146, 1996.

304. De Mello WC: Impaired regulation of cell communication by β-adrenergic receptor activation in the failing heart. *Hypertension* 27:265, 1996.

305. Wu J-R, Chang H-R, Huang T-Y, et al: Reduction in lymphocyte β-adrenergic density in infants and children with heart failure secondary to congenital heart failure. *Am J Cardiol* 22:120, 1996.

305a. Akhter SA, Eckhart AD, Rockman HA, et al: In vivo inhibition of elevated myocardial β-adrenergic receptor kinase activity in hybrid transgenic mice restores normal β-adrenergic signaling and function. *Circulation* 100:648, 1999.

305b. Cho M-C, Rao M, Koch WJ, et al: Enhanced contractility and decreased β-adrenergic receptor kinase-1 in mice lacking endogenous norepinephrine and epinephrine. *Circulation* 99:2702, 1999.

305c. Moniotte S, Kobzik L, Feron O, et al: Upregulation of β_3 adrenoceptors and altered contractile response to inotropic amines in human failing myocardium. *Circulation* 103:1649, 2001.

306. Sackner-Bernstein JD, Mancini DM: Rationale for treatment of patients with chronic heart failure with adrenergic blockade. *JAMA* 274:1462, 1995.

307. LeJemtel TH, Sonnenblick EH, Frishman WH: Diagnosis and management of heart failure. In: Fuster V, Alexander RW, O'Rourke RA, eds. *Hurst's The Heart,* 10th ed. New York: McGraw-Hill, 2000:687.

308. White DC, Hata JA, Shah AS, et al: Preservation of myocardial β-adrenergic receptor signaling delays the development of heart failure after myocardial infarction. *Proc Natl Acad Sci USA* 97:5428, 2000.

309. Manning BS, Shotwell K, Mao L, et al: Physiological induction of a β-adrenergic receptor kinase inhibitor transgene preserves β-adrenergic responsiveness in pressure-overload cardiac hypertrophy. *Circulation* 102:2751, 2000.

310. Shad AS, White DC, Emani S, et al: In vivo ventricular gene delivery of a β-adrenergic receptor kinase inhibitor to the failing heart reverses cardiac dysfunction. *Circulation* 103:1311, 2001.

311. Podlowski S, Luther HP, Morwinski R, et al: Agonistic anti-β_1-adrenergic receptor autoanti-bodies from cardiomyopathy patients reduces the β_1-adrenergic receptor expression in neonatal rat cardiomyocytes. *Circulation* 98:2470, 1998.

312. Francis GS, Goldsmith SR, Cohn JN: Relationship of exercise capacity to resting left ventricular performance and basal plasma norepinephrine levels in patients with congestive heart failure. *Am Heart J* 104:725, 1982.

313. Viquerat CE, Daly P, Swedberg K, et al: Endogenous catecholamine levels in congestive heart failure: relation to severity of hemodynamic abnormality. *Am J Med* 78:455, 1985.

314. Stanek B, Frey B, Hulsmann M, et al: Prognostic evaluation of neurohumoral plasma levels before and during beta blocker therapy in advanced left ventricular dysfunction. *J Am Coll Cardiol* 38:436, 2001.

315. Frishman WH: Multifactorial actions of β-adrenergic blocking drugs in ischemic heart disease. *Circulation* 67(Suppl I):I–11, 1983.

316. Daley PA, Sole MJ: Myocardial catecholamines and the pathophysiology of heart failure. *Circulation* 82(Suppl I):I–35, 1990.

317. Henderson EB, Kahn JK, Corbett JR, et al: Abnormal I123 metaiodobenzylguanidine myocardial washout and distribution may reflect myocardial adrenergic derangement in patients with congestive heart failure. *Circulation* 78:1192, 1988.

318. Cruikshank JM, Neil-Dwyer G, Degaute JP, et al: Reduction of stress/catecholamine induced cardiac necrosis by beta I-selective blockade. *Lancet* 2:585, 1987.

319. Pauletto P, Vescove G, Scannapieco G, et al: Cardioprotection by beta blockers: molecular and structural aspects in experimental hypertension. *Drugs Exp Clin Res* 16(3):1055, 1990.

320. Shizukuda Y, Buttrick PM, Geenen DL, et al: β-Adrenergic stimulation causes cardiocyte apoptosis: influence of tachycardia and hypertrophy. *Am J Physiol* 275:H961, 1998.

321. Iwai-Kanai E, Hasegawa K, Araki M, et al: α- and β-adrenergic pathways differentially regulate cell type-specific apoptosis in rat cardiac myocytes. *Circulation* 100:305, 1999.

322. Podrid PJ, Fuchs T, Candinas R: Role of the sympathetic nervous system in the genesis of ventricular arrhythmias. *Circulation* 82 (Suppl I):I–103, 1990.

323. Wit AL, Cranefield PF: Triggered and automatic activity in the canine coronary sinus. *Circ Res* 41:433, 1977.

324. Engelmeier RS, O'Connell JB, Walsh R, et al: Improvement in symptoms and exercise tolerance by metoprolol in patients with dilated cardiomyopathy: a double-blind, randomized, placebo-controlled trial. *Circulation* 72:536, 1985.

325. Waagstein F, Bristow MR, Swedberg K, et al: Beneficial effects of metoprolol in idiopathic dilated cardiomyopathy. *Lancet* 342:1441, 1993.

326. Olsen SL, Gilbert EM, Renlund DG, et al: Carvedilol improves left ventricular function and symptoms in chronic heart failure: a double-blind randomized study. *J Am Coll Cardiol* 25:1225, 1995.

327. Metra M, Nardi M, Giubbini R, Dei Cas L: Effects of short- and long-term carvedilol administration on rest and exercise hemodynamic variables, exercise capacity, and clinical conditions in patients with idiopathic dilated cardiomyopathy. *J Am Coll Cardiol* 24:1678, 1994.

328. Krum H, Sackner-Bernstein J, Goldsmith RL, et al: Double-blind, placebo-controlled study of the long-term efficacy of carvedilol in patients with severe chronic heart failure. *Circulation* 92:1499, 1995.

329. Australia-New Zealand Heart Failure Research Collaborative Group: Effects of carvedilol, a vasodilator–β blocker, in patients with congestive heart failure due to ischemic heart disease. *Circulation* 92:212, 1995.

330. Eichhorn EJ, McGhie AA, Bendotto JB, et al: Effects of bucindolol on neurohormonal activation in congestive heart failure. *Am J Cardiol* 67:67, 1991.

331. Leizorovicz A, Lechat P, Cucherat M, Bugnard F: Bisoproprolol for the treatment of chronic heart failure: a meta analysis on individual data of two placebo-controlled studies—CIBIS and CIBIS II. *Am Heart J* 143:301, 2002.

332. Goldstein S: Benefits of β-blocker therapy for heart failure. Weighing the evidence. *Arch Intern Med* 162: 641, 2002.

333. Farrell MH, Foody JM, Krumholz HM: β-blockers in heart failure: clinical applications. *JAMA* 287: 890, 2002.

334. Packer M, Bristow MR, Cohn N, et al: Effect of carvedilol on morbidity and mortality in chronic heart failure. *N Engl J Med* 334:1349–1355, 1996.

335. Joglar JA, Acusta AP, Shusterman NH, et al: Effect of carvedilol on survival and hemodynamics in patients with atrial fibrillation and left ventricular dysfunction: retrospective analysis of the U.S. Carvedilol Heart Failure Trials Program. *Am Heart J* 142:498, 2001.

336. Fowler MB, Vera-Llonch M, Oster G, et al for the U.S. Carvedilol Heart Failure Study Group: influence of carvedilol on hospitalizations in heart failure: incidence, resource utilization and costs. *J Am Coll Cardiol* 37:1692, 2001.

337. Yancy CW, Fowler MB, Colucci WS, et al for the U.S. Carvedilol Heart Failure Study Group: Race and the response to adrenergic blockade with carvedilol in patients with chronic heart failure. *N Engl J Med* 344:1358, 2001.

338. Kumar A, Choudhary G, Antonio C, et al: Carvedilol titration in patients with congestive heart failure receiving inotropic therapy. *Am Heart J* 142:512, 2001.

339. Hjalmarson A, Goldstein S, Fagerberg B, et al: for the MERIT-HF Study Group: Effects of controlled-release metoprolol on total mortality, hospitalizations, and well-being in patients with heart failure. The Metoprolol CR/XL Randomized Intervention Trial in Congestive Heart Failure (MERIT-HF). *JAMA* 283:1295, 2000.

340. Prakash A, Markham A: Metoprolol. A review of its use in chronic heart failure. *Drugs* 60:647, 2000.

340a. Ghali JK, Piña IL, Gottlieb SS, et al: Metoprolol CR/XL in female patients with heart failure. Analysis of the experience in Metoprolol Extended-release Randomized Intervention Trial in Heart Failure (MERIT-HF). *Circulation* 105:1585, 2002.

340b. Gottlieb SS, Fisher ML, Kjekshus J, et al: Tolerability of β-blocker initiation and titration in the Metoprolol CR/XL Randomized Intervention Trial in Congestive Heart Failure (MERIT-HF). *Circulation* 105:1182, 2002.

341. Gilbert EM, Sandoval A, Larrabee P, et al: Lisinopril lowers cardiac adrenergic drive and increases beta-receptor density in the failing human heart. *Circulation* 88:472, 1993.

342. Whyte K, Jones CR, Howie CA, et al: Haemodynamic, metabolic, and lymphocyte beta 2-adrenoceptor changes following chronic beta-adrenoceptor antagonism. *Eur Heart J* 32:237, 1987.

342a. Lowes BD, Gilbert EM, Abraham MT, et al: Myocardial gene expression in dilated cardiomyopathy treated with beta blocking agents. *N Engl J Med* 346:1357, 2002.

343. Luchner A, Burnett JC Jr, Jougasaki M, et al: Augmentation of the cardiac natriuretic peptides by beta-receptor antagonism: evidence from a population-based study. *J Am Coll Cardiol* 32:1839, 1998.

344. Floras J, Jones J, Hassan O, Sleight P: Effects of acute and chronic beta-adrenergic blockade on baroreflex sensitivity (abstr). *J Am Coll Cardiol* 11:148A, 1988.

345. Shimoyama H, Sabbah HN, Rosman H, et al: Effect of β blockade on left atrial contribution to ventricular filling in dogs with moderate heart failure. *Am Heart J* 131:772, 1996.

346. Kubo H, Margulies KB, Piacentino V, et al: Patients with end-stage congestive heart failure treated with β-adrenergic receptor antagonists have improved ventricular myocyte calcium regulatory protein abundance. *Circulation* 104:1012, 2001.

346a. Reiken S, Gaburjakova M, Gaburjakova J, et al. β-Adrenergic receptor blockers restore cardiac calcium release channel (ryanodine receptor) structure and function in heart failure. *Circulation* 104:2843, 2001.

346b. Doi M, Yano M, Kabayashi S, et al: Propranolol prevents the development of heart failure by restoring FKBP 12.6-mediated stabilization by ryanodine receptor. *Circulation* 105:1374, 2002.

347. Jonas M, Reicher-Reiss H, Boyko V, et al: Usefulness of beta blocker therapy in patients with non-insulin dependent diabetes mellitus and coronary artery disease. *Am J Cardiol* 27:1233, 1996.

348. Swan DA, Bell B, Oakley CM, Goodwin J: Analysis of symptomatic course and prognosis and treatment of hypertrophic obstructive cardiomyopathy. *Br Heart J* 33:671-685, 1971.

349. Hubner PJB, Ziady GM, Lane GK, et al: Double-blind trial of propranolol and practolol in hypertrophic cardiomyopathy. *Br Heart J* 35:116–123, 1973.

350. Epstein SE, Henry WL, Clark CE, et al: Asymmetric septal hypertrophy. *Ann Intern Med* 81:650–680, 1974.

351. Jeresaty RM: Mitral valve prolapse syndrome. *Prog Cardiovasc Dis* 15:623–652, 1973.

352. Slater EE, DeSanctis RW: Dissection of the aorta. *Med Clin North Am* 63:141–154, 1979.

353. Rios AS, Silber EN, Bavishi N, et al: Effect of long-term β blockade on aortic root compliance in patients with Marfan syndrome. *Am Heart J* 137:1057, 1999.

354. Rossi-Foulkes R, Roman MJ, Rosen SE, et al: Phenotypic features and impact of beta blocker or calcium antagonist therapy on aortic lumen size in the Marfan Syndrome. *Am J Cardiol* 83:1364, 1999.

355. Shimizu W, Antzelevitch C: Differential effects of beta-adrenergic agonists and antagonists in LQT1, LQT2 and LQT3 models of the long QT syndrome. *J Am Coll Cardiol* 35:778, 2000.

356. Moss AJ, Zareba W, Hall WJ, et al: Effectiveness and limitations of β blocker therapy in congenital long QT syndrome. *Circulation* 101:616, 2000.

357. Dorostkar PC, Eldar M, Belhassen B, Scheinman MM: Long-term follow-up of patients with long QT syndrome treated with β blockers and continuous pacing. *Circulation* 100:2431, 1999.

358. Hedblad B, Wikstrand J, Janson L, et al: Low-dose metoprolol CR/XL and fluvastatin slow progression of carotid intima-media thickness. Main results from the β Blocker Cholesterol-Lowering Asymptomatic Plaque Study (BCAPS). *Circulation* 103:1721, 2001.

359. Magsino CH Jr, Hamouda W, Bapna V, et al: Nadolol inhibits reactive oxygen species generation by leukocytes and linoleic acid oxidation. *Am J Cardiol* 86:443, 2000.

359a. The Propranolol Aneurysm Trial Investigators: propranolol for small abdominal aortic aneurysms: results of a randomized trial. *J Vasc Surg* 35:72, 2002.

360. Mahananda N, Bhuripanyo K, Kangkagate C, et al: Randomized, double-blind, placebo-controlled trial of oral atenolol in patients with unexplained syncope and positive upright tilt table test results. *Am Heart J* 130:1250, 1995.

361. Cox MM, Perlman BA, Mayor MR, et al: Acute and long-term beta-adrenergic blockade for patients with neurocardiogenic syncope. *J Am Coll Cardiol* 26:1293, 1995.

362. Iskos D, Dutton J, Scheinman MM, Lurie KG: Usefulness of pindolol in neurocardiogenic syncope. *Am J Cardiol* 82:1121, 1998.

363. Madrid AH, Ortego J, Rebollo JG, et al: Lack of efficacy of atenolol for the prevention of neurally mediated syncope in a highly symptomatic population: a prospective, double-blind, randomized and placebo-controlled study. *J Am Coll Cardiol* 37:554, 2001.

364. Poldermans D, Boersma E, Bax JJ, et al for the Dutch Echocardiographic Cardiac Risk Evaluation Applying Stress Echocardiography Study Group: the effect of bisoprolol on peri-operative mortality and myocardial infarction in high-risk patients undergoing vascular surgery. *N Engl J Med* 341:1789, 1999.

365. Lee TH: Reducing cardiac risk in noncardiac surgery (editorial). *N Engl J Med* 341:1838, 1999.

366. Shammash JB, Trost JC, Gold JM, et al: Perioperative β blocker withdrawal and mortality in vascular surgical patients. *Am Heart J* 141:148, 2001.

366a. Averbach AD, Goldman L: β-blockers and reduction of cardiac events in noncarddiac surgery. Clinical applications. *JAMA* 287:1445, 2002.

366b. Ferguson TB, Jr, Coombs LP, Peterson ED, for the Society of Thoracic Surgeons national adult cardiac surgery Database: preoperative β-blocker use and mortality and morbidity following CABG surgery in North America. *JAMA* 287:2221, 2002.

366c. Schmidt M, Lindenauer PK, Fitzgerald JL, Benjamin EM: Forcasting the impact of a clinical practice guideline for perioperative β-blockers to reduce cardiovascular morbidity and mortality. *Arch Intern Med* 162:63, 2002.

367. Sharma SK, Kini A, Marmur JD, Fuster V: Cardioprotective effect of prior β blocker therapy in reducing creatine kinase-MB elevation after coronary intervention. Benefit is extended to improvement in intermediate-term survival. *Circulation* 102:166, 2000.

368. Vetrovec GW: Acute and delayed benefits of β blockers during coronary intervention. True, true and unrelated (editorial). *Circulation* 102:147, 2000.

368a. Chan AW, Quinn MJ, Bhatt DL, et al: Mortality benefit of beta-blockade after successful elective percutaneous coronary intervention. *J Am Coll Cardiol* 40:669, 2002.

368b. Ellis SG, Brener SJ, Lincoff M, et al: β-blockers before percutaneous coronary intervention do not attenuate postprocedural creatine kinase isoenzyme rise. *Circulation* 104:2685, 2001.

369. Frishman WH, Kowalski M, Nagnur S, et al: Cardiovascular considerations in using topical, oral, and intravenous drugs for the treatment of glaucoma and ocular hypertension. Focus on β-adrenergic blockade. *Heart Disease* 3:386, 2001.

370. Drugs for migraine. *Med Lett Drugs Ther* 37:17, 1995.

371. Gironell A, Kulisevky J, Barbanoj M, et al: A randomized placebo-controlled comparative trial of gabapentin and propranolol in essential tremor. *Arch Neurol* 56:475, 1999.

372. Villanueva C, Balanzo J, Novella MT, et al: Nadolol plus isosorbide mononitrate compared with sclerotherapy for the prevention of variceal bleeding. *N Engl J Med* 334:1624, 1996.

373. Sarin SK, Lamba GS, Kumar M, et al: Comparison of endoscopic ligation and propranolol for the primary prevention of variceal bleeding. *N Engl J Med* 340:988, 1999.

374. Friedman LM: How do the various beta-blockers compare in type, frequency and severity of their adverse effects? *Circulation* 67(Suppl I):89, 1983.

375. Frishman W, Silverman R, Strom J, et al: Clinical pharmacology of the new beta-adrenoceptor blocking drugs. Part IV. Adverse effects: choosing a β-adrenoceptor blocker. *Am Heart J* 98:256, 1979.

376. Frishman WH: Beta-adrenergic receptor blockers: adverse effects and drug interactions. *Hypertension* 11(Suppl II):II21, 1988.

377. Frishman WH, Kostis J: The significance of intrinsic sympathomimetic activity in beta-adrenoceptor blocking drugs: update. *Cardiovasc Rev Rep* (Classics of the Decade Series) 12(12):46, 1991.

378. Frishman W, Kostis J, Strom J, et al: Clinical pharmacology of the new beta-adrenergic blocking drugs. Part VI. A comparison of pindolol and propranolol in treatment of patients with angina pectoris: the role of intrinsic sympathomimetic activity. *Am Heart J* 98:526, 1979.

379. Giudicelli JF, Lhoste F: β-Adrenoceptor blockade and atrioventricular conduction in dogs: role of intrinsic sympathomimetic activity. *Br J Clin Pharmacol* 13(Suppl 2):167, 1982.

380. Magjlessi-Simon G, Mary-Krause M, Fillette F, et al: Persistent transient myocardial ischemia despite beta-adrenergic blockade predicts a higher risk of adverse cardiac events in patients with coronary artery disease. *J Am Coll Cardiol* 27:1586, 1996.

381. Frishman WH, Klein N, Strom J, et al: Comparative effects of abrupt propranolol and verapamil withdrawal in angina pectoris. *Am J Cardiol* 50:1191, 1982.

382. Morimoto S-i, Shimizu K, Yamada K, et al: Can β blocker therapy be withdrawn from patients with dilated cardiomyopathy? *Am Heart J* 137:456, 1999.

383. George RB, Manocha K, Burford JG, et al: Effects of labetalol in hypertensive patients with chronic obstructive pulmonary disease. *Chest* 83:457, 1983.

384. Benson MK, Berrill WT, Cruickshank JM, et al: A comparison of four adrenoceptor antagonists in patients with asthma. *Br J Clin Pharmacol* 5:415, 1978.

385. Frohlich ED, Tarazi RC, Dustan HP: Peripheral arterial insufficiency: a complication of beta-adrenergic blocking therapy. *JAMA* 208:2471, 1969.

386. Lundvall J, Jarhult J: Beta-adrenergic dilator component of the sympathetic vascular response in skeletal muscle. *Acta Physiol Scand* 96:180, 1976.

387. Simpson FO: β-Adrenergic receptor blocking drugs in hypertension. *Drugs* 7:85, 1974.

388. Radack K, Deck C: β-Adrenergic blocker therapy does not worsen intermittent claudication in subjects with peripheral arterial disease. *Arch Intern Med* 151:1769, 1991.

389. Thadani U, Whitsett TL: Beta-adrenergic blockers and intermittent claudication. *Arch Intern Med* 151:1705, 1991.

390. Hiatt WR, Stoll S, Nies A: Effect of beta-adrenergic blockers on the peripheral circulation in patients with peripheral vascular disease. *Circulation* 72:1226, 1985.

391. Reveno WS, Rosenbaum H: Propranolol and hypoglycaemia. (letter to editor). *Lancet* 1:920, 1968.

392. Allison SP, Chamberlain MI, Miller JE: Effects of propranolol on blood sugar, insulin and free fatty acids. Diabetologia 5:339, 1969.

393. Sharma AM, Pischon T, Hardt S, et al: β-Adrenergic receptor blockers and weight gain. A systematic analysis. *Hypertension* 37:250, 2001.

394. Deacon SP, Barnett D: Comparison of atenolol and propranolol during insulin-induced hypoglycaemia *BMJ* 2:272, 1976.

395. Lloyd-Mostyn RH, Oram S: Modification by propranolol of cardiovascular effects of induced hypoglycaemia. *Lancet* 1:1213, 1975.

396. Fogari R, Zoppi A, Corradi L, et al: β Blocker effects on plasma lipids during prolonged treatment of hypertensive patients with hypercholesterolemia. *J Cardiovasc Pharmacol* 33:534, 1999.

397. Dimmitt SB, Williams PD, Croft KD, Beilin LJ: Effects of β-blockers on the concentration and oxidizability of plasma lipids. *Clin Sci* 94:573, 1998.

398. Perez-Stable EJ, Halliday R, Gardiner PS, et al: The effects of propranolol on cognitive function and quality of life: a randomized trial among patients with diastolic hypertension. *Am J Med* 108:359, 2000.

399. Jacob H, Brandt LJ, Farkas P, Frishman WH: Beta-adrenergic blockade and the gastrointestinal system. *Am J Med* 74:1042, 1983.

400. Stephen SA: Unwanted effects of propranolol. *Am J Cardiol* 18:463, 1966.

401. Nawabi IU, Ritz ND: Agranulocytosis due to propranolol. *JAMA* 223:1376, 1973.

402. Lydakis C, Lip GYH, Beevers M, Beevers DG: Atenolol and fetal growth in pregnancies complicated by hypertension. *Am J Hypertens* 12:541, 1999.

403. Bailey R, Neale TJ: Rapid clonidine withdrawal with blood pressure overshoot exaggerated by beta-blockade. *BMJ* 1:942, 1976.

404. Agabiti-Rosei E, Brown JJ, Lever AF, et al: Treatment of phaeochromocytoma and clonidine withdrawal hypertension with labetalol. *Br J Clin Pharmacol* 3(Suppl 3):809, 1976.

405. Wright P: Untoward effect associated with practolol administration: oculomucocutaneous syndrome. *BMJ* 1:595, 1975.

406. Blaufarb I, Pfeifer TM, Frishman WH: β Blockers: drug interactions of clinical significance. *Drug Safety* 13(6):359, 1995.

407. Opie LH, Frishman WH: Adverse cardiovascular drug interactions and complications. In: Fuster V, Alexander RW, O'Rourke RA, eds. *Hurst's The Heart*, 10th ed. New York: McGraw-Hill, 2001:2251.

408. Which beta blocker? *Med Lett* 43:9, 2001.

CHAPTER 8

Cholinergic and Anticholinergic Drugs

B. Robert Meyer

William H. Frishman

The term *parasympathetic nervous system* refers to those portions of the peripheral autonomic nervous system that begin as preganglionic fibers in one of three distinct regions of the central nervous system (CNS), exit the CNS in either the cranial or the sacral regions, and have their postganglionic fibers distributed in a variety of organs throughout the body. One of the three sites of origin for parasympathetic fibers is the midbrain. Fibers originating here join the third cranial nerve and course to the ciliary ganglion. At this ganglion they synapse, and postganglionic fibers innervate the iris and ciliary body. The second site of origin for the parasympathetic system is in the medulla. Fibers originating here join the seventh, ninth, and tenth cranial nerves to exit the CNS. These preganglionic fibers distribute in the pattern of each of these nerves. Fibers in the tenth nerve (the vagus) are distributed to ganglia associated with various visceral organs, including the heart and gastrointestinal tract. The third and final source of parasympathetic outflow is in the sacral portion of the spinal cord. Preganglionic fibers from this site lead to connections with the bladder, bowel, and pelvic organs.[1]

The anatomic organization of the parasympathetic system differs from that of the sympathetic system. The preganglionic fibers of the parasympathetic system extend from their sites of origin in the CNS to the end organ they are innervating. Ganglia of the parasympathetic system are relatively smaller than those of the sympathetic system, and the postganglionic fibers that emerge from these ganglia are short and localized to a specific organ. The sympathetic system has preganglionic fibers that synapse in large paravertebral ganglia and has an extensive and diffuse postganglionic network that distributes to multiple organs of the body.[1]

Inherent in the structural organization of the parasympathetic system is the ability to act at specific organs to cause very specific responses via localized discharges. In general, where the sympathetic system tends to diffusely stimulate activity through its widespread postganglionic network, the effects of the parasympathetic system are to act at specific organs to accommodate periods of rest and recovery. The system lowers heart rate, increases gastrointestinal motility, stimulates bladder emptying, increases biliary contraction, and lowers blood pressure. The parasympathetic nervous system is exclusively cholinergic in character (using acetylcholine as a transmitter), whereas in the sympathetic system the postganglionic fibers are almost exclusively adrenergic. Acetylcholine receptors were first recognized as being of two basic types in 1914, when Dale[2] noted that while acetylcholine could stimulate all types of cholinergic receptors, certain effects could be blocked by the administration of atropine. Effects that are blocked by atropine are termed *muscarinic effects,* named after a substance isolated from the poisonous mushroom *Amanita muscaria,* which produces these pharmacologic properties. These effects correspond almost directly to the actions of the parasympathetic system. After atropine blockade, higher doses of acetylcholine can elicit another constellation of effects that appear to be very similar to the properties of nicotine. Dale called these *nicotinic effects.*[1,2]

Modern investigation into the muscarinic receptors that constitute the parasympathetic system has demonstrated that there are at least five major subtypes of muscarinic receptors (Table 8-1).[3–7] All muscarinic receptors act via G proteins. Types 1, 3, and 5 activate a G protein that in turn stimulates phospholipase C. Phospholipase C then hydrolyzes phosphatidyl inositol. Ultimately activation of these receptors leads to increased intracellular calcium concentration. Type 2 and 4 receptors activate a different G protein that inhibits adenylate cyclase, activates K^+ channels, and may also suppress voltage controlled Ca^{2+} channels.

The most important subgroup of muscarinic receptors for the cardiovascular system are the M2 or cardiac receptors.[8] Activation of these receptors and alteration of potassium transport produces the negative chronotropic and inotropic effects noted in Table 8-1. Most muscarinic receptors are located in the specialized conduction tissue of the heart, and direct innervation of the myocardium itself is sparse. Effects of muscarinic stimulation lead to a decreased rate of spontaneous depolarization of the sinoatrial (SA) node, a consequent delay in the achievement of threshold potential, and a slowing of spontaneous firing. The rate of conduction in the atrioventricular (AV) node is also decreased, and the refractory period to repetitive stimulation is prolonged. The effects of muscarinic receptors on the contractility of the ventricle are substantially less intense than on the conduction system.[9] Blockade of cholinergic receptors produces positive inotropic effects; negative inotropic effects with cholinergic stimulation can be demonstrated in experimental situations. The clinical relevance of the aforementioned effects remains unknown.[1,9,10] All effects of muscarinic stimulation are enhanced in the context of activation of the sympathetic nervous system. M3 receptors have vasodilatory properties. Since direct muscarinic innervation of the vasculature has not been demonstrated and since acetylcholine is a local neurotransmitter, the exact role of these receptors as part of the parasympathetic nervous system is debatable. It appears that the pharmacologic effect of M3 receptors is mediated by receptor-mediated local release of nitric oxide.[11,12]

Drugs that act at muscarinic receptors can do so by a number of mechanisms to produce their effects. The most common mechanisms of action and the relevant drugs are shown in Table 8-2.

TABLE 8-1. Types of Muscarinic Receptors

Receptor	Location	Effect	Mechanism	Agonists	Antagonist
M1 (neural)	Cortex, hippocampus	Memory?	Stimulates phospholipase C	Acetylcholine Oxytremorine McNA343	Atropine Pirenzepine
	Gastric parietal cells Enteric ganglia	Gastric acid secretion GI motility	Increased intracellular Ca^{2+}		
M2 (cardiac)	SA Node	Slowed spontaneous depolarization	Inhibition of adenylate cyclase	Acetylcholine	Atropine Gallamine AF-DX 116
	Atrium	Shortened action potential duration, decreased contractile force	Activation of K^+ channels		
	AV Node Ventricle	Decreased speed of conduction Decreased contractile force			
M3	Smooth muscle Vascular endothelium Secretory glands	Contraction Vasodilatation Increased secretion	Increased phospholipase C	Acetylcholine Vasodilation via nitric oxide	Atropine Hexahydrosiladifenidol
M4	CNS	?	Like M2 via adenylate cyclase	Acetylcholine	?Himbacine
M5	CNS	?	?Increased phospholipase C	Acetylcholine	?

DRUGS THAT ENHANCE MUSCARINIC ACTIVITY

Choline Esters

Acetylcholine itself is not a useful drug. It has been used in heart failure patients in experimental studies to assess peripheral vascular function (endothelial release of nitric oxide). It has also been used in patients with coronary artery disease during angiography to assess endothelial function.[12a] Its pharmacologic properties are nonselective and include the stimulation of all muscarinic and nicotinic sites. Therefore an attempt has been made to develop synthetic analogues of acetylcholine that would have greater selectivity for specific subpopulations of muscarinic receptors. The only clinically useful agents that have thus far emerged from this effort are bethanechol and methacholine. Bethanechol is relatively selective for the urinary bladder and gastrointestinal tract. It has very little activity at M2 receptors in the heart. Methacholine is potentially useful in the diagnosis of reactive airway disease and has some activity at cardiac receptors as well. Pilocarpine is a naturally occurring muscarinic agent that has agonist properties principally at muscarinic receptors

in the eye and in the gastrointestinal tract.[13,14] Selective M1 receptor agonists have been developed for use in patients with Alzheimer's disease with little evidence to date for their effectivness.[15]

Anticholinesterase Agents

The effects of acetylcholine at postsynaptic sites are a function of the concentration of the transmitter at the postsynaptic receptor site. The compound is inactivated by the enzyme acetylcholinesterase, which is readily demonstrable at high concentrations at the postsynaptic sites. Some of the enzyme is bound to the membrane at the synaptic cleft itself and some floats free in the medium. Acetylcholine effects can be enhanced and prolonged by the inhibition of the action of acetylcholine-esterase. Clinically available anticholinesterases are listed in Table 8-2. These agents reversibly inhibit cholinesterase activity at all receptor sites; therefore their pharmacologic effects reflect not only muscarinic but also nicotinic actions. All of these drugs also inhibit the activity of butyrylcholinesterase. This pseudo-cholinesterase is present in many sites of the body, including the liver

TABLE 8-2. Mechanisms of Action of Drugs Active at Muscarinic Receptors

Mechanism of Action	Effect	Drug	Comments
Choline esters	Mimic effect of acetylcholine at receptors	Bethanechol Methacholine	Moderate selectivity (see text).
Anticholinesterases	Enhance effect of acetylcholine at receptors	Edrophonium Physostigmine Pyridostigmine Neostigmine Rivastigmine Donepezil Tacrine	Nicotinic and muscarinic effects both present.
Muscarinic receptor antagonists	Compete for binding at postsynaptic receptor	Atropine Scopolamine	Minimal structural selectivity for different muscarinic receptors. Selectivity reflects distribution/density of receptors. Selectivity may be enhanced by route of administration.

and plasma. Anticholinesterase drug effects constitute an enhancement of the vagal stimulus on the heart. This leads to a shortening of the effective refractory period, a decrease in SA- and AV-nodal conduction time and a diminution of cardiac output. This is modified somewhat by effects at nicotinic receptors. In addition, with persistent stimulation, a paradoxical decrease in effect will occur. Therefore, with high doses and longer duration of action, a paradoxical decrease in acetylcholine effect can be seen. All of these agents have significant potential for noncardiac effects, including gastrointestinal (increased contraction, acidity, propulsion), skeletal muscle (enhanced activity), and pulmonary effects (enhanced bronchoconstriction).[16]

The anticholinesterase with the shortest duration of action is edrophonium.[17,18] When given intravenously, it has an onset of effect within 30 to 60 s and a duration of effect that is generally less than 10 min, although longer durations of action may be seen in some susceptible individuals. Given this pharmacodynamic profile, edrophonium has been used for the acute diagnosis of myasthenia gravis and for the diagnosis and acute termination of paroxysmal supraventricular tachycardia. Cardiac disease is listed by the manufacturer of edrophonium as a reason for caution in its use, and the U.S. Food and Drug Administration (FDA) has not approved the drug for use in the management of cardiac disease. However, many clinicians have used the drug's capacity to produce acute and intense muscarinic effects as a way of diagnosing atrial arrhythmias after other routine measures have failed. Occasionally edrophonium is used for the acute control of heart rate; for example, slowing heart rate in the context of an evaluation of demand pacemaker functioning. As a single dose, edrophonium should not exceed 10 mg. In older or sicker patients, the maximal dose may need to be reduced to 5 to 7 mg. When the goal of therapy is to gradually decrease heart rate, the drug may be administered in 2-mg boluses up to a total dosage of 10 mg. Significantly higher doses of the drug have been used safely in other clinical contexts.[19–21]

Recent articles have suggested that the diagnostic use of edrophonium in cardiovascular disease may be extended to include its administration during tilt-table testing as part of the evaluation for possible vasovagal syncope.[22] It is also used in the diagnostic evaluation of patients with atypical chest pain syndromes, where response to acid infusion and edrophonium administration may identify those with esophageal sources of pain.[23]

Edrophonium is a quaternary drug whose affinity is limited to peripheral nervous system synapses. In contrast, the new cholinesterase inhibitors that have been introduced for the treatment of Alzheimer's disease (tacrine, donepezil, rivastigmine, galantamine) cross the blood-brain barrier to inhibit cholinesterase metabolism in the CNS.[24–26]

Other anticholinesterases include physostigmine, pyridostigmine, neostigmine, and amebonium. These drugs have generally not been found to have any significant role in the management of cardiovascular disease. However, they are used in other areas of medicine; therefore it is important to be familiar with the indications for their use and their potential cardiac side effects. Perhaps the most important use for some of these drugs is in the immediate reversal of neuromuscular blockade during general anesthesia. They will reverse the effects of nondepolarizing muscular blocking agents such as tubocurarine, metocurine, gallamine, vecuronium, atracurium, and pancuronium. When titrated appropriately with close monitoring of their effects on neuromuscular blockade, the cardiac effects of these drugs are generally not a problem. On occasion, however, they may produce the syndrome of excessive parasympathetic effect. Since they have no effect on the muscle blockade produced by depolarizing agents such as succinylcholine or decamethonium, these drugs should not be used in that context.[17,18]

Amebonium, pyridostigmine, and neostigmine are commonly used for the management of myasthenia gravis.[27] They may also be used to improve bladder function postoperatively.

Physostigmine is used in topical ophthalmic medications for the treatment of glaucoma. Since this drug is a tertiary amine and penetrates into the CNS more than other agents in this class, there has been sporadic interest in its potential use in enhancing cholinergic transmission in the CNS for patients with Alzheimer's disease.[17]

DRUGS THAT DIMINISH MUSCARINIC ACTIVITY

Muscarinic Receptor Antagonists

Atropine is the best known of the muscarinic receptor antagonists. Atropine has a dose-related effect upon muscarinic receptors. At its lowest doses, a relatively selective effect on salivary secretion and sweating is demonstrated; at higher doses, it exhibits cardiac effects and more diffuse anticholinergic effects that include nicotinic as well as muscarinic blockade. Atropine's dose-response curve is described in Table 8-3.[28] It has been reported that Chinese individuals show an increased sensitivity to atropine that is independent of resting vagal and sympathetic tone.[29] At low doses (<0.5 mg), it may produce a paradoxical and usually mild slowing of heart rate. The mechanism for this mild bradycardia has been debated. It has been attributed by some authors to a central stimulation of vagal afferents. At higher doses, atropine causes a progressive vagolytic effect on the heart, with increased heart rate, decreased refractory period of the AV node, and increased AV conduction velocity. Atropine is indicated for use in the acute treatment of severe symptomatic bradycardia, particularly in the context of acute myocardial infarction. On rare occasions, where it may be hypothesized that endogenous sympathetic activity is suppressed by parasympathetic effects of vagal stimulation, atropine has been thought to precipitate ventricular arrhythmias.[29a] For this reason it is clear that the drug should not be used casually; its use should be restricted to cases of severe symptomatic bradycardias.[28,30]

Since atropine will counteract bradycardia or heart block produced by acetylcholine or its analogues, it can be used to counteract the cardiac effects of any syndromes in which vagal nerve

TABLE 8-3. Dose-Effect Relationship for Atropine

Dose	Pharmacologic Effect
0.0–0.5 mg	Mild bradycardia, dry mouth, decreased sweating.
0.5–1.0 mg	Cardioacceleration, very dry mouth, some pupillary dilation.
1.0–2.0 mg	Tachycardia (potentially symptomatic) very dry mouth, pupillary dilation, blurred vision.
>3.0 mg	All of the preceding, except more marked, and including erythematous, hot skin, increased intestinal tone, urinary retention. At highest doses excitement and agitation leading to delirium or ultimately to coma, accompanied by fevers and scarlet skin.

stimulation plays an important role. The drug can therefore block the bradycardia and hypotension seen in vasovagal syndromes. Since atropine is available only as a parenteral injection and because its effects are relatively brief, it is useful only for acute reversal of bradyarrhythmias and has no role in chronic management of these conditions.

A selective muscarinic antagonist for the M2 receptor is available (triptamine), which has the potential for use in treating cholinergic bradycardia.

Atropine has also been investigated recently for its potential utility as an adjunct to dobutamine-stress echocardiography. Atropine has been given as a secondary medication for the enhancement of cardiac response where dobutamine infusion has limited success in producing the desired tachycardia, particularly for patients receiving beta-blockers.[31-34,34a]

There are other drugs with muscarinic blocking effects like those of atropine, but they have not had a significant role in cardiovascular therapy. Instead, their use has been largely confined to delivery systems designed to provide therapeutic benefit without cardiac effects. Ipratropium bromide (Atrovent) and tiotropium (Spirval) are quaternary ammonium compounds with atropine-like effects that are commonly used as inhalational agents for the reversal of cholinergically-mediated bronchoconstriction. Ipratropium bromide has had its greatest clinical utility in the management of patients with chronic obstructive pulmonary disease (COPD).[35] As a quaternary ammonium compound, ipratropium is very inefficiently absorbed from the pulmonary vascular bed. Approximately 1% of a dose is absorbed systemically. Most of this is probably secondary to oral absorption of swallowed drug. It is possible that, on rare occasions, systemic effects from this drug might be seen.[36,37]

Scopolamine continues to be available as a parenteral drug but is very rarely used. Its most common use at this time is in a transdermal patch preparation that delivers a low, continuous dose of drug over a 2- to 3-day period for the treatment of motion sickness. On occasion—either due to changes in the permeability of skin, excessive dosing (several patches at once), or from careless handling of the patches—a significant systemic effect from this drug can be seen.[28,38,39] Transdermal scopolamine has been investigated as an antiarrhythmic drug in patients with acute myocardial infarction and congestive heart failure, but it is not indicated for these conditions.[40]

REFERENCES

1. Hoffman BB, Taylor P: Neurotransmission: The autonomic and somatic motor nervous systems. In: Hardman JG, Limbird LE, eds. *Goodman & Gilman's The Pharmacological Basis of Therapeutics,* 10th ed. New York: McGraw-Hill, 2001:115.
2. Dale HH: The action of certain esters and ethers of choline, and their relation to muscarine. *J Pharmacol Exp Ther* 6:147, 1914.
3. Caulfield MP: Muscarinic receptors: Characterization, coupling and function. *Pharmacol Ther* 58:319, 1993.
4. Bonner TI, Buckley NJ, Young AC, Brann MR: Identification of a family of muscarinic receptor genes. *Science* 237:527, 1987.
5. Hammer R, Berrie CP, Birdsall NJ, et al: Pirenzepine distinguishes between different subclasses of muscarinic receptors. *Nature* 283:90, 1980.
6. Levine RR, Birdsall NJM, eds: Symposium: Subtypes of muscarinic receptors: V. *Life Sci* 52:405, 1993.
7. Levine RR, ed: Symposium: Subtypes of muscarinic receptors: VI. *Life Sci* 56:801, 1995.
8. Oberhauser V, Schwertfeger E, Rutz T, et al: Acetylcholine release in human heart atrium. Influence of muscarinic autoreceptors, diabetes, and age. *Circulation* 103:1638, 2001.
9. Brodde OE, Michel MC: Adrenergic and muscarinic receptors in the human heart. *Pharmacol Rev* 51:651, 1999.
10. Landzberg JS, Parker JD, Gautheir DF, Colucci WS: Effects of intracoronary acetylcholine and atropine on basal and dobutamine stimulated left ventricular contractility. *Circulation* 89:164, 1994.
11. Moncada S, Palmer RMJ, Higgs EA: Nitric oxide: Physiology, pathophysiology, and pharmacology. *Pharmacol Rev* 43:109, 1991.
12. Furchgott RF: The role of endothelium in the responses of vascular smooth muscle to drugs. *Annu Rev Pharmacol Toxicol* 24:175, 1984.
12a. Tio RA, Monnink SHJ, Amoroso G, et al: Safety evaluation of routine intracoronary acetylcholine infusion in patients undergoing a first diagnostic coronary angiogram. *J Investig Med* 50:133, 2002.
13. Goyal RK: Identification, localization, and classification of muscarinic receptor subtypes in the gut. *Life Sci* 43:2209, 1988.
14. Wein AJ: Practical uropharmacology. *Urol Clin North Am* 18:269, 1991.
15. Eglen RM, Choppin A, Dillon MP, Hegde S: Muscarinic receptor ligands and their therapeutic potential. *Curr Opin Chem Biol* 3:426, 1999.
16. Taylor P: Anticholinesterase agents. In: Hardman JG, Limbird LE, eds. *Goodman & Gilman's The Pharmacological Basis of Therapeutics,* 10th ed. New York: McGraw-Hill, 2001:175.
17. Morris RB, Cronnelly R, Miller RD, et al: Pharmacokinetics of edrophonium and neostigmine when antagonizing d-tubocurarine neuromuscular blockade in man. *Anaesthesiology* 54:399, 1981.
18. Morris RB, Cronnelly R, Miller RD, et al: Pharmacokinetics of edrophonium in anephric and renal transplant patients. *Br J Anaesth* 53:399, 1981.
19. American Society of Hospital Pharmacists: *AHFS Drug Information 1994.* Bethesda MD: American Hospital Formulary Service, American Society of Hospital Pharmacists, 1994.
20. McCarthy GH, Mirackhur RK, Maddineni VR, McCoy EP: Dose-responses for edrophonium during antagonism of vecuronium block in young and older adult patients. *Anaesthesia* 50:503, 1995.
21. Kiajima T, Ishii K, Ogata H: Edrophonium as an antagonist of vecuronium-induced neuromuscular block in the elderly. *Anaesthesia* 50:359, 1995.
22. Lurie KG, Dutton J, Mangat R, et al: Evaluation of edrophonium as a provocative agent for vasovagal syncope during head-up tilt-table testing. *Am J Cardiol* 72:1286, 1993.
23. Rokkas T, Anggiansah A, McCullagh M, Owen WJ: Acid perfusion and edrophonium provocation tests in patients with chest pain of undetermined etiology. *Dig Dis Sci* 37:1212, 1992.
24. Dooley M, Lamb HM: Donepezil: A review of its use in Alzheimer's disease. *Drugs Aging* 16:199, 2000.
25. Mayeux R, Sano M: Treatment of Alzheimer's disease. *N Engl J Med* 341:1670, 1999.
26. Corey-Bloom J, Anand R, Veach J: A randomized trial evaluating the efficacy and safety of ENA 713 (rivastigmine tartrate), a new acetylcholinesterase inhibitor, in patients with mild to moderately severe Alzheimer's disease. *Int J Psychopharmacol* 1:55, 1998.
27. Drachman DB: Myasthenia gravia. *N Engl J Med* 330: 1797, 1994.
28. Brown JH, Taylor P: Muscarinic receptor agonists and antagonists. In: Hardman JG, Limbird LE, eds. *Goodman & Gilman's The Pharmacological Basis of Therapeutics,* 10th ed. New York: McGraw-Hill, 2001:155.
29. Zhou HH, Adedoyin A, Wood AJ: Differing effect of atropine on heart rate in Chinese and white subjects. *Clin Pharm Ther* 52:120, 1992.
29a. Marine JE, Watanabe MA, Smith TW, Monahan KM: Effects of atropine on heart rate turbulence. *Am J Cardiol* 89:767, 2002.
30. Wellstein A, Pitschener HF: Complex dose-response curves of atropine in man explained by different functions of M1 and M2 cholinoreceptors. *Naunyn Schmiedebergs Arch Pharmacol* 338:861, 1988.
31. Pican E, Mathias W, Pingitore A, et al: Safety and tolerability of dobutamine-atropine stress echocardiography: A prospective, multicentre study. *Lancet* 344:1190, 1994.
32. Poldermans D, Fioretti PM, Boersma E: Safety of dobutamine-atropine stress echocardiography in patients with suspected or proven coronary artery disease. *Am J Cardiol* 73:456, 1994.
33. McNeill AJ, Fioretti PM, El-Said SM, et al: Enhanced sensitivity for detection of coronary artery disease by addition of atropine to dobutamine stress echocardiography. *Am J Cardiol* 70:41, 1992.

34. Poldermans D, Fioretti PM, Boersma E: Dobutamine-atropine stress echocardiography in elderly patients unable to perform an exercise test: Hemodynamic characteristics, safety, and prognostic value. *Arch Intern Med* 154:2681, 1994.

34a. Meisner JS, Shirani J, Alaeddini J, et al: Use of pharmaceuticals in noninvasive cardiovascular diagnosis. *Heart Dis* 4:315, 2002.

35. van Noord JA, Bantje TA, Eland ME, et al: A randomised controlled comparison of tiotropium and ipratropium in the treatment of chronic obstructive pulmonary disease. The Dutch Tiotropium Study Group. *Thorax* 55:289, 2000.

36. Chapman KR: The role of anticholinergic bronchodilators in adult asthma and chronic obstructive pulmonary disease. *Lung* 168(Suppl): 295, 1990.

37. Gross NJ: Ipratropium bromide. *N Engl J Med* 319:486–494, 1988.

38. Wilkinson JA: Side effects of transdermal scopolamine. *J Emerg Med* 5:389, 1987.

39. Ziskind AA: Transdermal scopolamine-induced psychosis. *Postgrad Med* 84:73, 1988.

40. LaRovere MT, DeFerrari GM: New potential uses for transdermal scopolamine (hyoscine). *Drugs* 50:769, 1995.

Calcium Channel Blockers

William H. Frishman

Domenic A. Sica

The calcium-channel blockers are a heterogeneous group of drugs with widely variable effects on heart muscle, sinus node function, atrioventricular (AV) conduction, peripheral blood vessels, and coronary circulation.[1–5] Ten of these drugs—nifedipine, nicardipine, nimodipine, nisoldipine, felodipine, isradipine, amlodipine, verapamil, diltiazem, and bepridil—are approved in the United States for clinical use. Other agents under investigation that are available for clinical use outside the United States include barnidipine,[6] benidipine,[7] cilnidipine,[8] clevidipine,[9] lacidipine,[10] lercanidipine,[11] and manidipine.[12]

PHYSIOLOGIC BACKGROUND

Calcium ions play a fundamental role in the activation of cells. An influx of calcium ions into the cell through specific ion channels is required for myocardial contraction, for determining peripheral vascular resistance through calcium dependent-regulated tone of vascular smooth muscle, and for helping to initiate the pacemaker tissues of the heart, which are activated largely by the slow calcium current.[2]

The concept of calcium-channel inhibition originated in 1960, when it was noted that prenylamine, a newly developed coronary vasodilator, depressed cardiac performance in canine heart-lung preparations.[13] Initial studies with verapamil showed that it also exerted negative inotropic effects on the isolated myocardium in addition to having vasodilator properties.[14] These potent negative inotropic effects seemed to differentiate these drugs from the classic coronary vasodilators, such as nitroglycerin and papaverine, which have little if any myocardial depressant activity. Unlike beta-adrenergic antagonists, many of the calcium antagonists depress cardiac contractility without altering the height or contour of the monophasic action potential and thus can interfere with excitation-contraction coupling.[15] Reversible closure of specific calcium ion channels in the membrane of the mammalian myocardial cell was suggested as the explanation of these observed effects.[16]

Subsequently, the effects of verapamil on atrial and ventricular intracellular potentials were studied.[17] Antiarrhythmic compounds were classified into local anesthetics, which decreased the maximum rate of depolarization; beta blockers; and a third class, which prolonged the duration of the cardiac action potential.[18] However, none of these electrophysiologic actions could explain the antiarrhythmic effect of verapamil.[18] Thus, a fourth class of antiarrhythmic drug, typified by verapamil, was proposed, with effects separate from those of sodium channel inhibitors and beta blockers.[17] It has been shown that the antiarrhythmic actions and negative inotropic effects of verapamil are mediated predominantly through interference with calcium conductance.[17]

CHEMICAL STRUCTURE AND PHARMACODYNAMICS

Structure of the Calcium-Channel Blockers

The structures of some of the available calcium-channel blockers are shown in Fig. 9-1. Diltiazem is a benzothiazepine derivative that is structurally unrelated to other vasodilators.[1] Nifedipine is a dihydropyridine derivative unrelated to the nitrates, which is lipophilic and is inactivated by light.[1,19] Nicardipine, amlodipine, felodipine, isradipine, nisoldipine, and nimodipine are also dihydropyridine derivatives similar in structure to nifedipine. Verapamil ([+] verapamil) has some structural similarity to papaverine.[1]

Bepridil, which is currently available for treatment of angina pectoris, is not related chemically to other cardioactive drugs.[20]

Differential Effects on Slow Channels

The most important characteristic of all calcium-channel blockers is their ability to selectively inhibit the inward flow of charge-bearing calcium ions when the calcium ion channels become permeable. Previously, the term *slow channel* was used, but it has recently been recognized that the calcium ion current develops faster than previously thought and that there are at least two types of calcium channels, the L and T.[21] The conventional calcium channel, which has been known to exist for a long time, is called the L channel. It is blocked by all the calcium-channel antagonists and has its permeability increased by catecholamines. The T-type channel appears at more negative potentials than the L-type and probably plays an important role in the initial depolarization of sinus and AV nodal tissue. The function of the L-type channel is to admit the substantial amount of calcium ions required for initiation of contraction via calcium-induced calcium release from the sarcoplasmic reticulum. Mibefradil is the first calcium-channel blocker that has selective blocking properties on the T-type channel in addition to its blocking effects on the L-type channel.[22,23] Specific blockers for the T-type channel are not yet available, but they could be expected to inhibit the sinus and AV nodes profoundly.[21]

Bepridil possesses all the characteristics of the traditional calcium antagonists. In addition, the drug appears to affect the sodium

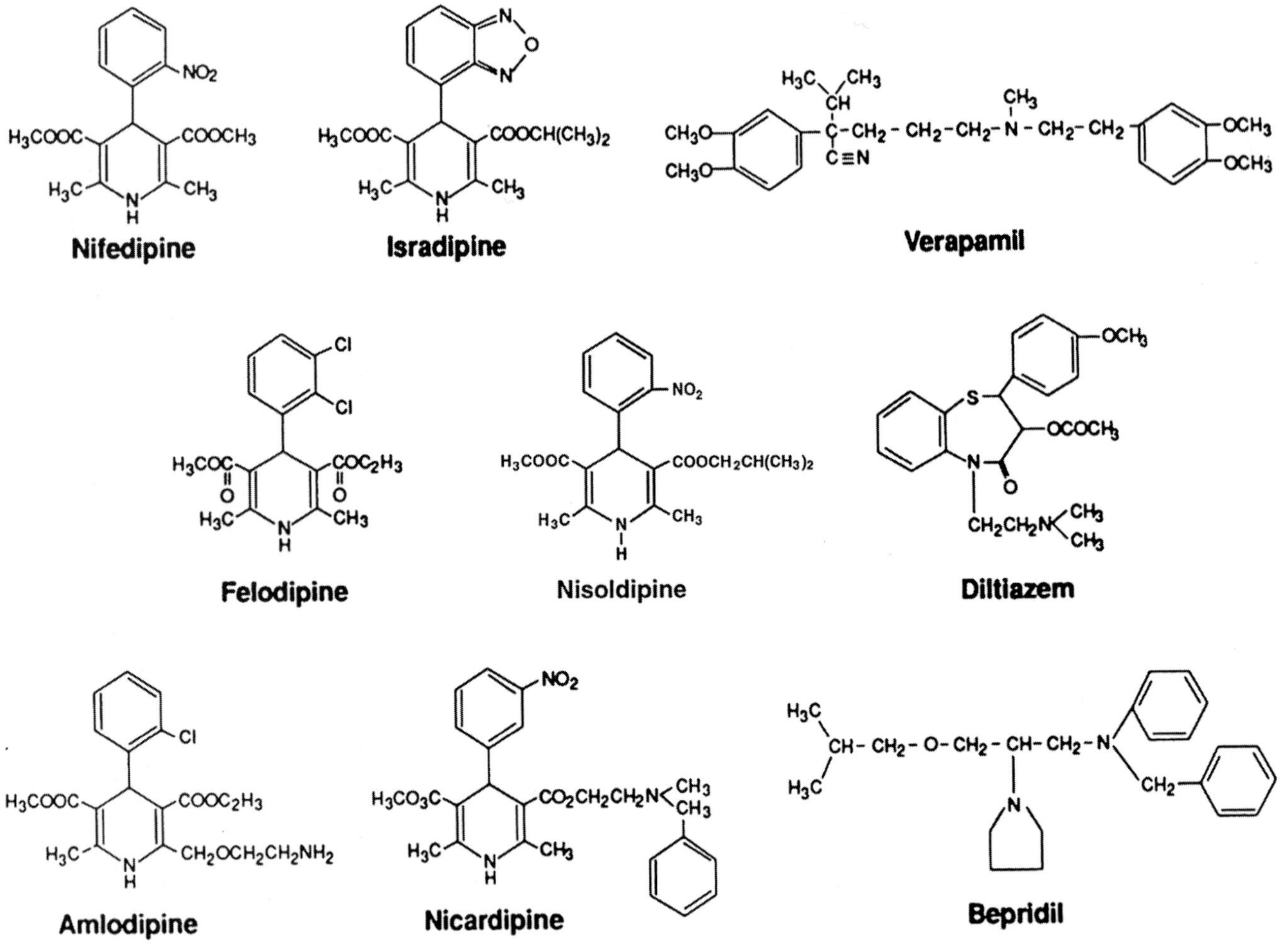

FIGURE 9-1. Chemical structures of diltiazem (a benzothiazepine derivative), nifedipine, felodipine, isradipine, amlodipine, nicardipine, nisoldipine (dihydropyridine derivatives), verapamil (structurally similar to papaverine), and bepridil (structure unlike other cardioactive drugs).

channel (fast channel) and possibly the potassium channel, producing a quinidine-like effect. Bepridil specifically inhibits maximal upstroke velocity (dV/dt_{max})—that is, the influx of sodium in appropriate load dosages. The effect of bepridil on the maximum rate of depolarization has been examined; the action potential height is not changed; however, the action potential duration is extended in a quinidine-like manner.[24]

CARDIOVASCULAR EFFECTS

Effects on Muscular Contraction

Calcium is the primary ionic link between neurologic excitation and mechanical contraction of cardiac, smooth, and skeletal muscle.[2] Actin and myosin are the protein filaments that slide past one another in the adenosine triphosphate (ATP)–dependent contractile process of all muscle cells. In myocardial cells, the regulatory proteins tropomyosin and troponin inhibit this process. When the myocardial cell membrane repolarizes, calcium enters the cell (L channel) and triggers the release of additional calcium from internal stores within the sarcoplasmic reticulum. Calcium released from this large intracellular reservoir then initiates contraction by combining with the inhibitors troponin and tropomyosin. Previously hidden

active sites on actin molecules are then available for binding by myosin.[2]

Effects on Coronary and Peripheral Arterial Blood Vessels

The contraction of vascular smooth muscle such as that found in the coronary arteries is slightly different from the contraction of cardiac and skeletal muscles (Table 9-1 and Fig. 9-2). Myosin must be phosphorylated, and calmodulin is the regulatory protein to which calcium binds.[2] In addition, vascular smooth muscle cells have significantly less intracellular calcium stores than do myocardial cells and so rely more heavily on the influx of extracellular calcium.[2]

The observation that calcium-channel blockers are significantly more effective in inhibiting contraction in coronary and peripheral arterial smooth muscle than in cardiac and skeletal muscle is of great clinical importance. This differential effect is explained by the observation that arterial smooth muscle is more dependent on external calcium entry for contraction, whereas cardiac and skeletal muscle rely on a recirculating internal pool of calcium.[2] Because calcium-entry blockers are membrane-active drugs, they reduce the entry of calcium into cells and therefore exert a much larger effect on vascular wall contraction.[2,25] This preferential effect allows

TABLE 9-1. Pharmacologic Effects of Calcium-Channel Blockers

	Heart Rate		Conduction		Myocardial Contractility	Peripheral Vasodilator	CO	Coronary BF	MVO$_2$ Demand
	Acute	Chronic	SA Node	AV Node					
Diltiazem	↓	↓	↓	↓	↓	↓	V	↑	↓
Bepridil	↓	↓	↓	↓	V	—	V	↑	↓
Verapamil	↑	↓	↓	↓	↓↓	↓	V	↑	↓
Amlodipine	↑	↑−	—	—	↓	↓↓	↑−	↑	↓
Felodipine	↑	↑−	—	—	—	↓↓	↑−	↑	↓
Isradipine	↑	↑−	—	—	—	↓↓	↑−	↑	↓
Nicardipine	↑	↑−	—	—	—	↓↓	↑−	↑	↓
Nifedipine	↑	↑−	—	—	↓	↓↓	↑−	↑	↓
Nimodipine	↑	↑−	—	—	—	V	↑−	↑	↓
Nisoldipine	↑	↑−	—	—	—	↓↓	↑−	↑	↓

SA = sinoatrial; AV = atrioventricular; CO = cardiac output; BF = blood flow; MVO$_2$ = myocardial oxygen; ↑ = increase; ↓ = decrease; − = no change; V = variable.

Source: Reproduced with permission from Frishman et al.[158]

calcium-entry blockers to dilate coronary and peripheral arteries in doses that do not severely affect myocardial contractility or have little if any effect on skeletal muscle.

It has been shown recently that dihydropyridines can induce the release of nitric oxide (NO) from the vascular endothelium of various blood vessels.[26–33] In addition, in several preparations, including micro- and macrovasculature, the sensitivity of the vasorelaxing effects of the dihydropyridines to inhibitors of NO synthase, such as L-N^G-nitroarginine (LNNA) or L-nitro-arginine-methyl-ester (L-NAME), has been shown. These findings on a dual mode of action of dihydropyridines—i.e., the direct relaxing effect by inhibition of the smooth muscle L-type calcium ion channel and the indirect relaxing effect by the release of NO from vascular endothelium—may explain the highly potent vasodilatory actions of these drugs.[33a] In addition, an antiendothelin action of calcium-channel blockers has also been described,[34] as well as an inhibitory effect on matrix metalloproteinase-1.[35]

Effects on Veins

The calcium-channel blockers seem to be less active in veins than in arteries and are ineffective at therapeutic doses (in contrast to nitrates) for increasing venous capacitance.[36]

Effects on Myocardial Contractility

Force generation during cardiac muscle contraction depends in part on calcium influx during membrane depolarization (see Table 9-1).[37] In isolated myocardial preparations, all calcium-channel antagonists have been demonstrated to exert potent negative inotropic effects.[38] In guinea pig atria exposed to drug concentration of 1026 mol/L, the order of potency for depressing the maximal rate of force development during constant pacing was found to be nifedipine > verapamil-diltiazem.[39] In dog papillary muscle, developed tension was also decreased most markedly by nifedipine; the relative potencies (on a weight basis) of verapamil and diltiazem were 1/15 and 1/40, respectively.[40] The negative inotropic effect of the calcium-channel antagonists are dose-dependent.[41] The excitation-contraction coupling of vascular smooth muscle is three to ten times more sensitive to the action of calcium-channel antagonists than is that of myocardial fibers.[38,41] Hence the relatively low doses of these drugs used in vivo to produce vasodilatation or beneficial antiarrhythmic effects may not produce significant negative inotropic effects.[41,42] Furthermore, in intact animals and human beings, the intrinsic negative inotropic properties of these compounds are greatly modified by a baroreceptor-mediated reflex augmentation of beta-adrenergic tone consequent to vasodilatation and a decrease in blood pressure.[43,44] Nifedipine and other dihydropyridines, which exert the

FIGURE 9-2. Calcium-ion–dependent regulation of muscle tone in vascular smooth muscle. Calcium-ion (Ca^{2+}) entry can occur in response to electrical stimulation through the voltage-dependent channel, receptor activation through the adrenergic-receptor–mediated channel, or both. On entry into the cell, the cellular free calcium ions bind to the calcium-binding protein calmodulin. This calmodulin-calcium-ion complex in turn activates myosin kinase, which causes phosphorylation of the light chain of myosin. Phosphorylation then activates the binding of actin to myosin and leads to contraction. Intracellular calcium ion levels are reduced through energy-dependent membrane pumps that promote calcium efflux, which involves sodium-calcium countertransport. (*Reproduced with permission from Frishman et al.*[70])

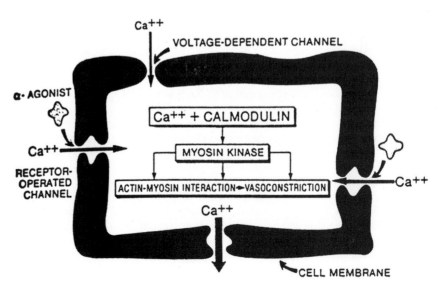

greatest vasodilator effects among these agents, accordingly produce the strongest reflex beta-adrenergic response and the one most likely to offset the negative inotropic activity of the drugs and lead to enhancement of ventricular performance.[45] Although this mechanism plays an important role in patients with normal or nearly normal left ventricular function, it is unlikely to play a similar role in patients with severe congestive heart failure (CHF), in whom the baroreceptor sensitivity is markedly attenuated.[42,46] Regarding the newer calcium-channel blockers, the hemodynamic profile of amlodipine was compared with those of verapamil and diltiazem in conscious normotensive rats.[47] Verapamil and diltiazem were negatively inotropic. Amlodipine decreased left ventricular contractility only at the highest dose used.

Electrophysiologic Effects

While verapamil, nifedipine, diltiazem, and bepridil all depress cardiac contractility with only quantitative differences (see Table 9-1), their effects on the electrophysiology of the heart are different qualitatively.[48–50] Local anesthetic actions of bepridil, diltiazem, and particularly verapamil may account for some of these differences.[51] Nifedipine and other dihydropyridines have a more selective action at the slow channels, whereas verapamil and diltiazem, at least at higher doses, also inhibit currents in the fast channels in the manner of the local anesthetics.[52] Bepridil has definite class I antiarrhythmic properties.

Verapamil and diltiazem prolong the conduction and refractoriness in the AV node; the A-H interval is lengthened more than is the H-V interval.[54,54] In therapeutic concentrations, there are no demonstrable actions on the rate of depolarization or the repolarization phases of the action potentials in atrial, ventricular, and Purkinje fibers.[50] The rate of discharge of the sinus node, which depends on the calcium ion current, is depressed by all calcium-channel blockers. In vivo, this effect can be compensated or overcompensated for by activation of baroreceptor reflexes, which increase sympathetic nervous activity.[50]

The antiarrhythmic actions of verapamil and diltiazem relate to their effects on nodal cardiac tissues.[50] In sinoatrial (SA) and AV nodal cells, the drugs modify slow-channel electropotentials in three ways: (1) there is a decrease in the rate of rise and slope of diastolic slow depolarization and an increase in the membrane threshold potential, which reduces the rate of firing in the cell[55]; (2) the action potential upstroke is decreased in amplitude, which slows conduction[56]; and (3) the duration of the action potential is increased.[55] These electrophysiologic effects are dose-related, and above the clinical range electrical standstill may occur in SA- and AV-nodal cells.[53] These observations and others support the concept that slow-channel activity is important in the generation of pacemaker potential in the SA node.

Verapamil and diltiazem also exert a depressant effect on the AV node and in low concentrations prolong the effective refractory period.[56,57] Unlike beta-adrenergic blocking drugs and vagomimetic interventions, which depress AV node transmission by altering autonomic impulse traffic, verapamil and diltiazem prolong AV-nodal refractoriness directly.[57] However, verapamil may have additional vagomimetic effects.[50]

Bepridil has a modest depressant effect on heart rate and intranodal and infranodal conduction, accompanied by a significant increment in the effective and functional refractory periods of the AV node. However, unexpected findings that cannot be explained solely on the basis of slow-channel inhibition of the myocardium include lengthening of the QTc interval and significant prolongation of the atrial and ventricular effective refractory periods.

Effects on Nonvascular Tissues

Calcium ions are required for contraction in all smooth muscles, and these drugs can inhibit contractions in the gastrointestinal tract.[58] Calcium is also important in excitation-secretion coupling. However, there is no evidence that, in clinical doses, these drugs have significant effects on the endocrine glands.[59,60] Although antiadrenergic effects of some calcium-entry blockers have been suggested, further studies are needed.[48,61,62]

Some calcium-entry blockers may partially inhibit adenosine diphosphate (ADP)- and epinephrine-induced platelet aggregation and thromboxane release from platelets.[63–65] There are good experimental data that verapamil and diltiazem and, to a lesser extent, nifedipine and amlodipine can inhibit platelet aggregation in vitro.[3,66,67] The drugs appear to be more efficacious in attenuating aggregation when they are present in the reaction mixture before aggregation begins. This can, however, interrupt or slow the rate of aggregation if added after the beginning of the reaction. In addition, the effect of aspirin in attenuating platelet aggregation appears to be potentiated in vitro in the presence of diltiazem. This has led to considerable speculation as to how much this effect may contribute to the efficacy of calcium-channel blockers in the treatment of unstable angina. There has been at least one report of patients with unstable angina in which those treated with verapamil demonstrated decreased platelet aggregability and thromboxane A2 levels.[3] If this is true in vivo, it would substantially support the use of some of these agents as first-line drugs for the treatment of unstable angina.

PHARMACOKINETICS

Although calcium-entry blockers are classified together, there are differences in their pharmacokinetic properties (Tables 9-2 and 9-3).[1,68–70] Differences in completeness of gastrointestinal absorption, amount of first-pass hepatic metabolism, protein binding, extent of distribution in the body, and the pharmacologic actions of different metabolites may influence the clinical usefulness of these drugs in different patients.[1,68]

Since many of the calcium-channel blockers are relatively short-acting, they are now available in various sustained-release delivery systems diffusion type (diltiazem, verapamil), bioerosion (diltiazem, nifedipine, nicardipine), osmosis (verapamil, isradipine, nifedipine), and diffusion-erosion (felodipine).[71–73] Nisoldipine was approved as a once-daily therapy in the coat-core formulation[74] and verapamil in two different delayed-onset sustained-release drug delivery systems.[75,75a] Diltiazem is currently being evaluated in a delayed-onset sustained-release formulation, and nitrendipine in a transdermal formulation.[75b,75c]

After administration of a certain oral dose, the calcium-entry blocking drugs, which are largely metabolized in the liver, show larger interindividual variation in circulating plasma levels.[68,69,76,77] In angina pectoris and hypertension, wide individual differences also exist in the relation between plasma concentrations of calcium-entry blockers and the associated therapeutic effect.[76,77]

TABLE 9-2. Pharmacokinetics of Calcium-Channel Blockers and Sustained-Release Preparations

Agent	Trade Name	Absorption (Percent)	Bioavailability (Percent*)	Protein Binding (Percent)	VOD (L/kg)	$t_{1/2}\,\beta$ (h)	Clearance (mL/min/kg)	Time to Peak Plasma Concentration (h)
Diltiazem	Cardizem	>90	35–60	78	5.0	4.1–5.6	15	2–3
Diltiazem SR	Cardizem SR	>90	35–60	78	5.0	5.7	15	6–11
Diltiazem IV	Cardizem		100	78	5.0	3.4	15	
Diltiazem CD	Cardizem CD	>95	40	70–80	5.0	5–8	15	10–14
Diltiazem XR	Dilacor XR	>95	40	70–80	5.0	5–10	15	4–6
Diltiazem ER	Tiazac	>90	40	70–80	5.0	4–9.5	15	6–11
Verapamil	Calan, Isoptin	>90	10–20	90	4.3	6±4 IV 8±6 PO	13±7	1–2
Verapamil SR	Calan SR, Isoptin SR	>90	10–20	90	4.3	4.5–12	13±7	1–2
	Verelan, Verelan PM	>90	20–35	90	162–380 L	12	—	7–9
Coer Verapamil	Covera	>90	20–30	90	—	6–12	—	11
Verapamil IV			100			2–5		
Nifedipine	Procardia, Adalat	>90	65	90	1.32	5	500–600	0.5
Nifedipine CC	Adalat CC	>90	84–89	92–98	1.32	—	500–600	2–2.5
Nifedipine GITS	Procardia XL	>90	85	>95	1.32	3.8–16.9	500–600	6 to plateau
Nicardipine	Cardene	>90	30	>90	0.6	1 IV	14	0.5–2.0
Nicardipine SR	Cardene SR	>90	35	>95		8.6	0.6	1–4 immediate
Nicardipine IV	Cardene		100	>90	9.3			
Amlodipine	Norvasc	>90	60–65	>95	21	35–45	7	6–12
Isradipine	Dynacirc	90–95	17	97	2.9	8.8	10	1.5
Isradipine GITS	Dynacirc CR							
Felodipine ER	Plendil	>95	15–25	>99	10	15.1±2.6	12	2.5–5
Bepridil	Vascor	>90	60	>95	80	33		5.3
Nimodipine	Nimotop	>90	13	>95	0.94	8–9		0.6
Nisoldipine	Sular	87	5	>99		7–12		6–12

VOD = volume of distribution; SR = sustained-release; IV = intravenous; CD, XR, CC, XL = extended release; PO = oral; GITS = gastrointestinal therapeutic system.

*Extraction ratio.

Source: Adapted from Frishman WH, Sonnenblick EH: Calcium channel blockers. In: Schlant RC, Alexander RW, eds. *Hurst's The Heart,* 8th ed. New York: McGraw Hill, 1994:1291.

Various dihydropyridine calcium-channel blockers (felodipine, nifedipine, nisoldipine) should not be administered with grapefruit juice or Seville orange juice, as it has been shown to interfere with the drug's metabolism, resulting in about a threefold mean increase in C_{max} and an almost twofold mean increase in area under the plasma concentration-time curve (AUC).[78–80]

The pharmacokinetics of calcium-channel blockers are minimally impacted by renal failure. Furthermore, the drugs are not dialyzable. The predictability of the kinetic profile of the calcium-channel blockers in renal failure simplifies their use in end-stage renal disease.[80a]

CLINICAL APPLICATIONS

The calcium-channel blockers are available in the United States for the treatment of patients with angina pectoris (diltiazem, nifedipine, amlodipine, nicardipine, verapamil, bepridil), for chronic treatment of systemic hypertension (verapamil, isradipine, diltiazem, amlodipine, nicardipine, nisoldipine, felodipine), for the management of hypertensive emergencies and perioperative hypertension (intravenous nicardipine), for treatment and prophylaxis of supraventricular arrhythmias (verapamil, diltiazem), and for reducing morbidity and mortality in patients with subarachnoid

hemorrhage (nimodipine). These drugs are also being evaluated and used for a multitude of other cardiovascular and noncardiovascular conditions.

Angina Pectoris

The antianginal mechanisms of calcium-entry blockers are complex (Table 9-4).[1,2,81–86] The drugs exert vasodilator effects on the coronary and peripheral vessels as well as depressant effects on cardiac contractility, heart rate, and conduction; all these actions may be important in mediating the antianginal effects of the drugs.[2,81–85] These drugs are not only mild dilators of epicardial vessels not in spasm but they also markedly attenuate sympathetically mediated and ergonovine-induced coronary vasoconstriction; these actions provide a rational basis for effectiveness of the drugs in vasospastic ischemic syndromes.[2,84] In patients with exertional angina pectoris, the peripheral vasodilator actions of diltiazem and verapamil and the inhibitory effects on the sinus node serve to attenuate the increases in double product that normally accompany and serve to limit exercise.[82,87]

Stable Angina Pectoris

Multiple double-blind placebo-controlled studies have clearly confirmed the efficacy of diltiazem,[77,85–90] nifedipine,[77,91–93] amlodipine,[94–98] nicardipine,[99,100] verapamil,[101–105] and bepridil[106–107]

TABLE 9-3. Additional Pharmacokinetic Characteristics of Calcium-Channel Blockers

Agent	Dosage Oral	Dosage IV	Onset of Action (min) Oral	Onset of Action (min) IV	Therapeutic PC (ng/mL)	Site of Metabolism	Active Metabolites	Excretion (%)
Diltiazem	30–90 mg q 6–8 h	75–150 μg/kg 10–20 mg	<30	<10	50–200	Deacetylation *N*-deacetylation *O*-demethylation Major hepatic first-pass effect	Yes	60 (fecal) 2–4 (unchanged in urine)
Diltiazem SR	60–120 mg q 12 h		30–60		50–200			Yes
Diltiazem IV		0.25 mg/kg (20 mg)						
Diltiazem CD	180–360 mg q 24 h		30–60		50–200		Yes	
Diltiazem XR	180–540 mg q 24 h		30–60		40–200		Yes	
Diltiazem ER	120–540 mg q 24 h				40–200		Yes	
Verapamil	80–120 mg q 6–12 h	150 μg/kg 10–20 mg	<30	<5	>100	*N*-dealkylation *O*-demethylation Major hepatic first-pass effect	Yes	15 (fecal) 70 (renal) 3–4 (unchanged in urine)
Verapamil SR	240–480 mg q 12 or 24 h		<30		>50		Yes	15 (fecal) 70 (renal) 3–4 (unchanged in urine)
Verelan (Verapamil SR)	120–480 mg q 24 h				>50		Yes	16 (fecal) 70 (renal) 3–4 (unchanged in urine)
Verelan PM	200–400 mg q 24 h							
Coer Verapamil	180–540 mg q 24 h		4–5 h				Yes	16 (fecal) 70 (renal) 3–4 (unchanged in urine)
Verapamil IV		5–10 mg (0.075– 0.15 mg/kg)						
Nifedipine	10–40 mg q 6–8 h	5–15 μg/kg	<20	3 SL	25–100	A hydroxycarbolic acid and a lactone with no known activity Major hepatic first-pass effect	No	20–40 (fecal) 50–80 (renal) <0.1 (unchanged in urine)
Nifedipine CC	30–90 mg/day		<60		25–100		No	
Nifedipine GITS	30–180 mg q 24 h		2 h				No	
Nicardipine	10–20 mg tid	1.15 mg/h	<20	<5	28–50	Major hepatic first-pass effect	No	30 (fecal) 60 (renal) <1 (unchanged in urine)
Nicardipine SR	30–60 mg bid		20		28–50			35 (fecal) 60 (renal) <1 (unchanged in urine)
Nicardipine IV		5–15 mg/h	4–5 h	<2–3	60–800	Hepatic	No	
Nimodipine	60 mg q 4 h		<30		7	Major hepatic first-pass effect	No	
Nisoldipine ER	20–40 mg q 24 h					Hepatic hydroxylation	Yes	80 (renal) <1 (unchanged in urine)

(continued)

TABLE 9-3. (*Continued*) Additional Pharmacokinetic Characteristics of Calcium-Channel Blockers

Agent	Dosage Oral	Dosage IV	Onset of Action (min) Oral	Onset of Action (min) IV	Therapeutic PC (ng/mL)	Site of Metabolism	Active Metabolites	Excretion (%)
Amlodipine	5–10 mg q 24 h		90–120 in vitro		6–10	Oxidation Extensive but slow hepatic metabolism	No	20–25 (fecal) 60 (renal) 10 (unchanged in urine)
Isradipine	2.5–10 mg q 12 h		120			Hepatic deesterification and aromatization	No	30 (fecal) 70 (renal) 0 (unchanged in urine)
Isradipine CR	5–20 mg q 24 h		2–3 h					25–30 (fecal) 60–65 (renal)
Felodipine ER	5–20 mg q 24 h		2–5 h		2–20 nmol/L	Hepatic microsomal P450 system oxidation Major hepatic first-pass effect	No	10 (fecal) 60–70 (renal) <0.5 (unchanged in urine and feces)
Bepridil	200–400 mg		30–60		1200–3500		Yes	70 (renal) 20 (fecal)

PC = plasma concentrations; bid = twice daily; tid = thrice daily; SL = sublingual; nd = no data.

Source: Adapted with permission from Frishman WH, Sonnenblick EH: Calcium channel blockers. In: Schlant RC, Alexander RW, eds. *Hurst's The Heart,* 8th ed. New York: McGraw Hill, 1994:1291.

in stable angina pectoris, with patients showing a reduction in chest pain attacks and nitroglycerin consumption and improved exercise tolerance.[108] Calcium-entry blockers, for the most part, appear to be as safe and effective as beta blockers and nitrates when used as monotherapies.[108–113] They can also be used as single-dose therapies in hypertensive patients with angina.[108,113,114]

In choosing between a calcium-channel antagonist and a beta-adrenergic blocking drug in the management of patients with effort-related symptoms, it is apparent that some patients do better with one drug than with the other, although beta blockers are considered the preferred first-line therapy.[115] Unfortunately, little is known about how to predict with confidence the superior agent in a specific patient without a therapeutic trial. However, verapamil and diltiazem can be used as effective alternatives in patients who remain symptomatic despite therapy with beta blockers and as first-time

antianginal drugs in patients with contraindications to beta blockade; the use of nifedipine as a first-line drug in its original formulation was limited by the reflex tachycardia and potential aggravation of angina that accompanied its use.[77,112,116] However, this is not a problem with the nifedipine gastrointestinal therapeutic system (GITS) formulation or with amlodipine.[89]

Diltiazem is also approved as a once-daily treatment for angina pectoris in a sustained-delivery formulation.[117] A delayed-release, sustained-release formulation of verapamil has been compared to atenolol, amlodipine, and the combination of amlodipine plus atenolol in patients with angina pectoris, and has been shown to be as effective in improving exercise tolerance and markers of silent ischemia.[118]

Bepridil is available in doses of 200 to 400 mg once daily for use in patients with angina pectoris who are refractory to other

TABLE 9-4. Hemodynamic Effects of Calcium-Entry Blockers on Myocardial Oxygen Supply and Demand*

	Verapamil	Nifedipine	Diltiazem	Bepridil
Demand				
Wall tension	↑↔	↔ reflex	↔	↔
Systolic blood pressure	↓	↓	↓	↔
Ventricular volume	↑	↔	↔	↔
Heart rate	↓↔	↑ reflex	↓↔	↓↔
Contractility	↓↓	↓	↓	↓
Supply				
Coronary blood flow	↑	↑↑	↑	↑
Coronary vascular resistance	↓	↓↓	↓	↓
Spasm	↓	↓	↓	↓
Diastolic perfusion time	↑↔	↓	↑↔	↑↔
Collateral blood flow	↔	↑	↑	↔

↑ = increase; ↓ = decrease; ↔ = no apparent effect.

*Heart rate may increase sharply but decreases with long-term use.

Source: Adapted from Frishman WH, Sonnenblick EH: Calcium channel blockers. In: Schlant RC, Alexander RW, eds. *Hurst's The Heart,* 8th ed. New York: McGraw Hill, 1994:1291.

antianginal drug therapy.[119] Close monitoring of patients with this drug is necessary at the onset of therapy because a small percentage of patients can have a prolongation of the QT interval on the ECG. Bepridil can be combined with a beta blocker if necessary.[119]

The comparative effects of abrupt withdrawal of verapamil and propranolol in patients with angina pectoris have been studied.[61] Ten percent of patients with stable effort-related symptoms experienced a severe clinical exacerbation of the anginal syndrome upon withdrawal of propranolol; no patient experienced rebound symptoms when verapamil was abruptly discontinued.[61] There also appear to be no major withdrawal reactions with nifedipine and diltiazem.[77]

Angina at Rest

Patients with angina at rest have a wide spectrum of disorders, ranging from those with variant angina (ST-segment elevation) associated with angiographically normal coronary arteries to those with unstable angina with ST-segment depression or elevation associated with multivessel coronary artery disease.[82,85,108,114] Studies suggest that the coronary vasospasm and/or thrombosis plays a major role in the pathogenesis of ischemia in most patients with angina at rest, regardless of the coronary anatomy.[82,108] In clinical trials, calcium-channel antagonists were effective in this syndrome because of their ability to block spontaneous and drug-induced spasm.[120–127]

The comparative efficacy of verapamil and propranolol was assessed in a randomized blind crossover trial in rest angina. Only verapamil reduced symptomatic and asymptomatic episodes of ischemia. These findings are consistent with the concept that coronary vasospasm plays a crucial role in patients with angina at rest; in contrast, rather than providing any benefit, propranolol may exacerbate vasospastic phenomena.[128]

Another study assessed the comparative efficacy of verapamil and nifedipine. Both verapamil and nifedipine proved equally effective, and neither drug depressed ventricular function at rest or during exercise.[129] Accordingly, in the management of patients with variant angina, the choice of a calcium antagonist is likely to be determined not so much by which drug is more effective but by which agent is better tolerated by an individual patient.

The usefulness of calcium-channel antagonists as an adjunctive therapy in the long-term management of unstable angina was demonstrated in a double-blind, placebo-controlled, randomized clinical trial showing that the addition of nifedipine to patients receiving nitrates and propranolol can reduce the number of patients with unstable anginal syndromes requiring surgery for relief of pain; the incidence of sudden death and myocardial infarction was similar in the two groups.[130] However, clinical benefits were largely

TABLE 9-5. Hemodynamic Effects of Calcium-Entry Blockers, Beta Blockers, and Combination Treatment

	Calcium Blockers	Beta Blockers	Combination
Heart rate	↓↔↑ reflex	↓	↓↔
Contractility	↓↔ reflex	↓	↓↔
Wall tension	↓	↔	↓
Systolic blood pressure	↓	↓	↓
Left ventricular volume	↓↔	↑	↑↔
Coronary resistance	↓	↑↔	↓↔

↑ = increase; ↓ = decrease; ↔ = no change.

Source: Reproduced with permission from Frishman WH: Beta-adrenergic blockade in the treatment of coronary artery disease. In: Hurst JW, ed. *Clinical Essays on the Heart.* New York: McGraw-Hill, 1984:48.

TABLE 9-6. Hemodynamic Rationale for Combining Nitrates and Calcium-Channel Blockers in Angina Pectoris

	Nitrates	Calcium-Channel Blockers	Combination
Heart rate	↑ reflex	↓↔↑	↔↑ reflex
Blood pressure	↓	↓	↓↓?
Heart size	↓/0	↓↔↑	0
Contractility	↑ reflex	↓	0
Venomotor tone	↓	0	↓
Peripheral resistance	↓	↓	↓↓?
Coronary resistance	↓	↓	↓↓?
Coronary blood flow	↑	↑	↑↑?
Collateral blood flow	↑	↑	↑↑?

↑ = increase; ↓ = decrease; ↓↓? = questionable additive effects; ↔ = no change.

Source: Reproduced with permission from Frishman WH: Beta-adrenergic blockade in the treatment of coronary artery disease. In: Hurst JW, ed. *Clinical Essays on the Heart.* New York: McGraw-Hill, 1984:48.

confined to patients whose pain was accompanied by ST-segment elevation. Current guidelines suggest that calcium-channel blockers be used as adjunctive therapy in patients with unstable angina.[130a]

Combination Therapy in Angina Pectoris

Combination therapy with nitrates and/or beta blockers may be more efficacious for the treatment of angina pectoris than one drug used alone.[82,85,119,131,132] The hemodynamic effects of a calcium blocker/beta-blocker combination are shown in Table 9-5. Because adverse effects can occur from this combination (heart block, severe bradycardia, congestive heart failure), patients must be carefully selected and observed.[133,134] The hemodynamic effects of combined nitrate/calcium-channel blocker therapy are shown in Table 9-6. Hypotension should be avoided. Different calcium-channel blockers may also be combined (nifedipine with verapamil or diltiazem) with added benefit; however, compared with monotherapy, side effects may be prohibitive.[77]

Arrhythmias

Sinus Tachycardia

In an intensive care setting, intravenous diltiazem has been used successfully to treat sinus tachycardia in critically ill patients with contraindications to β blockers or in whom β blockers were contraindicated.[134a]

Atrial Fibrillation

Except in rare situations, verapamil and diltiazem are ineffective in converting acute and chronic atrial fibrillation to normal sinus rhythm, and verapamil does not prevent long-term tachycardia-induced atrial electrical remodeling[135,136] (Table 9-7). However, both diltiazem and verapamil (oral and intravenous) are effective for decreasing and controlling ventricular rate during atrial fibrillation by prolonging AV-nodal conduction and refractoriness and thereby increasing AV block both at rest and during exercise.[137,138] Clinical trials with verapamil in patients with atrial fibrillation have shown that its ability to decrease ventricular rate appears to be unrelated to the chronicity of the arrhythmia, its etiology, or the patient's age.[139–142a] Verapamil appears to be more effective than digoxin in slowing the rapid ventricular rate in response to physical activity.[143]

TABLE 9-7. Effects of Diltiazem and Verapamil in Treatment of Common Arrhythmias

Effective	Ineffective
Sinus tachycardia	Nonparoxysmal automatic atrial tachycardia
Supraventricular tachycardia	
AV-nodal reentrant PSVT	Atrial fibrillation and flutter in WPW syndrome (ventricular rate may not decrease)
Accessory pathway reentrant	
PSVT SA-nodal reentrant PSVT	Ventricular tachyarrhythmias*
Atrial reentrant PSVT	
Atrial flutter (ventricular rate decreases but arrhythmia will only occasionally convert)	
Atrial fibrillation (ventricular rate decreases but arrhythmia will only occasionally convert)	

AV = atrioventricular; PSVT = paroxysmal supraventricular tachycardia; SA = sinoatrial; WPW = Wolff-Parkinson-White syndrome.

*There is only limited experience in this area.

Source: Reproduced with permission from Frishman and LeJemtel.[50]

Either diltiazem and verapamil can be used orally in combination with digoxin in treating rapid heart rates in patients with acute and chronic atrial fibrillation and flutter.[50]

It has been demonstrated that verapamil treatment can maintain normal sinus rhythm in patients undergoing electrocardioversion for atrial fibrillation.[144] Pretreatment with diltiazem has been shown to prevent atrial arrhythmias after thoracic surgery.[145]

Paroxysmal Supraventricular Tachycardia (SVT)

Virtually all cases of SVT due to intranodal reentry and those related to circus movement type of tachycardia in preexcitation respond promptly and predictably to intravenous verapamil or diltiazem, whereas only about two-thirds of ectopic atrial tachycardias convert to sinus rhythm after adequate doses of the drug (see Table 9-7).[50,146,147] Intravenous verapamil and diltiazem are highly efficacious in treating reentry paroxysmal SVT regardless of etiology or age.[50,147] The recommended dosage range of verapamil for terminating paroxysmal SVT in adults is 0.075 to 1.5 mg/kg infused over 1 to 3 min and repeated at 30 min.[50] In patients with myocardial dysfunction, the dose should be reduced. Children have safely been treated with a regimen of 0.075 to 0.15 mg/kg.[50] The recommended dose of diltiazem is 0.25 mg/kg infused over 2 min, repeated at 0.35 mg/kg after 15 min.

There have been few clinical studies comparing intravenous verapamil and diltiazem with other standard regimens in the treatment of paroxysmal SVT.[148] However, in a number of clinical situations, verapamil and diltiazem may offer an advantage over either digitalis preparations or beta-adrenergic blockers. For instance, verapamil would be preferable in cases where there is an urgent need to terminate paroxysmal SVT, since it can produce therapeutic responses within 3 min of infusion, whereas the effects of digoxin are not evident for approximately 30 min.[50] Also, if drug therapy fails to achieve normal sinus rhythm, the short duration of action of verapamil and diltiazem permit earlier cardioversion without some of the dangers that accompany electrical cardioversion during digoxin therapy. Verapamil and diltiazem also offer distinct advantages over beta-adrenergic blocking drugs in patients whose arrhythmias are associated with chronic obstructive lung disease and/or peripheral vascular disease.[50]

Oral verapamil has been approved for prophylaxis against paroxysmal SVT in doses of 160 to 480 mg per day, and the treatment experiences have yielded favorable results.[149] Diltiazem is not yet approved in oral form as an antiarrhythmic agent.

Atrial Flutter

The immediate effect of intravenous verapamil and diltiazem in atrial flutter in most patients is an increase in AV block that slows the ventricular response, rarely followed by a return to sinus rhythm (see Table 9-7).[50,141] In some, the response occurs through the development of atrial fibrillation with a controlled ventricular response.[50] A single intravenous dose of verapamil or diltiazem has been found to be of diagnostic value in differentiating rapid atrial flutter from paroxysmal SVT when these two arrhythmias are indistinguishable on the ECG. If the rhythm is atrial flutter, the AV block increases immediately, revealing the true nature of the arrhythmia.[139] Oral verapamil has also been used to convert paroxysmal atrial flutter and reduce the rapid ventricular rates associated with this arrhythmia.[149]

Preexcitation

Verapamil and diltiazem have been found to induce reversion of most cases of accessory pathway supraventricular tachycardia.[146] Using intracardiac recordings of electrical activity during programmed electrical stimulation of the heart, data have become available regarding the actions of verapamil on the electrophysiologic properties of the accessory pathway in overt cases of the Wolff-Parkinson-White (WPW) syndrome.[150,151] The drug has a minimal effect on the antegrade and retrograde conduction times and on the refractory period.[50,55,152] Verapamil and diltiazem, therefore, terminate accessory pathway paroxysmal supraventricular tachycardia in the same manner as they do AV-nodal reentrant paroxysmal SVT: by slowing AV-nodal conduction and increasing refractoriness. The minimal effect of verapamil and diltiazem on the electrophysiologic properties of the bypass tract is consistent with the observation that the drug is ineffective in atrial fibrillation, complicating WPW syndrome, in which fibrillatory impulses, as with digoxin, conduct predominantly through the anomalous pathway.[139] Under these circumstances, radiofrequency catheter ablation of the accessory pathways appears to be the therapy of choice.[153]

Ventricular Arrhythmias

Intravenous verapamil and diltiazem have no apparent benefit in ventricular arrhythmias except in acute myocardial infarction.[55,154] Oral verapamil has no demonstrated role in the management of ventricular tachyarrhythmias. However, bepridil, with its class I antiarrhythmic activity, has been shown to be effective in the short- and long-term control of ventricular arrhythmias. Dihydropyridines do not appear to have a proarrhythmic effect in patients with myocardial ischemia.[155]

Precautions in Treating Arrhythmias

A diseased SA node is much more sensitive to slow-channel blockers and may be depressed to the point of atrial standstill.[156] Sinus arrest can also occur without overt evidence of sick sinus syndrome.[50] Calcium-channel blockade also may suppress potential AV-nodal escape rhythms that need to arise if atrial standstill occurs.[50] In patients with the brady-tachy form of sick sinus syndrome, either digoxin or beta-adrenoceptor blocking drugs should probably not be combined with either verapamil or diltiazem in the prophylaxis of tachyarrhythmias unless a demand ventricular pacemaker is first inserted.[50]

Systemic Hypertension

Calcium-channel blockers are effective in the treatment of systemic hypertension and hypertensive emergencies.[70,157,158] Calcium-channel blocking drugs can be considered potential first-line therapy for initiating treatment in many patients with chronic hypertension.[159] A vast experience in the United States has been collected using verapamil,[75,158,159] diltiazem,[160,161] nifedipine,[162,163] amlodipine,[164] nicardipine,[165,166] felodipine,[167] nisoldipine,[73] lercanidipine, and isradipine[168] in patients with hypertension. Verapamil, nicardipine, nifedipine, nisoldipine, felodipine, and diltiazem are available in the United States in both conventional and sustained-release oral formulations, allowing once- and twice-daily dosing. Verapamil is available in unique delayed-onset sustained-release delivery systems[75,75a] to provide a peak blood level at the time of blood pressure elevation during awakening. Diltiazem may soon become available in a similar formulation.

Multiple studies have been carried out evaluating the effects of calcium-channel blockers in elderly patients with isolated systolic hypertension.[169] The Systolic Hypertension in Europe Study (SYST-EUR) was limited to patients 60 years of age and older with a resting systolic pressure of 160 to 219 mm Hg and a diastolic pressure <95 mm Hg. Patients were randomized to receive nitrendipine or placebo. If additional blood pressure control was necessary, patients received an (ACE) converting enzyme inhibitor and then a diuretic. Compared to placebo, nitrendipine therapy was associated with significant reductions in the rate of stroke, major cardiovascular events, and cognitive disorders.[170-172] Based on this study, the guidelines presented in the sixth report of the Joint National Committee on Detection, Evaluation and Treatment of High Blood Pressure (JNV-VI) include the use of dihydropyridine calcium antagonists in addition to thiazide diuretics as first-line treatment for ISH in the elderly.[172a]

The Systolic Hypertension in China (SYST-CHINA) study also looked at nitrendipine as a first-line treatment modality compared to placebo in elderly patients with ISH.[173] Compared to placebo, nitrendipine was associated with a reduction in stroke events, major cardiovascular events, and mortality.

The Stage I Systolic Hypertension in the Elderly was a pilot trial that enrolled elderly patients (>55 years of age) with mild (stage 1) systolic hypertension (140–155 mm Hg), a population not studied in SHEP, SYST-EUR, or SYST-CHINA. Felodipine was compared to placebo in an attempt to reduce systolic blood pressure by 10%. Felodipine was shown to be more effective than placebo in reducing blood pressure. In addition, the drug was shown to reduce ventricular wall thickness and improve ventricular function.[174] Amlodipine has also been shown to be as useful as chlorthalidone in reducing blood pressure in patients with stage I hypertension.[174a]

A number of studies have been completed comparing various calcium-channel blockers to other antihypertensive drugs in older subjects with combined systolic and diastolic hypertension. The Swedish Trial in Old Patients with Hypertension (STOP-2) enrolled 6600 patients ranging in age from 70 to 84 years with a supine blood pressure of 180/105 mm Hg or higher. The original STOP trial[174b] compared the effects of diuretics and beta blockers in elderly hypertensives in terms of cardiovascular morbidity and mortality. STOP-2[175] compared these two treatments with a calcium-channel

blocker (felodipine or isradipine) or an ACE inhibitor (enalapril or lisinopril). There was no difference between the three treatment groups with respect to the combined endpoints of fatal stroke, fatal myocardial infarction, and other cardiovascular diseases.[175,176] There was a lower incidence of nonfatal myocardial infarction and congestive heart failure in the ACE inhibitor group compared to the other treatment modalities. In the International Nifedipine Study Intervention as a Goal in Hypertension Treatment (INSIGHT),[177] 6321 elderly patients aged 55 to 80 years were randomized to double-blind treatment with either long-acting nifedipine GITS or the combination drug co-amilozide (hydrochlorothiazide and amiloride). The study end points were overall cardiovascular morbidity and mortality, and both treatments appeared equally effective in preventing vascular events. In the Nordic Diltiazem Study (NORDIL),[178] 10,881 patients aged 50 to 74 years with systemic hypertension were randomized to receive first-line therapy with either diltiazem, diuretics, or a beta blocker. Diltiazem was as effective as the other treatments in reducing the incidence of combined study end points of stroke, myocardial infarction, and other cardiovascular death. Another smaller study was conducted among Japanese patients 60 years or older [National Interventional Cooperative Study in Elderly Hypertensives (NICS-EH)].[179] Inclusion criteria were systolic blood pressure 160 to 220 mm Hg and diastolic blood pressure <115 mm Hg after a 4-week placebo period and no history of cardiovascular complications. The number of cardiovascular events was low owing to the small sample size and to the inclusion criteria. There was no difference in combined cardiovascular end points. In the Prospective Randomized Evaluation of Diltiazem CD Trial (PREDICT) study, 8000 patients 55 years of age or above were randomized to receive either diltiazem or chlorthalidone. The results have not been published to date.

Studies have demonstrated the efficacy of calcium-channel blockers used alone or in combination in elderly patients when compared to alternative medications.[179-183]

The HOT trial studied 18,000 patients aged 50 to 80 years. The study examined whether maximal reduction of diastolic blood pressure with antihypertensive drugs and aspirin could cause a further reduction in cardiovascular events (myocardial infarction or stroke) or be associated with harm (J-curve hypothesis).[184] Felodipine, a long-acting dihydropyridine, was used as the first-line treatment for all patients and aspirin (75 mg) or placebo was also given. An ACE inhibitor, a beta blocker, and a thiazide diuretic could be given to achieve the desired diastolic blood pressure goal. The study results showed that maximal protection with antihypertensive therapy was seen when a diastolic blood pressure of 82.6 mm Hg was achieved; in diabetic patients, an additional reduction in diastolic blood pressure (below 80 mm Hg) was needed to achieve maximal benefit. A J-curve response was not observed despite major reductions in blood pressure. The HOT study had greater success in achieving blood pressure targets among the oldest subjects, with a low incidence of medication side effects.

The Antihypertensive and Lipid-Lowering Treatment to Prevent Heart Attack Trial (ALLHAT), sponsored by the National Heart, Lung, and Blood Institute, is one of the largest prospective, randomized studies ever undertaken. The study enrolled 40,000 patients over the age of 55 years. The goal of the study is to compare four antihypertensive interventions—long-acting calcium antagonist (amlodipine), ACE inhibitor (lisinopril), diuretic (chlorthalidone), and alpha blocker (doxazosin)—in terms of their ability to reduce coronary disease. One-half of the patients also receive pravastatin to test the benefits of lowered cholesterol in older patients. A recent report from the trial showed that doxazosin was less effective than chlorthalidone in reducing cardiovascular events, despite blood pressure control. The blinded follow-up is still ongoing to compare lisinopril, amlodipine, and chlorthalidone.[185]

The Controlled-Onset Verapamil Investigation of Cardiovascular Events (CONVINCE) trial[186] was designed to compare a delayed/slow-release verapamil delivery system to atenolol or hydrochlorothiazide in 15,000 hypertensive patients aged 55 years of age or above. The study was stopped by the sponsor for cost reasons, and the accumulated data from the trial showed no advantage of using verapamil delivery system on morbid and mortal cardiovascular events.[169] (Data presented at the American Society of Hypertension, 17th Annual Scientific Meeting, May 14–18, 2002, New York, NY.)

The calcium-channel blockers reduce both systolic and diastolic pressures with minimal side effects, including orthostasis.[158] They can cause left ventricular hypertrophy to regress in patients with hypertension.[187,188] These drugs may also exhibit antiadrenergic and natriuretic activities and can normalize the abnormal coronary vasomotion often observed in hypertensive patients.[189–192] They can be combined with other antihypertensive drugs if necessary (beta blockers, ACE inhibitors, and diuretics).[158,163]

There is also a growing experience with combination calcium-channel blocker therapy in hypertension.[193] Innovative combination antihypertensive formulations have been evaluated in clinical trials and are now available: enalapril/extended-release diltiazem, benazepril/amlodipine,[194] trandolapril/extended-release verapamil,[195] and extended-release felodipine/enalapril.[196]

Calcium-channel blockers are equally effective in both black and white patients[197] and in the young as well as the old.[158,197] Women may have greater blood pressure lowering effects than men with comparable doses of drug.[198] They do not lower the pressures of normotensive patients.[158] These drugs may be most useful in patients with low-renin, salt-dependent forms of hypertension.[199,200] In addition, they have been shown to be useful in treating patients with hypertension following heart transplant.[201]

Hypertension with Concomitant Diabetes

Compared with placebo, nitrendipine has been shown to reduce the risk for subsequent cardiovascular events and mortality. In the SYST-EUR study,[170] 10.5% of patients had diabetes mellitus. Among those, systolic blood pressure was slightly higher than among patients without diabetes. Compared with placebo, the relative risk reduction for fatal and nonfatal strokes was 73%, for cardiovascular mortality was 76%, which clearly exceeded the benefit seen in nondiabetic patients.[202] Although not statistically significant, there was a 57% reduction in relative risk for myocardial infarction. In line with these findings are the results of the SYST-CHINA, trial with a large risk reduction among the subgroup of patients with diabetes.[173]

Although calcium-channel blockers in diabetic subjects are associated with a clear risk reduction compared with placebo, the results of studies where calcium-channel blockers were compared with other blood pressure–lowering drugs, in particular ACE inhibitors, appear to be less favorable. In the Appropriate Blood Pressure Control in Diabetes (ABCD) trial,[203] nisoldipine was compared with enalapril among patients with non-insulin-dependent diabetes with or without hypertension. Among the primary aims of the study was to test the effect of the calcium-channel blocker nisoldipine on risk of cardiovascular events. The trial was terminated early because in

the subgroup of patients with hypertension receiving nisoldipine, there was a significant excess in myocardial infarction. Compared with enalapril, the secondary endpoint fatal and nonfatal myocardial infarction was strongly increased 25 vs 5.

Similarly, in the Fosinopril Versus Amlodipine Cardiovascular Events Randomized Trial (FACET),[204] compared with fosinopril, patients randomized to calcium-channel blockers had a twofold excess in combined cardiovascular end points (27 vs 14). However, in a subanalysis of the STOP-2 trial[176] that included a large number of patients with diabetes mellitus, the potential disadvantage of calcium-channel; blockers compared with other treatments was less impressive.

Compared with placebo, calcium antagonists apparently reduce the risk for clinical end points among patients with diabetes and hypertension; but in head-to-head comparison, there is evidence that ACE inhibitors are superior to calcium blockers in reducing cardiovascular end points and for reducing the rate of progression of renal disease.[204a] However the superiority of other treatments over calcium blockers may be small or even absent.

Hypertension with Heart Disease

Despite the widespread use of calcium-channel blockers for the treatment of systemic hypertension, there are still questions regarding their relative cardioprotective efficacy compared to other antihypertensive agents.[205–208] The major hypertensive trials comparing calcium-channel blockers to placebo and other antihypertensives are summarized in Table 9-8.

In 1995, there were two published reports suggesting an increased risk of myocardial infarction and mortality in hypertensive patients receiving the short-acting calcium-channel blockers (verapamil, diltiazem, nifedipine) as treatment compared with patients receiving other antihypertensive therapies which included diuretics and beta blockers.[209,210] These reports were case-control studies that have built into their experimental design significant methodologic flaws. A great debate appeared in the medical literature regarding the safety of calcium-channel blockers as a class for treating hypertension.[211–216] Based on the available evidence, the U.S. Food and Drug Administration (FDA) has advised physicians not to use the short-acting calcium-channel blockers for treating hypertension, but it placed no restrictions on the first-line supplementary use of sustained-release calcium-channel blocker formulations or longer-acting formulations available for this indication where there appears to be no apparent harm with their use.[217,218,204a]

In the treatment of hypertension, dihydropyridine calcium-blockers appear to be as efficacious as diuretics in reducing cardiovascular and cerebrovascular morbidity and mortality. In hypertensive patients with angina, beta blockers should be the initial treatment of choice, with calcium blockers used as an add-on treatment or as an alternative monotherapy in individuals intolerant of beta blockers. In patients with hypertension and heart failure, ACE inhibitors, beta blockers, and diuretics are the treatment of choice, with calcium blockers as a possible add-on treatment. In patients with diabetes, there is strong evidence for the use of ACE inhibitors or angiotensin II blockers over calcium blockers. The ACE inhibitors seem also to provide a greater venoprotective effect than calcium blockers in hypertensive patients.[219]

In patients without evidence of coronary artery disease, heart failure, renal disease, or diabetes, calcium-channel blockers can be considered a front-line therapy with efficacy similar to that of other antihypertensive agents. The results of the ALLHAT study should

TABLE 9-8. Study Characteristics and Relative Risks for Different Endpoints Comparing CCB with Placebo and Other Blood Pressure-Lowering Drugs

Study	n	Comparison	Age (mean)	Sex (male), %	Diabetes Mellitus (%)	Cerebrovascular Disease at Baseline (%)	CHD at Baseline (%)	Mean Follow-up Time (years)	RR* (95% CI) Stroke	RR (95% CI) Myocardial Infarction	RR (95% CI) Cardiovascular Mortality	RR (95% CI) Noncardiovascular Mortality	RR (95% CI) Total Mortality
Ca antagonist compared with placebo:													
STONE	1,632	Nifedipine vs placebo	66	47	0	0	0	2.5	0.43 (0.24–0.77)	0.94 (0.13–6.66)	0.78 (0.35–1.73)	0.32 (0.11–1.03)	0.57 (0.30–1.08)
SYST-EUR	4,695	Nitrendipine vs placebo	70	33	10	2	12	2.5	0.58 (0.40–0.83)	0.70 (0.44–1.09)	0.73 (0.52–1.03)	0.99 (0.69–1.43)	0.85 (0.66–1.10)
SYST-China	2,394	Nitrendipine vs placebo	67	64	4	2	10	2.7	0.62 (0.42–0.91)	1.08 (0.39–2.84)	0.67 (0.43–1.07)	0.70 (0.42–1.16)	0.66 (0.47–0.93)
Compared with active treatment:													
STOP-2	6,614	Isradipine/felodipine vs AEC-I vs beta blockers and/or diuretics	76	33	11	4	8	5.0	0.91 (0.77–1.09)	1.25 (1.03–1.52)	0.95 (0.78–1.12)	1.00 (0.82–1.22)	0.97 (0.84–1.11)
INSIGHT	6,321	Slow-release nifedipine vs diuretics	65	46	21	—	6	3.5	0.91 (0.65–1.26)	1.27 (0.91–1.79)	1.16 (0.80–1.69)	0.97 (0.75–1.26)	1.03 (0.83–1.27)
NORDIL	10,881	Diltiazem vs diuretics/beta blocker	60	49	7	3	5	4.5	0.81 (0.66–1.01)	1.19 (0.95–1.47)	1.16 (0.90–1.49)	0.89 (0.68–1.17)	1.03 (0.85–1.24)
MIDAS	883	Isradipine vs hydrochlorothiazid	58	78	—	—	<5	3.0	2.00 (0.50–8.08)	1.20 (0.36–3.96)	1.00 (0.20–4.97)	0.83 (0.25–2.74)	0.88 (0.34–2.31)
NICS-EH	414	Nicardipine vs trichlormethiazide	70	33	—	0	0	3.4	0.74 (0.25–2.17)	1.00 (0.14–7.13)	1.00 2 v 0 CV-deaths	1.00 0 v 2 non-CV deaths	1.00 (0.14–7.13)
VHAS	1,414	Verapamil vs chlorthalidone	54	49	—	—	<5	2.0	0.75 (0.17–3.36)	1.00 (0.29–3.47)	1.25 (0.33–4.68)	no non-CV deaths	1.25 (0.33–4.68)
Diabetes mellitus: **Ca antagonist compared with placebo:**													y
SYST-EUR (subgroup)	492	Nitrendipine vs placebo		35	100	—	—	ca 2.5	0.30 (0.11–0.85)	0.43 (0.17–1.07)	0.28 (0.10–0.79)	1.05 (0.44–2.52)	0.56 (0.29–1.07)
Compared with active treatment													
ABCD	470	Nisoldipine vs enalapril	58	67	100	3	25	3.0	1.60 (0.61–4.20)	3.26 (1.50–7.09)	1.87 (0.68–5.16)	0.87 (0.31–2.44)	1.31 (0.64–2.70)
FACET	380	Amlodipine vs fosinopril	63	68	100	—	—	ca 3.0	2.56 (0.79–8.30)	1.31 (0.56–3.06)	—	—	1.24 (0.33–4.70)
STOP-2 (subgroup)	919	Isradipine/felodipine vs AEC-I vs beta blockers and/or diuretics	76	40	100	5	9	ca 5.0	0.81 (0.51–1.29)	1.66 (1.03–2.70)	0.80 (0.52–1.23)	0.92 (0.51–1.65)	0.82 (0.56–1.19)

Ca = calcium; CV = cardiovascular; RR = relative risk.

*Relative risk, approximated by unadjusted odds ratios.

Source: Reproduced with permission from Muntwyler J, Follath F: Calcium channel blockers in treatment of hypertension. *Prog Cardiovasc Dis* 44:207, 2001.

provide important information regarding the exact role for calcium-channel blockers in the treatment of hypertension.[220]

Hypertensive Emergencies and Perioperative Hypertension

Some of the calcium-channel blockers have also been shown to be beneficial and safe in patients with severe hypertension and hypertensive crises.[158,221–223] Single oral, sublingual, and intravenous doses of these drugs have rapidly and smoothly reduced blood pressure in adults and children without causing significant untoward effects.[162,221–224] The absolute reduction in blood pressure with treatment appears to be inversely correlated with the height of the pretreatment blood pressure level, and few episodes of hypotension have been reported.[221] Continuous hemodynamic monitoring of patients does not seem necessary in most instances.[221] Intravenous nicardipine is approved for clinical use in the treatment of hypertensive emergencies and perioperative hypertension. Its clinical utility compared with other parenteral treatments including other intravenous calcium blockers (clevidipine) is still to be determined.[9,225–227]

Silent Myocardial Ischemia

In addition to their favorable effects in relieving painful episodes of myocardial ischemia, the calcium blockers are also effective in relieving transient myocardial ischemic episodes (detected by ECG) that are unrelated to symptoms (silent myocardial ischemia).[228–230] Diltiazem,[77] nifedipine (low-dose), amlodipine,[97] and verapamil alone and in combination with beta blockers and nitrates have all been shown to be effective in reducing the number of ischemic episodes and their duration.[231–233] The prognostic importance of relieving silent myocardial ischemia with calcium blockers and other treatments was evaluated in a study sponsored by the National Heart Lung and Blood Institute, the Asymptomatic Coronary Ischemia Pilot (ACIP).[234–236]

Myocardial Infarction

Several experimental studies have indicated that nifedipine, verapamil, and diltiazem can reduce the size of myocardial necrosis induced in experimental ischemia.[237–239] Ischemia can lead to diminished ATP production, which can eventually affect the sodium and calcium ion pumps, with the ultimate consequence of calcium ion accumulation in the cytoplasm and calcium overload in the mitochondria. Calcium-channel blockers can diminish myocardial oxygen consumption and inhibit the influx of calcium ions to the myofibrils and thus favorably influence the outcome of experimental coronary occlusion.[48,237] These experimental observations have suggested the use of calcium-channel blockers for reducing or containing the extent of myocardial infarction during acute coronary artery occlusions in human beings and as an adjunct to cardioplegia during open heart surgery. However, there have been no adequate studies in human beings to support these approaches.

Compared with the established protective actions of some beta-blocking drugs used intravenously or orally in prolonging life and reducing the risk of nonfatal reinfarction in survivors of an acute myocardial infarction,[240] the results with calcium-channel blockers (diltiazem, lidoflazine, nifedipine, verapamil) have not been as favorable.[239,241–253] The results of a meta-analysis looking at the effects of immediate-release nifedipine in patients surviving myocardial infarction even suggested the potential for harm,[254] which also prompted a debate in the literature [213,218,219] regarding the safety of calcium-channel blockers as a treatment class for patients surviving myocardial infarction.

The plausibility of these mortality results with calcium blockers are supported by a failure to show a beneficial effect on infarct size, development of myocardial infarctions, or reinfarctions in most trials of patients with myocardial infarctions or unstable angina.[250] A trial using diltiazem in patients with non-Q-wave infarction reported a reduction in recurrent myocardial infarction in the diltiazem-treated patients but no reduction in mortality.[245] In a larger trial with diltiazem in infarction survivors, no favorable effects on mortality were seen.[249] A subgroup of patients with left ventricular dysfunction did worse with diltiazem therapy than with placebo; however, diltiazem therapy appeared effective in patients with relatively normal left ventricular function.[249] Similarly, a more recent study did show benefit of verapamil compared with placebo in infarction survivors, with less benefit observed in patients with left ventricular dysfunction.[250]

A double-blind study was completed comparing oral diltiazem and aspirin with aspirin alone [Incomplete Infarction Trial of European Research Collaborators Evaluating Prognosis Post-Thrombolysis (INTERCEPT)] in patients with myocardial infarction who had received thrombolytic therapy. The study enrolled 874 subjects and treatment with diltiazem did not reduce the cumulative occurrence of cardiac death, nonfatal reinfarction, or refractory ischemia during a 6-month follow up, but it did reduce composite end points of nonfatal cardiac events, particularly the need for myocardial revascularization.[255] In another study, intravenous diltiazem was given as an adjunct to thrombolysis in acute myocardial infarction and shown to have protective effects, with no effect on coronary artery patency and left ventricular function and perfusion.[256]

Prophylactic use of calcium-channel blockers to improve patient survival following myocardial infarction cannot be recommended as a first-line therapy unless there are specific indications for using these drugs.[241,251,252,257] However, in patients with contraindications to beta-adrenergic blockade, one can consider using verapamil or diltiazem in survivors of myocardial infarction who have good ventricular function.[252,258] Bepridil use may put postinfarction patients at an increased risk.[259]

Hypertrophic Cardiomyopathy

Propranolol remains the therapeutic agent of choice[260] for symptomatic patients with hypertrophic cardiomyopathy. The beneficial effects produced by propranolol derive from its blocking of sympathetic stimulation of the heart.[261,262]

Clinical studies have shown that the administration of verapamil can also improve exercise capacity and symptoms in many patients with hypertrophic cardiomyopathy.[263–266] The exact mechanism by which verapamil produces these beneficial effects is not known. Acute and chronic verapamil administration reduces left ventricular outflow obstruction, but examination of indices of left ventricular systolic function during chronic therapy shows that this effect does not result from a reduction in left ventricular hypercontractility.[263] Since patients with hypertrophic cardiomyopathy also exhibit abnormal diastolic function, it is likely that improvement in diastolic filling may be responsible in part for the benefit conferred by verapamil.[263] Enhanced early diastolic filling and improvement in the diastolic pressure-volume relation might be expected to result in an increase in left ventricular end-diastolic volume, which would decrease the Venturi forces that act to move the anterior mitral valve leaflet across the outflow tract toward the septum.[263] This decrease would cause a diminution of obstruction, reducing left ventricular pressure and myocardial wall stress and thus raising the threshold at which symptoms occur.[263]

In a large study of patients with hypertrophic cardiomyopathy refractory to beta blockers,[263] verapamil proved to be effective on a long-term basis, with almost 50% of patients showing either a significant improvement in exercise tolerance, an improvement in symptoms, or a reduction in myocardial ischemia.[264] Approximately 50% of patients who were considered to be candidates for surgery because of moderately severe symptoms unresponsive to propranolol showed significant improvement on verapamil, and surgery was no longer considered necessary.[263]

Other studies have reported that chronic administration of verapamil can not only improve symptoms in patients with hypertrophic cardiomyopathy but also reduce the left ventricular muscle mass and the ventricular septal thickness measured by echocardiographic and ECG analyses.[265] Verapamil and nifedipine were shown to improve the impaired left ventricular filling characteristics.[267,268] This beneficial effect on left ventricular diastolic relaxation has not occurred after propranolol.[267]

There may be serious and fatal complications of verapamil treatment in patients with hypertrophic cardiomyopathy.[263] These complications result from the accentuated hemodynamic or electrophysiologic effects of the drug. It is not clear whether the fatal complications occur as a result of verapamil-induced reduction in blood pressure with a resultant increase in left ventricular obstruction or the negative inotropic effects of the drug.[263] Verapamil probably should not be used in patients with clinical congestive heart failure. The loss of sequential atrial ventricular depolarization caused by the electrophysiologic effects of the drug could also compromise cardiac function. The adverse electrophysiologic effects are often transient; however, they could prevent the use of larger drug doses that might provide better relief.[263]

If the calcium-entry blocking effects of verapamil are responsible for its therapeutic actions in hypertrophic cardiomyopathy, other drugs in this class may also be useful. However, the results of a double-blind trial comparing verapamil with nifedipine indicated that verapamil is more effective than nifedipine in improving exercise tolerance and clinical symptoms.[269] Diltiazem was recently shown to improve active diastolic function in patients with hypertrophic cardiomyopathy; however, certain patients had a marked increase in outflow obstruction.[270]

Congestive Cardiomyopathy

The potent systemic vasodilatory actions of nifedipine and other dihydropyridine calcium-entry blockers make them potentially useful as afterload-reducing agents in patients with left ventricular failure.[39,46,271,272] Unlike other vasodilatory drugs, however, nifedipine also exerts a direct negative inotropic effect on the myocardium that is consistent with its ability to block transmembrane calcium transport in cardiac muscle cells.[39,40] The successful use of nifedipine as a vasodilator in patients with left ventricular failure would be dependent on its effect to reduce ventricular afterload exceeding its direct negative inotropic actions, thereby leading to an improvement in hemodynamics and forward flow.[87]

Studies evaluating the effect on hemodynamics of nifedipine used in combination with other vasodilators in patients with heart failure have uniformly demonstrated significant reductions in systemic vascular resistance, usually associated with increases in cardiac output.[87,273] It has been found that resting ejection fractions also rise with nifedipine therapy.[274,275] Reflex increases in heart rate have been reported,[274] but most investigators have found heart rate to remain the same[275,276] and, in isolated cases, to fall.[277] Left ventricular filling pressures usually decrease[275,276] or do not change significantly,[277] but there are instances where pulmonary capillary wedge pressures rise with the use of nifedipine in heart failure.[278,279] Patients with left ventricular dysfunction and nearly normal levels of left ventricular afterload—that is, disproportionately low wall stress—and those with intrinsic fixed mechanical interference to forward flow, such as aortic stenosis, appear most likely to have unfavorable hemodynamic responses to nifedipine therapy.[46] Most of the published data have dealt only with the acute hemodynamic effects of the agent after single sublingual dosing, with little work done on the use of nifedipine as chronic oral therapy for left ventricular failure.

There is a promising experience in clinical trials with the newer dihydropyridine calcium blockers amlodipine and felodipine in patients with congestive cardiomyopathy.[280–284a] A study has demonstrated the efficacy and safety of diltiazem in patients with idiopathic cardiomyopathy.[285]

Although evidence is incomplete, there are indications that a cardiac tissue renin-angiotensin system may counteract the actions of calcium-channel blockers, especially in patients with heart failure.[46] However, since calcium-channel blocking drugs are potent vasodilators, particularly on the arterial circulation, the combination of an ACE inhibitor and a calcium-channel blocker might appear to be useful in further augmenting vasodilation, thus improving myocardial perfusion and ejection fraction. Hence, the Third Vasodilator-Heart Failure Trial (V-HeFT III) was conducted to test the efficacy of the combination of felodipine, enalapril, digoxin, and a diuretic in patients with congestive heart failure.[286] The end points evaluated were exercise tolerance, quality of life, left ventricular function, levels of plasma norepinephrine and atrial natriuretic factor, and reduction in occurrence of arrhythmias and mortality.[286a] A similar pilot multicenter, placebo-controlled study was carried out using amlodipine in addition to ACE inhibitors, digoxin, and diuretics. This study, known as the Prospective Randomized Amlodipine Survival Evaluation (PRAISE), indicated no clear overall mortality or harm from the use of the drug in patients with severe congestive heart failure.[287] Contrary to the prior experiences of the investigators, there appeared to be little beneficial effect in the large subgroup of patients who had coronary artery disease and a barely significant reduction in morbidity and mortality in the minority of patients who did not have coronary artery disease.[288]

The investigation was followed up in a study comparing amlodipine to placebo in a study of 1800 patients having cardiomyopathy without coronary artery disease who were receiving digoxin, diuretics, and ACE inhibitors (PRAISE II), with no additional benefit from the calcium blocker being observed (Data presented at the 51st Annual Scientific Sessions of the American College of Cardiology, Atlanta, GA. March 17–20, 2002). Finally, mibefradil, a nondihydropyridine calcium blocker with little negative inotropic activity, was evaluated in a double-blind, placebo-controlled trial of 2000 patients with class II to III heart failure (New York Heart Association) who were already receiving standard heart failure therapies [Mortality Assessment in Congestive Heart Failure (MACH-1 Study)].[289]

The study demonstrated no benefit of mibefradil. The potential interaction with antiarrhythmic drugs, especially amiodarone, and drugs associated with torsades may have contributed to poor outcomes early in the study.

In a retrospective analysis of the Studies of Left Ventricular Dysfunction where enalapril was compared with placebo in patients with class I to III heart failure, it was observed that those patients who were receiving concomitant immediate-release calcium-channel blocker treatment had a higher mortality than subjects who were receiving concomitant beta-blocker therapy.[290]

Use of long-acting dihydropyridine calcium blockers as adjunctive vasodilator therapy in patients with left ventricular failure should be considered only if additional clinical reasons for their administration exist—that is, angina pectoris, systemic hypertension, and aortic regurgitation,[291] particularly if these conditions play important contributory roles in the development or exacerbation of left ventricular dysfunction. Some investigators now propose that calcium antagonists may provide some benefit to patients with predominant diastolic ventricular dysfunction,[292] but more clinical data are needed to substantiate this claim.[293,294]

Aortic Regurgitation

Dihydropyridine calcium blockers have been used successfully as arterial vasodilators in patients with chronic asymptomatic aortic and mitral regurgitation. These beneficial hemodynamic effects may postpone the need for valve replacement.[295]

Primary Pulmonary Hypertension

Primary pulmonary hypertension is an entity characterized by excessive pulmonary vasoconstriction and increased pulmonary vascular resistance induced by unknown stimuli.[296] Recently, it was suggested that endothelial cell dysfunction and injury may be responsible for the disease process.[297] Typically, the affected patient is a young to middle-age woman presenting with fatigue, dyspnea, chest discomfort, or syncope. Despite many attempts to develop effective therapy, the results of drug treatment have been generally unsatisfactory, and the syndrome continues to bear a poor prognosis.[296]

Based on the currently available data, it may be concluded that some calcium-channel antagonists provide beneficial responses in selected patients with pulmonary hypertension.[296,298,299] In general, patients with less severe pulmonary hypertension appear to respond better than do those with more advanced disease.[300] Furthermore, early treatment may serve to attenuate progression of the disease.

In patients with chronic hypoxia-induced pulmonary vasoconstriction, the use of calcium-channel blockers may be associated with a worsening of ventilation/perfusion mismatching secondary to inhibition of hypoxic pulmonary vasoconstriction.[301]

Cerebral Arterial Spasm and Stroke

A major complication of subarachnoid hemorrhage is cerebral arterial spasm, which may occur several days after the initial event.[302] Such a spasm may be a focal or diffuse narrowing of one or more of the larger cerebral vessels, which may cause additional ischemic neurologic deficits. Although the exact etiology of this spasm is unknown, a combination of various blood constituents and neurotransmitters has been postulated to produce a milieu that enhances the reactivity of the cerebral vasculature.[302] The final pathway for the vasoconstriction, however, involves an increase in the free intracellular calcium concentration.[303] Accordingly, it is reasonable to postulate that the calcium-channel antagonists may have a beneficial effect in reducing cerebral spasm.[304]

Although verapamil and nifedipine have been shown to prevent cerebral arterial spasm in experimental studies,[305,306] nimodipine and nicardipine, both nifedipine analogues, have demonstrated a preferential cerebrovascular action in this disorder.[307–309] The lipid-solubility of nimodipine enables it to cross the blood-brain barrier; this may account for its more potent cerebrovascular effects. In a multicenter placebo-controlled study involving 125 patients,[302] it was demonstrated that nimodipine significantly reduced the occurrence of severe neurologic deficits following angiographically demonstrated cerebral arterial spasm. All patients had a documented subarachnoid hemorrhage and a normal neurologic status within 96 h of entry into the study. Although 8 of the 60 placebo-treated patients developed a severe neurologic deficit, only 1 of 55 nimodipine-treated patients suffered such an outcome. Nimodipine is now approved for the improvement of neurologic outcome by reducing the incidence and severity of ischemic deficits in patients with subarachnoid hemorrhage from ruptured congenital aneurysms who are in good neurologic condition after ictus. The recommended dose is 60 mg by mouth every 4 h for 21 consecutive days.

Subsequent investigations have suggested that increased cellular calcium concentration may be implicated in neuronal death after ischemia.[310,310a] Nimodipine administered to laboratory animals after global cerebral ischemia had a more favorable effect on neurologic outcome than did placebo.[311] The results of a prospective double-blind placebo-controlled trial of oral nimodipine administered to 186 patients within 24 h of an acute ischemic stroke showed a reduction in both mortality and neurologic deficit with active treatment. The benefit was confined predominantly to men.[310] However, subsequent studies where nimodipine therapy was begun up to 48 h after the onset of symptoms revealed no benefit of therapy.[312,313]

Migraine and Dementia

Classic migraine is characterized by prodromal symptoms with transient neurologic deficits. Cerebral blood flow is reduced during these prodromes and then is increased during the subsequent vasodilatory phase, causing severe headache.[314] Because the entry of calcium ions into the smooth muscle cells is the final common pathway that controls vasomotor tone, calcium antagonists may prevent or ameliorate the initial focal cerebral vasoconstriction.[315]

Results from controlled studies have demonstrated that 80 to 90% of patients with vascular headaches benefit from nimodipine, confirming the selectivity of this agent for the cerebral blood vessels.[316] Verapamil and nifedipine have also been reported to be effective in the prophylaxis of migraine but are less selective for the cephalic blood vessels and thus cause more systemic side effects.[316–318] Relief from the migraine prodrome usually began 10 to 14 days after initiation of the drugs but could be delayed 2 to 4 weeks.[319] Cerebral vascular resistance was decreased by all three established calcium antagonists, but only nimodipine reduced the cerebral vasoconstriction induced by inhalation of 100% oxygen.[316] None of the calcium-entry blocking drugs are effective against muscle contraction or tension headaches.

Multiple clinical trials are now being carried out to examine the effects of calcium-entry blockers on the progression of dementing illness, both vascular and Alzheimer types. Preliminary results have shown equivocal benefit from treatment.[320] However, the

SYST-EUR trial showed a reduction in the incidence of cognitive decline in elderly patients receiving nitrendipine for isolated systolic hypertension compared to placebo.[171]

Other Vascular Uses

Amaurosis Fugax

Hypoperfusion of the retinal circulation may lead to a brief loss of vision in one eye, a syndrome known as amaurosis fugax.[321] This brief loss of sight has been attributed to embolism from the heart or great vessels or to carotid occlusive disease. In a small group of patients with amaurosis but no signs of emboli or carotid hypoperfusion, administration of aspirin or warfarin did not relieve symptoms.[322] However, oral doses of either verapamil or nifedipine abolished attacks. In several patients, the attacks returned when the calcium-blocking agent was discontinued.

High-Altitude Pulmonary Edema

Hypoxic pulmonary hypertension appears to play a role in the pathogenesis of high-altitude pulmonary edema. Nifedipine has been used for the emergency treatment of this condition, its benefit coming from its ability to reduce pulmonary artery pressure.[323,324]

Raynaud's Phenomenon

Raynaud's phenomenon is characterized by well-demarcated ischemia of the digits with pallor or cyanosis ending abruptly at one level on the digits.[325] Nifedipine has been shown to decrease the frequency, duration, and intensity of vasospastic attacks in approximately two-thirds of patients with primary or secondary Raynaud's phenomenon.[326,327] Patients with primary Raynaud's phenomenon usually demonstrate the most improvement; digital ulcers have been reported to heal in patients with scleroderma. Doses of 10 to 20 mg of nifedipine thrice daily have been used (see Chap. 50). Felodipine and isradipine are as effective as nifedipine. Diltiazem, 60 to 360 mg daily, was also useful in patients with primary or secondary Raynaud's phenomenon in multiple placebo-controlled trials.[325]

Atherosclerosis

Atherosclerosis develops through numerous and interrelated processes involving the accumulation of cholesterol, calcium, and matrix materials in the major arteries and at lesion sites. Many of the intracellular and extracellular processes involved in atherosclerotic plaque formation require calcium, and it has been suggested that large deposits of cholesterol may trigger physiologic changes in membranes that favor uptake of calcium into the vascular smooth muscle.[328]

The results of controlled studies employing angiography have suggested that some calcium-channel blockers may retard the progression of atherosclerosis in humans.[329-352] In the International Nifedipine Trial on Atherosclerosis Coronary Therapy (INTACT) study,[329] it was shown that nifedipine reduced the formation of new lesions when compared with placebo. However, nifedipine had no effect on the progression or regression of already existing coronary lesions, and an increased mortality compared to placebo was observed.

There is a suggestion from available experimental and clinical data that calcium blockers have an atherosclerotic plaque stabilizing action.[333] However, in a recent study with amlodipine, it was shown that the drug had no demonstrable effects on the progression of coronary atherosclerosis or the risk of major cardiovascular events.[334]

The administration of nicardipine for 24 months also had no effect on the progression or retardation of advanced stenoses in patients with coronary atherosclerosis as confirmed by arteriography.[330] However, the drug did appear to retard the progression of small lesions. Diltiazem was shown to retard the development of coronary artery disease in heart transplant recipients,[335] an action independent of the drug's blood pressure–lowering effect.

In the Multicenter Isradipine Diuretic Atherosclerosis Study (MIDAS),[336,337] which was a 3-year, double-blind, randomized trial designed to compare the effectiveness of isradipine and hydrochlorothiazide in retarding the progression of atherosclerotic lesions in the carotid arteries, no apparent benefit was seen with either treatment. A similar study to MIDAS is now being carried out with lacidipine, a new dihydropyridine calcium antagonist, in the 4-year European Lacidipine Study on Atherosclerosis (ELSA).[338]

Calcium blockers have also been used to treat patients with intermittent claudication and mesenteric insufficiency.[339]

Other Cardiovascular Uses

Diltiazem has been used as part of an ice-cold cardioplegia solution in patients undergoing coronary surgical procedures.[340] The addition of diltiazem appeared to preserve high-energy phosphate levels with an improvement in hemodynamics in the postoperative period.[340] Concomitant use of nifedipine appears to reduce the incidence of myocardial infarction and transient ischemia in patients undergoing bypass surgery.[341]

Intracoronary diltiazem has been used to reduce the severity and delay the onset of ischemic pain in patients undergoing percutaneous transluminal angioplasty.[342] Calcium blockers have also been used as a long-term treatment to prevent restenosis following balloon angioplasty with questionable benefit (see Chap. 39).[343,344] They have also been used to prolong graft patency in patients with radial artery coronary bypass grafts with no benefit seen.[345]

It has been shown that coronary artery vasospasm may be an important pathophysiologic mechanism in explaining some types of experimental cardiomyopathy. Experimentally, verapamil has been shown to reduce vasospasm in response to myocarditis and by this mechanism to prevent the development of cardiomyopathy.[346]

Calcium blockers (diltiazem and verapamil) have also been found to preserve the functioning of human renal transplants.[347-349] The drugs dilate the preglomerular afferent arterioles and appear to possess inherent immunosuppressive properties and the ability to ameliorate the nephrotoxic effects of cyclosporine.[350,351]

ADVERSE EFFECTS

In addition to their widely varying effects on cardiovascular function, these agents also have differing spectra of adverse effects (Table 9-9).[1,82] Immediate-release nifedipine is associated with a very high incidence of minor adverse effects (approximately 40%), but serious adverse effects are uncommon.[352] The most frequent adverse effects reported with nifedipine and other dihydropyridines include headache, pedal edema, flushing, paresthesias, gingival hyperplasia and dizziness; the most serious adverse effects of this drug include exacerbation of angina, which may occur in up to 10% of patients, and occasional hypotension.[77,112,116,352a] These side effects are reduced in number with the new long-acting formulation

TABLE 9-9. Adverse Effects of Calcium-Channel Blockers

	Overall	Headache	Dizziness	GI	Flushing	Paresthesia	Decreased SA and/or AV Conduction	CHF	Hypotension	Pedal Edema	Worsening of Angina
Diltiazem	5	+	+	+	+	0	3+	+	+	+	0
Diltiazem SR	5	+	+	+	+	0	3+	+	+	+	0
Verapamil	8	+	+	3+	0	0	3+	2+	+	+	0
Verapamil SR	8	+	+	3+	0	0	3+	2+	+	+	0
Bepridil	15	0	2+	3+	0	0	+	+	0	0	0
Amlodipine	15	2+	+	+	+	+	0	0	+	2+	0
Isradipine	15	2+	2+	+	+	+	0	0	+	2+	0
Nifedipine	20	3+	3+	+	3+	+	0	+	+	2+	+
Nifedipine GITS	10	+	+	+	+	+	0	+	+	+	0
Nicardipine	20	3+	3+	+	3+	+	0	0	+	2+	+
Nimodipine	15	+	+	+	+	0	0	+	+	+	0
Nisoldipine	15	2+	+	+	+	0	2+	0	+	2+	0
Felodipine	20	2+	2+	+	2+	+	0	0	+	2+	0

GI = gastrointestinal; SA = sinoatrial node; AV = atrioventricular node; CHF = congestive heart failure; 0 = no report; + = rare; 2+ = occasional; 3+ = frequent; SR = sustained-release; GITS = gastrointestinal therapeutic system.

Source: Adapted with permission from Frishman et al.[158]

of nifedipine[353] and may also be fewer in number with some of the new dihydropyridine calcium antagonists.[353a] The side effect of pedal edema is often reduced when dihydropyridines are combined with ACE inhibitors.

Diltiazem and verapamil can exacerbate sinus node dysfunction and impair AV nodal conduction, particularly in patients with underlying conduction system disease.[1,82] The most frequent adverse effect of verapamil is constipation.[1,82] The drug may also worsen congestive heart failure, particularly when used in combination with beta blockers or disopyramide.[1,82] There have been recent reports of verapamil-induced parkinsonism.[354] Most of the adverse effects noted with diltiazem have been cardiovascular, with occasional headache and gastrointestinal complaints.[1,82] The side effects of calcium blockers may increase considerably when these agents are used in combination.[77]

An increased risk of gastrointestinal hemorrhage in older patients has been reported with calcium-channel blockers, as well as intraoperative bleeding during coronary artery bypass surgery.[355,356] An increased risk of developing cancer in older subjects has also been reported.[357] These findings have not been confirmed by subsequent studies.[358–362]

Bepridil, which has class I antiarrhythmic properties, has the potential to induce malignant ventricular arrhythmias. In addition, because of its ability to prolong the QT interval, bepridil can cause torsades de pointes–type ventricular tachycardia. Because of these properties, bepridil should be reserved for patients in whom other antianginal agents do not offer a satisfactory effect.[363]

Drug Withdrawal

Serious problems that appear to be related to heightened adrenergic activity[61] have been reported with abrupt withdrawal of long-term beta-blocker therapy in patients with angina. Clinical experiences with the withdrawal of calcium-entry blockers suggest that although patients with angina get worse after treatment when a calcium-entry blocker is stopped abruptly, there is no evidence of an overshoot in anginal symptoms.[61,77]

Drug Overdose

Calcium-entry blocker overdosage has been described with increasing frequency. The cardiovascular problems associated with this condition are hypotension, left ventricular conduction, bradycardia, nodal blocks, and asystole. Treatment approaches are described in Table 9-10.[364–365]

TABLE 9-10. Cardiovascular Toxicity with Calcium-Channel Blockers and Recommendations for Treatment

Effects*	Suggested Treatment
Profound hypotension	10% calcium gluconate or calcium chloride; norepinephrine or dopamine
Severe LV dysfunction	10% calcium gluconate or calcium chloride; isoproterenol or dobutamine; glucagon; milrinone, norepinephrine or dopamine
Profound bradycardia	Atropine sulfate (not always effective)
Sinus bradycardia	10% calcium gluconate or calcium chloride
SA- and AV-nodal block	Isoproterenol or dobutamine
Asystole	External cardiac massage and cardiac pacing (if above measures fail)

AV = atrioventricular; LV = left ventricular; SA = sinoatrial.

*These effects are seen more frequently in patients who have underlying myocardial dysfunction and/or cardiac conduction abnormalities and who are receiving concomitant beta-adrenergic blocker treatment.

Source: Reproduced with permission from Frishman et al.[365]

Drug-Drug Interactions

There are few data on the interactions of diltiazem with other drugs.[1,77] Rifampin severely reduces the bioavailability of oral verapamil by enhancing the first-pass liver metabolism of the drug. Both nifedipine and verapamil increase serum digoxin levels, an observation not made with diltiazem (see Chap. 48). Verapamil has been reported to increase serum digoxin levels by approximately 70%.[78,366,367] apparently by decreasing renal clearance,[366] nonrenal clearance, and the volume of distribution.[367,368] Studies of the time course of this effect show that it begins with the first dose and reaches steady state within 1 to 4 weeks. Nifedipine also has been reported to increase serum digoxin concentrations in patients but to a lesser extent (about 45%).[369] The mechanism for this interaction is not clear. Verapamil[367] and diltiazem[370] have additive effects on AV conduction in combination with digitalis. They can be used to cause further decreases in heart rate compared with digitalis alone when patients are in atrial fibrillation.

Combinations of propranolol with nifedipine or verapamil have been extensively studied for the therapy of angina pectoris.[82] Several studies have shown improved efficacy for the combination of atenolol and nifedipine compared with any of the drugs used alone.[371] Hemodynamic studies have shown mild negative inotropic effects of verapamil in patients on a beta blocker.[133] There are also slight decreases in heart rate, cardiac output, and left ventricular ejection fraction.[133] Combinations of nifedipine and propranolol or metoprolol and of verapamil and propranolol are well tolerated by patients with normal left ventricular function, but there may be a greater potential for hemodynamic compromise in patients with impaired left ventricular function with combined verapamil-propranolol treatment.[133] Combinations of diltiazem, nifedipine, or verapamil with nitrates are well tolerated and clinically useful.[82] When diltiazem is combined with nifedipine, blood levels of nifedipine increase significantly, which may contribute to an increased frequency of adverse reactions with this combination.[77] The combination of verapamil and nifedipine is less effective in lowering pressure than diltiazem plus nifedipine, perhaps related to the diltiazem-nifedipine pharmacokinetic interaction.[372]

CONCLUSION

Each of the calcium antagonists exerts its effects through inhibition of slow-channel–mediated calcium ion transport. However, many of the drugs appear to accomplish this by different mechanisms and with differing effects on various target organs. These differences allow the clinician to select the particular drug most suitable for the specific needs of the patient. In addition, the side-effect profiles of these drugs (with little overlap between them) assure that most patients will tolerate at least one of these agents.

REFERENCES

 1. Keefe D, Frishman WH: Clinical pharmacology of the calcium-channel blocking drugs. In: Packer M, Frishman WH, eds. *Calcium Channel Antagonists in Cardiovascular Disease.* Norwalk, CT: Appleton-Century-Crofts, 1984:3–19.
 2. Braunwald E: Mechanism of action of calcium-channel blocking agents. N *Engl J Med* 307:1618, 1983.
 3. Frishman WH, Sonnenblick EH: Beta-adrenergic blocking drugs and calcium channel blockers. In: Alexander RW, Schlant RC, Foster V, eds. *Hurst's The Heart*, 9th ed. New York: McGraw Hill, 1998: 1583–1618.
 4. Frishman WH: Current status of calcium channel blockers. *Curr Probl Cardiol* 19(11):637, 1994.
 5. Frishman WH, Cheng-Lai A, Chen J, eds. *Current Cardiovascular Drugs*, 3rd ed. Philadelphia: Current Medicine, 2000.
 6. Malhotra HS, Plosker GL: Barnidipine. *Drugs* 61:989, 2001.
 7. Tomoda F, Takata M, Kagitani S, et al: Effects of a novel calcium antagonist, benidipine hydrochloride, on platelet responsiveness to mental stress in patients with essential hypertension. *J Cardiovasc Pharmacol* 34:248, 1999.
 8. Sakata K, Shirotani M, Yoshida H, et al: Effects of amlodipine and cilnidipine on cardiac sympathetic nervous system and neurohormonal status in essential hypertension. *Hypertension* 33:1447, 1999.
 9. Schwieler JH, Ericsson H, Löfdahl P, et al: Circulatory effects and pharmacology of clevidipine, a novel ultra short acting and vascular selective calcium antagonist, in hypertensive humans. *J Cardiovasc Pharmacol* 34:268, 1999.
10. Sánchez M, Sobrino J, Ribera L, et al: Long-acting lacidipine versus short-acting nifedipine in the treatment of asymptomatic acute blood pressure increase. *J Cardiovasc Pharmacol* 33:479, 1999.
11. Epstein M: Lercanidipine: A novel dihydropyridine calcium channel blocker. *Heart Dis* 3:398, 2001.
12. Cheer SM, McClellan K: Manidipine. A review of its use in hypertension. *Drugs* 61:1777, 2001.
13. Lindner E: Phenyl-propyl-diphenyl-prophyl-amin, a new substance with a dilating action in the coronary vessels. *Arzneim Forsch* 10:569, 573, 1960.
14. Haas H, Hartfelder G: A-Isopropyl-a(N-methyl-N-homoveratryl)-y aminopropyl)-3,4-dimethoxyphenylacetonitrol, a substance with vasodilating properties. *Arzneim Forsch* 12:549, 1962.
15. Fleckenstein A, Kammermeier H, Doring H, et al: On the action mechanism of new coronary dilators with oxygen sparing myocardial effects—Prenylamin and Iproveratril. *Z Kreislauf Forsch* 56:716, 839, 1967.
16. Fleckenstein A: Control of myocardial metabolism by verapamil: Sites of action and therapeutic effects. *Arzneim Forsch* 20:1317, 1970.
17. Singh BN, Vaughan-Williams EM: A fourth class of antidysrhythmic action? Effect of verapamil on ouabain toxicity, on atrial and ventricular intracellular potentials, and on other features of cardiac function. *Cardiovasc Res* 6:109, 1972.
18. Vaughan Williams EM: Classification of antiarrhythmic drugs. In: Sande E, Flensted-Jensen E, Olsen KH, eds. *Symposium on Cardiac Arrhythmia*s. Elsinor, Denmark: AB Astra, 1979:449–501.
19. Ebel VS, Schutz H, Hornitschek A: Studies on the analysis of nifedipine considering in particular transformation products formed by light exposure. *Arzneim Forsch* 28:2188, 1978.
20. Benet LZ: Pharmacokinetics and metabolism of bepridil. *Am J Cardiol* 55:8C, 1985.
21. Opie LH: Calcium channel blockers. In: Opie LH, Gersh BJ, eds. *Drugs for the Heart*, 5th ed. Philadelphia: Saunders, 2001:53–83.
22. Mishra SK, Hermsmeyer K: Selective inhibition of T-type Ca^{2+} channels by RO 40–5967. *Circ Res* 7:144, 1994.
23. de Curzon OP, Ghaleh B, Hittinger L, et al: Beneficial effects of the T- and L-type calcium channel antagonist, mibefradil, against exercise-induced myocardial stunning in dogs. *J Cardiovasc Pharmacol* 35:240, 2000.
24. Schwartz A, Matlib A, Balwierczak J, Lathrop DA: Pharmacology of calcium antagonists. *Am J Cardiol* 55:3C, 1985.
25. Braunwald E: Calcium-channel blockers: Pharmacologic considerations. *Am Heart J* 104:665, 1982.
26. Dhein S, Salameh A, Berkels R, Klaus W: Dual mode of action of dihydropyridine calcium antagonists. A role for nitric oxide. *Drugs* 58:397, 1999.
27. Kitakaze M, Asanuma H, Takashima S, et al: Nifedipine-induced coronary vasodilation in ischemic hearts is attributable to bradykinin- and NO-dependent mechanisms in dogs. *Circulation* 101:311, 2000.
28. Kitakaze M, Node K, Minamino T, et al: A Ca channel blocker, benidipine, increases coronary blood flow and attenuates the severity of myocardial ischemia via NO-dependent mechanisms in dogs. *J Am Coll Cardiol* 33:242, 1999.
29. Kobayashi N, Kobayashi K, Hara K, et al: Benidipine stimulates nitric oxide synthase and improves coronary circulation in hypertensive rats. *Am J Hypertens* 12:483, 1999.

30. Zhang X-p, Xu X, Nasjletti A, Hintze TH: Amlodipine enhances NO production induced by an ACE inhibitor through a kinin-mediated mechanism in canine coronary microvessels. *J Cardiovasc Pharmacol* 35:195, 2000.

31. Brovkovych V, Kalinowski L, Muller-Peddinghaus R, Malinski T: Synergistic antihypertensive effects of nifedipine on endothelium. Concurrent release of NO and scavenging of superoxide. *Hypertension* 37:34, 2001.

32. Berkels R, Egink G, Marsen TA, et al: Nifedipine increases endothelial nitric oxide bioavailability by antioxidative mechanisms. *Hypertension* 37:240, 2001.

33. Zhang X-P, Loke KE, Mital S, et al: Paradoxical release of nitric oxide by an L-type calcium channel antagonist, the R^+ enantiomer of amlodipine. *J Cardiovasc Pharmacol* 39:208, 2002.

33a. Taddei S, Virdis A, Ghiadoni L, et al: Restoration of nitric oxide availability after calcium antagonist treatment in essential hypertension. *Hypertension* 37:943, 2001.

34. Wei C, Burnett JC Jr: Inhibition by calcium antagonism of circulating and renal endothelin in experimental congestive heart failure. *Am J Physiol* 278:H263, 2000.

35. Ikeda U, Hojo Y, Ueno S, et al: Amlodipine inhibits expression of matrix metalloproteinase-1 and its inhibitor in human vascular endothelial cells. *J Cardiovasc Pharmacol* 35:887, 2000.

36. van Breeman C, Mangel A, Fahim M, et al: Selectivity of calcium antagonistic action in vascular smooth muscle. *Am J Cardiol* 49:507, 1982.

37. Millard RW, Lathrop DA, Grupp G, et al: Differential cardiovascular effects of calcium channel blocking agents: Potential mechanisms. *Am J Cardiol* 49:499, 1982.

38. Fleckenstein A: Specific pharmacology of calcium in myocardium, cardiac pacemakers, and vascular smooth muscle. *Annu Rev Pharmacol Toxicol* 17:149, 1977.

39. Henry PD, Borda L, Schuchleib R: Chronotropic and inotropic effects of vasodilators. In: Lichtlen PR, Kimura E, Taira N, eds. *International Adalat Panel Discussion: New Experimental and Clinical Results.* Amsterdam: Exerpta Medica, 1979:14–21.

40. Cohn JN, Franciosa JA: Vasodilatory therapy of cardiac failure. *N Engl J Med* 297:27, 1977.

41. Kohlhardt M, Krause H, Kubler M, et al: Kinetics of inactivation and recovery of the slow inward current in the mammalian ventricular myocardium. *Pflugers Arch* 355:1, 1975.

42. Himori N, Ono H, Taira N: Simultaneous assessment of effects of coronary vasodilators on the coronary blood flow and the myocardial contractility by using the blood perfused canine papillary muscle. *Jpn J Pharmacol* 26:427, 1976.

43. Singh BN, Hecht HS, Nademanee K, et al: Electrophysiologic and hemodynamic effects of slow channel blocking drugs. *Prog Cardiovasc Dis* 25:103, 1982.

44. Braunwald E, Stone PH, Antman EM, et al: Calcium channel blocking agents in the treatment of cardiovascular disorders: II. Hemodynamic effects and clinical applications. *Ann Intern Med* 93:886, 1980.

45. Ellrodt G, Chew CYC, Singh BN: Therapeutic implications of slow channel blockade in cardiocirculatory disorders. *Circulation* 62:669, 1980.

46. Landau AJ, Gentilucci M, Cavusoglu E, Frishman WH: Calcium antagonists for the treatment of congestive heart failure. *Coron Artery Dis* 5:37, 1994.

47. Veniant M, Clozel JP, Hess P, et al: Hemodynamic profile of RO 40-5967 in conscious rats: Comparison with diltiazem, verapamil and amlodipine. *J Cardiovasc Pharmacol* 18 (Suppl 10):S55, 1991.

48. Zsoter TT, Church JG: Calcium antagonists—pharmacodynamic effects and mechanism of action. *Drugs* 25:93, 1983.

49. Mitchell LB, Schroeder JS, Mason JW: Comparative clinical electrophysiologic effect of diltiazem, verapamil and nifedipine—a review. *Am J Cardiol* 49:629, 1982.

50. Frishman WH, LeJemtel T: Electropharmacology of calcium channel antagonists in cardiac arrhythmias. *Pace* 5:402, 1982.

51. Singh BN, Nademanee K, Baky S: Calcium antagonists. *Drugs* 25:125, 1983.

52. Nayler WG, Poole-Wilson PH: Calcium antagonists: Definition and mode of action. *Basic Res Cardiol* 76:1, 1981.

53. Yamaguchi I, Obayashi K, Mandel WJ: Electrophysiologic effects of verapamil. *Cardiovasc Res* 12:597, 1978.

54. Schmitt R, Kleinbluesen CH, Belz GG, et al: Hemodynamic and hormonal effects of the novel calcium antagonist RO 40-5967 in patients with hypertension. *Clin Pharmacol Ther* 52:314, 1992.

55. Singh BN, Collet J, Chew CYC: New perspectives in the pharmacologic therapy of cardiac arrhythmias. *Prog Cardiovasc Dis* 22:243, 1980.

56. Wit A, Cranefield P: The effects of verapamil on the sinoatrial and atrioventricular nodes of the rabbit and the mechanisms by which it arrests reentrant AV nodal tachycardia. *Circ Res* 35:413, 1974.

57. Zipes DP, Fischer JC: Effects of agents which inhibit the slow channel on sinus node automaticity and atrioventricular conduction in the dog. *Circ Res* 34:184, 1974.

58. Findling R, Frishman W, Javed MT, et al: Calcium channel blockers and the gastrointestinal tract. *Am J Ther* 3:383, 1996.

59. Schoen RE, Frishman WH, Shamoon H: Hormonal and metabolic effects of calcium-channel antagonists in man. *Am J Med* 84:492, 1988.

60. Shamoon H, Baylor P, Kamobosos D, et al: Influence of oral verapamil on glucoregulatory hormones in man. *J Clin Endocrinol Metabol* 60:536, 1985.

61. Frishman WH, Klein N, Strom J, et al: Comparative effects of abrupt withdrawal of propranolol and verapamil in angina pectoris. *Am J Cardiol* 50:1191, 1982.

62. McCall D: Excitation-contraction coupling in cardiac and vascular smooth muscle: Modification by calcium entry blockade. *Circulation* 75(Suppl V):V3, 1987.

63. Pumphrey CW, Fuster V, Dewanjee MK, et al: Comparison of the antithrombotic action of calcium antagonist drugs with dipyridamole in dogs. *Am J Cardiol* 51:591, 1983.

64. Mehta JL: Influence of calcium-channel blockers on platelet function and arachidonic acid metabolism. *Am J Cardiol* 55:158B, 1985.

65. Frishman WH, Miller KP: Platelets and antiplatelet therapy in ischemic heart disease. *Curr Probl Cardiol* 11:72, 1986.

66. Sanguigni V, Gallu M, Sciarra L, et al: Effect of amlodipine on exercise-induced platelet activation in patients affected by chronic stable angina. *Clin Cardiol* 22:575, 1999.

67. Tzivoni D: End organ protection by calcium channel blockers. *Clin Cardiol* 24:102, 2001.

68. McAllister RG: Clinical pharmacology of slow channel blocking agents. *Prog Cardiovasc Dis* 25:83, 1982.

69. Kates R: Calcium antagonists—pharmacokinetic properties. Drug 25:113, 1983.

70. Frishman WH, Stroh JA, Greenberg SM, et al: Calcium-channel blockers in systemic hypertension. *Curr Prob Cardiol* 12:287, 1987.

71. Brogden RN, McTavish D: Nifedipine gastrointestinal therapeutic system (GITS). *Drugs* 50:495, 1995.

72. Katz B, Rosenberg A, Frishman WH: Controlled-release drug delivery systems in cardiovascular medicine. *Am Heart J* 129:359, 1995.

73. Mitchell J, Frishman W, Heiman M: Nisoldipine: A new dihydropyridine calcium-channel blocker. *J Clin Pharmacol* 33:46, 1993.

74. Plosker GL, Faulds D: Nisoldipine coat-core. *Drugs* 52:232, 1996.

75. White WB: A chronotherapeutic approach to the management of hypertension. *Am J Hypertens* 9:29S, 1996.

75a. Prisant LM, Black HR, Messerli FH, et al: Results of a community-based trial of a chronotherapeutic verapamil formulation (abst). *Am J Hypertens* 15:58A, 2002.

75b. Tipre D, Vavia P. Optimization and stability study of an EUDRAGITE $100^{®}$ based transdermal therapeutic system of nitrendipine. *Drug Deliv Technol* 2:46, 2002.

75c. Glasser SP, Neutel JM, Albert KS, et al: Efficacy and safety of diltiazem HCL extended release dosed at nighttime (10 p.m.) compared to placebo and to morning dosing (8 a.m.) in moderate to severe hypertension. Presented at the American Society of Hypertension 17th Annual Scientific Meeting, May 14–18, 2002, New York, NY.

76. Frishman WH, Kirstein E, Klein M, et al: Clinical relevance of verapamil plasma levels in stable angina pectoris. *Am J Cardiol* 50:1180, 1982.

77. Frishman WH, Charlap S, Kimmel B, et al: Diltiazem compared to nifedipine and combination treatment in patients with stable angina: Effects on angina, exercise tolerance and the ambulatory ECG. *Circulation* 77:774, 1988.

78. Sica DA, Gehr TWB: Calcium-channel blockers and the cytochrome P450 system. In: Epstein M, ed: *Calcium Antagonists in Clinical Medicine*, 3rd ed. Philadelphia: Hanley and Belfus, 2002:93.

79. Bailey DG, Arnold JMO, Munoz C, Spence JD: Grapefruit juice felodipine interaction: Mechanism, predictability and effect of naringin. *Clin Pharmacol Ther* 53:637, 1993.

80. Malhotra S, Bailey DG, Paine MF, Watkins PB: Seville orange juice-felodipine interaction: Comparison with dilute grapefruit juice and involvement of furocoumarins. *Clin Pharmacol Ther* 69:14, 2001.

80a. Sica DA, Gehr TWB: Calcium-channel blockers and end-stage renal disease. In: Epstein M, ed. *Calcium Antagonists in Clinical Medicine*, 3rd ed. Philadelphia: Hanley and Belfus, 2002:701.

81. Singh BN, Chew CYC, Josephson MA, et al: Hemodynamic mechanisms underlying the antianginal actions of verapamil. *Am J Cardiol* 50:886, 1982.

82. Frishman WH, Sonnenblick EH: Cardiovascular uses of calcium-channel blockers. In: Messerli F, ed. *Current Cardiovascular Drug Therapy*, 2nd ed. Philadelphia: Saunders, l996:891.

83. Braun S, van der Wall EE, Emanuelsson H, Kobrin I, on behalf of the Mibefradil International Study Group: Effects of a new calcium antagonist, mibefradil (RO 40-5967), on silent ischemia in patients with stable chronic angina pectoris: A multicenter placebo-controlled study. *J Am Coll Cardiol* 27:317, 1996.

84. Landau AJ, Frishman WH, Alturk A: The pharmacological management of myocardial ischemia. *Curr Opin Cardiol* 8:629, 1993.

85. Theroux P, Taeymans Y, Waters D: Calcium antagonists: Clinical use in the treatment of angina. *Drugs* 25:178, 1983.

86. Opie LH: Calcium channel antagonists in the treatment of coronary artery disease: Fundamental pharmacological properties relevant to clinical use. *Prog Cardiovasc Dis* 38(4):273, 1996.

87. Abrams J, Frishman WH, Bates SM, et al: Pharmacologic options for treatment of ischemic disease. In: Antman EM, ed. *Cardiovascular Therapeutics*, 2nd ed. Philadelphia: Saunders, 2002:97.

88. Hossack KF, Pool PE, Steele P: Efficacy of diltiazem in angina of effort—a multicenter trial. *Am J Cardiol* 49:567, 1982.

89. Straus WE, McIntyre KM, Parisi AR, Shapiro W: Safety and efficacy of diltiazem hydrochloride for the treatment of stable angina pectoris. Report of a cooperative trial. *Am J Cardiol* 49:560, 1982.

90. Weiner DA, Cutler SS, Klein MD: Efficacy and safety of sustained release diltiazem in stable angina pectoris. *Am J Cardiol* 57:6, 1986.

91. Moskowitz RM, Piccini PA, Nacarelli GV, et al: Nifedipine therapy for stable angina pectoris: Preliminary results of effects on angina frequency and treadmill exercise response. *Am J Cardiol* 44:811, 1979.

92. Mueller HS, Chahine RA: Interim report of multicenter double-blind placebo-controlled studies of nifedipine in chronic stable angina. *Am J Med* 71:645, 1981.

93. Wallace WA, Wellington KL, Chess MA, et al: Comparison of nifedipine gastrointestinal therapeutic system and atenolol on antianginal efficacies and exercise hemodynamic responses in stable angina pectoris. *Am J Cardiol* 73:23, 1994.

94. Cavoretto D, Repossini A, Alamanni F, et al: Amlodipine in residual stable exertional angina pectoris after coronary artery bypass surgery: A randomised, placebo-controlled, double-blind, crossover study. *Clin Drug Invest* 10:22, 1995.

95. Bernink PJLM, de Weerd P, ten Cate FJ, et al: An 8 week double-blind study of amlodipine and diltiazem in patients with stable exertional angina pectoris. *J Cardiovasc Pharmacol* 17(Suppl 1):S53, 1991.

96. Singh S, Doherty J, Udhoji V, et al: Amlodipine versus nadolol in patients with stable angina pectoris. *Am Heart J* 11:1137, 1989.

97. Deanfield JE, Detry J-MRG, Lichtlen PR, et al for the CAPE Study Group: Amlodipine reduces transient myocardial ischemia in patients with coronary artery disease: Double-blind Circadian Anti-ischemia Program in Europe (CAPE Trial). *J Am Coll Cardiol* 24:1460, 1994.

98. Pehrsson SK, Tolagen K, Ulvenstam G: Efficacy and safety of amlodipine compared with diltiazem in patients with stable angina pectoris. *Clin Drug Invest* 11:313, 1996.

99. Kaufman P, Vassalli G, Utzinger U, Hess OM: Coronary vasomotion during dynamic exercise: Influence of intravenous and intracoronary nicardipine. *J Am Coll Cardiol* 26:624, 1995.

100. Pepine CJ, Lambert CR: Usefulness of nicardipine for angina pectoris. *Am J Cardiol* 59:13J, 1987.

101. Bala Subramanian V, Parmasivan R, Lahiri A, et al: Verapamil in chronic stable angina—a controlled study with computerized multi-stage treadmill exercise. *Lancet* 1:841, 1980.

102. Weiner DA, Klein MD: Verapamil therapy for stable exertional angina. *Am J Cardiol* 50:1153, 1982.

103. Weiner DA, Klein MD, Cutler SS: Evaluation of sustained-release verapamil in chronic stable angina pectoris. *Am J Cardiol* 59:215, 1987.

104. Scheidt S, Frishman WH, Packer M, et al: Long-term effectiveness of verapamil in stable and unstable angina pectoris: One year follow-up of patients treated in placebo-controlled double-blind randomized clinical trials. *Am J Cardiol* 50:1185, 1982.

105. Cutler NR, Anders RJ, Jhee SS, et al: Placebo-controlled evaluation of three doses of a controlled-onset, extended-release formulation of verapamil in the treatment of stable angina pectoris. *Am J Cardiol* 75:1102, 1995.

106. Shapiro W, DiBianco R, Thadani U, and other members of the Bepridil Collaborative Study Group: Comparative efficacy of 200, 300 and 400 mg of bepridil for chronic stable angina pectoris. *Am J Cardiol* 55:3C, 1985.

107. Singh BN for the Bepridil Collaborative Study Group: Comparative efficacy and safety of bepridil and diltiazem in chronic stable angina pectoris refractory to diltiazem. *Am J Cardiol* 68:306, 1991.

108. Opie LH: Calcium channel antagonists in the management of anginal syndromes: Changing concepts in relation to the role of coronary vasospasm. *Prog Cardiovasc Dis* 38:291, 1996.

109. Livesley B, Catley PF, Campbell RC, Oram S: Double-blind evaluation of verapamil, propranolol and isosorbide dinitrate against placebo in the treatment of angina pectoris. *Br Med J* 1:375, 1973.

110. Frishman WH, Klein NA, Strom JA, et al: Superiority of verapamil to propranolol in stable angina pectoris—a double-blind, randomized crossover trial. *Circulation* 65(Suppl I):151, 1982.

111. Kenmure ACF, Scruton JH: A double-blind controlled trial of the antianginal efficacy of nifedipine compared with propranolol. *Br J Clin Pract* 8:49, 1980.

112. Bala Subramanian V, Bowles MJ, Khurmi NS, et al: Comparative effectiveness of verapamil and nifedipine in stable angina pectoris. *Am J Cardiol* 50:1173, 1982.

113. Frishman WH, Klein N, Klein P, et al: Comparison of oral propranolol and verapamil for combined systemic hypertension and angina pectoris: A placebo-controlled double-blind randomized crossover trial. *Am J Cardiol* 50:1164, 1982.

114. Frishman WH, Charlap S: Calcium-channel blockers for combined systemic hypertension and myocardial ischemia. *Circulation* 75:V154, 1988.

115. Kizer JR, Kimmel SE: Epidemiologic review of the calcium channel blocker drugs. An up-to-date perspective on the proposed hazards. *Arch Intern Med* 161:1145, 2001.

116. Boden WE, Korr KS, Bough KW: Nifedipine-induced hypotension and myocardial ischemia in refractory angina pectoris. *JAMA* 253:1131, 1985.

117. Stone PH, Gibson RS, Glasser SP, et al: Comparison of propranolol, diltiazem, and nifedipine in the treatment of ambulatory ischemia in patients with stable angina: Differential effects on ambulatory ischemia, exercise performance, and anginal symptoms. *Circulation* 82:1962, 1990.

118. Frishman WH, Glasser S, Stone P, et al: Comparison of controlled-onset extended-release verapamil to amlodipine and amlodipine plus atenolol on exercise performance and ambulatory ischemia in patients with chronic stable angina pectoris. *Am J Cardiol* 83:507, 1999.

119. Frishman WH, Charlap S, Farnham J, et al: Combination propranolol and bepridil therapy in angina pectoris. *Am J Cardiol* 55:43C, 1985.

120. Johnson SM, Mauritson DR, Willerson JT, et al: A controlled trial of verapamil for Prinzmetal's variant angina. *N Engl J Med* 304:862, 1981.

121. Mehta J, Conti CR: Calcium channel antagonists in the treatment of unstable angina. *Am J Cardiol* 50:919, 1982.

122. Antman E, Muller JE, Goldberg S, et al: Nifedipine therapy for coronary artery spasm experience in 127 patients. *N Engl J Med* 302:1269, 1980.

123. Schroeder JS, Feldman RL, Giles TD, et al: Multiclinic controlled trial of diltiazem for Prinzmetals angina. *Am J Med* 72:227, 1982.

124. Goldberg S, Reichek N, Wilson J, et al: Nifedipine in the treatment of Prinzmetals (variant) angina. *Am J Cardiol* 44:804, 1979.

125. Prida XE, Gelman JS, Feldman RL, et al: Comparison of diltiazem alone and in combination in patients with coronary artery spasm. *J Am Coll Cardiol* 9:412, 1987.

126. Chahine RA, Feldman RL, Giles TD, et al: Randomized placebo controlled trial of amlodipine in vasospastic angina. *J Am Coll Cardiol* 21:1365, 1993.

127. McIvor ME, Undemir C, Lawson J, Reddinger J: Clinical effects and utility of intracoronary diltiazem. *Cath Cardiovasc Diag* 35:287, 1995.

128. Parodi O, Simonetti I, LAbbate A, et al: Comparative effectiveness of verapamil and propranolol in angina at rest. *Am J Cardiol* 50:923, 1982.

129. Johnson SM, Mauritson DR, Willerson JT, et al: Comparison of verapamil and nifedipine in the treatment of variant angina pectoris: preliminary observations in 10 patients. *Am J Cardiol* 47:1295, 1981.

130. Gerstenblith G, Ouyang P, Achuff S, et al: Nifedipine in unstable angina: a double-blind randomized trial. *N Engl J Med* 306:885, 1982.

130a. ACC/AHA Task Force on Practice Guidelines (Committee on Management of Patients with Unstable Angina): ACC/AHA Guideline update for the management of patients with unstable angina and non-ST-segment elevation myocardial infarction. www.acc.org/clinical/guidelines/unstable.pdf. 2002.

131. Pehrsson SK, Ringqvist I, Ekdahl S, et al: Monotherapy with amlodipine or atenolol versus their combination in stable angina pectoris. *Clin Cardiol* 23:763, 2000.

132. Emanuelsson H, Egstrup K, Nikus K, et al: Antianginal efficacy of the combination of felodipine-metoprolol 10/100 mg compared with each drug alone in patients with stable effort-induced angina pectoris: A multicenter parallel group study. *Am Heart J* 137:854, 1999.

133. Packer M, Leon MB, Bonow RO, et al: Hemodynamic and clinical effects of combined therapy with verapamil and propranolol in ischemic heart disease. *Am J Cardiol* 50:903, 1982.

134. Packer M, Frishman WH: Calcium channel antagonists in perspective. In: Packer M, Frishman WH, eds. *Calcium Channel Antagonists in Cardiovascular Disease.* Norwalk, CT: Appleton-Century-Crofts, 1984:xvii.

134a. Gabrielli A, Gallagher J, Caruso LJ, et al: Diltiazem to treat sinus tachycardia in critically ill patients. A four-year experience. *Crit Care Med* 29:1874, 2001.

135. Lee S-H, Yu W-C, Cheng J-J, et al: Effect of verapamil on long-term tachycardia-induced atrial electrical remodeling. *Circulation* 101:200, 2000.

136. Pandozi C, Bianconi L, Calo L, et al: Postcardioversion atrial electrophysiologic changes induced by oral verapamil in patients with persistent atrial fibrillation. *J Am Coll Cardiol* 36:2234, 2000.

137. Pritchett ELC: Management of atrial fibrillation. *N Engl J Med* 326:1264, 1992.

138. Ellenbogen KA, Dias VC, Plumb VJ, et al: A placebo-controlled trial of continuous intravenous diltiazem infusion for 24-h heart rate control during atrial fibrillation and atrial flutter: A multicenter trial. *J Am Coll Cardiol* 18:891, 1991.

139. Schamroth L, Krikler DM, Garrett C: Immediate effects of intravenous verapamil in cardiac arrhythmias. *Br Med J* 1:660, 1972.

140. Heng MK, Singh BN, Roche AHG, et al: Effects of intravenous verapamil on cardiac arrhythmias and on the electrocardiogram. *Am Heart J* 90:487, 1975.

141. Klein HO, Pauzner H, DiSegni E, et al: The beneficial effects of verapamil in chronic atrial fibrillation. *Arch Intern Med* 139:747, 1979.

142. Weiner I: Verapamil therapy for atrial flutter and fibrillation. In: Packer M, Frishman WH, eds. *Calcium Channel Antagonists in Cardiovascular Disease.* Norwalk, CT: Appleton-Century-Crofts, 1984:257–268.

142a. Pass RH, Liberman L, Al-Fayaddh M, et al: Continuous intravenous diltiazem infusion for short-term ventricular rate control in children. *Am J Cardiol* 86:559, 2000.

143. Klein HO, Kaplinsky E: Comparative effectiveness of verapamil and digoxin in atrial fibrillation. *Am J Cardiol* 50:894, 1982.

144. De Simone A, Stabile G, Vitale DF, et al: Pretreatment with verapamil in patients with persistent or chronic atrial fibrillation who underwent electrical cardioversion. *J Am Coll Cardiol* 34:810, 1999.

145. Amar D, Roistacher N, Rusch VW, et al: Effects of diltiazem prophylaxis on the incidence and clinical outcome of atrial arrhythmias after thoracic surgery. *J Thorac Cardiovasc Surg* 120:790, 2000.

146. Krikler DM, Spurrell RAJ: Verapamil in the treatment of paroxysmal supraventricular tachycardia. *Postgrad Med J* 50:447, 1974.

147. Singh BN, Nademanee D, Baky S: Calcium antagonists: Uses in the treatment of cardiac arrhythmias. *Drugs* 25:125, 1983.

148. Hartel G, Hartikainen M: Comparison of verapamil and practolol in paroxysmal supraventricular tachycardia. *Eur J Cardiol* 4:87, 1976.

149. Mauritson DR, Winniford MD, Walker WS, et al: Oral verapamil for paroxysmal supraventricular tachycardia: A long term, double-blind, randomized trial. *Ann Intern Med* 96:409, 1982.

150. Spurrell RAJ, Krikler DM, Sowton GE: The effect of verapamil on the electrophysiological properties of the anomalous atrioventricular connections in Wolff-Parkinson-White syndrome. *Br Heart J* 36:256, 1974.

151. Matsuyama E, Konishi T, Okazaki H, et al: Effects of verapamil on accessory pathway properties and induction of circus movement tachycardia in patients with the Wolff-Parkinson-White syndrome. *J Cardiovasc Pharmacol* 3:11, 1981.

152. Shigenobu K, Schneider JA, Sperelakis N: Verapamil blockade of slow Na1 and Ca11 responses in myocardial cells. *J Pharmacol Exp Ther* 190:280, 1974.

153. Ruskin J: Catheter ablation for supraventricular tachycardia (editorial). *N Engl J Med* 324:1660, 1991.

154. Gotsman M, Lewis B, Bakst A, et al: Verapamil in life-threatening tachyarrhythmias. *S Afr Med J* 46:2017, 1972.

155. Lichtlen PR, Fisher LD, and the CAPE Study Group: Analysis of arrhythmias in the Circadian Anti-ischaemia Program in Europe (CAPE) Study. *Eur Heart J* 1(Suppl I):17, 1999.

156. Carrasco HA, Fuenmayor A, Barboza J, et al: Effect of verapamil on normal sino-atrial node dysfunction and on sick sinus syndrome. *Am Heart J* 96:760, 1978.

157. Cummings DM, Amadio P, Nelson L, Fitzgerald JM: The role of calcium channel blockers in the treatment of systemic hypertension. *Arch Intern Med* 151:250, 1991.

158. Frishman WH, Stroh JA, Greenberg SM, et al: Calcium-channel blockers in systemic hypertension. *Med Clin North Am* 72:449, 1988.

159. Halperin AK, Icenogel MV, Kapsner CO, et al: A comparison of the effects of nifedipine and verapamil on exercise performance in patients with mild to moderate hypertension. *Am J Hypertens* 6:1025, 1993.

160. Frishman WH, Zawada ET, Smith LK, et al: A comparative study of diltiazem and hydrochlorothiazide as initial medical therapy for mild to moderate hypertension. *Am J Cardiol* 59:615, 1987.

161. Materson BJ, Reda DJ, Cushman WC, et al: Single-drug therapy for hypertension in men: A comparison of six antihypertensive agents with placebo. *N Engl J Med* 328:914, 1993.

162. Frishman WH, Garofalo JL, Rothschild A, et al: Multicenter comparison of the nifedipine gastrointestinal system and long-acting propranolol in patients with mild to moderate systemic hypertension receiving diuretics: A preliminary experience. *Am J Med* 83:15, 1987.

163. Ferlinz J: Nifedipine in myocardial ischemia, systemic hypertension and other cardiovascular disorders. *Ann Intern Med* 105:714, 1986.

164. Johnson BF, Frishman WH, Brobyn R, et al: A randomized placebo controlled, double-blind comparison of amlodipine and atenolol in patients with essential hypertension. *Am J Hypertens* 5:727, 1992.

165. Charlap S, Kimmel B, Laifer L, et al: Twice daily nicardipine in the treatment of patients with mild to moderate hypertension. *J Clin Hypertens* 2:271, 1986.

166. Taylor SH, Frais MA, Lee P, et al: A study of the long-term efficacy and tolerability of oral nicardipine in hypertensive patients. *Br J Clin Pharmacol* 20(Suppl 1):139S, 1985.

167. Todd PA, Faulds D: Felodipine: A review of the pharmacology and therapeutic use of the extended-release formulation in cardiovascular disorders. *Drugs* 44:251, 1992.

168. Hamilton BP: Treatment of essential hypertension with PN 200-110 (isradipine). *Am J Cardiol* 59:141, 1987.

169. Frishman WH, Qureshi A: Calcium antagonists in elderly patients with systemic hypertension. In: Epstein M, ed. *Calcium Antagonists in Clinical Medicine*, 3rd ed. Philadelphia: Hanley and Belfus, 2002:489.

170. Staessen JA, Fagard R, Thijs L, et al: Randomized double-blind comparison of placebo and active treatment for older patients with isolated systolic hypertension. *Lancet* 350:757, 1997.

171. Forette F, Seux M-L, Staeseen JA, et al: Prevention of dementia in randomized double-blind, placebo-controlled systolic hypertension in Europe (SYST-EUR). *Lancet* 352:1347, 1998.

172. Staessen JA, Thijs L, Fagard RH, et al: Calcium channel blockade and cardiovascular prognosis in the European trial on Isolated Systolic Hypertension. *Hypertension* 32:410, 1998.

172a. The Sixth Report of the Joint National Committee on Detection, Evaluation and Treatment of High Blood Pressure (JNC-VI). *Arch Intern Med* 157:2413, 1997.

173. Wang JG, Staessen JA, Gong L, et al: Chinese trial on Isolated Systolic Hypertension in the Elderly. Systolic Hypertension in China (SYST-CHINA) Collaborative Group. *Arch Intern Med* 160:211, 2000.

174. Black HR, Elliott WJ, Weber MA, et al for the Stage I Systolic Hypertension (SISH) Study Group: One-year study of felodipine or placebo for stage 1 isolated systolic hypertension. *Hypertension* 38:1118, 2001.

174a. Grimm RH Jr., Black H, Rowen R, et al: Amlodipine versus chlorthalidone versus placebo in the treatment of stage I isolated systolic hypertension. *Am J Hypertens* 15:31, 2002.

174b. Dahlof B, Lindholm LH, Hansson L, et al: Morbidity and mortality in the Swedish Trial in Old Patients with Hypertension (STOP-Hypertension). *Lancet* 338:1281, 1991.

175. Hansson L, Lindholm LH, Ekbom I, et al: Randomized trial of old and new antihypertensive drugs in elderly patients: Cardiovascular mortality and morbidity in the Swedish Trial of Old Patients with Hypertension-2 Study. *Lancet* 354:1751, 1999.

176. Lindholm LH, Hansson L, Ekbon T, et al: Comparison of antihypertensive treatments in preventing cardiovascular events in elderly diabetic patients: Results from the Swedish Trial in Old Patients with Hypertension-2 (STOP Hypertension-2 Study Group). *J Hypertension* 18:1671, 2000.

177. Brown MJ, Palmer CR, Castaigne A, et al: Morbidity and mortality in patients randomized to double-blind treatment with long-acting calcium channel blocker or diuretic in the International Nifedipine GITS Study: Intervention as a Goal in Hypertension Treatment (INSIGHT). *Lancet* 356:366, 2000.

178. Hansson L, Hedner T, Lund-Johansen P, et al: Randomized trial of effects of calcium antagonists compared with diuretics and beta blockers on cardiovascular morbidity and mortality in hypertension: The Nordic Diltiazem (NORDIL) Study. *Lancet* 356:359, 2000.

179. Randomized double-blind comparison of a calcium antagonist and a diuretic in elderly hypertensives. National Intervention Cooperative Study in Elderly Hypertensives Study Group. *Hypertension* 34:1129, 1999.

180. Ogihara T, Practitioner's Trial on the Efficacy of Anitihypertensive Treatment in the Elderly Hypertensive (The PATE-Hypertension Study) in Japan. *Am J Hypertens* 13:461, 2000.

181. Chan P, Lin CN, Tomlinson B, et al: Additive effects of diltiazem and lisinopril in the treatment of elderly patients with mild to moderate hypertension. *Am J Hypertens* 10(7 Pt 1):743, 1997.

182. Gong L, Zhang W, Zhu Y, et al: Shanghai trial of nifedipine in the elderly (STONE). *J Hypertens* 14:1237, 1996.

183. Liu L, Wang JG, Gong L, et al: for the Systolic Hypertension in China (Syst-China) Collaborative Group: Comparison of active treatment and placebo for older Chinese patients with isolated systolic hypertension. *J Hypertens* 16:1823, 1998.

184. Hansson L, Zanchetti A, Carruthers SG, et al: Effects of intensive blood-pressure lowering and low-dose aspirin in patients with hypertension: Principal results from the Hypertension Optimal Treatment (HOT) randomized trial. *Lancet* 351:1755, 1998.

185. ALLHAT Officers and Coordinators: Major cardiovascular events in hypertensive patients randomized to doxazosin vs chlorthalidone. The Antihypertensive and Lipid-Lowering Treatment to Prevent Heart Attack Trial (ALLHAT). *JAMA* 283:1967, 2000.

186. Black HR, Elliott WJ, Neaton JD, et al: Rationale and design for the Controlled Onset Verapamil Investigation of Cardiovascular Endpoints (CONVINCE). *Control Clin Trials* 19:370, 1998.

187. Hachamovitch R, Strom JA, Sonnenblick EH, Frishman WH: Left ventricular hypertrophy in hypertension and the effects of antihypertensive drug therapy. *Curr Probl Cardiol* 13(6):371, 1988.

188. Frishman WH, Skolnick AE: Effects of calcium blockade on hypertension-induced left ventricular hypertrophy. *Circulation* 80(Suppl IV):151, 1989.

189. Buhler F, DeLeeuw PW, Doyle A, et al: Calcium metabolism and calcium-channel blockers for understanding and treating hypertension. *Am J Med* 77(6B):1, 1984.

190. Fioretto P, Frigato F, Velussi M, et al: Effects of angiotensin converting enzyme inhibitors and calcium antagonists on atrial natriuretic peptide release and action and on albumin excretion rate in hypertensive insulin-dependent diabetic patients. *Am J Hypertens* 5:837, 1992.

191. Zanetti-Elshater F, Pingitore R, Beretta-Piccoli C, et al: Calcium antagonists for treatment of diabetes-associated hypertension: Metabolic and renal effects of amlodipine. *Am J Hypertens* 7:36, 1994.

192. Frielingsdorf J, Seiler C, Kaufmann P, et al: Normalization of abnormal coronary vasomotion by calcium antagonists in patients with hypertension. *Circulation* 93:1380, 1996.

193. Sica DA: Combination calcium channel blocker therapy in the treatment of hypertension. *J Clin Hypertens* 3:322, 2001.

194. Frishman WH, Ram CVS, McMahon FG, et al: Comparison of amlodipine and benazepril monotherapy to combination therapy in patients with systemic hypertension: A randomized, double-blind, placebo-controlled, parallel group study. *J Clin Pharmacol* 35:1060, 1995.

195. Messerli F, Frishman WH, Elliott W, and the Trandolapril Study Group: Additive effects of verapamil and trandolapril in the treatment of hypertension. *J Hypertens* 11(3 Pt 1):322, 1998.

196. Haria M, Plosker GL, Markham A: Felodipine/metoprolol. A review of the fixed dose controlled release formulation in the management of essential hypertension. *Drugs* 59:141, 2000.

197. Zing W, Ferguson RK, Vlasses PH: Calcium antagonists in elderly and black hypertensive patients: Therapeutic controversies. *Arch Intern Med* 151:2154, 1991.

198. Kloner RA, Sowers JR, DiBona GF, et al for the Amlodipine Cardiovascular Community Trial Study Group: Sex- and age-related antihypertensive effects of amlodipine. *Am J Cardiol* 77:713, 1996.

199. Buhler FR, Hulthen UL, Kiowski W, et al: Greater anti-hypertensive efficacy of the calcium channel inhibitor verapamil in older and low renin patients. *Clin Sci* 63:439S, 1982.

200. Erne P, Bolli P, Bertel O, et al: Antihypertensive monotherapy with calcium antagonists relates to older age, liver pretreatment renin and higher blood pressure: Comparison of nifedipine and verapamil. *Hypertension* 5(Suppl II):97, 1983.

201. Brozena SC, Johnson MR, Ventura H, et al: Effectiveness and safety of diltiazem or lisinopril in treatment of hypertension after heart transplantation. *J Am Coll Cardiol* 27:1707, 1996.

202. Tuomilehto J, Rastenyte D, Birkenhager WH, et al: Effects of calcium-channel blockade in older patients with diabetes and systolic hypertension. Systolic Hypertension in Europe Trial Investigators. *N Engl J Med* 340:677, 1999.

203. Estacio RO, Jeffers BW, H iatt WR, et al: The effect of nisoldipine as compared with enalapril on cardiovascular outcomes in patients with non-insulin-dependent diabetes and hypertension. *N Engl J Med* 338:645, 1998.

204. Tatti P, Pahor M, Byington RP, et al: Outcome results of the Fosinopril Versus Amlodipine Cardiovascular Events Randomized Trial (FACET) in patients with hypertension and NIDDM. *Diabetes Care* 21:597, 1998.

204a. Opie LH, Schall R: Evidence-based evaluation of calcium channel blockers for hypertension. *J Am Coll Card* 39:315, 2002.

205. Pahor M, Psaty BM, Alderman MH, et al: Health outcomes associated with calcium antagonists compared with other first-line antihypertensive therapies: A meta-analysis of randomised controlled trials. *Lancet* 356:1949, 2000.

206. Massie BM: The safety of calcium-channel blockers. *Clin Cardiol* 21(Suppl II):II-12, 1998.

207. Abascal V, Larson MG, Evans JC, et al: Calcium antagonists and mortality risk in men and women with hypertension in the Framingham Heart Study. *Arch Intern Med* 158:1882, 1998.

208. Opie LH, Yusuf S, Kubler W: Current status of safety and efficacy of calcium channel blockers in cardiovascular diseases: A critical analysis based on 100 studies. *Prog Cardiovasc Dis* 43:171, 2000.

209. Psaty BM, Heckbert SR, Koepsell TD, et al: The risk of myocardial infarction associated with antihypertensive drug therapies. *JAMA* 274:620, 1995.

210. Pahor M, Guralnik JM, Corti C, et al: Long-term survival and use of antihypertensive medications in older persons. *J Am Geriatr Soc* 43:1191, 1995.

211. Furberg CD, Psaty BM: Calcium antagonists: Not appropriate as first-line antihypertensive agents. *Am J Hypertens* 9:122, 1996.

212. Yusuf S: Calcium antagonists in coronary artery disease and hypertension: time for reevaluation? *Circulation* 92:1079, 1995.

213. Furberg CD, Psaty BM: Should dihydropyridines be used as first-line drugs in the treatment of hypertension? The con side (commentary). *Arch Intern Med* 155:2157, 1995.

214. Epstein E: Calcium antagonists should continue to be used for first-line treatment of hypertension (commentary). *Arch Intern Med* 155:2150, 1995.

215. Epstein M: Calcium antagonists: Still appropriate as first-line antihypertensive agents. *Am J Hypertens* 9:110, 1996.

216. Laragh JH, Held C, Messerli F, et al: Calcium antagonists and cardiovascular prognosis: A homogeneous group? *Am J Hypertens* 9:99, 1996.

217. Braun S, Boyko V, Behar S, et al: Calcium antagonists and mortality in patients with coronary artery disease: A cohort study of 11,575 patients. *J Am Coll Cardiol* 28:7, 1996.

218. Messerli F: What happened to the calcium antagonist controversy? *J Am Coll Cardiol* 28:12, 1996.

219. Sica DA, Douglas JG: The African American Study of Kidney Disease and Hypertension (AASK): New findings. *J Clin Hypertens* 3:244, 2001.

220. Furberg CD, Psaty BM, Pahor M, Alderman MH: Clinical implications of recent findings from the Antihypertensive and Lipid-Lowering Treatment to Prevent Heart Attack Trial (ALLHAT) and other studies in hypertension. *Ann Intern Med* 135:1074, 2001.

221. Frishman WH, Weinberg P, Peled H, et al: Calcium-entry blockers for the treatment of severe hypertension and hypertensive emergencies. *Am J Med* 77(2B):35, 1984.

222. Beer N, Gallegos I, Cohen A, et al: Efficacy of sublingual nifedipine in the acute treatment of systemic hypertension. *Chest* 79:571, 1981.

223. Ellrodt AG, Ault M, Riedinger MS, et al: Efficacy of sublingual nifedipine in hypertensive emergencies. *Am J Med* 79(4A):19, 1985.

224. Grossman E, Messerli F, Grodzicki: Should a moratorium be placed on sublingual nifedipine capsules given for hypertensive emergencies and pseudoemergencies. *JAMA* 276:1332, 1996.

225. Wallin JD, Fletcher E, Ram CVS, et al: Intravenous nicardipine for the treatment of severe hypertension. *Arch Intern Med* 149(12):2662, 1989.

226. IV Nicardipine Study Group: Efficacy and safety of intravenous nicardipine in the control of postoperative hypertension. *Chest* 99:393, 1991.

227. Abdelwahab W, Frishman W, Landau A: Management of hypertensive urgencies and emergencies. *J Clin Pharmacol* 35:747, 1995.

228. Frishman WH, Teicher M: Antianginal drug therapy for silent myocardial ischemia. *Med Clin North Am* 72:185, 1988.

229. Deedwania PC, Carbajal EV: Silent myocardial ischemia: A clinical perspective. *Arch Intern Med* 151:2373, 1991.

230. White WB, Black HR, Weber MA, et al: Comparison of effects of controlled onset extended release verapamil at bedtime and nifedipine gastrointestinal therapeutic system on arising on early morning blood pressure, heart rate, and heart rate–blood pressure product. *Am J Card* 81:424, 1998.

231. Epstein SE, Quyyumi Aa, Bonow RO: Myocardial ischemia—silent or symptomatic. *N Engl J Med* 318:1038, 1988.

232. Ardissino D, Savonitto S, Egstrup K, et al: Transient myocardial ischemia during daily life in rest and exertional angina pectoris and comparison of effectiveness of metoprolol versus nifedipine. *Am J Cardiol* 67:946, 1991.

233. Stone PH, Gibson RS, Glasser SP, et al: Comparison of propranolol, diltiazem and nifedipine in the treatment of ambulatory ischemia in patients with stable angina. Differential effects on ambulatory ischemia, exercise performance, and anginal symptoms. *Circulation* 82:1962, 1990.

234. Chaitmam BR, Stone PH, Knatterud GL, et al: Impact of anti-ischemia therapy on 12-week rest electrocardiogram and exercise test outcomes. The ACIP Investigators. *J Am Coll Cardiol* 26:585, 1995.

235. Rogers WJ, Bourassa MG, Andrews TC, et al: Asymptomatic Cardiac Ischemia Pilot (ACIP) Study: Outcome at 1 year for patients with asymptomatic cardiac ischemia randomized to medical therapy or revascularization. *J Am Coll Cardiol* 26:594, 1995.

236. Pratt CM, McMahon RP, Goldstein S, et al: Comparison of subgroups assigned to medical regimens used to suppress cardiac ischemia [The Asymptomatic Cardiac Ischemia Pilot (ACIP) Study]. *Am J Cardiol* 77:1302, 1996.

237. Nayler WG: Cardioprotective effects of calcium ion antagonists in myocardial ischemia. *Clin Invest Med* 3:91, 1980.

238. Melin JA, Becker LC, Hutchins GM: Protective effect of early and late treatment with nifedipine during myocardial infarction in the conscious dog. *Circulation* 69:131, 1984.

239. Skolnick AE, Frishman WH: Calcium channel blockers in myocardial infarction. *Arch Intern Med* 149:1669, 1989.

240. Frishman WH, Furberg CD, Friedewald WT: β-Adrenergic blockade in survivors of acute myocardial infarction. *N Engl J Med* 310:830, 1984.

241. Crea F, Deanfield J, Crean P, et al: Effects of verapamil in preventing early postinfarction angina and reinfarction. *Am J Cardiol* 55:900, 1985.

242. Sirnes PA, Overskeid K, Pedersen TR, et al: Evolution of infarct size during the early use of nifedipine in patients with acute myocardial infarction: The Norwegian Nifedipine Multicenter Trial. *Circulation* 70:638, 1984.

243. Wilcox RG, Hampton JR, Banks DC, et al: Trial of early nifedipine in acute myocardial infarction: The TRENT Study. *BMJ* 293:1204, 1986.

244. The Danish Study Group on Verapamil in Myocardial Infarction: verapamil in acute myocardial infarction. *Eur Heart J* 5:516, 1984.

245. Gibson RS, Boden WE, Theroux P, et al: Diltiazem and reinfarction in patients with non-Q-wave-myocardial infarction. *N Engl J Med* 315:423,1986.

246. Muller JE, Morrison J, Stone PH, et al: Nifedipine therapy for patients with threatened and acute myocardial infarction: A randomized, double-blind, placebo-controlled comparison. *Circulation* 69:740, 1984.

247. Neufeld HN: Calcium antagonists in secondary prevention after acute myocardial infarction: The Secondary Prevention Reinfarction Nifedipine Trial (SPRINT). *Eur Heart J* 7(Suppl B):51, 1986.

248. DeGeest, Kesteloot H, Piessens J: Secondary prevention of ischemic heart disease: Along-term controlled lidoflazine study. *Acta Cardiol* 24(Suppl):7, 1979.

249. The Multicenter Diltiazem Postinfarction Trial Research Group: The effect of diltiazem on mortality and reinfarction after myocardial infarction. *N Engl J Med* 319(7):385, 1988.

250. The Danish Study on Verapamil in Myocardial Infarction: The effect of verapamil on mortality and major events after myocardial infarction: The Danish Verapamil Infarction Trial II (DAVIT II). *Am J Cardiol* 66:779, 1990.

251. Yusuf S, Held P, Furberg CD: Update of effects of calcium antagonists in myocardial infarction or angina in light of the second Danish Verapamil Infarction Trial (DAVIT II) and other recent studies. *Am J Cardiol* 67:1295, 1991.

252. Frishman WH, Skolnick AE: Secondary prevention post-infarction: The role of β-adrenergic blockers, calcium-channel blockers and aspirin. In: Gersh BJ, Rahimtoola SH, eds. *Acute Myocardial Infarction*, 2nd ed. New York: Chapman & Hall, 1997:766–796.

253. Rengo F, Carbonin P, Pahor M, et al: A controlled trial of verapamil in patients after acute myocardial infarction: Results of the Calcium Antagonist Reinfarction Italian Study (CRIS). *Am J Cardiol* 77:365, 1996.

254. Furberg CD, Psaty BM, Meyer JV: Nifedipine: Dose-related increase in mortality in patients with coronary heart disease. *Circulation* 92:1326, 1995.

255. Boden WE, van Gilst WH, Scheldewaert RG, et al for the Incomplete Infarction Trial of European Research Collaborators Evaluating Prognosis post-Thrombolysis (INTERCEPT): Diltiazem in acute myocardial infarction treated with thrombolytic agents: A randomised placebo-controlled trial. *Lancet* 355:1751, 2000.

256. Theroux P, Gregoire J, Chin C, et al: Intravenous diltiazem in acute myocardial infarction. Diltiazem as adjunctive therapy to activase (DATA) trial. *J Am Coll Cardiol* 32: 620, 1998.

257. Sleight P: Calcium antagonists during and after myocardial infarction. *Drugs* 51:216, 1996.

258. Gibson RS, Hansen JF, Messerli F, et al: Long-term effects of diltiazem and verapamil on mortality and cardiac events in non-Q-wave acute myocardial infarction without pulmonary congestion: Post hoc subset analysis of the Multicenter Diltiazem Postinfarction Trial and the Second Danish Verapamil Infarction Trial studies. *Am J Cardiol* 86:275, 2000.

259. Jollis JG, Simpson RJ Jr, Chowdhury MK, et al: Calcium channel blockers and mortality in elderly patients with myocardial infarction. *Arch Intern Med* 159:2341, 1999.

260. Pelliccia F, Cianfrocca C, Romeo F, et al: Hypertrophic cardiomyopathy: Long-term effects of propranolol versus verapamil in

preventing sudden death in low-risk patients. *Cardiovasc Drugs Ther* 4:1515, 1990.

261. Cohen LS, Braunwald E: Amelioration of angina pectoris in idiopathic hypertrophic subaortic stenosis with beta-adrenergic blockade. *Circulation* 35:847, 1967.

262. Seiler C, Hess OM, Schoenbeck M, et al: Long term follow up of medical versus surgical therapy for hypertrophic cardiomyopathy. A retrospective study. *J Am Coll Cardiol* 17:634, 1991.

263. Rosing DR, Bonow RO, Packer M, et al: Verapamil therapy for the management of hypertrophic cardiomyopathy. In: Packer M, Frishman WH, eds. *Calcium Channel Antagonists in Cardiovascular Disease.* Norwalk, CT: Appleton-Century-Crofts, 1984:313–342.

264. Udelson JE, Bonow RO, OGara PT, et al: Verapamil prevents silent myocardial perfusion abnormalities during exercise in asymptomatic patients with hypertrophic cardiomyopathy. *Circulation* 79:1052, 1989.

265. Kaitenbach M, Hopf R, Kober G, et al: Treatment of hypertrophic obstructive cardiomyopathy with verapamil. *Br Heart J* 42:35, 1979.

266. Rosing DR, Kent KM, Maron BJ, et al: Verapamil therapy—a new approach for the pharmacologic treatment of hypertrophic cardiomyopathy: II. Effects on exercise capacity and symptomatic status. *Circulation* 60:1208, 1979.

267. Bonow RO, Rosing DR, Bacharach SL, et al: Effects of verapamil on left ventricular systolic function and diastolic filling in patients with hypertrophic cardiomyopathy. *Circulation* 64:787, 1981.

268. Lorell BH, Paulus WJ, Grossman W, et al: Modification of abnormal left ventricular diastolic properties by nifedipine in patients with hypertrophic cardiomyopathy. *Circulation* 65:499, 1982.

269. Rosing DR, Cannon RO, Watson RM, et al: Comparison of verapamil and nifedipine effects on symptoms and exercise capacity in patients with hypertrophic cardiomyopathy. *Circulation* 66(Suppl II):II-24, 1982.

270. Betocchi S, Piscione F, Losi M-A, et al: Effects of diltiazem on left ventricular systolic and diastolic function in hypertrophic cardiomyopathy. *Am J Cardiol* 78:451, 1996.

271. Packer M: Calcium channel blockers in chronic heart failure. *Circulation* 82:2254, 1990.

272. Charlap S, Frishman WH: Calcium antagonists and heart failure. *Med Clin North Am* 73:339, 1989.

273. Elkayam U, Amin J, Mehra A, et al: A prospective, randomized, double-blind, crossover study to compare the efficacy and safety of chronic nifedipine therapy with that of isosorbide dinitrate and their combination in the treatment of chronic congestive heart failure. *Circulation* 82:1954, 1990.

274. Losardo AA, Klein NA, Beer N, et al: Beneficial effects of sublingual nifedipine in patients with ischemic heart disease and depressed left ventricular function. *Angiology* 33:811, 1982.

275. Klugmann S, Salvi A, Camerini F: Haemodynamic effects of nifedipine in heart failure. *Br Heart J* 43:440, 1980.

276. Polese A, Fiorentini C, Olivari MT, Guazzi M: Clinical use of a calcium antagonistic agent (nifedipine) in acute pulmonary edema. *Am J Med* 66:825, 1979.

277. Fifer MA, Colucci WS, Lorell BH, et al: Comparison of hemodynamic responses to nifedipine in heart failure: Comparison with nitroprusside. *J Am Coll Cardiol* 5:731, 1985.

278. Packer M, Lee WH, Medina N, et al: Prognostic importance of the immediate hemodynamic response to nifedipine in patients with severe left ventricular dysfunction. *J Am Coll Cardiol* 10:1303, 1987.

279. Elkayam U, Weber L, McKay C, et al: Spectrum of acute hemodynamic effects of nifedipine in severe congestive heart failure. *Am J Cardiol* 546:560, 1985.

280. Cleophas TJ, van Marum R: Meta-analysis of efficacy and safety of second-generation dihydropyridine calcium channel blockers in heart failure. *Am J Cardiol* 87:487, 2001.

281. Perna GP, Valle G, Cianfrone N, et al: Amlodipine in ischaemic left ventricular dysfunction with mild to moderate heart failure. *Clin Drug Invest* 16:289, 1998.

282. Kukin ML, Freudenberger RS, Mannino MM, et al: Short-term and long-term hemodynamic and clinical effects of metoprolol alone and combined with amlodipine in patients with chronic heart failure. *Am Heart J* 138:261, 1999.

283. Krombach RS, Clair MJ, Hendrick JW, et al: Amlodipine therapy in congestive heart failure: Hemodynamic and neurohormonal effects at rest and after treadmill exercise. *Am J Cardiol* 84:3L, 1999.

284. Udelson JE, DeAbate A, Berk M, et al for the Amlodipine Exercise Trial Investigators: Effects of amlodipine on exercise tolerance, quality of life, and left ventricular function in patients with heart failure from left ventricular systolic dysfunction. *Am Heart J* 139:503, 2000.

284a. Mital S, Loke KE, Slater JP, et al: Synergy of amlodipine and angiotensin converting enzyme inhibitors in regulating myocardial oxygen consumption in normal canine and failing human hearts. *Am J Cardiol* 83:92H, 1999.

285. Figulla HR, Gietzen F, Zeymer U, et al: Diltiazem improves cardiac function and exercise capacity in patients with idiopathic dilated cardiomyopathy. *Circulation* 94:346, 1996.

286. Boden WE, Ziesche S, Carson PE, et al for the V-HeFT III Investigators: Rationale and design of the Third Vasodilator-Heart Failure Trial (V-HeFT III): Felodipine as adjunctive therapy to enalapril and loop diuretics with or without digoxin in chronic congestive heart failure. *Am J Cardiol* 77:1078,1996.

286a. Smith RF, Germanson T, Judd D, et al: Plasma norepinephrine and atrial natriuretic peptide in heart failure: Influence of felodipine in the Third Vasodilator Heart Failure Trial. V-HeFT III Investigators. *J Card Fail* 6:97, 2000.

287. OConnor CM, Belkin RN, Carson PE, et al: Effect of amlodipine on mode of death in severe chronic heart failure: The PRAISE Trial. *Circulation* 92:676, 1996.

288. Packer M, O'Connor CM, Ghali JK, et al: Effect of amlodipine on morbidity and mortality in severe chronic heart failure. *N Engl J Med* 335:1107, 1996.

289. Levine TB, Bernink PJLM, Caspi A, et al: Effect of mibefradil, a T-type calcium channel blocker, on morbidity and mortality in moderate to severe congestive heart failure. The MACH-1 Study. *Circulation* 101:758, 2000.

290. Kostis JB, Wilson AC, Cosgrove NM, Lacy CR: Effect of calcium channel blockers on the incidence of myocardial infarction in patients with left ventricular dysfunction (abstr). *J Am Coll Cardiol* 27(Suppl A): 36B, 1996.

291. Scognamiglio R, Rahimtoola S, Fasoli G, et al: Nifedipine in symptomatic patients with severe aortic regurgitation and normal left ventricular function. *N Engl J Med* 331:689, 1994.

292. Muntinga HJ, van der Vring JAFM, Niemeyer MG, et al: Effect of mibefradil on left ventricular diastolic function in patients with congestive heart failure. *J Cardiovasc Pharmacol* 27:652, 1996.

293. Sotaro JF, Zaret BL, Schulman DS, et al: Usefulness of verapamil for congestive heart failure associated with abnormal left ventricular diastolic filling and normal left ventricular systolic performance. *Am J Cardiol* 66:981, 1990.

294. Nishikawa N, Masuyama T, Yamamoto K, et al: Long-term administration of amlodipine prevents decompensation to diastolic heart failure in hypertensive rats. *J Am Coll Cardio* 38:1539, 2001.

295. Sondergaard L, Aldershvile J, Hildebrandt P, et al: Vasodilatation with felodipine in chronic asymptomatic aortic regurgitation. *Am Heart J* 139:667, 2000.

296. Fein SA, Frishman WH: The pathophysiology and management of primary pulmonary hypertension. *Cardiol Clin* 5:563, 1987.

297. Loscalzo J: Endothelial dysfunction in pulmonary hypertension (editorial). *N Engl J Med* 327:117, 1992.

298. Rich S, Kaufman E, Levy PS: The effect of high doses of calcium channel blockers on survival in primary pulmonary hypertension. *N Engl J Med* 327:76, 1992.

299. Ricciardi MJ, Bossone E, Bach DS, et al: Echocardiographic predictors of an adverse response to a nifedipine trial in primary pulmonary hypertension. Diminished left ventricular size and leftward ventricular septal bowing. *Chest* 116:1218, 1999.

300. Packer M: Vasodilator therapy for primary pulmonary hypertension. Limitations and hazards. *Ann Intern Med* 103:258, 1985.

301. Neely CF, Stein R, Matot I, et al: Calcium blockage in pulmonary hypertension and hypoxic vasoconstriction. *New Horizons* 4:99, 1996.

302. Allen GS, Ahn HS, Preziosi TJ, et al: Cerebral arterial spasm—A controlled trial of nimodipine in patients with subarachnoid hemorrhage. *N Engl J Med* 308:619, 1983.

303. Towart R: The pathophysiology of cerebral vasospasm and pharmacological approaches to its management. *Acta Neurochir (Wien)* 62:253, 1982.

304. Bussey HI, Talbert RL: Promising uses of calcium-channel blocking agents. *Pharmacotherapy* 4:137, 1984.

305. Allen GS, Bahr AL: Cerebral arterial spasm: X. Reversal of acute and chronic spasm in dogs with orally administered nifedipine. *Neurosurgery* 4:43, 1979.

306. Allen GS, Banghart SB: Cerebral arterial spasm: IX. In vitro effects of nifedipine on serotonin, phenylephrine and potassium-induced contractions of canine basilar and femoral artery. *Neurosurgery* 4:37, 1979.

307. Tettenborn D, Dycka J: Prevention and treatment of delayed ischemic dysfunction in patients with aneurysmal subarachnoid hemorrhage. *Stroke* 21(Suppl IV):IV85, 1990.

308. Wadworth AN, McTavish D: Nimodipine: A review of its pharmacological properties, and therapeutic efficacy in cerebral disorders. *Drugs Aging* 2:262, 1992.

309. Feigin VL, Rinkel GJ, Algra A, et al: Calcium antagonists in patients with subarachnoid hemorrhage: A systematic review. *Neurology* 50:876, 1998.

310. Gelmers HJ, Gorter K, DeWeerdt CJ, Wiezer HJA: A controlled trial of nimodipine in acute ischemic stroke. *N Engl J Med* 318:203, 1988.

310a. Weinberger J, Terashita D: Drug therapy of neurovascular disease. *Heart Dis* 1:163, 1999.

311. Steen PA, Gisvold SE, Milde JH, et al: Nimodipine improves outcome when given after complete cerebral ischemia in primates. *Anesthesiology* 62:406, 1985.

312. Trust Study Group: Randomised, double-blind, placebo-controlled trial of nimodipine in acute stroke. *Lancet* 336:1205, 1990.

313. The American Nimodipine Study Group: Clinical trial of nimodipine in acute ischemic stroke. *Stroke* 23:3, 1992.

314. Edmeads J: Cerebral blood flow in migraine. *Headache* 17:148, 1977.

315. Meyer JS: Calcium channel blockers in the prophylactic treatment of vascular headache. *Ann Intern Med* 102:395, 1985.

316. Meyer JS, Hardenberg J: Clinical effectiveness of calcium entry blockers in prophylactic treatment of migraine and cluster headaches. *Headache* 23:266, 1983.

317. Leone M, D'Amico LM, Frediani F, et al: Verapamil in the prophylaxis of episodic cluster headache: A double-blind study versus placebo. *Neurology* 54:1382, 2000.

318. Solomon GD, Steele JG, Spaccavento LJ: Verapamil prophylaxis of migraine: A double-blind placebo-controlled study. *JAMA* 250:2500, 1983.

319. Meyer JS, Dowell R, Mathew NJ, et al: Clinical and hemodynamic effects during treatment of vascular headaches with verapamil. *Headache* 24:313, 1984.

320. Morich FJ, Bieber F, Lewis JM, et al: Nimodipine in the treatment of probable Alzheimers disease. *Clin Drug Invest* 11:185, 1996.

321. Burger SK, Saul RF, Selhorst JB, et al: Transient monocular blindness caused by vasospasm. *N Engl J Med* 325:870, 1991.

322. Winterkorn JMS, Kupersmith MJ, Wirtschafter JD, et al: Brief report: treatment of vasospastic amaurosis fugax with calcium-channel blockers. *N Engl J Med* 329:396, 1993.

323. Bartsch P, Maggiorini M, Ritter M, et al: Prevention of high altitude pulmonary edema by nifedipine. *N Engl J Med* 325:1284, 1991.

324. Maggiorini M, Mélot C, Pierre S, et al: High-altitude pulmonary edema is initially caused by an increase in capillary pressure. *Circulation* 103:2078, 2001.

325. Coffman JD: Raynaud's phenomenon. *Hypertension* 17:593, 1991.

326. Rodeheffer RJ, Rommer JA, Wigley F, et al: Controlled double-blind trial of nifedipine in the treatment of Raynaud's phenomenon. *N Engl J Med* 308:880, 1983.

327. Raynaud's Treatment Study Investigators: Comparison of sustained-release nifedipine and temperature biofeedback for treatment of primary Raynaud phenomenon: results from a randomized clinical trial with 1-year follow up. *Arch Intern Med* 160:1101, 2000.

328. Ram CV: Antiatherosclerotic and vasculoprotective actions of calcium antagonists. *Am J Cardiol* 66:29I, 1990.

329. Lichtlen PR, Hugenholtz PG, Rafflenbeul W, et al: Retardation of angiographic progression of coronary artery disease by nifedipine. *Lancet* 335:1109, 1990.

330. Waters D, Lesperance J, Francetich M, et al: A controlled clinical trial to assess the effect of a calcium channel blocker on the progression of coronary atherosclerosis. *Circulation* 82:1940, 1990.

331. Mancini GBJ: Antiatherosclerotic effects of calcium channel blockers. *Prog Cardiovasc Dis* 45:1, 2002.

332. Motro M, Shemesh J: Calcium channel blocker nifedipine slows down progression of coronary calcification in hypertensive patients compared with diuretics. *Hypertension* 37:1410, 2001.

333. Mason RP: Mechanisms of atherosclerotic plaque stabilization for a lipophilic calcium antagonist amlodipine. *Am J Cardiol* 88 (Suppl): 2M, 2001.

334. Pitt B, Byington RP, Furberg CD, et al: Effect of amlodipine on the progression of atherosclerosis and the occurrence of clinical events. *Circulation* 102:1503, 2000.

335. Schroeder JS, Gao S-Z, Alderman EL, et al: A preliminary study of diltiazem in the prevention of coronary artery disease in heart transplant recipients. *N Engl J Med* 328:164, 1993.

336. Borhani NO, Bond MG, Sowers JR, et al: The Multicenter Isradipine Diuretic Atherosclerosis Study: A study of the antiatherogenic properties of isradipine in hypertensive patients. *J Cardiovasc Pharmacol* 18(Suppl 3):515, 1991.

337. Borhani NO, Mercuri M, Borhani PA, et al: Final outcome results of the multicenter isradipine diuretic atherosclerosis study (MIDAS). *JAMA* 276:785, 1996.

338. Einecke D: ELSA studies progression of atherosclerosis: Calcium antagonist arrests the process more than a beta blocker. *MMW Fortschr Med* 143:6, 2001.

339. Schwartz ML, Rotmensch HH, Frishman WH, Vlasses P: Potential applications of calcium-channel antagonists in the management of noncardiac disorders. In: Packer M, Frishman WH, eds. *Calcium Channel Antagonists in Cardiovascular Disease.* Norwalk, CT: Appleton-Century-Crofts, 1984:371–382.

340. Cristakis GT, Fremes SE, Weisel RD, et al: Diltiazem cardioplegia: A balance of risk and benefit. *J Thorac Cardiovasc Surg* 91:647, 1986.

341. Seitelberger R, Zwolfer W, Huber S, et al: Nifedipine reduces the incidence of myocardial infarction and transient ischemia in patients undergoing coronary bypass grafting. *Circulation* 83:460, 1991.

342. Piessens J, Brzostek T, Stammen F, et al: Effect of intravenous diltiazem on myocardial ischemia during percutaneous transluminal coronary angioplasty. *Am J Cardiol* 64:1103, 1989.

343. Hillegass WB, Ohman EM, Leimberger JD, et al: A meta-analysis of randomized trials of calcium antagonists to reduce restenosis after coronary angioplasty. *Am J Cardiol* 23:835, 1994.

344. Bestehorn HP et al: VESPA abstract (Verapamil high dose early administration slow release for prevention of major cardiovascular events and restenosis after angioplasty). XXII Congress of the European Society of Cardiology, 2000.

345. Gaudino M, Glieca F, Luciani N, et al: Clinical and angiographic effects of chronic calcium channel blocker therapy continued beyond first postoperative year in patients with radial artery grafts. Results of a prospective randomized investigation. *Circulation* 104(Suppl I):I-64, 2001.

346. Factor SM, Minase T, Cho S, et al: Microvascular spasm in the cardiomyopathic Syrian hamster: A preventable cause of focal myocardial necrosis. *Circulation* 66:342, 1982.

347. Neumayer HH, Wagner K: Prevention of delayed graft function in cadaver kidney transplants by diltiazem: outcome of two prospective, randomized clinical trials. *J Cardiovasc Pharmacol* 10(Suppl):S170, 1987.

348. Wagner K, Albrecht S, Neumayer HH: Prevention of post-transplant acute tubular necrosis by the calcium antagonist diltiazem: A prospective randomized study. *Am J Nephrol* 7:287, 1987.

349. Palmer BF, Dawidson I, Sagalowsky A, et al: Improved outcome of cadaveric renal transplantation due to calcium channel blockers. *Transplantation* 52:640, 1991.

350. Schrier RW, Arnold PE, VanPutten VJ, et al: Cellular calcium in ischemic acute renal failure: Role of calcium entry blockers. *Kidney Int* 32:313, 1987.

351. Epstein M: Calcium antagonists and renal protection: Current status and future perspectives. *Arch Intern Med* 152:1573, 1992.

352. Terry RW: Nifedipine therapy in angina pectoris: Evaluation of safety and side effects. *Am Heart J* 104:681, 1982.

352a. Ellis JS, Seymour RA, Steele JG, et al: Prevalence of gingival overgrowth induced by calcium channel blockers: A community-based study. *J Periodontol* 70:63, 1999.

353. Vetrovec GW, Parker VE, Cole S, et al: Nifedipine gastrointestinal therapeutic system in stable angina pectoris: results of a multicenter open-label, crossover comparison with nifedipine. *Am J Med* 83(B):24, 1987.

353a. Ram C, Verkata S: Usefulness of lercanidipine, a new calcium antagonist, for systemic hypertension. *Am J Cardiol* 89:214, 2002.

354. Padrell MD, Navarro M, Faura CC, Horga JF: Verapamil-induced parkinsonism. *Am J Med* 99:436, 1995.

355. Pahor M, Gurainik JM, Furberg CD, et al: Risk of gastrointestinal haemorrhage with calcium antagonists in hypertensive persons over 67 years old. *Lancet* 347:1061, 1996.

356. Garcia Rodriguez LA, Cattaruzzi C, Grazia Troncon M, Agostinis L: Risk of hospitalization for upper gastrointestinal tract bleeding associated with ketorolac, other nonsteroidal anti-inflammatory drugs, calcium antagonists, and other antihypertensive drugs. *Arch Intern Med* 158:33, 1998.

357. Cohen HJ, Pieper CF, Hanlon JT, et al: Calcium channel blockers and cancer. *Am J Med* 108: 210, 2000.

358. Lindholm LH, Anderson H, Ekbom T, et al: Relation between drug treatment and cancer in hypertensives in the Swedish Trial in Old Patients with Hypertension 2: A 5-year, prospective, randomised, controlled trial. *Lancet* 358:539, 2001.

359. Mason RP: Calcium channel blockers, apoptosis and cancer: Is there a biologic relationship? *J Am Coll Cardiol* 34:1857, 1999.

360. Messerli FH, Grossman E: Do calcium antagonists increase the risk for malignancies (editorial comment)? *J Am Coll Cardiol* 31:809, 1998.

361. Vezina RM, Lesko SM, Rosenberg L, Shapiro S: Calcium channel blocker use and the risk of prostate cancer. *Am J Hypertens* 11:1420, 1998.

362. Sorensen HT, Olsen JH, Mellemkjaer L, et al: Cancer risk and mortality in users of calcium channel blockers. A cohort study. *Cancer* 89:165, 2000.

363. Funk-Brentano C, Coudray P, Planellas J, et al: Effects of bepridil and diltiazem on ventricular repolarization in angina pectoris. *Am J Cardiol* 66:812, 1990.

364. Kenny J: Treating overdose with calcium channel blockers. *BMJ* 308:992, 1994.

364a. Boyer EW, Shannon M: Treatment of calcium-channel blocker intoxication with insulin infusion (correspondence). *N Engl J Med* 344:1721, 2001.

365. Frishman WH, Klein NA, Charlap S, et al: Recognition and management of verapamil poisoning. In: Packer M, Frishman WH, eds. *Calcium Channel Antagonists in Cardiovascular Disease.* Norwalk, CT: Appleton-Century-Crofts, 1984:365–370.

366. Klein HO, Lang R, Weiss E, et al: The influence of verapamil on serum digoxin concentrations. *Circulation* 65:998, 1982.

367. Schwartz JB, Keefe D, Kates RE, et al: Acute and chronic pharmacodynamic interaction of verapamil and digoxin in atrial fibrillation. *Circulation* 65:1163, 1982.

368. Pedersen KE, Dorph-Pedersen A, Hvidt S, et al: Digoxin-verapamil interaction. *Clin Pharmacol Ther* 30:311, 1981.

369. Belz GG, Aust PE, Munkes R: Digoxin plasma concentrations and nifedipine. *Lancet* 1:844, 1981.

370. Mitchell LB, Jutzy KR, Lewis SJ, et al: Intracardiac electrophysiologic study of intravenous diltiazem and combined diltiazem-digoxin in patients. *Am Heart J* 103:57, 1982.

371. Dargie HJJ for the TIBET Study Group: Medical treatment of angina can favourably affect outcome (abstr). *Eur Heart J* 14(Suppl):304, 1993.

372. Saseen JJ, Carter BL, Brown TER, et al: Comparison of nifedipine alone and with diltiazem or verapamil in hypertension. *Hypertension* 28:109, 1996.

The Renin-Angiotensin Axis: Angiotensin-Converting Enzyme Inhibitors and Angiotensin-Receptor Blockers

Domenic A. Sica

Todd W.B. Gehr

William H. Frishman

Over the past two decades, the renin-angiotensin-aldosterone (RAA) axis has been increasingly viewed as an important effector system for hypertension, cardiovascular disease, and cardiorenal disease; thus, it has become an important target for pharmacologic intervention. Of those drugs known to interrupt the RAA axis, by far, the greatest treatment experience exists for angiotensin-converting enzyme (ACE) inhibitors.[1-3]

ACE inhibitors have earned an important place in medical therapy since captopril, the initial compound in this class, was released in 1981. This compound proved to be an extremely effective blood-pressure (BP)-lowering agent as demonstrated in a wide range of renin-dependent models of hypertension.[2] The ACE inhibitor field thereafter quickly mushroomed so that there are currently 10 ACE inhibitors available in the United States.[3,4] Losartan, the first angiotensin-receptor blocker (ARB), was released in 1995, and there currently are seven ARBs on the United States market. In addition to their vasodepressor properties, ACE inhibitors and, in sequence, ARBs were quickly recognized for their ability to slow progressive renal, cardiac, and/or vascular disease processes. Thus, it was a logical step in their development to seek additional indications in the areas of congestive heart failure (CHF), post-myocardial infarction (post-MI), and diabetic nephropathy (Tables 10-1 and 10-2). More recently, a therapeutic indication for the treatment of the high-risk vascular disease in patients without discernible left ventricular dysfunction has emerged for the ACE-inhibitor ramipril.[5] A full description of the tissue-protective properties of ACE inhibitors and ARBs exceeds the scope of this chapter. The reader is referred to a number of comprehensive thematic reviews on this topic.[2,6-15]

MECHANISM OF ACTION

An understanding of how ACE inhibitors and ARBs work requires an appreciation of how each class interacts with the RAA axis and how they differ from other compounds, such as beta-blockers, that diminish RAA axis activity. For example, ACE inhibitors alter RAA axis activity by decreasing plasma angiotensin-II production as do beta-blockers; beta-blockers decrease plasma renin activity (PRA), whereas ARBs curb angiotensin-II effect by blocking the type I angiotensin-receptor (AT_1-R).[16,17]

The locus of activity of ACE inhibitors within the RAA axis is at ACE. ACE is pluripotent in that it catalyzes both the conversion of angiotensin-I to angiotensin-II and facilitates the degradation of bradykinin and a range of other vasoactive peptides.[18]

Although ACE inhibitors effectively curb the genration of angiotensin-II from angiotensin-I, they do not prevent the generation of angiotensin-II by non-ACE–dependent pathways.[19] These alternate pathways depend on chymase and other tissue-based proteases to produce angiotensin-II,[20] a process, which to a large extent represents the dominant mode of angiotensin-II generation in myocardial and vascular tissue.[21,22] The long-term administration of ACE inhibitors is frequently marked by a gradual rise in angiotensin-II levels, termed *angiotensin escape,* presumably due to an upregulation in the productive capacity of these alternative pathways.[22-24] In this regard, another facet of angiotensin-II effect is of importance. Within the RAA axis a negative feedback loop exists wherein downstream components of this cascade act to suppress upstream activity; thus, by its presence, angiotensin-II operationally shuts this system down. When an ACE inhibitor is administered, by virtue of its temporarily diminishing angiotensin-II, there is a disinhibition of renin secretion from the juxtaglomerular apparatus.[25] As this controlling influence dissipates, the concentration of both PRA and angiotensin-I increase.[26] This increase in PRA and angiotensin-I levels thus emerge as potential sources of substrate for alternative pathway action and therein angiotensin-II escape. The rise in angiotensin-I, which accompanies ACE inhibition, seems to derive from an enhanced release of active renin rather than an accumulation of angiotensin-I[27] and is effectively blunted by β-adrenergic antagonism.[28]

Because ACE inhibitors reduce angiotensin-II levels transiently (day's → weeks)[19,23,24] other mechanisms for their BP-lowering effect need to be considered, particularly if the pattern of BP response to ACE inhibition is probed. When first administered, ACE inhibitors transiently reduce BP in parallel with the degree of RAA axis activation.[29] With long-term therapy, any relationship between the fall in BP and the pretreatment levels of angiotensin-II fades.[30] This latter observation makes renin profiling of little practical value in predicting the degree to which an ACE inhibitor will reduce BP in a particular patient[31]; instead, the BP response achieved shortly after beginning an ACE inhibitor appears to provide a better indication of any long-term response. This pattern of response and

TABLE 10-1. FDA-Approved Indications for ACE Inhibitors

Drug	HTN	CHF	Diabetic Nephropathy	High-Risk Patients Without Left-Ventricular Dysfunction
Captopril	•	• (post-MI)*	•	
Benazepril	•			
Enalapril	•	•†		
Fosinopril	•	•		
Lisinopril	•	• (post-MI)*		
Moexipril	•			
Perindopril	•			
Quinapril	•	•		
Ramipril	•	• (post-MI)		•
Trandolapril	•	• (post-MI)		

*Captopril and lisinopril are indicated for CHF treatment both post-myocardial infarction and as adjunctive therapy in general heart failure therapy.

†Enalapril is indicated for asymptomatic left-ventricular dysfunction.

limited predictive value of pretherapy PRA values is similar with the ARBs.[32]

The persistence of the antihypertensive effect of ACE inhibitors despite angiotensin-II escape, argues for an active BP reducing role of alternative vasodepressor systems, such as bradykinin, although most such studies with bradykinin have only evaluated the short-term BP contribution of its effect.[33,34] How ACE inhibitors interact with the kallikrein-kinin system, though, is a matter of considerable interest. ACE processes several vasoactive peptides other than angiotensin-II, one of which is bradykinin. Therefore, in theory, ACE inhibitor administration should elevate tissue and/or circulating bradykinin levels, although the reproducibility of such measurements has proven methodologically complex.[35–37] Bradykinin also appears to increase with ARB administration, although by a different mechanism. ARBs, although they block the AT_1 receptor, conversely lead to stimulation of the AT_2 receptor because their administration is followed by a reactive rise in angiotensin-II levels.[38] AT_2-receptor stimulation then appears to be associated with increased bradykinin, nitric oxide, and cyclic GMP (guanosine monophosphate) levels at least in renal interstitial fluid, although the significance of these changes is unclear.[39]

The rise in bradykinin, which accompanies ACE inhibitor administration, also stimulates the production of endothelium-derived relaxing factor and the release of prostacyclin (PGI_2), although the exact contribution of prostaglandins to the antihypertensive effect of ACE inhibitors is still unknown.[40,41] ARBs have been studied in a rather limited fashion relative to their having any effect on components of the prostaglandin axis.[42] Although circulating levels of prostaglandin E_2 (PGE_2) and PGI_2 metabolites are not significantly changed following ACE-inhibitor administration, it has been recognized for some time that nonsteroidal anti-inflammatory drugs (NSAIDs) blunt the BP-lowering effect of ACE inhibitors (see "Class and Agent-Specific Drug Interactions" later in this chapter).[43,44] Low-dose aspirin (100 mg/d or less) has no significant effect on ACE inhibitor or ARB-induced BP reduction.[45] Higher doses, generally above 236 mg/d, can occasionally blunt the antihypertensive response to ACE inhibitors.[46,47]

A percentage of ACE inhibitor and ARB effect is also considered to be due to their reducing activity in the sympathetic nervous system (SNS).[48] This is attributable to a change in both central and peripheral SNS activity as well as to an attenuation of sympathetically mediated vasoconstriction, although these have not been consistent findings.[49] ACE inhibitors are poorly differentiable as to their individual effect on the SNS, which may relate to differences amongst the various class members in tissue compartmentalization and/or penetration through the blood-brain barrier.[50] In the instance of ARBs there is little to distinguish one compound from the other in their central nervous system effects. Where differences are noted between the various compounds in this class confounding variables such as route of administration, dose amount, duration of dosing and a compound's ability to cross the blood-brain barrier have limited the generalizability of the findings.[51,52] Alternatively, there is emerging evidence to suggest a differential effect of the ARB eprosartan on reducing SNS activity; however, this still requires additional study.[53] ACE inhibitors and ARBs also do not alter circulatory reflexes and/or baroreceptor function; thus, they do

TABLE 10-2. FDA-Approved Indications for Angiotensin-Receptor Blockers

Drug	HTN	CHF	Diabetic Nephropathy	Post-myocardial Infarction*	High-Risk Patients Without Left-Ventricular Dysfunction*
Candesartan	•				
Eprosartan	•				
Irbesartan	•		•		
Losartan	•		•		
Olmesartan	•				
Telmisartan	•				
Valsartan	•	•			

*FDA-approved indications for ARB therapy in these disease states are anticipated in the near future.

not increase heart rate when BP is lowered.[54,55] This latter property explains why both of these drug classes are seldom accompanied by postural hypotension.

ACE inhibitors and ARBs also improve endothelial function, facilitate vascular remodeling, and favorably alter the viscoelastic properties of blood vessels.[56–58] These additional properties of both ACE inhibitors and ARBs may provide an explanation for the observation that the long-term BP reduction with these drug classes generally exceeds that observed in the short-term.[59] Finally, the heptapeptide angiotensin 1–7, which can be formed directly from angiotensin-I by at least three endopeptidases, is a bioactive component of the RAA axis that may offset the actions of angiotensin-II.[60–62] ACE hydrolyzes angiotensin 1–7 to inactive peptide fragments, a process, which is blocked by ACE inhibition. The counter-regulatory role of angiotensin 1–7 to the pressor and proliferative actions of angiotensin-II relates, in part, to its interaction with kinins.[62]

PHARMACOLOGY

ACE Inhibitors

The first orally active ACE inhibitor was the drug captopril, which was released in 1981. Captopril is a sulfhydryl-containing compound, with a rapid and not particularly prolonged duration of action. Subsequently, the more long-acting compound enalapril maleate became available. Enalapril is a prodrug requiring in vivo hepatic and intestinal wall esterolysis to yield the active diacid inhibitor enalaprilat. All ACE inhibitors are administered as prodrugs with the exception of lisinopril and captopril.[63] It was originally believed that the formation of the active diacid metabolite of an ACE inhibitor, such as enalapril, could be inhibited in the presence of hepatic impairment, such as in advanced CHF, but this has proven not to be the case.[64] The extent of absorption, the degree of hydrolysis, and the bioavailability of enalapril in CHF patients appear to be similar to those values observed in normal subjects with the exception of the rates of absorption and hydrolysis being slightly slower in CHF.[65]

ACE inhibitors are structurally heterogeneous. All ACE inhibitors reduce the activity of ACE but do so by the binding to ACE of different chemical side groups. The chemical structure of this ligand serves as a criterion for dividing the ACE inhibitors into three classes. For example, the active chemical side group or ACE ligand for captopril is a sulfhydryl moiety and for fosinopril it is a phosphinyl group; each of the remaining ACE inhibitors contains a

carboxyl group. The side group on an ACE inhibitor is one factor, which has been suggested as being responsible for differing pharmacologic responses amongst these compounds.[66] Thus, the sulfhydryl group on captopril is purported to act as a recyclable free-radical scavenger and for this reason, captopril has been suggested to differentially retard the process of atherogenesis and/or protect from myocardial infarction and diabetes;[67] however, this has not been clinically substantiated. In addition, captopril directly stimulates prostaglandin synthesis, whereas other ACE inhibitors accomplish this indirectly by increasing bradykinin activity.[68] Alternatively, the sulfhydryl side group found on captopril is believed to lead to a higher rate of skin rash—usually in the form of maculopapular rashes—and dysgeusia.[69] The presence of a phosphinyl group on fosinopril has been offered as the reason for its low incidence of cough[70,71] and its ability to improve diastolic dysfunction.[72,73] In the instance of the latter, the phosphinyl group may facilitate the myocardial penetration and/or retention of fosinopril and thereby improve myocardial energetics.[74]

Although ACE inhibitors can be distinguished by differences in absorption, protein binding, half-life, and metabolic disposition, they behave quite similarly, in how they lower BP (Table 10-3).[63,75,76] Rarely, beyond the issue of frequency of dosing, should these pharmacologic subtleties govern selection of an agent.[3,76] This being said, two pharmacologic considerations for the ACE inhibitors—route of systemic elimination and tissue-binding—have generated considerable recent debate and warrant specific discussion.[77,78]

Pharmacokinetics

There is no evidence for accumulation of the prodrugs ramipril, enalapril, fosinopril, trandolapril, or benazepril in chronic renal failure (CRF), which suggests that they undergo intact biliary clearance or that the metabolic conversion of these drugs to their active diacid is unaffected by renal failure.[80–85] These findings have been offered by some as evidence for a dual route of elimination for these compounds. Technically, this is true, but it is irrelevant to dosing of ACE inhibitors in CRF because these prodrug forms are marginally active. True dual-route-of-elimination ACE inhibitors are those whose active diacid is both hepatically and renally cleared. Only the active diacids of the ACE inhibitors fosinopril and trandolapril undergo any significant degree of hepatic clearance.[83,84] For all other ACE inhibitors, elimination is almost exclusively renal with varying degrees of filtration and tubular secretion occurring.[77] Tubular secretion as a mode of elimination for ACE inhibitors is compound

TABLE 10-3. Pharmacokinetic Parameters of ACE Inhibitors

Drug	Onset/Duration (hours)	Peak Hypotensive Effect (hours)	Protein* Binding (%)	Effect of Food on Absorption	Serum Half-Life	Elimination†
Benazepril	1/24	2–4	>95	None	10–11	Renal/some biliary
Captopril	0.25/dose-related	1–1.5	25–30	Reduced	<2	Renal, as disulfides
Enalapril	1/24	4–6	50	None	11	Renal
Fosinopril	1/24	2–6	95	None	11	Renal = hepatic
Lisinopril	1/24	6	10	None	13	Renal
Moexipril	1/24	4–6	50	Reduced	2–9	Renal/some biliary
Perindopril	1/24	3–7	10–20	Reduced	3–10	Renal
Quinapril	1/24	2	97	Reduced	2	Renal > hepatic
Ramipril	1–2/24	3–6	73	Reduced	13–17	Renal
Trandolapril	2–4/24	6–8	80–94	None	16–24	Renal > hepatic

*Protein binding may vary for the prodrug and the active diacid of an ACE inhibitor.

†The concept of renal elimination of an ACE inhibitor takes into account both prodrug elimination and that of the active diacid where such is applicable.

TABLE 10-4. Pharmacologic Properties of Various Angiotensin-Converting Enzyme Inhibitors in Plasma and Tissue

Tissue Potency[*]	ACE Inhibitor Potencies (mmol/L $\times 10^{-9}$, ID_{50})[†]	Enzymatic (IC_{50})[‡]	Inhibition	Radioligand (DD_{50})[†]	Displacement	Plasma Half-Life[#]	Relative Lipid Solubility[§]
High							
Quinaprilat	0.07		5.5×10^{-11}		4.5×10^{-11}	25	++
Benazeprilat	NA		1.3×10^{-9}		4.8×10^{-11}	11	+
Ramiprilat	0.08		1.9×10^{-9}		7.0×10^{-11}	>50	++
Perindoprilat	0.40	NA		NA		10	++
Lisinopril	NA		4.5×10^{-9}		1.7×10^{-10}	12	NA
Enalaprilat	1.00		4.5×10^{-9}		1.1×10^{-9}	11	+
Fosinoprilat	NA		1.6×10^{-8}		5.1×10^{-10}	11.5	+++
Low							
Captopril	15.00	NA		NA		2	+

NA = not available.

[*] Radioligand binding studies using the active drug moiety.[92–94]

[†] ID_{50} is the inhibitor concentration required to displace 50% of ^{125}I-531A bound to human plasma.[95]

[‡] Comparison of 50% inhibition of enzymatic activity (IC_{50}) with 50% displacement of ^{125}I-351A (DD_{50}) from human plasma ACE.[95]

[#] Values cited for quinaprilat and ramiprilat are for dissociation from tissue ACE; i.e., terminal half-life.[96]

[§] Lipid solubility based on log P logarithm of the octanol/water partition coefficient of the active drug moiety, except for captopril; + signs represent increased lipid solubility.[95]

Source: Adapted with permission from Dzau et al.[78]

specific and occurs via the organic anion secretory pathway.[86,87] This property of combined renal and hepatic elimination minimizes accumulation of these compounds in CRF, once dosing to steady state has occurred.[84,88,89] To date, a direct adverse effect from ACE-inhibitor accumulation has not been identified, although cough has been suggested but not proven to be an ACE-inhibitor concentration-dependent side-effect. It is probable, however, that the longer drug concentrations remain elevated—once a response occurs—the more likely BP will remain reduced. Thus, the major adverse consequence of drug accumulation may be that of prolonged hypotension and its organ-specific sequelae.[90]

Tissue Binding

The second controversial pharmacologic feature of the ACE inhibitors relates to the concept of tissue binding.[78,91] The physico-chemical differences amongst ACE inhibitors, including binding affinity, potency, lipophilicity, and depot effect, allow for the arbitrary classification of ACE inhibitors according to tissue-ACE affinity.[78,92–96] The degree of functional in vivo inhibition of tissue ACE produced by an ACE inhibitor parallels two compound properties: the inhibitor's binding affinity and the free-inhibitor concentration within the tissue under survey. The free-inhibitor concentration, in turn, represents the dynamic equilibrium state, which arises from the shuttling of ACE inhibitor to the tissue and its subsequent washout and return into the blood. Free-inhibitor tissue concentrations are driven by traditional pharmacologic variables, including dose frequency and amount, absolute bioavailability, plasma half-life, tissue penetration, and subsequent retention at the tissue level. Bioavailability and half-life in blood can easily be determined and are important in the initial choice of an ACE-inhibitor dose. When blood levels of an ACE inhibitor are high—typically in the first third to half of the dosing period—tissue retention of an ACE inhibitor is unlikely to significantly impact functional ACE inhibition. However, as ACE-inhibitor blood levels drop toward the end of the dosing period, two factors appear to be crucial in prolonging functional ACE inhibition: (a) inhibitor-binding affinity and (b) tissue retention, which will directly influence the concentration of the free inhibitor in tissue.

The rank order of potency for several ACE inhibitors has been determined by using competition analyses[92,93,97,98] and by direct binding of tritium-labeled ACE inhibitors to tissue-ACE (Table 10-4).[99] The potency is quinaprilat = benazeprilat > ramiprilat > perindoprilat > lisinopril > enalaprilat > fosinopril > captopril.[92–95] The process of tissue retention of ACE inhibitors has also been studied. Isolated organ bath studies examining the duration of ACE inhibition after the removal of ACE inhibitor from the external milieu shows that functional inhibition of ACE lasts well beyond (two to five times longer) the time predicted solely on the basis of inhibitor dissociation rates or binding affinity.[99] The rank order of tissue retention is quinaprilat > lisinoprilat > enalaprilat > captopril and reflects both the binding affinity and lipophilicity of these inhibitors.[78]

The question arises as to whether the degree of tissue-ACE inhibition may extend to differences in efficacy amongst various ACE inhibitors. This is a very different question than whether an ACE inhibitor displays tissue-protective effects independent of the degree to which it lowers BP, as suggested by the HOPE Study.[5] Clearly, a reduction in angiotensin-II and increased nitric oxide bioavailability may represent mechanisms by which ACE inhibitors confer vascular protection. Consequently, endothelial function may be regarded as a surrogate marker for vascular protection. The effects of ACE inhibitors on endothelium-dependent relaxation appear to differ among several reports and appear to be dependent on the agents used and the construct of the experimental design. It should be noted that consistent improvement in endothelial function is reported with those ACE inhibitors with higher tissue-ACE affinity, such as quinapril and ramipril. Despite the appealing nature of these relationships there have been few direct head-to-head trials between ACE inhibitors, which are highly tissue bound and those ACE inhibitors with more limited tissue binding. In situations where such comparisons have occurred, the results do not convincingly support the claim of overall superiority for lipophilic ACE inhibitors.[100,101]

Application of Pharmacologic Differences

Because in the treatment of hypertension there is very little that truly separates one ACE inhibitor from another, the cost of an ACE inhibitor has become a dominant issue.[102] Allowing pricing to be a major factor behind the selection of an ACE inhibitor ignores the fact that only a small number of ACE inhibitors have been studied specifically for their ability to protect end organs. *Class effect* is a phrase often invoked to legitimatize use of a less-costly ACE inhibitor when a higher priced agent in the class was the one specifically studied in a disease state, such as CHF or diabetic nephropathy.[5,103–105] The concept of class effect may be best suited for application to the use of ACE inhibitors in the treatment of hypertension. Therein, little appears to distinguish one ACE inhibitor from another. Alternatively, it is less certain as to what represents true dose equivalence amongst ACE inhibitors when they are being used to treat proteinuric renal disease or CHF. In the treatment of proteinuric renal disease, the dose-response relationship for an ACE inhibitor and proteinuria reduction is poorly explored, a situation made more complex by the observation that the antiproteinuric effects of ACE inhibitors are greater in patients the higher the baseline urine protein excretion.[106] Because there are very few hard end-point studies in nephropathic patients with ACE inhibitors, it would seem reasonable, at least for now, to use cost as a criterion for selection of an ACE inhibitor.

Alternatively, in the case of CHF, BP normalization and/or reduction in urine protein excretion are not specific treatment goals. Rather, dose titration is attempted to a presumed maximal tissue-effect dose because improvement in the morbidity and mortality of CHF with ACE inhibitors is dose-dependent, although the differences are relatively modest between different doses of a specific ACE inhibitor.[107–112] Thus, the success of an ACE inhibitor in CHF may derive from many neurohumoral and tissue-based changes, and not just from changes in angiotensin-II consequent to inhibition of ACE.[110] Because not all ACE inhibitors have been thoroughly studied in CHF, or for that matter are clinically approved for CHF use (Table 10-1), particularly relative to secondary neurohumoral response parameters, it is less likely that specific doses of different ACE inhibitors are truly interchangeable in the treatment of CHF.

Angiotensin-Receptor Blockers

The ARBs are a relatively new class of drugs employed in the treatment of hypertension. These agents work selectively at the AT_1-receptor subtype, the receptor that mediates all of the known physiologic effects of angiotensin-II that are believed to be relevant to cardiovascular and cardiorenal homeostasis. Similar to ACE inhibitors, the ARBs each have a unique pharmacologic profile.[113] The pharmacologic differentiation of the various ARBs is a topic of growing relevance in that the ability to reduce BP may differ amongst the individual drugs comprising this class.[114,115] Since the release of the first ARB losartan (Cozaar) in 1995, six other compounds have been developed and are now marketed in the United States. These compounds include candesartan (Atacand), eprosartan (Teveten), irbesartan (Avapro), olmesartan (Benicar), telmisartan (Mycardis), and valsartan (Diovan). These compounds are now commonly given together with hydrochlorothiazide (HCTZ) as fixed-dose combination antihypertensive products. Currently available information does not suggest that any specific pharmacologic differences exist for an ARB if it were to be administered alone or together with HCTZ in a fixed-dose combination product.[116]

TABLE 10-5. Bioavailability of the Angiotensin-Receptor Blockers

Drug	Bioavailability (%)	Food Effect
Candesartan cilexetil[117,118]	15	No
Eprosartan[119–122]	6–29	AUC ↓ ≈ 25%
Irbesartan[123,124]	60–80	No
Losartan[125,126]	33	AUC ↓ ≈ 10%
Olmesartan[127]	29	
Telmisartan[128,129]	42–58	AUC ↓ 6–24%
Valsartan[130,131]	25	AUC ↓ ≈ 50%

Pharmacokinetics

Bioavailability

The bioavailability of the individual ARBs is quite variable (Table 10-5).[117–131] Three of the ARBs are administered in a prodrug form—losartan, candesartan cilexetil, and olmesartan medoxomil—although technically speaking, losartan is an active compound, albeit one ultimately converted to its more potent E-3174 metabolite. The bioavailability of eprosartan is low ($\approx$13%), a phenomenon that is not due to high first-pass elimination.[120] Eprosartan absorption is to a degree saturable over the dose range of 100 to 800 mg, most likely due to the physicochemical properties of the drug.[122] Irbesartan demonstrates a bioavailability profile with an absorption range between 60% and 80% and is without a food effect.[123,124] Losartan has a moderate bioavailability ($\approx$33%), with 14% of an administered dose being transformed to the E-3174 metabolite.[125,126] Telmisartan appears to have a saturable first-pass effect for its absorption; thus, the higher the dose the greater the absolute bioavailability.[127,128] Unfortunately, the most pertinent absorption characteristic of individual AT_1-RAs, day-to-day variability in bioavailability, is not routinely reported.

Dose Proportionality

The concept of dose proportionality is one important to any consideration of dose escalation for an antihypertensive agent in order to obtain BP control. One pattern of dose proportionality is displayed by irbesartan. In this regard, the results of two double-blind, placebo-controlled studies involving 88 healthy subjects show irbesartan to display, linear, dose-related pharmacokinetics for its area-under-the-curve (AUC) with escalating doses over a dose range from 10 to 600 mg. The maximum plasma concentration (C_{max}) over this same dose range was related to the dose in a linear but less than dose-proportional manner. Increases in plasma AUC and C_{max} in subjects receiving 900 mg of irbesartan were smaller than predicted from dose proportionality.[132,133] Possible explanations for this phenomenon are that intestinal absorption is dose limited, perhaps due to saturation of a carrier system at high drug concentrations, or that the dissolution characteristics of a compound are dose-dependent.[134] In the instance of irbesartan, that the terminal half-life of irbesartan is unchanged with higher irbesartan doses suggests that the intestinal absorption of irbesartan may saturate with increasing doses but that its metabolism and excretion are not so dose limited. Each of these proposed mechanisms may explain the absence of dose proportionality at doses above 400 mg that is observed with the ARB eprosartan.[122] It should be noted that the absence of dose proportionality for various of the ARBs, at doses, which are rarely employed clinically, has little, if any, relevance to the use of these compounds in the treatment of hypertension.

Volume of Distribution

The ARBs typically have a volume of distribution (V_D), which approximates extracellular fluid (ECF) volume, in part, in relationship to the extensive protein binding of these compounds. For example, the V_D for losartan and its E-3174 metabolite, are 34 L and 12 L,[135,136] respectively, while the V_D for candesartan, olmesartan, valsartan, and eprosartan are $\approx$10 (0.13 L/kg body weight), 30 L, 17 L, and 13 L, respectively.[119,137–139] Alternatively, telmisartan and irbesartan have the highest V_D of any of the ARBs, with values of 500 and 53 to 93/L (data on file, Bristol-Myers Squibb), respectively. That telmisartan has a V_D that is so high likely relates to a loose binding relationship with its predominant protein carrier, albumin.[129] To date, the clinical significance of ARBs having a high V_D remains unclear. Moreover, the V_D of the ARBs in disease states, such as renal failure, is unreported. Parenthetically, it has been suggested though that the greater the V_D for an ARB, the more likely it is that extravascular AT_1-receptors can be accessed and, therefore, at least in theory, the more profound the vasodepressor response.

Protein Binding

The protein binding of the ARBs is typically well in excess of 90%.[129,140–143] The exception to this pharmacologic characteristic is the ARB irbesartan, which has the highest plasma free fraction (4 to 5%) (data on file, Bristol-Myers Squibb). In general, none of the ARBs binds to red blood cells in a pharmacokinetically significant fashion.[129] Furthermore, the extent of protein binding for the ARBs remains fairly constant over a wide concentration range. Typically, protein binding dictates the V_D for a compound and, in fact, irbesartan demonstrates a V_D somewhat higher than that of the other ARBs, with the exception of telmisartan.[129] The significance of high protein binding for any ARB remains to be determined.

Metabolism and Active Metabolite Generation

There are two ways to view metabolic conversion of an ARB. First, it may be a step required in order to produce an active metabolite; such is the case with losartan,[144–146] candesartan cilexitil,[147] and olmesartan medoxomil.[139] Alternatively, metabolic conversion may factor into the conversion of a compound to a physiologically inactive metabolite, as in the case of irbesartan.[132] Losartan, an active substrate molecule, is converted via the P450 isozyme system (2C9 and 3A4) to its more active metabolite, E-3174,[144–146] whereas candesartan cilexetil, a prodrug, is hydrolyzed to the active compound candesartan in the course of absorption from the gastrointestinal tract.[147]

The metabolic conversion of candesartan cilexetil, an ester prodrug, seems not to be impacted to any degree by either disease states, genetic variation in metabolism, or chronic dosing.[147] The metabolic conversion of losartan to E-3174 has also been evaluated. First, variants of CYP2C9 have been identified. The presence of certain of these variants decreases the conversion of losartan to its active E-3174 metabolite. To date, less than 1% of the population of patients exposed to therapy with losartan has this abnormal genetic profile for the metabolism of losartan. Thus, it is unlikely that a metabolic polymorphism for losartan breakdown will ever be found in sufficient numbers of patients to matter clinically.[146]

It has also been suggested that known inhibitors of the P450 system and, more specifically, inhibitors of the P450 2C9 and 3A4 isozymes, such as fluconazole[148] and ketoconazole,[149] might interfere with the conversion of losartan to its E-3174 metabolite.[150] In theory, such drugs might interfere with both the rate and the extent of metabolism of losartan to its active E-3174 metabolite. Consequently, BP control might then become more difficult to achieve and/or maintain if losartan-treated patients were simultaneously treated with such enzyme inhibitors. Although this hypothesis seemed attractive initially, the available data does not support it. Drug-drug interactions of this nature are difficult to predict in broad population bases; thus, if a losartan-treated patient is simultaneously treated with inhibitors of either the P450 2C9 and/or 3A4 isozymes, BP should be closely monitored.[148] A final consideration with losartan is its degree of interaction with grapefruit juice. Although not formally tested as to its influencing the BP-lowering effect of losartan, grapefruit juice given together with losartan will reduce its conversion to E3174 as well as activate P-glycoprotein, which, in sum significantly increases the $AUC_{losartan}/AUC_{E-3174}$ ratio.[151]

Telmisartan is exclusively metabolized by conjugation to glucuronic acid. This lack of cytochrome P450 (CYP)-dependent metabolism distinguishes telmisartan from other ARBs.[129] Irbesartan undergoes metabolism to several glucuronidated or oxidated metabolites via the P450 2C9 pathway with metabolism by the P450 3A4 pathway being negligible. The primary circulating metabolite is irbesartan glucuronide, which represents approximately 6% of circulating metabolites. These metabolites do not possess relevant pharmacologic activity.[152,153]

Route of Elimination

It is well recognized that the systemic clearance of a compound is dependent on the integrity of both renal and hepatic function. As a result, if renal and/or hepatic dysfunction exists in a patient, repeated dosing of an antihypertensive compound will inevitably lead to drug accumulation and the occasional need to dose adjust in order to lessen concentration-related side effects. The ARBs have been studied only recently as to their renal and/or hepatic handling (Table 10-6). All these drugs undergo a significant degree of hepatic elimination with the exception of olmesartan, candesartan, and the E-3174 metabolite of losartan, which are 40%, 60%, and 50% hepatically cleared, respectively.[127,154,155] Irbesartan and telmisartan undergo the greatest degree of hepatic elimination amongst the ARBs, with each having >95% of their systemic clearance to be hepatic.[156,157] Valsartan and eprosartan each undergo about 70% hepatic clearance.[158–160] On the surface, the mode of elimination for an ARB may seem like a trivial issue. In reality, it proves to be an important variable in the renally compromised patient and may, in fact, dictate various elements of the change in renal function that occasionally occurs in the renal failure patient. In those who develop acute renal failure upon receipt of a hepatically cleared ARB, the duration of any renal failure episode is tempered by the quick hepatic disposition of the compound, a process that does not occur when the compound in question is mainly renally cleared.[90]

TABLE 10-6. Mode of Elimination for ARBs

Drug	Renal	Hepatic
Candesartan[154]	60	40
Eprosartan[159,160]	30	70
Irbesartan[156]	1	99
Losartan[155]	10	90
E-3174[155]	50	50
Olmesartan[127]	40	60
Telmisartan[157]	1	99
Valsartan[158]	30	70

To date, very few studies have assessed the BP-lowering effect of ARBs in the renally compromised patient.[161–166] In the studies reported to date, the BP-lowering effect of these compounds is evident in the renal failure patient, and in certain instances, may be quite significant. Dose adjustment, or more so, cautious use, in CRF is advocated with some of the ARBs—such as valsartan and olmesartan—that are partially renally cleared. This is more so because of presumed heightened sensitivity to these compounds rather than any specific adverse effects. A final consideration with the ARBs is that they are not dialyzable.[167] Additional experience is needed with the ARBs before definitive statements can be made concerning their efficacy in the renal failure population and whether relevant drug accumulation occurs with those ARBs, which undergo significant renal clearance, as is the case with the E-3174 metabolite of losartan, candesartan, and olmesartan.

Receptor Binding and Half-Life

The half-life ($t_{1/2}$) of a compound is a pure pharmacokinetic term that often correlates poorly with the duration of effect of a compound. This has typically been the case with antihypertensive compounds, including both ACE inhibitors and the ARBs. The discrepancy between the pharmacokinetic and pharmacodynamic $t_{1/2}$ of a compound derives from the fact that the predominant site of drug action for many compounds is to be found somewhere other than the vascular compartment. Because of the inability to sample at these extravascular sites of action for many drugs, the more meaningful tissue-based $t_{1/2}$ cannot be determined. This is particularly the case for the ARBs, because AT_1-receptors are found in multiple locations outside the vascular compartment and blocking AT_1-receptors at these alternative locations may, in an as-of-yet undefined fashion, influence the manner in which BP is reduced.

With the above in mind, the pharmacokinetic $t_{1/2}$ of an ARB will roughly approximate its duration of effect. Several of the ARBs, such as candesartan, olmesartan, telmisartan, and irbesartan, are observed to be once-daily compounds in pharmacokinetic terms. The true impact of pharmacologic $t_{1/2}$ for these compounds probably lies more so in the fact that drug is available for a longer period of time and thereby binds to additional AT_1-receptors as they are formed during a dosing interval. This phenomenon becomes obvious if the pressor response to angiotensin-II is evaluated. For example, a 300-mg dose of irbesartan maintains almost 60% inhibition of the pressor response to angiotensin-II, 24 hours after the dose is administered.[58,59] This observation, although interpretable in several ways, suggests that drug half-life has a role in duration of response.[168,169] Such data at best provide guidelines for therapy because patient responses are typically highly individualized.

Application of Pharmacologic Differences/Receptor Affinity

Receptor affinity is just one of several factors that determine the action of an ARB. An ARB demonstrates *insurmountable* or *noncompetitive* blockade if incrementally higher concentrations of angiotensin-II cannot overcome receptor blockade. The terms *surmountable, competitive, insurmountable,* and *noncompetitive* are often used interchangeably and often in an inconsistent fashion.[170,171] Surmountable antagonism implies that receptor blockade can eventually be overcome if high enough concentrations of angiotensin-II are made available. *Surmountable* antagonists shift concentration-response curves parallel one to the other and rightward without diminishing the maximal response to an agonist. Losartan behaves

as a surmountable antagonist. In the case of *competitive* antagonism, mass action kinetics exists and agonists and antagonists individually compete for receptor binding. Eprosartan functions as a *competitive* antagonist. *Noncompetitive,* irreversible antagonism is a phenomenon of loss of receptor numbers occurring by a process of chemical modification.

Insurmountable antagonism mimics *noncompetitive* antagonism. *Insurmountable* antagonists bind to their receptor in a semi-irreversible fashion, which differs from the permanent binding that occurs with *noncompetitive* antagonists. An *insurmountable* antagonist releases from its receptor slowly; thus, its drug-receptor dissociation constant can be quite prolonged. *Insurmountable* antagonists elicit a parallel shift of the agonist concentration-response curves with a depression in the maximal agonist response that is not overcome by increasing concentrations of the agonist. Valsartan, irbesartan, telmisartan, and the E-3174 metabolite of losartan exhibit this form of antagonism.

Insurmountable antagonists can also elicit nonparallel shifts of the agonist concentration-response curves, again depressing the maximal response to the agonist, a process that still is not overcome by increasing concentrations of the agonist. Candesartan demonstrates this form of *insurmountable* antagonism.[172–174] To date, the specific mode of receptor occupancy and/or differential pharmacokinetic features of an ARB have not been clearly linked with the varying BP responses to these drugs; thus, the actual basis for the superior efficacy of drugs, such as candesartan and irbesartan, as compared with losartan in terms of reduction in BP and maintenance of antihypertensive efficacy between doses, is not clear.[175] Instead, compound-specific differences in angiotensin-II receptor blockade, a surrogate for the BP-lowering response of these drugs, can be explained by differences in dosing, as was recently shown, wherein the effects of 160-mg or 320-mg doses of valsartan hardly differed from those obtained with recommended doses of irbesartan and candesartan.[176]

HEMODYNAMIC EFFECTS

A number of well-described hemodynamic effects occur with the administration of an ACE inhibitor (Table 10-7).[3] Although not comprehensively examined in a head-to-head fashion with ACE inhibitors, ARBs seem to exhibit quite similar hemodynamic profiles with the occasional difference, which may be study-design dependent.[177] The underlying disease being treated frequently dictates the magnitude change in many of these hemodynamic parameters. This is particularly evident in the treatment of CHF and/or renal failure, wherein hemodynamic responses may be exaggerated and linked to the degree to which BP drops. In addition, many of these hemodynamic changes are accentuated in the presence of an activated RAA axis, as may occur with diuretic therapy and/or a low-salt diet. The latter is a well-established risk factor for the occurrence of *first-dose hypotension* with an ACE inhibitor and/or an ARB.[178]

In the treatment of hypertension the observed reduction in BP with an ACE inhibitor or an ARB is not accompanied by either a decrease in cardiac output or an increase in heart rate.[17,54,179] Occasionally, cardiac output increases with ACE inhibitor therapy, particularly if cardiac output is reduced before therapy has begun.[180] The fall in peripheral vascular resistance that accompanies ACE inhibitor therapy is occasionally accompanied by a decrease

TABLE 10-7. Predominant Hemodynamic Effects of ACE Inhibitors and ARBs

Hemodynamic Parameter	Effect	Clinical Significance
Cardiovascular		
Total peripheral resistance	Decreased	
Mean arterial pressure	Decreased	
Cardiac output	Increased or no change	These parameters contribute to a
Stroke volume	Increased	general decrease in systemic
Preload and afterload	Decreased	blood pressure
Pulmonary artery pressure	Decreased	
Right atrial pressure	Decreased	
Diastolic dysfunction	*Improved*	
Renal		
Renal blood flow	Usually increased	Contributes to the renoprotective
Glomerular filtration rate	Variable, usually unchanged but may ↓ in renal failure	effect of these agents
Efferent arteriolar resistance	*Decreased*	
Filtration fraction	*Decreased*	
Peripheral Nervous System		
Biosynthesis of noradrenaline	Decreased	Enhances blood pressure-lowering
Reuptake of adrenaline	Inhibited	effect and resets baroreceptor
Circulating catecholamines	Decreased	function

in cardiac filling pressures.[54] Angiotensin-II can actively modulate both coronary vascular tone and blood flow, particularly if the RAA axis is activated. In turn, treatment with an ACE inhibitor can correct angiotensin-II–mediated reductions in coronary blood flow.[181] Several small trials, which have typically been of short duration, have assessed the effects of ACE inhibitors on severity of angina and/or on objective measures of myocardial ischemia, and have generated conflicting results.[182,183]

In addition, ACE inhibitors lower BP without diminishing cerebral blood flow.[184] This phenomenon is believed to represent a favorable effect of ACE inhibition on cerebral autoregulatory ability and is potentially of relevance to the treatment of hypertension in the elderly.[185] Furthermore, ACE inhibitors decrease capacitance vessel tone, which may explain why ACE inhibitors can alleviate the peripheral edema associated with calcium-channel blocker (CCB) therapy.[186,186a] ACE inhibitors do not limit the peak heart-rate response to exercise, although they do effectively reduce the peak BP response.[187] The addition of a diuretic to an ACE inhibitor does not alter the hemodynamic profile of ACE inhibition except in the instance of exercise, in which case, the exercise-related increase in cardiac output may be blunted.[188]

ACE inhibitors and ARBs routinely increase effective renal plasma flow (ERPF) while maintaining glomerular filtration rate (GFR). The rise in ERPF evoked by these two drug classes is characterized by a preferential vasodilatation of the post-glomerular or efferent arteriolar vascular bed.[8,177,189] The functional consequence of these renal hemodynamic changes is a drop in the filtration fraction (GFR/ERPF), a well-accepted marker for a reduction in angiotensin-II effect on the kidney. When glomerular filtration is heavily reliant on efferent arteriolar tone, as in CHF, dehydration, and/or renal artery stenosis, and an ACE inhibitor or an ARB is administered, the GFR may suddenly and precipitously fall.[90,190]

BLOOD PRESSURE-LOWERING EFFECT

Diuretics and beta-blockers are commonly employed as first-step therapy for hypertension, although ACE inhibitors and, more

recently, ARBs are increasingly viewed as a suitable first-step alternative.[191–193] The enthusiasm for the use of ACE inhibitors is not purely a matter of efficacy because they have a pattern of efficacy comparable to (and no better than) most other drug classes, with response rates from 40 to 70% in Stage I or Stage II hypertension.[194] A similar range of response rates is reported with ARBs. In head-to-head BP trials comparing ACE inhibitors and ARBs, there appears to be scant difference between the two drug classes.[195] Clinical trial results, obviously, do not reflect conditions in actual practice where the favorable side-effect profile of ACE inhibitors and ARBs and their highly touted end-organ protection features seem to dominate the thinking of many practitioners. In this regard, ACE inhibitors are extensively used because they are well tolerated and drugs that patients will continue to take over a long period.[196] The same can be said for ARBs, a drug class with a tolerability profile, which is superior to that of the ACE inhibitors.[197]

The enthusiasm for these two drug classes must be put in proper perspective because in uncomplicated nondiabetic hypertensive patients a number of drug classes given at low doses can prove effective and well tolerated at a fraction of the cost of ACE inhibitors and ARBs. Alternatively, increasing evidence supports the preferential use of ACE inhibitors and, more recently, ARBs in the diabetic and/or at risk cardiac/renal patient with either established atherosclerotic disease or proteinuria,[5,198–200] and offers a positive view of these drugs that is not available from prior comparator trials with ACE inhibitors.[201,202] For many of these at-risk cardiac/renal patients the recommendations for ACE inhibitor use are not based on the BP-lowering ability of these drugs, but rather on proposed tissue-based anti-inflammatory and antiproliferative effects, which are probably class and not agent-specific.[5,200]

There are very few predictors of the BP response to ACE inhibitors or ARBs. When hypertension is accompanied by significant activation of the RAA axis, such as in renal artery stenosis, the response to an ACE inhibitor or an ARB can be immediate and profound.[203,204] In most other cases, there is a limited relationship between the pre- and/or posttreatment PRA value, which is used as a marker of RAA axis activity, and the vasodepressor response to an ACE inhibitor or an ARB. Certain patient types demonstrate lower

TABLE 10-8. ACE Inhibitors: Dosage Strengths and Treatment Guidelines

Drug	Trade Name	Usual Total Dose and/or Range: *Hypertension* (Frequency per Day)	Usual Total Dose and/or Range: *Heart Failure* (Frequency per Day)	Comment	Fixed-Dose Combination*
Benazepril	Lotensin	20–40(1)	Not FDA approved for heart failure		Lotensin HCT, Lotrel
Captopril	Capoten	12.5–100 (2–3)	18.75–150 (3)	Generically available	Capozide†
Enalapril	Vasotec	5–40 (1–2)	5–40 (2)	Generic and intravenous	Vaseretic
Fosinopril	Monopril	10–40 (1)	10–40 (1)	Renal and hepatic elimination	Monopril-HCT
Lisinopril	Prinivil, Zestril	2.5–40 (1)	5–20 (1)	Generically available	Prinizide, Zestoretic
Moexipril	Univasc	7.5–30 (1)	Not FDA approved for heart failure		Uniretic
Perindopril	Aceon	2–16 (1)	Not FDA approved for heart failure		
Quinapril	Accupril	5–80 (1)	10–40 (1–2)		Accuretic
Ramipril	Altace	2.5–20 (1)	10 (2)	Indicated in high-risk vascular patients	
Trandolapril	Mavik	1–8 (1)	1–4 (1)	Renal and hepatic elimination	Tarka

*Fixed-dose combinations in this class typically contain a thiazide-like diuretic or a calcium-channel blocker.

†Capozide is indicated for first-step treatment of hypertension.

response rates to ACE inhibitor and ARB monotherapy including low-renin, salt-sensitive individuals such as the diabetic, African American or elderly hypertensive.[4,205] The low-renin state, characteristic of the elderly hypertensive, differs from other low-renin forms of hypertension in that it develops not as a response to volume expansion, but rather because of senescence-related changes in the activity of the axis.[206] The elderly generally respond well to ACE inhibitors at conventional doses,[185] although senescence-related renal failure, which slows the elimination of these drugs, complicates interpretation of dose-specific treatment successes. The elderly hypertensive, with systolic-predominant hypertension, also responds well to ARBs.[207] African American hypertensives, who as a group tend to have reduced activity in the RAA axis, are perceived as being poorly responsive to ACE inhibitor monotherapy when compared to whites[208] yet, in many instances, if careful dose titration occurs, BP will eventually be reduced with either monotherapy[209] or an appropriately constructed multidrug regimen based on ACE-inhibitor therapy.[210] This response pattern suggests that eliminating even small amounts of activity in the RAA axis is important to BP control.

All 10 ACE inhibitors are currently FDA-approved for the treatment of hypertension. The Joint National Committee (JNC) on the Detection, Evaluation, and Treatment of High Blood Pressure and the World Health Organization/International Society of Hypertension now recognize ACE inhibitors as an option for first-line therapy in patients with essential hypertension, especially in those with diabetes who also have renal disease/proteinuria and in patients with CHF.[1,211] The advisory position for ACE inhibitor use is currently in a state of flux and should become clearer when the results of the Antihypertensive and Lipid Lowering Treatment to Prevent Heart Attack Trial (ALLHAT) become available in late 2002. Therein, lisinopril is being compared to chlorthalidone in a large trial being conducted in older hypertensives with one or more established cardiovascular-renal (CVR) risk factors. Considerable dosing flexibility exists with the available ACE inhibitors. Enalaprilat is the sole ACE inhibitor available in an intravenous form (Table 10-8).[3] The dosing frequency for ACE inhibitors is somewhat arbitrary and

should consider the fact that these drugs may begin to lose their effect at the end of the dosing interval necessitating a second dose. Likewise, in the treatment of CHF, ACE inhibitors indicated for once daily dosing might require split dosing if BP drops excessively with an administered dose.

Results from a number of head-to-head trials support the comparable antihypertensive efficacy and tolerability of the various ACE inhibitors. However, there are differences amongst the ACE inhibitors as to the time to onset of effect and/or the time to maximum BP reduction, which may relate to the absorption characteristics of the various compounds. These differences, however, do not translate into different response rates *if* comparable doses of the individual ACE inhibitors are given. Typical confounding variables, which confuse the interpretation of the findings in BP studies with ACE inhibitors, have included differences in study design/methodology, as well as dose frequency and/or amount. ACE inhibitors labeled as "once-daily," vary in their ability to reduce BP for a full 24 hours, as defined by a trough:peak ratio >50%.[212] Unfortunately, the trough:peak ratio, as an index of duration of BP control, is oftentimes prone to misrepresent the true BP reduction seen with a compound.[213] As stated previously, dosing instructions for many of these compounds include the proviso to administer a second-daily dose if the antihypertensive effect has dissipated by the end of the dosing interval.

The question is often raised as to what to do if an ACE inhibitor fails to normalize BP. One approach is simply to raise the dose; however, the dose-response curve for ACE inhibitors, like most antihypertensive agents, is fairly steep at the beginning doses, and thereafter shallow to flat.[214] Responders to ACE inhibitors typically do so at doses well below those necessary for prolonged 24-hour suppression of ACE. In addition, the maximal vasodepressor response to an ACE inhibitor does not occur until several weeks after therapy is begun and may involve factors, such as vascular remodeling, above and beyond inhibition of ACE.[58] Thus, only with complete failure to respond to an ACE inhibitor should an alternative drug class be substituted. If a partial response has occurred, then therapy with an ACE inhibitor can be continued in anticipation of an

TABLE 10-9. Angiotensin-Receptor Blockers: Dosage Strengths and Treatment Guidelines

Drug	Trade Name	Usual Dosage, (Frequency per Day)	Comment	Fixed-Dose Combinations
Candesartan	Atacand	2–32 (1)		Atacand-HCT
Eprosartan	Teveten	400–800 (1)		
Irbesartan	Avapro	75–300 (1)	Indicated in diabetic nephropathy	Avalide
Losartan	Cozaar	25–100 (1)	Indicated in diabetic nephropathy; uricosuric	Hyzaar
Olmesartan	Benicar	10–40 (1)		
Telmesartan	Micardis	20–80 (1)		Micardis-HCT
Valsartan	Diovan	80–320 (1)	Indicated in congestive heart failure	Diovan-HCT

additional drop in BP over the next several weeks. Alternatively, an additional compound such as a diuretic, CCB, or peripheral alpha-blocker can be combined with an ACE inhibitor to effect better BP control (see Chap. 21).

Virtually all of the previous comments directed to the pharmacotherapeutic response to ACE inhibitors apply to the ARB class of drugs (Table 10-9). This includes considerations of predictors of response, onset and duration of response, the structure of their dose-response curves, and their capacity to have a late onset additional BP response. A number of head-to-head studies have been conducted between different ARBs.[59,215–218] The results of these comparisons suggest that candesartan cilexetil, irbesartan, and olmesartan may be more effective than the prototype ARB, losartan.[59,215–218] Moreover, studies mimicking the common event of a missed or delayed dose of antihypertensive medication, show that the antihypertensive effect of candesartan cilexetil extends well beyond the 24-hour dosing interval, while the effect of losartan declines rapidly over this period.[216,219]

Few studies have allowed the direct comparison of more than two ARBs.[220] Exceptions to this include a meta-analysis of randomized controlled trials by Conlin et al[221] and a crossover study by Fogari et al.[222] Both of these studies compared the efficacy of losartan, valsartan, irbesartan, and candesartan at low doses (50, 80, 150, and 8 mg, respectively) and after titration to double these doses. This meta-analysis revealed no differences among these drugs in their ability to reduce BP, either at the starting dose or after forced or elective titration.[221] In the crossover study, valsartan and irbesartan reduced BP more effectively than losartan when the drugs were used at their respective starting doses, although the difference was not maintained following elective dose titration.[222] In attempting to evaluate real or perceived differences amongst the ARBs while a meta-analysis can be useful in determining dose-response relationships for individual drugs, randomized, prospective, double-blind, head-to-head comparative studies remain the most accurate way to compare efficacy between drugs and would seem to favor several of the more recent additions to the ARB class over losartan.[223] Recently the FDA allowed an additional labeling claim for candesartan as being superior to losartan in its antihypertensive efficacy.

ACE INHIBITORS AND ARBS IN COMBINATION WITH OTHER AGENTS

To date, there appears to be little difference in the BP-lowering effect between ACE inhibitors and ARBs given in combination with other drug classes including diuretics and CCBs. Because of the paucity of published information for ARBs given in combination with other antihypertensive medication classes—with the exception of diuretic therapy—this section emphasizes the available combination therapies with ACE inhibitors. The BP-lowering effect of an ACE inhibitor is enhanced with the simultaneous administration of a diuretic, particularly in the African American hypertensive.[224,225] This pattern of response has spurred the development of a number of fixed-dose combination products, comprised of an ACE inhibitor and low to moderate doses of thiazide-type diuretics.[226] The rationale for combining these two drug classes derives from the observation that the sodium depletion produced by a diuretic increases activity in the RAA axis. Consequently, BP shifts to an angiotensin-II dependent mode, which is the optimal circumstance for an ACE inhibitor to reduce BP. Even very-low-dose diuretic therapy, such as 12.5-mg of HCTZ, can evoke this synergistic response, suggesting that even subtle alterations in sodium balance are sufficient to bolster the effect of an ACE inhibitor[225] (see Chaps. 11 and 21). Noteworthy is the observation that the addition of a diuretic to either an ACE inhibitor or an ARB eliminates the racial disparity in response to both ACE inhibitors and ARBs.[205,227]

ACE inhibitors have been given together with beta-blockers. The rationale behind this combination is that the beta-blocker will presumably abort the rise in PRA induced by an ACE inhibitor.[226,228] It was presumed that by preventing this hyperreninemic response that the ACE inhibitor response might be more robust. Although this hypothesis originally seemed attractive, in practice only a modest additional vasodepressor response occurs when these two drug classes are combined.[229] When BP substantively falls after addition of a beta-blocker to an ACE inhibitor, it is generally because pulse rate has been reduced in a patient whose BP is pulse rate dependent. Alternatively, the addition of a peripheral α-antagonist, such as doxazosin, to an ACE inhibitor can be followed by a significant additional BP response.[230] The mechanism behind this additive response remains to be more fully elucidated.[231] Finally, the BP-lowering effect of an ACE inhibitor is considerably enhanced by the coadministration of a CCB.[186,226,232,233]

This additive response occurs whether the CCB being given is a dihydropyridine (e.g., felodipine or amlodipine)[186,232] or a nondihydropyridine, such as verapamil.[233] The potency of this combination has provided the practical basis for the development of a number of fixed-dose combination products comprised of an ACE inhibitor and a CCB.[226] Adding an ACE inhibitor to a CCB is also useful in that the ACE inhibitor component of the combination attenuates the peripheral edema that accompanies CCB therapy.[186a,234]

The efficacy of both ACE inhibitors and ARBs as antihypertensive agents is well-documented. Quite logically, this has led to the belief that in combination these two drug classes may reduce BP better than if either were to be given alone. In contradistinction to the wealth of information on monotherapy with these drugs, there is strikingly little information about the efficacy of combined ACE inhibitor and ARB therapy.[235–240] Moreover, the trials currently published are not generalizable because in many instances, they involve a small number of patients and employ study designs with inherent limitations. For example, in one clinical trial, 20 patients received monotherapy with benazepril for 6 weeks. If average awake ambulatory diastolic BPs remained >85 mm Hg, subjects were randomized to either valsartan 80 mg/d or matching placebo in a blinded manner for 5 weeks while continuing to receive background benazepril. The patients then crossed over to the alternative regimen for a second 5-week period. Valsartan added to benazepril reduced BP by $6.5 \pm 12.6/4.5 \pm 8.0$ mm Hg (systolic/diastolic) over placebo for average awake ambulatory BP. Nocturnal systolic and diastolic BPs were also similarly reduced by $7.1 \pm 9.4/5.6 \pm 6.5$.[239] Until more substantive supporting information is forthcoming, the combination of an ACE inhibitor and an ARB should have a limited role in the treatment of hypertension.[240a]

Finally, a number of studies have demonstrated the utility of ACE inhibitors in the management of hypertensive patients, otherwise unresponsive to multidrug combinations.[241,242] Typically, such combinations have included a diuretic as well as either minoxidil, a CCB and/or a peripheral alpha-blocker. The key to this approach, as with two-drug combination therapy with ACE inhibitors, is to combine agents with different mechanisms of action. In addition, if an acute reduction in BP is desired, it can be achieved with either oral or sublingual captopril in that its onset of action is as soon as 15 minutes after its administration.[243] An additional option for the management of hypertensive emergencies is that of parenteral therapy with enalaprilat.[244] Compounds that interrupt RAA axis activity, such as ACE inhibitors, should be administered cautiously in patients suspected of a marked activation of the RAA axis (e.g., prior treatment with diuretics). In such subjects, sudden and extreme drops in BP have occasionally been observed with the first dose of an ACE inhibitor.[245]

ACE INHIBITORS AND ARBS IN HYPERTENSION ASSOCIATED WITH OTHER DISORDERS

ACE inhibitors effectively regress left ventricular hypertrophy (LVH) in the face of prolonged lowering of BP.[246–249] ARBs seem to have a similar effect on LVH, although fewer studies of a long-term nature have been conducted with compounds in this drug class.[250,250a] This is an important feature in that the presence of LVH portends a significant future risk of sudden death or myocardial infarction (MI).[251] The question of whether LVH regression is associated with a positive outcome has been answered with the completion of the Losartan Intervention for End-Point Reduction in Hypertension study (LIFE). The main LIFE study randomized 9193 patients aged 55 to 80 years with essential hypertension (baseline casual blood pressure 160 to 200/95 to 115 mm Hg) and electrocardiographic LVH (according to Cornell voltage-duration or Sokolow-Lyon voltage criteria) to a >4-year, double-blind treatment with losartan versus atenolol. This study showed a substantially reduced rate of stroke in the losartan-treated group despite comparably reduced BP readings in both the losartan and atenolol treatment groups.[250a,252]

A primary composite outcome of death, stroke, and cardiovascular morbidity showed a significant benefit in favor of losartan. There was also a greater effect on LVH regression with losartan compared to atenolol.[250a,252] ACE inhibitors and ARBs can be safely used in patients with coronary artery disease. Although they do not specifically vasodilate coronary arteries, they do improve hemodynamic factors, which dictate myocardial oxygen consumption and thereby reduce the risk of ischemia (Table 10-7). For example, ACE inhibitors do not reflexly increase myocardial sympathetic tone in hypertensive patients with angina, as can occur with other antihypertensives.[253]

ACE inhibitors and ARBs are also useful in the treatment of either isolated systolic hypertension or systolic-predominant forms of hypertension, which, in part, relates to their ability to improve arteriolar compliance.[254,255] In addition, ACE inhibitors are useful in the treatment of patients of cerebrovascular disease because they maintain cerebral autoregulatory ability despite their reducing BP.[184,256] This is particularly important in the treatment of the elderly hypertensive.[185] ACE inhibitors dilate both small and large arteries, can be used safely in patients with peripheral vascular disease, and may, on occasion, lessen intermittent claudication symptomatology.[257,258] As an example, of the 9297 patients in the HOPE study, 4051 had peripheral arterial disease, defined by a history of peripheral arterial disease, claudication, or an ankle-brachial index of less than 0.90. These patients had a similar reduction in the primary end-point when compared with those without peripheral arterial disease, thus demonstrating that an ACE inhibitor ramipril was effective in lowering the risk of fatal and nonfatal ischemic events among patients with peripheral arterial disease.[5]

ACE inhibitors and ARBs are also touted as agents of choice in the diabetic hypertensive patient, whether or not they have diabetic renal disease. Such enthusiasm needs to be tempered by the realization that these compounds, when administered as monotherapy, do not effectively reduce BP in many diabetics. This may relate to the fact that many diabetics have a low-renin, volume-expanded form of hypertension, which is generally less responsive to either an ACE inhibitor or an ARB. This efficacy hurdle can be overcome by addition of a diuretic to the treatment regimen or, alternatively, a different antihypertensive drug class may be considered for use. This rationale for therapy changes when the diabetic demonstrates evidence for renal involvement with their diabetes. The final results of the African American Study of Kidney Disease and Hypertension (AASK) demonstrated an advantage of the ACE inhibitor ramipril over the β-blocker metoprolol and the calcium antagonist amlodipine in preventing adverse renal outcomes in black patients with hypertension and diabetes.[258a] Therein, the data is now very impressive in support of ACE inhibitors and even more so with ARBs being a major element of the treatment regimen, although many times they must be given in conjunction with other antihypertensive medications to effect BP control in this typically difficult to manage population.[259,260] A final consideration with ACE inhibitors in the hypertensive diabetic relates to their effect on hyperlipidemia and/or insulin resistance. In this regard, ACE inhibitors and ARBs have failed to demonstrate an unambiguous effect on serum lipids and/or insulin resistance,[261–264] although in both the Captopril Prevention Project (CAPPP) and the HOPE studies, the ACE inhibitors captopril and ramipril, respectively, were found to decrease the incidence of new-onset type 2 diabetes mellitus.[201,265] Similarly, the incidence of new-onset diabetes (type 2) was decreased with losartan in the LIFE trial.[250a]

END ORGAN EFFECTS

Stroke

Given the significant public health impact of stroke and the identification of both nonmodifiable (age, gender, race/ethnicity) and modifiable (BP, diabetes, lipid profile, and lifestyle) risk factors, early prevention strategies are increasingly considered. When a patient and, in particular, a diabetic suffers a stroke, the focus of care becomes the prevention of secondary events. This can be accomplished with antiplatelet and lipid-lowering therapy, as well as by reducing BP. Despite the clear risk reduction with effective implementation of these preventative strategies, new approaches are needed. In particular, it is unclear whether the benefit gained from BP reduction is unique to the agent employed or a simple consequence of improvement in the hemodynamic profile.[266]

The Perindopril Protection Against Recurrent Stroke (PROGRESS) study reported for the first time that antihypertensive therapy with a combination of the ACE inhibitor, perindopril, and the thiazide diuretic indapamide reduced the recurrence of stroke even in patients with normal BP.[267] In this study, 6105 hypertensive and nonhypertensive patients who had stroke and no major disability within the past 5 years were randomized to a 4-mg dose of perindopril with or without a 2.5-mg dose of indapamide. After 4 years of follow-up (40% received perindopril alone and 60% combination therapy) there was a considerable disparity in the BP findings between these two treatment groups. In the subgroup of patients receiving perindopril and indapamide, BP was reduced by 12/5 mm Hg and the risk of stroke was reduced by 43%. Perindopril monotherapy reduced BP by 5/3 mm Hg, and yielded no significant reduction in the risk of stroke.[267] Based on the degree of BP reduction in the perindopril group, a 20% reduction in stroke risk would have been anticipated; thus, the findings in PROGRESS are somewhat enigmatic. A similar observation was made in the CAPPP trial where—despite its design problems—fatal or nonfatal stroke was 1.25-times more common in patients randomized to captopril, than in those assigned to conventional therapy with diuretics and/or beta-blockers.[201] Nevertheless, the beneficial effect of combination therapy with perindopril and indapamide is consistent with prior studies that showed a positive effect of diuretics on recurrent stroke rate.

In contradistinction to the PROGRESS study, the HOPE study provided compelling evidence that treatment with the ACE inhibitor ramipril, can further reduce the risk of stroke in high-risk patients without left ventricular dysfunction by mechanisms above-and-beyond reduction in BP.[5] Ramipril at a dose of 10 mg/d achieved a significant 32% reduction in total stroke and recurrent strokes were reduced by 33%. In a subanalysis of this trial, nonfatal stroke was reduced by 24%, and fatal stroke by 61%.[267a] Interestingly, in the HOPE study, ramipril was given at night and therefore its peak effect—be it hemodynamic or otherwise—occurred in the morning hours, a time when strokes occur more frequently.[268] Based on the HOPE study, the recently published American Heart Association guidelines for the primary prevention of stroke recommend ramipril to prevent stroke in high-risk patients and in patients with diabetes and hypertension.[269] Thus, it would appear that ACE inhibitor therapy—and in ACE inhibitor-intolerant patients, ARB treatment—is warranted if primary prevention is contemplated in a high-risk patient or secondary prevention is being considered in a patient already having sustained a cerebrovascular event. The positive results with losartan in the LIFE trial as relate to stroke adds a different layer of complexity to the selection process of

an antihypertensive agent.[250a,252] Recently the SCOPE (Study on Cognition and Progress in the Elderly) found a significant (28%) reduction in non-fatal strokes in elderly subjects with mild hypertension when treated with candesartan. Lowering blood pressure in this study did not interfere with cognitive function.

Renal

JNC VI recommends the use of ACE inhibitors in patients with hypertension and chronic renal disease to both control hypertension and to slow the rate of progression of CRF.[1] With the growing amount of data supporting the renal protective effects of ARBs, it is likely that ACE inhibitors and ARBs will be used interchangeably for this purpose.[198,199,270] Irrespective of the drug class being used to lower BP, the most important element in the management of the patient with hypertension and CRF remains tight BP control. JNC VI recommendations advise a goal blood pressure of 130/85 mm Hg, with even a lower value of 125/75 mm Hg being recommended for patients with proteinuria in excess of 1 g/d. Because of the volume dependency of the hypertension in this group of patients, ACE inhibitor and ARB therapy alone do not always provide the desired level of BP control. For example, in the Reduction of Endpoints in Non-Insulin-Dependent Diabetes Mellitus with the Angiotensin II Antagonist Losartan (RENAAL) study and Irbesartan Diabetic Nephropathy Trial (IDNT), the average number of medications required to achieve BP control, which was 140/90 and 135/85, respectively, in these studies, was three plus the study medication.[198,199] Thus, it is not uncommon in the treatment of these patients that diuretics and/or other drugs, such as CCBs, are added to the treatment regimen.[198]

Proteinuria has emerged as a robust marker for renal disease in diabetes as well as being an independent risk factor for cardiovascular disease.[271] Microalbuminuria typically augurs the development of progressive diabetic nephropathy and it is now routinely measured in all diabetics. Not only is screening for microalbuminuria recommended in diabetes but it is also suggested for others at increased risk for renal or CVR disease. The National Kidney Foundation's PARADE task force recently reviewed the evidence relating proteinuria and renal and cardiovascular risk leading to their recommendation that therapies used to treat hypertension should also target reductions in proteinuria.[272] Therapies directed at proteinuria reduction in nondiabetic renal disease are also recommended.[7] ACE inhibitors and ARBs have a number of renal effects, which culminate in substantial reductions in proteinuria and are obvious first choices for hypertensive patients with micro- or macroalbuminuria (Table 10-10).

ACE inhibitors have proven useful in the setting of established type 1 insulin-dependent diabetes mellitus (IDDM) nephropathy,[273] non-insulin-dependent diabetes mellitus (NIDDM) nephropathy,[274] normotensive type 1 IDDM patients with microalbuminuria,[275] and a variety of nondiabetic renal diseases.[276–286] Not all studies have demonstrated beneficial effects of ACE inhibitors. The Ramipril Efficacy in Nephropathy (REIN) study failed to detect a renoprotective effect in type 2 diabetic nephropathy patients treated with ramipril. Interestingly, those patients treated with ramipril lost renal function at a significantly faster rate than patients treated with a conventional non-ACE inhibitor-based regimen.[280] ACE inhibitor regimens shown to slow the rate of CRF progression include captopril 25 mg tid, enalapril 5 to 10 mg/d, benazepril 10 mg/d, and ramipril 2.5 to 5 mg/d.[3] It is presumed that renal failure increases the pharmacologic effect of these doses by reducing the renal clearance of the ACE inhibitor.[79]

TABLE 10-10. Effects of Angiotensin-Converting Enzyme Inhibitors on Proteinuria and Progression of Renal Disease in Diabetics and Nondiabetics*

Reference	Patients	Design	Drug	UAE	GFR	SCr	CL$_{cr}$	Arterial BP
Mathiesen et al[283]	44 type 1 DM, microalbuminuria	Open-label, randomized, prospective	Captopril 25–100 mg/d	↓†	0‡	NE	NE	0
Ahmad et al[281]	103 type 2 DM, persistent microalbuminuria	Prospective, randomized, single-blind, placebo-controlled	Enalapril 10 mg/d	↓†	0	NE	NE	0
Nielsen[291]	43 type 2 DM, persistent macroalbuminuria	Prospective, randomized, double and then single-blind	Lisinopril 10–20 mg/d vs atenolol 50–100 mg//d	Greater ↓ with lisinopril	↔	↔	↔	Similar reductions in both treatment limbs
Bakris[290]	52 type 2 DM with persistent proteinuria	Randomized, prospective	Lisinopril vs atenolol vs verapamil or diltiazem	↓ that was comparable in lisinopril and CCB groups	↔	↔	↔	Similar reductions in all three treatment limbs
UKPDS[292]	758 type 2 DM some with microalbuminuria	Randomized, prospective	Captopril vs atenolol	↓ that was comparable in captopril and atenolol groups	↔	↔	↔	Similar reductions in both treatment limbs
REIN[280]	352 nephropathic patients	Randomized, prospective	Ramipril vs conventional therapy	Greater ↓ with ramipril	↓ with ramipril only in nondiabetics			Similar reductions in both treatment limbs
HOPE[294]	980 patients with mild renal insufficiency with or without proteinuria	Randomized, prospective, double-blind	Ramipril 10 mg vs placebo	NE	NE	NE	NE	Greater cardiovascular event rate in placebo group despite minimal reduction in BP
Fogari et al[289]	51 type 2 DM, persistent proteinuria >300 and <2000 mg/d	Randomized, prospective	Ramipril 5 mg vs nitrendipine 20 mg	↓	0	NC	NC	Similar reductions in both treatment limbs

(continued)

TABLE 10-10. (*Continued*) Effects of Angiotensin-Converting Enzyme Inhibitors on Proteinuria and Progression of Renal Disease in Diabetics and Nondiabetics*

Reference	Patients	Design	Drug	UAE	GFR	SCr	Cl_cr	Arterial BP
Estacio et al[293]	470 type 2 DM with or without proteinuria	Prospective, randomized, double-blind	Enalapril *vs* Nisoldipine	↔	↔	↔	↔	Similar reductions in both treatment limbs
Lebovitz et al[288]	121 type 2 DM, persistent macroalbuminuria	Prospective, randomized, single-blind, positive control	Enalapril 10 mg/d	↓†	Enalapril slowed GFR decline			Equivalent reduction in treatment groups
Lewis et al[273]	409 type 1 DM, DN	Prospective, randomized, placebo-controlled	Captopril 25 mg tid	↓†	NE	↓†	NE	↓†
EUCLID[284]	530 type 1 DM, normoalbuminuria/microalbuminuria	Double-blind, randomized, placebo-controlled	Lisinopril 10–20 mg/d	↓†	NE	NE	NE	↓†
Ravid et al[282]	94 type 2 DM, microalbuminuria	Randomized, placebo-controlled	Enalapril 10 mg/d	↓†	NE	0	NE	0
Ravid et al[286]	156 type 2 DM	Randomized, double-blind, placebo-controlled	Enalapril 10 mg/d	↑†	NE	NE	↓†	0
Viberti et al[275]	92 type 1 DM, microalbuminuria	Randomized, double-blind, placebo-controlled	Captopril 50 mg bid	↓†	↓†	NE	NE	0
Sano et al[285]	52 type 2 DM, persistent microalbuminuria	Randomized	Enalapril 5 mg/d	↓†	NE	NE	0	0

BP = blood pressure; CCB = calcium-channel blocker; Cl_cr = creatinine clearance; DM = diabetes mellitus; DN = diabetic nephropathy; GFR = glomerular filtration rate; NC = no change; NE = not evaluated; SCr = serum creatinine; UAE = urinary albumin excretion.

*Compared with baseline.

†Statistically significant difference.

‡No statistically significant difference.

TABLE 10-11. Studies with Angiotensin-Receptor Blockers in Diabetic Nephropathy

	IDNT[199]	IRMA 2[270]	RENAAL[198]	MARVAL[287]
Study Design	IRB 300 mg vs AML 10 mg vs PLA	IRB 150 mg vs 300 mg vs PLA	LOS 50–100 mg vs AML	VAL 80 mg vs AML
N	1715	590	1513	332
Patient Type	HT/Type 2 Diabetes/Nephropathy	HT/Type 2 Diabetes/Microalbuminuria	Type 2 Diabetes/Nephropathy	Type 2 Diabetes/ Microalbuminuria/SBP <180 and/or DBP <105 mm Hg
Duration	Mean 2.6 years	2 years	Mean 3.4 years	24 weeks
End-points	Primary composite: doubling of serum creatinine/ESRD/death	Time to onset of nephropathy with UAER >200 μg/min/30% greater than baseline	Primary composite: doubling of serum creatinine/ ESRD/death	$\cong$UAER
Results	Risk of primary end-point 20% lower with IRB vs PLA; 23% lower vs AML — lower doubling of serum creatinine ESRD with IRB; no. difference in deaths	IRB was renoprotective; 5.2% reached end-point in 300-mg groups; 9.7% reached end-point in 150-mg group vs 14.9% in PLA ($P = .08$)	Risk of primary end-point lowered by 15% ($P = .02$) with LOS — lower doubling of serum creatinine ESRD with LOS; no. difference in deaths	VAL significantly lowered UAER (44%) vs AML (17%) ($P < .001$)

AML = amlodipine; DBP = diastolic blood pressure; ESRD = end-stage renal disease; HT = hypertension; IRB = irbesartan; LOS = losartan; PLA = placebo; UAER = urinary albumin excretion rate; SBP = systolic blood pressure; VAL = valsartan.

ARBs have also been found in recently published clinical trials to be useful in the setting of type 2 diabetes, both in established diabetic nephropathy with proteinuria[198,199] and in microalbuminuric diabetic patients.[270,287–294] Results of these trials are quite reminiscent of results observed in type 1 diabetic nephropathy treated with captopril. ARB regimens used in these trials included irbesartan 150 to 300 mg/d, losartan 50 to 100 mg/d, and valsartan 80 to 160 mg/d (Table 10-11). Therapies directed at reducing the production or effects of angiotensin-II have a variety of potentially beneficial effects on the kidney. ACE inhibitors transiently reduce GFR secondary to their ability to reduce glomerular capillary pressures.[295,296] Such decrements in GFR—ordinarily in the order of a 10 to 15% drop—are readily reversible and actually predictive of the degree of long-term renal protection.[297] Current practice considerations would suggest that there is not a specific level of renal function at which either an ACE inhibitor or an ARB cannot be started; rather, if significant hyperkalemia accompanies the use of these drugs that may be the basis for their being at least temporarily discontinued.

As already mentioned, reduction in proteinuria has been employed as a marker for the beneficial effects of these therapies. Reducing proteinuria may, in and of itself, also favorably affect the progression rate of the renal failure process.[298] The renoprotective effect of ACE inhibitors is most evident in patients with heavy proteinuria (>3 g/d) who, if left untreated, generally progress quite rapidly. ACE inhibitors and ARBs also modify tissue-based growth factors, such as transforming growth factor (TGF)-β, which are activated by prior/ongoing renal disease and are stimulated by the presence of angiotensin-II.[299] Inhibition of these tissue-based processes may further slow the progression of renal disease. There may be differences in the tissue-based effects of ACE inhibitors and ARBs, because the effect of ACE inhibitors on renal hemodynamics might be limited by the non-ACE-dependent generation of angiotensin II.[177,300]

Three factors are potential modifiers of the renal response to ACE inhibitors. First, a low sodium intake enhances the antiproteinuric effect of ACE inhibitors.[301] Second, short-term studies suggest that dietary protein restriction complements the ACE-inhibitor effect on protein excretion in nephrotic patients. This would seem to imply that combining ACE inhibitors and protein restriction might prove more effective than an ACE inhibitor alone in slowing the

progression of renal failure.[302] A third factor is that of inherited variation in ACE activity. Two common forms of the ACE gene I (insertion) and D (deletion) give rise to three potential genotypes: II, ID, and DD. The DD phenotype is associated with higher circulating ACE levels and a greater pressor response to the infusion of angiotensin-I as compared to the II phenotype, with the ID phenotype displaying intermediate characteristics.[303,304] These phenotypic characteristics can be expected to be relevant to the response to ACE inhibition. The finding that DD patients are at increased risk for myocardial infarction and ischemic cardiomyopathy first established the clinical significance of the inherited variation in ACE activity.[305] In this regard, recent work suggests that GFR declines more rapidly in DD than II patients and that such patients do not demonstrate significant reductions in proteinuria or slowing in the rate of progression of renal failure when administered ACEIs.[306,307] These three factors, which clearly modify the response to an ACE inhibitor, may also modify the response to ARBs, although ACE gene polymorphism should not be as important in defining the effect of ARBs.

Cardiac

Data from both placebo-controlled and open trials suggest that ACE inhibitors substantially reduce the risk of death and hospitalization for CHF while improving its symptomatology making ACE inhibitors first-line therapy for the treatment of CHF.[10,308,309] By modifying production of angiotensin-II these agents interrupt the neurohumoral deterioration characteristic of CHF.[109,110,310] While statistically significant reductions in mortality have been observed with enalapril, similar trends have been observed with other ACE inhibitors, including captopril, ramipril, quinapril, trandolapril, and lisinopril.[10,311] Furthermore, these agents have demonstrated efficacy and tolerability in the treatment of CHF based on the end-points of improved exercise tolerance and symptomatology. Although ACE inhibitors are almost universally recommended as a cost-effective strategy for the treatment of CHF, physician-prescribing practice is such that only $\approx$50% of those patients eligible for treatment with ACE inhibitors actually receive them.[312,313] Moreover, the dosages used in "real-world practice" are substantially lower than those

TABLE 10-12. Effect of Angiotensin-Receptor Blockers on Mortality Rates in Heart Failure

Study	Agent	End-Point	ARB	ACEI or Placebo	Risk Reduction	P
ELITE[321]	Losartan	Combined mortality/HF hospitalization	33/352	49/370	0.32 (−0.04–0.55)	0.075
ELITE II[322]	Losartan	All-cause mortality	280/1578	250/1574	1.13* (0.95–1.35)	0.16
Val-HeFT[319]	Valsartan	All-cause mortality	495/2511	484/2499[†]	1.02 (0.9–1.15)	0.800
Val-HeFT[319]	Valsartan	Combined morbidity and mortality	723/2511	801/2459[†]	0.87 (0.79–0.96)	0.035

ACEI = angiotensin-converting enzyme inhibitor; ARB = angiotensin-receptor blocker; ELITE = Evaluation of Losartan in the Elderly; HF = heart failure; Val-HeFT = Valsartan-Heart Failure Trial.

*Hazards ratio.

[†]Placebo results.

proven efficacious in randomized, controlled trials, with evaluations reporting only a minority of patients achieving target doses and/or an overall mean dose achieved to be less than one-half of the target dose. Factors predicting the use and optimal dose administration of ACE inhibitors include variables relating to the setting (previous hospitalization, specialty clinic follow-up), the physician (cardiology specialty vs family practitioner or general internist), the patient (increased severity of symptoms, male, younger), and the drug (lower frequency of administration).[314]

Enalapril, captopril, lisinopril, and trandolapril significantly reduce morbidity and mortality rates in patients with MI and a wide range of ventricular function. There are presently insufficient data to determine whether clinically significant differences exist among the ACE inhibitors in the post-MI setting, given the paucity of head-to-head trials among these agents and the fact that the studies discussed above varied in length and duration.[311,315] Currently, only captopril, lisinopril, ramipril, and trandolapril are approved specifically in post-MI left ventricular dysfunction, although enalapril is approved in asymptomatic left ventricular dysfunction. However, as in patients with CHF, numerous ACE inhibitors have demonstrated benefits in patients after MI, suggesting, to a certain degree, a class effect.[316] Thus, ACE inhibitors are indicated in all patients with acute MI who can tolerate them. In a hemodynamically stable patient after an MI, an oral ACE inhibitor should be initiated, generally within 24-hours of the event, particularly if the MI is anterior and associated with depressed left ventricular function. The hemodynamic effects and overall benefit of ACE inhibition are seen early, with 40% of the 30-day increase in survival observed in days 0 to 1, 45% in days 2 to 7, and approximately 15% after day 7.[317] The benefits of ACE inhibitor therapy in the postmyocardial infarction period appear not to be the result of a substantial decline in arrhythmic mortality.[318] ARBs have been studied in CHF (Table 10-12)[319–322B] and are currently under study in the postmyocardial infarction patient.[323,324] In the double-blind OPTIMAAL (Optimal Trial in Myocardial Infarction with the Angiotensin II Antagonist Losartan), losartan was compared with Captopril and a non-significant difference in total mortality in favor of Captupril was observed.[324] The ARBs do not appear to differ substantially from ACE inhibitors in symptomatic relief, improvement in exercise tolerance, and/or in favorably influencing morbidity and mortality. The combination of an ACE inhibitor and an ARB, as occurred in the Valsartan-Heart Failure Trial (Val-HeFT), improved morbidity but not mortality, and the exact best way to combine an ACE inhibitor with an ACE inhibitor in the management of CHF remains to be determined. Concomitant use of Valsartan with an ACE inhibitor and a beta blocker is not recommended based on the Val-Heft valsartan is now indicated for the treatment of heart failure (NYHA class II–IV) in patients who are intolerant of ACE inhibitors.

Several dosing strategies are effective in reducing morbidity and mortality in patients with systolic left ventricular dysfunction. Most importantly, a systematic effort must be made to reach target doses shown to be effective in the randomized trials having used ACE inhibitors in CHF. Emerging data seems to suggest that the doses of ACE inhibitors used in clinical practice are less effective than the relatively high doses used in the randomized trials.[111,325] Dose ranges used in community practice are typically in the 50 mg and 10 mg/d range for captopril and enalapril, respectively; whereas, randomized trials saw their success to be associated with captopril and enalapril doses approaching 150 and 40 mg/d, respectively. Until convincing evidence otherwise becomes available, the treatment of CHF should include sequential dose titration of the ACE inhibitor used. Such titration should strive to reach those doses shown to be successful in the randomized clinical trials. The ability to reach these doses in the CHF patient can sometimes be a vexing issue because a major deterrent is the development of systemic hypotension and/or a decline in GFR.[326] Thus, reaching goal ACE inhibitor doses necessitates a keen understanding of the critical relationship between volume status, blood pressure, and the final desired ACE-inhibitor dose. Probably the single most important variable, which allows effective dose titration, is this understanding of the relationship between volume status and BP.[326]

OTHER CLINICAL USES

ACE inhibitors have been used in the diagnosis of renal artery stenosis (captopril-stimulated renography) and primary hyperaldosteronism.[368] Patients suspected of having renovascular occlusive disease by clinical criteria are administered a dose of rapid-acting ACE inhibitor, such as oral captopril or intravenous enalaprilat 1 to 2 h prior to injection of a nuclear imaging tracer. Subtle differences in intraglomerular pressure between the two kidneys are amplified by the sudden decline in local and circulatory angiotensin-II levels that result from the administration of the ACE inhibitor. It has been reported that the diagnostic sensitivity of captopril-stimulated nuclear renography is 90 to 100%.[368] Regarding hyperaldosteronism, it has been shown that patients with adrenal adenomas do not show a decline in aldosterone levels with an ACE inhibitor, in contrast to patients with the hyperplastic type whose aldosterone levels usually decline by approximately 50%.[368]

ACE inhibitors have also been used to treat altitude polycythemia as well as another form of secondary polycythemia that follows renal transplantation.[369] The drugs have been used as treatment to prevent postangioplasty restenosis (see Chap. 40), although with little or no benefit being demonstrated in multiple clinical trials.[370]

CANCER AND ACE INHIBITORS

It went largely unnoticed in the prospective Studies of Left Ventricular Dysfunction (SOLVD) study that patients with left ventricular dysfunction treated with enalapril showed a slightly higher incidence of malignancy than did those patients receiving placebo (OR 1.59; CI 0.90 to 2.82). In this study, there were 38 gastrointestinal malignancies in the enalapril group as compared with 22 in the placebo group (OR 1.7).[327] Since the SOLVD study, several case reports have linked ACE inhibitors to the development of malignancies. For example, pemphigus vulgaris, which can be seen in association with internal malignancies, is a known adverse effect of captopril. One case report linked enalapril for the first time to pemphigus vegetans with a simultaneously occurring internal malignancy.[328] In a further case report, Kaposi's sarcoma appeared in a 70-year-old woman 8 months after starting captopril. Upon stopping the captopril, there was a marked reduction in both the cutaneous and gastric lesions of this disease, suggesting a cause-and-effect relationship between the captopril and the malignancy.[329]

A subsequent study disputed these findings in that it was shown that captopril inhibited angiogenesis in Kaposi's sarcoma.[330] These limited data are in contrast to a greater body of evidence supporting the lack of a cancer risk with ACE inhibitors. In the recent large-scale HOPE trial, 9297 high-risk patients who were treated either with ramipril or placebo for a mean of 5 years had similar numbers of deaths from noncardiovascular causes in both groups.[5] In addition, several other retrospective studies investigating the possible association between various antihypertensives and cancer risk failed to detect such a relationship with the use of ACE inhibitors.[331–333] Finally, the Scottish retrospective cohort study by Lever et al, who compared 1599 patients taking ACE inhibitors and 3648 on other antihypertensive drugs, demonstrated a risk reduction for female sex-specific and lung cancers.[334] Thus, the overall evidence available to date suggests that ACE inhibitors have a neutral cancer risk in hypertension[335] and might conceivably decrease the risk.[336] There are a limited number of long-term trials with ARBs; accordingly, no statement can be made about the risk or not of malignancy with this drug class.

SIDE EFFECTS OF ACE INHIBITORS AND ARBS

Soon after their release, a syndrome of "functional renal insufficiency" was observed to occur as a class effect with ACE inhibitors,[337] a process little different than what is occasionally seen with the ARBs.[13] This phenomenon was initially recognized in patients with either a solitary kidney and renal artery stenosis, or in the setting of bilateral renal artery stenosis. Since these original reports, this phenomenon has been repeatedly observed. Predisposing conditions to this process include dehydration, CHF, and/or microvascular renal disease, as well as the aforementioned macrovascular renal disease.[337] The mechanistic theme common to all of these conditions is a fall in afferent arteriolar flow. When this occurs, glomerular filtration temporarily drops. In response to this reduction in glomerular flow local release of angiotensin-II occurs, which then preferentially constricts the efferent or postglomerular arteriole. When the efferent arteriole constricts, upstream hydrostatic pressures within the glomerular capillary bed are restored despite the initial and frequently continuing decline in afferent arteriolar flow. The abrupt removal of angiotensin-II, as occurs with either an ACE inhibitor or an ARB, dilates the efferent arteriole. An offshoot of these hemodynamic changes is a sudden change in glomerular hemodynamic pressures and a plummeting of glomerular filtration.

This phenomenon of "functional renal insufficiency" is best treated by discontinuation of the offending agent, either an ACE inhibitor or an ARB, careful volume repletion if intravascular volume contraction exists, and, if suspected, investigation for the presence of renal artery stenosis.[326] An additional side effect with ACE inhibitors is that of hyperkalemia.[338] Relevant degrees of hyperkalemia with ACE inhibitor occur in predisposed patients, such as diabetic or CHF patients with renal failure receiving potassium-sparing diuretics or potassium supplements. Typically, though, hyperkalemia is not that common with ACE inhibitors[339] and is even less common with the ARBs.[340] Alternatively, ACE inhibitors and ARBs are known to lessen the degree of hypokalemia produced by diuretic therapy[341]

A dry, irritating, nonproductive cough is a common complication with ACE inhibitors, with its incidence variously estimated at between 0% and 44%.[342] Cough is a class phenomenon with ACE inhibitors and has ostensibly been attributed to increased bradykinin levels or other vasoactive peptides such as Substance P, which may play a second-messenger role in triggering the cough reflex.[343] Although numerous therapies have been tried, few have eliminated ACE inhibitor-induced cough with any lasting success. Most times the cough gradually disappears within 2 weeks after the offending agent is stopped. Alternatively, ARBs have been infrequently associated with cough, whether the cough incidence is determined in preselected patients having previously experienced ACE inhibitor-related cough or in parallel-limb treatment studies directly comparing an ACE inhibitor to an ARB.[195] ACE inhibitor-related nonspecific side effects are generally uncommon with the exception of taste disturbances, leukopenia, skin rash, and dysgeusia, which are almost exclusively seen in captopril-treated patients.[344] The sulfhydryl-group found on captopril has been implicated in these abnormalities. Alternatively, the ARBs have demonstrated a favorable safety and tolerability profile, which appears to be equivalent to that observed with placebo. To date, no clear class-specific adverse effect has been attributed to the ARBs.[197] In fact, certain side effects, such as headache, may occur less frequently with ARBs than with placebo, which is probably a consequence of better BP reduction with an ARB than with placebo.[345,345a]

Angioneurotic edema is a potentially life-threatening complication of ACE inhibitors that is more common in blacks.[346] The incidence rate ranges from 0.1 to 0.5% amongst ACE-inhibitor users and it can occur quite unpredictably. Amongst all-cause factors for angioedema, ACE inhibitors are causal 20% of the time.[347] Typically, it is not a first-dose phenomenon. It is easily recognized because of its characteristic involvement of the mouth, tongue, and upper airway.[348,349] ACE inhibitor-induced angioedema of the intestine can also occur. This typically presents with acute abdominal symptoms with or without facial and/or oropharyngeal swelling, and is more common in females.[350] Angioedema also occurs with ARBs, but much less frequently.[351] The mechanism of angioedema with ARBs is unknown, although in ARB-treated patients who develop angioedema, up to one-third had previously developed angioedema on an ACE inhibitor.[352] Because patients with previous ACE inhibitor–induced angioedema are at increased risk for recurrent angioedema with an ARB, these drugs should not be considered a safe substitute in patients with previous ACE inhibitor-induced angioedema.[353] ARB use can be considered in a patient having previously experience angioedema, but only if compelling indications exist, such as progressive CHF and/or proteinuric renal disease, and only then with appropriate patient instruction.

A final issue with ACE inhibitors and ARBs is their capacity to cause birth defects. These drugs are not teratogenic; rather, their use during the second and third trimester of pregnancy can cause oligoamnios, neonatal anuria, hypocalvaria, pulmonary hypoplasia, and/or fetal or neonatal death in that the maturing fetus is heavily reliant on angiotensin-II for proper development.[354–356] Unintended pregnancy remains common in young women; thus, in women of gestational age, a clinician must be alert to this possibility when the treatment of hypertension is contemplated and an agent is to be selected. This is particularly so with ACE inhibitors and/or ARBs.[357] If ACE inhibitors or ARBs are required or are being incidentally used when a women is nursing, there is minimal entry of these compounds into breast milk. Although not all ACE inhibitors or ARBs have been submitted to formal study, in most cases, breast milk selectively restricts the passage of these drugs.[358]

CLASS AND AGENT-SPECIFIC DRUG INTERACTIONS

Several class specific drug interactions occur with drugs in these two classes (see Chap. 48). For example, the concurrent administration of lithium with either an ACE inhibitor or an ARB is associated with a greater likelihood of lithium toxicity.[359,360] Potassium supplements or potassium-sparing diuretics, when given with either ACE inhibitors or ARBs, increase the probability of developing hyperkalemia. NSAIDs, such as indomethacin, reduce the antihypertensive effects of ACE inhibitors and ARBs as well, although the latter has been less-well studied.[361] NSAIDs also attenuate the natriuretic response seen with both ACE inhibitors and ARBs.[362] Finally, both ACE inhibitors and NSAIDs can lead to functional renal insufficiency, particularly in those taking diuretics. This combination of drugs should be administered with extreme care to highly vulnerable patients, such as the elderly.[363]

The issue of whether aspirin attenuates the effects of an ACE inhibitor in hypertension and/or CHF has been a matter of some controversy.[364] To whatever extent the improvement in symptoms and survival rendered by treatment with ACE inhibitors is attributable to their effects on the circulation and the kidneys, this benefit can be rescinded by concomitant administration of aspirin.[365] There is a wealth of data that suggests an important interaction between aspirin and ACE inhibitors in patients with chronic stable cardiovascular disease. An interaction is biologically plausible because there is considerable evidence that ACE inhibitors exert important effects through increasing the production of vasodilator prostaglandins, whereas aspirin blocks their production through inhibition of cyclooxygenase, even at low doses. There is some evidence that low-dose aspirin may also raise systolic and diastolic BP.[366] There is also considerable evidence that aspirin may entirely neutralize the clinical benefits of ACE in patients with CHF, possibly by blocking endogenous vasodilator prostaglandin production and/or by enhancing the vasoconstrictor potential of endothelin. In patients requiring treatment for CHF, if possible, aspirin should be avoided and the integrity of prostaglandin metabolism respected; the more severe the CHF the more compelling the argument. As an alternative in these patients antiplatelet therapy should be considered with agents that do not block the cyclooxygenase system.[364]

Finally, combining an ACE inhibitor with allopurinol is associated with a higher risk of hypersensitivity reactions with several reports of the Stevens-Johnson syndrome described with the combination of captopril and allopurinol.[367] Quinapril reduces the absorption of tetracycline by $\approx 35\%$, which may be due to the high magnesium content of quinapril tablets. To date, no drug-drug interactions have been described relative to the absorption of ARBs.

CONCLUSION

ACE inhibitors and ARBs are commonly used in the treatment of hypertension and of an increasing number of end-organ diseases. These compounds reduce BP by mechanisms involving change in the quantity and/or effect of angiotensin-II and by increasing bradykinin. Moreover, there is increasing evidence that these compounds also alter sympathetic outflow although in a compound-specific manner. Early belief held that these drugs were minimally effective in low-renin forms of hypertension, such as in the case of African American hypertensives. More recently, it has become clear that the African American hypertensive can respond well to these drugs, although with some interindividual variability in the pattern of response. A number of ACE inhibitors and ARBs are available, with distinctions between individual members of each drug class sometimes being quite subtle. Pharmacologic properties proposed as distinguishing features for both ACE inhibitors and ARBs include their tissue and receptor-binding potential and whether their mode of elimination is renal or renal/hepatic. ACE inhibitors, and more recently ARBs, are of clearly proven benefit in slowing the progression of CRF, and both drug classes have a major influence on the morbidity and mortality that attends progressive CHF. ACE inhibitors are generally without significant side effects other than cough, which, unfortunately, can occur in a significant number of patients receiving these drugs. Alternatively, ARBs are virtually side-effect free, which is a substantial advantage supporting the expanded use of drugs in this class.

REFERENCES

1. The Sixth Report of the Joint National Committee on Prevention, Detection, Evaluation, and Treatment of High Blood Pressure. *Arch Intern Med* 157:2413–2446, 1997.
2. Brunner HR, Waeber B, Nussberger J: Angiotensin-converting enzyme inhibitors. In: Messerli F, ed. *Cardiovascular Drug Therapy.* 2nd ed. Philadelphia: WB Saunders, 1996:690–711.
3. Sica DA, Gehr TWB: Angiotensin-converting enzyme inhibitors. In: Oparil S, Weber M, eds. *Hypertension, A Companion to the Kidney,* 1st ed. Philadelphia: WB Saunders, 2000:599–608.
4. Cheng A, Frishman WH: Use of angiotensin-converting enzyme inhibitors as monotherapy and in combination with diuretics and calcium channel blockers. *J Clin Pharmacol* 38:477–491, 1998.
5. Yusuf S, Sleight P, Pogue J, et al: Effects of an angiotensin-converting enzyme inhibitor, ramipril, on cardiovascular events in high-risk patients. The Heart Outcomes Prevention Evaluation Study Investigators. *N Engl J Med* 342:145–153, 2000.
6. Giatras I, Lau J, Levey SS: Effect of angiotensin-converting enzyme inhibitors on the progression of nondiabetic renal disease: A meta-analysis of randomized trials. *Ann Intern Med* 127:337–345, 1997.
7. Jafar TH, Schmid CH, Landa M, et al: Angiotensin-converting enzyme inhibitors and progression of nondiabetic renal disease. A meta-analysis of patient-level data. *Ann Intern Med* 135:73–87, 2001.
8. Navis G, Faber HJ, de Zeeuw D, de Jong PE: ACE inhibitors and the kidney. *Drug Saf* 15:200–211, 1996.
9. Navis G, de Jong PE, de Zeeuw D: Optimizing the renal response to ACE inhibition: A strategy toward more effective long-term renoprotection. *Adv Nephrol* 27:57–66, 1998.
10. Garg R, Yusuf S, for the Collaborative Group on ACE Inhibitor Trials. Overview of randomized trials of angiotensin-converting enzyme

inhibitors on mortality and morbidity in patients with heart failure. *JAMA* 273:1450–1456, 1995.

11. Lonn EM, Yusuf S, Jha P, et al: Emerging role of angiotensin-converting enzyme inhibitors in cardiac and vascular protection. *Circulation* 90:2056–2069, 1994.

12. Sica DA: Class effects of angiotensin-converting enzyme inhibitors. *Am J Manage Care* 6(Suppl 3):S85–S108, 2000.

13. Toto R: Angiotensin II subtype 1-receptor blockers and renal function. *Arch Intern Med* 161:1492–1499, 2001.

14. Carson P, Giles T, Higginbotham M, Hollenberg N, et al: Angiotensin receptor blockers: Evidence for preserving target organs. *Clin Cardiol* 24:183–190, 2001.

15. Jamali AH, Tang WH, Khot UN, Fowler MB: The role of angiotensin receptor blockers in the management of chronic heart failure. *Arch Intern Med* 161:667–672, 2001.

16. Johnston C, Risvanis J: Preclinical pharmacology of angiotensin II receptor antagonists: Update and outstanding issues. *Am J Hypertens* 10:306S–310S, 1997.

17. Burnier M: Angiotensin II type 1-receptor blockers. *Circulation* 103:904–912, 2001.

18. Carretero OA, Scicli AG: The kallikrein-kinin system as a regulator of cardiovascular and renal function. In: Brenner BM, Laragh JH, eds. *Hypertension: Pathophysiology, Diagnosis, and Management.* 2nd ed. New York: Raven Press, 1995:983–999.

19. Juillerat L, Nussberger J, Menard J, et al: Determinants of angiotensin II generation during converting enzyme inhibition. *Hypertension* 16:564–572, 1990.

20. Urata H. Nishimura H, Ganten D: Chymase-dependent angiotensin II forming system in humans. *Am J Hypertens* 9:277–284, 1996.

21. Petrie MC, Padmanabhan N, McDonald JE, et al: Angiotensin-converting enzyme and non-ACE dependent angiotensin II generation in resistance arteries from patients with heart failure and coronary heart disease. *J Am Coll Cardiol* 37:1056–1061, 2001.

22. Ennezat PV, Berlowitz M, Sonnenblick EH, Le Jemtel TH: Therapeutic implications of escape from angiotensin-converting enzyme inhibition in patients with chronic heart failure. *Curr Cardiol Rep* 2:258–262, 2000.

23. Swedberg K, Eneroth P, Kjekshus J, Wilhelmsen L: Hormones regulating cardiovascular function in patients with severe congestive heart failure and their relation to mortality. CONSENSUS Trial Study Group. *Circulation* 82:1730–1736, 1990.

24. Mooser V, Nussberger J, Juillerat L, et al: Reactive hyperreninemia is a major determinant of plasma angiotensin II during ACE inhibition. *J Cardiovasc Pharmacol* 15:276–282, 1990.

25. Vander AJ, Geelhoed GW: Inhibition of renin secretion by angiotensin II. *Proc Soc Exp Biol Med* 120:399–403, 1965.

26. Grima M, Ingert C, Michel B, et al: Renal tissue angiotensins during converting enzyme inhibition in the spontaneously hypertensive rat. *Clin Exp Hypertens* 19:671–685, 1997.

27. Nussberger J, Brunner DB, Waeber A, et al: Lack of angiotensin I accumulation after converting enzyme blockade with enalapril or lisinopril in man. *Clin Sci (Lond)* 72:387–389, 1987.

28. Staessen J, Fagard R, Lijnen P, et al: The hypotensive effect of propranolol in captopril-treated patients does not involve the plasma renin-angiotensin-aldosterone system. *Clin Sci (Lond)* 61:441S–444S, 1981.

29. Hodsman GP, Isles CG, Murray GD, et al: Factors related to the first dose hypotensive effect of captopril: Prediction and treatment. *Brit Med J* 286:832–834, 1983.

30. Case DB, Atlas SA, Laragh JH, et al: Use of first dose response or plasma renin activity to predict the long-term effect of captopril: Identification of triphasic pattern of blood pressure response. *J Cardiovasc Pharmacol* 2:339–346, 1980.

31. Brunner HR, Waeber B, Nussberger J: Does pharmacological profiling of a new drug in normotensive volunteers provide a useful guide to antihypertensive therapy? *Hypertension* 5(Supple III):101–107, 1983.

32. Ikeda LS, Harm SC, Arcuri KE, et al: Comparative antihypertensive effects of losartan 50 mg and losartan 50 mg titrated to 100 mg in patients with essential hypertension. *Blood Press* 6:35–43, 1997.

33. Gainer JV, Morrow JD, Loveland A, et al: Effect of bradykinin-receptor blockade on the response to angiotensin-converting enzyme inhibitor in normotensive and hypertensive subjects. *N Engl J Med* 339:1285–1292, 1998.

34. Squire IB, O'Kane KP, Anderson N, Reid JL: Bradykinin B (2) receptor antagonism attenuates blood pressure response to acute angiotensin-converting enzyme inhibition in normal men. *Hypertension* 36:132–136, 2000.

35. Su JB, Barbe F, Crozatier B, et al: Increased bradykinin levels accompany the hemodynamic response to acute inhibition of angiotensin-converting enzyme in dogs with heart failure. *J Cardiovasc Pharmacol* 34:700–710, 1999.

36. Ogihara T, Maruyama A, Hata T, et al: Hormonal responses to long-term converting enzyme inhibition I hypertensive patients. *Clin Pharmacol Ther* 30:328–335, 1981.

37. Gavras I: Bradykinin-mediated effects of ACE inhibition. *Kidney Int* 42:1020–1029, 1992.

38. Mazzolai L, Maillard M, Rossat J, et al: Angiotensin II receptor blockade in normotensive subjects: A direct comparison of three AT1 receptor antagonists. *Hypertension* 33:850–855, 1999.

39. Siragy HM, de Gasparo M, El-Kersh M, Carey RM: Angiotensin-converting enzyme inhibition potentiates angiotensin II type 1-receptor effects on renal bradykinin and cGMP. *Hypertension* 38:183–186, 2001.

40. Rodriguez-Garcia JL, Villa E, Serrano M, et al: Prostacyclin: Its pathogenic role in essential hypertension and the class effect of ACE inhibitors on prostaglandin metabolism. *Blood Press* 8:279–284, 1999.

41. Waeber B, Nussberger J, Brunner HR: Angiotensin-converting enzyme inhibitors in hypertension. In: Laragh JH, Brenner BM, eds. *Hypertension: Pathophysiology, Diagnosis, and Management.* 2nd ed. New York: Raven Press, 1995:2861–2875.

42. Quest DW, Gopalakrishnan V, McNeill JR, Wilson TW: Effect of losartan on angiotensin II-mediated endothelin and prostanoid excretion in humans. *Am J Hypertens* 13:1288–1294, 2000.

43. Salvetti A, Abdel-Hag B, Magagna A, et al: Indomethacin reduces the antihypertensive effect of enalapril. *Clin Exp Hypertens* 9:559–567, 1987.

44. Johnson AG: NSAIDs and increased blood pressure. What is the clinical significance? *Drug Saf* 17:277–289, 1997.

45. Nawarskas JJ, Townsend RR, Cirigliano MD, Spinler SA: Effect of aspirin on blood pressure in hypertensive patients taking enalapril or losartan. *Am J Hypertens* 12:784–789, 1999.

46. Nawarskas JJ, Spinler SA: Does aspirin interfere with the therapeutic efficacy of angiotensin-converting enzyme inhibitors in hypertension or congestive heart failure. *Pharmacotherapy* 18:1041–1052, 1998.

47. Guazzi MD, Campodonico J, Celeste F, et al: Antihypertensive efficacy of angiotensin-converting enzyme inhibition and aspirin counteraction. *Clin Pharmacol Ther* 63:79–86, 1998.

48. Balt JC, Mathy MJ, Pfaffendorf M, van Zwieten PA: Inhibition of angiotensin II-induced facilitation of sympathetic neurotransmission in the pithed rat: A comparison between losartan, irbesartan, telmisartan, and captopril. *J Hypertens* 19:465–473, 2001.

49. Lang CC, Stein M, He HB, et al: Angiotensin-converting enzyme inhibition and sympathetic activity in healthy subjects. *Clin Pharmacol Ther* 59:668–674, 1996.

50. Ranadive SA, Chen AX, Serajuddin AT: Relative lipophilicities and structural-pharmacological considerations of various angiotensin-converting enzyme (ACE) inhibitors. *Pharm Res* 9:1480–1486, 1992.

51. Gohlke P, Weiss S, Jansen A, et al: AT1 receptor antagonist telmisartan administered peripherally inhibits central responses to angiotensin II in conscious rats. *J Pharmacol Exp Ther* 298:62–70, 2001.

52. Culman J, von Heyer C, Piepenburg B, et al: Effects of systemic treatment with irbesartan and losartan on central responses to angiotensin II in conscious, normotensive rats. *Eur J Pharmacol* 367:255–265, 1999.

53. Krum H: Differentiation in the angiotensin II receptor 1 blocker class on autonomic function. *Curr Hypertens Rep* 3(Suppl 1):S17–S23, 2001.

54. Fagard R, Amery A, Reybrouck T, et al: Acute and chronic systemic and hemodynamic effects of angiotensin-converting enzyme inhibition with captopril in hypertensive patients. *Am J Cardiol* 46:295–300, 1980.

55. Yee KM, Struthers AD: Endogenous angiotensin II and baroreceptor dysfunction: A comparative study of losartan and enalapril in man. *Br J Clin Pharmacol* 46:583–588, 1998.

56. Vanhoutte PM: Endothelial dysfunction and inhibition of converting enzyme. *Eur Heart J* 19(Supple J):J7–J15, 1998.

57. Schiffrin EL, Park JB, Pu Q: Effect of crossing over hypertensive patients from a beta-blocker to an angiotensin receptor antagonist on resistance artery structure and on endothelial function. *J Hypertens* 20:71–78, 2002.

58. Schiffrin EL: Effects of antihypertensive drugs on vascular remodeling: Do they predict outcome in response to antihypertensive therapy? *Curr Opin Nephrol Hypertens* 10:617–624, 2001.

59. Oparil S, Guthrie R, Lewin AJ, et al: An elective-titration study of the comparative effectiveness of two angiotensin II-receptor blockers, irbesartan and losartan. Irbesartan/Losartan Study Investigators. *Clin Ther* 20:398–409, 1998.

60. Souza Dos Santos RA, Passaglio KT, Pesquero JB, et al: Interactions between angiotensin-(1–7), kinins, and angiotensin II in kidney and blood vessels. *Hypertension* 38:660–664, 2001.

61. Chappell MC, Allred AJ, Ferrario CM: Pathways of angiotensin-(1–7) metabolism in the kidney. *Nephrol Dial Transplant* 16(Suppl 1):22–26, 2001.

62. Santos RA, Campagnole-Santos MJ, Andrade SP: Angiotensin-(1–7): An update. *Regul Pept* 91:45–62, 2000.

63. White CM: Pharmacologic, pharmacokinetic, and therapeutic differences among ACE inhibitors. *Pharmacotherapy* 18:588–599, 1998.

64. Cody R: Optimizing ACE inhibitor therapy of congestive heart failure: Insights from pharmacodynamic studies. *Clin Pharmacokinet* 24:59–70, 1993.

65. Dickstein K: Pharmacokinetics of enalapril in congestive heart failure. *Drugs* 32(Suppl 5):40–44, 1986.

66. Herman AG: Differences in structure of angiotensin-converting enzyme inhibitors might predict differences in action. *Am J Cardiol* 70:102C–108C, 1992.

67. Salvetti A: Newer ACE inhibitors: A look at the future. *Drugs* 40:800–828, 1990.

68. Zusman RM: Effects of converting-enzyme inhibitors on the renin-angiotensin-aldosterone, bradykinin, and arachidonic acid-prostaglandin systems: Correlation of chemical structure and biological activity. *Am J Kidney Dis* 10(Suppl 1):13–23, 1987.

69. Chalmers D, Whitehead A, Lawson DH: Postmarketing surveillance of captopril for hypertension. *Br J Clin Pharmacol* 34:215–223, 1992.

70. Punzi HD: Safety update: Focus on cough. *Am J Cardiol* 72:45H–48H, 1993.

71. Sharif MN, Evans BL, Pylypchuk GB: Cough induced by quinapril with resolution after changing to fosinopril. *Ann Pharmacother* 28:720–722, 1994.

72. Zusman RM: Angiotensin-converting enzyme inhibitors: More different than alike? *Am J Cardiol* 72:25H–36H, 1993.

73. Zusman RM, Christensen DM, Higgins J, Boucher CA: Effects of fosinopril on cardiac function in patients with hypertension. Radionuclide assessment of left ventricular systolic and diastolic performance. *Am J Hypertens* 5:219–223, 1992.

74. Sica DA: Angiotensin-converting enzyme inhibitors: Fosinopril. In: Messerli F, ed. *Cardiovascular Drug Therapy.* 2d ed. Philadelphia: WB Saunders 1996:801–809.

75. Brockmeier D: Tight binding influencing the future of pharmacokinetics. *Methods Find Exp Clin Pharmacol* 20:505–516, 1998.

76. Reid JL: From kinetics to dynamics: Are there differences between ACE inhibitors? *Eur Heart J* 18(Suppl E):E14–E18, 1997.

77. Hoyer J, Schulte K-L, Lenz T: Clinical pharmacokinetics of angiotensin-converting enzyme inhibitors in renal failure. *Clin Pharmacokinet* 24:230–254, 1993.

78. Dzau VJ, Bernstein K, Celermajer D, et al: The relevance of tissue angiotensin-converting enzyme: Manifestations in mechanistic and end-point data. *Am J Cardiol* 88(Suppl 9):1L–20L, 2001.

79. Sica DA: Kinetics of angiotensin-converting enzyme inhibitors in renal failure. *J Cardiovasc Pharmacol* 20(Supp 10):S13–S20, 1992.

80. Ebihara A, Fujimura A: Metabolites of antihypertensive drugs. An updated review of their clinical pharmacokinetic and therapeutic implications. *Clin Pharmacokinet* 21:331–343, 1991.

81. Kelly JG, Doyle GD, Carmody M, et al: Pharmacokinetics of lisinopril, enalapril and enalaprilat in renal failure: Effects of haemodialysis. *Br J Clin Pharmacol* 26:781–786, 1988.

82. Schunkert H, Kindler J, Gassmann M, et al: Pharmacokinetics of ramipril in hypertensive patients with renal insufficiency. *Eur J Clin Pharmacol* 37:249–256, 1989.

83. Hui KK, Duchin KL, Kripalani KJ, et al: Pharmacokinetics of fosinopril in patients with various degrees of renal function. *Clin Pharmacol Ther* 49:457–467, 1991.

84. Danielson B, Querin S, LaRochelle P, et al: Pharmacokinetics and pharmacodynamics of trandolapril after repeated administration of 2 mg to patients with chronic renal failure and healthy control subjects. *J Cardiovasc Pharmacol* 23(Suppl 4):S50–S59, 1994.

85. Kaiser G, Ackermann R, Sioufi A: Pharmacokinetics of a new angiotensin-converting enzyme inhibitor, benazepril hydrochloride, in special populations. *Am Heart J* 117:746–751, 1989.

86. Noormohamed FH, McNabb WR, Lant AF: Pharmacokinetic and pharmacodynamic actions of enalapril in humans: Effect of probenecid pretreatment. *J Pharmacol Exp Ther* 253:362–368, 1990.

87. Lin JH, Chen IW, Ulm EH, Duggan DE: Differential renal handling of angiotensin-converting enzyme inhibitors enalaprilat and lisinopril in rats. *Drug Metab Dispos* 16:392–396, 1998.

88. Sica DA, Cutler RE, Parmer RJ, et al: Comparison of the steady-state pharmacokinetics of fosinopril, lisinopril, and enalapril in patients with chronic renal insufficiency. *Clin Pharmacokinet* 20:420–427, 1991.

89. Greenbaum R, Zucchelli P, Caspi A, et al: Comparison of the pharmacokinetics of fosinoprilat with enalaprilat and lisinopril in patients with congestive heart failure and chronic renal insufficiency. *Br J Clin Pharmacol* 49:23–31, 2000.

90. Sica DA, Deedwania PC: Renal considerations in the use of angiotensin-converting enzyme inhibitors in the treatment of congestive heart failure. *Cong Heart Fail* 3:54–59, 1997.

91. Brown NJ, Vaughn DE: Angiotensin-converting enzyme inhibitors. *Circulation* 97:1411–1420, 1998.

92. Fabris B, Jackson B, Kohzuki M, et al: Increased cardiac angiotensin-converting enzyme in rats with chronic heart failure. *Clin Exp Pharmacol Physiol* 17:309–314, 1990.

93. Johnston CI, Fabris B, Yamada H, et al: Comparative studies of tissue inhibition by angiotensin-converting enzyme inhibitors. *J Hypertens* 7(Suppl):S11–S16, 1989.

94. Fabris B, Chen BZ, Pupic V, et al: Inhibition of angiotensin-converting enzyme (ACE) in plasma and tissue. *J Cardiovasc Pharmacol* 15(Suppl 2):S6–S13, 1990.

95. Opie LH: ACE Inhibitors: Specific agents and pharmacokinetics. In: Opie LH, ed. *Angiotensin-Converting Enzyme Inhibitors: Scientific Basis for Clinical Use.* New York: Authors' Publishing House, 1994:171–247.

96. Jackson EK, Garrison JC: Renin and angiotensin. In: Hardman JG, Limbird L, eds. *Goodman & Gilman's The Pharmacological Basis of Therapeutics.* New York: McGraw-Hill, 1999:743–746.

97. Johnston CI, Fabris B, Yoshida K: The cardiac renin-angiotensin system in heart failure. *Am Heart J* 126:756–760, 1993.

98. Fabris B, Yamada H, Cubela R, et al: Characterization of cardiac angiotensin-converting enzyme and in vivo inhibition following oral quinapril to rats. *Br J Pharmacol* 100:651–655, 1990.

99. Kinoshita A, Urata H, Bumpus FM, Husain A: Measurement of angiotensin I-converting enzyme inhibition in the heart. *Circ Res* 73:51–60, 1993.

100. Leonetti G, Cuspidi C: Choosing the right ACE inhibitor. A guide to selection. *Drugs* 49:516–535, 1995.

101. Ruddy MC, Kostis JB, Frishman WH: Drugs that affect the renin-angiotensin system. In: Frishman W, Sonnenblick E, eds. *Cardiovascular Pharmacotherapeutics.* New York: McGraw-Hill, 1998:131–192.

102. Briscoe TA, Dearing CJ: Clinical and economic effects of replacing enalapril with benazepril in hypertensive patients. *Am J Health Syst Pharm* 53:2191–2193, 1996.

103. The SOLVD investigators. Effect of enalapril on survival in patients with reduced left ventricular ejection fractions and congestive heart failure. *N Engl J Med* 325:293–302, 1991.

104. Lewis EJ, Hunsicker LG, Bain RP, Rohde RD: The effect of angiotensin-converting enzyme inhibition on diabetic nephropathy. The Collaborative Study Group. *N Engl J Med* 329:1456–1462, 1993.

105. Sica DA: The HOPE Study: ACE inhibitors — are their benefits a class effect or do individual agents differ? *Curr Opin Nephrol Hypertens* 10:597–601, 2001.

106. Jafar TH, Stark PC, Schmid CH, et al: Proteinuria as a modifiable risk factor for the progression of non-diabetic renal disease. *Kidney Int* 60:1131–1140, 2001.

107. Wilson Tang WH, Vagelos RH, et al: Neurohormonal and clinical responses to high- versus low-dose enalapril therapy in chronic heart failure. *J Am Coll Cardiol* 39:70–78, 2002.

108. Packer M, Poole-Wilson PA, Armstrong PW, et al: Comparative effects of low and high doses of the angiotensin-converting enzyme inhibitor, lisinopril, on morbidity and mortality in chronic heart failure. ATLAS Study Group. *Circulation* 100:2312–2318, 1999.

109. Massie B: Neurohormonal blockade in chronic heart failure. How much is enough? Can there be too much? *J Am Coll Cardiol* 39:79–82, 2002.

110. Tang WH, Vagelos RH, Yee YG, et al: Neurohormonal and clinical responses to high- versus low-dose enalapril therapy in chronic heart failure. *J Am Coll Cardiol* 39:70–78, 2002.

111. Van Veldhuisen DJ, Genth-Zotz S, Brouwer J, et al: High- versus low-dose ACE inhibition in chronic heart failure. A double-blind, placebo-controlled study of imidapril. *J Am Coll Cardiol* 32:1811–1818, 1998.

112. The American College of Cardiology/American Heart Association Task Force on Practical Guidelines (Committee on Evaluation and Management of Heart Failure) Guidelines for the evaluation and management of heart failure. *Circulation* 92:2764–2784, 1995.

113. Sica DA: Pharmacology and clinical efficacy of angiotensin-receptor blockers. *Am J Hypertens* 14:242S–247S, 2001.

114. Kassler-Taub K, Littlejohn T, Elliott W, et al: Comparative efficacy of two angiotensin II receptor antagonists, irbesartan and losartan, in mild-to-moderate hypertension. *Am J Hypertens* 11:445–453, 1998.

115. Oparil S, Guthrie R, Lewin AJ, et al: An elective-titration study of the comparative effectiveness of two angiotensin II-receptor blockers, irbesartan and losartan. *Clin Ther* 20:398–409, 1998.

116. Israili ZH: Clinical pharmacokinetics of angiotensin II (AT1) receptor blockers in hypertension. *J Hum Hypertens* 14(Suppl 1):S73–S86, 2000.

117. Atacand (candesartan cilexetil). Product information. Wilmington, DE: AstraZeneca; 1998.

118. Riddell JG: Bioavailability of candesartan is unaffected by food in healthy volunteers administered candesartan cilexetil. *J Hum Hypertens* 11(Suppl 2): S29–S30, 1997.

119. Tenero D, Martin D, Ilson B, et al: Pharmacokinetics of intravenously and orally administered eprosartan in healthy males: Absolute bioavailability and effect of food. *Biopharm Drug Disp* 19:351–356, 1998.

120. Cox PJ, Bush BD, Gorycki PD, et al: The metabolic fate of eprosartan in healthy volunteers. *Exp Toxicol Pathol* 48(Suppl II):75–82, 1996.

121. Bottorff MB, Tenero DM: Pharmacokinetics of eprosartan in healthy subjects, patients with hypertension, and special populations. *Pharmacotherapy* 19:73S–78S, 1999.

122. Chapelsky MC, Martin DE, Tenero DM, et al: A dose proportionality study if eprosartan in healthy male volunteers. *J Clin Pharmacol* 38:34–39, 1998.

123. Vachharajani NN, Shyu WC, Chando TJ, et al: Oral bioavailability and disposition characteristics of irbesartan, an angiotensin antagonist, in healthy volunteers. *J Clin Pharmacol* 38:702, 1998.

124. Vachharajani NN, Shyu WC, Mantha S, et al: Lack of effect of food on the oral bioavailability of irbesartan in healthy male volunteers. *J Clin Pharmacol* 38:433–436, 1998.

125. Lo MW, Goldberg MR, McCrea JB, et al: Pharmacokinetics of losartan, an angiotensin II receptor antagonist, and its active metabolite, EXP3174 in humans. *Clin Pharmacol Ther* 58:641–649, 1995.

126. Cozaar (losartan). Product information. West Point, PA: Merck & Co; 1995.

127. Laeis P, Puchler K, Kirch W: The pharmacokinetic and metabolic profile of olmesartan medoxomil limits the risk of clinically relevant drug interactions. *J Hypertens* 19(Suppl 1):S21–S32, 2001.

128. Mycardis (telmisartan). Product information. Ridgefield, CT: Boehringer Ingelheim Pharmaceuticals; 1998.

129. Stangier J, Schmid J, Turck D et al: Absorption, metabolism, and excretion of intravenously and orally administered [14C] telmisartan in healthy volunteers. *J Clin Pharmacol* 40:1312–1322, 2000.

130. Flesch G, Muller P, Lloyd P: Absolute bioavailability and pharmacokinetics of valsartan, an angiotensin II receptor antagonist, in man. *Eur J Clin Pharmacol* 52:115–120, 1997.

131. Diovan (valsartan). Product information. East Hanover, NJ: Novartis Pharmaceuticals; 1998.

132. Gillis JC, Markham A: Irbesartan. A review of its pharmacodynamic and pharmacokinetic properties and therapeutic use in the management of hypertension. *Drugs* 54:885–902, 1997.

133. Marino MR, Langenbacher K, Ford NF, et al: Pharmacokinetics and pharmacodynamics of irbesartan in healthy subjects. *J Clin Pharmacol* 38:246–255, 1998.

134. Ludden TM: Nonlinear pharmacokinetics: Clinical implications. *Clin Pharmacokinet* 20:429–446, 1991.

135. Lo MW, Goldberg MR, McCrea JB, et al: Pharmacokinetics of losartan, an angiotensin II receptor antagonist, and its active metabolite, EXP3174 in humans. *Clin Pharmacol Ther* 58:641–649, 1995.

136. Lo MW, Toh J, Emmert SE, et al: Pharmacokinetics of intravenous and oral losartan in patients with heart failure. *Clin Pharmacol Ther* 38:525–532, 1998.

137. van Lier JJ, Heiningen PNM, Sunzel M: Absorption, metabolism and excretion of 14C-candesartan and 14C-candesartan cilexetil in healthy volunteers. *J Hum Hypertens* 11(Suppl 2):S27–S28, 1997.

138. Criscione L, Bradley WA, Buylamayer P, et al: Valsartan: Preclinical and clinical profile of an antihypertensive angiotensin II antagonist. *Cardiovasc Drug Rev* 13:230–250, 1995.

139. Bergmann K, Laeis P, Puchler K, et al: Olmesartan medoxomil: Influence of age, renal and hepatic function on the pharmacokinetics of olmesartan medoxomil. *J Hypertens* 19(Suppl 1):S33–S40, 2001.

140. Christ DD: Human plasma protein binding of the angiotensin II receptor antagonist losartan potassium (DuP 753/MK 954) and its pharmacologically active metabolite EXP3174. *J Clin Pharmacol* 35:515–520, 1995.

141. Martin DE, Chapelsky MC, Ilson B, et al: Pharmacokinetics and protein binding of eprosartan in healthy volunteers and in patients with varying degrees of renal impairment. *J Clin Pharmacol* 38:129–137, 1998.

142. Colussi DM, Parisot C, Rossolino ML, et al: Protein binding of valsartan, a new angiotensin receptor antagonist. *J Clin Pharmacol* 37:214–221, 1997.

143. van Lier JJ, Heiningen PNM, Sunzel M: Absorption, metabolism and excretion of 14C-candesartan and 14C-candesartan cilexetil in healthy volunteers. *J Hum Hypertens* 11(Suppl 2):S27–S28, 1997.

144. Yun CH, Lee HS, Lee H, et al: Oxidation of the angiotensin II receptor antagonist losartan (DuP 753) in human liver microsomes; role of cytochrome P4503A (4) in formation of the active metabolite EXP3174. *Drug Metab Dispos* 23:285–289, 1995.

145. Stearns RA, Chakravarty PK, Chen R, et al: Biotransformation of losartan to its active carboxylic acid metabolite in human liver microsomes. Role of cytochrome P4502C and 3A subfamily members. *Drug Metab Dispos* 23:207–215, 1995.

146. McCrea JB, Cribb A, Rushmore T, et al: Phenotypic and genotypic investigations of a healthy volunteer deficient in the conversion of losartan to its active metabolite E-3174. *Clin Pharmacol Ther* 65:348–352, 1999.

147. Hubner R, Hogemann AM, Sunzel M, et al: Pharmacokinetics of candesartan after single and multiple doses of candesartan cilexetil in young and elderly healthy volunteers. *J Hum Hypertens* 11(Suppl 2):S19–S25, 1997.

148. Kazierad DJ, Martin DE, Blum RA, et al: Effect of fluconazole on the pharmacokinetics of eprosartan and losartan in healthy male volunteers. *Clin Pharmacol Ther* 62:417–425, 1997.

149. McCrea JB, Low MW, Furtek CI, et al: Ketoconazole does not effect the systemic conversion of losartan to E-3174. *Clin Pharmacol Ther* 59:A169, 1996.

150. Yasar U, Tybring G, Hidestrand M, et al: Role of CYP2C9 polymorphism in losartan oxidation. *Drug Metab Dispos* 29:1051–1056, 2001.

151. Zaidenstein R, Soback S, Gips M, et al: Effect of grapefruit juice on the pharmacokinetics of losartan and its active metabolite E3174 in healthy volunteers. *Ther Drug Monit* 23:369–373, 2001.

152. Chando TJ, Everett DW, Kahle AD, et al: Biotransformation of irbesartan in man. *Drug Metab Dispos* 26:408–417, 1998.

153. Marino MR, Hammett JL, Ferreira I, et al: Lack of effect of nifedipine on the pharmacokinetics of irbesartan in healthy male subjects (abstr.). *J Clin Pharmacol* 37:872, 1997.

154. de Zeeuw D, Remuzzi G, Kirch W: The pharmacokinetics of candesartan cilexetil in patients with renal or hepatic impairment. *J Hum Hypertens* 11(Suppl 2):S37–S42, 1997.

155. Sica DA, Shaw WC, Lo MW, et al: The pharmacokinetics of losartan in renal insufficiency. *J Hypertens* 13(Suppl 1):S49–S52, 1995.

156. Sica DA, Marino MR, Hammett JL, et al: The pharmacokinetics of irbesartan in renal failure and maintenance hemodialysis. *Clin Pharmacol Ther* 62:610–618, 1997.

157. Stangier J, Su CA, Brickl R, Franke H: Pharmacokinetics of single-dose telmisartan 120 mg given during and between hemodialysis in subjects with severe renal insufficiency: Comparison with healthy volunteers. *J Clin Pharmacol* 40:1365–1372, 2000.

158. Prasad P, Mangat S, Choi L, et al: Effect of renal function on the pharmacokinetics of valsartan. *Clin Drug Invest* 13:207–214, 1997.

159. Kovacs SJ, Tenero DM, Martin DE, et al: Pharmacokinetics and protein binding of eprosartan in hemodialysis-dependent patients with end-stage renal disease. *Pharmacotherapy* 19:612–619, 1999.

160. Martin DE, Chapelsky MC, Ilson B, et al: Pharmacokinetics and protein binding of eprosartan in healthy volunteers and in patients with varying degrees of renal impairment. *J Clin Pharmacol* 38:129–137, 1998.

161. Toto R, Shultz P, Jaij L, et al: Efficacy and tolerability of losartan in hypertensive patients with renal impairment. *Hypertension* 31:684–691, 1998.

162. Cooper M, Anzalone D, Townes L, et al: Safety and efficacy of irbesartan in patients with hypertension and renal insufficiency (abstr.). *Am J Hypertens* 11:102A, 1998.

163. De Rosa ML, de Cristofaro A, Rossi M, et al: Irbesartan effects on renal function in patients with renal impairment and hypertension: a drug-withdrawal study. *J Cardiovasc Pharmacol* 38:482–489, 2001.

164. Pedro P, Gehr TWB, Brophy D, Sica DA: The pharmacokinetics and pharmacodynamics of losartan in continuous ambulatory peritoneal dialysis. *J Clin Pharmacol* 40:389–395, 2000.

165. Saracho R, Martin-Malo A, Martinez I, et al: Evaluation of the losartan in hemodialysis (ELHE) study. *Kidney Int* 54(Suppl 68):S125–S129, 1998.

166. Tepel M, van der Giet M, Zidek W: Efficacy and tolerability of angiotensin II type 1 receptor antagonists in dialysis patients using AN69 dialysis membranes. *Kidney Blood Press Res* 24:71–74, 2001.

167. Sica DA, Gehr TW, Fernandez A: Risk-benefit ratio of angiotensin antagonists versus ACE inhibitors in end-stage renal disease. *Drug Saf* 22:350–360, 2000.

168. Brunner HR: The new angiotensin II receptor antagonist, irbesartan. Pharmacokinetic and pharmacodynamic considerations. *Am J Hypertens* 10:311S–317S, 1997.

169. Mazzolai L, Maillard M, Rossat J, et al: Angiotensin II receptor blockade in normotensive subjects. A direct comparison of three AT1-receptor antagonists. *Hypertension* 33:850–855, 1999.

170. Hodges JC, Hamby JM, Blankey CJ: Angiotensin II receptor binding inhibitors. *Drugs Fut* 17:575–593, 1992.

171. Dickinson KE, Cohen RB, Skwish S, et al: BMS 180560, an insurmountable inhibitor of angiotensin-II stimulated responses: Comparison with losartan and EXP-3174. *Br J Pharmacol* 113:179–189, 1994.

172. Liu YJ, Shankley NP, Welsh NJ, et al. Evidence that the apparent complexity of receptor antagonism by angiotensin II analogues is due to a reversible and syntopic action. *Br J Pharmacol* 106:233–241, 1992.

173. Ojima M, Inada Y, Shibouta Y, et al: Candesartan (CV-11974) dissociates slowly from the angiotensin AT1 receptor. *Eur J Pharmacol* 319:137–146, 1997.

174. McConnaughey MM, McConnaughey JS, Ingenito AJ: Practical considerations of the pharmacology of angiotensin receptor blockers. *J Clin Pharmacol* 39:547–559, 1998.

175. Hansson L: The relationship between dose and antihypertensive effect for different AT1-receptor blockers. *Blood Press Suppl* 3:33–39, 2001.

176. Maillard MP, Wurzner G, Nussberger J, et al: Comparative angiotensin II receptor blockade in healthy volunteers: The importance of dosing. *Clin Pharmacol Ther* 71:68–76, 2002.

177. Hollenberg NK: Renal implications of angiotensin receptor blockers. *Am J Hypertens* 14:237S–241S, 2001.

178. Hodsman GP, Isles CG, Murray GD, et al: Factors related to first-dose hypotensive effect of captopril: Prediction and treatment. *Br Med J* 286:832–834, 1983.

179. Muiesan G, Alicandri CL, Agabiti-Rosei E, et al: Angiotensin-converting enzyme inhibition, catecholamines, and hemodynamics in essential hypertension. *Am J Cardiol* 46:1420–1424, 1980.

180. Saragoca MA, Homsi E, Ribeiro AB, et al: Hemodynamic mechanism of blood pressure response to captopril in human malignant hypertension. *Hypertension* 5(Suppl I):53–59, 1983.

181. Magrini F, Shimizu M, Roberts N, et al: Converting-enzyme inhibition and coronary blood flow. *Circulation* 75:1168–1174, 1987.

182. Yusuf S, Lonn E: Anti-ischemic effects of ACE inhibitors: Review of current clinical evidence and ongoing clinical trials. *Eur Heart J* 19(Suppl J):J36–J44, 1998.

183. Pitt B: The role of ACE-inhibitors in patients with coronary artery disease. *Cardiovasc Drugs Ther* 15:103–105, 2001.

184. Waldemar G, Ibsen H, Strandgaard S, et al: The effect of fosinopril sodium on cerebral blood flow in moderate essential hypertension. *Am J Hypertens* 3:464–470, 1990.

185. Israili ZH, Hall WD: ACE Inhibitors: Differential use in elderly patients with hypertension. *Drugs Aging* 7:355–371, 1995.

186. Gradman AH, Cutler NR, Davis PJ, et al: Combined enalapril and felodipine extended release for systemic hypertension. Enalapril-Felodipine ER Factorial Study Group. *Am J Cardiol* 79:431–435, 1997.

186a. Messerli FH, Weir MR, Neutal JM: Combination therapy of amlodipine/benazepril versus monotherapy of amlodipine in a practice-based setting. *Am J Hypertens* 15:550, 2002.

187. Morioka S, Simon G, Cohn JN: Cardiac and hormonal effects of enalapril in hypertension. *Clin Pharmacol Ther* 34:583–589, 1988.

188. Omvik P, Lund-Johansen P: Combined captopril and hydrochlorothiazide therapy in severe hypertension: Long-term haemodynamic changes at rest and during exercise. *J Hypertens* 2:73–80, 1984.

189. Hollenberg N, Raij L: Angiotensin-converting enzyme inhibition and renal protection. *Arch Intern Med* 153:2426–2435, 1993.

190. Toto RD, Mitchell HC, Lee HC, et al: Reversible renal insufficiency due to angiotensin-converting enzyme inhibitors in hypertensive nephrosclerosis. *Ann Intern Med* 115:513–519, 1991.

191. Siegel D, Lopez J, Meier J: Pharmacologic treatment of hypertension in the Department of Veterans Affairs during 1995 and 1996. *Am J Hypertens* 11:1271–1278, 1998.

192. Doyle JC, Mottram DR, Stubbs H: Prescribing of ACE inhibitors for cardiovascular disorders in general practice. *J Clin Pharm Ther* 23:133–136, 1998.

193. Sica DA: Old antihypertensive agents—diuretics and beta-blockers: Do we know how and in whom they reduce blood pressure? *Curr Hypertens Rep* 1:296–304, 1999.

194. Materson BJ, Reda DJ, Cushman WC, et al: Single-drug therapy for hypertension in men. A comparison of six antihypertensive agents with placebo. *N Engl J Med* 328:914–921, 1993.

195. Elliott WJ: Therapeutic trials comparing angiotensin-converting enzyme inhibitors and angiotensin II receptor blockers. *Curr Hypertens Rep* 2:402–411, 2000.

196. Caro JJ, Speckman JL, Salas M, et al: Effect of initial drug choice on persistence with antihypertensive therapy: The importance of actual practice data. *CMAJ* 160:41–46, 1999.

197. Mazzolai L, Burnier M: Comparative safety and tolerability of angiotensin II receptor antagonists. *Drug Saf* 21:23–33, 1999.

198. Brenner BM, Cooper ME, de Zeeuw D, et al: Effects of losartan on renal and cardiovascular outcomes in patients with type 2 diabetes and nephropathy. *N Engl J Med* 345:861–869, 2001.

199. Lewis EJ, Hunsicker LG, Clarke WR, et al: Renoprotective effect of the angiotensin-receptor antagonist irbesartan in patients with nephropathy due to type 2 diabetes. *N Engl J Med* 345:851–860, 2001.

200. Halkin A, Keren G: Potential indications for angiotensin-converting enzyme inhibitors in atherosclerotic vascular disease. *Am J Med* 112:126–134, 2002.

201. Hansson L, Lindholm L, Niskanen L, et al: Effect of angiotensin-converting-enzyme inhibition compared with conventional therapy on cardiovascular morbidity and mortality in hypertension: The Captopril Prevention Project (CAPPP) randomised trial. *Lancet* 353:611–616, 1999.

202. UK Prospective Diabetes Study Group. Efficacy of atenolol and captopril in reducing risk of macrovascular and microvascular complications in Type II diabetes. *BMJ* 317:713–720, 1998.

203. Smith RD, Franklin SS: Comparison of effects of enalapril plus hydrochlorothiazide versus standard triple therapy on renal function in renovascular hypertension. *Am J Med* 79(Suppl 3C):14–23, 1985.

204. Maillard JO, Descombes E, Fellay G, Regamey C: Repeated transient anuria following losartan administration in a patient with a solitary kidney. *Ren Fail* 23:143–147, 2001.

205. Flack JM, Saunders E, Gradman A, et al: Antihypertensive efficacy and safety of losartan alone and in combination with hydrochlorothiazide in adult African Americans with mild to moderate hypertension. *Clin Ther* 23:1193–1208, 2001.

206. Weidmann P, De Myttenaere-Bursztein S, Maxwell MH: Effect of aging on plasma renin and aldosterone in normal man. *Kidney Int* 8:325–333, 1975.

207. Sica DA: The importance of the sympathetic nervous system and systolic hypertension in patients with hypertension: Benefits in treating patients with increased cardiovascular risk. *Blood Press Monit* 5(Suppl 2):S19–S25, 2000.

208. Weinberger MH: Blood pressure and metabolic responses to hydrochlorothiazide, captopril, and the combination in black and white mild-to-moderate hypertensive patients. *J Cardiovasc Pharmacol* 7(Suppl 1):52–55, 1985.

209. Weir MR, Gray JM, Paster R, et al: Differing mechanisms of action of angiotensin-converting enzyme inhibition in black and white hypertensive patients. *Hypertension* 25:124–130, 1995.

210. Agodoa LY, Appel L, Bakris GL, et al: Effect of ramipril vs amlodipine on renal outcomes in hypertensive nephrosclerosis: A randomized controlled trial. *JAMA* 285:2719–2728, 2001.

211. 1999 World Health Organization-International Society of Hypertension Guidelines for the Management of Hypertension. Guidelines Subcommittee. *J Hypertens* 17:151–183, 1999.

212. Zannad F: Trandolapril: how does it differ from other angiotensin-converting enzyme inhibitors? *Drugs* 46(Suppl 2):172–182, 1993.

213. Omboni S, Fogari R, Palatini P, et al: Reproducibility and clinical value of the trough-to-peak ratio of the antihypertensive effect. Evidence from the Sample Study. *Hypertension* 32:424–429, 1998.

214. Sica DA, Gehr TWB: Dose-response relationship and dose adjustments. In: Izzo JL, Black HR, eds. *Hypertension Primer.* 2d ed. Baltimore, MD: Lippincott, Williams & Wilkins, 1999:342–344.

215. Gradman AH, Lewin A, Bowling BT, et al: Comparative effects of candesartan cilexetil and losartan in patients with systemic hypertension. Candesartan Versus Losartan Efficacy Comparison (CANDLE) Study Group. *Heart Dis* 1:52–57, 1999.

216. Mancia G, Dell'Oro R, Turri C, Grassi G: Comparison of angiotensin II receptor blockers: Impact of missed doses of candesartan cilexetil and losartan in systemic hypertension. *Am J Cardiol* 84:28S–34S, 1999.

217. Oparil S, Williams D, Chrysant SG, et al: Comparative efficacy of olmesartan, losartan, valsartan, and irbesartan in the control of essential hypertension. *J Clin Hypertens* 3:283–291, 2001.

218. Vidt DG, White WB, Ripley E, et al: A forced titration study of antihypertensive efficacy of candesartan cilexetil in comparison to losartan: CLAIM Study II. *J Hum Hypertens* 15:475–480, 2001.

219. Meredith PA: Clinical comparative trials of angiotensin II type 1 (AT1)-receptor blockers. *Blood Press Suppl* 3:11–17, 2001.

220. Oparil S: Are there meaningful differences in blood pressure control with current antihypertensive agents? *Am J Hypertens* 15:14S–21S, 2002.

221. Conlin PR, Spence JD, Williams B, et al: Angiotensin II antagonists for hypertension: Are there differences in efficacy? *Am J Hypertens* 13:418–26, 2000.

222. Fogari R, Mugellini A, Zoppi A, et al: A double-blind crossover study of the antihypertensive efficacy of angiotensin II-receptor antagonists and their activation of the renin-angiotensin system. *Curr Ther Res Clin Exp* 61:669–679, 2000.

223. Hansson L: The relationship between dose and antihypertensive effect for different AT1-receptor blockers. *Blood Press Suppl* 3:33–39, 2001.

224. Veteran's Administration Cooperative Study Group on Antihypertensive Agents. Low-dose captopril for the treatment of mild to moderate hypertension. *Hypertension* 5(Suppl III):139–144, 1983.

225. Neutel JM, Black HR, Weber MA: Combination therapy with diuretics: An evolution of understanding. *Am J Med* 101:61S–70S, 1996.

226. Sica DA: Rationale for fixed-dose combinations in the treatment of hypertension: The cycle repeats. *Drugs* 62:443–462, 2002.

227. Veteran Administration Cooperative Study Group on Antihypertensive Agents. Racial differences in response to low-dose captopril are abolished by the addition of hydrochlorothiazide. *Br J Clin Pharmacol* 14:97S–101S, 1982.

228. Hansson L: Beta blockers with ACE inhibitors—a logical combination? *J Hum Hypertens* 3:97–100, 1989.

229. Belz GG, Essig J, Erb K, et al: Pharmacokinetic and pharmacodynamic interactions between the ACE inhibitor cilazapril and beta-adrenoreceptor antagonist propranolol in healthy subjects and in hypertensive patients. *Br J Clin Pharmacol* 27(Suppl 2):317S–322S, 1989.

230. Black HR, Sollins JS, Garofalo JL: The addition of doxazosin to the therapeutic regimen of hypertensive patients inadequately controlled with other antihypertensive medications: A randomized, placebo-controlled study. *Am J Hypertens* 13:468–474, 2000.

231. Sica DA: Doxazosin and congestive heart failure. *Congest Heart Fail* 8:178, 2002.

232. Frishman WH, Ram CV, McMahon FG, et al., for the Benazepril/-Amlodipine Study Group. Comparison of amlodipine and benazepril monotherapy to amlodipine plus benazepril in patients with systemic hypertension: A randomized, double-blind, placebo-controlled, parallel-group study. *J Clin Pharmacol* 35:1060–1066, 1995.

233. DeQuattro V, Lee D: Fixed-dose combination therapy with trandolapril and verapamil SR is effective in primary hypertension. *Am J Hypertens* 10(Suppl 2):138S–145S, 1997.

234. Pool J, Kaihlanen P, Lewis G, et al: Once-daily treatment of patients with hypertension: A placebo-controlled study of amlodipine and benazepril vs amlodipine or benazepril alone. *J Hum Hypertens* 15:495–498, 2001.

235. Schulte KL, Fischer M, Meyer-Sabellak W: Efficacy and tolerability of candesartan cilexetil monotherapy or in combination with other antihypertensive drugs. Results of the AURA study. *Clin Drug Invest* 18:453–460, 1999.

236. Azizi M, Guyene TT, Chatellier G, et al: Additive effects of losartan and enalapril on blood pressure and plasma active renin. *Hypertension* 29:634–640, 1997.

237. Azizi M, Linhart A, Alexander J, et al: Pilot study of combined blockade of the renin-angiotensin system in essential hypertensive patients. *J Hypertens* 18:1139–1147, 2000.

238. Weir MR, Weber MA, Neutel JM, et al: Efficacy of candesartan cilexetil as add-on therapy in hypertensive patients uncontrolled on background therapy: A clinical experience trial. ACTION Study Investigators. *Am J Hypertens* 14:567–572, 2001.

239. Stergiou GS, Skeva II, Baibas NM, et al: Additive hypotensive effect of angiotensin-converting enzyme inhibition and angiotensin-receptor antagonism in essential hypertension. *J Cardiovasc Pharmacol* 35:937–941, 2000.

240. Taylor AA: Is there a place for combining angiotensin-converting enzyme inhibitors and angiotensin-receptor antagonists in the treatment of hypertension, renal disease or congestive heart failure? *Curr Opin Nephrol Hypertens* 10:643–648, 2001.

240a. Sica DA, Elliott WJ: Angiotensin-converting enzyme inhibitors and angiotensin receptor blockers in combination: Theory and practice. *J Clin Hypertens* 3:383, 2001.

241. Bevan EG, Pringle SD, Walker PC, et al: Comparison of captopril, hydralazine and nifedipine as third drug in hypertensive patients. *J Hum Hypertens* 7:83–88, 1993.

242. Dufloux JJ, Prasquier R, Chatellier G, et al: Effects of captopril and minoxidil on left ventricular hypertrophy in resistant hypertensive patients: A 6-month double-blind comparison. *J Am Coll Cardiol* 16:137–142, 1990.

243. Damasceno A, Ferreira B, Patel S, et al: Efficacy of captopril and nifedipine in black and white patients with hypertensive crisis. *J Hum Hypertens* 11:471–476, 1997.

244. Hirschl MM, Binder M, Bur A, et al: Impact of the renin-angiotensin-aldosterone system on blood pressure response to intravenous enalaprilat in patients with hypertensive crises. *J Hum Hypertens* 11:177–183, 1997.

245. Sica DA: Dosage considerations with perindopril for hypertension. *Am J Cardiol* 88(Suppl 1):13–18, 2001.

246. Schlaich MP, Schmieder RE: Left ventricular hypertrophy and its regression: Pathophysiology and therapeutic approach. *Am J Hypertens* 11:1394–1404, 1998.

247. Dahlöf B, Pennert K, Hansson L: Reversal of left ventricular hypertrophy in hypertensive patients. Meta-analysis of 109 treatment studies. *Am J Hypertens* 5:95–110, 1992.

248. Schmieder RE, Martus P, Klingbeil A, et al: Reversal of left ventricular hypertrophy in essential hypertension. A meta-analysis of randomized double-blind studies. *JAMA* 275:1507–1513, 1996.

249. Gottdiener JS, Reda DJ, Massie BM, et al., for the VA Cooperative Study Group on Antihypertensive Agents. Effect of single-drug therapy on reduction of left ventricular mass in mild to moderate hypertension. Comparison of six antihypertensive agents. *Circulation* 95:2007–2014, 1997.

250. Dahlof B: Left ventricular hypertrophy and angiotensin II antagonists. *Am J Hypertens* 14:174–182, 2001.

250a. Dahlof B, Devereux RB, Kjeldsen SE, et al: Cardiovascular morbidity and mortality in the Losartan Intervention for Endpoint reduction in hypertension study (LIFE): A randomised trial against atenolol. *Lancet* 359:995, 2002.

251. Koren MJ, Devereux RB, Casale PN, et al: Relation of left ventricular mass and geometry to morbidity and mortality in uncomplicated essential hypertension. *Ann Intern Med* 114:345–352, 1991.

252. Lindholm LH, Ibsen H, Dahlof B, et al: Cardiovascular morbidity and mortality in patients with diabetes in the Losartan Intervention for Endpoint reduction in hypertension study (LIFE): A randomised trial against atenolol *Lancet* 359:1004, 2002.

253. Daly P, Mettauer B, Rouleau JL, et al: Lack of reflex increase in myocardial sympathetic tone after captopril: Potential antianginal mechanism. *Circulation* 71:317–325, 1985.

254. Chrysant SG: Vascular remodeling: The role of angiotensin-converting enzyme inhibitors. *Am Heart J* 135:S21–30, 1998.

255. Schiffrin EL, Park JB, Pu Q: Effect of crossing over hypertensive patients from a beta-blocker to an angiotensin receptor antagonist on resistance artery structure and on endothelial function. *J Hypertens* 20:71–78, 2002.

256. Frei A, Muller-Brand J: Cerebral blood flow and antihypertensive treatment with enalapril. *J Hypertens* 4:365–368, 1986.

257. Roberts DH, Tsao Y, McLoughlin GA, et al: Placebo-controlled comparison of captopril, atenolol, labetalol, and pindolol in hypertension complicated by intermittent claudication. *Lancet* 2:650–653, 1987.

258. Regensteiner JG, Hiatt WR: Current medical therapies for patients with peripheral arterial disease: A critical review. *Am J Med* 112:49–57, 2002.

258a. Wright JT: The AASK Trial. Presented at the American Society of Hypertension 17th Annual Scientific Meeting. New York: NY, May 14–18, 2002.

259. Preston RA: Renoprotective effects of antihypertensive drugs. *Am J Hypertens* 12:19S–32S, 1999.

260. Sica DA, Bakris GL: Current concepts of pharmacotherapy in hypertension: Type 2 diabetes: RENAAL and IDNT—the emergence of new treatment options. *J Clin Hypertens* 4:52–57, 2002.

261. Malini P, Stochi E, Ambrosioni E, et al: Long-term antihypertensive, metabolic and cellular effects of enalapril. *J Hypertens* 2(Suppl 2):101–105, 1984.

262. Lithell HO, Pollare T, Berne C: Insulin sensitivity in newly detected hypertensive patients: Influence of captopril and other antihypertensive agents on insulin sensitivity and related biological parameters. *J Cardiovasc Pharmacol* 15(Suppl 5):S46–S52, 1990.

263. Tillmann HC, Walker RJ, Lewis-Barned NJ, et al: A long-term comparison between enalapril and captopril on insulin sensitivity in normotensive non-insulin dependent diabetic volunteers. *J Clin Pharmacol Ther* 22:273–278, 1997.

264. Julius S, Majahalme S, Palatini P: Antihypertensive treatment of patients with diabetes and hypertension. *Am J Hypertens* 14:310S–316S, 2001.

265. Yusuf S, Gerstein H, Hoogwerf B, et al: Ramipril and the development of diabetes. *JAMA* 286:1882–1885, 2001.

266. Sacco RL: Reducing the risk of stroke in diabetes: What have we learned that is new? *Diabetes Obes Metab* 4(Suppl 1):27–34, 2002.

267. Randomised trial of a perindopril-based blood-pressure-lowering regimen among 6,105 individuals with previous stroke or transient ischaemic attack. *Lancet* 358:1033–1041, 2001.

267a. Bosch J, Yusuf S, Pogue J, et al: Use of ramipril in preventing stroke: Double blind randomised trial. *BMJ* 324:699, 2002.

268. Svensson P, de Faire U, Sleight P, et al: Comparative effects of ramipril on ambulatory and office blood pressures: A HOPE substudy. *Hypertension* 38:E28–E32, 2001.

269. Goldstein LB, Adams R, Becker K, et al: Primary prevention of ischemic stroke: A statement for healthcare professionals from the Stroke Council of the American Heart Association. *Stroke* 32:280–299, 2001.

269a. Sever P: The SCOPE trial. *J Renin-Angiotensin-Aldosterone System* 3:2, 2002.

270. Parving HH, Lehnert H, Brochner-Mortensen J, et al: The effect of irbesartan on the development of diabetic nephropathy in patients with type 2 diabetes. *N Engl J Med* 345:870–878, 2001.

271. Keane WF: Proteinuria: Its clinical importance and role in progressive renal disease. *Am J Kidney Dis* 35(Suppl 1):S97–S105, 2000.

272. Keane WF, Eknoyan G: Proteinuria, albuminuria, risk, assessment, detection, elimination (PARADE): A position paper of the National Kidney Foundation. *Am J Kidney Dis* 33:1004–1010, 1999.

273. Lewis EJ, Hunsicker LG, Bain RP, Rohde RD: The effect of angiotensin-converting-enzyme inhibition on diabetic nephropathy: The Collaborative Study Group. *N Engl J Med* 329:1456–1462, 1993.

274. Ravid M, Lang R, Rachmani R, et al: Long-term renoprotective effect of angiotensin-converting enzyme inhibition in non-insulin dependent diabetes mellitus. A 7-year follow-up study. *Arch Intern Med* 156:286–289, 1996.

275. Viberti G, Mogensen CE, Groop LC, Pauls JF: Effect of captopril on progression to clinical proteinuria in patients with insulin-dependent diabetes mellitus and microalbuminuria: European Microalbuminuria Captopril Study Group. *JAMA* 271:275–279, 1994.

276. Maschio G, Alberti D, Janin G, et al: Effect of the angiotensin-converting enzyme inhibitor benazepril on the progression of chronic renal insufficiency. *N Engl J Med* 334:939–945, 1996.

277. Uhle BU, Whitworth JA, Shahinfar S, et al: Angiotensin-converting enzyme inhibition in nondiabetic progressive renal insufficiency: A controlled double-blind trial. *Am J Kidney Dis* 27:489–495, 1996.

278. The Gisen Group: Randomized placebo-controlled trial of effect of ramipril on decline in glomerular filtration rate and risk of terminal renal failure in proteinuric, non-diabetic nephropathy. *Lancet* 349:1857–1863, 1997.

279. Giatras I, Lau J, Levey As, et al., for the Angiotensin-Converting Enzyme Inhibition and Progressive Renal Disease Study Group. Effect of angiotensin-converting enzyme inhibitors on the progression of nondiabetic renal disease: A meta-analysis of randomized trials. *Ann Intern Med* 127:337–347, 1997.

280. Ruggenenti P, Perna A, Gherardi G, et al: Chronic proteinuric nephropathies: Outcomes and response to treatment in a prospective cohort of 352 patients with different patterns of renal injury. *Am J Kidney Dis* 35:1155–1165, 2000.

281. Ahmad J, Siddiqui MA, Ahmad H: Effective postponement of diabetic nephropathy with enalapril in normotensive type 2 diabetic patients with microalbuminuria. *Diabetes Care* 20:1576–1581, 1997.

282. Ravid M, Savin H, Jutrin I, et al: Long-term stabilizing effect of angiotensin-converting enzyme inhibition on plasma creatinine and on proteinuria in normotensive type II diabetic patients. *Ann Intern Med* 118:577–581, 1993.

283. Mathiesen ER, Hommel E, Giese J, Parving H: Efficacy of captopril in postponing nephropathy in normotensive insulin dependent diabetic patients with microalbuminuria. *BMJ* 303:81–87, 1991.

284. The EUCLID Study Group. Randomized placebo-controlled trial of lisinopril in normotensive patients with insulin-dependent diabetes and normoalbuminuria and microalbuminuria. *Lancet* 349:1787–1792, 1997.

285. Sano T, Kawamura T, Matsumae H, et al: Effects of long-term enalapril treatment on persistent microalbuminuria in well-controlled hypertensive and normotensive NIDDM patients. *Diabetes Care* 17:420–424, 1994.

286. Ravid M, Brosh D, Levi Z, et al: Use of enalapril to attenuate decline in renal function in normotensive, normoalbuminuric patients with type 2 diabetes mellitus. *Ann Intern Med* 128:982–988, 1998.

287. Wheeldon NM, Viberti G, for the MARVAL Trial. Microalbuminuria reduction with valsartan (abstr.). *Am J Hypertens* 14:0–6, 2001.

288. Lebovitz HE, Wiegmann TB, Cnaan A, et al: Renal protective effect of enalapril in hypertensive NIDDM: Role of baseline albuminuria. *Kidney Int* 45(Suppl):S150–S155, 1994.

289. Fogari R, Zoppi A, Corradi L, et al: Long-term effects of ramipril and nitrendipine on albuminuria in hypertensive patients with type II diabetes and impaired renal function. *J Hum Hypertens* 13:47–53, 1999.

290. Bakris GL, Copley JB, Vicknair N, et al: Calcium channel blockers versus other antihypertensive therapies on progression of NIDDM associated nephropathy. *Kidney Int* 50:1641–1650, 1996.

291. Nielsen FS, Rossing P, Gall MA, et al: Long-term effect of lisinopril and atenolol on kidney function in hypertensive NIDDM subjects with diabetic nephropathy. *Diabetes* 46:1182–1188, 1997.

292. UK Prospective Diabetes Study Group. Tight blood pressure control and risk of macrovascular and microvascular complications in type 2 diabetes: UKPDS 38. UK Prospective Diabetes Study Group. *BMJ* 317:703–713, 1998.

293. Estacio RO, Jeffers BW, Gifford N, Schrier RW: Effect of blood pressure control on diabetic microvascular complications in patients with hypertension and type 2 diabetes. *Diabetes Care* 23(Suppl 2):B54–B64, 2000.

294. Mann JF, Gerstein HC, Pogue J, et al: Renal insufficiency as a predictor of cardiovascular outcomes and the impact of ramipril: The HOPE randomized trial. *Ann Intern Med* 134:629–636, 2001.

295. Zatz R, Dunn BR, Meyer TW, et al: Prevention of diabetic glomerulopathy by pharmacological amelioration of glomerular capillary hypertension. *J Clin Invest* 77:1925–1930, 1986.

296. Bakris GL, Weir MR: Angiotensin-converting enzyme inhibitor-associated elevations in serum creatinine: Is this a cause for concern? *Arch Intern Med* 160:685–693, 2000.

297. Apperloo AJ, de Zeeuw D, de Jong PE: A short-term antihypertensive-treatment induced drop in glomerular filtration rate predicts long-term stability of renal function. *Kidney Int* 51:793–797, 1997.

298. Abbate M, Zoja C, Corna D, et al: In progressive nephropathies, overload of tubular cells with filtered proteins translates glomerular permeability dysfunction into cellular signals of interstitial inflammation. *J Am Soc Nephrol* 9:1213–1224, 1998.

299. Peters H, Border WA, Noble NA: Targeting TGF-β overexpression in renal disease: Maximizing the antifibrotic action of angiotensin II blockade. *Kidney Int* 54:1570–1580, 1998.

300. Osei SY, Price DA, Laffel LMB, et al: Effect of angiotensin II antagonist eprosartan on hyperglycemia-induced activation of intrarenal renin-angiotensin system in healthy humans. *Hypertension* 36:122–126, 2000.

301. Heeg JE, de Jong PE, van der Hem GK, et al: Efficacy and variability of the antiproteinuric effect of ACE inhibition by lisinopril. *Kidney Int* 36:272–279, 1989.

302. Gansevoort RT, de Zeeuw D, de Jong PE: Additive antiproteinuric effect of ACE inhibition and a low protein diet in human renal disease. *Nephrol Dial Transplant* 10:497–504, 1995.

303. Rigat B, Hubert C, Alhenc-Gelas F, et al: An insertion-deletion polymorphism in the angiotensin I converting enzyme gene accounting for half the variance of serum enzyme levels. *J Clin Invest* 86:1343–1346, 1990.

304. Ueda S, Elliott, Morton JJ, et al. Enhanced pressor response to angiotensin I in normotensive men with the deletion genotype (DD) for angiotensin-converting enzyme. *Hypertension* 25:1266–1269, 1995.

305. Cambien F, Poirier O, Lecerf L, et al: Deletion polymorphism in the gene for angiotensin-converting enzyme is a potent risk factor for myocardial infarction. *Nature* 359:641–644, 1992.

306. van Essen GG, Rensma PL, de Zeeuw D, et al: Association between angiotensin-converting enzyme gene polymorphism and failure of renoprotective therapy. *Lancet* 347:94–95, 1996.

307. Parving HH, Jacobsen P, Tarnow L, et al: Effect of deletion polymorphism of angiotensin-converting enzyme gene on progression of diabetic nephropathy during inhibition of angiotensin-converting enzyme. Observational follow-up study. *BMJ* 313:591–594, 1996.

308. ACC/AHA Guidelines for the evaluation and management of chronic heart failure in the adult: Executive summary. *Circulation* 104:2996–3007, 2001.

309. Liu P, Arnold M, Belenkie I, et al: The 2001 Canadian Cardiovascular Society consensus guideline update for the management and prevention of heart failure. *Can J Cardiol* 17(Suppl E):5E–25E, 2001.

310. Remme WJ: Effect of ACE inhibition on neurohormones. *Eur Heart J* 19(Suppl J):J16–J23, 1998.

311. Flather MD, Yusuf S, Kober L, et al: Long-term ACE-inhibitor therapy in patients with heart failure or left-ventricular dysfunction: A systematic overview of data from individual patients. ACE-Inhibitor Myocardial Infarction Collaborative Group. *Lancet* 355:1575–1581, 2000.

312. Stafford RS, Saglam D, Blumenthal D: National patterns of angiotensin-converting enzyme inhibitor use in congestive heart failure. *Arch Intern Med* 157:2460–2464, 1997.

313. Philbin EF, Andreou C, Rocco TA, et al: Patterns of angiotensin-converting enzyme inhibitor use in congestive heart failure in two community hospitals. *Am J Cardiol* 77:832–838, 1996.

314. Bungard TJ, McAlister FA, Johnson JA, Tsuyuki RT: Underutilization of ACE inhibitors in patients with congestive heart failure. *Drugs* 61:2021–2033, 2001.

315. Domanski MJ, Exner DV, Borkowf CB, et al: Effect of angiotensin-converting enzyme inhibition on sudden cardiac death following acute myocardial infarction. A meta-analysis of randomized clinical trials. *J Am Coll Cardiol* 33:598–604, 1999.

316. Megarry M, Sapsford R, Hall AS, et al: Do ACE inhibitors provide protection for the heart in the clinical setting of acute myocardial infarction? *Drugs* 54(Suppl 5):48–58, 1997.

317. Indications for ACE inhibitors in the early treatment of acute myocardial infarction: Systematic review of individual data from 100,000 patients in randomised trials. *Circulation* 97:2202–2212, 1998.

318. Naccarella F, Naccarelli GV, Maranga SS, et al: Do ACE inhibitors or angiotensin II antagonists reduce total mortality and arrhythmic mortality? A critical review of controlled clinical trials. *Curr Opin Cardiol* 17:6–18, 2002.

319. Cohn JN, Tognoni G: A randomized trial of the angiotensin-receptor blocker valsartan in chronic heart failure. *N Engl J Med* 345:1667–1675, 2001.

320. Pitt B: Clinical trials of angiotensin receptor blockers in heart failure: What do we know and what will we learn? *Am J Hypertens* 15:22S–27S, 2002.

321. Pitt B, Segal R, Martinez FA, et al: Randomised trial of losartan versus captopril in patients over 65 with heart failure (Evaluation of Losartan in the Elderly Study, ELITE). *Lancet* 349:747–752, 1997.

322. Pitt B, Poole-Wilson PA, Segal R, et al: Effect of losartan compared with captopril on mortality in patients with symptomatic heart failure: Randomised trial—the Losartan Heart Failure Survival Study ELITE II. *Lancet* 355:1582–1587, 2000.

322a. Coats AJS: Angiotensin type-1 receptor blockers in heart failure. *Prog Cardiovasc Dis* 44:231, 2002.

322b. McMurray J, Pfeffer MA: New therapeutic options in congestive heart failure. Part II. *Circulation* 105:2223, 2002.

323. Pfeffer MA, McMurray J, Leizorovicz A, et al: Valsartan in acute myocardial infarction trial (VALIANT): Rationale and design. *Am Heart J* 140:727–750, 2000.

324. Dickstein K, Kjekshus J, et al: Effects of losartan and captopril on mortality and morbidity in high-risk patients after acute myocardial infarction: The OPTIMAAL randomised trial. *Lancet* 360:752, 2002.

325. Packer M, Poole-Wilson PA, Armstrong PW, et al: Comparative effects of low and high doses of the angiotensin-converting enzyme inhibitor, lisinopril, on morbidity and mortality in chronic heart failure. ATLAS Study Group. *Circulation* 100:2312–2318, 1999.

326. Schoolwerth AC, Sica DA, Ballermann BJ, Wilcox CS: Renal considerations in angiotensin-converting enzyme inhibitor therapy: A statement for healthcare professionals from the Council on the Kidney in Cardiovascular Disease and the Council for High Blood Pressure Research of the American Heart Association. *Circulation* 104:1985–1991, 2001.

327. The SOLVD investigators: Effect of enalapril on survival in patients with reduced left ventricular ejection fractions and congestive heart failure. *N Engl J Med* 325:293–302, 1991.

328. Bastiaens MT, Zwan NV, Verschueren GL, et al: Three cases of pemphigus vegetans: Induction by enalapril—association with internal malignancy. *Int J Dermatol* 33:168–171, 1994.

329. Larbre JP, Nicolas JF, Collet P, et al: Kaposi's sarcoma in a patient with rheumatoid arthritis possible responsibility of captopril in the development of lesions. *J Rheumatol* 18:476–477, 1991.

330. Vogt B, Frey FJ: Inhibition of angiogenesis in Kaposi's sarcoma by captopril. *Lancet* 349:1148, 1997.

331. Meier CR, Derby LE, Jick SS, Jick H: Angiotensin-converting enzyme inhibitors, calcium channel blockers, and breast cancer. *Arch Intern Med* 160:349–353, 2000.

332. Stahl M, Bulpitt CJ, Palmer AJ, et al: Calcium channel blockers, ACE inhibitors, and the risk of cancer in hypertensive patients: A report from the Department of Health Hypertension Care Computing Project (DHCCP). *J Hum Hypertens* 14:299–304, 2000.

333. Pahor M, Guralnik JM, Salive ME, et al: Do calcium channel blockers increase the risk of cancer? *Am J Hypertens* 9:695–699, 1996.

334. Lever AF, Hole DJ, Gillis CR, et al: Do inhibitors of angiotensin-I-converting enzyme protect against risk of cancer? *Lancet* 352:179–184, 1998.

335. Sorensen HT, Mellemkjaer L, et al: Angiotensin-converting enzyme inhibitors and the risk of cancer: A population-based cohort study in Denmark. *Cancer* 92:2462–2470, 2001.

336. Friis S, Felmeden DC, Lip GY: Antihypertensive therapy and cancer risk. *Drug Saf* 24:727–739, 2001.

337. Textor SC: Renal failure related to angiotensin-converting enzyme inhibitors. *Semin Nephrol* 17:67–76, 1997.

338. Textor SC, Bravo EL, Fouad FM, Tarazi RC: Hyperkalemia in azotemic patients during angiotensin-converting enzyme inhibition and aldosterone reduction with captopril. *Am J Med* 73:719–725, 1982.

339. Garcia NH, Baigorria ST, Juncos LI: Hyperkalemia, renal failure, and converting-enzyme inhibition: An overrated connection. *Hypertension* 38:639–644, 2001.

340. Bakris GL, Siomos M, Richardson D, et al: ACE inhibition or angiotensin receptor blockade: impact on potassium in renal failure. VAL-K Study Group. *Kidney Int* 58:2084–2092, 2000.

341. Griffing GT, Sindler BH, Aurecchia SA, Melby JC: Reversal of diuretic-induced secondary hyperaldosteronism and hypokalemia by enalapril (MK-421): A new angiotensin-converting enzyme inhibitor. *Metabolism* 32:711–716, 1983.

342. Israili ZH, Hall WD: Cough and angioneurotic associated with angiotensin-converting enzyme inhibitor therapy: A review of the literature and pathophysiology. *Ann Intern Med* 117:234–242, 1992.

343. Chan WK, Chan TY, Luk WK: A high incidence of cough in Chinese subjects treated with angiotensin-converting enzyme inhibitors. *Eur J Clin Pharmacol* 44:299–300, 1993.

344. Chalmers D, Dombey SL, Lawson DH: Post-marketing surveillance of captopril (for hypertension): A preliminary report. *Br J Clin Pharmacol* 24:343–349, 1987.

345. Bensenor IM, Lotufo PA: Headache, hypertension, and irbesartan therapy. *Arch Intern Med* 161:775–776, 2001.

345a. Etminan M, Levine MA, Tomlinson G, Rochon PA: Efficacy of angiotensin II receptor antagonists in preventing headache: A systematic overview and meta-analysis. *Am J Med* 112:642, 2002.

346. Gibbs CR, Lip GYH, Beevers DG: Angioedema due to ACE inhibitors: Increased risk in patients of African origin. *Br J Clin Pharmacol* 48:861–865, 1999.

347. Herkner H, Temmel AF, Mullner M, et al: Different patterns of angioedema in patients with and without angiotensin-converting enzyme inhibitor therapy. *Wien Klin Wochenschr* 113:167–171, 2001.

348. Vleeming W, van Amsterdam JG, Stricker BH, et al: ACE inhibitor-induced angioedema. *Drug Saf* 18:171–188, 1998.

349. Brown NJ, Snowden M, Griffin MR: Recurrent angiotensin-converting enzyme inhibitor-associated angioedema. *JAMA* 278:232–233, 1997.

350. Oudit G, Girgrah N, Allard J: ACE inhibitor-induced angioedema of the intestine: Case report, incidence, pathophysiology, diagnosis and management. *Can J Gastroenterol* 15:827–832, 2001.

351. Chiu AG, Krowiak EJ, Deeb ZE: Angioedema associated with angiotensin II receptor antagonists: Challenging our knowledge of angioedema and its etiology. *Laryngoscope* 111:1729–1731, 2001.

352. Warner KK, Visconti JA, Tschampel MM: Angiotensin II receptor blockers in patients with ACE inhibitor-induced angioedema. *Ann Pharmacother* 34:526–528, 2000.

353. Fuchs SA, Koopmans RP, Guchelaar HJ, et al: Are angiotensin II receptor antagonists safe in patients with previous angiotensin-converting enzyme inhibitor–induced angioedema? *Hypertension* 37:1e, 2001.

354. Pryde PG, Sedman AB, Nugent CE, et al: Angiotensin-converting enzyme inhibitor fetopathy. *J Am Soc Nephrol* 3:1575–1582, 1993.

355. Burrows RF, Burrows EA: Assessing the teratogenic potential of angiotensin-converting enzyme inhibitors in pregnancy. *Aust N Z J Obstet Gynaecol* 38:306–311, 1998.

356. Lambot MA, Vermeylen D, Noel JC: Angiotensin-II-receptor inhibitors in pregnancy. *Lancet* 357:1619–1620, 2001.

357. Magee LA: Treating hypertension in women of childbearing age and during pregnancy. *Drug Saf* 24:457–474, 2001.

358. Shannon ME, Malecha SE, Cha AJ: Angiotensin-converting enzyme inhibitors (ACEIs) and angiotensin II receptor blockers (ARBs) and lactation: An update. *J Hum Lact* 16:152–155, 2000.

359. Zwanzger P, Marcuse A, Boerner RJ, et al: Lithium intoxication after administration of AT1 blockers. *J Clin Psychiatry* 62:208–209, 2001.

360. Correa FJ, Eiser AR: Angiotensin-converting enzyme inhibitors and lithium toxicity. *Am J Med* 93:108–109, 1992.

361. Conlin PR, Moore TJ, Swartz SL, et al: Effect of indomethacin on blood pressure lowering by captopril and losartan in hypertensive patients. *Hypertension* 36:461–465, 2000.

362. Fricker AF, Nussberger J, Meilenbrock S, et al: Effect of indomethacin on the renal response to angiotensin II receptor blockade in healthy subjects. *Kidney Int* 54:2089–2097, 1998.

363. Adhiyaman V, Asghar M, Oke A, et al: Nephrotoxicity in the elderly due to co-prescription of angiotensin-converting enzyme inhibitors and nonsteroidal anti-inflammatory drugs. *J R Soc Med* 94:512–514, 2001.

364. Cleland JG, John J, Houghton T: Does aspirin attenuate the effect of angiotensin-converting enzyme inhibitors in hypertension or heart failure? *Curr Opin Nephrol Hypertens* 10:625–31, 2001.

365. Hall D: Controversies in heart failure. Are beneficial effects of angiotensin-converting enzyme inhibitors attenuated by aspirin in patients with heart failure? *Cardiol Clin* 19:597–603, 2001.

366. Mahe I, Meune C, Diemer M, et al: Interaction between aspirin and ACE inhibitors in patients with heart failure. *Drug Saf* 24:167–182, 2001.

367. Samanta A, Burden AC: Fever, myalgia, and arthralgia in a patient on captopril and allopurinol. *Lancet* 1:679,1984.

368. Ruddy MC, Kostis JB, Frishman WH: Drugs that affect the renin-angiotensin system. In: Frishman WH, Sonnenblick EH, eds. *Cardiovascular Pharmacotherapeutics*. New York: McGraw Hill, 1997:131.

369. Plata R, Cornejo A, Arratia C, et al: Angiotensin-converting enzyme inhibition therapy in altitude polycythaemia: A prospective randomised trial. *Lancet* 359:663–66, 2002.

370. Frishman WH, Chiu R, Landzberg BR, Weiss M: Medical therapies for the prevention of restenosis after percutaneous coronary interventions. *Curr Probl Cardiol* 23:533–640, 1998.

Diuretic Therapy in Cardiovascular Disease

Todd W.B. Gehr

Domenic A. Sica

William H. Frishman

Modern diuretic therapy grew out of two apparently unrelated endeavors in the 1930s: the development of sulfanilamide, the first effective antibacterial drug, and the identification of the enzyme carbonic anhydrase. Clinical experience with sulfanilamide showed that this drug increased urine flow as well as sodium (Na^+) and potassium (K^+) excretion. The recognition that sulfanilamide inhibited carbonic anhydrase fueled attempts to synthesize compounds that might be more specific inhibitors of carbonic anhydrase. One such compound was acetazolamide. Unfortunately, the diuretic effect of acetazolamide was self-limited, lasting no more than a few days. One consequence of the search for inhibitors of carbonic anhydrase was the discovery of a series of potent diuretic compounds with greater long-term effectiveness. The prototype of these diuretics was chlorothiazide, which became available in 1958 and ushered in the modern era of diuretic therapy.[1]

Diuretics remain important therapeutic tools. First, they are capable of reducing blood pressure (BP), while simultaneously decreasing the morbidity and mortality that attends the hypertensive state. Diuretics are currently recommended as first-line therapy for the treatment of hypertension by the Joint National Commission on Detection, Evaluation, and Treatment of Hypertension of the National High Blood Pressure Education Program (JNC).[2] In addition, they remain an important element of the treatment regimen for congestive heart failure (CHF) in that they improve the congestive symptomatology, which characterizes the more advanced stages of CHF. This chapter reviews the mechanism of action of the various diuretic classes and the physiologic adaptations that accompany their use, and establishes the basis for their use in the treatment of hypertension and CHF. In addition, commonly encountered side effects with diuretics are elaborated on.

INDIVIDUAL CLASSES OF DIURETICS

The predominant site(s) of action of various diuretic classes along the nephron are depicted in Fig. 11-1. The range of diuretic classes available all have differing pharmacokinetics and, in many instances, pharmacodynamic responses dependent on both the nature and extent of underlying disease (Table 11-1).[3]

Carbonic Anhydrase Inhibitors

The administration of a carbonic anhydrase inhibitor ordinarily produces a brisk alkaline diuresis. By inhibiting carbonic anhydrase, these compounds decrease the generation of intracellular H^+, which is a necessary prerequisite for the absorption of Na^+; therein lies their primary diuretic effect.[4] Although carbonic anhydrase inhibitors work at the proximal tubule level, where the bulk of Na^+ reabsorption occurs, their final diuretic effect is typically rather modest being blunted by reabsorption more distally in other nephron segments.[5,6] Acetazolamide is currently the only carbonic anhydrase inhibitor employed primarily for its diuretic action. It is readily absorbed and is eliminated by tubular secretion. Its use is limited by its transient action and because prolonged use causes metabolic acidosis, amongst other side effects. Acetazolamide (250 to 500 mg daily) can be carefully used in patients with CHF who have developed metabolic alkalosis from thiazide or loop diuretic use and who cannot tolerate the volume load associated with the Cl^- repletion required for correction of the alkalemic state. Topiramate, a recently released anticonvulsant, inhibits carbonic anhydrase and is associated with the development of metabolic acidosis.[7]

Osmotic Diuretics

Mannitol is a polysaccharide diuretic given intravenously that is freely eliminated by glomerular filtration. Mannitol is poorly reabsorbed along the length of the nephron and thereby exerts a dose-dependent osmotic effect. This osmotic effect traps water and solutes in the tubular fluid, thus increasing Na^+ and water excretion. The half-life for plasma clearance of mannitol depends on the level of renal function but usually is between 30 and 60 min, thus its diuretic properties are quite transient. Because mannitol also expands extracellular volume and can precipitate pulmonary edema in patients with CHF, it is contraindicated in these patients. Moreover, excessive mannitol administration, particularly when the glomerular filtration rate (GFR) is reduced, can cause dilutional hyponatremia and/or acute renal failure.[8,9] The latter seems to be dose-dependent and typically corrects with elimination of mannitol as may be accomplished with hemodialysis.

Loop Diuretics

Loop diuretics act predominantly at the apical membrane in the thick ascending limb of the loop of Henle where they compete with chloride for binding to the $Na^+/K^+/2Cl^-$ cotransporter thereby inhibiting Na^+ and Cl^- reabsorption.[10] Besides this primary action, loop diuretics also have a variety of other effects on other nephron

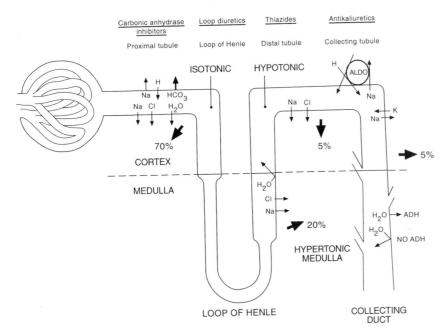

FIGURE 11-1. Schematic of the nephron illustrating the handling of water and electrolytes by the different segments and the major nephron sites of diuretic action. Heavy arrows represent the approximate percentage of sodium reabsorbed by the various nephron segments.

segments. Loop diuretics reduce Na^+ reabsorption in the proximal tubule by weakly inhibiting carbonic anhydrase and through poorly defined mechanisms independent of carbonic anhydrase inhibition.[11] Loop diuretics also have effects in the distal tubule,[12] descending limb of the loop of Henle,[13] and collecting duct.[14] Although the action of loop diuretics in these other nephron segments is quantitatively minor, as compared with their effects in the thick ascending limb, these actions serve to blunt the expected increase in more distal reabsorption, which is triggered with the use of these potent diuretics. Other clinically important effects of loop diuretics include an impairment in both free water excretion during water loading and free water absorption during dehydration,[15] a 30% increase in fractional calcium excretion,[16] a substantial increase in magnesium excretion,[17] and a transient increase followed by a decrease in urate excretion.[18]

In addition to their effects on water and electrolyte excretion, loop diuretics modulate renal prostaglandin synthesis, particularly that of prostaglandin E_2 (PGE_2).[19] The increased angiotensin-II generation following the administration of loop diuretics coupled with the increased synthesis of vasodilatory PGE_2 probably accounts for the marked redistribution of renal blood flow from the inner to the outer cortex of the kidney.[19] Despite these alterations in renal blood flow distribution, both total renal blood flow and GFR are preserved after loop diuretic administration to normal subjects.[20]

Loop diuretics in clinical use include furosemide, bumetanide, torsemide, and ethacrynic acid. The loop diuretics are highly protein bound and, therefore, are minimally filtered by the glomerulus. They typically access the tubular lumen by secretion via an organic anion transporter localized to the proximal tubule. The urinary diuretic concentration best represents the fraction of drug delivered to the

TABLE 11-1. Pharmacokinetics of Diuretics

Diuretic	Oral Bioavailability %	Normal Subjects	Half-Life Renal Insufficiency (hours)	CHF
Loop				
Furosemide	10–100	1.5–2	2.8	2.7
Bumetanide	80–100	1	1.6	1.3
Torsemide	80–100	3–4	4–5	6
Thiazide				
Bendroflumethazide	ND	2–5	ND	ND
Chlorthalidone	64	24–55	ND	ND
Chlorothiazide	30–50	1.5	ND	ND
Hydrochlorothiazide	65–75	2.5	Increased	ND
Hydroflumethazide	73	6–25	ND	6–28
Indapamide	93	15–25	ND	ND
Polythiazide	ND	26	ND	ND
Trichlormethiazide	ND	1–4	5–10	ND
Distal				
Amiloride	?	17–26	100	ND
Triamterene	>80	2–5	Prolonged	ND
Spironolactone	?	1.5	No change	ND
Active metabolites	?	>15	ND	ND

ND = not determined.

Source: Adapted with permission from Brater DC.[3]

medullary thick ascending limb and significantly correlates with the natriuretic response following diuretic administration.[3]

Furosemide is the most widely used diuretic in this class.[21] Furosemide is somewhat erratically absorbed with a bioavailability of 49% ± 17% and a range of 12 to 112%.[22] The coefficients of variation for absorption for different furosemide products varies from 25 to 43%; thus, switching from one formulation to another will not likely result in any predictable change in patient response to furosemide.[22] Furosemide is an organic anion compound that is highly bound to albumin in plasma, which gains entry to the tubular lumen through a probenecid-sensitive proximal tubular secretory mechanism.[23] Furosemide protein binding may be influenced by accumulated uremic toxins and/or fatty acids, although this is of poorly defined clinical significance.[24] Secretion of furosemide as well as other loop diuretics may be impaired by the presence of elevated levels of endogenous organic acids such as those seen in chronic renal failure (CRF), and by other drugs that share the same transporter such as salicylates and nonsteroidal anti-inflammatory drugs (NSAIDs). Following an oral dose of furosemide to normal subjects, the onset of action is within 30 to 60 min, peak effect occurs within 2 h, and its duration of action is approximately 6 h. The relationship between renal furosemide excretion and its natriuretic effect is best described by a sigmoidal shaped dose-response curve (Fig. 11-2).[25] This same pharmacokinetic-pharmacodynamic relationship based on urinary diuretic delivery applies to the other loop diuretics.[3] Alterations in this normal dose-response relationship can occur in a variety of pathophysiologic states such as CHF[26] and volume depletion.[27] The nonsteroidal anti-inflammatory agent indomethacin also alters this relationship through its inhibition of prostaglandin synthesis.[28] This relationship appears not to be perturbed by increased amounts of urinary protein as is seen in the nephrotic syndrome; thus urinary protein binding of loop diuretics is not a major mechanism for the diuretic resistance of the nephrotic syndrome.[29]

Bumetanide is 40 times more potent than furosemide and, like the other loop diuretics, is available in both oral and intravenous forms. In normal subjects, the bioavailability of bumetanide is 80% and the onset of diuretic effect occurs within 30 min, with a peak effect within 1 h. The duration of action of oral bumetanide is between 3 and 6 h and its half-life is between 1 and 3.5 h.[30] In healthy subjects, 60% of bumetanide is excreted unchanged in the urine and the remaining drug is hepatically metabolized via the cytochrome P450 pathway. Because of this extrarenal metabolism, bumetanide does not accumulate in renal failure, although renal disease does impair tubular delivery.[31] In contrast, in patients with hepatic disease, the plasma half-life of bumetanide is prolonged and more drug ultimately reaches the tubular fluid.[32]

Torsemide is the newest member of the loop diuretic class. It is rapidly absorbed and is 80 to 90% bioavailable. Maximal sodium excretion occurs within the first 2 h after either IV or oral administration. Only 20% of the drug is excreted unchanged in the urine and the remaining 80% undergoes hepatic metabolism.[33] In healthy subjects, the half-life of torsemide is 3.3 h, but is prolonged to 8 h in cirrhotic patients.[34] When selecting an oral agent in patients with CHF, oral torsemide may be particularly advantageous because its absorption is not reduced and is much less variable than is the case with oral furosemide.[35] In fact, torsemide disposition in CHF patients is comparable to that of normal subjects. Compared with furosemide-treated patients, torsemide-treated patients are less likely to be readmitted for CHF and for all cardiovascular-renal (CVR) causes, and are less fatigued.[36] As with furosemide, however, torsemide pharmacodynamics in CHF patients is typical for this group of patients, with a shift of the dose-response relationship downward and to the right.

Thiazides

The major site of action of the thiazide diuretics is the early distal convoluted tubule where they inhibit the coupled reabsorption of Na^+ and Cl^-.[37] The water-soluble thiazides such as hydrochlorothiazide (HCTZ) also inhibit carbonic anhydrase and, at high doses, further increase Na^+ excretion by this mechanism.[38] Thiazides also inhibit NaCl and fluid reabsorption in the medullary collecting duct.[39] Besides these effects on Na^+ excretion, the thiazides also impair urinary diluting capacity without affecting urinary concentrating mechanisms,[40] reduce Ca^{2+} and urate excretion,[41,42] and increase Mg^{2+} excretion.[43]

HCTZ is the most widely prescribed drug in this diuretic class. It is well absorbed, with a bioavailability of 71%. The onset of diuresis with HCTZ generally occurs within 2 h, peaks between 3 and 6 h, and continues for as long as 12 h.[44] The half-life of HCTZ is prolonged in patients with decompensated CHF and/or renal insufficiency.[45]

FIGURE 11-2. Pharmacokinetic (A) and pharmacodynamic (B) detetminants of loop diuretic response. The broken line represents an altered dose-response relationship, as is observed in a typical diuretic resistant state. Diuretic delivery necessary to achieve a threshold response can vary substantially in diuretic resistance.

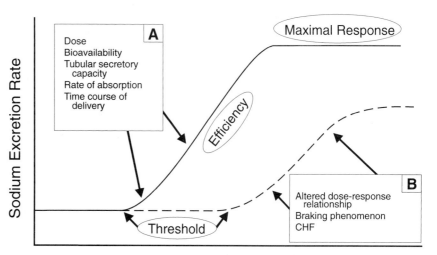

Large doses of thiazide diuretics in the order of 100 to 200 mg/d will initiate a diuresis in patients with chronic renal failure, although the magnitude of the diuretic response will be a function of the GFR, and thereby the filtered load, as well as the site at which these drugs work.[46]

Metolazone is a quinazoline diuretic and is similar to the thiazides both in structure and locus of action.[47] Although its major site of action is in the distal tubule, metolazone has a minor inhibitory effect on proximal Na^+ reabsorption through a carbonic anhydrase-independent mechanism.[48] Metolazone is also lipid soluble and has a longer duration of action and thereby more readily accesses the tubular lumen during states of renal insufficiency, unlike the thiazides.[49] These unique properties in combination probably account for the enhanced natriuretic efficacy of metolazone and its effectiveness in diuretic-resistant states when given together with a loop diuretic. Metolazone is available in different formulations, with some being very poorly and slowly absorbed. If the unpredictability of metolazone absorption is not recognized its failure to elicit a diuretic response may incorrectly be attributed to the severity of the underlying illness.

Distal Potassium-Sparing Diuretics

Potassium-sparing diuretics can be divided into two distinct classes: competitive antagonists of aldosterone, such as spironolactone, and those that do not interact with aldosterone receptors, such as amiloride and triamterene. These agents all act on the principal cells in the late distal convoluted tubule, the initial connecting tubule, and the cortical collecting duct, where they inhibit active Na^+ reabsorption. The inhibition of Na^+ entry into the cell causes a reduction in the activity of the basolateral Na^+, K^+-ATPase, which, in turn, reduces intracellular K^+ concentration. The resulting fall in the electrochemical gradient for K^+ and H^+ reduces the subsequent secretion of each of these cations.[50,51] Because these drugs are capable of producing only a modest natriuresis, their clinical utility lies elsewhere in their ability to reduce the excretion of K^+ and net acid, especially when distal fluid delivery is enhanced by more proximally acting diuretics or in states of hyperaldosteronism.[52] These agents all reduce Ca^{2+} and Mg^{2+} excretion.[17]

Spironolactone is a lipid-soluble K^+-sparing diuretic that is readily absorbed and highly protein bound. It has a 20-h half-life for elimination and takes 10 to 48 h to become maximally effective.[53,54] It is also metabolized to active metabolites.[55] Spironolactone is of particular use during states of reduced renal function because access to its site of action is not dependent on GFR, although its tendency to cause hyperkalemia in renal failure patients limits its use.

Eplerenone is a new aldosterone receptor antagonist that selectively binds to the aldosterone receptor. However, as compared with spironolactone, it has a lower affinity for the androgen and progesterone receptors. The molecular structure of eplerenone replaces the 17-α-thioacetyl group of spironolactone with a carbomethyl group, conferring excellent selectivity for the aldosterone receptor over steroid receptors.[56,56a] The drug has been evaluated against placebo and other antihypertensive drugs in more than 4000 patients with mild to moderate hypertension, and has a favorable efficacy and safety profile.[56] Similarly, the drug has been used in patients with heart failure after an acute myocardial infarction. The drug will soon be available for clinical use in the United States.

Amiloride is poorly absorbed and is actively secreted into the tubular lumen[57] where it works at the apical membrane. It has a duration of action of about 18 h. Triamterene, on the other hand, is well absorbed and is hydroxylated to active metabolites. The half-life of triamterene and its metabolites ranges from 3 to 5 h.[58] It also depends on active secretion to gain access to its site of action. Triamterene accumulates in cirrhotic patients owing to a reduction in hydroxylation and biliary secretion.[59] Both triamterene and amiloride accumulate in renal-failure patients,[60] and are associated with worsening of renal function, particularly when given with NSAIDs.[61]

Adaptation to Diuretic Therapy

Diuretic-induced inhibition of Na^+ reabsorption in one nephron segment elicits important adaptations in other nephron segments, which not only limits their antihypertensive and fluid-depleting actions but also contributes to the development of side effects. Although a portion of this diuretic resistance is a normal consequence of diuretic use, profound diuretic resistance is frequently encountered in patients with a variety of clinical disorders such as CHF, cirrhosis and/or renal insufficiency. An understanding of the mechanisms surrounding adaptation to diuretic therapy is necessary if this effect is to be minimized and side effects limited.

The first dose of a diuretic normally produces a brisk diuresis, which is quickly followed by a new equilibrium state in which daily fluid and electrolyte excretion matches intake and body weight stabilizes. In nonedematous patients given either a thiazide or a loop diuretic, this adaptation or *braking phenomenon* occurs within 1 to 2 days and limits weight loss to 1 to 2 kg.[27]

This braking phenomenon has been clearly demonstrated in normal subjects given the loop diuretics furosemide or bumetanide.[62–64] Furosemide administered to subjects ingesting a high-salt diet (270 mmol/24 h) produced a brisk natriuresis, which resulted in a negative Na^+ balance for the ensuing 6 h. This was followed by an 18-h period when Na^+ excretion was reduced to levels considerably below the level of Na^+ intake resulting in a positive Na^+ balance. This postdiuresis Na^+ retention balanced the initial natriuresis ending in a neutral Na^+ balance and in the aggregate no weight loss. After three successive days of furosemide administration, a similar pattern of Na^+ loss and retention was demonstrated. In fact, this same result is seen after even a month of furosemide administration.[20] However, if salt intake is kept very low, Na^+ balance will remain negative after a single dose of furosemide, even though the initial natriuresis is, to a degree, blunted. This occurs despite an abrupt decline in Na^+ excretion to very low levels, although not low enough to restore Na^+ balance because of the degree to which salt intake is reduced. This effect persists for the 3 days of furosemide use and results in loss of body weight. Administration of bumetanide to subjects on a "no added salt" diet (120 mmol/d) also leads to a negative Na^+ balance state that is curtailed by postdiuretic Na^+ retention and a blunted natriuretic effect.

The pathophysiology of this braking phenomenon is complex. The relationship between natriuresis and furosemide excretion rate is shifted to the right in those subjects receiving a low-salt diet indicating a blunting of the tubular responsiveness to the diuretic (see Fig. 11-2).[62–64] The importance of extra-cellular fluid (ECF) volume depletion in postdiuretic Na^+ retention has been clearly shown, although there clearly is a ECF volume-independent component to the Na^+ retention.[65] The etiology does not seem to be related to aldosterone either, as spironolactone therapy has little effect on the Na^+ retention.[20] Using Li^+ as a marker of proximal Na^+ handling, Na^+ retention has been ascribed to a reduced delivery of Na^+ from the proximal tubule and an increase in the fractional reabsorption of Na^+ in the distal tubule.[66] Structural hypertrophy in the distal nephron has also been clearly shown in rats receiving prolonged infusions of loop diuretics.[67,68] These structural changes are associated with enhanced rates of distal nephron Na^+ and Cl^- absorption and K^+ secretion, which is independent of aldosterone.[69] These nephron adaptations may contribute to postdiuretic Na^+ retention and to tolerance in humans, and could explain the Na^+ retention that can persist for up to 2 weeks after diuretic therapy is discontinued.[70,71]

Neurohumoral Response to Diuretics

An immediate (within minutes) increase in plasma renin activity (PRA) and plasma aldosterone concentration occurs in response to a diuretic dose that is independent of volume depletion or sympathetic nervous system (SNS) activation.[72,73] This rise in PRA is caused by inhibition of NaCl reabsorption at the macula densa[72] in conjunction with loop-diuretic-related stimulation of renal prostacyclin release.[73] This first-wave of neurohumoral effects although transient increases afterload and for a short period of time may reduce the effectiveness of a diuretic.[74] Following this initial rise diuretics cause a more sustained increase in PRA and aldosterone specifically due to an increase in SNS activity and a diminution in ECF volume. Diuretics also increase the renal production of prostaglandins, which is the probable explanation for the reduction of preload and the decrease in ventricular filling pressures that occur within 5 to 15 min of loop diuretic administration.[73–76] Inhibition of prostaglandin synthesis with NSAIDs diminishes the natriuretic response with all classes of diuretics.[77–79] Although the SNS is stimulated by loop diuretics as manifested by increases in plasma catecholamine concentrations and an increase in heart rate, α_1-receptor blockade with prazosin does not modify the natriuretic effect of furosemide.[61] β-Receptor blockade with propranolol blunts the component of diuretic-induced renin release related to ECF volume depletion.[72] Neurohumoral activation by diuretics remains an important consideration in the overall effect of diuretics in hypertension and CHF.

DIURETICS IN HYPERTENSION

Hypertension (HTN) is loosely defined by a systolic blood pressure (SBP) $\geq$140 mm Hg and/or a diastolic blood pressure (DBP) $\geq$90 mm Hg and is one of the most common disorders in the United States, with more than 50 million people affected.[2] Hypertension is definitionally dependent and if you add to this figure those patients with borderline HTN, this number grows larger. Both cardiovascular and cerebrovascular events, renal disease and all-cause mortality increases in a continuous fashion with increases in SBP and DBP. SBP is more predictive of morbidity and mortality than is DBP.[80] In its most recent report, JNC VI advocated the use of diuretics and beta-blockers as preferred first-line therapy for uncomplicated hypertension.[2] This position was adopted based on a number of outcome studies that used diuretics or beta-blockers and that reported therapy-related reductions in stroke and cardiovascular endpoints. All JNC documents dating to the original JNC I—published in 1977—have advocated a similar position favoring the early use of diuretics in the management of hypertension.

Mechanism of Action

The exact means by which diuretics lower BP is not known, although these agents have been used for more than 40 years. The effect of diuretics on BP may be separated into three sequential phases: acute, subacute, and chronic (Fig. 11-3), which correspond to periods of roughly 1 to 2 weeks, several weeks, and several months, respectively.[81] In the acute phase of response to diuretics, the major hypotensive effect of these agents is to reduce ECF volume and thereby decrease cardiac output. The initial response to diuretic therapy in a patient receiving a "no added salt" diet (100 to 150 mmol/d) is a negative Na^+ balance of from 100 to 300 mmol, which occurs in the first 2 to 4 days of treatment. Plasma Na^+ concentrations remain normal, and the loss of body Na^+ translates into a 1 to 2 L

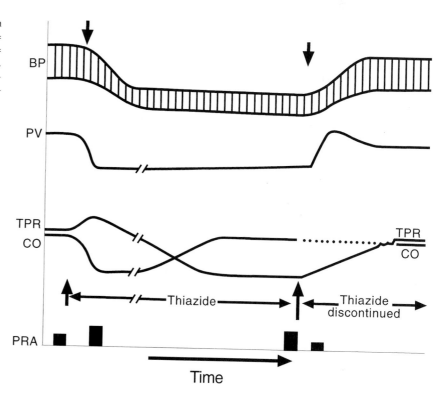

FIGURE 11-3. Effects of thiazide administration in an "idealized" patient. BP = blood pressure; CO = cardiac output; PRA = plasma renin activity; PV = plasma volume; TPR = total peripheral resistance. (*Modified from Moser M. Diuretics in the management of hypertension. Med Clin North Am 71:935–946, 1987.*)

decrease in ECF volume. Direct measurements of hypertensive patients treated with diuretics show a 12% decrease in ECF.[82] There is a similar reduction in plasma volume, which suggests that the acute volume loss arises proportionally from both the plasma and interstitial compartments.[83] The decrease in plasma volume reduces venous return and diminishes cardiac output, thereby producing the initial vasodepressor response.[84] The change in plasma volume variably stimulates both the SNS and the renin-angiotensin-aldosterone (RAA) axis. The degree to which these systems are activated may govern the magnitude of the acute BP decrease observed with diuretics. It has also been shown in hypertensive patients that diuretics can restore nocturnal BP decline in a manner similar to Na^+ restriction, which suggests that the kidneys and sodium metabolism play a role in the circadian rhythm of BP.[85]

Over time, these effects on volume and cardiac output lessen in importance, although BP remains lowered. During the first few weeks of treatment, plasma volume returns to slightly less than pretreatment levels, despite the continued administration of a diuretic.[73] Thus, the chronic vasodepressor effect of diuretics is less an issue of volume reduction than it is a process coupled to a persistent reduction in total peripheral resistance (TPR). The subacute phase of BP reduction with diuretics seems to be a transitional period during which both of these factors prevail.[84,86] There is no simple explanation for the drop in TPR that accompanies long-term diuretic use. The decrease in TPR during prolonged therapy has been attributed to several factors, including changes in the ionic content of vascular smooth-muscle cells, altered ion gradients across smooth-muscle cells, and changes in membrane-bound ATPase activity. The ability of diuretics to reduce BP seems to be critically linked to the presence of functioning renal tissue; thus, a thiazide diuretic does not reduce BP in patients undergoing maintenance hemodialysis.[87]

Understanding these mechanistic aspects of diuretic actions is important to the practical treatment of hypertension. The early action of diuretics to reduce ECF volume is optimized if dietary Na^+ is restricted at the beginning of therapy. This limits the repercussions of the breaking phenomenon, which inevitably occurs with continued diuretic use. Some limitation of dietary Na^+ intake may also be relevant to how diuretics maintain reduced TPR over the long-term. It is believed that changes in Na^+/Ca^{2+} balance in vascular smooth muscle cells arise from the short-term volume contraction seen during the first several days of thiazide diuretic therapy. How this phenomenon of volume contraction actually translates into a reduction in TPR is very poorly worked out. Whatever the mechanism, it can be very long-lived, because a residual BP-reduction can be seen several weeks after the withdrawal of thiazide diuretics.[88]

Another consideration in the ability of a diuretic to reduce BP over the long-term relates to the natriuretic pattern of diuretics. For example, when long-term therapeutic responses to HCTZ and furosemide are compared in hypertensive patients, SBP and DBP are more consistently reduced with HCTZ.[89] One explanation offered for this difference is the diuretic pattern of each agent. The natriuresis produced by a thiazide diuretic can be fairly prolonged but is generally modest at best, whereas a loop diuretic produces a brisk early diuretic response that rapidly falls off. The latter pattern of diuretic response is often accompanied by a significant postdiuretic period of Na^+ and water retention. When these two processes are summed, the result may be that the loop diuretic produces minimal volume loss despite its greater immediate potency. This period of antinatriuresis is of less consequence with the relatively less potent thiazide diuretic. In the end, a thiazide diuretic may be able to maintain a mild state of volume contraction more efficiently than a loop diuretic.[90] An exception to this may be found with the response to the loop diuretic torsemide. Small doses of this compound may cause significant BP reduction, a vasodepressor process that seems to be independent of the observed degree of diuresis.[91]

Diuretics in Clinical Trials

By the mid 1990s, evidence about the effects of BP-lowering regimens mainly based on diuretics and beta-blockers was available from a series of randomized controlled clinical trials involving more than 47,000 hypertensive patients.[92–105] Systematic overviews and/or meta-analyses of these trials showed that reductions in BP of about 10 to 12 mm Hg systolic and 5 to 6 mm Hg diastolic conferred relative risk reductions in stroke risk of 38% and a risk of coronary heart disease of 16% within just a few years of beginning therapy.[97–99,102–104,106] The size of these effects were similar in major subgroups of trials and patients, and seemed to be largely independent of differences in disease event rates amongst study patients. The few studies that directly compared diuretics and beta-blockers detected no clear differences in the risk of stroke or coronary artery disease.[104] However, it was shown in elderly patients with hypertension that first-line diuretic therapy reduces cerebrovascular events, coronary artery disease, and stroke, cardiovascular and all-cause mortality, in contrast to first-line beta-blockers that only reduced cerebrovascular events.[107]

In 1995, many studies of BP-lowering drugs were identified as planned or ongoing. Most of these trials had been designed to detect large differences in relative risk and had insufficient power to detect small to moderate differences between the studied regimens. To maximize the information acquired by these and future trials, a collaborative program of prospectively designed overviews was developed. The first publication of these overviews occurred in 2000.[106] Overviews of trials comparing angiotensin-converting enzyme (ACE)-inhibitor-based regimens with diuretic or beta-blocker-based regimens in hypertensive patients provide no evidence that the benefits of ACE inhibitors are any different than those conferred by diuretics or beta-blockers (Fig. 11-4).[108–110] Overviews of trials comparing calcium antagonists with diuretic- or beta-blocker-based regimens provide some evidence of differences in the effects of the two regimens on cause-specific outcomes with the risk for stroke being significantly less with calcium antagonists than with diuretics (Fig. 11-5). There was no evidence of differences between the treatment effects of calcium antagonists regimens based on dihydropyridine versus nondihydropyridine agents.[109,111,112]

The Antihypertensive and Lipid-Lowering Treatment to Prevent Heart Attack Trial (ALLHAT) is a randomized clinical outcome trial of antihypertensive and lipid-lowering therapy in a diverse population (including substantial numbers of women and minorities) of 42,419 high-risk hypertensives aged 55 years or older with a planned mean follow-up of 6 years. ALLHAT results are anticipated in the latter part of 2002. This trial is comparing three classes of antihypertensive therapy, the alpha-blocker doxazosin, the calcium-channel blocker amlodipine, and the ACE inhibitor lisinopril to the thiazide-type diuretic chlorthalidone. The study was terminated for the doxazosin arm of the study approximately 2 years early because of its inferiority to chlorthalidone with regard to two combined endpoints—coronary revascularization and angina—and the development of CHF.[113] This important trial will hopefully clarify which type or types of antihypertensive therapy is most beneficial in terms of cardiovascular morbidity and mortality and will importantly influence the therapeutic positioning of diuretics over the next decade.

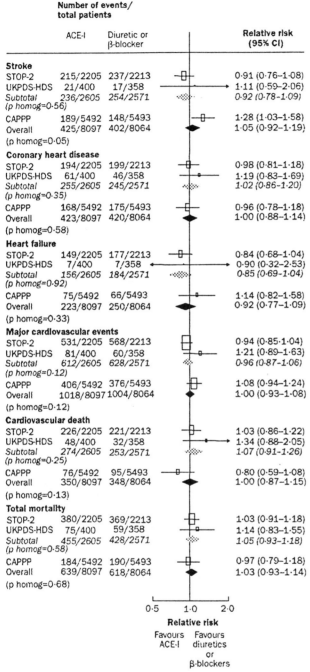

FIGURE 11-4. Comparisons of ACE-inhibitor-based therapy with diuretic-based or beta-blocker-based therapy. ACE-I = ACE inhibitor; p homog = p value from χ^2 test for homogeneity. (*Reprinted from Blood Pressure Lowering Treatment Trialists' Collaboration. Effects of ACE inhibitors, calcium antagonists, and other blood-pressure-lowering drugs: Results of prospectively designed overviews of randomised trials. Lancet 355:1955–1964, 2000.*)

Regression of Left Ventricular Hypertrophy with Diuretic Therapy

Left ventricular mass has been recognized as a powerful independent risk factor for cardiovascular morbidity.[114,115] Antihypertensive therapy, with the exception of direct vasodilators, is effective in regressing left ventricular hypertrophy (LVH).[115,116] In 1991, Moser and Setaro compiled an overview of all studies evaluating

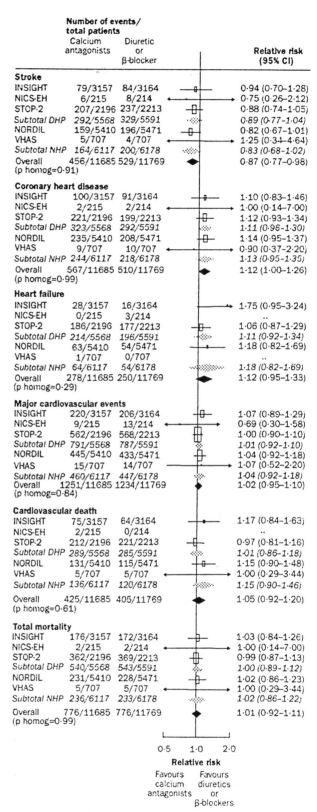

FIGURE 11-5. Comparisons of calcium-antagonist-based therapy with diuretic-based or beta-blocker-based therapy. DHP = dihydropyridine; NHP = nondihydropyridine; p homog = p value from χ^2 test for homogeneity. (*Reprinted from Blood Pressure Lowering Treatment Trialists' Collaboration. Effects of ACE inhibitors, calcium antagonists, and other blood-pressure-lowering drugs: Results of prospectively designed overviews of randomised trials. Lancet 355:1955–1964, 2000.*)

LVH regression in diuretic-treated hypertensive patients, which supported the efficacy of diuretics in regressing left ventricular mass.[117] Two meta-analyses have been undertaken specifically looking at LVH regression with different antihypertensive agents.[118,119] Using echocardiography, Dahlof et al. analyzed 109 studies comprising 2357 patients.[118] Diuretics were associated with an 11.3% reduction in LV mass; however, this was primarily due to a reduction in LV volume. Alternatively, the reduction of LV mass associated with ACE inhibitors was 15%, beta-blockers 8%, and calcium channel blockers 8.5% with structural changes largely reflected by a reversal of posterior and intraventricular septal thickness. Another analysis of 39 trials of diuretics, beta-blockers, calcium-channel blockers (CCBs), and ACE inhibitors showed that LV mass was related to the treatment-induced decline in BP, and, in particular, SBP. Reductions in LV mass of 13%, 9%, 6%, and 7% occurred with ACE inhibitors, CCBs, beta-blockers, and diuretics, respectively.[119] Accordingly, diuretics are comparable to most other drug classes in their ability to regress left ventricular mass.[120,121] Significant reductions in LVH with antihypertensive therapy has not yet been shown in prospective randomized trials to be related to reduced cardiovascular morbidity and mortality. These trials are sorely needed.

Responsive Patient Populations

When used alone in the nonedematous patient, thiazide diuretics are as efficacious as most other classes of drugs.[122] Although it is imprudent to offer universal recommendations about antihypertensive care on the basis of race alone, this is still done routinely. That said, black and elderly hypertensives typically respond better to diuretics than do non-black and younger patients.[122,123] The same can be said for other salt-sensitive forms of hypertension, such as that seen in diabetic patients.

Elderly

Five studies were specifically performed in the elderly hypertensive (age >60 years): the Systolic Hypertension in Elderly Program (SHEP),[100] the Swedish Trial in Old Patients (STOP),[101] the Medical Research Council Trial in the treatment of older adults (MRC-2),[104] the European Working party on High Blood Pressure in the Elderly (EWPHE),[103] and the trial of Coope and Warrender.[123] Significant reductions in stroke similar to that observed in younger patients and greater benefits in terms of protection from myocardial infarction and CHF were demonstrated in these older patients. In addition, diuretics have been shown to improve the quality of life as assessed by exercise capacity.[124]

Four clinical trials, with a total of 34,676 patients, have compared diuretics with beta-blockers: the International Prospective Primary Prevention Study in Hypertension (IPPPSH),[125] Heart Attack Primary Prevention in Hypertension Research Group (HAPPHY),[105] Medical Research Council (MRC), and MRC-2.[104] These two drug classes were comparable with regard to the incidence of stroke. With regards to myocardial infarction, two studies favored either diuretic or beta-blockers over the other although differences between these classes were quite small.

Three multicenter prospective clinical trials have been specifically performed in the elderly: the SHEP,[100] STOP,[101] and MRC-2 trials.[104] All three trials found significant reductions in cerebrocardiovascular morbidity and mortality associated with diuretic and/or beta-blocker therapy. Just to highlight one of these trials, the SHEP trial was a double-blind, placebo-controlled trial comprised of 4736

men and women with isolated systolic hypertension (ISH) who were older than 60 years of age.[100,126] Patients were randomized to receive a low-dose of the diuretic chlorthalidone as initial therapy; beta-blockers were then added as needed to reach goal BP. At the end of the 5-year follow-up period, 46% of the subjects had adequate BP control using only a low dose of chlorthalidone. Another 23% of patients were controlled with the addition of a beta-blocker. Outcome included a statistically significant 36% reduction in strokes and nonstatistically significant reductions in MI of 27% and overall mortality of 13%. Results of these trials clearly establish the benefit of low-dose diuretics and/or beta-blockers for the treatment of ISH in the elderly and have been the basis for current treatment recommendations advocating diuretic therapy in uncomplicated forms of hypertension.

Blacks

In black patients, hypertension is more prevalent at a younger age, is usually more severe, and is associated with a greater incidence of cardiac, central nervous system (CNS), and renal complications than occur in white patients.[127–129] Although the pathogenesis of hypertension has not been clearly defined, the majority of blacks fall into the low-renin category. This low-renin status cannot be explained by volume expansion alone, because no consistent relationship between these two factors has been found in this population.[130] In addition, the INTERSALT study, a multicenter, cross-sectional study that evaluated the relationship between electrolytes and BP, was unable to correlate excessive salt intake as a contributing factor to the development of hypertension in blacks.[129] Although not fully resolved as of yet there appears to be an important emerging role for potassium intake in the BP patterns expressed in normotensive and hypertensive blacks.[131,132]

Nonetheless, black patients respond very well to diuretics.[133–135] It has been reported that between 40% and 67% of young black patients and between 58% and 80% of elder blacks respond to monotherapy with diuretics.[134] As a rule, diuretics are more effective than beta-blockers, ACE inhibitors, or angiotensin-receptor blockers (ARBs) in blacks.[133–136] However, when diuretics are added to any of these antihypertensive drug classes in black patients, their efficacy is substantially improved.[134–137]

Diuretic therapy has been associated with reductions in morbidity and mortality in blacks. Black patients made up approximately half of the study participants in the Veterans Administration Cooperative Study and the Hypertension Detection and Follow-Up Program (HDFP), both of which were diuretic-based studies.[97,98] In the VA study, diuretic treatment was associated with a reduction in morbid events from 26 to 10% in black patients.[97] In the HDFP study, there was an 18.5% mortality reduction for black men and a 27.8% mortality reduction for black women.[98] However, the ability of diuretics to delay or prevent renal dysfunction in hypertensive blacks was put into question by the Multiple Risk Factor Intervention Trial (MRFIT), which did not show a benefit in this regard.[138]

General Considerations

Diuretics are likely to find their largest future use as "sensitizing" agents. Their primary modes of sensitization derive from volume depletion-related neurohumoral activation. In this regard, even subtle degrees of volume contraction or RAA-axis activation, as produced by low-dose thiazide-type diuretics, can enhance the effect of coadministered antihypertensive compounds.[139] This additive effect has rekindled interest in the use of fixed-dose combination antihypertensive therapy in the primary management of essential hypertension (see Chap. 21).[139] The concept of using two drugs at low doses for BP control is not necessarily of recent vintage. It has however, gathered new support because it is increasingly evident that most patients who receive such treatment not only achieve their target BP pressures but do so with a minimum of side effects.[140,141]

The dose-response relationship for the antihypertensive effect of diuretics has been fully characterized over the past decade. In the process, many of the supposed negative attributes of diuretics have been shown not to exist. In the early days of diuretic use, doses were unnecessarily high. At that time, the concept "if a little is good, a lot is better" was a routine part of practice. It was soon recognized that the dose-response relationship for a thiazide-type diuretic, such as HCTZ, was extremely flat beyond a dosage of 25 mg/d. Much of the early negative biochemical and metabolic experience with diuretics occurred with the very high dosages (100 to 200 mg/d) routinely used in the early days. When it was found that the blood pressure reduction with HCTZ was similar whether the dosage was 12.5 or 25 to 100 mg/d, diuretics were "back in the game."[107,142]

As practice patterns shifted to a low-dose strategy for thiazide-type diuretics, it was soon apparent that the frequency of the metabolically negative side effects had dramatically diminished: thus, such entities as hypokalemia, hypomagnesemia, glucose intolerance, and hypercholesterolemia are much less common with low-dose diuretics.[139,142] When the strong end-organ protection data for diuretics are combined with the fact that these agents produce few side effects at low doses, a compelling argument can be made for the use of diuretics as initial therapy for most persons with uncomplicated mild-to-moderate hypertension.[107]

DIURETICS IN CONGESTIVE HEART FAILURE

Diuretic use remains a vital part of the treatment of CHF. CHF is extremely common with an estimated 500,000 new cases diagnosed each year in the United States. The prevalence of heart failure is increasing as the population ages and patients with CHF survive longer. CHF is the leading discharge diagnosis in persons older than 65 years of age, thus having an enormous economic impact. Up to the middle 1970s, the treatment of CHF was limited to dietary salt restriction, diuretics, and digitalis. Since then, the therapeutic options have grown dramatically and therapy has had a beneficial impact on survival in these patients. Use of diuretics depends on the circumstances causing the CHF but they prove to be most efficacious in patients with chronic CHF. Unfortunately, the pharmacokinetics and pharmacodynamics of diuretics are altered in the setting of CHF, which may limit their overall efficacy. Such diuretic resistance often can be overcome with the judicious use of loop diuretics or combinations of diuretic classes. The following section briefly reviews the pathophysiology of CHF and highlights mechanisms of diuretic resistance and strategies to overcome this resistance.

Pathophysiology of CHF

All forms of CHF are caused by systolic and/or diastolic dysfunction. Systolic dysfunction is characterized by dilatation of the left ventricular cavity and a reduction in ejection fraction. Diastolic dysfunction is characterized by a normal or small left ventricular cavity with a thickened ventricular wall and normal or increased ejection fraction. Systolic dysfunction is most commonly caused by ischemic disease or idiopathic cardiomyopathies.[143] Diastolic

dysfunction is most commonly seen in the elderly and in patients with a history of hypertension. Systolic and diastolic dysfunction often coexist and either one may predominate in any one particular patient. Heart failure is often a dynamic process best exemplified by patients with poorly controlled hypertension in whom diastolic dysfunction predominates early in the course of the disease but is inevitably followed by systolic dysfunction if left untreated.[144]

The hemodynamic derangements associated with CHF provoke a complex array of biologic responses. Systemic neurohumoral activation cause significant effects on preload, afterload and heart rate and lead to many of the symptoms associated with CHF. Activation of biologic systems within the myocardium also plays a significant role in the remodeling of the failing ventricles and vasculature. It is now felt that this remodeling process plays a central role in the pathophysiology of CHF.[145,146]

Myocardial remodeling is characterized by a progressive change in ventricular chamber geometry.[144] At the molecular level, it is associated with hypertrophy and apoptosis of myocytes, side-by-side slippage of myocytes, regression to a molecular phenotype characterized by the expression of fetal genes and proteins, and alterations in the quantity and composition of extracellular matrix.[145,146] Many of these alterations can be induced by exposure of myocardial cells to mechanical stress, angiotensin-II, norepinephrine, endothelin, inflammatory cytokines, and reactive oxygen species.[147,148] From a clinical perspective, agents, such as ACE inhibitors or beta-blockers, that reverse this remodeling process show the greatest benefits in the treatment of CHF.[148]

Hemodynamic alterations that accompany CHF result in systemic vasoconstriction and increases in left ventricular afterload. This increase in afterload causes further reductions in systolic function, increases pulmonary vascular tone, elevates pulmonary venous pressure, and, eventually, left ventricular failure. The increased vascular tone in CHF reflects the activation of neurohumoral systems, especially the SNS and the RAA axis.[147,148] Attenuation of endothelium-dependent vasodilatation and increases in endothelin production may also contribute to the systemic and pulmonary vasoconstriction.[146,149—152] Arterial vasodilators, particularly ACE inhibitors and ARBs, increase stroke volume and cardiac output without causing a reduction in systemic BP and are the "backbone" of therapy for CHF.

As already alluded to, neurohumoral activation is a consistent finding in patients with CHF. Elevated SNS activity is reflected by increased sympathetic nerve traffic and increased levels of urinary and plasma catecholamines. These alterations are reflected in an attenuation in the contractile and chronotropic responses to β-adrenergic stimulation.[146] The sympathetic nervous system appears to be activated even in patients with asymptomatic disease and may contribute to the progression of CHF.[148]

The renin-angiotensin-aldosterone system (RAS) is also activated in CHF patients, as evidenced by increased plasma concentrations of renin, angiotensin, and aldosterone.[146] It has also been recognized that tissue components of the RAS are independently activated and that this activation contributes to myocardial and vascular remodeling.[146] Angiotensin-II also plays an important role in the kidney, where it effects glomerular hemodynamics and Na^+ reabsorption. In states of mildly reduced renal perfusion, such as CHF, angiotensin-II is important in maintaining glomerular filtration by its effect on efferent arteriolar tone. In severe CHF, however, angiotensin-II concentrations become markedly elevated causing afferent arteriolar constriction and glomerular mesangial cell contraction, both of which contribute to a further reduction in the GFR.[146,153]

Na$^+$ reabsorption is increased both by a direct effect of angiotensin-II on proximal tubular Na$^+$ reabsorption and through stimulation of aldosterone with its effects on increasing distal Na$^+$ reabsorption.[154] Although diuretics are important in countering this excessive Na$^+$ retention, they also stimulate angiotensin-II production and should typically be combined with agents that disrupt the RAS. Although ACE inhibitors have a major impact on the symptomatic relief and progression of CHF, the exact mechanism behind their beneficial effect remains elusive (see Chap. 10). ACE inhibitors also inhibit the degradation of bradykinin, which stimulates nitrous oxide, an important mediator of a number of endothelial functions. It is not clear to what extent the positive effects of ACE inhibitors reflect a reduction in angiotensin-II levels, an increase in bradykinin levels, or both. At the tissue level, angiotensin-II can also be generated by non-ACE pathways; thus, its production is not completely inhibited by ACE inhibitors. ARBs, a class of drug that also has beneficial effects in CHF, will hopefully refine the thinking on this issue.[155]

Circulating levels of endothelin, arginine vasopressin (AVP), and atrial natriuretic peptide (ANP) are also commonly elevated in patients with CHF. Levels of endothelin correlate with pulmonary vascular resistance in CHF.[156] AVP is stimulated despite the presence of a low serum Na$^+$ and plasma osmolality as is commonly seen in CHF patients.[157] AVP contributes to hyponatremia and possibly the vasoconstriction in severe CHF.[158] ANP is a renal vasodilator that acts as a counterregulatory factor that opposes the actions of several vasoconstrictors. Endothelin-receptor inhibitors, AVP-receptor antagonists, and brain natriuretic peptide (BNP) are currently undergoing intense investigation in the treatment of CHF.

Diuretics in CHF

Diuretics are useful in the long-term management of chronic stable CHF patients who have continuing salt and water retention despite dietary Na$^+$ restriction. They are also useful in patients who experience acute decompensation of their CHF. Intravenous diuretics can improve the hemodynamic profile of decompensated CHF rapidly but they also can be associated with further deterioration. In a study of 15 patients with severe acutely decompensated CHF, intravenous furosemide led to an abrupt increase in systemic vascular resistance and BP, and to a decrease in cardiac performance parameters.[159] This deleterious effect reversed itself over 2 h, coinciding with, but not necessarily relating to, the onset of diuresis. This phenomenon of acute decompensation is likely dose-dependent; thus, caution needs to be exercised in acutely decompensated CHF as to the amount of furosemide administered. In patients with compensated CHF and severe edema, loop diuretics can be important add-on therapy to ACE inhibitors. In a study of 13 patients with severe edema secondary to CHF, furosemide therapy increased stroke volume owing to a reduction in systemic vascular resistance and afterload.[160] In a double-blind study comparing a loop diuretic or cardiac glycoside with placebo, symptoms and pulmonary capillary wedge pressure were improved to a similar extent by both drug classes.[161] However, patients treated with diuretics were more likely to develop a decreased effective blood volume and symptoms such as orthostatic hypotension, weakness and prerenal azotemia. Therefore, salt-depleting therapy requires a continual assessment of effective blood volume and adjustments in dietary salt intake and/or diuretic dose to optimize cardiac performance.

Mild CHF often responds to dietary salt restriction (100 to 150 mmol/d) and/or low doses of a thiazide diuretic. As CHF worsens, the GFR also decreases and patients become less respon-

sive to thiazide diuretics. This usually occurs as the GFR falls below 30-mL/min (plasma creatinine concentration of 2 to 4 mg/dL). Larger, more frequent doses of loop diuretics and tighter control of dietary salt intake may then be required as the disease progresses.

Factors Influencing Diuretic Efficacy

Alterations in Pharmacokinetics

CHF modifies diuretic disposition. Although diuretic pharmacokinetics are usually unaltered in mild CHF, with severe CHF major abnormalities occur. Although the absolute absorption of furosemide and bumetanide is normal in CHF patients, the time required to reach peak serum diuretic concentrations after oral dosing is significantly delayed.[162] The delayed absorption can reduce the peak diuretic concentrations in plasma and urine, thus diminishing diuretic tubular delivery and thereby efficacy.[163] Impaired drug absorption is thought to be related to reduced gastric and intestinal motility, edematous bowel wall, and/or decreased splanchnic blood flow.

As renal plasma flow declines in CHF, so will the delivery of furosemide or other loop diuretics to their site of action in the loop of Henle. The secretion of furosemide is reduced when the GFR falls below 30-mL/min because of the accumulation of endogenous organic acids that compete with furosemide for secretion by the organic anion transporter.[164] At this level of renal insufficiency, loop diuretics must be administered in higher doses in order to circumvent factors, which limit tubular secretion.

Alterations in Pharmacodynamics

The relationship between natriuresis and excretion of loop diuretics is not altered in mild CHF,[165] but the dose-response curve is shifted rightward in more advanced CHF (Fig. 11-6).[166] The factors behind this shift in diuretic responsiveness are numerous, including structural adaptations that occur in the distal nephron, as well as excessive activation of the RAS and SNS. ACE inhibitors can sometimes reestablish a diuresis in resistant CHF patients by

FIGURE 11-6. Sodium excretory response following furosemide infusions in acute renal failure (ARF) or congestive heart failure (CHF) patients. Despite the flatness of the dose-response curves, the majority of the patients responded with an increment in urine volume/sodium excretion, having failed prior bolus therapy.

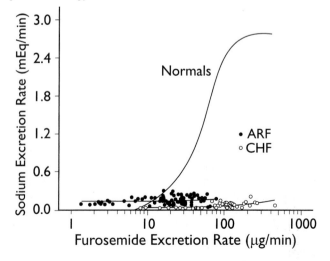

inhibiting the generation of angiotensin-II and thereby favorably altering afterload and/or renal blood flow.[167] Conversely, if the BP drop is excessive with an ACE inhibitor, the diuretic response can be attenuated.[168]

Diuretic Dosing in CHF

Because of alterations in diuretic pharmacokinetics and pharmacodynamics patients with CHF often appear to be resistant to diuretics.[169] The first step in evaluating a CHF patient for diuretic resistance is to assess the level of dietary salt and fluid intake. At steady state, dietary salt intake can be assessed from the measurement of 24-h Na^+ excretion. Patients ingesting a high-salt diet will overwhelm the capacity of the diuretic to produce a net diuresis and weight loss. If this is the case a dietitian may be necessary in order to suitably reduce daily Na^+ intake to 100 mmol/d or less. Before labeling the patient as truly diuretic resistant, it is also important to ensure that the patient is compliant with their diuretic dosing (usually twice a day dosing is necessary) and that the patient is not taking medication that interferes with the action of diuretics such as NSAIDs.[170] Once these factors are eliminated from consideration changes in diuretic doses or route of administration and diuretic combinations should be considered.

In CHF patients refractory to standard furosemide doses, high-dose therapy may prove efficacious. Daily doses of between 500 and 2000 mg of intravenous furosemide were administered to 20 patients with CHF and refractory edema. With this regimen, a diuresis was established, body weight was reduced, and the CHF class was improved. Similar studies have reported improved furosemide efficacy in refractory CHF where high-doses of oral furosemide were employed.[171] When moderate to severe renal impairment is present in decompensated CHF, a brief trial of high-dose furosemide is reasonable. Gerlag and Van Meijel treated patients with renal insufficiency (mean GFR, 32 mL/min) and refractory CHF with high-dose oral and IV furosemide over a 4-week period. Patients experienced a mean reduction in weight of 11.1 kg and an improvement in New York Heart Association (NYHA) classification.[172]

Continuous IV administration of loop diuretics is another effective method of overcoming diuretic resistance in CHF patients. In a randomized crossover study comparing continuous infusion versus bolus bumetanide in patients with severe renal insufficiency (mean GFR, 17 mL/min), Rudy et al observed a greater net Na^+ excretion during continuous infusion despite comparable total 14-h drug excretion.[173] The rate of urinary bumetanide excretion remained constant when infused. With intermittent administration, peak bumetanide excretion was observed within the first 2 h and tapered thereafter. In a similar study employing furosemide, a continuous IV infusion of furosemide (loading dose of 30 to 40 mg followed by infusion at a rate of 2.5 to 3.3 mg/h for 48 h) was compared to intermittent IV bolus administration (30 to 40 mg every 8 h for 48 h) in NYHA class III and class IV heart failure.[174] A significantly greater diuresis and natriuresis was observed using continuous furosemide infusion as compared with intermittent administration; this was accomplished at a lower peak furosemide concentration. When continuously infused, the pattern of furosemide delivery produced more efficient drug utilization. In a recent study examining the cost of care for 17 elderly patients with class IV CHF continuous intravenous furosemide infusion resulted in a successful diuresis of between 9 and 20 L over an average of 3.5 days. The length of stay for these patients was an average of 2.3 days shorter when compared to a contemporary group of class III and

class IV CHF patients who were managed with conventional dosing of furosemide, and resulted in significant cost savings.[175]

Combinations of diuretic classes have frequently by used in CHF patients refractory to loop diuretics alone. Because of structural adaptation occurring in the distal nephron with prolonged loop diuretic therapy the combination of a distal diuretic and loop diuretic is particularly effective in these patients. The combination of bumetanide and metolazone (a thiazide) produces a synergistic diuretic effect.[176] During prolonged furosemide therapy, the responsiveness to a thiazide is augmented.[177] Numerous reports have demonstrated a profound diuresis (1 to 2 L daily) accompanied by clinical improvement, following the addition of metolazone to furosemide in CHF patients previously resistant to furosemide therapy alone.[177-180] Metolazone is particularly effective because its duration of action is prolonged, it is lipophilic, and it remains effective in states of renal impairment. However, in a study comparing metolazone with a short-acting thiazide, both used in combination with a loop diuretic, no significant difference in sodium excretion or urine output was observed between the two drugs.[158] Spironolactone has also been used in combination with loop diuretics and has been associated with an improvement in diuretic response in CHF patients.[181] Above and beyond the known diuretic properties of spironolactone, it was recently shown that, as an aldosterone-receptor antagonist, spironolactone blocks a wide-range of deleterious tissue-based effects attributable to aldosterone, which include augmentation of vascular and myocardial fibrosis.[181a,b] Accordingly, spironolactone is increasingly advocated as adjunct therapy in CHF.[181c,182] The basis for this therapeutic recommendation is the Randomized Aldactone Evaluation Study (RALES).[183] In the RALES trial, spironolactone was shown to reduce the risk of all-cause mortality in NYHA class IV CHF patients treated with standard ACE inhibitor and diuretic therapy. It was recently demonstrated that aldosterone levels may often be elevated in CHF patients despite the use of ACE inhibitors.[183a] In the future, diuretic combinations, including loop and distal tubular diuretics, as well as aldosterone receptor inhibitors, may be routinely used in patients with CHF.

Other Pharmacologic Approaches to Diuresis

Other approaches to diuresis include the use of dopamine agonists (see Chap. 26), vasopressin antagonists (see Chap. 35), adenosine antagonists (see Chap. 32), natriuretic peptides (see Chap. 27), and neutral endopeptidase inhibitors (see Chap. 27).

ADVERSE EFFECTS OF DIURETICS

Hyponatremia

Severe diuretic-induced hyponatremia is a serious complication of diuretic therapy.[184] Elderly females treated with thiazide diuretics are most commonly affected, and the condition is usually seen within the first 2 weeks of therapy.[185] Elderly females seem to exhibit an exaggerated natriuretic response to a thiazide diuretic yet have a diminished capacity to excrete free water. These individuals also may have a low solute intake, which further diminishes their capacity for free water elimination.

Thiazide diuretics are more likely to cause hyponatremia than are loop diuretics because they increase Na^+ excretion and prevent maximal urine dilution while preserving the kidney's concentrating capacity. Loop diuretics inhibit salt transport in the renal medulla and prevent the generation of a maximal osmotic gradient and actually can be used in hyponatremic subjects to increase free water clearance.[186] CHF-related hyponatremia is more often a consequence of neurohumoral activation than a consequence of diuretic use, although diuretic use undoubtedly contributes to its development.

Mild asymptomatic hyponatremia can be treated by withholding diuretics, restricting free water intake and restoring K[+] losses.[187] Severe, symptomatic hyponatremia complicated by seizures is an emergency requiring intensive therapy, although steps should be taken to avoid rapid or overcorrection of the hyponatremia, because central pontine myelinolysis has occurred under these circumstances. The risks of ongoing hyponatremia must be weighed against those of too rapid a correction and current recommendations are that plasma Na[+] should be corrected by no more than 12 to 20 mmol in the first 24 h.[188,189] Controversy continues, however, in this area of therapy.

Hypokalemia and Hyperkalemia

Hypokalemia is a common finding in patients treated with loop and/or thiazide diuretics.[190] During the first week of therapy with a thiazide diuretic, plasma K[+] in subjects not taking K[+] supplements fell by an average of 0.6 mmol/L as compared with 0.3 mmol/L in those taking furosemide.[190] Mechanisms that contribute to hypokalemia during thiazide or loop diuretic use include augmented flow-dependent K[+] secretion in the distal nephron, a fall in luminal Cl[−] concentration in the distal tubule, metabolic alkalosis, and/or stimulation of aldosterone and/or vasopressin release, both of which promote distal K[+] secretion (Fig. 11-7).[191−194]

The clinical significance of diuretic-induced hypokalemia remains controversial, although mild degrees of diuretic-induced hypokalemia can be associated with increased ventricular ectopy.[195−197] The MRFIT trial found a significant inverse relationship between the serum K[+] concentration and the frequency of ventricular premature contractions (VPCs).[197] This relationship, however, has not been observed in all trials,[198−200] possibly because of the short duration of many of these trials. In the MRC study involving 324 patients with mild hypertension, 287 of whom underwent ambulatory electrocardiogram (ECG) monitoring, after 8 weeks of therapy, diuretic use was not associated with an increased frequency

of VPCs, whereas after 24-months, there was a significant difference in VPCs in those patients receiving diuretics as compared with those patients receiving placebo (20% vs 9%).[200] These VPCs were significantly correlated with the serum K[+] concentration. Patients with LVH, CHF, or myocardial ischemia are at a particularly high risk of developing lethal ventricular arrhythmias in the setting of K[+] depletion.[201−203]

Despite a concern about diuretic-related increases in cardiac risk, in part, due to electrolyte abnormalities, recent clinical trials including SHEP, STOP, and MRC, have shown that low-dose diuretic therapy is actually associated with a 20 to 25% reduction in cardiovascular events.[100,101,104] Perhaps the use of lower doses of thiazides or combination therapy with a K[+]-sparing diuretic explains these favorable results as compared with earlier trials, such as MRFIT, in which higher doses of diuretics were employed and VPCs were more frequent. However, in the SHEP trial, patients with hypokalemia did not achieve the benefit of treatment seen in normokalemic patients.[204]

Comparative effects on sudden cardiac death of different doses and combinations of diuretics have been reported.[205,206] The risk of cardiac arrest among patients receiving combined thiazide and K[+]-sparing diuretic therapy was lower than that found in patients treated with thiazides alone (odds ratio 0.3:1). Compared with low-dose thiazide therapy (25 mg/d), intermediate-dose thiazide therapy (50 mg/d) was associated with moderate increase in the risk of cardiac arrest (odds ratio 1.7:1) and high-dose (100 mg/d) was associated with an even greater increase in risk (odds ratio 3.6:1). In contrast with K[+]-sparing diuretics, the addition of K[+] supplements to thiazide therapy had little effect on the risk of sudden cardiac death (odds ratio 0.9:1). Among patients receiving only one antihypertensive medication, the risk of cardiac arrest was not higher with diuretic treatment than with beta-blockers (odds ratio 1:1). Serum K[+] concentrations <3 mmol/L occur infrequently with thiazide diuretics, and when found, are more common with loop diuretics or carbonic anhydrase inhibitors.[207] Profound hypokalemia with serum K[+] concentrations <2.5 mmol/L can lead to diffuse muscle weakness, including diaphragmatic paralysis, rhabdomyolysis, and acute renal failure.[208,209]

Distal K[+]-sparing diuretics and spironolactone can cause dangerous hyperkalemia. Hyperkalemia is usually encountered in patients predisposed to this complication, those with a reduction in

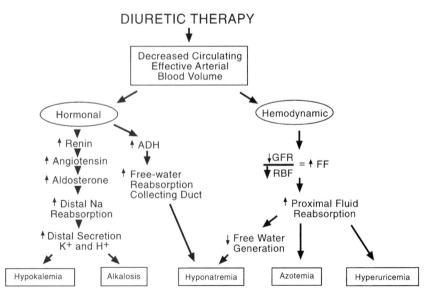

DIURETIC THERAPY

FIGURE 11-7. Adaptive changes to conserve salt and water in states of extracellular volume depletion resulting in side effects related to diuretic use.

their GFR (especially the elderly or those given potassium chloride supplements or salt substitutes), those on an ACE inhibitor or a NSAID, or in other situations that predispose to hyperkalemia such as acidosis, hyporeninemic hypoaldosteronism, or heparin therapy.[52]

Hypomagnesemia

Loop diuretics inhibit magnesium (Mg) reabsorption in the loop of Henle, a site where approximately 30% of the filtered load of Mg is reabsorbed. Potassium-sparing diuretics, including spirono-lactone, diminish the increase in Mg excretion that accompanies thiazide or loop diuretic use.[17,210] Prolonged therapy with thiazides and loop diuretics reduces plasma Mg concentration by an average of 5 to 10%, although patients occasionally develop severe hypomagnesemia.[211] Cellular Mg depletion occurs in 20 to 50% of patients during thiazide therapy and can be present despite a normal serum Mg concentration. This complication is more common in the elderly and in those patients receiving prolonged, high-dose diuretic therapy.[212] Hypomagnesemia often coexists with diuretic-induced hyponatremia and hypokalemia disorders that cannot be fully reversed until the underlying Mg deficit is corrected.[213] In one study, 41% of patients with hypokalemia were found to also have low serum Mg concentrations.[214] Two studies report hypomagnesemia in 19 to 37% of CHF patients treated with loop diuretics.[215,216] The data regarding the association of hypomagnesemia with an increased prevalence of ventricular premature contractions, sudden death, and overall cardiovascular survival are conflicting, and a definite causal relationship is lacking. Associated symptoms of hypomagnesemia include depression, muscle weakness, refractory hypokalemia, hypocalcemia, atrial fibrillation. Many of these abnormalities and, in particular, refractory hypokalemia and hypocalcemia, correct promptly with Mg administration.[211,214]

Acid-Base Changes

Thiazides and loop diuretics can both cause a metabolic alkalosis. The generation of this metabolic alkalosis is due primarily to a contraction of the ECF space caused by urinary loss of a relatively HCO_3-free fluid.[217] The maintenance of the alkalosis probably involves increased net acid excretion in response to hypokalemia, mineralocorticoid excess, and continued Na^+ delivery to the distal nephron sites of H^+ secretion.[217,218] Diuretic-induced metabolic alkalosis is best managed by administration of potassium and/or sodium chloride, although sodium chloride administration may not be feasible in the CHF patient who is already volume overloaded. In these cases, a potassium-sparing diuretic or, on rare occasions, a carbonic anhydrase inhibitor, such as acetazolamide, may be considered. Metabolic alkalosis also impairs the natriuretic response to loop diuretics and may contribute to diuretic resistance in the CHF patient.[219]

Spironolactone, as well as amiloride and triamterene, can cause hyperkalemic metabolic acidosis, which in elderly patients, or in those patients with renal impairment or CHF, can occasionally be severe and of a life-threatening nature.[220]

METABOLIC ABNORMALITIES

Hyperglycemia

Prolonged thiazide diuretic therapy impairs glucose tolerance and may occasionally precipitate diabetes mellitus.[221–223] Hy-perglycemia and carbohydrate intolerance have been linked to diuretic-induced hypokalemia, which inhibits insulin secretion by β cells, and reduces ECF volume and cardiac output. These aberrations are compounded by increases in SNS activity, which decreases peripheral glucose use. Short-term metabolic studies, epidemiologic studies, and a variety of clinical trials suggest a causal link between the use of thiazide diuretics and subsequent development of type 2 diabetes. However, these studies were compromised by small numbers of patients, relatively limited follow-up periods, varying definitions of new-onset diabetes, inadequate comparison groups, selection criteria that limited the generalizability of the findings, and study designs that precluded interclass comparisons amongst antihypertensive drug classes.[224]

For example, in one study non-insulin-dependent diabetics given HCTZ for only 3 weeks increased their fasting serum glucose concentration by 31%; when combined with propranolol, the increase was 53%.[225]

Diuretic-associated glucose intolerance appears to be dose-related, less common with loop diuretics,[222] and reversible on withdrawal of the agent, although the data on reversibility in HCTZ-treated patients appears conflicting. Ramsay and colleagues reviewed this issue and found several studies that support unaltered glucose homeostasis by using low-dose HCTZ therapy (25 to 50 mg/d).[225] However, they also report three long-term trials that note abnormalities in glucose homeostasis with HCTZ doses of between 12.5 and 50 mg/d. Recently, Gress et al conducted a large, prospective, cohort study that included 12,250 adults who did not have diabetes and that was designed to examine the independent relationship between the use of antihypertensive medications and the subsequent development of type 2 diabetes. After appropriate adjustment for confounders, patients with hypertension who were taking thiazide diuretics were found not to be at greater risk for subsequent diabetes development than patients who were not receiving antihypertensive therapy. The doses of thiazide diuretic given in the cohort study by Gress et al were not reported; thus, because of the perceived variability of this effect, blood glucose should be monitored during thiazide therapy, particularly in obese or diabetic patients.[226] Consequently, long-term thiazide therapy can be viewed as causing only small changes, if any at all, in fasting serum glucose concentration, an effect that might be reversed with the concomitant use of potassium-sparing diuretics.[227]

Hyperlipidemia

The short-term administration of either loop diuretics or of thiazides increases the plasma cholesterol concentrations by 4 to 14% and raises the levels of low-density and very-low-density lipoproteins and triglycerides,[228,229] an effect that may be simply related to mild volume depletion.[230] Long-term clinical trials have reported unchanged cholesterol levels after 1 year of diuretic therapy.[231,232] Moreover, data from the HDFP Study indicate that hypertensive subjects with baseline cholesterol values of >250 mg/dL, treated with diuretics, experience a decline in cholesterol levels from the second to the fifth years of treatment.[98]

Hyperuricemia

Thiazide therapy increases serum urate concentrations by approximately 35%, an effect related to decreased urate clearance.[233] Decreased urate clearance may be related to increased reabsorption secondary to diuretic-related ECF volume depletion.[42] Hyperuricemia is dose-related and does not usually precipitate a gouty attack unless the patient has an underlying gouty tendency or serum urate concentrations exceed 12 to 14 mg/dL.[234] In the MRC trial, patients receiving thiazide diuretics had significantly more withdrawals for gout than did placebo-treated patients (4.4 vs 0.1 per 1000 patient years).[104] If a gouty attack occurs, diuretic therapy should be discontinued. If this is not feasible then the lowest clinically effective dose should be given and the degree of volume contraction limited. An additional alternative in the gouty patient requiring diuretic therapy is that of allopurinol. However, allopurinol should be used cautiously in patients receiving HCTZ because the incidence of hypersensitivity reactions is higher with this combination.[235]

Other Adverse Effects

Impotence

In the MRC trial in which 15,000 hypertensive subjects received either placebo, thiazide, or a beta-blocker for 5 years, impotence was 22-fold and 4-fold higher in those receiving a thiazide compared to placebo or a beta-blocker, respectively.[221] Another smaller trial reported on by Chang et al confirmed a higher frequency of decreased libido, difficulty in gaining and sustaining an erection, and difficulty in ejaculating in patients receiving a thiazide.[236] Multivariate analysis suggested that these findings were not mediated by low serum potassium levels or by low blood pressure. The exact mechanism of diuretic-related impotence is not known. Patients on diuretics with impotence can respond favorably to sildenafil.[236a]

Ototoxicity

The association of ototoxicity and loop diuretics is well established.[237] Loop diuretics are direct inhibitors of the $Na^+/K^+/2Cl^-$ cotransport system, which also exists in the marginal and dark cells of the stria vascularis, which are responsible for endolymph secretion; thus, the ototoxicity of these agents may be indirect, due to changes in ionic composition and fluid volume within the endolymph.

Loop diuretic-induced ototoxicity usually occurs within 20 min of infusion and is typically reversible, although permanent deafness has been reported. Ototoxicity has been seen with ethacrynic acid, furosemide, and bumetanide with both IV and oral administration. The frequency appears to be higher with furosemide than with bumetanide.[238,239] Patients with renal failure and those receiving concomitant aminoglycoside therapy are at greatest risk of developing ototoxicity.[240]

Ototoxicity is clearly related to both the rate of infusion and to peak serum concentrations. Heidland and Wigand conducted audiometric studies during the infusion of furosemide at a constant rate of 25 mg/min and reported reversible hearing loss in two-thirds of patients.[241] Fries and colleagues found no hearing loss in renal-failure patients receiving between 500 and 1000 mg over 6 h.[242] Plasma levels of furosemide greater that 50 μg/mL are associated with a greater incidence of auditory disturbances, and Brown and colleagues found patients with levels greater than 100 μg/mL to be at risk for permanent deafness.[243,244] In general, the rate of furosemide infusion should not exceed 4 mg/min and serum concentrations should be maintained below 40 μg/mL.

Drug Allergy

Photosensitivity dermatitis occurs rarely during thiazide or furosemide therapy.[245] HCTZ more commonly causes photosensitivity than do the other thiazides.[246] Diuretics may occasionally cause a more serious generalized dermatitis and, at times, even a necrotizing vasculitis. Cross-sensitivity with sulfonamide drugs may occur with all diuretics, with the exception of ethacrynic acid. Severe necrotizing pancreatitis is an additional serious, life-threatening complication of thiazide therapy.[247] Acute allergic interstitial nephritis with fever, rash, and eosinophilia, although an uncommon complication of diuretics, is one that may result in permanent renal failure if the drug exposure is prolonged.[248] It may develop abruptly or some months after therapy is begun with a thiazide diuretic or, less commonly, with furosemide.[249] Ethacrynic acid is chemically dissimilar from the other loop diuretics and can be safely substituted in diuretic-treated patients who experience a number of these allergic complications.

Carcinogenesis

Two reports suggest an increased risk of renal cell carcinoma and colon cancer with long-term diuretic therapy,[250,251] but further confirmation is necessary.

ADVERSE DRUG INTERACTIONS

Besides those interactions already reviewed, other drug-diuretic interactions may occur with diuretics (see Chap. 48). Loop diuretics are known to potentiate aminoglycoside nephrotoxicity.[252] By causing hypokalemia, diuretics increase digitalis toxicity.[253] Plasma lithium concentrations can increase with thiazide therapy if significant volume contraction occurs; this is due to increased reabsorption of fluid and lithium in the proximal tubule.[254] However, some diuretics, such as chlorothiazide or furosemide, with significant carbonic anhydrase inhibitory effect decrease proximal fluid reabsorption and increase lithium clearance, thus leading to a fall in lithium levels.[255,256] Whole-blood lithium should be closely monitored in all patients being administered lithium in conjunction with diuretics. Furosemide can potentiate the myotoxic effects of clofibrate through the displacement of clofibrate from plasma protein binding sites.[257]

NSAIDs can both antagonize the effects of diuretics and predispose diuretic-treated patients to renal insufficiency. The combination of indomethacin and triamterene may be particularly dangerous in that acute renal failure can be precipitated.[258] A reversible form of renal insufficiency may also develop when excessive diuresis occurs in ACE-inhibitor-treated CHF patients. Risk factors for this form of functional renal insufficiency include hyponatremia, diabetes and the use of long-acting ACE inhibitors.[259,260] This response may be exaggerated if NSAIDs are also added to the mix of medications.[261] Na^+ balance plays an important role in modulating the BP response to ACE inhibitors in CHF. Patients with Na^+ and volume depletion before ACE inhibitors are started are at a higher risk of developing first-dose hypotension.[262]

REFERENCES

1. Dustan H, Rocella EJ, Garrison H: Controlling hypertension. A research success story. *Arch Intern Med* 156:1926, 1996.
2. The Sixth Report of the Joint National Committee on Prevention, Detection, Evaluation, and Treatment of High Blood Pressure. *Arch Intern Med* 153:154, 1997.
3. Brater DC: Diuretic therapy. *N Engl J Med* 339:387, 1998.
4. Ichikawa I, Kon V: Role of peritubular capillary forces in the renal action of carbonic anhydrase inhibitor. *Kidney Int* 30:828, 1986.

5. Eveloff J, Warnock DG: Renal carbonic anhydrase. In: Dirks JH, Sutton RA, eds. *Diuretics: Physiology, Pharmacology and Clinical Use*. Philadelphia: WB Saunders, 1986:49–65.

6. Cogan MG, Maddox DA, Warnock DG, et al: Effect of acetazolamide on bicarbonate reabsorption in the proximal tubule of the rat. *Am J Physiol* 237:F447, 1979.

7. Ko CH, Kong CK: Topiramate-induced metabolic acidosis: Report of two cases. *Dev Med Child Neurol* 43:701, 2001.

8. Kirschenbaum MA: Severe mannitol-induced hyponatremia complicating transurethral prostatic resection. *J Urol* 121:687, 1979.

9. Weaver A, Sica DA: Mannitol-induced acute renal failure. *Nephron* 45:233, 1987.

10. O'Grady SM, Palfrey HC, Field M: Characteristics and function of Na-K-2Cl cotransport in epithelial tissues. *Am J Physiol* 252:C177, 1987.

11. Radtke HW, Rumrich G, Kinne-Saffran E, Ulrich KJ: Dual action of acetazolamide and furosemide on proximal volume absorption in the rat kidney. *Kidney Int* 1:100, 1972.

12. Duarte CG, Chomety F, Giebisch G: Effect of amiloride, ouabain, and furosemide on distal tubular function in the rat. *Am J Physiol* 221:632, 1971.

13. Jung KY, Endou H: Furosemide acts on short loop of descending thin limb, but not on long loop. *J Pharmacol Exp Ther* 253:1184, 1990.

14. Wilson DR, Honrath U, Sonnenberg H: Furosemide action on collecting ducts: Effect of prostaglandin synthesis inhibition. *Am J Physiol* 244:F666, 1983.

15. Earley LE, Friedler RM: Renal tubular effects of ethacrynic acid. *J Clin Invest* 43:1495, 1964.

16. White MG, van Gelder J, Eastes G: The effect of loop diuretics on the excretion of Na+, Ca^{2+}, Mg^{2+}, and Cl$^-$. *J Clin Pharmacol* 21:610, 1981.

17. Ryan MP, Devane J, Ryan MG, Counihan TB: Effects of diuretics on the renal handling of magnesium. *Drugs* 28(Suppl 1):167, 1984.

18. Steele TH, Oppenheimer S: Factors affecting urate excretion following diuretic administration in man. *Am J Med* 47:564, 1969.

19. Gerber JG: Role of prostaglandins in the hemodynamic and tubular effects of furosemide. *Fed Proc* 42:1707, 1983.

20. Loon NR, Wilcox CS, Unwin RJ: Mechanism of impaired natriuretic response to furosemide during prolonged therapy. *Kidney Int* 36:682, 1989.

21. Benet LZ: Pharmacokinetics/pharmacodynamics of furosemide in man: A review. *J Pharmacokinet Biopharm* 7:1, 1979.

22. Murray MD, Haag KM, Black PK, et al: Variable furosemide absorption and poor predictability of response in elderly patients. *Pharmacotherapy* 17:98, 1997.

23. Bowman RH: Renal secretion of [^{35}S]furosemide and depression by albumin binding. *Am J Physiol* 229:93, 1975.

24. Takamura N, Maruyama T, Otagiri M: Effects of uremic toxins and fatty acids on serum protein binding of furosemide: Possible mechanism of the binding defect in uremia. *Clin Chem* 43:2274, 1997.

25. Chennavasin P, Seiwell R, Brater DC, et al: Pharmacodynamic analysis of the furosemide-probenecid interaction in man. *Kidney Int* 16:187, 1979.

26. Brater DC, Day B, Burdette A, et al: Bumetanide and furosemide in heart failure. *Kidney Int* 26:183, 1984.

27. Wilcox CS, Mitch WE, Kelly RA, et al: Response of the kidney to furosemide. I. Effects of salt intake and renal compensation. *J Lab Clin Med* 102:450, 1983.

28. Chennavasin P, Seiwell R, Brater DC: Pharmacokinetic-dynamic analysis of the indomethacin-furosemide interaction in man. *J Pharmacol Exp Ther* 215:77, 1980.

29. Agarwal R, Gorski JC, Sundblad K, Brater DC: Urinary protein binding does not affect response to furosemide in patients with nephrotic syndrome. *J Am Soc Nephrol* 11:1100, 2000.

30. Knoben JE, Anderson PO, eds. Diuretics. In: *Clinical Drug Data*. 6th ed. IL: Drug Intelligence Publications; 1988:611–616.

31. Voelker JR, Brown-Cartwright D, Anderson S, et al: Comparison of loop diuretics in patients with chronic renal insufficiency: Mechanism of difference in response. *Kidney Int* 32:572, 1987.

32. Marcantonio LA, Auld WH, Murdoch WR, et al: The pharmacokinetics and pharmacodynamics of the diuretic bumetanide in hepatic and renal disease. *Br J Clin Pharmacol* 15:245, 1983.

33. Rudy DW, Gehr TW, Matzke GR, et al: The pharmacodynamics of IV and oral torsemide in patients with chronic renal insufficiency. *Clin Pharmacol Ther* 56:39, 1994.

34. Schwartz S, Brater C, Pound D, et al: Bioavailability, pharmacokinetics, and pharmacodynamics of torsemide in patients with cirrhosis. *Clin Pharmacol Ther* 54:90, 1993.

35. Vargo DL, Kramer WG, Black PK, et al: Bioavailability, pharmacokinetics, and pharmacodynamics of torsemide and furosemide in patients with congestive heart failure. *Clin Pharmacol Ther* 57:601, 1995.

36. Murray MD, Deer MM, Ferguson JA, et al: Open-label randomized trial of torsemide compared with furosemide therapy for patients with heart failure. *Am J Med* 111:513, 2001.

37. Ellison DH, Velazquez H, Wright FS: Thiazide-sensitive sodium chloride cotransport in early distal tubule. *Am J Physiol* 253:F546, 1987.

38. Beyer KH: Chlorothiazide. *Br J Clin Pharmacol* 13:15, 1982.

39. Wilson DR, Honrath U, Sonnenberg H: Thiazide diuretic effect on medullary collecting duct function in the rat. *Kidney Int* 23:711, 1983.

40. Seldin DW, Eknoyan G, Suki WN, et al: Localization of diuretic action from the pattern of water and electrolyte excretion. *Ann N Y Acad Sci* 139:328, 1966.

41. Giles TD, Sander GE, Roffidal LE, et al: Comparative effects of nitrendipine and hydrochlorothiazide on calciotropic hormones and bone density in hypertensive patients. *Am J Hypertens* 5:875, 1992.

42. Weinman EJ, Eknoyan G, Suki WN: The influence of the extracellular fluid volume on the tubular reabsorption of uric acid. *J Clin Invest* 55:283, 1975.

43. Leary WP, Reyes AJ: Diuretic-induced magnesium losses. *Drugs* 28(Suppl 1):182, 1984.

44. Welling PG: Pharmacokinetics of the thiazide diuretics. *Biopharm Drug Dispos* 7:501, 1986.

45. Beermann B, Groschinsky-Grind M: Clinical pharmacokinetics of diuretics. *Clin Pharmacokinet* 5:221, 1980.

46. Knauf H, Mutschler E: Diuretic effectiveness of hydrochlorothiazide and furosemide alone and in combination in chronic renal failure. *J Cardiovasc Pharmacol* 26:394, 1995.

47. Stern A: Metolazone, a diuretic agent. *Am Heart J* 91:262, 1976.

48. Suki WN, Dawoud F, Eknoyan G, et al: Effects of metolazone on renal function in normal man. *J Pharmacol Exp Ther* 180:6, 1972.

49. Craswell PW, Ezzat E, Kopstein J, et al: Use of metolazone, a new diuretic, in patients with renal disease. *Nephron* 12:63, 1973.

50. Wingo CS: Cortical collecting tubule potassium secretion: Effect of amiloride, ouabain, and luminal sodium concentration. *Kidney Int* 27:886, 1985.

51. Wingo CS: Potassium secretion by the cortical collecting tubule: Effect of Cl gradients and ouabain. *Am J Physiol* 256:F306, 1989.

52. Brater DC: Clinical utility of the potassium-sparing diuretics. *Hosp Form Man* 19:79, 1984.

53. McInnes GT: Relative potency of amiloride and spironolactone in healthy man. *Clin Pharmacol Ther* 31:472, 1982.

54. Rahn KH. Clinical pharmacology of diuretics. *Clin Exp Hypertens* 5:157, 1983.

55. Andriulli A, Arrigoni A, Gindro T, et al: Canrenone and androgen receptor-active materials in plasma of cirrhotic patients during long-term K-canrenoate or spironolactone therapy. *Digestion* 44:155, 1989.

56. Burgess E, Niegowska J, Tan K-W, et al: Antihypertensive effect of eplerenone and enalapril in patients with essential hypertension (abst.). *Am J Hypertens* 15:23A, 2002.

56a. Epstein M, Buckalew V, Martinez F, et al: Antiproteinuric efficacy of eplerenone, enalapril and eplerenone/enalapril combination therapy in diabetic hypertensives with micro albuminuria (abst.) *Am J Hypertens* 15:24A, 2002.

57. Somogyi AA, Hovens CM, Muirhead MR, Bochner F: Renal tubular secretion of amiloride and its inhibition by cimetidine in humans and in an animal model. *Drug Metab Dispos* 17:190, 1989.

58. Mutschler E, Gilfrich HJ, Knauf H, et al: Pharmacokinetics of triamterene. *Clin Exp Hypertens* 5:249, 1983.

59. Villeneuve JP, Rocheleau F, Raymond G: Triamterene kinetics and dynamics in cirrhosis. *Clin Pharmacol Ther* 35:831, 1984.

60. Knauf H, Mohrke W, Mutschler E: Delayed elimination of triamterene and its active metabolite in chronic renal failure. *Eur J Clin Pharmacol* 24:453, 1983.

61. Sica DA, Gehr TW: Triamterene and the kidney. *Nephron* 51:454, 1989.

62. Kelly RA, Wilcox CS, Mitch WE, et al: Response of the kidney to furosemide. II. Effect of captopril on sodium balance. *Kidney Int* 24:233, 1983.

63. Wilcox CS, Guzman NJ, Mitch WE, et al: Na+ and BP homeostasis in man during furosemide: Effects of prazosin and captopril. *Kidney Int* 31:135, 1987.

64. Wilcox CS, Loon NR, Ameer B, et al: Renal and hemodynamic responses to bumetanide in hypertension: effects of nitrendipine. *Kidney Int* 36:719, 1989.

65. Almeshari K, Ahlstrom NG, Capraro FE, et al: A volume-independent component to post-diuretic sodium retention in man. *J Am Soc Nephrol* 3:1878, 1993.

66. Frolich JC, Hollifield JW, Dormois JC, et al: Suppression of plasma renin activity by indomethacin in man. *Circ Res* 39:447, 1976.

67. Ellison DH, Velazquez H, Wright FS: Adaptation of the distal convoluted tubule of the rat. Structural and functional effects of dietary salt intake and chronic diuretic infusion. *J Clin Invest* 83:113, 1989.

68. Kim J, Welch WJ, Cannon JK, et al: Immunocytochemical response of type A and type B intercalated cells to increased sodium chloride delivery. *Am J Physiol* 262:F288, 1992.

69. Stanton BA, Kaissling B: Adaptation of distal tubule and collecting duct to increase Na+ delivery. II. Na+ and K+ transport. *Am J Physiol* 255:F1269, 1988.

70. Loon NR, Wilcox CS, Unwin RJ: Mechanism of impaired natriuretic response to furosemide during prolonged therapy. *Kidney Int* 36:682, 1989.

71. Idiopathic edema: Role of diuretic abuse. *Kidney Int* 19:881, 1981.

72. Imbs JL, Schmidt M, Velly J, et al: Comparison of the effect of two groups of diuretics on renin secretion in the anesthetized dog. *Clin Sci Mol Med* 52:171, 1977.

73. Wilson TW, Loadholt CB, Privitera PJ, et al: Furosemide increases urine 6-keto-prostaglandin $F_{1\alpha}$. Relation to natriuresis, vasodilation, and renin release. *Hypertension* 4:634, 1982.

74. Kraus PA, Lipman J, Becker PJ: Acute preload effects of furosemide. *Chest* 98:124, 1990.

75. Ciabattoni G, Pugliese F, Cinotti GA, et al: Characterization of furosemide-induced activation of the renal prostaglandin system. *Eur J Pharmacol* 60:181, 1979.

76. Dikshit K, Vyden JK, Forrester JS, et al: Renal and extrarenal hemodynamic effects of furosemide in congestive heart failure after acute myocardial infarction. *N Engl J Med* 288:1087, 1973.

77. Favre L, Glasson P, Riondel A, et al: Interaction of diuretics and non-steroidal anti-inflammatory drugs in man. *Clin Sci (Colch)* 64:407, 1983.

78. Tiggeler RG, Koene RA, Wijdeveld PG: Inhibition of frusemide-induced natriuresis by indomethacin in patients with nephrotic syndrome. *Clin Sci Mol Med* 52:149, 1977.

79. Kirchner KA, Brandon S, Mueller RA, et al: Mechanism of attenuated hydrochlorothiazide response during indomethacin administration. *Kidney Int* 31:1097, 1987.

80. Black HR, Kuller LH, O'Rourke MF, et al: The first report of the Systolic and Pulse Pressure (SYPP) Working Group. *J Hypertens* 17(Suppl 5):S3, 1999.

81. Roos JC, Boer P, Koomans HA, et al: Haemodynamic and hormonal changes during acute and chronic diuretic treatment in essential hypertension. *Eur J Clin Pharmacol* 19:107, 1981.

82. Van Brummelen P, Man in't Veld AI, Schalekamp MADH: Hemodynamic changes during long-term thiazide treatment of essential hypertension in responders and non-responders. *Clin Pharmacol Ther* 27:328, 1980.

83. Tarazi RC, Dustan HP, Frohlich ED: Long-term thiazide therapy in essential hypertension. *Circulation* 41:709, 1970.

84. Conway J, Lauwers P: Hemodynamic and hypotensive effects of long-term therapy with chlorothiazide. *Circulation* 21:21, 1960.

85. Uzu T, Kimura G: Diuretics shift circadian rhythm of blood pressure from nondipper to dipper in essential hypertension. *Circulation* 100:1635, 1999.

86. Shah S, Khatri I, Freis ED: Mechanism of antihypertensive effect of thiazide diuretics. *Am Heart J* 95:611, 1978.

87. Bennett WM, McDonald WJ, Kuehnel E, et al: Do diuretics have antihypertensive properties independent of natriuresis? *Clin Pharmacol Ther* 22:499, 1977.

88. Kelly DA, Hamilton S: A placebo-controlled trial to evaluate the antihypertensive efficacy and acceptability of indapamide. *Curr Med Res Opin* 5:137, 1977.

89. Holland OB, Gomez-Sanchez CE, Kuhnert LV, et al: Antihypertensive comparison of furosemide with hydrochlorothiazide for black patients. *Arch Intern Med* 139:1015, 1979.

90. Sica DA, Gehr TWB: Diuretic combination in refractory edema states: Pharmacokinetic and pharmacodynamic relationships. *Clin Pharmacokinet* 30:229, 1996.

91. Dunn CJ, Fitton A, Brogden RN: Torasemide. An update of its pharmacological properties and therapeutic efficacy. *Drugs* 49:121, 1995.

92. Collins R, Peto R, MacMahon S, et al: Blood pressure, stroke, and coronary heart disease. Part 2: Short-term reductions in blood pressure: Overview of randomised drug trials in their epidemiological context. *Lancet* 335:827, 1990.

93. MacMahon S, Rodgers A: The effects of antihypertensive treatment on vascular disease: reappraisal of the evidence in 1994. *J Vasc Med Biol* 4:265, 1993.

94. Collins R, MacMahon S: Blood pressure, antihypertensive drug treatment and the risks of stroke and of coronary heart disease. *Br Med Bull* 50:272, 1994.

95. Gueyffier F, Boutitie F, Boissel JP, et al: Effect of antihypertensive drug treatment on cardiovascular outcomes in women and men: A meta-analysis of individual patient data from randomised controlled trials. *Ann Intern Med* 126:761, 1997.

96. Psaty B, Smith N, Siscovick D, et al: Health outcomes associated with antihypertensive therapies used as first-line agents: A systematic review and meta-analysis. *JAMA* 277:739, 1997.

97. Veterans Administration Cooperative Study Group on Antihypertensive Agents: Effects of treatment on morbidity in hypertension. II. Results in patients with diastolic blood pressure averaging 90 through 114 mm Hg. *JAMA* 213:1143, 1970.

98. Hypertension Detection and Follow Up Program Cooperation Group. Five-year findings of the Hypertension Detection and follow up program. I. Reduction in mortality of patients with high blood pressure, including mild hypertension. *JAMA* 242:2562, 1979.

99. Management Committee: The Australian therapeutic trial in mild hypertension. *Lancet* I:1261, 1980.

100. SHEP Cooperative Research Group: Prevention of stroke by antihypertensive drug treatment in older patients with isolated systolic hypertension. Final results of the Systolic Hypertension in the Elderly Program (SHEP). *JAMA* 265:3255, 1991.

101. Dahlof B, Lindholm LH, Hansson L, et al: Morbidity and mortality in the Swedish Trial in Old Patients with Hypertension (STOP-Hypertension). *Lancet* 338:1281, 1991.

102. Wright JM, Lee CH, Chambers GK: Systematic review of antihypertensive therapies: Does the evidence assist in choosing a first-line drug? *CMAJ* 161:25, 1999.

103. Amery A, Birkenhager W, Brixko R, et al: Mortality and morbidity results from the European Working Party on High Blood Pressure in the Elderly Trial. *Lancet* 1:1349, 1985.

104. MRC Working Party: Medical Research Council trial of treatment of hypertension in older adults: Principal results. *BMJ* 304:405, 1992.

105. Wilhelmsen L, Berglund G, Elmfeld D, et al: Beta-blockers versus diuretics in hypertensive men: Main results from the HAPPHY trial. *J Hypertens* 5:561, 1987.

106. Blood Pressure Lowering Treatment Trialists Collaboration. Effects of ACE inhibitors, calcium antagonists, and other blood-pressure-lowering drugs: Results of prospectively designed overviews of randomised trials. *Lancet* 355:1955, 2000.

107. Messerli FH, Gorssman E, Goldbourt U: Are β blockers efficacious as first-line therapy for hypertension in the elderly? A systematic review. *JAMA* 279:1902, 1998.

108. Hansson L, Lindholm LH, Niskanen L, et al: Effect of angiotensin-converting-enzyme inhibition compared with conventional therapy on cardiovascular morbidity and mortality in hypertension: The Captopril Prevention Project (CAPPP) randomised trial. *Lancet* 353:611, 1999.

109. Hansson L, Lindholm LH, Ekbom T, et al: Randomised trial of old and new antihypertensive drugs in elderly patients: Cardiovascular mortality and morbidity the Swedish Trial in Old Patients with Hypertension-2 study. *Lancet* 354:1751, 1999.

110. UK Prospective Diabetes Study Group. Efficacy of atenolol and captopril in reducing risk of macrovascular and microvascular complications in type 2 diabetes: UKPDS 39. *BMJ* 317:713, 1998.

111. Brown MJ, Palmer CR, Castaigne A, et al: Morbidity and mortality in patients randomised to double-blind treatment with a long-acting calcium-channel blocker or diuretic in the International Nifedipine GITS study: Intervention as a Goal in Hypertension Treatment (INSIGHT). *Lancet* 356:366, 2000.

112. Hansson L, Hedner T, Lund-Johansen P, et al: Randomised trial of effects of calcium antagonists compared with diuretics and β-blockers on cardiovascular morbidity and mortality in hypertension: The Nordic Diltiazem (NORDIL) study. *Lancet* 356:359, 2000.

113. ALLHAT Collaborative Research Group: Major cardiovascular events in hypertensive patients randomized to doxazosin vs chlorthalidone: The antihypertensive and lipid-lowering treatment to prevent heart attack trial (ALLHAT). *JAMA* 283:1967, 2000.

114. Hachamovitch R, Strom JA, Sonnenblick EH, Frishman WH: Left ventricular hypertrophy in hypertension and the effects of antihypertensive drug therapy. *Curr Probl Cardiol* 13:371, 1988.

115. Levy D, Garrison RJ, Savage DD, et al: Prognostic implications of echocardiographically determined left ventricular mass in the Framingham Heart Study. *N Engl J Med* 322:156, 1990.

116. Moser M, Hebert PR: Prevention of disease progression, left ventricular hypertrophy and congestive heart failure in hypertension treatment trials. *J Am Coll Cardiol* 27:1214, 1996.

117. Moser M, Setaro JF: Antihypertensive drug therapy and regression of left ventricular hypertrophy: A review with a focus on diuretics. *Eur Heart J* 12:1034, 1991.

118. Dahlof B, Pennert K, Hansson L: Reversal of left ventricular hypertrophy in hypertensive patients. A meta-analysis of 109 treatment studies. *Am J Hypertens* 5:95, 1992.

119. Schmieder RE, Martus P, Klingbeil A: Reversal of left ventricular hypertrophy in essential hypertension. *JAMA* 275:1507, 1996.

120. Neaton JD, Grimm RH Jr, Prineas, et al: Treatment of mild hypertension study (TOMHS): Final results. *JAMA* 270:713, 1993.

121. Gosse P, Sheridan DJ, Zannad F, et al: Regression of left ventricular hypertrophy in hypertensive patients treated with indapamide SR 1.5 mg versus enalapril 20 mg: The LIVE study. *J Hypertens* 18:1465, 2000.

122. Materson BJ, Reda DJ, Cushman WC, et al: Single-drug therapy for hypertension in men. A comparison of six antihypertensive agents with placebo. *N Engl J Med* 328:914, 1993.

123. Coope J, Warrender TS: Randomized trial of treatment of hypertension in elderly in primary care. *Br Med J* 293:1145, 1986.

124. Hampton JR: Comparative efficacy of diuretics: Benefit versus risk: Results of clinical trials. *Eur Heart J* 13(Suppl G):85, 1992.

125. The IPPPSH Collaborative Group: Cardiovascular risk and risk factors in a randomised trial of treatment based on the beta blocker oxprenolol: The International Prospective Primary Prevention Study in Hypertension (IPPPSH). *J Hypertens* 3:379, 1985.

126. Pahor M, Shorr RI, Somes GW, et al: Diuretic-based treatment and cardiovascular events in patients with mild renal dysfunction enrolled in the Systolic Hypertension in the Elderly Program. *Arch Intern Med* 158:1340, 1998.

127. Prineas RJ, Gillium RF: United States epidemiology of hypertension in blacks. In: Hall WB, Saunders E, Shulman NB, eds. *Hypertension in Blacks: Epidemiology, Pathophysiology and Treatment.* Chicago: Year Book Medical Publishers, 1985:17–36.

128. Frohlich ED, Messerli FH, Dunn FG, et al: Greater renal vascular involvement in the black patient with essential hypertension: A comparison of systemic and renal hemodynamics in black and white patients. *Miner Electrolyte Metab* 10:173, 1984.

129. INTERSALT Cooperative Research Group: INTERSALT: An international study of electrolyte excretion and blood pressure. Results of 24 h urinary sodium and potassium excretion. *BMJ* 297:319, 1988.

130. Chrysant SG, Danisa K, Kem DC, et al: Racial differences in pressure, volume and renin interrelationships in essential hypertension. *Hypertension* 1:136, 1979.

131. Wilson DK, Sica DA, Miller SB: Effects of potassium on blood pressure in salt-sensitive and salt-resistant black adolescents. *Hypertension* 34:181, 1999.

132. Whelton PK, He J, Cutler JA, et al: Effects of oral potassium on blood pressure. Meta-analysis of randomized controlled clinical trials. *JAMA* 277:1624, 1997.

133. Freis ED: Age and antihypertensive medication (hydrochlorothiazide, bendroflumethiazide, nadolol and captopril). *Am J Cardiol* 61:117, 1988.

134. Veterans Administration Cooperative Study Group on Antihypertensive Drugs: Comparison of propranolol and hydrochlorothiazide for the initial treatment of hypertension. I. Results of short term titration with emphasis on racial differences in response. *JAMA* 248:1996, 1982.

135. Moser M, Lunn J: Responses to captopril and hydrochlorothiazide in black patients with hypertension. *Clin Pharmacol Ther* 32:307, 1982.

136. Sica DA: Fixed-dose combination therapy. Is it rational? *Drugs* 48:16, 1994.

137. Flack JM, Saunders E, Gradman A, et al: Antihypertensive efficacy and safety of losartan alone and in combination with hydrochlorothiazide in adult African Americans with mild to moderate hypertension. *Clin Ther* 23:1193, 2001.

138. Walker WG, Neaton JD, Cutler JA, et al: Renal function change in hypertensive members of the Multiple Risk Factor Intervention Trial: Racial and treatment effects. *JAMA* 268:3085, 1992.

139. Sica DA: Rationale for fixed-dose combinations in the treatment of hypertension: the cycle repeats. *Drugs* 62:443, 2002.

140. Hansson L, Zanchetti A, Carruthers SG, et al: Effect of intensive blood-pressure lowering and low-dose aspirin in patients with hypertension: Principal results of the Hypertension Optimal Treatment (HOT) randomised trial. *Lancet* 351:1755, 1998.

141. Frishman WH, Bryzinski BS, Coulson LR, et al: A multifactorial trial design to assess combination therapy in hypertension: Treatment with bisoprolol and hydrochlorothiazide. *Arch Intern Med* 154:1461, 1994.

142. Moser M: Why are physicians not prescribing diuretics more frequently in the management of hypertension? *JAMA* 270:1813, 1998.

143. Vasan RS, Larson MG, Benjamin EJ, et al: Congestive heart failure in subjects with normal versus reduced left ventricular ejection fraction: Prevalence and mortality in a population-based cohort. *J Am Coll Cardiol* 33:1948, 1999.

144. Cohn JN: Structural basis for heart failure: Ventricular remodeling and its pharmacological inhibition (editorial). *Circulation* 91:2504, 1995.

145. Colucci WS: Molecular and cellular mechanisms of myocardial failure. *Am J Cardiol* 80:15L, 1997.

146. LeJemtel TH, Sonnenblick EH, Frishman WH: Diagnosis and management of heart failure. In: Fuster V, Alexander RW, O'Rourke RA, eds. *Hurst's The Heart.* 10th ed. New York: McGraw-Hill, 2001:687–724.

147. Givertz MM, Colucci WS: New targets for heart-failure therapy: Endothelin, inflammatory cytokines, and oxidative stress. *Lancet* 352(Suppl 1):S134, 1998.

148. Francis GS, Benedict C, Johnstone DE, et al: Comparison of neuroendocrine activation in patients with left ventricular dysfunction with and without congestive heart failure: A substudy of the Studies Of Left Ventricular Dysfunction (SOLVD). *Circulation* 82:1724, 1990.

149. Bank AJ, Lee PC, Kubo SH: Endothelial dysfunction in patients with heart failure: Relationship to disease severity. *J Card Fail* 6:29, 2000.

150. Katz SD, Khan T, Zeballos GA, et al: Decreased activity of the L-arginine-nitric oxide metabolic pathway in patients with congestive heart failure. *Circulation* 99:2113, 1999.

151. Sam F, Colucci WS: Role of endothelin-1 in myocardial failure. *Proc Assoc Am Physicians* 111:417, 1999.

152. Moraes DL, Colucci WS, Givertz MM: Secondary pulmonary hypertension in heart failure: The role of the endothelium in pathophysiology and management. *Circulation* 102:1718, 2000.

153. Ichikawa I, Yoshioka T, Fogo A, Kon V: Role of angiotensin II in altered glomerular hemodynamics in congestive heart failure. *Kidney Int Suppl* 30:S123, 1990.

154. Eiskjaer H, Bagger JP, Danielsen J, et al: Mechanisms of sodium retention in heart failure: Relation to the renin-angiotensin-aldosterone system. *Am J Physiol* 260:F883, 1991.

155. Rakugi H, Ogihara T: Review of randomized trials of angiotensin receptor blockers in the treatment of patients with congestive heart failure. *Nippon Rinsho* 59:2051, 2001.

156. Cody RJ, Haas GJ, Binkley PF, et al: Plasma endothelin correlates with the extent of pulmonary hypertension in patients with chronic congestive heart failure. *Circulation* 85:504, 1992.

157. Szatalowicz VL, Arnold PE, Chaimovitz C, et al: Radioimmunoassay of plasma arginine vasopressin in hyponatremic patients with congestive heart failure. *N Engl J Med* 305:263, 1981.
158. Goldsmith SR: Vasopressin as vasopressor. *Am J Med* 82:1213, 1987.
159. Francis GS, Siegel RM, Goldsmith SR, et al: Acute vasoconstrictor response to intravenous furosemide in patients with chronic congestive heart failure. Activation of the neurohumoral axis. *Ann Intern Med* 103:1, 1985.
160. Wilson JR, Reichek N, Dunkman WB, Goldberg S: Effect of diuresis on the performance of the failing left ventricle in man. *Am J Med* 70:234, 1981.
161. Bauer U, Haerer W, Fehske KJ, et al: Hemodynamic effects of piretanide and methyldigoxine in congestive heart failure: Long-term results of a placebo-controlled randomized double blind study. In: Puschett J, Greenberg A, eds. *Diuretics III: Chemistry, Pharmacology, and Clinical Applications.* New York: Elsevier Science Publishing, 1990:316–321.
162. Vasko MR, Cartwright DB, Knochel JP, et al: Furosemide absorption altered in decompensated congestive heart failure. *Ann Intern Med* 102:314, 1985.
163. Brater DC, Seiwell R, Anderson S, et al: Absorption and disposition of furosemide on congestive heart failure. *Kidney Int* 22:171, 1982.
164. Rose HJ, Pruitt AW, McNay JL: Effect of experimental azotemia on renal clearance of furosemide in the dog. *J Pharmacol Exp Ther* 196:238, 1976.
165. Cook JA, Smith DE, Cornish LA, et al: Kinetics, dynamics, and bioavailability of bumetanide in healthy subjects and patients with congestive heart failure. *Clin Pharmacol Ther* 44:487, 1988.
166. Brater DC, Day B, Burdette A, et al: Bumetanide and furosemide in heart failure. *Kidney Int* 26:183, 1984.
167. Dzau VJ, Colucci WS, Williams GH, et al.: Sustained effectiveness of converting-enzyme inhibition in patients with severe congestive heart failure. *N Engl J Med* 302:1373, 1980.
168. McLay JS, McMurray JJ, Bridges AB, et al: Acute effects of captopril on the renal actions of furosemide in patients with chronic heart failure. *Am Heart J* 26:879, 1993.
169. Kramer BK, Schweda F, Riegger GAJ: Diuretic treatment and diuretic resistance in heart failure. *Am J Med* 106:90, 1999.
170. Brater DC, Anderson S, Baird B, et al: Effects of ibuprofen, naproxen, and sulindac on prostaglandins in men. *Kidney Int* 27:66, 1985.
171. Marangoni E, Oddone A, Surian M, et al: Effect of high-dose furosemide in refractory congestive heart failure. *Angiology* 41:862, 1990.
172. Gerlag PG, van Meijel JJ: High-dose furosemide in the treatment of refractory congestive heart failure. *Arch Intern Med* 148:286, 1988.
173. Rudy DW, Voelker JR, Greene PK, et al: Loop diuretics for chronic renal insufficiency: A continuous infusion is more efficacious than bolus therapy. *Ann Intern Med* 115:360, 1991.
174. Lahav M, Regev A, Ra'anani P, et al: Intermittent administration of furosemide vs. continuous infusion preceded by a loading dose for congestive heart failure. *Chest* 102:725, 1992.
175. Howard PA: Aggressive diuresis for severe heart failure in the elderly. *Chest* 119:807, 2001.
176. Brater DC, Presley RH, Anderson SA: Mechanisms of the synergistic combination of metolazone and bumetanide. *J Pharmacol Exp Ther* 233:70, 1985.
177. Epstein M, Lepp BA, Hoffman DS, et al: Potentiation of furosemide by metolazone in refractory edema. *Curr Ther Res* 21:656, 1977.
178. Channer KS, Richardson M, Crook R, et al: Thiazides with loop diuretics for severe congestive heart failure. *Lancet* 335:922, 1990.
179. Kiyingi A, Field MJ, Pawsey CC, et al: Metolazone in treatment of severe refractory congestive heart failure. *Lancet* 335:29, 1990.
180. Channer KS, McLean KA, Lawson-Matthew P, et al: Combination diuretic treatment in severe heart failure: A randomised controlled trial. *Br Heart J* 71:146, 1994.
181. Van Viet AA, Danker AJM, NAFTA JJ, Overheat FW: Spironolactone in congestive heart failure refractory to high-dose loop diuretic and low-dose angiotensin converting enzyme inhibitor. *Am J Cardiol* 71:21A, 1993.
181a. Farquharson CAJ, Struthers AD: Spironolactone increases nitric oxide bioactivity, improves endothelial vasodilator dysfunction and suppresses vascular angiotensin I/angiotensin II conversion in patients with chronic heart failure. *Circulation* 101:594, 2000.
181b. Weber KT: Aldosterone in congestive heart failure. *N Engl J Med* 345:1689, 2001.
181c. Rocha R, Williams GH: Rationale for the use of aldosterone antagonists in congestive heart failure. *Drugs* 62:723, 2002.
182. Bauersachs J, Heck M, Fraccarollo D, et al: Addition of spironolactone to angiotensin-converting enzyme inhibition in heart failure improves endothelial vasomotor dysfunction. *J Am Coll Card* 39:351, 2002.
183. Pitt B, Zannad F, Rime WJ et al: The effect of spironolactone on morbidity and mortality in patients with severe heart failure. *N Engl J Med* 341:709, 1999.
183a. Jorde UP, Vittorio T, Katz SD, et al: Elevated plasma aldosterone levels despite complete inhibition of the vascular angiotensin-converting enzyme in chronic heart failure, *Circulation* 106:1055, 2002.
184. Ayus JC: Diuretic-induced hyponatremia (editorial). *Arch Intern Med* 146:1295, 1986.
185. Ashraf N, Locksley R, Arieff AI: Thiazide-induced hyponatremia associated with death or neurologic damage in outpatients. *Am J Med* 70:1163, 1981.
186. Szatalowicz VL, Miller PD, Lacher JW, et al: Comparative effect of diuretics on renal water excretion in hyponatraemic oedematous disorders. *Clin Sci (Colch)* 62:235, 1982.
187. Sonnenblick M, Friedlander Y, Rosin AJ: Diuretic-induced severe hyponatremia. Review and analysis of 129 reported patients. *Chest* 103:601, 1993.
188. Sterns RH: "Slow" correction of hyponatremia: A break with tradition? *Kidney* 23:1, 1991.
189. Berl T: Treating hyponatremia: What is all the controversy about? [see comments]. *Ann Intern Med* 113:417, 1990.
190. Morgan DB, Davidson C: Hypokalemia and diuretics: An analysis of publications. *Br Med J* 280:905, 1980.
191. Khuri RN, Strieder WN, Giebisch G: Effects of flow rate and potassium intake on distal tubular potassium transfer. *Am J Physiol* 228:1249, 1975.
192. Velazquez H, Wright FS: Control by drugs of renal potassium handling. *Ann Rev Pharmacol Toxicol* 26:293, 1986.
193. Stanton BA, Giebisch G: Effects of pH on potassium transport by renal distal tubule. *Am J Physiol* 242:F544, 1982.
194. Wilcox CS: Diuretics and potassium. In: Hoffman JF, Giebisch G, eds. *Current Topics in Membranes and Transport.* Orlando, FL: Academic Press, 1987:250–331.
195. Freis ED, Papademetriou V: How dangerous are diuretics? *Drugs* 30:469, 1985.
196. Holland OB, Nixon JV, Kuhnert L: Diuretic-induced ventricular ectopic activity. *Am J Med* 70:762, 1981.
197. MacMahon S, Collins G, Rautaharju P, et al: Electrocardiographic left ventricular hypertrophy and effects of antihypertensive drug therapy in hypertensive patients in the Multiple Risk Factor Intervention Trial. *Am J Cardiol* 63:202, 1989.
198. Madias J, Madias N, Gavras H: Nonarrhythmogenicity of diuretic-induced hypokalemia: Its evidence in patients with uncomplicated essential hypertension. *Arch Intern Med* 144:2171, 1984.
199. Papademetriou V, Fletcher R, Khatri IM, et al: Diuretic-induced hypokalemia in uncomplicated systemic hypertension. Effect of plasma potassium correction in cardiac arrhythmias. *Am J Cardiol* 52:1017, 1983.
200. Medical Research Council, Working Party on Mild to Moderate Hypertension: Ventricular extrasystole during thiazide treatment: Substudy of MRC Mild Hypertension Trial. *Br Med J* 287:1249, 1983.
201. Kafka H, Langevin L, Armstrong P: Serum magnesium and potassium in acute myocardial infarction: Influences on ventricular arrhythmia. *Arch Intern Med* 147:465, 1987.
202. Packer M: Potential role of potassium as a determinant of morbidity and mortality in patients with systemic hypertension and congestive heart failure. *Am J Cardiol* 65:45E, 1990.
203. Dargie HJ, Cleland J, Leckie B, et al: Relation of arrhythmias and electrolyte abnormalities to survival in patients with severe chronic heart failure. *Circulation* 75(Suppl IV):IV98, 1987.
204. Franse LV, Pahor M, DiBari M, et al: Hypokalemia associated with diuretic use and cardiovascular events in the Systolic Hypertension in the Elderly Program. *Hypertension* 35:1025, 2000.
205. Siscovick DS, Raghunathan TE, Psaty BM, et al: Diuretic therapy and the risk of primary cardiac arrest. *N Engl J Med* 330:1852, 1994.

206. Cooper HW, Dries DL, Davis CE, et al: Diuretics and risk of arrhythmic death in patients with left ventricular dysfunction. *Circulation* 100:1311, 1999.

207. Seigel D, Hulley SB, Black DM, et al: Diuretics, serum and intracellular electrolyte levels, and ventricular arrhythmias in hypertensive men. *JAMA* 267:1083, 1992.

208. Knochel JP, Schlein EM: On the mechanism of rhabdomyolysis in potassium depletion. *J Clin Invest* 51:1750, 1972.

209. Relman AS, Schwartz WB: The nephropathy of potassium depletion: A clinical and pathological entity. *N Engl J Med* 255:195, 1956.

210. Quamme GA: Effect of furosemide on calcium and magnesium transport in the rat nephron. *Am J Physiol* 241:F340, 1981.

211. Kroenke K, Wood DR, Hanley JF: The value of serum magnesium determination in hypertensive patients receiving diuretics. *Arch Intern Med* 147:1553, 1987.

212. Petri M, Cumber P, Grimes L, et al: The metabolic effects of thiazide therapy in the elderly: A population study. *Age Aging* 15:151, 1986.

213. Dyckner T, Wester PO: Effects of magnesium infusions in diuretic induced hyponatraemia. *Lancet* 1:585, 1981.

214. Whang R, Oei TO, Aikawa JK, et al: Predictors of clinical hypomagnesemia. Hypokalemia, hypophosphatemia, hyponatremia, and hypocalcemia. *Arch Intern Med* 144:1984.

215. Wester PO, Dyckner T: Intracellular electrolytes in cardiac failure. *Acta Med Scand* 707(Suppl):33, 1986.

216. Eichhorn EJ, Tandon PK, DiBianco R, et al: Clinical and prognostic significance of serum magnesium concentration in patients with severe chronic congestive heart failure: The PROMISE study. *J Am Coll Cardiol* 21:634, 1993.

217. Cannon PJ, Heineman HO, Albert MS, et al: "Contraction" alkalosis after diuresis of edematous patients with ethacrynic acid. *Ann Intern Med* 62:979, 1965.

218. Schlueter WA, Batlle DC. Effect of loop diuretics on urinary acidification. In: Puschett J, Greenberg A, eds. *Diuretics III: Chemistry, Pharmacology, and Clinical Applications.* New York: Elsevier Science Publishing, 1990:174–182.

219. Loon NR, Wilcox CS, Nelson R, Mounts M: Metabolic alkalosis impairs the response to bumetanide. *Kidney Int* 33:200A, 1988.

220. Levine DZ: Acid-base complications induced by diuretics. In: Puschett J, Greenberg A, eds. *Diuretics III: Chemistry, Pharmacology, and Clinical Applications.* New York: Elsevier Science Publishing, 1990:228–233.

221. Report of Medical Research Council Working Party on Mild to Moderate Hypertension. Adverse reactions to bendrofluazide and propranolol for the treatment of mild hypertension. *Lancet* 2:539, 1981.

222. Furman BL: Impairment of glucose intolerance produced by diuretics and other drugs. *Pharmacol Ther* 12:613, 1981.

223. Dornhorst A, Powell SH, Pensky J: Aggravation by propranolol of hyperglycaemic effect of hydrochlorothiazide in type II diabetics without alteration of insulin secretion. *Lancet* 1:123, 1985.

224. Sowers JR, Bakris GL: Antihypertensive therapy and the risk of type 2 diabetes mellitus. *N Engl J Med* 342:969, 2000.

225. Ramsay LE, Yeo WW, Jackson PR: Influence of diuretics calcium antagonists and alpha-blockers on insulin sensitivity and glucose tolerance in hypertensive patients. *J Cardiovasc Pharmacol* 20(Suppl 11):S49, 1992.

226. Gress TW, Nieto FJ, Shahar E, et al: Hypertension and antihypertensive therapy as risk factors for type 2 diabetes mellitus. *N Engl J Med* 342:905, 2000.

227. Jeunemaitre X, Charru A, Chatellier G, et al: Long-term metabolic effects of spironolactone and thiazides combined with potassium-sparing agents for treatment of essential hypertension. *Am J Cardiol* 62:1072, 1988.

228. Bloomgarden ZT, Ginsberg-Fellner F, Rayfield EJ, et al: Elevated hemoglobin A1c and low-density lipoprotein cholesterol levels in thiazide-treated diabetic patients. *Am J Med* 77:823, 1984.

229. Frishman WH, Clark A, Johnson B: Effects of cardiovascular drugs on plasma lipids and lipoproteins. In: Frishman WH, Sonnenblick EH, eds. *Cardiovascular Pharmacotherapeutics.* New York: McGraw-Hill, 1997:1515–1559.

230. Ruppert M, Overlack A, Kolloch R, et al: Neurohormonal and metabolic effects of severe and moderate salt restriction in non-obese normotensive adults. *J Hypertens* 11:743, 1993.

231. Mantel-Teeuwisse AK, Kloosterman JM, Maitland-van der Zee AH, et al: Drug-Induced lipid changes: A review of the unintended effects of some commonly used drugs on serum lipid levels. *Drug Saf* 24:443, 2001.

232. Lakshman MR, Reda DJ, Materson BJ, et al: Diuretics and β blockers do not have adverse effects at 1 year on plasma lipid and lipoprotein profiles in men with hypertension. *Arch Intern Med* 159:551, 1999.

233. Ljunghall S, Backman U, Danielson BG, et al: Effects of bendroflumethiazide on urate metabolism during treatment of patients with renal stones. *J Urol* 127:1207, 1982.

234. Wait WW, Wade WE, Cobb HH: The effect of three different diuretic regimens on serum uric acid in an ambulatory hypertensive population. *Hosp Pharm* 23:50, 1993.

235. Lang PG Jr: Severe hypersensitivity reactions to allopurinol. *South Med J* 72:1361, 1979.

236. Chang SW, Fine R, Siegel D, et al: The impact of diuretic therapy on reported sexual function [see comments]. *Arch Intern Med* 151:2402, 1991.

236a. Melman A, Christ GJ: The hemodynamics of erection and the pharmacotherapies of erectile dysfunction. *Heart Dis* 4:252, 2002.

237. Rybak LP: Ototoxicity of loop diuretics. *Otolaryngology Clin* 26:829, 1993.

238. Rybak LP: Pathophysiology of furosemide ototoxicity. *J Otolaryngol* 11:127, 1982.

239. Tuzel IH: Comparison of adverse reactions to bumetanide and furosemide. *J Clin Pharmacol* 21:615, 1981.

240. Reineck HJ: Diuretic use in renal failure. In: Eknoyan G, Martinez-Maldonado M, eds. *The Physiological Basis of Diuretic Therapy in Clinical Medicine.* Orlando, FL: Grune & Stratton, 1986:298.

241. Heidland A, Wigand ME: The effect of furosemide at high doses on auditory sensitivity in patients with uremia. *Klin Wochenschr* 48:1052, 1970.

242. Fries D, Pozet N, Dubois N, et al: The use of large doses of frusemide in acute renal failure. *Postgrad Med J* 47:(Suppl):18, 1971.

243. Beermann B, Dalen E, Lindstrom B, Rosen A: On the fate of furosemide in man. *Eur J Clin Pharmacol* 9:51, 1975.

244. Brown CG, Ogg CS, Cameron JS, Bewick M: High-dose furosemide in acute reversible intrinsic renal failure. *Scot Med J* 19(Suppl):35, 1974.

245. Addo HA, Ferguson J, Frain Bell W: Thiazide-induced photosensitivity: A study of 33 subjects. *Br J Dermatol* 116:749, 1987.

246. Diffey BL, Langtry J: Phototoxic potential of thiazide diuretics in normal subjects. *Arch Dermatol* 125:1355, 1989.

247. Frommer JP, Wesson DE, Eknoyan G: Side effects and complications of diuretic therapy. In: Eknoyan G, Martinez-Maldonado M, eds. *The Physiological Basis of Diuretic Therapy in Clinical Medicine.* Orlando, FL: Grune & Stratton, 1986:293–309.

248. Schwarz A, Krause PH, Kunzendorf U, et al: The outcome of acute interstitial nephritis: Risk factors for the transition from acute to chronic interstitial nephritis. *Clin Nephrol* 54:179, 2000.

249. Magil AB, Ballon HS, Cameron EC, Rae A: Acute interstitial nephritis associated with thiazide diuretics. Clinical and pathologic observations in three cases. *Am J Med* 69:939, 1980.

250. Grossman E, Messerli FH, Goldbourt U: Does diuretic therapy increase the risk of renal cell carcinoma? *Am J Cardiol* 83:1090, 1999.

251. Tenenbaum A, Grossman E, Fisman EZ, et al: Long-term diuretic therapy in patients with coronary disease: Increased colon cancer-related mortality over a 5-year follow up. *J Hum Hypertens* 15:373, 2001.

252. Lawson DH, Macadam RF, Singh MH, et al: Effect of furosemide on antibiotic-induced renal damage in rats. *J Infect Dis* 126:593, 1972.

253. Shapiro S, Slone D, Lewis GP, et al: The epidemiology of digoxin toxicity. A study in three Boston hospitals. *J Chronic Dis* 22:361, 1969.

254. Petersen V, Hvidt S, Thomsen K, et al: Effect of prolonged thiazide treatment on renal lithium clearance. *Br Med J* 3:143, 1974.

255. Boer WH, Loomans HA, Dorhout Mees EJ: Effects of thiazides with and without carbonic-anhydrase inhibiting activity on free water and lithium clearance. In: Puschett J, Greenberg A, eds. *Diuretics III: Chemistry, Pharmacology, and Clinical Applications.* New York: Elsevier Science Publishing, 1990:31–33.

256. Shirley DG, Walter SJ, Sampson B: A micropuncture study of renal lithium reabsorption: Effects of amiloride and furosemide. *Am J Physiol* 263:F1128, 1992.

257. Bridgman JF, Rosen SM, Thorp JM: Complications during clofibrate treatment of nephrotic-syndrome hyperlipoproteinaemia. *Lancet* 2:506, 1972.

258. Weinberg MS, Quigg RJ, Salant DJ, Bernard DB: Anuric renal failure precipitated by indomethacin and triamterene. *Nephron* 40:216, 1985.

259. Packer M, Lee WH, Kessler P, et al: Identification of hyponatremia as a risk factor for the development of functional renal insufficiency during converting enzyme inhibition in severe chronic heart failure. *J Am Coll Cardiol* 10:837, 1987.

260. Packer M Lee WH, Medina, et al: Functional renal insufficiency during long-term therapy with captopril and enalapril in severe chronic heart failure. *Ann Intern Med* 106:346, 1987.

261. Schlondorff D: Renal prostaglandin synthesis: Sites of production and specific actions of prostaglandins. *Am J Med* 81:1, 1985.

262. Sica DA: Dosage considerations with perindopril for systemic hypertension. *Am J Cardiol* 88(Suppl 7):13i, 2001.

CHAPTER 12

Magnesium, Potassium, and Calcium as Potential Cardiovascular Disease Therapies

Domenic A. Sica

William H. Frishman

Erdal Cavusoglu

Both deficiency states and abnormalities in the metabolism of the electrolytes magnesium, potassium, and calcium have been considered as etiologic factors in systemic hypertension, ischemic heart disease, congestive heart failure (CHF), stroke, atherosclerosis, diabetes mellitus, asthma, and/or a variety of arrhythmias. In experimental animals, either deficit replacement and/or simple supplementation of these cationic substances has been shown to both prevent and treat these cardiovascular maladies. In this chapter, magnesium, potassium, and calcium are discussed as potential cardiovascular disease therapies.

MAGNESIUM

Magnesium (Mg) is the second most common intracellular cation in the human body, second only to potassium, with a free cytosolic concentration of around 0.5 mmol/L.[1] Mg is also the fourth most abundant cation in the body.[2] It is distributed in three major body compartments: approximately 65% in the mineral phase of bone, about 34% in muscle, and 1% in plasma and interstitial fluid. Unlike plasma calcium, which is 40% protein-bound, only approximately 20% of plasma Mg is protein-bound. Consequently, changes in plasma protein concentrations have less effect on plasma Mg than on plasma calcium. Mg is a cofactor in well over 300 different enzymatic reactions in the body and is of particular importance for those enzymes that use nucleotides as cofactors or substrates.[1,3] This is because, as a rule, it is not the free nucleotide but its Mg complex that is the actual cofactor or substrate. Mg is important in many cell membrane functions, including the gating of calcium ion channels, mimicking many of the effects of calcium-channel blockade.[4] Mg is a necessary cofactor for any biochemical reaction involving ATP and is essential for the proper functioning of the sodium-potassium and calcium ATPase pumps, which are critical to the maintenance of a normal resting membrane potential.[4] Intracellular Mg ion deficiency can lead to abnormalities in myocardial membrane potential, which then serves as a trigger for cardiac arrhythmias.[5] Deficiency states or abnormalities in Mg metabolism also play important roles in ischemic heart disease, CHF, sudden cardiac death, diabetes mellitus, preeclampsia-eclampsia, and/or hypertension.[4,6]

Cardiovascular Effects of Mg

The Mg ion has numerous properties that could theoretically benefit the cardiovascular system. Mg modulates the contraction and tone of vascular smooth muscle cells, thus reducing systemic vascular resistance, and thereby decreasing blood pressure.[7–9] Mg also dilates coronary and cerebral arteries and is effective in the relief of coronary vasospasm.[10–13] Mg slows heart rate, preserves mitochondrial function and high-energy phosphate levels, and serves as an antiarrhythmic.[12,14] In addition, Mg possesses both antiplatelet and anticoagulant properties[15–17] and antiatherosclerotic properties,[4,18] the ability to improve endothelial function,[19] and the capacity to protect against the formation of oxygen free radicals.[4,20] Mg deficiencies or metabolic abnormalities can cause abnormalities in cardiovascular function, as outlined in Fig. 12-1.

Role of Mg in Ischemic Heart Disease and Myocardial Infarction

For many years Mg deficiency has been loosely tied to both ischemic heart disease and myocardial infarction (MI).[12] Although innumerable animal and human studies have attempted to establish a definitive role for Mg deficiency in both the incidence and limitations in the management of ischemic heart disease, much confusion still remains in this regard. Epidemiologic studies comparing death rates from ischemic heart disease from geographically diverse areas have attempted to link low Mg concentrations in soil and water with a higher cardiovascular mortality.[21,22] Several autopsy series dating back to the 1970s have also suggested that patients dying of acute MI tended to have reduced myocardial Mg concentrations compared with those dying from noncardiac causes.[23,24] A series of basic science studies have since demonstrated that acute ischemia is, in fact, associated with a dramatic increase in the efflux of Mg from the injured myocyte as well an increase in cellular calcium and sodium content.[25–27] Moreover, low myocardial Mg concentrations have been demonstrated in chronic ischemic heart disease.[24] In addition, Mg deficiency has been etiologically involved with many of the known risk factors for coronary artery disease (CAD), such as diabetes mellitus, hypertension, and hyperlipidemia.[12]

Studies in animal models of ischemia and infarction have suggested a beneficial role for Mg. It has been theorized that Mg protects against reperfusion injury by limiting cellular calcium overload.[28]

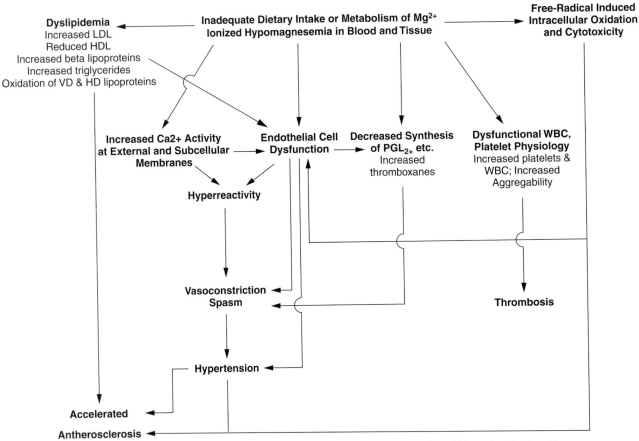

FIGURE 12-1. Hypothetical scheme whereby inadequate dietary intake or metabolism of Magnesium (Mg) could lead to vasospasm, hypertension, atherosclerosis, and intravascular thrombosis. (*Reproduced with permission from Altura and Altura.*[4])

Reports of the use of Mg in acute MI in humans date back to as early as the 1950s. Mg administration was found to have beneficial effects in patients with MI in several small studies, and an early overview on this topic suggested that the morbidity and mortality rate was lower with Mg therapy.[29]

The beneficial effects of intravenous (IV) Mg sulfate (MgSO$_4$) (8 mmol over 5 min followed by 65 mmol over 24 h) given immediately to patients with suspected acute MI, were initially documented in a large prospective double-blind trial—the Leicester Intravenous Mg Intervention Trial (LIMIT-2).[30] In this study the mortality rate was 7.8% in the MgSO$_4$ treatment arm versus 10.3% in the placebo group. The side effects of Mg treatment in this study were minimal and included transient flushing, related to the speed of injection of the loading dose, and an increased incidence of sinus bradycardia.[30] However, the routine administration of Mg during acute MI has been discontinued largely on the basis of the Fourth International Study of Infarct Survival (ISIS-4), which included 58,050 patients and found that Mg administration did not decrease 35-day mortality when compared to controls.[31] The timing of the loading of Mg dose in relation to thrombolytic therapy or spontaneous reperfusion has been offered as an explanation for the opposing results in LIMIT-2 and ISIS-4.[32] Early treatment appears essential, as serum Mg concentrations must be raised by the time of reperfusion, since injury is immediate.[33] This observation accords with the 25% reduction in early left ventricular failure in the Mg group of LIMIT-2.[33] Other studies using an earlier IV Mg loading dose (8 mmol MgSO$_4$ over

5 min plus 65 mmol over the next 24 h) have also failed to demonstrate a significant difference in cardiac arrhythmias compared to control therapy.[34]

Mg administration may have a greater therapeutic role in those patients experiencing an acute MI who are unable to receive thrombolytic therapy, a population with an inherently high in-hospital mortality rate.[35–36a] A 48-h infusion of MgSO$_4$ in this group of patients has been shown to significantly reduce the incidence of arrhythmias, CHF, and conduction disturbances compared with placebo. Left ventricular ejection fraction 72 h and 1 to 2 months after admission and in-house survival rates were higher in patients who received MgSO$_4$.[37] Similarly, a beneficial effect of Mg therapy has been reported in patients with unstable angina undergoing bypass grafting.[38]

The use of Mg in the preoperative and early postoperative periods is also highly effective in reducing the incidence of atrial fibrillation after elective coronary artery bypass grafting[39]; other studies, though, have been unable to confirm these cardioprotective effects.[40,41] For example, MgSO$_4$ given IV before, during, and after reperfusion did not decrease myocardial damage and did not improve short-term clinical outcome in patients with acute MI treated with direct angioplasty.[42]

The discrepancy in the results of these studies has dampened the enthusiasm for routine use of Mg in the management of patients with acute MI. The disparate results between these two large clinical trials (LIMIT-2 and ISIS-4) remain puzzling. However, the ISIS-4 trial was not specifically designed to test the hypothesis that Mg might limit reperfusion injury, and the time factor in which Mg is given needs to be further clarified. It is also important to determine whether those patients with Mg deficiency are the ones who benefit or whether Mg should be used as a true cardioplexic agent in the non-Mg-deficient individual. At this time, Mg therapy cannot be recommended as routine treatment in the management of acute MI.[32] The current American College of Cardiology/American Heart association guidelines for the treatment of patients with acute MI currently recommend IV Mg only for correction of documented Mg deficiency and for the treatment of the torsades de pointes–type of ventricular tachycardia.[43] Ongoing studies, such as the Mg in Coronaries (MAGIC) study, may help define a future role for Mg in ischemic heart syndromes.[44]

Mg in Diabetes and Congestive Heart Failure

Mg deficiency occurs in association with various medical disorders but is particularly common in diabetes mellitus,[1,45–49] CHF,[14,50,51] and following diuretic use.[52] Recognition of potassium deficiency and/or its correction follows fairly standard guidelines in these conditions; alternatively, the circumstances are much different for Mg, since serum Mg values reflect total body stores poorly.[1] Potassium repletion in a hypokalemic patient can prove difficult unless underlying Mg deficiency is first corrected.[49] Hypocalcemia is another common sequela to hypomagnesemia and can prove resistant to treatment owing to hypomagnesemia-related defects in parathyroid release and/or action.[53] This form of hypocalcemia responds to small amounts of supplemental Mg but can redevelop unless full repletion of the underlying Mg deficit is accomplished.[54]

The incidence of diuretic-related hypokalemia and/or hypomagnesemia, in either CHF and/or hypertension can be considerably lessened by using potassium-sparing diuretics, angiotensin converting enzyme (ACE) inhibitors, or angiotensin-receptor blockers (ARBs).

Excessive glycosuria is the main cause of Mg deficiency in diabetes mellitus, and its severity is inversely correlated with the level of glycemic control.[48] Fat and protein mobilization during acute hyperglycemia-associated metabolic decompensation, as well as other factors, also plays a role in diabetes-related hypomagnesemia. Hypomagnesemia can be both a cause and effect of hyperglycemia and is associated with insulin resistance.[47] The prevalence and severity of Mg deficiency can be influenced by other conditions, particularly CHF[14,50,51] and diuretic use.[49,52] In these cases, multiple electrolyte imbalances can develop simultaneously, predicting poor patient survival.[55] Hyponatremia is closely associated with a poor prognosis, hypokalemia with increased ventricular dysrhythmias, and hypomagnesemia with arrhythmias and the aforementioned refractory hypokalemia and/or hypocalcemia.[50] However, Mg deficiency has yet to be established as an independent cardiovascular mortality risk factor in such conditions.[56]

Mg in Arrhythmias

There is an inverse correlation between myocardial irritability and serum Mg concentrations, which is well illustrated in CHF.[57,58] For example, 0.2 mEq/kg of MgSO$_4$ given over 1 h to CHF patients reduced ectopic beats in a 6-h postdosing monitoring period,[57] and MgCl given as a 10-min bolus (0.3 mEq/kg) followed by a 24-h maintenance infusion (0.08 mEq/kg/h) also succeeded in reducing hourly ectopic beats. Noteworthy was the fact that Mg

concentrations 30 min and 24 h after the bolus were 3.6 ± 0.1 and 4.2 ± 0.1 mg/dL, respectively. Oral Mg replacement (15.8 mmol MgCl/day for 6 weeks) has also reduced ventricular irritability during the chronic phase of CHF treatment despite the fact that serum Mg changed insignificantly (0.87 ± 0.07 to 0.92 ± 0.05 mmol/L).[59] The risk of hypomagnesemia is particularly high in individuals concurrently receiving digitalis, as this association has an additive effect on arrhythmia development.[60,61]

As previously stated, Mg is an essential cofactor for the Na$^+$ K$^+$-ATPase enzyme. Mg deficiency impairs the function of this enzyme, which, in turn, lowers intracellular potassium concentrations. As a consequence of this, the resting membrane potential becomes less negative, thereby lowering its threshold for the development of arrhythmias.[62,63] In addition to its effect on the Na$^+$ K$^+$-ATPase pump, Mg has been shown to have profound effects on the several different types of potassium channels that are known to exist within cardiac cells.[64] Studies in animals appear to support the theory that Mg increases cellular resistance to the development of arrhythmias. For example, Mg infusion has been shown to raise the threshold for both ventricular premature contractions and the induction of ventricular fibrillation in normal denervated (heart-lung preparations) and whole-animal digitalis-treated hearts.[65] Moreover, considerable evidence exists linking Mg deficiency with an increased incidence of both supraventricular and ventricular arrhythmias.[66–69]

Evidence of the salutary effects of IV Mg in treating both supraventricular and ventricular tachyarrhythmias has been available for many years.[12] In addition, numerous anecdotal reports have been published attesting to the utility of Mg in cases of refractory ventricular arrhythmias, although most of these cases were probably associated with Mg deficiency. Interestingly, potassium-sparing diuretics, compounds that also exhibit Mg-sparing effects, do not carry the same increased risk for sudden cardiac death observed with non-potassium-sparing diuretics.[70] Despite these observations and the theoretical benefits of Mg with regard to the development of arrhythmias, there has actually been no controlled study designed to evaluate the specific efficacy of Mg as an antiarrhythmic agent in the treatment of ventricular arrhythmias. Furthermore, it is unclear whether the potential effectiveness of Mg in these situations represents a pharmacologic effect of Mg or whether it merely reflects repletion of an underling deficiency state. Whatever its potential role in the management of ventricular fibrillation,[71,72] supraventricular arrhythmias,[39] and "run-of-the-mill" ventricular arrhythmias,[12] Mg clearly does have a time-honored and proven place in the treatment of ventricular arrhythmias associated with digoxin toxicity.[73–76]

Mg in Hypertension

A number of studies have observed some form of hypomagnesemia (serum and/or tissue) in hypertensive patients with significant inverse correlations between Mg concentration and blood pressure.[4,8,77] Dietary Mg appears to be of some importance to this relationship. Epidemiologic studies have linked hypertension and hypertensive heart diseases, as well as ischemic heart disease, with "soft water," low in Mg, and protection from cardiovascular disease with "hard water," high in Mg,[8] with an inverse relationship between dietary Mg and the level of blood pressure.[78–80] This reduction in serum or tissue Mg might be enough to induce peripheral vasoconstriction and thereby raise blood pressure, although the exact mechanism triggering this change in vascular tone is not known.[4,8,77]

The therapeutic value of Mg in the treatment of hypertension was suggested as early as 1925, when Mg infusions were found to be effective in treating malignant hypertension. Considering the inexpensive nature of the agent and the fact that it is easy to handle, Mg is theoretically a useful adjunctive if not primary treatment modality for hypertension. However, this has not proven to be the case in most patients, although successful drug therapy of hypertension appears to be associated with elevations in the levels of intracellular free Mg in erythrocytes.[81] Ingestion of foodstuffs with a high content of Mg may have an effect on blood pressure, though Mg-enriched diets also typically contain higher amounts of the vasodepressor cations potassium and calcium.[82,83] Mg supplementation, though has not been found to affect blood pressure in a primary prevention of hypertension study in 698 patients treated for 6 months with 360 mg of Mg diglycine.[84]

However, the results of studies where Mg was used to treat hypertension have demonstrated conflicting results regarding blood pressure reduction.[85–89] Methodologic issues and heterogeneity of study populations likely explain the inconsistency in treatment results.[8] Nevertheless, Mg supplementation may more consistently be of benefit in certain patient subsets, including blacks, obese patients, those with insulin resistance, patients with hypertriglyceridemia, those with severe or malignant forms of hypertension, situations wherein Mg was supplemented long term, and/or hypertensive patients receiving thiazide diuretics.[90] Also, in many forms of secondary hypertension as well as in preeclampsia, Mg is effective in reducing blood pressure.[91,92] Taken together, these data suggest that Mg is at best weakly hypotensive. The use of Mg supplementation with diuretics, especially thiazide diuretics, is advisable to prevent intracellular Mg and potassium depletion.

Mg in Stroke

Mg exhibits a range of neuronal and vascular actions that may ameliorate ischemic central nervous system (CNS) insults, including stroke. Significant neuroprotection with Mg has been observed in different models of focal cerebral ischemia, with infarct volume reduction from 25 to 61%.[93] Maximal neuroprotection is evident at readily attainable serum concentrations, and neuroprotection is still seen when administration is delayed up to 6 h and in some cases 24 h after the onset of ischemia.[94] Several small trials have reported a reduced incidence of death or dependence with administration of Mg, but confidence intervals are wide, and more definitive data from ongoing large trials are needed before specific recommendations can be made for the use of Mg in the victim of acute stroke.

Clinical Use of Mg

There is a high incidence of Mg deficiency in hospitalized patients, particularly in those with other conditions that may aggravate Mg deficiency, such as poor nutrition and multisystem disorders. This is particularly important in patients receiving treatment with a myriad of medications—such as diuretics[51,52] and aminoglycoside antibiotics[95]—which increase urinary losses of Mg (Table 12-1).

Difficulty in establishing the diagnosis of Mg deficiency is due to the lack of reliable laboratory tests and the minimal or often absent clinical manifestations accompanying this disturbance.[1] When present, clinical manifestations are nonspecific and confined to mental changes or neuromuscular irritability. Tetany, one of the most striking and better-known manifestations, is only rarely found; instead, less specific signs such as tremor, muscle twitching, bizarre movements, focal seizures, generalized convulsions, delirium, or coma are more common findings.[96] Mg deficiency should be

TABLE 12-1. Causes of Hypomagnesemia

GI tract losses
   Chronic diarrhea
   Malabsorption syndromes
   Laxative abuse
   Pancreatitis
   Specific Mg malabsorption
   Prolonged nasogastric suctioning
Renal excretion
   Acute renal failure
   Renal tubular acidosis
   Postobstructive diuresis
   Primary renal tubular Mg wasting
   Drug-induced (acetazolamide, alcohol, aminoglycosides, amphotericin B, carbenicillin, chlorthalidone, cisplatin, digoxin, ethacrynic acid, furosemide, mannitol, methotrexate, pentamidine, theophylline, thiazides)
Nutritional deficiencies
   Malnutrition
   Mg-free parenteral feedings
   Long-term alcohol abuse
Endocrine disorders
   Hyperaldosteronism
   Hyperparathyroidism
   Hyperthyroidism
   Diabetes mellitus
   Ketoacidosis (diabetic, alcoholic)
   Hypoparathyroidism
   Syndrome of inappropriate secretion of antidiuretic hormone
   Bartter's syndrome
Redistribution
   Insulin treatment for diabetic ketoacidosis
   High-catecholamine states
   Major trauma or stress
   Hungry-bone syndrome
Multiple mechanisms
   Chronic alcoholism
   Alcohol withdrawal
   Major burns
   Liquid protein diet

Source: Reproduced with permission from Tosiello.[46]

suspected when other electrolyte abnormalities coexist since it tends to cluster with abnormalities such as hypocalcemia and hypokalemia.[97] Electrocardiographic (ECG) changes—such as prolongation of the QT and PR intervals, widening of the QRS complex, ST-segment depression, and low T waves as well as supraventricular and ventricular tachyarrhythmias—should also raise the index of suspicion for Mg deficiency.[98,99]

Once hypomagnesemia is suspected, the measurement of serum Mg concentration continues to be the routine test for detection of hypomagnesemia.[1] While a low level is helpful and is typically indicative of low intracellular stores, normal serum Mg values can still be observed in the face of significant body deficiencies of Mg; thus, serum Mg determinations are an unreliable measure of total body Mg balance.[2] Intracellular Mg measurements, as well as other technologies, are available, but remain clinically impractical. A more practical measure of Mg balance is the "Mg loading test," which at the same time is both therapeutic and diagnostic.[100] This test consists of the parenteral administration of $MgSO_4$ and a timewise assessment of urinary Mg retention, which can be accomplished on an outpatient basis in as short a time as 1 h.[101] Individuals in a state of normal Mg balance eliminate at least 75% of an administered load.

TABLE 12-2. Available Forms of Magnesium

Salt	Chemical Formula	Molecular Weight	Percent Mg	mEq/g	mmol/g
Sulfate	$MgSO_4 \cdot 7H_2O$	246.5	10%	8.1	4
Chloride	$MgCl_2 \cdot 6H_2O$	203.23	12%	9.8	4.9
Oxide	MgO	40.3	60%	49.6	25
Lactate	$C_6H_{10}MgO_6$	202.45	12%	9.8	4.9
Citrate	$C_{12}H_{10}Mg_3O_{14}$	451	16%	4.4	2.2
Hydroxide	$Mg(OH)_2$	58.3	42%	34	17
Gluconate			5.8%	4.8	2.4

This approach is recommended in all patients with a high index of suspicion for hypomagnesemia, particularly in those with ischemic heart disease or cardiac arrhythmias. Repletion of an Mg deficit should occur cautiously in anuric individuals and in those with significant renal impairment.[70] In mild deficiency states, Mg balance can often be reestablished by simply eliminating the causative factors and allowing the Mg content in a normal diet to repair the deficit. Parenteral Mg administration, however, is the most effective way to correct a hypomagnesemic state and should be the route used when replacement is necessary during medical emergencies. Total body deficits of Mg in the depleted patient are typically 1 to 2 mEq/kg of body weight. A recommended regimen is 2 g of $MgSO_4$ (16.3 mEq) given IV over 30 min, followed by a constant infusion rate providing between 32 and 64 mEq/day until the deficit is presumed corrected. A variety of oral Mg salts are available for clinical use (Table 12-2). Mg oxide is commonly employed, but this salt form is poorly soluble and acts as a cathartic, thereby decreasing absorption. Mg gluconate is the preferred salt form for oral therapy, as this agent possesses a high degree of solubility and does not cause diarrhea. Mg carbonate is poorly soluble and does not appear to be as effective in reversing hypomagnesemia as the gluconate salt. Oral Mg is not recommended for therapy during acute situations, since the high doses necessary almost always cause significant diarrhea. The intramuscular route for Mg administration is a useful but painful means of delivery and should be avoided as long as IV access is available.

Conclusion

Deficiency states or abnormalities in Mg metabolism also play important roles in ischemic heart disease, CHF, sudden cardiac death, diabetes mellitus, preeclampsia-eclampsia, and/or hypertension. How best to use Mg in these conditions, either individually or collectively, remains to be determined. Of similar importance is the effect of diuretic therapy on Mg balance and the difficulty in accurately identifying the presence and degree of a deficiency state. Therefore presumptive therapy in patients at risk for Mg deficiency-related complications should be considered.

POTASSIUM

Potassium (K^+) has a diverse relationship with cardiovascular disease.[101a] This includes issues as varied as its dietary intake, such deficiency states as may occur with diuretic therapy, and finally the consideration of specific K^+ membrane channels, which have an important cardiovascular role. For example, a relationship between a high dietary intake of K^+ and a reduced risk of cardiovascular disease has been suggested by both animal experiments and clinical investigations.[102–105] Conversely, diuretic-induced hypokalemia carries with its development an increased cardiovascular risk.[106,107] Finally, drugs affecting membrane K^+ channels have also been shown to favorably impact a variety of cardiovascular conditions (see Chap. 28).[108]

K^+ in Systemic Hypertension

In experimental animals prone to cardiovascular events, high dietary K^+ appears to protect against the development of stroke, cardiac hypertrophy, and/or systemic hypertension.[109–112] Observational population studies have shown a direct correlation between arterial blood pressure levels and dietary and/or urinary Na^+/K^+ ratios and an inverse relationship with urinary K^+.[112–115] The urinary Na^+/K^+ is typically more strongly correlated with blood pressure than either Na^+ or K^+ excretion alone.[110] The negative relationship between K^+ intake and blood pressure is more sharply defined for hypertensives than normotensives and for those with a family history of hypertension.[116] In particular, hypertension is more strongly associated with lower K^+ intake in black adults than in white adults with similar Na^+ intake.[117]

K^+ has multiple potential vasodepressor effects in humans, which support its use as a blood pressure–lowering agent[110] (Table 12-3). K^+ supplementation in humans has a natriuretic action even in the presence of elevated aldosterone and can decrease cardiac output.[110,118,119] K^+ can increase kallikrein and augment nitric oxide production by the endothelium, both factors that could lower blood pressure.[110] K^+ administration has also been shown to attenuate sympathetic activity and to decrease the amount and effect of several vasoactive hormones.[110] K^+ may have a direct systemic vasodilatory action by enhancing $Na^+ K^+$-ATPase activity and improving the compliance of large arteries.[110] Finally, K^+ intake may have a substantial influence on diurnal patterns of blood pressure responses. An increase in the intake of dietary K^+ converts nocturnal dipping status from nondipping to dipping in salt-sensitive normotensive adolescent blacks.[120]

TABLE 12-3. Proposed Mechanisms of Blood Pressure Reduction with Potassium

1. Direct natriuretic effect and conversion of salt-sensitive hypertension to salt-resistant hypertension
2. Increased renal kallikrein and eicosanoid production
3. Increased nitric oxide (increased vasodilatory response to acetylcholine)
4. Attenuation of sympathetic activity
5. Decreased amount and effect of plasma renin activity (PRA) and blunted rise in PRA following K^+-related natriuresis
6. Direct arterial effect—enhanced activity of $Na^+ K^+$-ATPase
7. Enhanced vascular compliance
8. Conversion of nocturnal nondipping to dipping blood pressure status

In clinical trials, oral K^+ supplementation (as opposed to dietary K^+) has been shown to lower blood pressure in hypertensive patients on a normal or high Na^+ intake.[121–124] The effect of oral K^+ supplementation on blood pressure is particularly prominent in patients with a low dietary intake of K^+.[123,124] Similar observations have also been made in elderly hypertensive subjects,[124–126] Fotherby and Potter having observed reductions in 24-h blood pressure of 6/3 mm Hg and clinic blood pressure of 10/6 mm Hg after 4 weeks of supplementation with 60 mmol of K^+.[126] In patients on salt-restricted diets, K^+ supplementation is less effective in reducing elevated blood pressure, suggesting that this form of treatment is most effective in the management of salt-sensitive hypertension.[124,127,128]

Dietary K^+ (60 mEq/day) has also been examined as a blood pressure–lowering supplement in patients already receiving antihypertensive drugs, such as diuretics[129] or beta blockers,[130] providing additional effectiveness in reducing blood pressure.

In summary, there is good evidence to suggest that dietary K^+ supplementation can cause a mild reduction in blood pressure, especially in hypertensive patients on high-Na^+ diets. It is still not known for how long the blood pressure–lowering effect of K^+ is maintained. In diuretic-treated patients who become hypokalemic, K^+ supplementation can correct the deficiency while at the same time further reducing blood pressure.[129] Rather than recommending K^+ supplements for the entire population of hypertensive patients or more particularly for those patients at risk for developing hypertension, biological markers need to be identified that might predict a response to K^+ supplements. A recent Canadian consensus panel offers commentary on aspects of this issue. This panel advises that the daily dietary intake of K^+ should be 60 mmol or greater and that dietary K^+ supplementation above this amount is not indicated as a means of preventing an increase in blood pressure in normotensive subjects.[131]

K^+ in Stroke

A protective effect of K^+ intake on risk of stroke has been recognized for a number of years, dating to the initial report by Khaw and Barrett-Connor.[111,132] More recently, in the National Health Professionals Study, K^+ intake was also shown to relate inversely to the risk of stroke.[133] This finding was further corroborated in a review by Fang et al. of the first National Health and Nutrition Examination Survey (NHANES-I), although the inverse association between K^+ intake and stroke mortality was detected only among black men and hypertensive males in this study.[134] The study by Fang et al. examined stroke mortality only and did not adjust for dietary factors that might confound the risk relation between K^+ and stroke—such as dietary intake of fiber, calcium, or vitamin C—which may explain its ethnicity- and gender-related findings.[134] As regards the relationship between K^+ intake and stroke, Bazzano et al. evaluated data from the NHANES-I Epidemiologic Follow-Up Study and also detected an independent association between low dietary K^+ intake and an increased hazard of stroke.[135] The relationship between decreased K^+ intake and stroke occurrence is not mechanistically resolved. It is possible, though not definitively proven, that the reduction in blood pressure that accompanies a high K^+ intake[119,127,128] and/or a more primary effect in slowing the atherosclerotic process may contribute to the positive effects of this nutritional factor.[103] The FDA has approved a health claim that "diets containing foods that are good sources of K^+ and low in fat may reduce the risk of high blood pressure and stroke."[135a]

K^+ in the Prevention of Atherosclerosis

It is currently believed that the development of the atherosclerotic lesion is initiated by the oxidation of low-density lipoproteins (LDLs) within the intimal layer of arteries.[136] Oxidized LDLs are then phagocytized by macrophages and monocytes, leading to the development of the lipid-laden foam cell, which is the prototypic cell of atherosclerosis. These foam cells lead to the formation of the fatty streak, the first microscopically visible element of the atherosclerotic plaque. Fatty streaks are of no clinical significance. In fact, many of them disappear spontaneously. However, certain of the fatty streaks progress into true atherosclerotic, fibrofatty plaques. Then endothelial cell injury occurs, leading to endothelial cell dysfunction. Subsequently, hemodynamic stress and/or induction of an inflammatory state triggers the release of platelet-derived growth factor from platelets and/or macrophages, which determines the transition of a fatty streak to a fibrous plaque. Ultimately, the transformation, proliferation and migration of subintimal smooth muscle cells lead to the development of the atherosclerotic lesion, with its well-described consequences.

Recent data suggest that the protective effect of K^+ on the atherosclerotic process may relate to its effect on the function of those cells involved in lesion formation as described above[102] (Fig. 12-2). Increases in K^+ have been shown in vitro to inhibit the formation of free radicals from both vascular endothelial cells and macrophages. This inhibitory effect on free radical formation could lead to a significant reduction in lesion formation in individuals with a high K^+ intake. Indeed, studies in animals have demonstrated reduced cholesterol content in the aorta of rats given large amounts of K^+.[137] In addition to its effect on free radical formation, elevation of K^+ has been shown to inhibit proliferation of vascular smooth muscle cells and to inhibit both platelet aggregation and arterial thrombosis. Thus, through a variety of mechanisms, elevations in K^+ could, at least theoretically, slow both the initiation and progression of the atherosclerotic lesion as well as the occurrence of thrombosis in the atherosclerotic vessel wall.[102,103,138] By these actions, small elevations of K^+ related to high levels of dietary intake could account for the apparent protection against cardiovascular diseases of atherosclerotic origin observed in primitive cultures with diets rich in K^+ and low in Na^+.

Electrophysiologic Effects

Hypokalemia

Hypokalemia reduces the rate of repolarization of the cardiac cell, leading to a prolongation of the recovery time.[139] In addition, hypokalemia causes the slope of phase 3 of the transmembrane action potential to become less steep. As a result, there is an increase in the interval during which the difference between the transmembrane potential and the threshold potential is small. Consequently, the period of increased excitability is prolonged and the appearance of ectopic atrial and/or ventricular beats is facilitated. A decrease in the extracellular K^+ concentration increases the difference in K^+ concentration across the cell membrane and tends to hyperpolarize the cell during diastole.[139]

Electrocardiographically, hypokalemia produces a flattening or inversion of the T wave with concomitant prominence of the U wave. This generally occurs without any significant change in the QT interval, although if the T wave fuses with the U wave, the QT interval may prove difficult to measure.[140] When hypokalemia is severe, the QRS complex may widen slightly in a diffuse manner. The

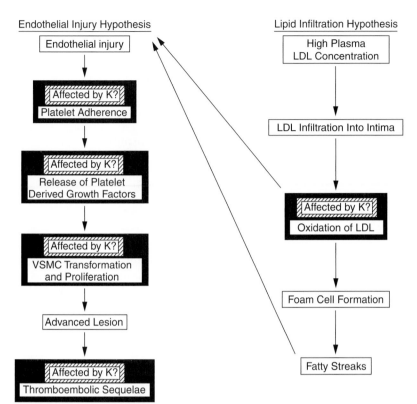

FIGURE 12-2. Combined endothelial injury–lipid infiltration hypothesis for atherosclerotic lesion formation and points at which increases in K^+ concentration may impede lesion development.[136]

ECG pattern of hypokalemia is not specific, and a similar pattern may be seen following the administration of digitalis, antiarrhythmic agents, or phenothiazines, and/or in patients with ventricular hypertrophy or bradycardia.

K^+ Supplementation

General Considerations

K^+ may be administered for multiple reasons. First, in diuretic-treated patients, it is given to replace a total body deficit, which may be as much as 300 to 400 mEq. Such replacement may be followed by a lower rate of cardiovascular events, as has been observed in a wide-range of diuretic-treated patients.[106,107,141] Second, K^+ may be given in a temporizing fashion to patients with hypokalemia attributable to transcellular shifts of K^+, wherein there is no total body deficit but a perceived need to treat a low serum K^+ value. This is not uncommonly the case in patients with high endogenous levels of catecholamines and, in particular, the beta$_2$ agonist epinephrine,[142] or in those receiving beta$_2$ agonists, such as asthmatics[143] or postcode patients.[144] Additionally, subjects with salt-sensitive hypertension may see a beneficial response to K^+ supplementation.[121,124] Furthermore, dietary K^+ may be as effective as supplementation, although the data in this regard are not as abundant. Finally, some investigators have proposed that the small elevations of serum K^+ concentration related to high levels of dietary K^+ intake might be enough to inhibit free radical formation, smooth muscle proliferation, and thrombus formation. In this way, the rate of progression to atherosclerotic lesions may be slowed and thrombosis in atherosclerotic vessels diminished.[102,103]

The issues surrounding K^+ replacement in clinical practice have recently been carefully articulated.[145]

Oral Therapy

If a patient consumes a diet that is deficient in K^+-rich foods (i.e., fruits and vegetables), dietary alterations may be sufficient to correct his or her hypokalemia. Such dietary modifications can provide 40 to 60 mEq/day of K^+ although generally in the form of K^+ citrate or acetate, which is somewhat less effective than K^+ chloride in correcting diuretic-induced hypokalemia. Salt substitutes provide another economical alternative to prescription K^+ supplements, although their bitter taste may dissuade patients from continuous use. They contain 7 to 14 mEq K^+/g (5 g equals approximately 1 teaspoon). K^+ supplements are usually given as K^+ chloride, available in either liquid or tablet formulations, although there are other forms as well (Table 12-4). The most common side effect of K^+ supplements is gastric irritation. The non-chloride-containing K^+ supplements provide an alternative for those unable to tolerate the K^+ chloride preparations or in whom K^+ depletion occurs in the setting of metabolic acidosis. As severe hyperkalemia can occur as a consequence of oral supplementation, serum K^+ levels should always be monitored during therapy.[146] This is particularly relevant to the patient also receiving ACE inhibitors, angiotensin receptor blockers, and/or spironolactone.[147]

Intravenous Therapy

K^+ can be administered intravenously in patients with severe hypokalemia and in those unable to tolerate oral preparations. A detailed discussion of the approximation of a K^+ deficit is beyond the scope of this chapter, although in the absence of an independent factor causing transcellular K^+ shifts, the magnitude of the deficit in body stores of K^+ correlates with the degree of hypokalemia (see Chap. 28). However, in the absence of ECG changes and with a K^+ level greater than 2.5 mEq/L, K^+ can generally be safely administered at a rate of up to 10 mEq/h in concentrations as

TABLE 12-4. Oral K⁺ Formulations*

Supplements	Attributes
Controlled-release microencapsulated tablets	Disintegrate better in the stomach than encapsulated microparticles; less adherent and less cohesive
Encapsulated controlled-release microencapsulated particles	Fewer erosions than wax-matrix tablets
K⁺ chloride elixir	Inexpensive, tastes bad, poor compliance; few erosions, immediate effect
K⁺ chloride (effervescent tablets) for solution	Convenient, more expensive than elixir, immediate effect
Wax-matrix extended-release tablets	Easier to swallow, more gastrointestinal tract erosions compared with microencapsulated formulations

*Other K⁺ formulations: K⁺ gluconate, K⁺ citrate, K⁺ acetate, and K⁺ carbonate, for use in hyperchloremia and hypokalemia. All K⁺ formulations are readily absorbed.

Source: Adapted with permission from Cohn et al.[145]

high as 30 mEq/L. However, higher concentrations (200 mmol/L) and rates of delivery (20 mmol/h) have been shown to be well tolerated.[148,149] Maximum daily administration should rarely exceed 100 to 200 mEq. If the serum K⁺ level is under 2 mEq/L and is associated with either ECG changes and/or neuromuscular symptoms, K⁺ can be administered intravenously at a rate of 40 mEq/h and at concentrations as high as 60 mEq/L. This should be accompanied by continuous ECG monitoring as well as measurement of serum K⁺ levels every several hours. In cases of life-threatening hypokalemia, K⁺ should initially be given in glucose-free solutions, as glucose may further lower K⁺.[150]

Conclusion

K⁺ has traditionally been used as a replacement in hypokalemia related to systemic illness and drug use.[151] Mg must often be gvien together with K⁺ to successfully correct hypokalemia. Recent evidence is mounting that K⁺ could be used to prevent and/or treat a range of cardiovascular diseases, such as hypertension and atherosclerosis, with favorable effects on morbidity and mortality.[101a,150a]

CALCIUM

Abnormalities in calcium (Ca^{2+}) homeostasis, like those in Mg and K⁺, appear to play an important role in the pathogenesis of cardiovascular disease.[77,152]

Cardiovascular Effects of Calcium

Calcium in Systemic Hypertension

Ca^{2+} metabolism is linked closely to the regulation of systemic blood pressure, and Ca^{2+} supplementation has been proposed as a treatment for systemic hypertension even though data on the association between dietary Ca^{2+} intake and blood pressure have been inconsistent.[153] Increased cytosolic concentrations of free Ca^{2+} found within vascular smooth muscle cells are thought to be responsible for the increased contractility of vessels characteristic of hypertension.[77] In animal models, acute intracellular Ca^{2+} overload of vascular smooth muscle cells can spark hypercontractility.[77] Hypertension can then develop if a general increase in systemic arteriolar tone ushers in a rise in peripheral resistance. Furthermore, with progressive elevation of intracellular Ca^{2+}, the structural

integrity of both arterial and arteriolar walls is compromised. Thus, in various animal models, Ca^{2+} overload initiates lesions of an arteriosclerotic character.[77,154] The increased concentrations of free Ca^{2+} within vascular smooth muscle cells could be secondary to alterations in Ca^{2+} entry, binding, or extrusion from the cells.[77,152] Studies on human cells have shown changes related to all three of these potential mechanisms.

Beyond the probability that an increased intracellular Ca^{2+} is involved in the pathogenesis of hypertension, there are other recognized relationships between Ca^{2+} and hypertension.[155] These include the relationship between serum Ca^{2+} levels and blood pressure,[77] the effect of dietary and supplemental Ca^{2+} on blood pressure, obesity,[156] and the renal excretion of Ca^{2+} and/or endogenous parathyroid hormone (PTH) in patients with hypertension.[90,155]

Serum Calcium and Hypertension

Hypertension is more common in the presence of hypercalcemia and, in many but not all studies, there appears to be a direct relationship between the total serum Ca^{2+} level and blood pressure.[155] However, the relationship between serum ionized Ca^{2+} and blood pressure does not appear to be as strong. Nevertheless, there are sufficient data to suggest a vasoconstrictive effect of increasing extracellular Ca^{2+} levels, presumably by a stimulation of catecholamine release and/or a direct vascular effect.[157]

Increased Renal Excretion of Calcium

Compared with normotensive subjects, hypertensive individuals excrete more Ca^{2+} both under basal circumstances[158] and during Na⁺ loading.[159] This may be due to the increase in Ca^{2+} excretion known to occur following intravascular volume expansion, with the resultant rise in Na⁺ excretion. Alternatively, it may be secondary to a decreased binding of Ca^{2+} to kidney cells.[155] Whatever the precise mechanism, it is known that patients with volume-expanded forms of hypertension excrete Ca^{2+} in excess.[155]

Increased Levels of Parathyroid Hormone

Hypertensive patients tend to have increased levels of plasma PTH, most likely as a homeostatic response to their urinary Ca^{2+} leak.[152] Although not nearly as high as those seen with primary hyperparathyroidism, these elevated PTH levels could exert a pressor effect and thereby cause or contribute to hypertension, a finding that is particularly prominent in women.[160,161]

Observational Studies and Clinical Trials with Calcium Supplements

There have been over 30 reports on observational studies of Ca^{2+} and hypertension, with the majority demonstrating an inverse relationship between dietary Ca^{2+} intake and the level of blood pressure.[90] However, clinical trials of Ca^{2+} supplementation (1–2 g/day for up to 4 years) have been less consistent in this regard, with only approximately two-thirds of such studies demonstrating any beneficial effect of supplemental Ca^{2+} on blood pressure.[155,162,163] The rationale for supplemental Ca^{2+} therapy is based on the assumption that PTH levels are elevated in response to low levels of ionized Ca^{2+}, resulting from the hypercalciuria seen in some forms of volume-expanded hypertension.[161] Additional Ca^{2+}, by raising plasma calcium, would tend to suppress PTH and thereby lower blood pressure. Indeed, in selected populations of hypertensives characterized by either increased urinary Ca^{2+} excretion, low ionized Ca^{2+}, or increased PTH levels, Ca^{2+} supplements often cause a significant fall in blood pressure. In addition, increased Ca^{2+} intake acts to increase Na^+ excretion in the urine and may lower blood pressure by this mechanism.[155] However, in unselected populations of hypertensives, most clinical studies have shown little or no effect of Ca^{2+} supplementation on blood pressure.[155,163,164] Furthermore, even those patients with lower serum Ca^{2+} and higher PTH levels, who may benefit from calcium supplementation, may do so with the potential risk of developing kidney stones in a dose-dependent manner, although the risk of calcium oxalate stone formation does not increase significantly in postmenopausal women with osteoporosis given calcium carbonate.[165] In contrast, studies in pregnant women have shown that Ca^{2+} supplementation can provide important reductions in both systolic and diastolic blood pressure and can reduce their risk of developing preeclampsia.[166,167]

In summary, based on the available data, Ca^{2+} supplementation or an increased intake of Ca^{2+} through enriched foods cannot be recommended as a treatment for the general hypertensive population or for the prevention of hypertension.[131] Individual patients, such as pregnant women, may benefit from this approach, but there are currently no screening methods for identifying those patients in the general population who would benefit from Ca^{2+} supplementation.

Calcium and Myocardial Contractility

Ca^{2+} is of fundamental importance to the process of myocardial contraction.[168] The initial event is activation of Na^+ channels, resulting in rapid Na^+ influx and membrane depolarization. As a consequence, voltage-gated, dihydropyridine-sensitive sarcolemmal Ca^{2+} channels are opened, allowing an influx of Ca^{2+} into the myocyte. There is a close proximity between sarcolemmal Ca^{2+} channels and Ca^{2+} channels of the sarcoplasmic reticulum, which is pertinent in that Ca^{2+} then stimulates the junctional sarcoplasmic reticulum to release Ca^{2+} via a ryanodine-sensitive calcium-release channel. The sum of the released Ca^{2+} represents a substantial increase in the free intracellular Ca^{2+}, which then diffuses into the myofibrils to combine with troponin. Troponin, in its Ca^{2+}-free state, inhibits the interaction of myosin and actin. With the rise in intracellular Ca^{2+}, troponin is bound to Ca^{2+}, and this inhibition disappears. Actin then combines with myosin, leading to the split of ATP by a Ca^{2+}-dependent ATPase. The energy that is released from this process is then transformed into mechanical work leading to the interaction of actin and myosin filaments and the resultant shortening of myofibrils.[168]

Recently, there has been much interest in the cellular abnormalities of Ca^{2+} homeostasis in the failing human heart. Studies of animal models and myocardium from patients with heart failure have demonstrated abnormalities of cytosolic Ca^{2+} handling, myofilament Ca^{2+} sensitivity, and myocyte energetics. Many of these metabolic abnormalities have been shown to be the result of alterations in the activity or number of myocyte enzymes and transport channels that are important in excitation-contraction coupling.[169] While a great deal of research work remains to be done in this area, it is becoming evident that cardiac dysfunction is intimately associated with Ca^{2+} handling abnormalities in cardiac cells.[170] A discussion of agents used to increase Ca^{2+} at the myosin-actin interaction sites and Ca^{2+} sensitivity at those sites for the treatment of congestive heart failure is provided in Chap. 13. Ca^{2+} supplementation itself has been poorly studied as a possible treatment for congestive heart failure.

Calcium Use in Cardiac Arrest

As described above, Ca^{2+} plays an essential role in excitation-contraction coupling,[168] and for many years intravenous calcium chloride was administered in cardiac resuscitation efforts in patients with bradyasystolic arrest.[171] It is no longer used for this indication, since no survival benefit has been observed[172,172a], and there is evidence that Ca^{2+} may induce cerebral vasospasm[173,174] and impact the extent of reperfusion injury in the heart and brain.[175,176]

Calcium Use in Arrhythmia

Intravenous calcium can slow the heart rate and has been used to treat tachycardias. The drug must be used cautiously, however, in patients receiving digoxin because it can precipitate digitalis toxicity and ventricular arrhythmias related to afterdepolarization. Afterdepolarizations are membrane potential voltage oscillations that are dependent on a preceding action potential. There are two types of afterdepolarizations. Early afterdepolarizations (EADs) occur during phase 2 or 3 of the action potential, whereas delayed afterdepolarizations (DADs) occur after the resting membrane potential has been reestablished (phase 4). DADs have been shown in vitro to occur in the setting of digitalis toxicity or catecholamine excess as well as in hypertrophied myocardium and in Purkinje cells after myocardial infarction.[177] DADs appear to result from the oscillatory release of Ca^{2+} ions from sarcoplasmic reticulum during conditions of Ca^{2+} overload. The clinical significance of DADs and triggered activity is not completely clear, but this mechanism has been etiologically invoked to explain at least some ventricular arrhythmias. While much remains to be learned, it seems likely that DADs will emerge as an important mechanism of human arrhythmia.

Decreases in extracellular Ca^{2+} concentration can increase the action potential duration, resulting from an increase in duration and a decrease in amplitude of phase 2 of the cardiac action potential. Hypocalcemia may cause a clinically insignificant decrease in the QRS duration; cardiac arrhythmias are uncommon. Intravenous calcium has been used to treat intoxications from Ca^{2+}-channel blockers (see Chap. 9) complicated by bradyarrhythmia and hypotension.

Clinical Use of Calcium

A number of Ca^{2+} salts are available (Table 12-5). Each has a different amount of elemental Ca^{2+} per administered gram. Ca^{2+} supplements are generally administered in conjunction with meals two to three times daily. The solubility of the various Ca^{2+} salts is quite

TABLE 12-5. Available Forms of Calcium

Calcium Salt	% Calcium	mEq/g Calcium
Calcium acetate	25	12.5
Calcium carbonate	40	20
Calcium citrate	21	10.5
Calcium glubionate	6.5	3.3
Calcium gluconate	9	4.5
Calcium lactate	13	6.5
Calcium phosphate, dibasic	23	11.5
Calcium phosphate, tribasic	39	19.5

varied. For example, calcium carbonate, although attractive as a therapy in that it is 40% elemental Ca^{2+} by weight, is poorly absorbed, which limits its utility. Ca^{2+} citrate and glubionate tend to be better absorbed.

In cases where hypocalcemia persists despite adequate calcium supplementation, a vitamin D supplement may be required to enhance Ca^{2+} absorption. Intravenous Ca^{2+} is available as several different salts including calcium chloride (27.2 mg/mL), Ca^{2+} gluceptate (18 mg/mL), and Ca^{2+} gluconate (9 mg/mL). Calcium chloride is the preferred formulation because it produces more predictable levels of ionized Ca^{2+} in plasma, though it can be quite venotoxic and should be used carefully whenever adequate vascular access is in question.[178]

Conclusion

Except for specific situations, such as calcium entry blocker overdose, pregnancy, and hypocalcemia, treatment with Ca^{2+} is not recommended for the prevention and treatment of cardiovascular disease. Dietary Ca^{2+}, however, should be maintained for the purpose of general health maintenance.

REFERENCES

1. Saris NE, Mervaala E, Karppanen H, et al: Magnesium: An update on physiological, clinical, and analytical aspects. *Clin Chim Acta* 294: 1, 2000.
2. Reinhart RA: Magnesium metabolism: A review with special reference to the relationship between intracellular content and serum levels. *Arch Intern Med* 148:2415, 1988.
3. Wacker WE, Parisi AF: Magnesium metabolism. *N Engl J Med* 278:658, 1968.
4. Altura BM, Altura BT: Role of magnesium in the pathogenesis of hypertension updated: relationship to its actions on cardiac, vascular smooth muscle, and endothelial cells. In: Laragh JN, Brenner BM, eds. *Hypertension: Pathophysiology, Diagnosis and Management.* New York: Raven Press, 1995:1213.
5. Reinhart RA: Clinical correlates of the molecular and cellular actions of magnesium on the cardiovascular system. *Am Heart J* 121:1513, 1991.
6. Fox C, Ramsoomair D, Carter C: Magnesium: Its proven and potential clinical significance. *South Med J* 94:1195, 2001.
7. Mroczek WJ, Lee WR, Davidov ME: Effect of magnesium sulfate on cardiovascular hemodynamics. *Angiology* 28:720, 1977.
8. Laurant P, Touyz RM: Physiological and pathophysiological role of magnesium in the cardiovascular system: Implications in hypertension. *J Hypertens* 18: 1177, 2000.
9. Iseri LT, French JH: Magnesium: nature's physiologic calcium blocker. *Am Heart J* 108:188, 1984.
10. Vigorito C, Giordano A, Ferraro P, et al: Hemodynamic effects of magnesium sulfate on the normal human heart. *Am J Cardiol* 67:1435, 1991.
11. Turlapaty PD, Altura BM: Magnesium deficiency produces spasms of coronary arteries: Relationship to etiology of sudden death ischemic heart disease. *Science* 208:198, 1980.
12. Arsenian MA: Magnesium and cardiovascular disease. *Prog Cardiovasc Dis* 35:271, 1993.
13. Satake K, Lee JD, Shimizu H, et al: Relation between severity of magnesium deficiency and frequency of anginal attacks in men with variant angina. *J Am Coll Cardiol* 28:897, 1996.
14. Cermuzynski L, Gebalska J, Wolk R, Makowska E: Hypomagnesemia in heart failure with ventricular arrhythmias. Beneficial effects of magnesium supplementation. *J Intern Med* 247:78, 2000.
15. Adams JH, Mitchell JR: The effect of agents which modify platelet behavior and of magnesium ions on thrombosus formation in vivo. *Thromb Haemost* 42:603, 1979.
16. Anstall HB, Huntsman RG, Lehman H, et al: The effect of magnesium on blood coagulation in human subjects. *Lancet* 1:814, 1959.
17. Shechter M: The role of magnesium as antithrombotic therapy. *Wien Med Wochenschr* 150:343, 2000.
18. Sherer Y, Bitzur R, Cohen H, et al: Mechanisms of action of the anti-atherogenic effect of magnesium: Lessons from a mouse model. *Magnes Res* 14:173, 2001.
19. Shechter M, Sharir M, Labrador MJ, et al: Oral magnesium therapy improves endothelial function in patients with coronary artery disease. *Circulation* 102:2353, 2000.
20. Kharb S, Singh V: Magnesium deficiency potentiates free radical production associated with myocardial infarction. *J Assoc Physicians India* 48:484, 2000.
21. Leary WP, Reyes AJ, Lockett CJ, et al: Magnesium and deaths ascribed to ischaemic heart disease in South Africa. A preliminary report. *S Afr Med J* 64:775, 1983.
22. Yamori Y, Mizushima S: A review of the link between dietary magnesium and cardiovascular risk. *J Cardiovasc Risk* 7:31, 2000.
23. Chipperfield B, Chipperfield JR: Heart-muscle magnesium, potassium, and zinc concentrations after sudden death from heart-disease. *Lancet* 2:293, 1973.
24. Johnson CJ, Peterson DR, Smith EK: Myocardial tissue concentrations of magnesium and potassium in men dying suddenly from ischemic heart disease. *Am J Clin Nutr* 32:967, 1979.
25. Abraham AS, Bar-On E, Eylath U: Changes in the magnesium content of tissues following myocardial damage in rats. *Med Biol* 59:99; 1981.
26. Chang C, Bloom S: Interrelationship of dietary magnesium intake and electrolyte homeostasis in hamsters: I. Severe magnesium deficiency, electrolyte homeostasis, and myocardial necrosis. *J Am Coll Nutr* 4:173, 1985.
27. Shen AC, Jennings RB: Myocardial calcium and magnesium in acute ischemic injury. *Am J Pathol* 67:417, 1972.
28. Steurer G, Yang P, Rao V, et al: Acute myocardial infarction, reperfusion injury, and intravenous magnesium therapy: Basic concepts and clinical implications. *Am Heart J* 132: 478, 496, 1996.
29. Teo KK, Yusuf S, Collins R, et al: Effects of intravenous magnesium in suspected acute myocardial infarction: Overview of randomised trials. *BMJ* 303:1499, 1991.
30. Woods KL, Fletcher S, Roffe C, Haider Y: Intravenous magnesium sulphate in suspected acute myocardial infarction: Results of the second Leicester Intravenous Magnesium Intervention Trial (LIMIT-2). *Lancet* 339:1553, 1992.
31. ISIS-4: A randomized factorial trial assessing early oral captopril, oral mononitrate, and intravenous magnesium sulphate in 58,050 patients with suspected acute myocardial infarction. ISIS-4 (Fourth International Study of Infarct Survival) Collaborative Group. *Lancet* 345:669, 1995.
32. Ziegelstein RC, Hilbe JM, French WJ, et al: Magnesium use in the treatment of acute myocardial infarction in the United States (Observations from the Second National Registry of Myocardial Infarction). *Am J Cardiol* 87:7, 2001.
33. Woods KL, Fletcher S: Long-term outcome after intravenous magnesium sulphate in suspected acute myocardial infarction: The second Leicester Intravenous magnesium Intervention Trial (LIMIT-2). *Lancet* 343:816, 1994.
34. Roffe C, Fletcher S, Woods KL: Investigation of the effects of intravenous magnesium sulphate on cardiac rhythm in acute myocardial infarction. *Br Heart J* 71:141, 1994.

35. Shechter M, Hod H, Kaplinsky E, Rabinowitz B: The rationale of magnesium as alternative therapy for patients with acute myocardial infarction without thrombolytic therapy. *Am Heart J* 132:483, 1996.

36. Antman EM: Magnesium in acute myocardial infarction: Overview of available evidence. *Am Heart J* 132:487, 1996.

36a. Woods KL, Abrams K: The importance of effect mechanism in the design and interpretation of clinical trials: The role magnesium in acute myocardial infarction. *Prog Cardiovasc Dis* 44:267, 2002.

37. Shechter M, Hod H, Chouraqui P, et al: Magnesium therapy in acute myocardial infarction when patients are not candidates for thrombolytic therapy. *Am J Cardiol* 75:321, 1995.

38. Caspi J, Rudis E, Bar I, et al: Effects of magnesium on myocardial function after coronary artery bypass grafting. *Ann Thorac Surg* 59:942, 1995.

39. Toraman F, Karabulut EH, Alhan HC, et al: Magnesium infusion dramatically decreases the incidence of atrial fibrillation after coronary artery bypass grafting. *Ann Thorac Surg* 72:1256, 2001.

40. Kinoshita K, Oe M, Tokunaga K: Superior protective effect of low-calcium, magnesium-free potassium cardioplegic solution on ischemic myocardium. Clinical study in comparison with St. Thomas' Hospital solution. *J Thorac Cardiovasc Surg* 101:695, 1991.

41. Demmy TL, Haggerty SP, Boley TM, Curtis JJ: Lack of cardioplegia uniformity in clinical myocardial preservation. *Ann Thorac Surg* 57:648, 1994.

42. Santoro GM, Antoniucci D, Bolognese L, et al: A randomized study of intravenous magnesium in acute myocardial infarction treated with direct coronary angioplasty. *Am Heart J* 140:891, 2000.

43. Ryan TJ, Antman EM, Brooks NH, et al: ACC/AHA guidelines for the management of patients with acute myocardial infarction. A report of the American College of Cardiology/American Heart Association Task Force on Practice Guidelines (Committee on Management of Acute Myocardial Infarction). *Circulation* 100:1016, 1999.

44. The MAGIC Steering Committee: Rationale and design of the magnesium in coronaries (MAGIC) study: A clinical trial to reevaluate the efficacy of early administration of magnesium in acute myocardial infarction. *Am Heart J* 139:10, 2000.

45. Jackson CE, Meier DW: Routine serum magnesium analysis. Correlation with clinical state in 5,100 patients. *Ann Int Med* 69:743, 1968.

46. Tosiello L: Hypomagnesemia and diabetes mellitus. A review of clinical implications. *Arch Intern Med* 156:1143, 1996.

47. Lima MD, Cruz T, Pousada JC, et al: The effect of magnesium supplementation in increasing doses on the control of type 2 diabetes. *Diabetes Care* 21:682, 1998.

48. Sjogren A, Floren CH, Nilsson A: Magnesium, potassium and zinc deficiency in subjects with type II diabetes mellitus. *Acta Med Scand* 224:461, 1988.

49. Agus ZS: Hypomagnesemia. *J Am Soc Nephrol* 10:1616, 1999.

50. Leier CV, Dei Cas L, Metra M: Clinical relevance and management of the major electrolyte abnormalities in congestive heart failure: Hyponatremia, hypokalemia, and hypomagnesemia. *Am Heart J* 128:564, 1994.

51. Cohen N, Alon I, Almoznino-Sarafian D, et al: Metabolic and clinical effects of oral magnesium supplementation in furosemide-treated patients with severe congestive heart failure. *Clin Cardiol* 23:433, 2000.

52. Wester PO, Dyckner T: Diuretic treatment and magnesium losses. *Acta Med Scand* 647(Suppl):145, 1981.

53. Chase LR, Slatopolsky E: Secretion and metabolic efficiency of parathyroid hormone in patients with severe hypomagnesemia. *J Clin Endocrinol Metab* 38:363, 1974.

54. Leicht E, Schmidt-Gayk H, Langer HJ, et al: Hypomagnesaemia-induced hypocalcaemia: Concentrations of parathyroid hormone, prolactin and 1,25-dihydroxyvitamin D during magnesium replenishment. *Magnes Res* 5:33, 1992.

55. Wester PO: Electrolyte balance in heart failure and the role for magnesium ions. *Am J Cardiol* 70:44C, 1992.

56. Eichhorn EJ, Tandon PK, DiBianco R, et al: Clinical and prognostic significance of serum magnesium concentration in patients with severe chronic congestive heart failure: The PROMISE Study. *J Am Coll Cardiol* 21:634, 1993.

57. Gottlieb SS, Fisher ML, Pressel MD, et al: Effects of intravenous magnesium sulfate on arrhythmias in patients with congestive heart failure. *Am Heart J* 125:1645, 1993.

58. Sueta CA, Clarke SW, Dunlap SH, et al: Effect of acute magnesium administration on the frequency of ventricular arrhythmia in patients with heart failure. *Circulation* 89:660, 1994.

59. Bashir Y, Sneddon JF, Staunton HA, et al: Effects of long-term oral magnesium chloride replacement in congestive heart failure secondary to coronary artery disease. *Am J Cardiol* 72:1156, 1993.

60. Cohen L, Kitzes R: Magnesium sulfate and digitalis-toxic arrhythmias. *JAMA* 249:2808, 1983.

61. Crippa G, Sverzellati E, Giorgi-Pierfranceschi M, Carrara GC: Magnesium and cardiovascular drugs: Interactions and therapeutic role. *Ann Ital Med Int* 14:40, 1999.

62. Dyckner T, Wester PO: Ventricular extrasystoles and intracellular electrolytes before and after potassium and magnesium infusions in patients on diuretic treatment. *Am Heart J* 97:12, 1979.

63. McLean RM: Magnesium and its therapeutic uses: A review. *Am J Med* 96:63, 1994.

64. Hirahara K, Matsubayashi T, Matsuura H, Ehara T: Intracellular magnesium depletion depresses the delayed rectifier potassium current in guinea pig ventricular myocytes. *Jpn J Physiol* 48:81, 1998.

65. Ghani MF, Rabah M: Effect of magnesium chloride on electrical stability of the heart. *Isr Heart J* 94:600, 1977.

66. Bigg RP, Chia R: Magnesium deficiency. Role in arrhythmias complicating acute myocardial infarction? *Med J Aust* 1:346, 1981.

67. Dyckner T, Wester PO: Magnesium deficiency contributing to ventricular tachycardia. Two case reports. *Acta Med Scand* 212:89, 1982.

68. Iseri LT: Magnesium and cardiac arrhythmias. *Magnesium* 5:111, 1986.

69. Tsuji H, Venditti FJ Jr., Evans JC, et al: The association of levels of serum potassium and magnesium with ventricular premature complexes (the Framingham Heart Study). *Am J Cardiol* 74: 232, 1994.

70. Hoes AW, Grobbee DE, Lubsen J, et al: Diuretics, β-blockers, and the risk for sudden cardiac death in hypertensive patients. *Ann Intern Med* 123:481, 1995.

71. Allegra J, Lavery R, Cody R, et al: Magnesium sulfate in the treatment of refractory ventricular fibrillation in the prehospital setting. *Resuscitation* 49:245, 2001.

72. Allen BJ, Brodsky MA, Capparelli EV, et al: Magnesium sulfate therapy for sustained monomorphic ventricular tachycardia. *Am J Cardiol* 15:64:1202, 1989.

73. Specter MJ, Schweizer E, Goldman RH: Studies on magnesium's mechanism of action in digitalis-induced arrhythmias. *Circulation* 52:1001, 1975.

74. Cohen L, Kitzes R: Magnesium sulfate and digitalis-toxic arrhythmias. *JAMA* 249:2808, 1983.

75. Ramee SR, White CJ, Svinarich JT, et al: Torsades de pointes and magnesium deficiency. *Am Heart J* 109:164, 1985.

76. Tzivoni D, Banai S, Schuger C, et al: Treatment of torsades de pointes with magnesium sulfate. *Circulation* 77:392, 1988.

77. Shingu T, Matsuura H, Kusaka M, et al: Significance of intracellular free calcium and magnesium and calcium-regulating hormones with sodium chloride loading in patients with essential hypertension. *J Hypertens* 9:1021, 1991.

78. McCarron DA: Calcium and magnesium nutrition in human hypertension. *Ann Intern Med* 98:800, 1983.

79. Joffres MR, Reed DM, Yano K: Relationship of magnesium intake and other dietary factors to blood pressure: The Honolulu Heart Study. *Am J Clin Nutr* 45:469; 1987.

80. Peacock JM, Folsom AR, Arnett DK, et al: Relationship of serum and dietary magnesium to incident hypertension: The Atherosclerosis Risk in Communities (ARIC) Study. *Ann Epidemiol* 9:159, 1999.

81. Resnick LM, Gupta RK, Laragh JH: Intracellular free magnesium in erythrocytes of essential hypertension: Relation to blood pressure and serum divalent cations. *Proc Natl Acad Sci U S A* 81: 6511, 1984.

82. Vollmer WM, Sacks FM, Ard J, et al: Effects of diet and sodium intake on blood pressure: Subgroup analysis of the DASH-Sodium Trial. *Ann Intern Med* 135:1019, 2001.

83. Ascherio A, Hennekens C, Willett WC, et al: Prospective study of nutritional factors, blood pressure, and hypertension among US women. *Hypertension* 27:1065, 1996.

84. Yamamoto ME, Applegate WB, Klag MJ, et al: Lack of blood pressure effect with calcium and magnesium supplementation in adults with high-normal blood pressure. Results from Phase I of the Trials of Hypertension Prevention (TOHP). Trials of Hypertension Prevention (TOHP) Collaborative Research Group. *Ann Epidemiol* 5:96, 1995.

85. Lind L, Lithell H, Pollare T, Ljunghall S: Blood pressure response during long-term treatment with magnesium is dependent on magnesium status. A double-blind, placebo-controlled study in essential hypertension and in subjects with high normal blood pressure. *Am J Hypertens* 4:674, 1991.

86. Cappuccio FP, Markandu ND, Benynon GW, et al: Lack of effect of oral magnesium on high blood pressure: A double blind study. *BMJ* 291:235, 1985.

87. Henderson DG, Schierup J, Schodt J: Effect of magnesium supplementation on blood pressure and electrolyte concentrations in hypertensive patients receiving long-term diuretic treatment. *BMJ* 293:664, 1986.

88. Nowson CA, Morgan TO: Magnesium supplementation in mild hypertensive patients on a moderately low sodium diet. *Clin Exp Pharmacol Toxicol* 16:299, 1989.

89. Ferrara LA, Iannuzzi R, Castaldo A, et al: Long-term magnesium supplementation in essential hypertension. *Cardiology* 81:25, 1992.

90. Harlan WR, Harlan LC: Blood pressure and calcium and magnesium intake. In: Laragh JH, Brenner BM, eds. *Hypertension: Pathophysiology, Diagnosis and Management.* New York: Raven Press, 1995:1143.

91. Lu JF, Nightingale CH: Magnesium sulfate in eclampsia and preeclampsia: Pharmacokinetic principles. *Clin Pharmacokinet* 38:305, 2000.

92. Witlin AG, Sibai BM: Magnesium sulfate in preeclampsia and eclampsia. *Obstet Gynecol* 92:883, 1998.

93. Muir KW: Magnesium for neuroprotection in ischaemic stroke: Rationale for use and evidence of effectiveness. *CNS Drugs* 15:921, 2001.

94. Lampl Y, Gilad R, Geva D, et al: Intravenous administration of magnesium sulfate in acute stroke: A randomized double-blind study. *Clin Neuropharmacol* 24:1, 2001.

95. Elliott C, Newman N, Madan A: Gentamicin effects on urinary electrolyte excretion in healthy subjects. *Clin Pharmacol Ther* 67:16, 2000.

96. Kingston ME, Al-Siba'i MB, Skooge WC: Clinical manifestations of hypomagnesemia. *Crit Care Med* 14:950, 1986.

97. Gettes LS: Electrolyte abnormalities underlying lethal and ventricular arrhythmias. *Circulation* 85(Suppl I):I70, 1992.

98. Chen WC, Fu XX, Pan ZJ, Qian SZ: ECG changes in early stage of magnesium deficiency. *Am Heart J* 104:1115, 1982.

99. Iseri LT, Freed J, Bures AR: Magnesium deficiency and cardiac disorders. *Am J Med* 58:837, 1975.

100. Gullestad L, Midtvedt K, Dolva LO, et al: The magnesium-loading test: Reference values in healthy subjects. *Scand J Clin Lab Invest* 54:23, 1994.

101. Rob PM, Dick K, Bley N, et al: Can one really measure magnesium deficiency using the short-term magnesium loading test? *J Intern Med* 246:373, 1999.

101a. Sica DA, Struthers AD, Cushman WC, et al: Importance of potassium in cardiovascular disease. *J Clin Hypertens* 4:1, 2002.

102. Young DB: Control, cardiovascular, and renal effects of potassium. In: Laragh JH, Brenner BM, eds. *Hypertension: Pathophysiology, Diagnosis and Management.* New York: Raven Press, 1995:1503.

103. Young DB, Lin H, McCabe RD: Potassium's cardiovascular protective mechanisms. *Am J Physiol* 268:R825, 1995.

104. Fang J, Madhavan S, Alderman MH: Dietary potassium intake and stroke mortality. *Stroke* 31:1532, 2000.

105. Bazzano LA, he J, Ogden LG, et al: Dietary potassium intake and risk of stroke in US men and women. National Health and Nutrition Examination Survey I Epidemiologic Follow-Up Study. *Stroke* 32:1473, 2001.

106. Cohen HW, Madhavan S, Alderman MH: High and low serum potassium associated with cardiovascular events in diuretic-treated patients. *J Hypertens* 19:1315, 2001.

107. Franse LV, Pahor M, DiBari M, et al: Hypokalemia associated with diuretic use and cardiovascular events in the Systolic Hypertension in the Elderly Program. *Hypertension* 35:1025, 2000.

108. Sanguinetti MC: Modulation of potassium channels by antiarrhythmic and antihypertensive drugs. *Hypertension* 19:228, 1992.

109. Singh H, Linas SL: Potassium therapy and hypertension. *Miner Electrolyte Metab* 19:57, 1993.

110. Morris RC Jr, Sebastian A: Potassium-responsive hypertension. In: Laragh, JH, Brenner BM, eds. *Hypertension: Pathophysiology, Diagnosis and Management,* 2nd ed. New York: Raven Press, 1995:2715.

111. Tobian L: The protective effects of high-potassium diets in hypertension, and the mechanisms by which high-NaCl diets produce hypertension—a personal view. In: Laragh JH, Brenner BM, eds. *Hypertension: Pathophysiology, Diagnosis and Management,* 2nd ed. New York: Raven Press, 1995:299.

112. Siani A, Strazzullo P: Relevance of dietary potassium intake to antihypertensive drug treatment. In: Laragh JH, Brenner BM, eds. *Hypertension: Pathophysiology, Diagnosis and Management,* 2nd ed. New York: Raven Press, 1995:2727.

113. Khaw KT, Barrett-Connor E: Dietary potassium and blood pressure in a population. *Am J Clin Nutr* 39: 963; 1984.

114. Khaw KT, Rose G: Population study of blood pressure and associated factors in St. Lucia, West Indies. *Int J Epidemiol* 11:372, 1982.

115. Reed D, McGee D, Yano K, Hankin J: Diet, blood pressure, and multicollinearity. *Hypertension* 7:405, 1985.

116. Pietinen PI, Wong O, Altschul AM: Electrolyte output, blood pressure, and family history of hypertension. *Am J Clin Nutr* 32:997, 1979.

117. Grim CE, Luft FC, Miller JZ, et al: Racial differences in blood pressure in Evans County, Georgia: Relationship to sodium and potassium intake and plasma renin activity. *J Chronic Dis* 33:87, 1980.

118. Fujita T, Ando K: Hemodynamic and endocrine changes associated with potassium supplementation in sodium-loaded hypertensives. *Hypertension* 6:184, 1984.

119. Young DB, McCaa RE, Pan YJ, Guyton AC: The natriuretic and hypotensive effects of potassium. *Circ Res* 38(Suppl 2):84, 1976.

120. Wilson DK, Sica DA, Miller SB: Effects of potassium on blood pressure in salt-sensitive and salt-resistant black adolescents. *Hypertension* 34:181, 1999.

121. Cappuccio FP, MacGregor GA: Does potassium supplementation lower blood pressure? A meta-analysis of published trials. *J Hypertens* 9:465, 1991.

122. Kawano Y, Minami J, Takishita S, Omae T: Effects of potassium supplementation on office, home, and 24-h blood pressure in patients with essential hypertension. *Am J Hypertens* 11:1141, 1998.

123. Gu D, He J, Wu X, et al: Effect of potassium supplementation on blood pressure in Chinese: A randomized, placebo-controlled trial. *J Hypertens* 19:1325, 2001.

124. Whelton PK, He J, Cutler JA, et al: Effects of oral potassium on blood pressure. Meta-analysis of randomized controlled clinical trials. *JAMA* 277:1624, 1997.

125. Smith SR, Klotman PE, Svetkey LP: Potassium chloride lowers blood pressure and causes natriuresis in older patients with hypertension. *J Am Soc Nephrol* 2:1302, 1992.

126. Fotherby MD, Potter JF: Potassium supplementation reduces clinic and ambulatory blood pressure in elderly patients. *J Hypertens* 10:1403, 1992.

127. Svetkey LP, Simons-Morton D, Vollmer WM, et al: Effects of dietary patterns on blood pressure: subgroup analysis of the Dietary Approaches to Stop Hypertension (DASH) randomized clinical trial. *Arch Intern Med* 159:285, 1999.

128. Sacks FM, Svetkey LP, Vollmer WM, et al: Effects on blood pressure of reduced dietary sodium and the Dietary Approaches to Stop Hypertension (DASH) diet. DASH-Sodium Collaborative Research Group. *N Engl J Med* 344:3, 2001.

129. Kaplan NM, Carnegie A, Ruskin P, et al: Potassium supplementation in hypertensive patients with diuretic-induced hypokalemia. *N Engl J Med* 312:746, 1985.

130. Salvetti A, Bishisao E, Caiazza A, et al: The combination of a low Na/high K salt with metoprolol in the treatment of mild-moderate hypertension. A multicenter study. *Am J Hypertens* 1:201S, 1988.

131. Burgess E, Lewanczuk R, Bolli P, et al: Lifestyle modifications to prevent and control hypertension. 6. Recommendations on potassium, magnesium and calcium. Canadian Hypertension Society, Canadian Coalition for High Blood Pressure Prevention and Control, Laboratory Centre for Disease Control at Health Canada, Heart and Stroke Foundation of Canada. *Can Med Assoc J* 160(Suppl 9):S35, 1999.

132. Khaw KT, Barrett-Connor E: Dietary potassium and stroke-associated mortality. A 12-year prospective population study. *N Engl J Med* 316:235, 1987.

133. Ascherio A, Rimm EB, Hernan MA, et al: Intake of potassium, magnesium, calcium, and fiber and risk of stroke among US men. *Circulation* 98:1198, 1998.

134. Fang J, Madhavan S, Alderman MH: Dietary potassium intake and stroke mortality. *Stroke* 31:1532, 2000.

135. Bazzano LA, He J, Ogden LG, et al: Dietary potassium intake and risk of stroke in US men and women: National Health and Nutrition Examination Survey I epidemiologic follow-up study. *Stroke* 32:1473, 2001.

135a. US FDA Center for Food Safety and Applied Nutrition Health claim notification for potassium-containing foods. Available at http://vm.cfsan.fda.gov/dms/helm/k.html. Accessed 4/20/02.

136. Steinberg D, Parthasarathy S, Carew TE, et al: Beyond cholesterol. Modifications of low-density lipoprotein that increase its atherogenicity. *N Engl J Med* 320:915, 1989.

137. Tobian L, Jahner TM, Johnson MA: High potassium diets markedly reduce atherosclerotic cholesterol ester deposition in aortas of rats with hypercholesterolemia and hypertension. *Am J Hypertens* 3:133, 1990.

138. Young DB, Ma G: Vascular protective effects of potassium. *Semin Nephrol* 19:477, 1999.

139. Rardon DP, Fisch C: Electrolytes and the heart. In: Schlant RC, Alexander RW, eds. *Hurst's The Heart,* 8th ed. New York: McGraw Hill, 1994:768.

140. Surawicz B: Electrolytes, hormones, temperature, and miscellaneous factors. In: *Electrophysiologic Basis of ECG and Cardiac Arrhythmias.* Baltimore: Williams & Wilkins, 1995:426.

141. Wahr JA, Parks R, Boisvert D, et al: Preoperative serum potassium levels and perioperative outcomes in cardiac surgery patients. Multicenter Study of Perioperative Ischemia Research Group. *JAMA* 281:2203, 1999.

142. Reid JL, Whyte KF, Struthers AD: Epinephrine-induced hypokalemia: The role of beta adrenoceptors. *Am J Cardiol* 57:23F, 1986.

143. Newhouse MT, Chapman KR, McCallum AL, et al: Cardiovascular safety of high doses of inhaled fenoterol and albuterol in acute severe asthma. *Chest* 110:595, 1996.

144. Salerno DM, Murakami M, Elsperger KJ: Effects of pretreatment with propranolol on potassium, calcium, and magnesium shifts after ventricular fibrillation in dogs. *J Lab Clin Med* 114:595, 1989.

145. Cohn JN, Kowey PR, Whelton PK, Prisant LM: New guidelines for potassium replacement in clinical practice: A contemporary review by the National Council on potassium in Clinical Practice. *Arch Intern Med* 160:2429, 2000.

146. Perzella MA: Drug-induced hyperkalemia: Old culprits and new offenders. *Am J Med* 109:307, 2000.

147. Schepkens H, Vanholder R, Billiouw JM, Lameire N: Life-threatening hyperkalemia during combined therapy with angiotensin-converting enzyme inhibitors and spironolactone: An analysis of 25 cases. *Am J Med* 110:438, 2001.

148. Kruse JA, Clark VL, Carlson RW, Geheb MA: Concentrated potassium chloride infusions in critically ill patients with hypokalemia. *J Clin Pharmacol* 34:1077, 1994.

149. Kruse JA, Carlson RW: Rapid correction of hypokalemia using concentrated intravenous potassium chloride infusions. *Arch Intern Med* 150:613, 1990.

150. Famularo G, Corsi FM, Giacanelli M: Iatrogenic worsening of hypokalemia and neuromuscular paralysis associated with the use of glucose solutions for potassium replacement in a young woman with licorice intoxication and furosemide abuse. *Acad Emerg Med* 6:960, 1999.

150a. He FJ, MacGregor GA: Beneficial effects of potassium. *BMJ* 323:497, 2001.

151. Gennari FJL Hypokalemia. *N Engl J Med* 339:451, 1998.

152. Hatton DC, Young EW, Bukoski RD, McCarron DA: Calcium metabolism in experimental genetic hypertension. In: Laragh JH, Brenner BM, eds. *Hypertension: Pathophysiology, Diagnosis and Management.* New York: Raven Press, 1995:1193.

153. Oparil S: Diet-micronutrients—special foods. In: Oparil S, Weber M, eds. *Hypertension: A Companion to the Kidney.* Philadelphia: Saunders, 2000:433.

154. Fleckenstein-Grun G, Frey M, Thimm F, et al: Calcium overload—an important cellular mechanism in hypertension and arteriosclerosis. *Drugs* 44(Suppl 1):23, 1992.

155. Sowers JR, Standley PR, Tuck ML, Ram JL: Calcium and calcium-regulatory hormones in hypertension. In: Laragh JH, Brenner BM, eds. *Hypertension: Pathophysiology, Diagnosis and Management.* New York: Raven Press, 1995:1155.

156. Zemel MB: Calcium modulation of hypertension and obesity: Mechanisms and implications. *J Am Coll Nutr* 20 (Suppl 5): 428S, 2001.

157. Sica DA, Harford AM, Zawada ET: Hypercalcemic hypertension in hemodialysis. *Clin Nephrol* 22:102, 1984.

158. Quereda C, Orte L, Sabater J, et al: Urinary calcium excretion in treated and untreated essential hypertension. *J Am Soc Nephrol* 7:1058, 1996.

159. Yamakawa H, Suzuki H, Nakamura M, et al: Disturbed calcium metabolism in offspring of hypertensive parents. *Hypertension* 19:528, 1992.

160. Jorde R, Sundsfjord J, Haug E, Bonaa KH: Relation between low calcium intake, parathyroid hormone, and blood pressure. *Hypertension* 35:1154, 2000.

161. Jorde R, Bonaa KH, Sundsfjord J: Population based study on serum ionized calcium, serum parathyroid hormone, and blood pressure. The Tromso study. *Eur J Endocrinol* 141:350, 1999.

162. Bucher HC, Cook RJ, Guyatt GH, et al: Effects of dietary calcium supplementation on blood pressure. A meta-analysis of randomized controlled trials. *JAMA* 275:1016, 1996.

163. Allender PS, Cutler JA, Follmann D, et al: Dietary calcium and blood pressure: A meta-analysis of randomized clinical trials. *Ann Intern Med* 124:825, 1996.

164. Griffith LE, Guyatt GH, Cook RJ, et al: The influence of dietary and nondietary calcium supplementation on blood pressure: An updated meta-analysis of randomized controlled trials. *Am J Hypertens* 12:84, 1999.

165. Domrongkitchaiporn S, Ongphiphadhanakul B, Stitchantrakul W, et al: Risk of calcium oxalate nephrolithiasis after calcium or combined calcium and calcitriol supplementation in postmenopausal women. *Osteoporosis Int* 11:486, 2000.

166. Bucher HC, Guyatt GH, Cook RJ, et al: Effect of calcium supplementation on pregnancy-induced hypertension and preeclampsia: A meta-analysis of randomized controlled trials. *JAMA* 275:1113, 1996.

167. Niromanesh S, Laghaii S, Mosavi-Jarrahi A: Supplementary calcium in prevention of pre-eclampsia. *Int J Gynaecol Obstet* 74:17, 2001.

168. LeWinter MM, Osol G: Normal physiology of the cardiovascular system. In: Fuster V, Alexander RW, O'Rourke RA, eds. *Hurst's the Heart,* 10th ed. New York: McGraw Hill, 2001:63–94.

169. Figueredo VM, Camacho SA: Basic mechanisms of myocardial dysfunction: Cellular pathophysiology of heart failure. *Curr Opinion Cardiol* 9:272, 1994.

170. Dhalla NS, Afzal N, Beamish RE, et al: Pathophysiology of cardiac dysfunction in congestive heart failure. *Can J Cardiol* 9:873, 1993.

171. Ornato JP, Gonzalez ER, Morkunas AR, et al: Treatment of presumed asystole during pre-hospital cardiac arrest: Superiority of electrical countershock *Am J Emer Med* 3:395, 1985.

172. Stempien A, Katz AM, Messineo FC: Calcium and cardiac arrest. *Ann Intern Med* 105:603, 1986.

172a. Kelsch T, Kikuchi K, Vahdat S, Frishman WH: Innovative pharmaco logic approaches to cardiopulmonary resuscitation. *Heart Dis* 3:46, 2001.

173. Kirsch JR, Dean JM, Rogers MC: Current concepts in brain resuscitation. *Arch Intern Med* 146:1413, 1986.

174. Dembo DH: Calcium in advanced life support. *Crit Care Med* 9:358, 1981.

175. Follette DM, Fey K, Buckberg GD, et al: Reducing postischemic damage by temporary modification of reperfusate calcium, potassium, pH, and osmolarity. *J Thorac Cardiovasc Surg* 82:221, 1981.

176. Zimmerman AN, Hulsmann WC: Paradoxical influence of calcium ions on the permeability of the cell membrane of the isolated rat heart. *Nature* 211:646,1966.

177. Hessen SE, Michelson EL: Mechanisms of ventricular arrhythmias: From laboratory to bedside. *Am Coll Cardiol Curr J Rev* 4:11, 1995.

178. White RD, Goldsmith RS, Rodriguez R, et al: Plasma ionic calcium levels following injection of chloride, gluconate, and gluceptate salts of calcium. *J Thorac Cardiovasc Surg* 71:609, 1976.

Inotropic Agents

Edmund H. Sonnenblick

Thierry H. LeJemtel

William H. Frishman

BACKGROUND

The life expectancy of patients with congestive heart failure (CHF) is shortened or at best unchanged by long-term exposure to currently available positive inotropic agents.[1,1a] All positive inotropic agents currently available enhance myocardial contractility by increasing intracellular Ca^{2+} concentration. Rising intracellular Ca^{2+} promotes afterpotential depolarizations and, thereby, ventricular arrhythmia and sudden death. Accordingly, the use of positive inotropic agents for the treatment of chronic heart failure is not as widespread as in the past and is now limited to specific indications. Moreover cardiac glycosides, the only oral inotropic agents, are now administered at doses that mostly reverse the autonomic dysfunction associated with CHF and minimally affect myocardial contractility.[2] The low doses of cardiac glycosides that are now routinely recommended are most likely responsible for their neutral effect on mortality. The use of intravenous inotropic agents such as dobutamine and milrinone is limited to patients who, despite optimal manipulation of cardiac loading conditions, are in a low-cardiac-output state in the absence of severe functional mitral regurgitation.[3] In the presence of severe functional mitral regurgitation, further manipulations of loading conditions can improve forward cardiac output without the risk of triggering ventricular arrhythmia that often plagues positive inotropic therapy.[4] Currently, the use of dobutamine is reserved for patients with severely decompensated CHF who are not improved by intravenous administration of loop diuretics and natriuretic peptides in addition to optimal oral doses of angiotensin converting enzyme (ACE) inhibitors, nitrates, and digoxin and not concomitantly treated with beta-blocking agents.[5] The aim of short-term dobutamine therapy is to achieve an improvement in left ventricular (LV) performance that is sustained after discontinuation of therapy. The mechanisms that mediate the sustained improvement in LV performance are not fully elucidated but appear to be predominantly related to reversal of peripheral abnormalities and not to sustained increase in myocardial contractility.[6] The metabolic cost of enhancing myocardial contractility with dobutamine leads to a twofold increase in myocardial blood flow in experimental preparations of heart failure. When the presence of severe coronary artery disease hinders the required increase in myocardial blood flow, dobutamine may promote myocardial ischemia and loss of cardiac myocytes, as evidenced by a rising level of troponin I.

Long-term administration of dobutamine is routinely used as a bridge to transplantation in patients who develop a low-output syndrome while awaiting cardiac transplantation.[7] The use of lower doses of dobutamine than those previously administered seems to have reduced the likelihood that the initial improvement in LV performance attenuates with time, a phenomenon referred to as tachyphylaxis.

The indications and aim of short-term administration of milrinone are similar to those of dobutamine (Table 13-1). The metabolic cost of enhancing myocardial contractility with milrinone is offset by the concomitant decrease in LV wall tension that results from its substantial vasodilating properties. Thus, milrinone is the preferred positive inotropic agent in patients with decompensated CHF who exhibit clinical or laboratory evidence of active myocardial ischemia or in patients with known critical coronary artery obstructions. Since milrinone acts downstream from the beta-adrenergic receptors, it also the preferred inotropic agent for patients with decompensated CHF who are receiving beta-adrenergic blockade. Last, in view of its arteriolar and venous relaxing properties, milrinone is preferable to dobutamine in patients with decompensated CHF and severe pulmonary hypertension.

From this brief introduction of currently available positive inotropic agents, it is clear that the problem of heart failure and its evolution cannot be solved by long-term inotropic stimulation. Thus, the major use of positive inotropic agents is in the acute temporary enhancement of cardiac output and reduction of LV filling pressures when all other interventions have failed. The cost of increasing contractility, in terms of increased energy requirements and potentially lethal arrhythmias, limits their long-term benefits while not addressing the primary limitations of ongoing myocardial cell loss or excessive loading of the ventricles.

Cardiac glycosides, dobutamine and other beta-adrenergic sympathetic agonists, as well as phosphodiesterase (PDE) inhibition with milrinone, are discussed in greater detail below.

DIGITALIS GLYCOSIDES

Digitalis glycosides have had a long and venerable history in the treatment of CHF. In 1785, William Withering[8] reported on his use of the digitalis leaf as a purported diuretic agent to treat anasarca, presumably due to CHF (see Chap. 11). Indeed, the major effects of digitalis were thought to be on the kidneys, although important effects on heart rate were noted. Only in the latter part of the nineteenth century did it become apparent that there was a direct

TABLE 13-1. Indications for Parenteral Inotropes

Bridge to transplantation
Acute decompensation with low cardiac output
Short-term following cardiac surgery
Maximal medical therapy—not a candidate for transplantation,
    revascularization, or valvular repair
Bridge to beta blockers

action of digitalis glycosides to increase cardiac contractility,[9] while in the earlier part of the twentieth century its effects on the peripheral circulation and the autonomic nervous system were noted.[10]

Pharmacologic Action

Digitalis glycosides have important effects on multiple systems in addition to augmenting myocardial contractility.[11,12] Electrophysiologically, digitalis glycosides speed conduction in the atrium while inhibiting conduction through the atrioventricular node. In the normal circulation, digitalis glycosides also produce generalized arteriolar vasoconstriction; they also affect the central nervous system by enhancing parasympathetic and reducing sympathetic nervous system activation. Digitalis sensitizes baroreflexes to decrease efferent sympathetic activity, which acts to reduce sinus node activity and thus reduce heart rate. The increase in baroreflex sensitization also increases parasympathetic tone, while central vagal nuclei are also stimulated. The broad enhancement of parasympathetic activity with digitalis glycosides contributes to slow the heart rate and to control supraventricular arrhythmias. As discussed below, in the failing state, the effects of sympathetic withdrawal may be dominant, so as to reduce arterial vascular resistance, while in the normal circulation arterial vasoconstriction may be dominant. Integration of these various actions adds to the inotropic activity of digitalis glycosides and their therapeutic usefulness.

The action of digitalis glycosides to increase contractility and alter the electrophysiology of heart muscle occurs through inhibition of the enzyme Na^+ K^+-ATPase on the surface membrane of myocardial cells, which results in an increase in the amount of Ca^{2+} to activate contraction.[13,14] The Na^+ K^+-ATPase is an energy-requiring "sodium pump," which extrudes three Na^+ ions that enter the cell during depolarization in exchange for two potassium ions, thus creating an electrical current and a negative resting potential.[15] Contraction is brought about by an action potential that depolarizes the surface membrane of the cell. This action potential is created by a rapid inward current of Na^+ into the cell that opens Ca^{2+} channels, permitting Ca^{2+} to enter the cell. This, in turn, releases substantially more Ca^{2+} from stores in the sarcoplasmic reticulum within the cell and thereby activates the contractile mechanism by binding to a component of the troponin-tropomyosin system, which had been maintaining the resting state. With Ca^{2+} bound to troponin, actin and myosin can interact to produce force and shortening. The greater the amount of activating Ca^{2+}, the greater the force and shortening.[14,15] When Ca^{2+} is released from troponin and taken up by the sarcoplasmic reticulum, relaxation occurs.[14] The relatively small amount of Ca^{2+} that enters the cell with activation is ultimately removed by an electrogenic Na^+-Ca^{2+} exchange which extrudes one Ca^{2+} for three Na^+ ions. When intracellular Na^+ is increased, less exchange occurs and the net amount of intracellular Ca^{2+} is increased. Thus, by inhibiting the Na^+ K^+-ATPase, digitalis glycosides produce a decrease in intracellular K^+ and an increase in intracellular Na^+, which increases intracellular Ca^{2+} (Fig. 13-1).[14,15]

In general, the main pathway by which all inotropic agents, including digitalis glycosides, increase contractility is by increasing the amount of Ca^{2+} available for activation.[16] This is the case in normal as well as failing myocardium. In the failing heart, there appears to be a decrease in the Ca^{2+} released into the cytosol with activation.[17,18] The inotropic effects of digitalis glycosides are apparently due to an increase in intracellular Ca^{2+} that augments Ca^{2+} stores in the sarcoplasmic reticulum, resulting in a subsequent increase in the extent of myocyte activation.

The electrophysiologic actions of digitalis glycosides are complex, since they are intimately related to autonomic actions as well as K^+ effects and also the type of cardiac tissue affected.[19] In pacemaker cells in the atria, there is little effect except for increased automaticity at toxic levels. In the sinoatrial node and atrioventricular conduction system, the refractory period is prolonged. At toxic levels, conduction block can be produced through decreasing resting potential, which results in slowed conduction.[19] At toxic levels of glycoside, the Purkinje system may become autonomous due to decreased resting potentials. All of these effects are magnified by decreased extracellular K^+, so that toxicity is enhanced by a low serum K^+ and reduced by an increased K^+.[19]

At therapeutic levels, the effects of digitalis glycosides reflect the direct electrophysiologic actions of the drug and the indirect actions of neurohormonal stimuli. In the atria, increased parasympathetic tone decreases the refractory period, which overrides the direct digitalis effect to prolong the refractory period. Increased parasympathetic stimulation may reduce automaticity through hyperpolarization of pacemaker cells, while sinus node activity, which is not affected directly by digitalis, is reduced through both increased parasympathetic and decreased sympathetic tone.[14]

Toxic levels of digitalis glycosides tend to exaggerate the parasympathetic augmentation, which may actually lead to atrial arrhythmias. Sympathetic activity may increase at toxic levels,[20] which, added to the direct actions of digitalis glycosides, can potentially result in life-threatening ventricular tachyarrhythmias.

In addition to effects on heart muscle to increase contractility and on vascular smooth muscle to increase contraction, digitalis glycosides exert significant actions on the autonomic nervous system, and these effects may provide a major part of purported beneficial actions.[12,21,22] These effects include both stimulation and inhibition and may vary with dose of drug and underlying state of disease. In addition, short- and long-term effects may differ and alter ultimate efficacy. Relatively low doses of digitalis glycosides increase parasympathetic tone through apparent increased sensitivity of the efferent limb of both ventricular and arterial baroreceptors.[12] Increased sensitivity of arterial baroreceptors enhances efferent parasympathetic activity while leading to withdrawal of reflex sympathetic tone,[21] resulting in sinus bradycardia as well as arterial and venous dilatation. This indirect effect is opposite to the direct effect of glycosides to produce smooth muscle vasoconstriction. Added effects of this sympathetic withdrawal include increased renal blood flow, renin release inhibition, and decreased antidiuretic hormone (ADH) release.[23] Release of acetylcholine by vagal fibers is also thought to inhibit norepinephrine release from nerve endings as well as to reduce beta-receptor responses.[21]

The overall effects of digitalis glycoside in the healthy individual are the result of the sum of its actions on the heart, the circulation, and the central nervous system, so that it is difficult to differentiate direct from indirect effects of glycosides in many instances. Digitalis glycosides increase myocardial contractility directly in both the

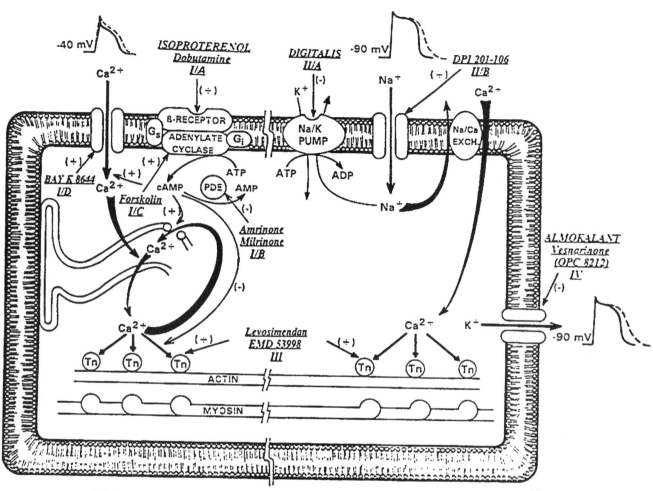

FIGURE 13-1. Diagram of various inotropic sites of action on and within the cardiac cell. While catecholamines act at cell surface receptors, agents such as amrinone and milrinone (PDE III inhibitors) act within the cell to augment adenylate cyclase. Calcium sensitizers increase the Ca^{2+} sensitivity of troponin (Tn) in the contractile system itself. (*Reproduced with permission from Varro A, Papp JG: Classification of positive inotropic actions based on electrophysiologic characteristics: Where should calcium sensitizers be placed? J Cardiovasc Pharmacol 26(Suppl 1):S32, 1995.*)

normal and failing heart, although the effects are relatively greater in the latter situation. However, hemodynamic results differ. In the absence of CHF, where both sympathetic and parasympathetic tone are minimal, digitalis glycosides increase peripheral arterial resistance directly, with a concomitant modest increase in arterial pressure accompanied by a shift in blood volume to the splanchnic bed, with a decline in venous return and cardiac output.[12] In contrast, with CHF, with withdrawal of elevated sympathetic nerve activity and increased parasympathetic tone, a fall in peripheral arterial resistance occurs with an increase in cardiac output.[24,25] In terms of the heart, a decrease in ventricular filling pressure also occurs while stroke volume increases. These effects are increased by enhancing parasympathetic tone in the failing circulation, which may mimic some of the beneficial effects of beta blockers and unloading agents, as noted elsewhere.

Whether the effects of digitalis glycosides are always beneficial, and if so, at what dose, remains controversial. Studies in the elderly and in patients with myocardial infarction have demonstrated an increased threat of digitalis toxicity without careful monitoring.[26] However, in the presence of severe failure [New York Heart

Association (NYHA) class III], withdrawal of digoxin has resulted in substantial and rapid clinical deterioration despite concomitant therapy, including ACE inhibitors and diuretics.[27–29] When used in mild CHF, digitalis glycosides have increased ejection fraction, while ACE inhibitors were largely effective only in increasing exercise performance.[30,31] These beneficial effects are observed whether the patients were in atrial fibrillation or in sinus rhythm.[31,32] The placebo-controlled multicenter Digitalis Investigation Group study, comprising over 7000 patients with CHF, showed that digoxin did not affect mortality but reduced hospitalization for heart failure when compared to control. Digoxin therapy was also shown to improve both ventricular function and patients' symptoms.[33]

Digitalis Preparations: Structure, Pharmacokinetics, and Metabolism

All cardiac glycosides contain a ring structure termed an aglycone, to which are attached up to four sugar molecules at the C3 position (Fig. 13-2). The aglycone itself is formed by a steroid nucleus to

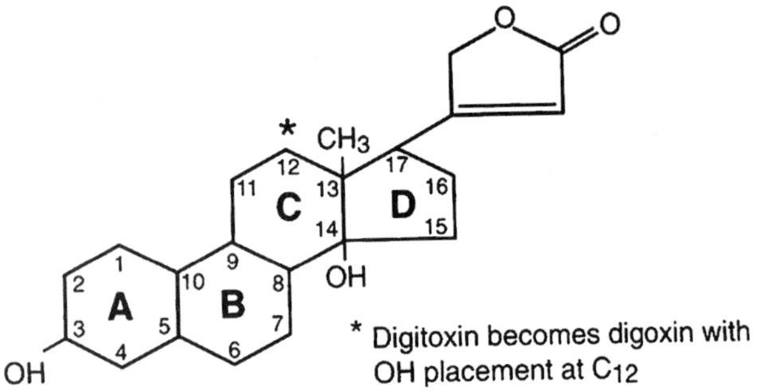

FIGURE 13-2. Structure of the digitalis molecule.

which a beta unsaturated lactone ring is attached at the C17 position. Hydroxyl groups are generally found at C3 and C14, while a glucose moiety is generally attached through the C3 hydroxyl group. At present, digoxin and digitoxin are the glycosides that are used clinically; they differ structurally only by the presence in digoxin of a hydroxyl group in the C12 position. Cardiac activity, which correlates with the binding of drug to $Na^+ K^+$-ATPase on the cell surface sarcolemma, depends on the unsaturated lactone ring, the hydroxyl at C14, and a cis configuration in carbons 8 to 17 in the aglycone ring. As the number of sugars on C3 is reduced, water-solubility increases and hepatic metabolism rather than renal excretion is favored. Thus, digoxin is excreted primarily by the kidneys while digitoxin is metabolized in the liver.[34] Digitoxin is 90% bioavailable, as compared to 60% for digoxin. A major difference between these agents is that digoxin is 25% protein-bound while digitoxin is 93% bound, such that the half-life of digoxin is 1.7 days and that of digitoxin is quite long at 7.0 days.

At present, digoxin and digitoxin are the only glycosides readily available in the United States, and digoxin is used in most instances. Digoxin has an onset of action from 30 min to 2 h when given orally and 5 to 30 min when given intravenously. Peak action occurs in 6 to 8 h when given orally and in 1 to 4 h when given intravenously. The plasma half-life of digoxin is 32 to 48 h, and 50 to 70% is renally cleared as an intact molecule.[34] Renal impairment may delay excretion of digoxin, which may lead to its accumulation and the development of toxicity. Digitoxin has a much longer half-life of several days and is metabolized largely by the liver.

Clinical Use

A loading dose for both digoxin and digitoxin is necessary to reach a stable state rapidly, although with digoxin this is attained in 5 to 7 days with only a maintenance dose. While intravenous digoxin is available, the oral dosage is generally adequate except in urgent settings. The average loading dose of digoxin is 1.0 to 1.5 mg. given in divided doses over 24 h, with a maintenance dose of 0.125 to 0.25 mg a day. These doses are commonly halved in the elderly or in patients with renal insufficiency. The maintenance dose commonly needs adjustment in order to regulate resting heart rate in atrial fibrillation (between 55 and 70 beats per minute). In sinus rhythm, the dose is more uncertain and a desired serum level of around 1.0 mg/mL should be sought.

As noted previously, the beneficial effects of augmented parasympathetic tone and sympathetic withdrawal may be obtained with relatively small doses of digitalis while not encountering potentials of toxicity.[34a,34b] Thus, the issue of dosage of digoxin remains unsettled relative to the benefit sought.

Digitoxin requires a loading dose, since steady state on maintenance dosing is attained only after several weeks. The loading dose is about 1.0 mg in divided doses with maintenance of 0.1 to 0.15 mg a day. The advantage of digitoxin is its hepatic excretion in the presence of renal insufficiency and the lessened impact of poor patient compliance due to its much longer duration of action. Its disadvantage is the long time required for washout should toxicity occur or be suspected.

The serum level of digoxin can be affected by several other drugs.[35] Cholestyramine, kaolin-pectin, neomycin, and bran can decrease digoxin absorption. Erythromycin, omeprazole, and tetracycline can increase digoxin absorption. Thyroxine can increase the volume of distribution of digoxin and enhance renal clearance. Quinidine increases serum digoxin levels, doubling levels in most patients over 1 to 2 days. The mechanism remains unclear, but if digoxin intake is not reduced, toxicity can occur. Verapamil reduces renal excretion and can increase serum digoxin levels by as much as 50% over a period of time. Amiodarone and propafenone appear to have a similar effect. With concurrent verapamil, amiodarone, and propafenone use, digoxin doses should be halved. Other antiarrhythmic agents do not exhibit interactions with digoxin.

Both thiazides and loop diuretics may lead to K^+ depletion, which augments myocardial sensitivity to digitalis glycosides and leads to arrhythmias, often requiring oral K^+ replacement or the use of K^+-sparing diuretics such as amiloride. This may lead to arrhythmias of digoxin toxicity at even relatively low serum digoxin levels. Spironolactone, which inhibits the effects of aldosterone and thus serves to save K^+, may also have an opposing effect to reduce renal clearance of digoxin, thus raising its serum level.[35]

In general, digoxin is used most commonly and thus is the focus of the remaining discussion.

Digoxin in the Treatment of Congestive Heart Failure

As noted above, digoxin has its most beneficial hemodynamic actions when substantial ventricular depression is evident along with CHF. In this circumstance, it augments myocardial performance while reflexly reducing peripheral resistance.[25] Slowing of the heart rate—whether via enhanced parasympathetic tone and reduced sympathetic activity to reduce sinus rate or via control of heart rate in atrial fibrillation (as discussed below)—will greatly benefit ventricular filling and reduce pulmonary congestion. Thus the actions of digitalis glycosides affect not only the performance of the depressed myocardium but have a central action to favorably alter the neurohumoral milieu that may impact adversely on the heart and circulation.[36] In the treatment of CHF, digoxin is generally employed along with diuretics, beta blockers, and vasodilator agents. By reducing peripheral resistance, digoxin and peripheral vasodilators act in a complementary manner.[36a]

In acute heart failure—characterized by acute pulmonary edema, severe limitations of cardiac output, and perhaps hypotension—more rapidly acting inotropic agents such as intravenous dobutamine or milrinone may be required along with loop diuretics, natriuretic peptides, and vasodilators. This situation may occur in the setting of rapid deterioration of the patient with CHF or following a large myocardial infarction.[37] In this circumstance, the main aim is to increase cardiac output and reduce filling pressure as a setting for longer-term stabilization.

While rapidly acting inotropic agents are being used, digitalization may be begun cautiously for its longer-term effects. In the setting of myocardial infarction, the situation is more complex.[38] Due to a fear that arrhythmias may be induced or oxygen consumption increased, which may be detrimental, digoxin is generally avoided in the first few days following the infarction; in the longer term, however, digitalization, especially if dosing is carefully controlled, may be of value along with other agents, especially ACE inhibitors. In the absence of clear CHF with only lower ejection fraction (NYHA class I–II), digitalis has had an apparent adverse effect on long-term mortality[37] and should be avoided. For chronic CHF, digoxin is of use over the long term when administered in association with loop diuretics and ACE inhibitors. Benefits are most evident in patients with NYHA Class III or IV CHF. In this circumstance, the response of the circulation is characterized by a decrease in venous pressure and ventricular filling pressure and an increase in cardiac output. Heart rate is slowed and ejection fraction tends to rise, while peripheral resistance falls with little or no change in arterial pressure. These salutary effects are attributed to a combination of augmented myocardial contractility and restoration of baroreceptor sensitivity, which results in enhanced parasympathetic and decreased sympathetic tone. Myocardial oxygen consumption tends to be reduced in heart failure due to a decrease in heart size, and thus ventricular wall tension, and a slowing of heart rate. Earlier concepts supported the view that digoxin was of greatest benefit when atrial fibrillation was present and controlled. It is now clear that efficacy is also present when the patient with heart failure is in sinus rhythm.[32] Withdrawal of digoxin from such patients has led to rapid deterioration even when both diuretics and ACE inhibitors were used.[27] While digoxin has been associated with an increase in ejection fraction, vasodilators have shown more significant increments in exercise performance.[30] These considerations would justify the combined use of these agents. However, whereas the use of ACE inhibitors may well be indicated when the ejection is reduced but symptoms are limited (classes I and II), digoxin should probably be reserved for use with more overt symptoms (classes III and IV).

While digoxin can be given once a day without tolerance or tachyphylaxis, the dose is a matter of issue. In general, a serum level of 0.5 to 1.5 ng/mL is felt to be therapeutic.[34] This level may vary from patient to patient, and clear dose-response relation has not been established. Indeed, some of the greatest benefits may be gained from lower doses (e.g., 0.125 mg a day), which may induce the neurohumoral benefits of lower sympathetic and higher parasympathetic tone while reducing the incidence of possible toxic side effects, as discussed below. There appear to be no adverse effects from digoxin usage in terms of mortality in patients with CHF,[33] and substantially increased morbidity is noted when the drug is withdrawn.[27,28,31] Effects on mortality with digoxin are complicated by the fact that the nature and progression of the underlying process, which has led to failure in the first place, may well be the ultimate determinant of mortality. If morbidity is reduced substantially with digoxin, as demonstrated,[33] a neutral effect on ultimate mortality, as has been demonstrated, would be acceptable. This was demonstrated in the Digitalis Investigation Group Study, a controlled trial in patients with CHF sponsored by the National Institutes or Health (NIH), which showed no effect on survival compared to placebo, a reduction in hospitalizations, and a low incidence of digoxin toxicity.[33]

Digoxin has been of limited value in the treatment of right-sided heart failure, as may occur in cor pulmonale or left-to-right shunts. Digoxin also has limited value in the face of acute LV failure due to acute myocardial infarction. After the first few days of an

infarction have passed, longer-term digoxin use has been employed, as it would be in any form of chronic failure, but its effects on mortality have remained controversial. Nevertheless, since mortality may be increased by giving digoxin postinfarction, especially when clear evidence of heart failure is absent, its use is best reserved for those with overt CHF.

Digitalis Toxicity

Digoxin levels can be readily measured in the serum by immunologic techniques, and the therapeutic level is thought to be 1.0 to 2.0 ng/mL.[39] Administration of other drugs may change the serum level by altering either absorption or elimination and may contribute to toxicity, as noted previously. For example, verapamil and quinidine may increase plasma levels. Drugs like spironolactone and canrenone can also falsely lower the measured concentration of digoxin.[39a]

The signs and symptoms of digitalis toxicity have been amply described, although some may be very subtle.[20,39–41] These include nausea and anorexia, which may lead to weight loss, fatigue, and visual disturbances. Psychiatric disturbances may occur less commonly; they may include delirium, hallucinations, or even seizures. Electrocardiographic alterations occur with variable degrees of atrioventricular (AV) block and ventricular ectopy. Sinus bradycardia, junctional rhythm, paroxysmal tachycardia with variable AV block, Wenckebach AV block, and ventricular tachycardia leading to ventricular fibrillation may be seen. Such arrhythmias are potentiated by hypokalemia as well as digitalis-mediated enhanced parasympathetic tone. They may be life-threatening in the presence of severe heart failure and should be avoided or controlled as much as possible.

The diagnosis of digitalis toxicity is suggested by signs and symptoms as well as electrocardiographic alterations and is supported by an elevated serum digoxin level.[20,41,42] Certainty of the diagnosis may only be made with drug withdrawal accompanied by subsidence of these findings. With the therapeutic level of digoxin between 1.0 and 2.0 ng/mL, digitalis toxicity levels would be unlikely but not excluded; levels beyond 3.0 ng/mL would suggest toxicity, while levels below 1.5 ng/mL when not complicated by hypokalemia would suggest other problems. It is important to note that only steady-state serum drug concentrations show any relationship with cardiac glycoside toxicity. Thus, for example, in monitoring serum digoxin concentration, the samples should be collected at least 6 to 8 h after drug administration.[43] Nevertheless, there is considerable crossover between patients reflecting variable sensitivity, such that withdrawal of digoxin on suspicion is always advisable for treatment as well as diagnosis. This is especially true since some patients experience profound vagal responses with relatively small amounts of digoxin.

While withdrawal of digoxin and correction of hypokalemia as a potentiating cause may be adequate treatment of digitalis toxicity in most instances, a temporary pacemaker may be required for severe bradycardia or complete heart block. Lidocaine is useful to treat ventricular ectopy or ventricular tachycardia. Dilantin has also been used, while quinidine, which may displace digoxin from binding sites and thus raise serum digoxin levels further, should be avoided. Amiodarone and intravenous magnesium have also been successfully utilized for this purpose.

In the presence of massive digoxin overdosage, most commonly associated with suicide attempts, digitalis-specific antibodies (digoxin-specific Fab fragments) have been remarkably effective.[20,44] In general, such an approach in the usual therapeutic setting is unnecessary but provides a backup to more conservative approaches, if they are not proceeding well, such as normalizing serum K^+ and withholding digoxin.

Digoxin reduction should be considered and individualized in the elderly patient with renal insufficiency.[45] Since electrical conversion is accompanied by ventricular arrhythmias, reduction of dosage 1 to 2 days before the procedure is advisable.

CATECHOLAMINES

In general, positive inotropism is based on enhancing the delivery of Ca^{2+} to the contractile system so as to increase force and shortening. Increasing Ca^{2+} in the serum will effect this transiently, while, as noted previously, digitalis glycosides increase Ca^{2+} for activation by inhibiting sarcolemmal Na^+ K^+-ATPase. Catecholamines increase activating Ca^{2+} via beta-adrenergic receptors and the adenylate cyclase system (see Fig. 13-1).

Beta receptors are located in the sarcolemma and comprise a complex structure that spans the membrane.[46] The beta receptor is connected with G proteins (see Fig. 13-1) that either activate (Gs) or inhibit (Gi) a secondary system, adenylate cyclase, which, when activated by Gs, induces the formation of $3'$-$5'$ cyclic adenosinemonophosphate (cyclic AMP). Cyclic AMP, in turn, activates certain protein kinases, which lead to intracellular phosphorylation of proteins that enhance both the entry and removal of intracellular Ca^{2+}.[47] When more Ca^{2+} is provided to the troponin tropomyosin system, a greater interaction between actin and myosin occurs, increasing force and shortening. Increasing the rate of Ca^{2+} removal from the cytoplasm speeds the rate of relaxation.

In the normal heart, norepinephrine is synthesized and stored in sympathetic nerve endings that invest the entire heart, atria, conduction system, and ventricle.[48] When activated, these nerve endings are depolarized and norepinephrine is released from granules in nerve endings into myocardial clefts containing beta-adrenergic receptors, which, when activated, turn on the sequence of events noted above. This not only enhances Ca^{2+} entry into the myocyte to augment contraction but also phosphorylates phospholamban, which enhances relaxation.[47] Subsequently, most of the released norepinephrine is taken back up and re-stored in the sympathetic nerve endings. Released norepinephrine is also inactivated by two enzymes, catechol-O-methyltranferase (COMT) and monoamine oxidase (MAO), and the products are excreted largely by the kidneys.[47]

In very severe heart failure, stores of norepinephrine in the ventricle are largely depleted and the sympathetic nerve endings fail to take up norepinephrine normally.[49] At the same time, circulating norepinephrine released from peripheral sympathetic nerve endings may be increased, especially in severe failure.[50] In less severe heart failure, the decreased norepinephrine levels may reflect enhanced release due to increased sympathetic nerve activity.[51]

In both the normal and failing myocardium, activation of the adenylate cyclase system can augment contractility. Agents that do this may be divided into two categories. The first comprises the catecholamines (e.g., norepinephrine, epinephrine) and their synthetic derivatives (e.g., dobutamine, isoproterenol), which act via cell-surface adrenergic receptors.[47] The second includes agents that inhibit the breakdown of cyclic AMP by inhibition of PDE type III (e.g., amrinone, milrinone, and enoximone).[52] Other agents, such as

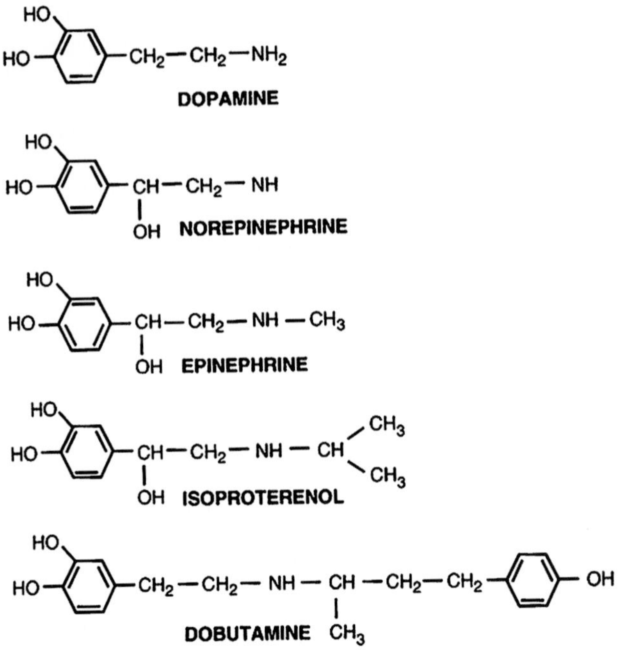

FIGURE 13-3. Structure of catecholamines.

levosimendan, increase myofibrillar sensitivity to calcium and then further augment contraction.[53]

Catecholamines constitute an endogenous hormonal system exerting reflex control of the heart and circulation. Their effects depend on localized controlled neural release and receptor specificity in terms of action.

Dopamine is the naturally occurring precursor of both norepinephrine and epinephrine (Fig. 13-3).[54] While epinephrine is released from the adrenal medulla, norepinephrine is the primary mediator in the heart and peripheral circulation.[47]

The actions of both endogenous and exogenous catecholamines depends on their activation of specific alpha- and beta-adrenergic receptors (Table 13-2).[47] Alpha receptors include alpha$_1$ receptors, which are postsynaptic and are located in vascular smooth muscle and in the myocardium. In smooth muscle, they mediate vasoconstriction; in the heart, they have weak positive inotropic and negative chronotropic effects. Alpha$_2$ receptors are presynaptic; when stimulated, they decrease norepinephrine release from peripheral nerve endings as well as sympathetic outflow from the central nervous system. Alpha receptors may also mediate vasoconstriction in specific peripheral vascular beds.

Beta-adrenergic receptors can be divided into two types: beta$_1$ and beta$_2$. Beta$_1$ receptors are located in the myocardium, where they mediate positive inotropic, chronotropic, and dromotropic effects.[51] They are activated primarily by norepinephrine released from neurons in the heart. Beta$_2$ receptors are located in vascular smooth muscle, where they mediate vasodilatation, and in the sinoatrial node, where they are chronotropic. In general, beta$_2$ receptors are activated by circulating catecholamines released from peripheral sites, such as the adrenal medulla.

Another type of receptor has been termed the *dopaminergic receptor,* which is localized to the mesenteric and renal circulations and mediates arterial vasodilatation (drugs that act on peripheral dopaminergic receptors are discussed in Chap. 26). The physiologic and pharmacologic action of various catecholamines depends on

TABLE 13-2. Adrenergic Receptor Activity of Sympathomimetic Amines

	α_1	β_1	β_2	Dopaminergic	Dose
Dopamine	+++	++	+	++++	<2 μg/kg/min—vasodilation effects on peripheral dopaminergic receptors 2–10 μg/kg/min—inotropic effects, β_1-receptor activation 5–20 μg/kg/min—peripheral vasoconstriction, α effects
Norepinephrine	++++	++++	0	0	Initiate with 8–12 μg/min; maintain 2–4 μg/min
Epinephrine	+++	++++	++	0	
Isoproterenol	0	++++	++++	0	0.5–5 μg/min
Dobutamine	+++	++++	++	0	Start at 2–3 μg/kg/min and titrate upward

which receptor they activate, both in the heart and periphery (Table 13-3).

Norepinephrine has potent alpha$_1$ and beta$_1$ activity. When norepinephrine is released from cardiac nerve endings, as occurs in normal exercise, myocardial contractility and heart rate are augmented. When norepinephrine is administered exogenously, its major action is to stimulate alpha$_1$ receptors, leading to marked peripheral arterial vasoconstriction. Thus, norepinephrine has been used to reverse severe hypotension in order to preserve blood flow to vital organs. Continued administration of norepinephrine may produce ischemic renal damage due to sustained renal vasoconstriction. For the failing heart, this peripheral vasoconstriction also provides an undesirable added pressure load (afterload) and altered oxygen consumption,[55] which tends to vitiate the potential benefits of beta$_1$ stimulation.

Dopamine[54] has alpha$_1$ and beta$_1$ activity but also stimulates dopaminergic receptors in the renal vasculature to produce arterial dilation and increased renal blood flow. Its beta$_1$ effects in the heart occur largely through the release of endogenous norepinephrine, which may be largely depleted in the failing heart. As doses of dopamine are increased, conversion to norepinephrine also occurs, which tends to produce relatively more pressor effects than myocardial inotropic stimulation. Dopamine may also depress minute ventilation in patients with heart failure.[56] As such, the benefits of dopamine administration, if any, are at low doses (e.g., 0.02 mg/kg/min), where they may induce renal arterial vasodilatation in association with administration of other more potent inotropic agents (e.g., dobutamine). Low-dose dopamine can also be used in combination with norepinephrine to blunt norepinephrine-induced renal vasoconstriction.[57]

TABLE 13-3. Physiologic and Pharmacologic Actions of Catecholamine Receptors

Receptor	Receptor Activity	Primary Location
β_1	Positive inotropic and chronotropic action; increased AV conduction	Heart (atria, ventricle AV node)
β_2	Peripheral vasodilation	Arterioles, arteries, veins, bronchioles
α_1	Arteriolar vasoconstriction	Arterioles
α_2	Presynaptic inhibition of norepinephrine release	Sympathetic nerve endings, CNS
Dopaminergic	Renal and mesenteric vasodilation, natriuresis, diuresis	Kidneys

A recent randomized, placebo-controlled study showed that the administration of low-dose dopamine by continuous infusion to critically ill patients provided no significant protection from renal dysfunction.[58]

Dobutamine[59,60] (see Fig. 13-3) is a synthetic variant of the catecholamines whose structure has been altered to optimize hemodynamic response in the dog, characterized by an increase in cardiac output and a decrease in ventricular filling pressure with little change in heart rate. Since arterial pressure also rises modestly, peripheral vascular resistance must of necessity fall. The positive inotropic activity of dobutamine is mediated by direct stimulation of beta$_1$ adrenergic receptors in the myocardium (see Tables 13-2 and 13-3). It is unclear why heart rate does not increase concomitantly. The increased arterial pressure resulting from enhanced cardiac output may increase baroreceptor activity and thereby offset the rise in heart rate induced by beta-adrenergic stimulation. Given the capacity of dobutamine to increase cardiac output and reduce filling pressure without substantial heart rate change, dobutamine has been widely used to treat severe acute LV failure in the absence of profound hypotension, which is poorly responsive to diuretics, natriuretic peptides, and vasodilators, as may be seen following a very large myocardial infarction or in acute decompensation in the course of chronic CHF. In the presence of severe hypotension, the beta$_2$ stimulation of dobutamine may be harmful and administration of an alpha$_1$-stimulating vasoconstrictor such as norepinephrine or a higher dose of dopamine may also be necessary in order to increase arterial peripheral resistance.

Dobutamine infusion is generally begun at 2 μg/kg/min and titrated to optimize cardiac output while reducing LV filling pressure. Tachycardia is carefully avoided so as not to increase ischemia. The effects on myocardial oxygen consumption (MVO$_2$) are complex.[60] Enhanced contractility increases MVO$_2$, while the resulting decrease in LV wall tension tends to reduce it. The net result is most often an increase in MVO$_2$. However, a rise in systolic arterial pressure coupled to a reduction in LV filling pressure may enhance myocardial perfusion in the absence of tachycardia. The major side effects of dobutamine are an excessive increase in heart rate with high rates of infusion and ventricular arrhythmias, both of which may mandate dose reduction and even drug discontinuation.[61] Tachyphylaxis may also occur to a variable degree. In general, once hemodynamic benefits are attained, dobutamine is slowly withdrawn. In some cases this has not been possible and sustained administration becomes necessary, which may require portable pumps for administration.[61a,b] The outcome in this circumstance is generally dire.

In chronic CHF, the patient is commonly maintained on vasodilators such as ACE inhibitors, loop diuretics, and digoxin. Nevertheless, episodes of acute decompensation may intervene, characterized by increased pulmonary congestion and edema as well as reduced renal function with increasing fluid accumulation. Intermittent infusion of dobutamine in conjunction with amiodarone may result in steady clinical benefits in patients with heart failure refractory to standard medical treatment.[62]

PDE INHIBITORS AND OTHER AGENTS

The adenylate cyclase cyclic AMP system can also be activated beyond the beta receptor. Hormones such as glucagon activate the system and can increase myocardial contractility acutely despite beta$_1$ blockade.[63] While useful in overcoming beta-adrenergic blockade if necessary, glucagon may induce gastric atony and nausea, which has limited its more generalized use.

Amrinone and milrinone (Fig. 13-4) are prototypes of a class of cardiotonic agents that activate the adenylate cyclase system through inhibition of the enzyme that breaks down cyclic AMP: PDE III.[64,65] PDE III inhibitors decrease the breakdown of cyclic AMP in the myocardium and increase cyclic guanidine monophosphate (cyclic GMP) in vascular smooth muscle, resulting in an increase in myocardial contractility as well as arterial and venous vasodilatation. Other members of this class of drugs include enoximone. Presently, only amrinone and milrinone have been approved by the U.S. Food and Drug Administration (FDA) for treatment of acute heart failure. The mechanisms by which vasodilation occurs is not completely understood. Increased cyclic AMP induces phosphorylation of myosin light-chain kinase, which decreases sensitivity to calcium and calmodulin.[66] In the heart, inotropism may relate not only to increased cyclic AMP–mediated calcium availability for contraction and increased rates of its removal for relaxation but also to increased sensitivity of the contractile system for calcium.[67] Both amrinone and milrinone,[65] which are available as intravenous agents, have substantial ability to augment cardiac output while reducing both right and LV filling pressures. The lowering of filling pressures is greater than that seen with dobutamine. Dilatation of the pulmonary vasculature is also a very useful therapeutic effect. Arterial pressure tends to be reduced while an increase in heart rate may occur. Since dobutamine increases cyclic AMP and milrinone reduces its breakdown, the combination of these agents is substantially more potent than either agent alone.[65] When either dobutamine or milrinone is utilized, ectopic activity may be increased, which requires careful supervision in their use.

PDE III inhibitors are also orally active and produce the same hemodynamic improvement as seen with intravenous use. However, in longer-term oral use, increased mortality was seen with the use

FIGURE 13-4. Structures of milrinone and amrinone.

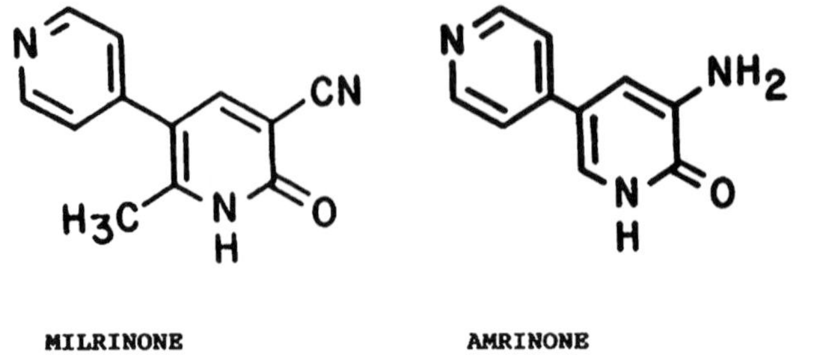

MILRINONE   **AMRINONE**

of milrinone, especially in the presence of class IV heart failure.[68] This increased mortality may have been due to the relatively short duration of action of this agent ($1\frac{1}{2}$ h half-life) which leads to large peaks and valleys in dosing and concomitant arrhythmias. For the time being, this has vitiated clinical study of these agents, but more stringent control of the use of this class of agents as adjuncts to other agents may ultimately increase their value.

Milrinone

Intravenous milrinone therapy is commonly initiated with a bolus of 50 μg/kg, immediately followed by a continuous infusion at a rate of 0.375 to 0.75 μg/kg/min. Initiation of milrinone therapy with a loading bolus has the advantage of producing immediate hemodynamic improvement. However, the loading bolus may precipitate ventricular arrhythmias and/or systemic hypotension. In clinical conditions that do not require immediate improvement of LV performance, as in patients with decompensated CHF, initiating milrinone therapy without a bolus is preferable to avoid the risk of precipitating ventricular arrhythmias or hypotension. Whether or not a bolus is administered, IV milrinone produces identical hemodynamic improvement 2 h after initiation of therapy.[69] The IV bolus of milrinone is particularly useful to evaluate the reversibility of pulmonary hypertension in patients with severe CHF who are being screened for cardiac transplantation. The rapid onset of the direct relaxant effect of milrinone on the pulmonary vasculature is well suited to test pulmonary vascular reactivity.[70] Milrinone decreases pulmonary vascular resistance by increasing cardiac output. In contrast to nitroprusside and nitric oxide, which also decrease pulmonary vascular resistance, milrinone does not affect the transpulmonary pressure gradient. The milrinone-induced increase in cardiac output presumably lowers pulmonary vascular resistance by recruiting accessory vessels in the pulmonary circulation as well as flow-mediated pulmonary vasodilatation.

Besides its positive inotropic action, milrinone substantially increases Ca^{2+} ATPase activity in the sarcoplasmic reticulum (SR) and thereby LV relaxation in the canine pacing model of heart failure.[71] Increased SR Ca^{2+} ATPase activity is due to a selective inhibition by milrinone of SR membrane-bound PDE III. Increased SR Ca^{2+} ATPase activity mediates the well-documented lusitropic action of milronone.[72] Of note, while the positive inotropic action of milrinone is limited by reduced cAMP and PDE levels in the failing cardiac myocyte, the lusitropic effect is completely preserved due to a compartmentalized modulation of cyclic AMP in the failing heart.[72]

The clinical effects of intermittent or long-term administration of milrinone in patients with severe CHF are controversial.[73–75] Uncontrolled reports have suggested its usefulness in reducing the use of mechanical LV device in patients awaiting cardiac transplantation.[76–79] A recent controlled trial of intermittent administration of milrinone failed to document any clinical benefits.[79a] It is clear that not every patient with severe CHF is improved by long-term administration of milrinone. However, most heart failure/cardiac transplantation specialists have seen few patients who undoubtedly improved while receiving long-term milrinone therapy. Attempts have also been made to use milrinone to increase the tolerability of beta-blocker initiation by counteracting the myocardial depressant action of catecholamine withdrawal. Thus, this mode of therapy should be tailored to the individual response of patients and initiated only when other FDA-approved therapeutic modalities at the appropriate dosages have failed.

Positive Inotropic Agents under Investigation

Enoximone is an imidazolone derivative that selectively inhibits the SR-associated typeof III PDE. Thus, the mechanisms of action of enoximone are similar to those of milrinone. However, the relative dose responses of the inotropic and vasodilating actions of enoximone and milrinone differ. At low doses, enoximone exhibits a more balanced inotropic and vasodilator effect than does milrinone.[80] The therapeutic efficacy of enoximone at lower doses than those initially investigated is currently under evaluation in three randomized, placebo-controlled trials in Europe and the United States. In particular, the use of low-level inotropic stimulation with enoximone to facilitate initiation of beta-adrenergic blockade in patients with tenuous CHF is under investigation (ESSENTIAL study).[81]

Other type III PDE inhibitors that have been under investigation include toborinone and olprinone.[82,83]

Levosimendan has both positive inotropic and vasodilator properties, and improves LV performance in patients with decompensated heart failure.[84] It increases myocardial contractility via calcium sensitization through a calcium-dependent interaction with troponin C.[85,86] The calcium dependency of levosimendan prevents impairment of myofilament relaxation observed with calcium sensitizers that are calcium-independent. The vasodilator action of levosimendan is attributed to opening of the ATP-sensitive potassium channels. In addition, levosimendan blocks the release of endothelin. While levosimendan is a potent and highly selective inhibitor of PDE III, this action does not contribute, at least at low doses, to its inotropic and vasodilator properties. In contrast to specific type III PDE inhibitors, such as milrinone or enoximone, the positive inotropic effect of levosimendan in cardiac tissue is not attenuated by disease.

In plasma, over 95% of levosimendan is bound to plasma proteins. Approximately one-third of an IV bolus of levosimendan is excreted via the urine over 24 h and one-third is excreted in feces over 72 h. Levosimendan has two active metabolites, OR-1855 and OR-1896, that have inotropic, chronotropic, and vasodilator properties and a long duration of action. These metabolites are likely to prolong the hemodynamic effects of levosimendan after disappearance of the parent drug.

To date, several clinical trials have been conducted in central Europe and Russia with levosimendan.[87–89] Preliminary findings from these trials and pilot studies in the United States[84,90,91] that involved patients with acute and chronic heart failure appear promising. In a recent randomized study, it was shown that in patients with severe low-output failure, levosimendan improved hemodynamic performance more effectively than dobutamine and was associated with a lower mortality rate. Another rare study (REVIVE) is now in progress.

A similar agent, pimobendan, has also been evaluated in clinical trials, and it was observed that the drug inhibited the production of proinflammatory cytokines in a murine model of myocarditis.[92]

Other calcium sensitizing drugs are in development.[93]

Clinical Use

The clinical development of vesnarinone has been brought to a halt. Vesnarinone is a noncatecholamine, nonglycosidic, orally active 2(IH) quinalone derivative that has a unique and complex mechanism of action.[94] It is a mild inhibitor of type III PDE, thereby leading to increased intracellular potassium, and also affects numerous myocardial ion channels, resulting in the prolongation of the opening time of sodium channels and a decrease in the delayed outward and inward rectifying potassium current (see Fig. 13-1). In vitro, it also has demonstrated significant effects on cytokine production which may theoretically account for some of its observed clinical benefits.[95] Indeed, hemodynamic studies of vesnarinone in humans with CHF show very little effect on ventricular function.[94] Nevertheless, placebo-controlled studies in patients with heart failure have suggested a benefit in morbidity and mortality with a 60-mg dose.[96,97] However, there is increased mortality with vesnarione at the 120-mg daily dose, suggesting a narrow therapeutic window for the drug.[97] Its predominant toxic side effect is a 2% incidence of reversible neutropenia.[98,99] Subsequently, a placebo-controlled, randomized trial of 30 and 60 mg of vesnarinone was stopped due to increased mortality with the drug.[100]

Sodium-channel modulators (BDF 9198) are under investigation for heart failure. The sensitivity of the failing human myocardium to sodium-channel modulators is increased when compared with nonfailing myocardium, suggesting an alteration in sodium homeostasis in human heart failure.[101]

NEW APPROACHES TO ENHANCE MYOCARDIAL CONTRACTILITY

Besides the novel positive inotropic agents that are currently under investigation, interventions based on gene therapy are now proposed to increase myocardial contractility (see also Chap. 41).[102] Overexpression of SR Ca^{2+} ATPase (SERCA2a) in ventricular myocytes of patients with end-stage heart failure results in faster contraction velocity and enhanced relaxation velocity.[103,104] Diastolic Ca^{2+} decreases in failing cardiomyocytes overexpressing SERCA2a. Overexpression of SERCA2a also normalizes the frequency response of failing myocytes with increasing contraction at increasing frequencies.[103] Using an intracoronary approach to overexpress beta-adrenergic receptors (β-AR) in the myocardium results in a substantial increase in LV performance 1 week after delivery of the β-AR gene.[105] Similarly, adenoviral gene transfer of the vasopressin 2 receptor (V2R) into the myocardium increases contractility in vivo.[106] Although the above-mentioned findings are promising, gene transfer therapy with the aim of enhancing myocardial contractility in patients with CHF will require long-term validation in animals before such an approach can be considered in humans.[107]

CONCLUSION

Inotropic agents still play a role in the management of patients with acutely decompensated CHF that is refractory to optimal standard therapy. Their hemodynamic effects are compared with other classes of drugs used to treat acute CHF in Table 13-4. Dobutamine and milrinone can be used in combination with vasodilator drugs and diuretics to maximize hemodynamic benefit. There is now conclusive evidence that when used properly, digoxin is both safe and effective when added to diuretics and ACE inhibitors.

TABLE 13-4. Relative Hemodynamic Effects of Agents in Heart Failure

	Ventricular Filling Pressure	Peripheral Vascular Resistance	Cardiac Output	BP	Ejection Fraction
Inotropic agents					
Digoxin	↓	↓	↑	—	↑
Dobutamine	↓/NC	↓↓	↑↑	↑	↑↑
Norepinephrine	↓/NC	↑↑	↑/NC	↑↑	↑/NC
Dopamine	↓/NC	↑	↑	↑	↑/NC
Inodilators					
Milrinone	↓↓	↓↓	↑↑	↓	↑
Diuretics	↓↓	↑/NC	↓/NC	↓/NC	—
Vasodilators					
NTG—oral	↓↓	↓↓	—	↓/NC	—
IV	↓↓↓	↓↓↓	—	↓/NC	—
Nitroprusside	↓↓	↓↓↓	↑	↓	—
Hydralazine	↓/NC	↓↓	↑	↓/NC	—
ACE inhibitors	↓↓	↓↓	↑/NC	↓	—
β blockers	↓	↓/NC	↑/NC	NC/↓	↑

↑ = increase; ↓ = decrease; ACE = angiotensin converting enzyme; NC = no change; NTG = nitroglycerin.

REFERENCES

1. Warner Stevenson L: Inotropic therapy for heart failure. *N Engl J Med* 339:1848, 1998.
1a. A report of the American College of Cardiology/American Heart Association Task Force on Practice Guidelines (Committee to Revise the 1995 Guidelines for the Evaluation and Management of Heart Failure: ACC/AHA Guidelines for the evaluation and management of chronic heart failure in the adult: Executive summary). *J Am Coll Cardiol* 38:2101, 2001.
2. LeJemtel TH, Sonnenblick EH, Frishman WH: Diagnosis and management of heart failure. In: Fuster V, Alexander RW, O'Rourke RA, eds. *Hurst's The Heart,* 10th ed. New York: McGraw-Hill, 2000:687.
3. Ferguson DW: Digitalis and neurohormonal abnormalities in heart failure and implications for therapy. *Am J Cardiol* 69:24G, 1992.
4. Felker GM, O'Connor CM: Inotropic therapy for heart failure: An evidence-based approach. *Am Heart J* 142:393, 2001.
5. Burger AJ, Elkayam U, Neibaur MT, et al: Comparison of the occurrence of ventricular arrhythmias in patients with acutely decompensated congestive heart failure receiving dobutamine versus nesiritide therapy. *Am J Cardiol* 88:35, 2001.
6. Patel MB, Kaplan IV, Patni RN, et al: Sustained improvement in flow mediated vasodilation after short-term administration of dobutamine in patients with severe congestive heart failure. *Circulation* 99:60, 1999.
7. Drazner MH, Solomon MA, Thompson B, Yancy CW: Tailored therapy using dobutamine and nitroglycerin in advanced heart failure. *Am J Cardiol* 84:941, 1999.
8. Withering W: *An Account of the Foxglove, And Some of Its Medical Uses: With Practical Remarks on Dropsy and other Diseases.* London: GGJ and J Robinson, 1785.
9. Fothergill JM: *Digitalis: Its Mode of Action.* London, 1871.
10. Dock W, Tainter ML: The circulatory changes after full therapeutic doses of digitalis, with critical discussion of views on cardiac output. *J Clin Invest* 8:467, 1929.
11. Fisch C: William Withering: An account of the foxglove and some of its medical uses, 1785–1985. *J Am Coll Cardiol* 5:1A, 1985.
12. Gillis RA, Quest JA: The role of the nervous system in the cardiovascular effects of digitalis. *Pharmacol Rev* 31:19, 1980.
13. Rahimtoola SH, Tak T: The use of digitalis in heart failure. *Curr Probl Cardiol* 21:785, 1996.
14. Fozzard HA, Sheets MF: Cellular mechanism of action of cardiac glycosides. *J Am Coll Cardiol* 5:10A, 1985.
15. Charlemagne D: Molecular and cellular level of action of digitalis. *Herz* 18:79, 1993.
16. Scholz H: Inotropic drugs and their mechanisms of action. *J Am Coll Cardiol* 4:389, 1984.
17. Siri FM, Krueger JW, Nordin C, et al: Depressed intracellular calcium transients and contraction in myocytes from hypertrophied and failing guinea pig hearts. *Am J Physiol* 261:H514, 1991.
18. Li P, Park C, Micheletti R, Li B, et al: Myocyte performance during evolution of myocardial infarction in rats: Effects of propionyl-L-carnitine. *Am J Physiol* 268:H1702, 1995.
19. Rosen MR: Cellular electrophysiology of digitalis toxicity. *J Am Coll Cardiol* 5:22A, 1985.
20. Smith TW, Antman EM, Friedman PL, et al: Digitalis glycosides: Mechanisms and manifestations of toxicity. Parts I, II, III. *Prog Cardiovasc Dis* 26:413, 495; 27:21, 1984.
21. Wantanabe AM: Digitalis and the autonomic nervous system. *J Am Coll Cardiol* 5:35A, 1985.
22. Newton GE, Tong JH, Schofield AM, et al: Digoxin reduces cardiac sympathetic activity in severe congestive heart failure. *J Am Coll Cardiol* 28:155, 1996.
23. Wenger T, Butler VP Jr., Haber E, Smith TW: Digoxin-specific antibody treatment of digitalis toxicity. In: Erdmann E, Greeff K, Skou JC, eds. *Update in Cardiac Glycosides 1785–1985.* New York: Springer-Verlag, 1986:377–388.
24. Braunwald E, Ross J Jr, Sonnenblick EH: *Mechanisms of Contraction of the Normal and Failing Heart,* 2nd ed. Boston: Little, Brown, 1976.
25. Mason DT, Braunwald E, Karsh RB, Bullock FA: Studies on digitalis. X: Effects of ouabain on forearm vascular resistance and venous tone in normal subjects and in patients with heart failure. *J Clin Invest* 43:532, 1964.
26. Eberhardt RT, Frishman WH, Landau A, et al: Increased mortality incidence in elderly individuals receiving digoxin therapy: Results of the Bronx Longitudinal Aging Study. *Cardiol Elderly* 3:177, 1995.
27. Packer M, Gheorghiade M, Young JB, et al: Withdrawal of digoxin from patients with chronic heart failure treated with angiotensin-converting-enzyme inhibitors. RADIANCE Study. *N Engl J Med* 329:1, 1993.
28. Uretsky BF, Young JB, Shahidi FE, et al: Randomized study assessing the effect of digoxin withdrawal in patients with mild to moderate chronic congestive heart failure: Results of the PROVED Trial. *J Am Coll Cardiol* 22:955, 1995.
29. Adams KF Jr, Gheorghiade M, Uretsky BF, et al: Clinical predictors of worsening heart failure during withdrawal from digoxin therapy. *Am Heart J* 135:389–397, 1998.
30. Captopril-Digoxin Multicenter Research Group: Comparative effects of therapy with captopril and digoxin in patients with mild to moderate heart failure. *JAMA* 259:539, 1988.
31. Tauke J, Goldstein S, Gheorghiade M: Digoxin for chronic heart failure: A review of the randomized controlled trials with special attention to the PROVED and RADIANCE Trials. *Prog Cardiovasc Dis* 37:49, 1994.

32. Kraus F, Rudolph C, Rudolph W: Efficacy of digitalis in patients with chronic congestive heart failure and sinus rhythm: An overview of randomized, double-blind, placebo-controlled studies. *Herz* 18:95, 1993.

33. The Digitalis Investigation Group: The effect of digoxin on mortality and morbidity in patients with heart failure. *N Engl J Med* 336:525, 1997.

34. Wirth KE: Relevant metabolism of cardiac glycosides. In: Erdmann E, Greeff K, Skou JC, eds. *Update in Cardiac Glycosides, 1785–1985.* New York: Springer-Verlag, 1986:257–262.

34a. Adams KF Jr., Gheorghiade M, Uretsky BF, et al: Clinical benefits of low serum digoxin concentrations in heart failure. *J Am Coll Cardiol* 39:946, 2002.

34b. van Veldhuisen DJ: Low-dose digoxin in patients with heart failure: Less toxic and at least as effective? *J Am Coll Cardiol* 39:954, 2002.

35. Marcus FI: Pharmacokinetic interactions between digoxin and other drugs. *J Am Coll Cardiol* 5:82A, 1985.

36. Sonnenblick EH, LeJemtel TH: Heart failure: Its progression and its therapy. *Hosp Pract* 28:121, 1993.

36a. Hauptman PJ, Kelly RA: Digitalis. *Circulation* 99:1265, 1999.

37. Muller JE, Turi ZG, Stone PH, et al for the MILIS Group: Digoxin therapy and mortality following confirmed or suspected myocardial infarction: experience in the MILIS Study. In: Erdmann E, Greeff JC, Skou JC, eds. *Update in Cardiac Glycosides 1785–1985.* New York: Springer-Verlag, 1986:493.

38. Spargias KS, Hall AS, Ball SG: Safety concerns about digoxin after acute myocardial infarction. *Lancet* 354:391, 1999.

39. Lewis RP: Clinical use of serum digoxin concentrations. *Am J Cardiol* 69:97G, 1992.

39a. Steimer W, Muller C, Eber B: Digoxin assays: Frequent, substantial and potentially dangerous interference by spironoactone, canrenone, and other steroids. *Clin Chem* 48:507, 2002.

40. Kelley RA, Smith TW: Recognition and treatment of digitalis toxicity. *Am J Cardiol* 69:108G, 1992.

41. Marcus FI: Digitalis. In: Schlant RC, Alexander RW, eds. *Hurst's The Heart,* 8th ed. New York: McGraw-Hill, 1994:573–588.

42. Williamson KM, Thrasher KA, Fulton KB, et al: Digoxin toxicity. An evaluation in current clinical practice. *Arch Intern Med* 158:2444, 1998.

43. Cardiac glycosides interact with many drugs. *Drugs Ther Perspect* 6(3):11, 1995.

44. Eddleston M, Rajapakse S, Rajakanthan SJ, et al: Anti-digoxin Fab fragments in cardiotoxicity induced by ingestion of yellow oleander: A randomised controlled trial. *Lancet* 355:767, 2000.

45. Marik PE, Fromm L: A case series of hospitalized patients with elevated digoxin levels. *Am J Med* 105:110, 1998.

46. Benovic JL, Bouvier M, Caron MG, Lefkowitz RJ: Regulation of adenyl cyclase-coupled β-adrenergic receptors. *Am Rev Cell Biol* 4:405, 1988.

47. Hoffman BB, Taylor P: Neurotransmission. In: Hardman JG, Limbird LE, eds. *Goodman & Gilman's The Pharmacological Basis of Therapeutics,* 10th ed. New York: McGraw-Hill, 2001:115–153.

48. Kelly RB: Storage and release of neurotransmitters. *Cell/Neuron* 72(Suppl. 72):443, 1993.

49. Spann JF, Sonnenblick EH, Cooper T, et al: Cardiac norepinephrine stores and the contractile state of the heart. *Circ Res* 19:317, 1966.

50. Francis GS, Goldsmith SR, Levine TB, et al: The neurohumoral axis in congestive heart failure. *Ann Intern Med* 101:370, 1984.

51. Insel PA: Adrenergic receptors—evolving concepts and clinical implications. *N Engl J Med* 334:580, 1996.

52. Movsesian MA: Beta-adrenergic receptor agonists and cyclic nucleotide phosphodiesterase inhibitors: Shifting the focus from inotropy to cyclic adenosine monophosphate *J Am Coll Cardiol* 34:318–324, 1999.

53. Pagel PS, Haikala H, Pentikainen PJ, et al: Pharmacology of levosimendan: A new myofilament calcium sensitizer. *Cardiovasc Drugs Rev* 14:286, 1996.

54. Goldberg LI, Rajfer SI: Dopamine receptors: Applications in clinical cardiology. *Circulation* 72:245, 1985.

55. Leclerc KM, Steele NP, Levy WC: Norepinephrine alters exercise oxygen consumption in heart failure patients. *Med Sci Sports Exerc* 32:2029, 2000.

56. van de Borne P, Oren R, Somers VK: Dopamine depresses minute ventilation in patients with heart failure. *Circulation* 98:126, 1998.

57. Hoogenberg K, Smit AJ, Girbes ARJ: Effects of low-dose dopamine on renal and systemic hemodynamics during incremental norepinephrine infusion in healthy volunteers. *Crit Care Med* 26:260, 1998.

58. Australian and New Zealand Intensive Care Society (ANZICS) Clinical Trials Group: Low-dose dopamine in patients with early renal dysfunction: A placebo-controlled randomised trial. *Lancet* 356:2139, 2000.

59. Ruffolo RR Jr.: Review: The pharmacology of dobutamine. *Am J Med Sci* 294:244, 1987.

60. Sonnenblick EH, Frishman WH, LeJemtel TH: Dobutamine: A new synthetic cardioactive sympathetic amine. *N Engl J Med* 300:17, 1979.

61. Tisdale JE, Patel R, Webb CR, et al: Electrophysiologic and proarrhythmic effects of intravenous inotropic agents. *Progr Cardiovasc Dis* 38:167, 1995.

61a. Oliva F, Latini R, Politi A, et al for the DICE (Dobutamina nell'Insufficienza Cardiaca Estrema) Investigators: Intermittent 6-month low-dose dobutamine infusion in severe heart failure: DICE Multicenter Trial. *Am Heart J* 138:247, 1999.

61b. Silver MA: Intermittent inotropes for advanced heart failure: Inquiring minds want to know. *Am Heart J* 138:191, 1999.

62. Nanas JN, Kontoyannis DA, Alexopoulos GP, et al: Long-term intermittent dobutamine infusion combined with oral amiodarone improves the survival of patients with severe congestive heart failure. *Chest* 119:1173, 2001.

63. Parmley WW, Sonnenblick EH: A role for glucagon in cardiac therapy. *Am J Med Sci* 258:224, 1969.

64. Braunwald E, Sonnenblick EH, Chakrin LW, Schwarz RP Jr., eds. *Milrinone Investigation: A New Inotropic Therapy for Congestive Heart Failure.* New York: Raven Press, 1984.

65. Grose R, Strain J, Greenberg M, LeJemtel TH: Systemic and coronary effects of intravenous milrinone and dobutamine in congestive heart failure. *J Am Coll Cardiol* 7:1107, 1986.

66. Harris AL, Silver PJ, Lemp BM, Evans DB: The vasorelaxant effects of milrinone and other vasodilators are attenuated by ouabain. *Eur J Pharmacol* 145:133–139, 1988.

67. Nielsen-Kudsk JE, Aldershvile J: Will calcium sensitizers play a role in the treatment of heart failure? *J Cardiovasc Pharmacol* 26 (Suppl 1):577, 1995.

68. Packer M, Carver JR, Rodeheffer RJ, et al: Effect of oral milrinone on mortality in severe chronic heart failure. *N Engl J Med* 325:1468, 1991.

69. Baruch L, Patacsil P, Hameed A, et al: Pharmacodynamic effects of milrinone with and without a bolus loading infusion. *Am Heart J* e6:141, 2000.

70. Givertz MM, Hare JM, Loh E, et al: Effect of bolus milrinone on hemodynamic variables and pulmonary vascular resistance in patients with severe left ventricular dysfunction: A rapid test for reversibility of pulmonary hypertension. *J Am Coll Cardiol* 28:1775, 1996.

71. Yano M, Kohno M, Ohkusa T, et al: Effect of milrinone on left ventricular relaxation and Ca^{2+} uptake function of cardiac sarcoplasmic reticulum. *Am J Physiol* 279:H1898, 2000.

72. Tanigawa T, Yano M, Kohno M, et al: Mechanism of preserved positive lusitropy by cAMP-dependent drugs in heart failure. *Am J Physiol* 278:H313, 2000.

73. Hatzizacharias A, Makris T, Krespi P, et al: Intermittent milrinone effect on long-term hemodynamic profile in patients with severe congestive heart failure. *Am Heart J* 138:241, 1999.

74. Milfred-LaForest SK, Shubert J, Mendoza B, et al: Tolerability of extended duration intravenous milrinone in patients hospitalized for advanced heart failure and the usefulness of uptitration of oral angiotensin-converting enzyme inhibitors. *Am J Cardiol* 84:894, 1999.

75. Ewy GA: Inotropic infusions for chronic congestive heart failure. Medical miracles or misguided medicinals? *J Am Coll Cardiol* 33:572, 1999.

76. Cesario D, Clark J, Maisel A: Beneficial effects of intermittent home administration of the inotrope/vasodilator milrinone in patients with end-stage congestive heart failure: A preliminary study. *Am Heart J* 135:121, 1998.

77. Mehra MR, Ventura HO, Kapoor C, et al: Safety and clinical utility of long-term intravenous milrinone in advanced heart failure. *Am J Cardiol* 80:61, 1997.

78. Canver CC, Chanda J: Milrinone for long-term pharmacologic support of the status of heart transplant candidates. *Ann Thorac Surg* 69:1823, 2000.

79. Cusick DA, Pfeifer PB, Quigg RJ: Effects of intravenous milrinone followed by titration of high-dose oral vasodilator therapy on clinical outcome and rehospitalization rates in patients with severe heart failure. *Am J Cardiol* 82:1060, 1998.

79a. Cuffe MS, Califf RM, Adams KF Jr. et al: Short-term intravenous milrinone for acute exacerbation of chronic heart failure. A randomized, controlled trial. *JAMA* 287:1541, 2002.

80. Lowes BD, Higginbotham M, Petrovich L, et al: Low-dose enoximone improves exercise capacity in chronic heart failure. *J Am Coll Cardiol* 36:501, 2000.

81. Shakar SF, Bristow MR: Low-level inotropic stimulation with type III phosphodiesterase inhibitors in patients with advanced symptomatic chronic heart failure receiving β-blocking agents. *Curr Cardiol Rep* 3:224, 2001.

82. Sugiyama A, Satoh Y, Hashimoto K: Electropharmacologic effects of a new phosphodiesterase III inhibitor, toborinone (OPC-18790), assessed in an in vivo canine model. *J Cardiovasc Pharmacol* 38:268, 2001.

83. Yu Y, Mizushige K, Ueda T, et al: Effect of olprinone, phosphodiesterase III inhibitor, on cerebral blood flow assessed with technetium-99m-ECD SPECT. *J Cardiovasc Pharmacol* 35:422, 2000.

84. Slawsky MT, Colucci WS, Gottlieb SS, et al: Acute hemodynamic and clinical effects of levosimendan in patients with severe heart failure. *Circulation* 102:2222, 2001.

85. Lehtonen L: Levosimendan: A promising agent for the treatment of hospitalized patients with decompensated heart failure. *Curr Cardiol Rep* 2:233, 2000.

86. Figgitt DP, Gillies PS, Goa KL: Levosimendan. *Drugs* 61:613, 2001.

87. Folláth F, Hinkka S, Jäger D, et al: Dose-ranging and safety with intravenous levosimendan in low-output heart failure: Experience in three pilot studies and outline of the levosimendan infusion versus dobutamine (LIDO) trial. *Am J Cardiol* 83:21I, 1999.

88. Ukkonen H, Saraste M, Akkila J, et al: Myocardial efficiency during levosimendan infusion in congestive heart failure. *Clin Pharmacol Ther* 68:522, 2000.

89. Harjola V-P, Peuhkurinen K, Nieminen MS, et al: Oral levosimendan improves cardiac function and hemodynamics in patients with severe congestive heart failure. *Am J Cardiol* 83:4I, 1999.

90. Nijhawan N, Nicolosi AC, Montgomery MW, et al: Levosimendan enhances cardiac performance after cardiopulmonary bypass: A prospective, randomized placebo-controlled trial. *J Cardiovasc Pharmacol* 34:219, 1999.

91. Hosenpud JD, for the Oral Levosimendan Study Group: Levosimendan, a novel myofilament calcium sensitizer, allows weaning of parenteral inotropic therapy in patients with severe congestive heart failure. *Am J Cardiol* 83:9I, 1999.

91a. Follath F, Cleland JGF, Just H, et al: Efficacy and safety of intravenous levosimendan compared with dobutamine in severe low-output heart failure (the LIDO study): A randomised double-blind study. *Lancet* 360:196, 2002.

92. Iwasaki A, Matsumori A, Yamada T, et al: Pimobendan inhibits the production of proinflammatory cytokines and gene expression of inducible nitric oxide synthase in a murine model of viral myocarditis. *J Am Coll Cardiol* 33:1400, 1999.

93. Dorigo P, Floreani M, Santostasi G, et al: Pharmacological characterization of a new Ca^{2+} sensitizer. *J Pharmacol Exp Ther* 295:994, 2000.

94. Cavusoglu E, Frishman WH, Klapholz M: Vesnarinone: A new inotropic agent for treating congestive heart failure. *J Card Fail* 1:249, 1995.

95. Matsumori A, Shioi T, Yamada T, et al: Vesnarinone, a new inotropic agent, inhibits cytokine production by stimulated human blood from patients with heart failure. *Circulation* 89:955, 1994.

96. OPC 8212 Multicenter Research Group: A placebo-controlled, randomized, double-blind study of OPC 8212 in patients with mild chronic heart failure. *Cardiovasc Drugs Ther* 4:419, 1990.

97. Feldman AM, Bristow MR, Parmley WW, et al for the Vesnarinone Study Group: Effects of vesnarinone on morbidity and mortality in patients with heart failure. *N Engl J Med* 329:149, 1993.

98. Bertolet BD, White BG, Pepine CJ: Neutropenia occurring during treatment with vesnarinone. *Am J Cardiol* 74:968, 1994.

99. Furusawa S, Ohashi Y, Asanoi H: Vesnarinone-induced granulocytopenia: Incidence in Japan and recommendations for safety. *J Clin Pharmacol* 36:477, 1996.

100. Cohn JN, Goldstein SO, Greenberg BH et al: A dose-dependent increase in mortality with vesnarinone among patients with severe heart failure. *N Engl J Med* 339:1810, 1998.

101. Müller-Ehmsen J, Brixius K, Schwinger RHG: Positive inotropic effects of a novel Na+-channel modulator BDF 9198 in human non-failing and failing myocardium. *J Cardiovasc Pharmacol* 31:684, 1998.

102. McMurray J, Pfeffer MA: New therapeutic options in congestive heart failure, Part II. *Circulation* 105:2223, 2002.

103. del Monte F, Harding SE, Schmidt U, et al: Restoration of contractile function in isolated cardiomyocytes from failing human hearts by gene transfer of SERCA2a. *Circulation* 100:2308, 1999.

104. del Monte F, Williams E, Lebeche D, et al: Improvement in survival and cardiac metabolism after gene transfer of sarcoplasmic reticulum Ca^{2+}-ATPase in a rat model of heart failure. *Circulation* 104:1424, 2001.

105. Maurice JP, Hata JA, Shah AS, et al: Enhancement of cardiac function after adenoviral-mediated in vivo intracoronary $β_2$-adrenergic receptor gene delivery. *J Clin Invest* 104:21, 1999.

106. Weig H-J, Laugwitz K-L, Moretti A, et al: Enhanced cardiac contractility after gene transfer of V2 vasopressin receptors in vivo by ultrasound-guided injection or transcoronary delivery. *Circulation* 101:1578, 2000.

107. Marbán E: Gene therapy for common acquired diseases of the heart. The Sirens' song (editorial). *Circulation* 101:1498, 2000.

CHAPTER 14

The Organic Nitrates and Nitroprusside

Jonathan Abrams

William H. Frishman

The organic nitrates and sodium nitroprusside (NP) make up a class of drugs known as the nitrovasodilators. The common denominator of these agents is the production of nitric oxide (NO) within vascular smooth muscle cells and platelets[1-4] (Fig. 14-1). Nitric oxide activates the enzyme guanylate or guanylyl cyclase, which in turn results in an accumulation of intracellular cyclic guanosine $3'$ $5'$ monophosphate or cGMP. Cyclic GMP in turn activates a cGMP-dependent protein kinase, which has been shown to mediate vasorelaxation via phosphorylation of proteins that regulate intracellular Ca^{2+} levels. Smooth muscle–cell relaxation is induced by cGMP through fluxes in intracellular calcium. In the platelet, increases in cGMP exert an antiaggregatory action and thus decreased platelet activation, resulting in less thrombosis.[5,6] The predominant actions of the nitrovasodilators are the hemodynamic perturbations resulting from vascular dilatation. In contrast to the majority of vasodilating agents available to the clinician, the nitrates and NP relax the venous capacitance bed as well as arteries and arterioles. The role of the antiplatelet and antithrombotic actions of these compounds remains somewhat controversial, although much recent evidence supports a true benefit for nitrate-induced decreases in platelet-thrombus activation.[5-8]

Nitroglycerin (NTG) has been utilized in medicine for well over 100 years. This drug, initially employed for anginal chest pain, became a mainstay of the homeopathic tradition in the early part of the twentieth century.[9] For the past three decades or more, NTG and the organic nitrates have been widely used for the acute and chronic therapy of ischemic chest pain. More recently, these compounds have been employed in patients with acute and post-myocardial infarction (MI) and, importantly, as adjunctive therapy in congestive heart failure. NP, available only as an intravenous agent, is effective in the treatment of severe or acute hypertension, acute or chronic congestive heart failure, and pulmonary edema. As a general rule, NP is not used to alleviate myocardial ischemia.

Attenuation of nitrate effects, or nitrate tolerance, is the major obstacle to successful utilization of these drugs in clinical practice. There does not appear to be a significant degree of tolerance to the actions of NP, however. In recent years, a wide variety of nitrate formulations and compounds has become available (Table 14-1), whereas some older nitrate compounds (e.g., pentaerythritol tetranitrate) are no longer in use.

THE ORGANIC NITRATES

Mechanisms of Action

Cellular

NTG, isosorbide dinitrate (ISDN), and 5-isosorbide mononitrate (ISMN) are metabolized by vascular tissue at or near the plasma membrane of smooth muscle cells of veins and arteries (see Fig. 14-1). It was previously believed that nitrates underwent a stepwise dinitration process that resulted in S-nitrosothiol (SNO) via the production of nitrite ion (NO_2^-). However, it now appears that these compounds may form NO directly through an enzymatic process that does not necessarily involve nitrite production as an intermediary.[10] Furthermore, the obligatory role of SNOs remains controversial (see Fig. 14-1). Nitrates can be converted to SNO but are dominantly a direct precursor of SNO. Both NO and SNO can activate guanylate or guanylyl cyclase, leading to the production of cGMP, a second messenger that relaxes vascular smooth muscle cells.[1-4]

The enzymatic conversion of the nitrovasodilators is not homogenous; NP and SNO appear to require different enzymes or "receptors," which presumably accounts for some of the differences in the hemodynamic spectrum among these agents and could also relate to the different susceptibility to tolerance among the organic nitrates, NP or SNO. Intracellular chemical processes also result in NO formation in a nonenzymatic manner; this is much less important for the organic nitrates than for NP. In the platelet, increases in cGMP have been correlated with the degree of vasodilation in the coronary arteries.[11] Presumably, nitrate platelet activation is modulated via cGMP-induced processes.

Nitrate Tolerance

Whereas the precise mechanisms of tolerance remain the subject of intense investigation,[11a] it is now known that NO production and cGMP responses become attenuated in the setting of nitrate tolerance.[11b] Furthermore, the obligatory role of thiols during nitrate activation remains controversial as regards tolerance phenomena. Although it now seems clear that intracellular glutathione or cysteine stores remain adequate, and thiol deficiency per se is not a factor in tolerance development,[12] thiol or –SH groups are critical to SNO and thionitrate formation. Furthermore, a thiol moi-

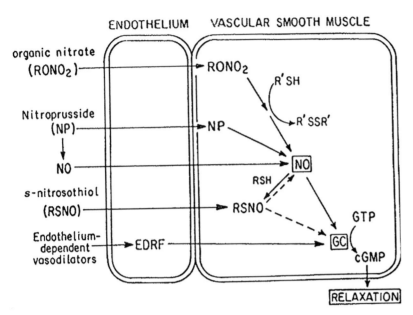

FIGURE 14-1. Nitrovasodilators, endothelium-dependent vasodilators, and vascular smooth muscle relaxation. *Abbreviations:* NO = nitric oxide; EDRF = endothelium-derived relaxing factor; R9SH and RSH = two distinct pools of intracellular sulfhydryl groups; R9SSR9 = disulfide groups; GC = guanylate cyclase. (*Reproduced with permission from Kowaluk E, Fung H-L: Pharmacology and pharmacokinetics of nitrates. In: Abrams J, Pepine C, Thadani U, eds. Medical Therapy of Ischemic Heart Disease: Nitrates, Beta Blockers, and Calcium Antagonists. Boston: Little Brown, 1992:152.*)

ety is a component of the enzyme that converts nitrates to NO.[10] Thus, tolerance development may in part be related to thiols within the vascular smooth muscle cell in relationship to the production of SNO or the nitrate enzyme(s) responsible for NO formation. Fung hypothesized that nitrates may oxidize SH proteins, resulting in thionitrate production. This compound can act as a potent oxidant for intracellular proteins, perhaps initiating a cascade of events resulting in abnormalities of nitric oxide synthase (NOS), activation of vasoconstrictors, and interference with the conversion of 1-arginine to NO. (Fung H-L, personal communication). Munzel and coworkers have documented endothelial cell production of free radicals and the subsequent activation of protein kinase leading to endothelin and angiotensin II production (see below). Recently, it was reported that nitrate tolerance was associated with increased activity of the cGMP phosphodiesterase, which decreases cGMP levels necessary for mediating vasorelaxation via phosphorylation of proteins that regulate intracellular Ca^{2+} levels.[12a] These phenomena contribute to a vasoconstrictor milieu, for which oxidant stress is the probable cause.

Nitrate Effects on the Regional Circulations

Administration of NTG or other nitrates in sufficient dosage results in dilatation of veins and large- to moderate-size arteries, with a fall in vascular impedance. At high concentrations nitrates dilate the smaller arteries, and at very high doses nitrates can relax arterioles and the microcirculation.[13] Venodilatation is seen at low nitrate concentrations and is near maximal at moderate dosage (Fig. 14-2). Interesting studies by Harrison's group have suggested that the enzymes responsible for nitrate conversion to NO apparently are not present in the coronary microvessels, thus limiting the degree of increase in coronary blood flow and decrease in coronary vascular resistance that can be achieved with NTG through dilatation of these small coronary vessels.[3,14] Nitroprusside, on the other hand, directly forms NO in the microcirculation and readily relaxes the resistance vessels[13]; this can cause a fall in distal coronary bed pressure and may also allow for a coronary steal phenomenon in vessels beyond a coronary atherosclerotic obstruction.[15] (See below for discussion of NP.)

TABLE 14-1. Nitrate Formulations: Dosing Recommendations and Pharmacokinetics

	Usual Dose(mg)*	Onset of Action (min)	Effective Duration of Action
Sublingual NTG	0.3–0.6	2–5	20–30 min
Sublingual ISDN	2.5–10.0	5–20	45–120 min
Buccal NTG	1–3 bid tid	2–5	30–300 min[†]
Oral ISDN	10–60 bid tid	15–45	2–6 h
Oral ISDN-SR	80–120 once daily	60–90	10–14 h
Oral ISMN	20 bid[‡]	30–60	3–6 h
Oral ISMN-SR	60–120 qd	60–90	10–14 h
NTG ointment	0.5–2.0 tid	15–60	3–8 h
NTG patch	0.4–0.8 mg/h[§]	30–60	8–12 h

ISDN = isosorbide dinitrate; ISMN = isosorbide mononitrate; SR = sustained release; NTG = glyceryltrinitrate (nitroglycerin).

*Higher doses are often required in heart failure.

[†] Effect persists only while tablet intact in buccal cavity.

[‡] Two daily doses 7 h apart (e.g., 8 A.M., 2 P.M.).

[§] Patch should be removed daily for 10–12 h.

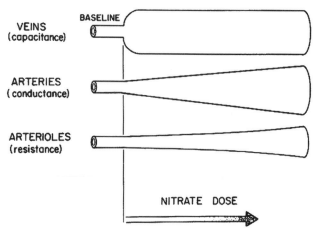

FIGURE 14-2. Vasodilatory actions of organic nitrates in the major vascular beds. Note that the venous or capacitance system dilates maximally with low doses of organic nitrates. Increasing the amount of drug does not cause appreciable additional venodilatation. Arterial dilatation and enhanced arterial conductance begin with low doses of nitrate. With further vasodilatation, appearing with increasing dosage at high plasma concentrations, the arteriolar or resistance vessels dilate, resulting in a decrease in systemic and regional vascular resistance. (*Reproduced with permission from Abrams J: Hemodynamic effects of nitroglycerin and long acting nitrates. Am Heart J 110:216–224, 1985.*)

Nitrates dilate the epicardial coronary arteries and, to a lesser degree, the smaller or distal coronary vessels.[3,13,16] Coronary blood flow transiently increases and then declines below baseline as myocardial energy needs decrease. Systemic venous relaxation in the extremities and splanchnic circulation results in sequestration of the circulating blood volume away from the heart and lungs, with a fall in cardiac output.[16,17] Nitrates also relax the splanchnic and mesenteric arterial beds, possibly contributing to the decrease in blood flow return to the heart.[18] Renal blood flow is marginally affected by NTG; it may decrease to a modest degree.[19] The cerebrovascular bed dilates with nitrates, and blood volume in the brain may increase. Thus, these agents are contraindicated when intracranial pressure is elevated.

An important clinical action of nitrates relates to the pulmonary circulation. These drugs consistently lower pulmonary venous and pulmonary capillary pressure, which contributes significantly to their efficacy in heart failure as well as myocardial ischemia. Relaxation of the pulmonary arterial bed is beneficial to subjects with secondary pulmonary hypertension; nitrates do not generally have a useful role in primary pulmonary hypertension.

Hemodynamic Correlates of Clinical Nitrate Efficacy

Table 14-2 indicates the presumed mechanisms of action for the various clinical conditions for which these agents are prescribed.[20] The traditional view has been that nitrate-induced reversal and/or prevention of myocardial ischemia are due to reductions in myocardial oxygen consumption related to reduced cardiac chamber size and decreased systolic and diastolic pressures within the heart.[16] These alterations are predominantly related to the venous and arterial vasodilating actions discussed above. The presumed paradigm is a major nitrate induced decrease in cardiac work to match available coronary blood supply. However, in recent years much evidence has contributed to the view that the organic nitrates have important actions in increasing regional or nutrient coronary blood flow, particularly to areas of myocardial ischemia. In addition to epicardial coronary artery dilatation, prevention or reversal of coronary

TABLE 14-2. Mechanisms of Action of Nitrates: Relationship to Clinical Indications

Acute attacks and prophylaxis of stable angina pectoris	Decreased myocardial oxygen consumption
	Decreased LV dimension
	Decreased LV filling pressure
	Decreased LV systolic pressure
	Decreased vascular impedance
	Increased coronary blood supply
	Epicardial coronary artery dilation
	Coronary stenosis enlargement
	Improved coronary endothelial function
	Dilation of coronary collaterals or small distal coronary vessels
Unstable angina	Same as above, plus antiplatelet, antithrombotic action
Acute myocardial infarction	Same as above, plus antiplatelet, antithrombotic action
Congestive heart failure	Decreased LV and RV dimensions (little data in CHF)
Systolic dysfunction	Decreased LV and RV filling-pressure
	Decreased systemic vascular resistance
	Decreased arterial pressure
	Decreased PA and RA pressure
	Improved endothelial function
	CAD patients: increased coronary blood flow
	Decreased mitral regurgitation
Diastolic dysfunction	Decreased LV filling pressure
Hypertension	Decreased systolic blood pressure
	Decreased systemic vascular resistance
	Decreased LV preload—uncertain importance

CAD = coronary artery disease; CHF = congestive heart failure; LV = left ventricular; PA = pulmonary artery; RA = right atrial; RV = right ventricular.

artery vasoconstriction or spasm, increased coronary collateral size and flow, enhanced distal vessel and collateral caliber when constrictor forces predominate,[21] coronary atherosclerotic stenosis enlargement,[22] and improved coronary endothelial function[3,13,23] are all mechanisms that may interact in a favorable fashion to alleviate or prevent ischemia by directly enhancing coronary blood supply to myocardium downstream from a fixed or dynamic coronary obstruction[16,20] (see Table 14-2).

In congestive heart failure, the beneficial effects and rationale for the nitrates are more obvious and are related to a predictable lowering of left-and right-ventricular filling pressures as well as the unloading actions that arise from decreased arterial pressure and impedance to left ventricular ejection.[24] These afterload-reducing actions contribute to a modest increase in stroke volume and cardiac output in subjects with impaired left ventricular systolic function, in contradistinction to the typical nitrate-induced fall in forward cardiac output in the normal heart. In addition, NTG appears to improve impaired vascular endothelial function common to heart failure.[25]

Nitroglycerin: The Exogenous Endothelium-Derived Relaxing Factor

Normal endothelial function is vasodilator- and platelet-antiaggregatory. In the presence of even mild coronary atherosclerosis, the dilating actions of the endothelium are impaired in both the coronary and systemic circulations. Thus, diminished vasodilation to physiologic stimuli (e.g., shear stress, platelet release products) as well as impaired platelet antiadhesion and aggregation responses are present in many to most individuals with clinically evident coronary artery disease (CAD). Vasoconstrictor responses to exercise, mental stress, cold pressor testing, as well as with the administration of endothelium-dependent dilator stimuli (e.g., acetylcholine, bradykinin) have been well documented in CAD subjects. Diminished availability of NO and prostacyclin, as well as increased endothelin and angiotensin II expression are common in such individuals; increased superoxide anions plays a major role in inducing the endothelial dysfunction common to CAD.[26] Stenotic constriction or collapse is an advanced manifestation of impaired endothelial function and may substantially contribute to the precipitation of myocardial ischemia in patients with angina or silent ischemia[27] NTG prevents or reverses this phenomenon, which has been documented with acetylcholine administration[28] as well as exercise.[27]

In congestive heart failure, disordered endothelial vasodilator activity is also common, importantly contributing to the vasoconstrictor state common to heart failure.[24,25,29] Enhanced sensitivity to catecholamines is part of the abnormal vascular physiology found in association with endothelial dysfunction; this phenomenon should be viewed as deleterious in heart failure as well as CAD.

Nitrates, as donors of NO, have been called exogenous endothelium-derived relaxing factor (ERDF) agents; these drugs improve responses to a variety of stimuli in the presence of endothelial dysfunction. Thus, in the patient with CAD, it has been postulated that administration of organic nitrates can partially or completely normalize impaired endothelial-related vasodilation[3,23,30,31] and, presumably but as yet unproved, restore endothelium-modulated antiplatelet activity toward normal. In fact, in some studies vascular responses to administered NTG appear to be more robust in the setting of endothelial dysfunction than in the normal state.[13,30,31] Nitrates may also improve endothelial function in heart failure.[25] However, in spite of suggestive favorable data from studies where nitrates are administered acutely, recent reports have suggested that in the presence of unequivocal nitrate tolerance, endothelial dysfunction may actually be induced, perhaps due to impaired eNOS activity and other intracellular perturbations of the nitric oxide cascade.[32–36]

CLINICAL INDICATIONS FOR NITRATES

The major cardiovascular conditions for which nitrates are effective are listed in Table 14-2. The role of NTG and the other organic nitrates in CAD is well established. Treatment and prophylaxis of anginal attacks as well as prevention of chest pain in chronic angina pectoris are the most important uses of these drugs. More problematic is the usefulness of nitrates in uncomplicated acute MI. Although sublingual or intravenous NTG are excellent drugs for recurrent ischemic chest pain, hypertension, or heart failure in the setting of an acute infarct, there is considerable uncertainty as to the benefits of routine 24- or 48-h infusions of NTG or the use of any nitrate when obvious clinical indications are absent in the setting of acute infarction. In spite of promising but limited animal and human data,[37–40a] the European megatrials GISSI-3 (Gruppo Italiano per lo Studio della Supravivenza nellInfarcto Miocardico) and ISIS-4 (Fourth International Study of Infarct Survival) have failed to show an important role for early administration of nitrates weeks after an acute MI and continued use for the next 5 to 6 weeks.[41,42]

There is a suggestion that NTG pretreatment in patients undergoing angioplasty can protect the myocardium against ischemia. The mechanism proposed is a delayed preconditioning mimetic effect of NTG.[43,44]

Nitrates are underutilized in congestive heart failure. These drugs are effective in improving symptoms and exercise tolerance[24] and, in conjunction with the angiotensin converting enzyme (ACE) inhibitors, are useful for the treatment of symptomatic heart failure.[45–48] Large doses are often required in these patients. Nitrate resistance, as well as the necessity to use huge amounts of these drugs, has been described in advanced heart failure.[49,50] In the first Veterans Administration cooperative heart failure mortality study, the combination of ISDN 40 mg four times daily and hydralazine 300 mg per day reduced mortality.[51] However, the combination of hydralazine and oral ISDN subsequently proved to be less effective in improving survival in heart failure patients than the ACE inhibitor enalapril.[52]

Intravenous NTG is an effective formulation for lowering blood pressure in the setting of acute hypertension or for the control of mean arterial pressure during a variety of delicate surgical procedures. This agent has been successfully employed for post–coronary bypass patients with elevated blood pressure. Oral nitrates, while utilized extensively in the early part of this century for hypertension, are not part of contemporary conventional therapy of systemic hypertension, in part because of the appearance of tolerance to the systolic pressure–lowering effects of these drugs. A report from France indicates a potential benefit for oral ISDN in systolic hypertension of the elderly.[53]

There is also available experimental evidence to suggest that NTG may be useful in reversing cerebral vasospasm in patients with subarachnoid hemorrhage.[54]

NITRATE FORMULATIONS AND NITRATE PHARMACOKINETICS

Three organic nitrate compounds—NTG, ISDN, and ISMN—are currently used throughout the world and have been shown to provide

TABLE 14-3. Factors That Influence Nitrate Tolerance

Induce Tolerance	Prevent Tolerance
Continuous or prolonged nitrate exposure (e.g., transdermal patches, intravenous)	Intermittent dosing
	Small doses
	Infrequent dosing
Large doses	Short-acting formulations
Frequent dosing	Provision of adequate nitrate-free
Sustained-action formulations	interval
No or brief nitrate-free interval	

benefits in angina pectoris and congestive heart failure. There does not appear to be any difference in clinical efficacy among these compounds. Choice of formulation, dosage, use of a tolerance-avoidance regimen, and physician experience and bias are major factors influencing which nitrate is prescribed for which patient. Tolerance is a problem for all nitrate formulations except for sublingual NTG and ISDN or transmucosal NTG, which are not designed to be administered continuously. Appropriately designed dosing regimens can prevent the appearance of significant nitrate tolerance but limited available data suggest that attenuation of nitrate's hemodynamic action may begin to appear within hours of nitrate administration (see Tables 14-1 and 14-3).

Nitroglycerin

The classic prototype nitrate is NTG, which is available in many formulations (see Table 14-1). This molecule has a very short half-life of several minutes; cessation of an intravenous NTG infusion or removal of a transdermal patch results in a rapid fall in NTG plasma levels within 20 to 40 min. The metabolism of NTG occurs within the vascular wall (see Fig. 14-1). Veins take up NTG more avidly than arteries. It is not useful or practical to measure NTG plasma levels in clinical practice; this assay is technically difficult, and the relationship between plasma NTG level and effect changes as tolerance develops. Early studies with sublingual NTG suggest that the therapeutic NTG level is at least 1 ng/mL[51]; plasma concentrations with the NTG patch are substantially lower. The minimum recommended dose of the patch is 0.4 mg/h, with larger amounts often being more effective, particularly in heart failure. Several recent studies confirm a true anti-ischemic action of these agents,[56–58] which must be administered in an on-off fashion. The patch should be applied continuously for only 12 to 14 h each day. Rebound angina and vasoconstriction are possible adverse effects of intermittent therapy.[59,60] Several dosing systems for NTG have been available to physicians but are not widely used and may not be available in many pharmacies. These include the buccal or transmucosal formulation, NTG ointment, and oral sustained-release NTG capsules. Ointment and buccal NTG are effective but difficult for patients to use. NTG ointment is recommended for hospitalized or home-bound patients with nocturnal angina or symptomatic congestive heart failure. Oral NTG has virtually no reliable data supporting its effectiveness.

Isosorbide Dinitrate

Isosorbide dinitrate (ISDN) is perhaps the most widely used long-acting nitrate in the world. It is available in short-acting and sustained release formulations; the majority of clinical studies in the literature have employed short-acting oral ISDN. Table 14-4 outlines the relevant pharmacokinetic features of ISDN and ISMN. Sustained-release ISDN should be used only once daily. In Europe, intravenous ISDN is commercially available. Sublingual or chewable ISDN have long been utilized for acute attacks of chest pain or angina prophylaxis, but these formulations are infrequently prescribed in the United States.

When ISDN is administered, the parent compound is converted to two active metabolites, 2- and 5-isosorbide mononitrate.[61] The latter is a pharmacologically active molecule that is commercially synthesized, and available in short-acting and sustained-release formulations. A dose of the parent compound ISDN results in plasma concentrations of all three molecules (Fig. 14-3).[62] ISDN has a short half-life of 50 to 60 min and rapidly disappears from the circulation. ISMN has a much longer half-life of 4 to 6 h and accounts for the protracted nitrate effects following administration of ISDN. Approximately 50 to 60% of ISDN is converted to 5-ISMN. Thus, although only 20 to 25% of ISDN itself is bioavailable when taken orally, a substantial component of the administered dose becomes pharmacologically active as 5-ISMN (see Table 14-4).

Isosorbide 5-Mononitrate

The 5-mononitrate is the most recent nitrate formulation released in the United States. It was initially available only in the short acting form; to avoid tolerance, short-acting 5-ISMN is recommended to be taken in a twice-daily regimen, with 7 to 8 h between doses (see Table 14-1).[63,64] Earlier Scandinavian and European experience suggested that a q 12 h regimen was satisfactory to avoid tolerance, but American trials with this compound indicated that a longer overnight interval was necessary to avoid attenuation of clinical effectiveness.[63,64] Sustained-release 5-ISMN is effective on a once-daily basis.[65] A minimum of 60 mg per day is recommended; a large American multicenter trial suggested that higher doses, such as 120 or 240 mg daily, may be necessary for sustained antianginal efficacy without tolerance[66] (Fig. 14-4). A 50-mg once-daily, immediate-release/sustained-release ISMN formulation is now available, which appears to maintain antianginal efficacy without tolerance.[67,68]

TABLE 14-4. Pharmacokinetics of Isosorbide Dinitrate and 5-Mononitrate

	ISDN	5-ISMN
Bioavailability	20–25%*	100%
Half-life	30–60 min	4–5 h
Metabolites	2-ISMN, 5-ISMN	None
Plasma levels	Low	High
Formulations†	IV, SL, oral, oral sustained release ointment, spray	Oral, oral sustained release,

*Extensive hepatic first-pass effect.

†Only oral and sublingual compounds available in the United States.

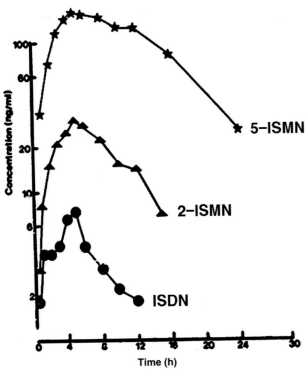

FIGURE 14-3. Pharmacokinetics of ISDN. Concentrations of ISDN (closed circles), 5-ISMN (stars), and 2-ISMN (triangles) following injection of 40 mg radiolabeled oral ISDN. Note that the relative duration of activity of the parent compound ISDN is substantially shorter than that of 5-ISMN; 5-ISMN is responsible for much of the later action oral ISDN. The half-life of ISDN is under 1 h; whereas the half-life of 5-ISMN is 4 to 5 h. The biologic activity of the 2-ISMN compound is believed to be rather weak and clinically unimportant. (*Modified with permission from Chasseaud LF: Newer aspects of the pharmacokinetics of organic nitrates. Z Kardiol 72:20–23, 1983.*)

SUGGESTIONS FOR NITRATE DOSING

It is important to start nitrate therapy with small doses and to carefully increase to a predetermined endpoint or maximally tolerated amount over time. Headache and dizziness are the limiting symptoms with nitrate administration. Some individuals are extremely sensitive to organic nitrates; others experience little to no side effects. Many if not most patients are under dosed with long-acting nitrates, at least with respect to clinical trial data. For instance, 10 mg of oral ISDN, 30 or 60 mg of ISMN-SR, or 0.2 to 0.4 mg/h of the NTG patch are less likely to be clinically effective doses. If the angina is well controlled with these relatively low doses, it is satisfactory to continue such a regimen. However, the physician should be sure that the more desirable clinical response has been achieved; if so, higher amounts of the nitrate should be tried. In congestive heart failure, the dosage of nitrates to achieve a significant hemodynamic effect is usually considerably higher than in patients with normal left ventricular function. Often patients who are troubled with nitrate headaches with initial nitrate dosing can be effectively treated with analgesics (aspirin, acetaminophen) to control the headache symptoms, which usually decrease or disappear over time. Nitrate hypotension is best handled by reducing the dose; concomitant therapy with calcium channel antagonists or ACE inhibitors or hypovolemia increase the likelihood of dizziness and/or syncope owing to low blood pressure following nitrate administration.

ADVERSE EFFECTS

In addition to headache and hypotension-related dizziness, nitrates can occasionally cause nausea. Patients with congestive heart failure tolerate large doses of nitrates surprisingly well. Rare cases of nitrate syncope have been reported, as have marked vasovagal responses and even AV block. Nitrates should be given with great care in the setting of right ventricular infarction complicating inferior myocardial infarction, as these drugs lower right ventricular filling pressure and can further depress cardiac output. Nitrates should also not be used with sildenafil because of a major hypotensive effect with this combination.[69] Intravenous NTG has been suggested to interfere with the actions of heparin, resulting in increased heparin requirements to achieve the desired prolongation of the activated clotting time.[70–72] This interaction remains controversial. One report suggests that NTG may impair tissue plasminogen activator activity during thrombolysis,[73] and a recent report suggested that nitroglycerin might have adverse effects on atherosclerotic plaque irritability by activating matrix metalloproteinase activity.[73a] These effects may explain the lack of a positive association between nitroglycerin therapy and beneficial effects on plaque progression or coronary event rates, despite nitroglycerin's vasodilator activity.[73a] In general, the organic nitrates are well-tolerated drugs with little serious adverse sequelae. Headache, the most problematic symptom related to nitrate therapy, can be controlled in many patients. However, upward of 20 to 30% of individuals cannot tolerate long-acting nitrate therapy.

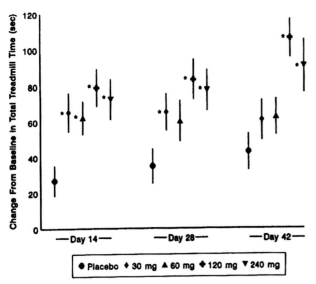

FIGURE 14-4. Randomized double-blind trial of sustained-release ISMN in 313 patients with angina. Four ISMN doses and placebo were tested with serial treadmills over a 6-week period. These are the data at 4 h after dosing. (*Reproduced with permission from Chrysant*).[66]

NITRATE TOLERANCE

Clearly, the most vexing issue regarding nitrate therapy is the attenuation of nitrate efficacy with repeated dosing. This subject has an

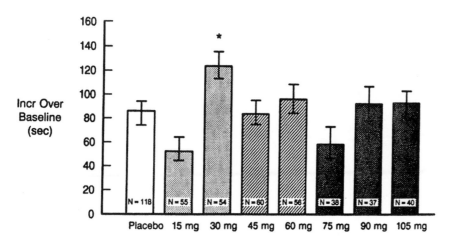

FIGURE 14-5. High-dose transdermal nitroglycerin in angina. Chronic exercise tolerance data after 8 weeks of double-blind therapy. All groups showed an increase (Incr) in treadmill performance over baseline at the end of the trail. Only the 30 mg/24 h group demonstrated a nominally statistically significant increase that was greater than placebo; $P < .05$ over placebo. (*Reproduced with permission from Steering Committee.*)[78]

enormous literature[11–12,74–93] and continues to engender considerable controversy. However, almost all experts agree that tolerance will predictably appear when protolerant dosing regimens are utilized. Dozens of high-quality clinical and basic research studies underscore the magnitude of this problem. The rapid onset of tolerance can be substantiated after several repeated doses of oral nitrate given with too short an interdose interval.[83,84] Major attenuation of nitrate action in angina has been repeatedly demonstrated with continuous 24-h application of transdermal NTG[78,85]; in fact, an antianginal effect can no longer be detected by the second day of continuous patch therapy, even when very large doses are used (Fig. 14-5 demonstrates 8 week data).[78] Similar findings have been demonstrated for intravenous NTG, as well as the oral agents ISDN and ISMN, when these drugs are not administered in a tolerance-avoidance regimen. Table 14-3 lists the cardinal principles for avoiding nitrate tolerance. Table 14-1 outlines the recommended dosing schedules for the available nitrates. Intravenous NTG administered for the acute ischemic syndromes of unstable angina pectoris or acute myocardial infarction should not be abruptly terminated so as to avoid tolerance; rebound phenomena are well known, and sudden withdrawal of intravenous NTG may be dangerous in this setting, even if some degree of hemodynamic tolerance is present.

The conundrum of nitrate tolerance remains incompletely resolved. Recent data confirm that endothelial vasodilator function is markedly impaired during nitrate tolerance.[32–36,86,87,92,93] The precise cause of this abnormality remains controversial. Abnormalities of 1-arginine availability, NOS function, and particularly excessive oxidant stress have all been postulated as potential mechanisms, based on a variety of experimental observations.[32–36,80–88,92,93] Table 14-5 lists a variety of hypotheses regarding nitrate tolerance. Older research suggested that nitrate tolerance is related to poor sulfhydryl or thiol group availability, plasma volume expansion, and/or neurohumoral activation of the renin-angiotensin system. Several recent studies suggest that antioxidants, such as vitamin C, can prevent or reverse nitrate tolerance[89–91]; however, this approach remains as yet an unproven hypothesis. There is some evidence that not all organic nitrates have a comparable ability or potential to induce nitrate tolerance.

Much data suggest that during experimentally induced NT, there is an enhanced vasoconstrictor milieu, related in part to increased oxidant stress.[34–36,80,88–91,93] Abnormalities of vascular and endothelial function, modulated through activation of protein kinase C, include endothelial cell expression of angiotensin II and endothelin, along with increased amounts of peroxynitrate, an oxidant formed by interaction of O_2^- anions with NTG.[11a,32–36,80,86–93] ACE inhibitors can modify the development of nitrate-concomitant tolerance by an endothelium-dependent mechanism involving mainly an enhanced nitric oxide availability via the B_2-kinin receptor.[94] Parker et al have documented major perturbations of endothelial vasodilator function in the setting of induced nitrate tolerance, as well as easily demonstrated coronary vasoconstriction to acetylcholine after a NTG patch is removed in the setting of nitrate tolerance (Fig. 14-6).[33,36] These investigators have hypothesized abnormalities of NOS function as a contributor to the endothelial dysfunction in nitrate tolerance.[33,92] Folic acid supplementation has recently been suggested to prevent NT, presumed to be related to increased tetrahydrobiopterin availability, resulting in enhanced eNOS function.[92] Tolerance is clearly multifactorial, and a clinical solution is not yet available.[93] For the more interested reader, a variety of reviews and commentaries are available.[11a,74–77,81,82,93,95]

Clinical Implications of Nitrate Tolerance

In addition to the loss of the desired actions of nitrates for specific cardiovascular disorders, NT may be associated with other adverse disturbances in vascular function, including withdrawal chest pain and/or ischemia as well as reflex vasoconstriction of coronary arteries or atherosclerotic stenoses.[96] Several recent reports suggest that long-term nitrate use may result in adverse clinical outcomes in patients with CAD.[97,98] At the very least, the disappointing results of the large ISIS-4[42] and GISSI-3[41] postinfarction trials could in part be related to heretofore unsuspected abnormalities of vascular

TABLE 14-5. Proposed Mechanisms of Nitrate Tolerance

Sulfhydryl depletion: inadequate generation of reduced –SH or cysteine groups required for organic nitrate biotransformation to NO.

Desensitization of soluble guanylate cyclase; impaired activity of the enzyme guanylate cyclase.

Counterregulatory neurohormonal activation: nitrate-induced increases in catecholamines, arginine vasopressin (AVP), plasma renin, aldosterone, and angiotensin II activity, with resultant vasoconstriction and fluid retention.

Plasma volume shifts: increased intravascular blood volume related to decreased capillary pressure.

Oxygen free radical destruction of nitric oxide with production of peroxynitrates resulting in enhanced sensitivity to vasoconstrictors, especially angiotensin II).

Upregulation of PDE 1A1 expression resulting in decreased formation of cGMP.

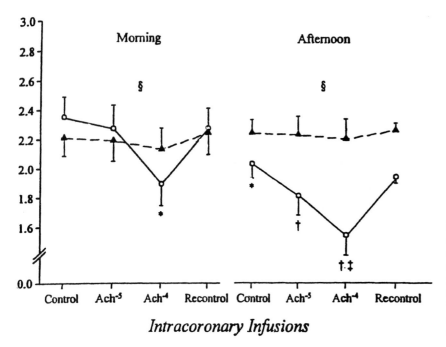

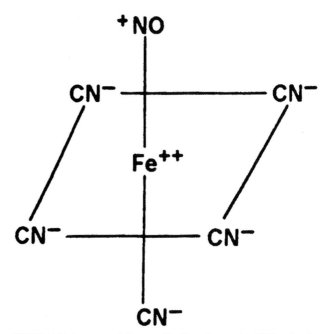

FIGURE 14-6. Change in luminal diameter of the left anterior descending artery (LAD) during intracoronary infusions of acetylcholine (Ach) and nitroglycerin. Ach^{-5} and Ach^{-4} indicate 10^{-5} and 10^{-4} mol/L respectively. O = nitroglycerin group; ▲ = nonnitroglycerin group; $^*P < .01$ versus morning control; $^†P < .01$ versus afternoon control; $^‡P < .01$ versus morning Ach^{-4}; $^§P < .01$ GTN group versus non-GTN group.

endothelial function induced by conventional nitrate dosing. Intermittent dosing strategies may reduce or attenuate the likelihood of nitrate tolerance, but it is possible or even likely that even shorter periods of nitrate exposure (e.g., less than 12–14 h) may initiate intracellular and endothelial mechanisms leading to unwanted alterations in eNOS function and endothelial function modulated by a reduced availability of nitric oxide. There may be decreased nitric oxide synthesis as well as enhanced nitric oxide degradation induced by a variety of mechanisms.[32–36,80,86–95] Thus, as some have suggested, chronic nitrate therapy for angina or heart failure may sow the seeds for unwanted outcomes with respect to long-term morbidity and even mortality.[33–36,59,60,95–98] This would be a remarkable reversal of our concepts about these drugs and their utility in clinical cardiovascular disease; randomized clinical trial data are required to truly validate these concepts but are unlikely to become available in the future.

NITROPRUSSIDE

NP is an inorganic nitrovasodilator that results in abundant NO availability in vascular smooth muscle cells. It is likely that NP has antiplatelet activity, but there are limited data in this regard. NP is a ferrocyanide compound with a nitroso-moiety (Fig. 14-7). Cyanide molecules are released as the molecule undergoes metabolism to NO, but in general, plasma cyanide and thiocyanate concentrations at clinically utilized dosage are too low to cause toxicity in subjects with normal renal function. NP provides NO throughout the vasculature; metabolic conversion to NO does not depend on enzymatic conversion to NO to any significant degree.[3] Thus, NO is abundantly available in the microcirculation following NP infusion; these distal small vessels have a decreased capacity to metabolize the NTG molecule.[3,14] This is an important dissimilarity between the two compounds, as their spectrum of vasodilatation differs significantly.[20] Because NP has a potent effect on the small resistance vessels of the heart, there is a greater possibility for a coronary steal phenomenon than with NTG. NP induces relaxation

of the microcirculation throughout the myocardium, potentially allowing for diversion of nutrient coronary blood flow away from regions of ischemia distal to a coronary obstruction. NP appears to dilate collateral vessels to a lesser degree than NTG, which could exacerbate a potentially deleterious diversion of blood from ischemic zones (see below.) NP is a potent venodilator. On the arterial side, it is more hemodynamically active than NTG, particularly regarding the smaller arterioles and resistance vessels. In general, there is a more equivalent degree of venous and arterial vasodilatation with NP than NTG, which has more dominant venodilator than arterial action, particularly at lower doses.[20]

FIGURE 14-7. Structure of nitroprusside. Note the cyanide (CN) molecules and the nitroso (NO) group.

Indications for Nitroprusside

NP is a drug used exclusively in critical care settings and operating rooms. It is a highly effective vasodilator of great potency. NP was investigated extensively in the early days of vasodilator therapy for acute myocardial infarction and congestive heart failure.[99] Its balanced venous and arterial actions make it an ideal drug for the immediate therapy of acute and/or severe heart failure associated with high ventricular filling pressure and low stroke volume. The drug is also a first-line choice for treatment of severe hypertension and is probably preferable to intravenous NTG in this capacity because of its greater arterial dilator potency. At very high NTG concentrations, the hemodynamic activity of intravenous NTG is quite similar to NP.

A series of animal and human investigations have suggested a potential hazard for the use of NP in nonhypertensive ischemic states, such as acute myocardial infarction and unstable angina pectoris. Decreases in regional myocardial blood flow and collateral flow, associated with increased ischemia, have been demonstrated in human and canine studies when NP was compared to intravenous NTG.[15,100] One early animal investigation suggested a more potent vasodilating action on the smaller coronary vessels than NTG, which was more active in the larger coronary arteries.[101] Another trial successfully treated patients with immediate post–coronary bypass grafting hypertension with NP or intravenous NTG.[102] Two conflicting trials of NP in the setting of acute myocardial infarction were published in 1982.[103,104] In the VA cooperative study, NP offered no advantage to patients given a 48-h infusion of NP versus placebo, when the infusion was instituted a mean of 17 h after onset of chest pain (Fig. 14-8).[103] However, a retrospective analysis suggested that patients treated early (within

FIGURE 14-8. Intravenous nitroprusside in acute myocardial infarction. There were approximately 400 patients in each group, NP versus placebo. Cumulative percentage of patients surviving after early treatment (within 9 h of onset of acute myocardial infarction) and late treatment (later than 9 h). (*Reproduced with permission from Cohn JN, Franciosa JA, Francis GS, et al: Effect of short-term infusion of sodium nitroprusside on mortality rate in acute myocardial infarction complicated by left ventricular failure. N Engl J Med 306:1129–1135, 1982.*)

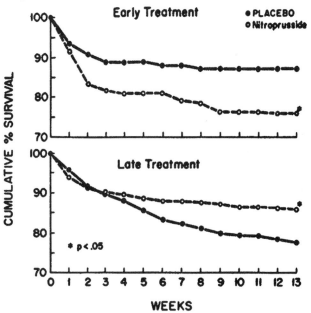

TABLE 14-6. Indications for Nitroprusside

Severe hypertension
Acute pulmonary edema
Severe congestive heart failure
Acute and/or severe mitral or aortic regurgitation
Acute myocardial infarction complications: Heart failure or uncontrolled hypertension
Use extreme caution: Hypotension or borderline systolic blood pressure
Acute myocardial ischemia in the absence of heart failure
Renal insufficiency

9 h of onset of symptoms) fared less well with NP than with placebo, whereas subjects treated later had a decreased mortality rate (see Fig. 14-8). It was speculated that the former group may have had lower left ventricular filling pressures during the first day or two, and thus may have been exposed to a NP-induced risk of hypoperfusion of the coronary bed or a coronary steal phenomenon; the late-treated cohort presumably had more patients with left ventricular dysfunction and elevated filling pressures, and in these subjects NP would have been of benefit when compared with placebo. However, another study from the Netherlands demonstrated a decrease in mortality in acute MI patients randomized to NP.[104] The reasons for the different results are unknown, although it has been speculated that the latter study included a number of hypertensive subjects who may have derived additional benefits from NP which may have affected the final outcome.[105] In any case, this dilemma has not been resolved, and there have not been subsequent confirming studies. Warnings about the use of NP in acute MI are not new,[105] and current guidelines for the therapy of myocardial infarction include intravenous NTG but not NP.[106] Tables 14-6 and 14-7 list the indications and precautions that accompany the use of NP.

Dosage

The infusion of NP should begin at 0.5 to 1 μg/kg/min, increasing to no more than 10 μg/kg/min. Most experts recommend reducing the mean or systolic arterial pressure by 10%, thereby avoiding central aortic hypotension. Meticulous care must be given to the patient with actual or potential myocardial ischemia, so as to prevent an excessive central aortic pressure decrease. NP must be given with appropriate precautions, including protection from ambient light to prevent an accelerated release of NO and cyanide. The infusion should be limited in duration to 48 h, as NP toxicity can occur over time as the cumulative dose increases. Renal and hepatic insufficiencies are risk factors for adverse reactions to NP, with excessive concentrations of cyanide and thiocyanate, the metabolic by-product of NP metabolism. Thiocyanate toxicity should be suspected in patients receiving NP who develop abdominal pain, mental status changes, or convulsions. Cyanide toxicity can be manifest by a reduction in cardiac output and metabolic or lactic acidosis. Methemoglobinemia can be observed as a relatively pure manifestation of NP toxicity.

TABLE 14-7. Precautions in the Use of Nitroprusside

Exposure of NP solution to light
Prolonged infusion (more than 48 h)
Renal insufficiency
Infusion rates greater than 10 μg/kg/min
Measure thiocyanate levels in high-risk subjects (prolonged infusion, azotemia)

CONCLUSION

The available nitrovasodilators remain important cardiovascular drugs for the management of patients with ischemic heart disease, emergent hypertension, and congestive heart failure. Their actions appear to simulate many of the normal vascular physiologic processes involved in vasodilation and have provided tremendous insights into the pathophysiology of vascular disease. Nevertheless, nitrate tolerance remains a fascinating and complex subject, and recent work implicating tolerance-induced endothelial dysfunction raises more questions than answers. Informed and judicious use of the nitrates and NP should provide benefit for many individuals with cardiovascular disease.[108]

REFERENCES

1. Fung H-L, Chung S-J, Bauer JA, et al: Biochemical mechanism of organic nitrate action. *Am J Cardiol* 70:4B, 1992.
2. Kukovetz WR, Holzmann S, Schmidt K: Cellular mechanisms of action therapeutic nitric oxide donors. *Eur Heart J* 12(suppl E):16, 1991.
3. Harrison DG, Bates JN: The nitrovasodilators: New ideas about old drugs. *Circulation* 87:1461, 1993.
4. Torfgard KE, Ahlner J: Mechanisms of action of nitrates. *Cardiovasc Drugs Ther* 8:701, 1994.
5. Loscalzo J: Antiplatelet and antithrombotic effects of organic nitrates. *Am J Cardiol* 70:18B, 1992.
6. Diodati J, Theroux P, Latour J-G, et al: Effects of nitroglycerin at therapeutic doses on platelet aggregation in unstable angina pectoris and acute myocardial infarction. *Am J Cardiol* 66:683, 1996.
7. Folts JD, Stamler J, Loscalzo J: Intravenous nitroglycerin infusion inhibits blood flow responses caused by periodic platelet thrombus formation in stenosed canine coronary arteries. *Circulation* 83:2122, 1991.
8. Lam JYT, Chesebro JH, Fuster V: Platelets, vasoconstriction and nitroglycerin during arterial wall injury: A new antithrombotic role for an old drug. *Circulation* 78:712, 1988.
9. Fye WB: Nitroglycerin: A homeopathic remedy. *Circulation* 73:21, 1986.
10. Seth P, Fung H-L: Biochemical characterization of a membrane-bound enzyme responsible for generating nitric oxide from nitroglycerin in vascular smooth muscle cells. *Biochem Pharmacol* 64:1481, 1993.
11. Watanabe H, Kakihana M, Ohtsuka S, et al: Platelet cyclic GMP. A potentially useful indicator to evaluate the effects of nitroglycerin and nitrate tolerance. *Circulation* 88:29, 1993.
11a. Parker JD, Gori T: Tolerance to the organic nitrates: New ideas, new mechanisms, continued mystery. *Circulation* 104:2263, 2001.
11b. Sage PR, de la Lande IS, Stafford I: Nitroglycerin tolerance in human vessels. Evidence for impaired nitroglycerin bioconversion. *Circulation* 102:2810, 2000.
12. Boesgaard S, Aldershvile J, Lofts S, et al: Nitrate tolerance in vivo is not associated with depletion of arterial or venous thiol levels. *Circ Res* 74:115, 1994.
12a. Kim D, Rybalkin SD, Pi X, et al: Upregulation of phosphodiesterase 1A1 expression is associated with the development of nitrate tolerance. *Circulation* 104:2338, 2001.
13. Bassenge E: Coronary vasomotor responses: Role of endothelium and nitrovasodilators. *Cardiovasc Drugs Ther* 8:601, 1994.
14. Kurz MA, Lamping KG, Bates JN, et al: Mechanisms responsible for the heterogeneous coronary microvascular response to nitroglycerin. *Circ Res* 68:847, 1991.
15. Chiariello M, Gold HK, Leinbach RC, et al: Comparison between the effects of nitroprusside and nitroglycerin on ischemic injury during acute myocardial infarction. *Circulation* 54:766, 1976.
16. Abrams J: Mechanisms of action of the organic nitrates in the treatment of myocardial ischemia. *Am J Cardiol* 70:30B, 1992.
17. Loos D, Schneider R, Schorner W: Changes in regional body blood volume caused by nitroglycerin. *Z Kardiol* 72(Suppl 3):29, 1983.
18. Vatner SF, Pagani M, Rutherford JD, et al: Effects of nitroglycerin on cardiac performance and regional blood flows distribution in conscious dogs. *Am J Physiol* 234(3):H244, 1978.
19. Leier CV, Huss P, Bambach D, et al: Central and regional hemodynamic effects of intravenous isosorbide dinitrate, nitroglycerin and nitroprusside in patients with congestive heart failure. *Am J Cardiol* 48:1115, 1981.
20. Abrams J: Beneficial actions of nitrates in cardiovascular disease. *Am J Cardiol* 77:31C, 1996.
21. Pupita G, Maseri A, Kaski JC, et al: Myocardial ischemia caused distal coronary-artery constriction in stable angina pectoris. *N Engl J Med* 323:514, 1990.
22. Brown BG, Bolson EL, Dodgett T: Dynamic mechanisms in human coronary stenosis. *Circulation* 70:917, 1984.
23. Bassenge E, Zanzinger J: Nitrates in different vascular beds, nitrate tolerance, and interactions with endothelial function. *Am J Cardiol* 70:23B, 1992.
24. Dupuis J: Nitrates in congestive heart failure. *Cardiovasc Drugs Ther* 8:501, 1994.
25. Schwarz M, Katz SD, Demopoulos L, et al: Enhancement of endothelium dependent vasodilation by low-dose nitroglycerin in patients with congestive heart failure. *Circulation* 89:1609, 1994.
26. Luscher TF, Noll G: The endothelium in coronary vascular control, update 3. In: Braunwald E, ed. *Heart Disease*. Philadelphia: Saunders, 1995:1.
27. Gage JE, Hess OM, Murakami T, et al: Vasoconstriction of stenotic coronary arteries during dynamic exercise in patients with classic angina pectoris: Reversibility by nitroglycerin. *Circulation* 73:865, 1986.
28. Ludmer PL, Selwyn AP, Shook TL, et al: Paradoxical vasoconstriction induced by acetycholine in atherosclerotic arteries. *N Engl J Med* 315:1046, 1986.
29. Paulus WJ: Endothelial control of vascular and myocardial function in heart failure. *Cardiovasc Drugs Ther* 8:437, 1994.
30. Rafflenbeul W, Bassenge E, Lichtlen P: Competition between endothelium-dependent and nitroglycerin-induced coronary vasodilation. *Z Kardiol* 78(Suppl 2):45, 1989.
31. Luscher TF: Endothelium-derived nitric oxide: The endogenous nitrovasodilator in the human cardiovascular system. *Eur Heart J* 12(Suppl E):2, 1991.
32. Münzel T, Giaid A, Kurz S, et al: Evidence for a role of endothelin 1 and protein kinase C in nitroglycerin tolerance. *Proc Natl Acad Sci USA* 92:5244, 1995.
33. Gori T, Mak SS, Kelly S, Parker JD: Evidence supporting abnormalities in nitric oxide synthase function induced by nitroglycerin in humans. *J Am Coll Cardiol* 38:1096, 2001.
34. Münzel T, Sayegh H, Freeman BA, et al: Evidence for enhanced vascular superoxide anion production in nitrate tolerance. A novel mechanism underlying tolerance and cross-tolerance. *J Clin Invest* 95 (1):187, 1995.
35. Heizer T, Just H, Brockhoff C et al: Long-term nitroglycerin treatment is associated with supersensitivity to vasoconstrictors in men with stable coronary artery disease: Prevention by concomitant treatment with captopril. *J Am Coll Cardiol* 31(1):83, 1998.
36. Caramori PR, Adelman AG, Azevedo ER, et al: Therapy with nitroglycerin increases coronary vasoconstriction in response to acetylcholine. *J Am Coll Cardiol* 32(7):1969, 1998.
37. Jugdutt BI, Tymchak WJ, Burton JR: Preservation of left ventricular geometry and function after late reperfusion and intravenous nitroglycerin in acute transmural myocardial infarction. *Circulation* 84:II-683, 1991.
38. McDonald KM, Francis GS, Matthews J, et al: Long-term oral nitrate therapy prevents chronic ventricular remodeling in the dog. *J Am Coll Cardiol* 21:514, 1993.
39. Jugdutt BI, Warnica JW: Intravenous nitroglycerin therapy to limit myocardial infarct size, expansion, and complications: Effect on timing, dosage and infarct location. *Circulation* 78:906, 1988.
40. Yusuf S, Collins R, MacMahon S, Peto R: Effect of intravenous nitrates on mortality in acute myocardial infarction: An overview of the randomized trials. *Lancet* 2:1088, 1988.
40a. Beltrame JF, Stewart S, Leslie S, et al: Resolution of ST segment elevation following intravenous administration of nitroglycerin and verapamil. *Am J Cardiol* 89:452, 2002.

41. Gruppo Italiano per lo Studio della Supravivenza nellInfarcto Miocardico (GISSI-3): Effects of lisinopril and transdermal glyceryl trinitrate singly and together on 6-week mortality and ventricular function after acute myocardial infarction. *Lancet* 343:1115, 1994.

42. ISIS-4 (Fourth International Study of Infarct Survival) Collaborative Group (ISIS-4): A randomized factorial trial assessing early oral captopril, oral mononitrate, and intravenous magnesium sulphate in 58,050 patients with suspected acute myocardial infarction. *Lancet* 345:669, 1995.

43. Leesar MA, Stoddard MF, Dawn B, et al: Delayed preconditioning-mimetic action of nitroglycerin in patients undergoing coronary angioplasty. *Circulation* 103:2935, 2001.

44. Heusch G: Nitroglycerin and delayed preconditioning in humans. Yet another new mechanism for an old drug? *Circulation* 103:2876, 2001.

45. Abrams J: Nitrates and nitrate tolerance in congestive heart failure. *Coron Artery Dis* 4:27, 1993.

46. Mehra A, Ostrzega E, Shotan A, et al: Persistent hemodynamic improvement with short-term nitrate therapy in patients with chronic congestive heart failure already treated with captopril. *Am J Cardiol* 70:1310, 1992.

47. Parker JD, Parker JO: Effect of therapy with an angiotensin converting enzyme inhibitor on hemodynamic and counterregulators responses during continuous therapy with nitroglycerin. *J Am Coll Cardiol* 21:1445, 1993.

48. Elkayam U, Johnson JV, Shotan A, et al: Double-blind, placebo-controlled study to evaluate the effect of organic nitrates in patients with chronic heart failure treated with angiotensin-converting enzyme inhibition. *Circulation* 99:2652, 1999.

49. Elkayam U, Mehra A, Shotan A, Ostrzega E: Nitrate resistance and tolerance: Potential limitations in the treatment of congestive heart failure. *Am J Cardiol* 70:98B, 1992.

50. Abrams J: The mystery of nitrate resistance. *Am J Cardiol* 68: 1393, 1991.

51. Cohn JN, Archibald DG, Ziesche S, et al: Effect of vasodilator therapy on mortality in chronic congestive heart failure: Results of a Veterans Administration Cooperative Study. *N Engl J Med* 314:1547, 1986.

52. Cohn JN, Johnson G, Ziesche S, et al: A comparison of enalapril with hydralazine-isosorbide dinitrate in the treatment of chronic congestive heart failure. *N Engl J Med* 325:303, 1991.

53. Duchier J, Iannascoli F, Safor M: Antihypertensive effect of sustained release isosorbide dinitrate for isolated systolic systemic hypertension in the elderly. *Am J Cardiol* 60:99, 1987.

54. Ito Y, Isotani E, Mizuno Y, et al: Effective improvement of the cerebral vasospasm after subarachnoid hemorrhage with low-dose nitroglycerin. *J Cardiovasc Pharmacol* 35:45, 2000.

55. Armstrong PW, Armstrong JA, Marks GS: Blood levels after sublingual nitroglycerin. *Circulation* 59:585, 1979.

56. Mahmarian JJ, Fenimore NL, Marks GF, et al: Transdermal nitroglycerin patch therapy reduces the extent of exercise-induced myocardial ischemia: Results of a double-blind, placebo-controlled trial using quantitative thallium-201 tomography. *J Am Cardiol* 24:25, 1994.

57. Fallen EL, Nahmia SC, Scheffel A, et al: Redistribution of myocardial blood flow with topical nitroglycerin in patients with coronary arterial disease. *Circulation* 91:1381, 1995.

58. Parker JO, Amies MH, Hawkinson RW, et al: Intermittent transdermal nitroglycerin therapy in angina pectoris: Clinically effective without tolerance or rebound. *Circulation* 91:1368, 1995.

59. DeMots H, Glasser SP: Intermittent transdermal nitroglycerin therapy in the treatment of chronic stable angina. *J Am Coll Cardiol* 13:786, 1989.

60. Freedman SB, Daxini BV, Noyce D, Kelly DT: Intermittent transdermal nitrates do not improve ischemia in patients taking beta-blockers or calcium antagonists: Potential role of rebound ischemia during the nitrate-free period. *J Am Coll Cardiol* 25:349, 1995.

61. Bogaert MG: Clinical pharmacokinetics of nitrates. *Cardiovasc Drugs Ther* 8:693, 1994.

62. Schaumann W: Pharmacokinetics of isosorbide dinitrate and isosorbide-5-mononitrate. *Int J Clin Pharmacol Ther Toxical* 27:445, 1989.

63. Parker JO and the Isosorbide-5-Mononitrate Study Group: Eccentric dosing with isosorbide-5-mononitrate in angina pectoris. *Am J Cardiol* 73:871, 1993.

64. Abrams J: The role of nitrates in coronary heart disease. *Arch Intern Med* 155:357, 1995.

65. Gunasekara NS, Noble S: Isosorbide 5-mononitrate. A review of a sustained-release formulation (Imdur) in stable angina pectoris. *Drugs* 57:261, 1999.

66. Chrysant SG, Glasser SP, Bittar N, et al: Efficacy and safety of extended release isosorbide mononitrate for stable effort angina pectoris. *Am J Cardiol* 72:1249, 1993.

67. Prakash A, Markham A: Long-acting isosorbide mononitrate. *Drugs* 57:93, 1999.

68. Waller DG: Optimal nitrate therapy with a once-daily sustained-release formulation of isosorbide mononitrate. *J Cardiovasc Pharmacol* 34 (Suppl 2):S21, 1999.

69. Webb DJ, Miurhead GJ, Wulff M, et al: Sildenafil citrate potentiates the hypotensive effect of nitric oxide donor drugs in male patients with stable angina. *J Am Coll Cardiol* 36:25, 2000.

70. Col J, Col-Debeys C, Lavenne-Pardonge E, et al: Propylene glycol induced heparin resistance during nitroglycerin infusion. *Am Heart J* 110:171, 1986.

71. Becker RC, Jeanne CM, Corrao JM, et al: Intravenous nitroglycerin induced heparin resistance: A qualitative antithrombin III abnormality. *Am Heart J* 119:1254, 1990.

72. Bode V, Weizel D, Franz G, et al: Absence of drug interaction between heparin and nitroglycerin: Randomized placebo-controlled crossover study. *Arch Intern Med* 150(10):2117, 1990.

73. Nicolini FA, Ferrini D, Ottani F, et al: Concurrent nitroglycerin therapy impairs tissue-type plasminogen activator–induced thrombolysis in patients with acute myocardial infarction. *Am J Cardiol* 74:662, 1994.

73a. Death AK, Nakhla S, McGrath KCY, et al: Nitroglycerin upregulates matrix metalloproteinase expression in human macrophages. *J Am Coll Cardiol* 39:1943, 2002.

74. Parker JO: Nitrate tolerance. *Am J Cardiol* 60:44H, 1987.

75. Mangione NJ, Glasser SP: Phenomenon of nitrate tolerance. *Am Heart J* 128:137, 1994.

76. Elkayam V: Tolerance to organic nitrates: Evidence, mechanisms, clinical relevance, and strategies for prevention. *Ann Intern Med* 114: 667, 1991.

77. Fung H-L, Bauer JA: Mechanisms of nitrate tolerance. *Cardiovasc Drugs Ther* 94-8:489, 1993.

78. Steering Committee, Transdermal Nitroglycerin Cooperative Study: Acute and chronic antianginal efficacy in continuous twenty-four hour application of transdermal nitroglycerin. *Am J Cardiol* 68:1263, 1991.

79. Thadani U, Fung H-L, Darke AC, Parker JO: Oral isosorbide dinitrate in angina pectoris: Comparison of duration of action and dose response relationship during actue and sustained therapy. *Am J Cardiol* 49:411, 1982.

80. Münzel T, Mollnau H, Hartmann M et al: Effects of a nitrate-free interval on tolerance, vasoconstrictor sensitivity and vascular superoxide production. *J Am Coll Cardiol* 36(2):628, 2000.

81. Abrams J, Elkayam U, Thadani U, Fung H: Nitrate tolerance: An historical overview. *Am J Cardiol* 81(1A):3-14A, 1998.

82. Glasser S: Prospects for therapy of nitrate tolerance. *Lancet* 353:1545, 1999.

83. Elkayam U, Roth A, Mehra A, et al: Randomized study to evaluate the relation between oral isosorbide dinitrate dosing interval and the development of early tolerance to its effect on left ventricular filling pressure in patients with chronic heart failure. *Circulation* 84:2040, 1991.

84. Frishman WH: Tolerance, rebound and time-zero effect of nitrate therapy. *Am J Cardiol* 70:436, 1992.

85. Ferratini M, Pirelli S, Merlini P, et al: Intermittent transdermal nitroglycerin monotherapy in stable exercise-induced angina: A comparison with a continuous schedule. *Eur Heart J* 10:998, 1989.

86. Abou-Mohamed G, Kaesemeyer WH, Caldwell RB, Caldwell RW: Role of L-arginine in the vascular actions and development of tolerance to nitroglycerin. *Br J Pharmacol* 130(2):211, 2000.

87. Gruhn N, Aldershvile J, Boesgaard S: Tetrahydrobiopterin improves endothelium-dependent vasodilation in nitroglycerin-tolerant rats. *Eur J Pharmacol* 416(3):245, 2001.

88. Milone SD, Pace-Asciak CR, Reynaud D, et al: Biochemical, hemodynamic, and vascular evidence concerning the free radical hypothesis of nitrate tolerance. *J Cardiovasc Pharmacol* 33(5):685, 1999.

89. Dikalov S, Fink B, Skatchkov M, Bassenge E: Comparison of glyceryl trinitrate-induced with pentaerythrityl tetranitrate-induced in vivo

formation of superoxide radicals: Effect of vitamin C. *Free Radic Biol Med* 27(1–2):170, 1999.

90. Bassenge E, Fink N, Skatchkov M, Fink B: Dietary supplement with vitamin C prevents nitrate tolerance. *J Clin Invest* 102(1):67, 1998.

91. Watanabe H, Kakihana M, Ohtsuka S, Sugishita Y: Randomized, double-blind, placebo-controlled study of the preventive effect of supplemental oral vitamin C on attenuation of development of nitrate tolerance. *J Am Coll Cardiol* 31(6):1323, 1998.

92. Gori T, Burstein JM, Ahmed S, et al: Folic acid prevents nitroglycerin-induced nitric oxide synthase dysfunction and nitrate tolerance. *Circulation* 104:1119, 2001.

93. Loscalzo J: Folate and nitrate-induced endothelial dysfunction: A simple treatment for complex pathology. *Circulation* 104:1086, 2001.

94. Berkenboom G, Fontaine D, Unger P, et al: Absence of nitrate tolerance after long-term treatment with ramipril: An endothelium-dependent mechanism. *J Cardiovasc Pharmacol* 34:517, 1999.

95. Munzel T: Does Nitroglycerin therapy hit the endothelium? (editorial). *J Am Coll Cardiol* 38:1102, 2001.

96. Hebert D, Lam JYT: Nitroglycerin rebound associated with vascular, rather than platelet, hypersensitivity. *J Am Coll Cardiol* 36:2311, 2000.

97. Kanamasa K, Hayashi T, Takenaka T, et al: Continuous long-term dosing with oral slow-release isosorbide dinitrate does not reduce incidence of cardiac events in patients with healed myocardial infarction. *Clin Cardiol* 24:608, 2001.

98. Nakamura Y, Moss AJ, Brown MW, et al: Long-term nitrate use may be deleterious in ischemic heart disease: A study using the databases from two large-scale post-infarction studies. Multicenter Myocardial Ischemia Research Group. *Am Heart J* 138:577, 1999.

99. Miller RR, Vismara LA, Zelis R, et al: Clinical use of sodium nitroprusside in chronic ischemic heart disease: Effect on peripheral vascular resistance and venous tone on ventricular volume, pump and mechanical performance. *Circulation* 51:328, 1975.

100. Mann T, Cohn P, Holman BL, et al: Effect of nitroprusside on regional myocardial blood flow in coronary artery disease: Results in 25 patients and comparison with nitroglycerin. *Circulation* 52:732, 1978.

101. Macho P, Vatner SF: Effects of nitroglycerin and nitroprusside on large and small coronary vessels in conscious dogs. *Circulation* 64:1101, 1981.

102. Flaherty JT, Magee PA, Gardner TJ, et al: Comparison of intravenous nitroglycerin and sodium nitoprusside for the treatment of acute hypertension developing after coronary artery bypass surgery. *Circulation* 65:1172, 1981.

103. Cohn JN, Franciosa JA, Francis GS, et al: Effect of short-term infusion of sodium nitroprusside on mortality rate in acute myocardial infarction complicated by left ventricular failure. *N Engl J Med* 306:1129, 1982.

104. Durrer JD, Lie KI, van Chapelle FJL, Durrer D: Effect of sodium nitroprusside on mortality in acute myocardial infarction. *N Engl J Med* 306:1121, 1982.

105. Flaherty JT: Role of nitrates in acute myocardial infarction. In: Abrams J, Pepine C, Thadani U, eds. *Medical Therapy of Ischemic Heart Disease.* Boston, Little Brown, 1992:309.

106. Ryan TJ, Antman EM, Brooks NH, et al: ACC/AHA Guidelines for the management of patients with acute myocardial infarction. *Circulation* 100:1016, 1999.

107. Abrams J, Frishman WH, Bates SM, et al: Pharmacologic options for treatment of ischemic disease. In: Antman EM, ed. Cardiovascular Therapeutics, 2/e. Philadelphia: WB Saunders, 2002:97–153.

108. Darius H: Role of nitrates for the therapy of coronary artery disease patients in the years beyond 2000. *J Cardiovasc Pharmacol* 34(Suppl 2): S15, 1999.

CHAPTER 15

Antiadrenergic Drugs with Central Action and Neuron Depletors

Lawrence R. Krakoff

Drugs that reduce arterial pressure by interrupting the sympathetic nervous system are among the oldest antihypertensive agents. One of the first such agents to be shown effective in clinical trials was reserpine, derived from *Rauwolfia serpentina*—i.e., of herbal origin.[1] Medicinal chemistry and pharmacology led to the discovery of the autonomic ganglion blockers and guanethidine, all introduced before 1965. Methyldopa became available and widely prescribed in the 1960s. Clonidine, an alpha$_2$-receptor agonist, emerged in the 1970s; several similar drugs were then developed (guanabenz and guanfacine). Guanethidine was the first peripheral adrenergic neuron depletor. New neuron depletors were developed during the past few decades: bethanidine and guanadrel. Most of the drugs mentioned remain available for use in cardiovascular therapy, primarily as antihypertensive agents.[2–4] The ganglionic blockers, however, are either no longer available or are rarely prescribed.

A new class of drugs, the imidazole receptor agonists, acting at central I-1 receptor sites, are dealt with separately in Chap. 30.

This chapter focuses primarily on two groups of antiadrenergic drugs: (1) those whose action lies primarily within the central nervous system and (2) peripheral adrenergic neuron depletors. These drugs have all been used to treat hypertension, but some have been studied in congestive heart failure or have properties useful in cardiac arrhythmia management. The use of these agents for noncardiovascular indications (mainly anesthesia and pain management) is not included in this chapter.

CENTRALLY ACTING AGENTS: RESERPINE, METHYLDOPA, AND ALPHA$_2$ AGONISTS

The major pharmacologic features of the centrally acting agents covered in this chapter are given in Table 15-1. Most of the therapeutic effects of these drugs can be explained by effects within the brain's cardiovascular regulatory centers. Likewise the predominant adverse effects of these drugs are best related to their central action. Some other drug classes have minor central effects (the beta receptor blockers and some alpha$_1$-receptor blockers). These agents are discussed in other chapters.

Reserpine

Reserpine is a distinct antihypertensive drug that has both central and peripheral actions. Once absorbed, reserpine enters central and peripheral adrenergic and serotoninergic neurons. where it specifically eliminates amine storage granules. This action causes irreversible depletion of neurotransmitters through intraneuronal metabolism by monoamine oxidase. Blood pressure falls due to the sustained deficit in catecholamine release. Reserpine is rapidly eliminated from the circulation; its metabolism is poorly characterized. However, because of the time necessary for regeneration of new intraneuronal amine storage granules, there is a prolonged pharmacologic effect. After administration of reserpine is stopped, it may take weeks or even months for full adrenergic neuronal functional recovery.

Reserpine is an effective antihypertensive agent but has many adverse effects. Fatigue, depression, nasal congestion, and gastric hyperacidity have often often observed. Depression may occur insidiously months after initiation of treatment and can be severe, even leading to suicide. Reserpine causes salt/water retention, offsetting its antihypertensive effect (pseudotolerance) and then requiring the addition of a diuretic for control of pressure. Early retrospective studies implicated reserpine in breast cancer, but data from prospective studies show only a weak association between reserpine and breast cancer.[4a]

At present, reserpine is rarely used as monotherapy for hypertension. In combination with a thiazide-type diuretic, low-dose reserpine (0.1 mg daily) is highly effective for the reduction of pressure with an acceptable side effect experience.[5] Reserpine was employed as additional therapy to low-dose chlorthalidone in a treatment subgroup of the SHEP trial.[6] This study demonstrated the benefit of antihypertensive drug treatment for prevention of both fatal and nonfatal cardiovascular disease in elderly patients with isolated systolic hypertension.

Alpha Methyldopa

Alpha methyldopa is an antiadrenergic antihypertensive agent with multiple actions at central and peripheral sites. Originally developed as an inhibitor of dopa-decarboxylase, alpha methyldopa was conceived as a drug that would inhibit catecholamine synthesis (preventing the enzymatic conversion of dihydroxyphenylalanine, dopa, to dopamine by dopa decarboxylase). However, this effect was far too small to account for methyldopa's antihypertensive effect, as dopa decarboxylase is not a rate-limiting enzyme but is usually present in excess in a variety of tissues. Later studies led to the recognition that alpha methyldopa could be converted to alpha methyldopamine, a false neurotransmitter but also an alpha$_2$ agonist, with the central and peripheral actions of the other members of this group. More recently, it has been proposed that conversion of alpha methyldopa to alpha methyl epinephrine (by *N*-methylation) may also participate

TABLE 15-1. Major Features of the Centrally Acting Antiadrenergic Drugs

Name	Mechanism of Action	Usual Dose Range, Frequency	More Frequent Adverse Effects	Comments
Reserpine	Aminergic neuron depletor	0.05–0.1 mg	Sedation, fatigue nasal congestion, depression	Effective at low doses with diuretic
Alpha methyldopa	Mixed action: inhibits dopa decarboxylase, false transmitter	250–500 mg twice or three times a day	Fatigue, dizziness positive Coombs test Rare—hepatitis	Use generally limited to hypertension of pregnancy
Alpha methyldopa ester	Same as above	Intravenous form: 250–500 mg every 6–8 hours	Sedation	Same as above
Clonidine oral	Alpha$_2$ agonist	0.1–0.3 mg two to three times daily	Fatigue, dry mouth	Withdrawal overshoot hypertension
Clonidine TTS* skin patch	Alpha$_2$ agonist	One patch each week	Skin reactions	May be useful for less compliant patients
Guanabenz	Alpha$_2$ agonist	4–16 mg once or twice daily	Fatigue, dry mouth	Withdrawal overshoot hypertension
Guanfacine	Alpha$_2$ agonist	1–3 mg daily	Fatigue, dry mouth	Withdrawal overshoot hypertension

*Transdermal delivery system.

in this drug's hypotensive action. Alpha methyldopa is effective for only a portion of the day after administration of a single oral dose. It is usually prescribed as a twice-a-day agent.

Alpha methyldopa is an effective antihypertensive agent when given by mouth or intravenously. Prolonged treatment with alpha methyldopa is often associated with salt and water retention, reversing the antihypertensive effect (pseudotolerance), which then requires addition of a diuretic agent. The intravenous formulation is an ester of the parent drug and has been used for hypertensive emergencies, including toxemia of pregnancy.

Adverse effects related to alpha methyldopa are fatigue, somnolence, possible memory impairment, and diminished sexual function (reduced libido and impotence). Several of these are common to other centrally active agents. Unique to alpha methyldopa, however, are (1) a positive Coombs test (owing to appearance of an antibody directed against red cell Rh determinants), which occasionally causes significant hemolysis, and (2) a drug-induced hepatitis with fever, eosinophilia, and increased serum levels of hepatic enzymes, and (3) drug-induced lupus. The acute drug-induced hepatitis is self-limited, once alpha methyldopa is discontinued. There have been several case reports and small series of patients with chronic hepatitis and even cirrhosis found after many years of exposure to alpha methyldopa. Whether these cases were truly drug-induced or the consequence of undetected viral hepatitis (e.g., prior to the discovery of hepatitis C virus) is not certain. One drug surveillance study has reported an association of alpha methyldopa with acute pancreatitis.[7]

At present, alpha methyldopa is used as monotherapy or with hydralazine for pregnancy-related hypertension. Treatment of essential hypertension with alpha methyldopa as a single agent has become uncommon. While the combination of a thiazide-type diuretic with alpha methyldopa can reduce blood pressure, there are few recent studies evaluating this approach, either in comparison with other strategies or for outcomes.[7a] Thus, alpha methyldopa has become a "niche" drug for hypertension in pregnancy.[8]

Alpha$_2$-Receptor Agonists: Clonidine and Related Drugs

The classic alpha$_2$-receptor agonists have been well studied for their various effects. They reduce sympathetic tone within the brainstem by stimulating alpha$_2$ receptors on neurons of vasomotor centers that inhibit outflow of impulses to spinal preganglionic neurons. In addition, they may also achieve their effect by stimulating recently described imidazole receptors. In peripheral postganglionic noradrenergic neurons, stimulation of presynaptic alpha$_2$ receptors diminishes release of transmitter—a feedback system for control of intrasynaptic norepinephrine concentration. Thus, alpha$_2$ agonists reduce arterial pressure by both central and peripheral effects. However, at post- or nonsynaptic sites on cardiac or smooth muscle cells, alpha$_2$ receptors may be stimulated by alpha$_2$ agonists, causing an increase in pressure.[9] Thus a transient rise in pressure may occur within the first hour after a single dose of clonidine is given. Thereafter, blood pressure falls to well below pretreatment levels in parallel with a demonstrable decrement in sympathetic neural function. Clonidine's pressor effect accounts for occasional reports of hypertensive crises due to massive overdose of the drug when used in anesthesia.[10]

The reduction of sympathetic (noradrenergic) function due to administration of alpha$_2$-receptor agonists has been the basis of a clinically useful assessment, the clonidine suppression test. In this test, normal subjects and those with essential hypertension have a >40% reduction in plasma norepinephrine, 2 to 3 h after clonidine is given.[11,12] Patients with pheochromocytomas have little change in plasma norepinephrine concentration after clonidine is given, providing the rationale for the clonidine suppression test as a diagnostic assessment for these tumors.[13–15] Several forms of suspected neurogenic hypertension have been evaluated by the clonidine suppression test. Those with hypertension and neurovascular compression of the ventrolateral medulla oblongata (by magnetic resonance imaging) tend to have high baseline plasma norepinephrine, compared to those without vascular compression, but responses to clonidine are similar.[16] In a small series of four patients with hypertension associated with lumbosacral paraplegia, clonidine suppression of norepinephrine was >35% in three but <5% in one.[17]

Clonidine is the prototype alpha$_2$ agonist. Guanabenz and guanfacine are similar to clonidine but have longer durations of action. All the alpha$_2$ agonists are effective antihypertensive drugs as monotherapy[18] or in combination with a thiazide-type diuretic.[19] Both resting and exercise-induced blood pressure are decreased by these agents.[20] The available alpha$_2$ agonists have a similar pattern of adverse effects: sedation, dry mouth, and a tendency to overshoot or produce rebound hypertension on withdrawal. In sleep studies, clonidine has been found to reduce rapid-eye-movement (REM) sleep, presumably a detrimental effect, when compared with the beta blocker atenolol.[21] Clonidine has also been studied in sleep apnea, with inconsistent effects.[22] However, a case report describes severe somnolence with respiratory acidosis associated with clonidine treatment of a patient with known sleep apnea syndrome. Yohimbine, the alpha$_2$-receptor antagonist, was given and was thought to be beneficial in reversing the coma.[23]

Alpha$_2$ agonists are active as oral preparations. Clonidine, in addition, is effective as a transdermal delivery system (TTS), which releases medication at a relatively constant rate over 7 days. Some studies suggest that clonidine TTS is associated with fewer adverse effects, compared with tablets. This preparation may be useful for selected noncompliant patients who do not like to take pills. For patients already taking clonidine tablets and who must have surgery with general anesthesia, the TTS formulation can be used to maintain control of blood pressure and avoid rebound hypertension during the perioperative period, when medications cannot be given by mouth. Prolonged use of the TTS patch can cause a skin reaction severe enough that a change to alternative therapy becomes necessary.[23a]

Clonidine has been studied in congestive heart failure as a strategy to reduce the sympathetic activation often found in this disorder. Short-term studies suggest that reduction of sympathetic activity by clonidine may be beneficial in congestive heart failure.[24–27a] There is, however, evidence that presynaptic downregulation of norepinephrine release by alpha$_2$ agonists is impaired in congestive heart failure, which may limit the effectiveness of clonidine as treatment.[28] Outcome studies evaluating alpha$_2$ agonists in congestive heart failure have not been reported as of this writing.

In addition, oral clonidine has been shown to be effective in controlling rapid ventricular rates in patients with new-onset atrial fibrillation with an efficacy comparable to that of standard agents.[29]

PERIPHERAL NEURON DEPLETORS

Guanethidine, bethanidine, and guanadrel enter peripheral noradrenergic nerve terminals via amine uptake channels, where these drugs bind to norepinephrine storage vesicles, inhibiting transsynaptic release of transmitter. In addition, norepinephrine stores are depleted by displacement from vesicles and intraneuronal metabolism by monoamine oxidase. Both cardiac and vascular postganglionic sympathetic neurons are depleted by these drugs. Unlike reserpine, the peripheral neuron depletors do not damage or eliminate storage vesicles. Consequently, sympathetic neurotransmission returns to normal as drug concentration falls, with dissociation of the drug-vesicle complex. Duration of action is longest for guanethidine, about 24 h, and shorter for bethanidine and guanadrel, 6 to 10 h. Usual doses of these drugs are given below.

- Guanethidine: 10 to 50 mg daily
- Bethanidine: 25 to 50 mg once or twice daily
- Guanadrel: 10 to 50 mg twice daily

Reduction of sympathetic transmitter release during treatment with the neuron depletors affects basal or resting blood pressure but is much more prominent during standing or exercise, when sympathetic activity is normally increased. Orthostatic hypotension and/or exercise weakness, even syncope, have often been observed during treatment. It is therefore necessary to monitor both supine and standing blood pressures when these agents are used as antihyper-

tensive therapy. Bradycardia and possibly heart block may occur as a result of diminished cardiac adrenergic transmission. Other effects of reduced peripheral sympathetic function that may be observed during treatment with these agents are (1) retrograde ejaculation, (2) diarrhea-like change in bowel function, and (3) loss of normal adrenergic pupillary responses. Because the peripheral neuron depletors enter the nerve terminal via norepinephrine uptake, their action is prevented by drugs such as cocaine or tricyclic antidepressants (e.g., imipramine). This unique drug interaction accounts for the reversal of blood pressure control in patients receiving the peripheral neuron depletors when tricyclics are given concurrently.

The peripheral neuron depletors may be effective for treatment of hypertension as monotherapy or together with low-dose diuretics. This drug class has not been studied in congestive heart failure. In general, because of their prominent adverse effects, the peripheral neuron depletors have nearly disappeared from clinical use in the United States.

EFFECTIVENESS OF CENTRAL-ACTING DRUGS AND PERIPHERAL NEURON DEPLETORS

Assessment of antihypertensive drugs includes, as a primary measure, whether they have been found to prevent cardiovascular mortality and morbidity in randomized clinical trials. In this context, reserpine and alpha methyldopa deserve attention. Reserpine, in combination with a thiazide diuretic and hydralazine, reduced major trial end points compared to placebo in the Veterans Administration trial for severe and moderate hypertension.[29a] In the SHEP trial, reserpine was a second-step drug, given in addition to chlorthalidone for the treatment of isolated systolic hypertension in the elderly.[6] Methyldopa was used for active therapy in combination with a thiazide diuretic in several clinical trials of mild to moderate hypertension that are now considered pivotal in establishing the benefit of antihypertensive drug treatment.[30] However, there is insufficient evidence to conclude that either reserpine or alpha methyldopa is beneficial as monotherapy or are superior to other drug classes when used in addition to a diuretic. The other available centrally acting agents, the alpha$_2$ agonists, have infrequently been employed in the large, randomized clinical outcome trials.

Both the ganglionic blockers and guanethidine were evaluated for treatment of severe or malignant hypertension. Observational studies suggested that reduction of pressure in such patients was beneficial in comparison with historical controls or untreated patients by altering the rapidly fatal course of those with the highest blood pressure levels and evidence of extensive target-organ damage.

SPECIAL CONSIDERATIONS

Pregnancy

Few antihypertensive drugs have been thoroughly studied in pregnancy. The cumulative observations with alpha methyldopa over the past decades suggest that it is a safe and effective agent for use in pregnancy-induced hypertension or for treatment of hypertensive women who become pregnant.[31] In these settings, alpha methyldopa has the legitimacy of an extensive but largely uncontrolled clinical experience. However, the value of drug treatment for mild to moderate hypertension in pregnancy has never been fully established by randomized clinical trials. Recent systematic reviews focusing on this issue imply that the issue remains unresolved.[32,33]

Alcohol Withdrawal

The cessation of alcohol intake in those who drink to excess, alcohol withdrawal syndrome, is a hyperadrenergic state in which tachycardia, cardiac arrhythmias, and hypertensive episodes may accompany the agitation and other signs and symptoms of the disorder. The cardiovascular features of the alcohol withdrawal syndrome are due to centrally mediated activation of the sympathetic nervous system. Alpha$_2$ receptors may be downregulated, since the hypotensive response to clonidine during early alcohol withdrawal is less than that of age-matched controls.[34] Nonetheless, clonidine may be effective for reducing blood pressure and heart rate, if needed, during treatment of alcohol withdrawal. The sedative effect of clonidine is also beneficial in this situation but of lesser magnitude than that of the benzodiazepines.[35]

SUMMARY OF CURRENT AND RECOMMENDED USE

Most of the approved antihypertensive drugs reviewed in this chapter will have little or no role to play in the management of the majority of patients with essential hypertension, having been largely replaced by more recently developed drug classes. However, the long-term safety record for these drugs cannot be discounted. If hypertensive patients are well controlled on these older agents and have no related adverse effects, there is no compelling rationale for changing medication.

REFERENCES

1. Mashour NH, Lin GI, Frishman WH: Herbal medicine for the treatment of cardiovascular disease. *Arch Intern Med* 158:2225, 1998.
2. Oates JA, Brown NJ: Antihypertensive agents and the drug therapy of hypertension. In: Hardman JG, Limbird LE, eds. *Goodman & Gilman's The Pharmacological Basis of Therapeutics*, 10th ed. NY: McGraw-Hill, 2001:871–900.
3. Drugs for hypertension. *Med Lett* 43:17, 2001.
4. Materson BJ: Central and peripheral sympatholyticsL. In: Izzo JL, Black HR, eds. *Hypertension Primer,* 2nd ed. Dallas: American Heart Association 1999:370.
4a. Grossman E, Messerli FH, Goldbourt U: Carcinogenicity of antihypertensive therapy. *Curr Hypertens Rep* 4:195, 2002.
5. Kronig B, Pittrow DB, Kirch W, et al: Different concepts in first-line treatment of essential hypertension. Comparison of a low-dose reserpine-thiazide combination with nitrendipine monotherapy. German Reserpine in Hypertension Study Group. *Hypertension* 29:651, 2001.
6. SHEP Cooperative Research Group: Prevention of stroke by antihypertensive drug treatment in older persons with isolated systolic hypertension: Final results of the Systolic Hypertension in the Elderly Program SHEP. *JAMA* 265:3255, 1991.
7. Eland IA, van Puijenbroek EP Sturkenboom MJ, et al: Drug-associated acute pancreatitis: 21 years of spontaneous reporting in The Netherlands. *Am J Gastroenterol* 94:2417, 1999.
7a. Hall DR, Odendaal HJ: The addition of a diuretic to anti-hypertensive therapy for early severe hypertension in pregnancy. *Intl J Gynecol Obstet* 60:63, 1998.
8. Lindheimer MD, Akbari A: Hypertension in pregnant women. In: Oparil S, Weber MA, eds. *Hypertension: A Companion to Brenner and Rector's The Kidney.* Philadelphia: Saunders, 2000:688.
9. Brahmbhatt R, Baggaley P, Hockings B: Normalization of blood pressure in a patient with severe orthostatic hypotension and supine hypertension using clonidine. *Hypertension* 37:E24, 2001.
10. Frye CB, Vance MA: Hypertensive crisis and myocardial infarction following massive clonidine overdose. *Ann Pharmacother* 34:611, 2000.
11. Bravo EL, Tarazi RC, Fouad FM, et al: Clonidine-suppression test: A useful aid in the diagnosis of pheochromocytoma. *N Engl J Med* 305:623, 1981.
12. Hui TP, Krakoff LR, Felton K, Yeager K: Diuretic treatment alters clonidine suppression of plasma norepinephrine. *Hypertension* 8:272, 1986.
13. Bravo EL, Gifford RW Jr: Pheochromocytoma: Diagnosis, localization and management. *N Engl J Med* 311:1298, 1984.
14. Grossman E, Goldstein DS, Hoffman A, Keiser HR: Glucogan and clonidine testing in the diagnosis of pheochromocytoma. *Hypertension* 17:733, 1991.
15. Manelli M, Ianni L, Cilotti A, Conti A: Pheochromocytoma in Italy: A multicentric retrospective study. *Eur J Endocrinol* 141:619, 2001.
16. Makino Y, Kawano Y, Okuda N, et al: Autonomic function in hypertensive patients with neurovascular compression of the ventrolateral medulla oblongata. *J Hypertens* 17:1257, 2001.
17. Roche WJ, Nwofia C, Gittler M, et al: Catecholamine-induced hypertension in lumbosacral paraplegia: Five case reports. *Arch Phys Med Rehabil* 81:222, 2000.
18. Materson BJ, Reda DJ, Cushman WC, et al: Single-drug therapy for hypertension in men: A comparison of six antihypertensive agents with placebo. *N Engl J Med* 328:914, 1993.
19. Materson BJ, Reda DJ, Cushman WC, Henderson WG: Results of combination anti-hypertensive therapy after failure of each of the components. Department of Veterans Affairs Cooperative Study Group on Anti-hypertensive Agents. *J Hum Hypertens* 9:791, 1995.
20. Dziedzic SW, Elijovich F, Felton K, et al: Effect of guanabenz on blood pressure responses to posture and exercise. *Clin Pharm Ther* 33:151, 1983.
21. Danchin N, Genton P, Atlas P, et al: Comparative effects of atenolol and clonidine on polygraphically recorded sleep in hypertensive men: A randomized, double-blind, crossover study. *Int J Clin Pharmacol Ther* 33:52, 1995.
22. Issa FG: Effect of clonidine in obstructive sleep apnea. *Am Rev Respir Dis* 145:435, 1992.
23. Robege JR, Kimball ET, Warren J: Clonidine and sleep apnea syndrome interaction: Antagonism with yohimbine. *J Emerg Med* 16:727, 2001.
23a. Murphy M, Carmichael AJ: Transdermal drug delivery systems and skin sensitivity reactions. Incidence and management. *Am J Clin Dermatol* 1:361, 2000.
24. Manolis AJ, Olympios C, Sifaki M, et al: Combined sympathetic suppression and angiotensin-converting enzyme inhibition in congestive heart failure. *Hypertension* 29:525, 2001.
25. Manolis AJ, Olympios C, Sifaki M, et al: Suppressing sympathetic activation in congestive heart failure: A new therapeutic strategy. *Hypertension* 26:719, 1995.
26. Azevedo ER, Newton GE, Parker JD: Cardiac and systemic sympathetic activity in response to clonidine in human heart failure. *J Am Coll Cardiol* 33:186, 1999.
27. Grassi G, Turri C, Seravalle G, et al: Effects of chronic clonidine administration on sympathetic nerve traffic and baroreflex function in heart failure. *Hypertension* 38:286, 2001.
27a. Gavras I, Manolis AJ, Gavras H: The alpha$_2$-adrenergic receptors in hypertension and heart failure: Experimental and clinical studies. *J Hypertens* 19:2115, 2001.
28. Aggarwal A, Esler MD, Socratous F, Kaye DM: Evidence for functional presynaptic alpha-2 adrenoceptors and their down-regulation in human heart failure. *J Am Coll Cardiol* 37:1246, 2001.
29. Simpson CS, Ghali WA, Sanfilippo AJ, et al: Clinical assessment of clonidine in the treatment of new-onset rapid atrial fibrillation: A prospective, randomized clinical trial. *Am Heart J* 142:300, 2001.
29a. Effects of treatment on morbidity in hypertension. Results in patients with diastolic blood pressures averaging 115 through 129 mm Hg. *JAMA* 202:1028, 1967.
30. Collins R, Peto R, MacMahon S, et al: Blood pressure, stroke, and coronary heart disease: Part 2. Short-term reductions in blood pressure: Overview of randomized drug trials in their epidemiological context. *Lancet* 335:827, 1990.
31. August P: Management of pregnant hypertensive patients. In: Izzo JL Jr, Black HR, eds. *Hypertension Primer*, 2nd ed. Dallas: American Heart Association, 1999:427.

32. Abalos E, Duley L, Steyn DW, Henderson-Smart DJ: Antihypertensive drug therapy for mild to moderate hypertension during pregnancy (Cochrane Review). The Cochrane Library, 2001.

33. Magee LA, Duley L: Oral beta-blockers for mild to moderate hypertension during pregnancy (Cochrane Review). The Cochrane Library 2001.

34. Fahlke C, Berggren U, Balldin J: Cardiovascular responses to clonidine in alcohol withdrawal: Are they related to psychopathology and mental well-being? *Alcohol* 1:231, 2000.

35. Adinoff B: Double-blind study of alprazolam, diazepam, clonidine, and placebo in the alcohol withdrawal syndrome: Preliminary findings. *Alcohol Clin Exp Res* 18:873, 1994.

Nonspecific Antihypertensive Vasodilators

Lawrence R. Krakoff

Increased systemic vascular resistance has been considered a hemodynamic characteristic of arterial hypertension. In established essential hypertension and various forms of secondary hypertension, raised systemic vascular resistance is nearly always found when diastolic pressure is elevated. Nonetheless, reduced compliance of medium-sized and large arteries may also contribute to increased systolic pressure and wide pulse pressures in middle-aged and elderly hypertensives.[1] Both increased systemic vascular resistance and reduced arterial compliance (increased stiffness) may be partly due to activation of vascular smooth muscle. It is not surprising, then, that drugs which relax vascular smooth muscle, as a direct effect—i.e., vasodilators, specifically hydralazine—were among the first to be developed for treatment of hypertension. Other vasodilators, minoxidil and diazoxide, more recently defined as K(ATP)channel hyperpolarizers, have been developed and have found some use as antihypertensive agents.[2]

It became evident during the initial assessment of vasodilators that their antihypertensive effect led to activation of sympathetic baroreflexes, with tachycardia and increased cardiac output, in compensation for the reduction in peripheral (systemic) vascular resistance. Furthermore, fluid-volume retention and activation of the renin-angiotensin system were also a consequence of unopposed nonspecific systemic arteriolar vasodilation. By the 1970s, the orally active nonselective vasodilators became recognized as third-line antihypertensive drugs, to be used only in combination with diuretics and antiadrenergic agents, usually beta-receptor blockers, as the triple-drug regimen for severe hypertension. With the availability of angiotensin converting enzyme (ACE) inhibitors, angiotensin II type 1 receptor antagonists, and calcium-entry blockers, the hydralazine and K(ATP) hyperpolarizers have become less used as third- to fourth-line, last-resort drugs.[3,4] There are, however, a few specific places where these vasodilators may play more specific or important therapeutic roles, as described in this chapter.

PHARMACOLOGY AND CLASSIFICATION OF THE NONSPECIFIC VASODILATORS

Hydralazine

1-Hydrazinophthalazine (hydralazine) was one of the first available orally active vasodilators. The hydrazine (HN–NH2) in position 1 of the double-ringed phthalazine confers activity as a vasodilator.[2] Hydralazine is a direct arteriolar vasodilator, independent of any receptor blockade. Its mechanism of action remains somewhat unclear but seems to be dependent on endothelial cells and may be related to the formation of nitric oxide and/or hyperpolarization of

vascular smooth muscle cells and interruption of intracellular calcium action.

Hydralazine lowers systemic vascular resistance with activation of sympathetic reflexes, increased heart rate, and cardiac output on a neurogenic basis. The reflex-mediated changes in cardiac function after hydralazine treatment can be prevented by beta-receptor antagonists.[5] Chronic administration of hydralazine stimulates renin release, raising plasma renin activity. Salt and water retention with gain in weight are also observed. While the half-life of hydralazine, reflected by plasma concentrations, is 1 to 2 h, the antihypertensive effect may last for 6 to 12 h. The drug should be taken taken two to three times daily at 8- to 12-h intervals.

After absorption from the gastrointestinal tract, hydralazine is acetylated in the liver, to a varying degree. Slow and fast acetylators are represented almost equally in the population of the United States. Hydralazine is relatively less bioavailable for slow acetylators, who require higher oral doses for equal antihypertensive effect. Extrahepatic metabolism also occurs and accounts for the drug's elimination after reaching the circulation.

Adverse effects of hydralazine may be divided into two categories: (1) those related to the hemodynamic effect of the drug and (2) those specifically linked to its unique biochemical characteristics. Headaches, flushing, tachycardia, palpitations, angina-like chest discomfort or true angina of myocardial ischemia, dizziness, and orthostatic hypotension are the consequences of the vasodilating action of hydralazine and the significant sympathetic reflex activation as a physiologic response. In contrast, the hydralazine lupus syndrome, serum-sickness like reaction, hemolytic anemia, and glomerulonephritis syndromes seem best related to hydralazine itself and are more likely to occur in slow acetylators, often white women. Many patients treated with hydralazine who develop positive antinuclear antibodies do not proceed to symptomatic lupus. However, with so many alternative drugs, there is little basis for continuing antinuclear antibody (ANA)-positive patients on hydralazine in most situations. Vitamin B_6 (pyridoxal-responsive)-dependent polyneuropathy is a rare adverse effect of sustained hydralazine administration explainable by a direct chemical combination of the drug with pyridoxine, reducing supply of the cofactor for many enzymes. Both hydralazine lupus syndromes and polyneuropathy usually occur during treatment with doses more than 50 mg daily.

Hydralazine is effective for essential hypertension, pregnancy-induced hypertension, and congestive heart failure.

For treatment of essential hypertension, hydralazine is a third- or fourth-line drug to be added when a diuretic and a beta blocker and/or ACE inhibitor have not achieved control. Although hydralazine must be given two to three times a day (hindering compliance), the drug is inexpensive and may be necessary for use in those health care systems that have limited financial resources.[6] Otherwise, the once-a-day, long-acting calcium-channel blockers (nifedipine in controlled-release formulations, amlodipine, and felodipine) have largely replaced hydralazine in the multidrug combinations used to treat more severe or refractory hypertension.

Intramuscular or intravenous hydralazine remains useful for the treatment of hypertensive emergencies and severe pregnancy-induced hypertension, including toxemia.[7–9] Its value for mild to moderate hypertension in pregnancy is not established.[10] In studies of congestive heart failure, before the availability of the ACE inhibitors, hydralazine therapy used alone and in combination with isosorbide dinitrate was beneficial, especially when compared to the alpha$_1$-receptor blocker prazosin.[11] The advent of the ACE inhibitors and other strategies for the treatment of heart failure has rendered the use of hydralazine somewhat problematic.[12] Studies need to be done to determine whether there is any additional benefit from giving hydralazine to patients with heart failure already receiving diuretics, digoxin, ACE inhibitors, or angiotensin-receptor blockers and beta blockers.

ATP-K1 Channel Openers: Minoxidil and Diazoxide

The powerful arteriolar vasodilators minoxidil and diazoxide were developed in the 1970s for use in the treatment of severe and refractory hypertension and hypertensive emergencies. Minoxidil became a part of the triple drug regimen for treatment of severe hypertension, especially for patients who were unresponsive or had significant adverse reactions to hydralazine. Diazoxide, given as an intravenous bolus, was used for hypertensive emergencies as an alternative to sodium nitroprusside.

Minoxidil is a prodrug that becomes active with sulfation of an N–O site by a hepatic sulfotransferase. Minoxidil and diazoxide activate K(ATPase) channels, causing hyperpolarization of smooth muscle cell membranes with relaxation (vasodilation). Other K(ATPase) channel activators—nicorandil, cromokalim, aprikalim, bimakalim, and emakalim (see Chap. 28)—have been assessed as coronary artery vasodilators.[13] Some of the ATP-K1 channel activators inhibit release of insulin from pancreatic islet beta cells (long recognized as an effect of diazoxide), antagonizing the effect of the sulfonylureas at the K1 channel. Experimental studies suggest that diazoxide is the most potent agent for inhibition of hypoglycemia due to a sulfonylurea, with pinacidil having a detectable but lesser effect.[14,15]

ATP-K1 channel openers cause a profound nonselective reduction in systemic vascular resistance. Sympathetic reflexes are activated, causing tachycardia, increased cardiac output, and an increase in plasma norepinephrine. Beta-receptor blockade diminishes both the degree of tachycardia and the increase in cardiac output.[16] These drugs cause fluid retention in part by activation of the renin-angiotensin aldosterone system (pseudotolerance) and by intrarenal proximal and distal tubular mechanisms.[17] Sustained use of minoxidil may lead to increased pulmonary artery pressures—i.e., pulmonary hypertension—perhaps the result of the prolonged hyperdynamic state resulting from reduced precapillary vascular resistance and an arteriovenous shunt–like state. Other side effects of minoxidil include adverse effects on myocardial repolarization and peripheral effusions.[18]

The currently available ATP-K1 channel openers, minoxidil and diazoxide, are used only for severe hypertension when other agents are ineffective. At a dose of 5 to 20 mg once or twice daily, minoxidil in combination with a beta-receptor blocker and a potent diuretic (most often a loop-active agent such as furosemide) is almost always effective in reducing blood pressure. Weight gain, despite diuretic use, often occurs. Hair growth is inevitable and is usually cosmetically disfiguring.

Diazoxide is given by intravenous injection for hypertensive emergencies at doses of 150 to 300 mg (or reduced doses in children) by bolus injection or rapid intravenous infusion. Hypotension can occur, as the response to a given dose is unpredictable. Prolonged use of diazoxide often causes hyperglycemia due to inhibition of insulin release, an effect explained by activation of ATP-K1 channels.

Pinacidil has not been approved by the U.S. Food and Drug Administration. This drug has been studied as an antihypertensive agent and is very similar to minoxidil with regard its hemodynamic effects and pattern of adverse reactions.[19]

SUMMARY: EFFECTIVENESS AND CURRENT USE OF VASODILATORS

Hydralazine remains an effective third- or fourth-line drug for treatment of some patients with refractory hypertension, pregnancy-related severe hypertension, and perhaps selected patients with congestive heart failure. Minoxidil's use as an antihypertensive is limited to those with the most refractory hypertension who are willing to accept its adverse effects. Diazoxide may still be useful for hypertensive emergencies. However, with so many more promising agents now available, it is highly likely that both minoxidil and diazoxide will fall by the wayside in near future.

REFERENCES

1. McVeigh GE, Bratteli, CW, Morgan DJ, et al: Age-related abnormalities in arterial compliance identified by pressure pulse contour analysis: Aging and arterial compliance. *Hypertension* 33:1392, 1999.
2. Oates JA: Antihypertensive agents and the drug therapy of hypertension. In: Hardman JG, Limbird LE, Gilman AG, eds. *Goodman & Gilman's The Pharmacological Basis of Therapeutics.* New York: McGraw Hill 1996:780–808.
3. The Sixth Report of the Joint National Committee on Prevention, Detection, Evaluation, and Treatment of High Blood Pressure. *Arch Intern Med* 157:2413, 1997.
4. Guidelines Subcommittee: 1999 World Health Organization—International Society of Hypertension Guidelines for the Management of Hypertension. *J Hypertens* 17:151, 1999.
5. Warltier DC, Zyvoloski MG, Gross GJ, Brooks HL: Comparative actions of dihydropyridineslow channel calcium blocking agents in conscious dogs: Systemic and coronary hemodynamics with and without combined beta adrenergic blockade. *J Pharmacol Exp Ther* 230:367, 1984.
6. Seedat YK: Hypertension in developing nations in Sub-Saharan Africa. *J Hum Hypertens* 14:739, 2001.
7. Duley L, Henderson-Smart DJ: Drugs for rapid treatment of very high blood pressure during pregnancy (Cochrane Review). The Cochrane Library, 2000.
8. Ram CVS: Director vasodilators. In: Izzo JL Jr, Black HR, eds. *Hypertension Primer,* 2nd ed. Dallas, American Heart Association, 1999:385.
9. Calhoun DA: Hypertensive crisis. In: Oparil S, Weber MA, eds. *Hypertension: A Companion to Brenner and Rector's The Kidney.* Philadelphia: Saunders, 2000:715.
10. Abalos E, Duley L, Steyn DW, Henderson-Smart DJ: Antihypertensive drug therapy for mild to moderate hypertension during pregnancy (Cochrane Review). The Cochrane Library, 2001.
11. Cohn JN, Archibald DG, Ziesche S, et al: Effect of vasodilator therapy on mortality in chronic congestive heart failure: Results of a Veterans Administration Cooperative Study. *N Engl J Med* 314:1547, 1986.

12. Cohn JN, Johnson G, Ziesche S, et al: A comparison of enalapril with hydralazine-isosorbide dinitrate in the treatment of chronic congestive heart failure. *N Engl J Med* 325:303, 1991.

13. Haeusler G, Lues I: Therapeutic potential of potassium channel activators in coronary heart disease. *Eur Heart J* 15(Suppl C):82, 1994.

14. Clapham JC, Trail BK, Hamilton TC: K^+ channel activators, acute glucose tolerance and glibenclamide-induced hypoglycemia in the hypertensive rat. *Eur J Pharmacol* 257:79, 1994.

15. Links TP, Smit AJ, Reitsma WD: Potassium channel modulation: Effect of pinacidil on insulin release in healthy volunteers. *J Clin Pharmacol* 35:291, 1995.

16. Stone CK, Wellington KL, Willick A, et al: Acute hemodynamic effects of pinacidil in hypertensive patients with and without propranolol treatment. *J Clin Pharmacol* 31:333, 1991.

17. Krusell LR, Jespersen LT, Thomsen K, Pedersen OL: Proximal renal tubular pressure-natriuresis in essential hypertensives following acute vasodilation. *Blood Press* 2:40, 1993.

18. Sica DA, Gehr TW: Direct vasodilators and their role in hypertension management. *J Clin Hypertens* 3:110, 2001.

19. Fletcher AE, Battersby C, Adnitt P, et al: Quality of life on antihypertensive therapy: A double-blind trial comparing quality of life on pinacidil and nifedipine in combination with a thiazide diuretic. *J Cardiovasc Pharmacol* 20:108, 1992.

Antiarrhythmic Drugs

Tatjana N. Sljapic

Peter R. Kowey

Eric L. Michelson

Cardiac arrhythmias form a spectrum from clinically insignificant rhythms to life-threatening and lethal arrhythmias. Effective pharmacologic treatment of arrhythmias requires an understanding of the underlying mechanism of arrhythmia as well as the pharmacokinetics, pharmacodynamics, and electropharmacology of available antiarrhythmic medications. Whereas mechanisms have been established with some certainty for a number of arrhythmias, for many the mechanisms remain to be elucidated. Interrelationships between cardiac anatomy, nature and extent of structural heart disease, severity of functional impairment, cellular electrophysiology, metabolic fluxes, and factors such as ischemia and autonomic state are only beginning to be understood. Moreover, a profound revolution in our understanding of electrophysiology and electropharmacology is just emerging, based on major advances in genomics and molecular cardiology.[1,1a] Finally, the interface of advances in diagnostic techniques, interventional procedures, and devices must be integrated into any consideration of antiarrhythmic drugs in clinical practice. With these diverse factors acting within each patient, it should come as no surprise that antiarrhythmic drug action is often unpredictable[1b] and must be applied empirically to individual patients.

CLASSIFICATION

Several different classifications of antiarrhythmic drugs have been proposed in the past. A useful classification scheme should relate drug class, cellular electrophysiologic effects, and utility of various antiarrhythmic agents in specific clinical situations. Today, the most widely used classification system is a modification of the one proposed by Vaughn Williams[1c] (Table 17-1). It classifies drugs according to their effects on action potentials in individual cells. In this scheme, class I drugs block sodium channels responsible for the fast response in atrial, ventricular, and Purkinje tissues, depressing conduction velocity. Class I drugs are further divided into three subclasses based on (1) the kinetics of association and dissociation of the drug with the sodium channel, (2) the strength of channel blockade, and (3) the effects on repolarization. Class II drugs are beta-adrenergic receptor antagonists. Class III agents prolong cardiac repolarization, predominantly by blocking potassium channels during phases 2 and 3 of the action potential, thereby increasing tissue refractoriness. Class IV drugs block calcium channels, depressing the slow response in sinus nodal, atrioventricular (AV) nodal, and

perhaps in other cells. Admittedly, such a classification is a considerable oversimplification and does not account for autonomic nervous system effects or the action of agents such as digoxin or adenosine, for example, all of which need to be considered in discussing antiarrhythmic drugs. In addition, it has become clear that a single antiarrhythmic drug may have multiple effects on cardiac cells. For example, sotalol has beta-blocking activity (class II) and also significantly prolongs the action potential duration (class III). Amiodarone has been shown to have class I, II, III, and IV effects and perhaps other effects as well. Similarly, individual stereoisomers of drugs may have diverse effects. For example, the dextro isomer of sotalol possesses class III activity with only minimal beta-blocking activity, while the levo isomer possesses both beta-blocking and class III activity. Finally, many drugs undergo metabolism to electrophysiologically active metabolites, which may have electrophysiologic effects that differ from those of the parent compound. Procainamide, a class Ia drug, is metabolized in the liver to N-acetylprocainamide (NAPA), a drug with significant class III effects. A more recent classification scheme, called the Sicilian gambit, attempts to relate the various clinical effects of antiarrhythmic drugs to specific anatomic or physiologic weak points of target arrhythmias,[2] based on an understanding of ion channels and receptors and modulators of membrane activity. Although scientifically based and clinically oriented and therefore more appealing, it is not clear that this new classification will be more useful than the Vaughn Williams classification.

Successful clinical application of antiarrhythmic agents requires not only an understanding of the cellular electrophysiology of the drugs and a thorough understanding of their pharmacology but also knowledge of drug-drug interactions, hemodynamic effects, and the ancillary properties of these agents. Failure to consider these factors often results in drug inefficacy or toxicity. This chapter presents most antiarrhythmic drugs currently available in the United States. The pharmacology, electrophysiology, pharmacokinetics, antiarrhythmic effects, drug interactions, hemodynamic properties, side effects, indications, and dosing are presented. A complete discussion of these agents is beyond the scope of this chapter, and data for recently released drugs are often incomplete and based to a large measure on animal data and preliminary data from clinical studies. Adverse effects reported for new agents represent those effects seen in highly selected patient populations and are subject to investigator interpretation; they may not be representative of those seen in clinical practice. It should also be noted that virtually all antiarrhythmic

TABLE 17-1. Modified Vaughn Williams Classification of Antiarrhythmic Drugs

Main Electrophysiologic Properties		Examples
I	Ia Sodium-channel blockade	Quinidine
	Intermediate channel kinetics	Procainamide
	Repolarization lengthened	Disopyramide
	Ib Sodium-channel blockade	Lidocaine
	Rapid channel kinetics	Mexiletine
		Tocainide
	Ic Sodium-channel blockade	Flecainide
	Slow channel kinetics	Propafenone
		Moricizine
II	Beta-adrenergic blockade	Propranolol
		Esmolol
		Acebutolol
III	Potassium-channel blockade	Sotalol*
	Sodium-channel activation	Amiodarone
		Ibutilide
		Dofetilide
IV	Calcium-channel blockade	Verapamil
		Diltiazem

*Also major class II properties.

drugs have the potential to depress automaticity, conduction, and contractility; all have potential proarrhythmic effects. One characteristic form of proarrhythmia is the occurrence of polymorphic ventricular tachycardia in association with QT prolongation, known as torsades de pointes. In addition, in many cases, there is relatively little information available on the effects of various drugs on abnormal myocardium or in patients with more advanced cardiac pathologies.

Antiarrhythmic drugs must also be considered potential cardiac toxins. A physician treating a patient with an arrhythmia hopes the drug is more toxic to tissue involved with the arrhythmia than to the rest of the heart or patient. Often this is not the case, as the therapeutic index of these drugs can be quite low. In addition, noncardiac side effects are frequent. Achievement of therapeutic drug levels does not guarantee efficacy or eliminate the risk of toxicity. Furthermore, agents effective for the acute management of arrhythmias may not be effective for chronic prophylaxis. The failure to reduce or paradoxically increase mortality also exists with antiarrhythmic drugs, as demonstrated by the Cardiac Arrhythmia Suppression Trial (CAST).[3] Thus, antiarrhythmic therapy should be used cautiously and ideally should be reserved for those situations that significantly affect a patient's duration or quality of life. At the very least, it is incumbent upon practitioners to have a knowledge of the full prescribing information for drugs approved for use in the United States, so as to maximize the chance of benefit while minimizing the risk of harm. For most drugs, only limited information is available in special populations, such as pediatric and pregnant patients, and additional caution is warranted.

OVERVIEW OF OPTIMAL ANTIARRHYTHMIC MANAGEMENT

Although a complete discussion of the clinical use of antiarrhythmic drugs is beyond the scope of this chapter, the following generalizations for commonly occurring arrhythmias may be made.

Atrial Fibrillation

Atrial fibrillation is the most common sustained tachyarrhythmia encountered in clinical practice. Management goals include (1) prevention of thromboembolism and stroke, (2) control of ventricular rate, and (3) restoration and maintenance of sinus rhythm. Consensus guidelines have been published that provide a framework for the evidence-based management of patients with atrial fibrillation.[4] Almost all patients with atrial fibrillation—paroxysmal, persistent, or permanent—should be anticoagulated with warfarin to reduce the risk of thromboembolism. Exceptions include those patients with a contraindication to warfarin and those younger than 65 years of age with no structural heart disease (lone atrial fibrillation). Aspirin therapy may be useful for patients with a contraindication to warfarin. Control of ventricular rate by slowing impulse conduction through the AV node has been achieved for more than a century with digitalis preparations. Although effective at rest, digitalis is unable to control ventricular rate adequately during exercise or other clinical states with elevated levels of catecholamines. In many patients, better control may be achieved by utilizing beta-blocking agents or calcium channel blockers such as verapamil or diltiazem. Intravenous agents such as esmolol or diltiazem can be used to rapidly achieve rate control; longer-acting drugs can then be used for chronic therapy. Other antiarrhythmics, such as class Ic drugs and amiodarone also slow the ventricular rate. Patients with excessive tachycardia due to inadequate rate control (average heart rate over the day above 80 beats per minute and the maximum heart rate more than 110% of the maximum predicted heart rate for that patient) may develop cardiomyopathy with progression to congestive heart failure. Patients whose heart rate is uncontrollable using combinations of agents (i.e., digoxin and verapamil or propranolol) should be considered for catheter ablative techniques and permanent pacemaker implantation. Antiarrhythmic drugs are useful to restore sinus rhythm and lessen the duration between episodes of atrial fibrillation. Agents used for these purposes include class Ia drugs (quinidine, procainamide, and disopyramide); class Ic drugs (propafenone and flecainide); class II agents; and class III agents (sotalol, amiodarone, and dofetilide). In general, antiarrhythmic drugs do not eliminate recurrent episodes of atrial fibrillation but can increase the duration of sinus rhythm between recurrences. Beta-blocking drugs are especially useful for this purpose in patients immediately after cardiac surgery. Class III agents (amiodarone, sotalol, and dofetilide) are being used more frequently for control of atrial fibrillation. Ibutilide, a class III agent, is used in bolus fashion to chemically cardiovert patients to sinus rhythm. It has been effective in approximately 40 to 70% of patients. Nonpharmacologic techniques for control of atrial fibrillation are rapidly being developed and include radiofrequency catheter ablation/isolation of pulmonary vein foci, catheterbased or surgical MAZE procedure, and tachy/brady device–based therapies. A large multicenter study has been conducted by the National Institutes of Health (NIH) to determine whether optimized antiarrhythmic drug therapy administered to maintain sinus rhythm in patients having episodes of atrial fibrillation/flutter has an impact on total mortality and disabling stroke when compared to optimized therapy that merely controls heart rate in patients with atrial fibrillation/flutter [atrial fibrillation follow-up investigation of rhythm management (AFFIRM)].[5] Preliminary results indicate that in these selected patients who tolerated atrial fibrillation sufficiently well that they were candidates for rate control, a strategy of rhythm control with the currently available antiarrhythmic drugs did not result in better outcomes. Effective anticoagulation was important for reduction of stroke risk with both approaches. Among available treatments, amiodarone was the most effective in maintaining sinus rhythm.

Atrial Flutter

In many ways, management of atrial flutter is similar to that of atrial fibrillation. Acute control of ventricular rate is usually achieved through intravenous therapy, using either a beta-blocking agent such as esmolol or propranolol or a calcium-channel blocking drug such as verapamil or diltiazem. Infusions of esmolol or diltiazem may be preferred due to their short half-life, which permits finer control of ventricular rate with a faster offset in case hypotension or excessive bradycardia develops. Chronic control of ventricular rate with atrial flutter is difficult, but similar types of agents, given orally, are commonly used. Digoxin alone is rarely sufficient except in patients with intrinsic AV nodal dysfunction. Direct current (DC) cardioversion or atrial overdrive pacing are the most rapid methods used to restore sinus rhythm, although pharmacologic conversion may become more frequent in the future. Ibutilide appears uniquely able to rapidly terminate established atrial flutter in a majority of patients.[6] The risk of embolization and stroke after conversion from atrial flutter appears to be less than with atrial fibrillation, although the majority of clinicians also anticoagulate patients with atrial flutter. Oral antiarrhythmic drugs—such as quinidine, procainamide, disopyramide, sotalol, amiodarone, dofetilide, flecainide, moricizine, and propafenone—may be used to restore and maintain sinus rhythm. Particular care must be used when administering class Ia or Ic agents to patients with atrial flutter. These drugs may slow the atrial rate, whereas the anticholinergic effects of some of these agents may facilitate AV nodal conduction, resulting in an acceleration of ventricular rate. Occasionally, 1:1 conduction of the flutter impulse may occur, resulting in a ventricular rate between 220 and 250 beats per minute, which may cause hemodynamic compromise. This complication may be averted by ensuring adequate AV nodal blockade prior to instituting therapy with these agents. Amiodarone slows AV conduction in addition to other antiarrhythmic properties and may be used as a single agent. Administration of adenosine to patients with atrial flutter will increase AV block, allowing visualization of flutter waves. AV conduction may paradoxically improve after adenosine administration and has also caused 1:1 AV conduction. Nonpharmacologic therapy for atrial flutter is increasingly being used,[6a] Radiofrequency catheter ablation of the isthmus of atrial tissue between the tricuspid valve and inferior vena cava annulus is effective at preventing recurrences of atrial flutter. Alternatively, for intractable cases, ablation of the AV junction to create complete heart block with insertion of a permanent pacemaker may be performed.

AV-Nodal Reentrant Tachycardia

After atrial fibrillation and atrial flutter, AV-nodal reentrant tachycardia is the most common form of supraventricular tachycardia. This arrhythmia is caused by a reentrant circuit within the AV node and perinodal tissues. Therefore pharmacologic therapies are directed toward the AV node. Acute management includes vagal maneuvers such as carotid sinus massage or Valsalva. Administration of adenosine or verapamil intravenously will universally terminate this arrhythmia. Similarly, intravenous beta blockers, diltiazem, or verapamil can be effective. Agents useful for long-term pharmacologic management include digoxin, beta-adrenergic-receptor antagonists,

and calcium-channel antagonists such as verapamil or diltiazem. In unusual cases propafenone, flecainide, or amiodarone may be useful. Patients with this arrhythmia are also effectively being treated with radiofrequency catheter modification of the AV-nodal slow pathway.

AV-Reentrant Tachycardia (Wolff-Parkinson-White Syndrome)

Patients with Wolff-Parkinson-White (WPW) syndrome have an anatomic fiber of myocardium which directly connects the atria and ventricles. This fiber may conduct cardiac impulses unidirectionally from atria to ventricles or from the ventricles to atria, but bidirectional impulse conduction is also common. Because of the presence of dual pathways (the normal AV conduction system being the antegrade or retrograde limb) for impulse conduction from atria to ventricles, reentrant arrhythmias are possible. The most common tachycardia, orthodromic reciprocating tachycardia, utilizes the bypass tract in a retrograde (ventriculoatrial) direction and generally results in a narrow QRS tachycardia. Atrial fibrillation or flutter commonly occurs in conjunction with the WPW syndrome; if the accessory pathway is capable of antegrade (AV) conduction, an irregular rhythm with both wide and narrow QRS complexes, often at rapid rates (if the antegrade effective refractory period of the accessory pathway is short), will occur. Rarely, such patients will develop ventricular fibrillation (VF) from exceedingly rapid ventricular rates. The least common arrhythmia, antidromic reciprocating tachycardia, utilizes the bypass tract in an antegrade direction and results in a regular wide-complex arrhythmia resembling ventricular tachycardia (VT). Any of the above arrhythmias should be terminated using synchronized DC cardioversion if hemodynamic collapse is present. Patients with a narrow QRS tachycardia are best treated with vagal maneuvers, followed, if necessary, by intravenous adenosine, esmolol, diltiazem, or verapamil. Caution should be used with adenosine in patients with known WPW syndrome, since adenosine may produce atrial fibrillation. If rapid antegrade conduction over the bypass tract is possible, hemodynamic collapse may occur. A DC defibrillator should always be immediately available whenever adenosine is used. Patients with wide complex tachycardias and WPW syndrome should be treated as if they had VT. Intravenous procainamide or ibutilide is the therapy of choice if cardioversion is not required. Digoxin should not be used to treat patients with a bypass tract capable of antegrade conduction as it may accelerate impulse conduction over the tract.

The need for chronic pharmacologic therapy for patients with WPW syndrome has almost been completely eliminated by the success of radiofrequency catheter ablation. When necessary, patients without antegrade bypass-tract conduction may often be treated with either a beta blocker or calcium-channel blocking drug. Patients with antegrade bypass tract conduction or those with arrhythmia recurrences during therapy with beta-blockers or calcium-channel blocking drugs should be treated with a class Ia, Ic, or III drug. Flecainide, propafenone, quinidine, procainamide, disopyramide, or moricizine may be used, often in conjunction with a beta-blocking agent. Sotalol, with beta-blocking and class III activity, may also be used. Amiodarone, while effective, is rarely necessary.

Atrial Tachycardia

Atrial tachycardia is an uncommon supraventricular tachycardia caused by abnormal automaticity or reentry within the atria.

Patients with structural heart disease, especially after surgical correction of congenital heart disease, have reentrant atrial tachycardias due to atrial suture lines. Automatic atrial tachycardias are often self-limited and may disappear after several months to years. Patients with atrial tachycardias are often symptomatic, and pharmacologic treatment is justified. Long-standing tachycardias, with heart rates in excess of 130 beats per minute, may produce a dilated cardiomyopathy and congestive heart failure.

Innapropriate sinus tachycardia is an uncommon disorder, still poorly understood. Abnormal autonomic influence on the sinus node, either excessive sympathetic tone or reduced vagal tone, is one possible explanation.[7] The first-line therapy should be pharmacologic, including beta-blockers, calcium-channel blockers, and class Ia or Ic agents.

Automatic tachycardias are sometimes amenable to treatment with beta-blocking or calcium-channel blocking drugs such as propranolol or verapamil. In more resistant cases, class Ic drugs such as flecainide or propafenone may be helpful. Some cases of atrial tachycardia are refractory to pharmacologic therapy and require catheter ablation for control. Reentrant atrial tachycardias often require therapy with class Ia, Ic, or III antiarrhythmic drugs. Sotalol, flecainide, and amiodarone are often used. Unlike automatic arrhythmias, reentrant arrhythmias rarely are self-limited, requiring therapy for life. Patients with these arrhythmias often undergo catheter ablation to avoid lifelong antiarrhythmic drug therapy. Multifocal atrial tachycardia appears to result from a diffuse increase in atrial automaticity. It is commonly seen in patients with severe lung disease and may be facilitated by theophylline, inhaled or oral beta-adrenergic stimulants, and possibly digoxin. Therapy with either verapamil or metoprolol has been shown to be helpful, although any long-term therapy should include improving underlying lung function.[8]

Ventricular Tachycardia

VT is a heterogeneous collection of ventricular tachyarrhythmias caused by several different arrhythmia mechanisms that occur in patients with varying degrees of structural heart disease.[8a] Most commonly, VT is a reentrant arrhythmia occurring in a patient with coronary artery disease, prior myocardial infarction, and frequently left ventricular (LV) dysfunction. Hemodynamic collapse is a common result of VT that is not self-terminating; sudden cardiac death is often the final result.

Occasionally, VT may be hemodynamically tolerated. In these individuals, intravenous infusion of lidocaine, procainamide, or amiodarone may result in the slowing and often termination of arrhythmia. Ventricular overdrive pacing is also effective, but synchronized DC cardioversion (with appropriate sedation and anesthesia) is the quickest method to restore a normal rhythm. However, most episodes of VT terminate spontaneously and produce no symptoms. Optimal management of these patients is currently unknown.

Intravenous lidocaine, procainamide, bretylium, and amiodarone are useful acutely for the prevention of VT recurrences. Class III agents sotalol and amiodarone are increasingly being used as chronic therapy for symptomatic VT. Other useful agents include mexiletine, quinidine, procainamide, disopyramide, propafenone, flecainide, and moricizine. All these agents have appreciable cardiac and noncardiac side effects, and depending on the method used to judge efficacy, each may be effective in only 10 to 30% of patients. It does appear certain that whatever pharmacologic agent is employed must be proved effective, either by suppression of ambient ectopy,

by Holter monitoring, or by means of electrophysiologic testing. VT with a continuously changing QRS morphology occurring in the setting of a prolonged QT interval (torsades de pointes) is a unique form of VT. This arrhythmia is often due to effects of antiarrhythmic drugs that prolong the action potential (classes Ia and III). Although this form of VT often terminates spontaneously, VF and sudden death may occur. Acute therapy consists of normalization of potassium and magnesium levels, along with acceleration of the heart rate to 110 to 120 beats per minute by pacing or infusion of isoproterenol. Chronic therapy consists of elimination of all agents that prolong the duration of action potentials. If it is necessary to treat other arrhythmias, amiodarone appears safe for use in patients with torsades de pointes despite its ability to markedly prolong the QT interval. Torsades de pointes can also occur as a familial form of arrhythmia as a result of mutations to DNA encoding either the cardiac sodium- or potassium-channel proteins.

Unusual forms of VT may occur in apparently structurally normal hearts. VT with left bundle branch morphology and an inferior frontal plane axis often originates from the right ventricular outflow tract. This arrhythmia is often catecholamine-sensitive; it is frequently induced by exercise. Beta-blocker drugs, calcium-channel blockers, or catheter ablation is usually effective. Another unique type of VT, idiopathic LV VT, has a right-bundle-branch QRS morphology with a superior frontal-plane axis. This VT is often responsive to verapamil; catheter ablation is also effective. However, most patients with right-bundle superior axis VT will not have the verapamil-sensitive type. It is also worth noting that verapamil should not be administered to patients during VT except when the VT is known by prior electrophysiologic testing to be verapamil-sensitive. Administration of verapamil to patients with VT and coronary artery disease has resulted in hypotension and several deaths. Implantable cardioverter-defibrillators (ICDs) are currently being increasingly used for patients with recurrent hemodynamically destabilizing VT as well as for primary prophylaxis in patients with history of coronary artery disease (CAD), LV systolic dysfunction, nonsustained VT (NSVT), and inducible VT during programmed electrical stimulation. In a large randomized trial of patients with CAD, ejection fraction (EF) below 40%, NSVT, and inducible VT, ICD therapy significantly reduced the incidence of arrhythmic death and total mortality.[9] Other therapies, such as endocardial resection and catheter ablative techniques may be useful in selected patients.

Ventricular Fibrillation

Immediate DC countershock is the appropriate response to VF. After a hemodynamically stable rhythm has been restored, antiarrhythmic therapy may be useful to prevent recurrences of this lethal arrhythmia.[9a] Acceptable intravenous medications include lidocaine, procainamide, bretylium, and amiodarone. Adjunctive therapies, such as relief of myocardial ischemia and correction of electrolyte imbalance are often helpful. Small doses of an intravenous beta-blocking agent—such as propranolol, metoprolol, or esmolol—can have a surprisingly beneficial effect as well. Patients with frequent recurrences of VF whose intrinsic rhythm is relatively bradycardic may be helped by temporary atrial or ventricular pacing at heart rates of approximately 100 to 120 beats per minute. Chronic antiarrhythmic drug therapy for the prevention of recurrences of VF should ideally be guided by either serial electrophysiologic testing or serial Holter monitoring to ensure drug efficacy. Common choices include sotalol or amiodarone. Empiric therapy with amiodarone has been evaluated as one therapy arm in the multicenter Antiarrhythmic Drug Versus Implantable Defibrillator (AVID) study. In this study 1016 patients with CAD, EF < 40%, and VF or VT with syncope/hemodynamic compromise were randomized to empiric therapy with amiodarone plus Holter/EP (electrophysiologic)-guided sotalol versus ICD. ICD therapy has proven to be effective in reducing arrhythmic but not total mortality as compared with antiarrhythmic drugs, and this benefit was most prominent in patients with EF <35%.[10] Of course, implantable cardioverter defibrillators do not prevent recurrences of ventricular tachyarrhythmias, but immediately resuscitate patients when these arrhythmias are detected. Often combined therapy of an ICD with antiarrhythmic drug therapy is necessary in patients with frequent episodes of ventricular tachyarrhythmias.[11] Unfortunately, no currently available primary antiarrhythmic drug therapy has been demonstrated to substantially reduce the incidence of sudden cardiac death, a major cause of mortality. Only beta-blockers, when used as adjunctive therapy in patients with heart failure or recent myocardial infarction, have shown a significant benefit.

CLASS Ia AGENTS

Class Ia drugs block the sodium channel and fast response, predominantly in atrial, ventricular, and Purkinje tissue. The maximum rate of rise of phase 0 of the action potential is depressed, slowing conduction velocity. The potency of channel blockade is moderate, and repolarization (action potential duration) is prolonged. In addition, the drugs kinetics of channel association and dissociation may be on the order of several seconds, and consequently, drug effects are typically more profound at more rapid heart rates. Class Ia antiarrhythmic drugs are effective for many atrial and ventricular tachyarrhythmias.

Quinidine

Pharmacologic Description

Quinidine, an optical isomer of quinine, is an alkaloid derived from cinchona bark. First described by van Heynigen in 1848, quinidine was given its present name by Louis Pasteur in 1853. Use of cinchona in patients with atrial fibrillation was described by Jean Baptiste de Senac of Paris in 1749.

Electrophysiologic Action

Quinidine is a prototypic class Ia antiarrhythmic agent. It decreases the slope of phase 0 of the action potential, decreases the amplitude of the action potential, and slows conduction velocity in atrial, ventricular, and Purkinje tissue.[12] In addition, quinidine delays repolarization, thereby increasing the duration of action potentials. Electrocardiographic effects include prolongation of the QT as well as corrected QT (QTc) and QRS intervals. QRS prolongation greater than 35 to 50% of baseline is usually associated with toxicity.

Pharmacokinetics and Metabolism

Quinidine is currently available as quinidine sulfate, quinidine gluconate, and quinidine polygalacturonate. The bioavailability of quinidine ranges from 47 to 96%, averaging 75%.[13] The milligrams of quinidine base in different preparations vary, and thus should be considered in dosing, particularly when switching formulations. The

bioavailability of the gluconate preparation is 10% less than that of the quinidine sulfate. After oral ingestion of quinidine sulfate, peak plasma concentrations occur within 60 to 90 min. The gluconate preparation is more slowly absorbed, with peak levels occurring 4 h after dosing. The elimination half-life ranges between 6 and 8 h. The clearance of quinidine is decreased in patients with significant hepatic insufficiency and with advancing age.[14,15] Smaller maintenance doses are required in these patients. Advanced renal disease has only minimal effects on quinidine clearance.[16] Approximately 90% of quinidine is bound to plasma proteins. Several cardioactive metabolites have been identified including (3S)-3-hydroxyquinidine, (3OH) quinidine and quinidine-N-oxide (QNO).[17] Although these metabolites are less active than the parent compound (approximately 25% and 4% for 3OH-Q and QNO, respectively), in approximately one-fourth of patients their concentrations may approach or even exceed that of quinidine and contribute significantly to the overall electrophysiologic effects of the drug. As these metabolites are not measured in all assays, quinidine levels may underestimate the potential activity of the drug under steady-state conditions.

Hemodynamic Effects

Quinidine is an alpha-adrenergic receptor antagonist that lowers peripheral vascular resistance. Whereas large oral doses can produce hypotension through this mechanism, the problem is most common with intravenous dosing. Although quinidine directly depresses myocardial contractility, clinically significant myocardial depression usually does not occur except with large intravenous doses.

Antiarrhythmic Effects

Quinidine can suppress a wide variety of supraventricular and ventricular arrhythmias. In life-threatening ventricular tachyarrhythmias, quinidine has shown long-term efficacy in 15 to 30% of patients with VT or cardiac arrest when guided by electrophysiologic testing.[18,19] Quinidine can also terminate atrial flutter or fibrillation in many patients, especially when these conditions are of recent onset and if the atria are not enlarged. Quinidine also has vagolytic effects, which can enhance AV-nodal conduction. In some patients, this can result in an increased ventricular rate with some atrial tachyarrhythmias, such as atrial flutter, unless an AV-nodal blocking agent is also given. Typically, therapeutic levels range from 3 to 6 μg/mL.

Side Effects

Gastrointestinal side effects are common, with diarrhea and nausea the most bothersome. Quinidine may cause tinnitus, blurred vision, dizziness, light-headedness, and tremor, a syndrome known as cinchonism. Rarely, severe antibody-mediated thrombocytopenia, pancytopenia, or hemolytic anemia may occur. Side effects may require cessation of therapy in as many as 30% of patients.[20] Up to 3 to 4% of patients receiving quinidine may develop quinidine syncope, a form of proarrhythmia usually caused by rapid polymorphic VT associated with prolongation of the QT interval (torsades de pointes). Other cases have been attributed to sinus pauses or first-dose hypotension related in part to alpha-adrenergic receptor blockade. The risk of serious proarrhythmia is greatest during the first few days of dosing, during bradycardia or hypokalemia. Many advocate the initiation of quinidine therapy in the hospital with electrocardiographic (ECG) monitoring, particularly in patients with cardiac dysfunction.

Interactions

Drugs that alter the kinetics of hepatic enzyme systems—such as phenobarbital, phenytoin, and rifampin—can increase hepatic metabolism of quinidine and reduce its concentration. Cimetidine, on the other hand, decreases hepatic metabolism of quinidine, increasing the plasma concentration.[21] In addition, the concomitant administration of amiodarone increases the concentration of many antiarrhythmic drugs, including quinidine. Quinidine increases serum levels of digoxin by decreasing digoxin clearance, volume of distribution, and affinity of tissue receptors for digoxin, and thus may contribute to digoxin toxicity.[22,23] Digitoxin levels are also increased. Recently quinidine has been shown to be a potent inhibitor of cytochrome P450db1, a genetically determined polymorphic enzyme responsible for the oxidative metabolism of many drugs by the liver. Because of inhibition of this enzyme system, quinidine substantially decreases the metabolism of some drugs, such as encainide and propafenone,decreasing the concentration of their metabolites while increasing the concentrations of the parent compounds.[24,25]

Indications and Dosage

Quinidine is indicated for the treatment of incapacitating atrial, AV-nodal, and ventricular tachyarrhythmias. The usual adult dose of quinidine sulfate is 200 to 400 mg four times daily, or less frequently with longer-acting preparations. Intravenous quinidine gluconate is occasionally used in special situations such as the electrophysiology laboratory and may be given using a dose of 6 to 10 mg/kg at a rate of 0.3 to 0.5 mg/kg/min with frequent checks of blood pressure and ECG parameters. In some patients, efficacy can be enhanced by the concomitant use of class Ib or class II antiarrhythmic drugs, such as mexiletine, propafenone, and propranolol.[25a]

Procainamide

Pharmacologic Description

Procainamide hydrochloride is an amide analogue of procaine hydrochloride, a local anesthetic agent. It was introduced in 1951 for the treatment of both supraventricular and ventricular arrhythmias.[26–29]

Electrophysiologic Action

Procainamide is a class Ia antiarrhythmic agent. It decreases phase 0 of the action potential, decreases the amplitude of the action potential, and slows conduction velocity in atrial, ventricular, and Purkinje tissue. In addition, procainamide increases the effective refractory periods of atrial and ventricular cells.[30] Its major electrophysiologic effects on myocardial tissues are similar to those of quinidine. Normal sinus node automaticity is not affected. Procainamide is less vagolytic than quinidine and does not induce an adrenergic blockade. The major metabolite of procainamide, N-acetylprocainamide (NAPA), has different electrophysiologic effects, predominantly prolonging the duration of the action potential, a class III effect. ECG effects of procainamide include prolongation of the QT, QTc, and QRS intervals.

Pharmacokinetics and Metabolism

Procainamide is currently available in parenteral (intravenous or intramuscular) as well as regular and sustained-release tablet and capsule formulations. The bioavailability of procainamide is approximately 83%. Following ingestion of regular release tablets, peak plasma levels are obtained within 60 to 90 min.[31]

Approximately 15% of procainamide is bound to plasma proteins.[32] In adults, the elimination half-life varies between 2.5 and 4 h. Elimination is more rapid in children, averaging 1.7 h.[33] Approximately 50% of procainamide is excreted unchanged by the kidney. Of the remainder, a variable portion undergoes hepatic acetylation to NAPA, a cardioactive metabolite. Depending on a patients genetically determined acetylator phenotype, 16 to 22% (slow acetylators) or 24 to 33% (fast acetylators) of procainamide is metabolized to NAPA. Elimination of NAPA is approximately 85% dependent on the kidney, with an elimination half-life of 7 to 8 h. Small amounts of NAPA may be deacetylated to procainamide.[34]

Hemodynamic Effects

Procainamide can depress myocardial contractility but is usually well tolerated hemodynamically even by patients with moderately severe cardiac dysfunction. When given intravenously, hypotension may result from vasodilatation due to a mild ganglionic blocking action.

Antiarrhythmic Effects

Procainamide can effectively suppress a variety of atrial, AV-nodal, and ventricular tachyarrhythmias, including 20 to 30% of patients with sustained ventricular tachyarrhythmias. It is the drug of choice in the acute medical treatment of wide-complex tachycardias including atrial fibrillation with ventricular preexcitation (WPW syndrome). A mild vagolytic effect may result in an increased ventricular rate due to enhanced AV-nodal conduction when given for supraventricular tachyarrhythmias such as atrial flutter. Suppression of ventricular arrhythmias has been shown to occur at plasma levels between 4 and 10 mg/mL of procainamide, but higher levels may be required for suppression of sustained ventricular tachyarrhythmias. In addition, the contribution of NAPA to efficacy cannot always be ascertained.[35] Procainamide has been used extensively with electrophysiologic testing for life-threatening ventricular arrhythmias and cardiac arrest.[18] Failure to respond to procainamide during electrophysiologic testing in these cases often predicts failure with other individual antiarrhythmic agents as well.[36,37]

Side Effects

Major side effects of procainamide are gastrointestinal, with nausea, vomiting, anorexia, or diarrhea occurring in up to 30% of patients. A bitter taste, dizziness, mental depression, and psychosis have also been reported. Drug-induced fever, rash, and hepatitis may occur. Agranulocytosis, sometimes fatal, has been described.[38] Most patients will develop a positive antinuclear antibody titer if exposed to the drug for prolonged intervals. Of these, up to 30% can develop a drug-induced systemic lupus like syndrome. Slow acetylators may be at increased risk of procainamide-induced lupus due to increased production of a hydroxylamine metabolite, which appears to be important in the pathogenesis of this syndrome.[39,40] Recently, procainamide-induced lupus anticoagulants have been described, which may increase the risk of thrombosis in some patients.[41–43] As in the case of quinidine, new-onset polymorphic VT in the setting of QT prolongation has been reported. Procainamide usually causes only minimal depression of cardiac function with chronic dosing, but hypotension is not uncommon with rapid intravenous infusions.

Interactions

Unlike quinidine, procainamide does not significantly alter the pharmacokinetics of digoxin. Trimethoprim and cimetidine decrease renal clearance of procainamide and NAPA, resulting in increased plasma levels of both. Concomitant administration of amiodarone also increases procainamide levels.[44–46]

Indications and Dosage

Procainamide is indicated for the treatment of incapacitating atrial, AV-nodal, and ventricular tachyarrhythmias. An average oral daily dose for patients under 50 years of age is 30 to 60 mg/kg, divided into equal doses given every 3, 4, or 6 h. Various sustained-release formulations facilitate dosing on a two-, three-, or four-times-per-day basis with lower peak and higher trough levels. In addition, efficacy may be enhanced in some patients with concomitant use of other agents, including beta-blockers. Older patients or patients with renal insufficiency require smaller doses. Intravenous therapy can be initiated with loading infusion of up to 20 mg/kg given at a rate not to exceed 50 mg/min. Frequent blood pressure and ECG checks are required. A maintenance intravenous dose is approximately 30 to 60 mg/kg/min in a patient with normal renal function.

Disopyramide

Pharmacologic Description

Disopyramide phosphate was first noted to have antiarrhythmic properties in 1962.[47] It was subsequently released for clinical use in the United States in 1978. As currently available, disopyramide exists as a racemic combination of d and l enantiomers.

Electrophysiologic Action

The electrophysiologic effects of disopyramide are similar to those of other class Ia agents, such as quinidine and procainamide.[47] It produces a rate-dependent decrease in the rate of rise of phase 0 of the action potential, slows conduction velocity, and prolongs the effective refractory period more than it prolongs the action potential duration. Disopyramide may prolong the action potential duration to a greater extent in normal cells than in cells from infarcted regions of the heart.[48] The different enantiomers of disopyramide have differing electrophysiologic effects: the d enantiomer prolongs action potential duration while the l enantiomer shortens it.[49] The d enantiomer has approximately one-third the vagolytic properties as the l enantiomer. Disopyramide exerts strong anticholinergic effects which tend to counteract some of its direct electrophysiologic effects, particularly in the sinus and AV nodes. In humans, AV-nodal conduction is minimally affected by disopyramide.[49–51] However, in the denervated (transplanted) heart, AV-nodal conduction is markedly depressed.[52] Disopyramide can either increase or decrease the sinus rate, depending on prevailing cholinergic tone.[53] ECG effects of disopyramide include prolongation of the QRS, QT, and QTc intervals.

Pharmacokinetics and Metabolism

Disopyramide is available in regular and sustained-release capsule formulations. An intravenous preparation is undergoing clinical investigation. After an oral dose, disopyramide is almost completely absorbed with peak plasma concentrations occurring within 2 h.[54,55] Peak levels occur from 4 to 6 h after ingestion of sustained-release disopyramide capsules.[56] The elimination half-life is 6 to 9 h, with 40 to 60% excreted unchanged by the kidney.[57,58] Approximately 50% of disopyramide is excreted unchanged in the urine; an additional 20% is excreted as the mono-n-dealkylated metabolite, with another 10% excreted as other metabolites.[56] Protein binding is highly variable, ranging from 40 to 90%, depending on plasma concentration.[59] At higher doses, a greater concentration of drug is unbound, resulting in a greater pharmacologic effect than would be predicted based on the total plasma level. The clinical significance of this effect is unknown. Alpha-1-acid glycoprotein accounts for the majority of protein binding with albumin accounting for only 5 to 10% of the total.

Hemodynamic Effects

Disopyramide causes significant depression of myocardial contractility, with reductions in systemic blood pressure, stroke index, and cardiac index.[60] Systemic vascular resistance and right atrial pressure increase. Patients with LV dysfunction tolerate disopyramide poorly. In a retrospective study among patients with preexisting congestive heart failure, 55% of patients given disopyramide had clinically significant worsening of their heart failure.[61] In contrast, only 3% of patients without a history of congestive heart failure developed this complication during disopyramide therapy. The drug has been used as a treatment for hypertrophic cardiomyopathy, both as a monotherapy and in combination with beta-blockers.

Antiarrhythmic Effects

Like other class Ia antiarrhythmic drugs, disopyramide is effective in a variety of supraventricular and ventricular tachyarrhythmias.[62] Disopyramide can suppress premature ventricular contractions, with plasma concentrations in the range of 3 to 8 mg/mL, but is less effective with sustained VT as assessed by electrophysiologic testing.[63–67] Disopyramide has been combined with other antiarrhythmic agents, such as mexiletine, for increased efficacy in treating ventricular arrhythmias with fewer side effects.[68] Disopyramide has been used successfully for the treatment of atrial flutter and atrial fibrillation, including patients with the WPW syndrome.[69–71] Disopyramide may also be effective for preventing inducible and spontaneous neurally mediated syncope due to its negative inotropic and anticholinergic properties.[72]

Side Effects

Disopyramide significantly depresses myocardial contractility and must be used with caution if at all in patients with LV dysfunction. Anticholinergic side effects are frequent, and in up to 10% of patients may necessitate discontinuation of the drug. These symptoms include dry mouth, blurred vision, and particularly in older men, urine retention. Disopyramide can also precipitate acute angle-closure glaucoma.[52] Gastrointestinal symptoms are uncommon. As with other drugs that prolong ventricular repolarization and the QT interval, disopyramide can induce polymorphic VT (torsades de pointes).[73,74] Rare side effects include rash, cholestatic jaundice, psychosis, and agranulocytosis. Hypoglycemia occurs infrequently, apparently owing to increased pancreatic secretion of insulin.[75]

Interactions

Drugs that induce hepatic enzymes, such as phenytoin and phenobarbital, increase hepatic metabolism of disopyramide and result in lower serum levels. Disopyramide does not induce hepatic enzymes, however. Disopyramide does not alter serum digoxin levels. Erythromycin has been reported to increase disopyramide levels, with development of potentially fatal ventricular arrhythmias.[76] The potent negative inotropic effects of disopyramide warrant additional caution in patients with possible cardiac dysfunction requiring therapy with beta-blockers or calcium-channel blockers for indications such as ischemic heart disease.

Indications and Dosage

Disopyramide is indicated for the prevention or suppression of premature ventricular contractions and VT. It has also been used to treat atrial arrhythmias. The usual adult oral dose is 300 to 1600 mg daily, divided into three or four equal doses. Dosage must be reduced in elderly patients and in patients with renal insufficiency. The controlled-release capsules may be given every 12 h.

CLASS Ib AGENTS

Class Ib drugs also block sodium channels, but to a lesser degree than class Ia drugs. The association and disassociation kinetics are more rapid than in class Ia drugs, typically less than 1 s. In addition, repolarization tends to be mildly shortened. Class Ib drugs often suppress premature ventricular contractions but are only occasionally effective as monotherapy for life-threatening ventricular tachyarrhythmias. Class Ib drugs, as a class, are generally ineffective for atrial arrhythmias.

Lidocaine

Pharmacologic Description

Initially synthesized in 1943, lidocaine is widely used as a local anesthetic agent. Its antiarrhythmic properties were noted in the 1950s, but its use did not become common until the advent of coronary care units in the 1960s.[77]

Electrophysiologic Action

Lidocaine is classified as a class Ib antiarrhythmic drug. The action potential duration and effective refractory period of Purkinje and ventricular tissues are shortened. At high concentrations, it depresses the rate of rise of phase 0 of the action potential and decreases conduction velocity in Purkinje fibers.[78] Lidocaine has minimal effects on AV and intraventricular conduction except at high concentrations (above 30 mg/mL).[79,80] In patients with severe His-Purkinje system disease, lidocaine may precipitate complete AV block.[81] Lidocaine decreases phase 4 diastolic depolarizations in Purkinje tissue and decreases automaticity. Consequently, lidocaine may depress both the sinus node and potential subsidiary escape pacemakers, rarely causing asystolic pauses. Lidocaine increases the VF threshold. In abnormal myocardium, the effects of lidocaine in depressing conduction may be more pronounced.

Pharmacokinetics and Metabolism

Lidocaine is almost completely absorbed after oral administration, but approximately 70% is rapidly metabolized by hepatic first-pass biotransformation.[82] Less than 10% of an administered dose is recovered unchanged in the urine. For this reason, the drug is almost always given parenterally; however rectal administration is feasible, as is intramuscular administration, particularly in the pre-hospital phase of the management of acute myocardial infarction.[82] Lidocaine is approximately 60 to 80% protein-bound, depending on the concentration of alpha$_1$-acid glycoprotein in the serum.[83,84] During acute myocardial infarction, serum levels of alpha$_1$-acid glycoprotein are increased, resulting in more drug bound to alpha$_1$-acid glycoprotein and less free (active) drug.[84] Thus, higher total lidocaine levels may be required during acute myocardial infarction.

Lidocaine is almost completely cleared by the liver, with clearance proportional to hepatic blood flow.[85] The mean elimination half-life of lidocaine in humans is 1.5 to 2 h, which is increased in the elderly, patients with reduced cardiac output, and patients with hepatic disease.[77,85–87] Elimination is also delayed during prolonged infusions in patients with acute myocardial infarction, the mechanism of which is not understood.[88] The two principal metabolites are glycinexylidide and monoethylglycinexylidide (MEGX), both of which have weaker antiarrhythmic effects in humans than does lidocaine but can contribute measurably to the central nervous system toxicity of lidocaine.[89] Both metabolites are renally excreted, and glycinexylidide may accumulate in patients with renal failure.

Hemodynamic Effects

At usual doses, lidocaine causes minimal hemodynamic effects. Minimal decreases in cardiac output, arterial blood pressure, heart rate, and ventricular contractility have been reported.

Antiarrhythmic Effects

Lidocaine can be effective for the suppression of ventricular tachyarrhythmias, particularly in patients with myocardial ischemia.. Prophylactic use of lidocaine after myocardial infarction, once a common practice, has been abandoned as prophylactic use of any class Ia agents after myocardial infarction has been associated with increased mortality.[90,91] It also appears to reduce the incidence of VF.[91] Therapeutic plasma concentrations range from 2 to 5 μg/mL.

Side Effects

Adverse effects of lidocaine almost always involve the central nervous system. Early, transient effects include paresthesias, dizziness, and drowsiness, which can be managed by interrupting the drug temporarily. Later, more persistent effects include hallucinations, confusion, somnolence, and muscle tremor, which presage impending seizures, respiratory, or cardiac arrest.[92] Rarely, lidocaine can depress sinus node function or precipitate heart block in patients with severe His-Purkinje system disease; it can also inhibit escape rhythms from His-Purkinje tissue. Adverse effects of lidocaine are common when the plasma concentration exceeds 6 μg/mL.

Interactions

Lidocaine is highly dependent on hepatic metabolism for elimination. Drugs that alter hepatic metabolism cause marked changes in lidocaine pharmacokinetics. Propranolol, metoprolol, cimetidine and halothane decrease lidocaine clearance.[93–95]

Indications and Dosage

Lidocaine is indicated for the acute management of ventricular arrhythmias, such as those associated with acute myocardial infarction or cardiac surgery. It may be administered intravenously as a bolus of 0.7 to 1.4 mg/kg at a rate of 25 to 50 mg min. If necessary, this dose may be repeated in 5 min followed by a continuous infusion of 0.014 to 0.057 mg/kg (1–4 mg/min). Alternative loading and maintenance infusion regimens have also been advocated, typically entailing a total of 2 to 4 mg/kg in divided doses over 30 min. Lidocaine may be given by intramuscular injection of 300 to 400 mg (4.3 mg/kg) for use during acute myocardial infarction.[96] The deltoid muscle is the preferred injection site. Lidocaine has also been used in combination with other agents including procainamide, bretylium, and beta-blockers.

Tocainide

Pharmacologic Description

Tocainide hydrochloride is a primary amine analogue of lidocaine. Minor side-chain differences from lidocaine enable it to avoid substantial first-pass metabolism in the liver, thus allowing oral administration. Its antiarrhythmic effects were described in 1976 and it was approved for oral use in the United States in 1984.[97,98] As currently available, tocainide is supplied as a racemic mixture of enantiomers d-tocainide and l-tocainide.

Electrophysiologic Action

Tocainide produces dose-dependent decreases in sodium and potassium conductance, thus depressing myocardial excitability. It suppresses the amplitude and rate of depolarization of the action potential and may shorten the action, potential duration, and to a lesser extent the effective refractory period of Purkinje tissue.[99,100] Tocainide increases the fibrillation threshold in normal and ischemic tissue.[101] AV conduction and sinus node automaticity are usually unaffected by tocainide. Tocainide usually produces no significant ECG changes.[102,103] However, the QT interval may decrease.[104] The individual enantiomers of tocainide may be more effective for ventricular arrhythmias induced by programmed electrical stimulation than the racemic combination.[105]

Pharmacokinetics and Metabolism

Following oral administration, the bioavailability of tocainide approaches 100%. Peak plasma concentrations appear between 0.5 and 2 h.[106] Between 10 and 50% of tocainide is bound to plasma proteins.[107] Approximately 40% is excreted unchanged in the urine. The elimination half-life averages 13 to 15 h in healthy subjects but can vary between 9 and 37 h.[98,106,108] Elimination is delayed in the presence of renal insufficiency but only minimally changed in the presence of hepatic disease.

Hemodynamic Effects

Intravenous tocainide produces small degrees of LV depression with no apparent change in cardiac output. Small increases in aortic and pulmonary artery pressures have been observed, probably secondary to increases in vascular resistance. In patients with moderate to severe LV dysfunction, including those receiving beta-blocking drugs, hemodynamic changes are often minimal, although more marked and additive effects may occur.[109,110] In one study, congestive heart failure was precipitated by tocainide in approximately 1.5% of patients.[111]

Antiarrhythmic Effects

Tocainide is a modestly effective agent for suppressing premature ventricular contractions in a number of patients, with approximately 90% suppression in some patients at plasma concentrations of 8.5 mg/mL.[98,111] Typically, 30 to 75% of patients will have significant suppression of premature ventricular contraction. Tocainide is at times effective in suppressing premature ventricular contractions in patients who are unresponsive to class Ia agents, and the response to lidocaine may be predictive of the response to tocainide.[112–116] Response to lidocaine appears to be a sensitive but nonspecific predictor of efficacy with tocainide.[113] Thus, lidocaine failure is often predictive of tocainide inefficacy, while lidocaine efficacy does not necessarily predict tocainide success. Only a small percentage of patients with life-threatening ventricular arrhythmias will respond to tocainide when assessed by electrophysiologic testing.[117,118]

However, the drug may be synergistically effective when combined with class Ia drugs.[119] Dosing tocainide at 600 mg orally twice daily produces levels effective in suppressing premature ventricular contractions in many patients (4 to 10 μg/mL).[108]

Side Effects

Side effects are common with tocainide, having been reported in 20 to 40% of patients. Typically gastrointestinal and central nervous system side effects occur, including nausea, dizziness, tremor, vomiting, paresthesia, tremor, ataxia, and confusion. These effects usually occur with high plasma concentrations and may be minimized by dividing doses and taking the medication with meals to delay absorption. Skin rash occurs not infrequently. Rarely, more serious adverse effects occur, such as pulmonary fibrosis, a lupus like syndrome, or hematologic abnormalities chiefly agranulocytosis.[116,120]

Interactions

Tocainide has no significant effects on warfarin or digoxin. Concomitant use with beta-blocking drugs is safe in most patients. Rifampin has been reported to increase elimination, resulting in reduced plasma levels of tocainide.[121] Cimetidine, but not ranitidine, results in decreased bioavailability of tocainide.[122]

Indications and Dosage

Tocainide is specifically indicated for the treatment of life-threatening ventricular tachyarrhythmias, although it is only infrequently effective for this purpose. It has the same efficacy profile as mexiletine, but its potentially serious systemic side effects have restricted its use. It should not be used as first line therapy, but only for symptomatic VT resistant to other therapies. Tocainide is available as tablets of 400 and 600 mg. Total daily doses of 800 to 2400 mg are usually administered as divided doses two to four times daily. The dosage should be reduced in the presence of renal insufficiency. Plasma levels above 3 μg/mL are associated with efficacy, while levels above 10 μg/mL are associated with increased side effects.[123]

Mexiletine

Pharmacologic Description

Mexiletine hydrochloride is a drug closely related in structure to lidocaine. Initially developed as an anticonvulsant, mexiletine has been recognized to have antiarrhythmic properties since 1972.[124,125] Used in Europe to treat ventricular arrhythmias since 1976, it became available in the United States in 1986.

Electrophysiologic Action

Mexiletine decreases the rate of rise of phase 0 of the action potential and shortens the action potential's duration.[124–126] The effective refractory period is decreased in Purkinje tissue but not in ventricular muscle.[127] The slope of phase 4 diastolic depolarization is decreased. The electrophysiologic effects of mexiletine are similar to those of other class Ib agents. Usually, no significant changes occur in the PR, QRS, QT, or QTc intervals with either intravenous or oral mexiletine.[128] In patients with normal His-Purkinje function, no significant changes are observed after mexiletine. Patients with His-Purkinje system disease may develop prolongation of conduction and rarely block, however. In addition, prolongation of QRS duration has been reported with mexiletine toxicity.[129]

Pharmacokinetics and Metabolism

Mexiletine is highly bioavailable, with approximately 90% absorption.[130] Absorption occurs in the alkaline environment of the proximal small bowel. Peak plasma levels occur in 2 to 3 h but may be delayed in clinical situations, such as acute myocardial infarction or diabetes mellitus, in which gastric emptying is delayed. Some 50 to 60% of mexiletine is protein-bound. Mexiletine is extensively metabolized in the liver; only 10% is excreted unchanged by the kidney.[130] Several metabolites have minor electrophysiologic activity, the most potent (N-methylmexiletine) having less than 20% of the effect of the parent compound. In healthy subjects, the average elimination half-life is 10 h, ranging from 8 to 12 h.[131–133] Renal insufficiency has minimal effect on elimination half life, whereas hepatic insufficiency or reduced hepatic blood flow reduces mexiletine clearance.[130,134]

Hemodynamic Effects

Mexiletine generally has minimal negative inotropic effects at therapeutic levels. Small decreases in blood pressure and LV contractility with increased LV end diastolic pressure have been observed in some studies. Administered orally, mexiletine produced no changes in LV EF, blood pressure, heart rate, or exercise capacity.[135]

Antiarrhythmic Effects

Mexiletine may be used to suppress frequent and high-grade ventricular arrhythmias, including those that have failed to respond to class Ia antiarrhythmic drugs. Used alone, mexiletine is only infrequently effective in suppressing life-threatening ventricular arrhythmias.[136,137] Combination therapy with class Ia antiarrhythmic agents can be more effective than either agent alone, with potentially less toxicity.[137–140] Mexiletine is effective in suppressing warning ventricular arrhythmias in a number of patients with acute myocardial infarction.[141,142] The antiarrhythmic response to lidocaine may be used as a sensitive but nonspecific predictor of mexiletine efficacy.[116,143] Thus, failure to respond to intravenous lidocaine is a strong predictor of mexiletine inefficacy, while lidocaine efficacy only weakly predicts mexiletine efficacy. Similarly, the response to either tocainide or mexiletine is not necessarily predictive of the response to the other. Plasma concentrations of 0.5 to 2.0 mg/mL are associated with efficacy in many patients.

Side Effects

Side effects are common with mexiletine, occurring in up to 40 to 60% of patients in some series.[128] The most frequent side effects are related to the central nervous system or the gastrointestinal tract and include nausea, vomiting, dizziness, tremor, ataxia, slurred speech, blurred vision, memory impairment, and personality changes. Skin rash and hepatitis occur infrequently. Rarely, seizures have been reported. Gastrointestinal side effects may be reduced by administering the drug with food or by reducing the dosage. Adverse cardiac effects are rare, but worsening of congestive heart failure and proarrhythmic effects have been reported.

Interactions

No specific adverse effects have been reported to date from combining mexiletine with other cardiotonic agents, such as beta-blocking drugs or other antiarrhythmics. Significant alkalinization of the urine by drugs may decrease renal clearance and result in elevated blood levels. Drugs such as phenobarbital or phenytoin, which induce hepatic enzymes, enhance mexiletine metabolism; cimetidine reduces metabolism and results in increased mexiletine levels.

Indications and Dosage

Mexiletine is indicated for the suppression of incapacitating ventricular arrhythmias, including VT. Effective oral regimens usually require 200 to 400 mg every 8 h. Doses should be given with food to minimize side effects. Dosages may be increased or decreased by 50 to 100 mg at intervals of at least 2 to 3 days. An intravenous preparation is not available in the United States and is associated with a relatively high incidence of side effects. Intravenous therapy has been given as a loading dose of 400 mg over 40 min with 600 to 900 mg per day for maintenance therapy.

CLASS Ic AGENTS

Class Ic drugs are potent sodium-channel blocking agents. They have little effect on repolarization and have long half-time kinetics of channel association and dissociation, usually greater than 20 to 30 s. Thus, drug effects are potentiated at moderate to rapid heart rates. They are effective for a variety of atrial and ventricular tachyarrhythmias. As a class, the Ic drugs are highly effective in suppressing chronic ventricular ectopy. Unfortunately, the marked slowing of conduction induced by these agents is an efficient mechanism to induce ventricular proarrhythmia. This effect is most marked in patients with significant structural heart disease but may occur in normal individuals, especially in the setting of rapid heart rates, such as those produced by exercise.

Moricizine

Pharmacologic Description

Moricizine is a phenothiazine derivative first synthesized in the Soviet Union.[144,145]

Electrophysiologic Action

Intravenous moricizine (3 mg/kg) produces both a reduction in the upstroke velocity of phase 0 and a reduction in the action potential duration, effects similar to those of other class Ib antiarrhythmic agents.[144] In contrast to class Ib agents, however, moricizine has prolonged sodium channel recovery kinetics, similar to class Ic agents. Moricizine does not decrease the slope of phase 4 depolarization in automatic Purkinje fibers unless the fibers are ischemic. Voltage clamp experiments have shown that moricizine reduces the fast sodium current by decreasing maximal conduction of sodium ions. In humans, intravenous moricizine (1.5 to 2 mg/kg) lengthens the P wave to low right atrial (PA), atrial to His bundle (AH), and PR intervals. The sinus rate, QT and His bundle to ventricular (HV) intervals, as well as the effective refractory periods of the atrium, AV node, and ventricle were not affected in early studies.[146,147] The refractoriness of an accessory pathway or of the retrograde fast pathway of dual AV-nodal pathways is increased by moricizine, however. Using an oral dose of 10 mg/kg, slight prolongation of the HV interval was noted, whereas at a higher dose of 15 mg/kg, the PR and QRS intervals were prolonged.[148,149] In patients with sinus node dysfunction, moricizine given intravenously (2 mg/kg) has caused prolongation of the sinus node recovery time and second-degree sinus exit block.[150] Although some properties are similar to those of other class Ib agents, in aggregate moricizine behaves more like a class Ic drug.

Pharmacokinetics and Metabolism

Moricizine is well absorbed when given orally, with peak plasma concentrations occurring 1 to 1.5 h after dosing.[145] The drug undergoes extensive metabolism, with less than 1% of the drug recovered in the urine and feces.[145] Active metabolites have not been identified thus far. After a single oral dose, the elimination half-life is approximately 2 to 5 h.[151] In patients with cardiac disease, the steady-state elimination half-life averages 10 h, but it may be prolonged to 47 h in patients with renal insufficiency. Antiarrhythmic effects of the drug may not be noted for up to 24 h after dosing, an effect that is not completely understood. Therefore plasma levels may provide little guidance for antiarrhythmic efficacy, and in fact several studies have reported little correlation between plasma concentration and drug toxicity in the form of proarrhythmia.[152,153]

Hemodynamic Effects

Hemodynamic data in humans are incomplete; however, moricizine appears to have minimal effect on most hemodynamic parameters.[154,155] Moricizine does not appear to depress myocardial contractility in dogs. In patients with preexisting LV dysfunction, moricizine may cause decompensation, however.[156] In one study, the failure to increase cardiac index by 1.0 L/min/m² or to increase stroke work during bicycle exercise not only predicted patients likely to decompensate but also predicted those patients unlikely to have an antiarrhythmic response.[156]

Antiarrhythmic Effects

Moricizine may be effective for the treatment of both supraventricular and ventricular arrhythmias.[144–147,150,154,157–159] With doses ranging from 2.4 to 15 mg/kg per day, moricizine was effective in reducing premature ventricular contractions in 50 to 60% of patients, comparing favorably with disopyramide in one study.[145,150,156,158] Moricizine appears less effective in the treatment of life-threatening ventricular tachyarrhythmias and has demonstrated an excessive cardiac mortality rate during the first 2 weeks of exposure in patients with ischemic cardiomyopathy and recent myocardial infarction.[148,152,160,161] Unlike other class Ib antiarrhythmic agents, when given intravenously, moricizine has shown efficacy in terminating and preventing initiation of both AV-nodal supraventricular tachycardias and reciprocating bypass tract tachycardias by slowing retrograde fast-pathway conduction.[146,147] Recently, it has also been shown safe, well tolerated, and effective in maintaining sinus rhythm in patients with chronic atrial fibrillation and systolic dysfunction.[162]

Side Effects

Moricizine appears to be a generally well-tolerated antiarrhythmic agent. Nausea, vomiting, diarrhea, and dizziness as well as mild anxiety reactions have been reported. Nervousness, perioral numbness, vertigo, confusion, dry mouth, blurred vision, headache, and insomnia have occurred.[163] Worsening of sinus node dysfunction may occur, and the drug may cause hypotension or worsening of congestive heart failure.[150] Some patients have had transient elevation of hepatic transaminase enzyme levels. Rarely, diaphoresis and memory loss have been reported with long-term therapy. Proarrhythmia reportedly occurred in approximately 3.2% of patients in one review and was reportedly relatively unrelated to dose.[153] Sinusoidal VT, occasionally induced with exercise, has been reported.

Interactions

Serum digoxin levels may increase 10 to 15% during acute but not chronic dosing in cardiac patients with normal renal function. Other drug interactions have not been reported, but this has not been completely investigated.

Indications and Dosage

At doses of 150 to 250 mg every 8 h, moricizine appears effective for the treatment of atrial and ventricular ectopy. Doses may be given every 8 to 12 h. Therapeutic drug levels appear to be 0.2 to 1.5 mg/mL. The role of moricizine in the treatment of life-threatening ventricular arrhythmias remains undefined.

Flecainide

Pharmacologic Description

Flecainide acetate, a fluorobenzamide, is a derivative of procainamide first synthesized in 1972. Its antiarrhythmic effects were first reported in 1975 and it was released for the treatment of ventricular arrhythmias in the United States in 1985.[164] Subsequently it has been approved for the treatment of supraventricular tachyarrhythmias including atrial flutter and atrial fibrillation in patients with structurally normal hearts.

Electrophysiologic Action

Flecainide exhibits potent sodium channel blocking action, depressing phase 0 of the action potential and slowing conduction in a frequency- and dose-dependent manner throughout the heart. His-Purkinje tissue and ventricular muscle are affected the most, followed by atrial muscle, accessory AV pathways, and AV-nodal tissue. In most studies, the action potential duration is not significantly affected. Sinus rate, sinoatrial conduction, and sinus node recovery times are usually not affected by flecainide.[165] However, patients with sinus node dysfunction may have significant increases in the corrected sinus node recovery time.[166] Flecainide produces a concentration-dependent increase in PR, QRS, and intraatrial conduction intervals as well as prolongation of the ventricular effective refractory period.[167,168] An intravenous dose of 2 mg/kg (mean level 335 mg/L) produced a mean QRS increase of 23%.[168] The QT interval increases, reflecting QRS prolongation, with minimal to no change in the JT interval.

Pharmacokinetics and Metabolism

Flecainide is well absorbed (95%), with peak plasma concentrations occurring 2 to 4 h after dosing. Flecainide is 30 to 40% bound to plasma proteins, independent of drug level, over a range of 0.015 to 3.4 μg/mL.[169] Clinically important drug interactions based on protein-binding effects would therefore not be expected. In healthy subjects, 30% (range 10 to 50%) of flecainide is excreted unchanged in the urine.[169] Approximately 70% of flecainide is metabolized in the liver. The major metabolite (meta-O-dealkylated flecainide) is approximately 20% as potent as the parent compound, while the minor metabolite (meta-O-dealkylated lactam of flecainide) is electrophysiologically inactive. The average elimination half-life is 20 h after repeated doses, but is highly variable and ranges between 12 and 27 h.[170,171] Steady-state levels are not obtained for 3 to 5 days. Since flecainide is extensively metabolized, the relationship between flecainide elimination and creatinine clearance is complex. Reduced doses must be used in patients with renal insufficiency or hepatic insufficiency.[172,173]

Hemodynamic Effects

Flecainide produces dose-dependent depression of cardiac contractility and cardiac output.[174,175] Oral treatment is generally well tolerated, but patients with LV dysfunction may develop new or worsening congestive heart failure. Flecainide should not be used in patients with LV dysfunction.[176,177]

Antiarrhythmic Effects

Flecainide is effective in suppressing both supraventricular and ventricular tachyarrhythmias and premature contractions.[170,178–188] Flecainide is able to suppress chronic premature ventricular contractions by more than 75% and repetitive forms by more than 90% in most patients, including patients resistant to other antiarrhythmic drugs.[167,186,187] Among patients with life-threatening ventricular tachyarrhythmias, flecainide is reported to prevent induction of VT in 15 to 25%.[185,188,189] Flecainide has shown efficacy in the prevention and treatment of atrial fibrillation and arrhythmias in patients with ventricular preexcitation or accessory pathways.[178–183] Flecainide is most effective in suppressing chronic ectopy in patients with preserved LV function without VT. Patients with LV dysfunction or clinically documented VT are at increased risk for proarrhythmic side effects. Flecainide has been shown to increase cardiac mortality among patients with ventricular ectopy after acute myocardial infarction.[3] Therapeutic levels of flecainide are 0.2 to 1.0 μg/mL; higher levels are associated with an increasing incidence of toxicity.

Side Effects

Most side effects of flecainide are neurologic and cardiac. Neurologic effects include blurred vision, headache, dizziness, paresthesias, and tremor. Skin rash, abdominal pain, diarrhea, and impotence have been reported. Cardiac effects are not uncommon and include worsening of arrhythmia, slowed conduction or heart block, and aggravation of congestive heart failure.[190] Worsening of ventricular arrhythmias occurs in up to 10% or more of patients, more commonly in patients with LV dysfunction and clinical VT. Some episodes of VT induced by flecainide have been resistant to electrical cardioversion.[191] Acute and chronic elevations of the pacing threshold have been reported by some investigators.[192]

Interaction

Small increases in serum digoxin concentrations have been noted with flecainide administration. Both flecainide and propranolol concentrations increase mildly with coadministration of both agents. No clinically important interactions have been reported. The concomitant administration of flecainide and a beta-blocker or calcium-channel antagonist can be expected to have additive cardiac depressant effects.

Indications and Dosage

Flecainide is indicated for the treatment of life-threatening ventricular arrhythmias, such as sustained VT, as well as resistant supraventricular arrhythmias in patients with normal ventricular function. In patients with normal renal and hepatic function, treatment may be begun with 100 mg every 12 h. Dose adjustments should be no larger than 50 mg per dose every 4 days to minimize toxicity. Total daily doses of 200 to 300 mg are associated with efficacy in most patients. Patients with LV dysfunction or a history of VT should have therapy initiated using smaller dosages with continuous electrocardiographic monitoring in a hospital environment.

Propafenone

Pharmacologic Description

Propafenone hydrochloride, an antiarrhythmic agent structurally similar to beta-blocking drugs, was first synthesized in 1970. Commercially available since 1977 in Europe, propafenone is approved in the United States for the treatment of life-threatening ventricular arrhythmias and supraventricular arrhythmias in patients with structurally normal hearts. Propafenone exists as a racemic mixture of d propafenone and l-propafenone.

Electrophysiologic Action

Propafenone blocks the fast inward sodium current in atrial, ventricular, and His-Purkinje tissue, decreasing the rate of rise of phase 0 of the action potential.[193,194] The blocking effect is concentration-dependent, with ischemic tissue being more susceptible.[194] In patients with ventricular preexcitation or bypass tracts, propafenone decreases conduction velocity and increases refractoriness of the accessory pathway.[195,196] Sinus node automaticity may be depressed, especially in the presence of preexisting sinus node dysfunction. Propafenone possesses weak beta-adrenergic and calcium-channel antagonist activities. Both stereoisomers appear to have equal sodium channel blocking ability while d-propafenone is responsible for the clinically observed beta-blockade.[197] Propafenone suppresses delayed afterdepolarizations in ischemic Purkinje fibers. Endocardial pacing thresholds are increased.[198] Electrocardiographic effects include prolongation of the PR and QRS intervals without significant change of the QT interval.[199,200]

Pharmacokinetics and Metabolism

Absorption of propafenone is almost complete after oral dosing, with peak plasma levels obtained in 2 to 3 h, but extensive first-pass metabolism reduces systemic bioavailability to approximately 12%. The availability appears to vary with the dose, so that higher doses have increased bioavailability, probably due to saturation of hepatic microsomal enzymes with larger doses.[201] About 77 to 79% of propafenone is protein-bound, with alpha$_1$-acid glycoprotein being the major binding protein. The metabolism of propafenone is polymorphic and segregates with the debrisoquin metabolic phenotype.[202] Extensive metabolizers form two major metabolites: 5 hydroxypropafenone and N-depropyl-propafenone. Poor metabolizers have high levels of propafenone and therefore more beta-blocking effect and minimal levels of active metabolites. Overall, however, electrophysiologic effects appear similar in both groups given comparable doses. Elimination of propafenone is mostly hepatic; less than 1% is recovered intact in the urine. The average elimination half-life ranges from 3.6 to 7.2 h.[199–201] In patients with hepatic disease, the elimination half-life is prolonged, averaging 14 h. Doses must be decreased in these patients.

Hemodynamic Effects

Propafenone has negative inotropic effects. In several studies occasional patients with depressed cardiac function have had hemodynamic deterioration.[203,204] Most patients experience no change in resting LV EF, although EF may decrease with exercise.[205] One study using intravenous propafenone (2 mg/kg) showed a slight depression of cardiac index with increased pulmonary vascular resistance but no change in systemic arterial pressure.[206] Thus, caution is necessary if propafenone is used in patients with LV dysfunction.

Antiarrhythmic Effects

Propafenone appears effective in treating both supraventricular and ventricular arrhythmias. As other class Ic antiarrhythmic agents, propafenone is effective in suppressing frequent premature ventricular contractions, including complex forms.[65,204,207,208] It is less effective in treating life-threatening ventricular arrhythmias, but even in this difficult population, up to 25% of patients may respond.[199,200,206,209] Propafenone has also been shown to be effective in treating supraventricular tachyarrhythmias, such as atrial fibrillation or flutter, including patients with the WPW syndrome.[195,196,210–212] Propafenone should be used cautiously in patients with recent myocardial infarction in view of the recent CAST findings showing increased mortality in this population when treated with other class Ic drugs (flecainide or encainide).[3]

Side Effects

Approximately 21 to 32% of patients experience adverse reactions to propafenone; 3 to 7% require discontinuation of the medication. Worsening of ventricular arrhythmias was reported to occur in 6.1% of 1579 patients in early clinical trials of propafenone. Patients at highest risk include those with LV dysfunction and those with pre-existing sustained VT. Noncardiac side effects are predominantly gastrointestinal or related to the central nervous system. Dizziness, light-headedness, nausea, vomiting, or a metallic taste occur most frequently. Central nervous system effects and effects related to beta-adrenergic blockade may be more frequent in individuals with a poor metabolizer phenotype.[196]

Interactions

Propafenone in a dose of 300 mg every 8 h orally increases digoxin levels an average of 83%; the magnitude of increase seems related to the dose of propafenone. Significant increases in plasma warfarin concentrations and prothrombin times have been reported.[213] Propafenone concentrations may increase with concomitant cimetidine therapy. Propafenone also decreases metoprolol elimination, resulting in increased beta-adrenergic blockade. Quinidine in low doses effectively stops hepatic metabolism of propafenone, converting rapid metabolizers to poor metabolizers. The clinical significance of this interaction is unknown.

Indications and Dosage

Propafenone is approved for the treatment of ventricular arrhythmias. Therapy for both supraventricular and ventricular arrhythmias may be initiated using a dosage of 150 mg three times a day; doses up to 900 mg (occasionally 1200 mg) daily have been used. High dose oral propafenone (600 mg) has also been shown to be very safe and effective in restoring sinus rhythm in patients with recent onset atrial fibrillation with conversion rates of up to 76% at 8 h after treatment.[214] Intravenous propafenone has been evaluated for supraventricular and ventricular arrhythmias at doses such as 2 mg/kg followed by a maintenance infusion, but this formulation remains investigational in the United States. A new sustained-release formulation has been proven safe and effective and will be available soon for clinical use.

CLASS II AGENTS

Class II drugs are beta-adrenergic blocking agents.[215] Different beta-blockers will vary with respect to lipid solubility, membrane-stabilizing effect, relative specificity for the beta₁ receptor, cardioselectivity, and partial agonist activity (intrinsic sympathomimetic activity). As a class, beta blockers are useful for the treatment of many atrial and AV-nodal arrhythmias (see Chap. 7). In addition, some beta blockers may reduce ventricular ectopy. Several beta-blocking agents have been shown to reduce mortality when administered after acute myocardial infarction and may be useful as primary or adjunctive agents in some patients with or at risk for life-threatening ventricular tachyarrhythmias.

Propranolol

Pharmacologic Description

Propranolol hydrochloride is a nonselective beta-adrenergic-receptor blocking agent. It is indicated in the United States for the treatment of supraventricular and ventricular arrhythmias. It is also indicated for the treatment of hypertrophic cardiomyopathy, acute myocardial infarction, angina pectoris, hypertension, and numerous noncardiac conditions such as migraine headache and essential tremor.

Electrophysiologic Action

The electrophysiologic effects of propranolol relate primarily to its beta-blocking activity, an effect almost entirely mediated by its l stereoisomer.[216] Propranolol is a competitive nonselective beta-blocker. Beta₁ receptors predominate in cardiac tissue, blockade of which produce an increase in the sinus node cycle length and slowing of AV nodal conduction. At high concentrations, propranolol depresses the inward sodium current in Purkinje fibers, the so-called membrane-stabilizing or quinidine-like effect. This effect generally occurs only at concentrations several times that required for beta-blockade and thus is probably insignificant clinically. Propranolol can shorten the duration of action potentials acutely in Purkinje fibers and to a lesser extent in atrial and ventricular muscle.[215,217] With chronic administration, the action potential may lengthen. ECG effects include a slowing of sinus rate and an increase in the PR interval with minimal or no change in QRS and QTc intervals.[218] The effective refractory period is minimally increased.

Pharmacokinetics and Metabolism

Propranolol is almost completely absorbed after oral administration but undergoes extensive first-pass metabolism in the liver, resulting in a bioavailability of approximately 30%. Peak clinical effects occur between 60 and 90 min after oral dosing.[219] The average biologic half-life is 4 h. A long-acting formulation is also available for once-daily use. Elimination is hepatic and is proportional to hepatic blood flow. With oral dosing, a total of 160 to 240 mg daily is considered necessary for achieving effective beta-blockade, although smaller doses are often used in antiarrhythmic regimens. With intravenous dosing, a total dose of 0.2 mg/kg achieves effective beta-blockade, with activity evident almost immediately.

Hemodynamic Effects

Propranolol is a negative inotropic agent by virtue of its beta-blocking action. It may precipitate or worsen congestive heart failure. By blocking beta₂ receptors in the peripheral circulation, propranolol may increase vascular resistance.

Antiarrhythmic Effects

Propranolol is an effective agent for the treatment of supraventricular arrhythmias such as atrial tachycardia. It will slow the ventricular response to atrial fibrillation/flutter and may terminate arrhythmias requiring participation of the AV node, such as AV-nodal reciprocating tachycardias and those associated with the WPW syndrome and accessory pathways. Propranolol has a variable effect on the rapid ventricular response to atrial fibrillation due to accessory pathway conduction. Propranolol can be effective in treating arrhythmias due to digitalis toxicity, thyrotoxicosis, and anesthesia and as adjunctive therapy for pheochromocytoma.[215] Ventricular premature contractions may be suppressed by propranolol, but it is infrequently effective as a single agent in the treatment of life-threatening ventricular tachyarrhythmias. Propranolol may be more effective in preventing rapid polymorphic VTs or VF than monomorphic VT when assessed by electrophysiologic testing.[220] Propranolol can be an effective adjunctive agent in combination with other agents, with caution to avoid additive depressant effects on conduction and contractility. Beta blockers have also been used successfully in some patients with congenital QT prolongation and associated ventricular tachyarrhythmias, including torsades de pointes. Therapeutic plasma levels for propranolol are highly variable but often range from 50 to 100 ng/mL.

Side Effects

Common side effects include bradycardia, hypotension, claudication, Raynaud's phenomenon, and AV block.[219] Worsening of heart failure or asthma may occur. Propranolol is lipophilic and easily penetrates the blood-brain barrier, contributing to central nervous system adverse effects such as vivid dreams, insomnia, mental depression, and possibly fatigue and impotence. Insulin-dependent diabetics may be at increased risk for hypoglycemia. Sudden discontinuation of beta-blockade may worsen angina pectoris and may even precipitate acute myocardial infarction.

Interactions

Negative inotropic drugs such as verapamil or disopyramide should be used cautiously with propranolol in patients with LV dysfunction. Propranolol and verapamil in combination may occasionally precipitate AV block. Antacids containing aluminum hydroxide significantly reduce absorption of propranolol. Phenytoin, phenobarbital, and rifampin accelerate hepatic metabolism of propranolol, resulting in reduced serum concentrations; cimetidine increases serum concentrations of propranolol. Propranolol, by decreasing cardiac output, can reduce the systemic clearance of lidocaine, theophylline, and antipyrine.

Indications and Dosage

Arrhythmic indications for propranolol include supraventricular arrhythmias and arrhythmias associated with thyrotoxicosis or digitalis toxicity as well as arrhythmias associated with increased catecholamine states. Propranolol may be effective for ventricular ectopy and some ventricular tachyarrhythmias. Propranolol, along with other beta-blocking agents, has been shown to reduce cardiovascular mortality for at least 2 to 3 years after acute myocardial infarction. As a class, these drugs are the only antiarrhythmic agents shown to reduce mortality in patients following acute myocardial infarction. Intravenous doses should be given under ECG monitoring beginning with 0.25 to 1.0 mg using up to 0.2 mg/kg total dose. Oral dosages are highly variable, ranging from 20 to 240 mg daily or more, divided into three or four intervals for antiarrhythmic therapy. Longer-acting preparations may allow once- or twice-daily dosing. Doses of 180 to 240 mg daily in two or three divided doses are recommended to reduce mortality after myocardial infarction.[219]

Acebutolol

Pharmacologic Description

Acebutolol hydrochloride is a relatively cardioselective $beta_1$-adrenergic receptor antagonist with mild intrinsic sympathomimetic activity. It is available in the United States for the treatment of hypertension and ventricular arrhythmias.

Electrophysiologic Action

The electrophysiologic effects of acebutolol are predominantly are related to its $beta_1$-receptor blocking activity. At rest, the sinus cycle length increases minimally owing to intrinsic sympathomimetic activity. The sinus response to exercise is markedly blunted, however. Although acebutolol possesses membrane-stabilizing activity (sodium-channel blocking ability) in high concentrations, this effect does not appear to be important clinically.[221] ECG effects consist of prolongation of the PR interval (AH interval) with minimal if any change in the QTc interval. The QRS duration is unchanged.

Pharmacokinetics and Metabolism

Following oral administration, acebutolol is well absorbed from the gastrointestinal tract but undergoes extensive first-pass metabolism, resulting in an absolute bioavailability of 40% (range 20 to 60%). The major metabolite, an N-acetyl derivative (diacetolol), is approximately equally active but is more cardioselective than the parent compound. Acebutolol is 26% bound to plasma proteins.[222] Peak plasma concentrations of acebutolol are reached 2.5 h after oral ingestion, whereas peak levels of diacetolol occur at 3.5 h. The elimination half-life of acebutolol is 3 to 4 h, whereas the half-life for diacetolol is 8 to 13 h. Forty percent of acebutolol is eliminated by the kidneys; diacetolol is almost entirely renally excreted. In the presence of renal impairment, plasma concentrations of acebutolol are not significantly changed, but concentrations of diacetolol increase two- to threefold. Therefore dose reduction is necessary with renal insufficiency.

Acebutolol and diacetolol are hydrophilic; therefore only minimal concentrations of these compounds are found within the central nervous system.

Hemodynamic Effects

Like propranolol, acebutolol decreases heart rate and cardiac contractility. The potential for heart rate slowing is somewhat less with acebutolol owing to its partial agonist activity. Blood pressure reduction typically is proportional to baseline pressure, but hypotension may occur in previously normotensive individuals.

Antiarrhythmic Effects

The beta-blocking activity of acebutolol is approximately 25% that of propranolol on a milligram-to-milligram basis. Acebutolol can suppress premature ventricular contractions, including complex forms, in many patients. Patients with exercise-induced arrhythmias may respond favorably to acebutolol. Acebutolol is also effective for various supraventricular arrhythmias, especially those related to excess catecholamine states or those which require participation of the AV node, such as AV-nodal and AV reciprocating tachycardias. A randomized, double blind, placebo-controlled trial including 600 post-MI patients (APSI trial), demonstrated that a rather low dose of acebutolol, 200 mg twice daily, decreased cardiovascular mortality by 58%.[223]

Side Effects

Side effects related to acebutolol are similar to those of other beta-blocking agents. Patients with congestive heart failure, hypotension, severe peripheral vascular disease, brittle diabetes mellitus, or bronchospastic lung disease should not be treated with acebutolol, despite its partial agonist activity. Similarly, acebutolol may depress sinus node and AV-nodal function. Fatigue, headache, reversible mental depression, skin rash, agranulocytosis, development of antinuclear antibodies, alopecia, and Peyronie's disease have been reported.

Interactions

Although specific interactions have not been reported with acebutolol, caution should be used if it is given with other drugs known to depress automaticity, conduction, or cardiac contractility or other drugs known to interact with beta-blockers.

Indications and Dosage

Acebutolol is indicated for treatment of ventricular premature contractions. It is also effective for some supraventricular arrhythmias. The initial antiarrhythmic dosage usually is 200 mg twice daily, with total daily doses up to 600 to 1200 mg necessary in some patients.[222]

Esmolol

Pharmacologic Description

Esmolol hydrochloride, a phenoxypropanolamine, is a beta$_1$-selective adrenergic-receptor blocking agent. Esmolol is similar in chemical structure to the beta blocker metoprolol but contains an ester linkage on the para position of the phenyl ring. Because of this ester linkage, esmolol has an ultrashort plasma half-life of 9 min. It has no appreciable intrinsic sympathomimetic or membrane-stabilizing activity. On a milligram-to-milligram basis, esmolol is approximately 1/50th as potent as propranolol.

Electrophysiologic Action

Electrophysiologic effects of esmolol are those typical of beta-blockade. Esmolol increases the sinus node's cycle length and slows AV-nodal conduction.[224] AV-nodal refractoriness is increased as a result of decreased sympathetic tone. Thus esmolol may be effective when used to slow the ventricular response to atrial fibrillation or atrial flutter, or in treating arrhythmias requiring participation of the AV node, such as reciprocating tachycardias.[225,226] Electrocardiographic effects consist of prolongation of the PR interval with no significant changes in QRS or QTc duration.

Pharmacokinetics and Metabolism

Esmolol is rapidly metabolized by hydrolysis of the ester linkage, chiefly by esterases in the cytosol of red blood cells.[226] The distribution half-life of esmolol is 2 min; the elimination half-life is 9 min, necessitating continuous infusion or repeated boluses for sustained effects. Metabolism of esmolol results in a negligible amount of methanol and an acid metabolite.[227] Less than 2% of esmolol is

recovered in the urine. The metabolite has about 1/1500th the beta-blocking activity of esmolol and is eliminated with a half life of 3.7 h in individuals with normal renal function. Unlike that of many other agents with ester groups, the metabolism of esmolol is unaffected by plasma cholinesterase.[225] With continuous high-dose infusion of esmolol, levels of methanol approximate endogenous methanol levels with concentrations reaching only 2% of those associated with methanol toxicity. Esmolol is about 55% bound to plasma proteins, while the acid metabolite is only 10% bound.

Hemodynamic Effects

Esmolol produces a dose-dependent decrease in heart rate, cardiac contractility, cardiac output, and blood pressure. Recovery of these effects is nearly complete within 15 to 30 min after discontinuation of the infusion. In clinical trials, approximately 10 to 30% of patients (particularly those with borderline-low or low-normal pretreatment blood pressures) treated with esmolol developed transient hypotension, defined as a systolic pressure less than 90 mm Hg or a diastolic pressure less than 50 mm Hg.[226] Twelve percent of patients were symptomatic.

Antiarrhythmic Effects

Esmolol has been used mainly in acute settings to control the ventricular response to supraventricular arrhythmias. In a multicenter double-blind, randomized study, esmolol was as effective as propranolol, resulting in at least a 20% reduction in ventricular rate in 72% of patients.[228] Conversion to sinus rhythm occurred in 14%. In other studies, esmolol compared favorably with verapamil, with a significantly greater percentage of conversion to sinus rhythm.[229]

Side Effects

The principal side effect of esmolol is hypotension. Other side effects are typical of beta blockers and include increased heart failure, dyspnea, bradycardia, decreased peripheral perfusion, nausea, vomiting, irritation at the infusion site, and headache. To avoid phlebitis, esmolol should not be infused using concentrations in excess of 10 mg/mL. For a typical patient requiring 50 to 150 mg/kg/min, 20 to 60 mL/h of fluid administration is required, necessitating attention to volume status.

Interactions

Esmolol can be very effective when used in combination with digoxin, and the effects on the AV node are additive. Concomitant administration of esmolol and morphine results in a 46% increase in steady-state levels of esmolol. Esmolol prolongs the metabolism of succinylcholine-induced neuromuscular blockade by 5 to 8 min. Esmolol should be administered with caution in patients prone to bradycardia, AV block, or hypotension or patients on other medications likely to potentiate these effects.

Indications and Dosage

Esmolol is indicated for the acute management and rapid control of ventricular rate in patients with atrial fibrillation or atrial flutter and in some patients with noncompensatory sinus tachycardia. Therapy is usually initiated with a loading dose of 500 μg/kg over 1 min, followed by a maintenance infusion of 25 to 50 μg/kg/min. Dose titration can be performed after 5 min and consists of additional boluses of 500 μg/kg over 1 min, followed by an increase in the maintenance infusion by 25 to 50 μg/kg/min. Most patients are controlled with a maintenance infusion of 50 to 200 μg/kg/min. Esmolol may also be useful in the management of acute myocardial ischemia or infarction, although this has not been studied extensively.[230] The effects of prolonged infusions of esmolol (longer than 48 h) also have not been fully evaluated.

CLASS III AGENTS

Class III drugs prolong the duration of action potential and increase refractoriness. The effect is often mediated by blockade of potassium channels during phase 2 or 3 of the action potential. Some newer agents prolong the duration of the action potential by activating sodium channels during the plateau phase.

Amiodarone

Pharmacologic Description

Amiodarone hydrochloride, an iodinated benzofuran derivative, was initially developed as a vasodilating agent for the treatment of angina pectoris. Thirty-seven percent of its molecular weight is iodine. It was subsequently found to have potent antiarrhythmic properties in 1970.[231] It has been used extensively for the treatment of supraventricular and ventricular arrhythmias, especially in Argentina, Israel, and Europe. Both oral and intravenous preparations are available in the United States for the treatment of life-threatening ventricular arrhythmias.

Electrophysiologic Action

Amiodarone has been shown to have class I, II, III, and IV effects. It is a weak, noncompetitive inhibitor of alpha- and beta-adrenergic receptors. Its predominant action on cardiac tissue consists of prolongation of the duration of the action potential and increases in refractoriness.[231] Amiodarone has only slight effects on the rate of rise of phase 0 of the action potential. Conduction velocity is decreased, however, apparently owing to effects on resistance to passive current flow rather than effects on the inward sodium current.[232] In automatic cells, amiodarone decreases the slope of phase 4 of the action potential, decreasing the depolarization rate of these cells. Amiodarone has differential effects on the two components of cardiac rectifier K^+ current, depending on the length of treatment.[232a] ECG effects consist of a slowing of the sinus rate and prolongation of the PR, QRS, and QT intervals. Amiodarone also prolongs the refractory period of accessory AV pathways in patients with bypass tracts or the WPW syndrome.[233] The time course of onset of antiarrhythmic action varies, with effects on the sinus and AV nodes occurring within 2 weeks of therapy, while prolongation of the ventricular functional refractory period, QT prolongation, and ventricular antiarrhythmic effects are not maximal for up to 10 weeks.[234]

Pharmacokinetics and Metabolism

When the drug is administered orally, absorption of amiodarone is slow and erratic. Bioavailability ranges from 22 to 65% in most patients.[235] Peak plasma concentrations occur between 3 and 7 h after a single oral dose. Even with loading doses, maximal antiarrhythmic effects may not appear for several days to months.[234,235a] Amiodarone is 95% protein-bound and has a large but variable volume of distribution of approximately 60 L/kg. Amiodarone and its major metabolite, desethylamiodarone, are highly lipophilic and accumulate throughout the body, including liver, adipose tissue, lung, myocardium, kidney, thyroid, skin, eye, and skeletal muscle. Elimination is principally hepatic via biliary excretion. Enterohepatic recirculation may occur. The elimination of amiodarone is biphasic, with an initial half-life of 2.5 to 10 days; the terminal elimination half-life is 26 to 107 days, with most patients in the 40- to 55-day range. Desethylamiodarone has an elimination half-life averaging 61 days.

Hemodynamic Effects

With intravenous administration, amiodarone decreases heart rate, myocardial contractility, and systemic vascular resistance. Coronary vasodilatation may also occur. Rapid intravenous administration may produce profound hypotension, partly related to systemic vasodilation caused by the vehicle Tween-80.[236] Oral amiodarone usually does not worsen congestive heart failure, even in patients with severe LV dysfunction, although caution is warranted, especially with high doses used during drug loading, since some patients may show hemodynamic deterioration.[237]

Antiarrhythmic Effects

A large number of studies have documented the efficacy of amiodarone in suppressing supraventricular and ventricular arrhythmias even when other agents were ineffective. Amiodarone is very effective in chronic maintenance of sinus rhythm in patients with atrial fibrillation, although it is not approved for this indication in the United States.[237a,b] Daily doses of 200 to 400 mg have shown the efficacy of 53 to 79% for sinus rhythm maintenance.[238,239] It was more effective than sotalol or propafenone in the maintenance of sinus rhythm in patients with chronic paroxysmal or persistent atrial fibrillation.[240] The drug is often used in patients with life-threatening ventricular tachyarrhythmias who are unresponsive to other antiarrhythmic agents. In a composite of 10 reports from the literature, amiodarone prevented recurrent sustained VT or VF in 66% of 567 patients during a mean follow-up of 13 months.[235] The prognostic utility of electrophysiologic testing with amiodarone remains controversial. The ability to induce VT using programmed ventricular stimulation during therapy with amiodarone does not preclude a good outcome.[241,242] Patients rendered not inducible by amiodarone have a good outcome.[242] Induction of a hemodynamically well-tolerated ventricular tachyarrhythmia apparently suggests a relatively favorable prognosis. Suppression of ventricular ectopy on ambulatory monitoring by amiodarone is an unreliable indicator of success, whereas failure to suppress ventricular ectopy appears to indicate a worse prognosis. Therapeutic plasma concentrations are usually between 1.0 and 2.0 μg/mL with chronic dosing. Several trials have shown that amiodarone may improve mortality, or at least not worsen mortality, when used to treat patients after myocardial infarction or with LV dysfunction.[243–245] Whether amiodarone is superior in this regard to conventional beta-blocking drugs is unknown. Intravenous amiodarone is at least as effective as bretylium for VT or VF and is associated with fewer hemodynamic side effects.[246–249]

Side Effects

Almost every organ system is affected by amiodarone. Corneal microdeposits of brownish crystals are expected. They may result in blurred vision, halos, or a smoky hue, but reportedly disappear following cessation of therapy. Abnormal thyroid function tests are not uncommon, and in some cases clinical hypothyroidism or hyperthyroidism becomes evident.[250] A bluish-gray skin discoloration and photosensitivity may occur. Liver function abnormalities, neuropathy, and myositis have been reported. Occasionally severe hepatitis has occurred; two cases of fatal hepatic necrosis have been reported after rapid infusion of large intravenous doses. As many as 5 to 15% of patients treated with 400 mg per day will develop pulmonary toxicity. This usually resolves with discontinuation of therapy but may be fatal. Therapy with corticosteroids may be beneficial. Cardiac side effects include bradycardia, AV block, worsening of congestive heart failure, and rarely proarrhythmia. Torsades de pointes occurs only rarely, and a number of patients having this arrhythmia while on other drugs have not had this recur while on amiodarone. Intravenous amiodarone in concentrations of greater than 2.0 mg/mL should be infused only via a central venous catheter owing to a high incidence of peripheral vein phlebitis. Lower concentrations may be infused using a peripheral vein.

Interaction

Amiodarone interacts with many drugs, increasing the plasma concentrations of warfarin (100%), digoxin (70%), quinidine (33%), procainamide (55%), and NAPA (33%). Concentrations of phenytoin and flecainide have also been reported to increase. Appropriate caution should be exercised when using any of these agents along with amiodarone.

Indications and Dosage

The oral and newer intravenous formulations of amiodarone are indicated in the United States for the treatment of recurrent life-threatening ventricular arrhythmias that have not responded adequately to other agents. Because of the large volume of distribution, large loading doses are required initially. Typically, 1000 to 1600 mg is administered daily for 7 to 14 days, followed by 600 to 800 mg daily for the next 7 to 30 days. Long-term maintenance therapy usually requires 200 to 400 mg daily. Doses should be slowly reduced to the lowest level consistent with adequate arrhythmia control, since higher chronic doses are associated with an increased incidence of toxicity. Therapy with intravenous amiodarone is usually initiated with a bolus dose of 150 mg administered over 10 to 15 min, followed by a slower loading dose of 360 mg over 6 h (1 mg/min). Maintenance therapy is given at a dose of 0.5 mg/min. Concomitant oral therapy may be started simultaneously. Given the favorable mortality results with amiodarone and its efficacy in treating almost any cardiac arrhythmia, clinical use of amiodarone has increased.

Intravenous Amiodarone

Intravenous amiodarone is indicated for treatment and prophylaxis of frequently recurring VF and hemodynamically unstable VT. Peak serum concentration after a single 5-mg/kg 15-min infusion in healthy subjects range between 5 and 41 mg/L. Due to rapid distribution, serum concentrations decline to 10% of peak values within 30 to 45 min after the end of the infusion. It has been reported to produce negative inotropic and vasodilatory effects in animals and humans, with drug-related hypotension occurring in 16% of treated patients. Additional adverse effects were: bradycardia and AV block, VF (less than 2%), adult respiratory distress syndrome (ARDS) (2%) and torsades de pointes. The recommended starting dose of IV amiodarone is about 1000 mg over the first 24 h of therapy, delivered by the following infusion regimen: first rapid infusion—150 mg over the first 10 min, followed by a slow infusion of 360 mg over the next 6 h and a maintenance infusion of 540 mg over the remaining 18 h. Intravenous amiodarone is effective in suppressing refractory VT/VF and provides control of 60 to 80% of recurrent

VT/VF when conventional drugs as continuous oral therapy have failed.[251]

Intravenous amiodarone has increased survival to hospital admission in patients with out-of-hospital cardiac arrest due to refractory VT/VF and has been shown to be significantly more effective than lidocaine in improving survival to hospital for out-of-hospital cardiac arrest patients.[252,253] The most recent Advanced Cardiac Life Support (ACLS) guidelines suggest the use intravenous amiodarone (class IIb) at a dose of 300 mg IV as initial bolus, followed by a second dose of 150 mg IV if VF/pulseless VT recurs.[254]

Sotalol

Pharmacologic Description

Sotalol is a nonselective beta-adrenergic antagonist introduced in 1965 for the treatment of hypertension. It is without significant intrinsic sympathomimetic activity or membrane-stabilizing activity. Sotalol prolongs the action potential duration, however, accounting for its class III designation. The antiarrhythmic effects in humans were reported in 1970.[255]

The electrophysiologic effects of sotalol are those of beta-blockade and class III activity. Sotalol exists as a racemic mixture of d-sotalol and l-sotalol. The d-sotalol form has about 1/50th the beta-blocking activity of l-sotalol, but both are equally responsible for class III effects.[256] Sotalol causes an increase in the duration of the action potential and the refractory period of human atria, ventricles, AV node, Purkinje fibers, and accessory pathways.[257,258] Conduction velocity is reportedly not decreased by sotalol except for the beta-blocking effects on nodal tissues. ECG effects consist of increases in the PR, QT, and QTc intervals. QRS duration and the HV interval are unchanged.

Pharmacokinetics and Metabolism

Sotalol is rapidly absorbed following oral administration, with bioavailability varying from 60 to nearly 100%. Sotalol is not bound to plasma proteins, and more than 75% of an administered dose is recovered unchanged in the urine. No metabolites have been detected. The elimination half-life averages 10 to 15 h, permitting twice daily dosing.[259] Sotalol will accumulate in patients with renal but not hepatic insufficiency.

Hemodynamic Effects

Prolongation of the duration of the action potential allows more time for calcium ions to enter a cell, potentially increasing the inotropic state of the cell. Sotalol appears unique among beta-blocking agents in this regard. Studies in isolated muscle preparations, animals, and humans suggest that sotalol may cause less depression of contractility than other beta-blocking drugs.[260,261] Nevertheless, sotalol can reduce blood pressure and precipitate or worsen congestive heart failure in some patients.

Antiarrhythmic Effects

Sotalol has been used effectively for the treatment of supraventricular and ventricular tachyarrhythmias, including WPW syndrome. Sotalol has been effective in terminating many supraventricular arrhythmias or slowing the ventricular response to atrial fibrillation or flutter. In one study, oral sotalol produced a beneficial response in 31 of 33 patients with atrial arrhythmias.[262] Other studies have found sotalol effective in the treatment of life-threatening ventricular arrhythmias when assessed by electrophysiologic testing, including those refractory to class I antiarrhythmic agents.[263-267]

Polymorphic VT (torsades de pointes) in the setting of a prolonged QT interval has occurred with sotalol, often in association with either hypokalemia or renal insufficiency (high sotalol levels). Sotalol has also been shown to reduce defibrillation thresholds as well as the frequency of ICD shocks for VT/VF.[268,269]

Side Effects

Rates of bronchospasm, fatigue, impotence, depression, and headache are similar to those of other beta-blocking drugs. Sinus node slowing, AV block, hypotension, and worsening of congestive heart failure may occur. Rare cases of retroperitoneal fibrosis have been reported. Polymorphic VT is a potentially life-threatening adverse reaction to sotalol. Its incidence may be minimized by careful attention to electrolyte status as well as avoiding high serum concentrations or excessive bradycardia. Chronic oral therapy with sotalol can increase the serum level of cholesterol as in the case of other beta-blockers without partial agonist activity. The clinical significance of this effect is unknown.

Interactions

Significant drug interactions have not been reported. However, sotalol should be administered with caution with agents that produce hypokalemia or prolong the QT interval. In addition, sotalol should be used cautiously with drugs that depress cardiac contractility, especially in patients with LV dysfunction and those with contraindications to beta-blockers.

Indications and Dosage

Sotalol is effective for the treatment of supraventricular and ventricular tachyarrhythmias. Oral therapy is usually begun with 80 mg administered twice daily. Total daily doses greater than 480 mg should rarely be used. Dosage reduction is necessary in patients with mild to moderate renal insufficiency. Sotalol should probably not be used in patients with severe renal insufficiency. Intravenous doses of 0.2 to 1.0 mg/kg have been used in the acute treatment of arrhythmias. The d stereoisomer of sotalol (d-sotalol) was withdrawn from further clinical testing after it was shown to be associated with increased cardiac and all-cause mortality as compared with placebo in patients with history of myocardial infarction and reduced LV function.[270]

Ibutilide

Pharmacologic Description

Ibutilide fumarate, a class III antiarrhythmic agent that prolongs repolarization, was approved by the U.S. Food and Drug Administration (FDA) for intravenous use in the United States. Ibutilide is structurally similar to sotalol but is devoid of any clinically significant beta-adrenergic blocking activity.[271]

Electrophysiologic Action

Ibutilide affects the the duration of action potentials of atrial, ventricular, and His-Purkinje cells in a unique dose-dependent manner. At low concentrations, ibutilide prolongs the duration of action potentials, whereas at higher concentrations the duration decreases. Unlike other class III agents, such as sotalol or N-acetylprocainamide, ibutilide prolongs the duration of action potentials by activating an inward sodium current during the plateau phase of the action potential in addition to blocking an outward potassium current.

Pharmacokinetics and Metabolism

Ibutilide is well-absorbed after oral administration but, like lidocaine, is rapidly metabolized in the liver, such that oral bioavailability is small. Thus, oral administration does not appear practical. Ibutilide has a large volume of distribution (10 to 15 L/kg), with a terminal elimination half-life of between 6 and 9 h. Rapid distribution after IV administration accounts for the disappearance of QT prolongation several minutes after dosing.

Hemodynamic Effects

No significant effects on cardiac contractility have been seen in animal models. In addition, a study of hemodynamic function in patients with EFs both above and below 35% showed no clinically significant effects on cardiac output, mean pulmonary artery pressure, or pulmonary capillary wedge pressure at doses of up to 0.03 mg/kg.

Antiarrhythmic Effects

In animal studies and in phase 2 clinical trials, ibutilide has shown efficacy in prevention of induction of VT during programmed electrical stimulation. Ibutilide appears to decrease the defibrillation threshold in dogs.[272] In human studies, ibutilide has been investigated most extensively for its ability to terminate established atrial flutter or atrial fibrillation.[272a,272b,272c] Up to 60% of patients with atrial flutter and approximately 40% of those with atrial fibrillation will revert to sinus rhythm with 0.025 mg/kg of ibutilide given intravenously. Patients with more a recent onset of arrhythmia had a higher rate of conversion. Ibutilide pretreatment can also facilitate electrocardioversion of atrial fibrillation.[272c,272d]

Side Effects

To date, the most significant side effect observed in clinical trials of ibutilide is the development of polymorphic VT (torsades de pointes), which has occasionally become sustained and required cardioversion. It occurs in about 1.7% of patients treated and is dose-related. The risk of polymorphic VT is higher in patients with systolic dysfunction. Rare episodes of advanced-degree AV block and infra-His conduction block have been reported.

Interactions

Class Ia as well as class III antiarrhythmic drugs should not be given concomitantly with ibutilide infusion or within 4 h postinfusion because of their potential to prolong refractoriness. The potential for proarrhythmia may increase with the administration of ibutilide to patients who are being treated with drugs that prolong the QT interval, such as phenothiazines, tricyclic antidepressants, and certain antihistamine drugs.

Indications and Dosage

Ibutilide is indicated for the acute treatment (cardioversion) of recent onset atrial flutter or atrial fibrillation. Patients whose atrial arrhythmias were sustained longer than 90 days were not evaluated in clinical trials. A dose of 1 mg is administered over 10 min intravenously. After an additional 10 min, the dose may be repeated if needed. Patients weighing under 60 kg should have the dose reduced.

Dofetilide

Pharmacologic Description

Dofetilide has Vaughn Williams class III antiarrhythmic activity. The mechanism of action is the blockade of the cardiac ion channel carrying the rapid component of the delayed rectifier potassium current I_{Kr}. At all studied concentrations, dofetilide blocks only I_{Kr} with no relevant block of the other repolarizing potassium currents. It has no effect on sodium channels, alpha receptors, or beta receptors.

Electrophysiologic Action

Dofetilide increases the duration of action potentials in a predictable, concentration-dependent manner, primarily due to delayed repolarization. It increases the effective refractory period of both atria and ventricles. It does not have an effect on PR interval or QRS width. Dofetilide does not increase the electrical energy required to convert electrically induced VF, and it significantly reduces the defibrillation threshold in patients with VT and VF undergoing implantation of a cardioverter-defibrillator device.

Pharmacokinetics and Metabolism

The oral bioavailability of dofetilide is >90%, with maximum plasma concentration occurring at about 2 to 3 h. Oral bioavailability is not affected by food intake or antacid use. Steady-state concentration is reached within 2 to 3 days and half-life is about 10 h. Plasma protein binding is 60 to 70% and the volume of distribution is 3 L/kg. Eighty percent of the drug is excreted in urine unchanged and the remaining 20% comprises five minimally active metabolites. The half-life is longer and the clearance of dofetilide is decreased in patients with renal impairment.

Hemodynamic Effects

In hemodynamic studies, dofetilide had no effect on cardiac output, cardiac index, stroke volume index, systemic vascular resistance in patients with VT, mild to moderate congestive heart failure or angina, and either normal or low LV EF. There was no evidence of a negative inotropic effect related to dofetilide therapy in patients with atrial fibrillation. There was no increase in heart failure in patients with significant LV dysfunction or any significant change in blood pressure. Heart rate was decreased by 4 to 6 beats per minute in studies in patients.[273]

Dofetilide use is usually safe in patients with structural heart disease, including patients with impaired LV function (EF $\leq 35\%$) (Diamond CHF)[273a–c] or recent myocardial infarction (Diamond MI).[274]

Antiarrhythmic Effects

Dofetilide, like most other class III antiarrhythmic agents, has antifibrillatory activity in the atria; this property is of importance for the conversion and maintenance of sinus rhythm in patients with atrial fibrillation (AF)/atrial flutter (AFL).[274a–c] In a placebo-controlled blinded study, the conversion rate was 31% in AF patients, 54% in AFL patients, and 0% in those on placebo.[275]

Side Effects

Dofetilide can cause ventricular arrhythmia, primarily torsades de pointes associated with QT prolongation. Prolongation of the QT interval is directly related to the plasma concentration of dofetilide. Factors such as reduced creatinine clearance or dofetilide drug interactions will increase the plasma concentration of dofetilide. The risk of torsades de pointes can be reduced by controlling the plasma concentration through adjustment of the initial dofetilide dose according to creatinine clearance and by monitoring the ECG for excessive increases in the QT interval.

In patients with supraventricular arrhythmias, the overall incidence of torsades was 0.8%—3.3% in patients with congestive heart failure (CHF) and 0.9% in patients on dofetilide with recent myocardial infarction. The majority of the episodes of torsades de pointes occurred within the first 3 days of treatment. The rate of torsades de pointes was reduced when patients were dosed according to their renal function. Other adverse reactions reported were headache, chest pain, dizziness, and respiratory tract infection.

Interactions

The use of dofetilide in conjunction with other drugs which prolong the QT interval is not recommended. Such drugs include phenothiazines, cisapride, bepridil, tricyclic antidepressants, and certain oral macrolides. Class I or III antiarrhythmic should be withheld for at least three half-lives prior to dosing with dofetilide. In clinical trials, dofetilide was administered to patients previously treated with oral amiodarone only if serum amiodarone levels were below 0.3 mg/L or amiodarone had been withdrawn for at least 3 months.

Dofetilide is metabolized to a small degree by the CYP3A4 isoenzyme of the cytochrome P450 system and an inhibitor of this system could increase systemic dofetilide exposure. Concomitant use of the following drugs is contraindicated: cimeditine, verapamil, ketonazole, and trimethoprim alone or in combination with sulfamethoxazole.

Indication and Dosage

The use of dofetilide is indicated for the maintenance of normal sinus rhythm (delay in time to recurrence of atrial fibrillation/atrial flutter) in patients with AF/AFL of greater than 1 week's duration who have been converted to normal sinus rhythm. Because dofetilide can cause life-threatening ventricular arrhythmias, it should be reserved for patients in whom AF/AFL is highly symptomatic. Dofetilide is also indicated for the conversion of AF/AFL to normal sinus rhythm. Dofetilide has not been shown to be effective in patients with paroxysmal AF.

Therapy with dofetilide must be initiated (and if necessary reinitiated) in a setting that provides continuous ECG monitoring. Patients should continue to be monitored in this way for a minimum of 3 days. Additionally, patients should not be discharged within 12 h of electrical or pharmacologic conversion to normal sinus rhythm.

Because prolongation of QT interval and the risk of torsades de pointes are directly related to plasma concentrations of dofetilide, dose adjustment must be inidividualized according to calculated creatinine clearance and QTc. The QT interval should be used if the heart rate is <60 beats per minute. If the QTc >440 ms (500 ms in bundle branch block) or creatinine clearance <20 mL/min, dofetilide is contraindicated. The dose adjustment according to the creatinine clearance is shown in Table 17-2. During loading, a 12-lead ECG should be done 2 to 3 h after the dose and the QT checked.

If patients do not convert to normal sinus rhythm within 72 h of initiation of dofetilide therapy, electrical conversion should be considered, with subsequent monitoring for 12 h postcardioversion.

TABLE 17-2. Dofetilide Dose Adjustment According to Calculated Creatinine Clearance

Creatinine Clearance	Dofetilide Dose
<20 mL/min	Dofetilide is contraindicated
20–40 mL/min	125 μg bid
40–60 mL/min	250 μg bid
>60 mL/min	500 μg bid

NEW CLASS III AGENTS IN DEVELOPMENT

Azimilide

Pharmacologic Description

Azimilide dihydrochloride is a novel class III (I_{Kr} and I_{Ks} blocker) antiarrhythmic drug with weak beta-blocking activity. It is structurally different from other class III agents in that it lacks the methanesulfonamide. Whereas most class III antiarrhythmics are methanesulfonanilide derivatives and block only the rapidly activating I_{Kr} component, azimilide also blocks the slowly activating I_{Ks} component at micromolar concentrations, therefore retaining its antiarrhythmic activity in the presence of tachycardia.

Electrophysiologic Action

Azimilide increases the refractoriness of cardiac cells. In both animals and humans, it causes a dose-dependent increases in the QT interval and prolongation of atrial and ventricular refractory periods.[276] Azimilide has no significant effect on heart rate or on PR or QRS intervals. Electrophysiologic studies have shown that azimilide has little or no effect on sinus node function, AV-nodal conduction time, or His-Purkinje conduction time. In vitro studies have also shown that azimilide prolongs refractoriness over a wide range of cycle lengths, with positive rate and voltage dependence. It has alpha- and beta-adrenergic blocking activity and agonistic effect on muscarinic receptors. It was initially developed for the maintenance of sinus rhythm in patients with AF/AFL.

Hemodynamic Effects

Azimilide initially increases cardiac contractility and only at higher doses decreases heart rate and blood pressure.

Pharmacokinetics and Metabolism

The pharmacokinetics of azildimide is fairly predictable. The drug is completely absorbed after oral intake and the extent of absorption is not affected by food intake. It reaches peak effect after 5 to 7 h of administration and about 2 weeks are required to achieve steady state. The bioavailability of oral azimilide is >85%. It is approximately 94% bound to plasma protein, has a volume of distribution of 10 L/kg and a long half-life (about 4 days), allowing once-a-day dosing. Ninety percent of the drug is metabolized by the liver, with renal clearance accounting for only about 10% of total clearance.[277] It undergoes extensive biotransformation, with more than 10 metabolites detected.

Antiarrhythmic Effects

Azimilide has demonstrated efficacy in the supression of supraventricular and ventricular tachycardias. In a dog model, intravenous azimilide terminated AF and prevented its reinduction in 8 of 8 dogs.[278] Azimilide was also shown to be effective in converting AF to normal sinus rhythm in 13 of 14 dogs as opposed to dofetilide, which was effective in 6 of 12 dogs.[279] Studies in humans, of whom about 80% had some form of structural heart disease, have shown that the time to first symptomatic AF or AFL recurrence was significantly prolonged in the azimilide group (dosing regimen of 100 and 125 mg PO daily) compared to the placebo group.[280] The efficacy of intravenous azimilide in the termination and prevention of ventricular tachyarrhythmias has been investigated in a postinfarction dog model. At a dose of 10 mg/kg given within a week of myocardial infarction, it prevented sudden death in 8 of 12 dogs.[281]

Side Effects

In large trials done to date, more than 90% of patients began randomized therapy with azimilide as outpatients and the drug was well tolerated. It demonstrated a good safety profile in more than 800 patients with supraventricular tachyarrhythmias, most of whom had structural heart disease. The drug does cause a dose-dependent prolongation of the QT interval; 7 patients were required to withdraw from the protocol for QTc >525 ms, and torsades de pointes has been reported in 1 out of 280 patients treated. Additional side effects reported were neutropenia, skin rash, abnormalities in liver function tests, diarrhea and flu-like illness with weakness, dizziness, and paresthesias.[280]

Indications and Dosage

The efficacy and safety of azimilide is now being evaluated in the Azimilide Supraventricular Arrhythmia Program (ASAP). About 1000 patients (more than 70% with structural cardiovascular disease, including CAD, systolic dysfunction, or hypertension) have been randomized to receive either placebo or azimilide. All trials to date have been designed to allow outpatient initiation of the drug (in a significant percentage of patients). The efficacy of azimilide in preventing sudden cardiac death was also evaluated in the Azimilide Post-Infarction Survival Evaluation (ALIVE).[282] In this double-blind, placebo-controlled trial, azimilide had no effect on survival in patients at high risk for sudden cardiac death, namely those with recent myocardial infarction, low LV EF (15 to 25%) and a low heart rate variability (≤20 U).

The doses evaluated so far in large clinical trials for atrial fibrillation were 50, 100, and 125 mg daily. The assigned treatment regimen was given twice a day for 3 days (the loading period), following which the frequency was reduced to once-a-day dosing. Higher doses of the drug were associated with greater efficacy. Clinical data suggest that dose adjustments of azimilide for age, gender, liver/renal function, or concomitant use of digoxin or warfarin (Coumadin) were not necessary.[280]

Tedisamil

Pharmacologic Description

Tedisamil is a heterocyclic dihydrochloride derived from sparteine. It is a blocker of the early rapid repolarized I_{to} channel and I_{Kr} channel and was initially developed for its anti-ischemic properties. It is different from simpler molecules, such as dofetilide, d-sotalol, and other so-called pure class III drugs, because if blocks a complex aggregate of repolarizing myocardial ionic currents, has anti-ischemic properties, and slows the heart rate by a direct effect on the sinus node.

Electrophysiologic Action

Clinical trials have shown that the electrophysiology of tedisamil is that of a class III antiarrhythmic. The drug has been reported to block the I_{Kr} (delayed rectifier potassium) channel and the I_{tr} (transient outward current) channel. It prolongs the duration of action potentials in the atrial and ventricular myocardium, with corresponding increases in the atrial and ventricular effective refractory period (ERP).[283,284]

In humans, intravenous tedisamil (0.3 mg/kg) reduces heart rate by 12%, with a parallel prolongation of QTc interval (+10%) and LV monophasic actional potential (+16% at 90% repolarization).[285] This effect diminishes with increased atrial pacing rate, indicating a reverse use-dependent prolongation effect on LV repolarization and refractoriness.[285] The bradycardic effect of tedisamil is mainly due to prolongation of the repolarization phase in pacemaker cells of the sinus node and was noted under both resting and exercise conditions. It was readily observed at a dose of 8 mg intravenously and >100 mg by mouth.[286] The drug does not influence the atrial conduction time or the conduction through the AV node.

Pharmacokinetics

After single oral and intravenous administration, linear pharmacokinetics is observed. About 60% of the drug is absorbed after oral intake of a single dose, while multiple dosing increased oral bioavailability and higher plasma concentration of the drug was observed. Concurrent food intake does not produce a relevant change in tedisamil pharmacokinetics. It is 96% bound to plasma proteins and reaches its maximum plasma concentration between 1 and 2 h following oral administration. The mean plasma elimination half-life after oral or intravenous administration is between 9 and 12 h. The volume of distribution at steady state is 0.97 L/kg. No metabolites have been detected in humans. It is excreted renally as unchanged drug; in patients with renal dysfunction plasma concentration and elimination half-life are increased.[287]

Hemodynamic Effects

Tedisamil does not impair ventricular contractility; it decreases myocardial oxygen demand and can be used safely in patients with ischemic disease.[288] Filling pressure and dP/dT remain unchanged, with a decrease in heart rate, and LV pump function (EF, stroke volume, and LV efficiency) decreases slightly, by 3 to 13%, whereas LV volume increases (end-diastolic volume by 6%, end-systolic volume by 23%).[288] Bradycardic doses of tedisamil elevate arterial systolic blood pressure; in addition, the drug has diuretic and natriuretic properties.

Antiarrhythmic Effects

Tedisamil has antifibrillatory properties and has been shown effective for conversion of sustained AF to normal sinus rhythm in two different animal models of AF. The efficacy of tedisamil was dose-dependent, with a dose of 1g/kg being 100% effective in terminating AF. The drug was also shown to prevent reinduction of sustained AF 30 min after intravenous administration.[289] Animal data show efficacy in supressing ventricular tachyarrhythmias as well. In dogs studied approximately 8 days after anterior myocardial infarction, tedisamil suppressed programmed stimulation–induced ventricular tachyarrhythmias in 8 of 10 dogs and reduced the incidence of arrhythmias developing in response to acute myocardial ischemia compared with controls (5 of 10 vs. 30 of 40; $P = .027$).[290] In a separate study of isolated rabbit heart VF, 3 μM of tedisamil reduced the incidence of VF compared with controls (5 of 6 vs. 0 of 6; $P = .007$).[291]

Side Effects

The most important frequent adverse effects reported in clinical trials included dose-related incidence of diarrhea, mild increases in hepatic transaminase values and headache after oral administration in CAD patients, as well as transient burning at the site of infusion, metallic taste, and circumoral paresthesia after intravenous dosing.[286] Doses of 100 mg bid and greater produced a statistically significant prolongation of QTc of about 10%, but this effect was not clinically significant. Since tedisamil prolongs the QTc time at

higher doses, it was recommended that ECGs should be monitored closely and care should be taken that QT intervals do not exceed 550 ms.

Indications and Dosage

At doses of 50 to 100 mg twice a day, tedisamil was found to be a good antianginal agent. This was demonstrated in a prospective double-blind, placebo-controlled study of 203 patients with chronic stable angina. Tedisamil led to a prolongation of exercise duration and decreased the frequency of anginal attacks in a dose-dependent fashion.[286]

Tedisamil is available as an oral and parenteral formulation for investigational purposes. The safety and efficacy of intravenous tedisamil in the rapid conversion to normal sinus rhythm in patients with recent onset AF or AFL is being evaluated in an ongoing multicenter, double-blind, randomized, placebo-controlled trial, results of which are pending.

Dronedarone and EO 47/1

Dronedarone (SR33589) is a deiodinated benzofuran derivative structurally related to amiodarone. The short-term effects of dronedarone are similar to those of amiodarone. In animal studies, dronedarone inhibited ischemia-induced arrhythmias, reduced sinus rate, and had a sympatholytic effect characteristic of amiodarone.[292] Animal data have shown that despite the deletion of iodine from the molecule, the major electrophysiologic properties of dronedarone are very similar to those of amiodarone. It reduced sinus frequency in vivo and in vitro, with a significant prolongation of the duration of action potentials in the rabbit ventricular myocardium and a corresponding prolongation of ventricular ERP; it exhibited even less reverse-use dependency of repolarization than that found with amiodarone.[293]

Resting values of LVEF, fractional shortening, LV dP/dT and mean blood pressure remained unchanged after dronedarone administration, whereas resting heart rate was significantly and dose-dependently reduced in dogs with healed myocardial infarction.[294]

Dronedarone is in relatively early stages of development. It is available in both oral and intravenous forms for investigational use in therapy of atrial as well as ventricular arrhythmias. A placebo-controlled dose-finding safety and tolerability study of dronedarone in patients with ICDs and need for antiarrhythmic therapy is currently being conducted.

EO 47/1 is another intravenous amiodarone derivative that is being evaluated in patients with acute supraventricular or ventricular arrhythmia.[294a]

CLASS IV AGENTS

Class IV antiarrhythmic drugs are the nondihydropyridine calcium-channel blocking agents (see Chap. 9).

Verapamil

Pharmacologic Description

Verapamil hydrochloride, a synthetic papaverine derivative, was the first calcium-channel blocking agent to be used clinically. It is indicated for the treatment of supraventricular arrhythmias, control of ventricular rate at rest and during exercise in patients with

AF/AFL, as well in as certain forms of ventricular tachyarrhythmias that occur in patients with structurally normal hearts.

Electrophysiologic Action

The principal electrophysiologic effect of verapamil is inhibition of the slow inward calcium current. Verapamil prolongs the time-dependent recovery of excitability and the effective refractory period of AV-nodal fibers.[295] It has little effect on fibers in the lower AV node (NH region) and no effect on atrial or Purkinje action potentials, which are activated by a rapid sodium current. However, verapamil may be effective in suppressing triggered arrhythmias arising from ventricular or Purkinje tissue.[296] Expected ECG changes consist of prolongation of the PR interval with no significant change in QRS or QT duration. Verapamil may also depress sinus node function (automaticity and conduction), particularly when it is abnormal.

Pharmacokinetics and Metabolism

Verapamil is almost completely (more than 90%) absorbed after oral administration but undergoes extensive first-pass metabolism. Absolute bioavailability ranges from 20 to 35%, with peak plasma levels occurring 1 to 2 h after dosing.[297] Verapamil is 90% bound to plasma proteins. The l isomer of verapamil undergoes more rapid metabolism than the d isomer; the l-verapamil isomer is also more active electrophysiologically.[297] Twelve metabolites of verapamil have been identified; the major one, norverapamil, can reach concentrations equal to those of the parent compound with chronic dosing. The cardiovascular activity of norverapamil is approximately 20% that of verapamil. After single oral doses, the elimination half-life of verapamil varies from 3 to 7 h; with multiple doses, the half-life ranges from 3 to 12 h. Elimination half-life is usually prolonged with increasing age. In one study, the elimination half-life in patients over the age of 61 years was 7.4 h, compared with 3.8 h in individuals under 36 years of age.[298] The elimination of verapamil may also be prolonged in patients with atrial fibrillation or with hepatic dysfunction.

Hemodynamic Effects

Verapamil produces negative inotropic, dromotropic (AV and SA nodes), and chronotropic (SA node) effects. However, it is well tolerated in most individuals, even in those with LV dysfunction. Hypotension, bradycardia, AV block, and asystole have occurred on occasion. Simultaneous use of verapamil with a beta blocker may result in significant hypotension and depression of cardiac function. This risk is more pronounced with intravenous administration of verapamil.

Antiarrhythmic Effects

Verapamil will slow the ventricular response to atrial fibrillation and flutter even in patients with normal AV conduction.[299] Patients with atrial fibrillation and accessory AV pathways may experience increases in ventricular rate after verapamil administration, related to either a reflex increase in sympathetic tone following vasodilation or decreased AV-nodal conduction with less retrograde penetration of the bypass tract. Verapamil can slow and terminate most arrhythmias utilizing the AV node as part of the reentrant circuit, such as AV-nodal reentry or AV reciprocating tachycardia using an accessory pathway. Oral verapamil is consistently less effective than intravenous verapamil in terminating these arrhythmias, a difference that may be explained in part by the differences in bioavailability

and metabolism of the more active l isomer when the racemic mixture of d- and l-verapamil is given by these two routes.[297] Verapamil can be effective monotherapy for long-term control of ventricular rate in patients with AF or as adjunctive therapy in combination with digoxin. Verapamil is generally ineffective in treating reentrant VT but may be effective in certain ventricular tachyarrhythmias, usually seen in younger patients, presumedly due to triggered activity.[296] Verapamil may also be used to suppress or reduce the ventricular rate in patients with multifocal atrial tachycardia.

Side Effects

Intravenous verapamil may produce hypotension, bradycardia, AV block, and occasionally asystole. The risk of hypotension may be lessened by the prior administration of 1000 mg intravenous calcium chloride without interfering with the acute depressant effects of intravenous verapamil on AV-nodal conduction.[300] It should be avoided in patients with severe LV dysfunction and in those with wide QRS tachycardias in which VT or AF with preexcitation are considerations. Oral therapy is most commonly associated with constipation, but some patients complain of dizziness, fatigue, or ankle edema. Rarely, increases in liver aminotransferases have been observed.

Interactions

Verapamil reduces the clearance of digoxin by 35%, with an increase in serum digoxin concentrations of 50 to 75% within the first week of verapamil therapy.[297,301] Concomitant administration of verapamil and quinidine may result in significant hypotension, since both drugs antagonize the effects of catecholamines on alpha-adrenergic receptors. Other drugs with negative inotropic properties, such as disopyramide or flecainide, should be used cautiously with verapamil. Simultaneous administration of beta-blockers and verapamil may result in hypotension, bradycardia, or AV block. Verapamil appears to variably increase the bioavailability of metoprolol from 0 to 28%.[302]

Indications and Dosage

Verapamil is indicated for the termination of supraventricular tachycardias involving the AV node. It is also indicated to control the ventricular rate in patients with atrial fibrillation or flutter and normal AV conduction. Intravenous doses of 5 to 10 mg given over no fewer than 2 min are often effective. The dose may be repeated if necessary in 30 min. Alternatively, smaller doses (e g., 2.5 mg) repeated as indicated at more frequent intervals also may be effective. In contrast to certain class I and III antiarrhythmic agents, verapamil is rarely effective in converting AF/AFL to sinus rhythm. Oral therapy using doses of 160 to 480 mg per day, in three or four divided doses, can be effective for chronic control of ventricular response with AF or prophylaxis of paroxysmal supraventricular tachycardia. Sustained-release preparations may allow once- or twice-daily dosing in many patients.

Diltiazem

Pharmacologic Description

Diltiazem hydrochloride is a benzothiazepine derivative that blocks influx of calcium ions during cell depolarization in cardiac and vascular smooth muscle. It is indicated for therapy of supraventricular arrhythmias and for control of ventricular rate to atrial fibrillation and flutter.

Electrophysiologic Action

The principal electrophysiologic effect of diltiazem is inhibition of the slow inward calcium current. It prolongs the time-dependent recovery of excitability and the effective refractory period of AV-nodal fibers.[303,304] Expected ECG changes consist of prolongation of the PR (AH) interval with no significant change in QRS or QT duration. Diltiazem also may depress sinus node function (automaticity and conduction), particularly when it is abnormal.

Pharmacokinetics and Metabolism

Diltiazem binds to both alpha$_1$-acid glycoprotein (40%) and serum albumin (30%). Diltiazem is extensively metabolized in the liver by the cytochrome P450 system. Little diltiazem is renally eliminated. As such, diltiazem doses do not need to be adjusted in the presence of renal insufficiency or failure. The elimination half-life of intravenous diltiazem is approximately 3.4 h.

Hemodynamic Effects

Intravenous diltiazem produces negative inotropic, dromotropic, and chronotropic effects. Administered acutely, diltiazem lowers both systolic and diastolic blood pressure and systemic vascular resistance. Coronary artery vascular resistance also decreases, increasing coronary blood flow.

Antiarrhythmic Effects

Diltiazem increases AV-nodal conduction time and increases AV-nodal refractoriness. The effects of diltiazem on the AV node demonstrate use dependence, being more pronounced at faster heart rates. In addition, diltiazem slows the rate of depolarization of the sinus node. AV-nodal reentry and reciprocating tachycardia may be terminated by direct effects on the AV node.[305] Increased AV nodal refractoriness also slows the ventricular response to AF/AFL.

Side Effects

Hypotension is the most common side effect of diltiazem, occurring in approximately 4.3% of patients in clinical trials. Although the sinus rate decreases with intravenous diltiazem, sinus bradycardia or high-grade AV block occurs rarely. Elevations of serum aminotransferase enzyme levels occur rarely.

Interactions

Drugs that produce hypotension or interfere with sinus and AV-nodal function would be expected to produce synergistic effects with diltiazem. Agents that interfere or induce the hepatic microsomal enzyme system would be expected to alter diltiazem levels. Diltiazem increases propranolol levels by 50%.

Indications and Dosage

Intravenous diltiazem is indicated for temporary control of the rapid ventricular rate associated with supraventricular tachyarrhythmias such as AF/AFL, AV-nodal reentrant tachycardia, or reciprocating tachycardia utilizing an AV bypass tract. Diltiazem should not be used to treat patients with AF/AFL and AV bypass tracts. Initial therapy with intravenous diltiazem is usually administered as a bolus dose of 15 to 25 mg (0.25 mg/kg), followed by an infusion of between 5 to 15 mg/h. If ventricular rate control is not achieved after the first bolus, the bolus dose may be repeated in 15 min. An 11 mg/h infusion approximates the steady-state levels achieved with a 360 mg sustained-release preparation of diltiazem. Oral preparations are available in immediate-release tablets of between 30 to 120 mg used every 6 to 8 h and a sustained-release form of between 180 to 300 mg requiring only once-daily dosing. Although effective, oral forms of diltiazem are not approved for treatment of arrhythmias.[306,307]

UNCLASSIFIED ANTIARRHYTHMIC AGENTS

Adenosine and ATP

Pharmacologic Description

Adenosine is an endogenous compound found within every cell of the human body (see Chap. 32). It is approved by the FDA for use in the United States. Adenosine 5' triphosphate (ATP), a nucleotide, has been used in Europe since 1929. Adenosine and ATP have short half-lives, enabling multiple doses without danger of cumulative or long-lasting effects.

Electrophysiologic Action

Adenosine and ATP both exert negative chronotropic and dromotropic effects on the sinus and AV nodes. Both decrease the duration of action potentials and hyperpolarize atrial myocardial cells.[308] No direct effect on ventricular tissue has been demonstrated; however, catecholamine-enhanced ventricular automaticity may be suppressed by adenosine. The electrophysiologic effects of ATP, and to a lesser extent adenosine, may be mediated in part by a vagal reflex. ECG effects consist of slowing of the sinus rate and prolongation of the PR interval.

Pharmacokinetics and Metabolism

Both adenosine and ATP have half-lives of less than 10 s. ATP is metabolized to adenosine by extracellular enzymes. Adenosine is degraded by extracellular deaminases as well as by intracellular deaminases after it is rapidly transported into cells, forming inosine.

Hemodynamic Effects

Adenosine and ATP are potent vasodilators that tend to reduce systolic blood pressure. Hemodynamic effects are transient following single bolus doses of either agent, which are usually well tolerated. Adenosine is also a potent coronary artery vasodilator.

Antiarrhythmic Effects

Both adenosine and ATP are effective in terminating supraventricular tachyarrhythmias requiring participation of the AV-node, such as AV-nodal reentry or AV reciprocating tachycardia in patients with accessory pathways. In one study of 21 patients, ATP (100%) was more effective than verapamil (80%) in terminating paroxysmal AV nodal tachycardia.[309] Compared with verapamil, adenosine may be more likely to unmask latent ventricular preexcitation after termination of AV reentrant tachycardia in patients with WPW syndrome. It may also cause fewer hemodynamically significant arrhythmias after termination of AV reentrant tachycardia.[310] Overall, adenosine has been effective in 60% to more than 90% of patients in different small series, in part reflecting dosing regimens, patient selection, and arrhythmia mechanism. Occasionally, transient AF has been reported following administration of adenosine or ATP; therefore caution is warranted in administering these agents to patients with preexcitation.[311] In patients with various atrial tachyarrhythmias, including AF, adenosine will depress AV-nodal conduction, which can be useful diagnostically. ATP and adenosine can also be effective for certain types of VT in both animal models and humans, including catecholamine-sensitive tachyarrhythmias in young adults.[312] Further studies are required, however, to determine the efficacy and utility of adenosine and ATP in the treatment of ventricular tachyarrhythmias.

Side Effects

Both adenosine and ATP produce transient flushing and dyspnea following intravenous administration. Additional side effects, more prominent with ATP, include bronchospasm, dyspnea, vomiting, retching, cramps, headache, and rarely cardiac arrest. The reported difference in side effects may be related in part to the fact that ATP has been in clinical usage for over 50 years, whereas adenosine has been studied for only a short time. But, in addition ATP triggers a more marked vagal reflex. Side effects with either compound are transient, and the potential for long-lasting adverse effects is minimal. Nevertheless, the possibility of profound bradycardia, AV block, or AF, especially in WPW patients with accelerated accessory AV conduction, justifies appropriate caution. Selective adenosine agonists are currently being developed to avoid these problems.

Interactions

Numerous drugs affect adenosine transport or degradation, often potentiating the effect of adenosine, in experimental models. Examples include dipyridamole, digitalis, verapamil, and benzodiazepines. Aminophylline and other methylxanthines antagonize the effects of both adenosine and ATP in humans. In one documented case, a patient receiving sustained-release theophylline failed to respond to high-dose adenosine.[311]

Indications and Dosage

Adenosine and ATP are effective agents in the acute management of paroxysmal supraventricular and AV reciprocating tachycardias involving the AV node. Adenosine is usually administered in doses of 3 to 12 mg (3 mg/mL) by rapid intravenous bolus. ATP has been given in doses of 2 to 20 mg. To be maximally effective, these agents must be given as rapid intravenous bolus injections, administered directly in a free-flowing intravenous line; effects are more marked with injection into a central line. Injection into a circuitous line of peripheral tubing may be ineffective.

Digitalis

Pharmacologic Description

Digitalis glycosides are among the oldest antiarrhythmic agents still used today (see Chap. 13). Medicinal use of foxglove (digitalis) was mentioned by Welsh physicians as early as 1250. It was used to treat heart failure and arrhythmias in patients in 1775, and William Withering described his experiences with digitalis 10 years later in the classic monograph "An Account of the Foxglove and Some of Its Medical Uses"....[313] Digitalis preparations are steroid glycosides mostly derived from the leaves of the common flowering plants *Digitalis purpurea* (digitoxin) and *Digitalis lanata* (digoxin, lanatoside C, and deslanoside). Ouabain, a rapidly acting digitalis preparation, is derived from seeds of *Strophanthus gratus*. Digoxin and to a much lesser extent digitoxin are the most commonly used digitalis preparations.

Electrophysiologic Action

Digitalis glycosides produce electrophysiologic effects by a direct effect on myocardial cells as well as by indirect effects mediated by the autonomic nervous system. Digitalis preparations are specific inhibitors of a magnesium- and ATP-dependent sodium-potassium ATPase enzyme. Inhibition of this enzyme indirectly promotes an increased concentration of intracellular calcium ions. Increased intracellular calcium results in an increased force of myocardial contraction and also appears to be responsible for many of the arrhythmic effects seen with digitalis toxicity. Indirect effects result from a vagomimetic action and include negative chronotropic and dromotropic (AV node) effects. At toxic levels, digitalis results in increased sympathetic activity. Effective refractory periods of atrial and ventricular muscle generally decrease, while those of the AV node and Purkinje fibers increase. Refractory periods of accessory AV pathways may decrease in some patients, which can increase the rate of AV conduction in these patients with atrial fibrillation.[314] In most individuals, digitalis does not appreciably alter the sinus rate. Sinus rate may slow markedly in patients with heart failure treated with digitalis, however, owing in part to vagal effects and to withdrawal of sympathetic tone. ECG effects include prolongation of the PR (AH) interval with various changes in the ST segment and T wave, characteristically with concave coving of downward-sloping ST segments.

Pharmacokinetics and Metabolism

Digoxin is 60 to 80% bioavailable when administered orally in tablets. A capsule preparation of digoxin in solution is 90 to 100% bioavailable. In as many as 10% of patients, intestinal bacteria may degrade up to 40% of digoxin to cardioinactive products such as dihydrodigoxin, resulting in reduced digoxin serum levels. Digoxin is 20 to 25% protein-bound. Elimination is mostly renal, with a half-life averaging 36 to 48 h in normal individuals. Severe renal insufficiency can prolong the elimination half-life up to 4.4 days. Digitoxin is a less polar glycoside that constitutes the principal active ingredient of the digitalis leaf. Digitoxin is nearly completely bioavailable after oral administration and is approximately 95% bound to serum proteins. Elimination is predominantly hepatic with an elimination half-life averaging 7 to 9 days.

Hemodynamic Effects

Digitalis produces positive inotropic effects in both normal and failing hearts.[315] Cardiac output does not increase in normal individuals, however, owing to counteracting changes in preload and afterload.[316] Digitalis increases arterial and venous tone, increasing systemic vascular resistance.[317] Vascular resistance may increase prior to positive inotropic effects. Thus caution is required when digitalis is administered acutely in patients in whom an increase in vascular resistance would be deleterious. Rapid administration increases coronary vascular resistance, an effect which may be avoided by slow administration.[318] In addition, increased mesenteric vascular tone may possibly, on occasion, result in ischemic bowel necrosis.[319]

Antiarrhythmic Effects

Antiarrhythmic effects result predominantly from conduction slowing within the AV node. Thus digitalis is most useful in controlling the ventricular rate in patients with atrial fibrillation. It is somewhat less effective in adequately slowing AV conduction in patients with atrial flutter or atrial tachycardia or in cases where sympathetic tone is high. Addition of a beta blocker or calcium-channel antagonist such as verapamil or diltiazem typically results in additive electrophysiologic effects. Whether digitalis can reduce the frequency of these arrhythmias or facilitate their conversion to sinus rhythm has not been clearly established.[319a] Digitalis may also be effective in the chronic prophylactic or acute management of patients with AV-nodal reentrant tachycardia. Therapeutic plasma levels range from 0.8 to 2.0 ng/mL for digoxin and from 14 to 26 ng/mL for digitoxin.

Side Effects

Adverse reactions most commonly involve the heart, central nervous system, and gastrointestinal tract. Hypersensitivity reactions are rare, and gynecomastia occurs infrequently. Patients with abnormal AV-nodal function may experience heart block in the absence of toxicity. Digitalis toxicity results in many cardiac and noncardiac manifestations. Noncardiac effects include nausea, vomiting, abdominal pain, headache, and visual disturbances, especially a yellow-green color distortion. Ventricular premature contractions are perhaps the most common manifestation of cardiac toxicity; however, VT or fibrillation may occur. In addition, advanced-degree AV block, atrial tachycardia, and accelerated junctional rhythms are commonly seen. Combinations of enhanced automaticity (or triggered activity) with AV block (e.g., paroxysmal atrial tachycardia with AV block) are suggestive of digitalis toxicity. Toxicity may be treated with potassium if serum concentrations of potassium are low or normal, with monitoring to avoid high-grade AV block. Magnesium, lidocaine, propranolol, and temporary cardiac pacing may be helpful in selected cases, when withdrawal of digoxin is not sufficient to resolve toxicity. In some patients with WPW syndrome and accelerated AV conduction, digoxin may shorten the refractory period of the bypass tract, making rapid anomalous conduction more likely if atrial fibrillation occurs.[314] In cases of severe digoxin or digitoxin toxicity associated with life-threatening ventricular arrhythmias, hyperkalemia, and/or heart block, rapid reversal of toxicity is possible with the administration of bovine digoxin immune antigen-binding fragments (Fab).[320] Free levels of digoxin drop to undetectable levels within 1 min of administration, with favorable cardiac effects usually occurring within 30 min. Each vial of antigen fragments (40 mg) will bind approximately 0.6 mg of digoxin or digitoxin. The average dose of Fab used during clinical trials was 10 vials; however, up to 20 vials or more may be necessary in suicidal overdose situations. Antigen-binding fragments are excreted mainly by the kidneys with an elimination half-life averaging 15 to 20 h in patients with normal renal function. Patients with significant renal insufficiency must be observed closely for the reemergence of digitalis toxicity. The Fab fragments may not be excreted from the body in these patients but rather are degraded by other processes with subsequent liberation of previously bound digitalis.

Interactions

Concomitant administration of quinidine, verapamil, amiodarone, flecainide, or propafenone increases digoxin levels and may precipitate digitalis toxicity.[22,23,201] Potassium-depleting diuretics and corticosteroids may also precipitate digitalis toxicity. Antibiotics may increase digoxin absorption by reducing metabolism of digoxin by intestinal bacteria. Antacids and resins such as cholestyramine may reduce digoxin absorption. Concomitant administration of calcium channel antagonists or beta blockers may produce heart block when administered with digitalis preparations. Digitoxin metabolism may be enhanced by agents such as phenobarbital and phenytoin, which enhance hepatic microsomal enzyme activity.

Indications and Dosage

Digitalis preparations are indicated as antiarrhythmic agents to control the ventricular rate in patients with paroxysmal or chronic atrial fibrillation and in those with AV-nodal reentrant or AV reciprocating tachycardias. Complete digitalization of an adult typically requires 0.6 to 1.2 mg of digoxin administered in divided doses intravenously or orally; however, differences in bioavailability between preparations must be considered. Maintenance doses of digoxin usually range from 0.125 to 0.25 mg daily but must be substantially reduced in patients with renal insufficiency. When rapid digitalization is not required, therapy may be begun with maintenance therapy, with steady-state levels achieved in approximately 7 days in patients with normal renal function. Digitoxin may be useful in patients with renal insufficiency since its metabolism is not dependent on renal excretion. Digitalization may be accomplished by giving 0.2 mg digitoxin orally twice daily for 4 days. Maintenance therapy ranges from 0.1 to 0.3 mg daily.

Electrolytes

Although not traditionally considered antiarrhythmic agents, serum electrolytes can have a profound effect on many cardiac arrhythmias. Alterations in the concentration of sodium, potassium, magnesium, or calcium may exacerbate many cardiac arrhythmias. In some cases, arrhythmias may be entirely due to electrolyte imbalance, and correction of electrolyte imbalance may be all that is required to treat these patients. Electrolyte abnormalities may be particularly arrhythmogenic in the setting of hypoxemia, ischemia, high-catecholamine states, cardiac hypertrophy or dilatation, altered pH, and in the presence of digitalis. During myocardial infarction, hypokalemia increases the risk of VT and fibrillation.[321] In addition, hypokalemia diminishes the effectiveness of class I antiarrhythmic agents; it may also increase the risk of toxicity or proarrhythmia, especially with class Ia antiarrhythmic agents (torsades de pointes). Arrhythmias due to digitalis toxicity may often be treated successfully with potassium supplementation provided that the serum potassium concentration is not elevated, and with monitoring to avoid high-degree AV block. Hypokalemia, hypoxia, and high-catecholamine states also may cause or exacerbate abnormal atrial tachyarrhythmias, especially multifocal atrial tachycardia. In some patients, hypokalemia may be refractory to oral repletion unless concomitant magnesium replacement is undertaken.

Magnesium

Pharmacologic Description

Magnesium is the second most abundant intracellular cation (after potassium). It is involved as a cofactor in many diverse intracellular biochemical processes (see Chap. 12), including cellular energy production, protein synthesis, DNA synthesis, and maintenance of cellular electrolyte composition (potassium and calcium). All enzymatic reactions involving ATP have an absolute requirement for magnesium. Use of magnesium to treat cardiac arrhythmias was first documented by Zwillinger in 1935.[322] Until recently, its use in the treatment of arrhythmias has been largely ignored, with only occasional case reports being published. Magnesium deficiency has become more common with the widespread use of thiazide and loop diuretics.

Electrophysiologic Action

Magnesium's effects on the heart may be direct, or indirect via effects on potassium and calcium homeostasis. Magnesium increases the length of the sinus cycle, slows AV-nodal conduction, and slows intraatrial and intraventricular conduction.[323] It also increases the effective refractory periods of the atria, AV node, and ventricles.[324] Hypomagnesemia often produces opposite effects, such as sinus tachycardia and shortening of effective refractory intervals. Magnesium is essential for the proper functioning of sodium-potassium ATPase; thus magnesium deficiency reduces the ability of a cell to maintain a normal intracellular potassium concentration, producing intracellular hypokalemia. These alterations increase automaticity and excitability while reducing conduction velocity, predisposing to arrhythmogenesis. In addition, magnesium is a physiologic calcium-channel antagonist.[325] ECG effects of magnesium administration include prolongation of the PR and QRS intervals and a shortening of the QT interval. Magnesium deficiency may produce ST-segment and T-wave abnormalities; occasionally a prolonged QT interval and U wave are seen. In general, however, hypomagnesemia cannot be recognized with certainty on the ECG, and many of these changes may reflect hypokalemia, which is a commonly associated abnormality.

Pharmacokinetics and Metabolism

Magnesium is mostly contained within bones and soft tissues. Only 1% of total body magnesium is found in the serum. Thus, serum concentrations may not accurately reflect total body magnesium content.[326] Absorption of magnesium occurs in the small bowel, typically beginning within 1 h of ingestion and continuing at a steady rate for 2 to 8 h. The kidney is the principal organ responsible for the maintenance of magnesium homeostasis. In the presence of hypomagnesemia, urinary excretion decreases to less than 1 mEq per day. Parathyroid hormone and vitamin D may also be important in magnesium regulation. In the presence of normal renal function, hypermagnesemia is difficult to maintain.

Hemodynamic Effects

Administration of magnesium may cause an increase in stroke volume and coronary blood flow related to arterial dilatation, which may also result in mild blood pressure reduction. Cardiac output may decrease, however, owing in part to a decrease in heart rate.

Antiarrhythmic Effects

Antiarrhythmic effects of magnesium have been demonstrated for the treatment of both digitalis toxicity and polymorphic VT associated with a prolonged QT interval (torsades de pointes).[327,328] Accumulating evidence also suggests that magnesium may be beneficial in the treatment of VF and VT.[329–331] Correction of magnesium deficiency has been shown to reduce the frequency of ventricular ectopy.[332] Administration of magnesium sulfate in doses sufficient to double the serum magnesium concentration (65 mmol per day) significantly reduced the number of deaths and serious ventricular arrhythmias in patients with acute myocardial infarction in one study.[333]

Side Effects

Progressive increases in magnesium concentration produces hypotension, PR and QRS interval prolongation, and peaked T waves. At concentrations greater than 5.0 mmol/L, areflexia, respiratory paralysis, and cardiac arrest may occur. Hypermagnesemia most commonly occurs in patients with renal insufficiency.

Indications and Dosing

Magnesium may be beneficial in the treatment of many arrhythmias; however, arrhythmias secondary to magnesium deficiency, digitalis toxicity, and torsades de pointes appear especially responsive. Acute treatment of arrhythmias may be accomplished by the administration of 2 g of magnesium sulfate intravenously.[320] If necessary, an additional 2 g may be administered in 5 to 15 min. Doses should be administered over 1 to 2 min. Maintenance infusions may be used, with doses ranging from 3 to 20 mg/min.[320] Continuous electrocardiographic monitoring is required, and serum magnesium levels should be checked frequently, especially in patients with renal insufficiency. Oral therapy with magnesium chloride (e.g., two to six 500-mg tablets daily) or magnesium oxide (e.g., 400 to 800 mg daily) may be used to prevent or treat diuretic-induced magnesium depletion. Substitution or addition of potassium- and magnesium-sparing diuretics (e.g., spironolactone, amiloride, or triamterene) may also be beneficial.

REFERENCES

1. Members of the Sicilian Gambit: New approaches to antiarrhythmic therapy, Part 1. Emerging therapeutic applications of the cell biology of cardiac arrhythmias. *Circulation* 104:2865, 2001.
1a. Members of the Sicilian Gambit: New approaches to antiarrhythmic therapy, Part II. Emerging therapeutic applications of the cell biology of cardiac arrhythmias. *Circulation* 104:2990, 2001.
1b. Lau W, Newman D, Dorian P: Can antiarrhythmic agents be selected based on mechanism of action? *Drugs* 60:1315, 2000.
1c. Harrison DC: Antiarrhythmic drug classification: New science and practical applications. *Am J Cardiol* 50:185, 1985.
2. The Task Force of the Working Group on Arrhythmias of the European Society of Cardiology: The Sicilian gambit: A new approach to the classification of antiarrhythmic drugs based on their actions on arrhythmogenic mechanisms. *Circulation* 84:1831, 1991.
3. The Cardiac Arrhythmia Suppression Trial (CAST) Investigators: Preliminary report: Effect of encainide and flecainide on mortality in a randomized trial of arrhythmia suppression after myocardial infarction. *N Engl J Med* 321:406, 1989.
4. ACC/AHA/ESC Guidelines for the Management of Patients With Atrial Fibrillation: Executive summary. *Circulation* 104:2118, 2001.
5. Waldo AL: Management of atrial fibrillation: the need for AFFIRMative action. AFFIRM investigators. Atrial Fibrillation Follow-up investigation of Rhythm Management. *Am J Cardiol* 84(6):698, 1999.
6. Ellenbogen KA, Clemo HF, Stambler BS, et al: Efficacy of ibutilide for termination ofatrial fibrillation and flutter. *Am J Cardiol* 78(8A):42, 1996.
6a. Natale A, Newby KH, Pisano E, et al: Prospective randomized comparison of antiarrhythmic therapy versus first-line radiofrequency ablation in patients with atrial flutter. *J Am Coll Cardiol* 35:1898, 2000.
7. Bauernfeind RA, Amat-y-Leon F, Dhingra RC, et al: Chronic non-paroxysmal sinus tachycardia in otherwise healthy persons. *Ann Intern Med* 91:702, 1979.
8. Kastor J: Multifocal atrial tachycardia. *N Engl J Med* 322(24):1713, 1990.
8a. Cannom DS, Prystowsky EN: Management of ventricular arrhythmias. Detection, drugs and devices. *JAMA* 281:172, 1999.
9. Buxton AE, Lee K, Fisher JD, et al: A Randomized study of the prevention of sudden death in patients with coronary artery disease. *N Engl J Med* 341:1882, 1999.
9a. Kuck K-H, Cappato R, Siebels J: Randomized comparison of antiarrhythmic drug therapy with implantable defibrillators in patients resuscitated from cardiac arrest. The Cardiac Arrest Study Hamburg (CASH). *Circulation* 102:748, 2000.
10. The Antiarrhythmics versus Implantable Defibrillators(AVID) Investigators: A Comparison of antiarrhythmic-drug therapy with implantable defibrillators in patients resuscitated from near-fatal ventricular arrhythmias. *N Engl J Med* 337:1576, 1997.

11. Pacifico A, Hohnloser SH, Williams JH, et al: Prevention of implantable-defibrillator shocks by treatment with sotalol. d,l—Sotalol Implantable Cardioverter–Defibrillator Study Group. *N Engl J Med* 340(24)1885, 1999.
12. Hoffman BF, Rosen MR, Wit AL: Electrophysiology and pharmacology of cardiac arrhythmias: VII. Cardiac effects of quinidine and procainamide. *Am Heart J* 90:117, 1975.
13. Ueda CT, Williamson BJ, Dzindzio BS: Absolute quinidine bioavailability. *Clin Pharmacol Ther* 20:260, 1976.
14. Kessler KM, Humphries WC, Black M, Spann J: Quinidine pharmacokinetics in patients with cirrhosis receiving propranolol. *Am Heart J* 96:627, 1978.
15. Drayer DE, Hughes M, Lorenzo B, Reidenberg M: Prevalence of high (S)-3-hydroxyquinidine/quinidine ratios in serum, and clearance of quinidine in cardiac patients with age. *Clin Pharmacol Ther* 27:72, 1980.
16. Kessler KM, Lowenthal DT, Warner H, et al: Quinidine elimination in patients with congestive heart failure or poor renal function. *N Engl J Med* 290:706, 1974.
17. Uematsu T, Sato R, Vozeh S, et al: Relative electrophysiological potencies of quinidine, 3-OH quinidine and quinidine-N-oxide in guinea-pig heart. *Arch Intern Pharmacodyn Ther* 297:29, 1989.
18. DiMarco JP, Garan H, Ruskin JN: Efficacy of quinidine in the treatment of ventricular arrhythmias: The role of electrophysiologic testing. *Circulation* 64(Suppl IV):38, 1981.
19. Ruskin JN, DiMarco JP, Garan H: Out-of-hospital cardiac arrest: Electrophysiologic observations and selection of long-term antiarrhythmic therapy. *N Engl J Med* 303:607, 1980.
20. Lown B, Wolf M: Approaches to sudden death from coronary heart disease. *Circulation* 44:130, 1971.
21. Farringer JA, McWay-Hess K, Clementi WA: Cimetidine-quinidine interaction. *Clin Pharm* 3:81, 1984.
22. Leahey EB, Reiffel JA, Drusin RE, et al: Interaction between quinidine and digoxin. *JAMA* 240:533, 1978.
23. Schenck-Gustafsson K, Jogestrand T, Norlander R, Dahlqvist TR: Effect of quinidine on digoxin concentration skeletal muscle and serum in patients with atrial fibrillation: Evidence for reduced binding of digoxin in muscle. *N Engl J Med* 305:209, 1981.
24. Funck-Brentano C, Turgeon J, Woosley RL, Roden DM: Effect of low dose quinidine on encainide pharmacokinetics and pharmacodynamics: Influence of genetic polymorphism. *J Pharmacol Exp Ther* 249:134, 1989.
25. Funck-Brentano C, Kroener HK, Pavlou H, et al: Genetically determined interaction between propafenone and low dose quinidine: Role of active metabolites in modulating net drug effect. *Br J Clin Pharmacol* 27:435, 1989.
25a. Lau C-P, Chow MSS, Tse H-F, et al: Control of paroxysmal atrial fibrillation recurrence using combined administration of propafenone and quinidine. *Am J Cardiol* 86:1327, 2000.
26. Mark LC, Kayden HJ, Steele JM, et al: The physiological disposition and cardiac effects of procainamide. *J Pharmacol Exp Ther* 102:5, 1951.
27. Kinnsman JM, Hansen WR, McClendon RL: Procainamide (Pronestyl) in the treatment of cardiac arrhythmias. *Am J Med Sci* 222:365, 1951.
28. Miller H, Nathanson MH, Griffith GC: The action of procainamide in cardiac arrhythmias. *JAMA* 146:1004, 1951.
29. Berry K, Garlett EL, Bellet S, Gefter WI: Use of Pronestyl in the treatment of ectopic rhythms. *Am J Med* 11:431, 1951.
30. Josephson ME, Caracta AR, Ricciutti MA, et al: Electrophysiologic properties of procainamide in man. *Am J Cardiol* 33:596, 1974.
31. Manion CV, Lalka D, Baer DT, Meyer MB: Absorption, kinetics of procainamide in humans. *J Pharm Sci* 66:981, 1977.
32. Karlsson E: Clinical pharmacokinetics of procainamide. *Clin Pharmacokinet* 3:97, 1978.
33. Singh S, Gelband H, Mehta AV, et al: Procainamide elimination kinetics in pediatric patients. *Clin Pharmacol Ther* 32:607, 1982.
34. Kluger J, Leech S, Reidenberg MM, et al: Long-term antiarrhythmic therapy with acetylprocainamide. *Am J Cardiol* 48:1124, 1981.
35. Bigger JT, Heissenbuttel RH: The use of procainamide and lidocaine in the treatment of cardiac arrhythmias. *Prog Cardiovasc Dis* 11:515, 1969.
36. Waxman HL, Buxton AE, Sadowski LM, Josephson ME: The response to procainamide during electrophysiologic study for sustained ventricular tachyarrhythmias predicts the response to other medications. *Circulation* 67:30, 1983.
37. Rae AP, Sokoloff NM, Webb CR, et al: Limitations of failure of procainamide during electrophysiological testing to predict response to other medical therapy. *J Am Coll Cardiol* 6:410, 1985.
38. Ellrodt AG, Murata GH, Riedinger MS, et al: Severe neutropenia associated with sustained-release procainamide. *Ann Intern Med* 100:197, 1984.
39. Sim E: Drug-induced immune-complex disease. *Comp Inflamm* 6:119, 1989.
40. Adams LE, Sanders CE, Budinsky RA, et al: Immunomodulatory effects of procainamide metabolites: Their implications in drug-related lupus. *J Lab Clin Med* 113:482, 1989.
41. Asherson RA, Zulman J, Hughes GR: Pulmonary thromboembolism associated with procainamide induced lupus syndrome and anticardiolipin antibodies. *Ann Rheum Dis* 48:232, 1989.
42. Li GC, Greenberg CS, Currie MS: Procainamide-induced lupus anticoagulants and thrombosis. *South Med J* 81:262, 1988.
43. Heyman MR, Flores RH, Edelman BB, Carliner NH: Procainamide-induced lupus anticoagulant. *South Med J* 81:934, 1988.
44. Kosoglou T, Rocci ML, Vlasses PH: Trimethoprim alters the disposition of procainamide and N-acetylprocainamide. *Clin Pharmacol Ther* 44:467, 1988.
45. Lai MY, Jiang FM, Chung CH, et al: Dose dependent effect of cimetidine on procainamide disposition in man. *Int J Clin Pharmacol Ther Toxicol* 26:118, 1988.
46. Christian CD, Meredith CG, Speeg KV: Cimetidine inhibits renal procainamide clearance. *Clin Pharmacol Ther* 36:221, 1984.
47. Danilo P Jr, Hordoff AJ, Rosen MR: Effects of disopyramide on electrophysiologic properties of canine cardiac Purkinje fibers. *J Pharmacol Exp Ther* 201:701, 1977.
48. Sasyniuk BI, Kus T: Cellular electrophysiologic changes induced by disopyramide in normal and infarcted hearts. *J Int Med Res* 4 (Suppl I): 20, 1976.
49. Kidwell GA, Lima JJ, Schaal SF, Muir WW: Hemodynamic and electrophysiologic effects of disopyramide enantiomers in a canine blood superfusion model. *J Cardiovasc Pharmacol* 13:644, 1989.
50. Birkhead JS, Vaughan Williams EM: Dual effect of disopyramide on atrial and atrioventricular conduction and refractory periods. *Br Heart J* 39:657, 1977.
51. Morady F, Scheinman MM, Desai J: Disopyramide. *Ann Intern Med* 96:337, 1982.
52. Bexton RS, Hellestrand KJ, Cory-Pearce R, et al: The direct electrophysiologic effects of disopyramide phosphate in the transplanted human heart. *Circulation* 67:38, 1983.
53. Katoh T, Karagueuzian HS, Jordan J, Mandel JW: The cellular electrophysiologic mechanism of the dual actions of disopyramide on rabbit sinus node dysfunction. *Circulation* 66:1216, 1979.
54. Dubetz DK, Brown NN, Hooper WD, et al: Disopyramide: Pharmacokinetics and bioavailability. *Br J Clin Pharmacol* 6:279, 1978.
55. Hinderling PH, Garrett ER: Pharmacokinetics of the antiarrhythmic disopyramide in healthy humans. *J Pharmacokinet Biopharm* 4:199, 1976.
56. Capparelli EV, DiPersio DM, Zhao H, et al: Clinical pharmacokinetics of controlled-release disopyramide in patients with cardiac arrhythmias. *J Clin Pharmacol* 28:306, 1988.
57. Karim A: The pharmacokinetics of Norpace. *Angiology* 26:85, 1975.
58. Bonde J, Jensen NM, Pedersen LE, et al: Elimination kinetics and urinary excretion of disopyramide in human healthy volunteers. *Pharmacol Toxicol* 62:298, 1988.
59. Lima JJ, Boudoulas H, Blanford M: Concentration-dependence of disopyramide binding to plasma protein and its influence on kinetics and dynamics. *J Pharmacol Exp Ther* 219:741, 1981.
60. Leach AJ, Brown JE, Armstrong PW: Cardiac depression by intravenous disopyramide in patients with left ventricular dysfunction. *Am J Med* 68:839, 1980.
61. Podrid PJ, Schoeneberger A, Lown B: Congestive heart failure caused by oral disopyramide. *N Engl J Med* 302:614, 1980.
62. Yoshida Y, Hirai M, Yamada T, et al: Antiarrhythmic efficacy of dipyridamole in treatment of reperfusion arrhythmias. Evidence for cAMP-mediated triggered activity as a mechanism responsible for reperfusion arrhythmias. *Circulation* 101:624, 2000.

63. Jennings G, Jones MBS, Besterman EMM, et al: Oral disopyramide in prophylaxis of arrhythmias following myocardial infarction. *Lancet* 1:51, 1976.

64. Vismara LA, Mason DT, Amsterdam EA: Disopyramide phosphate: Clinical efficacy of a new oral antiarrhythmic drug. *Am Heart J* 16:330, 1974.

65. Jonason T, Ringqvist I, Bandh S, et al: Propafenone versus disopyramide for treatment of chronic symptomatic ventricular arrhythmias: A multicenter study. *Acta Med Scand* 223:515, 1988.

66. Ueda CT, Dzindzio BS, Vosik WM: Serum disopyramide concentrations and suppression of ventricular premature contractions. *Clin Pharmacol Ther* 36:326, 1984.

67. Vismara LA, Vera Z, Miller RR, Mason DT: Efficacy of disopyramide phosphate in the treatment of refractory ventricular tachycardia. *Am J Cardiol* 39:1027, 1977.

68. Kim SG, Mercando AD, Tam S, Fisher JD: Combination of disopyramide and mexiletine for better tolerance and additive effects for treatment of ventricular arrhythmias. *J Am Coll Cardiol* 13:659, 1989.

69. Della-Bella P, Tondo C, Marenzi G, et al: Facilitating influence of disopyramide on atrial flutter termination by overdrive pacing. *Am J Cardiol* 61:1046, 1988.

70. Karlson BW, Torstensson I, Jansson SO, Peterson LE: Disopyramide in the maintenance of sinus rhythm after electroconversion of atrial fibrillation: A placebo-controlled one-year follow-up study. *Eur Heart J* 9:284, 1988.

71. Fujimura O, Klein GJ, Sharma AD, et al: Acute effect of disopyramide on atrial fibrillation in the Wolff-Parkinson-White syndrome. *J Am Coll Cardiol* 13:1133, 1989.

72. Morillo CA, Leitch JW, Yee R, Klein GJ: A placebo-controlled trial of intravenous and oral disopyramide for prevention of neurally mediated syncope induced by head-up tilt. *J Am Coll Cardiol* 22(7):1843, 1993.

73. Meltzer RS, Robert EW, McMorrow M, Martin RP: Atypical ventricular tachycardia as a manifestation of disopyramide toxicity. *Am J Cardiol* 42:1049, 1978.

74. Nicholson WJ, Martin CE, Gracey JG, Knoch HR: Disopyramide induced ventricular fibrillation. *Am J Cardiol* 43:1053, 1979.

75. Nakabayashi H, Ito T, Igawa T, et al: Disopyramide induces insulin secretion and plasma glucose diminution: Studies using the in situ canine pancreas. *Metabolism* 38:179, 1989.

76. Ragosta M, Wiehl AC, Rosenfeld LE: Potentially fatal interaction between erythromycin and disopyramide. *Am J Med* 86:465, 1989.

77. Harrison DC, Sprouse JH, Morrow AG: The antiarrhythmic properties of lidocaine and procainamide. *Circulation* 28:486, 1963.

78. Harrison DC, Alderman EL: The pharmacology and clinical use of lidocaine as an antiarrhythmic drug. *Modern Treatment* 9:139, 1972.

79. Rosen KM, Lau SH, Weiss MB, Damato AN: The effect of lidocaine on atrioventricular and intraventricular conduction in man. *Am J Cardiol* 25:1, 1970.

80. Singh BN, Vaughn Williams EM: Effect of altering potassium concentration on the action of lidocaine and di phenylhydantoin on rabbit atrial and ventricular muscle. *Circ Res* 29:286, 1971.

81. Lichtstein E, Chadda KD, Gupta PK: Atrioventricular block with lidocaine therapy. *Am J Cardiol* 31:277, 1973.

82. DeBoer AG, Breimer DD, Mattie H, et al: Rectal bioavailability of lidocaine in man: Partial avoidance of first-pass metabolism. *Clin Pharmacol Ther* 26:701, 1979.

83. Drayer DE, Lorenzo B, Werns S, Reidenberg MM: Plasma levels, protein binding, and elimination data of lidocaine and active metabolites in cardiac patients of various ages. *Clin Pharmacol Ther* 34:14, 1983.

84. Routledge PA, Barchowsky A, Bjornsson TD, et al: Lidocaine plasma protein binding. *Clin Pharmacol Ther* 27:347, 1980.

85. Stenson RE, Constantino RT, Harrison DC: Interrelationships of hepatic blood flow, cardiac output, and blood levels of lidocaine in man. *Circulation* 43:205, 1971.

86. Rowland M, Thomson PD, Guichard A, Melmon KL: Disposition kinetics of lidocaine in normal subjects. *Ann NY Acad Sci* 179:383, 1971.

87. Thomson PD, Melmon KL, Richardson JA, et al: Lidocaine pharmacokinetics in advanced heart failure, liver disease, and renal failure in humans. *Ann Intern Med* 78:499, 1973.

88. LeLorier J, Grenon D, Latour Y, et al: Pharmacokinetics of lidocaine after prolonged intravenous infusion in uncomplicated myocardial infarction. *Ann Intern Med* 87:700, 1977.

89. Narang PK, Crouthamel WG, Carliner NH: Lidocaine and its active metabolites. *Clin Pharmacol Ther* 24:654, 1978.

90. Teo KK, Yusuf S, Furberg CD: Effects of prophylactic antiarrhythmic drug therapy in acute myocardial infarction. An overview of results from randomized controlled trials. *JAMA* 270(13):1589, 1993.

91. Yusuf S, Wittes J, Friedman L: Overview of results of randomized clinical trials in heart disease: I. Treatments following myocardial infarction. *JAMA* 260:2088, 1988.

92. Noneman JW, Jones MR: Lidocaine in drug treatment of cardiac arrhythmias. In: Goupd LA, ed. *Drug Treatment of Cardiac Arrhythmias.* Mt. Kisco, NY: Futura, 1983:193.

93. Ochs HR, Carstens G, Greenblatt DJ: Reduction in lidocaine clearance during continuous infusion and by coadministration of propranolol. *N Engl J Med* 303:373, 1980.

94. Feely J, Wilkinson GR, McAllister CB, Wood AJJ: Increased toxicity and reduced clearance of lidocaine by cimetidine. *Ann Intern Med* 96:592, 1982.

95. Boyce JR, Cervenko FW, Wright FJ: Effects of halothane on the pharmacokinetics of lidocaine in digitalis-toxic dogs. *Can Anaesth Soc J* 25:323, 1978.

96. Koster RW, Dunning AJ: Intramuscular lidocaine for prevention of lethal arrhythmias in the prehospitalization phase of acute myocardial infarction. *N Engl J Med* 313:1105, 1985.

97. McDevitt DG, Nies RS, Wilkinson GR, et al: Antiarrhythmic effects of a lidocaine cogener, tocainide, 2 amino-29, 69 propionoxylidide, in man. *Clin Pharmacol Ther* 19:396, 1976.

98. Winkle RA, Meffin PJ, Fitzgerald JW, Harrison DC: Clinical efficacy and pharmacokinetics of a new orally effective antiarrhythmic, tocainide. *Circulation* 54:884, 1976.

99. Moore EN, Spear JF, Horowitz LN, et al: Electrophysiological properties of a new antiarrhythmic drug–tocainide. *Am J Cardiol* 41:703, 1978.

100. Oshita S, Sada H, Kojima M, Ban T: Effects of tocainide and lignocaine on the transmembrane action potentials as related to external potassium and calcium concentrations in guinea pig papillary muscles. *Arch Pharmacol* 314:67, 1980.

101. Griffin J, Schnittger F, Peters PJ, et al: Effects of tocainide on ventricular fibrillation threshold. *Circulation* 56(Suppl III):158, 1977.

102. Schnittger J, Griffin JC, Hall RJ, et al: Effects of tocainde on ventricular fibrillation threshold: Comparison with lidocaine. *Am J Cardiol* 42:76, 1978.

103. Horowitz LN, Josephson ME, Farshidi A: Human electropharmacology of tocainide, a lidocaine cogener. *Am J Cardiol* 42:267, 1978.

104. Young MD, Hadidian Z, Horn ER, et al: Treatment of ventricular arrhythmias with oral tocainide. *Am Heart J* 100:1041, 1980.

105. Uprichard AC, Allen JD, Harron DW: Effects of tocainide enantiomers on experimental arrhythmias produced by programmed electrical stimulation. *J Cardiovasc Pharmacol* 11:235, 1988.

106. Gaffner C, Conradson T, Horvendahl S, Ryden L: Tocainide kinetics after intravenous and oral administration in healthy subjects and in patients with acute myocardial infarction. *Clin Pharmacol Ther* 27:64, 1980.

107. Elvin AT, Lalka D, Stroeckel K, et al: Tocainide kinetics and metabolism: Effects of phenobarbitone and substrates for glucuronyl transferase. *Clin Pharmacol Ther* 28:652, 1980.

108. Lalka D, Meyer MB, Duce BR, Elvin AT: Kinetics of the oral antiarrhythmic lignocaine cogener, tocainide. *Clin Pharmacol Ther* 19:757, 1976.

109. Nyquist O, Forssell G, Nordlander R, Schenck-Gustafsson K: Hemodynamic and antiarrhythmic effects of tocainide in patients with acute myocardial infarction. *Am Heart J* 100:1000, 1980.

110. Winkle RA, Anderson JL, Peters F, et al: The hemodynamic effects of intravenous tocainide in patients with heart disease. *Circulation* 57:787, 1978.

111. Ravid S, Podrid PJ, Lampert S, Lown B: Congestive heart failure induced by six of the newer antiarrhythmic drugs. *J Am Coll Cardiol* 14:1326, 1989.

112. Roden DM, Reele SB, Higgins SB, et al: Tocainide therapy for refractory ventricular arrhythmias. *Am Heart J* 100:15, 1980.

113. Maloney JD, Nissen RG, McColgan JM: Open clinical studies at a referral center: Chronic maintenance tocainide therapy in patients

with recurrent sustained ventricular tachycardia refractory to conventional antiarrhythmic agents. *Am Heart J* 100:1023, 1980.

114. Podrid PJ, Lown B: Tocainide for refractory symptomatic ventricular arrhythmias. *Am J Cardiol* 49:1279, 1982.

115. Winkle RA, Meffin PJ, Harrison DC: Long term tocainide therapy for ventricular arrhythmias. *Circulation* 57:1008, 1978.

116. Murray KT, Barbet JT, Kopelman HA, et al: Mexiletine and tocainide: A comparison of antiarrhythmic efficacy, adverse effects, and predictive value of lidocaine testing. *Clin Pharmacol Ther* 45:553, 1989.

117. Adhar GC, Swerdlow CD, Lance BL, et al: Tocainide for drug resistant sustained ventricular tachyarrhythmias. *J Am Coll Cardiol* 11:124, 1988.

118. Winkle RA, Mason JW, Harrison DC: Tocainide for drug resistant ventricular arrhythmias: Efficacy, side effects, and lidocaine responsiveness for predicting tocainide success. *Am Heart J* 100:1031, 1980.

119. Barbey JT, Thompson KA, Echt DS, et al: Tocainide plus quinidine for treatment of ventricular arrhythmias. *Am J Cardiol* 61:570, 1988.

120. Klein MD, Levine PA, Ryan TJ: Antiarrhythmic efficacy, pharmacokinetics and clinical safety of tocainide in convalescent myocardial infarction. *Chest* 77:726, 1980.

121. Rice TL, Patterson JH, Celestin C, et al: Influence of rifampin on tocainide pharmacokinetics in humans. *Clin Pharm* 8:200, 1989.

122. North DS, Mattern AL, Kapil RP, Lalonde RL: The effect of histamine-2 receptor antagonists on tocainide pharmacokinetics. *J Clin Pharmacol* 28:640, 1988.

123. Woosley RL, McDevitt DG, Nies AS, et al: Suppression of ventricular ectopic depolarization by tocainide. *Circulation* 56:980, 1977.

124. Singh BN, Vaughn Williams EM: Investigations of the mode of action of a new antidysrhythmic drug, Ko 1173. *Br J Pharmacol* 44:1, 1972.

125. Allen JD, Kofi Ekue JM, et al: The effect of Ko 1173, a new anticonvulsant agent, on experimental cardiac arrhythmias. *Br J Pharmacol* 45:561, 1972.

126. Weld FM, Bigger JT, Swistel D, et al: Electrophysiologic effects of mexiletine (Ko 1173) on bovine cardiac Purkinje fibres. *J Pharmacol Exp Ther* 210:222, 1979.

127. Arita M, Goto M, Nagamoto Y, Saikawa T: Electrophysiological actions of mexiletine (Ko 1173) on canine Purkinje fibers and ventricular muscle. *Br J Pharmacol* 67:143, 1979.

128. Campbell NPS, Pantridge JF, Adgey AAJ: Long-term antiarrhythmic therapy with mexiletine. *Br Heart J* 40:796, 1978.

129. Nora MO, Chandrasekaran K, Hammill SC, Reeder GS: Prolongation of ventricular depolarization: ECG manifestation of mexiletine toxicity. *Chest* 95:925, 1989.

130. Prescott LF, Clements JA, Pottage A: Absorption, distribution and elimination of mexiletine. *Postgrad Med J* 53(Suppl I):50, 1977.

131. Campbell NPS, Pantridge JF, Adgey AAJ: Mexiletine in the management of ventricular arrhythmias. *Eur J Cardiol* 6:245, 1977.

132. Middleton D: Baseline pharmacology, electrophysiology and pharmacokinetics of mexiletine. *Acta Cardiol* 25(Suppl): 45, 1980.

133. Talbot RG, Clark RA, Nimmo J, et al: Treatment of ventricular arrhythmias with mexiletine (Ko 1173). *Lancet* 2:399, 1973.

134. Horowitz JD, Anavekar SN, Morris PM, et al: Comparative trial of mexiletine and lidocaine in treatment of early ventricular tachyarrhythmias after acute myocardial infarction. *J Cardiovasc Pharmacol* 3:409, 1981.

135. Stein J, Podrid PJ, Lampert S, Hirshowitz GH: Long-term mexiletine for ventricular arrhythmia. *Am Heart J* 107:1091, 1984.

136. Poole JE, Werner JA, Brady GH, et al: Intolerance and ineffectiveness of mexiletine in patients with severe ventricular arrhythmias. *Am Heart J* 112:322, 1986.

137. Whitford EG, McGovern B, Schoenfeld MH, et al: Long-term efficacy of mexiletine alone and in combination with a class Ia antiarrhythmic drugs for refractory ventricular arrhythmias. *Am Heart J* 115:360, 1988.

138. Duff HJ: Mexiletine-quinidine combination: Enhanced antiarrhythmic and electrophysiologic activity in the dog. *J Pharmacol Exp Ther* 249:617, 1989.

139. Kim SG, Mercando AD, Tam S, Fisher JD: Combination of disopyramide and mexiletine for better tolerance and additive effects for treatment of ventricular arrhythmias. *J Am Coll Cardiol* 13:659, 1989.

140. Kim SG, Felder SD, Waspe LE, Fisher JD: Electrophysiologic effects and clinical efficacy of mexiletine used alone or in combination with class Ia agents for refractory recurrent ventricular tachycardias or ventricular fibrillation. *Am J Cardiol* 58:485, 1986.

141. Achuff SC, Campbell RWF, Pottage A, et al: Mexiletine in the prevention of ventricular arrhythmias in acute myocardial infarction. *Postgrad Med J* 53(Suppl I):163, 1977.

142. Campbell RWF, Dolder MA, Prescott LF, et al: Comparison of procaineamide and mexiletine in prevention of ventricular arrhythmias after acute myocardial infarction. *Lancet* 1:1257, 1975.

143. Zehender M, Geibel A, Tresse N, et al: Prediction of efficacy and tolerance of oral mexiletine by intravenous lidocaine application. *Clin Pharmacol Ther* 44:389, 1988.

144. Danilo P, Langan WB, Rosen MR, Hoffman BF: Effects of the phenothiazine analog, EN-313, on ventricular arrhythmias in the dog. *Eur J Pharmacol* 45:127, 1977.

145. Morganroth J, Pearlman AS, Dunkman WB, et al: Ethmozine: A new antiarrhythmic agent developed in the USSR: Efficacy and tolerance. *Am Heart J* 98:621, 1979.

146. Chazov EI, Shugushev KK, Rosenshtraukh LV: Ethmozine: I. Effects of intravenous drug administration on paroxysmal supraventricular tachycardia in the ventricular preexcitation syndrome. *Am Heart J* 108:475, 1984.

147. Chazov EI, Rosenshtraukh LV, Shugushev KK: Ethmozine: II. Effects of intravenous drug administration on atrioventricular nodal reentrant tachycardia. *Am Heart J* 108:483, 1984.

148. Doherty JU, Rogers DP, Waxman HG, Buxton AE: Electrophysiological properties of ethmozine in sustained ventricular tachycardia. *Circulation* 70(Suppl II):440, 1984.

149. Salerno DM, Sharkey PJ, Granrud G, et al: Efficacy, safety, and pharmacokinetics of high-dose ethmozine during short and long-term therapy. *Circulation* 70(Suppl II):440, 1984.

150. Shugushev KK, Rosenshtraukh LV, Smetnev AS: Electrophysiologic effects of ethmozine on sinus node function in patients with and without sinus node dysfunction. *Clin Cardiol* 9:443, 1986.

151. Whitney CC, Weinstein SH, Gaylord JC: High performance liquid chromatographic determination of ethmozine in plasma. *J Pharmacol Sci* 70:462, 1981.

152. Dorian P, Echt DS, Mead RH, et al: Ethmozine: Electrophysiology, hemodynamics, and antiarrhythmic efficacy in patients with life threatening ventricular arrhythmias. *Am Heart J* 112:327, 1986.

153. Morganroth J, Pratt CM: Prevalence and characteristics of proarrhythmia from moricizine (Ethmozine). *Am J Cardiol* 63:172, 1989.

154. Pratt CM, Yepsen SC, Taylor AA, et al: Ethmozine suppression of single and repetitive ventricular premature depolarizations during therapy: Documentation of efficacy and long-term safety. *Am Heart J* 106:85, 1983.

155. Singh SN, DiBianco R, Gottdiener JS, et al: Effect of miricizine hydrochloride in reducing chronic high frequency ventricular arrhythmia: Results of a prospective controlled trial. *Am J Cardiol* 53:745, 1984.

156. Seals AA, English L, Leon CA, et al: Hemodynamic effects of moricizine at rest and during supine bicycle exercise: Results in patients with ventricular tachycardia and left ventricular dysfunction. *Am Heart J* 112:36, 1986.

157. Mann DE, Luck JC, Herre JM, et al: Electrophysiologic effects of ethmozine in patients with ventricular tachycardia. *Am Heart J* 107:674, 1984.

158. Podrid PJ, Lyakishev A, Lown B, Mazur N: Ethmozine, a new antiarrhythmic drug for suppressing ventricular premature complexes. *Circulation* 61:450, 1980.

159. Pratt CM, Young JB, Francis MJ, et al: Comparitive effect of disopyramide and ethmozine in suppressing complex ventricular arrhythmias by use of a double-blind, placebo-controlled, longitudinal cross over design. *Circulation* 69:288, 1984.

160. Miura DS, Wynn J, Torres V, et al: Antiarrhythmic efficacy of ethmozine in patients with ventricular tachycardia as determined by programmed electrical stimulation. *Am Heart J* 111:661, 1986.

161. CAST II Investigators. Effect of the anatiarrhythmic agent moricizine on survival after myocardial infarction. *N Engl J Med* 327:227, 1992.

162. Geller JC, Geller M, Carlson MD, Waldo AL: Efficacy and safety of moricizine in the maintenance of sinus rhythm in patients with recurrent atrial fibrillation. *Am J Cardiol* 87(2):172, 2001.

163. Grubb BP: Moricizine: A new agent for the treatment of ventricular arrhythmias. *Am J Med Sci* 301:398, 1991.

164. Banitt EH, Coyne WE, Schmid JR, Mendel A: Antiarrhythmics. N-aminoalkylene) trifluoroethoxybenzamides and N-(aminoalkylene) trifluoroethoxynaphthamides. *J Med Chem* 18:1130, 1975.

165. Seipel L, Abendroth PR, Breithart G: Electrophysiologische Effekte des neuen Antiarrhythmikums Flecainid (R818) beim Menschen. *Z Kardiol* 70:524, 1981.

166. Vik-Mo H, Ohm O-J, Lund-Johansen P: Electrophysiologic effects of flecainide acetate in patients with sinus node dysfunction. *Am J Cardiol* 50:1090, 1982.

167. Hodess AB, Follanshee WT, Spear JF: Electrophysiological effects of a new antiarrhythmic agent, flecainide, in the intact canine heart. *J Cardiovasc Pharmacol* 1:427, 1979.

168. Hellestrand KJ, Bexton RS, Nathan AW, et al: Acute electrophysiologic effects of flecainide acetate on cardiac conduction and refractoriness in man. *Br Heart J* 48:140, 1982.

169. Conrad GJ, Ober RE: Metabolism of flecainide. *Am J Cardiol* 53:4B, 1982.

170. Anderson JL, Stewart JR, Perry BA, et al: Oral flecainide acetate for the treatment of ventricular arrhythmias. *N Engl J Med* 305:473, 1981.

171. Hodges M, Haugland JM, Granrud G, et al: Suppression of ventricular ectopic depolarizations by flecainide acetate, a new antiarrhythmic agent. *Circulation* 65:879, 1982.

172. Forland SC, Cutler RE, McQuinn RL, et al: Flecainide pharmacokinetics after multiple dosing in patients with impaired renal function. *J Clin Pharmacol* 28:727, 1988.

173. McQuinn RL, Pentikainen PJ, Chang SF, Conrad GJ: Pharmacokinetics of flecainide in patients with cirrhosis of the liver. *Clin Pharmacol Ther* 44:566, 1988.

174. Cohen AA, Daru V, Covelli G, et al: Hemodynamic effects of intravenous flecainide in acute uncomplicated myocardial infarction. *Am Heart J* 110:1193, 1985.

175. Jewitt DE: Hemodynamic effects of newer antiarrhythmic drugs. *Am Heart J* 100:984, 1980.

176. Webb CR, Morganroth J, Senior S, et al: Safety and efficacy of antiarrhythmic therapy with flecainide for patients with ventricular tachycardia and ventricular dysfunction. *Clin Res* 32:685A, 1984.

177. Josephson MA, Ikeda N, Singh BN: Effects of flecainide on ventricular function: Clinical and experimental correlations. *Am J Cardiol* 53:945B, 1984.

178. Van Wijk LM, den Heijer P, Crijns HJ, et al: Flecainide versus quinidine in the prevention of paroxysms of atrial fibrillation. *J Cardiovasc Pharmacol* 13:32, 1989.

179. Wafa SS, Ward DE, Parker DJ, Camm AJ: Efficacy of flecainide acetate for atrial arrhythmias following coronary artery bypass grafting. *Am J Cardiol* 63:1058, 1989.

180. Gavaghan TP, Koegh AM, Kelly RP, et al: Flecainide compared with a combination of digoxin and disopyramide for acute atrial arrhythmias after cardiopulmonary bypass. *Br Heart J* 60:497, 1988.

181. Van Wijk LM, Crijns HJ, van Gilst WH, et al: Flecainide acetate in the treatment of supraventricular tachycardias: Value of programmed electrical stimulation for long-term prognosis. *Am Heart J* 117:365, 1989.

182. Zee Cheng CS, Kim SS, Ruffy R: Flecainide acetate for treatment of bypass tract mediated reentrant tachycardia. *Am J Cardiol* 62:23D, 1988.

183. Kim SS, Smith P, Ruffy R: Treatment of atrial tachyarrhythmias and preexcitation syndrome with flecainide acetate. *Am J Cardiol* 62:29D, 1988.

184. The Cardiac Arrhythmia Pilot Study (CAPS) Investigators: Effects of encainide, flecainide, imipramine and moricizine on ventricular arrhythmias during the year after acute myocardial infarction: The CAPS. *Am J Cardiol* 61:501, 1988.

185. Capparelli EV, Kluger J, Regnier JC, Chow MS: Clinical and electrophysiologic effects of flecainide in patients with refractory ventricular tachycardia. *J Clin Pharmacol* 28:268, 1988.

186. Flecainide-Quinidine Research Group: Flecainide versus quinidine for treatment of chronic ventricular arrhythmias: A multicenter clinical trial. *Circulation* 67:1117, 1983.

187. Morganroth J, Price B: Flecainide vs quinidine: Efficacy and tolerance in patients with chronic stable ventricular ectopy. *Am J Cardiol* 49:1015, 1982.

188. Viswanathan PC, Bezzina CR, George AL Jr, et al: Gating-dependent mechanisms for flecainide action in SCH5A-linked arrhythmia syndromes. *Circulation* 104:1200, 2001.

189. Lal R, Chapman PO, Naccarelli GV, et al: Short- and long-term experience with flecainide acetate in the management of refractory life threatening ventricular arrhythmias. *J Am Coll Cardiol* 6:772, 1985.

190. Chimienti M, Cullen MT, Casadei G: Safety of long-term flecainide and propafenone in the management of patients with symptomatic paroxysmal atrial fibrillation: Report from the Flecainide and Propafenone Italian Study Investigators. *Am J Cardiol* 77:60A, 1996.

191. Reid PR, Griffith LSC, Platia EV, Ord SE: Evaluation of flecainide acetate in the management of patients at high risk of sudden cardiac death. *Am J Cardiol* 53:108B, 1983.

192. Hellestand KJ, Burnett PJ, Milne JR, et al: Effect of the antiarrhythmic agent flecainide acetate on acute and chronic pacing thresholds. *PACE* 6:892, 1983.

193. Kohlhardt M: Basic electrophysiological action of propafenone in heart muscle. In: Schlepper M, Olssen B, eds. *Cardiac Arrhythmias: Diagnosis, Prognosis and Therapy: Proceedings of 1st International Rhythmonorm Congress.* New York: Springer-Verlag, 1983:91.

194. Zeiler RH, Grough WB, El-Sherif N: Electrophysiologic effects of propafenone on canine ischemic cardiac cells. *Am J Cardiol* 54:424, 1984.

195. Rudolph W, Petri H, Kafka W, Hall D: Effects of propafenone on the accessory pathway in patients with WPW syndrome. *Am J Cardiol* 43:430, 1979.

196. Dubuc M, Kus T, Campa MA, et al: Electrophysiologic effects of intravenous propafenone in Wolff-Parkinson-White syndrome. *Am Heart J* 117:370, 1989.

197. Kroemer HK, Funck-Brentano C, Silberstein DJ, et al: Stereoselective disposition and pharmacologic activity of propafenone enantiomers. *Circulation* 79:1068, 1989.

198. Karagueuzian HS, Katoh T, McCullen A, et al: Electrophysiologic and hemodynamic effects of propafenone, a new antiarrhythmic agent, on the anesthetized, closed-chest dog: Comparative study with lidocaine. *Am Heart J* 107:418, 1984.

199. Chilson DA, Heger JJ, Zipes DP, et al: Electrophysiologic effects and clinical efficacy of oral propafenone therapy in patients with ventricular tachycardia. *J Am Coll Cardiol* 5:1407, 1985.

200. Connolly ST, Kates RE, Labsack CS, et al: Clinical efficacy and electrophysiology of oral propafenone for ventricular tachycardia. *Am J Cardiol* 52:1208, 1983.

201. Connolly SJ, Kates RE, Lebsack CS, et al: Clinical pharmacology of propafenone. *Circulation* 68:589, 1983.

202. Siddoway LA, Thompson KA, McAllister CB, et al: Polymorphism of propafenone metabolism and disposition in man: Clinical and pharmacokinetic consequences. *Circulation* 75:785, 1987.

203. Baker BJ, Dinh H, Kroskey D, et al: Effect of propafenone on left ventricular ejection fraction. *Am J Cardiol* 54:20D, 1984.

204. Podrid PJ, Cytryn R, Lown B: Propafenone: Noninvasive evaluation of efficacy. *Am J Cardiol* 54:53D, 1984.

205. Henze E, Roth J, Haerer W, et al: Long term inotropic effects of flecainide and propafenone. *Eur J Nucl Med* 13:568, 1988.

206. Shen EN, Sung RJ, Morady F, et al: Electrophysiologic and hemodynamic effects of intravenous propafenone in patients with recurrent ventricular tachycardia. *J Am Coll Cardiol* 3:1291, 1984.

207. Singh BN, Kaplinsky E, Kirsten E, Guerrero J: Effects of propafenone on ventricular arrhythmias: Double-blind, parallel, randomized, placebo-controlled dose-ranging study. *Am Heart J* 116:1542, 1988.

208. Dinh H, Baker BJ, deSoyza N, Murphy ML: Sustained therapeutic efficacy and safety of oral propafenone for treatment of chronic ventricular arrhythmias: A 2-year experience. *Am Heart J* 115(1Pt 1):92, 1988.

209. Prystowsky EN, Heger JJ, Chilson DA, et al: Antiarrhythmic and electrophysiologic effects of oral propafenone. *Am J Cardiol* 54:26D, 1984.

210. Musto B, DOnofrio A, Cavallaro C, Musto A: Electrophysiological effects and clinical efficacy of propafenone in children with recurrent paroxysmal supraventricular tachycardia. *Circulation* 78:863, 1988.

211. Connolly SJ, Hoffert DL: Usefulness of propafenone for recurrent paroxysmal atrial fibrillation. *Am J Cardiol* 63:817, 1989.

212. Aliot E, Denjoy I: Comparison of the safety and efficacy of flecainide versus propafenone in hospital out-patients with

294a. Domanovits H, Schillinger M, Lercher P, et al: E 047/1: A new class III antiarrhythmic agent. *J Cardiovasc Pharmacol* 35:716, 2000.

295. Wit AL, Cranefield PF: Verapamil inhibition of the slow response: A mechanism for its effectiveness against reentrant AV nodal tachycardia. *Circulation* 50(III):146, 1974.

296. Sung RJ, Shapiro WA, Shen EN, et al: Effects of verapamil on ventricular tachycardias possibly caused by reentry, automaticity, and triggered activity. *J Clin Invest* 72:350, 1983.

297. Hoon TJ, Bauman JL, Rodvold KA, et al: The pharmacodynamic and pharmacokinetic differences of the d and l isomers of verapamil: Implications in the treatment of paroxysmal supraventricular tachycardia. *Am Heart J* 112:396, 1986.

298. Abernethy DR, Schwartz JB, Todd EL, et al: Verapamil pharmacodynamics and disposition in young and elderly hypertensive patients: Altered electrocardiographic and hypotensive response. *Ann Intern Med* 105:329, 1986.

299. Waxman HL, Meyerburg RJ, Appel R, Sung: Verapamil for control of ventricular rate in paroxysmal supraventricular tachycardia and atrial fibrillation or flutter. *Ann Intern Med* 94:1, 1981.

300. Haft JI, Habbab MA: Treatment of atrial arrhythmias, effectiveness of verapamil when preceded by calcium infusion. *Arch Intern Med* 146:1085, 1986.

301. Klein HO, Kaplinsky E: Verapamil and digoxin: their respective effects on atrial fibrillation and their interaction. *Am J Cardiol* 50:894, 1982.

302. Keech AC, Harper RW, Harrison PM, et al: Pharmacokinetic interaction between oral metoprolol and verapamil for angina pectoris. *Am J Cardiol* 58:551, 1986.

303. Stark G, Schulze-Bauer C, Stark U, et al: Comparison of the frequency-dependent effects on the atrioventricular node of verapamil, amiodarone, digoxin, and diltiazem in isolated guinea pig hearts. *J Cardiovasc Pharmacol* 25:330, 1995.

304. Talajic M, Lemery R, Roy D, et al: Rate-dependent effects of diltiazem on human atrioventricular nodal properties. *Circulation* 86:870, 1992.

305. Dougherty AH, Jackman WM, Naccarelli GV, et al: Acute conversion of paroxysmal supraventricular tachycardia with intravenous diltiazem. *Am J Cardiol* 70:587, 1992.

306. Clair WK, Wilkinson WE, McCarthy EA, et al: Treatment of paroxysmal supraventricular tachycardia with oral diltiazem. *Clin Pharmacol Ther* 51:562, 1992.

307. Roy D: Efficacy of diltiazem in recurrent supraventricular tachyarrhythmias. *Can J Cardiol* 11:538, 1995.

308. Pelleg A: Cardiac cellular electrophysiologic actions of adenosine and adenosine triphosphate. *Am Heart J* 110:688, 1985.

309. Belhassen B, Glick A, Laniado S: Comparative clinical and electrophysiologic effects of adenosine triphosphate and verapamil on paroxysmal reciprocating junctional tachycardia. *Circulation* 77:795, 1988.

310. Garratt C, Linker N, Griffith M, et al: Comparison of adenosine and verapamil for termination of paroxysmal junctional tachycardia. *Am J Cardiol* 64:1310, 1989.

311. DiMarco JP, Sellers TD, Lerman BB, et al: Diagnostic and therapeutic use of adenosine in patients with supraventricular tachyarrhythmias. *J Am Coll Cardiol* 6:417, 1985.

312. Lerman BB, Belardinelli L, West GA, et al: Adenosine sensitive ventricular tachycardia: Evidence suggesting cyclic AMP–mediated triggered activity. *Circulation* 74:270, 1986.

313. Withering W: An account of the foxglove and some of its medical uses, with practical remarks on dropsy and other diseases. In: Willis FA, Keys TE, eds. *Classics of Cardiology*. New York: Henry Schuman, 1941:231.

314. Sellers TD, Bashore TM, Gallagher JJ: Digitalis in the preexcitation syndrome—analysis during atrial fibrillation. *Circulation* 56:260, 1977.

315. Cotten M de V, Stopp PE: Action of digitalis on the nonfailing heart of the dog. *Am J Physiol* 192:114, 1958.

316. Sonnenblick EH, Williams JF Jr, Glick G, et al: Studies on digitalis: XV. Effects of cardiac glycosides on myocardial force velocity relations in the nonfailing human heart. *Circulation* 34:532, 1966.

317. Mason DT, Braunwald E: Studies on digitalis: X. Effects of ouabain on forearm vascular resistance and venous tone in normal subjects and in patients in heart failure. *J Clin Invest* 43:532, 1964.

318. DeMots H, Rahimtoola SH, McAnulty JH, Porter GA: Effects of ouabain on coronary and systemic vascular resistance and myocardial oxygen consumption in patients without heart failure. *Am J Cardiol* 41:88, 1978.

319. Shanbour LL, Jacobson ED: Digitalis and the mesenteric circulation. *Am J Dig Dis* 17:826, 1972.

319a. Murgatroyd FD, Gibson SM, Baiyan X, et al: Double-blind placebo-controlled trial of digoxin in symptomatic paroxysmal atrial fibrillation. *Circulation* 99:2765, 1999.

320. Smith TW, Butler VP, Haber E, et al: Treatment of life-threatening digitalis intoxication with digoxin-specific Fab antibody fragments. *N Engl J Med* 307:1357, 1982.

321. Nordrehaug JE, Johannessen K, Von der Lippe G: Serum potassium concentration as a risk factor of ventricular arrhythmias early in acute myocardial infarction. *Circulation* 71:645, 1985.

322. Zwillinger L: Uber die Magnesiumwirkung auf das Hertz. *Klin Wochenschr* 14:1429, 1935.

323. Watanabe Y, Dreifus LS: Electrophysiological effects of magnesium and its interactions with potassium. *Cardiovasc Res* 6:79, 1972.

324. Chen H, Bando S, Nakaya Y: Alterations of cardiac conduction and refractoriness in humans following intravenous administration of magnesium sulfate. *Tokushima J Exp Med* 35:13, 1988.

325. Iseri LT, French JH: Magnesium: nature's physiologic calcium blocker. *Am Heart J* 108:188, 1984.

326. Reinhart RA: Magnesium metabolism: A review with special reference to the relationship between intracellular content and serum levels. *Arch Intern Med* 148:2415, 1988.

327. Specter MJ, Schweizer E, Goldman RH: Studies on magnesium's mechanism of action in digitalis-induced arrhythmias. *Circulation* 52:1001, 1975.

328. Tzivoni D, Banai S, Schuger C, et al: Treatment of torsades de pointes with magnesium sulfate. *Circulation* 77:392, 1988.

329. Scheinman MM, Sullivan RW, Hyatt KH: Magnesium metabolism in patients undergoing cardiopulmonary bypass. *Circulation* 39:I235, 1969.

330. Billman GE, Hoskins RS: Prevention of ventricular fibrillation with magnesium sulfate. *Eur J Pharm* 158:167, 1988.

331. Allen BJ, Brodsky MA, Capparelli EV, et al: Magnesium sulfate therapy for sustained monomorphic ventricular tachycardia. *Am J Cardiol* 64:1202, 1989.

332. Dyckner T, Wester PO: Ventricular extrasystoles and intracellular electrolytes before and after potassium and magnesium infusions in patients on diuretic treatment. *Am Heart J* 97:12, 1979.

333. Smith LF, Heagerty RF, Bing RF, Barnett DB: Intravenous infusion of magnesium sulphate after acute myocardial infarction: Effects on arrhythmias and mortality. *Int J Cardiol* 12:175, 1986.

CHAPTER 18

Antiplatelet and Antithrombotic Drugs

William H. Frishman

Robert G. Lerner

Michael D. Klein

Mira Roganovic

Remarkable advances have occurred in the management of ischemic heart disease with innovative antiplatelet, antithrombotic, and thrombolytic therapies leading the list of breakthrough drugs. In this chapter, antiplatelet drugs and antithrombotic drugs are reviewed, focusing on the management of cardiovascular diseases. The use of these agents for preventing postangioplasty restenosis are reviewed in Chap. 40.

Newer antiplatelet and antithrombotic drugs under clinical development are reviewed in the final portion of this chapter, except for the direct thrombin inhibitors, which are discussed earlier. The thrombolytic drugs are discussed in Chap. 19.

PLATELET PHYSIOLOGY

The chief function of blood platelets is to interact with the vascular endothelium and soluble plasma factors in the hemostatic process. Under normal physiologic conditions, platelets are mostly inert; an intact vascular wall prevents their adhesion to the subendothelial matrix. In response to vessel trauma, platelets will spontaneously adhere to newly exposed adhesive proteins, forming a protective monolayer of cells. Within seconds, these platelets will be activated by agonists such as thrombin, collagen, and adenosine 5'-diphosphate (ADP), causing them to change shape and to release stored vesicles. The constituents of the vesicles are mostly involved in the further activation of platelets and the propagation of the hemostatic process. Ultimately, these activated platelets will aggregate to form a hemostatic plug, closing the vent in the endothelium and preventing further loss of blood from the site.[1] Under certain pathologic conditions (i.e., rupture of an atherosclerotic plaque), these platelet aggregates can form thrombi and be associated with multiple cardiovascular ischemic events, including unstable angina and myocardial infarction (MI). This process is discussed in the following section.

Platelet Function

Platelet Adhesion

When the endothelial intima is interrupted by vascular trauma, the subendothelial protein matrix is exposed to circulating platelets and plasma coagulation factors. The major subendothelial glycoproteins involved in platelet adhesion are von Willebrand factor, collagen, and possibly fibronectin and/or vitronectin. Platelet adhesion to the von Willebrand factor ligand at high shear rates involves the platelet surface-receptor glycoprotein GP Ib. This receptor is exposed on the surface of nonactivated platelets and is the major receptor for platelet adhesion.[2] The process of platelet adhesion in hemostasis is unique in that it occurs without prior activation by platelet activators.

Platelet Activation

After the platelet monolayer is formed over the endothelial lesion, specific agonists induce platelet vesicle secretion and aggregation. The most physiologically important agonists include thrombin, ADP, collagen, and thromboxane A_2 (produced from arachidonic acid). All of these agonists probably act by a common pathway that leads to the increase of intraplatelet calcium concentrations through direct ion flux or the release of stored calcium.[3] For example, a common pathway is the ligand-receptor activation (by G proteins) of phospholipase C that cleaves phosphatidyl inositol biphosphate to inositol triphosphate (IP3) and diacylglycerol. IP3 then leads to the mobilization of stored calcium from the dense tubular system within the platelet cytosol and degranulation of platelets (Fig. 18-1).

Two important calcium-dependent processes include the phosphorylation of the myosin light chain and the activation of phospholipase A_2.[1] The phosphorylation of myosin (and actin polymerization) is involved in the physical changes that the platelet undergoes on stimulation, including the loss of its normal discoid shape, formation of pseudopodia, and centralization and exocytosis of storage granules. The activation of phospholipase A_2 leads to an increase in arachidonic acid, which is converted by cyclooxygenases into thromboxane A_2, a powerful prostaglandin agonist. The release of thromboxane A_2 (with thrombin and collagen) can lead to the release of ADP from platelet α granules. This ADP can, in turn, stimulate the arachidonic acid pathway and the further release of thromboxane A_2.[4] In this way, the platelet can further increase its own activation.

Platelet Aggregation

The final common pathway of all agonist-receptor interactions is the activation (by an unknown mechanism) of a specific receptor responsible for platelet aggregation. This receptor, GP IIb/IIIa,

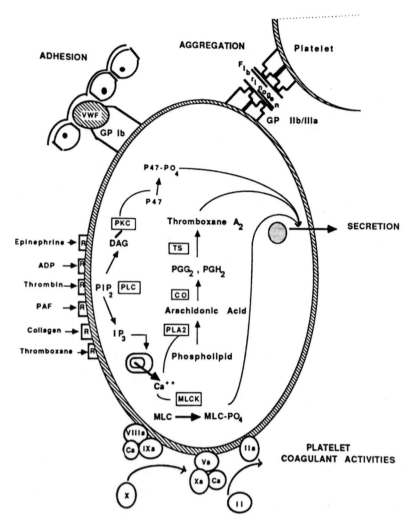

FIGURE 18-1. Platelet function. Adhesion to endothelial cells is mediated by GP Ib, which binds von Willebrand factor (VWF) on endothelial cells. Aggregation is mediated by GP IIb/IIIa bridged to GP IIb/IIIa on another platelet by fibrinogen. Various agonists, such as ADP and platelet-activating factor (PAF), interact with specific receptors and activate phospholipase C (PLC), probably through G proteins. This enzyme catalyzes the cleavage of phosphatidylinositol 4,5-bisphosphate (PIP_2) to IP_3, which mobilizes calcium from the dense tubular system to activate myosin light-chain kinase (MLCK), which phosphorylates myosin light chain (MLC). Calcium also activates phospholipase A2 (PLA_2) to release arachidonic acid from phospholipids, which, in turn, is converted by cyclooxygenase (CO) to prostaglandin (PG) G_2 and PGH_2 and then by thromboxane synthetase (TS) to thromboxane A_2. The other product of cleavage of PIP_2 is diacylglycerol (DAG), which stimulates protein kinase C (PKC) to phosphorylate intracellular protein P47 to P47-PO_4. The latter, thromboxane A_2 and MLC-PO_4, together stimulate secretion of productions of the dense α and lysosomal granules. Platelet coagulant activity is generated by coagulation factors (Roman numerals) to form tenase (VIII, IXa, and Ca) and prothrombinase (Va, Xa, and Ca) on platelet external membrane phospholipid to convert prothrombin (II) to thrombin (IIa). (*Courtesy of A. Koneti Rao, MD.*)

unlike the GP Ib receptor responsible for platelet adhesion, is active only after the platelet has been stimulated (and consequently after its intracellular calcium concentration has become increased). Also unique is that GP IIb/IIIa is found only on cells of megakaryocytic origin (i.e., platelets). The receptor has a high affinity for the tripeptide sequence arginine-glycine-aspartic acid (RGD), which is found in fibrinogen, von Willebrand factor, fibronectin, and vitronectin.[5] Fibrinogen, primarily because of its high concentration in the plasma, is the primary polypeptide involved in platelet aggregation. Because fibrinogen is a divalent dimer, it is able to link adjacent platelets. Other GPs, including fibronectin, von Willebrand factor, and thrombospondin, also may be involved in platelet aggregation after the initial binding to fibrinogen. The GP IIb/IIIa receptor is discussed in detail later.

The Role of Platelets in Ischemic Heart Disease

Thrombosis is often regarded as the pathologic extension of the normal hemostatic process. It involves the formation of a platelet aggregate, or thrombus, within vasculature that has not usually received external trauma. The presence of atherosclerotic vascular disease is highly correlated with the development and clinical presentation of platelet thrombi. Once formed, the thrombus may partially or totally occlude a vessel, resulting in the disruption of blood flow and tissue ischemia and necrosis. Thrombosis in the coronary arteries

may directly produce the clinical conditions of unstable angina and/or acute MI.

Atherosclerosis

There are two distinct phases of atherosclerotic progression. The first phase involves the primary progression of growth of multifocal intimal lesions from fatty streaks to fibrous plaques. The second phase is the development of platelet thrombosis as a result of plaque rupture or ulceration.[6] The second phase is most directly involved in the clinical manifestations of atherosclerosis and, therefore, is most commonly the target of pharmacologic intervention to prevent ischemic heart disease (IHD).

Atherosclerosis is a chronic disease that affects only medium to large arteries, primarily the coronary and cerebral arteries and the aorta. In a study of Macaca primates which were fed a high-lipid diet, it was determined that the initiating mechanism in the development of intimal lesions is the migration of monocytes/macrophage from the vessel lumen through an intact endothelium. This migration occurs without any platelet interaction. Often, these infiltrating macrophages exist as lipid-filled foam cells. Within 3 months the foam cells that have become lodged within the intima disrupt the endothelial cell layer. By the fourth month, the first sign of platelet interaction is visible; platelets have adhered to the subendothelial matrix exposed by microlesions in the endothelial layer. It therefore appears that platelets are more involved with the growth of atherosclerotic plaques than with their initiation.[7]

The earliest atherosclerotic lesions are the fatty streaks. The streaks appear as areas of yellow, oval discolorations ≤2 mm in diameter. They are composed primarily of lipid-filled foam cells (macrophages) that have infiltrated the intima. All human infants, regardless of the rate of future IHD within their population, have aortic fatty streaks by age 1 year of age.[6] Fatty streaks also appear universally in the coronary arteries by age 15 and in the cerebral arteries by the third and fourth decades.

Fibrous (or raised) plaques are believed to develop from fatty streaks. Unlike the streaks, the progression to plaque development is not universal in the population. Instead, the number of raised plaques in an individual person often reflects the prevalence of IHD in his or her particular geographic population. Patients with risk factors for coronary artery disease, such as increased cholesterol, smoking, and a familial pattern and history, appear to have an increased number of raised plaques at autopsy.

The fibrous plaques appear to develop at points of hemodynamic stress along the coronary artery (and especially at points of bifurcation). They are palpable above the surface of the intima and may be as long as 2 cm in the aorta. The plaques usually consist of a cholesterol-filled center surrounded by a layer of foam cells. Overlying the lipid layer is a fibromuscular cap composed of collagen, smooth muscle, and elastin with an intact endothelial wall separating the plaque from the vessel lumen. Advanced plaques appear to have a pool of free cholesterol in their center, leading to a decrease in plaque stability.

Thrombosis

It is believed that the clinical manifestations of IHD are not caused by the continued growth of fibrous plaques but by complications resulting from the eventual rupture and ulceration of these plaques.[7a] Plaque rupture occurs when the fibrous cap of the plaque is disrupted by physical stresses, and either tears or is removed completely.[8] As the atherosclerotic plaque growth advances, lipid-filled foam cells invade the smooth muscle/collagen cap, consequently reducing its strength. Advanced plaques may also contain a sizable pool of extracellular cholesterol within the plaque's core. These weak plaques with high lipid content are particularly inclined to rupture, exposing circulating platelets to the thrombogenic substances (collagen, tissue factor, and cholesterol) within. The damage to the endothelium also disrupts production of endogenous vasodilator and antiplatelet substances (i.e., nitric oxide and prostacyclin).

Platelets exposed to the subendothelial plaque material may undergo activation and subsequent aggregation to form a thrombus within the plaque itself (Fig. 18-2). Risk factors for development of a thrombus are related to the size of the fissure, the plasma fibrinogen levels, the rate of blood flow, and the rate of spontaneous platelet aggregation. These thrombi can continue to expand, leading to the enlargement of the plaque and the appearance of "de novo" arterial stenosis on the angiogram.[9]

Some plaques may heal from the fissure, whereas in other plaques, mural thrombi may develop and project into the lumen of the vessel. These thrombi have a high platelet component, causing the clot to appear white on examination. The intraluminal plaques may transiently reduce coronary blood flow leading to the ischemic condition of unstable angina, or they may break up into microemboli, causing focal areas of necrosis and possible arrhythmia. These mural thrombi have been visualized by coronary angioscopy in

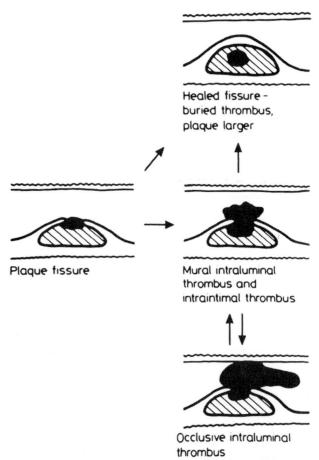

FIGURE 18-2. Proposed outcome of atherosclerotic plaque fissuring. *Left:* Initial plaque fissure. *(Top right):* Fissure is sealed, and incorporated thrombus undergoes fibrotic organization, contributing to progression of coronary disease. *Middle right:* Fissure leads to intraintimal and intraluminal thrombosis, resulting in partial or transient reduction of coronary flow as seen in unstable angina. *(Bottom right):* Fissure results in occlusive thrombosis, which if persistent, can lead to MI or sudden death, particularly in absence of collateral flow. *(Reproduced with permission from Ip et al.[11]).*

patients with unstable angina.[10] If the intraluminal clot grows rapidly, it may not allow time for the development of collateral flow. This predisposes the patient to an acute MI.[11] With acute coronary syndromes, platelets can remain activated for as long as 1 month after clinical stabilization, suggesting the need for long-term antiplatelet therapy.[12]

In patients who survive events caused by intraluminal thrombus formation, a natural fibrinolytic reaction normally occurs. Plasminogen is converted to the enzyme plasmin which breaks down the fibrinogen and fibrin component of the thrombus. Fibrinolytic therapy with tissue plasminogen activators has also proven effective. Yet fibrin debris that remains may contribute to further stenosis or to possible chronic total obstruction.

CONVENTIONAL ANTIPLATELET THERAPY

The efficacy of acetylsalicylic acid, or aspirin, as an antiplatelet agent has been thoroughly investigated, and it remains the most widely used and cost-efficient drug in the prevention of platelet aggregation.[13] Ticlopidine, an alternative drug with demonstrated

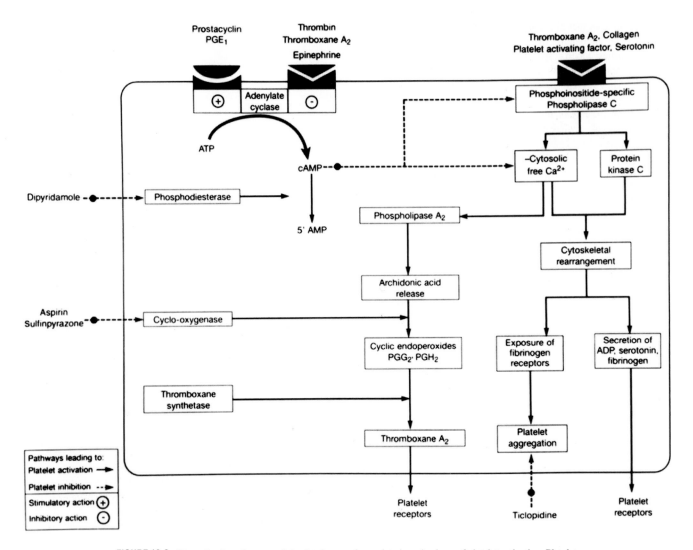

FIGURE 18-3. Sites of action of some antiplatelet drugs and associated mechanisms of platelet activation. Platelet activation results from mobilization of calcium, which in turn results from agonist binding to platelet receptor. $5'$-AMP $= 5'$-Adenosine monophosphate; ATP $=$ adenosine triphosphate; cAMP $=$ cyclic adenosine monophosphate; PG $=$ prostaglandin. (*Adapted from Saltiel E, Ward A: Ticlopidine: A review of its pharmacodynamic and pharmacokinetic properties, and therapeutic efficacy in platelet-dependent disease states. Drugs 34:222–262, 1987.*)

antithrombotic properties in the prevention of strokes is approved for use in aspirin-sensitive patients; however, its higher cost, its additional adverse side effects (particularly thrombotic thrombocytopenic purpura and agranulocytosis), and the essentially similar results obtained with aspirin, preclude its general use.[14] Clopidogrel, a similar drug, is now commonly used instead of ticlopidine because it has a lower incidence of side effects. Until recently, dipyridamole was regarded as an antiplatelet agent, but a significant antithrombotic benefit of the drug when used alone has not been demonstrated.[14]

Aspirin

By virtue of aspirin's antiplatelet properties, it has become an essential part of the treatment of ischemic cardiac syndromes.[15] Aspirin diminishes the production of thromboxane A_2 through its ability to irreversibly inhibit the cyclooxygenase activity of prostaglandin (PG)H synthase-1 and PGH synthase-2 known also as COX-1 and COX-2 (Fig. 18-3).[16]

As a result, platelets exposed to aspirin exhibit diminished aggregation in response to thrombogenic stimuli.[17,18] Aspirin's ability to inhibit cyclooxygenase is impressive, as only 30 mg/d is required to eliminate the production of thromboxane A_2 completely.[16] The cyclooxygenase is irreversibly inhibited and cannot be replaced by new protein synthesis because the platelet has no nucleus. As a result, because the body's reservoir of platelets is renewed only every 10 days, one dose of aspirin exhibits detectable inhibition of platelet aggregation for more than a week, although a clinical antithrombotic effect may be of lesser duration. Additionally, there is evidence that aspirin may reduce clotting ability by inhibiting the synthesis of vitamin K-dependent factors, and by stimulating fibrinolysis. These nonprostaglandin mechanisms are dose-dependent and less clearly defined.[19]

In addition to inhibiting platelet cyclooxygenase, aspirin also inhibits the production of prostacyclin by the vascular endothelium. Prostacyclin is a substance that promotes vasodilation and inhibits platelet aggregation. Because its inhibition would theoretically promote thrombosis, it has been postulated that the beneficial effects of aspirin are reduced because of reduced prostacyclin levels.[20] Unlike platelets, however, prostacyclin production recovers within hours after aspirin administration.[21] Various formulations of aspirin have been studied in an attempt to selectively inhibit thromboxane A_2 without inhibiting prostacyclin. It seems, however, that even low doses of conventionally formulated aspirin will inhibit them both.[21] Selective inhibition of thromboxane A_2 has been achieved using a low-dose (75 mg), sustained-release aspirin preparation. Platelets in the prehepatic circulation have their cyclooxygenase irreversibly inhibited. Because extensive first pass metabolism occurs, however, the endothelium in the systemic circulation is exposed to insufficient drug to inhibit prostacyclin production.[22] Whether this is related to the now well-established clinical benefit is unknown. It has been suggested that using the lowest effective dose is the most sensible strategy to maximize efficacy and minimize toxicity. The ASA and Carotid Endarterectomy trial reported a lower risk of stroke, MI, or death in patients taking 81 or 325 mg aspirin than in those patients taking 650 or 1300 mg.[23]

Aspirin in Chronic Stable Angina

One arm of the Physician's Health Study examined 383 male physicians with chronic stable angina.[24] The subjects were randomized to either 325 mg of aspirin every other day or to placebo. Treatment was over a 5-year period. Although no change in symptom frequency or severity was noted between the two groups, the occurrence of a first myocardial infarction was reduced by 87% in those subjects treated with aspirin. It seems likely that although there was no change in disease progression (as noted by unchanged symptomatology), the addition of aspirin reduced the risk of thrombosis in the event of plaque instability. This conclusion has been supported by data from Chesebro et al who noted that the use of aspirin and dipyridamole decreased the incidence of myocardial infarction and new atherosclerotic lesions without affecting the progression of old atherosclerotic plaques.[25] The Swedish Angina Pectoris Aspirin Trial (SAPAT) found that the addition of low-dose aspirin to sotalol treatment provided additional benefit in terms of cardiovascular events, including a significant reduction in the incidence of first myocardial infarction in patients with angina pectoris.[26]

Unstable Angina

Unstable angina represents the midpoint of the spectrum of ischemic cardiac syndromes, which spans chronic stable angina and myocardial infarction. Its pathogenesis lies in the rupture of an intracoronary plaque, which promotes platelet aggregation, thrombus formation and luminal compromise. Theoretically, because aspirin has potent antiplatelet properties, it should be beneficial in the treatment of unstable angina.

Numerous studies have examined the use of aspirin in patients with unstable angina, all of which have shown marked clinical benefit. The Veterans Administration study examined 1384 patients with unstable angina within 48 h of hospital admission.[27] These patients were randomized to receive either 325 mg of aspirin per day or placebo for 12 weeks. Death or nonfatal MI occurred in 11% of those treated with placebo compared to only 6.3% in the aspirin group (P <.004). Although treatment was limited to 12 weeks, 1-year mortality was reduced from 9.6% in the placebo group to 5.5% in those treated with aspirin (P <.01). Cairns et al randomized 555 patients with unstable angina within 8 days of admission to either 325 mg of aspirin four times a day or to placebo.[28] Treatment was for 48 h and nonfatal MI or cardiac death was reduced from 14.7 to 10.5% in those treated with aspirin (P <.07). Similarly, total

mortality was reduced from 10% with placebo to 5.8% in the aspirin group (P <.04). Theroux et al randomized 479 patients with unstable angina to 325 mg of aspirin two times per day or to placebo.[29] The patients were enrolled upon presentation to the hospital and were treated for 3 to 9 days. Nonfatal MI was reduced from 6.4% in the placebo group to 2.5% in those treated with aspirin (P <.04). Finally, the RISC study investigated the effects of a reduced dose of aspirin in unstable angina.[30] In the aspirin versus placebo arm, it enrolled 388 patients to receive either 75 mg of aspirin or placebo for 3 months. This study demonstrated a reduction in the rate of nonfatal MI or noncardiac death from 17% in the placebo group to 7.4% in aspirin group (P = .0042).

It is clear from the above studies, that aspirin is effective at reducing the morbidity and mortality of unstable angina with and without heparin.[31] Specifically, nonfatal MI and cardiac death were reduced by 50 to 70%. This benefit seemed to occur across a broad spectrum of daily doses, from 1300 mg/d in the study by Cairns (28), to only 75 mg/d in the RISC trial.[30] Because platelets are exquisitely sensitive to aspirin, this finding is not unexpected. A study of the effect of aspirin on C-reactive protein (CRP), a marker of risk in unstable angina, was carried out to assess whether the beneficial effects of aspirin were related to aspirin's ability to influence CRP release.[32] Serial blood samples for CRP and troponin I assay were obtained from 304 consecutive patients admitted with non-ST-elevation acute coronary syndromes. End-points were cardiac death and nonfatal myocardial infarction during follow-up for 12 months. Patients taking aspirin had lower troponin I concentrations throughout the sampling period, only 45 (26.0%) having concentrations >0.1 mg/L as compared with 48 (37.8%) patients not taking aspirin (P = .03). Maximum CRP concentrations were also lower in patients taking aspirin [8.16 mg/L (3.24 to 24.5)] than in patients not taking aspirin [11.3 mg/L (4.15 to 26.1)], although the difference was not significant. However, there was significant interaction (P = .04) between prior aspirin therapy and the predictive value of CRP concentrations for death and myocardial infarction at 12 months. Thus, odds ratios (95% confidence intervals) for events associated with an increase of 1 standard deviation in maximum CRP concentration were 2.64 (1.22 to 5.72) in patients not pretreated with aspirin as compared with 0.98 (0.60 to 1.62) in patients pretreated with aspirin. The authors concluded that the association between CRP and cardiac events in patients with unstable angina is influenced by pretreatment with aspirin, and that modification of the acute-phase inflammatory responses to myocardial injury is the major mechanism of this interaction.[32]

Primary Prevention of Myocardial Infarction

The rupture of an intracoronary atheromatous plaque causes the majority of MIs. This exposes subendothelial collagen to local blood products, which results in the attraction and activation of platelets. These activated platelets release growth factors and vasoactive compounds that produce vasoconstriction, further platelet aggregation, and, ultimately, the formation of an occlusive mural thrombus.

While aspirin was shown to improve outcomes in patients with unstable angina, its benefit in primary prevention of MI was largely unknown until the results of the US Physicians' Health Study were reported on. In this study, 22,071 male US physicians were randomized to either 325 mg of aspirin every other day or to placebo. Ninety-eight percent of those involved were free of cardiac-related symptoms and treatment took place over a 5-year period. While the frequency of angina, coronary revascularization, or death was unchanged between the two groups,[33] the incidence of MI was impressively reduced in the aspirin treated group. Specifically, the risk of fatal or nonfatal MI was reduced by 44%.[34]

The observations made in the US Physicians' Health Study were challenged by a similar study from Europe.[35] The British Physicians' Health Study was an uncontrolled trial that involved 5139 British male physicians, two-thirds of whom were treated with 500 mg of aspirin per day.[35] In contrast to the US study, there was no significant reduction in MI or total mortality. Criticisms of this trial were many and included its uncontrolled design, its smaller sample size, the higher dose of aspirin, its older subjects with poorer compliance, and its high confidence intervals. Its results, however, were sufficient to cast some doubt on aspirin's utility in the primary prevention of MI.

Any doubts as to aspirin's role in the primary prevention of MI were largely put to rest by a large, observational study of US nurses and their aspirin usage. In this study, aspirin usage by 87,000 US nurses was analyzed over a 6-year period.[36] All of the nurses involved were free of cardiac-related symptoms. The study showed that in women over the age of 50 years, ingestion of one to six 325-mg tablets of aspirin per week was associated with a 32% reduction in first myocardial infarction. This benefit was most striking in women with risk factors for coronary artery disease including tobacco use, hypercholesterolemia, and hypertension. In women who took more than seven tablets per week, however, there was no reduction in the rate of MI. In addition, women who took more than 15 tablets per week were at a significantly increased risk of hemorrhagic stroke.

It appears from the above studies that 325 mg of aspirin every other day is effective at preventing a first MI in asymptomatic individuals. An aspirin dose as low as 75 mg/d is the minimum dose that effectively reduces the risk of a first MI.[37] The benefit of aspirin is most pronounced in patients who are at high risk for coronary artery disease, specifically, older individuals with multiple cardiac risk factors. The corollary of this is that the risk-to-benefit ratio for aspirin use is lowest in healthy individuals and highest in high-risk individuals. Higher doses of aspirin do not appear to confer any additional benefit and most likely impart additional risk of developing hemorrhagic stroke. Despite its proven benefit, aspirin is still being underutilized in clinical practice.[38,38a]

Secondary Prevention of Myocardial Infarction

Seven prospective, randomized, placebo-controlled trials have examined the use of aspirin in the secondary prevention of myocardial infarction.[39–45] As a cumulative total, these studies have enrolled over 15,000 survivors of MI whose treatment consisted of various aspirin regimens, with doses ranging from 325 to 1500 mg/d. Patients were enrolled from 4 weeks to 5 years post-MI. When each of these trials was examined individually, no statistically significant decrease in mortality was observed. Because the numbers of patients in each study may have been too small to provide adequate statistical power, a meta-analysis of six of the trials was performed. This meta-analysis contained 10,703 patients and showed that when aspirin was compared with placebo, cardiovascular morbidity was reduced by 21%.[46] In another meta-analysis from the Antiplatelet Trialists Collaboration, the risk of developing a nonfatal reinfarction was shown to be reduced by 31% and death from vascular causes was reduced by 13% in those patients treated with aspirin during the 1- to 4-year follow-up period.[15] Finally, in a 23-month follow-up of 931 patients with acute infarction or unstable angina, 80% of subjects were found to use aspirin on a regular basis. Their cardiac death rate was markedly reduced compared to nonaspirin users and was not explicable by imbalances

in predictors of postinfarction risk, by concurrent drug therapy, or by preinfarction thrombolysis or angioplasty.[47]

In addition to the cardiac benefits demonstrated by the above studies, aspirin also seems to reduce the risk of stroke in post-MI patients. In a subset of the Antiplatelet Trialists Collaboration,[15] the risk of stroke in those patients treated with aspirin was examined. A 42% reduction in nonfatal strokes in the aspirin group was demonstrated, as compared to placebo treatment. With these results in mind, treatment of post-MI patients with low-dose aspirin (perhaps 75 mg/d) seems reasonable.[48] Although many of the above trials relied on pooled data and meta-analysis to demonstrate aspirin's benefit in the post-MI population, the data are compelling to that effect. Aspirin does not appear to increase the risk of nonfatal cerebrovascular accident (CVA), and will most likely reduce the risk of future cardiac events. The optimal dose of aspirin for long-term postinfarction prophylaxis is unclear at this time, and will need to be determined with future studies.

A recent meta-analysis of five randomized trials of primary prevention included 52,251 participants randomized to aspirin doses ranging from 75 to 650 mg/d; the mean overall stroke rate was 0.3% per year during an average follow-up of 4.6 years. Meta-analysis revealed no significant effect on stroke (relative risk = 1.08; 95% confidence interval, 0.95 to 1.24) contrasting with a decrease in myocardial infarction (relative risk = 0.74; 95% confidence interval, 0.68 to 0.82). The authors concluded that the effect of aspirin therapy on stroke differs between individuals based on the presence or absence of overt vascular disease, in contrast with the consistent reduction in myocardial infarction by aspirin therapy observed in all populations.[49]

Acute Myocardial Infarction

Localized coronary thrombosis due to the rupture of an unstable, intracoronary, atheromatous plaque is thought to be responsible for more than 90% of Q-wave myocardial infarctions.[50] Although thrombolytic agents break down the primary clot responsible for the acute event, substances liberated during this process can themselves promote platelet aggregation and reocclusion.[51] Although spontaneous recanalization may occur, thrombus reformation is common and may perpetuate the ischemic process. By virtue of aspirin's potent antiplatelet properties, it is an effective agent, when used either alone or with thrombolytic agents, at reducing the mortality from acute myocardial infarctions.

The Second International Study of Infarct Survival (ISIS-2) was a double-blind, placebo controlled trial that defined aspirin's role in the treatment of acute myocardial infarction.[52] ISIS-2 enrolled 17,187 patients with suspected acute myocardial infarction and randomized them to either intravenous streptokinase (1.5 million units over 60 min), aspirin (162 mg/d for 1 month), to both, or to neither. Five weeks after randomization, aspirin reduced the risk of nonfatal reinfarction by 51% and of vascular mortality by 23% when compared with placebo. The addition of intravenous streptokinase further reduced mortality in conjunction with aspirin. These results indicated that aspirin reduced mortality to a similar degree as did streptokinase alone and that when the two were combined, a cumulative benefit was observed. Aspirin's reduction in mortality also extended to groups treated with various heparin dosages, ranging from no heparin (288 vs 347 deaths), to subcutaneous heparin (338 vs 431 deaths) and to intravenous heparin (178 vs 238 deaths, $P < .001$). Mortality benefits were similar in both men and women and remained present after 24 months of follow-up. Importantly, treatment with aspirin did not result in any increased incidence of major bleeds (31 vs 33 bleeds) and seemed to decrease the risk of nonfatal CVA by 46% ($P = .003$). It seems clear that aspirin, with or without thrombolytic therapy, is effective at reducing the mortality and morbidity of an evolving MI.

Non-Q-wave MI results when an intracoronary occlusion is incomplete or occurs for only a short time. The pathophysiology of a non-Q-wave MI is similar to both unstable angina and to Q-wave MI in that a ruptured atheromatous plaque results in acute intracoronary thrombus formation. Although it seems likely that aspirin would confer a benefit in evolving non-Q-wave myocardial infarctions, no adequate trials have been performed to date in this subgroup of patients.

Current recommendations of the American College of Chest Physicians Sixth Consensus Conference are that all patients with acute MI who receive fibrinolytic therapy receive adjunctive treatment with aspirin (165 to 325 mg) on arrival to the hospital and daily thereafter. They further recommend that patients receive heparin or hirudin as an adjunct depending on their risk factor for systemic or venous thromboembolism and the fibrinolytic agent with which they are treated.[53]

Percutaneous Transluminal Coronary Angioplasty and Arterial Stenting

When percutaneous transluminal coronary angioplasty is performed, the intracoronary atheromatous plaque that is acted upon is "cracked" or "fissured" by the destructive action of balloon inflation. This results in the exposure of underlying subendothelial collagen to circulating blood products, which activates platelets and promotes thrombogenesis. It has been shown that the magnitude of platelet deposition after angioplasty is related to the depth of arterial injury[54] and that in animals, pretreatment with aspirin reduces the degree of thrombus formation.[55]

There have been two randomized, prospective trials that have evaluated the role of aspirin in preventing abrupt closure after angioplasty.[56,57] In these studies, aspirin (650 to 990 mg/d) and dipyridamole (225 mg/d) were started 24 h preangioplasty and continued indefinitely. They demonstrated that the incidence of abrupt closure was significantly reduced when compared with placebo. In another trial by Barnathan et al,[58] it was noted that when the coronary angiograms of patients undergoing angioplasty were analyzed retrospectively, the incidence of coronary thrombosis was significantly lower in those patients treated with either aspirin or aspirin plus dipyridamole. Finally, although aspirin does appear to lower the risk of acute thrombosis after angioplasty, it has not been shown to effect the rate of late restenosis.[54] With regards to coronary artery stenting, aspirin remains an important prophylactic treatment in preventing acute thrombosis, especially in combination with ticlopidine[59] or clopidogrel.[60] In a randomized trial of 700 patients with 899 lesions, after the placement of coronary-artery stents antiplatelet therapy with aspirin and clopidogrel was as safe and effective as aspirin and ticlopidine, while noncardiac events were significantly reduced with aspirin plus clopidogrel.[60]

Coronary Artery Bypass Surgery

In coronary artery bypass grafting (CABG) surgery, native coronary arteries whose blood flow is compromised by atherosclerotic blockages are "bypassed" using either venous or arterial conduits. The arterial conduit usually consists of either the left or right internal mammary arteries and the venous conduit is usually a reversed, saphenous vein from the leg. Although this surgery is one of the

mainstays of treatment for coronary artery disease, occlusion of the bypass vessels either acutely or over time, is not uncommon. It has been noted for example, that 40 to 50% of saphenous vein grafts will occlude within 10 years of their implantation.[61] Reasons for graft occlusion vary with the age of the conduit. "Acute" closure (less than 1 month after placement) is usually due to thrombosis, whereas "intermediate" closure (1 month to 1 year) is caused by accelerated intimal hyperplasia. Finally, "late" occlusion (more than 1 year) results from atherosclerosis within the bypass graft.[62]

Multiple studies have demonstrated a decreased incidence of early thrombosis when aspirin is used in the perioperative period.[63–66] Goldman et al[65] randomized 50 groups of CABG patients to receive either (a) aspirin 325 mg/d, (b) aspirin 325 mg tid, (c) aspirin 325 mg tid and dipyridamole 75 mg tid, (d) sulfinpyrazone 267 mg tid, or (e) placebo. This study demonstrated a significantly decreased risk of early thrombosis in all groups treated with aspirin [73% graft patency with placebo at 2 months vs 93% with aspirin, $P < .05$]. The addition of dipyridamole resulted in no additional benefit and sulfinpyrazone was ineffective in reducing the risk of thrombosis. Although those patients treated with aspirin had increased blood loss and need for reoperation, perioperative mortality was unchanged. The benefits noted in this study remained present after 1 year of follow-up.[66] In a follow up to this study, predictors of patency 3 years after CABG were analyzed. For a patient with patent vein grafts 7 to 10 days after the operation, predictors of 3-year graft patency are more closely related to operative techniques and underlying disease, and not to aspirin treatment.[67]

Despite the lack of effect on patency at 3 years, it is still recommended that aspirin should be given to all patients undergoing bypass surgery unless a clear contraindication exists. A dose of 325 mg/d is probably reasonable, as higher doses do not add any additional clinical benefit. The medication may be started preoperatively or within 48 h postoperatively if preoperative administration is not possible.[68,69]

Transient Ischemia Attack and Stroke

The capacity of aspirin in doses of 50 to 1500 mg/d, either alone or in combination with other antiplatelet agents (dipyridamole, sulfinpyrazone), to reduce the risk of recurrent cerebrovascular events[70] was studied in 10 trials involving approximately 8000 patients with stroke (CVA) or transient ischemic attacks (TIA).[71] Based upon these studies, treatment of 1000 patients with aspirin for 3 years will reduce fatal and nonfatal cardiovascular events including recurrent CVA by about one-fourth.[71] Optimal daily dose of aspirin for secondary prophylaxis in cerebrovascular disease remains somewhat controversial, but doses between 300 to 1200 mg/d are the recommended dose range.[72] The FDA published its rules for labeling aspirin products for over-the-counter human use and recommended aspirin doses from 50 to 325 mg/d for prevention of ischemic stroke.[73] The ASA and Carotid Endarterectomy trial suggested that low-dose aspirin is at least as effective as high-dose aspirin.[23]

The Clopidogrel Versus Aspirin in Patients at Risk of Ischemic Events (CAPRIE) study included 19,185 patients, 6431 entering the trial with stroke. There was a statistically nonsignificant relative risk reduction of 8% for stroke favoring clopidogrel.[74] The European Stroke Prevention Study 2 demonstrated that aspirin combined with sustained release dipyridamole was more effective than either alone in reducing the risk of stroke.[75] The results were independent of age. Based on this study, a combination formulation of aspirin and dipyridamole has been approved for clinical use.[75a]

Systemic Lupus Erythematosus

Prophylactic aspirin should be given to all patients with systemic lupus erythematosus to prevent both arterial and venous thrombotic manifestations, especially in patients with antiphospholipid antibodies.[76]

Venous Thromboembolism

Aspirin use has also been shown to reduce the risk of thromboembolism after major orthopedic surgery.[77] It has not been compared to low-molecular-weight heparin (LMWH) or evaluated in combination with LMWH.

Atrial Fibrillation

Aspirin has been used to reduce the hazard of thromboembolic stroke in nonvalvular atrial fibrillation (NVAF) and compared with the efficacy of warfarin.[78–80] Data from randomized trials support aspirin use for thromboembolism prophylaxis in younger NVAF patients (<60 years), especially in the absence of associated risk factors of hypertension, recent congestive heart failure, or remote thromboembolism.[81] A slightly greater hazard for intracranial bleeding with warfarin might make aspirin a suitable alternative to warfarin in selected other patients.[81] An ongoing clinical trial (SPAF III) was designed to evaluate the relative efficacy and safety of aspirin as an adjunct to low-intensity fixed-dose warfarin in preventing thromboembolism in high-risk NVAF patients. The trial is ongoing in low-risk patients. The trial was stopped prematurely in high-risk patients due to an excess of strokes in patients receiving aspirin plus low-dose warfarin.[82] The published results thus far support the use of conventional dose warfarin in the majority of patients with atrial fibrillation.

Adverse Effects and Drug-Drug Interactions

The most common side effect of aspirin treatment is gastrointestinal (GI) intolerance. In the Aspirin Myocardial Infarction Study in which patients with known peptic ulcer disease (PUD) were excluded, 24% of those treated with aspirin (1000 mg/d) reported GI intolerance as compared with 15% in the placebo group.[40] In the United Kingdom TIA Trial,[70] GI symptoms were reduced by 30% when the dose of aspirin was decreased from 1200 mg/d to 300 mg/d. Finally, in the Physicians' Health Study[34] (patients with known PUD were excluded), 325 mg of aspirin every other day resulted in only a 0.5% increase in GI symptoms when compared with placebo. GI intolerance due to aspirin, therefore, appears to occur in a dose-dependent manner and treatment with 325 mg/d appears to be well tolerated. Two forms of cyclooxygenase enzymes have been identified, one which produces the "good" prostaglandins that act in the stomach and other tissues (COX-1) and another (COX-2) which is involved in thromboxane formation.

Agents are now available to inhibit COX-2 while sparing COX-1, which could provide a stomach-sparing aspirin. The relative risk of GI bleeding with such drugs as compared with other NSAIDs is reduced.[83] However, a recent study would suggest that COX-2 inhibitors may have a prothrombotic effect in patients at risk for coronary artery disease. Therefore, until this issue is resolved, the COX-2 inhibitors cannot be used as aspirin substitutes for cardiovascular prophylaxis.

Bleeding complications are a common side effect of aspirin therapy. Specifically, the risk of developing a hemorrhagic event such as bruising, melena and epistaxis are all increased with aspirin use. The Physicians' Health Study[34] confirmed this by reporting that 27% of those treated with aspirin (325 mg every other day) experienced bleeding complications, as compared with only 20% in the placebo group. In the United Kingdom TIA Trial,[70] there was a significant increase in the risk of GI bleeding when the dose of aspirin was increased to 1200 mg/d. For these reasons, the risks and benefits of aspirin therapy need to be weighed against one another in patients who are at increased risk of bleeding. Furthermore, the dose of aspirin used should be as low as possible because higher doses do not appear to confer additional benefits, but do increase bleeding risk substantially.

Aspirin also possibly interferes with the clinical benefit of angiotensin-converting enzyme (ACE) inhibitors (see Chap. 10) and with furosemide in patients with heart failure.[84]

Aspirin Resistance

Aspirin does not block thromboxane A_2 in some patients, making them resistant to the protective effects of the drug. Patients taking aspirin who had high levels of thromboxane in their urine were found to have a 3 to 5 times higher risk of cardiovascular death than patients who had lower levels. High levels of 11-dehydrothromboxane B_2 in urine can identify patients who are resistant to aspirin. Those patients may benefit from alternative antiplatelet therapies or treatments that more effectively block thromboxane production.

Conclusion

Aspirin is effective at reducing the morbidity and mortality associated with ischemic cardiac syndromes.[85] In particular, it is effective as primary prevention against myocardial infarction in asymptomatic patients and in those with both chronic stable and unstable angina. It also reduces the risk of reinfarction in the peri- and post-MI period. Aspirin decreases the incidence of acute thrombosis after percutaneous transluminal coronary angioplasty (PTCA) and stenting, as well as reducing the risk of bypass graft thrombosis after CABG surgery. These benefits must by weighed against the increased risk of bleeding associated with aspirin therapy.[85a] In those patients who are at a low risk for bleeding complications and who fall into one of the above categories, 325 mg of aspirin—either daily or every other day—is recommended. In patients with a higher likelihood of bleeding, these risks and benefits need to be taken into account and therapy individualized.

Dipyridamole

Dipyridamole is a pyramidopyrimidine compound that can act as both a vasodilator and an antithrombotic. The drug inhibits platelet action in vitro only at doses that are higher than those commonly used in patients, but it has been clinically effective in reducing platelet adherence to prosthetic surfaces in vivo at lower doses when combined with other agents.[86] A number of mechanisms for its antiplatelet activity have been proposed, including either the inhibition of phosphodiesterase[87] or the indirect activation of adenylate cyclase through its effects on prostacyclin and/or the inhibition of adenosine uptake by the vascular endothelium.[88,89] The exact mechanism of action still requires further definition, although the common pathway involves elevated levels of intraplatelet cyclic adenosine monophosphate, a platelet inhibitory substance. The usual dose of dipyridamole is 400 mg/d in three to four divided doses. It is also used as a provocative agent in patients undergoing diagnostic testing for coronary artery disease.

Clinical Studies

Its primary use in man has been as an adjunct to anticoagulant therapy in the prevention of thromboembolic events in patients with prosthetic heart valves.[90] Although current American College of Chest Physicians' guidelines do not include dipyridamole as a first-line therapy in a patient with prosthetic heart valves, it is a useful adjunct to anticoagulant therapy. It is recommended as part of the therapy in a patient with a prosthesis related thromboembolic event,[91] especially in those patients with peptic ulcer disease where aspirin may need to be avoided. Dipyridamole is not associated with an excess of hemorrhage when combined with anticoagulant therapy.[64,90] Dipyridamole has also been used as part of the therapy for patients with prosthetic grafts.[92] Both experimental and clinical evidence suggests a superiority of an aspirin/dipyridamole combination to either drug used alone in terms of both platelet survival and graft patency.[83–86]

A controlled trial comparing aspirin and dipyridamole alone and in combination against placebo for secondary prevention of ischemic stroke in 6602 patients found an 18% reduction for aspirin alone, a 16% reduction for dipyridamole alone, and a 37% reduction with combination therapy. Although there was no effect on the death rate, there was also a significant reduction in TIAs. Bleeding was significantly more common in patients receiving aspirin.[75] A combination aspirin-dipyridamole formulation is now available for stroke prevention.

Controlled trials comparing aspirin to dipyridamole in patients with stable angina are few. The limited data suggest no statistically significant difference between aspirin and dipyridamole used together as compared with aspirin alone. No trial has shown a definitive superiority of combination therapy over aspirin alone in either stable coronary disease,[15,39,45] graft survival after coronary artery bypass, or in the need for emergency revascularization after angioplasty.[93]

Adverse Effects

The primary side effects of dipyridamole are gastrointestinal and consist of nausea and vomiting.[14] In rare cases, angina has been provoked through what is believed to be a coronary steal phenomenon.[94]

Ticlopidine

Ticlopidine is a thienopyridine compound that acts by blocking ADP receptors within the platelet membrane, and acts independently of arachidonic acid pathways. Ticlopidine produces a thrombasthenia-like state,[95] with a resultant reduction in platelet aggregation, a prolongation of the bleeding time, a decrease in platelet granule release, and a reduction in platelet and fibrin deposition on artificial surfaces.

Cerebrovascular and Peripheral Vascular Disease

Ticlopidine has been tested thoroughly in the prevention of cerebrovascular disease. When compared with placebo in 1000 patients as part of a study in secondary prevention after stroke, the administration of ticlopidine resulted in a 30% reduction in the relative risk of stroke, myocardial infarction, or vascular death.[96] When compared with aspirin in the TASS study, ticlopidine was found to be superior in terms of all cause mortality as well as nonfatal stroke. This benefit persisted throughout the 5-year duration of the trial.[97]

In patients with peripheral vascular disease and claudication, treatment with ticlopidine was associated with a reduction in mortality, myocardial infarction, and cerebrovascular events.[98] Patients with cerebrovascular and peripheral vascular disease appear to benefit from ticlopidine therapy in terms of stroke, myocardial infarction, and vascular events.

Cardiovascular Disease

Ticlopidine has been used in the therapy of patients after coronary artery bypass grafting. In a randomized trial involving 173 patients, ticlopidine therapy resulted in a reduction in vein graft closure at 1 year as compared with placebo.[99] The graft closure rate, as assessed by digital angiography at day 10, day 180, and day 360 was decreased in the ticlopidine group as compared to the placebo group. When used in the therapy of patients with electrocardiographic evidence of unstable coronary syndromes, the addition of ticlopidine to standard therapy was associated with a reduction in vascular death and nonfatal myocardial infarction, as well as the composite end-point of both fatal and nonfatal myocardial infarction.[100] In those patients who undergo coronary stent implantation, ticlopidine and aspirin have demonstrated a superiority over anticoagulant therapy with heparin and phenprocoumon.[101,102] In patients undergoing stenting, ticlopidine should be administered at a 500-mg loading dose and then given 250 mg twice daily for 10 to 14 days.

In patients with acute MI, the drug appears to be similar to aspirin as regards subsequent mortality, recurrent acute myocardial infarction (AMI), stroke, and angina.[103,104] The drug in combination with aspirin reduces the plasma levels of procoagulant tissue factor in patients with unstable angina.[105]

Adverse Events

Neutropenia can occur in up to 4% of patients receiving ticlopidine. It is generally reversible, although cases of agranulocytosis have been reported. It is recommended that during the first 2 months of therapy white blood cell counts should be checked. The most common side effects of the medication are gastrointestinal, occurring in about 12% of patients, and include nausea, vomiting, diarrhea, and dyspepsia. A rash has been reported within the first 3 months of ticlopidine treatment. Ticlopidine is associated with a risk of thrombotic thrombocytopenic purpura estimated at 0.02%.[106] Although this complication has also been reported with clopidogrel,[107] ticlopidine has been supplanted by clopidogrel because of an overall better safety profile.[107a]

Clopidogrel

Clopidogrel is a thienopyridine antiplatelet drug in the same class as ticlopidine. Similar to ticlopidine, clopidogrel is a prodrug that is not active in vitro but is active in vivo.[108,108a] It functions as an ADP-selective agent whose antiaggregating properties are several times higher than those of ticlopidine and are apparently due to the same mechanism of action (i.e., inhibition of ADP binding to its platelet receptor and triggering the release of thrombogenic factor-containing alpha granules).[108] In various experimental animal models, a single oral or intravenous administration of clopidogrel inhibited ADP-induced platelet aggregation for several days and potently reduced thrombus formation.[108]

Clinical Trials

Clopidogrel has been evaluated in a large phase III clinical trial (CAPRIE, Clopidogrel vs Aspirin in Patients at Risk of Ischemic Events), a randomized, blinded, clinical study comparing clopidogrel 75 mg/d with aspirin 325 mg/d in 19,000 patients who had suffered a recent ischemic stroke or MI, or who had symptomatic atherosclerotic peripheral vascular disease.[74] The study showed a more favorable effect on clinical outcomes with clopidogrel as compared to aspirin[74] and based on this study, clopidogrel was approved by the FDA. Clopidogrel is also of benefit when started with aspirin at the time patients present with acute coronary syndrome,[109–111] and may be a useful alternative in patients having aspirin resistance.

In addition to aspirin and glycoprotein IIb/IIIa integrin receptor blockers, clopidogrel has become an important drug for use in patients undergoing angioplasty and stenting to reduce thrombotic complications.[111a] In patients undergoing stenting, it should be given as a 300-mg oral loading dose followed by a maintenance dose of 75 mg twice daily for 14 to 30 days.[112,113] The drug is also as effective as aspirin and ticlopidine as an antiplatelet agent after MI, and can be combined with aspirin to achieve a greater antiplatelet effect.[109,114] In patients who had had prior cardiac surgery, clopidogrel was shown to be better than aspirin in reducing events with less bleeding.[115]

THE GP IIb/IIIa INTEGRIN GLYCOPROTEIN RECEPTOR ANTAGONISTS

Platelet aggregation is mediated by the GP IIb/IIIa receptor, a member of the integrin superfamily of membrane-bound adhesion molecules. Integrins are defined as subunit receptors composed of an α subunit (i.e., GP IIb) and a β subunit (i.e., GP IIIa) capable of mediating adhesive interactions between cells or matrix. Although integrins are distributed widely throughout the vasculature (see Chap. 39), where they are expressed on endothelial, smooth-muscle cells, and leukocytes, expression of the GP IIb/IIIa integrin is restricted to platelets.[116] It is the chief receptor responsible for platelet aggregation by its ability to bind soluble fibrinogen, forming bridges between platelets and leading, ultimately, to thrombus formation. GP IIb/IIIa is widely distributed on platelet surfaces (approximately 50,000 per cell) but remains unable to bind fibrinogen unless the platelet is first stimulated by agonists (such as ADP, thrombin, arachidonic acid, etc), and undergoes a conformational

change. It is believed that the adhesive binding pocket is somehow hidden until platelet activation, although this process is still unclear. Although fibrinogen is the peptide that mediates aggregation, mostly because of the large concentration of fibrinogen in plasma, GP IIb/IIIa is also capable of binding von Willebrand factor, fibronectin, and vitronectin.[2] It has been demonstrated that aggregation can be supported by von Willebrand factor in the absence of fibrinogen. Therefore, these molecules may also play a role in aggregation at high shear rates, such as is found in the coronary arteries.[117]

GP IIb/IIIa, a heterodimer of two subunits, was the first integrin to be identified and has served as a model for characterization of other integrins. It has been demonstrated by electron microscopy that the receptor is composed of a globular head and two flexible tails that are imbedded in the platelet membrane. The GP IIb subunit has calcium-binding sites that have homology with calmodulin.[116] In the presence of the calcium chelating agent ethylenediamine tetraacetic acid, the receptor function is lost and the integrin dissociates into its two individual subunits. Each subunit contains a portion of the head and a single tail (Fig. 18-4).

The GP IIb/IIIa domains responsible for binding adhesive proteins have been identified and in general are characterized by their ability to recognize the peptide sequence RGD. The RGD recognition sequence was originally described for fibronectin, but is now known to be present in fibrinogen, von Willebrand factor, vitronectin, and thrombospondin.[118] Fibrinogen is a symmetrical protein composed of two α chains, two β chains, and two γ chains. Both of its RGD sequences are located on the α chain at residues 95 to 97 and 572 to 574. Fibrinogen also contains a 12-amino acid residue that possesses the ability to bind to the GP IIb/IIIa receptor. This dodecapeptide (HHLGGAKQAGDV) is located at residues 400 to 411 on the fibrinogen gamma chain. It has been proposed that the RGD residues and the dodecapeptide competitively bind to GP IIb/IIIa. By initiating a conformational change in the receptor after binding, one recognition sequence on fibrinogen renders the other sequence inaccessible for binding.[116] This alteration in receptor shape may be a self-regulatory mechanism of the GP IIb/IIIa receptor.

If two activated platelets with functional GP IIb/IIIa receptors each bind to the same fibrinogen molecule, a fibrinogen bridge is

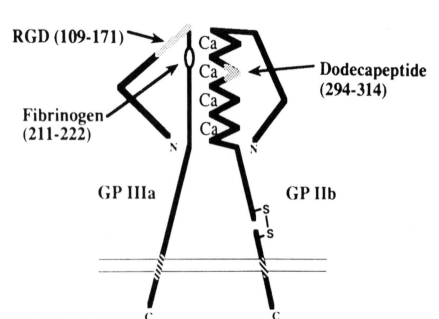

FIGURE 18-4. Structure of GP IIb/IIIa complex. Transmembrane domains are near carboxyl termini of GP IIb and GP IIIa. RGD peptides have been crosslinked to domain within amino acids 109 to 171 of GP IIIa, whereas dodecapeptide from the γ chain of fibrinogen crosslinks to domain within residues 294 to 314 of GP IIb. Third region in GP IIIa involved in fibrinogen binding corresponds to residues 211 to 222. (*Adapted from Charo et al. In: Colman RW et al. Hemostasis and Thrombosis: Basic principles and clinical practice. 3d ed. Philadelphia: JB Lippincott, 1994:489–507.*)

created between the two platelets (Fig. 18-5). When this process of aggregation is repeated thousands of times, a thrombus will form. Experiments indicate that the RGD peptides bind to the GP IIIa subunit at residues 109 to 171.[119] In contrast, the dodecapeptide binds to the GP IIb subunit at residues 294 to 314. Genetic defects in either of these two subunits can lead to the rare hemostatic disorder of Glanzmann's thrombasthenia. Patients with Glanzmann's thrombasthenia usually have a bleeding disorder during childhood. Although they have a normal platelet count, the GP IIb/IIIa receptor is either nonfunctional or absent. Platelet aggregation, in response to agonists such as thrombin, ADP, or arachidonic acid is, therefore, completely absent.[2]

GP IIb/IIIa Antagonists as Antiplatelet Agents

As discussed earlier in this chapter, aspirin is the most common antiplatelet drug in use today. However, it is a relatively weak drug, effective against only one of the many platelet activators, thromboxane A_2. Other drugs similar to clopidogrel, ticlopidine and hirudin, which are effective against ADP and thrombin, respectively, also are limited in their activity because of the platelet's ability to be activated by multiple agonists. Many patients with vascular disease take the current antiplatelet drugs and still sustain thromboembolic complications that often develop into ischemic conditions. Of importance, therefore, is the development of more effective antiplatelet agents. A drug able to inhibit platelet activation in response to all endogenous agonists would constitute a more effective therapy.

The binding of fibrinogen to activated platelets is the final step in platelet aggregation, and this binding is completely mediated by GP IIb/IIIa. Therefore, expression of the GP IIb/IIIa integrin is the final common pathway for platelet aggregation by *all* agonists. GP IIb/IIIa also is unique to platelets, and is the most abundant platelet surface glycoprotein. These factors make GP IIb/IIIa an extremely favorable target for therapeutic pharmacologic blockade.[118,120] A drug that could block the binding of fibrinogen to GP IIb/IIIa could theoretically abolish thrombosis resulting from vessel damage or atherosclerotic plaque rupture, regardless of the platelets degree of activation. Discussed below are three classes of GP IIb/IIIa antagonists: disintegrins, (naturally occurring GP IIb/IIIa blocking agents), monoclonal antibodies to the GP IIb/IIIa receptor, and synthetic peptide- and nonpeptide-receptor antagonists capable of blocking fibrinogen binding to platelets.

Natural GP IIb/IIIa Antagonists: Disintegrins

Several natural peptides derived from snake venoms have demonstrated the ability to block the GP IIb/IIIa receptor and prevent aggregation. Not surprisingly, these peptides, termed *disintegrins,* contain the same RGD sequence found in the endogenous adhesive proteins fibrinogen and von Willebrand factor. This tripeptide sequence enables the disintegrins to have a high affinity and specificity for all integrins, including GP IIb/IIIa.[121] The disintegrin family includes trigramin from the snake *Trimeresurus graminues,* bitistatin from *Bitis arietans,* and kistrin from the pit viper *Agkistrodon rhodostoma.* All of these peptides are 54 to 73 amino acids in length, and many exist in a cyclic conformation because of multiple disulfide bonds.[122]

Bitistatin and kistrin have demonstrated the ability to inhibit platelet aggregation and subsequent thrombosis in canine models when administered in conjunction with heparin.[123] Because the

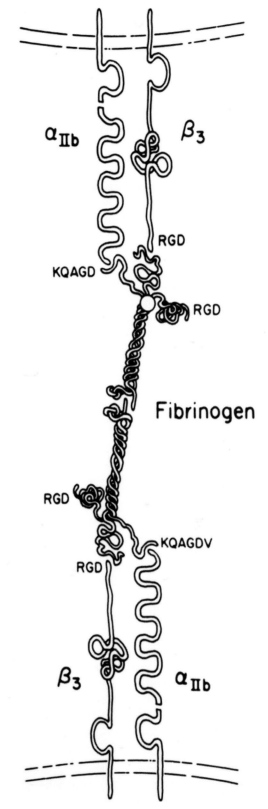

FIGURE 18-5. GP IIb/IIIa structure and interactions binding platelets by divalent fibrinogen. (*Reproduced with permission from Harker et al: In: Colman RW et al. Hemostasis and thrombosis: Basic principles and clinical practice. 3d ed. Philadelphia: JB Lippincott, 1994:1638–1660.*)

disintegrins have a short half-life, the antiplatelet effects are potentially reversible. Reversibility is important because of the risk of substantial, uncontrollable bleeding from tissue wounds (i.e., intravenous puncture sites).

A problem with most disintegrins is that they are not specific for GP IIb/IIIa, but are able to bind all RGD-dependent integrin receptors. This lack of specificity poses the potential for multiple negative side effects, including the blockade of adhesive proteins to endothelial cells and leukocytes. However, one disintegrin peptide has been identified that can uniquely bind to the GP IIb/IIIa receptor on the platelet membrane. Isolated from the pygmy rattlesnake *Sistrurus M. barbouri,* the disintegrin barbourin will not react with closely related integrins. This specificity appears to result from the substitution of a lysine (K) instead of the normal arginine (R) in the RGD sequence.[124] The KGD sequence of barbourin has become the model for new, cyclic, synthetic antiplatelet peptides (discussed later).

Although disintegrins have several properties that would be of benefit in a GP IIb/IIIa antagonist, such as high specificity (i.e., with KGD) and reversibility, their use also poses problems. They tend to induce transient thrombocytopenia (abnormal decrease in blood platelets), and are highly antigenic, capable of generating an immune response. These serious adverse effects have severely limited the potential use of disintegrins as therapeutic agents.

Murine Monoclonal Antibodies (7E3)

In 1983, Coller produced a mouse monoclonal antibody against the GP IIb/IIIa integrin receptor.[125] Coller later developed an additional antibody called 7E3 which more rapidly bound to ADP activated platelets.[126] This antibody was subsequently used to make a human/mouse chimeric 7E3 Fab,[127] now known as abciximab.[128]

Monoclonal antibodies, first produced in the 1970s by Kohler and Milstein, are populations of identical immunoglobulins derived from a single plasma cell that have been fused with an "immortal" malignant cell line. These hybridomas have the capacity to produce millions of identical antibodies with an absolute specificity for a single protein epitope.[129] The Coller antibody 7E3, in its chimeric form, exhibits both a high-affinity and absolute specificity for the GP IIb/IIIa receptor, two properties that made abciximab an attractive therapeutic agent for the blocking of adhesive proteins.[130]

Abciximab is a highly effective antithrombotic agent, specifically in preventing arterial thrombi, in both canines and primates, including human beings. To eliminate the binding of fibrinogen to activated platelets, large doses of abciximab must be given to block GP IIb/IIIa receptor function effectively on all circulating platelets. However, by blocking all GP IIb/IIIa receptors and, consequently, inhibiting platelet aggregation, the risk of concurrent hemorrhage is increased. This bleeding risk is increased when combining antiplatelet therapy with invasive treatments such as coronary angioplasty or bypass surgery.

Studies in baboons demonstrate that monoclonal antibodies have the potential to prevent platelet thrombi from forming on synthetic fiber grafts in an arteriovenous fistula.[131] The positive results of these primate studies highlight the potential for monoclonal antibody use in antithrombotic therapy in human beings. 7E3 has been tested in the treatment of patients with unstable angina and to prevent restenosis after coronary balloon angioplasty. Gold et al[132] showed that 7E3 has the ability to block approximately 87% of GP IIb/IIIa receptors on platelets in human beings. In their study, a single injection of 7E3, 0.05 to 0.2 mg/kg, led to the absence of anginal symptoms (chest pain) for ≥12 h in all patients tested, and in most cases (10 of 16 patients), freedom from pain for 72 h. As expected, a large dose (0.2 mg/kg) of 7E3 prolonged the bleeding time from 6.3 min to >30 min.

In patients with IHD who received 7E3 as a bolus injection, the effect on ADP-induced platelet aggregation and bleeding time is dose dependent, with the maximal effect achieved at a dose of 0.25 mg/kg.[133] A delayed and variable decrease in platelet fibrinogen levels is also observed.[134] After an intravenous bolus dose of 0.25 mg/kg, blockade of GP IIb/IIIa receptors and inhibition of platelet function were maintained in patients receiving a maintenance infusion of 10 μg/min, but not in those receiving 5 μg/min.[133] Approximately 40 to 50% of GP IIb/IIIa receptor blockade is required for inhibition of platelet aggregation.[135] Fluorescence flow cytometry studies reveal that platelets are uniformly coated with the drug within 30 min of infusion. Surface-bound antibody is still present on platelets 14 days after its administration, suggesting that antibody may be transferred to new platelets (platelet life span of approximately 10 days) or to megakaryocytes. Within 4 to 6 days of completion of a 24- to 72-h intravenous infusion of the antibody, platelet-bound antibody concentrations are reduced by 50% and platelet function recovers over a 48-h period.[133,136] After administration of an intravenous bolus, the antibody is cleared rapidly from the plasma, with an initial half-life of <10 min and second phase half-life of about 30 min. Less than 5% of the antibody can still be found in the plasma after 2 h. Free concentrations in plasma remain relatively constant during continuous infusion of antibody at a rate of 10 μg/min for 96 h, with concentrations in plasma levels decreasing rapidly the first 6 h after treatment, and more slowly after that.[130] It is likely that the antibody is metabolized in a manner comparable to that of other natural proteins.[130]

In an early randomized, placebo-controlled study of 60 patients with unstable angina, the addition of 7E3 to standard medical therapy (heparin and aspirin) appeared to be safe and effective in reducing major cardiovascular events during the hospital stay.[137] The antibody was administered as a 0.25 mg/kg bolus followed by a 10 μg/min infusion for 18 to 24 h until 1 h after completion of a second angiography and percutaneous transluminal coronary angioplasty (Table 18-1).

It has been shown, experimentally, that approximately 70% of platelet deposition at the site of balloon injury is GP IIb/IIIa-dependent, and the remaining 30% results from non-GP IIb/IIIa-mediated platelet subendothelial adhesion.[138] In human beings, it appears that 7E3 can result in blockade of >80% of receptors and can reduce platelet aggregation to <20%.[139] The drug also can suppress the levels of circulating inflammatory markers after angioplasty.

The results of a larger study demonstrated the effectiveness of 7E3 in the prevention of postangioplasty restenosis. The Evaluation of 7E3 for the Prevention of Ischemic Complications (EPIC) study highlighted the importance of the GP IIb/IIIa receptor in abrupt vessel closure after high-risk coronary angioplasty and atherectomy.[140,141] A random population (2099 patients) scheduled to undergo these procedures, received either a bolus and infusion of placebo, a bolus of 0.25 mg/kg 7E3 and a 12-h infusion of placebo, or a bolus and infusion of 7E3.[140] Results were measured as the risk of experiencing a composite primary end-point (which included death, nonfatal MI or unplanned invasive revascularization procedures) by 30 days. Data indicated that, as compared with those patients given placebo, patients who received administration of the bolus and infusion of 7E3 had a 35% risk reduction in the composite-event rate.

TABLE 18-1. Randomized Double-Blind, Placebo-Controlled Trials of 7E3 Fab Evaluating Reduction of Ischemic Complications in Patients at High Risk Undergoing PTCA

| Trial | No. of Patients | Dosage Regimen | Results (% of patients) | | | | | |
			Death	Nonfatal MI	Urgent PTCA	Urgent PTCA	Ischemic Complications*	Overall
EPIC[140][†]	708	7E3 Fab 0.25 mg/kg IV bolus ≥10 min before PTCA; then 10 μg/min IV × 12 h	1.7	5.2	0.8	2.4	8.3	7E3 Fab > placebo
	695	7E3 Fab 0.25 mg/kg IV bolus ≥10 min before PTCA; then placebo	1.3	6.3	3.6	2.3	11.4	
	696	Placebo	1.7	8.6[#]	4.5[§]	3.6	12.8[#]	
Simoons et al[137][‡]	30	7E3 Fab 0.25 mg/kg IV bolus; then 10 μg/min IV × 18–24 h[¶]	0	3.3	0	0	3.3	7E3 Fab > Placebo
	30	Placebo	3.3	13.3	6.78	10.0	23.3[#]	

EPIC = Evaluation of 7E3 for the Prevention of Ischemic Complications; IV = intravenous; PTCA = percutaneous transluminal coronary angioplasty or directional atherectomy; > = 7E3 Fab significantly superior to placebo in preventing ischemic complications.

*Composite primary study end-point, comprising death, nonfatal MI, and recurrent ischemia requiring urgent intervention.

[†]Events occurring ≤30 days of randomization.

[#]$p \leq 0.03$ compared with 7E3 Fab recipients.

[§]$p < 0.001$ compared with 7E3 Fab recipients.

[‡]Events before hospital discharge.

[¶]Until 1 h after PTCA completion.

Source: Adapted from Faulds D, Sorkins EM: Abciximab (c7E3Fab). *Drugs* 48:590, 1994.

Patients who received only a 0.25 mg/kg bolus of 7E3 (and placebo infusion) still showed a 10% reduction in the risk of experiencing a primary end-point (Table 18-1, Fig. 18-6). On the basis of the results of the EPIC trial and other pharmacologic studies, the 7E3 antibody, abciximab, was approved for use in patients undergoing high-risk angioplasty. The drug is now also approved for unstable angina. The FDA-approved dose is 0.25 mg/kg bolus and 10 μg/min infusion for 18 to 24 h before percutaneous coronary intervention (PCI) and continued for 1 h after PCI. This may not be the optimal dose and a 12 h infusion after PCI is recommended.[142]

In addition, during a 6-month follow-up period, the number of ischemic events was reduced by 26% in patients who received the 7E3 antibody, suggesting a long-term benefit against clinical coronary artery stenosis.[141] Table 18-2 summarizes additional studies with the drug.

Although these results demonstrate the importance of pharmacologic blockade of GP IIb/IIIa as therapy for ischemic events, the use of abciximab results in several negative complications. In 14% of the patients in the EPIC trial who received both the 7E3 bolus and infusion, a significant amount of bleeding, twice the number of major bleeding episodes in the placebo group, occurred and often required transfusion. The bleeding usually occurred at the site of vascular puncture in the groin. The increased bleeding time is compounded because the antibodies are inherently long-lived and do not dissociate from platelets during the platelets' survival time in the plasma. Thus, the inhibitory effect on systemic platelet aggregation is nonreversible and may last several days. This situation may prove to be deleterious for patients with unstable conditions that may require unplanned invasive procedures. Thrombocytopenia and pseudothrombocytopenia have been described with the use

FIGURE 18-6. Probability of no urgent repeated percutaneous revascularization procedures in three treatment groups (Kaplan-Meier plots). Events began to occur shortly after index procedure in placebo group, between 6 and 12 h after procedure in group given bolus of c7E3 Fab, and even later in group given bolus and infusion; *y* axis is truncated at 97% to demonstrate differences in this end-point, which occurred with low frequency. (*Reprinted with permission of EPIC Investigators.*[140])

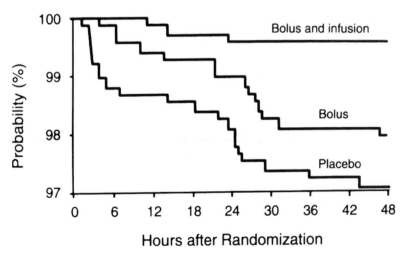

TABLE 18-2. Additional Studies with 7E3 Fab (Abciximab)

Indication	Phase	No. of Patients	Results and Comments
Angioplasty[146]	3	1500	EPILOG; improved clinical outcomes with 7E3 Fab; primary end results.
Unstable angina[146]	3	1050	CAPTURE; improved clinical outcomes with 7E3 Fab.
Angioplasty	2	103	PROLOG; completed; heparin and ReoPro dose-ranging study showing additional safety with weight-adjusted heparin
Unstable angina[137]	2	60	Safe; no excessive bleeding; lower incidence of ischemic events vs heparin.

EPILOG = Evaluation in PTCA to Improve Long-Term Outcome with ReoPro GP IIb/IIIa Blockade; CAPTURE = Chimeric Anti-Platelet Antibody Therapy in Unstable Angina Refractory to Standard Treatment; PROLOG = pilot study for EPILOG.

of abciximab[143] and altered leukocyte adhesion has been observed when it is combined with ticlopidine.[144] Last, the use of large doses of monoclonal antibodies could stimulate the proliferation of neutralizing antibodies and, therefore, may restrict 7E3 therapy to a single use. Despite these complications, the positive results obtained by monoclonal antibody blockade of GP IIb/IIIa receptors have furthered the development of high-affinity, synthetic, peptide antagonists.

The EPILOG trial (Evaluation of PTCA to Improve Long term Outcomes by 7E3 GPIIb/IIIa Receptor Blockade Trial) evaluated the use of both high- and low-risk PTCA with 7E3.[145] The original study design called for the enrollment of 4800 patients (Table 18-2) who were to be randomized to either placebo/high-dose heparin (ACT >300), 7E3/high-dose heparin, or to 7E3/low-dose heparin. The trial was double blind and placebo controlled with an interim analysis to be done after 1500 patients. After the interim analysis, the study was terminated prematurely for the following reasons. In those patients treated with 7E3, a three-time decrease in CPK levels was noted, as well as a 68% reduction in the combined end-point of MI and death. Additionally, in contrast to the results from the EPIC trial, bleeding complications in the 7E3/low-dose heparin group were not significantly different than with placebo (<2% with treatment, 3.1% placebo). These reductions in the rate of bleeding complications may have been due to the use of early sheath removal in the EPILOG trial.

Finally, the use of abciximab (7E3) in patients who developed unstable angina with ECG changes before scheduled PTCA was evaluated in the CAPTURE trial (Chimeric c7E3 Antiplatelet Therapy in Unstable Angina Refractory to Standard Therapy).[146] In this trial, patients who were scheduled for PTCA the following day and who developed unstable angina/ECG changes the night before were randomized to standard therapy with or without 7E3. The medication was continued into the PTCA the next day. Although 1200 patients were to be enrolled, the trial was stopped prematurely after only 1050 patients because of strongly favorable results in those treated with abciximab.[145,146] Specifically, the primary end-points of MI—death and recurrent PTCA—were reduced from 16.4 to 10.8% in the treatment group. Additionally, the incidence of MI was reduced from 9.4 to 4.9% and the secondary end-points of emergent CABG/repeat PTCA/emergent stent placement were all significantly reduced in those patients who received abciximab. No increased risk of intracranial bleeding was noted, although the incidence of major bleeding was increased from 1.7 to 2.8%.

When abciximab was used as an adjunct to standard therapy for unstable angina, there was no additional benefit on outcomes in patients not undergoing invasive procedures.[147] Patients receiving abciximab plus stenting, however, have better outcomes than with thrombolysis in MI patients.[148] Abciximab has also been combined with thrombolytic agents in acute MI[149] with no additional benefit observed when compared to thrombolytics used alone.[150] The drug has been used as an alternative to thrombolysis when lytic therapy is unsuccessful.[151]

A recent placebo-controlled trial showed that the early administration of abciximab in patients with acute myocardial infarction improves coronary patency before stenting, the success rate of the stenting procedure, the rate of coronary patency at 6 months, left ventricular function, and clinical outcomes.[152]

It is now well accepted that abciximab improves outcome when used in conjunction with PCI in high-risk patients with acute coronary syndromes, and that the early use of IIb/IIIa inhibitors before percutaneous coronary revascularization may qualify the discrepancies in earlier trials.[153,154]

Synthetic Peptide and Nonpeptide Antagonists

As an alternative to monoclonal antibodies, researchers have attempted to develop small synthetic peptides with the ability to block fibrinogen from binding to the GP IIb/IIIa platelet receptor.[155] The goal of this effort has been to create a peptide with the same affinity and specificity exhibited by monoclonal antibodies, but without the negative side effects of prolonged bleeding time, immunogenicity, and irreversibility. In many cases, the synthetic peptides were modeled on the "disintegrin" or natural antiplatelet antagonists, but were smaller and therefore less immunogenic. By using the RGD binding sequence found in circulating adhesive proteins, researchers have developed a series of modified RGD analogues capable of binding to GP IIb/IIIa. One modification includes the addition of disulfide bonds for the creation of cyclic peptides. The cyclic conformation has not only rendered the peptides more stable in plasma, but also has imparted a higher affinity for the integrin receptor.[156] Another modification has been to substitute lysine (K) in the RGD sequence for arginine (R). This substitution creates a peptide similar to the disintegrin barbourin (discussed earlier in this chapter), which has absolute specificity for GP IIb/IIIa integrin.

The cyclic heptapeptide eptifibatide (Integrelin) is now approved for use in acute coronary syndromes[157] on the basis of the PURSUIT trial.[158] The recommended dose for acute coronary syndromes is 180 µg/kg bolus followed by an infusion of 2.0 µg/kg/min for 72 to 96 h. The approved dose for PCI on the basis of the IMPACT-II trial[159] is a bolus of 135 µg/kg followed by an infusion of 0.5 µg/kg/min for 20 to 24 h. However, a dose based on the

ESPRIT trial[160,161] is now recommended, which is two 180 μg/kg boluses 10 min apart, and a 2.0 μg/kg/min infusion for 18 to 24 h.

The nonpeptide tirofiban (Aggrastat) is approved for use in acute coronary syndromes at a dose of 0.4 μg/kg/min for 30 min and then 0.1 μg/kg/min for 48 to 108 h.[162,163] When tirofiban was used in patients with coronary syndromes undergoing invasive therapy, a more favorable outcome was observed compared with conservative therapy.[164]

A comparison trial of two platelet glycoprotein IIb/IIIa inhibitors, tirofiban and abciximab, for the prevention of ischemic events with percutaneous coronary revascularization demonstrated that tirofiban offered less protection from major ischemic events than did abciximab.[165]

Although the peptide antagonists to the GP IIb/IIIa integrin appear to compensate for the shortcomings of the monoclonal antibodies (i.e., decreased bleeding time, reversibility and nonimmunogenicity), they have one major limitation: none is orally bioavailable in human beings. Currently, all antagonists, peptide or monoclonal antibody, must be administered intravenously. Therefore, their therapeutic use is limited to acute thrombotic situations, such as maintenance of coronary flow after angioplasty or thrombolysis (with tissue plasminogen activator or streptokinase). To be effective as preventative therapy (i.e., for unstable angina and MI), an orally active form must be available. This drug must maintain low concentrations in plasma to prevent spontaneous hemorrhage, but should also maximally inhibit platelet aggregation. A prototype, orally active glycoprotein IIb/IIIa receptor nonpeptide inhibitor has been developed, SC-54684A (xemilofiban), and has undergone Phase I and II testing in patients, including in patients who had previously received abciximab.[166] Xemilofiban is an ester prodrug that is converted to an active moiety (SC-54701A). However, in the EXCITE trial, when xemilofiban was used in patients undergoing PCI, there was increased bleeding and no reduction in ischemic events.[167]

Orbofiban is an oral glycoprotein IIb/IIIa inhibitor that was studied in 10,288 patients with acute coronary syndromes. Despite a benefit that was observed among patients who underwent percutaneous coronary intervention, the trial was terminated prematurely because of an unexpected increase in 30-day mortality in the orbofiban treated group.[168]

Sibrafiban, another oral agent, showed no additional benefit over aspirin for secondary prevention of major ischemic events after an acute coronary syndrome, and was associated with more dose-related bleeding.[169] A second sibrafiban study that combined aspirin with low-dose sibrafiban did not show improved outcomes after acute coronary syndromes and caused more bleeding as compared with aspirin alone. There was a trend toward increased mortality in this group and a significant increase in a high-dose arm.[170]

A lotrafiban trial was also stopped because of increased mortality.[171]

In a meta-analysis of oral glycoprotein IIb/IIIa inhibitor trials,[172] the authors found a highly significant excess in mortality that was consistent across four trials with three different oral glycoprotein IIb/IIIa inhibitor agents, and that was associated with a reduction in the need for urgent revascularization and no increase in myocardial infarction. The authors believed that these findings suggest the possibility for a direct toxic effect with these agents that is related to a prothrombotic mechanism.

The several hypotheses put forward to explain the increased mortality associated with the use of oral glycoprotein IIb/IIIa inhibitors[125] include: (a) induction of a binding configuration of the glycoprotein IIb/IIIa receptor by drug cycling on and off;

(b) activation of myocyte caspase causing apoptosis; (c) increased plaque hemorrhage; and (d) a proinflammatory effect.

Conclusion

Antiplatelet therapy is an effective treatment for patients with coronary and cerebral vascular diseases. Aspirin is effective in reducing mortality risk in survivors of acute MI, and aspirin, ticlopidine, and clopidogrel are useful in preventing strokes in persons at high-risk. The development of monoclonal antibodies and intravenous peptide and nonpeptide compounds that bind to the GP IIb/IIIa receptor in activated platelets show great potential for treating patients undergoing coronary angioplasty to prevent short- and long-term complications and for treating patients with unstable angina and myocardial infarction. The clinical development of oral glycoprotein IIb/IIIa inhibitor agents suitable for long-term use has been disappointing and is an area for future research.

OTHER ANTICOAGULANTS AND DIRECT ANTITHROMBINS

In this section, the anticoagulant drugs heparin, heparin derivatives, and warfarin are reviewed, along with a discussion of the new direct thrombin inhibitors hirudin, hirulog, argatroban, melagatran, and ximelagatran.

Heparin

Mechanisms of Action

Heparin, a glycosaminoglycan, is composed of alternating residues of D-glucosamine and iduronic acid. Its principal anticoagulant effect depends upon a critical pentasaccharide with high-affinity binding to antithrombin III (ATIII).[173] When bound to the critical pentasaccharide, ATIII changes its configuration so that it can directly inhibit activated factor X (Xa). If the polysaccharide chain is long enough (>18 saccharides), the heparin/ATIII complex can also bind thrombin and inactivate its active site. Heparin catalyzes the inactivation of thrombin by ATIII (Fig. 18-7) by providing a template to which both thrombin (factor IIa) and the naturally occurring serine protease inhibitor, ATIII can bind.[174] Additionally, heparin catalyzes thrombin inactivation via a specific pathway involving heparin cofactor II, a mechanism requiring higher heparin doses but not involving the ATIII-binding pentasaccharide.[175] In contradistinction to direct thrombin inhibitors that impede thrombin activity, heparin indirectly inhibits both thrombin activity and thrombin generation; the heparin-ATIII complex also inhibits other anticoagulation proteases, including factors IXa, Xa, XIa, XIIa.[176]

The molecular weight of heparin ranges from 5000 to 30,000, with a mean value of 15,000, and containing an average of approximately 50 saccharide chains. Heparin's pharmacokinetic properties in anticoagulant activity are heterogenous for two reasons: First, its plasma clearance is influenced by molecular size with larger-sized molecules being cleared more rapidly than smaller-sized molecules, resulting in an increased antifactor Xa to antifactor IIa (thrombin) activity ratio. Second, the anticoagulant activity of heparin is also influenced by molecular chain length; only about one-third of standard unfractionated heparin molecules in clinical usage are sufficiently long (containing >18 saccharides) to possess the ability to inhibit thrombin via ATIII-mediated anticoagulant action.[175]

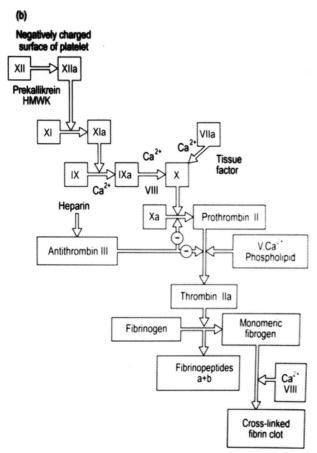

FIGURE 18-7. Antithrombin III inactivates factors Xa and thrombin (IIa). This effect is enhanced by heparin.

Pharmacokinetics

Because it is not absorbed orally, heparin is given either subcutaneously or intravenously. When given in sufficient doses, the safety and efficacy of both routes are comparable for treating venous thrombosis[175,177] if the reduced bioavailability of subcutaneous heparin is taken into account.[178] At clinically therapeutic doses, a substantial proportion of heparin is cleared via the dose-dependent rapid pathway. Hence, the anticoagulant response to heparin is not linear but increases disproportionately both in intensity and duration with larger heparin doses. The apparently biologic half-life of heparin increases from 30 min to 60 min to 150 min after bolus intravenous doses of 25, 100, and 400 U/kg, respectively.[175]

Pharmacodynamics

The intensity of heparin anticoagulant effect is monitored by the activated partial thromboplastin time (aPTT) test, which is sensitive to both antithrombin (antifactor IIa) and antifactor IXa and Xa effects. Experimental data have suggested than an aPTT of 1.5 times control could prevent venous thrombus extension. When heparin is used clinically, however, consideration must be given to (a) interpatient variability in plasma and tissue binding that alters heparin pharmacokinetics; (b) potential increases in factor VIII (occurring as part of an acute phase reaction in seriously ill patients) that can blunt the aPTT response to a given heparin level; and (c) the variable potency of commercially employed aPTT reagents. It has been recommended that the therapeutic range for each aPTT

reagent be calibrated to be the equivalent to a heparin level of 0.2 to 0.4 U/mL by protamine titration or to an antifactor Xa level of about 0.3 to 0.7 U/mL.[175]

Clinical Use: Venous Thrombosis

Randomized clinical trials have established the efficacy of heparin usage in venous thrombosis.[179] Heparin may be given in an initial intravenous bolus of 5000 U, or a weight-adjusted bolus, followed by at least 30,000 U/24 h by continuous infusion with additional heparin dose adjustments to maintain a therapeutic aPTT range.[175] Heparin's effectiveness is dependent on using an adequate starting dose and maintenance infusion that produce an adequate anticoagulant effect, measured either by aPTT or by heparin levels, provided that the heparin level is >0.3 U/mL antifactor Xa activity.[175,179]

Orthopedic and General Surgery

Heparin has been recommended for routine usage in the prevention of venous thromboembolism, especially in surgical patients undergoing elective hip or knee repair or replacement who are at high risk for perioperative venous thrombosis and pulmonary embolism.[180] The prevalence of venous thromboembolism following total knee or hip replacement surgery has been summarized as between 45% and 84%, and that following hip fracture surgery as being between 36% and 60%, with a corresponding pulmonary embolism rate of 2 to 30% and 4 to 24%, respectively.[180] A meta-analysis comparing the efficacy of LMWH to low-dose unfractionated heparin (LDUH) indicated that LMWH was more effective in suppressing venous thromboembolism.[181]

Elective neurosurgery and acute spinal cord-injury patients also have a high risk for venous thromboembolism, averaging 24%.[180] Although there has been concern regarding intracranial or intraspinal bleeding, a recent study has demonstrated the efficacy and safety of both LDUH and LMWH prophylaxis.[182]

Acute Myocardial Infarction and Unstable Angina

Heparin has been used in acute MI patients to prevent venous thromboembolism, mural thrombosis,[48,183] and systemic embolism. Amongst acute MI patients not treated with antithrombotic agents, the incidence of deep-vein thrombosis (DVT) is about 24%.[180] Subcutaneous LDUH in doses of 5000 to 7500 U twice daily and high-dose intravenous heparin 40,000 U/d reduce DVT without adverse bleeding events.[180] In the contemporary acute MI patient, heparin anticoagulation, coupled with aspirin and other antiplatelet therapy, has become a mainstay of treatment. However, no benefit was seen on early coronary patency in MI patients receiving heparin before primary angioplasty.[184] In acute coronary syndromes, it has been used to reduce the frequency of unstable angina. It has also become a standard adjunct to thrombolytic drugs despite definitive proof of its efficacy,[185] where it is used concurrently with either tissue plasminogen activator (t-PA), tenecteplase (TNK-tPA), reteplase, or anisoylated plasminogen streptokinase activator complex (APSAC), or subsequent to streptokinase, thereby, minimizing thrombolytic drug activation of the coagulation system during fibrinolysis.[186] The increased plasmin generated during fibrinolytic drug therapy mediates both platelet activation and plasmin mediated-prothrombinase activity,[187] requiring ancillary antithrombotic drug treatment.

Studies examining the efficacy of heparin therapy for the treatment of MI in the thrombolytic era are reviewed next. The SCATI[188] study examined 711 patients randomized to receive either subcutaneous heparin or no heparin as part of the therapy for MI. Approximately half of the patients received thrombolytic therapy with streptokinase. In the heparin plus thrombolytic group and in the heparin-alone group, a reduction in mortality associated with heparin was noted. In addition, a trend toward a reduction in the number of postinfarction ischemic episodes was noted in those patients who received thrombolytic therapy plus heparin. Heparin therapy was clearly effective either alone or as an adjunct to thrombolytic therapy in the treatment of acute MI. In a larger trial, the GISSI-2[189] study, subcutaneous heparin therapy was not associated with a statistically significant difference in mortality, reinfarction, or unstable angina. It did, however, highlight an excess of bleeding. The International Study Group,[190] which incorporated some of the GISSI-2 data, examined 20,891 patients who underwent thrombolytic therapy with either APSAC or streptokinase. The group that received subcutaneous heparin experienced an excess of bleeding episodes without the benefit of a reduction in reinfarction or stroke. In addition, the Third International Study of Infarct Survival[191] examined 41,300 patients treated with thrombolytic therapy. The addition to aspirin of heparin resulted in an excess of transfused or major bleeding, with only a trend toward a reduction in reinfarction, and with no differences in mortality or stroke. However, a meta-analysis of the data from the ISIS and GISSI trials support a decrease in mortality during the treatment period.[191] This mortality benefit came at the expense of increased bleeding. Taken together with a review of prior data on the use of heparin as adjuvant therapy for MI published in 1985,[192] heparin did not appear to significantly influence the rates of reinfarction or death.

A few trials using heparin have demonstrated an improved patency rate of the infarct-related artery up to 3 days after thrombolysis for acute MI. The HART[193] study, in which 205 patients received t-PA plus either heparin or aspirin, demonstrated improved 18-h patency of the infarct-related artery associated with heparin therapy. There were no significant differences amongst the two groups in terms of patency at 7 days or in terms of hemorrhagic events. Examination of the data from either the TAMI[194] or the GUSTO (Global Use of Strategies to Open Occluded Coronary Arteries)[195] trials did not demonstrate an effect of heparin on mortality, reinfarction, major hemorrhage, infarct-related artery patency, or reocclusion. These angiographic trials highlighted the fact that heparin may improve coronary patency in some patients, with improvement being greatest in those patients not treated or undertreated with aspirin.

In all, the data available with heparin as adjunctive therapy for MI does not support its routine use with streptokinase.[48] Anticoagulant therapy should be reserved for use in those patients who are at higher risk for further events—specifically, those patients with

atrial fibrillation, heart failure, or who have suffered a large MI. The data regarding the use of heparin with t-PA is even more limited. However, the short duration of activity, the more specific fibrinolytic effect, and the angiographic data lends some support to its use with t-PA.

Randomized clinical trials have compared the effectiveness of intravenous heparin (an indirect thrombin inhibitor) with intravenous hirudin (a direct thrombin antagonist). In the TIMI (Thrombolysis in Myocardial Infarction) 9B study, heparin (5000 U/h and 1000 U/h) and hirudin (0.1 mg/kg/h and 0.1 mg/kg/h) were found to be equally effective and to have similar major hemorrhagic side effects (4 to 5%) when used as adjuncts to t-PA or streptokinase to preventing unsatisfactory thrombotic outcomes in AMI patients.[196]

Dosing

There are several methods for optimizing intravenous heparin dose adjustments. These nomograms have been used for the treatment of both venous thromboembolism and AMI patients.[197] A weight-based heparin nomogram has also been recommended in the current treatment guidelines for unstable angina.[198] Such algorithms are convenient to use, are successful in achieving therapeutic aPTT levels in an expeditious manner, and reduce thromboembolism.[199]

Side Effects

Bleeding is the major side effect associated with heparin use,[200] and is partly a function of the drug's complex pharmacokinetics, its use in severely ill patients who are often on other antithrombotic or fibrinolytic agents, and the numerous other actions of heparin on a variety of processes besides anticoagulation.[201]

Of special concern, however, is heparin-induced thrombocytopenia (HIT). Two mechanisms for HIT have been elucidated: an early reversible nonimmune thrombocytopenia, possibly related to weak platelet activation by the drug, and a late, serious immune thrombocytopenia with immunoglobulin G (IgG)-mediated platelet activation and thrombotic complications.[175,202] Immune-related HIT was seen in 1% and 3% of patients receiving LDUH for 7 and 14 days, respectively, but was not observed with LMWH.[201] When present, HIT becomes manifest 5 to 15 days after initiating heparin therapy, but may arise within hours in patients previously exposed to heparin within the prior 3 to 6 months.[175] In vitro studies suggest that LMWH can cross-react to activate platelets in serum from HIT patients.[203]

Low-Molecular-Weight Heparins (LMWH)

LMWH are fragments of commercial-grade standard heparin produced by enzymatic or chemical depolymerization with a resultant molecular weight of 4000 to 6500 (Table 18-3). Because smaller

TABLE 18-3. Low-Molecular-Weight Heparins

Generic Name	Brand Name	Mean & Range Molecular Weight	Anti-Xa to Anti-IIa Ratio	Plasma Half-Life (min)
Ardeparin	Normiflow	5000		
Certroparin	Sandoparin	6000 (5000–9000)	2.0/1.0	270
Dalteparin*	Fragmin	5000 (2000–9000)	2.7/1.0	119–139
Enoxaparin*	Lovenox	4500 (3000–8000)	3.8/1.0	129–180
Naroparin	Fraxiparine	4500 (2000–8000)	3.2/1.0	132–162
Parnaparin	Flaxum	—	—	—
Reviparin	Clivarine	3900 (2000–4500)	5.0/1.0	—
Tinzaparin*	Innohep	4500 (3000–6000)	2.8/1.0	111

* FDA approved.

heparin molecules (MW <4000) are not able to bind to thrombin (factor II) and antithrombin III (AT-III) simultaneously, LMWH have a diminished ability to accelerate the inactivation of thrombin by AT-II. However, LMWH retains its ability to catalyze the inhibition of factor Xa by AT-III. Therefore, as contrasted to standard heparin (average molecular weight 12,000 to 15,000) with an anti-Xa/anti-IIa inhibitory ratio of 1:1, commercial LMWH has anti-Xa/anti-IIa ratios of 2:1 to 4:1 when tested in vitro. The persistence of anti-IIa activity by LMWH emanates from the larger oligosaccharide chains in its polydispersed spectrum.[204]

Other properties that distinguish LMWH from standard heparin include lack of inhibition of activity by platelet factor IV (PF4), a potent inhibitor of standard heparin release during coagulation;[205] persistence of inactivation of Xa bound to platelet membranes in the prothrombinase complex, a feature lacking in standard heparin; and lack of LMWH binding by plasma proteins, histidine-rich glycoprotein, fibronectin, vitronectin, and von Willebrand factor, as opposed to the plasma binding of standard heparin, which partially neutralizes its anti-Xa inhibition.[206] In addition, unfractionated heparin (UH) binds to endothelium, monocytes, and osteoclasts. The diminished binding of LMWH to osteoclasts may account for the decreased incidence of osteoporosis as compared to that seen with the prolonged use of UH.

These features of LMWH, which distinguished it from standard heparin, can result in certain clinical advantages: (a) a more predictable dose response with patient variability to a fixed dose; (b) a long half-life and reduced bleeding for equivalent antithrombotic effects; (c) enhanced safety and efficacy in the treatment of patients with venous thrombosis. Table 18-3 lists several LMWHs.[207]

Clinical Trials

A meta-analysis of the relevant randomized clinical trials comparing UH with LMWH examined total mortality, pulmonary embolism mortality, rates of recurrent venous thromboembolism (RVTE), change in venography scores, and incidence of bleeding.[208] LMWH significantly reduced short-term and pulmonary embolism mortality, while causing less major bleeding as contrasted to UH. Longer-term mortality and serious bleeding rates were influenced by case mix and efficacy of subsequent oral anticoagulation, but were still favorably influenced by LMWH as compared to UH, with a relative risk of 0.30 (95% CI 0.3 to 0.4; $P = .0006$) for mortality and 0.42 (95% CI 0.2 to 0.9; $P < .01$) for major bleeding.[208] Additional data favoring the safety of LMWH versus UH were provided from a study of 3809 patients undergoing major abdominal surgery with heparin prophylaxis for ≥ 5 days perioperatively.[209] The 4-week incidence of major bleeding was reduced from 141 to 93 ($P < .058$), and major hematoma from 2.7 to 1.4%, when LMWH was compared to UH. Individual trials and a meta-analysis show that LMWH use in venous thromboembolism is associated with a decreased mortality as compared to UH. This decreased mortality incidence appears to be seen only in cancer patients, and is the subject of new trials.

Acute Ischemic Stroke

Thrombolytics have a place in the treatment of acute stroke, but full-dose anticoagulation with either UH or LMWH is generally not recommended, except possibly for prevention of recurrence in cardioembolic stroke.[210] The International Stroke Trial compared aspirin, subcutaneous heparin, both, or neither and found no significant advantage from heparin, but a higher rate of bleeding with higher doses of the drug.[211]

Kay et al,[212] in a randomized double-blind, placebo-controlled trial, compared the effect of two dosages of LMWH with placebo. Three hundred and twelve patients with acute ischemic stroke were randomized within 48 h of symptoms to high-dose nadroparin (4100 antifactor Xa IU subcutaneously twice daily), low-dose nadroparin (4100 IU subcutaneously once daily), or placebo subcutaneously for 10 days. The primary end-point at 6 months of death and dependency of living were analyzed for 306 patients. A significant favorable dose-dependent effect of LMWH on outcomes was noted as follows: high-dose group 45%, low-dose group 52%, and placebo 65% ($P = .005$). No statistically significant differences in hemorrhagic transformation of the infarct was noted between the three groups. LMWH improved the 6-month outcome of acute ischemic stroke. However, it has been pointed out that these findings could not be duplicated in a very similar trial that used the same agent.[210]

Myocardial Infarction

LMWH can be used as an alternative to weight-adjusted UH in patients with acute MI undergoing thrombolysis. In a recent trial, tenecteplase plus enoxaparin reduced the frequency of ischemic complications of an acute MI as compared to UH. The tenecteplase-enoxaparin combination was also shown to be as effective as tenecteplase plus abciximab, but easier to administer to patients.[213,214]

Unstable Angina

The use of antithrombotic agents for unstable angina, a process that results from platelet aggregation and thrombus formation, has been well studied. Gurfinkel et al,[215] in a prospective, single-blind, randomized trial of patients with unstable angina, compared the effects of nadroparin calcium, a LMWH (214 IU/kg anti-Xa subcutaneous bid), and ASA versus UH and ASA (200 mg/d) versus ASA (200 mg/d) alone in 211 patients. Primary outcomes were recurrent angina, acute MI, urgent revascularization, major bleeding, and death. There was a significant benefit with the use of LMWH and ASA versus UH and ASA in the rate of recurrent angina, 21% versus 44%, respectively.

FRISC (Fragmin During Instability with CAD) was a multicenter study that randomized 1506 patients with unstable angina to LMWH (120 IU/kg subcutaneously every 12 h up to day 6 and then 7500 U every day at home until day 40) or placebo. At day 6, there were differences between the LMWH and placebo groups in the occurrence of new MI and death (1.8% and 4.7%, respectively) and severe angina (7.8% and 13.9%, respectively). The benefit continued through day 40. By day 150 no differences were noted between the two groups. FRIC, another multicenter, randomized study, enrolled 1482 patients with unstable angina. Patients were randomized to UH (5000 U intravenous bolus, 1000 U/h infusion, and then 1250 U subcutaneous bid) versus LMWH (120 IU/kg every 12). Therapy continued for 6 weeks. The initial data at 7 days indicated that there were no differences between groups in death, MI, urgent revascularization, non-Q-wave MI, or unstable angina.[216]

In a study of thrombolytic therapy with enoxaparin plus aspirin versus UH plus aspirin, enoxaparin plus aspirin was more effective in reducing the incidence of ischemic events in patients with unstable angina or non-Q-wave myocardial infarctions in the early stage.[217] This greater efficacy was sustained at a 1 year follow-up.[218] A recent meta-analysis shows no difference in efficacy or safety between UH and LMWH in aspirin-treated patients with acute coronary syndromes. Both therapies halve the risk of MI and death. There is no evidence to support the use of LMWH after 7 days.[219] The American College of Chest Physicians Consensus Conference now recommends that unstable angina be treated with aspirin or an alternative antiplatelet agent combined with intravenous heparin (about 75 U/kg intravenous bolus, initial maintenance 1250 U/h intravenous, aPTT 1.5 to 2 times control) or LMWH (dose regimen from trial), dalteparin (120 IU/kg subcutaneous every 12 h), enoxaparin (1 mg/kg subcutaneous bid), nadroparin (either 86 anti-Xa IU/kg bid for 4 to 8 days or the same dose given intravenously then subcutaneously bid for 24 days) for at least 48 h, or until the unstable pain pattern resolves.[220] The newest ACC/AHA guidelines for managing acute coronary syndromes also recommend LMWH as an alternative to UH.[198]

The SYNERGY Trial is the largest study currently planned for the acute therapy of patients with non-ST-segment elevation acute coronary syndromes, and is comparing enoxaparin to UH. The primary efficacy endpoint is death or non-fatal MI 30 days after enrollment.[220a]

Prevention of Venous Thromboembolism after Knee Arthroplasty

In patients undergoing major knee surgery, 60 to 70% develop DVT.[221] Proximal DVT occurs in 20% of these patients. Initially, pneumatic compression cuffs and warfarin were used as prophylaxis. In a double-blind, randomized trial, Levine et al[222] compared the use of ardeparin (Normiflo), a LMWH, and compression stockings with stockings alone for the prevention of thromboembolism postoperation. The study group received ardeparin 0.005 mL/kg subcutaneously every 12 h. At day 14, venography was performed. Of the patients receiving LMWH, 28 of 90 (31%) were found to have DVT and 2 (2%) were proximal DVT, whereas 60 of the 104 patients with compression stockings alone (58%) developed DVT and 16 (15%) were proximal. One patient in each group developed pulmonary embolism. There was no difference in the rate of major bleeding between groups. LMWH was found to be safe and effective.

Leclerc et al[223] compared the use of the LMWH enoxaparin with placebo in patients undergoing knee replacement. The incidence of distal and proximal DVT in the placebo group was 45% and 20%. The LMWH group only had a 19% incidence of distal DVT and no proximal DVT. In a recent randomized, double-blind trial by Leclerc, enoxaparin and warfarin were compared. Patients undergoing knee replacement were randomized to enoxaparin (30 mg subcutaneously every 12 h) or warfarin [dose adjusted to keep the international normalized ratio (INR) between 2.0 and 3.0]. The primary end-point was the incidence of DVT as per bilateral venography. The secondary end-point was the incidence of hemorrhage. The incidence of DVT was 36.9% for the enoxaparin group and 51.7% for the warfarin group. There was no difference in the incidence of major bleeding, 1.8% versus 2.1%, respectively, or proximal DVT.

Other studies[224] have compared LMWH to warfarin in patients undergoing knee arthroplasty (Table 18-4). All but one of the studies showed that fixed-dose LMWH was more effective than adjusted-dose warfarin in preventing DVT postoperatively. Hull et al[224] compared Logiparin (tinzaparin) subcutaneously every day to warfarin. The incidence of DVT was 45% versus 55%, respectively. The high incidence of DVT in the LMWH group was believed to be secondary to the daily dosing required instead of the usual twice-a-day dosing regimen. The American College of Chest Physicians

Consensus Conference reviewed six randomized trials that directly compared oral anticoagulants with LMWH in total knee replacement and found total DVT rates of 46.2% and 31.5%, respectively, with some increase in bleeding.[225] However, because one high-quality study found a 3-month cumulative incidence of only 0.8%,[226] it was concluded that adjusted-dose warfarin was also effective after total-knee replacement.

Acute Proximal Deep-Vein Thrombosis

Acute proximal DVT is associated with the risk of pulmonary embolism and recurrent thromboembolism. Management of this condition has traditionally required a hospitalization of 5 to 7 days for treatment with UH and initiation of oral anticoagulation with warfarin. Recent studies compared the use of LMWH to UH in hospital for the treatment of proximal DVT. Hull et al randomized 418 patients to receive either UH or LMWH (Logiparin, now called tinzaparin, 175 U/kg subcutaneously once daily) and demonstrated a significantly lower recurrence and bleeding rate with LMWH, as well as a decreased mortality rate.[227] Subsequent studies took this type of treatment to the outpatient setting. Levine et al[228] randomized 253 patients to receive UH intravenously and 247 patients to receive LMWH (enoxaparin 1 mg/kg subcutaneous bid) for the management of acute proximal DVT. There was, however, no statistically significant difference in recurrent thromboembolism or major bleeding between the two groups. There was a major difference in the average length of hospitalization, 1.1 days for the LMWH group and 6.5 days for the UH group. Similarly, Koopman et al[229] randomized 198 patients to receive UH intravenously and 202 patients to receive weight-dosed nadroparin-Ca (Fraxiparine) subcutaneously twice a day. Rates of recurrent thromboembolism and major bleeding were low and similar between the two groups. Again, there was a significant reduction the length of hospitalization for the LMWH group. The outpatient treatment of proximal DVT with LMWH is safe and effective. Gould et al conducted a meta-analysis of 11 randomized, controlled studies comparing LMWH to UH for the acute treatment of DVT and confirmed the finding of Hull et al that there was a significant decrease in mortality with LMWH and similar rates of recurrence and bleeding.[230] Subset analysis suggests that this decrease in mortality was seen only in cancer patients with DVT and new trials are addressing this issue.

Restenosis after Percutaneous Transluminal Coronary Angioplasty

Anticoagulants are important after PTCA because they reduce thrombus formation, which is responsible for acute closure and late restenosis (see Chap. 40). Heparin inhibits smooth-muscle cell migration and proliferation in vitro. It alters the binding of specific growth factors such as platelet-derived growth factor (PDGF) and epidermal growth factor (EGF). In experimental animal models, heparin has reduced neointimal hyperplasia and restenosis following vascular injury. Three clinical trials analyzing the effects of LMWH on restenosis were done. The ERA Trial, a double-blind multicenter study, examined the effects of enoxaparin 40 mg subcutaneous every day versus placebo for 1 month post-PTCA.[231] The angiographic and clinical restenosis rate at 6 months was similar for both groups. The restenosis rate was 52% for the LMWH group and 51% for the placebo group. The EMPAR (Enoxaparin and Maxepa for the Prevention of Angioplasty Restenosis Trial) studied the effects of LMWH and omega-3 polyunsaturated fatty acid on restenosis. The angiographic restenosis rate at 4 months was 47%

TABLE 18-4. Comparative Studies of Warfarin and Low-Molecular-Weight Heparin after Knee Arthroplasty

Study	Intensity	Warfarin n/n(%)				Regimen	Low-Molecular-Weight Heparin n/n(%)			
		DVT	Proximal DVT	Wound Hematoma	Major Bleeding		DVT	Proximal DVT	Wound Hematoma	Major Bleeding
Hull et al[224]	INR 2.0–3.0	152/277 (55)	34/277 (12)	19/324 (6)	3/321 (1)	Tinzaparin 75 U/kg/d	116/258 (45)	20/258 (8)	28/317 (9)	9/317 (3)
RD Heparin Group (*J Bone Joint Surg* 76:1174, 1994)	Prothrombin time ratio, 1.2–1.5	60/147 (41)	15/147 (10)	NA	NA	Ardeparin 90 U/kg/d	41/149 (28)	7/149 (5)	NA	NA
				NA	NA	Ardeparin 50 U/kg twice daily	37/150 (25)	9/150 (6)	NA	NA
Spiro et al (*Blood* 84:246A, 1994)	INR 2.0–3.0	72/122 (59)	16/122 (13)	6/176 (3)	4/176 (2)	Exoxaparin 30 mg twice daily	41/108 (38)	3/108 (3)	12/173 (7)	9/173 (5)
Heit et al (*Thromb Haemost* 73:978A, 1995)	INR 2.0–3.0	81/222 (36)	15/222 (7)	NA	NA	Ardeparin 50 U twice daily	58/230 (25)	14/230 (6)	NA	NA
Leclerc[223]	INR 2.0–3.0	109/211 (52)	22/211 (10)	18/334 (5)	6/334 (2)	Enoxaparin 30 mg twice daily	76/206 (37)	24/206 (12)	18/336 (5)	7/336 (2)

DVT = deep venous thrombosis; INR = international normalized ration; NA = not available.

Source: Values are the number of patients with events/number of patients studied (%). Leclerc.[223]

for the treatment group and 46% for the placebo group.[232] FACT,[233] a multicenter double-blind randomized trial, compared Fraxiparine with aspirin post-PTCA. The 3-month angiographic restenosis rate was similar for both groups, 41% and 38%, respectively. There was no difference in the 6-month clinical-event rates for death, acute MI, and repeat revascularization. One study examined whether intramural enoxaparin before balloon-expandable stenting decreases the in-stent restenosis rate when compared to the use of intravenous unfractionated heparin. Late lumen loss and in-stent stenosis were lower in the enoxaparin group than in the heparin group.[234]

Management of Intermittent Claudication

Several small studies have demonstrated clinical improvement using LMWH in patients with intermittent claudication and Raynaud's phenomenon.[235] Mannarino et al[236] randomized 44 patients into a double-blinded controlled study evaluating LMWH versus placebo. Patients were treated for 6 months with daily subcutaneous injections of either LMWH or placebo. After 6 months of treatment, the LMWH group had a 25% improvement in pain-free walking time ($P < .05$) with no adverse bleeding effects. Although patients were clinically improved, no angiographic changes were found. Calabro et al[237] randomized 36 patients in a double-blinded study to receive either LMWH or placebo for a period of 6 months. Patients receiving LMWH had statistically significant increases in claudication time and absolute claudication distance, and in the time interval free of pain. These small studies showing clinical improvement using LMWH versus placebo suggest that LMWH may have a role in the management of intermittent claudication (see Chap. 50), but larger and more definitive studies are needed.

Another small study tested the hypothesis that low-molecular weight heparin would be more effective than aspirin and dipyridamole in maintaining graft patency in patients undergoing femoropopliteal bypass grafting.[238] Patients were randomized to receive either a daily injection of 2500 IU LMWH or 300 mg aspirin with 100 mg dipyridamole for 3 months. Ninety-four patients were randomized to LMWH and 106 were randomized to aspirin and dipyridamole. Patients were stratified according to indication for surgery and were followed up for 1 year. Benefit was confined to those having salvage surgery. For those having surgery for claudication, there was no significant benefit. No major bleeding events occurred in either group. The authors concluded that LMWH is better than aspirin and dipyridamole in maintaining femoropopliteal-graft patency in patients with critical limb ischaemia undergoing salvage surgery.[238] This study also suffers from small numbers of patients, and LMWH has not yet gained a standard role in the management of intermittent claudication.

Thromboembolic Prophylaxis in Patients with Atrial Fibrillation

The increased risk of arterial embolism associated with chronic atrial fibrillation is well known. Both aspirin and oral anticoagulation with warfarin reduce the incidence of embolic events in patients with chronic nonrheumatic atrial fibrillation.[239] Harenberg et al[240] randomized 75 patients with nonrheumatic atrial fibrillation to receive either the LMWH CY 216 or to receive no specific treatment. Patients with a history of cerebral or peripheral embolism were included in the study. Overall mortality in the control group was 43%; it was 7.5% in the treatment group. The number of embolic events was reduced in the treatment group from 20 to 8.6%. The most striking difference was seen in the group of patients with a history

of prior cerebral embolism. In the 15 patients from this subset who were treated with LMWH, one extracerebral nonfatal embolism occurred, while 3 of the 7 patients with prior stroke who received no treatment experienced fatal reembolism. No major bleeding complications were reported in either group. Further studies to evaluate the efficacy and safety of LMWH versus oral anticoagulation are necessary, particularly in patients with prior embolic events. There is no evidence that LMWH is superior to aspirin for the treatment of acute ischemic stroke in patients with atrial fibrillation.[241] The use of LMWH as bridging therapy to warfarin with cardioversion or other procedures is attractive from an economic point of view.[242] This approach has been carried out in small trials, but it requires further study.[243]

Thromboprophylaxis for Hemodialysis

Standard UH is used to prevent clotting in the membrane filter during hemodialysis. As many azotemic patients have increased risk for bleeding complications, due to abnormal platelet function, an alternative to UH is being sought in LMWHs in the hope of reducing bleeding complications in hemodialysis patients. Several preliminary studies have demonstrated adequate antithrombosis with fewer hemorrhagic effects.[244] An additional benefit of LMWH prophylaxis is a decrease in lipid blood levels. Schmitt and Schneider[245] switched 22 patients on chronic hemodialysis from UH to the LMWH dalteparin. They found significant decreases in total cholesterol, LDL cholesterol, apolipoprotein B, and a minor decrease in HDL cholesterol levels. Triglycerides increased during the first 2 months of LMWH therapy, but then normalized to previous levels. Hyperlipidemia presents a high risk for developing cardiovascular disease and LMWH may become the antithrombotic of choice in hemodialysis patients if further trials indicate its safety, efficacy, and significant lipid-lowering effects. Recent small studies have found no difference in lipid profiles over 24 weeks of LMWH or UH for hemodialysis, and small or no differences in anticoagulant efficacy, so that the increased cost of LMWH has resulted in UH still being the standard product used for both standard and venovenous hemodialysis.[246]

Angina

Preliminary studies suggest that LMWHs may play a role in the control of stable angina but no definitive recommendation can be made just yet. Melandri et al[247] conducted a randomized, double-blind, placebo-controlled trial of 29 patients with stable exercise-induced angina pectoris proven angiographically coronary artery disease. Patients aged 40 to 79 years received either 6400 U of the LMWH parnaparin or placebo subcutaneously. All patients were treated with beta-blockers and calcium-channel blockers, nitrates, and aspirin. Treadmill exercise testing was conducted at the beginning and repeated at the end of the 3-month treatment period with myocardial ischemia being defined as ST depression >1 mm. Exercise time to ischemia (ST depression) was increased in the treatment group from 285 to 345 seconds. There was no significant increase in the placebo group. The time to the onset of symptoms was nonsignificantly increased in the treatment group, although there was a significant improvement ($P = .016$) in terms of the Canadian Cardiovascular Society classification for angina reflecting subjective improvement in symptoms.

Cost-Effectiveness

Cost minimization analyses have addressed the issue of the higher cost of LMWH versus UH.[248] These analyses show that the higher medication cost of LMWH was outweighed by the reduction in cost attributable to a reduced incidence of DVT (deep vein thrombosis), PE (pulmonary embolism), and major and minor bleeding associated with LMWH, both for general and orthopedic surgical patients undergoing perioperative heparin thromboembolic prophylaxis.[248,249]

Danaparoid

The heparin analogue danaparoid sodium is a mixture of sulfated glycosaminoglycans of porcine origin. Danaparoid consists of heparan sulfate ($\approx$84%), dermatan sulfate ($\approx$12%) and a small amount of chondroitin sulfate ($\approx$4%).[250] The drug is FDA-approved for prophylaxis of postoperative DVT in patients undergoing elective hip replacement surgery. In contrast to LMWHs, which have an 80 to 90% incidence of cross-reactivity in HIT, danaparoid has a cross-reactivity rate of approximately 10%. Although danaparoid is effective for total DVT prophylaxis, it does not offer a significant advantage over comparators for prophylaxis of the more clinically important proximal DVT. For this reason, its high cost prohibits routine use for this indication. It has been used as an option in patients who have documented HIT and still require anticoagulation. However, new agents (see below) have now been approved that have no cross-reactivity with the antibodies found in HIT.

Hirudin (Direct Thrombin Inhibition)

The rationale for developing direct thrombin inhibitors came from the realization that: (a) the acute coronary syndromes, MI, and unstable angina are the result of plaque rupture and in situ thrombosis;[251] and (b) thrombin plays a central role in the activation of clotting factors V and VIII, platelet activation and aggregations, cross-linking of fibrin, and stabilization of the hemostatic plug. Therefore, investigators have looked to thrombin and thrombin-inhibitors as prime targets for anticoagulant drug therapy.

Brief Review of Thrombin's Action

Thrombin is a key regulator of the hemostatic process responsible for the conversion of fibrinogen to fibrin. Thrombin is generated from prothrombin through the action of activated factors V, X, calcium, and phospholipid. Thrombin not only acts to catalyze the conversion of fibrinogen to fibrin, it also acts with factor XIII to cross-link and stabilize the clot.[1] It amplifies the clotting cascade by activating other clotting factors, and acts as a potent agonist for platelet activity and recruitment. In terms of its interaction with the endothelial surface, it can act as a vasodilator in areas where the endothelial surface has not been damaged, but it can also be a potent vasoconstrictor when it comes into contact with injured or denuded endothelial surfaces. This action is dependent on endothelin release. In addition, it stimulates the release of platelet-derived growth factor, interleukin 1, and, therefore, may be an important mediator of smooth-muscle growth and proliferation;[252,253] thus, it possibly plays an important role in subacute coronary artery closure and in postangioplasty restenosis.

Shortfalls of Heparin

The search for more potent and more direct antagonists to the clotting cascade was brought about by the realization that heparin actions are incomplete, unpredictable, and dependent upon cofactors not consistently found from patient to patient. Heparin's shortfalls have included a dependence on ATIII and cofactor II for its anticoagulant effect;[254] varied activity from preparation to preparation; binding to plasma proteins, leukocytes, and osteoclasts; and an inability to inactivate clot-bound thrombin.[254]

Meticulous monitoring of the anticoagulant effect is necessary to retain heparin in a therapeutic range for several reasons. First, heparin is a heterogenous mixture of molecules, each with variable biologic effects. Second, the concentrations of cofactors ATIII and cofactor II vary from individual to individual.[254,254a] Third, heparin can be bound by a number of plasma proteins with variable concentrations from individual to individual with a resultant difference in the amount of heparin available to exert an anticoagulant effect.[255] In addition, activated platelets release platelet factor 4 and heparinase, both of which can act to counter the anticoagulant activity of heparin.[255,256] Finally, much of the active thrombin is clot bound which protects it from inactivation by heparin.[254a] Thus, the nidus for clot formation and propagation cannot be activated.

In contrast, the direct thrombin inhibitors are ATIII independent, provide a stable, anticoagulant effect, and are able to inhibit clot-bound thrombin.[254a,255]

Properties and Mechanism of Action

Hirudin is a 65-amino-acid polypeptide that was originally isolated from leech salivary glands and is now available as a recombinant product derived from yeast.[257]

Hirudin is a specific inhibitor of thrombin that binds to both the active and substrate recognition sites of thrombin.[257] The attachment of hirudin to thrombin is not limited to these two sites, and other areas of contact have been described.[257] Hirudin is specific for thrombin, and does not inhibit other serine proteases.[258] While binding is not covalent, the process of deattachment is slow and for most purposes is irreversible.[259] This is in contrast to many of the other direct thrombin inhibitors, where binding to thrombin is not as extensive. Lepirudin is one of several recombinant hirudins. It is FDA-approved for use in patients with HIT on the basis of two clinical trials.[260,261]

Argatroban and melagatran also are potent thrombin inhibitors.[262,263] Argatroban is safe and effective for patients requiring anticoagulation who either have HIT or a prior episode of HIT,[263,264] and was approved recently for clinical use in patients with HIT. Before administering argatroban, heparin should be discontinued. The recommended dose of argatroban is 2 μg/kg/min administered as a continuous infusion. Therapy with argatroban is monitored using the aPTT and the dose of the drug should not exceed 10 μg/kg/min.

Although melagatran has complete subcutaneous bioavailability and low interindividual variability with parental administration, its oral bioavailability is low. To improve the oral bioavailability of melagatran, it has been converted into an orally absorbable prodrug, H376/95 (ximelagatran). Subcutaneous melagatran combined with oral H376/95 has shown promise as a therapeutic modality in patients with DVT; additional studies are in progress.[265]

Thrombin aptamers bind to the substrate recognition site, and demonstrate potent thrombin inhibition with a short half-life.[264] Alternate antithrombin strategies include the development of factor Xa inhibitors that can block thrombin formation (e.g., fondaparinux: see Other Anticoagulation Approaches).[266,267,267a]

Myocardial Infarction

Trials in MI have demonstrated the efficacy and safety of hirudin. In the TIMI 5 trial, which involved 246 patients, hirudin was associated with a significant reduction in the composite end-point of death, reinfarction, congestive heart failure (CHF), or shock.[268] Hirudin use was associated with improved patency of the infarct related artery at 18 to 36 h. Major hemorrhage occurred in 23% of heparin-treated patients, and in 17% of hirudin-treated patients. The HIT trial also showed a low incidence of spontaneous hemorrhage and low incidence of reocclusion with low doses of hirudin.[269] HIT also showed that higher doses of hirudin were associated with cerebral bleeds.[269] The TIMI 6 data confirmed the results of TIMI 5, with favorable trends in the incidence of death, reinfarction, and shock without increases in major hemorrhage.[270] In the phase III clinical trials, TIMI 9A and GUSTO 2A, an excess of cerebral hemorrhage associated with hirudin was revealed without a clear mortality benefit.[271–273] TIMI 9B also did not demonstrate a superiority to heparin in terms of efficacy or safety.[196] More recently, the GUSTO 2B data did not reveal an advantage of hirudin over heparin in the composite end-point of death or reinfarction at 30 days.[274] However, treatment with hirudin resulted in fewer adjustments of anticoagulant doses, and a significant reduction in the combined end-point at 48 h. In patients with unstable angina, hirudin improved the minimal luminal diameter of the culprit artery to a greater extent than does heparin, and slightly reduced the incidence of MI.[270]

Percutaneous Transluminal Coronary Angioplasty

There have been a number of trials comparing heparin to hirudin and hirulog in patients undergoing angioplasty (see Chap. 40). In a pilot trial involving 113 patients, coronary flow 24 h postprocedure was 100% for hirudin and 91% for heparin.[274] The end-point of ischemia on 24-h Holter monitor, myocardial infarction, and the composite end-point of death, myocardial infarction, and coronary artery bypass were reduced in the hirudin group.[274] The HELVETICA[275] trial involved more than 1000 patients and compared angiographic evidence of restenosis at 6 months postangioplasty. This trial revealed no significant differences in restenosis. However, the incidence of death, myocardial infarction, and repeat intervention within the first 24 h was less with hirudin. The rates of major bleeds were similar. Hirulog reduces bleeding complications after angioplasty, but is ineffective in reducing important clinical events.[276]

Monitoring Therapy and Dose

There are a number of issues that should be considered in the dosing and monitoring of hirudin activity. Hirudin levels can be monitored using both the aPTT and the thrombin time.[277] The thrombin time is the most accurate indicator of hirudin activity. However, the assay system may be too cumbersome for routine clinical use.[277] The aPTT system is the most widely used system despite the fact that the aPTT values may not be completely reliable. A number of studies have found the aPTT is insensitive at both high and low doses of hirudin.[278] In addition, the dose range of heparin that has been effective in the treatment of cardiovascular disease was determined empirically, which may not be true for hirudin.[279] Antithrombotic doses of hirudin that appear to be equipotent with heparin prolong the aPTT to a lesser degree in animal and human models.[280] However, clinical studies in man have demonstrated efficacy for hirudin, as well as hirulog.[280a] Weight-adjusted dosing with a target aPTT of 65 to 90 seconds was effective and safe in the TIMI 6 trial.[270] In TIMI 9A,[271] a hirudin dose of 0.6 mg/kg bolus with an infusion rate of 0.2 mg/kg/h was excessive. GUSTO 2B[274] evaluated a dose of hirudin at 0.1 mg/kg bolus and infusion of 0.1 mg/kg/min and found

that it was safe and effective, but not superior to heparin. The dosage regimen approved for clinical use in the United States for patients with HIT and associated thromboembolic disease is 0.4 mg/kg as a bolus dose followed by a 0.15 mg/kg/h infusion for 2 to 10 days.

Adverse Effects

The major reported complication with hirudin has been bleeding. Initial trials have demonstrated efficacy and safety of use as compared with heparin. Unlike heparin, however, hirudin does not have a commercially available antagonist. If significant bleeding occurs, the clinician should be familiar with the therapies available to neutralize the effects of hirudin. Some studies have suggested that activated prothrombin complex concentrates may be useful. The mechanism of this reversal has not been elucidated; presumably, the production of thrombin generated by the activated complexes overcomes the effects of hirudin.[281] Recombinant factor VIIa also restores platelet function and reverses the bleeding effect of hirudin. Lastly, either monoclonal antibodies or plasma infusions have been used to neutralize the effects of hirudin. In addition, physical methods of removing hirudin from the circulation are available; these include hemofiltration and hemodialysis.[281]

Other Direct Thrombin Inhibitors

Other direct thrombin inhibitors have been developed. Hirulog, also known as bivalirudin, binds at both the active and substrate recognition sites of thrombin, and does not exhibit other multiple areas of contact.[282] In addition, there is evidence that it is degraded at the active site, making it a less-potent thrombin inhibitor.[282] Bivalirudin has been used as an adjunct to thrombolytic therapy, with initial results indicating favorable trends in terms of vessel patency, clinical events, and bleeding complications.[282a] The drug is FDA-approved for use as an anticoagulant in patients with unstable angina undergoing PTCA, on the basis of trials showing that it is as effective as heparin, while causing less bleeding.[276,282a–d] The recommended dose of bivalirudin is 1 mg/kg as an IV bolus followed by a 4-h infusion at a rate of 2.5 mg/kg/h. After the completion of the initial 4-h infusion, an additional infusion may be initiated at a rate of 0.2 mg/kg/h for up to 20 h.

Warfarin

Mechanism of Action

Warfarin is a vitamin K antagonist that blocks the cyclic interconversion of vitamin K_{H2} and its 2,3 epoxide by inhibiting two regulatory enzymes, vitamin K epoxide reductase and vitamin K reductase.[283] Vitamin K_{H2} is an essential cofactor for the carboxylation of glutamate residues on N-terminal portions of inactive coagulant proenzymes (factors II, VII, IX, X) in a reaction that is catalyzed by a vitamin K-dependent carboxylase. Because γ-carboxylation of vitamin K-dependent coagulation enzymes is a requisite step in the ability of the enzymes to bind metals, undergo conformational changes, bind to cofactors, and become activated, warfarin impedes the activity of these essential reactions in the coagulation pathway.[283]

Pharmacokinetics

Warfarin, a racemic mixture of R and S isoforms, undergoes rapid and extensive gastrointestinal absorption, reaching maximal plasma concentrations in 90 min.[283] In the blood, it has a half-life

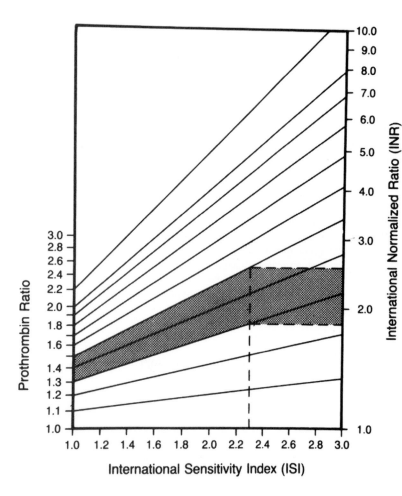

FIGURE 18-8. Relationship between the prothrombin time ratio and the INR for thromboplastin reagents over a range of ISI values. The example shown is for a prothrombin time (PT) ratio of 1.3 to 1.5 for a thromboplastin preparation with an ISI of 2.3. From the formula $INR = PT^{ISI}$, the INR is calculated as $1.3^{2.3}$ to $1.5^{2.3}$, or 1.83 to 2.54. (*Modified with permission from Hirsh J, Polker L, Deykin D, et al: Optimal therapeutic range for anticoagulants. Chest 95(Suppl 2):55–115, 1989.*)

of 36 to 42 h[283] and is extensively bound to plasma proteins, principally albumin. Only 1 to 3% of warfarin circulates in the free state, but it rapidly accumulates in the liver where it is metabolized microsomally to inactive catabolites, the R isomers are metabolized to warfarin alcohols and excreted in the urine, and the S isomers are oxidized and eliminated via the bile.[283] Numerous drugs and disease entities that alter warfarin absorption, plasma protein binding, liver microsomal activity, or basal vitamin K levels can increase or decrease warfarin anticoagulant intensity[283,284] (see Chap. 48). Because many of these agents may be prescribed concurrently with warfarin, adjustment in the daily anticoagulant dose will be necessary to avoid inadequate or excessive anticoagulation. A dietary inventory, including all drug and vitamin supplementation, is equally important: massive amounts of dietary vitamin K can increase warfarin resistance;[283] dietary vitamin K deficiency, malabsorption problems, liquid paraffin laxatives, hypocholesterolemic bile-binding resins can reduce warfarin absorption or increase warfarin excretion;[283] and large doses of vitamin E used as an antioxidant can antagonize vitamin K action.[283] Moreover, variations in dose response to warfarin can occur during extended periods of anticoagulation, variations that may have one or several patient, medication, or laboratory causes.[283,285]

Laboratory Monitoring of Warfarin

Historically, the most commonly used test to monitor warfarin anticoagulation has been the prothrombin time. This test is sensitive to reduced activity of factors II, VII, and X, but not to reduced activity of factor IX.[286] Interpretation of the prothrombin

time results, while satisfactory for individual patient measurement, has been complicated, however, because thromboplastin reagents in standard usage vary in their sensitivity to the reduction of vitamin K-dependent clotting factors.[286,287] Hence, the prothrombin-time result can reflect very different degrees of anticoagulation when different thromboplastins are used as reagents.

Efforts to resolve the problem of variability in thromboplastin sensitivity have led to the adoption of the INR system, based upon a World Health Organization International Reference Thromboplastin Reagent. The INR is the prothrombin time ratio obtained by testing a given anticoagulated patient plasma sample using the WHO Reference Thromboplastin. The INR for any prothrombin time ratio (PTR) measured with any thromboplastin reagent can be calculated if the International Sensitivity Index (ISI) of the reagent is known, where $INR = $ measured PTR^{ISI}.[287] Figure 18-8 shows the relationship between PTR and INR for thromboplastins reagents of differing ISI. The INR value is the preferred method for expressing the degree of anticoagulation with warfarin, for comparing various results of clinical trials using warfarin, and for setting standard ranges of anticoagulation for specific clinical entities.[288]

Certain caveats regarding the use of an INR measurement system should be kept in mind, however.[289] First, during induction of warfarin anticoagulation the prothrombin time (PT) may more accurately define warfarin effect because the INR standard is based on ISI values derived from patients anticoagulated for at least 6 weeks, when factors II, VII, and X are all decreased in activity. During the initial 2 to 3 days of warfarin therapy, the PT increase is mainly attributable to decreased functional factor VII and, to a lesser extent,

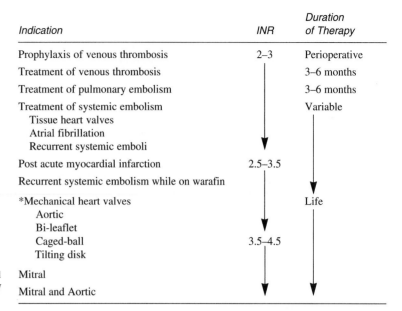

Indication	INR	Duration of Therapy
Prophylaxis of venous thrombosis	2–3	Perioperative
Treatment of venous thrombosis		3–6 months
Treatment of pulmonary embolism		3–6 months

Treatment of systemic embolism
  Tissue heart valves
  Atrial fibrillation
  Recurrent systemic emboli
		Variable

Post acute myocardial infarction	2.5–3.5	
Recurrent systemic embolism while on warafin		

*Mechanical heart valves
  Aortic
  Bi-leaflet
  Caged-ball
  Tilting disk
	3.5–4.5	Life

Mitral		
Mitral and Aortic		

FIGURE 18-9. Therapeutic goals for warfarin therapy. (Adapted with permission from *Chest* 108:2315, 1995; 371S, 1995, and *N Engl J Med* 333:54, 1995.)

factor X. Second, the naturally occurring anticoagulant protein C is also decreased by warfarin anticoagulation. During the early stages of warfarin anticoagulation, protein C falls rapidly just as factor VII does. Thus, there is a period when the full impact of anticoagulation is not manifest, but a natural protective mechanism has been diminished. This is particularly important when considering switching from argatroban or lepirudin to warfarin anticoagulation in the treatment of HIT.[290] Third, individual thromboplastin reagents vary in their sensitivity to differing proportionate reductions in the activity of the three of four vitamin K-dependent procoagulant factors impeded by warfarin. Fourth, the calculated INR value is less accurate when the PT is measured with insensitive thromboplastin having high ISI values.[291] Despite these limitations, expert panels continue to recommend the INR as a grading system for warfarin dosing during both induction and maintenance anticoagulation, especially when sensitive thromboplastin (INR ≤1.5) reagents are used, careful calibration of laboratory automated clot detectors are employed, and mean normal PT is calculated according to recommended guidelines.[289,292]

Warfarin Dosing: Initiation of Treatment

Upon inception of warfarin, a measurable anticoagulation effect is delayed until circulating factors II, VII, and X are cleared and replaced by dysfunctional vitamin K-dependent factors with fewer carboxyglutamate residues.[289] An initial anticoagulant effect will occur within 24 h as factor VII (half-time 6 to 7 h) is cleared. Peak anticoagulation action of warfarin is delayed for 72 to 96 h because of the longer half-time of factors II (50 h), IX (24 h), and X (36 h).[293] Warfarin suppression of the anticoagulant activity of proteins C (half-time 8 h) and S (30 h) may also contribute to the initial delay in anticoagulant effect.[283]

Selection of an initial warfarin dose will depend upon an appraisal of the age[283] and nutritional status of the patient and concomitant medical conditions and drugs that could alter warfarin impact on anticoagulation. Expeditious but safe anticoagulation is also an economic concern for hospitalized patients with decreased inpatient length of stay. For rapid effect, a dose of 10 mg warfarin can be given on day 1. If the INR is <1.5 on day 2, an additional

10 mg can be given. If the INR is >1.5 on day 2, then a smaller warfarin dose may be given (5.0 to 7.5 mg). By day 3, an INR of <1.5 suggests a higher-than-average maintenance dose (≥5 mg), an INR of 1.5 to 2.0 suggests an average maintenance dose (4 to 6 mg), and an INR of >2.0 suggests a lower-than-average maintenance dose is needed. When urgent anticoagulation is required, intravenous heparin should be utilized concurrently for 3 to 4 days.

When less-urgent outpatient anticoagulation is desired, warfarin can be initiated at 5 mg/d. In many patients, an INR of 2.0 can be attained in about 4 to 5 days.[289] Daily maintenance doses will depend upon the clinical condition being treated and the targeted INR range.

Warfarin Dosing: Maintenance Therapy

Chronic warfarin therapy is used in the prevention of venous and arterial thromboembolism. Specific clinical indications, generally recommended INR ranges, and duration of therapy are outlined in Fig. 18-9, and are summarized in greater detail in a consensus report on antithrombotic therapy and a detailed report of anticoagulation in patients with artificial cardiac valves.[289,294] The use of specialized anticoagulation clinics can enhance the quality of care receiving warfarin treatment by assuring that the INR remains within the desired range. Thromboembolic strokes arising from inadequate anticoagulation and serious bleeding adverse events stemming from excessive anticoagulation are thereby kept to a minimum.[295]

Persistent questions regarding the optimal benefit-risk ratio of specific or combined drug therapy with warfarin and aspirin in the treatment of arterial thromboembolism have been recently addressed.[296] Three hundred and seventy cardiac surgical patients receiving a mechanical or tissue valve replacement were randomized to 100-mg delayed-release enteric aspirin or placebo, in addition to warfarin adjusted to an INR of 3.0 to 4.5.[297] Combined aspirin-warfarin therapy reduced total and cardiovascular mortality and major systemic and cerebral emboli, with an additional overall risk reduction of 61% (9.9% per year for placebo-warfarin, 3.9% per year for aspirin-warfarin), albeit with increased minor bleeding events. The average INR values in these patients was 3.0 to 3.1, and the average warfarin dose was 5.5 to 5.8 mg/d. Low-dose aspirin and low-dose warfarin studies have been carried out to test the efficacy and safety of such combinations with no apparent benefit seen. Clinical experience with well-controlled adequate warfarin anticoagulation continues to be the mainstay of treatment for prosthetic valve patients[298,299] and for patients with rheumatic mitral valve disease who have either a history of systemic embolism or who have paroxysmal or chronic atrial fibrillation.[300] Warfarin is also recommended as a prophylaxis in patients with nonrheumatic atrial fibrillation.[301] Recent recommendations have stratified such patients according to the presence of risk factors for embolization, including left ventricular systolic dysfunction, history of prior embolism, hypertension, or age older than 75 years. Warfarin is recommended for patients with any of these high-risk factors, while aspirin or warfarin is recommended for lower-risk patients.[301]

Further studies using a case control methodology indicate that amongst patients with nonrheumatic atrial fibrillation, warfarin anticoagulation prophylaxis is highly effective against ischemic stroke at an INR of ≥ 2.0.[302] Adjusted odds ratio for ischemic stroke rose to 1.5 at INR 1.8 and more precipitously at lower INRs. Secondary stroke prevention in nonvalvular atrial fibrillation patients was also found to be effective at INR of ≥ 2.0, while hemorrhagic risk increased at INRs above 4.5.[303] In older patients, low-intensity warfarin (INR 1.5 to 2.1) appears to be safer than conventional-intensity treatment.[304] While higher INRs are required for mechanical heart valves, adverse bleeding events also increase at INR levels of ≥ 4.5.[300]

Clinical Recommendation for Myocardial Infarction

Data from the prethrombolytic era demonstrates significant reductions in pulmonary embolism, stroke, and, in one case, reductions in mortality associated with anticoagulant use after MI.[305] A meta-analysis of several trials from this era reveals reductions in the combined end-point of mortality and nonfatal reinfarction.[306] Recently, the ASPECT trial demonstrated a 50% reduction in reinfarction, and a 40% reduction in stroke associated with the use of warfarin after MI.[307] A number of studies from the thrombolytic era support the use of warfarin after MI, particularly in the prevention of embolic events in those patients who are at high risk (anterior wall myocardial infarction, atrial fibrillation, significant left ventricular dysfunction).[48,306,308] The Warfarin Aspirin Reinfarction Study (CARS) examined the effect of low-dose warfarin in combination with aspirin in the long-term treatment of the postinfarction patient. Warfarin doses of up to 3 mg/d in combination with aspirin 80 mg/d, did not improve mortality when compared to aspirin 160 mg/d. In fact, the combination group showed a stroke rate that was higher than that observed in the aspirin group alone.[309] At this juncture, we would recommend the use of oral anticoagulants in those patients who have suffered an anterior MI, have significant left ventricular dysfunction, atrial fibrillation, or history of a thromboembolic event.[48,309]

Unstable Angina

The Antithrombotic Therapy in Acute Coronary Syndromes (ATACS) trial showed that the long-term combination of aspirin plus warfarin was superior to aspirin alone in preventing ischemic events.[310]

Prosthetic Valves

There are clear indications for anticoagulation after the placement of prosthetic heart valves. For those patients with bioprosthetic heart valves in the aortic position, we do not recommend routine anticoagulation. However, evidence exists for a high rate of embolic events in the first 3 months, and some recommend anticoagulants for the first 3 months postoperatively.[311] For those patients with bioprosthetic valves in the mitral position, the rate of embolic events range from 0.4 to 1.9% per year in those patients without atrial fibrillation, without prior history of emboli, and without enlarged atria.[311] However, given a thromboembolic rate of up to 80% within the first 3 months of replacement, all patients after mitral valve replacement should be anticoagulated for the first 3 months.[311] However, it remains unclear whether these patients should be anticoagulated long-term. If atrial fibrillation has become evident, left atrial thrombus is present, or there is a history of embolic events, then these patients should probably be anticoagulated.

Those patients with mechanical heart valves should be anticoagulated regardless of location. Those patients with a prosthetic valve in the mitral position are more likely to have a thromboembolic event as compared to those patients with a prosthetic valve in the aortic position.[311] Other risk factors for high rates of thromboembolic events include patients with prior thromboembolic events, atrial fibrillation, enlarged left atria, ball-and-cage type valves, and dual-valve replacement. Given that there are data for the different types of valves, each with its own optimal regimen, our recommendations are bound to be oversimplified.[312] For those patients without a prior embolic event, we recommend a PT ratio of 2.5 to 3.5, with a slightly higher INR for those patients with a ball-and-cage valve.[313] For those patients with a prior embolic event, aspirin at an initial dose of 80 mg or dipyridamole at a dose of 400 mg/d should be added.[314] Although the risk of bleeding will be greater[315] if significant bleeding occurs in patients with prosthetic valves, anticoagulation can be stopped for up to 2 weeks with a low risk of thromboembolism.[316]

Atrial Fibrillation

There have been several randomized, placebo-controlled trials of anticoagulant therapy in atrial fibrillation.[80,317,318] The current recommendations for anticoagulant therapy can be divided into several major groups. Those patients with valvular disease and atrial fibrillation should be anticoagulated. Those patients younger than age 75 years with nonvalvular atrial fibrillation without structural heart disease, and without risk factors for heart disease, can be managed without anticoagulant therapy, and, in many cases, without aspirin.[318] Those patients who are older than 75 years of age should be anticoagulated.[80,318,319] However, the decision to treat should be balanced with the risk of an age-related increase in bleeds.[80,318,320] For those patients who are older than 65 years and younger than 75 years, the presence of risk factors plays a major role in the decision to anticoagulate.[80,318,319] Those patients with either a prior thromboembolic event, hypertension, diabetes, existing coronary disease, or reduced left ventricular function are at increased risk of a thrombotic event.[80,318,319] Those patients with none of these risk factors are at a risk of thromboembolic events of 2 to 4% per year, and the benefit of therapy with oral anticoagulants as compared to aspirin is much reduced.[80,318–320] In the Stroke Prevention in Atrial Fibrillation Trial II, there was no significant difference between aspirin therapy and warfarin therapy for some patients.[80] Lastly, patients with atrial fibrillation complicating thyrotoxicosis are at increased risk of thromboembolism and should be anticoagulated.[321]

Angioplasty and Thrombolysis

In a clinical trial of warfarin started before PCI and continued for 1 year, there was also a reduction in early and long-term ischemic events.[322]

Adverse Effects

The main complication associated with warfarin therapy is bleeding. The risk of bleeding is directly related to the intensity of therapy, with higher anticoagulant levels being associated with the greatest risk of hemorrhage.[283,323] The risk of bleeding is also reported to be associated with advancing age, prior history of gastrointestinal bleeding, prior stroke, and concomitant use of aspirin and other nonsteroidal anti-inflammatory agents.[283,320] If bleeding does occur, anticoagulation can be stopped.

Additional adverse events with warfarin have been described, the most important of which is warfarin-induced skin necrosis.[324] The mechanism is still unclear; however, an association with both protein C and protein S deficiencies have been described.[324] In addition, a similarity between these lesions and those seen in neonatal purpura fulminans (complicating homozygous protein C deficiency) has been noted. The lesion is caused by thrombosis of venules and capillaries in subcutaneous fatty tissue. In this group of patients, anticoagulation with warfarin must be overlapped with heparin, and warfarin therapy is begun at very low doses (0.03 mg/kg).[324] Lastly, warfarin therapy should be avoided in pregnancy. Specifically, it is associated with birth defects, central nervous system abnormalities, and fetal bleeding.[325]

ANTIPLATELET DRUGS IN DEVELOPMENT

This section reviews specific inhibitors of thromboxane A_2 (TXA_2) synthesis and/or action and the other antiplatelet strategies (Table 18-5).

Inhibitors of Thromboxane A_2 (TXA_2) Synthesis and Action

In platelets, cell-membrane phospholipids serve as the precursor to arachidonic acid formation through the action of phospholipase A_2 (PLA_2). Although the actual phospholipids that serve as the arachidonic acid precursor have never been properly established, arachidonic acid is stereospecifically numbered at the 2 position. Therefore, it is accepted that arachidonic acid is derived from the S_N2 position of intracellular phospholipids. The enzyme cyclooxygenase oxygenates arachidonic acid to prostaglandin G_2 (PGG_2), which is rapidly converted to prostaglandin H_2 (PGH_2) by the peroxidase activity of cyclooxygenase (Fig. 18-10). From here PGH_2 undergoes cell-specific isomerization and or reduction to create the major biologically active prostanoids PGD_2, PGE_2, PGF_2, prostacyclin (PGI_2), or thromboxane A_2. TXA_2 is the predominant cyclooxygenase product formed from arachidonic acid in human platelets.

TABLE 18-5. New Antiplatelet Treatments

1. Thromboxane (TXA_2) synthase inhibitors
2. Thromboxane receptor inhibitors (TXA_2/PGH_2)
3. Dual TXA_2 synthase–TXA_2/PGH_2 receptor inhibitors
4. Platelet glycoprotein lb integrin inhibitors
5. von Willebrand factor inhibitors
6. Platelet purinoceptor antagonists
7. Prostacyclin and analogues
8. Recombinant CD39
9. Nitroester of aspirin (NCX4016)
10. Trapidil
11. Triflusal

TXA_2 is neither stored in platelets nor is it formed in the absence of activation.[326]

Arachidonic acid metabolism also takes place in the vessel wall, where the major product is prostacyclin. PGI_2 actions include that of a platelet inhibitor and vasodilator. Arachidonic acid metabolism is identical in the vessel wall to its metabolism in platelets except for the last step, which, in endothelium leads to prostacyclin (by prostacyclin synthase) formation, and in platelets leads to TXA_2 formation (by thromboxane synthase).

TXA_2 mediates its actions by binding to specific receptors located on platelet membranes. At one time it was thought that all of the biological activities of the arachidonic acid cascade were attributable to TXA_2 and that PGH_2 was confined to the role of a simple metabolic precursor. However, it has become clear that PGH_2 can exert the same effects as TXA_2 on platelets. In fact, the affinity of PGH_2 for the thromboxane receptor is actually greater than is the affinity of TXA_2, and it is actually a more powerful platelet aggregator. The importance of this unique quality of PGH_2 will become apparent later when thromboxane synthase inhibition is discussed. While it would appear that PGH_2 exerts its action by binding to the TXA_2 receptor, a distinct receptor subtype specific to PGH_2 cannot be ruled out.[327]

Binding of TXA_2 to the TXA_2/PGH_2 receptor elicits biological responses in platelets. TXA_2 is both a potent platelet-aggregating substance and a vasoconstrictor. It is thought to stimulate platelet aggregation by mobilizing intracellular calcium from the dense tubular system. This release of Ca^{2+} has two distinct biological phases. The first phase is that it further activates phospholipase A_2, causing enhanced activation of arachidonic acid which leads to increased production of TXA_2. The second phase is that it activates the myosin light chain leading to platelet contraction. This leads to secretion of ADP and serotonin; two strong platelet aggregators. It is also thought that TXA_2 inhibits the production of adenylate cyclase, which leads to a reduction of intracellular cyclic AMP. Cyclic AMP inhibits both platelet secretion and aggregation by reducing intracellular Ca^{2+} levels, and its concentration depends on the activity of both adenyl cyclase and phosphodiesterase. Any reduction in adenyl cyclase activity or inhibition of phosphodiesterase would lead to decreased intracellular cyclic AMP and increased platelet activity. The latest findings in the field of prostacyclin and TXA_2 modulators under clinical evaluation have been recently reviewed.[282e]

As discussed earlier, aspirin exerts its antiplatelet effects by acetylating, and thereby inactivating, the enzyme cyclooxygenase that inhibits TXA_2 production. Because platelets do not contain a nucleus and cannot generate more cyclooxygenase, the inhibition of TXA_2 is permanent for the life of the platelet. The antiplatelet benefit of aspirin is complicated by its capacity to block cyclooxygenase in the endothelium, thus preventing the production of PGI_2. Endothelial cells can regenerate cyclooxygenase within a few hours after being inhibited by aspirin. It has been reported that 95% inhibition of the capacity to produce TXA_2 must be achieved before a therapeutic antiplatelet effect is achieved. This then requires an aspirin dose above that necessary to preserve PGI_2 production. The optimal drug is one that inhibits platelet TXA_2 while preserving PGI_2 production in the vascular endothelium. An even better approach would be to use a drug that inhibits platelet TXA_2 production and increases production of PGI_2 by directly inhibiting TXA_2 synthase, thus shunting the substrates to be acted upon by PGI_2 synthase and increasing the production of PGI_2. The following discussion will describe this pharmacologic approach taken to directly inhibit TXA_2 synthase or to directly blocking the actions on the TXA_2 receptor itself.

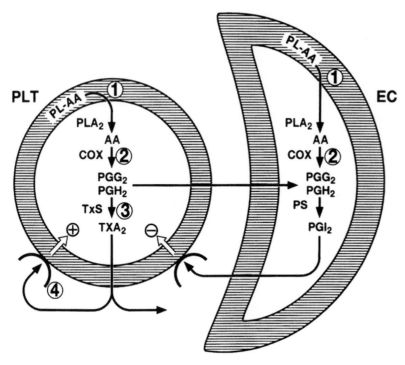

FIGURE 18-10. Platelet (PLT)-endothelial cell (EC) interactions mediated by arachidonic acid (AA) metabolites. Activators of each cell type induce the phospholipase A_2 (PLA_2)-mediated hydrolysis of free AA from membrane phospholipid (PL) pools. Arachidonic acid is converted in each cell type by cyclooxygenase (COX) to prostaglandin endoperoxides PGG_2 and PGH_2. Endoperoxides are metabolized to thromboxane A_2 (TXA_2) by thromboxane synthase (TxS) in platelets and to PGI_2 by prostacyclin synthase (PS) in endothelial cells. TXA_2 binds to platelet receptors to stimulate platelet activation; PGI_2 binds to separate platelet receptors to inhibit platelet activation. (These eicosanoids likewise exert opposing actions on vascular tone, with TXA_2 causing vasoconstriction and PGI_2 causing vasorelaxation.) Endothelial cells can also use platelet-derived endoperoxides as substrate for PS. Antiplatelet agents have targeted AA mobilization from membrane PL pools (1), AA oxygenation by COX (2), thromboxane synthase (3), or TXA_2 receptors (4). (*Adapted with permission from Schafer A: Antiplatelet therapy. Am J Med 101:199–209, 1996.*)

Thromboxane Synthase Inhibitors

To make inhibition of TXA_2 more specific, drugs were designed that are specific inhibitors of thromboxane synthase, the enzyme that converts PGH_2 into thromboxane A_2 (Fig. 18-1). By inhibiting production of TXA_2 without interfering with the production of PGH_2, these drugs indirectly increase the formation of endothelial cell-produced PGI_2. Adding to the antithrombotic effect, this production of prostacyclin precursors by activated platelets occurs at the site of vessel injury where they can exert their greatest influence.

Activated platelets release PGH_2, which is taken up by endothelial cells and converted to PGI_2 by PGI_2 synthase. It was suggested that normal patients treated with thromboxane synthase inhibitors had as much as a threefold increase in circulating PGI_2.[327] Despite this laboratory finding, early clinical studies with these drugs have been disappointing. In 1990, Fiddler and Lumley reviewed the clinical studies of TXA_2 synthase inhibitors and TXA_2 receptor blockers that had been tested over the previous 10 years. The prototype TXA_2 synthase inhibitor dazoxiben was studied in several separate trials in patients with stable angina, with little or no clinical benefit.[328] It should be noted, however, that TXA_2 and its metabolites do not appear to be elevated in patients with stable angina, possibly accounting for the negative findings.[328] There were three small studies demonstrating the effect of dazoxiben on peripheral vascular disease, that showed mixed results at best. These results are disappointing, especially because Reilly et al had demonstrated previously an increased production of TXA_2 in nine patients with peripheral vascular disease. They also demonstrated that the administration of a TXA_2 synthase inhibitor displayed incomplete inhibition of TXA_2 synthesis and evidence for continued platelet activation in vivo.[329] Studies using dazoxiben have been performed in a variety of clinical situations, including cardiopulmonary bypass, hemodialysis, adult respiratory distress syndrome (ARDS), and Raynaud's disease with similar disappointing results. One of the explanations given for the failure of thromboxane synthase inhibitors to provide clinical benefit is that certain endoperoxides accumulate in the presence of thromboxane synthase inhibition (such as PGH_2), which can substitute for TXA_2 and cause platelet aggregation (Fig. 18-11). The affinity of PGH_2 for the platelet receptor is higher than the affinity of TXA_2 and it is even more potent than TXA_2 in inducing platelet aggregation. Because the receptor that TXA_2 acts on is also acted by PGH_2 (with greater affinity) it has been named the TXA_2/PGH_2 receptor.

TXA_2/PGH_2 Receptor Antagonists

Whether or not TXA_2/PGH_2 receptor blockade offers any significant clinical advantage was also reviewed by Fiddler and Lumley.[328] They reported on a number of TXA_2/PGH_2 receptor blockers in a variety of clinical conditions thought to be associated with increased TXA_2 production. Receptor antagonists showed no clinical benefit with exercise-induced angina. This result is consistent with a 1986 report that showed a lack of elevation of TXA_2 metabolites in these patients. In addition, the drug BM13.177 (a TXA_2/PGH_2 receptor antagonist), when administered intravenously, actually induced resting myocardial ischemia in 50% of patients studied. This was thought to be due to a coronary steal mechanism.[330]

In peripheral vascular disease, AH23848 (a TXA_2/PGH_2 receptor antagonist) was compared with aspirin in a double-blind, placebo-controlled trial in which platelet accumulation on mature Dacron aortobifemoral grafts was evaluated. Because TXA_2 and its metabolites are elevated in this disease state, it would stand to reason that a TXA_2 receptor blocker would inhibit peripheral vascular disease. Unlike aspirin, AH23848 significantly reduced platelet deposition on the grafts.[331]

Dual TXA_2 Inhibition and TXA_2/PGH_2 Receptor Antagonism

Two independent studies were done with compounds designed to have a dual effect—TXA_2 synthase inhibition and TXA_2/PGH_2 receptor antagonism. The compounds were shown to both inhibit the

FIGURE 18-11. Representation of the arachidonic acid cascade and drugs used in the present study to block the formation or action of thromboxane A$_2$ (TXA$_2$). Aspirin, by blocking cyclooxygenase, prevents further metabolism of arachidonic acid, thus inhibiting both thromboxane A$_2$ and prostaglandin (PG) formation. Selective inhibitors of thromboxane A$_2$ synthase prevent the conversion of PGH$_2$ to thromboxane A$_2$ without reducing the synthesis of PGI$_2$. In fact, the excess of PGH$_2$ formed in the presence of thromboxane A$_2$ synthase inhibition may be shunted toward the synthesis of PGD$_2$, PGE$_2$, and PGI$_2$ (*hatched arrows*). In addition, PGH$_2$ itself may directly stimulate the same receptor shared with thromboxane A$_2$ (*light gray arrow*). Finally, the effects of thromboxane A$_2$ can be prevented by selective thromboxane A$_2$/PGH$_2$-receptor antagonists. (*Adapted with permission from Golino P, Ambrosio G, Villari B, et al: Endogenous prostaglandin endoperoxides may alter infarct size in the presence of thromboxane synthase inhibition: Studies in a rabbit model of coronary artery occlusion-reperfusion. J Am Coll Cardiol 21(2):493–501, 1993.*)

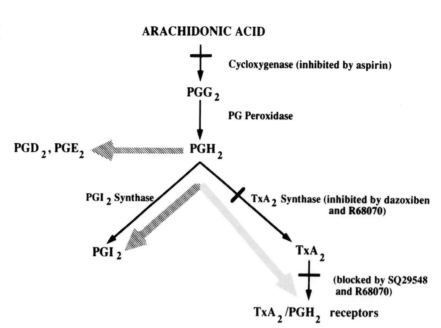

production of TXA$_2$ and to increase the production of the antithrombogenic prostaglandin PGI$_2$. The compounds were also shown to inhibit platelet aggregation, induced by various proaggregatory stimuli.[332,333] Another such agent deserving of further study appears to be BM-531.[334] Hoet et al studied a combined TXA$_2$/PGH$_2$ receptor antagonist and TXA$_2$ synthase inhibitor (R68070), and compared it with aspirin, in an in vivo setting.[335] They found that while aspirin and R68070 both significantly inhibited TXA$_2$-dependent reactions, R68070 was more powerful than aspirin in prolonging the bleeding time. In addition, serum PGI$_2$ was completely inhibited by aspirin, while being stimulated by R68070. These results suggested that R68070, by virtue of its ability to increase PGI$_2$ production, could be a more powerful platelet inhibitor than aspirin.[335]

Although there is a relative paucity of clinical trials in human subjects testing the effectiveness of combined TXA$_2$ synthase inhibition/receptor antagonism, there are in vivo studies reporting its effectiveness in inhibiting thrombosis.

A comparison of aspirin, a 5HT$_2$ (5-hydroxytryptamine-2) antagonist (ZM 170809) and a combined TXA$_2$ synthase inhibitor/receptor antagonist (ZD 1542) as adjuncts to t-PA was reported on by McAuliffe et al.[336] Tissue plasminogen activator (t-PA) with either aspirin, ZM 170809, ZD 1542, or saline was given to dogs with thrombosed left-circumflex coronary arteries. They found that both ZD 1542 and ZM 170809 significantly reduced the time taken to lyse the thrombus as compared with the saline group. Aspirin did not offer any benefit to using t-PA alone. In addition, they found that the number of dogs in which the artery reoccluded was significantly less in the group receiving ZM 170809 or ZD 1542 than in the aspirin or control groups.

Evidence from both in vivo and in vitro studies shows that the effects of thrombolytic therapy can be inhibited by enhanced platelet activation. All the studies described show the effectiveness of TXA$_2$ synthase inhibitors/receptor blockers such as picotamide in preventing thrombosis following thrombolysis. Most of the studies show that having a TXA$_2$ synthase inhibitor combined with a TXA$_2$/PGH$_2$ receptor blocker is far superior to either therapy alone. Platelet activation leads to the release of proaggregatory and vasoconstricting substances such as 5HT$_2$ and TXA$_2$. Because both 5HT$_2$ and TXA$_2$ act independently, a combination of both therapies would be

expected to act in synergy with one another. Further studies evaluating the effects of TXA$_2$ inhibition combined with 5HT$_2$ inhibition need to be performed.

Because TXA$_2$ synthase inhibitors/receptor blockers have proven themselves in animal experiments as superior to aspirin as an adjunct in thrombolytic therapy, clinical studies using this treatment in human patients undergoing thrombolysis and angioplasty were performed.

Timmermans et al compared the standard therapy of aspirin and a calcium-channel antagonist with ridogrel (a dual TXA$_2$ synthase inhibitor/receptor blocker) in 30 patients undergoing PTCA.[337] Each patient was given ridogrel during PTCA and then followed up at 6 months. None of the patients had early reocclusion, as opposed to 5.6% of patients treated with the standard therapy who underwent PTCA during this period. Serum TXA$_2$ was almost completely suppressed, and PGF$_1$ was significantly elevated as early as 2 h after receiving ridogrel.[337] Subsequent studies using dual-TXA$_2$ synthase inhibitor/receptor blocker drugs for preventing postangioplasty restenosis have shown no apparent benefit (see Chap. 40).

Clearly there needs to be more in vivo human studies that test the effects of TXA$_2$ inhibition and its effects on thrombolysis. There is already a great abundance of information characterizing aspirin and its effects on thrombolysis. As mentioned previously, ISIS-2 convincingly demonstrated the benefit of aspirin as cojoint treatment in patients undergoing thrombolysis. If TXA$_2$ synthase inhibitors/receptor blockers are going to have a major role in this field, there must be studies comparing the effects of TXA$_2$ synthase inhibition/receptor blockade with aspirin. The Ridogrel Versus Aspirin Patency Trial (RAPT) compared the efficacy of ridogrel with that of aspirin for enhancing coronary reperfusion in approximately 900 patients with acute myocardial infarction receiving thrombolytic therapy.[338] Coronary patency as determined by angiography did not differ greatly in the two groups (70.5% vs 73.7%). However, over a long-term follow up, there was a significant (32%) decrease in the incidence of new ischemic events in the patients who took ridogrel, in contrast to the patients who took aspirin. These results indicate that ridogrel is not superior to aspirin in potentiating thrombolysis and preventing rethrombosis, but it may be more effective than aspirin in preventing new ischemic events in the weeks to months after myocardial infarction. Although ridogrel did not prove to be superior to aspirin in the setting of an acute myocardial infarction, it is safe and well tolerated. Therefore, ridogrel could be a perfectly acceptable alternative to aspirin in patients with an acute myocardial infarction who cannot tolerate aspirin because of allergy.[339] However, for patients who have no adverse reaction to aspirin, ridogrel has no apparent benefit. A more recent study by Tranchesi et al[340] confirmed the findings of the RAPT study.

Miscellaneous Uses

There have been a number of recent reports assessing the role of TXA_2 synthase inhibitors/receptor blockers in other cardiovascular diseases. Ritter et al[341] studied the effects of ridogrel in patients with uncomplicated essential hypertension. Although excretion of TXA_2 metabolites was decreased and vasodilatory prostaglandin metabolites were increased, blood pressure did not differ significantly between ridogrel and placebo treatment periods. This study confirmed the findings of an earlier study by Kudo that showed that OKY-0469, a TXA_2 synthase inhibitor/receptor blocker, had no effect on blood pressure, but did augment the hypotensive effect of captopril.[342]

TXA_2 may, by virtue of its being a potent vaso- and bronchoconstrictor as well as platelet aggregator, be an important mediator in circulatory shock. Patel et al studied the effects of SQ-29548, a potent TXA_2 receptor blocker in a rat model of circulatory shock. They found that in combination with leukotriene receptor antagonism, SQ-29548 caused a significant prolongation in survival time, and a prolongation of circulatory compensation.[343]

Conclusion

Aspirin is of great benefit in a number of cardiovascular conditions with minimal side effects. It has been thoroughly studied and is extremely cost-effective. For TXA_2 synthase inhibitors/receptor blockers to replace aspirin, they must demonstrate superior effectiveness for these same cardiovascular conditions. Several studies in experimental animals show TXA_2 synthase inhibitors/receptor blockers to be superior to aspirin as an adjunct to thrombolysis. These results, however, were not duplicated in humans studies. Quite the contrary; recent studies show no benefit of ridogrel over aspirin in potentiating fibrinolysis and preventing rethrombosis. This could be explained by a number of different mechanisms. Ridogrel has only modest receptor antagonism and the loss of vasodilator function in the endothelium in an evolving myocardial infarction could be used to explain the lack of efficacy in these patients. The discussion made no distinction between the various TXA_2 synthase inhibitors/receptor antagonists, but it is possible that a drug with more potent receptor blocking properties could prove to be more effective than aspirin, TXA_2 synthase inhibitors/receptor blockers are potent inhibitors of TXA_2 production and powerful preservers of PGI_2 production by various in vivo and in vitro studies. Yet, clinically, their effectiveness is limited. An effective inhibition of the arachidonic acid pathway is not associated with enhanced clinical effectiveness. Clearly, other pathways of platelet activation not affected by arachidonic acid must be involved, as demonstrated by the efficacy of specific antithrombotic therapies aimed at the GP IIb/IIIa fibrinogen receptor. Given the cost, paucity of clinical trials, and lack of clinical benefit, when compared to aspirin, one cannot help but to conclude that there is little place for TXA_2 inhibition at this time in the treatment and prevention of cardiovascular disorders.

Glycoprotein Ib Antagonists

Circulating platelets will adhere to the subendothelial vasculature matrix during vascular injury by the attachment of the platelet GP Ib glycoprotein to von Willebrand factor.[344] The binding of GP Ib receptors can also make the GP IIb/IIIa receptors functional for platelet aggregation. The vascular biology of the GP Ib-IX-V complex was recently reviewed.[344] The authors point out that the GP Ib-IX-V complex regulates shear dependent adhesion and aggregation of platelets and may provide a suitable target for therapeutic intervention.

Monoclonal antibodies against both GP Ib and von Willebrand factor have antithrombotic actions in animal models.[345] Clinical studies still need to be done.

Another novel approach to inhibit thrombogenesis may be by targeting adhesive proteins, such as P-selectin, and their interaction with leukocytes and tissue factor.[346]

P_2T-Purinoceptor Antagonists

The P_2T-purinoceptor [now called P2Y(12)][347] antagonist FPL67085 (now AR-C67085MX) and others are currently in clinical development as infusible antithrombotic agents for acute use. They are potent selective inhibitors of ADP-induced platelet aggregation (similar to the mechanism of ticlopidine and clopidogrel).[348] ADP receptors and their inhibition were recently reviewed.[349]

Analogues of Prostacyclin

Prostacyclin and its analogues are potent inhibitors of platelet activation and are discussed in Chap. 25.

CD39

A new class of antiplatelet agents may be derived from the observation that CD39, an endothelial cell ectoenzyme, inhibits platelet activation by metabolizing ADP and ATP. A recombinant soluble form of CD39 has now been prepared and may be useful as an antithrombotic agent.[350]

Cilostazol

Cilostazol, a specific inhibitor of phosphodiesterase-3 (see Chap. 50), is an effective inhibitor of agonist and shear-stress-induced platelet aggregation.[351] Cilostazol has similar antiplatelet effects to ticlopidine. In combination with aspirin, it appears to be as effective as aspirin plus ticlopidine after primary angioplasty and stent implantation.[352]

Trapidil

Trapidil (triazolopyrimidine) is an antiplatelet agent that also acts as a platelet-derived growth factor agonist. It has been used with aspirin to reduce cardiovascular events in MI patients after thrombolysis or angioplasty.[353]

NCX 4016

NCX 4016, a nitroester of aspirin, displays antiaggregatory and antithrombotic activity by a dual mechanism of action involving inhibition of cyclooxygenase and release of nitric oxide. In animal studies, it reduces infarct size,[354] and may reduce restenosis after PTCA.[354a]

Triflusal

Triflusal is an antiplatelet drug that is similar and structurally related to aspirin, but which has several notable differences in its mechanism of action. In a clinical trial following acute MI, it had comparable efficacy and fewer complications than aspirin.[355]

OTHER ANTICOAGULATION APPROACHES

A new generation of anticoagulants are being developed (Table 18-6), some of which were recently approved for clinical use.

Tissue Factor Pathway Inhibitors

Tissue factor (TF), a low-molecular-weight glycoprotein, is a major regulator of coagulation through the extrinsic coagulation cascade. TF is located away from the luminal surface of the blood vessels and is present in the adventitia and in the media, though less so in the latter. It was found that advanced atheromatous lesions, especially the lipid core, are rich in TF produced by monocyte-derived macrophages. Upon plaque rupture, TF is exposed to the circulating blood and initiates the coagulation cascade with thrombus formation leading to unstable coronary syndromes.[356,357] Tissue factor pathway inhibitor (TFPI) is a naturally occurring multivalent coagulation inhibitor that binds and makes an inactive complex consisting of TF, TFPI, factor VIIa, and factor Xa, inhibiting the TF-dependent coagulation cascade. In normal arteries, TFPI is found in the endothelium and its presence increased in atherosclerotic vessels.[358] The effects of TFPI can be reversed by an infusion of rVIIa.[359]

Anti-TF antibodies and recombinant TFPI have been studied in several animal models. These studies show that local irrigation with TFPI at the time of arterial intervention on an animal atherosclerotic artery can inhibit intimal hyperplasia and thrombus formation.[360,361] Recently, it was reported that adenoviral gene transfer of TFPI to balloon-injured atherosclerotic arteries in rabbits could decelerate the hyperplastic response to injury in the absence of changes in the hemostatic system.[362]

A nematode anticoagulant protein, NAPc2, binds to a noncatalytic site in both factors X and Xa, and inhibits factor VIIa within the factor VIIa/TF complex. Because it binds to factor Xa, the drug has a very long half-life. Studies are now in progress evaluating NAPc2 for the prevention of venous thrombosis in patients who are at high risk for venous thromboembolic disease.

In addition, a soluble, mutant form of TF has been expressed that has reduced function for factor VIIa-mediated activation of factor X. Also available is an active site-blocked factor VIIa (factor VIIA),

TABLE 18-6. New Antithrombotic Treatments

1. New low-molecular-weight heparins
2. Heparinoids (e.g., Danaparoid)
3. Direct thrombin inhibitors (e.g., hirudin, hirulog)
4. Tissue factor pathway inhibitors (TFPI)
5. Factor Xa inhibitors (fondaparinux)
6. Protein C
7. Thrombomodulin
8. Antithrombin III

which acts as an anticoagulant by competing with factor VIIa for TF binding.[265]

Factor Xa Inhibitors

The direct thrombin inhibitors do not affect thrombin generation and may not inhibit all available thrombin.[363] The inhibition of factor Xa can prevent thrombin from being generated while at the same time disrupting the thrombin feedback loop which amplifies additional thrombin[363,364] production.

Selective inhibition of factor Xa with the recombinant tick anticoagulant peptide (TAP) was shown to be a useful adjunct to thrombolytics in animals undergoing electrically induced coronary thrombosis.[363] TAP has potential use in treating heparin-resistant arterial thrombosis and as an adjunct treatment with thrombolysis.[363]

TAP appears to be more effective than TFPI in maintaining arterial patency after thrombolysis. Synthetic inhibitors of factor Xa have been synthesized, which can be used both intravenously and orally (e.g., DX-9065a, SEL2711), as effective inhibitors of arterial and venous thrombus formation in several animal models.[365] Another novel synthetic inhibitor of factor Xa, ZK-807834, decreases early arterial reocclusion after thrombolysis in dogs and improves 24-h patency,[366] without increasing bleeding as compared with heparin/aspirin. ZK-807834 also appeared more effective than TAP.

Another novel approach to factor Xa inhibition has been taken by synthesizing the critical pentasaccharide of heparin that is the binding site of heparin to antithrombin III.[367,367a] This agent, previously known as SR90107A/ORG 31540, is now called fondaparinux. It has been used successfully as a prophylactic anticoagulant for the prevention of deep-vein thrombosis during hip surgery[368] and as a treatment for deep-vein thrombosis.[369] It is now approved by the FDA for prophylaxis to prevent venous thromboembolic disease in total hip replacement, total knee replacement, and hip fracture surgery at a dose of 2.5 mg daily by subcutaneous injection.[370–373] In clinical trials in orthopedic surgery, fondaparinux was started 6 h postoperatively and shown to be more effective than LMWH. When used in patients undergoing coronary angioplasty, administration of the pentasaccharide led to the inhibition of thrombin generation without modification of the aPTT and activated clotting time. Vessel closure rate was similar to rates seen in prior trials. Additional clinical trials are underway.

Although the results with fondaparinux were better than with LMWH, it is possible that the improved results were because of the timing of dosing in close proximity to surgery instead of the next day, and not because of an inherent superiority of fondaparinux to LMWH.[374] Others believe that the difference is due to the longer duration of action of fondaparinux.[375] It should be noted that the aPTT is not affected by this dose of fondaparinux and clinical monitoring is not recommended.[376] Additional clinical data support its potential benefits in arterial thrombotic disorders.[377]

Protein C

Protein C is a natural anticoagulant that when activated selectively degrades the coagulation cofactors Va and VIIIa, thereby inhibiting thrombosis.[378] Activated protein C interrupts the feedback actions of thrombin on the coagulation cascade. The action of activated protein C is enhanced by protein S, another vitamin K-dependent plasma protein.[379] A deficiency or reduced response to activated protein C is associated with an increased risk for vascular diseases.

Protein C can be isolated from plasma or obtained by use of recombinant technology. Its antithrombotic activity has been demonstrated in animals, but it is associated with significant bleeding.[380]

A novel protein C activator has been identified, which when infused into monkeys, can cause dose-dependent, reversible anticoagulation without consumption of fibrinogen, coagulation factors, or platelet activation, and without prolongation of the bleeding time.

Reduced levels of activated protein C are found in the majority of patients with sepsis. In sepsis, due to the inflammatory cytokines (TNF-α, IL-β, IL-6), thrombomodulin is down regulated, resulting in a decreased level of activated protein C, thereby increasing thrombosis and decreasing fibrinolysis. It is also found that activated protein C has anti-inflammatory properties by inhibiting production of inflammatory cytokines.[381] Recombinant activated protein C is now approved for clinical use to reduce the coagulation and inflammatory changes in severe sepsis, while reducing mortality.[382]

Synthetic Oral Antithrombin

Another approach currently under development is the use of synthetic oral antithrombin. Melagatran is a synthetic antithrombin with antithrombotic effect that must be given intravenously.[383] An oral prodrug H 376/95, also called ximelagatran, has been synthesized and is undergoing clinical development.[384]

Oral Heparin

An additional approach to oral anticoagulation is the development of agents that enhance the intestinal absorption of heparin. These agents have been administered to humans and show anticoagulant activity.[385] The same approach to an oral LMWH might show promise.

Thrombomodulin

Thrombomodulin is an endothelial cell-surface protein that complexes with thrombin, causing it to lose its coagulant activity while promoting the production of the endogenous anticoagulant protein C.[363,386] Thrombomodulin is present on the endothelial cells of most blood vessels including those of the heart. Studies show that mutations in the promoter region of the thrombomodulin gene may constitute a risk factor for arterial thrombosis.[387] Novel recombinant soluble human thrombomodulin, ART-123, activates the protein C pathway in healthy volunteers,[388] and prolongs the thrombin time, prothrombin time, and aPPT.

High circulating levels of thrombomodulin were found in patients with sepsis[389] and organ dysfunction. Purified soluble thrombomodulin from human urine (MR-33) has been studied in rat disseminated intravascular coagulation (DIC) models and shown to improve hematologic abnormalities without excessive prolongation of the aPTT and bleeding time. Clinical trials evaluating MR33 for the treatment of DIC are now in progress.[390]

Antithrombin III

Antithrombin is a natural plasma protein that inactivates free thrombin and factor Xa. Concentrations of human plasma antithrombin C462 are available; they are given with heparin to maximize the inhibition of factor Xa and thrombin. Numerous studies of antithrombin

supplementation in sepsis have been reported over the last 20 years. Since 1993, four placebo-controlled randomized studies have been performed in Europe showing a 22% reduction in 30-day all-cause mortality.[391]

Preliminary trials of antithrombin supplementation with heparin treatment during PTCA[392] and cardiopulmonary bypass,[393] have shown less activation of coagulation and a reduction in restenosis.

Antithrombin therapy is now clinically approved for the treatment of antithrombin deficiency during periods of increased thrombotic risk.

Conclusion

New anticoagulants that may provide advantages over conventional anticoagulants are available, but the safety and efficacy of these new approaches need to be established in clinical trials.

REFERENCES

1. Colman RW, Marder VJ, Salzman EW, Hirsh J: Overview of hemostasis. In: Colman RW, Hirsh J, Marder VJ, Salzman EW, eds. *Hemostasis and Thrombosis: Basic Principles and Clinical Practice*. 3d ed. Philadelphia: JB Lippincott, 1994:3.
2. Bennett JS: Mechanisms of platelet adhesion and aggregation: An update. *Hosp Prac* 15:70, 1992.
3. Detwiler TC, Charo IP, Feinman RD: Evidence that calcium regulates platelet function. *Thromb Haemost* 40:207, 1978.
4. Coller BS: Blood elements at surfaces: Platelets. *Ann N Y Acad Sci* 516:362, 1987.
5. Hirsh J, Salzman EW, Marder VJ, Colman RW: Overview of the thrombotic process and its therapy. In: Colman RW, Hirsh J, Marder VJ, Salzman EW, eds. *Hemostasis and Thrombosis: Basic Principles and Clinical Practice*. 3d ed. Philadelphia: JB Lippincott, 1994: 1151.
6. Davies MJ: Mechanisms of thrombosis in atherosclerosis. In: Colman RW, Hirsh J, Marder VJ, Salzman EW, eds. *Hemostasis and Thrombosis: Basic Principles and Clinical Practice*. 3d ed. Philadelphia: JB Lippincott, 1994:1224.
7. Faggiotto A, Ross R, Harker L: Studies of hypercholesterolemia in the nonhuman primate. I. Changes that lead to fatty streak formation. *Arteriosclerosis* 4:323, 1984.
7a. Mann JM, Davies MJ: Vulnerable plaque: Relation of characteristics to degree of stenosis in human coronary arteries. *Circulation* 94:928, 1996.
8. Richardson PD, Davies MJ, Born GBR: Influence of plaque configuration and stress distribution of fissuring of coronary atherosclerotic plaques. *Lancet* 2:941, 1989.
9. Steering Committee of the Physician's Health Study Research Group: Final Report on the Aspirin Component of the Ongoing Physician's Health Study. *N Engl J Med* 321:129, 1989.
10. Lee G, Garcia JM, Corso PJ, et al: Correlation of coronary angioscopic to angiographic findings in coronary artery disease. *Am J Cardiol* 58:238, 1986.
11. Ip JH, Fuster V, Israel D, Chesbro JH: Evolution, progression, and clinical manifestation of atherosclerosis. In: Colman RW, Hirsh J, Marder VJ, Salzman EW, eds. *Hemostasis and Thrombosis: Basic Principles and Clinical Practice*. 3d ed. Philadelphia: JB Lippincott, 1994:1379.
12. Ault KA, Cannon CP, Mitchell J, et al: Platelet activation in patients after an acute coronary syndrome: Results from the TIMI-12 trial. *J Am Coll Cardiol* 33:634, 1999.
13. Frishman WH, Miller KP: Platelets and antiplatelet therapy in ischemic heart disease. *Curr Probl Cardiol* 11:73, 1986.
14. Frishman WH, Cheng-Lai A, Chen J, eds: *Current Cardiovascular Drugs*. 3d ed. Philadelphia: Current Medicine, 2000:85.
15. Antiplatelet Trialist's Collaboration: Secondary prevention of vascular disease by prolonged anti-platelet treatment. *BMJ* 296:320, 1988.
16. Awtry EH, Loscalzo J: Aspirin. *Circulation* 101:1206, 2000.
17. Schafer AI: Antiplatelet therapy. *Am J Med* 101:199, 1996.

18. Miller, KP, Frishman WH: Platelets and anti-platelet therapy in ischemic heart disease. *Med Clin North Am* 72:117, 1988.

19. Patrono C, Coller B, Dalen JE, et al: Platelet-active drugs: The relationships among dose, effectiveness, and side effects. *Chest* 119(Suppl 1):39S, 2001.

20. Moncada S, Vane JR: The role of prostacyclin in vascular tissue. *Fed Proc* 38:66, 1979.

21. Preston FE, Whipps S, Jackson CA, et al: Inhibition of prostacyclin and platelet thromboxane A2 after low-dose aspirin. *N Engl J Med* 304:76, 1981.

22. Clarke RJ, Mayo G, Price P, et al: Suppression of thromboxane A_2 but not of systemic prostacyclin by controlled-release aspirin. *N Engl J Med* 324:1137, 1991.

23. Taylor DW, Barnett HJ, Haynes RB, et al: Low-dose and high-dose acetylsalicylic acid for patients undergoing carotid endarterectomy: A randomised controlled trial. ASA and Carotid Endarterectomy (ACE) Trial Collaborators. *Lancet* 353:2179, 1999.

24. Ridker PM, Manson JE, Graziano M, et al: Low-dose aspirin therapy for chronic stable angina: A randomized, placebo-controlled clinical trial. *Ann Intern Med* 114:835, 1991.

25. Chesebro JH, Webster MWI, Smith HC, et al: Antiplatelet therapy in coronary disease progression: Reduced infarction and new lesion formation. *Circulation* 80(Suppl 11):266, 1989.

26. Juul-Moller S, Edvardsson N, Jahnmatz B, et al: Double-blind trial of aspirin in primary prevention of myocardial infarction in patients with stable chronic angina pectoris. The Swedish Angina Pectoris Aspirin Trial (SAPAT) Group. *Lancet* 340:1421, 1992.

27. Lewis HD, Davis JW, Archibald DG, et al: Protective effects of aspirin against myocardial infarction and death in men with unstable angina. *N Engl J Med* 309:396, 1983.

28. Cairns JA, Gent M, Singer J, et al: Aspirin, sulfinpyrazone, or both in unstable angina. N Engl J Med 313:1369, 1985.

29. Theroux P, Quimet H, McCans J, et al: Aspirin, heparin, or both to treat acute unstable angina. *N Engl J Med* 320:1014, 1989.

30. The RISC Group: Risk of myocardial infarction and death during treatment with low-dose aspirin and intravenous heparin in men with unstable coronary artery disease. *Lancet* 336:827, 1990.

31. Oler A, Whooley MA, Oler J, Grady D: Adding heparin to aspirin reduces the incidence of myocardial infarction and death in patients with unstable angina. *JAMA* 276:811, 1996.

32. Kennon S, Price CP, Mills PG, et al: The effect of aspirin on C-reactive protein as a marker of risk in unstable angina. *J Am Coll Cardiol* 37:1266, 2001.

33. Manson JE, Grobbee DE, Stampfer MJ, et al: Aspirin in the primary prevention of angina pectoris in a randomized trial of United States physicians. *Am J Med* 89:772, 1990.

34. Steering Committee of the Physicians' Health Study Research Group: Final report on the aspirin component of the ongoing Physicians' Health Study. *N Engl J Med* 321:129, 1989.

35. Peto R, Gray R, Collins R, et al: Randomized trial of prophylactic daily aspirin in British male doctors. *BMJ* 296:313, 1988.

36. Manson JE, Stampfer MJ, Colditz GA, et al: A prospective study of aspirin use and primary prevention of cardiovascular disease in women. *JAMA* 266:521, 1991.

37. de Gaetano G: Collaborative Group of the Primary Prevention Project (PPP): Low-dose aspirin and vitamin E in people at cardiovascular risk: A randomised trial in general practice. *Lancet* 357:89, 2001.

38. Stafford RS: Aspirin use is low among United States outpatients with coronary artery disease. *Circulation* 101:1097, 2000.

38a. Jackson EA, Sivasubramian R, Spencer FA, et al: Changes over time in the use of aspirin in patients hospitalized with acute myocardial infarction (1975-1997): A population-based prospective. *Am Heart J* 144:259, 2002.

39. The Persantine-Aspirin Reinfarction Study Research Group: Persantine and aspirin in coronary artery disease. *Circulation* 62:449, 1980.

40. The Aspirin Myocardial Infarction Study Research Group: The aspirin myocardial infarction study: final results. *Circulation* 62 (Suppl V):V79, 1980.

41. Breddin K, Loew D, Lechner K, et al: The German-Austrian Aspirin Trial: A comparison of acetylsalicylic acid, placebo and phenprocoumon in secondary prevention of myocardial infarction. *Circulation* 62(Suppl V):V63, 1980.

42. Elwood PC, Cochrane AL, Burr ML, et al: A randomized controlled trial of acetylsalicylic acid in the secondary prevention of mortality from myocardial infarction. *Br Med J* 1:436, 1974.

43. Elwood PC, Sweetnam PM: Aspirin and secondary mortality after myocardial infarction. *Circulation* 62(Suppl V):V53, 1980.

44. The Coronary Drug Project Research Group: Aspirin in coronary heart disease. *Circulation* 62(Suppl V):V59, 1980.

45. Climt CR, Knatterud GL, Stamler J: Persantine-Aspirin Reinfarction Study II. Secondary coronary prevention with persantine and aspirin. *J Am Coll Cardiol* 7:251, 1986.

46. Aspirin after myocardial infarction. *Lancet* 1:1172, 1980.

47. Goldstein RE, Andrews M, Hall W, et al: Marked reduction in long-term cardiac deaths with aspirin after a coronary event. *J Am Coll Cardiol* 28:326, 1996.

48. ACC/AHA Guidelines for the Management of Patients with Acute Myocardial Infarction. Executive Summary and Recommendations. A Report of the American College of Cardiology/American Heart Association Task Force on Practice Guidelines (Committee on Management of Acute Myocardial Infarction). *Circulation* 100:1016, 1999.

49. Hart RG, Halperin JL, McBride R, et al: Aspirin for the primary prevention of stroke and other major vascular events: Meta-analysis and hypotheses. *Arch Neurol* 57:306, 2000.

50. De Wood MA, Spores J, Notske R, et al: Prevalence of total coronary occlusion during the early hours of transmural infarction. *N Engl J Med* 303:897, 1980.

51. Fitzgerald DJ, Catella R, Roy L, et al: Marked platelet activation in vivo after intravenous streptokinase in patients with acute myocardial infarction. *Circulation* 77:142, 1988.

52. ISIS-2 (Second International Study of Infarct Survival) Collaborative Group: Randomized trial of intravenous streptokinase, oral aspirin, both, or neither among 17,187 cases of suspected acute myocardial infarction: ISIS-2. *Lancet* 2:349, 1988.

53. Ohman EM, Harrington RA, Cannon CP, et al: Intravenous thrombolysis in acute myocardial infarction. *Chest* 119(Suppl 1):253S, 2001.

54. Frishman WH, Chiu R, Landzberg BR, Weiss M: Medical therapies for the prevention of restenosis after percutaneous coronary interventions. *Curr Probl Cardiol* 23:533, 1998.

55. Lam JYT, Chesebro JH, Steel PM, et al: Is vasopressin related to platelet deposition? Relationship in a porcine preparation of arterial injury in vivo. *Circulation* 75:243, 1987.

56. White CW, Chaitman B, Ticlopidine Study Group: Antiplatelet agents are effective in reducing the immediate complications of PTCA: Results from the ticlopidine multicenter trial (abstr.). *Circulation* 76(Suppl IV):IV-400, 1987.

57. Schwartz L, Bourassa MG, Lesperance J, et al: Aspirin and dipyridamole in the prevention of restenosis after percutaneous transluminal coronary angioplasty. *N Engl J Med* 318:1714, 1988.

58. Barnathan ES, Schwartz JS, Taylor L, et al: Aspirin and dipyridamole in the prevention of acute coronary thrombosis complicating coronary angioplasty. *Circulation* 76:125, 1987.

59. Hall P, Nakamura S, Maiello L, et al: A randomized comparison of combined ticlopidine and aspirin therapy versus aspirin therapy alone after successful intravascular ultrasound-guided stent implantation. *Circulation* 93:215, 1996.

60. Muller C, Buttner HJ, Petersen J, Roskamm H: A randomized comparison of clopidogrel and aspirin versus ticlopidine and aspirin after the placement of coronary-artery stents. *Circulation* 101(6):590, 2000.

61. Lytle W, Loop FD, Cosgrove DM, et al: Long-term (5 to 12 years) serial studies of internal mammary artery and saphenous vein coronary bypass grafts. *J Thorac Cardiovasc Surg* 89:248, 1985.

62. Spray TL, Roberts WC: Changes in saphenous veins used as aorto-coronary bypass grafts. *Am Heart J* 94:500, 1977.

63. Brown BG, Cukingnan RA, DeRouen T, et al: Improved graft patency in patients treated with platelet-inhibiting therapy after coronary bypass surgery. *Circulation* 72:138, 1985.

64. Chesebro JH, Fuster V, Elveback LR, et al: Effect of dipyridamole and aspirin on late vein-graft patency after coronary artery bypass operations. *N Engl J Med* 310:209, 1984.

65. Goldman S, Copeland J, Moritz T, et al: Improvement in early saphenous vein graft patency after coronary artery bypass surgery with antiplatelet therapy: Results of a Veterans Administration Cooperative study. *Circulation* 77:1324, 1988.

66. Goldman S, Copeland J, Moritz T, et al: Saphenous vein graft patency 1 year after coronary artery bypass surgery and effects of antiplatelet

therapy: Results of a Veterans Administration Cooperative study. *Circulation* 80:1190, 1989.

67. Goldman S, Zadina K, Krasnicka B, et al: Predictors of graft patency 3 years after coronary artery bypass graft surgery. Department of Veterans Affairs Cooperative Study Group No. 297. *J Am Coll Cardiol* 29:1563, 1997.

68. Yli-Mayry S, Huikuri HV, Korhonen UR, et al: Efficacy and safety of anticoagulant therapy started pre-operatively in preventing coronary vein graft occlusion. *Eur Heart J* 14(5):723, 1993.

69. Gavaghan TP, Gebski V, Baron DW: Immediate postoperative aspirin improves vein graft patency early and late after coronary artery bypass graft surgery. A placebo-controlled, randomized study. *Circulation* 83(5):1526, 1991.

70. UK-TIA Study Group: United Kingdom transient ischemic attack (UK-TIA) aspirin trial: interim results. *BMJ* 296:316, 1988.

71. Antiplatelet Trialist's Collaboration: Collaborative overview of randomized trials of antiplatelet therapy-I: Prevention of death, myocardial infarction, and stroke by prolonged antiplatelet therapy in various categories of patients. *BMJ* 308:81, 1994.

72. The UKTIA Study Group: United Kingdom Transient Ischemic Attack aspirin trial: Final results. *J Neurol Neurosurg Psychiatry* 54:1044, 1991.

73. *Fed Reg* 63:56802, 66015, 1998.

74. CAPRIE Steering Committee: A randomised, blinded, trial of clopidogrel versus aspirin in patients at risk of ischaemic events (CAPRIE). *Lancet* 348:1329, 1996.

75. Diener HC, Cunha L, Forbes C, et al: European Stroke Prevention Study. 2. Dipyridamole and acetylsalicylic acid in the secondary prevention of stroke. *J Neurol Sci* 143(1-2):1, 1996.

75a. Neill KK, Luer MS: Ischemic stroke prevention: An update on antiplatelet therapy. *Neurol Res* 24:381, 2002.

76. Wahl DG, Bounameaux H, de Moerloose P, Sarasin FP: Prophylactic antithrombotic therapy for patients with systemic lupus erythematosus with or without antiphospholipid antibodies. Do the benefits outweigh the risks? A decision analysis. *Arch Intern Med* 160:2042, 2000.

77. Pulmonary Embolism Prevention (PEP) Trial Collaborative Group: Prevention of pulmonary embolism and deep venous thrombosis with low-dose aspirin: Pulmonary Embolism Prevention (PEP) Trial. *Lancet* 355:1295, 2000.

78. Peterson P, Boysen G, Godfredsen J, et al: Placebo-controlled randomized trial of warfarin and aspirin for prevention of thromboembolic complications in chronic atrial fibrillation: The Copenhagen AFASAK Study. *Lancet* 1:175, 1989.

79. Stroke Prevention in Atrial Fibrillation Investigators: Final results. *Circulation* 84:527, 1991.

80. The Stroke Prevention in Atrial Fibrillation Investigators: A comparison of warfarin with aspirin for prevention of thromboembolism in atrial fibrillation: Results of the SPAFII Study. *Lancet* 343:687, 1994.

81. Golzari H, Cebul RD, Bahler RC: Atrial fibrillation restoration and maintenance of sinus rhythm and indications for anticoagulation therapy. *Ann Intern Med* 125:311, 1996.

82. Cleland JG, Cowburn PJ, Falk RH: Should all patients with atrial fibrillation receive warfarin? Evidence from randomized clinical trials. *Eur Heart J* 17(5):674, 1996.

83. Catella-Lawson F, Crofford LJ: Cyclooxygenase inhibition and thrombogenicity. *Am J Med* 110(Suppl 3A):28S, 2001.

84. Jhund PS, Davie AP, McMurray JJV: Aspirin inhibits the acute venodilator response to furosemide in patients with chronic heart failure. *J Am Coll Cardiol* 37:1234, 2001.

85. Handin RJ: Platelets and coronary artery disease. *N Engl J Med* 334:1126, 1996.

85a. Cleland JGF: Is aspirin "the weakest link" in cardiovascular prophylaxis? The surprising lack of evidence supporting the use of aspirin for cardiovascular disease. *Prog Cardiovasc Dis* 44:275, 2002.

86. Fusitani RM, Merdestgaard AG, Marcus CS, et al: Perioperative suppression of platelet adherence to small diameter polytetrafluoroethylene grafts. *J Surg Res* 44:455, 1998.

87. Best LC, McGuire MB, Jones PBB, et al: Mode of action of dipyridamole on human platelets. *Thromb Res* 16:367, 1979.

88. Mehta J, Mehta P, Pepine CJ, et al: Platelet function studies in coronary artery disease. Effect of dipyridamole. *Am J Cardiol* 47:1111, 1981.

89. Cructhley DJ, Ryan JW: Effects of aspirin and dipyridamole on the degradation of adenosine diphosphate by cultured cells derived from bovine pulmonary artery. *J Clin Invest* 66:29, 1989.

90. Chesebro JH, Fuster V, McGoon DC et al: Trial of warfarin plus dipyridamole or aspirin therapy in prosthetic heart valve replacement: danger of aspirin compared with dipyridamole. *Am J Cardiol* 51:1537, 1983.

91. Stein PD, Alpert JS, Bussey HI, et al: Antithrombotic therapy in patients with mechanical and biological prosthetic heart valves. *Chest* 119(Suppl):220S, 2001.

92. Pumphrey CW, Chesebro JH, Dewanjee MK: In vivo quantitation of platelet deposition on human peripheral arterial bypass grafts using indium-111-labeled platelets. *Am J Cardiol* 51:796, 1983.

93. Schwartz L, Bourassa MG, Lesperance J, et al: Aspirin and dipyridamole in the prevention of restenosis after percutaneous transluminal coronary angioplasty. *N Engl J Med* 318:1714, 1988.

94. Keltz T, Innerfeld M, Gitler B, Cooper JA: Dipyridamole-induced myocardial ischemia. *JAMA* 257:1515, 1987.

95. DiMinno G, Cerbone Am, Mattioli PM, et al: Functionally thromboasthenic state in normal platelets following the administration of ticlopidine. *J Clin Invest* 75:328, 1985.

96. Gent M, Blakely JA, Easton JD, et al: The Canadian American Ticlopidine Study in thromboembolic stroke. *Lancet* I:1215, 1989.

97. Hass WK, Easton JD, Adams HP, et al:. A randomized trial comparing ticlopidine hydrochloride with aspirin for the prevention of stroke in high risk patients. *N Engl J Med* 321:501, 1989.

98. Janzon L, Bergqvist D, Boberg J, et al: Prevention of myocardial infarction and stroke in patients with intermittent claudication: Effects of ticlopidine: Results from STIMS, the Swedish Ticlopidine Multicenter Study. *J Intern Med* 227:301, 1990.

99. Limet R, David JL, Magotteau P, et al: Prevention of aorta-coronary bypass graft occlusion. Beneficial effect of ticlopidine on early and late patency rates of venous coronary bypass surgery grafts: A double-blind study. *J Thorac Cardiovasc Surg* 94:773, 1987.

100. Balsano F, Rizzon P, Violi F, et al: Antiplatelet treatment with ticlopidine in unstable angina: a controlled multicenter trial. *Circulation* 82:17, 1990.

101. Schomig A, Neumann FJ, Kastrati A, et al: A randomized comparison of antiplatelet and anticoagulant therapy after the placement of coronary artery stents. *N Engl J Med* 334:1084, 1996.

102. Steinhubl SR, Ellis SG, Wolski K, et al, for the EPISTENT Investigators: Ticlopidine pretreatment before coronary stenting is associated with sustained decrease in adverse cardiac events. Data from the Evaluation of Platelet IIb/IIIa inhibitor for Stenting (EPISTENT) Trial. *Circulation* 103:1403, 2001.

103. Scrutinio D, Cimminiello C, Marubini E, et al, on behalf of the STAMI Group: Ticlopidine versus aspirin after myocardial infarction (STAMI) trial. *J Am Coll Cardiol* 37:1259, 2001.

104. Solet DJ, Zacharski LR, Plehn JF: The role of adenosine 5'-diphosphate receptor blockade in patients with cardiovascular disease. *Am J Med* 111:45, 2001.

105. Marco J, Ariens RAS, Fajadet J, et al: Effect of aspirin and ticlopidine on plasma tissue factor levels in stable and unstable angina pectoris. *Am J Cardiol* 85:527, 2000.

106. Steinhubl SR, Tan WA, Foody JM, Topol EJ: Incidence and clinical course of thrombotic thrombocytopenic purpura due to ticlopidine following coronary stenting. EPISTENT Investigators. Evaluation of Platelet IIb/IIIa Inhibitor for Stenting. *JAMA* 281:806, 1999.

107. Bennett CL, Connors JM, Carwile JM, et al: Thrombotic thrombocytopenic purpura associated with clopidogrel. *N Engl J Med* 342(24):1773, 2000.

107a. Taniuchi M, Kurz HI, Lasala JM: Randomized comparison of ticlopidine and clopidogrel after intracoronary stent implantation in a broad patient population. *Circulation* 104:539, 2001.

108. Jarvis B, Simpson K: Clopidogrel. A review of its use in the prevention of atherosclerosis. *Drugs* 60:347, 2000.

108a. Lerner RG, Frishman WH, Mohan KT: Clopidogrel. A new antiplatelet drug. *Heart Dis* 2:168, 2000.

109. Moshfegh K, Redondo M, Julmy F, et al: Antiplatelet effects of clopidogrel compared with aspirin after myocardial infarction: Enhanced inhibitory effects of combination therapy. *J Am Coll Cardiol* 36:699, 2000.

110. Mehta SR, Yusuf S, Peters RJG, et al, for the Clopidogrel in Unstable angina to prevent Recurrent Events trial (CURE) Investigators. Effects of pretreatment with clopidogrel and aspirin followed by long-term therapy in patients undergoing percutaneous coronary intervention: The PCI-CURE study. *Lancet* 358:527, 2001.

111. The Clopidogrel in Unstable Angina to Prevent Recurrent Events Trial Investigators. Effects of clopidogrel in addition to aspirin in patients with acute coronary syndromes without ST-segment elevation. *N Engl J Med* 345:494, 2001.

111a. Gaspoz J-M, Coxson PG, Goldman PA, et al: Cost effectiveness of aspirin, clopidogrel, or both for secondary prevention of coronary heart disease. *N Engl J Med* 346:1800, 2002.

112. Berger PB, Bell MR, Rihal CS, et al: Clopidogrel versus ticlopidine after intracoronary stent placement. *J Am Coll Cardiol* 34:1891, 1999.

113. Bertrand ME, Rupprecht H-J, Urban P, et al, for the CLASSICS Investigators: Double-blind study of the safety of clopidogrel with and without a loading dose in combination with aspirin compared with ticlopidine in combination with aspirin after coronary stenting. The Clopidogrel Aspirin Stent International Cooperative Study (CLASSICS). *Circulation* 102:624, 2000.

114. Dangas G, Mehran R, Abizaid AS, et al: Combination therapy with aspirin plus clopidogrel versus aspirin plus ticlopidine for prevention of subacute thrombosis after successful native coronary stenting. *Am J Cardiol* 87:470, 2001.

115. Bhatt DL, Chew DP, Hirsch AT, et al: Superiority of clopidogrel versus aspirin in patients with prior cardiac surgery. *Circulation* 103:363, 2001.

116. Phillips DR, Charo IF, Scarborough RM: GPIIb-IIIa: The responsive integrin. *Cell* 65:359, 1991.

117. Ikeda Y, Handa M, Kawano K, et al: The role of von Willebrand factor and fibrinogen in platelet aggregation under varying shear stress. *J Clin Invest* 87:1234, 1991.

118. Coller BS: Platelets and thrombolytic therapy. *N Engl J Med* 322:33, 1990.

119. D'Souza SE, Ginsberg MH, Burke TA, Plow EF: Localization of an arg-gly-asp recognition site within an integrin adhesion receptor. *Science* 242:91, 1988.

120. Frishman WH, Burns B, Atac B, et al: Novel anti-platelet therapies for treatment of patients with ischemic heart disease: Inhibitors of the platelet glycoprotein IIb/IIIa integrin receptor *Am Heart J* 130:877, 1995.

121. Lefkowitz J, Plow EF, Topol EJ: Platelet glycoprotein IIb/IIIa receptors in cardiovascular medicine. *N Engl J Med* 332:1553, 1995.

122. Shebuski RJ, Stabilito IJ, Sitko GR, Polokoff MH: Acceleration of a recombinant tissue-type plasminogen activator-induced thrombolysis and prevention of reocclusion by the combination of heparin and the arg-gly-asp-containing peptide bitistatin in a canine model of coronary thrombosis. *Circulation* 82:169, 1990.

123. Yasuda T, Gold HF, Leinbach RC, Y et al: Kistrin, a polypeptide GPIIb/IIIa receptor antagonist, enhances and sustains coronary arterial thrombolysis with recombinant tissue-type plasminogen activator in a canine preparation. *Circulation* 83:1038, 1991.

124. Scarborough RM, Rose JW, Hsu MA, et al: Barbourin: A GPIIb/IIIa-specific integrin antagonist from the venom of *Sistrurus M. barbouri*. *J Biol Chem* 266:9359, 1991.

125. Coller BS, Peerschke EI, Scudder LE, Sullivan CA: A murine monoclonal antibody that completely blocks the binding of fibrinogen to platelets produces a thrombasthenic-like state in normal platelets and binds to glycoproteins IIb and/or IIIa. *J Clin Invest* 72:325, 1983.

126. Coller BS: A new murine monoclonal antibody reports an activation dependent change in the conformation and/or microenvironment of the glycoprotein IIb/IIIa complex. *J Clin Invest* 76:101, 1985.

127. Knight DM, Wagner C, Jordan R, et al: The immunogenicity of the 7E3 murine monoclonal Fab antibody fragment variable region is dramatically reduced in humans by substitution of human for murine constant regions. *Mol Immunol* 32:1271, 1995.

128. Coller BS, Anderson K, Weisman HF: New antiplatelet agents: platelet GPIIb/IIIa antagonists. *Thromb Haemost* 74(1):302, 1995.

129. Kohler G, Milstein C: Continuous cultures of fused cells secreting antibody of predefined specificity. *Nature* 2567:495, 1975.

130. Faulds D, Sorkin EM. Abciximab (c7E3 Fab): A review of its pharmacology and therapeutic potential in ischemic heart disease. *Drugs* 48:583, 1994.

131. Hanson SR, Pareti FI, Ruggeri ZM, et al: Effects of monoclonal antibodies against the platelet glycoprotein IIb/IIIa complex on thrombosis and hemostasis in the baboon. *J Clin Invest* 81:149, 1988.

132. Gold HK, Gimple LW, Yasuda T, Coller BS: Pharmacodynamic study of F(ab')2 fragments of murine monoclonal antibody 7E3 directed against human platelet glycoprotein IIb/IIIa in patients with unstable angina pectoris. *J Clin Invest* 86:651, 1990.

133. Bhattacharya S, Jordan R, Machin S, et al: Blockade of human platelet GP IIb/IIIa receptor by a murine monoclonal antibody Fab fragment (7E3): Potent dose-dependent inhibition of platelet function. *Cardiovasc Drug Ther* 9:665, 1995.

134. Harrison P, Wilbourn B, Cramer E, et al: The influence of therapeutic blocking of GP IIb/IIIa on platelet α-granular fibrinogen. *Br J Haematol* 82:721, 1992.

135. Christopoulos C, Mackie I, Lahiri A, et al: Flow cytometric observations on the in vivo use of Fab fragments of a chimeric monoclonal antibody to platelet glycoprotein IIb-IIIa. *Blood Coag Fibrinolysis* 4:729, 1993.

136. Sweeney J, Holme S, Heaton A, et al: Infusion of a chimeric monoclonal Fab fragment (c7E3) against platelet glycoprotein IIb-IIIa potently inhibits platelet aggregation but does not affect in vivo platelet survival (abstr). *J Am Coll Cardiol* 21:253A, 1993.

137. Simoons ML, deBoer MJ, van den Brand MJBM, et al, and the European Cooperative Study Group: Randomized trial of GPIIb/IIIa platelet receptor blocker in refractory unstable angina. *Circulation* 89:596, 1994.

138. Kaplan AV, Leung LL-K, Leung W-H, et al: Roles of thrombin and platelet membrane glycoprotein IIb/IIIa in platelet-subendothelial deposition after angioplasty in an ex vivo whole artery model. *Circulation* 84:1279, 1991.

139. Tcheng JE, Ellis SG, George BS, et al: Pharmacodynamics of chimeric glycoprotein IIb/IIIa integrin antiplatelet antibody Fab 7E3 in high-risk coronary angioplasty. *Circulation* 90:1757, 1994.

140. EPIC Investigators: Use of a monoclonal antibody directed against the platelet glycoprotein IIb/IIIa receptor in high-risk coronary angioplasty. *N Engl J Med* 330:956, 1994.

141. Topol EJ, Califf RM, Weissman HF, et al, on behalf of EPIC Investigations. Randomized trial of coronary intervention with antibody against platelet IIb/IIIa integrin for reduction of clinical restenosis; results at six months. *Lancet* 343:881, 1994.

142. Coller BS: Anti-GPIIb/IIIa drugs: Current strategies and future directions. *Thromb Haemost* 86:427, 2000.

143. Dasgupta H, Blankenship JC, Wood GC, et al: Thrombocytopenia complicating treatment with intravenous glycoprotein IIb/IIIa receptor inhibitors: a pooled analysis. *Am Heart J* 140:206, 2000.

144. Fredrickson BJ, Turner NA, Kleiman NS, et al: Effects of abciximab, ticlopidine, and combined abciximab/ticlopidine therapy on platelet and leukocyte function in patients undergoing coronary angioplasty. *Circulation* 101:1122, 2000.

145. Lincoff AM: Results of the interim analysis of the EPILOG Trial. *J Am Coll Cardiol* 27(Suppl A):XXI, 1996.

146. Ferguson JJ: EPILOG and CAPTURE trials halted because of positive interim results. *Circulation* 93:637, 1996.

147. GUSTO IV-ACS Investigators: Effect of glycoprotein IIb/IIIa receptor blocker abciximab on outcome in patients with acute coronary syndromes without early coronary revascularisation. *Lancet* 357:1915, 2001.

148. Stone GW, Grines CL, Cox DA, et al: Comparison of angioplasty with stenting, with or without abciximab in acute myocardial infarction. *N Engl J Med* 346:957, 2002.

149. Gibson CM, deLemos J, Murphy SA et al, for the TIMI Study Group: Combination therapy with abciximab reduces angiographically evident thrombus in acute myocardial infarction. A TIMI 14 substudy. *Circulation* 103:2550, 2001.

150. The GUSTO V Investigators: Reperfusion therapy for acute myocardial infarction with fibrinolytic therapy or combination reduced fibrinolytic therapy and platelet glycoprotein IIb/IIIa inhibition: The GUSTO V randomised trial. *Lancet* 357:1905, 2001.

151. Cantor WJ, Kaplan AL, Velianou JL, et al: Effectiveness and safety of abciximab after failed thrombolytic therapy. *Am J Cardiol* 87:439, 2001.

152. Montalescot G, Barragan P, Wittenberg O, et al, ADMIRAL Investigators: Platelet glycoprotein IIb/IIIa inhibition with coronary stenting for acute myocardial infarction. *N Engl J Med* 344(25):1895, 2001.

153. Boden WE, McKay RG: Optimal treatment of acute coronary syndromes—an evolving strategy. *N Engl J Med* 344(25):1939, 2001.

154. Throckmorton DC: Future trials of antiplatelet agents in cardiac ischemia. *N Engl J Med* 344:1937, 2001.

155. Kouns WC, Kirchhofer D, Hadvary P, et al: Reversible conformational changes induced in glycoprotein IIb/IIIa by a potent and selective peptidomimetric inhibitor. *Blood* 80:2539, 1992.

156. Nichols AJ, Ruffolo RR, Huffman WF, et al: Development of GP IIb/IIIa antagonists as antithrombotic drugs. *Trends Pharmacol Sci* 13:413, 1992.

157. Goa KL, Noble S: Eptifibatide. A review of its use in patients with acute coronary syndromes and/or undergoing percutaneous coronary intervention. *Drugs* 57:439, 1999.

158. Schulman SP, Goldschmidt-Clermont PJ, Topol EJ, et al: Effects of integrelin, a platelet glycoprotein IIb/IIIa receptor antagonist, in unstable angina. A randomized multicenter trial. *Circulation* 94(9):2083, 1996.

159. Randomised placebo-controlled trial of effect of eptifibatide on complications of percutaneous coronary intervention: IMPACT-II. Integrilin to Minimise Platelet Aggregation and Coronary Thrombosis-II. *Lancet* 349(9063):1422, 1997.

160. The ESPRIT Investigators: Novel dosing regimen of eptifibatide in planned coronary stent implantation (ESPRIT): A randomised, placebo-controlled trial. *Lancet* 356(9247):2037, 2000.

161. O'Shea JC, Hafley GE, Greenberg S, et al, ESPRIT Investigators: Platelet glycoprotein IIb/IIIa integrin blockade with eptifibatide in coronary stent intervention: The ESPRIT trial: A randomized controlled trial. *JAMA* 285(19):2468, 2001.

162. The RESTORE Investigators: Effects of platelet glycoprotein IIb/IIIa blockade with tirofiban on adverse cardiac events in patients with unstable angina or acute myocardial infarction undergoing coronary angioplasty. *Circulation* 96(5):1445, 1997.

163. PRISM-PLUS Study Investigators: Inhibition of the platelet glycoprotein IIb/IIIa receptor with tirofiban in unstable angina and non-Q-wave myocardial infarction. Platelet Receptor Inhibition in Ischemic Syndrome Management in Patients Limited by Unstable Signs and Symptoms. *N Engl J Med* 339(16):1163, 1998.

164. Cannon CP, Weintraub WS, Demopoulos LA, et al, for the TACTICS—Thrombolysis in Myocardial Infarction 18 Investigators: Comparison of early invasive and conservative strategies in patients with unstable coronary syndromes treated with the glycoprotein IIb/IIIa inhibitor tirofiban. *N Engl J Med* 344:1879, 2001.

165. Topol EJ, Moliterno DJ, Herrmann HC, et al: Comparison of two platelet glycoprotein IIb/IIIa inhibitors, tirofiban and abciximab, for the prevention of ischemic events with percutaneous coronary revascularization. *N Engl J Med* 344(25):1888, 2001.

166. Kereiakes DJ, Runyon JP, Kleinman NS, et al: Differential dose-response to oral xemilofiban after antecedent intravenous abciximab. *Circulation* 94:906, 1996.

167. O'Neill WW, Serruys P, Knudtson M, et al: Long-term treatment with a platelet glycoprotein-receptor antagonist after percutaneous coronary revascularization. EXCITE Trial Investigators. Evaluation of Oral Xemilofiban in Controlling Thrombotic Events. *N Engl J Med* 342(18):1316, 2000.

168. Cannon CP, McCabe CH, Wilcox RG, et al: Oral glycoprotein IIb/IIIa inhibition with orbofiban in patients with unstable coronary syndromes (OPUS-TIMI 16) trial. *Circulation* 102(2):149, 2000.

169. The SYMPHONY Investigators: Comparison of sibrafiban with aspirin for prevention of cardiovascular events after acute coronary syndromes: A randomised trial. *Lancet* 355(9201):337, 2000.

170. Second SYMPHONY Investigators: Randomized trial of aspirin, sibrafiban, or both for secondary prevention after acute coronary syndromes. *Circulation* 103(13):1727, 2001.

171. Sorelle R: SmithKline Beecham halts tests of Lotrafiban, an oral glycoprotein IIb/IIIa inhibitor. *Circulation* 103:e9001, 2001.

172. Chew DP, Bhatt DL, Sapp S, Topol EJ: Increased mortality with oral platelet glycoprotein IIb/IIIa antagonists: A meta-analysis of phase III multicenter randomized trials. *Circulation* 103(2):201, 2001.

173. Rosenberg RD, Bauer KA: The heparin-antithrombin system: A natural anticoagulant mechanism. In: Coleman RW, Hirsh J, Marder VJ, et al, eds. *Hemostasis and Thrombosis: Basic Principles and Clinical Practice.* 3rd ed. Philadelphia: JB Lippincott, 1992:837.

174. Bjork I, Lindahl U: Mechanism of the anticoagulant action of heparin. *Mol Cell Biochem* 48:161, 1982.

175. Hirsh J, Warkentin TE, Shaughnessy SG, et al: Heparin and low-molecular-weight heparin: mechanisms of action, pharmacokinetics, dosing, monitoring, efficacy and safety. *Chest* 119(Suppl):64S, 2001.

176. Loscalzo J: Thrombin inhibitors in fibrinolysis: A Hobson's choice of alternatives. *Circulation* 94:863, 1996.

177. Hommes DW, Bura A, Mazzolai L, et al: Subcutaneous heparin compared with continuous intravenous heparin administration in the initial treatment of deep vein thrombosis: A meta-analysis. *Ann Intern Med* 116:279, 1992.

178. Hull RD, Raskob GE, Hirsh J, et al: Continuous intravenous heparin compared with intermittent subcutaneous heparin in the initial treatment of proximal-vein thrombosis. *N Engl J Med* 315:1098, 1996.

179. Levine M, Hirsh J, Gent M, et al: A randomized trial comparing activated thromboplastin time with heparin assay in patients with acute venous thromboembolism requiring large daily doses of heparin. *Arch Intern Med* 154:49, 1994.

180. Geerts WH, Heit JA, Clagett GP, et al: Prevention of venous thromboembolism. *Chest* 119(Suppl):132S, 2001.

181. Nurmohamed Mt, Rosendaal FR, Buller HR, et al: Low-molecular-weight heparin versus standard heparin in general and orthopedic surgery: A meta-analysis. *Lancet* 340:152, 1992.

182. Iorio A, Agnelli G: Low-molecular-weight and unfractionated heparin for prevention of venous thromboembolism in neurosurgery. A meta-analysis. *Arch Intern Med* 160:2327, 2000.

183. Turpie AGG, Robinson JG, Doyle DJ, et al: Comparison of high-dose with low-dose subcutaneous heparin to prevent left ventricular mural thrombosis in patients with acute transmural myocardial infarction. *N Engl J Med* 320:352, 1989.

184. Liem A, Zijlstra F, Ottervanger JP, et al: High-dose heparin as pretreatment for primary angioplasty in acute myocardial infarction: The Heparin in Early Patency (HEAP) Randomized Trial. *J Am Coll Cardiol* 35:600, 2000.

185. Mahaffey KW, Granger CB, Collins R, et al: Overview of randomized trials of intravenous heparin in patients with acute myocardial infarction treated with thrombolytic therapy. *Am J Cardiol* 77:551, 1996.

186. Eisenberg PR, Sherman LA, Jaffe AS: Paradoxic elevation of fibrinopeptide A after streptokinase: Evidence for continued thrombosis despite intense thrombolysis. *J Am Coll Cardiol* 10:527, 1987.

187. Eisenberg PR, Sobel BE, Jaffe AS: Activation of prothrombin accompanying thrombolysis with recombinant tissue-type plasminogen activator. *J Am Coll Cardiol* 19:1065, 1992.

188. The SCATI (Studio sulla Caliparina nell'Angina e nella Thrombosi Ventriculare nell'Infarto) Group: Randomized controlled trial of subcutaneous calcium-heparin in acute myocardial infarction. *Lancet* 2:182, 1989.

189. Gruppo Italiano per lo Studio della Streptochinase Nell'Infarcto Miocardico: GISSI 2: A factor randomized trial of alteplase and heparin versus no heparin among 12,490 patients with acute myocardial infarction. *Lancet* 336:65, 1990.

190. The International Study Group: In-hospital mortality and clinical course of 20,891 patients with suspected acute myocardial infarction randomized between alteplase and streptokinase with or without heparin. *Lancet* 336:71, 1990.

191. ISIS-3 Collaborative Group. ISIS-3: A randomised comparison of streptokinase vs tissue plasminogen activator vs anistreplase and of aspirin plus heparin vs aspirin alone among 41,299 cases of suspected acute myocardial infarction. *Lancet* 339:753, 1991.

192. Yusuf S, Collins R, Peto R, et al: Intravenous and intracoronary fibrinolytic therapy in acute myocardial infarction: Overview of results on mortality, reinfarction and side effects from 33 randomized controlled trials. *Eur Heart J* 6:556, 1985.

193. Bleich SD, Nichols TC, Schumacher RR, et al: Effect of heparin on coronary arterial patency after thrombolysis with tissue plasminogen activator in acute myocardial infarction. *Am J Cardiol* 66:1412, 1990.

194. Topol EJ, George BS, Kereiakes DJ, et al: A randomized controlled trial of intravenous tissue plasminogen activator and early intravenous heparin in acute myocardial infarction. *Circulation* 79:281, 1989.

195. The GUSTO Investigators: An international randomized trial comparing four thrombolytic strategies for acute myocardial infarction. *N Engl J Med* 329:673, 1993.

196. Antman EM for the TIMI 9B Investigators: Hirudin in acute myocardial infarction. Thrombolysis and thrombin inhibition in myocardial infarction (TIMI) 9B trial. *Circulation* 94:911, 1996.

197. Mungall DR, Anbe D, Forrester PL, et al: A prospective randomized comparison of the accuracy of computer-assisted versus GUSTO nomogram-directed heparin therapy. *Clin Pharmacol Ther* 55:591, 1994.

198. Braunwald E, Antman EM, Beasley JW, et al: ACC/AHA guidelines for the management of patients with unstable angina and

non-ST-segment elevation myocardial infarction: executive summary and recommendations. A report of the American College of Cardiology/American Heart Association Task Force on Practice Guidelines (Committee on the Management of Patients with Unstable Angina). *Circulation* 102:1193, 2000.

199. Raschke RA, Reilly BM, Guidry JR, et al. The weight-based heparin dosing nomogram compared with a standard care nomogram. *Ann Intern Med* 119:874, 1993.

200. Zidane M, Schram MT, Planken EW, et al: Frequency of major hemorrhage in patients treated with unfractionated intravenous heparin for deep venous thrombosis or pulmonary embolism. A study in routine clinical practice. *Arch Intern Med* 160:2369, 2000.

201. Engelberg H: Actions of heparin in the atherosclerotic process. *Pharmacol Rev* 48:327, 1996.

202. Warkentin TE, Kelton JG: Temporal aspects of heparin-induced thrombocytopenia. *N Engl J Med* 344:1286, 2001.

203. Warkentin TE, Levine MN, Hirsh J, et al: Heparin-induced thrombocytopenia in patients treated with low-molecular-weight heparin. *N Engl J Med* 332:1330, 1995.

204. Hirsh J, Levine MN: Low-molecular-weight heparin. *Blood* 79:1, 1992.

205. Lane DA, Denton J, Flynn AM, et al: Anticoagulant activities of heparin oligosaccharides and their neutralization by platelet factor IV. *Biochem J* 218:725, 1984.

206. Anderrson LO, Barrowcliffe TW, Holmer E, et al: Molecular weight dependency of the heparin potentiated inhibition of thrombin and activated factor X: Effect of heparin neutralization in plasma. *Thromb Res* 115:531, 1979.

207. Kakkar VV: Effectiveness and safety of low-molecular-weight heparins (LMWH) in the prevention of venous thromboembolism. *Thromb Haemost* 74:364, 1995.

208. Hirsh J, Siragusa S, Ginsberg JS: Low-molecular-weight heparins (LMWH) in the treatment of patients with acute venous thromboembolism. *Thromb Haemost* 74:360, 1995.

209. Kakkar VV, Cohen AT, Edmundson RA, et al: Low-molecular-weight heparins versus standard heparin for patients of venous thromboembolism after major abdominal surgery. *Lancet* 341:259, 1993.

210. Albers GW, Amarenco P, Easton JD, et al: Antithrombotic and thrombolytic therapy for ischemic stroke. *Chest* 119:300s, 2001.

211. International Stroke Trial Collaborative Group: The International Stroke Trial (IST): A randomised trial of aspirin, subcutaneous heparin, both, or neither among 19435 patients with acute ischaemic stroke. *Lancet* 349(9065):1569, 1997.

212. Kay R, Wong KS, Yu YL, et al: Low-molecular-weight heparin for the treatment of acute ischemic stroke. *N Engl J Med* 333:1588, 1995.

213. The Assessment of the Safety and Efficacy of a new Thrombolytic Regimen (ASSENT)-3 Investigators: Efficacy and safety of tenecteplase in combination with enoxaparin, abciximab, or unfractionated heparin in acute myocardial infarction: ASSENT-3. *Lancet* 358:605, 2001.

214. Llevadot J, Giugliano RP, Antman EM: Bolus fibrinolytic therapy in acute myocardial infarction. *JAMA* 286:442, 2001.

215. Gurfinkel EP, Manos EJ, Mejail RI, et al: Low-molecular-weight heparin versus regular heparin or aspirin in treatment of unstable angina and silent ischemia. *J Am Coll Cardiol* 26:313, 1995.

216. Low-molecular-weight heparin during instability in coronary artery disease, Fragmin during Instability in Coronary Artery Disease (FRISC) study group. *Lancet* 347:561, 1996.

217. Cohen M, Demers C, Gurfinkel EP, et al: A comparison of low-molecular-weight heparin with unfractionated heparin for unstable coronary artery disease. Efficacy and Safety of Subcutaneous Enoxaparin in Non-Q-Wave Coronary Events Study Group. *N Engl J Med* 337(7):447, 1997.

218. Goodman SG, Cohen M, Bigonzi F, et al: Randomized trial of low-molecular-weight heparin (enoxaparin) versus unfractionated heparin for unstable coronary artery disease: One-year results of the ESSENCE Study. Efficacy and Safety of Subcutaneous Enoxaparin in Non-Q Wave Coronary Events. *J Am Coll Cardiol* 36:693, 2000.

219. Elkelboom JW, Anand SS, Malmberg K, et al: Unfractionated heparin and low-molecular-weight heparin in acute coronary syndrome without ST elevation: A meta-analysis. *Lancet* 355:1936, 2000.

220. Cairns JA, Theroux P, Lewis HD Jr, et al: Antithrombotic agents in coronary artery disease. *Chest* 119(Suppl):228s, 2001.

220a. The SYNERGY Executive Committee: The SYNERGY Trial: Study design and rationale. *Am Heart J* 143:952, 2002.

221. Pineo GF, Hull RD: Prevention and treatment of venous thromboembolism. *Drugs* 52:71, 1996.

222. Levine M, Gent M, Hirsh J, et al: Ardeparin (low-molecular-weight heparin) vs. graduated compression stockings for the prevention of venous thromboembolism. *Arch Intern Med* 156:851, 1996.

223. Leclerc JR, Goerts WH, Desjardins L, et al: Prevention of venous thromboembolism after knee arthroplasty—a randomized, double-blind trial comparing enoxaparin with warfarin. *Ann Intern Med* 124:619, 1996.

224. Hull R, Raskob G, Pineo G, et al: A comparison of subcutaneous low-molecular-weight heparin with Warfarin sodium for prophylaxis against deep-vein thrombosis after hip or knee implantation. *N Engl J Med* 329:1370, 1993.

225. Geerts WH, Heit JA, Clagett CP, et al: Prevention of venous thromboembolism. *Chest* 119:132S, 2001.

226. Heit JA, Berkowitz SD, Bona R, et al: Efficacy and safety of low-molecular-weight heparin (ardeparin sodium) compared to warfarin for the prevention of VTE after total knee replacement surgery: A double-blind, dose-ranging study. *Thromb Haemost* 77:32, 1997.

227. Hull RD, Raskob GE, Pineo GF, et al: Subcutaneous low-molecular-weight heparin compared with continuous intravenous heparin in the treatment of proximal-vein thrombosis. *N Engl J Med* 326:975, 1992.

228. Levine M, Gent M, Hirsh J, et al: A comparison of low-molecular-weight heparin administered primarily at home with unfractionated heparin. Administered in the hospital for proximal deep-vein thrombosis. *N Engl J Med* 334:677, 1996.

229. Koopman M, Prandoni P, Piovella F, et al: Treatment of venous thrombosis with intravenous unfractionated heparin administered in the hospital as compared with subcutaneous low-molecular-weight heparin administered at home. *N Engl J Med* 334:682, 1996.

230. Gould MK, Dembitzer AD, Doyle RL, et al: Low-molecular-weight heparins compared with unfractionated heparin for treatment of acute deep venous thrombosis. A meta-analysis of randomized, controlled trials. *Ann Intern Med* 130:800, 1999.

231. Faxon DP, Spiro TE, Minor S, et al: Low-molecular-weight heparin in prevention of restenosis after angioplasty. Results of Enoxaparin Restenosis Trial (ERA). *Circulation*; 90:908, 1994.

232. Cairns JA, Gill J, Morton B, et al: Fish oils and low-molecular-weight heparin for the reduction of restenosis after percutaneous transluminal coronary angioplasty. The EMPAR Study. *Circulation* 94:1553, 1996.

233. Lablanche JM, McFadden EP, Meneveau N, et al: Effect of nadroparin, a low-molecular-weight heparin, on clinical and angiographic restenosis after coronary balloon angioplasty: The FACT study. Fraxiparine Angioplastic Coronaire Transluminate. *Circulation* 96:3396, 1997.

234. Kiesz RS, Buszman P, Martin JL, et al: Local delivery of enoxaparin to decrease restenosis after stenting: Results of initial multicenter trial: Polish-American Local Lovenox NIR Assessment study (The POLONIA study). *Circulation* 103:26, 2001.

235. Belch JJF: Pharmacotherapy of Raynaud's phenomenon. *Drugs* 52:682, 1996.

236. Mannarino E, Pasqualini L, Innocente S, et al: Efficacy of low-molecular-weight heparin in the management of intermittent claudication. *Angiology* 42:1, 1991.

237. Calabro A, Piarulli F, Milan D, et al: Clinical assessment of low-molecular-weight heparin effects in peripheral vascular disease. *Angiology* 44:188, 1993.

238. Edmondson RA, Cohen AT, Das SK, et al: Low-molecular-weight heparin versus aspirin and dipyridamole after femoropopliteal bypass grafting. *Lancet* 344:914, 1994.

239. Boston Area Anticoagulation Trial: The effect of low-dose warfarin on the risk of stroke in patients with non-rheumatic atrial fibrillation: The Boston Area Anticoagulation Trial for Atrial Fibrillation Investigators. *N Engl J Med* 323:1505, 1990.

240. Harenberg J, Weuster B, Pfitzer M, et al: Prophylaxis of embolic events in patients with atrial fibrillation using low-molecular-weight heparin. *Semin Thromb Hemost* 19(Suppl 1):116, 1993.

241. Berge E, Abdelnoor M, Nakstad PH, et al: Low-molecular-weight heparin versus aspirin in patients with acute ischaemic stroke and atrial fibrillation: A double-blind randomised study. *Lancet* 355:1205, 2000.

242. Murray RD, Deitcher SR, Shah A, et al: Potential clinical efficacy and cost benefit of a transesophageal echocardiography-guided low-molecular-weight heparin (enoxaparin) approach to antithrombotic therapy in patients undergoing immediate cardioversion from atrial fibrillation. *J Am Soc Echocardiogr* 14:200, 2001.

243. Camm AJ: Atrial fibrillation: Is there a role for low-molecular-weight heparin? *Clin Cardiol* 24(Suppl 3):I15, 2001.

244. Jeffrey RF, Khan AA, Douglas, JT, et al: Anticoagulation with low-molecular-weight heparin (Fragmin) during continuous hemodialysis in the intensive care unit. *Artif Organs* 17(8):717, 1993.

245. Schmitt Y, Schneider H: Low-molecular-weight heparin (LMWH): Influence on blood lipids in patients on chronic hemodialysis. *Nephrol Dial Transplant* 8(5):438, 1993.

246. Saltissi D, Morgan C, Westhuyzen J, Healy H: Comparison of low-molecular-weight heparin (enoxaparin sodium) and standard unfractionated heparin for haemodialysis anticoagulation. *Nephrol Dial Transplant* 11:2698, 1999.

247. Melandri G, Semprini F, Cervi V, et al: Benefit of adding low-molecular-weight heparin to the conventional treatment of stable angina pectoris. A double-blind, randomized, placebo-controlled trial. *Circulation* 88(6):2517, 1993.

248. Estrada CA, Mansfield CJ, Heudebert GR: Cost-effectiveness of low-molecular-weight heparin in the treatment of proximal deep vein thrombosis. *J Gen Intern Med* 15:108, 2000.

249. Hull RD, Raskob GE, Rosenbloom D, et al: Treatment of proximal vein thrombosis with subcutaneous low-molecular-weight heparin vs intravenous heparin. An economic perspective. *Arch Intern Med* 157:289, 1997.

250. Wilde MI, Markham A: Danaparoid: A review of its pharmacology and clinical use in the management of heparin induced thrombocytopenia. *Drugs* 54:903, 1997.

251. Chesebro J, Fuster V: Thrombosis in unstable angina. *N Engl J Med* 327:192, 1992.

252. Graham DJ, Alexander JJ: The effect of thrombin on bovine aortic endothelial and smooth muscle cells. *J Vasc Surg* 11:307, 1990.

253. Jones A, Geczy CL: Thrombin and factor Xa enhance the production of interleukin-1. *Immunology* 71:236, 1990.

254. Hirsh J: Heparin. *N Engl J Med* 324:1565, 1991.

254a. Hogg PJ, Jackson CM: Fibrin monomer protects thrombin from inactivation by heparin-antithrombin III: Implications for heparin efficacy. *Proc Natl Acad Sci USA* 86:3619, 1989.

255. Weitz JI, Huboda M, Massel D, et al: Clot-bound thrombin is protected from inhibition by heparin-antithrombin but is susceptible to inactivation by antithrombin III-independent inhibitors. *J Clin Invest* 86:385, 1990.

256. Loscalzo J, Melinick B, Handin R: The interaction of platelet factor 4 and glycosaminoglycans. *Arch Biochem Biophys* 240:446, 1985.

257. Greinacher A, Lubenow N: Recombinant hirudin in clinical practice. *Circulation* 103:1479, 2001.

258. Rydel TJ, Ravichandran KG, Tulinsky A, et al: The structure of a complex of recombinant hirudin and human alpha-thrombin. *Science* 249:277, 1990.

259. Stone SR, Hofsteenge J: Kinetics of the inhibition of thrombin by hirudin. *Biochemistry* 825:4622, 1986.

260. Greinacher A, Völpel H, Janssens U, et al: Recombinant hirudin (lepirudin) provides safe and effective anticoagulation in patients with the immunologic type of heparin-induced thrombocytopenia: A prospective study. *Circulation* 99:73, 1999.

261. Greinacher A, Janssens U, Berg G, et al: Lepirudin (recombinant hirudin) for parenteral anticoagulation in patients with heparin-induced thrombocytopenia. *Circulation* 100:587, 1999.

262. McKeage K, Plosker GL: Argatroban. *Drugs* 61:515, 2001.

263. Lewis BE, Wallis DE, Berkowitz SD, et al, ARG-911 Study Investigators: Argatroban anticoagulant therapy in patients with heparin-induced thrombocytopenia. *Circulation* 103:1838, 2001.

264. Chen JL: Argatroban: A direct thrombin inhibitor for heparin-induced thrombocytopenia and other clinical applications. *Heart Dis* 3:189, 2001.

265. Hirsh J: New anticoagulants. *Am Heart J* 142:S3, 2001.

266. Mellot MJ, Holahan MA, Lynch JJ, et al: Acceleration of recombinant tissue-type plasminogen activator-induced reperfusion and prevention of reocclusion by recombinant antistasin, a selective factor Xa inhibitor, in a canine model of femoral arterial thrombosis. *Circ Res* 70:1152, 1992.

267. Sitko GR, Ramjit DR, Stabilito II, et al: Conjunctive enhancement of enzymatic thrombolysis and prevention of thrombotic reocclusion with the selective factor Xa inhibitor, tick anticoagulant peptide. *Circulation* 85:805, 1992.

267a. Spencer FA, Becker RC: Novel inhibitors of factor Xa for use in cardiovascular disease. *Curr Cardiol Rep* 2:395, 2000.

268. Cannon CP, McCabe CH, Henry TD, et al: A pilot trial of recombinant desulfatohirudin compared with heparin in conjunction with tissue-type plasminogen activator and aspirin for acute myocardial infarction: Results of the Thrombolysis in Myocardial Infarction (TIMI) 5 Trial. *J Am Coll Cardiol* 23:993, 1994.

269. Neuhaus KL, Niederer W, Wagner J, et al: HIT (Hirudin for the Improvement of Thrombolysis) results of a dose escalation study (abstr.). *Circulation* 88:I-292, 1993.

270. Lee LV, for the TIMI 6 Investigators: Initial experience with hirudin and streptokinase in acute myocardial infarction: Results of the TIMI 6 trial. *Am J Cardiol* 75:7, 1995.

271. Antman EM, for the TIMI 9A Investigators: Hirudin in acute myocardial infarction: Safety report from the Thrombolysis and Thrombin Inhibition in Myocardial (TIMI) 9A trial. *Circulation* 90:1624, 1994.

272. The Global Use of Strategies to Open Occluded Coronary Arteries (GUSTO) IIa Investigators: A randomized trial of intravenous heparin versus recombinant hirudin for acute coronary syndromes. *Circulation* 90:1631, 1994.

273. Antman EM for the TIMI 9B Investigators: Hirudin in acute myocardial infarction: thrombolysis and thrombin inhibition in myocardial infarction: Thrombolysis and thrombin inhibition in myocardial infarction (TIMI) 9B trial. *Circulation* 94:911, 1996.

274. van den Boss AA, Deckers JW, Heyndricks GR, et al: Safety and efficacy of recombinant hirudin (CGP 39393) versus heparin in patients with stable angina undergoing coronary angioplasty. *Circulation* 88:2058, 1993.

275. Serruys PW, Deckers JW, Close P, on behalf of the HELVETICA study group: A double-blind, randomized heparin controlled trial evaluating acute and long-term efficacy of r-hirudin (CGP 39393) in patients undergoing coronary angioplasty (abstr). *Circulation* 90(Suppl I) [pt 2]:1394, 1994.

276. Bittl JA, Strony J, Brinker JA, et al: Treatment with bivalirudin (hirulog) as compared with heparin during coronary angioplasty for unstable and post-infarction angina. Hirulog Angioplasty Study Investigators. *N Engl J Med* 333:764, 1995.

277. Zoldhelyi P, Webster MWI, Fuster V, et al: Recombinant hirudin in patients with chronic, stable coronary artery disease: Safety, half-life, and effect on coagulation parameters. *Circulation* 88:2015, 1993.

278. Walenga JM, Hoppensteadt D, Koza MM, et al: Comparative studies on various essays for the laboratory evaluation of hirudin. *Semin Thromb Hemost* 17:103, 1991.

279. Lefkovits J, Topol EJ: Direct thrombin inhibitors in cardiovascular medicine. *Circulation* 90:1522, 1994.

280. Porta R, Pescador M, Mantovani M, Prino G: Quantitative comparison of recombinant hirudin's antithrombotic and anticoagulant activities with those of heparin. *Thromb Res* 57:639, 1990.

280a. Global Use of Strategies to Open Occluded Coronary Arteries (GUSTO) IIb Investigators: A comparison of recombinant hirudin with heparin for the treatment of acute coronary syndrome. *N Engl J Med* 335:775, 1996.

281. Fareed J, Walenga J, Hoppensteadt D, et al: Neutralization of recombinant hirudin: Some practical considerations. *Semin Thromb Hemost* 17:137, 1991.

282. Maraganore JM, Bourdon P, Jablonski J, et al: Design and characterization of Hirulogs: A novel class of bivalent peptide inhibitors of thrombin. *Biochemistry* 29:7095, 1990.

282a. Theroux P, Perez-Villa F, Waters D, et al: A randomized double-blind comparison of two doses of Hirulog or heparin as adjunctive therapy to streptokinase to promote early patency of the infarct-related artery in acute myocardial infarction. *Circulation* 91:2132, 1995.

282b. Fuchs J, Cannon CP: Hirulog in the treatment of unstable angina: Results of the Thrombin Inhibition in Myocardial Ischemia (TIMI) 7 trial. *Circulation* 92:727, 1995.

282c. Nawarskas JJ, Anderson JR: Bivalirudin: A new approach to anticoagulation. *Heart Dis* 3:131, 2001.

282d. Dogne JM, de Leval X, Delarge J, et al: New trends in thromboxane and prostacyclin modulators. *Curr Med Chem* 7(6):609, 2000.

283. Hirsh J: Oral anticoagulant drugs. *N Engl J Med* 324:1865, 1991.

284. Koch-Weser J, Sellers EM: Drug interactions with coumarin anticoagulants. *N Engl J Med* 285:487–498, 547, 1971.

285. Wells PS, Holbrook AM, Crowther NR, et al: Interactions of warfarin with drugs and food. *Ann Intern Med* 121:676, 1994.

286. Raskob GE, Pineo GE, Hull RD: The technique of administering oral anticoagulant therapy. *J Crit Illness* 6:923, 1991.

287. Hirsh J: Substandard monitoring of warfarin in North America. Time for change. *Arch Intern Med* 152:257, 1992.

288. Cook DJ, Guyatt GH, Laupacis A, et al: Clinical recommendations using levels of evidence for antithrombotic agents. *Chest* 108:227S, 1995.

289. Hirsh J, Dalen JE, Deykin D, et al: Oral anticoagulants. Mechanism of action, clinical effectiveness and optimal therapeutic range. *Chest* 108:231S, 1995.

290. Warkentin TE: Venous thromboembolism in heparin-induced thrombocytopenia. *Curr Opin Pulm Med* 6:343, 2000.

291. Moriarty HT, Lam-PO-Tang PR, Anastas N: Comparison of the thromboplastins using the ISI and INR system. *Pathology* 22:71, 1990.

292. Van den Bessellar AMHP, Lewis SM, Mannucci PM: Status of present and candidate international reference preparations (IRP) of thromboplastins for the prothrombin time: A report of the subcommittee for the control of anticoagulation. *Thromb Haemost* 69:85, 1993.

293. Hellemans J, Vorlat M, Verstraete M: Survival time of prothrombin in factors VII, IX, and X after complete synthesis blocking doses of coumarin derivatives. *Br J Haematol* 57:213, 1984.

294. Cannegeiter SC, Rosendaal FR: Optimal oral anticoagulation for patients with mechanical heart valves. *N Engl J Med* 333:11, 1995.

295. Cortelazzo S. Finazzi G, Viero P, et al: Thrombotic and hemorrhagic complications in patients with mechanical heart valve prosthesis attending an anticoagulation clinic. *Thromb Haemost* 69:316, 1993.

296. Rosendaal FR: The Scylla and Charybdis of oral anticoagulant treatment. *N Engl J Med* 335:587, 1996.

297. Turpie AG, Gent M, Laupacis A, et al: Comparison of aspirin with placebo in patients treated with warfarin after heart valve replacement. *N Engl J Med* 329:524, 1993.

298. Fihn SD: Aiming for safe anticoagulation. *N Engl J Med* 333:54, 1995.

299. Stein PD, Alpert JS, Bussey HI, et al: Antithrombotic therapy in patients with mechanical and biological prosthetic heart valves. *Chest* 119(Suppl 1):220S, 2001.

300. Salem DN, Daudelin HD, Levine HJ, et al: Antithrombotic therapy in valvular heart disease. *Chest* 119(Suppl 1):207S, 2001.

301. Albers GW, Dalen JE, Laupacis A, et al: Antithrombotic therapy in atrial fibrillation. *Chest* 119(Suppl 1):194S, 2001.

302. Hylek EM, Skates SJ, Sheehan MA, et al: An analysis of the lowest effective intensity of prophylactic anticoagulation for patients with non-rheumatic atrial fibrillation. *N Engl J Med* 335:540, 1996.

303. The European Atrial Fibrillation Trial Study Group: Optimal oral anticoagulant therapy in patients with non-rheumatic atrial fibrillation and recent cerebral ischemia. *N Engl J Med* 333:5, 1995.

304. Yamaguchi T, for Japanese Nonvalvular Atrial Fibrillation-Embolism Secondary Prevention Cooperative Study Group: Optimal intensity of warfarin therapy for secondary prevention of stroke in patients with nonvalvular atrial fibrillation. A multicenter, prospective, randomized trial. *Stroke* 31:817, 2000.

305. Veterans Administration Cooperative Study: Anticoagulants in acute myocardial infarction: results of a cooperative clinical trial. *JAMA* 225:724, 1973.

306. International Anticoagulant Review Group: Collaborative analysis of long-term anticoagulant administration after acute myocardial infarction. *Lancet* 1:203, 1970.

307. ASPECT Research Group: Effect of long-term oral anticoagulant treatment on mortality and cardiovascular morbidity after myocardial infarction. *Lancet* 343:400, 1994.

308. Smith P, Arnesen H, Holme I: The effect of warfarin on mortality and reinfarction after myocardial infarction. *N Engl J Med* 323:147, 1990.

309. Azar AJ, Cannegieter SC, Deckers JW, et al: Optimal intensity of oral anticoagulant therapy after myocardial infarction. *J Am Coll Cardiol* 27:1349, 1996.

310. Cohen M, Adams PC, Parry G, et al, and the Antithrombotic Therapy in Acute Coronary Syndromes Research Group: Combination antithrombotic therapy in unstable rest angina and non-Q-wave infarction in nonprior aspirin users. Primary end points analysis from the ATACS trial. *Circulation* 89:81, 1994.

311. Stein PD, Alpert JS, Bussey HI, et al: Antithrombotic therapy in patients with mechanical and biological prosthetic heart valves. *Chest* 119(Suppl 1):220s, 2001.

312. Cannegieter SC, Rosendaal FR, Wintzen AR, et al: Optimal oral anticoagulant therapy in patients with mechanical heart valves. *N Engl J Med* 333:11, 1995.

313. Chesebro JH, Fuster V: Optimal antithrombotic therapy for mechanical prosthetic heart valves. *Circulation* 94:2055, 1996.

314. Altman R, Rouvier J, Gurfinkel E, et al: Comparison of high-dose with low-dose aspirin in patients with mechanical heart valve replacement treated with oral anticoagulant. *Circulation* 94:2113, 1996.

315. Massel D, Little SH: Risks and benefits of adding anti-platelet therapy to warfarin among patients with prosthetic heart valves: A meta-analysis. *J Am Coll Cardiol* 37:569, 2001.

316. Collaborative Group of the Primary Prevention Project (PPP): Low-dose aspirin and vitamin E in people at cardiovascular risk: A randomised trial in general practice. *Lancet* 357:89, 2001.

317. Ezekowitz MD, Bridgers SL, James KE, et al, for the Veterans Affairs Stroke Prevention in Nonrheumatic Atrial Fibrillation Investigators: Warfarin in the prevention of stroke associated with nonrheumatic atrial fibrillation. *N Engl J Med* 327:1406, 1992.

318. Atrial Fibrillation Investigators: Risk factors for stroke and efficacy of anti-thrombotic therapy in atrial fibrillation: Analysis of pooled data from five randomized controlled trials. *Arch Intern Med* 154:1449, 1994.

319. The Stroke Prevention in Atrial Fibrillation Investigators: Predictors of thromboembolism in atrial fibrillation: I. Clinical features of patients at risk. *Ann Intern Med* 116:1, 1992.

320. Mungall D, White R: Aging and warfarin therapy. *Ann Intern Med* 117:878, 1992.

321. Presti CF, Hart RG: Thyrotoxicosis, atrial fibrillation and embolism revisited. *Am Heart J* 117:976, 1989.

322. ten Berg JM, Kelder JC, Suttorp MJ, et al: Effect of coumarins started before coronary angioplasty on acute complications and long-term follow up. A randomized trial. *Circulation* 102:386, 2000.

323. Palareti G, Leali N, Coccheri S, et al: Bleeding complications of oral anticoagulant treatment: An inception-cohort, prospective collaborative study (ISCOAT). *Lancet* 348:423, 1996.

324. Sun DK, Frishman WH, Grossman M: Adverse dermatologic effects of cardiovascular drug therapy. In Frishman WH, Sonnenblick EH (eds): Cardiovascular Pharmacotherapeutics. NY: McGraw Hill 1997; 1005–1037.

325. Hall JAG, Pauli RM, Wilson KM: Maternal and fetal sequelae of anticoagulation during pregnancy. *Am J Med* 68:122, 1980.

326. Smith WL: Prostanoid biosynthesis and mechanisms of action. *Am J Physiol* 263:F181, 1992.

327. Gresele P, Deckmyn H, Giuseppe G, et al: Thromboxane synthase inhibitors, thromboxane receptor antagonists and dual blockers in thrombotic disorders. *Trends Pharmacol Sci* 12:158, 1991.

328. Fiddler GI, Lumley P: Preliminary studies with thromboxane synthase inhibitors and thromboxane receptor blockers: A review. *Circulation* 81(Suppl I):I69, 1990.

329. Reilly, IA, Doran JB, Smith B, Fitzgerald GA: Increased thromboxane biosynthesis in a human preparation of platelet activation. Biochemical and functional consequences of selective inhibition of thromboxane synthase. *Circulation* 73:1300, 1986.

330. Terres W, Kupper W, Hamm CW: Resting myocardial ischemia after intravenous infusion of BM 13.177, a thromboxane receptor antagonist. *Thromb Res* 48:577, 1987.

331. Lane IF, Irwin JTC, Jennings SA, et al: A specific thromboxane receptor antagonist evaluated in vascular graft patients. *Br J Surg* 71:903, 1984.

332. Gresele P, Deckymn H, Arnout J, et al: Characterization of N,N'-bis(3-picolyl)-4-Methoxy-Isophtalamide (picotamide) as a dual thromboxane synthase inhibitor/thromboxane A_2 receptor antagonist in human platelets. *Thromb Haemost* 61(3):479, 1989.

333. DeClerk F, Beetens J, deChaffoy D, et al: R 68070: Thromboxane A_2/prostaglandin endoperoxide receptor blockade combined in one molecule. Biochemical profile in vitro. *Thromb Haemost* 61(1):35, 1989.

334. Dogne JM, Rolin S, de Leval X, et al: Pharmacology of the thromboxane receptor antagonist and thromboxane synthase inhibitor BM-531. *Cardiovasc Drug Rev* 19:87, 2001.

335. Hoet B, Falcon C, De Reys S, et al: R68070, a combined thromboxane/endoperoxide receptor antagonist and thromboxane synthase inhibitor, inhibits human platelet activation in vitro and in vivo: A comparison with aspirin. *Blood* 75(3):646, 1990.

336. McAuliffe SJG, Moors JA, Jones HB: Comparative effects of antiplatelet agents as adjuncts to tissue plasminogen activator in a dog model of occlusive coronary thrombosis. *Br J Pharmacol* 112:272, 1994.

337. Timmermans C, Vrolix M, VanHaecke J, et al: Ridogrel in the setting of percutaneous transluminal coronary angioplasty. *Am J Cardiol* 68:463, 1991.

338. The RAPT Investigators: The Ridgorel vs. Aspirin Patency Trial. Randomized trial of ridogrel, a combined thromboxane A$_2$ synthase inhibitor and thromboxane A$_2$/prostaglandin endoperoxide receptor antagonist vs. aspirin as adjunct to thrombolysis in patients with acute myocardial infarction. *Circulation* 89:588, 1994.

339. Hirsh J, Salzman EW, Harker L, et al: Aspirin and other platelet active drugs: Relationship among dose, effectiveness and side effects. *Chest* 95(2):12S, 1989.

340. Tranchesi B, Pileggi F, Vercammen E, et al: Ridogrel does not increase the speed and rate of coronary recanalization in patients with myocardial infarction treated with alteplase and heparin. *Eur Heart J* 15(5):660, 1994.

341. Ritter JM, Barrow SE, Doktor HS, et al: Thromboxane A$_2$ receptor antagonism and synthase inhibition in essential hypertension. *Hypertension* 22:197, 1993.

342. Kudo K, Abe K, Chiba S, et al: Role of thromboxane A$_2$ in the hypotensive effect of captopril in essential hypertension. *Hypertension* 11:147, 1988.

343. Patel JP, Beck LD, Briglia FA, et al: Beneficial effects of combined thromboxane and leukotriene receptor antagonism in hemorrhagic shock. *Crit Care Med* 23:231, 1995.

344. Berndt MC, Shen Y, Dopheide SM, et al: The vascular biology of the glycoprotein Ib-IX-V complex. *Thromb Haemost* 86(1):178, 2001.

345. Krupski WC, Bass A, Cadroy Y, et al: Antihemostatic and antithrombotic effects of monoclonal antibodies against von Willebrand factor in nonhuman primates. *Surgery* 112:433, 1992.

346. Furie B, Furie BC, Flaumenhaft R: A journey with platelet P-selectin: The molecular basis of granule secretion, signalling and cell adhesion. *Thromb Haemost* 86(1):214, 2001.

347. Jin J, Tomlinson W, Kirk IP, et al: The C6-2B glioma cell P2Y(AC) receptor is pharmacologically and molecularly identical to the platelet P2Y(12) receptor. *Br J Pharmacol* 133(4):521, 2001.

348. Ingall AH, Dixon J, Bailey A, et al: Antagonists of the platelet P2T receptor: A novel approach to antithrombotic therapy. *J Med Chem* 42(2):213, 1999.

349. Gachet C: ADP receptors of platelets and their inhibition. *Thromb Haemost* 86(1):222, 2001.

350. Gayle RB III, Maliszewski CR, Gimpel SD, et al: Inhibition of platelet function by recombinant soluble ecto-ADPase/CD39. *J Clin Invest* 101(9):1851, 1998.

351. Tanigawa T, Nishikawa M, Kitai T, et al: Increased platelet aggregability in response to shear stress in acute myocardial infarction and its inhibition by combined therapy with aspirin and cilostazol after coronary intervention. *Am J Cardiol* 85:1054, 2000.

352. Park S-W, Lee CW, Kim H-S, et al: Comparison of cilostazol versus ticlopidine therapy after stent implantation. *Am J Cardiol* 84:511, 1999.

353. Yasue H, Ogawa H, Tanaka H, et al, on behalf of the Japanese Antiplatelets Myocardial Infarction Study (JAMIS) Investigators: Effects of aspirin and trapidil on cardiovascular events after acute myocardial infarction. *Am J Cardiol* 83:1308, 1999.

354. Rossoni G, Manfredi B, DeGennaro Colonna V, et al: The nitro derivative of aspirin, NCX 4016, reduces infarct size caused by myocardial ischemia-reperfusion in the anesthetized rat. *J Pharmacol Exp Ther* 297:380, 2001.

354a. Napoli C, Aldini G, Wallace JL, et al: Efficacy and age-related effects of nitric oxide–releasing aspirin on experimental restenosis. *Proc Natl Acad Sci U S A* 99:1689, 2002.

355. Cruz-Fernandez JM, Lopez-Bescos L, Garcia-Dorado D, et al, and Triflusal in Myocardial Infarction (TIM) Investigators: Randomized comparative trial of Triflusal and aspirin following acute myocardial infarction. *Eur Heart J* 21:457, 2000.

356. Chesebro JH, Rauch U, Fuster V, Badimon JJ: Pathogenesis of thrombosis in coronary artery disease. *Haemostasis* 27(Suppl 1):12, 1997.

357. Toschi V, Gallo R, Lettino M, et al: Tissue factor modulates the thrombogenicity of human atherosclerotic plaques. *Circulation* 95:594, 1997.

358. Banai S, Gertz SD: Tissue factor as a therapeutic target in coronary syndromes. *Am J Cardiol* 763:87, 2001.

359. Friederich PW, Levi M, Bauer KA, et al: Ability of recombinant factor VIIa to generate thrombin during inhibition of tissue factor in human subjects. *Circulation* 103:2555, 2001.

360. Han X, Girard TJ, Baum P, et al: Structural requirements for TFPI-mediated inhibition of neointimal thickening after balloon injury in the rat. *Arterioscler Thromb Vasc Biol* 19:2563, 1999.

361. St. Pierre J, Yang LY, Tamirisa K, et al: Tissue factor pathway inhibitor attenuates procoagulant activity and up regulation of tissue factor at the site of balloon-induced arterial injury in pigs. *Arterioscler Thromb Vasc Biol* 19:2263, 1999.

362. Zoldhelyi P, Chen ZQ, Schelat HS, et al: Local gene transfer of tissue factor pathway inhibitor regulates intimal hyperplasia in atherosclerotic arteries. *Proc Natl Acad Sci U S A* 98:4078, 2001.

363. Weitz JI, Hirsh J: New anticoagulant drugs. *Chest* 119:95s, 2001.

364. Peter K, Graeber J, Kipriyanov S, et al: Construction and functional evaluation of a single-chain antibody fusion protein with fibrin targeting and thrombin inhibition after activation by factor Xa. *Circulation* 101:1158, 2000.

365. Hobbelem PMJ, VanDinther TG, Vogel GMT, et al: Pharmacological profile of the chemically synthesized antithrombin III binding fragment of heparin (pentasaccharide) in rats. *Thromb Haemost* 63:265, 1990.

366. Abendschein DR, Baum PK, Verhallen P, et al: A novel synthetic inhibitor of factor Xa decreases early reocclusion and improves 24-h patency after coronary fibrinolysis in dogs. *J Pharmacol Exp Ther* 296(2):567, 2001.

367. Petitou M, Duchaussoy P, Jaurand G, et al: Synthesis and pharmacological properties of a close analogue of an antithrombotic pentasaccharide (SR 90107A/ORG 31540). *J Med Chem* 40(11):1600, 1997.

367a. Keam SJ, Goa KL: Fondaparinux sodium. *Drugs* 62:1673, 2002.

368. Turpie AG, Gallus AS, Hoek JA: Pentasaccharide Investigators. A synthetic pentasaccharide for the prevention of deep-vein thrombosis after total hip replacement. *N Engl J Med* 344(9):619, 2001.

369. The Rembrandt Investigators: Treatment of proximal deep vein thrombosis with a novel synthetic compound (SR90107A/ORG31540) with pure anti-factor Xa activity. A phase II evaluation. *Circulation* 102:2726, 2000.

370. Eriksson BI, Bauer KA, Lassen MR, et al, for the Steering Committee of the Pentasaccharide in Hip-Fracture Surgery Study: Fondaparinux compared with enoxaparin for the prevention of venous thromboembolism after hip-fracture surgery. *N Engl J Med* 345:1298, 2001.

371. Bauer KA, Eriksson BI, Lassen MR, et al, for the Steering Committee of the Pentasaccharide in Major Knee Surgery Study: Fondaparinux compared with enoxaparin for the prevention of venous thromboembolism after elective major knee surgery. *N Engl J Med* 345:1305, 2001.

372. Lassen MR, Bauer KA, Eriksson BI, Turpie AGG: Postoperative fondaparinux versus preoperative enoxaparin for prevention of venous thromboembolism in elective hip-replacement surgery: A randomised double-blind comparison. *Lancet* 359(9319):1715, 2002.

373. Turpie AGG, Bauer KA, Eriksson BI, Lassen MR: Postoperative fondaparinux versus postoperative enoxaparin for prevention of venous thromboembolism in elective hip-replacement surgery: A randomised double-blind trial. *Lancet* 359(9319):1721, 2002.

374. Hull R, Pineo G: A synthetic pentasaccharide for the prevention of deep-vein thrombosis. *N Engl J Med* 345:291, 2001.

375. Doggrell SA: Fondaparinux versus enoxaparin for the prevention of venous thromboembolism. *Expert Opin Pharmacother* 3(4):455, 2002.

376. Walenga JM, Jeske WP, Samama MM, et al: Fondaparinux: A synthetic heparin pentasaccharide as a new antithrombotic agent. *Expert Opin Investig Drugs* 11(3):397, 2002.

377. Bauer KA, Hawkins DW, Peters PC, et al: Fondaparinux, a synthetic pentasaccharide: The first in a new class of antithrombotic agents—the selective factor Xa inhibitors. *Cardiovasc Drug Rev* 20(1):37, 2002.

378. Shibata M, Kumar SR, Amar A, et al: Anti-inflammatory, antithrombotic, and neuroprotective effects of activated protein C in a murine model of focal ischemic stroke. *Circulation* 103:1799, 2001.

379. Dalhbäck B: Protein S and C4b-binding protein: Components involved in the regulation of the protein C anticoagulant system. *Thromb Haemost* 66:49, 1991.

380. Arljots B, Bergqvist D, Dahlbäck B: Inhibition of microarterial thrombosis by activated protein C in a rabbit model. *Thromb Haemost* 72:415, 1994.

381. Esmon CT: Inflammation and thrombosis: Mutual regulation by protein C. *Immunologist* 6:84, 1998.

382. Bernard GR, Vincent JL, Laterre PF, et al: Recombinant human protein C Worldwide Evaluation in Severe Sepsis (PROWESS) study group. Efficacy and safety of recombinant human activated protein C for severe sepsis. *N Engl J Med* 344(10):699, 2001.

383. Eriksson BI, Carlsson S, Halvarsson M, et al: Antithrombotic effect of two low-molecular-weight thrombin inhibitors and a low-molecular weight heparin in a caval vein thrombosis model in the rat. *Thromb Haemost* 78(5):1404, 1997.

384. Gustafsson D, Nystrom J, Carlsson S, et al: The direct thrombin inhibitor melagatran and its oral prodrug H 376/95: Intestinal absorption properties, biochemical and pharmacodynamic effects. *Thromb Res* 101(3):171, 2001.

385. Baughman RA, Kapoor SC, Agarwal RK, et al: Oral delivery of anticoagulant doses of heparin. A randomized, double-blind, controlled study in humans. *Circulation* 98(16):1610, 1998.

386. Esmon CT: The roles of protein C and thrombomodulin in the regulation of blood coagulation. *J Biol Chem* 258:12238, 1983.

387. Ireland H, Kunz G, Kyriakoulis K, et al: Thrombomodulin gene mutations associated with myocardial infarction. *Circulation* 96:15, 1997.

388. Nakashima M, Uematsu T, Umemura K et al: A novel recombinant soluble human thrombomodulin, ART-123, activates the protein C pathway in healthy male volunteers. *J Clin Pharmacol* 38:540, 1998.

389. Kidokoro A, Iba T, Fukunaga M, Yagi Y: Alterations in coagulation and fibrinolysis during sepsis. *Shock* 5:223, 1996.

390. Ohmori Y, Takahashi Y: Thrombomodulin. *Nippon Yakurigaku Zasshi* 116:283, 2000.

391. Eisele B, Lamy M, Thijs LG, et al: Antithrombin III in patients with severe sepsis. *Intensive Care Med* 24:663, 1998.

392. Grip L, Blomback M, Egberg N, et al: Antithrombin III supplementation for patients undergoing PTCA for unstable angina pectoris. *Eur Heart J* 18:443, 1997.

393. Rossi M, Martinelli L, Storti S, et al: The role of antithrombin III in the perioperative management of the patient with unstable angina. *Ann Thorac Surg* 68:2231, 1999.

Thrombolytic Agents

Robert Forman

William H. Frishman

Thrombolytic agents are drugs administered to patients for dissolution by fibrinolysis of established blood clot by activating endogenous plasminogen. Although some of these agents have been available for more then 50 years, it was not until the 1980s that they came into wide use for the treatment of patients with acute myocardial infarction and other thrombotic states.

Thrombolytic agents act by converting the proenzyme plasminogen to the active enzyme plasmin (Fig. 19-1) by cleavage of the Arg-Val peptide bond.[1,2] Plasmin lyses fibrin clot and is a nonspecific serum protease that is capable of breaking down plasminogen factors V and VIII.[3,4] The action of plasmin is neutralized by circulating plasma inhibitors, primarily alpha$_2$ antiplasmin.[1] Endogenous thrombolysis is also inhibited by plasminogen activator inhibitor (PAI-1). Thrombolytics also affect platelet function in response to pathologic shear stress by inhibiting platelet aggregation in stenotic arteries.[4a]

SPECIFIC THROMBOLYTIC AGENTS

Streptokinase

Streptokinase is a single-chain polypeptide derived from beta-hemolytic streptococci. It is not an enzyme and thus has no enzymatic action on plasminogen. It binds with plasminogen in a 1:1 ratio, resulting in a conformational change in the plasminogen, which thus becomes an active enzyme.[4] This active plasminogen-streptokinase complex catalyzes the conversion of another plasminogen molecule to active plasmin. This activation of plasminogen is enhanced in the presence of fibrinogen but also other coagulation proteins, resulting in a systemic fibrinolytic state. In contrast to plasmin, the plasminogen-streptokinase complex is not rapidly neutralized by alpha$_2$ antiplasmin.[5]

Anistreplase

Anisoylated plasminogen streptokinase activator complex (APSAC) is a second-generation agent consisting of streptokinase bound in vitro to plasminogen by the insertion of an anisoyl group. This results in a much more stable enzyme complex, protecting it from plasmin inhibitors and resulting in a prolonged half-life thus permitting the agent to be administered as single bolus. APSAC is currently unavailable in the United States.

Urokinase

Urokinase is available in both single- and double-chain forms. The double-chain form was originally isolated from urine and more recently from human kidney cells in culture. Urokinase activates plasminogen directly and has no specific affinity for fibrin, activating both fibrin bound and circulating plasminogen.

Because urokinase is a naturally occurring product, it is not antigenic and is not neutralized by antibodies.

During recent inspections of Abbott Laboratories and its supplier of the human neonatal kidney cells used in the manufacture of Abbokinase (urokinase), the U.S. Food and Drug Administration (FDA) identified numerous significant deviations from the Current Good Manufacturing Practice regulations designed to help assure product safety.[6] The product has been temporarily withdrawn and will be re-released in the latter part of 2002.

Tissue Plasminogen Activator (tPA)

Single-chain tPA occurs naturally but is synthesized for commercial use using a recombinant DNA technique and is known as Alteplase. A double chain form of tPA, duteplase, was also synthesized and appeared to have similar activity when tested in vitro but this form is not commercially available. The tPA molecule has a binding site enabling it to bind specifically to fibrin in thrombus. Thus it should theoretically be clot-specific and not result in activation of generally circulating plasminogen. Plasminogen activator inhibitor (PAI-1) is important and under natural conditions neutralizes endogenous tPA but not with administration of therapeutic doses of tPA.[5]

The currently available thrombolytic agents are listed in Table 19-1. The doses listed are for patients with acute myocardial infarction.[7]

Reteplase

Recombinant plasmin activator, or reteplase, is a deletion mutant of naturally occurring tPA that has a kringle-2 domain and lacks the finger, epidermal growth factor, and kringle-1 domain. Its slower clearance permits Reteplase to be given as a double bolus injection.

Tenecteplase (TNK-tPA)

TNK-tPA is a genetically engineered variant of tPA with amino acid substitution at three sites. These substitutions lead to a longer

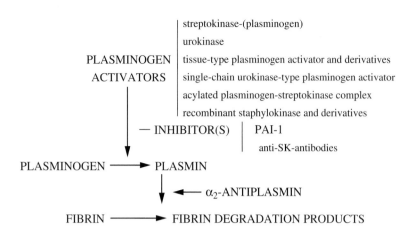

PLASMINOGEN ACTIVATORS
- streptokinase-(plasminogen)
- urokinase
- tissue-type plasminogen activator and derivatives
- single-chain urokinase-type plasminogen activator
- acylated plasminogen-streptokinase complex
- recombinant staphylokinase and derivatives

— INHIBITOR(S) | PAI-1
                | anti-SK-antibodies

PLASMINOGEN ⟶ PLASMIN
                ↓ ⟵ α₂-ANTIPLASMIN
FIBRIN ⟶ FIBRIN DEGRADATION PRODUCTS

FIGURE 19-1. Schematic representation of fibrinolytic system. Plasminogen is a proenzyme and is activated by plasminogen into the active enzyme plasmin. Plasmin degrades fibrin into fibrin degradation products. Fibrinolysis may be inhibited at the level of plasminogen activators by PAI-1 (plasminogen activator inhibitor) and anti-SK (streptokinase) antibodies or the level of plasmin by α_2-antiplasmin. (*Reproduced with permission from Collen.*[1])

half-life, increased fibrin specificity, and an increased resistance to plasminogen activator inhibitor.[7a,7b] The longer half-life of TNK-tPA makes it the only thrombolytic agent currently available that can be given as a single bolus injection.

FIBRIN SPECIFICITY

An agent that is fibrin specific is activated in the presence of fibrin clot and will not indiscriminately activate circulating plasminogen. Agents that are non–fibrin specific will activate circulating plasminogen, which is not indiscriminately clot bound. This may result in depletion of circulating plasminogen and lead to "plasminogen steal," leaching fibrin-bound plasminogen from the clot and reducing the intensity of the thrombolysis.[8]

USE IN ACUTE MYOCARDIAL INFARCTION

Enthusiasm for the use of thrombolytic agents with the ensuing trials only became popular after the pathophysiology of acute myocardial infarction was understood. Davies and Thomas observed in pathologic specimens that most cases with acute myocardial infarction were due to sudden occlusion of a coronary artery by a thrombus at the site of a ruptured atherosclerotic plaque.[9] DeWood and colleagues confirmed this by demonstrating an occlusive thrombus in over 85% of coronary angiograms performed in patients within the first 3 h of presentation with a transmural myocardial infarction.[10] A decade earlier Reimer established that a "wavefront"

of myocardial infarction progressed from the subendocardium to the subepicardium with a longer duration of temporary occlusion of a circumflex coronary artery in dogs.[11]

Rentrop and his colleagues in Germany demonstrated the successful dissolution of the offending coronary thrombus with the use of intracoronary streptokinase.[12,13] Subsequent trials utilizing intracoronary administration of streptokinase revealed significant improvement in survival, particularly in those patients in whom the thrombus was successfully lysed.[14–15a] However, it was not until intravenous thrombolytic agents were administered that large multicenter trials could be successfully undertaken.

Effect on Mortality

Intravenous administration of thrombolytic agents has been shown to significantly reduce the mortality rate of acute myocardial infarction by approximately 25%.[15a] The results of the larger multicenter randomized trials in which different intravenous thrombolytic agents were used are shown in Table 19-2.

The first large-scale trial conducted by the Gruppo Italiano per lo Studio della Streptochinasi nell 'Infarto Miocardico (GISSI) in 1986 convincingly showed that intravenous streptokinase administered within 6 h of acute myocardial infarction significantly reduced the 21-day mortality by 18%.[16] A similar 25% reduction in vascular mortality with the use of intravenous streptokinase was shown in the Second International Study of Infarct Survival (ISIS-2).[17] In this trial, patients were admitted with symptoms suggestive of acute myocardial infarction, and only 55% had significant ST-segment elevation. One smaller trial of Intravenous Streptokinase in Acute

TABLE 19-1. Thrombolytic Agents Currently Available in the United States

Characteristic	Streptokinase	tPA*	Reteplase	Tenecteplase
Molecular weight (daltons)	47,000	70,000	40,000	70,000
Plasma clearance time (min)	15–25	4–8	13–16	20–24
Fibrin specificity	Minimal	Moderate	Mild-moderate	High
Plasminogen binding	Indirect	Direct	Direct	Direct
Potential allergic reaction	Yes	No	No	No
Typical dose	1.5 million units	100 mg	20 million units	40 mg
Administration	1-h IV infusion	15 mg IV bolus, 0.75 mg/kg over 30 min (max 50 mg) then 0.5 mg/kg over 60 min (max 35 mg)	Double bolus: 10 million U then 10 million U 30 min later	Single bolus: according to weight <60 kg: 30 mg 60–69 kg: 35 mg 70–79 kg: 40 mg 80–89 kg: 45 mg ≥90 kg: 50 mg
Approximate cost ($)	340	2000	2000	2000

*Tissue plasminogen activator.

note the results from two separate surveys that were conducted outside the trials. The incidence of intracerebral hemorrhage in a group of nonrandomized patients admitted to 61 hospitals in Holland over 18 months was 1.0% (95% confidence limits, 0.62 to 1.3%).[81] Analysis of events from a Myocardial Infarction Triage and Intervention (MITI) Study,[82] where patients in the Seattle area with myocardial infarction were monitored, revealed an equal incidence of stroke in patients receiving thrombolysis (1.6%) as in patients who did not (2.2%). The incidence of hemorrhagic stroke was 1.1% among the patients who received thrombolysis compared with 0.4% among those who did not.

The incidence of intracranial hemorrhage was as high as 1.3% in the TIMI-II trial,[83] in which patients were treated with 150 mg of tPA. This was decreased to 0.4% when the dose of tPA was decreased to 100 mg; thus the larger dose of tPA is no longer used.

Although hypertension is generally regarded as a significant risk factor in the development of an intracranial bleed following administration of thrombolytic agents, this has not been proven from the trials or general surveys.[49,81] A multivariant logistic regression analysis found that only prior treatment with other anticoagulants, body weight less than 70 kg, and age greater than 65 years were associated with a significantly greater incidence of intracerebral bleeding.[49]

It was originally deemed that patients who had a cerebrovascular episode more than 6 months prior to the myocardial infarction would be at low risk for an intracerebral bleed. When such patients were randomized to receive tPA in the TIMI study, the incidence of cerebral hemorrhage remained very high, at 3.4%, compared with 0.5% in the later part of the trial, when such patients were excluded.[83]

There appears to be a small difference in hemorrhagic stroke according to the thrombolytic agent used. A significant difference in intracerebral bleeding was found in ISIS-3 trial[23] between patients who received tPA (0.7%) and those who received streptokinase (0.3%). This difference has been attributed to a higher dose of duteplase compared with a lower dose of alteplase, which is currently the form of tPA used today. In the GISSI-2 trial,[22] the incidence of hemorrhagic stroke was 0.3% in the tPA group and 0.25% in patients receiving streptokinase. However, in the GUSTO trial,[24] the incidence of hemorrhagic stroke was 0.7%, and significantly greater than 0.5% in patients receiving streptokinase. In patients over the age of 75, the incidence of hemorrhagic stroke was 2.08% in those treated with tPA and significantly greater than the 1.23% in the patients receiving streptokinase.[24] Thus it may be more judicious to use streptokinase in very elderly patients presenting with acute myocardial infarction.

Noncerebral Hemorrhage

Major noncerebral bleeds that require blood transfusion occurred more frequently in patients who received thrombolysis, with an excess of 7.3 per 1000 patients (1.1% in patients receiving thrombolysis and 0.4% in the patients in the control group.)[49]

Treatment of Bleeding with Thrombolysis

Massive bleeding accompanied by hemodynamic compromise, particularly if the bleeding site is not compressible, should be treated with coagulation factors and volume replacement.[84] If the patient is receiving heparin, it should be discontinued and protamine administered. In the absence of heparin therapy, a prolonged partial thromboplastin time will identify patients with a persistent fibrinolytic state. Such a patient should immediately receive 10 U of cryoprecipitate.[84] The fibrinogen level should be monitored only after the cryoprecipitate has been given; if that level is less than 100 mg/100 mL, the patient should receive an additional 10 U of cryoprecipitate. If bleeding persists after fibrinogen has been restored, 2 U of fresh frozen plasma should be given. If the bleeding continues to be uncontrolled, it is recommended that bleeding time be monitored.[84] If this is longer than 9 min, the patient should receive 10 U of platelets; if the bleeding time is less then 9 min, it is suggested that the patient receive an antifibrinolytic agent such as aminocaproic acid.

Cardiac Rupture

Myocardial rupture is a consequence of transmural myocardial necrosis and occurs in approximately 4% of patients admitted with acute myocardial infarction. It has been reasoned that early administration of thrombolytic therapy will reduce cardiac rupture by preventing transmural necrosis, whereas late thrombolysis, which promotes hemorrhage into a transmural myocardial infarct, will increase the incidence of myocardial rupture.[84] Honan et al.,[85] in a metanalysis of placebo-controlled trials in which thrombolysis was administered to 1638 patients, found that 58 patients had developed myocardial rupture. Regression-line analysis revealed that the incidence of myocardial rupture increased with the time interval between the onset of symptoms and the administration of the thrombolytic agent and that the odds ratio are greater than 1.0 of developing cardiac rupture when the thrombolytic agents are administered 11 h after the onset of symptoms. However, in the prospectively designed LATE study,[86] the incidence of myocardial rupture was greater with thrombolysis between 6 and 12 h compared with 12 and 24 h after the onset of symptoms.

Thus, it appears that the time course of rupture may be accelerated by thrombolysis but that the overall incidence may not be increased.

INDICATIONS AND CONTRAINDICATIONS TO THROMBOLYSIS

The indications for thrombolysis in patients with acute myocardial infarction are listed in Table 19-6 and the contraindications in Table 19-7. A more detailed discussion of the following items is provided in the earlier part of the text: time after myocardial infarction, site of

TABLE 19-6. Criteria for Thrombolysis in Acute Myocardial Infarction

Chest pain consistent with acute myocardial infarction lasting 30 min
Electrocardiographic changes:
    ST-segment elevation in at least two contiguous limb leads of 0.1 mV
        V_1–V_3 of 0.2 mV
        V_4–V_6 of 0.1 mV
    ST-segment depression in V_{1-3} with tall R in V_2 with diagnosis of posterior infarction
    New or presumed left bundle branch block
Time from onset of symptoms:
    <6 h: most beneficial
    6–12 h: intermediate benefit
    >12 h: least benefit; consider if chest pain present or staggered pain course in high-risk patients

TABLE 19-7. Contraindications to Thrombolytic Therapy

Absolute contraindications:
  Prior intracranial bleed
  Thromboembolic stroke within 2 months
  Neurosurgery within 1 month
  Active internal bleeding (excluding menstruation)
  Dissecting aortic aneurysm

Relative contraindications:
  Persistent hypertension ≥180/110 mm Hg despite therapy
  Recent puncture of noncompressible vessel
  Gastrointestinal and genitourinary bleeding within 1 month
  Bleeding diathesis
  Anticoagulant therapy
  Significant liver and renal disease
  Pericarditis
  Proliferative diabetic retinopathy
  Pregnancy
  Recent surgery or biopsy of internal organ within 2 weeks

myocardial infarction, non-Q-wave myocardial infarction, cardiogenic shock, elderly patients, and hypertension. The distinction between absolute and relative contraindications to thrombolysis becomes less important when a cardiac catheterization laboratory is available for the performance of immediate coronary angioplasty.

THROMBOLYSIS FOR CONDITIONS OTHER THAN ACUTE MYOCARDIAL INFARCTION

Obstructive Mechanical Prosthetic Valve

The incidence of thrombosis of mechanical mitral prostheses is greater than that in the aortic position, with an annual incidence of less than 0.5%. The operative mortality has been reported to be 11 to 12%,[87,88] but it was significantly higher, 17.5%, in patients with class IV New York Heart Association symptoms. Roudaut[89] and colleagues describe successful thrombolysis in 73% of 75 thrombotic events, with a 92% success rate in patients with functional class I and II and 63% in patients functional class III and IV symptoms. Embolic events occurred in 12 of the 64 patients, 4 of which were major. Thrombosis recurred in 11 patients in approximately 1 year. In a meta-analysis, thrombolysis was reported to be effective in 84%, and streptokinase appeared to be more effective than urokinase.[90]

Others have reported a very low rate of embolic events following thrombolysis in the presence of mobile thrombi. However, most believe that a mobile thrombus is a relative contraindication to thrombolysis. Successful thrombolysis is frequently achieved with one to three courses of thrombolytic agent on a daily basis, using streptokinase 60,000 to 100,000 U/h over 16 to 24 h or tPA with a 10-mg bolus followed by 90-mg infusion over 3 h.[91,92] It is advised that the patients continue taking warfarin during thrombolysis and receive heparin until such time as the international normalized ratio (INR) is therapeutic. If the patient requires emergent surgery, it is advantageous to use tPA rather than streptokinase, as the latter is associated with a systemic thrombolytic state and depletion of thrombin.

It has been recommended that patients who have obstructed prostheses with minimal clot seen on transesophageal echocardiography should receive thrombolysis, which has an expected success rate of 92%.[90,92] Surgery is also recommend for patients with large substantial clots or those who have class IV symptoms with obstructive prostheses.

Pulmonary Embolism

In the Urokinase Pulmonary Embolism Trial (UPET) conducted in the early 1970s, in which urokinase followed by heparin was compared with heparin alone in a total of 160 patients, there was a trend toward reduction in mortality and recurrent emboli in patients assigned to receive thrombolysis.[93] There was a significantly more rapid and complete dissolution of thrombi but also more bleeding complications in the patients receiving thrombolysis.

Unfortunately, the subsequent trials have utilized even fewer patients than in UPET. The PAIMS-2 trial in Italy showed that thrombolysis produced a more efficient dissolution of thrombus and more rapid reduction in pulmonary arterial pressure following 2 h of tPA infusion compared with heparin.[94] When tPA was compared with urokinase in the European Cooperative Study Group, it was observed that there was a more significant and rapid reduction in pulmonary vascular resistance at 2 h, but the results were similar at 6 h.[95]

In the series of trials carried out by Goldhaber et al.,[96] it was shown that, after tPA infusion, there was significantly greater clot lysis after 2 h when compared with urokinase administered over 24 h; at 24 h, however, there was no difference in clot lysis between these two groups.[97] Similar efficacy resulted when a condensed dose of urokinase was administered.[98] This group also demonstrated that there was significantly greater improvement in right ventricular systolic function as measured by echocardiography at 24 h when tPA was administered compared with heparin.[99] It has been shown that tPA administered via a pulmonary catheter or a peripheral vein resulted in similar rate of thrombolysis; thus thrombolytic agents did not have to be administered via a pulmonary catheter.[100]

The use of heparin and a thrombolytic agent were compared in a report from a multiple-center registry of 719 consecutive patients with major pulmonary embolism and specifically excluded patients who were hemodynamically unstable.[101] The mortality rate was 4.7% for 169 patients receiving thrombolytic treatment, whereas it was 11.1% for 555 patients receiving heparin. Although the groups were not similar, multivariate logistic regression analysis demonstrated that thrombolytic treatment was an independent predictor of survival. The patients receiving thrombolysis had a significantly higher rate of major hemorrhage: 21.9%, versus 7.8% of patients receiving heparin. Only 1.2% of the patients receiving thrombolysis developed intracranial hemorrhage.[101]

It has now become accepted practice to treat massive pulmonary embolism associated with hemodynamic instability with thrombolysis. The presence of right ventricular dysfunction seen on echocardiography is also considered an indication for thrombolysis.[102]

Regimens approved by the U.S. Food and Drug Administration (FDA) for the treatment of pulmonary embolism are as follows: streptokinase 250,000 U loading dose over 30 min followed by 100,000 U/h for 24 h; urokinase 4,400 U/kg loading dose over 10 min followed by 4,400 U/h for 12 to 24 h; and tPA 100 mg over 2 h. It is recommended that heparin not be given simultaneously with a thrombolytic agent.[96]

Ischemic Stroke

The use of thrombolytic agents in the treatment of ischemic stroke remains controversial. Earlier studies using streptokinase were prematurely stopped because of excess intracranial hemorrhage[103–105] or because treatment was of no benefit when tPA was used.[106] These trials treated patients up to 6 h after the onset of stroke.

In a subsequent study, patients were randomized to receive tPA or placebo within 3 h after the onset of stroke. After a computed tomographic scan had excluded intracranial hemorrhage, patients who received thrombolysis were 30 to 50% more likely to have minimal or no disability at 3 months.[107]

Thrombolysis with intravenous tPA is now accepted treatment when administered within 3 h of the onset of nonhemorrhagic ischemic stroke,[108,108a] with some consideration for its administration in the time window up to 6-h after onset of symptoms.[108b] In addition, a number of strategies combining antiplatelet and thrombolytic therapies for stroke are now being refined.[108c] Unfortunately only 5% of stroke patients receive intravenous thrombolysis in the United States.[108] Pro-urokinase has been given intraarterially in patients with middle cerebral artery occlusion up to 6 h after onset with significant success.[109]

Deep Venous Thrombosis

Standard treatment of deep venous thrombosis with heparin reduces the extension and embolization of thrombus but does not increase the rate of clot lysis. Thus permanent damage to the venous valvular system may ensue, with a resultant postthrombotic syndrome of pain, edema, stasis, and dermatitis.

Significantly faster resolution of deep venous thrombosis has been reported with the use of streptokinase, urokinase, and tPA, with approximately 45% complete resolution using a thrombolytic agent compared with 4% with heparin.[110-112] Complete lysis of thrombus may require several days of treatment and is less successful for older thrombi, particularly those beyond 7 days. However, using selective catheter infusion of a thrombolytic agent may improve the rate of thrombolysis. A more recent study reported that systemically administered thrombolytic agents resulted in higher recanalization and a lower incidence of postthrombotic syndrome.[112] Because of a 6% rate of major bleeding complications, they advised its use only in patients with limb-threatening situations.

Subclavian and axillary venous thromboses have been successfully treated with direct infusion of thrombolytic agents into the distal vein, and thrombectomy has generally been avoided. Those patients with primary thrombosis of the subclavian or axillary veins may require additional surgery to correct thoracic outlet syndrome.

The doses of thrombolytics used are as follows: streptokinase 2500 U bolus, followed by 100,000 U/h for up to 3 days; streptokinase 3 million U over 4 h; tPA 0.05 mg/kg/h for 8 to 24 h. For local or regional infusion: urokinase 100,000 U/day, tPA 20 mg/day.[112,113]

Thrombotic Arterial Occlusion

Patients with acute arterial occlusion of the lower limbs and pelvis are potential candidates for intraarterial infusion of thrombolytic agents. With acute ischemia that threatens the viability of the limb, surgery should be considered primarily and thrombolysis only if surgery is not feasible or the limb not threatened. Thrombolytic therapy should be infused by an intraarterially directed catheter into the occluded artery. This has been successfully performed using streptokinase, urokinase, and tPA and has resulted in fewer lower limb amputations and a significant increase clot lysis and recanalization.[114-116] Thrombolytic artery occlusion therapy has also been used as a treatment for mesenteric thrombosis.[116a]

A recent consensus statement indicated that catheter-directed thrombolysis was more likely to be superior to surgery if the guidewire could pass through the thrombus, the occlusion were less than 14 days old, the occlusion were thrombotic rather than embolic, and significant comorbid cardiopulmonary disease coexisted.[117]

Doses of catheter-directed thrombolytic agents used: urokinase 4,000 units/hour over 4 h, tPA 0.5 to 0.1 mg/kg/h for up to 12 h.

Arterial emboli are better removed by balloon catheter techniques or surgery, since thrombolysis in such instances has not been as successful.

Hemodialysis Catheters, Grafts and Fistulas, and Central Venous Catheters

Thrombolytic agents can be used to clear occluded central venous catheters. They have also been shown to be efficacious in treating occluded hemodialysis accesses that include native arteries and vascular grafts.[117a,117b]

NEW THROMBOLYTIC AGENTS

Staphylokinase (SAK)

Staphylokinase is a 136-chain amino acid protein produced by selective strains of *Staphylococcus aureus*. It forms an SAK-plasmin complex, which converts plasminogen to plasmin. It differs from streptokinase in that SAK is not bound to plasmin and is rapidly inhibited by C_2 antiplasmin.[118,119] In patients who received SAK in a dose-finding trial, a similar TIMI grade III patency rate of 62 to 65% was achieved across a threefold increment in dose (15, 30, and 45 mg).[120] An earlier study showed similar TIMI grade 3 flow rates but significantly less depletion of fibrinogen in patients receiving SAK compared with tPA, thus making SAK more fibrin-specific.[121]

SAK can induce neutralizing antibodies,[121] but protein engineering has significantly reduced its antigenicity without functional inactivation.[122] Modification of the SAK molecule has decreased its clearance five fold, which will permit it to be given by bolus injection.[122]

Lanoteplase (nPA)

Lanoteplase is a novel synthetic plasminogen activator that lacks fibronectin finger and epidermal growth factor domains. It is more potent that tPA, has a much longer plasma clearance, is less fibrin-specific, and can be administered as a single bolus.[123] At comparable lytic doses, both nPA and tPA have comparable effects on fibrinogen alpha$_2$ antiplasmin.

Administration of the highest doses of nPA resulted in a 90-min TIMI grade 3 flow rate of 57%, compared with 46% in patients receiving tPA ($P = .11$).[123] However, in this study, a relatively low TIMI 3 flow rate for the 107 patients who received tPA was reported. There was no difference in the 30-day survival or composite endpoint when the two agents were compared. In the In TIME-II (Intravenous nPA for Treatment of Infarcting Myocardium Early) study,[124] there was no difference in the 30-day survival of the 15,078 patients randomized in a 2:1 ratio to receive 120 U/kg nPA or tPA (6.75 versus 6.61%): however, the rate of hemorrhagic stroke was 0.64% with tPA versus 1.12% with nPA ($P = .004$).

Vampire Bat Salivary Activator (bat-PA)

The saliva of the vampire bat (*Desmodus rotundus*) contains four plasminogen activators (DSPAs) that are similar in structure to tPA. One of these, bat-PA, has been reported in animal experiments to accomplish similar reperfusion rates to tPA and to be highly fibrin specific, but it caused a greater number of bleeding episodes.[125,126]

Saruplase/Pro-urokinase (scu-PA)

The single-chain form of urokinase is also known as pro-urokinase (scu-PA) and Saruplase. The single-chain form occurs naturally and the agent is synthesized by recombinant DNA techniques. It is the only natural plasminogen activator that is a zymogen and hence inactive until its conversion to double-chain urokinase. This conversion requires clot-bound plasminogen, which is converted to clot-bound plasmin, which in turn converts other urokinase molecules to activate urokinase on the clot surface.[127]

Although two trials have shown a similarity in efficacy with alteplase[128] and streptokinase,[129,130] the European Medical Evaluation Agency (EMEA) has rejected saruplase for clinical use,[131] presumably because of a higher incidence of intracranial hemorrhage.

Pamitiplase and Amediplase

These two newer thrombolytic agents have been created by novel modification of tPA.[131–133] They both have longer half-lives and can be given by bolus injection, have fibrin specificity, and are currently in phase 2 studies in patients with acute myocardial infarction.[131]

CONCLUSION

Modification of the molecular structure of thrombolytic agents has improved their potency and fibrin specificity and delayed their plasma clearance. Addition of more potent antiplatelet regimens has also enhanced their thrombolytic efficacy. However, these modifications in treatment of patients with acute myocardial infarction have not always been translated into improved survival.

REFERENCES

1. Collen D: Fibrin-selective thrombolytic therapy for acute myocardial myocardial infarction. *Circulation* 93:857, 1996.
2. Robbins KC, Summaira L., Hsieh B, Shah RJ: The peptide chains of human plasmin. Mechanism of activation of human plasminogen to plasmin. *J Biol Chem* 242:2333, 1967.
3. Granger CB, Califf RM, Topol EJ: Thrombolytic therapy for acute myocardial infarction. *Drugs* 44:293, 1992.
4. Collen D, Verstrate M: Pharmacology of thrombolytic drugs. In: Schlant RC, Alexander RW, eds. *Hurst's The Heart*, 8th ed. New York: McGraw Hill, 1994:1327.
4a. Kamat SG, Michelson AD, Benoit SE, et al: Fibrinolysis inhibits shear stress-induced platelet aggregation. *Circulation* 92:1399, 1995.
5. Collen D: On the regulation of control of fibrinolysis. *Thromb Haemost* 43:77, 1980.
6. www.abbott.com. Important drug warning: Issued 1/25/1999.
7. Anderson HV, Willerson JT: Thrombolysis in acute myocardial infarction. *N Engl J Med* 329:703, 1993.
7a. Modi NB, Fox NL, Clow F-W, et al: Pharmacokinetics and pharmacodynamics of tenecteplase: Results from a phase II study in patients with acute myocardial infarction. *J Clin Pharmacol* 40:508, 2000.

7b. van de Werf F, Cannon CP, Luyten A, et al for the ASSENT-1 investigators: Safety assessment of single-bolus administration of TNK tissue-plasminogen activator in acute myocardial infarction: The ASSENT-1 trial. *Am Heart J* 137:786, 1999.
8. Torr SR, Nachowiak DA, Fujui S, Sobel BE: Plasminogen steal and clot lysis. *J Am Coll Cardiol* 19:1085, 1992.
9. Davies, MJ, Thomas, AC: Plaque fissuring—the cause of acute myocardial infarction, sudden ischemic death and crescendo angina. *Br Heart J* 53:363, 1985.
10. DeWood MA, Spokes J, Notske R, et al: Prevalence of total coronary occlusion during early hours of transmural myocardial infarction. *N Engl J Med* 303:897, 1980.
11. Reimer KA, Lowe JE, Rasmussen MM, Jennings RB: The wakefront phenomenon of ischemic cell death l. Myocardial infarct size versus duration of coronary occlusion in dogs. *Circulation* 56:786, 1977.
12. Rentrop P, Blanke H, Karsch KR, et al: Acute myocardial infarction: Intracoronary application of nitroglycerin and streptokinase. *Clin Cardiol* 2:354, 1979.
13. Rentrop P, Blanke H, Karsch KR, et al: Selective intracoronary thrombolysis in acute myocardial infarction and unstable angina. *Circulation* 63:307, 1981.
14. Kennedy JW, Ritchie JL, Davis KB, et al: The Western Washington randomized trial of intracoronary streptokinase in acute myocardial infarction. *N Engl J Med* 309:1477, 1983.
15. Kennedy JW, Ritchie JL, Davis KB, et al: The Western Washington randomized trial of intracoronary streptokinase in acute myocardial infarction. *N Engl J Med* 312:1073, 1985.
15a. van Domburg RT, Boersma E, Simoons ML: A review of the long term effects of thrombolytic agents. *Drugs* 60:293, 2000.
16. Gruppo Italiano per lo Studio della streptochinasi nell'infarto miocardico (GISSI): Effective intravenous thrombolytic treatment in acute myocardial infarction. *Lancet* 1:1397, 1986.
17. ISIS-2 (Second International Study of Infarct Survival) Collaborative Group: Randomized trial of intravenous streptokinase, oral aspirin, both or neither among 17,187 cases of suspected acute myocardial infarction: ISIS-2. *Lancet* 2:349, 1988.
18. The ISAM Study Group: A prospective trial of intravenous streptokinase in acute myocardial infarction (ISAM) mortality, morbidity, and infarct size at 21 days. *N Engl J Med* 314:1465, 1986.
19. AIMS Trial Study Group: Effect of intravenous APSAC on mortality after acute myocardial infarction: Preliminary report of a placebo-controlled clinical trial. *Lancet* 1:842, 1988.
20. AIMS Trial Study Group: Long-term effects of intravenous anistreplase in acute myocardial infarction: Final report of the AIMS study. *Lancet* 335:427, 1990.
21. Wilcox RG, Von der Lippe G., Olson G, et al: Trial of tissue plasminogen activator for mortality reduction in acute myocardial infarction: Anglo-Scandinavian Study of Early Thrombolysis (ASSET). *Lancet* 2:525, 1988.
22. Gruppo Italiano per lo Studio Della sopravvivenza nell'infarcto miocardico. GISSI-2: A factorial randomized trial of alteplase versus streptokinase and heparin versus no heparin among 12,490 patients with acute myocardial infarction. *Lancet* 336:65, 1990.
23. Third International Study of Infarct Survival Collaborative Group. ISIS-3: A randomized comparison of streptokinase versus tissue plasminogen activator versus anistreplase and of aspirin plus heparin versus aspirin alone among 41,299 cases of suspected acute myocardial infarction. *Lancet* 339:753, 1992.
24. The GUSTO Investigators: An international randomized trial comparing four thrombolytic strategies for acute myocardial infarction. *N Engl J Med* 329:673, 1993.
24a. Califf RM, White HD, Van de Werf F, et al: One-year results from the Global Utilization of Streptokinase and tPA for Occluded Coronary Arteries (GUSTO-1) trial. *Circulation* 94:1233, 1996.
25. Mueller HS, Rao AK, Forman SA: The TIMI Investigators thrombolysis in myocardial infarction (TIMI): Comparative studies of coronary reperfusion and systemic fibrinogenolysis with two forms of recombinant tissue-type plasminogen activator. *J Am Coll Cardiol* 10:479, 1987.
26. The Continuous Infusion versus Double-Bolus Administration of Alteplase (COBOLT) Investigators: A comparison of continuous infusion of alteplase with double-bolus administration for acute myocardial infarction. *N Engl J Med* 337:1124, 1997.

27. Bode C, Smalling RW, Berg G, et al for RAPID II Investigators; Randomized comparison of coronary thrombolysis achieved with double-bolus reteplase (recombinant plasminogen activators) and front-loaded, accelerated alteplase (recombinant tissue plasminogen activator) in patients with acute myocardial infarction. *Circulation* 946:891, 1996.

28. International Joint Efficacy Comparison of thrombolytics: Randomized, double-blind comparison of reteplase double-bolus administration with streptokinase in acute myocardial infarction (INJECT): Trial to investigate equivalence. *Lancet* 346:329, 1995.

29. Global Use of Strategies to Open Coronary Arteries (GUSTO III) Investigation: Comparison of reteplase with alteplase for acute myocardial infarction. *N Engl J Med* 337:1118, 1997.

30. Assessment of the Safety and Efficacy of a New Thrombolytic (ASSENT-2) Investigators: Single-bolus tenecteplase compared with front-loaded alteplase in acute myocardial infarction: The ASSENT-2 double-blind trial. *Lancet* 354:716, 1999.

31. EMERAS (Estudio Multicentrico Estreptoquinasa Republicas de America del Sur) Collaborative Group: Randomized trial of late thrombolysis in patients with suspected acute myocardial infarction. *Lancet* 342:767, 1993.

32. LATE Study Group: Late assessment of thrombolysis efficacy (LATE). Study with alteplase after onset of acute myocardial infarction. *Lancet* 342:759, 1993.

33. Chesboro JH, Knatterud G, Roberts R, et al: Thrombolysis in myocardial infarction (TIMI) trial, phase 1: A comparison between intravenous and tissue plasminogen activator and intravenous streptokinase. *Circulation* 76:142, 1987.

34. Dalen JE: Six and twelve month follow-up of phase 1 thrombolysis in myocardial infarction (TIMI) trial. *Am J Cardiol* 62:179, 1988.

35. The GUSTO angiographic investigators: The effects of tissue plasminogen activator, streptokinase, or both on coronary artery patency, ventricular function and survival after acute myocardial infarction. *N Engl J Med* 329:1615, 1993.

36. Gillis JC, Wagstaff AJ, Goa KL: Alteplase. Reapproval of its pharmacolgic properties and therapeutic uses in acute myocardial infarction. *Drugs* 50:101, 1995.

37. Rurors JA, McNeil AJ, Siddiqui RT, et al: Efficacy of 100-mg of double-bolus alteplase in achieving complete perfusion in the treatment of acute myocardial infarction. *J Am Coll Cardiol* 23:6, 1944.

38. Smalling RW, Bode C, Kalbfleisch J, et al and RAPID investigators: More rapid, complete, and stable coronary thrombolysis with bolus administration of reteplase compared with alteplase infusion in acute myocardial infarction. *Circulation* 91:2725, 1995.

39. Cannon CP, McCable CH, Gibson CM, et al and TIMI 10A investigators. TNK-tissue plasminogen activator in acute myocardial infarction. Results of thrombolysis in myocardial infarction (TIMI) 10A dose ranging trial. *Circulation* 95:351, 1997.

40. Cannon CP, Gibson CM, McCabe CH, et al for TIMI 10B investigators. TNK-tissue plasminogen activator compared with front loaded alteplase in a cute myocardial infarction. *Circulation* 98:2805, 1998.

40a. Goldman LE, Eisenberg MJ: Identification and management of patients with failed thrombolysis after acute myocardial infarction. *Ann Intern Med* 132:556, 2000.

41. Ohman EM, Califf RM, Topol EJ, et al: Consequences of reocclusion after successful reperfusion therapy in acute myocardial infarction. *Circulation* 82:781, 1990.

41a. Pilote L, Miller DP, Califf RM, et al: Determinants of the use of coronary angiography and revascularization after thrombolysis for acute myocardial infarction. *N Engl J Med* 335:1198, 1996.

42. Barbarsh GI, Birnbaum Y, Bogaerts K, et al: Treatment of reinfarction after thrombolytic therapy for acute myocardial infarction. An analysis of outcome and treatment choices in the Global Utilization of Streptokinase and Tissue Plasminogen Activator for Occluded Coronary Arteries (GUSTO I) and Assessment of the Safety of a New Thrombolytic (ASSENT 2) studies. *Circulation* 103:954, 2001.

43. White HD: Thrombolytic treatment for recurrent myocardial infarction. Avoid repeating streptokinase or anistreplase. *BMJ* 302:429, 1991.

44. Barbash GI, Hod H, Roth A. et al: Repeat infusions of recombinant tissue-type plasminogen activator in patients with acute myocardial infarction and recurrent myocardial ischemia. *J Am Coll Cardiol* 16:779, 1990.

45. Anderson JL, Karagounis LA, Becker LC, et al: TIMI perfusion grade 3 but not grade 2 results improve outcome after thrombolysis for myocardial infarction. Ventriculographic enzymatic, and electrocardiographic evidence from the TEAM-3 study. *Circulation* 87:1829, 1993.

46. Simes RJ, Topol EJ, Holmes DR: Link between angiographic substudy and mortality outcomes in a large randomized trial of myocardial reperfusion. Importance of early and complete infarct artery reperfusion. *Circulation* 91:1923, 1995.

47. Gibson CM, Murphy SA, Rizzo MJ et al: Relationship between TIMI frame count and clinical outcomes after thrombolytic administration. *Circulation* 99:1945, 1999.

48. Grines CL, DeMaria AN: Optimal utilization of thrombolytic therapy for acute myocardial infarction: Concepts and controversies. *J Am Coll Cardiol* 16:223, 1990.

49. Fibrinolytic Therapy Trialists (FTT) Collaborative Group: Indications for fibrinolytic therapy in suspected acute myocardial infarction: Collaborative overview of early mortality and major morbidity in results from all randomize trials of more than 1000 patients. *Lancet* 343:311, 1994.

50. The TIMI IIIB Investigators: Effects of tissue plasminogen activator and comparison of early invasive and conservative strategies in unstable angina and non-Q wave myocardial infarction. Results of the TIMI IIIB trial. *Circulation* 89:1545, 1994.

51. Braunwald E, Cannon PC: Non Q wave and ST segment depression myocardial infarction: Is there a role for thrombolytic therapy? *J Am Coll Cardiol* 27:1333, 1996.

52. Langes A, Goodman SG, Topol EJ, et al: Late assessment of thrombolytic efficacy (LATE) Study: Prognosis in patients with non-Q wave myocardial infarcts. *J Am Coll Cardiol* 27:1327, 1996.

53. Sgarbossa EB, Pinski SL, Barbagelata A, et al for GUSTO-1 investigators. Electrocardiographic diagnosis of evolving acute myocardial infarction in the presence of left bundle branch block. *N Eng J Med* 344:481, 1996.

54. Holmes DR, Bates ER, Kleinman NS, et al: Contemporary reperfusion therapy for cardiogenic shock: The GUSTO-1 trial experience. *J Am Coll Cardiol* 26:668, 1995.

55. Hochman JS, Sleeper LA, Webb JG, et al: Early revascularization in acute myocardial infarction complicated by cardiogenic shock. *N Eng J Med* 341:625, 1999.

55a. Berger AK, Radford MJ, Wang Y, Krumholz HM: Thrombolytic therapy in older patients. *J Am Coll Cardiol* 36:366, 2000.

55b. Ayanian JZ, Braunwald E: Thrombolytic therapy for patients with myocardial infarction who are older than 75 years. Do the risks outweigh the benefits? *Circulation* 101:2224, 2000.

56. Lenefsky EJ, Lundergan CF, Hodgson JMcB, et al: Increased left ventricular dysfunction in elderly patients despite successful thrombolysis. The GUSTO-1 angiographic experience. *J Am Coll Cardiol* 28:331, 1966.

57. Thiemann DZR, Coresh J, Schulman SP, et al: Lack of benefit for intravenous thrombolysis in patients with myocardial infarction who are older than 75 years. *Circulation* 101:2239, 2000.

58. White HD: Thrombolytic therapy in the elderly (editorial). *Lancet* 356:2028, 2000.

58a. Ridker PM, Hennekens CH: Age and thrombolytic therapy. *Circulation* 94:1807, 1996.

59. Antman EM, Giugliano RP, Gibson C.M., et al: Abciximab facilitates the rate and extent of thrombolysis. Results of the Thrombolysis in Myocardial Infarction (TIMI) 14 trial. *Circulation* 99:2720, 1999.

60. Neumann F-J, Zohlnhofer D, Fakhoury D, et al: Effect of glycoprotein IIb/IIIa. Receptor blockade on platelet/leukocyte interaction and surface expression of the leukocyte integrin Mac-1 in acute myocardial infarction. *J Am Coll Cardiol* 34:1420, 1999.

61. Ohman EM, Kleiman NS, Gacioch G, et al for IMPACT-AMI Investigators: Combined accelerated tissue plasminogen activator and platelet glycoproteins IIb/IIIa. Integrin receptor blockage with integrelin in acute myocardial infarction. Results of a randomized, placebo-controlled dose-ranging trial. *Circulation* 95:846, 1997.

62. Strategies for Patency Enhancement in the Emergency Department (SPEED) Group Trial of abciximab with and without low-dose reteplase for acute myocardial infarction. *Circulation* 101:2788, 2000.

63. Gibson CM., deLemos JA, Murphy SA, et al: Combination therapy with abciximab reduces angiographically evident thrombus in acute

myocardial infarction. A TIMI 14 Sub-study. *Circulation* 103:2550, 2001.

64. The GUSTO V Investigators. Reperfusion therapy for acute myocardial infarction with fibrinolytic therapy or combination reduced fibrinolytic therapy and platelet glycoprotein IIb/IIIa inhibition: The GUSTO V randomized Trial. *Lancet* 357:1905, 2001.

64a. Assessment of the Safety and Efficacy of a New Thrombolytic regimen (ASSENT-3) Investigators: Efficacy and safety of tenecteplas in combination with enoxaparin, abciximab or unfractionated heparin: The ASSENT-3 randomized trial in acute myocardial infarction. *Lancet* 358:605, 2001.

65. Eisenberg PR, Sherman LA, Jaffe AS: Paradoxical elevation of fibrinopeptide A: Evidence for continued thrombosis despite intensive fibrinolysis. *J Am Coll Cardiol* 10:527, 1987.

66. Aronson DL, Chang P, Kessler CM: Platelet-dependent thrombin generation after in vitro-fibrinolytic treatment. *Circulation* 85:1706, 1992.

67. Fitzgerald DJ, Catella F, Roy L, et al: Marked platelet activation in vivo after intravenous streptokinase in patients with acute myocardial infarction. *Circulation* 77:142, 1988.

67a. Keller NM, Feit F: Thrombolytic therapy in acute MI, Part 2: Update on adjuvants. *J Crit Illness* 13:646, 1998.

68. Handin, R.I.: Platelets and coronary artery disease. *N Engl J Med* 334:1126, 1996.

68a. Harding SA, Boon NA, Flapan AD: Antiplatelet treatment in unstable angina: Aspirin, clopidogrel, glycoprotein IIb/IIIa antagonist, or all three? *Heart* 88:11, 2002.

68b. Gaspoz JM, Coxson PG, Goldman PA, et al: Cost effectiveness of aspirin, clopidogrel, or both for secondary prevention of coronary heart disease. *N Engl J Med* 346:1800, 2002.

68c. Granger CB, Becker R, Tracy RP, et al for the GUSTO-I Hemostasis Substudy Group: Thrombin generation, inhibition and clinical outcomes in patients with acute myocardial infarction treated with thrombolytic therapy and heparin: Results from the GUSTO-I trial. *J Am Coll Cardiol* 31:497, 1998.

69. Topol EJ, George BS, Kareiakes DJ, et al: A randomized trial of intravenous tissue plasminogen activator and early intravenous heparin in acute myocardial infarction. *Circulation* 79:281, 1989.

70. Hsia JA, Hamilton WP, Kleinman N, et al: A comparison between heparin and low dose aspirin as adjunctive therapy with tissue plasminogen activator for acute myocardial infarction. *N Engl J Med* 323:1433, 1990.

71. DeBono DP, Simoons ML, Tijssen J: Effect of early intravenous heparin on coronary patency, infarct size, and bleeding complications after alteplase. Thrombolysis: Results of a randomized double-blind European Cooperative Study Group Trial. *Br Heart J* 67:122, 1992.

72. Hirsh J, Fuster V: Guide to anticoagulant therapy, part 1: Heparin. *Circulation* 89:1449, 1994.

73. International Study Group: In-hospital mortality and clinical course of 20,891 patients with suspected acute myocardial infarction randomized between alteplase and streptokinase. *Lancet* 336:71, 1990.

74. The SCATI (Studio sulla Calciparina nell'Angina e nella Trombosi Ventricolare nell' Infarto) Group: Randomized controlled trial of subcutaneous calcium heparin in acute myocardial infarction. *Lancet* 2:182, 1989.

75. The Global Use of Strategies to Open Occluded Coronary Arteries (GUSTO) IIa Investigators: Randomized trial of intravenous heparin versus recombinant hirudin for acute coronary syndromes. *Circulation* 90:1631, 1994.

76. Antman EM for TIMI9A Investigators: Hirudin in acute myocardial infarction safety report from the thrombolysis and thrombin inhibitors in myocardial infarction (TIMI) 9A trial. *Circulation* 90:1624, 1994.

77. Nehaus KL, Essen R, Tebbe U, et al: Safety observations from the pilot phase of randomized versus hirudin for improvement of thrombolysis (HIT-III) study. *Circulation* 90:1638, 1994.

77a. Jang I-K, Brown DFM, Giugliano RP, et al for the MINT Investigators: A multicenter, randomized study of argatroban versus heparin as adjunct to tissue plasminogen activator (TPA) in acute myocardial infarction: Myocardial Infarction with Novastan and TPA (MINT) Study. *J Am Col Cardiol* 33:1879, 1999.

78. American College of Cardiology/American Heart Association Task Force on Practice Guidelines: 1999 Update: ACC/AHA guidelines for management of patients with acute myocardial infarction: Executive summary and recommendations *Circulation* 100:1016, 1999.

78a. Patel SC, Mody A: Cerebral hemorrhage complications of thrombolytic therapy. *Prog Cardiovasc Dis* 42:217, 1999.

79. Berkowitz SD, Granger CB, Pieper KS, et al for the GUSTO I Investigators: Incidence and predictors of bleeding after contemporary thrombolytic therapy for myocardial infarction. *Circulation* 95:2508, 1997.

80. Sloan MA, Gore JM: Ischemic stroke and intracranial hemorrhage following thrombolytic therapy for acute myocardial infarction: Benefit analysis. *Am J Cardiol* 69:21A, 1991.

81. DeJaegere PP, Arnold AA, Balk AH, Simoons ML: Intracranial hemorrhage in association with thrombolytic therapy: Incidence and clinical predictive factors. *J Am Coll Cardiol* 19:289, 1992.

82. Longstreth WT, Litwin PE, Weaver WD, MITI project group: Myocardial infarction, thrombolytic therapy and stroke. A community-based study. *Stroke* 24:587, 1993.

83. Gore JM, Sloan M, Price TR, et al: Intracranial hemorrhage, cerebral infarction, and subdural hematoma after acute myocardial infarction and thrombolytic therapy in thrombolysis in myocardial infarction study. Thrombolysis in Myocardial Infarction. Phase II Pilot and Clinical Trial. *Circulation* 83:448, 1991.

84. Sane DE, Califf RM, Topol EJ, et al: Bleeding during thrombolytic therapy for acute myocardial infarction: Mechanisms and management. *Ann Interrn Med* 3:1012, 1989.

85. Honan MB, Harrell FE, Reiner KA, et al: Cardiac rupture, mortality and timing of thrombolytic therapy: A meta-analysis. *J Am Coll Cardiol* 16:359, 1990.

86. Becker RC, Charlesworth A, Wilcox RG, et al: Cardiac rupture associated with thrombolytic therapy: Impact of time to treatment in the Late Assessment of Thrombolytic Efficacy (LATE) Study. *J Am Coll Cardiol* 25:1063, 1995.

87. Deviri E, Sareli P, Wisenbaugh T, Cronje SL: Obstruction of mechanical heart valve prostheses: Clinical aspects and surgical management. *J Am Coll Cardiol* 17:646, 1991.

88. Kontos GJ, Schaft HV, Orszulak TA, et al: Thrombolytic obstruction of disc valves: Clinical recognition and surgical management. *Ann Thorac Surg* 48:60, 1989.

89. Roudaut R, Labbe T, Lorient-Roudaut MF, et al: Mechanical cardiac valve thrombosis: Is fibrinolysis justified? *Circulation* 86(Suppl. 2):II-8, 1992.

90. Hurrell DG, Schaft HV, Tajik AJ: Thrombolytic therapy for obstruction of mechanical prosthetic valves. *Mayo Clin Proc* 71:605, 1996.

91. Shapiro Y, Herz I, Vaturi M, et al. Thrombolysis is an effective and safe therapy in stuck bi-leaflet mitral valves in the absence of high-risk thrombi. *J Am Coll Cardiol* 35:1874, 2000.

92. Ozkan M, Kaymaz C, Kirma C et al: Intravenous thrombolytic treatment of mechanical prosthetic valve thrombosis: A study using serial transesophageal echocardiography. *J Am Coll Cardiol* 35:1881, 2000.

93. Sasahara AA, Myers TH, Cole CM, et al: The Urokinase Pulmonary Embolism Trial. A national cooperative study. *Circulation* 47:1, 1973.

94. Dalla-Volta S, Palla A, Santolicandro A, et al: PAIMS 2: Alteplase combined with heparin versus heparin in the treatment of acute pulmonary embolism. Plasminogen Activator Italian Multicenter Study 2. *J Am Coll Cardiol* 20; 520, 1992.

95. Meyer G, Sors H, Charbonnier B, et al: Effects of intravenous urokinase versus alteplase on total pulmonary resistance in acute massive pulmonary embolism: A European multicenter double-blind trial. *J Am Coll Cardiol* 19:239, 1992.

96. Goldhaber SZ: Contemporary pulmonary embolism thrombolysis. *Chest* 107:45, 1995.

97. Goldhaber SZ, Kessler CM, Heit JA, et al: A randomized control trial of recombinant tissue plasminogen activator versus urokinase in the treatment of acute pulmonary embolism. *Lancet* 2:193, 1988.

98. Goldhaber SZ, Kessler CM, Heit JA, et al: Recombinant tissue type plasminogen activator versus a novel dosing regimen of urokinase in acute pulmonary embolism: A randomized controller multicenter trial. *J Am Coll Cardiol* 20:20,1992.

99. Goldhaber SZ, Haire WD, Feldstein ML, et al: Alteplase versus heparin in acute pulmonary embolism: Randomized trial assessing right ventricular and pulmonary perfusion. *Lancet* 341:507, 1993.

100. Verstraete M, Miller GAH, Bounamcaux H, et al: Intravenous and intra pulmonary recombinant tissue - type plasminogen activator in the treatment of acute massive pulmonary embolism. *Circulation* 77:353, 1988.

101. Kanstantinedes S, Geibel A, Olschewski M, et al: Association between thrombolytic treatment and prognosis of hemodynamically stable patients with major pulmonary embolism. *Circulation* 96:882, 1997.

102. Goldhaber SZ: Pulmonary embolism thrombolysis. Broadening the paradigm for its administration. *Circulation* 96:716, 1997.

103. Hommel M, Boissel JP, Connu C, et al: Termination of trial: Streptokinase in severe acute ischemic stroke. *Lancet* 345:57, 1995.

104. Donnan GA, Hommel M, Davis SM, McNeil JJ: Streptokinase in acute ischemic stroke. *Lancet* 346:56, 1995.

105. The Multicenter Acute Stroke Trial—Europe Study Group: Thrombolytic therapy with streptokinase in acute ischemic stroke. *N Engl J Med* 335:145, 1996.

106. Hacke W, Kaste M, Fieschi C, et al: Intravenous thrombolysis with recombinant tissue plasminogen activator for acute hemispheric stroke. *JAMA* 274:1017, 1995.

107. The National Institute of Neurological Disorders and Stroke rt-PA Stroke Study Group: Tissue plasminogen activator for acute ischemic stroke. *N Engl J Med* 333:1581, 1995.

108. Wolf PA, Gotta JC: Cerebrovascular disease. *Circulation* 102:IV-75, 2000.

108a. Albers GW, Bates VE, Clark WM, et al: Intravenous tissue-type plasminogen activator for treatment of acute stroke. The Standard Treatment with Alteplase to Reverse Stroke (STARS) study. *JAMA* 283:1145, 2000.

108b. Ringleb PA, Schellinger PD, Schranz C, Hacke W: Thrombolytic therapy within 3 to 6 h after onset of ischemic stroke: Useful or harmful? *Stroke* 33:1437, 2002.

108c. Bednor MM: Combining antiplatelet and thrombolytic therapies for stroke. *Expert Opin Pharmacother* 3:401, 2002.

109. Furlan A, Higaohida R, Wechsler L, et al: Intra-arterial prourokinase for acute ischemic stroke: The PROACT II Study: A randomized control trial. *JAMA* 282:2003, 1999.

110. Francis CW, Marde VJ: Fibrinolytic therapy for venous thrombosis. *Progr Cardiovasc Dis* 34:193, 1991.

111. Comeroto AJ, et al: Venous thromboembolism. In: Rutherford RB, ed. *Vascular Surgery*, 4th ed. Philadelphia: Saunders, 1995:1800.

112. Schweizer J, Kirch W, Koch R, et al: Short- and long-term results after thrombolytic treatment of deep venous thrombosis. *J Am Coll Cardiol* 36:1336, 2000.

113. Wagstaff AJ, Gillis JC, Goa KL: Alteplase. A reappraisal of its pharmacology and therapeutic use in vascular disorders other than acute myocardial infarction. *Drugs* 50:289, 1995.

114. Hess H: Thrombolytic therapy in peripheral vascular disease. *Br J Surg* 77:1083, 1990.

115. Lonsdale RJ, Berridge DC, Earnshaw JJ: Recombinant tissue-type plasminogen activator is superior to streptokinase for local intra-arterial thrombolysis. *Br J Surg* 79:272, 1992.

116. The Stile Investigators: Results of a prospective randomized trial evaluating surgery versus thrombolysis for ischemia of the lower extremity. *Ann Surg* 220:251, 1994.

116a. Tabriziani H, Schieu A, Frishman WH, Brandt LJ: Drug therapies for mesenteric vascular disease. *Heart Dis* 4:306, 2002.

117. Trans Atlantic Intersociety Consensus (TASC): Management of peripheral vascular disease. *J Vasc Surg* 31:S151, 2000.

117a. New applications for thrombolytics: Alteplase in the periphery. *Formulary* 36(Suppl 4): 4, 2001.

117b. Clase CM, Crowther MA, Ingram AJ, Cina CS: Thrombolysis for restoration of patency to haemodialysis central venous catheters: A systematic review. *J Thromb Thrombolysis* 11:127, 2001.

118. Verstraete M, Lijnen HR, Collen D. Thrombolytic agents in development. *Drugs* 50:29, 1995.

119. Collen D, Lijnen HR: Staphylokinase, a fibrin specific plasminogen activator with therapeutic potential? *Blood* 84:680, 1994.

120. Armstrong PW, Burton JR, Palisaitis D, et al: Collaborative angiographic patency trial of recombinant staphylokinase (CAPTORS). *Am Heart J* 139:820, 2000.

121. Vanderschueren S, Barrlos L, Kerdsinchai P, et al. A randomized trial of recombinant staphylokinase versus alteplase for coronary artery patency in acute myocardial infarction. *Circulation* 92:2044, 1995.

122. Collen D, Sinnaeve P, Demarsin E, et al: Polyethylene glycol-derivatized cysteine-substitution variants of recombinant staphylokinase for single-bolus treatment of acute myocardial infarction. *Circulation* 102:1766, 2000.

123. den Heijer P, Vermeer F, Ambrosini E, et al on behalf of In TIME investigators: Evaluation of weight-adjusted single-bolus plasminogen activators in patients with myocardial infarction. A double-blind, randomized angiographic trial of lanoteplase versus alteplase. *Circulation* 98:2117, 1998.

124. The In TIME-II Investigators: Intravenous NPA for the treatment of infarcting myocardium early. In TIME-II, a double-blind comparison of single-bolus lanoteplase vs accelerated alteplase for treatment of patients with acute myocardial infarction. *Eur Heart J* 24:2005, 2000.

125. Gardell SJ, Ramjit DR, Stabilito II, et al: Effective thrombolysis without marked plasminemia after bolus intravenous administration of vampire bat salivary plasminogen activator in rabbits. *Circulation* 84:244, 1991.

126. Montoney M, Gardell SJ, Marder VJ: Comparison of the bleeding potential of vampire bat salivary plasminogen activator versus tissue plasminogen activator in an experimental rat model. *Circulation* 91:1540, 1995.

127. Lijnen HR, Nelles L, Holmes WE, et al: Biochemical and thrombolytic properties of a lower molecular weight form (comprising Leu 144 through Leu 411) of recombinant single-chain urokinase type plasminogen activator. *J Biol Chem* 163:5594, 1988.

128. Bar FW, Meyer J, Vermeer F, et al: Comparison of saruplase and alteplase in acute myocardial infarction. The Study of Europe with Saruplase and Alteplase in Myocardial Infarction. *Am J Cardiol* 97:727, 1997.

129. PRIMI Trial Study Group: Randomized double-blind trial of recombinant pro-urokinase against streptokinase in acute myocardial infarction. *Lancet* 1989; 1:863, 1989.

130. Tebbe U, Michels R, Adgey J, et al: Randomized double blind study comparing saruplase with streptokinase therapy in acute myocardial infarction: The COMPASS equivalence trial. *J Am Coll Cardiol* 31:487, 1998.

131. Armstrong PW, Collen D: Fibrinolysis for acute myocardial infarction. Current status and new horizons of pharmacological reperfusion. Part I. *Circulation* l03: 863, 2001.

132. Verstraete M: Search for more effective and safer thrombolytic agents. *Biomed Prog* 13:68, 2000.

133. Verstrate M: Third-generation thrombolytic drugs. *Am J Med* 109:52, 2000.

Lipid-Lowering Drugs

Neil S. Shachter

Peter Zimetbaum

William H. Frishman

A direct relationship between elevated serum cholesterol levels, especially elevated low-density-lipoprotein (LDL)-cholesterol levels, and the incidence of coronary artery disease (CAD) is now well established.[1–4] The lowering of LDL-cholesterol levels by means of diet and/or drug therapy has been shown to reduce the progression of coronary artery lesions (Fig. 20-1) and the incidence of clinical coronary artery events.[5–19] As predicted from the Framingham Study, a 10% decrease in cholesterol levels is associated with a 20% decrease in the incidence of combined morbidity and mortality related to CAD.[20,21] Elevations in triglycerides and reductions in high-density-lipoprotein (HDL)-cholesterol levels may also contribute to an increased CAD risk.[22–25]

Advances in the understanding of lipid metabolism and the development of new drugs and dietary strategies for the treatment of lipid and lipoprotein disorders have made effective therapy of hyperlipidemia, and thus coronary heart disease (CHD) risk intervention, an understandable and attainable goal.[20]

Gould et al.[18] performed a metanalysis of 35 randomized trials and assessed the relation of cholesterol lowering to benefit or harm as well as the effects of specific drug regimens on clinical outcomes such as CHD mortality, noncoronary mortality, and total mortality. The authors concluded that for every 10 mg/dL of cholesterol lowering, coronary disease mortality was reduced significantly by 13% and total mortality by 10%. Cholesterol lowering per se had no effect on noncoronary mortality. Their analysis also indicated that fibric acid derivatives increased noncoronary mortality by 30% and total mortality by 17%. Hormones such as estrogen and d-thyroxine, which patients were given in the past, may have increased coronary disease mortality in men by about 27%, noncoronary mortality by 55%, and total mortality by 33%. Other interventions—such as niacin, resins, statins, diet, and partial ileal bypass—had no specific adverse effects.

In the following introductory section, a framework for understanding the treatment of lipid disorders is presented. Recommendations are provided—based on the third expert panel report of the National Cholesterol Education Program (NCEP)[20]—regarding screening and dietary and drug interventions in human populations with hyperlipidemia at risk for premature CAD.

RATIONALE FOR THE TREATMENT OF HYPERLIPIDEMIA IN PREVENTION OF CORONARY ARTERY DISEASE

The basis for the treatment of hyperlipidemia is the theory that abnormalities in lipid and lipoprotein levels are risk factors for CAD and that the lowering of blood lipids can decrease the risk of disease and its complications.[20] Levels of plasma cholesterol and LDL-cholesterol have consistently been shown to be directly correlated with the risk of CAD.[22,26]

The results of the clinical trials with cholesterol and LDL-cholesterol–lowering interventions support the premise that cholesterol-lowering therapies aimed at reducing cholesterol by at least 20 to 25% produce clinically significant reductions in cardiovascular events in patients having preexisting vascular disease across a broad range of cholesterol values within 5 years of starting treatment. The greatest impact of cholesterol lowering still occurs in individuals with the highest baseline cholesterol levels.[27] The absolute magnitude of these benefits would be even greater in those individuals having other risk factors for CAD, such as cigarette smoking and hypertension.[27,28] These risk relationships are the basis for recommending lower cholesterol cut points and goals for those who are at high risk for developing clinical CHD.[20]

Thus, taking into consideration the recommendations of the NCEP[20] and data from recently published trials,[28,29] two general groups of patients that warrant aggressive therapy for hypercholesterolemia can be identified: those without evidence of CAD who are at high risk for developing CAD (primary prevention, target LDL <130 mg/dL) and those with known CAD or other atherosclerotic processes and high cholesterol (secondary prevention, target LDL <100 mg/dL). Patients with lesser degrees of risk are treated to less aggressive LDL targets (<160 mg/dL). The current guidelines have also identified a fourth group whose risk factors mark them as having a "coronary risk equivalent." Such patients are treated in keeping with the aggressive goals recommended for known CHD (now all atherosclerotic disease). The most important category is diabetes, but—due to the important influence of age on coronary risk—many older individuals with other risk factors also meet current criteria

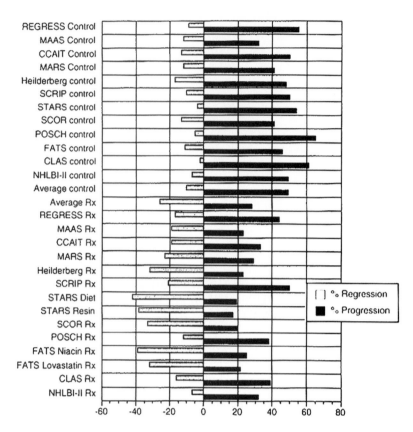

FIGURE 20-1. Arteriographic CAD regression trials. The percent of subjects classified as regression are to the left, and those classified as progression are to the right. The control groups are listed on top of the figure, and the treatment groups are on the bottom. (*Modified from Superko HR, Krauss RM: Coronary artery disease regression. Convincing evidence for the benefit of aggressive lipoprotein management. Circulation 90:1056, 1994.*)

for treatment to the target of <100 mg/dL LDL. Recommendations for the treatment of elevated triglycerides are less definitive.[20,30] Several prospective studies have shown a correlation between levels of plasma triglycerides and CAD.[31] Data from the Framingham Study, however, have indicated that when other risk factors—such as obesity, elevated serum cholesterol (or hypercholesterolemia), hypertension, and diabetes—are accounted for, triglycerides are not a potent independent risk factor for CAD.[32] However, there is a select group of patients with isolated hypertriglyceridemia who are at increased risk of CHD and who can be identified by a strong family history of premature CAD.[20,31] It should be kept in mind that, to some extent, the epidemiologic studies evaluating the independent risk associated with hypertriglyceridemia have been exercises of little relevance to clinical decision making. Clearly, once one adjusts for some of the risk factors that are causes of hypertriglyceridemia (obesity, diabetes, lack of exercise, little dietary fiber, family history, etc.), risks associated with the correlates of hypertriglyceridemia (other manifestations of the insulin resistance syndrome, such as hypertension) and the risks associated with the consequences of hypertriglyceridemia (low HDL, small dense LDL), then little measurable risk will remain. However, hypertriglyceridemia is a valuable marker of the insulin resistance syndrome, and therapy addressed at the bases of that syndrome will benefit all the causes and correlates of hypertriglyceridemia.[32] In addition, the level of plasma triglycerides is a primary determinant of the level of HDL, the most potent predictor of the risk of atherosclerotic disease; the two measurements exhibit a strong inverse correlation.[33] In general, the direction of causation is clearly that of the level of triglycerides determining the level of HDL, and most therapies that raise the level of HDL are, in fact, directed at modifying triglyceride metabolism. Therefore, whether triglycerides or HDL are the more important element in the physiologic mediation of atherosclerotic risk cannot be determined

from either epidemiologic studies or intervention trials. HDL is the more potent statistical predictor, but this is likely due to "ascertainment bias." Triglyceride levels are quite variable, while HDL levels are fairly stable, leading to greater predictive value for the HDL measurement. In part, this is likely due only to its being a more accurately ascertained surrogate for the level of plasma triglycerides. There is now evidence that by lowering triglyceride levels or raising HDL levels (or both), the risk of CAD will be diminished. The Veterans Affairs Low HDL Intervention Trial (VA-HIT), showed a significant reduction in coronary events in otherwise high-risk patients with normal LDL levels associated with the use of an agent (gemfibrozil) that markedly lowered triglycerides and modestly raised HDL but had no effect on the level of LDL.[24] However, similar benefit was not observed in another trial that used a related drug (Bezafibrate Infarction Prevention Study, or BIP).[30]

While CAD is the most important clinical manifestation of atherosclerosis, it bears emphasis that lipid-lowering therapy has been shown to decrease the incidence of all atherosclerotic diseases. Comprehensive metanalyses of the HMG-CoA reductase inhibitor trials have specifically confirmed the value of these agents in preventing stroke in hyperlipidemic subjects.[34,35]

RISK ASSESSMENT

For many years clinicians depended on total cholesterol and triglyceride measurements for patient management. More sophisticated lipoprotein measurements were available only in research facilities. Methodologic advances have made lipoprotein subclass and apolipoprotein determinations available from many clinical laboratories. As a result, LDL-cholesterol has been shown to be a more accurate predictor of CAD risk than total cholesterol.[20] Likewise, low levels of HDL-cholesterol have been demonstrated to be more powerful predictors of CAD than elevated total cholesterol.[22,23] Levels of plasma lipoprotein(a), apolipoproteins A-I and B, and the distribution of HDL subfractions (HDL2 and HDL3) are also accurate univariate predictors of CAD risk. However, in most cases, these measurements contribute little to the assessment of coronary risk provided by LDL, HDL, and triglyceride.[36] Mean serum cholesterol and calculated LDL-cholesterol values for various population groups have been reported and document a progressive decline in plasma cholesterol in the United States; this is consistent with the decreased mortality from atherosclerotic disease that has been observed simultaneously.[20,37] A number of nonlipid measurements (homocysteine and a variety of inflammatory markers, including C-reactive protein) can also contribute to the assessment of coronary risk. Only C-reactive protein, as measured by the high-sensitivity assay, appears to provide significant prediction independent of the traditional lipid risk factors.[38]

WHO SHOULD BE SCREENED FOR HYPERLIPIDEMIA?

The Third Report of the NCEP Expert Panel on Detection, Evaluation and Treatment of High Blood Cholesterol in Adults continues to suggest that total cholesterol be measured in all adults 20 years of age and older at least once every 5 years.[20] A controversy was raised when the American College of Physicians recommended only general cholesterol screening for middle-aged men—an approach that was vigorously challenged and did not receive acceptance.[39,40] An NCEP panel recommended that cholesterol screening should not be done routinely in children unless there was a history of familial hyperlipidemia or a family history of premature CAD. Cholesterol values in the general pediatric population may not always predict the future development of hypercholesterolemia in adults.[40a,41]

WHO SHOULD BE TREATED FOR HYPERCHOLESTEROLEMIA?

Ideally, a fasting lipid profile (total cholesterol, HDL-cholesterol, total triglycerides, calculated LDL) should be obtained in all cases. If this is not practicable, then screening cholesterol and HDL values should be obtained (Table 20-1). A total cholesterol above 200 mg/dL or an HDL-cholesterol below 40 mg/dL mandates obtaining a fasting lipid profile.[20] The presence of a high cholesterol should always be confirmed with a second lipid profile to make a more precise estimate of CAD risk.[20] The standard deviation of

TABLE 20-1. ATP III Classification of LDL, Total and HDL Cholesterol (mg/dL)

LDL-cholesterol	
<100	Optimal
100–129	Near or above optimal
130–159	Borderline high
160–189	High
≥190	Very high
Total cholesterol	
<200	Desirable
200–239	Borderline high
≥240	High
HDL cholesterol	
<40	Low
≥60	High

Source: Reproduced with permission from *JAMA* 285:2486, 2001.[20]

repeated measurements in an individual over time has been reported as 0.39 mm/L (15 mg/dL) for total cholesterol and 0.39 mm/L (15 mg/dL) for LDL-cholesterol. Patients should be maintained on the same diet during these initial determinations before therapy is instituted. Secondary causes of hypercholesterolemia (hypothyroidism, nephrotic syndrome, diabetes mellitus) should also be considered.[20]

The NCEP recommends an approach in adults based on LDL-cholesterol, which is shown in Tables 20–2 and 20–3. In most cases, management should begin with dietary intervention. When the response to diet is inadequate or when the target LDL is unlikely to be achieved by diet alone, the addition of pharmacologic therapy is recommended. Specific drug therapies are discussed in subsequent sections of this chapter.

WHO SHOULD BE TREATED FOR HYPERTRIGLYCERIDEMIA?

Interest in the link between serum triglyceride levels and CHD has grown in recent years. Triglyceride levels correlate positively with levels of LDL-cholesterol[42] and inversely with HDL.[30] Clinical trials with the triglyceride-lowering drugs, nicotinic acid,[6] and gemfibrozil[7,24] have shown a benefit on the frequency of coronary artery events compared with placebo therapy. However, therapy in these trials was not targeted to patients with primary hypertriglyceridemia. The currently recommended approach to the problem of hypertriglyceridemia is presented in the report of the NCEP.[20]

Normal triglycerides are defined as <150 mg/dL, borderline high triglycerides as 150 to 199 mg/dL, high triglycerides as 200 to 499 mg/dL, and very high triglycerides as >500 mg/dL. Most

TABLE 20-2. LDL Goals, Cutpoints for Therapeutic Lifestyle Changes (TLC) and Drug Therapy in Different Risk Categories

Therapy Risk Category	LDL Goal (mg/dL)	Initiate Lifestyle Changes	Initiate Drug Rx
CHD or CHD risk equivalents (10 yr risk >20%)	<100	≥100	≥130 (100–129: drug optional)
2+ Risk factors (10 yr risk ≤20%)	<130	≥130	10 yr risk 10%–20% ≥130 10 yr risk <10% ≥160
0–1 Risk factor	<160	≥160	≥190 (160–189: LDL-lowering drug optional)

Source: Reproduced with permission from *JAMA* 285:2486, 2001.[20]

TABLE 20-3. Major Risk Factors (Exclusive of LDL-Cholesterol) that Modify LDL Goals

- Cigarette smoking
- Hypertension (BP ≥140/90 mm Hg or on antihypertensive medication)
- Low HDL cholesterol (<40 mg/dL)*
- Family history of premature CHD
    CHD in male first degree relative <55 years
    CHD in female first degree relative <65 years
- Age (men ≥45 years; women ≥55 years)
- Diabetes (fasting glucose ≥127 mg/dL) in and of itself mandates an LDL goal of <100 mg/dL

*HDL cholesterol ≥60 mg/dL counts as a "negative" risk factor; its presence removes one risk factor from the total count.

Source: Adapted from *JAMA* 285:2486, 2001.

hypertriglyceridemia up to 5.65 mm/L (500 mg/dL) is primarily due to insulin resistance related to the "metabolic syndrome." Criteria for the diagnosis of this syndrome are shown in Table 20-4.[20] Common contributors to this syndrome include obesity (BMI >30 kg/m^2), overweight (BMI > 25 kg/m^2), physical inactivity, excess alcohol consumption, and high consumption of low-fiber carbohydrate sources (>60% of total energy). Other contributors to hypertriglyceridemia may include diabetes mellitus, hypothyroidism, marked obesity, chronic renal disease (failure or nephrotic syndrome), and certain drugs (glucocorticoids, estrogens, retinoids, and higher doses of either beta-adrenergic blocking agents or thiazide diuretics). Weight loss, exercise, dietary change (decreased saturated fat, increased omega-3 unsaturated oils, increased dietary fiber), reduction/elimination of triglyceride-raising drugs, and/or treatment of the primary disease process (e.g., improved glycemic control of diabetes) may be sufficient to reduce triglycerides.

Patients with familial combined hyperlipoproteinemia often have associated hypertriglyceridemia. Patients with this condition are at risk for premature CHD. These patients should have dietary treatment first and, if necessary, drugs.[20,30] Patients with borderline hypertriglyceridemia with clinical manifestations of CAD can be treated as if they had combined hyperlipoproteinemia, with lifestyle, LDL-lowering, and triglyceride-lowering therapies.[20,30]

TABLE 20-4. Clinical Identification of the Metabolic Syndrome

Risk Factor	Defining Level
Abdominal obesity* (waist circumference†)	
Men	>102 cm (>40 in.)
Women	>88 cm (>35 in.)
Triglycerides	>150 mg/dL
HDL-cholesterol	
Men	<40 mg/dL
Women	<50 mg/dL
Blood pressure	>130 / >85 mm Hg
Fasting glucose	>110 mg/dL

*Overweight and obesity are associated with insulin resistance and the metabolic syndrome. However, the presence of abdominal obesity is more highly correlated with the metabolic risk factors than is an elevated body mass index (BMI). Therefore the simple measure of waist circumference is recommended to identify the body weight component of the metabolic syndrome.

†Some male patients can develop multiple metabolic risk factors when the waist circumference is only marginally increased, e.g., 94 to 102 cm (37–40 in.). Such patients may have a strong genetic contribution to insulin resistance; they should benefit from changes in life habits, like men with categorical increases in waist circumference.

Source: Reproduced with permission from NCEP.[20]

TABLE 20-5. Major Causes of Reduced Serum HDL-Cholesterol

Cigarette smoking
Obesity
Lack of exercise
Androgenic and related steroids
Androgens
Progestational agents
Anabolic steroids
β-Adrenergic blocking agents
Hypertriglyceridemia
Genetic factors
Primary hypoalphalipoproteinemia

APPROACH TO LOW SERUM HDL CHOLESTEROL

A low serum HDL-cholesterol level is a strong lipoprotein predictor of CHD. [23] In one prospective study, after adjustment for other risk factors in predicting the risk of myocardial infarction, a change in one unit in the ratio of total to HDL-cholesterol was associated with a 53% change in risk.[22] However, it is still unclear how low HDL levels are linked to CAD. A recent trial of combined LDL-lowering and HDL-raising therapy showed benefit well beyond that anticipated from LDL lowering alone.[43] HDL metabolism is complex, and the utility of interventions to raise HDL will likely depend on the specific HDL-raising pathway that is targeted.[44] The major causes of reduced serum HDL-cholesterol are listed in Table 20-5. Clearly, attempts should be made to raise low HDL-cholesterol by hygienic means.[20] When a low HDL is associated with an increase in plasma triglycerides, as is typically the case, the latter deserves consideration for therapeutic modification.[20] However, when the HDL is reduced without hypertriglyceridemia or other associated risk factors, the utility of raising low HDL levels by drugs for primary prevention has not been adequately addressed in clinical trials.[20,24,44]

SPECIAL PROBLEMS

Diabetes Mellitus

The frequency of lipid abnormalities and the increased risk of CAD in diabetes has long been recognized. Prospective intervention studies in diabetic patients have demonstrated that the improvement of LDL with fenofibrate is associated with a reduced risk of morbidity and mortality from atherosclerosis.[45] In addition post hoc analyses of all the major statin trials and of the VA-HIT gemfibrozil trial have documented benefits that, on a percentage basis, are at least equal to those achieved in nondiabetic high-risk patients.[46–50] On the basis of these data and of data indicating that the risks of diabetes and of established CAD are comparable, the NCEP now considers diabetes a "CHD equivalent" and recommends that LDL-cholesterol be reduced to 2.58 mmol/L (100 mg/dL) in both men and women with diabetes.[20,52–53] Similar recommendations were previously endorsed by the American Diabetes Association. Of note, the elimination of marked hyperglycemia is an important factor in the control of the hypertriglyceridemia associated with diabetes, which may become severe enough to pose the risk of acute pancreatitits. However, tight control of plasma glucose has a very modest additional effect on plasma lipoprotein parameters and did not yield a statistically significant reduction in "macrovascular" disease endpoints in the large UKPDS study.[54]

Gender

Most clinical trials examining the effect of lipid-lowering therapy on the incidence of CAD have examined middle-aged males, owing to ease of recruitment in secondary prevention studies and increased statistical power in primary prevention studies. The rates of CHD are four times higher in middle-aged men than women and two times higher in elderly men. However, epidemiologic evidence supports a dyslipidemia-associated increase in risk similar to that in men and a similar approach to lifestyle, dietary, and/or drug therapy.[55] Such an approach is supported by the findings in those clinical trials that have included significant numbers of women.[56,57] Of note, despite the large difference in incidence rates at younger ages, because of the greater life expectancy of women, the contribution of atherosclerotic disease to total mortality is only modestly less in women than in men. The role of postmenopausal estrogen replacement therapy (see Chap. 36) remains controversial, despite the advantages suggested by the earlier observational literature and the apparently beneficial effects on the lipid profile.[58] The Heart and Estrogen/Progestin Replacement Study (HERS), a large secondary prevention trial, failed to detect any benefit despite a reduction in LDL-cholesterol and elevation in HDL-cholesterol.[59] This appeared to be due to an early increase in events, followed by a late decrease. This pattern has been interpreted as the consequence of the prothrombotic and proinflammatory effects of the regimen, followed by the emergence of its antiatherosclerotic effects, or due to negative effects specific to the progestin preparation that was used and others, but such interpretations

are entirely speculative. The increase in plasma triglycerides that has been known to accompany estrogen replacement therapy may have proatherosclerotic consequences.[60] An angiographic regression trial also showed no benefit from estrogen replacement, and a recent primary prevention trial (the Women's Health Initiative Trial) also showed no benefit with an estrogen-progestin combination.[61,61a]

Age

Children and Adolescents

The NCEP Expert Panel on Blood Cholesterol Levels in Children and Adolescents recommends the selective screening, in the context of regular health care, of children and adolescents who have a family history of premature cardiovascular disease or at least one parent with high cholesterol.[62] In children and adolescents from families with hypercholesterolemia or premature CAD, the NCEP established the following classifications for total cholesterol and LDL-cholesterol values. For total cholesterol, desirable levels are <4.40 mmol/L (<170 mg/dL), borderline levels 4.40 to 5.09 mm/L (170 to 199 mg/dL), and high levels >5.17 mm/L (>200 mg/dL) (Fig. 20-2).[62] For LDL-cholesterol, desirable levels are <2.84 mm/L (<110 mg/dL), borderline levels are 2.84 to 3.34 mm/L (110 to 129 mg/dL), and high levels >3.36 mm/L (>130 mg dL).[62]

For young individuals being screened because they have one parent with high cholesterol, the initial test may be measurement of total cholesterol. If the child's or adolescent's total cholesterol is high, a lipoprotein profile should be done.[62] If the total cholesterol

FIGURE 20-2. Classification based on total cholesterol (children and adolescents). * = defined as a history of premature (before age 55 years) cardiovascular disease in a parent or grandparent. (*Reproduced with permission from the NCEP Expert Panel.[62]*)

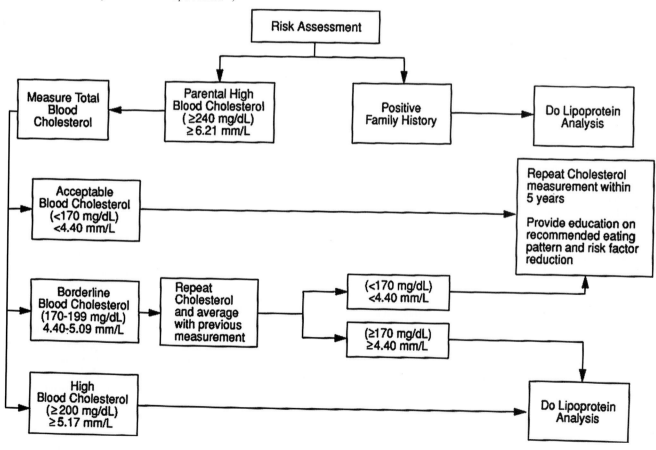

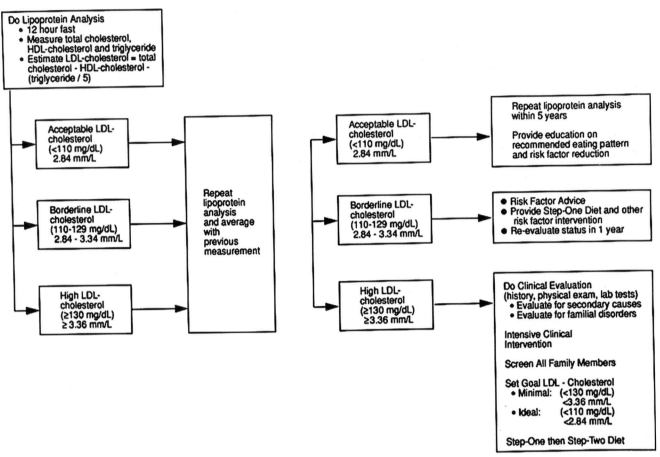

FIGURE 20-3. Classification based on low-density lipoprotein (LDL)-cholesterol (children and adolescents). (*Reproduced with permission from the NCEP Expert Panel.*[62])

level is borderline, a second measurement of total cholesterol should be taken, and if the average is borderline or high, a lipoprotein profile should be performed (Fig. 20-2). For young individuals being tested due to a documented history of premature atherosclerotic disease, a lipoprotein profile should, of course, be performed.[62]

Once the lipoprotein analysis has been obtained, it should be repeated to determine the average LDL-cholesterol level. The NCEP, as with adults, recommends a management approach to children and adolescents that is primarily based on LDL-cholesterol (Fig. 20-3).

Dietary therapy is the primary approach to treating children and adolescents with elevated blood cholesterol (Fig. 20-4).[62] Drug therapy is recommended in children aged 10 or older if the LDL-cholesterol remains above 4.91 mm/L (190 mg/dL) or if the LDL-cholesterol remains >4.14 mm/L (>160 mg/dL) and there are other cardiovascular risk factors present in the child or adolescent that cannot be controlled.[62] At the time these guidelines were issued, until longer-term safety data with other lipid-lowering drugs become available, the NCEP was comfortable recommending only bile acid sequestrants as drug therapy.[62] Clearly, in those rare children with homozygous familial hypercholesterolemia or with premature atherosclerotic disease due to severe heterozygous familial hypercholesterolemia, all therapies may be considered.

The Elderly

Increasing age in itself is a potent risk factor for CHD.[20] As a consequence, a progressively declining fraction of the risk for CHD can be attributed to dyslipidemia.[63,64] Nevertheless, while individu-

als over age 70 have not been carefully examined, there has been no evidence of a significant age-related decline in the effectiveness of lipid-lowering therapy in preventing cardiovascular endpoints in the available clinical studies that included older individuals.[56] Since the absolute risk of CHD increases with age and the benefits of lipid-lowering therapy are already evident after a year of therapy, a strong rationale emerges for the continued aggressive use of lipid-lowering therapy in the elderly.[56,64a] To cite an illustrative example: the Framingham algorithm incorporated into the third edition of the NCEP guidelines mandates a target LDL of <100 mg/dL for individuals whose risk is considered equivalent to that of known CAD. Such individuals who are male will have 15 or more "points" after applying the algorithm to their risk factor profile (23 for females). However, the algorithm assigns 13 points to men (and 16 to women) simply for an age between 75 and 79.[20]

Systemic Hypertension

A report from the Working Group on Management of Patients with Hypertension and High Blood Cholesterol emphasizes the synergistic effects of hypertension and hypercholesterolemia on the risk of developing cardiovascular disease.[65] Hypertension is more than randomly associated with dyslipidemia, since both conditions are commonly manifestations of the insulin resistance syndrome. In this regard, hypertension serves both as a cause of atherosclerotic disease and a marker of insulin resistance. In part because of this association, the risk associated with hypertension is not completely mitigated by

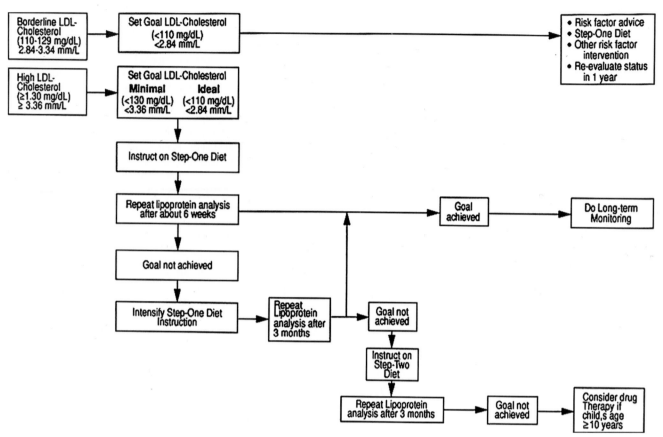

FIGURE 20-4. Dietary and drug treatment (children and adolescents). LDL = low-density lipoprotein. (*Reproduced with permission from the NCEP Expert Panel.*[62])

good blood pressure control, and the NCEP guidelines continue to count hypertension as a risk factor even in patients under good pharmacologic control.[20,66] Nonpharmacologic therapy—in the form of proper diet, exercise, and smoking cessation—is the foundation for the management of both hypertension and high cholesterol. Clinicians should use these nondrug measures as definitive or adjunctive therapy. The achievement of control using these strategies would lead to the elimination of hypertension as a factor to be considered in risk analyses. Pharmacologic agents can also be very beneficial in managing the risks. In selecting medications, it is important to consider benefits, costs, and potential untoward effects.[65,67]

Myocardial Infarction

The post–myocardial infarction setting is the paradigm of known atherosclerotic disease. Virtually all such patients require aggressive lipid lowering with the maintenance of an LDL-cholesterol <100 mg/dL.[20,68] All patients with known CAD should have a fasting lipoprotein analysis. If this is not accomplished promptly (within a few hours of presentation), the measured cholesterol levels will be artifactually depressed by the acute-phase response. Under these circumstances, the initial dosage of lipid-lowering therapy may have to be empiric, with the dosage adjusted subsequently based on the levels at least 3 months after the acute event, at which point the effects of the acute-phase response will have substantially resolved.[69] The value of the immediate institution of high-dose LDL-lowering therapy in the setting of acute myocardial infarction is an area of controversy. An observational study adjusted for possible confounders found a significantly lower incidence of short-term (30 days and

6 months) mortality in individuals discharged on lipid-lowering therapy.[70] A randomized trial of high-dose (80 mg) atorvastatin after presentation with acute non-Q-wave myocardial infarction or unstable angina found a significant decrease in rehospitalizations for ischemia within 16 weeks and a decrease in complicating stroke without any difference in death, recurrent myocardial infarction, or heart failure.[71]

Aggressive lipid-lowering therapy results in a marked reduction of cardiovascular thrombotic events, with only minimal change in the size of the coronary artery plaque; but exactly how this happens is still uncertain.[72] Once a plaque develops, it may remain stable for long periods of time. What triggers acute ischemic syndromes, such as myocardial infarction or unstable angina, is the development of lesion instability.[73,74] An unstable lesion has an increased tendency to rupture or crack. leading to exposure of the highly thrombogenic interior, with superimposed thrombosis and thereafter acute ischemic syndromes. Several studies have suggested that the lipid content of a plaque correlates with the risk of a subsequent rupture.[75,76] Most commonly, the crack occurs at the junction of the plaque and the normal intima. Progressive accumulation of lipids appears to promote macrophage accumulation, which destabilizes the plaque, leading to thinning and destruction of the fibrous cap and resulting in rupture at points of high pressure.[77] Thus, it has been suggested that limiting the lipid pool of the atherosclerotic plaque may prevent plaque thinning and facilitate the conversion of an unstable, vulnerable plaque to a stable one. Changes in plaque composition that predict vulnerability are not detectable by coronary angiography but have been shown to be detectable by specialized cardiac magnetic resonance imaging techniques.[78]

It is well established that atherosclerosis and hypercholesterolemia are associated with endothelial cell dysfunction, which may play a part in the pathogenesis of acute ischemic syndromes via an increased tendency to vasospasm and decreased secretion of prostaglandins, which suppress platelet aggregation. An important mediator of normal endothelial function is nitric oxide, which is released continuously, maintaining vascular tone and preventing platelet and leukocyte adhesion.[79] Hypercholesterolemia and coronary atherosclerosis have been shown to impair nitric oxide release, whereas aggressive lipid lowering can improve nitric oxide–mediated responses.[80,81] This likely represents an additional mechanism by which cholesterol reduction reduces the risk of myocardial infarction.

Coronary Artery Bypass Grafts

In an important observational study, investigators at the Montreal Heart Institute performed angiography 1 and 10 years after surgery to determine the patency of vein grafts in 82 patients who had undergone saphenous vein bypass surgery.[82] The 10-year examination confirmed that atherosclerotic changes are common in saphenous vein bypass grafts. At that time: of 132 grafts that were patent at the 1-year examination, only 50 (37.5%) showed no change at the 10-year examination, whereas evidence of atherosclerosis was found in 43 (33%) and complete occlusion in 30 (29.5%). Progressive atherosclerosis was identified as the single most important cause of occlusion in these grafts. When the investigators analyzed the relationship between cardiovascular risk factors and the development of atherosclerosis, they found no significant difference for smoking, hypertension, or diabetes between the group that developed disease and the group that did not. However, in a multivariate analysis, it was revealed that low HDL-cholesterol, high LDL-cholesterol, and high apolipoprotein B were the most significant predictors of atherosclerotic disease in grafts.[82] Almost 80% of those who did not develop disease had normal lipid levels and normal LDL and apolipoprotein B levels, in contrast to 8% of patients who developed disease.

There is now evidence that aggressive dietary and LDL-lowering drug therapy with niacin/colestipol and with the HMG-CoA reductase inhibitor lovastatin can slow down, arrest, and even reverse atherosclerotic disease in patients with saphenous vein coronary bypass grafts.[83–85] Detailed lipoprotein analysis of the patients in the study using lovastatin indicated that the beneficial effects were achieved, as expected, by LDL lowering and not via effects on triglyceride-rich lipoproteins and HDL.[10] However, a similar trial that used a triglyceride-lowering agent (gemfibrozil) in patients who have had coronary artery bypass grafts with low HDL also showed a beneficial effect on atherosclerosis progression.[11] Of note, internal thoracic artery and other arterial grafts have a significantly lower rate of atherosclerosis than saphenous vein grafts and are now performed whenever it is feasible.

Coronary Angioplasty

Restenosis after successful isolated coronary angioplasty has been observed in 25 to 40% of patients undergoing this procedure.[86] This incidence has been significantly reduced by the routine use of coronary stenting, but the problem of restenosis has not been eliminated.[87] Attempts have been made to decrease the incidence of restenosis using a wide array of pharmacologic interventions (see Chap. 40). Restenosis after angioplasty appears to result from the proliferation of intimal smooth-muscle cells.[88] Results of experiments in cholesterol-fed animals after balloon injury of the arterial wall have suggested that restenosis occurs primarily from the migration and proliferation of smooth muscle cells in response to platelet-derived growth factor released from platelets adherent to the site of deendothelialization.[89] Antiplatelet drugs and calcium-channel blocking drugs have had little or no benefit in reducing the rate of postangioplasty restenosis. A recent study with fluvastatin has shown benefit,[89a] and some positive results have been achieved with probucol and a related antioxidant compound, drugs not currently approved in the United States (see Chap. 40).[90,91] Local irradiation and specific drug-containing stents have been the most promising of the currently studied modalities.[92]

Heart Transplantation

Elevated plasma lipids as well as an increased risk of having accelerated CAD are commonly found in recipients of cardiac transplants.[93] Although many of the drugs used to treat and/or prevent rejection (high-dose steroids, cyclosporine) can raise LDL-cholesterol,[94] hypercholesterolemia has not been found to be a primary risk factor for developing graft atherosclerosis.[95] Pathologically, the CAD is often different from that seen in nontransplanted patients and is characterized as a diffuse, necrotizing vasculitis or, more commonly, intimal hyperplasia of the entire coronary arterial system.[93,96] It has been proposed that the development of CAD in transplant recipients may be a manifestation of chronic tissue rejection.[93]

Monitoring of lipids after cardiac transplantation is still worthwhile and intake of dietary fats and cholesterol should be modified.[93] Use of lipid-lowering drug therapy does carry with it an increased risk of potential complications. However, prospective studies with both pravastatin and simvastatin have shown a prominent benefit from lipid-lowering drug therapy in this population, without excessive risk.[97,98] Early administration of diltiazem is also indicated as part of a regimen to prevent graft vasculopathy.[99]

Cerebrovascular Disease

The results of recent trials indicate that lipid-lowering treatment can reduce the risk of stroke in patients with existing heart disease. The mechanism for risk reduction includes plaque stabilization and the retardation of plaque progression.[100]

Nephrotic Syndrome

The nephrotic syndrome is associated with increased levels of cholesterol and triglycerides. The elevated serum concentrations of LDL-cholesterol, other lipids, and apolipoprotein B in patients with uncomplicated nephrotic syndrome are due to reversible increases in lipoprotein production.[100a] These lipid disorders are difficult to treat, and they predispose patients to early-onset CAD. It has been suggested that the treatment guidelines adopted by the NCEP be extended to patients with unremitting nephrotic syndrome.[100b] Statins have been shown to reduce plasma concentrations of very low density lipoprotein (VLDL)- and LDL-cholesterol in patients with nephrotic syndrome with kinetic evidence of enhanced LDL receptor activity.[100c] In addition, statins may reduce renal protein excretion in hypertensive patients who are already receiving ACE inhibitors or angiotensin receptor blockers.

Calcific Aortic Stenosis

Hypercholesterolemia is associated with calcific aortic stenosis and may be implicated in its pathogenesis and progression.[101] A randomized controlled trial of cholesterol-lowering therapy in patients with calcific aortic stenosis is indicated at this time.[101a]

Conclusion

Hyperlipidemia, specifically elevations in plasma cholesterol and LDL-cholesterol, is associated with an increased risk of morbidity and mortality from CAD. Elevations in plasma triglycerides and lower HDL-cholesterol values may also contribute to increased risk. It is now clear that dietary and/or drug therapy of hypercholesterolemia can modify this risk favorably. Guidelines for selecting subjects for drug treatment have been established.[20] In the subsequent sections, pharmacologic interventions designed to treat hyperlipidemia and the associated cardiovascular disease risk are presented and discussed. These guidelines will continue to be refined as more information becomes available from clinical trials in a wide range of patient populations.

BILE ACID SEQUESTRANTS

The bile acid–binding resins cholestyramine and colestipol have long been among the drugs of first choice for hypercholesterolemia in patients without concurrent hypertriglyceridemia. Despite the mounting data on the safety, efficacy, and tolerability of HMG-CoA reductase inhibitors, this remains true for children, adolescents, and women who may become pregnant. Colesevelam, a newer bile acid sequestrant (BAS) with increased bile acid–binding specificity— and consequently a decrease in bulk, in gastrointestinal (GI) side effects, and the potential for vitamin and drug malabsorption—has reawakened interest in this class.[102]

Cholestyramine was originally used for treatment of pruritus caused by elevated concentrations of bile acids secondary to cholestasis. However, attention has focused on the ability of the BASs to lower the concentration of LDL-cholesterol in plasma. The resins have been extensively tested in large-scale, long-term follow-up clinical trials to explore their efficacy for such an application[103,104] These drugs are not absorbed in the GI tract and therefore have a limited range of systemic side effects. For this reason they are particularly useful for the treatment of pregnant women with hypercholesterolemia and are the drugs generally recommended in children with heterozygous familial hypercholesterolemia.[105] The disadvantage of the early sequestrants cholestyramine and colestipol lie in their mode of administration and the frequency of GI side effects.

Chemistry

Cholestyramine (Questran powder) is the chloride salt of a basic anion-exchange resin. The ion-exchange sites are provided by the presence of trimethylbenzylammonium groups in a large copolymer of styrene and divinyl benzene.[106] The resin is hydrophilic yet insoluble in water. It is given orally after being suspended in water or juice. It is not absorbed in the GI tract and not altered by digestive enzymes, permitting it to remain unchanged while traversing the intestines.

Colestipol (Colestid), supplied as the powder colestipol hydrochloride, is a basic anion-exchange copolymer made up of diethylenetriamine and 1 chloro-2,3-epoxypropane. It has approximately one out of its five amine nitrogens protonated (chloride form). Like cholestyramine, colestipol is not altered by digestive enzymes, nor is it absorbed in the digestive tract. It is supplied in powder form and is taken orally after being suspended in liquid.

Colesevelam is poly(allylamine hydrochloride) cross-linked with epichlorohydrin and alkylated with 1-bromodecane and (6-bromohexyl)-trimethylammonium bromide; it has been engineered to bind bile acids specifically. It is a nonabsorbed hydrophilic polymer that is unmodified by digestive enzymes. It is supplied in tablet form and taken orally.

Pharmacology

Bile acids are synthesized in the liver from cholesterol, their sole precursor. They are then secreted into the GI tract, where they interact with fat-soluble molecules, thereby aiding in the digestion and subsequent absorption of these substances. Bile acids are absorbed along with the fat-soluble molecules and are subsequently recycled by the liver via the portal circulation for resecretion into the GI tract. The bile acids remain in the enterohepatic circulation and never enter the systemic circulation.

Cholestyramine, colestipol, and colesevelam bind bile acids in the intestine. The complex thus formed is then excreted in the feces. By binding the bile acids, the resins deny the bile acids entry into the bloodstream and thereby remove a large portion of the acids from the enterohepatic circulation. The decrease in hepatic concentrations of bile acids allows a disinhibition of cholesterol 7a-hydroxylase, the rate-limiting enzyme in bile acid synthesis.[107,108] Also seen is an increase in activity of phosphatidic acid phosphatase, an enzyme responsible for the conversion of alpha-glycerol phosphate to triglyceride. The increased activity of this enzyme causes a shift away from phospholipid production and ultimately an increase in the triglyceride content and size of VLDL particles.[109] There is also evidence to suggest that the BASs cause an increase in the activity of HMG-CoA reductase, the rate-limiting enzyme in the hepatic cholesterol synthesis pathway.[110] Although cholesterol synthesis is increased when BASs are used, there is no rise in plasma cholesterol, presumably because of the immediate shunting of the newly formed cholesterol into the bile acid–synthesis pathway. The apparent shortage of cholesterol causes the hepatocyte cell surface receptors for LDL particles to be altered either quantitatively, by increasing in number, or qualitatively, by increasing their affinity for the LDL particle.[111] By sequestering the cholesterol-rich LDL particles, the liver decreases the plasma concentration of cholesterol.

Pharmacokinetics

Cholestyramine, colestipol, and colesevelam bind bile acids in the intestines, forming a chemical complex that is excreted in the feces. There is no chemical modification of the resins while in the GI tract; however, the chloride ions of the resins may be replaced by other anions with higher affinity for the resin. Colestipol and colesevelam are hydrophilic but virtually insoluble in water (99.75%). The high-molecular-weight polymers of cholestyramine, colestipol, and colesevelam are not absorbed in the GI tract. Less than 0.05% of ^{14}C-labeled colestipol or ^{14}C-labeled colesevelam is excreted in the urine.

Since the resins are not absorbed into the systemic circulation, any interactions that occur between the resins and other molecules occur in the intestines, usually with substances ingested at or near the time of resin ingestion. In the case of cholestyramine and colestipol, interaction between resins and fat-soluble substances, such as the fat-soluble vitamins, causes a decrease in absorption of these substances. Malabsorption of vitamin K, for instance, has been associated with a hypoprothrombinemia. It is therefore recommended that vitamins K and D be supplemented in patients on long-term resin therapy. Likewise, medications taken with or near the time of resin ingestion may be bound by the resin and not be absorbed. Drugs at risk include phenylbutazone, warfarin, chlorothiazide (acidic), propranolol (basic), penicillin G, tetracycline, phenobarbitol, thyroid and thyroxine preparations, and digitalis preparations. In the case of colesevelam, such interactions essentially do not occur, though modest and variable effects on verapamil absorption have been described.[111a]

The dose-response curves for the bile acid resins are nonlinear, with increases in the antihypercholesterolemic effect being minimal for doses >30 g per day. Furthermore, there tend to be compliance problems when large doses of resin are used, making doses >15 g twice daily inefficacious.[112] In the case of colesevelam, which has a lower dosing range, nonlinearity was evident in the 3.75-g dose, which had about twice (19%) the cholesterol-lowering efficacy of the 3-g dose (9%).[113]

Since the BASs are polymeric cations bound to chloride anions, continued ingestion of the resins imposes a chloride load on the body. This chloride load may cause a decrease in the urine pH and also an increase in the urinary excretion of chloride, which can reach 60% of the ingested resin load. Furthermore, there may be an increase in the excretion of calcium ions, which is dependent on the extent of chloride ion excretion. Because of this increase in calcium ion excretion, care should be taken, especially in treating a person at risk for osteoporosis, to limit the extent of calcium excretion by controlling the dietary chloride load.[114]

Clinical Experience

Numerous studies have shown the BASs cholestyramine and colestipol to be efficacious in lowering LDL and total cholesterol levels in the plasma.[115,116] Studies have further correlated the decreased levels of LDL-cholesterol with the slowing of progression of coronary atherosclerosis and a lowered incidence of coronary events.[103–106,117–121] Similarly, the use of BASs retards the progression of femoral atherosclerosis.[121a,b] Furthermore, studies of the lipoprotein content in resin-treated individuals have detected a qualitative effect that may contribute to the antiatherosclerotic effects of the drug.[122a,b] Sequestrants are limited to use in those patients having hypercholesterolemia that is not associated with severe hypertriglyceridemia. Therefore, unless bile acid resins are combined with other antihyperlipidemic drugs, their use is typically limited to treatment of individuals with isolated hypercholesterolemia.

Effects on LDL-Cholesterol

The Lipids Research Clinics Coronary Primary Prevention Trial (LRC-CPPT)[103] represents the most extensive study of BASs and their effects on lowering the incidence of symptomatic CAD. The study involved 3806 subjects with type II hyperlipoproteinemia with plasma cholesterol values >6.85 mm/L (>265 mg/dL). The subjects were placed either into a placebo group on a low-cholesterol diet or a

treatment group consisting of cholestyramine therapy (24 g per day) plus diet. Results showed that diet accounted for a 5% decrease in total cholesterol in both groups. The cholestyramine-treated group experienced a decrease in mean total cholesterol and LDL-cholesterol of 13.4 and 20.3%, respectively. These decreases were 9 and 13% lower than those in the placebo group for total and LDL-cholesterol, respectively (placebo total cholesterol decreased 8.5%, and LDL-cholesterol decreased 12.6%). The study then looked for correlations between lower cholesterol and the incidence of CHD. To do this, the researchers defined two primary endpoints that would be used as markers for CHD: death from CHD and nonfatal myocardial infarction. The study found an overall 19% reduction in the incidence of the primary endpoints for the treated group over the placebo group. This included a 24% lower incidence of death from CHD and a 19% reduction in nonfatal myocardial infarction.

Effects on Intermediate-Density Cholesterol Particles

Evaluation of a subset of the National Heart, Lung and Blood Institute (NHLBI) study group examined the effect of cholestyramine on intermediate-density cholesterol (IDL) particles.[116] The study found that the drug-induced changes of IDL mass seen 2 years into treatment were the best predictors of progression of CHD 5 years into treatment. Based on these findings, it was hypothesized that the major antiatherosclerotic effect of cholestyramine may not be its LDL-lowering and HDL-raising effect but rather an IDL-lowering effect caused by the binding of the IDL particles to the upwardly regulated LDL receptors on the hepatocytes. This hypothesis is based on the fact that IDL particles are able to bind to the LDL receptor.[117]

Effects on VLDL-Cholesterol and Triglycerides

As previously mentioned, cholestyramine has the tendency to increase synthesis of triglycerides, which may contribute to the observed increases in VLDL particle concentration. In a study comparing normotriglyceridemic, hypertriglyceridemic, and obese patients, the observed increase in VLDL-triglyceride seen with resin treatment was shown to be due to increased synthesis of the lipoprotein and not decreased catabolism.[123] For the above reason, bile acid–binding resins should be used only in patients with triglyceride levels <3.39 mm/L (<300 mg/dL); it is therefore important to determine not only a patient's LDL level but also the triglyceride level to distinguish hypercholesterolemia due to elevations in both LDL and VLDL.[124]

Effects on HDL-Cholesterol

In a study of 1907 patients enrolled in the LRC-CPPT, the HDL levels were found to be inversely proportional to the extent of CAD (as defined by the number of patients reaching the primary endpoint).[125] Each 0.30-mm/L (1-mg/dL) increase of HDL above the mean at baseline was associated with a 5.5% decrease in the chance of a definite CAD associated death or a nonfatal myocardial infarction. Furthermore, each 0.03-mm/L (1-mg/dL) increase of HDL from baseline during the course of the study was associated with a 4.4% risk reduction for the primary endpoints. There was a similar finding in the placebo group when diet appeared to induce an increase in HDL. Cholestyramine had its greatest antihypercholesterolemic effect in those patients with the highest HDL concentrations. It is important to keep in mind that the LRC-CPPT study was not designed to answer questions about HDL levels; therefore the above suppositions are not conclusive.

Clinical Use of Resins

Bile acid resins are indicated as adjunct therapy to diet for reduction of serum cholesterol in patients with primary hypercholesterolemia. Dietary therapy should precede resin usage and should address both the patient's specific type of hyperlipoproteinemia and his or her body weight, since obesity has been shown to be a contributing factor in hyperlipoproteinemia. Since resin use can cause a 5 to 20% increase in VLDL levels, it should be restricted to hypercholesterolemic patients with only slightly increased triglyceride levels. The increase in VLDL seen with resin use usually starts during the first few weeks of therapy and disappears 4 weeks after the initial rise. It is thought that excessive increases in the VLDL particles may dampen the LDL-lowering effect of the drug by competitively binding the upwardly regulated LDL receptors on the hepatocyte. The resins should, therefore, not be used in patients whose triglyceride levels exceed 3.5 mmol/L unless accompanied by a second drug that has antihypertriglyceride effects; some suggest not using resins if the triglyceride level exceeds 2.5 mmol/L. A general rule of thumb is that if the triglyceride level exceeds 7 mmol/L, the LDL concentration is seldom raised; therefore treatment with a bile acid resin would not be effective.

Both cholestyramine and colestipol are available as powders that must be mixed with water or fruit juice before ingestion; they are taken in two to three divided doses with or just after meals. BASs can decrease absorption of some antihypertensive agents, including thiazide diuretics and propranolol. As a general recommendation, all other drugs should be administered either 1 h before or 4 h after the BAS. The cholesterol-lowering effect of 4 g of cholestyramine appears to be equivalent to that of 5 g of colestipol. The response to therapy is variable in each individual, but a 15 to 30% reduction in LDL-cholesterol may be seen with colestipol given at 20 to 30 g per day or cholestyramine at 16 to 24 g per day. The fall in LDL concentration becomes detectable 4 to 7 days after the start of treatment and approaches 90% of maximal effect in 2 weeks. Initial dosing should be 4 to 5 g of cholestyramine or colestipol, respectively, two times daily. The drugs are also useful if they are administered once daily.[126] In patients who do not respond adequately to initial therapy, the dosing can be increased to the maximum mentioned above.

Dosing above the maximum dose does not increase the antihypercholesterolemic effect of the drug considerably but does increase side effects, and therefore decreases compliance. Since both resins are virtually identical in action, the choice of one over the other is based on patient preference, specifically taste and the ability to tolerate ingestion of bulky material.

To avoid some of the difficulties with use of the powders, colestipol is available in 1-g tablets that are swallowed whole.[127] In addition, colestipol is available in a flavored powdered form. Cholestyramine is also available in a low-calorie, lower-volume formulation that contains 1.4 cal per packet.[128]

If resin treatment is discontinued, cholesterol levels return to pretreatment levels within a month. In patients with heterozygous hypercholesterolemia who have not achieved desirable cholesterol levels on resin plus diet, the combination therapy of colestipol hydrochloride and nicotinic acid has been shown to provide further lowering of serum cholesterol, triglycerides, and LDL and cause an increase in serum HDL concentration.[121,122,129] Other drug combinations have been studied; of particular promise is the combination therapy of a BAS and HMG-CoA reductase inhibitor.[130,131]

Oral colesevelam can be administered alone or in combination with an HMG-CoA reductase inhibitor as an adjunctive therapy to diet and exercise for the reduction of elevated LDL-cholesterol. The recommended dose is three 625-mg tablets taken twice daily with meals or six tablets once a day with a liquid meal. The dose can be increased to seven tablets a day.

Adverse Effects of Resins

Since cholestyramine and colestipol are not absorbed in the body, the range of adverse effects is limited. A majority of patients' complaints stem from the resins' effect on the GI tract[132] and from subjective complaints concerning the taste, texture, and bulkiness of the resins. The most common side effect is constipation, which is reported in approximately 10% of patients on colestipol and 28% of patients on cholestyramine but is less common with colesevelam. This side effect is seen most commonly in patients taking large doses of the resin and most often in patients over 65 years of age. Although most cases of constipation are mild and self-limiting, progression to fecal impaction can occur. A range of 1 in 30 to 1 in 100 patients on colestipol and approximately 12% on cholestyramine experience abdominal distention and/or belching, flatulence, nausea, vomiting, and diarrhea. Peptic ulcer disease, GI irritation and bleeding, cholecystitis, and cholelithiasis have been reported in 1 of 100 patients taking colestipol but have not been shown to be purely drug-related.

Fewer than 1 of 1000 patients on colestipol experience hypersensitivity reactions such as urticaria or dermatitis. Asthma and wheezing were not seen with colestipol treatment but were reported with cholestyramine treatment in a small number of patients. In a small percentage of patients, muscle pain, dizziness, vertigo, anxiety, and drowsiness have been reported with both drugs. With cholestyramine treatment, hematuria, dysuria, and uveitis have also been reported. Resin therapy has been associated with transient and modest elevations of serum glutamic oxaloacetic transaminase and alkaline phosphatase. Some patients have shown an increase in iron-binding capacity and serum phosphorus along with an increase in chloride ions and a decrease in sodium ions, potassium ions, uric acid, and carotene.

Case reports have described hyperchloremic acidosis in a child taking cholestyramine suffering from ischemic hepatitis and renal insufficiency,[133] in a child with liver agenesis and renal failure,[134] and in a patient with diarrhea due to ileal resection.[135] For these reasons, those patients at risk for hyperchloremia should have serum chloride levels checked during the course of resin treatment.[136]

In the LRC-CPPT study, the incidence of malignancy in the cholestyramine-treated group was equal to that in the control group; however, the incidence of GI malignancy in the treated group was higher than in the nontreated group (21 versus 11, respectively), with more fatal cases in the treated group (eight deaths in the treated group versus one in the control group). In animal studies, cholestyramine was shown to increase the mammary tumerigenesis capabilities of 7,12-dimethylbenzanthracene (DMBA) in Wistar rats. In the rats treated with cholestyramine plus DMBA, there was a fivefold increase in the incidence of mammary cancer over control.[137] Owing to the resin's ability to disrupt the normal absorption of fat-soluble vitamins in the gut, there have been a number of reports concerning the occurrence of hypoprothrombinemic hemorrhage secondary to vitamin K malabsorption.[138] In both of the cases cited above, the patients responded to adjunctive vitamin K therapy. An early study showed that colestipol can bind T_4 in the gut and in vitro. This binding can theoretically upset the normal reabsorption of T_4 from the gut and thereby disrupt normal T_4 recycling, causing hypothyroidism. However, a subsequent study showed that for euthyroid patients, thyroid function tests remained normal throughout resin treatment.[139] It is advisable for patients on thyroid replacement therapy to avoid taking the replacement drug at the same time as the resin so as to avoid any malabsorption problems.

Colesevelam appears to have a better side-effect profile than cholestyramine and colestipol and fewer associated drug interactions. Compared to placebo, a significantly greater incidence of dyspepsia, constipation, and myalgia has been reported in clinical trials with cholestyramine and colestipol.

Conclusion

The BASs have been extensively studied and have been proved effective in reducing cholesterol levels in patients with primary hypercholesterolemia caused by increases in LDL-cholesterol (type IIa). Studies have shown that resins have the ability to slow the progression of atherosclerosis when used alone and in combination and to limit the clinical consequences of the disease. Because of their effectiveness and safety, BASs will continue to be a drug of first resource for certain patients who have hypercholesterolemia unresponsive to diet therapy. The newer agent, colesevelam, may possess the beneficial properties of the BASs, causing less constipation and vitamin/drug malabsorption. Further use of BASs will focus on combination therapy with other antihyperlipoproteinemic drugs, such as nicotinic acid or HMG-CoA reductase inhibitors. The use of these combination therapies will increase the range of the antihyperlipoproteinemic effect of the agents and allow for a decrease in dosage of the drugs used, thereby decreasing the incidence of side effects.

GEMFIBROZIL, FENOFIBRATE, AND OTHER FIBRIC ACID DERIVATIVES

Fibric acid derivatives (FADs) are a class of drugs that have been shown to inhibit the production of VLDL, while enhancing VLDL clearance, principally owing to decreased hepatic synthesis of the endogenous lipoprotein lipase inhibitor apolipoprotein C-III and, to some extent, via stimulation of lipoprotein lipase gene expression.[140] The drugs can reduce plasma triglycerides and concurrently raise HDL-cholesterol levels, primarily due to the effects of lower plasma triglycerides but, in part, also to a modest direct effect on the production of the principal HDL apolipoproteins, apolipoprotein A-I and apolipoprotein A-II. Their effects on LDL-cholesterol are less marked and more variable. FADs also modify intracellular lipid metabolism by increasing the transport of fatty acids into mitochondria and improving peroxisomal and mitochondrial fatty acid catabolism.[141] All effects of the currently available FADs are felt to be due to ligation and activation of the ligand-activated transcription factor peroxisome proliferator activated receptor (PPAR)-alpha.[141] PPARs (there are three: PPAR-alpha, PPAR-gamma, and PPAR-delta) heterodimerize with the retinoid X receptor (RXR) and bind to characteristic DNA sequence elements.[142]

In screening tests in rats carried out in 1962 and 1963, a series of arloxyisobutyric acids reduced plasma concentrations of total lipid and cholesterol.[143] The compound that combined maximal

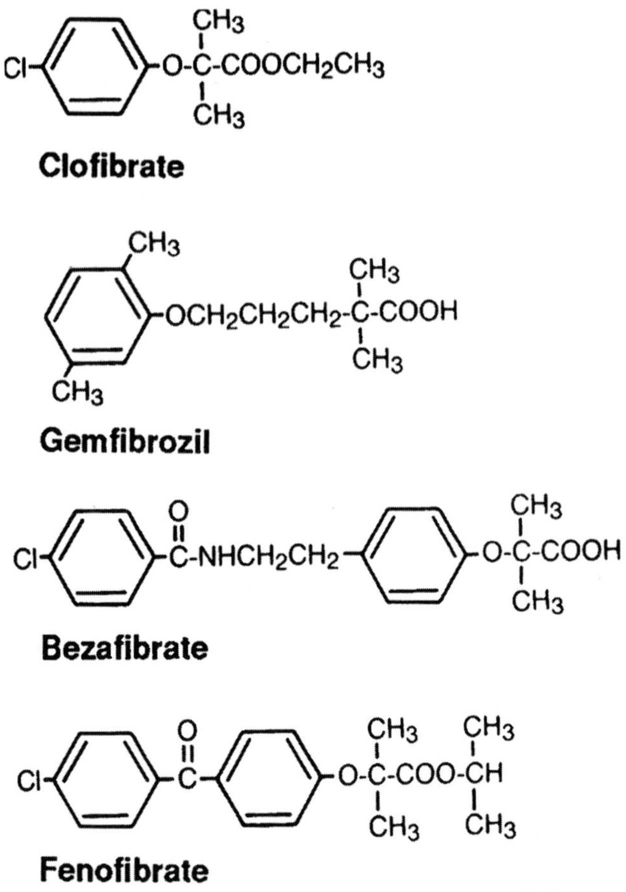

FIGURE 20-5. Chemical structures of some fibric acid derivatives.

effectiveness with relatively little toxicity was clofibrate. However, when the drug was used in the large World Health Organization trial to determine its effect on primary prevention of CHD, problems with the agent were identified. Although a decline in the rate of nonfatal myocardial infarction was observed, an increase in the rates of noncardiac death and overall mortality was also reported.[144]

There was also an observed increase in the frequency of GI diseases with the drug, specifically cholelithiasis.[145] A twofold increase in the rate of cholelithiasis was also reported with clofibrate as compared with placebo in the Coronary Drug Project.[144,145] During the 1960s and 1970s, many analogues of clofibrate were developed and tested for their hypolipidemic potential (Fig. 20-5). Of these, gemfibrozil and fenofibrate are currently marketed in the United States. The results of the Helsinki Heart Study[7,146,147] demonstrated the safety and efficacy of gemfibrozil as a lipid-modifying agent and its potential role for reducing the risk of CHD in patients with specific lipid and lipoprotein disorders. Other FADs—bezafibrate, ciprofibrate, etofibrate, and etophylline clofibrate—are available in Europe and many have been investigated in the United States.

This section reviews the clinical pharmacology of gemfibrozil and the other FADs, discusses the therapeutic experiences with these agents, and provides recommendations for their clinical use.

Pharmacokinetics

Gemfibrozil is well absorbed from the GI tract, with peak plasma levels seen 1 to 2 h after administration.[148] The plasma half-life is 1.5 h after a single dose and 1.3 h after multiple-dose therapy. The plasma drug concentration is proportional to dose and steady state and is reached after 1 to 2 weeks of twice-daily dosing. Gemfibrozil undergoes oxidation of the ring methyl group in the liver to form hydroxymethyl and carboxyl metabolites[148] (in total, there are four major metabolites). No reports as yet have described distribution of the drug into human breast milk or across the placenta. Two-thirds (66%) of the twice-daily dose is eliminated in the urine within 48 h, 6% is eliminated in the feces within 5 days of dosing,[148] and less than 5% of the drug is eliminated unchanged in the urine. Regardless of the dosing schedule, there is no drug accumulation with normal or impaired renal function.[148]

In vitro, gemfibrozil is 98% bound to albumin at therapeutic levels.[148] There have been reports that when gemfibrozil is combined with warfarin in vitro, a doubling of the unbound warfarin fraction ensues. Similarly, clofibrate has been found to potentiate the anticoagulant activity of warfarin.[149]

The other FADs behave in much the same way as gemfibrozil. Fenofibrate has been studied most extensively.[150] It is well absorbed after oral administration and is hydrolyzed to fenofibric acid, subsequently undergoing carbonyl reduction, which results in reduced fenofibric acid. Fenofibrate and reduced fenofibric acid are both active pharmacologically.[150] Sixty-five percent of fenofibrate is excreted into the urine, principally as fenofibryl glucuronide (<20% is excreted through the bile).[150] Drug elimination is completed within 24 to 48 h, and the half-life of the drug is approximately 4.9 h. Steady-state equilibrium is established within 2 to 3 days. Unlike gemfibrozil, the newer FADs—particularly ciprofibrate, fenofibrate, and bezafibrate—can accumulate in patients with renal and hepatic failure; therefoe dose adjustments may be necessary.[151–153] No pharmacokinetic interaction exists between fenofibrate and BAS.[150]

Mechanism of Action of Gemfibrozil and Other FADs

The PPAR-alpha transcription factor has a central role in coordinating fatty acid metabolism in the liver, kidney, heart, and muscle.[151] Much of current knowledge of the role of this transcription factor has emerged from studies on the effects of the fibrate drugs on individual lipoprotein components and cholesterol-triglyceride metabolic pathways.[148,154]

One direct action of FADs appears to be an increase in the level of plasma lipoprotein lipase (LPL).[155] LPL is deficient in patients with type I hyperlipoproteinemia, types I and II diabetes mellitus, hypothyroidism, heart failure, and nephrotic syndrome. LPL is increased by insulin treatment of diabetes mellitus, aerobic exercise, and FADs. LPL is the rate-limiting enzyme governing the removal of triglycerides from lipoproteins in the plasma.[156] It functions at the luminal surface of the vascular endothelium and depends on the presence of apolipoprotein C-II (apo C-II) on chylomicrons, VLDL, and HDL to activate its hydrolytic capacity.[156] The level of LPL has been found to be increased after the addition of gemfibrozil. Enhancement of LPL is also found with fenofibrate therapy.[157] Similarly, bezafibrate has been found to increase LPL activity. When coupled with the decrease in apo C-III, the catabolism of VLDL is dramatically increased.[158] An increase in lipoproteins containing both apo B and apo C-III has been shown to be an important discriminator of atherosclerotic risk in a number of clinical trials.[8,10,159–161] A decrease in these lipoproteins may be part of the antiatherosclerotic benefit of the FAD.

VLDL is produced in the liver and circulates in the plasma, where LPL hydrolyzes it to a VLDL remnant by removing triglyceride. The VLDL remnant is then either taken up by an apo E receptor–mediated process in the liver or converted to LDL. FADs have been shown to decrease the production of VLDL and to increase its fractional catabolic rate (FCR).[155]

Gemfibrozil has been studied predominantly in subjects with hypertriglyceridemia. The newer FADs have been studied both in subjects with hypertriglyceridemia and those with hypercholesterolemia. Although the FADs have similar triglyceride-lowering abilities, fenofibrate, bezafibrate, and ciprofibrate appear to have a greater cholesterol-lowering effect than gemfibrozil and clofibrate, which may relate to their having additional HMG-CoA reductase-inhibiting activity.[162]

In the hypertriglyceridemic state, there are alterations in the usual homogeneity of lipoprotein subfractions.[163] For instance, much of the LDL of hypertriglyceridemic patients contains a smaller amount of cholesterol ester and a greater amount of triglyceride than is usual.[155] Presumably, this aberration results from an exchange of triglyceride for cholesterol between VLDL and LDL. The triglyceride-enriched LDL is then hydrolyzed by hepatic triglyceride lipase, leading to a further reduction in size and increase in density of the LDL molecule. Thus, in the hypertriglyceridemic state, there are LDL fragments of normal composition coexisting with triglyceride-enriched and triglyceride depleted forms. The clinical consequences of this heterogenous LDL population are not yet apparent.

In the hypertriglyceridemic state, the production and fractional clearance of LDL are also increased.[163,164] Thus, patients with isolated hypertriglyceridemia may have low to normal LDL levels. Correction of the hypertriglyceridemic state with gemfibrozil restores the normal LDL population as well as reducing the production and catabolism of LDL. The result is often a slight increase in LDL levels. Similarly with fenofibrate or bezafibrate, when there are normal or low LDL levels, treatment increases levels of LDL.[165] Grundy and Vega offer the explanation that during fibrate therapy, the increased lipolysis of VLDL-triglyceride promotes increased hepatic uptake of VLDL remnants, leaving fewer receptors for clearance of LDL and thus increased plasma LDL.[155] It has been suggested that the short-term result of FAD therapy is an increased production of LDL-cholesterol secondary to increased VLDL catabolism and a resultant downregulation of hepatic LDL receptors.[153] As the VLDL levels decrease, the LDL-cholesterol content increases, establishing a more normal LDL particle. Regardless of the mechanism for changes in LDL levels, the importance of inhibiting production of VLDL as well as enhancing catabolism has been well documented.[166] Studies show that in the primary hypertriglyceridemic state, gemfibrozil increases LDL less than clofibrate, a drug that enhances VLDL catabolism without altering production.[166] Fenofibrate treatment of hypertriglyceridemic patients improves the conversion of VLDL to LDL and causes LDL levels to increase by 25% as VLDL levels decrease by 77%.[167] However, the drug also increases the clearance rate of apo B and causes a decrease in apo B levels of approximately 35%.[165] Thus these changes would be expected to be, on balance, antiatherogenic. Similar observations have been made with bezafibrate treatment of hypertriglyceridemia.[168]

The composition of HDL is also altered in hypertriglyceridemia. Normally, HDL2a, the cholesterol ester–rich subfraction, predominates in the circulation. HDL2a is transformed to HDL2b when it acquires triglyceride. HDL3 is formed from the removal of triglyceride from HDL2b by hepatic triglyceride lipase and LPL. HDL3 then acquires new cholesterol ester via lecithin cholesterol acetyl transferase (LCAT) and forms HDL2a. Hypertriglyceridemia markedly reduces HDL2a concentration and increases HDL2b concentrations. Essentially, hypertriglyceridemia decreases the cholesterol content of HDL. FAD therapy reverses this process, leading to increased cholesterol content of HDL.[155] Gemfibrozil has also been found to stimulate the synthesis of apo AI, the major apoprotein on HDL, without altering its catabolism. Similarly, fenofibrate and bezafibrate increase apo AI levels during treatment of hypertriglyceridemia. However, the levels of apo AI rarely increase to the extent that HDL rises.[170]

Finally, the hypertriglyceridemic state is thought to be associated with an increase in cholesterol synthesis.[171] One explanation for this is that hypertriglyceridemic LDL is altered and may present less cholesterol to the cells, thus leading to less effective downregulation of LDL receptors and less inhibition of HMG-CoA reductase. Consequently, cholesterol synthesis is increased. There is some evidence that FADs inhibit cholesterol synthesis.[172] From comparison studies conducted by Hunninghake and Peters, it would appear that the newer FADs—fenofibrate, bezafibrate, and ciprofibrate—are more effective than gemfibrozil and clofibrate in reducing cholesterol levels.[162] The results of animal studies appear to confirm that these new agents inhibit HMG-CoA reductase.[148] Although the older agents may have some minimal activity ininhibiting HMG-CoA reductase, the results of animal studies have shown much greater activity with the newer agents, such as bezafibrate, versus clofibrate.[173] In vivo, fenofibrate has been shown to decrease HMG-CoA reductase activity on human mononuclear cells in type IIa and IIb patients.[174] Similarly, bezafibrate has been found to inhibit HMG-CoA reductase activity from mononuclear cells of both normal and hypercholesterolemic patients.[175] Other data suggest an increased peripheral mobilization of cholesterol from tissues with FADs and feedback inhibition of hepatic cholesterol synthesis.[155]

FADs are also known to increase the secretion of cholesterol into bile and to decrease the synthesis of bile acids.[176] This effect is modulated by LDL receptor activity, with FADs increasing hepatic uptake of cholesterol, and subsequent secretion into the bile. In 1972, Grundy et al. first noticed this increased lithogenicity of bile accompanying clofibrate therapy.[172] Since then, other investigators have reported decreased fecal bile acid secretion and increased fecal excretion of neutral steroid with gemfibrozil therapy.[177] The net effect of decreased bile acid concentration and increased cholesterol concentration is a cholesterol supersaturation of bile, providing the potential nidus for gallstone formation. Studies with the newer FADs, especially fenofibrate, have shown variable results in terms of total bile acid synthesis and subsequent bile acid saturability.[178,179] European and American studies, so far, have shown no increase in gallstone formation in patients on fenofibrate therapy.[178] Thus, the newer FADs may have less potential for gallstone formation.

Patients with elevated cholesterol levels are believed to have increased platelet-mediated coagulation secondary to enhanced platelet reactivity and thromboxane A2 production.[180] A suggested pathogenesis is the ability of elevated LDL and cholesterol to alter the lipid membranes of platelets. Hypertriglyceridemia has also been associated with platelet hyperaggregability; however, the postulated defect in this condition is abnormal fibrinolysis.[181]

Carvalho et al. have demonstrated that patients with type II hyperlipoproteinemia have a platelet abnormality causing increased aggregation in response to mediators such as adenosine diphosphate and epinephrine.[180] After the onset of aggregation, these platelets release factors continue to accelerate the coagulation process, leading to increased fibrin formation. Data available thus far suggest that FADs might help correct the defective coagulation and fibrinolytic problems induced by hyperlipidemia.

Torstila et al. studied the effects of gemfibrozil on type II patients and found that plasma prekallikrein and kininogen levels increased by 10.5 and 18.5%, respectively.[182] Laustiola et al. observed that in patients with hypercholesterolemia who exercised, gemfibrozil caused a decrease in platelet reactivity and aggregability.[183] Sirtori et al.[184] also studied gemfibrozil's effect on platelet function and found no statistically significant effect on aggregation or thromboxane A2 levels. However, clofibrate and other FADs have been shown to decrease platelet aggregation in type II patients.

Fenofibrate and bezafibrate have been found to reduce platelet aggregation.[185] In a study of 62 patients with atherosclerotic vasculopathy and hyperfibrinogenemia, treatment with bezafibrate resulted in dose-dependent increases in fibrinolytic activity, with decreased fibrinogen, blood filterability, and platelet aggregation as compared with placebo.[186] It was recently demonstrated in young dyslipidemic male postinfarction patients in a placebo-controlled study, the Bezafibrate Coronary Atherosclerosis Intervention Trial (BECAIT), that bezafibrate therapy improved dyslipidemia, lowered plasma fibrinogen, and reduced the progression of focal coronary artery narrowing on coronary angiography. In addition, recurrent coronary events were reduced in the bezafibrate-treated group.[187] With regard to the myocardial microcirculation, Lesch et al.[188] found that when 35 patients were treated with fenofibrate, there was a significant decrease in platelet viscosity and erythrocyte aggregation. Moreover, in 8 of 12 patients in this study selected for thallium myocardial scintigraphy after 8 weeks, 2 showed global and 6 showed regional improvement in myocardial blood flow.[188] Thus, a reduction in fibrinogen concentration may lead to an improved coronary microcirculation.

Additionally, fenofibrate has been shown to decrease platelet-derived growth factor (PDGF) in vitro, which inhibits smooth muscle proliferation in rabbit aorta.[189] Thus, the FADs may directly inhibit atherosclerotic plaque formation.

An additional property unique to fenofibrate is the ability to decrease uric acid by 10 to 28% in 90 to 95% of all treated patients with an increase in renal uric acid secretion.[178] The exact mechanism and clinical significance of this observation is unclear.

Clinical Experience

The effects of FADs are largely dependent on the pretreatment lipoprotein classification of the patient.[162] In short, most patients respond to therapy with a decrease in triglyceride levels and an increase in HDL levels.[146,148] Hypertriglceridemic patients without hypercholesterolemia often have a slight increase in cholesterol and LDL levels. However, patients with hypercholesterolemia often have a decrease in their cholesterol and LDL levels. The predominant difference between gemfibrozil and the newer FADs is that the latter appear to lower LDL to a greater degree than does gemfibrozil.[162] As mentioned earlier, one explanation for this is that these new derivatives may also inhibit HMG-CoA reductase to some extent.

The clinical data for FADs are best summarized according to their effect on hypertriglyceridemic patients, subjects with combined hypertriglyceridemia and hypercholesterolemia, and subjects with only hypercholesterolemia.[190] Patients with type I chylomicronemia would benefit little from FADs because these individuals lack LPL, the enzyme responsible for the increased clearance mediated by the FADs.

The Helsinki Heart Study, a 5-year double-blind intervention trial, used gemfibrozil on 2051 middle-aged men, 8.8% of whom had isolated hypertriglyceridemia (type IV hyperlipidemia). In this subgroup there was a 5% increase in LDL with gemfibrozil compared with a 7% increase with placebo.[146] There was a 10% increase in HDL and a significant decrease in total cholesterol. Type IV patients experienced the greatest drop in triglycerides compared with type IIa or IIb subjects. There was a 2% incidence in cardiovascular endpoints in this treated group compared with 3.3% in the placebo group. A relationship between the decreased triglyceride levels and the decreased cardiovascular morbidity was not observed.[147] Instead, it was proposed that the elevated HDL, perhaps resulting from triglyceride lowering, conferred protection.

The Bezafibrate Coronary Atherosclerosis Intervention Trial was a small (81 patients) 5-year angiographic trial of bezafibrate. There was a small but statistically significant and unanticipated—given the small numbers—reduction in coronary events.[191] The Bezafibrate Infarction Prevention Study (BIP) was a much larger undertaking: 3090 patients divided between placebo and active drug who were followed for a mean of 6.2 years to assess an effect on clinical coronary endpoints. A modest decrease in ischemic endpoints did not reach statistical significance and there was no effect on mortality.[30] A posthoc subgroup analysis speculated that the very modest benefit detected in the group as a whole may have been due to its apparent concentration in the small number of individuals with plasma triglycerides over 200 mg/dL.[192] In contrast the Lopid Coronary Angiographic Trial (LOCAT), which used gemfibrozil in 372 men with prior coronary artery bypass graft surgery, did show a significant benefit in decreasing angiographic progression and new lesion development in both native vessels and saphenous vein grafts.[11] The VA-HIT study, which used gemfibrozil to detect an effect on clinical endpoints in over 2500 men with normal (<140 mg/dL) LDL and low HDL (<40 mg/dL), also showed a significant benefit with this agent, including a favorable effect on stroke incidence.[193] While specific differences with bezafibrate are possible, this difference may reflect the fact that VA-HIT patients had higher triglycerides levels (triglyceride levels up to 300 mg/dL were permitted) and were at higher risk than BIP patients, corresponding to the increased benefit in hypertriglyceridemic patients that was suggested in the post-hoc analysis of BIP.[193]

Clinical Use

It is well established that FADs are first-line therapy to reduce the risk of pancreatitis in patients with very high levels of plasma triglycerides. Results from the Helsinki Heart Study have also suggested that the hypertriglyceridemic patient with low HDL values can derive a cardioprotective effect from gemfibrozil.[146] Isolated low HDL levels are not as responsive to fibrate therapy.[194] Niacin therapy, when tolerated, may be preferable in these patients. Nevertheless, the benefit in decreased coronary endpoints demonstrated in such patients in the VA-HIT study is supportive of the use of gemfibrozil to reduce coronary risk in patients with isolated low HDL, despite the rather modest increase in HDL that was achieved.[24]

FADs, particularly the newer generation, decrease total cholesterol and LDL levels. However, in the absence of elevated triglycerides, they should not be first-line therapy for hypercholesterolemic patients. Type IIb patients are the subset most commonly seen in clinical practice that would benefit from FAD therapy. HMG-CoA reductase inhibitors combined with FADs are excellent therapy for

severe type IIb disease; however, the development of symptoms of myositis must be monitored. Bile acid resins plus gemfibrozil are also a reasonable combination for type IIb disease; however, HDL levels may drop slightly.

Gemfibrozil is approved for clinical use in the United States for the treatment of patients with very high serum triglycerides who are at risk of developing pancreatitis and for reducing the risk of clinical CAD in patients with type IIB hypercholesterolemia who are not symptomatic and who have low HDL-cholesterol and elevated LDL-cholesterol and triglyceride levels. The recommended dose for gemfibrozil is 600 mg before the morning meal and 600 mg before the evening meal.[148] Some patients may respond to 800 mg per day, but in most instances the therapeutic benefit is augmented with an increase to 1200 mg daily. Some patients derive benefit from increasing the dosage of gemfibrozil to 1600 mg daily.[195]

Fenofibrate tablets are approved for clinical use as adjunctive therapy to diet for the reduction of LDL-cholesterol, total cholesterol, triglycerides, and apo B in adult patients with primary hypercholesterolemia or mixed dyslipidemia (type IIA, IIB). The drug is also indicated as adjunctive therapy to diet for the treatment of patients with hypertriglyceridemia (types IV and V hyperlipidemia). For treatment of primary hypercholesterolemia or mixed hyperlipidemia, the initial dose of fenofibrate is 160 mg once daily. For patients with hypertriglyceridemia, the initial dose is 54 to 160 mg once daily. Dosage should be individualized according to the patient's response and should be adjusted as necessary following repeat lipid determinations at 4- to 8-week intervals. The maximum dose is 160 mg daily.

Bezafibrate and ciprofibrate are not approved for clinical use in the United States. Clofibrate is available for clinical use in the United States. The recommended daily dose of 2000 mg is usually divided into two to three daily doses.

Adverse Effects

Clofibrate, one of the earliest FADs, became unpopular because of its causative association with cholelithiasis and cholecystitis in the Coronary Drug Project.[145] The World Health Organization trial then reported a 29% increase in overall mortality in clofibrate-treated compared to placebo-treated subjects.[144] The mortality was principally due to postcholecystectomy complications, pancreatitis, and assorted malignancies. The Helsinki Heart Study reported a decrease in cardiovascular mortality but not overall mortality in gemfibrozil-treated subjects.[146] The reason for the similarity of overall mortality rates with placebo and gemfibrozil remains a mystery at this time. Obviously, these findings have led to careful scrutiny of currently used and tested FADs. The significant adverse effects noted in the Helsinki Heart Study included atrial fibrillation, acute appendicitis, dyspepsia, abdominal pain, and nonspecific rash.[146] The review of the European clinical trials of fenofibrate with 6.5 million patient-years shows a 2 to 15% adverse reaction rate, the most common adverse reactions being GI disturbances, dizziness and headache, muscle pains, and rash.[178] However, the only side effect significant in frequency was skin rash. In a United States multicenter study of fenofibrate in 227 patients,[196] there was a 6% increase in side effects from the drug, similar to the observations of the European studies. Three of four of the patients who withdrew from the U.S. fenofibrate study had skin rashes, the fourth had fatigue and impotence. Overall, the adverse experiences with bezafibrate have been similar to fenofibrate, with GI and neurologic disturbances, muscle aches, and rashes most commonly seen.[153,196]

In the Helsinki Heart Study, there was a 55% excess incidence of gallstones and a 64% excess incidence of cholecystectomy in the drug-treated compared with placebo-treated group.[146] Although European studies of fenofibrate may show some increased lithogenicity of the bile, there has been no increase in the incidence of gallstone formation, either during the trials or during postmarketing surveillance.[178]

The manufacturers of gemfibrozil and fenofibrate have reported mild depressions of hemoglobin, white blood cell count, and hematocrit with the drugs.[148] The Helsinki Heart Study did not find significant alterations in these parameters.[146]

The combination of fibrates and HMG-CoA reductase inhibitors has been repeatedly shown to predispose to rhabdomyolysis and, in some cases, renal failure.[197] The Helsinki Heart Study did not report any cases of myopathy in patients treated with only gemfibrozil.[146]

Fenofibrate therapy is associated with increases in liver function tests, leading to discontinuation of treatment in 1.6% of patients in double-blind trials. Like treatment with other fibrates, fenofibrate treatment may cause myopathy, especially in patients with impaired renal function, which interferes with the drug's excretion. Uric acid is noted to increase 10 to 28% on fenofibrate therapy[197a]; the clinical significance of this is unknown.

Conclusion

Gemfibrozil and fenofibrate can inhibit VLDL production and enhance VLDL clearance owing to stimulation of lipoprotein lipase activity. The drugs lower plasma triglyceride levels while raising HDL-cholesterol levels. They have variable effects on LDL levels, although the newer FADs may have greater cholesterol-lowering potential than gemfibrozil. The drugs are particularly useful in patients with very high triglycerides who are at risk of pancreatitis, and gemfibrozil specifically has been shown to reduce the risk of CAD complications in men with type IIb hyperlipoproteinemia.[198] How well these drugs protect against the complications of coronary vascular disease is still not known, and morbidity and mortality studies with the newer FADs still need to be done.

The FADs are well tolerated; however, there is a small risk of cholelithiasis with these drugs. Combination therapy with HMG-CoA reductase inhibitors may be associated with an increased incidence of myositis and rhabdomyolysis.

HMG-CoA REDUCTASE INHIBITORS

In 1987 the U.S. Food and Drug Administration (FDA) approved the marketing of lovastatin, a competitive inhibitor of HMG-CoA reductase, the rate-limiting enzyme step in cholesterol synthesis in the body. The pharmacology and clinical efficacy of this cholesterol-lowering drug and other drugs in this class that were also approved for marketing are reviewed in this section.

Lovastatin

Chemistry

Lovastatin (Mevinolin) is a fermentation product of the fungus *Aspergillus terreus*.[199] It is similar in structure to an earlier compound, mevastatin, a less potent inhibitor of HMG-CoA reductase, whose clinical development was limited by its possible cardiogenicity in animals.[200] The chemical structures of lovastatin

and some other HMG-CoA reductase inhibitors are shown in Fig. 20-6.

Pharmacology

Lovastatin, as a competitive inhibitor of HMG-CoA reductase, interferes with the formation of mevalonate, a precursor of cholesterol. Mevalonate also is a precursor of ubiquinone and dolichol, nonsterol substances essential for cell growth.[201] It was initially thought that the HMG-CoA reductase inhibitors might inhibit formation of these substances, but this is not the case.[201] Nonsterol synthesis does not appear to be inhibited by HMG-CoA reductase inhibitors.

Pharmacokinetics

Lovastatin is an inactive lactone (prodrug) that is hydrolyzed in the liver to an active β-hydroxyacid form. The prodrug was developed rather than the active hydroxyacid form because the prodrug undergoes more efficient shunting to the liver on first pass. The potential result of this enhanced liver uptake is lower peripheral drug concentrations and fewer systemic side effects.[202] This principal metabolite is the inhibitor of the enzyme HMG-CoA reductase. The dissociation constant of the enzyme inhibitor complex (Ki) is approximately 1029 mol/L.[203]

An oral dose of lovastatin is absorbed from the GI tract, with greater absorption at meals. The drug undergoes extensive first-pass metabolism in the liver, its primary site of action, with subsequent excretion of drug equivalents in the bile. It is estimated that only 5% of an oral dose reaches the general circulation as an active enzyme inhibitor. The drug is excreted via the bile (83%) and the urine (10%).[203,204]

Lovastatin and its β-hydroxyacid metabolite are highly bound to human plasma proteins.[204] Lovastatin crosses the blood-brain and placental barriers. The major active metabolites present in human plasma are the β-hydroxyacid of lovastatin, its 61-hydroxy derivative, and two unidentified metabolites. Peak plasma levels of both active and total inhibitors are attained 2 to 4 h after lovastatin ingestion. The half-life of the β-hydroxyacid is approximately 1 to 2 h. This rapid metabolism would seem to necessitate multiple doses per day. Clinical trials, however, have indicated that once- or twice-daily dosing is optimum. With a once-daily dosing regimen, within the therapeutic range of 20 to 80 mg per day, steady-state plasma concentration of total inhibitors after 2 to 3 days was about 1.5 times that of a single dose.[204] Single daily doses administered in the evening are more effective than the same dose given in the morning, perhaps because cholesterol is mainly synthesized at night (between 12 and 6 a.m.).[205] A substantial clinical effect of lovastatin is noted within 2 weeks and a maximal effect at 4 to 6 weeks; the effect dissipates completely 4 to 6 weeks after the drug is stopped. A tachyphylaxis effect has been suggested with prolonged use of statins.[206]

Clinical Experience

Several investigators have demonstrated that lovastatin lowers the cholesterol levels of normal and hypercholesterolemic animals.[199,207,208] These studies demonstrate that the increased LDL receptor activity and decreased LDL synthesis are responsible for the hypocholesterolemic effect of the drug. Several studies in humans have confirmed this observation.[207–210] This increase in LDL receptor activity occurs in response to a decrement in cholesterol synthesis by HMG-CoA reductase inhibition. LDL may be reduced

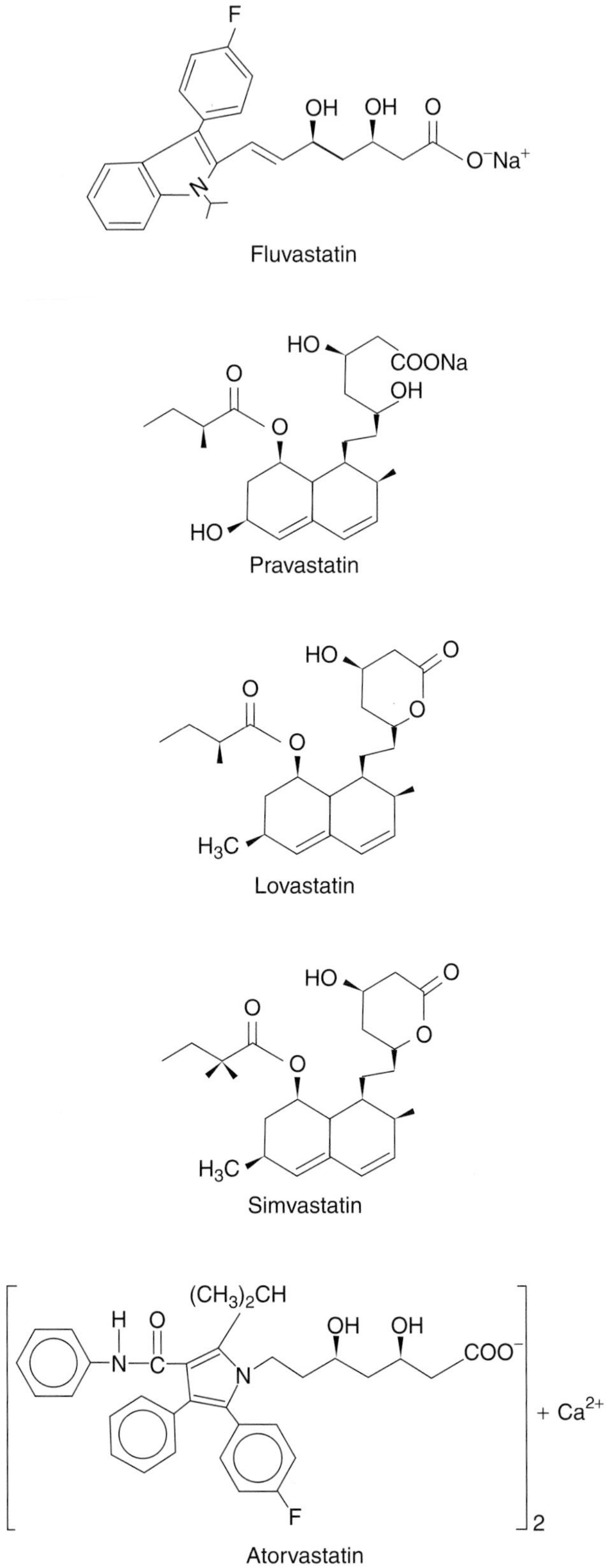

FIGURE 20-6. Chemical structures of fluvastatin, pravastatin, lovastatin, simvastatin, and atorvastatin.

by either its increased clearance from the plasma or its decreased production.

Clinical Endpoints

In a report from the Familial Atherosclerosis Treatment Study (CATS),[211] the combination of lovastatin 40 mg and colestipol 30 g daily was more effective than colestipol and diet alone in reducing LDL and raising HDL in patients with CAD and elevated apo B levels. There were also fewer cardiovascular events, less progression of coronary lesions, and more regression.

In the Monitored Atherosclerotic Regression Study (MARS),[212] patients whose cholesterol was 190 to 295 mg/dL and who were receiving lovastatin 80 mg per day and a cholesterol-lowering diet showed a slower rate of progression and an increase in the regression in coronary artery lesions, especially in more severe lesions, compared with placebo plus diet. These anatomic changes on coronary angiography with lovastatin were associated with a significant reduction in total cholesterol, LDL-cholesterol, and apo B levels, with a modest increase in HDL-cholesterol. In this study, lovastatin was also shown to reduce the progression of early, preintrusive atherosclerosis of the carotid artery as evaluated by B-mode ultrasonography.[213]

In the Canadian Coronary Atherosclerosis Intervention Trial (CCAIT), 331 patients with diffuse but not necessarily severe coronary atherosclerosis on coronary angiography and cholesterol between 220 and 300 mg/dL were randomized to receive either diet plus lovastatin (20, 40, and 80 mg), titrated to achieve an LDL-cholesterol below 130 mg/dL, or diet plus placebo.[214] Lovastatin treatment was shown to slow the progression of coronary atherosclerosis, especially of the milder lesions, and inhibited the development of new lesions. In a substudy analysis of female participants in CCAIT, lovastatin was shown to be effective in slowing the progression and neogenesis of coronary atherosclerotic lesions.[215]

The effects of lovastatin on atherosclerotic lesions in the carotid arteries was assessed in The Asymptomatic Carotid Artery Progression Study (ACAPS).[216,217] In this study, 919 asymptomatic men and women with early carotid atherosclerosis as defined by B-mode ultrasonography and LDL-cholesterol levels between 130 and 159 mg/dL were randomized to receive 20 to 40 mg of lovastatin or placebo. In addition, all patients received 80 mg of aspirin daily, and one-half were treated with 1 mg of warfarin daily.

Lovastatin reduced LDL-cholesterol levels and, after 3 years of follow-up, slowed the progression of mean intimal-medial thickness of the common carotid arteries and decreased mortality and major cardiovascular events.

As in the findings in ACAPS, FATS, MARS, and CCAIT, reductions in cardiac event rates were also observed with lovastatin compared with placebo.

The Air Force/Texas Coronary Atherosclerosis Prevention Study (AFCAPS/TexCAPS) was a double-blind placebo-controlled primary prevention study using lovastatin that targeted 5608 men and women with average LDL levels (mean 60th percentile) and low HDL level (25th percentile for men, 16th for women).[218] Its primary endpoint was the development of a first major acute coronary event (MI, unstable angina, or sudden cardiac death). The drug was well tolerated, with no clinical difference in liver enzyme abnormalities, myositis, etc. After a mean 5.2 years of follow-up, lovastatin reduced the incidence of the primary endpoint by 37% ($p < 0.001$), with a similar benefit on a variety of other atherosclerotic endpoints (coronary revascularizations, etc.), presumably via the noted 25% reduction in LDL and 6% increase in HDL. Mortality was limited in this relatively low-risk population, and the apparent benefit of treatment did not reach statistical significance. Most of these individuals would not have met criteria for therapy under the NCEP guidelines then in force. However, post hoc subgroup analysis revealed that the benefit was substantially confined to the two-thirds of subjects with HDL levels below 40 mg/dL.[218] Redefinition of the low-HDL risk factor from below 35 mg/dL to below 40 mg/dL would have led to most of these subjects meeting criteria for therapy under the guidelines. This analysis was a prominent factor in the redefinition of the low-HDL risk factor to <40 mg/dL in the current (third) edition of the guidelines.[20]

Clinical Use

Lovastatin is approved as an adjunct to diet for the reduction of elevated total and LDL-cholesterol in patients with primary hypercholesterolemia (type IIa and IIb) when the response to a diet restricted in saturated fat and cholesterol has not been adequate. In individuals without symptomatic cardiovascular disease, average to moderately elevated total cholesterol and LDL-cholesterol, and below average HDL-cholesterol, lovastatin is indicated to reduce the risk of myocardial infarction, unstable angina, and coronary revascularization procedures. The drug is also indicated for slowing the progression of atherosclerosis in patients with CHD.

Lovastatin doses as low as 5 mg twice daily produce significant reductions in serum cholesterol. Patients should be placed on a standard cholesterol-lowering diet prior to drug treatment.[218a] The recommended starting dose is 20 mg once daily given with the evening meal. The recommended dosing range is 20 to 80 mg daily in single or divided doses. Adjustments should be made at intervals of 4 weeks or more. A dose of 40 mg daily can be initiated in patients with cholesterol levels >7.76 mm/L (>300 mg/dL).

Twice-daily dosing appears to be the most effective treatment regimen, with daily evening doses being slightly less effective and daily morning doses least effective. Maximal and stable cholesterol reduction typically is achieved within 4 to 6 weeks of treatment initiation. A new extended-release formulation of lovastatin has been approved for once-daily clinical use.

In patients with high cholesterol, diet and lovastatin may not reduce cholesterol to the desired level. Niacin, BAS, and fibrates, in combination with lovastatin, may provide additional efficacy. A combination niacin-lovastatin formulation has been approved for clinical use.[218b,218c]

Adverse Effects

Several hypercholesterolemic agents are available, each having a significant side-effect profile.[218d] Lovastatin and other HMG-CoA reductase inhibitors have an acceptable rate of adverse reactions, but must to be used with some caution.[204,218e,218f]

In the published trials, approximately 2% of patients were withdrawn from treatment because of adverse reactions. GI side effects (diarrhea, abdominal pain, constipation, flatulence) are the most commonly reported adverse effects. Marked, persistent, but asymptomatic increases (to greater than three times the upper limit of normal) in serum transaminases have been reported in 2% of patients receiving the drug for 1 year. The increases are predominantly in serum glutamate pyruvate transaminase (SGPT) and serum glutamic-oxaloacetic transaminase (SGOT) rather than alkaline phosphatase, suggesting a hepatocellular, not cholestatic, effect.[219] These abnormalities rapidly return to normal after the discontinuation of the drug, and no permanent liver damage has been reported with the drug.[218d] Symptomatic hepatitis in patients without

underlying disease or other known hepatotoxic medications has been observed. It is recommended that liver function tests be performed before the initiation of treatment, at 6 and 12 weeks after initiation of therapy or elevations of dose, and semiannually thereafter.

The side effect of greatest concern with lovastatin is a myopathy, which appears to develop in three clinical patterns. The first, a moderate elevation in plasma creatinine kinase levels, is asymptomatic. Second, patients may develop muscle pain, primarily in the proximal muscle groups. CPK elevations may or may not be present. Finally, patients may develop a severe myopathy marked by extreme elevations in CPK, muscle pain with weakness, myoglobinuria and, rarely, acute renal failure.[219,219a,219b] This finding most often occurs in the setting of concurrent immunosuppressive therapy (cyclosporine), particularly when gemfibrozil, erythromycin, or niacin is added.[219,220] Similarly, the use of itraconazole, an antimycotic drug, has been shown to drastically increase plasma concentrations of lovastatin and lovastatin acid.[221] Inhibition of CYP3A4-mediated hepatic metabolism probably explains the increased toxicity of lovastatin caused not only by intraconazole but also by cyclosporine, erythromycin, and other inhibitors of CYP3A4. Cases of myopathy have been identified as early as a few weeks and as late as 2 or more years after the initiation of therapy. CPK elevations appear to correlate little with the severity of the symptoms, but if CPK levels rise or muscle pain develops, it is recommended that lovastatin be reduced. If levels rise drastically (>10 times the upper limits of normal) with muscle pain, therapy should be discontinued.

In a study of 11 cardiac transplant patients, all were treated with lovastatin and cyclosporine, monitored closely for 1 year, and were not treated with other hepatotoxic medications or lipid-lowering agents.[222] None developed any evidence of hepatic, muscle, or renal toxicity, and the authors concluded that in the absence of other effective therapy, cardiac transplantation should not be a contraindication to the use of lovastatin. Combinations of lovastatin with hepatotoxic agents, in the absence of cyclosporine, have also been reported to be associated with myositis.[223] The FDA has documented multiple cases of myopathy and rhabdomyolysis associated with lovastatin-gemfibrozil combination therapy and has discouraged the use of this regimen. Although the reason that myopathy has been associated with lovastatin is not well understood, it has been postulated that drugs which impair hepatic function may alter the first-pass extraction of lovastatin and produce elevated levels, which, in turn, may be responsible for the myotoxicity. Lovastatin may disrupt the proper assembly of membrane glycoproteins, the oxidation-reduction reactions of the mitochondrial respiratory chain, or the regulation of DNA replication.[224] Tobert does report, however, four cases of myositis with lovastatin monotherapy, but three of these patients had biliary stasis, leading to decreased clearance of the drug.[224a]

Several reports of bleeding, increase in prothrombin time, or both have been observed in patients on concomitant warfarin anticoagulation. Although these accounts have not been attributed to lovastatin, it is recommended that prothrombin time be carefully regulated in these patients, as in all patients receiving oral anticoagulation.[225]

In addition to reports of rashes during the clinical trials, there have been several accounts of serious hypersensitivity reactions during prescription use: anaphylaxis, arthralgia, a lupus-like syndrome, angioedema, urticaria, hemolytic anemia, leukopenia, and thrombocytopenia have all been reported. Twenty-five cases were considered serious, but all of these patients recovered with discontinuation of lovastatin therapy. Since these adverse effects were never reported during the clinical trials, it is likely that the incidence is significantly less than 1 per 1000. Sleep disturbances, characterized by insomnia or shortening of the sleep period, have also been described.[225]

Lovastatin (40 mg daily) and pravastatin (40 mg daily) were compared in a double-blind study of effects on quality of life and drug tolerability in men 20 to 65 years of age with primary hypercholesterolemia who received treatment for 12 weeks.[226] No significant differences between the two groups were observed in tolerability, health-related quality-of-life measures, or changes in lipid profile.

Simvastatin

Simvastatin (synvinolin) is a prodrug that is enzymatically hydrolyzed in vivo to its active form.[227] In clinical trials since 1985 and approved in 1992, simvastatin is synthesized chemically from lovastatin and differs from lovastatin by only one methyl group. Like lovastatin, it has a very high affinity for HMG-CoA reductase; but on a milligram-per-milligram basis, simvastatin is twice as potent.[228] Peak plasma concentrations of active inhibitor occur within 1.3 and 2.4 h.[229] One 12-week multicenter double-blind study comparing simvastatin to probucol found that a daily dose of simvastatin of 20 and 40 mg lowered LDL-cholesterol by 34% and 40%, respectively. Simvastatin also reduced total cholesterol, triglycerides, and apo B. HDL was increased.[230] As with lovastatin, interactions with warfarin and digoxin have been noted. Another multicenter study comparison with cholestyramine demonstrated that a low dose of simvastatin (10 mg) was sufficient to reduce total cholesterol by 21% and LDL by 30%, while HDL increased by 17%.[231] In comparisons of simvastatin to FADs and BAS, simvastatin produced greater reductions in total and LDL-cholesterol, whereas the latter had a greater effect on the serum triglycerides.[232,233] In a small study of patients with familial hypercholesterolemia, it was shown that 40 mg of simvastatin in combination with 12 g of cholestyramine reduced total cholesterol by 43% and LDL-cholesterol by 53%.[234]

The effects of simvastatin are achieved using a single evening dose.[235] Despite its potency, simvastatin has never been shown to disrupt adrenocortical function.[236] Side effects are predominantly headaches and dyspepsia, but asymptomatic myositis has also been noted.[230] It is interesting that some patients who experienced enzyme elevations with lovastatin and lovastatin rechallenge tolerated simvastatin well.[237]

Simvastatin has been shown to be useful in all the hypercholesterolemic conditions where other HMG-CoA reductase inhibitors are used.[227] On a milligram-per-milligram basis, it is about twice as potent as lovastatin. Simvastatin, 10 mg daily, or 20 mg of pravastatin or lovastatin usually produce about 25 to 30% reductions in LDL-cholesterol compared with about 20 to 25% reductions with 20 mg of fluvastatin. Lovastatin (80 mg), pravastatin (40 mg), or simvastatin (40 mg) generally decrease LDL-cholesterol by about 30 to 40%; maximum doses of fluvastatin (40 mg) decrease LDL-cholesterol by about 25%.[238] The maximum approved daily dose of simvastatin is 80 mg.

As a treatment for nephrotic hyperlipidemia, simvastatin was noted to be more effective and better tolerated than cholestyramine.[239] Simvastatin has also been evaluated for its effect on the cholesterol saturation index of gallbladder bile, a potential side effect of several hypocholesterolemic agents. A mean decline of 23% was noted in the 10 hypercholesterolemic patients studied, raising the possibility that an HMG-CoA reductase inhibitor may play a future role in the treatment of gallstones.[240]

Effect on Clinical Endpoints

Like lovastatin and pravastatin, simvastatin was shown to slow the progression of coronary atherosclerosis assessed by coronary angiography.[241,242] In the Multicentre Anti-Atheroma Study (MAAS), simvastatin, 20 mg daily, was compared with placebo in 381 patients with CAD receiving a similar lipid-lowering diet. Patients on simvastatin had a 23% reduction in total cholesterol, a 31% reduction in LDL-cholesterol, and a 9% increase in HDL cholesterol compared with placebo over 4 years. Patients on simvastatin had less progression and more regression of existing lesions and a lower rate of new lesion development.[241]

In a landmark secondary prevention study, The Scandinavian Simvastatin Survival Study (4S), simvastatin was shown to reduce mortality and morbidity in patients with known CAD and hypercholesterolemia.[56,243] In this study, 4444 patients with prior angina pectoris or myocardial infarction and elevated total serum cholesterol levels (220 to 320 mg/dL or 5.5 to 8.0 mm/L) were randomized in double-blind fashion to receive either simvastatin, 20 to 40 mg, or placebo and were followed for a median of 5.4 years (Fig. 20-7). All patients were on a cholesterol-lowering diet. Compared with placebo, simvastatin reduced total cholesterol 25% and LDL-cholesterol 35% and increased HDL cholesterol 8%. Compared with placebo, there were highly statistically significant reductions of all fatal coronary events by 42% with simvastatin; all fatal cardiovascular events were reduced by 35% (Fig. 20-8), and all-cause mortality was reduced by 30%. Patients over 60 years of age had a 27% reduction in mortality, essentially identical to the findings in the younger group. Results on secondary endpoints (myocardial infarction, revascularization, etc.) paralleled the results on mortality. There was also a 30% reduction in cerebrovascular events with simvastatin. Results in women were essentially the same as the results in men. In comparing placebo and simvastatin treatment, there was no difference in noncardiovascular mortality. Based on this

FIGURE 20-7. Kaplan-Meier curves for all-cause mortality. Number of patients at risk at the beginning of each year is shown below the horizontal axis. (*Reproduced with permission from The Scandinavian Simvastatin Survival Study Group.*[56])

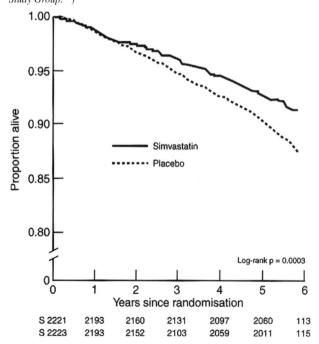

	0	1	2	3	4	5	6
S	2221	2193	2160	2131	2097	2060	113
S	2223	2193	2152	2103	2059	2011	115

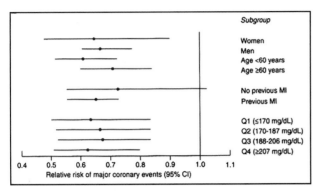

FIGURE 20-8. Relative risks [95% confidence interval (CI)] by age, gender, history of myocardial infarction (MI), and baseline low-density lipoprotein (LDL)-cholesterol quartile (Q1–Q4). The quartile limits were <4.39, 4.40 to 4.84, 4.85 to 5.34, and >5.35 mmol/L. Risk reduction = (1-relative risk) × 100%. (*Reproduced with permission from Kjekshus et al.*[243])

study, subsequent pharmacoeconomic analysis has demonstrated the cost-effectiveness of simvastatin in secondary prevention.[244]

The Heart Protection Study (HPS) enrolled 20,536 patients aged 40 to 80 years with CHD, noncoronary arterial disease, diabetes, and treated hypertension. Patients were randomized to simvastatin (40 mg daily), a vitamin cocktail (1600 mg E, 250 mg C, 20 mg beta carotene), or placebo. Patients were followed for 5 years. There was no effect from the vitamin therapy. Simvastatin caused a one-third reduction in the risk of myocardial infarction, stroke, coronary and noncoronary revascularization regardless of baseline cholesterol levels.[245]

Based on experimental studies, the suggestion has been made that simvastatin may reduce cardiovascular events beyond the effect on lipid lowering. The possibility of such effects is a continuing area of controversy. Simvastatin and other HMG-CoA reductase inhibitors have been shown to reduce factor VIIc activity and inhibit platelet activation[246,247] while reducing the propensity of LDL to oxidation.[247] In addition, the drug has been shown to depress blood clotting by inhibiting activation of prothrombin, thrombin factor V, and factor XIII.[248,249] A beneficial effect to statins has been associated with a lower risk of deep venous thrombosis.[250] Simvastatin was also shown to have a favorable action in causing regression of cardiac hypertrophy in an animal model of hypertrophic cardiomyopathy.[251]

Clinical Use

Similar to other marketed HMG-CoA reductase inhibitors, simvastatin is approved for use in patients with primary hypercholesterolemia and mixed dyslipidemia (Fredrickson types IIa and IIb). In addition, based on the results of the 4S study, the drug has also been approved in patients with CHD as long-term treatment for hypercholesterolemia and to reduce the risk of total mortality by reducing coronary death, the risk of nonfatal myocardial infarction, the risk for undergoing myocardial revascularization, and the risk of stroke or transient ischemic attack. In addition, the drug is approved for use in patients with hypertriglyceridemia (Frederickson type IV) and primary dyslipoproteinemia (Fredrickson type III). Simvastatin is administered orally as a single dose in the evening. The recommended starting dose is 20 mg daily, which is then titrated according to the individual patient's response at 4-week intervals to a maximum 80-mg daily dose. Simvastatin can be combined with FADs, niacin, and BASs—including colesevelam—to achieve maximal cholesterol lowering.[252] A combination formula of simvastatin and ezetimibe, a cholesterol absorption inhibitor (see Chap. 46) is now in clinical development.[252a,252b]

In patients with severe renal insufficiency or those receiving cyclosporine, the recommended starting dose is 5 mg daily, and close monitoring is required. Drug-drug interactions with amiodarone and verapamil require dosing adjustments. The dose of simvastatin should not exceed 20 mg/d. In patients taking fibrates, niacin or cyclosporin, the simvastatin dose should not exceed 10 mg/d. The low risk of liver enzyme abnormalities and their lack of clinical severity has led to less stringent requirements for liver function testing. Testing is now recommended prior to initiating or increasing the dose of therapy and twice during the subsequent year, with routine laboratory monitoring ceasing a year after the last dosage increment if liver function tests remain normal.

Adverse Effects

The side-effects profile of simvastatin is similar to that of lovastatin and other HMG-CoA reductase inhibitors. The rare occurrence of a lupus-like syndrome has recently been reported with both lovastatin and simvastatin.

Pravastatin

Pravastatin (Pravachol CS 514, SQ 3100, epstatin) is the 6 alpha-hydroxy acid form of compactin.[253] It is the first HMG-CoA reductase inhibitor to be administered in the active form and not as a prodrug. In vitro studies by Tsujita et al. demonstrated that pravastatin has a greater specificity for hepatic cells than lovastatin.[254] In vivo animal studies comparing pravastatin to lovastatin and simvastatin, however, found that the concentration of pravastatin in the liver was only half that of the latter two, whereas the concentrations in peripheral tissues were three to six times greater.[255]

Pravastatin was also found to be a specific inhibitor of hepatic HMG-CoA reductase in humans.[256] Other enzymes involved in cholesterol metabolism [alpha-hydroxylase, which governs bile acid synthesis and acyl-coenzyme A; cholesterol O-acetyltransferase (ACAT), which regulates cholesterol esterification] were not affected by treatment. Inhibition of hepatic HMG-CoA reductase activity by pravastatin results in an increased expression of hepatic LDL receptors, which explains the lowered plasma levels of LDL-cholesterol.[256]

Multiple studies have already been conducted on humans to establish efficacy and dosage.[257] Despite its short plasma half-life of approximately 2 h, a single daily dose of pravastatin has been shown to be as effective as twice-daily doses.[257] As with all HMG-CoA reductase inhibitors, the sustained duration of benefit relates to the relatively long half-life of plasma LDL and is independent of the systemic half-life of the drug, most of which is removed in the first pass through the liver in any event. As with other drugs in this class, administration of the drug in the evening rather than the morning appears to bring about greater cholesterol-lowering activity. Mabuchi et al.[258] treated patients with heterozygous FH with pravastatin, 10 and 20 mg. They found a 26 and 33% decrease in LDL, respectively. HDL was significantly increased. Nakaya et al.[259] also found that 5-, 20-, and 40-mg doses lowered the total serum cholesterol by 11.1, 18.8, and 25.3%, respectively, in hypercholesterolemic patients. The investigators reported some mild side effects but no myositis.

The efficacy and safety of pravastatin has been evaluated in various patient subgroups. A low dose (10 mg) of pravastatin daily was shown to be a safe and effective method of reducing total and LDL-cholesterol in hypercholesterolemic, hypertensive elderly patients who were receiving concurrent antihypertensive drug therapy.[260] The safety and efficacy of using lovastatin (20 and 40 mg) in the elderly was also confirmed in the Cholesterol Reduction in Seniors Program.[261] The effect of pravastatin on morbidity and mortality in the elderly is now being evaluated in the NIH-funded Antihypertensive Lipid Lowering Heart Attack Trial (ALLHAT). Pravastatin (20 mg daily) has been shown to be well tolerated and effective in lowering total cholesterol and LDL-cholesterol in patients with type I or II diabetes mellitus and hypercholesterolemia.[262] Finally, pravastatin (20 mg daily) has been found to be an effective and safe lipid-lowering agent, as have other drugs in this class, in African Americans with primary hypercholesterolemia and in the elderly.[263]

Lovastatin, simvastatin, and pravastatin have been directly compared, and the published data suggest that, at equipotent dosages, the drugs are approximately equal in efficacy with respect to reducing LDL-cholesterol.[264,265]

Effects on Clinical Endpoints

The benefit of using pravastatin to reduce morbidity and mortality in patients with CAD was first established in the Pravastatin Multinational Study.[266] In this 6-month trial, pravastatin treatment was demonstrated to reduce the incidence of serious cardiovascular events including myocardial infarction and unstable angina.

Four vascular regression trials using pravastatin have been completed, with the results reported on two of the trials.[267–270] PLAC-I (Pravastatin Limitation of Atherosclerosis in the Coronary Arteries)[267] and REGRESS (Regression Growth Evaluation Statin Study)[270] included patients with CAD to assess by serial angiography the effects of pravastatin on CAD. PLAC-II[268] was designed to evaluate the ability of pravastatin to retard the ultrasonographic 3-year progression of extracranial carotid artery in patients with known CAD. The KAPS (Kuopio Atherosclerosis Study) was a 3-year ultrasonographic study that evaluated the effects of pravastatin on the progression of carotid and femoral atherosclerosis.[269]

All the studies were placebo-controlled, and pravastatin doses of 20 to 40 mg were used as monotherapy. Patients receiving pravastatin in PLAC-1 had a 40 to 50% reduction in the progression of coronary lesions, a 28% reduction in LDL-cholesterol, and fewer nonfatal and fatal myocardial infarctions compared with placebo.[267] In PLAC-II, pravastatin-treated patients showed a 35% reduction of atherosclerosis in the common carotid artery and a 80% reduction in fatal and nonfatal infarctions compared with placebo.[268] In KAPS, there was a significant reduction in the progression of carotid atherosclerosis compared with placebo.[269] In REGRESS, there was a significant reduction in the progression of coronary atherosclerosis with pravastatin and a reduced rate of adverse cardiovascular events compared with placebo, including fewer myocardial infarctions, sudden deaths, strokes, and invasive coronary procedures.

In these four studies, a total of 1891 patients had been evaluated, and although the major objective was to assess regression of atherosclerosis with aggressive lipid lowering with pravastatin, a metanalysis was performed to assess the impact of treatment on clinical cardiovascular events[271] compared with placebo. The risk of fatal plus nonfatal myocardial infarctions was reduced by 62%, the risk of stroke reduced by 62%, and total mortality by 46%.

In a prospective study of patients with known cardiovascular disease, pravastatin was shown to reduce the level of the inflammatory biomarker C-reactive protein (CRP) in a largely LDL-cholesterol–independent manner, suggesting that statins may have anti-inflammatory in addition to lipid-lowering effects[272–274] that contribute to their clinical benefit in patients at risk for CAD.[275]

Pravastatin was also shown to have a blood pressure–lowering effect in patients with moderate hypercholesterolemia and

hypertension.[276] In addition, the drug improves endothelial function after acute coronary syndromes[277,278] and decreases thrombus formation.[279]

Pravastatin has been used in one large primary prevention and several secondary prevention studies with reported benefit on clinical cardiovascular outcomes. In the West of Scotland Prevention Study (WOSCOPS),[280] 6595 middle-aged men with no history of myocardial infarction and average plasma cholesterol values above 252 mg/dL were randomized to receive either placebo or 40 mg of pravastatin and followed for an average of almost 5 years. Pravastatin decreased LDL-cholesterol by 26% and increased HDL-cholesterol by 5%. Pravastatin treatment also significantly reduced the incidence of myocardial infarction and death from cardiovascular causes by 31% as well as decreasing a variety of other coronary endpoints without adversely affecting the risk of death from noncardiovascular causes. Total mortality was decreased by 22% (Fig. 20-9).[280]

The Cholesterol and Recurrent Events Study (CARE)[281] was designed to assess whether pravastatin treatment (40 mg daily) could reduce the sum of fatal CAD and nonfatal myocardial infarctions in patients who have survived a myocardial infarction yet have a total cholesterol below 240 mg/dL, a population different from that studied in 4S. Results indicated a significant benefit of pravastatin therapy on cardiovascular outcomes compared with placebo. The primary endpoint of fatal coronary event or myocardial infarction was reduced 24%, despite this being a population with somewhat lower than average LDL levels (139 mg/dL). A variety of other coronary endpoints was also significantly reduced as was stroke.[282] No significant effect on all-cause mortality was detected in this relatively low-risk group.[283] A post-hoc subgroup analysis showed that the benefit was confined to those patients having a baseline LDL-cholesterol above 125 mg/dL, an observation that led to a period of questioning of the NCEP guidelines target LDL of <100 mg/dL for patients with know atherosclerotic disease.[284] The NCEP target has been, in the main, supported by the literature and remains the consensus.[20]

The Long-term Intervention with Pravastatin in Ischemic Heart Disease trial (LIPID) was a relatively similar trial that evaluated placebo versus pravastatin, 40 mg, in patients who had either an acute myocardial infarction or an unstable angina episode and had cholesterol values of 155 to 271 mg/dL. The study looked at the effects of treatment on CAD mortality as the primary endpoint.[284,285,285a] Median LDL levels, at 150 mg/dL, were slightly higher. The primary endpoint was decreased by 24%, there were similar significant effects on other coronary endpoints, and all-cause mortality was decreased by 22% as well. In addition, a beneficial effect was seen on the risk of nonhemorrhagic stroke from any cause.[286]

An additional pravastatin study evaluating the use of HMG-CoA reductase inhibitors with or without vitamin E and marine polyunsaturated fats (fish oil) in 6000 patients with a history of myocardial infarction was stopped early due to the publication of the CARE and LIPID data.

Clinical Use

Pravastatin has a similar approval for treatment of hypercholesterolemia as other HMG-CoA reductase inhibitors and, in addition, is approved for both the primary and secondary prevention of complications related to CAD. The drug is also approved for the secondary prevention of stroke and ischemic attacks as well as the progression of coronary atherosclerosis. The drug is approved for use in patients with primary hypertriglyceridemia (Fredrickson type

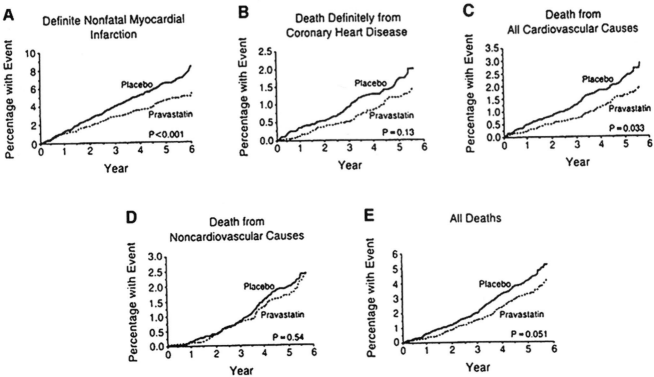

FIGURE 20-9. Kaplan-Meier analysis of time to a definite nonfatal myocardial infarction (*panel A*), death definitely from coronary heart disease (*panel B*), death from all cardiovascular causes (*panel C*), death from noncardiovascular causes (*panel D*), and death from any cause (*panel E*) according to treatment group. (*Reproduced with permission from Shepherd et al.[280]*)

IV), primary dyslipoproteinemia (Fredrickson type III), primary hypercholesterolemia (Fredrickson type IIa) and mixed dyslipidemia (Fredrickson type IIa). The recommended starting dose is 10 to 20 mg once daily at bedtime for primary hypercholesterolemia, with a usual dosing range of 10 to 40 mg daily. A 40-mg dose may be necessary to achieve the clinical benefits observed in the primary and secondary prevention trials done with the drug. Recently a pravastatin/aspirin co-package has become available for the long-term management to reduce the risk of cardiovascular events in patients with clinically evident coronary disease.

Similar to other HMG-CoA reductase inhibitors, the drug may be combined with other classes of lipid-lowering drugs. When combined with cholestyramine or colestipol, pravastatin should be administered 1 h before or 4 h after the bile-acid resin is given. Such precautions appear not to be necessary with colesevelam.

Adverse Effects

The adverse effect profile is similar to other HMG-CoA reductase inhibitors in use. Since the drug does not cross the blood brain barrier, it has been proposed to cause a lower incidence of sleep disturbances than either lovastatin or simvastatin.[287] A rare peripheral–neuropathic complication with both lovastatin and pravastatin has been described.

As with simvastatin, the low risk of liver enzyme abnormalities and their lack of clinical severity has led to less stringent requirements for liver function testing. The recommendation for liver function testing at 6 weeks has been eliminated as has the recommendation for semi-annual testing if liver function tests are normal at 12 weeks. twice a year, ceasing a year after the last dosage increment if liver function tests remain normal.

Fluvastatin

Fluvastatin was the first synthetic HMG-CoA reductase inhibitor, and it is structurally distinct from the fungal derivatives lovastatin, simvastatin, and pravastatin.[288] It was approved for clinical use in the United States for the treatment of primary hypercholesterolemia (type IIa and IIb). The drug also received approval as the fourth statin to slow the progression of coronary arteriosclerosis in patients with CHD, as part of a treatment to lower total and LDL-cholesterol to target rates. Using doses of 20 to 40 mg daily in patients with hypercholesterolemia, the drug was shown to reduce LDL-cholesterol by 19 to 31%, total cholesterol by 15 to 21%, with small declines in triglycerides of 1 to 12%. The drug raises HDL-cholesterol by 2 to 10%.[289] Maximal lipid-lowering effects of a dose are usually seen after 4 weeks of therapy and are sustained long term. On a milligram-to-milligram basis, the drug appears to be less potent in its lipid-lowering effects than other available HMG-CoA reductase inhibitors, and the recommended maximal dose has recently been increased to 80 mg daily in two divided doses.

Fluvastatin is well absorbed after oral administration and, like other HMG-CoA reductase drugs, undergoes extensive first-pass metabolism.[288] Its side-effect profile is similar to those of other HMG-CoA reductase inhibitors, and it may cause less myopathy and risk of rhabdomyolysis when used alone or with gemfibrozil, nicotinic acid, cyclosporine, and erythromycin.[288]

The drug has been combined with other lipid-lowering therapies—including cholestyramine, bezafibrate, and nicotinic acid—to achieve greater lipid-lowering effects[290,291]; it has been used safely in diabetic and hypertensive patients.[288]

Effects on Clinical Endpoints

Although many patients with known CAD have received fluvastatin, there are as yet no published survival studies with the drug. One study assessed the efficacy of high-dose fluvastatin (80 mg daily) in preventing restenosis after balloon angioplasty; no significant benefit was detected.[292] In another study, known as the Lipoprotein and Coronary Atherosclerosis Study (LCAS), the effects of fluvastatin versus placebo on long-term progression of atherosclerosis were assessed in patients with known CAD using serial coronary angiography.[293] Results from the LCAS demonstrated a benefit of fluvastatin treatment on the progression and regression of atherosclerosis. Recently the results of the prospective Lescol Intervention Prevention Study (LIPS) demonstrated that statin therapy initiated soon after successful percutaneous coronary intervention improved clinical outcomes.[64a] These data support the use of early lipid-lowering therapy in post-PCI patients regardless of baseline cholesterol level.

Fluvastatin has been evaluated as an anti-ischemic drug in patients immediately following myocardial infarction (Effects of Fluvastatin Administration Immediately after an Acute MI on Myocardial Ischemia—FLORIDA), with no benefit compared to placebo after 1 year.[294] The drug has been shown to lower total and LDL-cholesterol as well as dense LDL, a more atherogenic subfraction of LDL.[295]

Clinical Use

Fluvastatin (capsules and an extended-release tablet form of the drug[296]) is indicated as an adjunct to diet to reduce elevated total cholesterol, LDL-cholesterol, triglycerides, and apo B levels and to increase HDL cholesterol in patients with primary hypercholesterolemia and mixed dyslipidemia (Fredrickson types IIa and IIb). Both formulations are also indicated to slow the progression of coronary atherosclerosis in patients with CHD as part of a treatment strategy to lower total and LDL-cholesterol.

The recommended starting dose is 40 mg as one capsule or 80 mg as one extended-release tablet administered as a single dose in the evening or 80 mg in divided doses of the 40 mg capsules given twice daily. As in the case of other HMG-CoA reductase inhibitors, it takes at least 4 weeks to achieve the maximal effect. If fluvastatin is combined with cholestyramine, fluvastatin plasma levels drop considerably. Fluvastatin must be given at least 4 h after a cholestyramine dose.[288]

Atorvastatin

Atorvastatin is a newer synthetic HMG-CoA reductase inhibitor with a long half-life (14 h, 20 to 30 h for activity due to the presence of active metabolites) that is similar in structure to fluvastatin. Atorvastatin is twice as potent on a milligram-to-milligram basis as simvastatin and much more potent than fluvastatin in reducing total cholesterol and LDL-cholesterol.[297] Early investigations proposed that atorvastatin was unique in its ability to reduce triglycerides.[298] This has been less striking in subsequent studies; if such potency is present at all, the advantage is modest. In 1997, the drug was approved for clinical use in patients with types IIa and IIb hypercholesterolemia and homozygous familial hypercholesterolemia. Its side-effect profile appears to be similar to those of other HMG-CoA reductase inhibitors in doses up to 80 mg daily used once daily.[298,299]

In the ASAP trial, aggressive therapy with atorvastatin 80 mg was shown to produce less progression of noninvasively quantitated carotid atherosclerosis than lower-dose therapy with Simvastatin 40 mg.[300] The published long-term clinical experience with atorvastatin remains limited because of the recency of its introduction, though many trials are ongoing. The clinical endpoints evidence base is primarily based on two large relatively short-term studies. The Myocardial Ischemia Reduction with Aggressive Cholesterol Lowering (MIRACL) trial showed that the administration of atorvastatin 80 mg immediately after hospitalization for unstable angina or non-Q-wave myocardial infarction reduced the incidence of recurrent ischemic events over the first 16 weeks.[71] Patients who were treated with either simvastatin or pravastatin in the three major secondary prevention statin trials (4S, CARE, LIPID) or pravastatin or lovastatin in the two major primary prevention trials (WOSCOPS and AFCAPS/TexCAPS) did not show benefit at such an early time point. This may reflects differences in the biology of acute as opposed to chronic coronary syndromes, increased statistical power due to a high risk of short-term ischemic complications in unstable patients, or particular advantages of the high-dose atorvastatin regimen used. Other trials examining the benefits of initiating high-dose statin therapy early after an acute coronary event are ongoing. Of note, at high doses atorvastatin loses some of its effectiveness in raising HDL, an effect not seen with equipotent doses of simvastatin.[301] The clinical significance of this observation is unknown.

The Atorvastatin versus Revascularization Treatment study (AVERT) examined 341 patients with stable CAD who were referred for percutaneous transluminal coronary angioplasty.[302] Patients were randomly assigned to either atorvastatin 80 mg per day or to angioplasty followed by usual care, which did not exclude lipid-lowering therapy. Over 18 months of follow-up, the incidence of ischemic events was 36% lower in the atorvastatin group ($p = 0.048$, but not significant after statistical adjustment for interim analyses). The patients who received atorvastatin also had a longer time to the first ischemic event ($p = 0.03$). There was no "usual care" placebo group, and it is unclear to what extent the results in this study reflect the benefit of atorvastatin versus possible disadvantages of angioplasty in the study population.

There have been no primary or secondary CHD prevention trials of lipid-lowering therapy, specifically in a diabetic population. Two studies are now in place evaluating the effects of atorvastatin in diabetic patients [Atorvastatin as Prevention of Coronary Heart Disease in Patients with Type II Diabetes (ASPEN); Collaborative Atorvastatin Diabetes Study (CARDS)].[303]

Clinical Use

Atorvastatin is approved for reducing elevated total cholesterol, LDL-cholesterol, apo B, and triglyceride levels and to increase HDL cholesterol in patients with primary hypercholesterolemia and mixed dyslipidemia. In addition, the drug is approved for use in patients with primary dysbetalipoproteinemia and elevated triglyceride levels.

The recommended starting dose of atorvastatin is 10 mg once daily. The dosage range is 10 to 80 mg once daily. The drug can be administered as a single dose at any time of the day, with or without food.

Cerivastatin

Cerivastatin is a potent synthetic HMG-CoA reductase inhibitor that was studied in controlled trials and shown to be effective in reducing plasma total cholesterol and LDL-cholesterol in patients with heterozygous familial and nonfamilial forms of hypercholesterolemia, and in mixed hyperlipidemia.[304] Like other drugs in the class, it was approved for clinical use as an adjunct to diet for the reduction of elevated total and LDL-cholesterol levels in patients with primary hypercholesterolemia and mixed dyslipidemia (Fredrickson types IIa and IIb) when the response to dietary restriction of saturated fat and cholesterol and other nonpharmacologic measures alone has been inadequate. It was recommended that the drug be administered once daily in the evening using a 0.3-mg tablet. Higher doses were subsequently approved. After the introduction of these higher doses, an increased risk of rhabdomyolysis-associated mortality, particularly in the elderly and in patients on gemfibrozil, became evident relative to other statins. These events were relatively rare; but given the availability of many safer alternatives in the same class, cerivastatin was withdrawn from the market in 2001.[305]

Rosuvastatin

Rosuvastatin is a highly efficacious statin that is currently in the final stages of regulatory approval in the United States.[306–308] It appears to combine a number of the characteristics of the currently available statins. Like pravastatin, rosuvastatin is liver-selective, hydrophilic, and minimally metabolized via CYP3A4. Like atorvastatin, rosuvastatin has a prolonged half-life in systemic plasma of about 20 h and is quite potent. The maximum tested dose of 80 mg reduced LDL 65%, significantly more than is possible using current monotherapy however, the high dose was not well tolerated in some patients. Rosuvastatin also produced greater increases in HDL than is seen with high-dose atorvastatin. The 10 mg dose reduced LDL by approximately 50%. No long-term side effect, clinical endpoint, or angiographic data are yet available.

Conclusion

There has been an evolution of more rigorous and aggressive approaches to the primary and secondary prevention of CAD that have occurred in parallel with growing evidence for the safety and effectiveness of HMG-CoA reductase inhibitors in treating hypercholesterolemia and for reducing the incidence of cardiovascular morbidity and mortality in patients at greater risk.[64a] The HMG-CoA reductase inhibitors are the most effective agents for reducing both total and LDL-cholesterol and can be used in conjunction with other lipid-lowering treatments for achieving maximal lipid-lowering effectiveness in patients. HMG-CoA reductase inhibitors, to a variable extent, also produce modest increases in HDL that may be clinically significant and, in higher doses, also lower triglycerides. In addition, these drugs have been shown to have protective actions beyond the effects of cholesterol reduction (nitric oxide–mediated improvement of endothelial dysfunction, antioxidant effect, anti-inflammatory properties and anticoagulant and antihypertensive effects).[309–310b] The drugs have been shown to reduce the risk of hip fracture and dementia in elderly patients,[311–313] and may counteract the adverse effects of hormone replacement in post-menopausal women with coronary artery disease.[313a] In practice, inadequate utilization and, in particular, titration of HMG-CoA reductase inhibitor therapy continues to be a problem, and information regarding the safety record of HMG-CoA reductase inhibitor therapy and the benefits of this treatment on clinical outcomes must be disseminated more widely, both to clinicians and patients.[314,314a]

Statins need to be prescribed at the time of discharge after myocardial infarction in order to achieve a maximal benefit.[315,315a] Statin

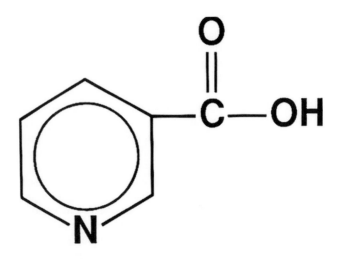

FIGURE 20-10. Chemical structure of nicotinic acid.

pretreatment in patients with acute coronary syndromes may be associated with improved clinical outcomes.[315b,315c] However, discontinuation of statins after onset of symptoms negates the beneficial effect.[315c]

NICOTINIC ACID (NIACIN)

Nicotinic acid (pyridine-3 carboxylic acid, or niacin) is a water-soluble B-complex vitamin (Fig. 20-10) that is used for the prophylaxis and treatment of pellagra. The substance functions in the body after conversion to either nicotinamide-adenine dinucleotide (NAD) or nicotinamide-adenine dinucleotide phosphate (NADP). In 1955, Altschul and colleagues demonstrated that large doses of nicotinic acid lower the concentration of plasma cholesterol in humans.[316] This property of nicotinic acid is not shared by nicotinamide and appears to have nothing to do with the role of these compounds as vitamins. Subsequently, nicotinic acid in high doses was shown to reduce triglycerides and have favorable effects in patients with various hyperlipoproteinemias. From the results of controlled clinical trials with nicotinic acid, there is evidence that cardiovascular morbidity can be reduced with long-term therapy. In this section, the clinical pharmacology of nicotinic acid as a lipid-lowering agent is reviewed and recommendations for its clinical use are presented.

Pharmacokinetics

Nicotinic acid is readily absorbed from the intestinal tract after the oral administration of pharmacologic doses.[317] The level of free nicotinic acid in plasma reaches a peak value between 30 and 60 min after a single dose of 1 g is ingested. Because nicotinic acid is rapidly eliminated, the doses necessary to achieve pharmacologic effects (2 to 8 g daily) are much greater than the amount needed for its physiologic functions as a vitamin. When large doses of the vitamin were given to rats by intraperitoneal injection, the half-life of the compound was found to be approximately 1 h in blood.[318] The half-life of nicotinic acid seems to be determined primarily by the rate of renal clearance of the unchanged compound when given in high doses. At lower doses, it is mainly excreted as its metabolites.[318]

The metabolic fate of nicotinic acid is complex and varies with the dose. Under normal conditions, metabolites of nicotinic acid found in the urine are mainly the products of catabolism of the pyridine nucleotides, the stored forms of the vitamin.[317] The primary route of metabolism is via methylation to N-methyl-nicotinamide, which is further oxidized to N-methyl-2- and -4-pyridone carboxamides. With pharmacologic doses, the excretion of nicotinuric acid, produced by the conjugation of nicotinic acid and glycine, is enhanced and seems to play a role as a detoxification product at these higher doses. Once the dose is large enough to overcome the production rate of nicotinuric acid, nicotinic acid is excreted largely unchanged.[318]

Pharmacology

Nicotinic acid in large doses lowers total plasma cholesterol and has been found to have beneficial effects on the levels of the major serum lipoproteins, including Lp(a).[318a] Specifically, it decreases the levels of VLDL triglyceride (VLDL-Tg) and LDL-cholesterol and causes an increase in the levels of HDL-cholesterol.[319] This lipid-altering activity is not shared by nicotinamide and seems to be unrelated to the role of nicotinic acid as a vitamin in the NAD and NADP coenzyme systems. Pharmacologic doses of nicotinic acid result in a rapid decrease in plasma triglyceride (Tg) levels, in part by lowering VLDL-Tg concentrations by 20 to more than 80%.[319] The magnitude of the reduction is related to the initial VLDL levels. Within 1 week of initiation of therapy, concentrations of LDL-cholesterol decrease. Typically, a 10 to 5% reduction in LDL-cholesterol is observed within 3 to 5 weeks of attaining full dosage. The magnitude of the drop is also related to the dose of nicotinic acid. In addition to these lipid-lowering effects, nicotinic acid raises HDL cholesterol concentrations.[319,320] Mobilization of cholesterol from peripheral tissues seems to occur after prolonged therapy, as evidenced by the regression of eruptive, tuboeruptive, tuberous, and tendon xanthomas.[319]

There are several mechanisms by which nicotinic acid alters serum lipoprotein levels. Nicotinic acid's actions as an antilipolytic agent may be related to its effects on lowering VLDL-Tg concentration. Nicotinic acid has been found to decrease lipolysis in adipose tissue, resulting in decreased levels of plasma free fatty acids.[321] After oral administration of 1 g of nicotinic acid, a significant depression of free fatty acids occurs, as well as a reduction in plasma glycerol levels. During fasting, free fatty acids released from adipose tissue serve as the major precursors for the formation of VLDL-Tg, which is synthesized mainly in the liver and serves as the major carrier of endogenous triglyceride.[319] The decrease in the release of free fatty acid from adipose tissue that is induced by nicotinic acid is thought to decrease uptake of free fatty acid by the liver and thereby reduce the hepatic synthesis of VLDL.[319]

Clinical Experience

As outlined above, nicotinic acid has been shown to have beneficial effects on all plasma lipoprotein fractions, including Lp(a), and was identified as one of the drug choices for the treatment of hypercholesterolemia by the Adult Treatment Panel of the NCEP.[20] Studies of the clinical efficacy of nicotinic acid fall into two main groups: those that examine the use of nicotinic acid in patients with known CHD and those that test its efficacy, often in combination with other lipid-lowering agents, in altering plasma lipoprotein levels in patients with various types of hyperlipoproteinemias.

The Coronary Drug Project, a long-term nationwide, double-blind, placebo-controlled study, looked at a number of lipid-altering regimens, including nicotinic acid and clofibrate, in male survivors of myocardial infarction.[145]

Over the follow-up period, nicotinic acid effected mean decreases in total serum cholesterol of 9.9% and in total triglycerides of 26.1%.[145] However, the incidence of all deaths in the follow-up period (8.5 years) was insignificantly lower than that in the placebo group (24.4 versus 25.4%). In contrast to the findings on total mortality, the incidence of definite, nonfatal myocardial infarction over the total follow-up period was 27% lower in the treatment group than in the control group (10.1 versus 13.9%). Also, during this period, the treatment group showed a 24% lower incidence of fatal or nonfatal cerebrovascular events than the placebo group. There was also a lower incidence of bypass surgery in the group receiving nicotinic acid (0.9 versus 2.7%).[145]

Investigators in the Coronary Drug Project conducted a follow-up study nearly 9 years after termination of the original trial.[322] With a mean total follow-up of 15 years, total mortality in the nicotinic acid group was found to be 11% lower than in the placebo group (52 versus 58.2%). The men in the study had presumably stopped taking the drug after the original mean follow-up of 6.2 years. The decreased mortality is primarily due to a decrease in CHD mortality, with smaller decreases in death due to cerebrovascular causes, other cardiovascular events, cancer, and other noncardiovascular and noncancer causes.

Explanations for this observed late benefit of nicotinic acid on mortality include the early decreases in incidence of nonfatal reinfarction and the cholesterol-lowering effects of nicotinic acid on the coronary arteries.[322] It seems that patients with the largest decreases in cholesterol at 1 year follow-up had lower subsequent mortality than did subjects with increases in cholesterol. Nearly 30% of the men in the nicotinic acid group adhered poorly to the treatment regimen (took less than 60% of the amount of drug called for by the protocol), yet there was a significant benefit in 15-year mortality. This suggests that less than optimal doses of nicotinic acid may nevertheless result in therapeutic benefits. Of course, statements regarding the efficacy of nicotinic acid as a primary prevention of CHD or whether the administration of nicotinic acid over longer periods of time would be beneficial or detrimental cannot be made based on the findings of this study.

In a Swedish study by Carlson et al.,[323] the effects of combined treatment with nicotinic acid (up to 3 g daily) and clofibrate (2 g daily) were examined in 558 survivors of MI randomly assigned to one of two groups 4 months after their acute events. Both groups received advice regarding diet, and the treatment group received both drugs as above. Subjects in the treatment group exhibited mean reductions in total serum cholesterol and serum triglycerides of 15 to 20 and 30%, respectively. Control group subjects showed insignificant reductions in these levels. There were no significant differences between the two groups with regard to total and CHD-related deaths. However, over a 4-year period, the number of nonfatal reinfarctions in the treatment group was reduced by 50% compared with the control group. In comparison, the Coronary Drug Project reported a 27% reduction in nonfatal reinfarctions in the nicotinic acid group and insignificant reductions in the clofibrate group. Considering the more modest decreases in serum cholesterol and triglycerides (6 and 10%, respectively) found in the Coronary Drug Project as compared with those observed in this study, it has been suggested that the rate of nonfatal reinfarction may be related to the degree of serum lipid lowering.[323]

The Cholesterol-Lowering Atherosclerosis Study (CLAS) employed a colestipol-nicotinic acid combination to test the hypothesis that aggressive lowering of LDL-cholesterol and raising of HDL-cholesterol reverses or retards the progression of atherosclerotic lesions.[8,324] The subjects, chosen to minimize the effects of other major nonlipid risk factors for atherosclerosis, included 162 normotensive nonsmoking men aged 40 to 59 years with previous coronary bypass surgery and fasting levels of total cholesterol in the range of 4.78 to 9.05 mm/L (185 to 350 mg dL).

The results of angiographic readings show that the treatment group's score distribution was significantly shifted toward lower scores than that of the control group, indicating less disease progression with colestipol-nicotinic acid treatment. In fact, 61% of the treatment group subjects improved or remained the same, and 16.2% showed regression of atherosclerotic lesions at 2 years. This differs from the results in the placebo control group of 39 and 2.4%, respectively. Regarding native vessels, treatment reduced the average number of lesions that progressed per subject and the percentage of subjects with new lesions.[8] Similarly, with respect to bypass grafts, the percentage of subjects either with new lesions or showing any adverse change in preexisting lesions was significantly lower in the treatment group. Recently reported were the results of a 7-year follow-up of a subpopulation from CLAS.[324] These findings suggest that, following coronary artery bypass surgery, patients should receive intensive interventions to improve blood lipid and lipoprotein levels.[323]

The results of the Familial Atherosclerosis Treatment Study (FATS) demonstrated a favorable effect of nicotinic acid plus colestipol on the progression of coronary atherosclerotic disease.[325] With the nicotinic acid-colestipol combination, 25% of patients showed progression of coronary lesions, 39% showed regression, and only two cardiovascular events occurred. In contrast, 10 cardiovascular events occurred in the control group, 46% of patients showed regional progression, and 11% showed regression of coronary lesions. Patients with disease, a family history of premature cardiovascular events, and elevated levels of apo B (3.23 mm/L or 125 mg/dL) were counseled on diet and assigned to one of three treatment regimens: nicotinic acid 4 g per day plus colestipol 30 g per day; lovastatin 40 mg per day plus colestipol; or colestipol alone (control). The combination regimens caused the greatest reductions in LDL and the greatest elevations in HDL. Bimonthly visits spanned 2.5 years between coronary angiograms. Favorable changes in clinical course and lesion severity appeared with the combination regimens.

A blinded, placebo-controlled larger (160 patients) angiographic regression trial of combination therapy was recently reported.[43] The effects of combination therapy with simvastatin and niacin or of an antioxidant vitamin cocktail (or of both) were evaluated in a population with known CAD and normal LDL levels (mean 125 mg/dL). The vitamin supplement (vitamin E, vitamin C, beta-carotene, and selenium) was without effect on lipid levels but was documented to decrease the susceptibility of LDL to in vitro oxidation. Simvastatin was titrated to obtain an LDL below 90 mg/dL and then slow-release niacin was added in the ultimate dose of 1 g twice a day. Patients whose HDL did not exhibit a desired increase (5 mg/dL at 3 months, 10 mg/dL by 12 months) were switched to crystalline niacin in higher doses. Simvastatin was backtitrated if the LDL fell below 40 mg/dL. Combined antioxidant therapy significantly blunted the benefit of the drug regimen, both on plasma lipids and on angiographic progression. Proximal coronary stenosis increased by a mean 3.9% in the placebo group, 1.8% in the antioxidant group, and 0.7% in the combined therapy group, but it decreased by 0.4% in

the group receiving drug therapy alone. In addition, there was a 90% decrease in the incidence of a first cardiovascular event (death, myocardial infarction, stroke, or revascularization) in this group. The endpoint was reached in 24% of the placebo-treated patients, 21% of the patients given antioxidants alone, 14% of those given both, and 3% of those given simvastatin and niacin alone. These benefits were out of proportion to the LDL lowering achieved (42%), particularly given the limited period of follow-up (38 months), and provide support for the potential value of HDL-raising therapy, in particular using niacin, in the management of coronary risk. The negative effect of combining vitamins with drug therapy cannot be considered established given the modest size and statistical power of this study. However, any benefits of vitamins alone on angiographic disease did not reach statistical significance and were not correlated with any effect on clinical endpoints.

Clinical Use

Nicotinic acid—through its beneficial effects on VLDL-Tg, LDL, and HDL-cholesterol levels—is indicated in most forms of hyperlipoproteinemia and for patients with depressed HDL. This includes patients with types II, III, IV, and V hyperlipoproteinemia. It is particularly useful in patients who have elevated plasma VLDL-Tg levels as a part of their lipid profile. It is important to remember that a diet low in cholesterol and saturated fats is the foundation of therapy for hyperlipoproteinemia.

Nicotinic acid is available in 100-, 125-, 250-, and 500-mg tablets as well as in a time-release form. The typical dose is 3 to 7 g daily given in three divided doses. Therapeutic effects of the drug are usually not manifest until the patient reaches a total daily dose of at least 3 g. A greater response may be attained with periodic increases in doses up to a maximum of 7 to 8 g daily, although the incidence of adverse effects also increases with higher doses. In general, it is best to use the lowest dose necessary to achieve the desired alterations in plasma lipoprotein levels. Unfortunately, many patients cannot tolerate therapeutic doses of nicotinic acid, the primary side effects being cutaneous flushing and GI disturbance. However, steps can be taken to minimize these untoward effects.

Nicotinic acid therapy should be initiated with a low-dosage regimen (100 mg daily), gradually increasing the dose every few days over a period of several weeks until the patient attains a dosage level of 3 g daily given in three divided doses. If, while increasing the dose, the patient develops any adverse effects, the dose should be cut back and then resumed at a more gradual pace. Taking the doses with meals decreases gastric irritation and cutaneous flushing.[326] Further, cutaneous flushing can be reduced or avoided by taking one aspirin tablet daily (more frequent administration is unnecessary, as one tablet will inhibit cyclooxygenase for up to 2 weeks).[326] It is interesting that tachyphylaxis to the flushing phenomenon often occurs within a few days,[8] although the bothersome episodes may recur if the patient misses two or three doses.[326] Once the initial maintenance dose is reached, it is important to evaluate for therapeutic effects by measuring plasma lipoprotein values. If the therapeutic effects are unsatisfactory, the dose should be increased by a further 1.0 to 1.5 g per day, with periodic increases to a maximum of 7 to 8 g daily as needed. Usually, when doses of 4 g daily are achieved, another lipid-lowering drug is added. Regardless of the dose, it is important to make several laboratory evaluations for potential adverse effects at regular intervals. These include assessment of liver function (bilirubin, alkaline phosphatase, and transaminase levels), uric acid levels, and serum glucose levels. Nicotinic acid is contraindicated in patients with active peptic ulcer disease. The drug may also impair glucose tolerance and is contraindicated in patients with diabetes that is difficult to control. Nicotinic acid is also associated with reversible elevations of liver enzymes and uric acid and should not be used in patients with hepatic disease or a history of symptomatic gout.[326]

Various sustained-release preparations of nicotinic acid are available without prescription. Timed-release forms of nicotinic acid were developed after it was noted that the incidence of cutaneous flushing was reduced when the drug was taken with meals, suggesting that this side effect is related to the rate of GI absorption.[327,328] In fact, patients taking the timed-release preparation do have a lower incidence of flushing than patients on unmodified nicotinic acid and require less frequent administration. However, this is outweighed by the far greater incidence of GI and constitutional symptoms experienced by patients on the timed-release form, including nausea, vomiting, diarrhea, fatigue, and decreased male sexual function.[327] In addition, the timed-release preparations appear to be associated with greater hepatotoxicity, even at low doses, including greater alkaline phosphatase and transaminase elevations.[329] In the doses required for the treatment of hyperlipidemia, they clearly have an increased potential for chemical hepatitis that can be severe.[329,330,330a]

A proprietary "intermediate release" formulation of nicotinic acid (Niaspan) that requires a prescription is also suitable for once-daily administration.[331] This preparation also appears to decrease side effects to some extent and is without an increased risk of hepatitis in its recommended dosing range (only up to 2 g daily).[331] Other newer delayed-release preparations are still undergoing evaluation for safety and efficacy.[43] A combination of a delayed-release nicotinic acid and lovastatin is now available for clinical use.[330,331] A clinical experience was reported with the use of a new form of nicotinic acid that employs a wax-matrix vehicle for sustained-release drug delivery.[332]

Adverse Effects

Despite the efficacy of nicotinic acid in beneficially altering serum lipoprotein levels, its use is limited by a variety of troublesome and sometimes serious side effects. Some studies have experienced as much as a 50% dropout rate as a result of drug-related side effects.[333]

The Coronary Drug Project, with 1100 subjects on nicotinic acid therapy, reported the common occurrences of cutaneous flushing and pruritus.[145] Other dermatologic side effects include dryness of skin, rash, and acanthosis nigricans, which are all reversible with cessation of therapy. The mechanism of the flushing is presumed to be related to the effect of nicotinic acid on vasodilatory prostaglandins and is frequently attenuated by pretreatment with aspirin. This vasodilatory effect in combination with antihypertensive therapy may potentially result in postural hypotension. The Coronary Drug Project also described an increased incidence of atrial fibrillation, and other transient cardiac arrhythmias were noted.[145] In addition, elevations in uric acid levels associated with an increased incidence of acute gouty arthritis were observed.

GI symptoms including diarrhea, nausea, vomiting, and abdominal pain were also frequent complaints encountered in the Coronary Drug Project.[145] Activation of peptic ulcer disease by nicotinic acid is a potential adverse effect,[319] but it was not observed in this large-scale study.

Liver function tests are frequently abnormal during nicotinic acid therapy. Generally, there is elevation in alkaline phosphatase and hepatic transaminases. Some studies have also noted elevations

in bilirubin, occasionally leading to jaundice. The elevations in transaminases are generally transient and reverse with decrease in dosage or cessation of therapy, and can be minimized by increasing the dosage in gradual increments when therapy is being initiated.[326] Unlike the elevations in hepatic enzymes associated with HMG-CoA reductase inhibitors, the elevations that occur with the use of nicotinic acid may be symptomatic. Several cases of niacin hepatitis progressing to fulminant hepatic failure have been described, most frequently with the time-release formulation, with biochemical, clinical, and histologic evidence of hepatocellular injury.[333a,334] This seems to be a dose-related hepatotoxicity rather than a hypersensitivity, occurring in almost all cases at doses greater than 3 g daily. In most cases, cessation of therapy leads to eventual resolution of abnormalities. Hyperglycemia and impaired glucose tolerance may occur with nicotinic acid therapy and often necessitates adjustments in diet and hypoglycemic therapy in diabetic patients.

The results of a recent study demonstrated that niacin is an effective treatment for hyperlipidemia in patients with diabetes and that its adverse effects on glycemic control are modest.[334a]

The Coronary Drug Project[145] noted a statistically significant increase in creatine phosphokinase (CPK) levels with nicotinic acid therapy, and there have been reports of associated reversible myopathy.[335] The combination of lovastatin and nicotinic acid has been causally implicated in at least one case of rhabdomyolysis.[336]

Conclusion

Nicontinic acid is a second or third choice for isolated hypercholesterolemia because of the troublesome side effects associated with the drug. However, patients who are consistent with their regimen will usually see side effects diminish after several months. Niacin has a therapeutic advantage as monotherapy in patients with combined hyperlipidemia when reduction of elevated concentrations of total plasma cholesterol, LDL-cholesterol, and triglyceride is needed and elevation of HDL. Niacin is uniquely potent in reducing Lp(a) compared to all other currently available agents. The drug is, therefore, potentially useful for the management of all types of hyperlipoproteinemia except type I; however, untoward adverse reactions must be carefully monitored.[337] The combination of nicotinic acid with a BAS resin, HMG-CoA reductase inhibitor, or gemfibrozil may allow for greater effectiveness in lowering the concentration of both LDL-cholesterol and/or triglycerides along with an increase in HDL, with an associated increased benefit in angiographic and clinical parameters of CAD.

PROBUCOL

Probucol, first introduced in the early 1970s, was advocated for its LDL-cholesterol–lowering properties and favorable side-effect profile. However, it was soon noted that, in most instances, this drug lowered HDL cholesterol more than it lowered LDL-cholesterol. Probucol was also challenged for its potential to prolong the electrocardiographic QT interval,[338] possibly leading to ventricular arrhythmias in nonhuman primates. However, it was recently shown that probucol is effective in decreasing the rate of restenosis after percutaneous transluminal coronary angioplasty (see Chap. 40).[339] In addition, experimental studies have shown the drug to have beneficial effects on ventricular remodeling in rats with heart failure.[339a]

DIETARY FIBER (PSYLLIUM)

In recent years, there has been a growing interest in the use of dietary fiber in health maintenance and disease prevention.[339b—d] Some researchers have speculated that a deficiency of fiber in the western diet might be contributing to the epidemics of diabetes mellitus, CAD, and colon cancer.[340]

Americans have become more health-conscious and aware of their diets. This awareness has probably contributed to the reported 30% decline in the death rate from CAD observed over the past 15 years.[341] In particular, fiber has been considered a possible dietary supplement for the control of systemic hypertension,[342] diabetes mellitus,[343] obesity,[344] and hyperlipidemia,[345] all known risk factors for the development of CAD.

Dietary fiber is a collective term for a variety of plant substances that are resistant to digestion by human GI enzymes.[346] Fiber may be obtained either from dietary sources or from extradietary supplements. The chemical components of naturally occurring dietary fiber include cellulose, lignins, hemicelluloses, pectins, gums, and mucilages. Dietary fibers can be classified into two major groups based on their water-solubility.[346] The structural or matrix fibers (lignins, cellulose, and some hemicelluloses) are insoluble. The natural gel-forming fibers (pectins, gums, mucilages, and the rest of the hemicelluloses) are soluble in humans.

Both soluble and insoluble fibers cause an increased bulk of softer stool due to their increased water-retaining capabilities. In addition, soluble fibers retard gastric emptying and decrease food absorption and digestion. In various experimental studies, soluble fibers such as pectin, guar gum, oat bran, and psyllium, have also been shown to reduce blood cholesterol levels.[347] Soluble fibers in general appear to be effective in proportion to their viscosity (rather than their precise chemical composition), which impairs the diffusion of luminal bile acids to the ileal sites where they are reabsorbed.[348] It should be noted that population studies have suggested that insoluble fibers and slowly absorbed carbohydrates, which do not directly reduce cholesterol, may be more effective in the reduction of coronary risk due to a therapeutic effect, by yet unknown mechanisms, on the insulin resistance syndrome or on other mediators of atherosclerosis risk (coagulation, etc.). This may simply relate to the correlation of increased insoluble dietary fiber with increased vegetable protein, which may be the actual therapeutic agent.[349]

Psyllium hydrophilic mucilloid, a well-known bulk laxative, is a potential cholesterol-lowering agent. Its effectiveness relates to its ability in delivering five times more soluble fiber than oat bran and its ease of administration as a dietary supplement to patients with hypercholesterolemia.

Psyllium is a soluble gel-forming fiber derived from the husks of blond psyllium seeds of the genus *Plantago,* plants grown in the Mediterranean region and in India. The processing of psyllium involves the initial separation of the seeds from the plant husks and then grinding the husks to make the final psyllium substance. The seed husk is then enriched with mucilloid, a hydrophilic substance that forms a gelatinous mass when mixed with water. The nonutilized seed extracts are marketed as health foods or as animal feed.[347] The chemical composition of psyllium is based on its being broken into an 85% mucilage polysaccharide and a 15% nonpolysaccharide component. The polysaccharide fraction is the active one and is made of 63% D-xylose, 20% L-arabinose, 6% rhamrose, and 9% D-galacturonic acid, as derived by acid hydrolysis and methylation analysis. Structural features of this component are those of a highly branched acidic arabinoxylan; xylan backbone with sugar 1:4 and 1:3 linkages.[350] The nonpolysaccharide component has nitrogen and other nonactive components.[350]

Several investigators have studied the activity of psyllium as a cholesterol-reducing agent. It is the universal impression from clinical trials that psyllium is a hypocholesterolemic agent[351] with and without a modified diet. However, there is still debate as to the degree of cholesterol reduction with psyllium.

Mechanism of Action

The mechanism by which psyllium and other soluble fiber lower serum cholesterol is currently uncertain. Available information suggests that one or more of the following mechanisms may be operative. First, psyllium has been shown prevent the normal reabsorption of bile acids in the gut.[352] A similar mechanism of action is also seen with cholestyramine and other BAS drugs. Second, soluble fibers such as psyllium may interfere with micelle formation in the proximal small intestine, resulting in decreased absorption of cholesterol and fatty acids.[352] Finally, short-chain fatty acids are produced by bacterial fermentation of soluble fiber in the colon. These fatty acids (predominantly propionate and acetate) are rapidly absorbed into the bloodstream and may inhibit hepatic cholesterol synthesis.[353] Short-chain fatty acids may also decrease hepatic cholesterol concentrations and secretions by interfering with compensatory mechanisms.[353]

Adverse Reactions and Drug Interactions

Psyllium and other soluble fibers are well tolerated by patients. In many of the clinical trials, treatment compliance was high. A possible reason for the acceptability of psyllium therapy is that patients will have well-formed stools and a low incidence of side effects.

Some patients placed on psyllium report abdominal distention, excessive gas, and flatulence, but these symptoms usually subside after a few weeks. Rarely, allergic reactions to psyllium have been described.[354]

Although there are reports indicating possible effects of psyllium and soluble fibers on reducing calcium, magnesium, zinc, copper, and iron absorption, other studies have contradicted these findings.[355] Animal studies have revealed the absence of teratogenic effects of psyllium. Some studies have revealed an effect of psyllium on the binding of sodium warfarin. Any potential problem can be avoided by separating the intake of psyllium and drug by 1 to 2 h. Finally, patients with congestive heart failure may be at risk from an excessive salt load with psyllium ingestion.

Clinical Recommendations

The current recommendation for fiber in the diet is 25 to 35 g per day for adults and 5 to 10 g per day for children. Fiber supplementation is widely accepted as part of achieving a healthful diet in adults and children.[356,357] This is in conjunction with a low-fat, low-cholesterol diet, which is considered to be prudent by the American Heart Association. The phase I diet in the treatment of hypercholesterolemia consists of no more than 300 mg of dietary cholesterol per day, with a maximum 30% total energy as fat. This diet has been shown to decrease cholesterol by varying amounts. With the addition of fiber, the cholesterol-lowering effect of this diet can be improved significantly.

The efficacy of psyllium in lowering cholesterol is consistent with that of many other soluble fibers. Studies have found that, in contrast to oat bran, 15 g of pectin added to the diet lowered cholesterol by an additional 11%. The addition of 100 g of oat bran to the diet has been shown to lower cholesterol by 19% and LDL-cholesterol by 11%.[358] However, the effectiveness of oat bran alone as a long-term hypercholesterolemic intervention has come into question.[358]

The efficiency of psyllium is revealed in its ability to achieve reductions in cholesterol in studies that have used only 10.2 g of the substance daily. It is concluded that psyllium is useful as an adjunct to dietary therapy in the treatment of patients with mild to moderate hypercholesterolemia. Clearly, cholestyramine and the HMG-CoA reductase inhibitors have greater efficacy than psyllium alone in reducing cholesterol. However, combining psyllium with the other drug treatments for lowering cholesterol appears to be quite useful.[359,360]

CONCLUSION

One of the most important breakthroughs in clinical medicine over the last 30 years has been the confirmation of the cholesterol hypothesis by the demonstration that lipid-lowering drug therapy could affect morbidity and mortality from CAD. The drugs will also serve as pharmacologic probes for helping to understand the pathogenesis of atherosclerosis and its major vascular complications.

REFERENCES

1. Stamler J, Wentworth D, Neaton J: Is the relationship between serum cholesterol and risk of death from coronary heart disease continuous and graded? *JAMA* 256:2823, 1986.
2. LaRosa JC, Hunninghake D, Bush D, et al: The cholesterol facts: A summary of the evidence relating dietary fats, serum cholesterol, and coronary heart disease. A joint statement by the American Heart Association and the National Heart, Lung and Blood Institute. *Circulation* 81:1721, 1990.
3. Verschuren WMM, Jacobs DR, Bloemberg BPM, et al: Serum total cholesterol and long-term coronary heart disease mortality in different cultures. Twenty-five year follow-up of the Seven Countries Study. *JAMA* 274:131, 1995.
4. Chien PC, Frishman WH: Lipid disorders. In: Crawford MH, ed. *Current Diagnosis and Treatment in Cardiology,* 2nd ed. New York: McGraw Hill, 2002:17.
5. Lipid Research Clinics Program: The Lipid Research Clinics Coronary Primary Prevention Trial Results: I. Reduction in the incidence of coronary heart disease. *JAMA* 251:351, 1986.
6. Canner PL, Berge KG, Wenger NK, et al: Fifteen year mortality in Coronary Drug Project patients: Long-term benefit with niacin. *J Am Coll Cardiol* 8:1245, 1986.
7. Frick MH, Elo MO, Haapa K, et al: Helsinki Heart Study: Primary prevention trial with gemfibrozil in middle-aged men with dyslipidemia. *N Engl J Med* 317:1237, 1987.
8. Blankenhorn DH, Nessim SA, Johnson RL, et al: Beneficial effects of combined colestipol-niacin therapy on coronary atherosclerosis and coronary venous bypass grafts. *JAMA* 257:3233, 1987.
9. The Post Coronary Artery Bypass Graft Investigators. The effect of aggressive and moderate lowering of low-density lipoprotein cholesterol levels and low-dose anticoagulation on obstructive changes in saphenous-vein coronary artery bypass grafts. *N Engl J Med* 336:153, 1997.
10. Alaupovic P, Fesmire JD, Hunninghake D, et al: The effect of aggressive and moderate lowering of LDL-cholesterol and low dose anticoagulation on plasma lipids, apolipoproteins and lipoprotein families in post coronary artery bypass graft trial. *Atherosclerosis* 146:369, 1999.
11. Frick MH, Syvänne M, Nieminen MS et al: Prevention of the angiographic progression of coronary and vein-graft atherosclerosis by gemfibrozil after coronary bypass surgery in men with low levels of HDL cholesterol. *Circulation* 96:2137, 1997.
12. Ornish D, Brown SE, Scherwitz LW, et al: Can lifestyle reverse coronary heart disease? *Lancet* 336:129, 1990.
13. Kane JP, Malloy MJ, Ports TA, et al: Regression of coronary atherosclerosis during treatment of familial hypercholesterolemia with combined drug regimens. *JAMA* 264:3007, 1990.
14. Brown G, Albers JJ, Fisher LD, et al: Regression of coronary artery disease as a result of intensive lipid-lowering therapy in men with high levels of apolipoprotein B. *N Engl J Med* 323:1289, 1990.
15. Buchwald H, Varco RL, Matts JP, et al: Effect of partial ileal bypass surgery on mortality and morbidity from coronary heart disease in patients with hypercholesterolemia. *N Engl J Med* 323:946, 1990.
16. Holme I: Cholesterol reduction and its impact on coronary artery disease and total mortality. *Am J Cardiol* 76:10C, 1995.
17. Haskell WI, Alderman EL, Fair JM, et al: The effects of intensive multiple risk factor reduction on coronary atherosclerosis and clinical cardiac events in men and women with coronary artery disease: The Stanford Coronary Risk Intervention Project (SCRIP). *Circulation* 89:975, 1994.
18. Gould AL, Rossouw JE, Santanello NC, et al: Cholesterol reduction yields clinical benefit. A new look at old data. *Circulation* 91:2274, 1995.
19. Grundy SM, Friedman D: Rationale for cholesterol-lowering strategies. *Curr Probl Cardiol* 20(5):281, 1995.
20. Executive Summary of the Third Report of the National Cholesterol Education Program (NCEP) Expert Panel on Detection, Evaluation and Treatment of High Blood Cholesterol in Adults (Adult Treatment Panel III). *JAMA* 285:2486, 2001.
21. Kannel WB, Castelli WP, Gordon T: Cholesterol in the prediction of atherosclerotic disease: New perspectives in the Framingham Study. *Ann Intern Med* 90:85, 1979.
22. Stampfer MJ, Sacks FN, Salvini S, et al: A prospective study of cholesterol, apolipoproteins, and the risk of myocardial infarction. *N Engl J Med* 325:373, 1991.
23. Gordon DJ, Probstfeld JL, Garrison RJ, et al: High-density lipoprotein cholesterol and cardiovascular disease: Four prospective American series. *Circulation* 79:8, 1989.
24. Rubins HB, Robins SJ, Collins D et al: Gemfibrozil for the secondary prevention of coronary heart disease in men with low levels of high-density lipoprotein cholesterol. *N Engl J Med* 341:410, 1999.
25. Hodis HN, Mack WJ: Triglyceride-rich lipoproteins and the progression of coronary artery disease. *Curr Opin Lipidol* 6:209, 1995.
26. Pasternak RC, Grundy SM, Levy D, Thompson PD: Task Force 3: spectrum of risk factors for coronary heart disease. *J Am Coll Cardiol* 27:978, 1996.
27. Kannel WB, Neaton JD, Wentworth D, et al: Overall and CHD mortality rates in relation to major risk factors in 325,348 men screened for the MRFIT. *Am Heart J* 112:825, 1986.
28. Gould AL, Roussouw JE, Santanello NC, et al: Cholesterol reduction yields clinical benefit. Impact of statin trials. *Circulation* 97:946–952, 1998.
29. Steinberg D, Gotto AM Jr: Preventing coronary artery disease by lowering cholesterol levels. Fifty years from bench to bedside. *JAMA* 282:2043, 1999.
30. Faergeman O: Hypertriglyceridemia and the fibrate trials. *Curr Opin Lipidol* 11:609, 2000.
31. Stampfer MJ, Krauss RM, Ma J, et al: A prospective study of triglyceride level, low-density lipoprotein particle diameter, and risk of myocardial infarction. *JAMA* 276:882, 1996.
32. Lemieux I, Pascot A, Couillard C, et al: Hypertriglyceridemic waist. A marker of the atherogenic metabolic triad (hyperinsulinemia; hyperapolipoprotein B; small, dense LDL) in men? *Circulation* 102:179, 2000.

33. Myers LH, Phillips NR, Havel RJ: Mathematical evaluation of methods for estimation of the concentration of the major lipid components of human serum lipoproteins. *J Lab Clin Med* 88:491, 1976.

34. Crouse JR III, Byington RP, Furberg CD: HMG-CoA reductase inhibitor therapy and stroke risk reduction: An analysis of clinical trials data. *Atherosclerosis* 138:11, 1998.

35. Warshafsky S, Packard D, Marks SJ, et al: Efficacy of 3-hydroxy-3-methylglutaryl coenzyme A reductase inhibitors for prevention of stroke. *J Gen Intern Med* 14:763, 1999.

36. Sharrett AR, Ballantyne CM, Coady SA, et al: Coronary heart disease prediction from lipoprotein cholesterol levels, triglycerides, lipoprotein(a), apolipoproteins A-I and B, and HDL density subfractions: The Atherosclerosis Risk in Communities (ARIC) Study. *Circulation* 104:1108, 2001.

37. Johnson CL, Rifkind BM, Sempos CT, et al: Declining serum total cholesterol levels among US adults. The National Health and Nutrition Examination Surveys. *JAMA* 269:3002, 1993.

38. Ridker PM, Stampfer MJ, Rifai N: Novel risk factors for systemic atherosclerosis. A comparison of C-reactive protein, fibrinogen, lipoprotein (a), and standard cholesterol screening as predictors of peripheral arterial disease. *JAMA* 285:2481, 2001.

39. American College of Physicians: Guidelines for using serum cholesterol, high-density lipoprotein cholesterol, and triglyceride levels as screening tests for preventing coronary heart disease in adults. *Ann Intern Med* 124:515, 1996.

40. Task Force on Risk Reduction, American Heart Association: Cholesterol screening in asymptomatic adults. No cause to change. *Circulation* 93:1067, 1996.

40a. Lauer RM, Clarke WR: Use of cholesterol measurements in childhood for the prediction of adult hypercholesterolemia. The Muscatine Study. *JAMA* 264:3034, 1990.

41. Newman TB, Browner WS, Hulley SB: The case against childhood cholesterol screening. *JAMA* 264:3039, 1990.

42. Phillips NR, Havel RJ, Kane JP: Levels and interrelationships of serum and lipoprotein cholesterol and triglycerides: association with adiposity and the consumption of ethanol, tobacco, and beverages containing caffeine. *Arteriosclerosis* 1:13, 1981.

43. Brown BG, Zhao X-Q, Chait A, et al: Simvastatin and niacin, antioxidant vitamins, or the combination for the prevention of coronary disease. *N Engl J Med* 345:1583, 2001.

44. von Eckardstein A, Assmann G: Prevention of coronary heart disease by raising high-density lipoprotein cholesterol? *Curr Opin Lipidol* 11:627, 2000.

45. Diabetes Atherosclerosis Intervention Study (DAIS) Investigators. Effect of fenofibrate on progression of coronary-artery disease in type 2 diabetes. *Lancet* 357:905, 2001

46. Betteridge D: Lipid-lowering trials in diabetes. *Curr Opin Lipidol* 12:619, 2001

47. Haffner SM, Alexander CM, Cook TJ et al: Reduced coronary events in simvastatin-treated patients with coronary heart disease and diabetes or impaired fasting glucose levels. Subgroup analysis in the Scandinavian Simvastatin Survival Study. *Arch Intern Med* 159:2661, 1999.

48. Goldberg R, Mellies MJ, Scaks FM, et al: Cardiovascular events and their reduction with pravastatin in diabetic and glucose-intolerant myocardial infarction survivors with average cholesterol levels. Subgroup analysis in the Cholesterol and Recurrent Events (CARE) Trial. *Circulation* 98:2513, 1998.

49. The Long-Term Intervention with Pravastatin in Ischaemic Disease (LIPID) Study Group: Prevention of cardiovascular events and death with pravastatin in patients with coronary heart disease and a broad range of initial cholesterol levels. *N Engl J Med* 339:1349, 1998.

50. Grover SA, Coupal L, Zowall H, Dorais M: Cost-effectiveness of treating hyperlipidemia in the presence of diabetes. Who should be treated? *Circulation* 102:722, 2000.

51. Haffner SM, Lehto S, Ronnemaa T, et al: Mortality from coronary heart disease in subjects with type 2 diabetes and in nondiabetic subjects with and without prior myocardial infarction. *N Engl J Med* 339:229, 1998

52. Howard BV, Robbins DC, Sievers ML, et al: LDL-cholesterol as a strong predictor of coronary heart disease in diabetic individuals with insulin resistance and low LDL. The Strong Heart Study. *Arterioscler Thromb Vasc Biol* 20:830, 2000.

53. American Diabetes Association: Management of dyslipidemia in adults with diabetes. *Diabetes Care* 25(Suppl 1):S74, 2002.

54. Anonymous: Intensive blood-glucose control with sulfonylureas or insulin compared with conventional treatment and risk of complications in patients with type 2 diabetes (UKPDS 33). UK Prospective Diabetes Study (UKPDS) Group. *Lancet* 352:837, 1998.

55. Lerner DJ, Kanner WB: Patterns of coronary heart disease morbidity and mortality in the sexes: a 26 year follow-up of the Framingham population. *Am Heart J* 111:383,1986.

56. Scandinavian Simvastatin Survival Study Group. Randomized trial of cholesterol lowering in 4444 patients with coronary heart disease: the Scandinavian Simvastatin Survival Study (4S). *Lancet* 344:1383, 1994.

57. Downs JR, Clearfield M, Weis S, et al: Primary prevention of acute coronary events with lovastatin in men and women with average cholesterol levels: Results of AFCAPS/TexCAPS. Air Force/Texas Coronary Atherosclerosis Prevention Study. *JAMA* 279:1615, 1998.

58. The Writing Group for the PEPI Trial. Effects of estrogen or estrogen/progestin regimens on heart disease risk factors in postmenopausal women. The Postmenopausal Estrogen Progestin Interventions (PEPI). *JAMA* 273:199, 1995.

59. Hulley S, Grady D, Bush T, et al: Randomized trial of estrogen plus progestin for secondary prevention of coronary heart disease in postmenopausal women. *JAMA* 280:605, 1998.

60. Wakatsuki A, Ikenoue N, Okatani Y, et al: Estrogen-induced small low density lipoprotein particles may be atherogenic in postmenopausal women. *J Am Coll Cardiol* 37:425, 2001.

61. Herrington DM, Reboussin DM, Brosnihan KB, et al: Effects of estrogen replacement on the progression of coronary artery atherosclerosis. *N Engl J Med* 343:522, 2000.

61a. Writing Group for the Women's Health Initiative Investigators: Risks and benefits of estrogen plus progestin in healthy postmenopausal women. Principal results from the Women's Health Initiative Randomized Controlled Trial. *JAMA* 288:321, 2002.

62. Report of the National Cholesterol Education Program Expert Panel on Blood Cholesterol Levels in Children and Adults. *Pediatrics* 89(3 Pt 2):525, 1992.

63. Rubin SM, Sidney S, Black DM, et al: High blood cholesterol in elderly men and the excess risk for coronary artery disease. *Ann Intern Med* 113:916, 1990.

64. Zimetbaum P, Frishman WH, Ooi WL, et al: Plasma lipids and lipoproteins and the incidence of cardiovascular disease in the old: The Bronx Longitudinal Aging Study. *Arteriol Thromb* 12:416, 1992.

64a. Lemaitre RN, Psaty BM, Heckbert SR, et al: Therapy with hydroxymethylglutaryl coenzyme A reductase inhibitors (statins) and associated risk of incident cardiovascular events in older adults: Evidence from the Cardiovascular Health Study. *Arch Intern Med* 162:1395, 2002.

65. Working Group on Management of Patients with Hypertension and High Blood Cholesterol: National Education Programs Working Group Report on the Management of Patients with Hypertension and High Blood Cholesterol. *Ann Intern Med* 114:224, 1991.

66. Bonaa KH, Thelle DS: Association between blood pressure and serum lipids in a population. *Circulation* 83(4):1305, 1991.

67. Frishman WH, Clark A, Johnson B: The effects of cardiovascular drugs on plasma lipids and lipoproteins. In: Frishman WH, Sonnenblick EH (eds). *Cardiovascular Pharmacotherapeutics.* New York: McGraw-Hill, 1997, p 1515.

68. Smith SC Jr, Blair SN, Bonow RO, et al: AHA/ACC guidelines for preventing heart attack and death in patients with atherosclerotic cardiovascular disease: 2001 update. *Circulation* 104:1577, 2001.

69. Ahnve S, Angelin B, Edhag O, et al: Early determination of serum lipids and apolipoproteins in acute myocardial infarction: Possibility for immediate intervention. *J Intern Med* 226:297, 1989.

70. Aronow HD, Topol EJ, Roe MT, et al: Effect of lipid-lowering therapy on early mortality after acute coronary syndromes: An observational study. *Lancet* 357:1063,2001.

71. Schwartz GG, Olsson AG, Ezekowitz MD, et al: Effects of atorvastatin on early recurrent ischemic events in acute coronary syndromes: The MIRACL study: a randomized controlled trial. *JAMA* 285:1711, 2001.

72. Rossouw JE: Lipid-lowering interventions in angiographic trials. *Am J Cardiol* 76:86C, 1995.

73. Falk E: Why do plaques rupture? *Circulation* 86(Suppl III):III30, 1992.

74. Fuster V, Badimon L, Badimon JJ, Chesebro JH: The pathogenesis of coronary artery disease and the acute coronary syndromes. *N Engl J Med* 326:310, 1992.

75. Richardson PD, Davies MJ, Born GV: Influence of plaque configuration and stress distribution on fissuring of coronary atherosclerotic plaques. *Lancet* 2:941, 1989.

76. OKeefe JH Jr., Conn RD, Lavie CJ Jr., Bateman TM: The new paradigm for coronary artery disease: altering risk factors, atherosclerotic plaques, and clinical prognosis. *Mayo Clin Proc* 71:957, 1996.

77. Farmer JA, Gotto AM Jr: Dyslipidemia and the vulnerable plaque. *Prog Cardiovasc Dis* 44:415, 2002.

78. Fayad ZA, Fuster V: Clinical imaging of the high-risk or vulnerable atherosclerotic plaque. *Circ Res* 89:305, 2001.

79. Schini VB, Vanhoutte P: Endothelium-derived vasoactive factors. In: Loscalzo J, Schaefer AI (eds). *Thrombosis and Hemorrhage.* Boston: Blackwell Science, 1994, p 349.

80. Egashira K, Hirooka Y, Kai H, et al: Reduction in serum cholesterol with pravastatin improves endothelium-dependent coronary vasomotion in patients with hypercholesterolemia. *Circulation* 89:2519, 1994.

81. Shiode N, Nakayama K, Morishima N, et al: Nitric oxide production by coronary conductance and resistance vessels in hypercholesterolemia patients. *Am Heart J* 131:1051, 1996.

82. Campeau L, Enjalbert M, Lesperance J, et al: The relation of risk factors to the development of atherosclerosis in saphenous vein bypass grafts and the progression of disease in the native circulation: A study 10 years after aortocoronary bypass surgery. *N Engl J Med* 311:1329, 1984.

83. Popma JJ, Sawyer M, Selwyn AP, Kinlay S: Lipid-lowering therapy after coronary revascularization. *Am J Cardiol* 86(Suppl H):18H, 2000.

84. Campeau L, Hunninghake DB, Knatterud GL, et al: Aggressive cholesterol lowering delays saphenous vein graft atherosclerosis in women, the elderly, and patients with associated risk factors. NHLBI post coronary artery bypass graft clinical trial. *Circulation* 99:3241, 1999.

85. Knatterud GL, Rosenberg Y, Campeau L, et al: Long-term effects on clinical outcomes of aggressive lowering of low-density lipoprotein cholesterol levels and low-dose anticoagulation in the post coronary artery bypass graft trial. *Circulation* 102:157, 2000.

86. Leimgruber PP, Roubin GS, Hollman J, et al: Restenosis after successful coronary angioplasty in patients with single vessel disease. *Circulation* 73:710, 1986.

87. Virmani R, Farb A: Pathology of in-stent restenosis. *Curr Opin Lipidol* 10:49, 1999.

88. Austin GE, Ratliff NB, Hollman J, et al: Intimal proliferation of smooth muscle cells as an explanation for recurrent coronary artery stenosis after percutaneous transluminal coronary angioplasty. *J Am Coll Cardiol* 6:369, 1985.

89. Ross R, Bowen-Pope D, Raines EW: Platelets, macrophages, endothelium and growth factors: Their effects upon cells and their possible roles in atherogenesis. *Ann NY Acad Sci* 454:254, 1985.

89a. Serruys PWJC, de Feyter P, Macaya C, et al for the Lescol Intervention Prevention Study (LIPS) Investigators: Fluvastatin for prevention of cardiac events following successful first percutaneous coronary intervention: A randomized controlled trial. *JAMA* 287:3215, 2002.

90. Meng CQ: Restenosis drug discovery—a formidable task. *Curr Opin Invest Drugs* 2:1237, 2001.

91. de Feyter PJ, Vos J, Rensing BJ: Anti-restenosis trials. *Curr Intervent Cardiol Rep* 2:326, 2000.

92. Chan AW, Moliterno DJ: In-stent restenosis: Update on intracoronary radiotherapy. *Cleve Clin J Med* 68:796, 2001.

93. Butman S: Hyperlipidemia after cardiac transplantation: Be aware and possibly wary of drug therapy for lowering of serum lipids. *Am Heart J* 121:1585, 1991.

94. Ballantyne CM, Podet EJ, Patsch WP, et al: Effects of cyclosporine therapy on plasma lipoprotein levels. *JAMA* 262:53, 1989.

95. Olivari MT, Homans DC, Wilson RF, et al: Coronary artery disease in cardiac transplant patients receiving triple-drug immunosuppressive therapy. *Circulation* 80(Suppl III):III-111, 1989.

96. Johnson DE, Gao SZ, Schroeder JS, et al: The spectrum of coronary artery pathological findings in human cardiac allografts. *J Heart Transplant* 8:349, 1989.

97. Kobashigawa JA, Katznelson S, Laks H, et al: Effect of pravastatin on outcomes after cardiac transplantation. *N Engl J Med* 333:621, 1995.

98. Wenke K, Meiser B, Thiery J, et al: Simvastatin reduces graft vessel disease and mortality after heart transplantation: A four-year randomized trial. *Circulation* 96:1398, 1997.

99. Kobashigawa J: What is the optimal prophylaxis for treatment of cardiac allograft vasculopathy? *Curr Control Trials Cardiovasc Med* 1:166, 2000.

100. Crouse JR: Effects of statins on carotid disease and stroke. *Curr Opin Lipidol* 10:535, 1999.

100a. Joven J, Villabona C, Vilella E, et al: Abnormalities of lipoprotein metabolism in patients with nephrotic syndrome. *N Engl J Med* 323:579, 1990.

100b. Keane WF, Kasiske BL: Hyperlipidemia in nephrotic syndrome. *N Engl J Med* 323:603, 1990.

100c. Vega GL, Grundy SM: Lovastatin therapy in nephrotic hyperlipidemia. Effects on lipoprotein metabolism. *Kidney Int* 33:1160, 1988.

101. Chui MCK, Newby DE, Panarelli M, et al: Association between calcific aortic stenosis and hypercholesterolemia: Is there a need for a randomized controlled trial of cholesterol-lowering therapy? *Clin Cardiol* 24:52, 2001.

101a. Rajamannan NM, Subramaniam M, Springett M, et al: Atorvastatin inhibits hypercholesterolemia-induced cellular proliferation and bone matrix production in the rabbit aortic valve. *Circulation* 105:2660, 2002.

102. Davidson MH, Dillon MA, Gordon B, et al: Colesevelam hydrochloride (Cholestagel). A new, potent bile acid sequestrant associated with a low incidence of gastrointestinal side effects. *Arch Intern Med* 159:1893, 1999.

103. Frishman WH, Ast M: Bile acid sequestrants. In: Frishman WH (ed). *Medical Management of Lipid Disorder. Focus on Prevention of Coronary Artery Disease.* Mt. Kisco: Futura Publ. Co. Inc., 1992:103–123.

104. Lipid Research Clinics Program: The Lipid Research Clinics Coronary Primary Prevention Trial Results: II. The relationship in reduction of incidence of coronary heart disease to cholesterol lowering. *JAMA* 251:365, 1984.

105. Glueck CJ: Pediatric primary prevention of atherosclerosis. *N Engl J Med* 314:175, 1986.

106. Witzum J: Drugs used in the treatment of hyperlipoproteinemias. In: Hardman JG, Limbird LE (eds). In: *Goodman & Gilman's The Pharmacological Basis of Therapeutics,* 9th ed, New York: McGraw Hill, 1996, pp 875–897.

107. Grundy SM, Ahrens EH, Salen S: Interruption of the enterohepatic circulation of bile acids in man: Comparative effects of cholestyramine and ileal exclusion on cholesterol metabolism. *J Lab Clin Med* 78:94, 1971.

108. Packard CJ, Shepherd J: The hepatobiliary axis and lipoprotein metabolism: Effects of bile acid sequestrants and ileal bypass surgery. *J Lipid Res* 23:1081, 1982.

109. Shepherd J: Mechanism of action of bile acid sequestrants and other lipid lowering drugs. *Cardiology* 76(Suppl 1):65, 1982.

110. Innis SM: The activity of HMG-CoA reductase and acyl- CoA cholesterol acyltransferase in hepatic microsomes in male, female and pregnant rats. The effect of cholestyramine treatment and the relationship of enzyme activity to microsomal lipid composition. *Biochim Biophys Acta* 875:355, 1986.

111. Shepherd J, Packard CJ, Bicker S, et al: Cholestyramine promotes receptor-mediated low-density lipoprotein catabolism. *N Engl J Med* 302:1219, 1980.

111a. Donovan JM, Stypinski D, Stiles MR, et al: Drug interactions with colesevelam hydrochloride, a novel, potent lipid-lowering agent. *Cardiovasc Drugs Ther* 14:681, 2000.

112. Illingworth RD: Lipid lowering drugs: An overview of indications and optimum therapeutic use. *Drugs* 33:259, 1987.

113. Davidson MH, Dillon MA, Gordon B, et al: Colesevelam hydrochloride (cholestagel): A new, potent bile acid sequestrant associated with a low incidence of gastrointestinal side effects. *Arch Intern Med* 159:1893, 1999.

114. Runeberg L, Miettinen TA, Nikkils EA: Effect of cholestyramine on mineral excretion in man. *Acta Med Scand* 192:71, 1972.

115. Brensike JF, Levy RI, Kelsey SF, et al: Effects of therapy with cholestyramine on progression of coronary arteriosclerosis: Results of the NHLBI type II coronary intervention study. *Circulation* 69:313, 1984.

116. Levy RI, Brensike JF, Epstein SE, et al: The influence of changes in lipid values induced by cholestyramine and diet on progression of coronary artery disease: Results of the NHLBI type II coronary prevention study. *Circulation* 69:325, 1984.

117. Krauss RM, Williams PT, Brensike J, et al: Intermediate-density lipoproteins and progression of coronary artery disease in hypercholesterolemic men. *Lancet* 2:62, 1987.

117a. Blankenhorn DH, Nessim SA, Johnson RL, et al: Beneficial effects of combined colestipol-niacin therapy on coronary atherosclerosis and coronary venous bypass grafts. *JAMA* 257:3233, 1987.

118. Cashin-Hemphill L, Mack WJ, Pogoda JM, et al: Beneficial effects of colestipol-niacin on coronary atherosclerosis. *JAMA* 264:3013, 1990.

119. Brown G, Albers JJ, Fisher LD, et al: Regression of coronary artery disease as a result of intensive lipid lowering therapy in men with high levels of apolipoprotein B. *N Engl J Med* 323:1289, 1990.

120. Kane JP, Malloy MJ, Ports TA, et al: Regression of coronary atherosclerosis during treatment of familial hypercholesterolemia with combined drug regimens. *JAMA* 264:3007, 1990.

121. Watts GF, Lewis B, Brunt JNH, et al: Effects of coronary artery disease on lipid-lowering diet or diet plus cholestyramine, in the St. Thomas Atherosclerosis Regression Study (STARS). *Lancet* 339:563, 1992.

121a. Duffield RGT, Lewis B, Miller NE, et al: Treatment of hyperlipidaemia retards progression of symptomatic femoral atherosclerosis: A randomized controlled trial. *Lancet* 2:639, 1983.

121b. Blankenhorn DH, Azen SP, Crawford DW, et al: Effects of colestipol-niacin therapy on human femoral atherosclerosis. *Circulation* 83:438. 1991.

122a. Marais AD: Therapeutic modulation of low-density lipoprotein size. *Curr Opin Lipidol* 11:597, 2000.

122b. Witzum JL, Schonfeld G, Weidman JW, et al: Bile sequestrant therapy alters the composition of low-density and high-density lipoprotein. *Metabolism* 28:221, 1979.

123. Beil U, Crouse JR, Einarsson K, Grundy SM: Effect of interruption of the enterohepatic circulation of bile acids on the transport of very low density lipoprotein triglycerides. *Metabolism* 31:438, 1982.

124. Crouse JR: Hypertriglyceridemia: A contraindication for use of bile acid binding resins. *Am J Med* 83:243, 1987.

125. Gordon DJ, Knoke J, Probstfield JL, et al, for the Lipid Research Clinics Program: High-density lipoprotein cholesterol and coronary heart disease in hypercholesterolemic men: The Lipid Research Clinics Coronary Primary Prevention Trial. *Circulation* 74:1217, 1986.

126. Lyons D, Webster J, Fowler G, et al: Colestipol at various dosage intervals in the treatment of moderate hypercholesterolemia. *Br J Clin Pharmacol* 37:59, 1994.

127. Tonstad S, Bing RF, Frohlich J, et al: Effectiveness of colestipol tablets vs granules in patients with moderate to severe hypercholesterolaemia. *Clin Drug Invest* 10:257, 1995.

128. Insull W, Marquis NR, Tsianco MC: Comparison of the efficacy of Questran Light, a new formulation of cholestyramine powder, to regular Questran in maintaining lowered plasma cholesterol levels. *Am J Cardiol* 67:501, 1991.

129. Kane JP, Malloy MJ, Tun P, et al: Normalization of low-density lipoprotein levels in heterozygous familial hypercholesterolemia with a combined drug regimen. *N Engl J Med* 304:251, 1981.

130. Hoogerbrugge N, Mol M, VanDormaal JJ, et al: Efficacy and safety of pravastatin, compared to and in combination with bile acid binding resins in familial hypercholesterolemia. *J Intern Med* 228:261, 1990.

131. Schrott HG, Stein EA, Dujoune CA, et al: Enhanced low-density lipoprotein cholesterol reduction and cost-effectiveness by low dose colestipol plus lovastatin combination therapy. *Am J Cardiol* 75:34, 1995.

132. Masclee AAM, Jansen JBMJ, Rovati LC, et al: Effect of cholestyramine and cholecystokinin receptor antagonist CR1505 (loxiglumide) on lower esophageal sphincter pressure in man. *Dig Dis Sci* 38:1889, 1993.

133. Pattison M, Lee SM: Life-threatening metabolic acidosis from cholestyramine in an infant with renal insufficiency (letter). *Am J Dis Child* 141:479, 1987.

134. Kleinman PA: Cholestyramine and metabolic acidosis (letter). *N Engl J Med* 290:861, 1974.

135. Hartline JV: Hyperchloremia, metabolic acidosis, and cholestyramine. *J Pediatri* 89:155, 1976.

136. Scheel PJ, Whelton A, Rossiter K, Watson A: Cholestyramine induced hyperchloremic metabolic acidosis. *J Clin Pharmacol* 32:536, 1992.

137. Melkem MF, Galoriet HF, Eskander ED, Rao KN: Cholestyramine promotes 7,12 dimethylbenzanthracene induced mammary cancer in Wistar rats. *J Cancer* 56:45, 1987.

138. Shosania AM, Grewar D: Hypoprothrombinemic hemorrhage due to cholestyramine therapy. *Can Med Assn J* 134:609, 1986.

139. Witztum JL, Jacobs LS, Schonfeld G: Thyroid hormone and thyrotropin levels in patients placed on colestipol hydrochloride. *J Clin Endocrinol Metab* 46:838, 1978.

140. Hertzd R, Bishara-Shieban J, Bar-Tana J: Mode of action of peroxisome proliferators as hypolipidemic drugs suppression of apolipoprotein C-III. *J Biol Chem* 270:13470, 1995.

141. Gervois P, Torra IP, Fruchart JC, et al: Regulation of lipid and lipoprotein metabolism by PPAR activators. *Clin Chem Lab Med* 38:3, 2000.

142. Staels B, Dallongeville J, Auwerx J, et al: Mechanism of action of fibrates on lipid and lipoprotein metabolism.*Circulation* 98:2088, 1998.

143. Thorp JM: Modification of metabolism and distribution of lipids by chlorphenoxyisobutyrate. *Nature* 194:948, 1962.

144. Report from the Committee of Principal Investigators: A cooperative trial in the primary prevention of ischaemic heart disease using clofibrate. *Br Heart J* 40:1069, 1978.

145. Coronary Drug Project Research Group: Clofibrate and niacin in coronary artery disease. *JAMA* 231:360, 1975.

146. Zimetbaum P, Frishman WH, Kahn S: Effects of gemfibrozil and other fibric acid derivatives on blood lipids and lipoproteins. In: Frishman WH (ed). Medical Management of Lipid Disorders: Focus on Prevention of Coronary Artery Disease. Mt. Kisco: Futura Publishing Co Inc. 1992:125–151.

147. Manninen V, Elo O, Frick H, et al: Lipid alterations and decline in the incidence of coronary heart disease in the Helsinki Heart Study. *JAMA* 260:41, 1988.

148. Spencer CM, Barradell LB: Gemfibrozil. *Drugs* 51:982, 1996.

149. Brown WV: Potential use of fenofibrate and other fibric acid derivatives in the clinic. *Am J Med* 83(5B):85, 1987.

150. Balfour JA, Heel RC: Fenofibrate: A review of its pharmacodynamic and pharmacokinetic properties and therapeutic use in dyslipidaemia. *Drugs* 40:260, 1990.

151. Grutzmacher P, Scheuermann EH, Siede W, et al: Lipid lowering treatment with bezafibrate in patients on chronic haemodialysis: Pharmacokinetics and effects. *Klin Wochenschr* 64(19):910, 1986.

152. Betteridge DJ: Ciprofibrate—a profile. *Postgrad Med J* 69(Suppl 1):S42, 1993.

153. Monk JP, Todd PA: Bezafibrate: a review of its pharmacodynamic and pharmacokinetic properties, and therapeutic use in hyperlipidaemia. *Drugs* 33:539, 1987.

153a. Auboeuf D, Rieusset J, Fajas L, et al: Tissue distribution and quantification of the expression of the peroxisome proliferator activated receptors and of LXR alpha mRNAs in human: Effect of obesity and NIDDM in adipose tissue. *Diabetes* 46:1319, 1997.

154. Shepherd J: Mechanism of action of fibrates. *Postgrad Med J* 69(Suppl 1):S34,1993.

155. Grundy SM, Vega GL: Fibric acids: Effects on lipids and lipoprotein metabolism. *Am J Med* 83(5B):9, 1987.

156. Eckel RH: Lipoprotein lipase: A multifunctional enzyme relevant to common metabolic disease. *N Engl J Med* 320:1060, 1989.

157. Heller F, Harvengt C: Effect of clofibrate, bezafibrate, fenofibrate and probucol on plasma lipolytic enzymes in normolipidemic subjects. *Eur J Clin Pharmacol* 25:57, 1983.

158. Gavish D, Oschry Y, Fainaru M, Eisenberg S: Changes in very low, low, and high density lipoproteins during lipid lowering (bezafibrate) therapy: Studies in type IIA and IIB hyperlipoproteinemia. *Eur J Clin Invest* 16(1):61, 1986.

159a. Gervaise, N, Garrigue MA, Lasfargues G, et al: Triglycerides, apo C3 and Lp B:C3 and cardiovascular risk in type II diabetes. *Diabetologia* 43:703, 2000.

160b. Luc G, Fievet C, Arveiler D, et al: Apolipoproteins C3 and E in apoB- and non apo B-containing lipoproteins in two populations at contrasting risk for myocardial infarction: the ECTIM study. *J Lipid Res* 37:508, 1996

161. Sacks FM, Alaupovic P, Moye LA, et al: VLDL, apolipoproteins B, CIII, and E, and risk of recurrent coronary events in the Cholesterol and Recurrent Events (CARE) trial. *Circulation* 102:1886–1892, 2000.

162. Hunninghake DB, Peters JR: Effects of fibric acid derivatives on blood lipid and lipoprotein levels. *Am J Med* 83(5B):44, 1987.

163. Eisenberg S, Gavish D, Oschry Y, et al: Abnormalities in very low, low and high density lipoproteins in hypertriglyceridemia. *J Clin Invest* 74:470, 1984.

164. Vega GL, Grundy SM: Kinetic heterogeneity of low density lipoproteins in primary hypertriglyceridemia. *Arteriosclerosis* 6:395, 1986.

165. Ginsberg HN: Changes in lipoprotein kinetics during therapy with fenofibrate and other fibric acid derivatives. *Am J Med* 83(5B):66, 1987.

166. Kasaniemi YA, Grundy SM: Influence of gemfibrozil and clofibrate on metabolism of cholesterol and plasma triglycerides in man. *JAMA* 251(17):2241, 1984.

167. Shepard J, Caslake MJ, Lorimer AR, et al: Fenofibrate reduces low density catabolism in hypertriglyceridemic subjects. *Arteriosclerosis* 5:162, 1985.

168. Packard CJ, Clegg RJ, Dominiczak MH, et al: Effect of bezafibrate on apolipoprotein B metabolism in type III hyperlipidemic subjects. *J Lipid Res* 27(9):930, 1986.

169. Eisenberg S: High density lipoprotein metabolism. *J Lipid Res* 25:1012, 1984.

170. Schwandt P, Weisweiler P: Effect of bezafibrate on the high density lipoprotein subfractions HDL2 and HDL3 in primary hyperlipoproteinemia type IV. *Artery* 7(6):464, 1980.

171. Kleinman Y, Eisenberg S, Oschry Y, et al: Defective metabolism of hypertriglyceridemic lipoprotein in cultured human skin fibroblasts. Normalization with bezafibrate. *J Clin Invest* 75:1796, 1985.

172. Grundy SM, Ahrens EGJ, Salen G, et al: Mechanism of action of clofibrate on cholesterol metabolism in patients with hyperlipidemia. *J Lipid Res* 13:531, 1972.

173. Hudson K, Mojumder S, Day AJ: The effect of bezafibrate and clofibrate on cholesterol ester metabolism in rabbit peritoneal macrophages stimulated with acetylated low density lipoproteins. *Exp Mol Pathol* 38(1):77, 1983.

174. Schneider A, Stange EF, Ditschuneit HH, Ditschuneit H: Fenofibrate treatment inhibits HMG-CoA reductase activity in mononuclear cells from hyperlipoproteinemic patients. *Atherosclerosis* 56(3):257, 1985.

175. Blasi F, Sommariva D, Cosentini R, et al: Bezafibrate inhibits HMG-CoA reductase activity in incubated blood mononuclear cells from normal subjects and patients with heterozygous familial hypercholesterolemia. *Pharmacol Res* 21(3):247, 1989.

176. Palmer RH: Effects of fibric acid derivatives on biliary lipid composition. *Am J Med* 83(5B):37, 1987.

177. Kasaniemi YA, Grundy SM: Clofibrate, caloric restriction, supersaturation of bile, and cholesterol crystals. *Scand J Gastroenterol* 18:897, 1983.

178. Blane GF: Review of European clinical experience with fenofibrate. *Cardiology* 76(Suppl 1):1, 1989.

179. Leiss O, Meyer-Krahmer K, Von Bergmann K: Biliary lipid secretion in patients with heterozygous familial hypercholesterolemia and combined hyperlipidemia. Influence of bezafibrate and fenofibrate. *J Lipid Res* 27(7):213, 1986.

180. Carvalho ACA, Colman RW, Lees RS: Platelet function in hyperlipoproteinemia. *N Engl J Med* 290:434, 1974.

181. Hamsten A, Wiman B, DeFaire U, Blomback M: Increased plasma levels of a rapid inhibitor of tissue plasminogen activator in young survivors of myocardial infarction. *N Engl J Med* 313:1557, 1985.

182. Torstila I, Kaukola S, Malkonen M, et al: Effect of gemfibrozil on plasma lipoproteins, apolipoproteins and the kallikrein-kinin system. *Proceedings of an International Symposium: 8th Asian Pacific Congress of Cardiology*. 1984, pp 36–42.

183. Laustiola K, Lassila R, Koskinen P, et al: Gemfibrozil decreases platelet reactivity in patients with hypercholesterolemia during physical stress. *Clin Pharm Ther* 43:302, 1988.

184. Sirtori CR, Franceschini G, Gianfranceschi G, et al: Effects of gemfibrozil on plasma lipoprotein-apolipoprotein distribution and platelet reactivity in patients with hypertriglyceridemia. *J Lab Clin Med* 110:279, 1987.

185. Kloer HU: Structure and biochemical effects of fenofibrate. *Am J Med* 83(5B):3, 1987.

186. Niort G, Bulgarelli A, Cassader M, Pagano G: Effect of short term treatment with bezafibrate on plasma fibrinogen, fibrinopeptide A, platelet activation, and blood filterability in atherosclerotic hyperfibrinogenemic patients. *Arteriosclerosis* 71(2–3):113, 1988.

187. Ericsson C-G, Hamsten A, Nilsson J, et al: Angiographic assessment of effects of bezafibrate on progression of coronary artery disease in young male postinfarction patients. *Lancet* 347:849, 1996.

188. Lesch M, Hoffken H, Schmidtsdorff A, et al: Effect of fenofibrate on fibrinogen concentration and blood viscosity. Consequences for myocardial microcirculation in coronary heart disease? *Dtsch Med Wochenschr* 114(24):939, 1989.

189. Gotto AM: The Helsinki Heart Study Trial. *Cardiol Bd Rev* 6(3 Suppl):47, 1989.

190. Faergeman O: Hypertriglyceridemia and the fibrate trials. *Curr Opin Lipidol* 11:609, 2000.

191. Ruotolo G, Ericsson CG, Tettamanti C, et al: Treatment effects on serum lipoprotein lipids, apolipoproteins and low density lipoprotein particle size and relationships of lipoprotein variables to progression of coronary artery disease in the Bezafibrate Coronary Atherosclerosis Intervention Trial (BECAIT). *J Am Coll Cardiol* 32:1648, 1998.

192. Mooney A: Treating patients with hypertriglyceridemia saves lives: Triglyceride revisited. *Curr Med Res Opin* 15:65, 1999.

193. Rubins HB, Davenport J, Babikian V, et al for the VA-HIT Study Group: Reduction in stroke with gemfibrozil in men with coronary heart disease and low HDL cholesterol. The Veterans Affairs HDL Intervention Trial (VA-HIT). *Circulation* 103:2828, 2001.

194. Gordon DJ, Rifkind BM: High density lipoprotein—the clinical implications of recent studies. *N Engl J Med* 321:1311, 1989.

195. Virtamo J, Manninen V, Malkonen M: A placebo controlled rising dose, double-blind trial with gemfibrozil in dieting patients with primary hyperlipoproteinemia. *Vasc Med* 2:22,1984.

196. Knopp R: Review of the effects of fenofibrate on lipoproteins, apoproteins, and bile saturability. U.S. Studies. *Cardiology* 76(Suppl 1):14, 1989.

197. Pierce LR, Gysowski DK, Gross TP: Myopathy and rhabdomyolitis associated with lovastatin-gemfibrozil combination therapy. *JAMA* 264:71, 1990.

197a. Ruth E, Vollmar J: Improvement in diabetes control by treatment with bezafibrate. *Dtsch Med Wochenschr* 107:1470, 1982.

198. Manninen V, Tenkanen L, Koskinen P, et al: Joint effects of serum triglycerides and LDL-cholesterol and HDL cholesterol concentrations on coronary heart disease risk in the Helsinki Heart Study: Implications for treatment. *Circulation* 85:37, 1992.

199. Alberts AW, Chen J, Kuron G, et al: Mevinolin: A highly potent competitive inhibitor of hydroxymethylglutaryl-coenzyme A reductase and a cholesterol-lowering agent. *Proc Natl Acad Sci U S A* 77:3957, 1980.

200. Endo A, Kuroda M, Tsijita Y: ML-236B and ML-236C, new inhibitors of cholesterogenesis produced by *Penicillium citrium*. *J Antibiot* 29:1346, 1976.

201. Brown MS, Goldstein JL: Multivalent feedback regulation of HMG-CoA reductase, a control mechanism coordinating isoprenoid synthesis and cell growth. *J Lipid Res* 21:505, 1980.

202. Alberts AW: Discovery, biochemistry and biology of lovastatin. *Am J Cardiol* 62(15):10J, 1988.

203. Tobert JA: New developments in lipid-lowering therapy. The role of inhibitors of hydroxymethylglutaryl coenzyme A reductase. *Circulation* 76:534, 1987.

204. Krukemyer JJ, Talbert RL: Lovastatin: A new cholesterol-lowering agent. *Pharmacotherapy* 7:198, 1987.

205. Parker TS, McNamara DJ, Brown C: Mevalonic acid in human plasma: relationship of concentration and circadian rhythm to cholesterol synthesis rates in man. *Proc Natl Acad Sci U S A* 79:3037, 1982.

206. Cromwell WC, Ziajka PE: Development of tachyphylaxis among patients taking HMG CoA reductase inhibitors. *Am J Cardiol* 86:1123, 2000.

207. Grundy SM: HMG-CoA reductase inhibitors for treatment of hypercholesterolemia. *N Engl J Med* 319:24, 1988.

208. Henwood JM, Heel AC: Lovastatin. *Drugs* 36:429, 1988.

209. Vega GL, Grundy SM: Treatment of primary moderate hypercholesterolemia with lovastatin (Mevinolin) and colestipol. *JAMA* 257:33, 1987.

210. Bradford RH, Shear CL, Chremos AN, et al: Expanded Clinical Evaluation of Lovastatin (EXCEL) study. Results: I. Efficacy in modifying plasma lipoproteins and adverse effect profile in 8245 patients with moderate hypercholesterolemia. *Arch Intern Med* 151:43, 1991.

211. Brown G, Albers JJ, Fisher LD, et al: Regression of coronary artery disease as a result of intensive lipid lowering therapy in men with high levels of apolipoprotein B. *N Engl J Med* 323:1289, 1990.

212. Blankenhorn DH, Azen SP, Kramsch DM, et al: Coronary angiographic changes with lovastatin therapy. The Monitored Atherosclerosis Regression Study (MARS). *Ann Intern Med* 119:969, 1993.

213. Hodis HN, Mack WJ, LaBree L, et al: Reduction in carotid arterial wall thickness using lovastatin and dietary therapy. A randomized, controlled clinical trial. *Ann Intern Med* 124:548, 1996.

214. Waters D, Higginson L, Gladstone P, et al: Effects of monotherapy with an HMG-CoA reductase inhibitor on the progression of coronary atherosclerosis as assessed by serial quantitative arteriography. The Canadian Coronary Atherosclerosis Intervention Trial. *Circulation* 89:959, 1994.

215. Waters D, Higginson L, Gladstone P, et al: Effects of cholesterol lowering on the progression of coronary atherosclerosis in women. A Canadian Coronary Atherosclerosis Intervention Trial (CCAIT) substudy. *Circulation* 92:2404, 1995.

216. Furberg CD, Adams HP, Applegate WB, et al: Effect of lovastatin on early carotid atherosclerosis and cardiovascular events. *Circulation* 90:1679, 1994.

217. Probstfield JL, Margitic SE, Byington RP, et al: Results of the primary outcome measure and clinical events from the Asymptomatic Carotid Artery Progression Study. *Am J Cardiol* 76:47C, 1995.

218. Downs JR, Clearfield M, Weis S, et al: Primary prevention of acute coronary events with lovastatin in men and women with average cholesterol levels. *JAMA* 279:1615, 1998.

218a. Cobb MM, Teitelbaum HS, Breslow JL: Lovastatin efficacy in reducing low-density lipoprotein cholesterol levels on high vs low fat diets. *JAMA* 265:997, 1991.

218b. Gupta EK, Ito MK: Lovastatin and extended-release niacin combination product. The first drug combination for the treatment of hyperlipidemia. *Heart Dis* 4:124, 2002.

218c. Kashyap ML, McGovern ME, Berra K, et al: Long-term safety and efficacy of a once-daily niacin/lovastatin formulation for patients with dyslipidemia. *Am J Cardiol* 89:672, 2002.

218d. Knodel LC, Talbert RL: Adverse effects of hypolipidaemic drugs. *Med Toxicol* 2:10, 1987.

218e. Davidson MH: Safety profile for the HMG-CoA reductase inhibitors. Treatment and trust. *Drugs* 61:197, 2001.

218f. Blais L, Desgagne A, LeLorier J: 3-Hydroxy-3-methylglutaryl coenzyme A reductase inhibitors and the risk of cancer. *Arch Intern Med* 160:2363, 2000.

219. Norman DJ, Illingworth DR, Munson J, Hosenpud J: Myolysis and acute renal failure in a heart transplant recipient receiving lovastatin (letter). *N Engl J Med* 318:46, 1988.

219a. Evans M, Rees A: The myotoxicity of statins. *Curr Opin Lipidol* 13:415, 2002.

219b. Pasternak RC, Smith SC Jr., Bairey-Merz CN, et al: ACC/AHA/NHLBT Clinical Advisory on the Use and Safety of Statins. *J Am Coll Cardiol* 40:567, 2002.

220. Frishman WH, Zimetbaum P, Nadelmann J: Lovastatin and other HMG CoA reductase inhibitors. *J Clin Pharmacol* 29:975, 1989.

221. Neuvonen PJ, Jalava K-M: Intraconazole drastically increases plasma concentrations of lovastatin and lovastatin acid. *Clin Pharmacol Ther* 60:54, 1996.

222. Kuo PC, Kirshenbaum JM, Gordon J, et al: Lovastatin therapy for hypercholesterolemia in cardiac transplant recipients. *Am J Cardiol* 64:631, 1989.

223. Pierce LR, Wysowski DK, Gross T: Myopathy and rhabdomyolysis associated with lovastatin-gemfibrozil combination therapy. *JAMA* 264:71, 1990.

224. Goldman JA, Fishman AB, Lee JE, Johnson RJ: The role of cholesterol-lowering agents in drug-induced rhabdomyolysis and polymyositis. *Arthritis Rheum* 32:358, 1989.

224a. Tobert JA: Efficacy and long-term adverse effect pattern of lovastatin. *Am J Cardiol* 62:28J, 1988.

225. Tobert JA, Shear CL, Cremos AN, Mantell GE: Clinical experience with lovastatin. *Am J Cardiol* 65:23F, 1990.

226. Weir MR, Berger ML, Weeks ML, et al: Comparison of the effects on quality of life and the efficacy and tolerability of lovastatin versus pravastatin. *Am J Cardiol* 77:475, 1996.

227. Plosker GL, McTavish D: Simvastatin: A reappraisal of its pharmacology and therapeutic efficacy in hypercholesterolemia. *Drugs* 50:334, 1995.

228. Stalenhoef AFH, Mol MJTM, Stuyt PMJ: Efficacy and tolerability of simvastatin (MK 733). *Am J Med* 87(4A):39S, 1989.

229. Quercia RA: Focus on simvastatin: a potent HMG CoA reductase inhibitor for the treatment of hypercholesterolemia. *Hosp Form* 24:559, 1989.

230. Pietro DA, Sidney A, Mantell G, et al: Effects of simvastatin and probucol in hypercholesterolemia (Simvastatin Multicenter Study Group II). *Am J Cardiol* 63:682, 1989.

231. Stein E, Kreisberg R, Miller V, et al: Multicenter group l: Effects of simvastatin and cholestyramine in familial and nonfamilial hypercholesterolemia. *Arch Intern Med* 150:341, 1990.

232. Tikkanan XJ, Bocanegra TS, Walker JF, Cook T, the Simvastatin Study Group: Comparison of low-dose simvastatin and gemfibrozil in the treatment of elevated plasma cholesterol. *Am J Med* 87(4A):47S, 1989.

233. Erkelens DW, Baggen MGA, Van Doormaal JJ, et al: Clinical experience with simvastatin compared with cholestyramine. *Drugs* 36(Suppl 3):87, 1988.

234. Dacol PG, Cattin L, Valenti M, et al: Efficacy of simvastatin plus cholestyramine in the two-year treatment of heterozygous hypercholesterolemia. *Curr Ther Res Clin Exp* 48:798, 1990.

235. Havel RJ: Simvastatin: A once a day treatment of hypercholesterolemia: Introduction to a symposium. *Am J Med* 87(4A):2S, 1989.

236. Mol MJT, Stalenhoef AFH: Adrenocortical function in patients with simvastatin. *Lancet* 335:412, 1990.

237. Stein E: Management of hypercholesterolemia: Guide to diet and drug therapy. *Am J Med* 87(4A):24S, 1989.

238. Illingworth DR, Stein EA, Knopp RH, et al: A randomized multicenter trial comparing the efficacy of simvastatin and fluvastatin. *Cardiovasc Pharmacol Ther* 1:23, 1996.

239. Rabelink AJ, Henle RJ, Erkelens DW, et al: Effects of simvastatin and cholestyramine on lipoprotein profile in hyperlipidaemia of nephrotic syndrome. *Lancet* 10:1335, 1988.

240. Duane WC, Hunninghake DB, Freeman ML, et al: Simvastatin, a competitive inhibitor of HMG-CoA reductase, lowers cholesterol saturation index of gallbladder bile. *Hepatology* 8(5):1147, 1988.

241. MAAS Investigators: Effect of simvastatin on coronary atheroma: The Multicentre Anti-Atheroma Study (MAAS). *Lancet* 344:633, 1994.

242. Corti R, Fayad ZA, Fuster V, et al: Effects of lipid-lowering by simvastatin on human atherosclerotic lesions. A longitudinal study by high-resolution, noninvasive magnetic resonance imaging. *Circulation* 104:249, 2001.

243. Kjekshus J, Pedersen TR for the Scandinavian Simvastatin Survival Study Group (4S): Reducing the risk of coronary events: Evidence from the Scandinavian Simvastatin Survival Study. *Am J Cardiol* 76:64C, 1995.

244. Pedersen TR, Kjekshus J, Berg K, et al: Cholesterol lowering and the use of healthcare resources. Results of the Scandinavian Simvastatin Survival Study. *Circulation* 93:1796, 1996.

245. Heart Protection Study Collaborative Group: MRC/BHF Heart Protection Study of cholesterol lowering with simvastatin in 20,536 high-risk individuals: A randomised placebo-controlled trial. *Lancet* 360:7, 2002.

246. Alessandri C, Basili S, Maurelli M, et al: Effect of hydroxy-methylglutaryl-coenzyme A reductase inhibitors on some blood coagulation parameters. *Curr Ther Res* 53:188, 1993.

247. Giroux LM, Davignon J, Naruszewicz M: Simvastatin inhibits the oxidation of low-density lipoproteins by activated human monocyte derived macrophages. *Biochim Biophys Acta* 1165:335, 1993.

248. Szczeklik A, Musial J, Undas A, et al: Inhibition of thrombin generation by simvastatin and lack of additive effects of aspirin in patients with marked hypercholesterolemia. *J Am Coll Cardiol* 33:1286, 1999.

249. Undas A, Brummel KE, Musial J, et al: Simvastatin depresses blood clotting by inhibiting activation of prothrombin, factor V and factor XIII and by enhancing factor Va inactivation. *Circulation* 103:2248, 2001.

250. Ray JG, Mamdani M, Tsuyuki RT, et al: Use of statins and the subsequent development of deep vein thrombosis. *Arch Intern Med* 161:1405, 2001.

251. Patel R, Nagueh SF, Tsybouleva N, et al: Simvastatin induces regression of cardiac hypertrophy and fibrosis and improves cardiac function in a transgenic rabbit model of human hypertrophic cardiomyopathy. *Circulation* 104:317, 2001.

252. Knapp HH, Schrott H, Ma P, et al: Efficacy and safety of combination simvastatin and colesevelam in patients with primary hypercholesterolemia. *Am J Med* 110:352, 2001.

252a. Bays H, Weiss S, Gagne C, et al: Ezetimibe added to ongoing statin therapy for treatment of primary hypercholesterolemia (abst.). *J Am Coll Cardiol* 39 (Suppl A): 245A, 2002.

252b. Davidson M, McGarry T, Bettis R, et al: Ezetimibe co-administered with simvastatin in 668 patients with primary hypercholesterolemia (abst.). *J Am Coll Cardiol* 39(Suppl A):226A, 2002.

253. McTavish D, Sorkin EM: Pravastatin. A review of its pharmacological properties and therapeutic potential in hypercholesterolaemia. *Drugs* 42:65, 1991.

254. Tsujita Y, Kuroda M, Simada Y, et al: CS 514, a competitive inhibitor of 3-hydroxy-3-methyl glutaryl coenzyme A reductase: Tissue selective inhibitor of steroid synthesis and hypolipidemic effects on various animal species. *Biochem Biophys Acta* 877:50, 1986.

255. Germershausen JI, Hunt VM, Bostedor RG, et al: Tissue selectivity of the cholesterol-lowering agents lovastatin, simvastatin and pravastatin in rats in vivo. *Biochem Biophys Res Commun* 158(3):667, 1989.

256. Reihner E, Rudling M, Stahlberg D, et al: Influence of pravastatin, a specific inhibitor of HMG CoA reductase, on hepatic metabolism of cholesterol. *N Engl J Med* 323:224, 1990.

257. Hunninghake DB, Knopp RH, Schonfeld G, et al: Efficacy and safety of pravastatin in patients with primary hypercholesterolemia. 1. A dose-response study. *Atherosclerosis* 85:81, 1990.

258. Mabuchi A, Kamon N, Fujita H, et al: The effects of CS 514 on serum lipoprotein, lipid and apolipoprotein levels in patients with familial hypercholesterolemia. *Metabolism* 36:475, 1987.

259. Nakaya N, Yasuhiko H, Hiromitsu T, et al: The effect of CS 514 on serum lipids and apolipoproteins in hypercholesterolemic subjects. *JAMA* 257(22):3088, 1987.

260. Chan P, Lee C-B, Lin T-S, et al: The effectiveness and safety of low dose pravastatin in elderly hypertensive hypercholesterolemic subjects on antihypertensive therapy. *Am J Hypertens* 8:1099, 1995.

261. LaRosa JC, Applegate W, Crouse JR, et al: Cholesterol lowering in the elderly. *Arch Intern Med* 154:529, 1994.

262. Raskin P, Ganda OP, Schwartz S, et al: Efficacy and safety of pravastatin in the treatment of patients with type I or type II diabetes mellitus and hypercholesterolemia. *Am J Med* 99:362, 1995.

263. Prisant LM, Downton M, Watkins LO: Efficacy and tolerability of lovastatin in 459 African-Americans with hypercholesterolemia. *Am J Card* 78:420, 1996.

264. The Simvastatin Pravastatin Study Group: Comparison of the efficacy, safety and tolerability of simvastatin and pravastatin for hypercholesterolemia. *Am J Cardiol* 71:1408, 1993.

265. The Lovastatin Pravastatin Study Group: A multicenter comparative trial of lovastatin and pravastatin in the treatment of hypercholesterolemia. *Am J Cardiol* 71:810, 1993.

266. Bekhoonek BD, McGovern ME, Markowitz JS, et al: Effects of pravastatin in patients with total serum cholesterol levels from 5.2 to 7.8 mmol/liter (200 to 300 mg/dL) plus two additional atherosclerotic risk factors. *Am J Cardiol* 72:1031, 1993.

267. Pitt B, Mancini J, Ellis SG, et al: Pravastatin Limitation of Atherosclerosis in the Coronary Arteries (PLAC I): Reduction in atherosclerosis progression and clinical events. *J Am Coll Cardiol* 26:1133, 1995.

268. Crouse JR III, Byington RP, Bond MG, et al: Pravastatin, lipids and atherosclerosis in the coronary arteries (PLAC II). *Am J Cardiol* 75:455, 1995.

269. Salonen R, Nyyssonen K, Porkkala E, et al: Kuopio Atherosclerosis Prevention Study (KAPS). A population-based primary preventive trial of the effect of LDL lowering on atherosclerotic progression in carotid and femoral arteries. *Circulation* 92:1758, 1995.

270. Jukema JW, Bruschke AVG, van Boven AJ, et al: Effects of lipid lowering by pravastatin on progression and regression of coronary artery disease in symptomatic men with normal to moderately elevated serum cholesterol levels. The Regression Growth Evaluation Statin Study (REGRESS). *Circulation* 91:2528, 1995.

271. Byington RP, Jukema JW, Salonen JT, et al: Reduction in cardiovascular events during pravastatin therapy. Pooled analysis of clinical events of the Pravastatin Atherosclerosis Intervention Program. *Circulation* 92:2419, 1995.

272. Albert MA, Danielson E, Rifai N, et al: Effect of statin therapy on C-reactive protein levels. The Pravastatin Inflammation/CRP Evaluation (PRINCE): A randomized trial and cohort study. *JAMA* 286:64, 2001.

273. Azar RR, Waters DD: PRINCE's prospects: Statins, inflammation, and coronary risk. *Am Heart J* 141:881, 2001.

274. Ridker PM, Rifai N, Pfeffer MA, et al: Long-term effects of pravastatin on plasma concentration of C-reactive protein. *Circulation* 100:230, 1999.

275. Horne BD, Muhlestein JB, Carlquist JF, et al: Statin therapy, lipid levels, C-reactive protein and the survival of patients with angiographically severe coronary artery disease. *J Am Coll Cardiol* 36:1774, 2000.

276. Glorioso N, Troffa C, Filigheddu F, et al: Effect of the HMG-CoA reductase inhibitors on blood pressure in patients with essential hypertension and primary hypercholesterolemia. *Hypertension* 34:1281, 1999.

277. Dupuis J, Tardif JC, Cernacek P, Theroux P: Cholesterol reduction rapidly improves endothelial function after acute coronary syndromes. The RECIFE (Reduction of Cholesterol in Ischemia and Function of the Endothelium) trial. *Circulation* 99:3227, 1999.

278. Kaesemeyer WH, Caldwell RB, Huang J, Caldwell RW: Pravastatin sodium activates endothelial nitric oxide synthase independent of its cholesterol-lowering actions. *J Am Coll Cardiol* 33:234, 1999.

279. Dangas G, Badimon JJ, Smith DA, et al: Pravastatin therapy in hyperlipidemia: effects on thrombus formation and the systemic hemostatic profile. *J Am Coll Cardiol* 33:1294, 1999.

280. Shepherd J, Cobbe SM, Ford I, et al: Prevention of coronary heart disease with pravastatin in men with hypercholesterolemia. *N Engl J Med* 333:1301, 1995.

281. Pfeffer MA, Sacks F, Moye LA, et al: Cholesterol and Recurrent Events: A secondary prevention trial for normolipidemic patients. *Am J Cardiol* 76:98C, 1995.

282. Plehn JF, Davis BR, Sacks FM, et al: Reduction of stroke incidence after myocardial infarction with pravastatin. The Cholesterol and Recurrent Events (CARE) study. *Circulation* 99:216, 1999.

283. Sacks FM, Pfeffer MA, Moye LA, et al: The effect of pravastatin on coronary events after myocardial infarction in patients with average cholesterol levels. *N Engl J Med* 335:1001, 1996.

284. Tonkin AM, Colquhoun D, Emberson J, et al: Effects of pravastatin in 3260 patients with unstable angina: results from the LIPID study. *Lancet* 355:1871, 2000.

285. Hunt D, Young P, Simes J, et al: Benefits of pravastatin on cardiovascular events and mortality in older patients with coronary heart disease are equal to or exceed those seen in younger patients: Results from the LIPID trial. *Ann Intern Med* 134:931, 2001.

285a. Simes RJ, Marschner IC, Hunt D, et al: Relationship between lipid levels and clinical outcomes in the Long-Term Intervention with Pravastatin in Ischemic Disease (LIPID) Trial. To what extent is the reduction in coronary events with pravastatin explained by on-study lipid levels? *Circulation* 105:1162, 2002.

286. White HD, Simes J, Anderson NE, et al: Pravastatin therapy and the risk of stroke. *N Engl J Med* 343:317, 2000.

287. Vgontzas AN, Kales A, Bixler EO, et al: Effects of lovastatin and pravastatin on sleep efficiency and sleep stages. *Clin Pharmacol Ther* 50:730, 1991.

288. Langtry HD, Markham A: Fluvastatin: A review of its use in lipid disorders. *Drugs* 57:583, 1999.

289. Davidson MH, FLUENT investigation group: Fluvastatin Long-Term Extension Trial (FLUENT): Summary of efficacy and safety. *Am J Med* 96:4S, 1994.

290. Jacotot B, Banga JD, Waite R, et al: Long-term efficacy with fluvastatin as monotherapy, and combined with cholestyramine (a 156 week multicenter study). *Am J Cardiol* 76(Suppl):41A, 1995.

291. Leitersdorf E, Muratti EN, Eliav O, et al: Efficacy and safety of a combination fluvastatin-bezafibrate treatment for familial hypercholesterolemia: Comparative analysis with a fluvastatin-cholestyramine combination. *Am J Med* 96:401, 1994.

292. Foley DP, Bonnier H, Jackson G, et al: Prevention of restenosis after coronary balloon angioplasty: Rationale and design of the Fluvastatin Angioplasty Restenosis (FLARE) trial. *Am J Cardiol* 73:5D, 1994.

293. Herd JA, Ballantyne C, Farmer JA, et al: Effects of fluvastatin on coronary atherosclerosis in patients with mild to moderate cholesterol elevations [Lipoprotein and Coronary Atherosclerosis Study (LCAS)]. *Am J Cardiol* 80:278, 1997.

294. Liem A, van Boven AJ: Effects of fluvastatin administered immediately after an acute MI on myocardial ischemia. Presented at the American Heart Association Scientific Sessions 2000, New Orleans, La. Nov 12–15, 2000.

295. Marz W, Scharnagl H, Abletshauser C, et al: Fluvastatin lowers atherogenic dense low-density lipoproteins in postmenopausal women with the atherogenic lipoprotein phenotype. *Circulation* 103:1942, 2001.

296. Sabia H, Prasad P, Smith HT, et al: Safety, tolerability, and pharmacokinetics of an extended-release formulation of fluvastatin administered once daily to patients with primary hypercholesterolemia. *J Cardiovasc Pharmacol* 37:502, 2001.

297. Nawrocki JW, Weiss SR, Davidson MH, et al: Reduction of LDL-cholesterol by 25% to 69% in patients with primary hypercholesterolemia by atorvastatin: A new HMG-CoA reductase inhibitor. *Arterioscler Thromb Vasc Biol* 15:678, 1995.

298. Bakker-Arkema RG, Davidson MH, Hgoldstein RJ, et al: Efficacy and safety of a new HMG-CoA reductase inhibitor, atorvastatin, in patients with hypertriglyceridemia. *JAMA* 275:128, 1996.

299. Cilla DD Jr, Gibson DM, Whitfield LR, Sedman AJ: Pharmacodynamic effects and pharmacokinetics of atorvastatin after administration in normocholesterolemic subjects in the morning and evening. *J Clin Pharmacol* 36:604, 1996.

300. Smilde TJ, van Wissen S, Wollersheim H, et al: Effect of aggressive versus conventional lipid lowering on atherosclerosis progression in familial hypercholesterolaemia (ASAP): A prospective, randomised, double-blind trial. *Lancet* 357:577, 2001.

301. Illingworth DR, Crouse JR 3rd, Hunninghake DB, et al: A comparison of simvastatin and atorvastatin up to maximal recommended doses in a large multicenter randomized clinical trial. *Curr Med Res Opin* 17:43, 2001.

302. Pitt B, Waters D, Brown WV, et al: Aggressive lipid-lowering therapy compared with angioplasty in stable coronary artery disease. Atorvastatin versus Revascularization Treatment Investigators. *N Engl J Med* 341:70, 1999.

303. Betteridge DJ, Colhoun H, Armitage J: Status report of lipid-lowering trials in diabetes. *Curr Opin Lipidol* 11:621, 2000.

304. Cheng-Lai A: Cerivastatin. *Heart Dis* 2:93, 2000.

305. Sica DA, Gehr TW: Rhabdomyolysis and statin therapy: Relevance to the elderly. *Am J Geriatr Cardiol* 11:48, 2002.

306. Davidson MH: Rosuvastatin: A highly efficacious statin for the treatment of dyslipidaemia. *Expert Opin Investig Drugs* 11:125, 2002.

307. McTaggart F, Buckett L, Davidson R, et al: Preclinical and clinical pharmacology of rosuvastatin, a new 3-hydroxy-3-methylglutaryl coenzyme A reductase inhibitor. *Am J Cardiol* 87(Suppl):28B, 2001.

308. Olsson AG: Statin therapy and reductions in low-density lipoprotein cholesterol: Initial clinical data on the potent new statin rosuvastatin. *Am J Cardiol* 87(Suppl):33B, 2001.

309. Davignon J, Laaksonen R: Low-density lipoprotein-independent effects of statins. *Curr Opin Lipidol* 10:543, 1999.

310. Gotto AM Jr., Farmer JA: Pleiotropic effects of statins: Do they matter? *Curr Opin Lipidol* 12:391, 2001.

310a. Alber HF, Dulak J, Frick M, et al: Atorvastatin decreases vascular endothelial growth factor in patients with coronary artery disease. *J Am Coll Cardiol* 39:1951, 2002.

310b. Yeung AC, Tsao P: Statin therapy. Beyond cholesterol lowering and anti-inflammatory effects. *Circulation* 105:2937, 2002.

311. Wang PS, Solomon DH, Mogun H, Avorn J: HMG-CoA reductase inhibitors and the risk of hip fractures in elderly patients. *JAMA* 283:3211, 2000.

312. Chan KA, Andrade SE, Boles M, et al: Inhibitors of hydroxymethylglutaryl-coenzyme A reductase and risk of fracture among older women. *Lancet* 355:2185, 2000.

313. Jick H, Zornberg GL, Jick SS, et al: Statins and the risk of dementia. *Lancet* 356:1627, 2000.

313a. Herrington DM, Vittinghoff E, Lin F, et al: Statin therapy, cardiovascular events, and total mortality in the Heart and Estrogen/Progestin Replacement Study (HERS). *Circulation* 105:2962, 2002.

314. Marcelino JJ, Feingold KR: Inadequate treatment with HMG-CoA reductase inhibitors by health care providers. *Am J Med* 100:605, 1996.

314a. Teo KK, Burton JR: Who should receive HMG CoA reductase inhibitors? *Drugs* 62:1707, 2002.

315. Aronow HD, Topol EJ, Roe MT, et al: Effect of lipid-lowering therapy on early mortality after acute coornary syndromes: An observational study. *Lancet* 357:1063, 2001.

315a. Stenestrand U, Wallentin L, for the Swedish Register of Cardiac Intensive Care (RIKS-HIA): Early statin treatment following acute myocardial infarction and 1-year survival. *JAMA* 285:430, 2001.

315b. Newby LK, Kristinsson A, Bhapkar MV, et al: Early statin initiation and outcomes in patients with acute coronary syndromes. *JAMA* 287:3087, 2002.

315c. Heeschen C, Hamm CW, Laufs U, et al: Withdrawal of statins increases event rates in patients with acute coronary syndromes. *Circulation* 105:1446, 2002.

316. Altschul R, Hoffer A, Stephen JD: Influence of nicotinic acid on serum cholesterol in man. *Arch Biochem* 54:558, 1955.

317. Fumagalli R: Pharmacokinetics of nicotinic acid and some of its derivatives. In: Gey KF, Caarlson LA (eds): *Metabolic Effects of Nicotinic Acid and Its Derivatives.* Bern: Hans Huber, 1971, pp 33–49.

318. Petrack B, Greengard P, Kalinsky H: On the relative efficacy of nicotinamide and nicotinic acid as precursors of nicotinamide adenine dinucleotide. *J Biol Chem* 241(10):2367, 1966.

318a. See M, Hoppichler F, Reavely D, et al: Relation of serum lipoprotein(a) concentration and apolipoprotein(a) phenotype to coronary heart disease in patients with familial hypercholesterolemia. *N Engl J Med* 322:1494, 1990.

319. Mahley RW, Bersot TP: Drug therapy for hypercholesterolemia and dyslipidemia. In: Hardman JG, Limbird LE (eds): *Goodman and Gilman's. The Pharmacological Basis of Therapeutics,* 10th ed. New York: McGraw Hill 2001:971–1002.

320. Alderman JD, Pasternak RC, Sacks FM, et al: Effect of a modified, well-tolerated niacin regimen on serum total cholesterol, high density lipoprotein cholesterol and the cholesterol to high density lipoprotein ratio. *Am J Cardiol* 64:725, 1989.

321. Arner P, Ostman J: Effect of nicotinic acid on acylglycerol metabolism in human adipose tissue. *Clin Sci* 64:235, 1983.

322. Canner PL, Berge KG, Wenger NK, et al: Fifteen year mortality in Coronary Drug Project patients: Long term benefit with niacin. *J Am Coll Cardiol* 8(6):1245, 1986.

323. Carlson LA, Danielson M, Ekberg I, et al: Reduction of myocardial reinfarction by the combined treatment with clofibrate and nicotinic acid. *Atherosclerosis* 28:81, 1977.

324. Azen SP, Mack WJ, Cashin-Hemphill L, et al: Progression of coronary artery disease predicts clinical coronary events. Long-term follow-up from the Cholesterol Lowering Atherosclerosis Study. *Circulation* 93:34, 1996.

325. Brown G, Albers JJ, Fisher LD, et al: Regression of coronary artery disease as a result of intensive lipid lowering therapy in men with high levels of apolipoprotein B. *N Engl J Med* 323:1289, 1990.

326. Witztum JL: Current approaches to drug therapy for the hypercholesterolemic patient. *Circulation* 80(5):1101, 1989.

327. Knopp RH, Ginsberg J, Albers JJ, et al: Contrasting effects of unmodified and time-release forms of niacin on lipoproteins in hyperlipidemic subjects: Clues to mechanism of action of niacin. *Metabolism* 34(7):642, 1985.

328. Goldberg A, Alagona P Jr., Capuzzi DM, et al: Multiple dose efficacy and safety of an extended-release form of niacin in the management of hyperlipidemia. *Am J Cardiol* 85:1100, 2000.

329. Etchason JA, Miller TD, Squires RW, et al: Niacin-induced hepatitis: A potential side effect with low-dose time-release niacin. *Mayo Clin Proc* 66:23, 1991.

330. Dalton TA, Berry RS: Hepatotoxicity associated with sustained-release niacin. *Am J Med* 93:102, 1992.

330a. Grundy SM, Vega GL, McGovern ME, et al: Efficacy, safety and tolerability of once-daily niacin for the treatment of dyslipidemia associated with Type 2 diabetes: Results of the Assessment of Diabetes Control and Evaluation of the Efficacy of Niaspan Trial. *Arch Intern Med* 162:1568, 2002.

331. Morgan JM, Capuzzi DM, Guyton JR, et al: Treatment effect of Niaspan, a controlled-release niacin in patients with hypercholesterolemia: A placebo-controlled trial. *J Cardiovasc Pharmacol Ther* 1:195, 1996.

332. Keenan JM, Fontaine PL, Wenz JB, et al: Niacin revisited. *Arch Intern Med* 151:1424, 1991.

333. Gibbons LW, Gonzalez V, Gordon N, Grundy S: The prevalence of side effects with regular and sustained-release nicotinic acid. *Am J Med* 99:378, 1995.

333a. Patterson DJ, Dew EW, Gyorkey F, Graham DY: Niacin hepatitis. *South Med J* 76(2):239, 1983.

334. Clementz GL, Holmes AW: Nicotinic-acid-induced fulminant hepatic failure. *J Clin Gastroenterol* 9(5):582, 1987.

334a. Elam MB, Hunninghake DB, Davis KB, et al: Effect of niacin on lipid and lipoprotein levels and glycemic control in patients with diabetes and peripheral arterial disease. The ADMIT Study: A randomized trial. *JAMA* 284:1263, 2000.

335. Litin SC, Anderson CF: Nicotinic-acid associated myopathy: A report of three cases. *Am J Med* 86:481, 1989.

336. Reaven P, Witztum JL: Lovastatin, nicotinic acid, and rhabdomyolysis (letter). *Ann Intern Med* 109:597, 1988.

337. Rader JI, Calvert RJ, Hathcock JN: Hepatic toxicity of unmodified and time-release preparations of niacin. *Am J Med* 92:77, 1992.

338. Walldius G, Erikson U, Olsson AG, et al: The effect of probucol on femoral atherosclerosis: The Probucol Quantitative Regression Swedish Trial (PQRST). *Am J Cardiol* 74:875, 1994.

339. Cote G, Tardif JC, Lesperance J, et al: Effects of probucol on vascular remodeling after coronary angioplasty. Multivitamins and Protocol Study Group. *Circulation* 99:30, 1999.

339a. Sia YT, Lapointe N, Parker TG, et al: Beneficial effects of long-term use of the antioxidant probucol in heart failure in the rat. *Circulation* 105:2549, 2002.

339b. Knopp RH, Superko HR, Davidson M, et al: Long-term blood cholesterol-lowering effects of a dietary fiber supplement. *Am J Prev Med* 17:18, 1999.

339c. Maki KC, Davidson MH, Malik KC, et al: Cholesterol lowering with high-viscosity hydroxypropylmethylcellulose. *Am J Cardiol* 84:1198, 1999.

339d. Wolk A, Manson JE, Stampfer MJ, et al: Long-term intake of dietary fiber and decreased risk of coronary heart disease among women. *JAMA* 281:1998, 1999.

340. Walker ARP: Dietary fiber and the pattern of diseases (editorial). *Ann Intern Med* 80:663, 1974.

341. Stamler J: Coronary heart disease: Doing the right things. *N Engl J Med* 312:1053, 1985.

342. Wright A, Burstyn PG, Gibney MJ: Dietary fiber and blood pressure. *Br Med J* 2:1541, 1979.

343. Anderson JW, Ward K: High-carbohydrate, high-fiber diets for insulin-treated men with diabetes mellitus. *Am J Clin Nutr* 32:2312, 1979.

344. Anderson JW: Dietary fiber and diabetes, in Vahouny GV, Kritchevsky D (eds): *Dietary Fiber in Health and Disease.* New York: Plenum Press, 1982, pp 151–165.

345. Miettinen TA: Dietary fiber and lipids. *Am J Clin Nutr* 45(Suppl): 1237, 1987.

346. Eastwood MA, Passmore R: Dietary fibre. *Lancet* 2:202, 1983.

347. Chan JKC, Wypyszyk V: A forgotten natural dietary fiber: Psyllium mucilloid. *Cereal Foods World* 33:919, 1988.

348. Jenkins DJA, Kendall CWC, Axelsen M, et al: Viscous and nonviscous fibres, nonabsorbable and low glycaemic index carbohydrates, blood lipids and coronary heart disease. *Curr Opin Lipidol* 11:49, 2000.

349. Jenkins DJ, Axelsen M, Kendall CW, et al: Dietary fibre, lente carbo-hydrates and the insulin-resistant diseases. *Br J Nutr* 83:S157, 2000.

350. Kennedy JF, Sandhu JS, Southgate DAT: Structural data for the car-bohydrate of ispaghula husk (ex Plantago ovata Forsk). *Carbohydr Res* 75:269, 1979.

351. Levin EG, Miller VT, Muesing RA, et al: Comparison of psyllium hydrophilic mucilloid and cellulose as adjuncts to a prudent diet in the treatment of mild to moderate hypercholesterolemia. *Arch Intern Med* 150:1822, 1990.

352. Pietinen P, Rimm EB, Korhonen P, et al: Intake of dietary fiber and risk of coronary artery disease in a cohort of Finnish men: The Al-pha Tocopherol, Beta-Carotene Cancer Prevention Study. *Circulation* 94:2320, 1996.

353. Chen WL, Anderson JW, Jennings D: Propionate may mediate the hypocholesterolemic effects of certain soluble plant fiber in choles-terol fed rats. *Proc Soc Exp Biol Med* 175:215, 1984.

354. Lantner RR, Espiritu BR, Zumerchik P, Tobin MC: Anaphylaxis fol-lowing ingestion of a psyllium-containing cereal. *JAMA* 264:2534, 1990.

355. Behall KM, Scholfield DJ, Lee K, et al: Mineral balance in adult men: Effect of 4 refined fibers. *Am J Clin Nutr* 46:307, 1987.

356. Kwiterovich PO Jr: The role of fiber in the treatment of hypercholes-terolemia in children and adolescents. *Pediatrics* 96(5, Pt 2 of 2):1005, 1995.

357. Rimm EB, Ascherio A, Giovannucci E, et al: Vegetable, fruit, and cereal fiber intake and risk of coronary heart disease among men. *JAMA* 275:447, 1996.

358. Davidson MH, Dugan LD, Burns JH, et al: The hypocholesterolemic effects of b-glucan in oatmeal and oat bran. A dose-controlled study. *JAMA* 265:1833, 1991.

359. Lipsky H, Gloger M, Frishman WH: Dietary fiber for reducing blood cholesterol. *J Clin Pharmacol* 30:699, 1990.

360. Spence JD, Huff MW, Heidenheim P, et al: Combination therapy with colestipol and psyllium mucilloid in patients with hyperlipidemia. *Ann Intern Med* 123:493, 1995.

CHAPTER 21

Combination Drug Therapy

Michael A. Weber

Joel M. Neutel

William H. Frishman

Almost all major cardiovascular diseases are treated with combination therapy. Conditions like congestive heart failure and angina pectoris are typically treated with three or more drugs and there is growing evidence that even prophylactic therapies designed to prevent thrombotic episodes may best be achieved with more than one agent. The main focus of this chapter, however, is to explore the use of combination therapy in systemic hypertension.

The well-established benefits of combination treatment as compared with single-agent treatment include greater efficacy, reduced or attenuated side effects, and convenience.[1–4,4a] However, new evidence from major hypertension trials with clinical end points has created a new imperative in the management of hypertension: the reduction of blood pressure below aggressive target levels. Current guideline recommendations (see later) have suggested the achievement of blood pressure values below 140/90 mm Hg in hypertensive patients in general; however, for those considered at high risk—including diabetics or those with evidence for renal or other target organ involvement—blood pressure should be 130/85 mm Hg or even lower. In most instances achieving these goals requires at least two antihypertensive agents and often three or more.

The studies that have helped influence this new attitude include the Hypertension Optimal Treatment (HOT) study,[5] The United Kingdom Prospective Diabetes Study (UKPDS),[6] and the Modification of Diet in Renal Disease (MDRD) study.[7] These clinical outcomes studies all emphasize that the achievement of low blood pressure levels during therapy might be just as important, if not more so, as basing therapy on appropriate pharmacologic agents.[8–10] One interesting example of this type has been the African American Study of Kidney Disease and Hypertension (AASK) study,[11] in which progression of renal disease in African-American hypertensive patients could be substantially slowed by therapy with an angiotensin converting enzyme (ACE) inhibitor. Even though ACE inhibitors generally have not been highly effective in reducing blood pressure in African-American patients, the use of combination therapy in this study achieved appropriate blood pressure goals and allowed these patients to benefit from the selective renal-protective effects of the ACE inhibitor.

Marketing surveys in the antihypertensive area indicate that physicians in general now understand the value of combination therapy. In particular, fixed combinations of such agents as ACE inhibitors and calcium-channel blockers are rapidly growing in use, and fixed combinations of angiotensin receptor blockers with diuretics now account for well over 30% of the use of these newer agents.

PRINCIPLES OF COMBINATION THERAPY

Drug combinations have been used traditionally to treat many cardiovascular conditions such as congestive heart failure angina pectoris, and hypertension. But the historical development of using multiple medications has differed for each condition. For example, digitalis was first used in the eighteenth century to provide clinical benefits for patients with congestive heart failure. Then, in the mid-1990s, diuretics were shown to produce symptomatic and functional advantages when used in addition to digitalis. More recently, physicians added an ACE inhibitor to digitalis and diuretic treatment to improve clinical findings and prolong survival, thereby completing a logical triad of drugs, each of which contributed in a separate but meaningful fashion. Most recently, adding beta blockers, spironolactone, and even angiotensin receptor blockers (ARBs) to ACE inhibitors has been shown to further enhance outcomes in congestive heart failure, providing a powerful illustration of the potential value of well-fashioned combination therapy.

Hypertension therapy, which is the main focus of this chapter, has almost always required drug combinations. Usually, more than one drug was required, because earlier classes of drugs either were not effective alone or doses that produced efficacious decreases in blood pressure, unfortunately, also produced unacceptable adverse side effects or events. Indeed, 30 years ago the pooling of low doses of as many as three separate agents into a single fixed-dose product was quite commonplace. SerApEs, for example, brought together reserpine, hydralazine, and hydrochlorothiazide; this fixed-combination product was popular with physicians, reasonably well tolerated by patients, and quite effective for reducing blood pressure.

The first attempt at a systematic method for treating hypertension was termed the "stepped-care" approach.[12] Very simply, it recommended that treatment of all hypertensive patients begin with a diuretic—albeit in higher doses than would be customary now. If the diuretic was not efficacious, then a second-step drug, typically a sympatholytic agent, could be added. If success was still not achieved, then a third-step drug, usually a vasodilator, would be superimposed upon the previous drugs. Yet further agents could be added, as necessary, to bring the blood pressure under control. At each step, the added medication would usually be increased to the maximum dose, often limited by side effects or adverse reactions.

EVOLUTION OF CARE

The stepped-care approach, employing separate drug prescriptions or the use of fixed combinations, became standard practice by the early 1970s. Almost immediately, though, conceptual challenges to this method of treatment began to appear. The most visible challenge came from the volume-vasoconstriction hypothesis advanced by Laragh.[13] It was postulated that essential hypertension was a heterogeneous condition where each patient had a different combination of both volume excess and vasoconstriction as the pathophysiologic cause of the high blood pressure. Thus, ideally, some patients should be treated with diuretics to reduce the volume-excess component, whereas other patients, whose excess vasoconstriction might be due largely to increased activity of the renin-angiotensin system, should be treated with drugs to inhibit renin release or to inhibit angiotensin II.

Laragh's group suggested that a simple measurement of plasma renin activity could guide the selection of a single agent from the drug class most likely to be beneficial. For instance, low plasma renin levels would suggest volume excess (treatable with diuretics) and high plasma renin levels would suggest increased activation of the renin-angiotensin system (treatable with ACE inhibitors or beta blockers). Of course, for the patients whose plasma renin levels fell into the middle range, presumably indicating the presence of both volume and vasoconstriction factors, it might be necessary to use a combination of these drugs. Also, at the time, it was reported that patients with different demographic backgrounds had different renin profiles and a tendency to respond preferentially to certain drug types. For example, patients who were white or relatively young tended to respond well to such agents as beta blockers, whereas African American patients and the elderly tended to respond well to diuretics.

As diagnostic and therapeutic strategies evolved, innovative new drug classes were created. Later-generation beta blockers, the calcium-channel blockers, the ACE inhibitors, and angiotensin II receptor blockers were all effective and produced relatively few adverse events or side effects. For these reasons, the Fourth Joint National Committee (JNC-IV) recommended individualizing therapy and encouraged physicians to search for the single agent that would best suit the needs of each individual patient.[14] Diuretics, beta blockers, calcium-channel blockers, and ACE inhibitors were all considered appropriate drugs with which to initiate the treatment of hypertension.

Despite this progress, however, the overall treatment of hypertension still has not progressed satisfactorily. The Third National Health and Nutrition Examination Survey (NHANES 3) revealed that only 24% of hypertensive patients in the United States had their blood pressures reduced below 140/90 mm Hg.[15] The growing number of drug classes and individual agents for the management of hypertension suggests that, as yet, there are no fully adequate solutions. Drug combinations, therefore, remain a staple of antihypertensive therapy now and for the foreseeable future.

A MATTER OF DEFINITION

Combination therapy involves multiple doses of multiple medications. Most commonly, physicians will start with a single agent, and, after making adjustments to its dose, will add further drugs while

adjusting the doses as necessary. Most of the discussion in this chapter assumes this approach. However, from the very origins of antihypertensive therapy, manufacturers have made available a variety of fixed combinations. The intent of these products has been to provide a simpler and more convenient way of taking more than one agent. By and large, these fixed-dose combinations have been only moderately successful in the marketplace. For example, it is estimated that fixed formulations of an ACE inhibitor and a diuretic are prescribed only 10% as frequently as the primary ACE inhibitor. The main objection to these products has been that they do not allow physicians to titrate the dose of each drug separately but rather compel them to prescribe the use of the two agents in a prefixed ratio. This objection has been particularly popular in academic medical centers, where physicians usually have not allowed fixed combinations on their formularies. The attitude of the U.S. Food and Drug Administration (FDA) toward these combinations also has not encouraged their use. The regulatory agency has insisted that physicians first titrate each separate component to an appropriate level, and then switch to the combination product only if the doses correspond to an available fixed combination. In reality, though, these products have gone through rigorous testing to ascertain the optimal doses of each agent within the combination. Apparently, most physicians find this a tedious approach and tend to construct their own multidrug combination regimens.

There have been exceptions to this rule. Combinations of two diuretics, hydrochlorothiazide and triamterene, with the trade names of Dyazide and Maxzide, have been widely accepted. Likewise, Ziac, which contains a diuretic and a beta blocker, Logimax, which contains a beta blocker and a calcium-channel blocker, and Lotrel, Teczem, Lexxel, and Tarka, which contain an ACE inhibitor and a calcium-channel blocker, have received attention because of the unusual nature of their dosing or their components.[16–18]

Manufacturers have sometimes selected names for these fixed combinations that differ totally from those of the individual components in order to create the impression of what they call "new types of dual-acting single entities." Market research data seem to confirm the success of these strategies. For example, in the United States during the 1993–1994 and 1994–1995 business years, the growth rates of total prescriptions for single-agent antihypertensives were 6 and 7%, respectively, whereas for fixed combinations they were 8 and 20%.

RATIONALE FOR COMBINATION THERAPY

Treating hypertension with combination therapy provides more opportunity for creative solutions to a number of problems. Five issues in combined therapy—some practical, some speculative—are listed in Table 21-1.

TABLE 21-1. Rationale for Combination Drug Therapy for Hypertension

Increased antihypertensive efficacy
    Additive effects
    Synergistic effects
Reduced adverse events
    Low-dose strategy
    Drugs with offsetting actions
Enhanced convenience and compliance
Prolonged duration of action
Potential for additive target organ protection

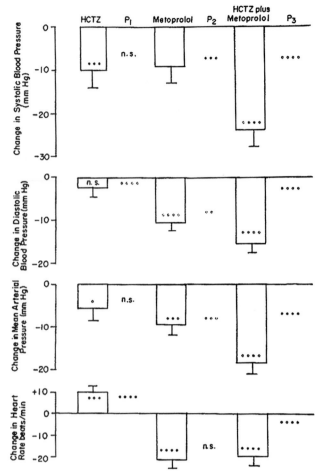

FIGURE 21-1. Changes in systolic, diastolic, and mean blood pressures and heart rate, measured in the upright position, during treatment with hydrochlorothiazide (HCTZ) 50 mg daily or metoprolol 100 to 400 mg daily or the combination of both in 20 patients with essential hypertension. Values are mean ± SE (*$P < .05$, **$P < .02$, ***$P < .01$, ***$P < .001$). P3 refers to difference between combination treatment and HCTZ alone. (*Reproduced with permission from Weber et al.*[19])

The most obvious benefit of drug combinations is the enhanced efficacy that fosters their continued widespread use. Theoretically, some drug combinations might produce synergistic effects that are greater than would be predicted by summing the efficacies of the component drugs. More commonly, combination therapy achieves a little less than the sum of its component-drug efficacies. In contrast, some combinations of drugs produce offsetting interactions that weaken rather than strengthen their antihypertensive effects, as previously seen with agents affecting peripheral-neuronal actions. For instance, guanethidine and reserpine produced this offsetting interaction; but since these agents are now used only rarely, this issue need not be considered further.

A second benefit of combination therapy concerns the avoidance of adverse effects. When patients are treated with two drugs, each drug can be administered in a lower dose that does not produce unwanted side effects but still contributes to overall efficacy. A third issue concerns convenience. Obviously, the multiple drugs of a combination regimen could be confusing and distracting to patients and could lead to poor treatment compliance. On the other hand, a well-designed combination pill that incorporates logical doses of two agents could enhance convenience and improve compliance.

Further potential value of combination treatment may result from the effects that two drugs have on each other's pharmacokinetics. Although this has not been well studied, there might be situations where the clinical duration of action of the participating drugs becomes longer when used in combination than when they are administered as monotherapies. Finally, it is interesting to consider the attributes of such agents as ACE inhibitors, angiotensin receptor blockers, and calcium-channel blockers that exhibit antigrowth or antiatherosclerotic actions in addition to their blood pressure–lowering properties. Is it possible that combinations of these newer agents may provide even more powerful protective effects on the circulation? Each of these five potentially important attributes of antihypertensive combination therapy is considered in more detail below.

EFFICACY OF COMBINATION THERAPY

The most common motivation for administering more than one antihypertensive agent is to increase overall efficacy. Most of the time, the effects of the two agents being used are approximately additive, although it is likely—in view of the theories of hypertension heterogeneity reviewed earlier—that one drug plays a predominant role in reducing the blood pressure. Sometimes, a form of synergy can be achieved.

The data shown in Figs. 21-1 and 21-2 come from a study in which each hypertensive patient was treated with three different

FIGURE 21-2. Changes in PRA and urinary aldosterone excretion during treatment with hydrochlorothiazide (HCTZ) 50 mg daily or metoprolol 100 to 400 mg daily or the combination of both in 20 patients with essential hypertension. Values are mean ± SE (*$P < .05$, **$P < .02$, ***$P < .01$, ****$P < .001$). P3 refers to difference between combination treatment and HCTZ alone. (*Reproduced with permission from Weber et al.*[19])

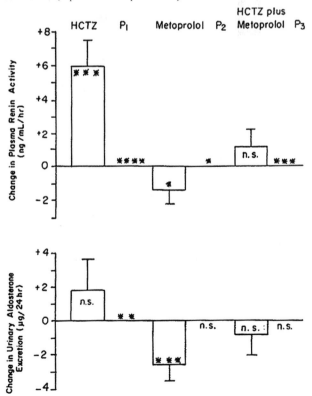

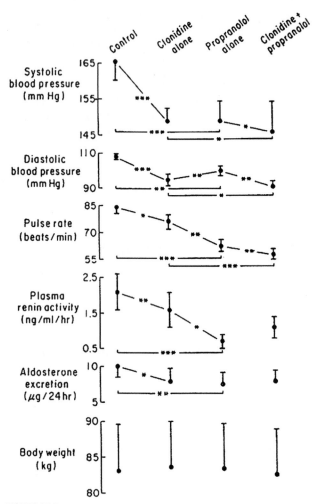

FIGURE 21-3. Clinical and biochemical values in eight patients with essential hypertension treated with clonidine (0.3 mg daily), propranolol (120 mg daily), or a combination of both. Values are mean ± SEM: (*) $P < .05$; (**) $P < .01$; (***) $P < .001$. (*Reproduced with permission from Weber et al.*[20])

regimens at different times: the beta blocker metoprolol, 100 to 400 mg daily alone; the diuretic hydrochlorothiazide, 50 mg daily alone; or both drugs in combination. The three active treatment periods were separated by periods of placebo treatment.[19] It is evident from Fig. 21-1 that metoprolol monotherapy in this predominantly Caucasian group was slightly more effective than the diuretic. The combination, in turn, was clearly more effective than either of the individual therapies. Of particular note, statistical testing, employing the pooled estimate of the within-sample variance derived from the error sum of squares, confirmed that the lower end of the 95% confidence limits of the decreases in systolic and diastolic blood pressure during combination therapy exceeded the sum of the blood pressure decreases produced by each drug alone. This finding suggests a synergistic effect, the mechanism of which might be explained by the data shown in Fig. 21-2. In these patients, the 50-mg diuretic dose, high by today's standards, had strong stimulatory effects on the renin-aldosterone axis. Metoprolol, on the other hand, had an inhibitory effect on this axis. Most importantly, the metoprolol appeared able to neutralize the renin-stimulating effects of hydrochlorothiazide during the combination therapy, thereby counteracting vasoconstrictor and other reactions to the diuretic. This mechanism appears to explain the excellent efficacy achieved when beta blockers, ACE inhibitors, and other antagonists of the renin axis are combined with a diuretic.

A contrasting situation is displayed in Fig. 21-3.[20] In this study, each patient was treated with three different therapies at different times with placebo periods in between: (1) propranolol, a beta blocker; (2) clonidine, a centrally acting sympatholytic; or (3) propranolol and clonidine combined. Each of the individual drugs was effective as monotherapy, and the two in combination were slightly better than either of the monotherapies but not equal to the predicted sum of effects of both drugs. It is noteworthy that each of these agents had inhibitory effects on renin and aldosterone but that their combined use did not potentiate this action. Thus, while these two drugs could be useful when administered together, this combination does not appear to offer the same logic and power of additive or synergistic effects seen when agents with disparate mechanisms are combined.

The principal antihypertensive drug classes in modern use are diuretics, beta blockers, calcium-channel blockers, ACE inhibitors, angiotensin II receptor antagonists, selective alpha blockers, centrally acting sympatholytic agents, and direct-acting vasodilators. This wide array of drug classes offers an enormous number of potential combinations. In reality, most fixed-combination products on the market employ a diuretic, mirroring the clinical practice of most physicians. Therefore the diuretic-containing formulations are discussed first and then, briefly, some nondiuretic combinations of interest are reviewed.

COMBINATIONS INVOLVING A DIURETIC

Before considering their role in combination therapy, it is helpful to define the way in which diuretics are now used most commonly. In general, the popularity of this class of agents has diminished in recent years. This is largely because of a perception among physicians that with diuretics, unwanted metabolic side effects—including changes in plasma lipids, glucose, uric acid, and potassium—might adversely increase the risk of cardiovascular events despite the antihypertensive efficacy of these agents. On the other hand, physicians have realized that alternative drug choices, while avoiding these metabolic effects, are often not successful in controlling blood pressure. Diuretic use, therefore, remains widespread, though often as a supplement to other drugs. Moreover, the diuretics are used mostly in doses far lower than when they were first used; 12.5 mg has become quite typical, especially when used as part of a combination, and doses as low as 6.25 mg can be effective when used in combinations. Most of the modern fixed-dose products that include diuretics have employed these lower doses.

Combination with ACE Inhibitors

Combining a diuretic with an ACE inhibitor is one of the most logical approaches to the treatment of hypertension. Diuretics work primarily by increasing renal clearance of sodium and water, thereby reducing intravascular volume, at least in the short term. For many patients, a diuretic alone is an effective way to reduce blood pressure. For example, monotherapy with diuretics is often effective in African-American patients and in the elderly.[21,22] The renin-angiotensin system of patients in these two groups often exhibits less of a reactive response to volume depletion and thus generates less compensatory angiotensin-mediated vasoconstriction. In contrast,

TABLE 21-2. Effects on Systolic and Diastolic Blood Pressures of Monotherapy with Placebo or Various Dosages of Losartan Followed by Combination Therapy with Hydrochlorothiazide

Treatment	No. of Patients	Mean (±SD) Systolic/Diastolic		
		Baseline	After 4 Weeks of Monotherapy	Additional Decrease after 2 Weeks of Combination Therapy with HCTZ 12.5 mg/day
Placebo	26	148.5 (14.7)/100.5 (3.8)	150.8 (12.9)/99.9 (5.9)	8.7 (11.4)/4.0 (6.4)
Losartan 50 mg qd	21	159.3 (16.6)/101.0 (4.9)	148.9 (16.5)/96.2 (7.9)	5.5 (14.0)/5.1 (7.8)
Losartan 100 mg qd	16	150.9 (14.0)/102.3 (4.7)	140.9 (15.7)/95.6 (7.6)	6.0 (7.5)/4.0 (6.1)
Losartan 50 mg bid	20	155.2 (13.8)/101.7 (4.1)	146.2 (12.6)/95.6 (6.4)	7.3 (10.4)/4.0 (6.9)

SD = standard deviation; HCTZ = hydrochlorothiazide; qd = once daily; bid = twice daily.

Source: Reproduced with permission from Weber et al.[32]

ACE inhibitors are often effective in white hypertensive patients[23,24] and in other settings where renin activity is relatively high. From a clinical perspective, diuretics and ACE inhibitors appear to have complementary properties. These attributes appear to be maximized when the two drug classes are used together, especially as the ACE inhibitors effectively prevent the counterproductive stimulation of the renin-angiotensin system produced by diuretics.

Clinical trials have confirmed that these complementary properties are highly effective. In patients whose blood pressures have responded only partly to initial treatment with an ACE inhibitor, addition of even a very small dose of diuretic is more effective in reducing blood pressure than major increases in the dose of the ACE inhibitor.[25–27]

Of practical importance, the combination of a diuretic with an ACE inhibitor appears to be effective in as many African-American patients as in white patients.[24,28] This has strong clinical implications beyond blood pressure itself, as discussed elsewhere in this book. ACE inhibitors are now believed to have powerful renal and cardiovascular protective properties, and the thoughtful use of diuretic/ACE inhibitor combinations will make it possible for African-American patients, who are particularly vulnerable to hypertensive renal disease, to benefit from these target-organ actions.

Finally, it should be stressed again that only small doses of diuretics are required in this type of combination treatment. In fact, most currently available fixed-dose combinations of ACE inhibitors and diuretics employ a dose of 12.5 mg of hydrochlorothiazide. It is possible, too, that the ACE inhibitors and diuretics may have offsetting metabolic effects. These are discussed briefly later in this chapter.

It was recently demonstrated in a multicenter study of 6105 patients with a history of stroke or transient ischemic attack that the combination of the diuretic indapamide and the ACE inhibitor perindopril reduced the risk of stroke by one-third when compared to placebo or monotherapy.[29] One out of 10 stroke survivors given the combination therapy avoided death, heart attack, or further stroke even without a history of hypertension.

Combination of Diuretics with Angiotensin Receptor Antagonists

Most of the theory underlying the successful pairing of diuretics with ACE inhibitors should also apply to diuretics with angiotensin-receptor antagonists.[30] Available agents work by selectively block-ing the angiotensin II receptor (AT_1), thereby interrupting most of the known hemodynamic, endocrine, and growth effects of the renin-angiotensin system.

Clinical trials with losartan have shown that the addition of hydrochlorothiazide in a dose of 12.5 mg can increase the antihypertensive response rate from approximately 50% to almost 80%.[31] Clearly, the effects of the AT_1 blocker and the diuretic in combination are additive. An example of this efficacy is shown in Table 21-2.[32] These data show that the addition of 12.5 mg of hydrochlorothiazide in patients receiving either placebo or a variety of losartan dosing regimens produces consistent beneficial effects. Indeed, the blood pressure decrements observed when the diuretic is added to the losartan treatments are virtually identical to those observed when the diuretic is added to placebo—suggesting that these two drugs have a true additive effect when given in combination. A very low dose of 6.25 mg of hydrochlorothiazide in combination with losartan was tested in only one study, and the results indicated that this dose may not be adequate to optimize efficacy.[31]

In clinical trials in patients with essential hypertension, adding hydrochlorothiazide 12.5 or 25 mg/day to valsartan 80 mg/day resulted in a greater blood pressure reduction than increasing the valsartan dose to 160 mg/day. Similarly, in African-American hypertensives, adding 12.5 mg of hydrochlorothiazide to valsartan 160 mg/day resulted in substantially greater blood pressure reduction than that achieved by increasing valsartan from 160 to 320 mg/day or by adding benazepril 20 mg/day.[32a] Efficacy of the valsartan/hydrochlorothiazide combination was maintained up to 3 years of treatment.[33] Similar findings have been observed with other diuretic AT_1 blocker combinations (i.e., hydrochlorothiazide/irbesartan, hydrochlorothiazide/telmisartan, hydrochlorothiazide/candesartan).[33a]

Combination of Diuretics with Beta Blockers

The combination of diuretics with beta blockers is highly efficacious and shares mechanisms in common with the ACE inhibitor/diuretic combinations. Earlier we discussed the combination of hydrochlorothiazide with metoprolol, pointing it out as an example of a synergistic relationship between two agents. Although illustrative, that particular example may not be typical of more modern diuretic usage, where doses are lower and stimulation of the renin system is less extreme. Beta blockers, as monotherapy, appear to be effective often in white patients and the young, although they can be effective in older patients as well.[34] These

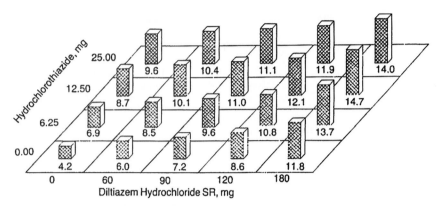

FIGURE 21-4. Estimated mean supine diastolic blood pressure reduction (in millimeters of mercury) in response to therapy. Each dose was administered twice a day. SR indicates slow-release. (*Reproduced with permission from Burris et al.*[45])

agents, however, do not appear to be very effective in low-renin hypertension. In fact, we have previously noted a paradoxical increase in blood pressure in low-renin patients treated with propranolol, perhaps reflecting the unmasking of vasoconstrictor, alpha-adrenergic activity resulting from the blockade of beta-receptors.[35]

Because beta blockers were introduced into widespread clinical use several years before the ACE inhibitors, most of the experience with beta blocker/diuretic combinations, especially fixed combinations, had been with relatively higher diuretic doses. Typically, hydrochlorothiazide was used in 25-mg doses. There is one unique and exciting recent exception to this rule: the fixed combination of a very low dose of the beta blocker bisoprolol with a dose of only 6.25 mg of hydrochlorothiazide. The implications of this special case are discussed later in this chapter.

Combination of Diuretics with Calcium-Channel Blockers

Unlike the ACE inhibitors and the beta blockers, the calcium-channel blockers have been theorized to be poor choices for combination with a diuretic. Since both the calcium-channel blockers and diuretics are thought to work best in similar populations, such as the elderly and African Americans, and to be most effective in low-renin hypertension, they might be too similar to provide additive effects. Acute administration of calcium-channel blockers has also been shown to produce measurable natriuresis, further suggesting that these two classes would not have complementary actions. Experience with different states of sodium loading has reinforced these prejudices. Dietary sodium restriction may attenuate the antihypertensive efficacy of calcium-channel blocker monotherapy, whereas sodium loading may actually enhance it.[36,37] In experimental rat models, sodium loading has been shown to increase the number of dihydropyridine receptors on cell membranes[38]; under these circumstances, the calcium-channel blockers appear to have increased effectiveness in limiting sympathetic stimulation.[39]

However, in practice, the combination of calcium-channel blockers and diuretics has worked very well in the clinical setting. All three major types of calcium-channel blockers currently available—verapamil, diltiazem, and the dihydropyridines—have been shown to produce additive effects when combined with a diuretic.[40–42] Indeed, some authors have shown that the addition of a calcium-channel blocker to a diuretic produces antihypertensive effects similar in amplitude to those observed when either beta blockers[43] or ACE inhibitors[44] were added to a diuretic.

Some of the pivotal studies of the effects of combining calcium-channel blockers and diuretics employed an innovative study design; the efficacies of a matrix of differing calcium-channel blocker and diuretic doses were compared with each other and with placebo so as to define the optimal composition of the combinations. The results of a study using this factorial design to evaluate diltiazem and hydrochlorothiazide are shown in Fig. 21-4.[45] Each of the drugs is more efficacious than placebo, and it is clear that their effects are additive when used in combination. It is also interesting that the low 6.25-mg diuretic dose contributes usefully to the combined effect, especially when used with the higher doses of diltiazem.[45] Documentation of the dose-response relationships of the drugs and their combinations can be accomplished by a response surface analysis, which is shown in Fig. 21-5.

Combination of Diuretics with Sympatholytics

A relatively large array of antihypertensive drugs, especially in the earlier days of antihypertensive drug development, was targeted primarily at the sympathetic nervous system. Some, such as clonidine and alpha-methyldopa, worked centrally to reduce sympathetic outflow. These agents could be effective as monotherapy but were more efficacious when combined with a diuretic.[46] Newer members of this class, most recently guanfacine, are actually designed to supplement a diuretic. Sympatholytic agents with more peripheral sites of action, including reserpine and guanethidine, benefited similarly from working in combination with a diuretic. It should be remembered that most of these drugs were developed, and became popular, during the era when the stepped-care approach was the standard and when the therapy of most hypertensive patients started with a diuretic. Alpha-methyldopa, clonidine, and reserpine, among others, were formulated in fixed combinations with diuretics as well as being available as monotherapies. The newer, selective alpha$_1$ blockers—notably prazosin, terazosin, and doxazosin—can also have their efficacy enhanced when combined with a diuretic agent.

Combination of Two Diuretics

It is rarely necessary to prescribe two diuretics at one time. This need usually occurs in the presence of renal insufficiency where refractory fluid retention might not respond adequately to usual or higher doses of a single diuretic. Under those circumstances, a loop diuretic or an agent such as metolazone might be combined with one of the more conventional thiazides.[46a]

The use of the combination of hydrochlorothiazide with the potassium-sparing diuretics triamterene, spironolactone, and amiloride has become ubiquitous. The two most common

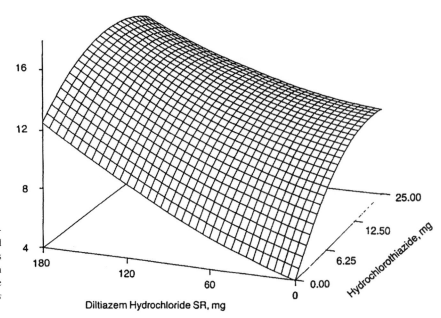

FIGURE 21-5. Response surface analysis of diastolic blood pressure in response to combination and monotherapy that demonstrates dose-relationships for hydrochlorothiazide and slow-release diltiazem hydrochloride. Each dose was administered twice a day. (*Reproduced with permission from Burris et al.*[45])

proprietary diuretic formulations in wide use are dyazide, which contains hydrochlorothiazide 25 mg and triamterene 50 mg; and maxzide, which contains hydrochlorothiazide 50 mg and triamterene 75 mg. Dyazide is provided as a capsule, whereas maxzide comes as a tablet that can be halved for a lesser dose. These products are so well accepted that they are, in effect, often considered to be single entities. The confidence of physicians in these formulations may be well placed, for there has been recent evidence that diuretics that are not combined with a potassium-sparing component may be associated with an increased risk of sudden cardiac death in hypertensive patients.[47]

OTHER ANTIHYPERTENSIVE COMBINATIONS

There is almost no limit to the number of ways in which different drug classes and individual agents can be combined effectively in the management of hypertension. Some of the more interesting examples of such combinations are considered below.

Hydralazine, the direct-acting vasodilator, is effective during chronic treatment almost only when used as part of a combination. Although it is a powerful arterial vasodilator, this drug stimulates two powerful reactive mechanisms: it produces marked fluid retention and it causes tachycardia, renin release, and other evidence of sympathetic activation. Therefore, for hydralazine to work effectively, it must be combined both with a diuretic and with a sympatholytic agent. For this reason, the stepped-care approach had always listed hydralazine as a third-step drug; it would be futile to administer it without a diuretic and sympatholytic drug already in place. Interestingly, the historical three-part fixed-dose combination SerApEs contained all three of these components: hydrochlorothiazide, reserpine, and hydralazine. This product is no longer available.

The newer drug classes have prompted innovative new combinations, and pharmaceutical manufacturers have been studying formulations pairing two nondiuretic drugs. Three current combination formulations are worth exploring. The first combines calcium-channel blockers with beta blockers. Since they have complementary actions, at least in terms of the patient demographics in which

they work best, beta blockers and calcium-channel blockers should work well together. One combination that already has completed pivotal early clinical trials couples felodipine, the calcium blocker, with metoprolol, the beta blocker. This product (brand name Logimax) is significantly more efficacious than either of its component drugs alone.[16,48] The data are shown in Fig. 21-6, indicating that decrements in both systolic and diastolic blood pressure are superior with the combination.

The development of Logimax highlights another issue in formulating fixed combinations: because each component drug is formulated to maximize its own constant delivery and duration of action, the marrying of the two agents requires rigorous engineering and testing to ensure that their essential pharmacokinetic properties are maintained.[49,50,50a]

The second nondiuretic combination to be discussed involves the coupling of a calcium-channel blocker with an ACE inhibitor. Fixed combinations of amlodipine and benazepril (Lotrel), verapamil and trandolapril (Tarka), felodipine ER and enalapril (Lexxel), and diltiazem and enalapril (Teczem) were released for hypertension therapy and are currently the only available nondiuretic, fixed-dose combination antihypertensives.[51-53] Their mechanistic logic is similar to that of an ACE inhibitor/diuretic combination. The calcium-channel blocker works best in low-renin hypertension as well as in a large percentage of African Americans and the elderly, and it appears to be effective in blocking actions of the sympathetic nervous system. The ACE inhibitor works best in high-renin hypertension, succeeds in a large percentage of white patients and the young, and is obviously effective at interrupting the renin-angiotensin system. Moreover, unlike a diuretic, the calcium-channel blocker should not cause any unwanted metabolic effects.[54,55] The effects of amlodipine alone, benazepril alone, their combination, and placebo have been compared in Fig. 21-7. The study employed ambulatory blood pressure monitoring and demonstrated that benazepril and amlodipine each provide consistent antihypertensive efficacy during the 24-h dosing interval. The combination clearly provides additive efficacy throughout the day.[56] The experience obtained during the development of this fixed-dose combination showed that its response rate, defined as either a reduction in diastolic blood pressure to less than 90 mm Hg or a fall of at

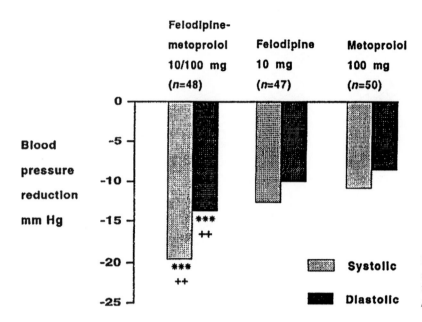

FIGURE 21-6. Mean supine systolic and diastolic blood pressure reductions after 12 weeks of treatment. [++]$P < .01$ vs. felodipine; [***]$P < .001$ vs. metoprolol. (*Reproduced with permission from Dahlof et al.*[48])

least 10 mm Hg, exceeded 80% in patients with mild-to-moderate hypertension.

The third combination, at first sight rather illogical, couples an ACE inhibitor with an angiotensin receptor antagonist. Since each of these agents appears to work primarily by interrupting the renin-angiotensin system, their effects should not be additive.[56a] Nevertheless, clinical trials with a combination of an ACE inhibitor and angiotensin receptor antagonist have been completed in patients with systolic and diastolic congestive heart failure, showing additive benefit,[57,58] and possibly will be expanded to include patients with hypertension.[59] In order to understand why these drugs might work well together, their respective actions must be delineated in more detail.

ACE inhibitors prevent the conversion of angiotensin I, which is functionally inactive, into angiotensin II, the effector hormone.

During chronic treatment with ACE inhibitors, however, it has been observed that plasma concentrations of angiotensin II, which are largely suppressed during the early stages of treatment, tend to rise toward their baseline values after several months. Despite this, the ACE inhibitors appear to retain much of their antihypertensive efficacy or, in the case of congestive heart failure, to sustain their beneficial hemodynamic and symptomatic effects and to reduce clinical events such as myocardial infarction. One possible explanation for this apparent discrepancy is that measurements of angiotensin II in the plasma are not an accurate reflection of the overall activity of angiotensin II at its sites of action within the circulation. Alternatively, ACE inhibitors are known to interrupt the action of the kininase enzyme that breaks down kinins; thus, ACE inhibitor treatment results in increased concentrations of bradykinin. Bradykinin has vasodilatory properties and also stimulates endothelial nitric oxide, which

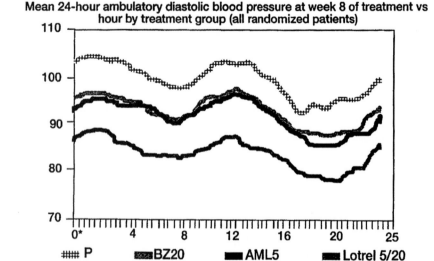

FIGURE 21-7. Whole-day ambulatory diastolic pressures during treatment with placebo, amlodipine, benazepril, or Lotrel in patients with mild-to-moderate hypertension. (*Reproduced from Ciba Geigy.*[66a])

TABLE 21-3. Multifactorial Trial with Bisoprolol, Hydrochlorothiazide, Placebo, and Combination: Mean Reduction (in mm Hg) from Baseline Sitting Diastolic Blood Pressure at 3 to 4 Weeks*

HCTZ,[†] mg/day	Bisoprolol, mg/day			
	0	2.5	10	40
0	3.8	8.4	10.9	12.6
6.25	6.4	10.8	13.4	15.2
25	8.4	12.9	15.4	17.2

*Entry criteria: sitting diastolic blood pressure 95 to 115 mm Hg.

[†]Hydrochlorothiazide.

Source: Reproduced with permission from Frishman et al.[61]

itself has vasodilatory and antigrowth properties. This stimulation of the bradykinin pathway may be a crucial part of the ACE inhibitor's efficacy.

In contrast to the ACE inhibitors, angiotensin II antagonists produce powerful and sustained blockade of the effects of angiotensin II at its receptors. For this reason, it could be conjectured that ACE inhibitors, with their recruitment of kinin and nitric oxide mechanisms, and angiotensin antagonists, with their powerful blockade of the renin-angiotensin system, could produce additive cardiovascular effects.

COMBINATION THERAPY: REDUCTION IN SIDE EFFECTS

For many antihypertensive drugs there is a difference between their dose/efficacy relationships and their dose/adverse events relationships. In treating hypertension, the dose-response curve for efficacy often flattens early; low doses can achieve a large fraction of the potential maximum effect. On the other hand, adverse symptomatic complaints most often become a major problem with doses in the middle to upper end of the range. For this reason, low doses are attractive when they provide a moderate level of efficacy while minimizing unwanted effects. If two drugs have additive efficacies, then putting them together at low doses should produce a powerful therapeutic response without inducing adverse effects.

The FDA went so far as to publish an opinion on how this approach could be translated into new therapeutic formulations.[60] In particular, they argued that there could be a basis for approving a low-dose fixed combination for the initial treatment of hypertension. Previously, the FDA had indicated combinations as later-step therapy, only to be used after monotherapies had proved inadequate.

To make a first-step approach valid for fixed-dose combination therapy, the FDA required that the two drug components must be drawn from classes known to have a dose-dependent increase in side effects and where the use of very low doses could thus be anticipated to provide better-tolerated therapy. By this reasoning, combinations of diuretics and beta blockers would be appropriate; whereas combinations of ACE inhibitors and calcium-channel blockers, both of which generally do not have dose-dependent side effects, would not qualify. A second criterion for approving the low-dose fixed combination was that each of the drugs involved, when tested as monotherapy in its proposed combination dose, should exhibit efficacy that would not differ meaningfully from that of placebo. Thus, a clinically useful antihypertensive effect would be achieved only if the two drugs were used in combination.

Low-Dose Strategy for Reducing Side Effects

The most successful development of such a combination has been with hydrochlorothiazide, in a dose of 6.25 mg, and bisoprolol, the long-acting cardioselective beta blocker. This combination product has the trade name of Ziac. The data used to justify the approval of this agent are shown in Table 21-3.[61] It is evident that the combinations of the low-dose components produce meaningful decreases in blood pressure, whereas the individual components have only small effects.[62] The JNC-VI recommends a low-dose combination treatment as an alternative first-line approach to the management of hypertension.[63]

In a further study, this formulation was compared, in double-blind fashion, with full doses of the ACE inhibitor enalapril and the calcium channel blocker amlodipine.[64,65] The combination decreased blood pressure at least as well as the full-dose monotherapies. Even more important, especially in support of the underlying rationale for this type of formulation, mild and serious clinical adverse events tended to occur less commonly with Ziac than with the other agents. Quality-of-life measurements confirmed that the low-dose combination performed at least as well as enalapril or amlodipine.[65]

Pharmacologic Interactions That Reduce Side Effects

From a practical point of view, most of the adverse effects of antihypertensive treatment can be divided into two main groups: those that cause symptomatic complaints and those that produce metabolic abnormalities in clinical test results—most commonly routine biochemistries. However, during combination therapy, even with full drug doses, it is possible for one agent to modify the adverse metabolic effects produced by the other agent while at the same time contributing to overall antihypertensive efficacy.

One of the best examples of complementary metabolic effects is produced when ACE inhibitors are given together with diuretics. The diuretics are known to produce hypokalemia, hyperuricemia, hyperglycemia, and possibly increased plasma concentrations of LDL-cholesterol. However, concomitant administration of an ACE inhibitor will moderate these changes enough to obviate the need to discontinue diuretic therapy or to introduce additional treatments to manage the unwanted metabolic effects.[66] More recently, the angiotensin receptor antagonist losartan also was noted to modify the adverse metabolic consequences of treatment with hydrochlorothiazide.[32]

A good example of how one drug attenuates a clinical finding produced by another is given in Table 21-4. This study with the calcium-channel blocker amlodipine and the ACE inhibitor

TABLE 21-4. How Combined Formulations Attenuate the Adverse Effects Produced by Individual Drugs

Adverse Experience	Lotrel (n = 760)	Amlodipine (n = 475)	Benazepril (n = 554)	Placebo (n = 408)
Edema*	2.1	5.1[†]	0.9	2.2
Cough	3.3[‡]	0.4	1.8	0.2
Headache	2.2	2.9	3.8	5.6[§]
Dizziness	1.3	2.3	1.6	1.5

*Edema refers to all edema, such as dependent edema, angioedema, facial edema. Adverse experiences not statisitcally significant unless noted.

[†]Statistically significant difference between Lotrel and amlodipine ($P < .01$).

[‡]Statistically significant difference between Lotrel and amlodipine and between Lotrel and placebo ($P < .001$).

[§]Statistically significant difference between Lotrel and placebo ($P < .01$).

Source: Reproduced from Ciba-Geigy,[66a] data on file.

benazepril examined their individual and combined effects on common adverse experiences, most importantly edema.[66a] It is well known that calcium-channel blockers can produce peripheral edema, which for some patients—most frequently women—can be bothersome. It is evident from these data, however, that when patients receive Lotrel, the fixed combination of amlodipine with benazepril, the frequency of edema is no different from that observed with placebo. The ACE inhibitor prevents the edema produced by the calcium-channel blocker. The best explanation for this finding is that calcium-channel blockers may produce edema because they primarily dilate the arterial side of the circulation. They have relatively minimal venous effects, thereby allowing plasma to pool peripherally. ACE inhibitors dilate both the arterial and venous circulations and thus are able to facilitate the central return of peripheral fluid accumulation. It is interesting, therefore, that the combination of a calcium-channel blocker with an ACE inhibitor not only enhances efficacy but also has an beneficial effect on the side-effect profile.[67,67a]

COMBINATION TREATMENT: CONVENIENCE AND INCONVENIENCE

Persuading patients to continue taking their antihypertensive medications on a long-term basis is one of the more difficult tasks in clinical medicine. Compliance with treatment tends to be poor and nearly 50% of patients started on drug therapy are lost to follow-up within a year. Explanations for this poor outcome include inadequate instructions to the patient, denial and other psychological responses, the side effects of the drugs, the cost of the drugs, and the burden of taking medications on a regular basis—often multiple drugs multiple times a day.

Combination treatment of hypertension, especially where more than two drugs are concerned, might easily have a deleterious effect on patient compliance. Clearly, such an approach may add to cost, complexity, and the likelihood of side effects. Patients find it discouraging to be dependent on this type of regimen when they may not have been taking any medications previously.

Fixed combinations potentially have some advantages. If efficacy can be achieved by two agents that happen to be part of a standard combined formulation, it is possible that this formulation alone might provide a satisfactory remedy for the hypertension. Combinations that pair an ACE inhibitor or a beta blocker with a diuretic appear to be efficacious in a majority of patients. More innovative products, including the low-dose formulation of bisoprolol with

hydrochlorothiazide, the calcium-channel blocker/ACE inhibitor combinations, and the formulation of metoprolol ER and felodipine ER might be yet further examples of approaches that could enhance treatment compliance. The instructions for using the newly available angiotensin antagonists (losartan, irbesartan, telmisartan, valsartan, olmesartan, candesartan, eprosartan) also exploit this approach. It is suggested that physicians start treatment with a single 50-mg dose of losartan; if this does not adequately control blood pressure, the recommendation is to switch immediately to the losartan/diuretic combination hyzaar. The goal is to facilitate efficacy without intimidating the patient with multiple monotherapy titration steps or with a need for multiple drugs. Finally, manufacturers of the fixed combinations have understood that one of the advantages of these formulations is that they can be priced competitively and be made available at a cost only minimally higher than that of the primary monotherapy.

EFFECTS ON DURATION OF ACTION

During the development of new antihypertensive agents or formulations, it is necessary to study pharmacokinetic interactions between the new drug and other drugs that might be used in the same patients. In general, drug-drug interactions among the antihypertensive classes are relatively minimal, and there has been no compelling need to alter doses or frequency of administration of the commonly prescribed agents.

This does not preclude the possibility that coadministration of two agents might sufficiently affect their biological duration of action to justify altering their clinical use. The short-acting ACE inhibitor captopril is a notable example. This drug typically must be given two or three times daily as monotherapy, but adding hydrochlorothiazide changes this. Ambulatory blood pressure recordings obtained during 24-h monitoring periods with this combination are shown in Fig. 21-8. Compared with placebo, the captopril/hydrochlorothiazide combination produced sustained reduction of blood pressure throughout the 24-h dosing interval when administered once daily. Like Ziac, the formulation has been approved as a first-line combination therapy.[2] There was slightly greater efficacy with twice daily administration, but it is clear that this combination, despite captopril's short duration of action, can provide true day-long efficacy.[68] Indeed, if data in this study are considered only from those patients who were effective responders to the therapy, there is virtually no difference between once-daily and twice-daily treatment (Fig. 21-9).

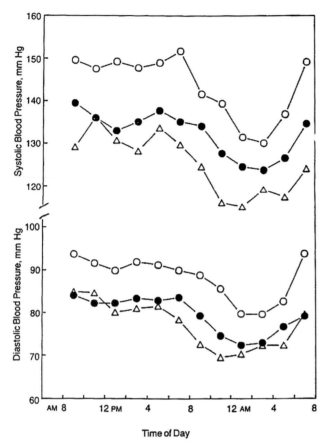

FIGURE 21-8. Whole-day systolic and diastolic blood pressures of subjects receiving placebo (open circles) and during once-daily (solid circles; $n = 13$) and twice-daily (triangles) therapy with captopril and hydrochlorothiazide. The total daily dose of captopril was 50 mg and of hydrochlorothiazide 15 mg throughout the study for all patients included in this figure. (*Reproduced with permission from Cheung et al.*[68])

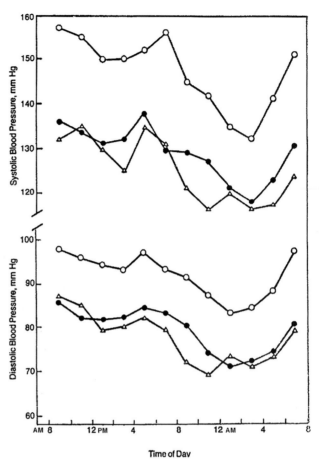

FIGURE 21-9. Whole-day systolic and diastolic mean blood pressures of treatment-responsive subjects receiving placebo (open circles) and during once-daily (solid circles; $n = 12$) and twice-daily (triangles; $n = 12$) therapy with captopril and hydrochlorothiazide. (*Reproduced with permission from Cheung et al.*[68])

The mechanism of this prolonged effect is not clear, but it is possible that captopril retains sufficient ACE-inhibitory capacity, even in its low serum levels toward the end of the dosing interval, to moderate the diuretic-related stimulation of the renin-angiotensin system. In response to research with this combination, the FDA has granted once-daily labeling for the fixed combination of captopril with hydrochlorothiazide.

Another attempt to exploit this type of relationship was far less successful. A collaboration between the manufacturers of captopril and the calcium-channel blocker diltiazem, was undertaken to evaluate the efficacy of a fixed combination of the two drugs. At the time this venture was undertaken, diltiazem was still made only in its original, immediate-release, short-acting formulation and was typically administered three times daily. There was hope of an interaction between these two short-acting agents that might make their combination effective when administered just once daily. But study results did not support this expectation. Although the formal findings were not published in the medical literature, preliminary data on the efficacy of the combination, as judged by blood pressure reduction at the end of the 24-h dosing interval, demonstrated no differences between combination therapy and monotherapy. Of course, this failure of the combination to demonstrate either pharmacokinetic or clinical advantages does not detract from the logic of an ACE inhibitor/calcium-channel blocker combination. As

discussed earlier, the combined use of long-acting ACE inhibitors and calcium-channel blockers offers an example of how this approach to combination therapy can be highly effective.

ADDITIVE VASCULOPROTECTIVE ACTIONS

The chief goals of antihypertensive therapy include preventing coronary events (infarction, arrhythmia, angina), major cardiovascular episodes, and strokes. Although controlling the blood pressure and reducing other known cardiovascular risk factors are pivotal in achieving these goals, additional strategies also are needed to provide optimal protection against cardiovascular disease. A variety of endocrine and paracrine factors—including the renin-angiotensin system, the sympathetic nervous system, and endothelin as well as other proteins and substances having effects on vascular growth and function—have become the targets of therapeutic intervention.

Both the ACE inhibitors and the calcium-channel blockers have been shown to have strong vasoprotective actions in animal models of atherosclerosis. It is likely that other drug classes, already available or in development, will also perform in this fashion. It is not yet proven that data from the laboratory will translate into human clinical benefits, but already a number of studies have reported significant reductions in myocardial infarctions when patients with a variety of cardiovascular conditions were treated with ACE inhibitors.[29,69–71] Calcium-channel blockers can also exhibit antiatherosclerotic effects in humans, although recent controversies involving the short-acting agents nifedipine and isradipine have raised clinical questions. Experiences with newer, long-acting agents appear more promising.

If each of these drug classes has apparent beneficial actions on the vascular wall, is it possible that their use in combination could provide an additional measure of atherosclerosis prevention? In the same way that combining drugs from two classes produces additive antihypertensive actions, could they also produce additive effects within vascular tissue? There are now clinical data available demonstrating that combination therapies might produce clinical effects that outweigh those produced with single-agent treatment.[29,57,58]

DUAL-ACTING MOLECULES

Traditionally we have regarded combination therapy as the concomitant use of two or more separate agents. But we have learned that there are some molecules that can produce two separate actions, each of which can complement the other. Currently there are at least two such agents, labetalol and carvedilol, that have been approved for the treatment of hypertension.

Labetalol is a molecule that possesses both alpha- and beta-adrenergic blocking properties. As described earlier, beta blockade is an effective approach to blood pressure reduction, and agents with this property work particularly well in white patients, the young, and hypertensives with higher plasma renin values. Alpha blockers are efficacious across all age groups and in African-American patients. For this reason, the alpha/beta blocker labetalol has been found to be efficacious in similar numbers of both white and African-American patients, whereas the beta blocker propranolol tends to be most effective in white patients.[72] Of more interest, beta-blocker monotherapy produces a somewhat adverse effect on the lipid profile, decreasing plasma concentrations of HDL cholesterol. In contrast, alpha blockers have a slightly beneficial effect on the lipid profile. During treatment with labetalol, these offsetting actions result in a neutral effect on lipid measurements.[73] Thus, this single molecule provides complementary benefits of alpha and beta blockade on both blood pressure reduction and adverse outcomes.

Carvedilol similarly has beta- and alpha-blocking activity. Its clinical effects are weighted more toward the alpha-blocking effect, and the drug appears to produce vasodilatory actions. Like labetalol, this newer agent provides antihypertensive efficacy across all ages, including the elderly, and all racial groups. Moreover, it has clear antianginal properties.[74] Of note, carvedilol appears to provide hemodynamic benefits in patients with congestive heart failure, and it may decrease the incidence of new cardiovascular events in these patients.[75–77]

Other innovative molecules are currently in development. One of the most visible of these are molecule entities that have been engineered to provide inhibitory effects on neutral endopeptidase (NEP) activity and also to function as ACE inhibitors (e.g., omapatrilat).[78] The NEP-inhibitory action allows this molecule to interrupt the breakdown of endogenous atrial natriuretic factor (ANF). Since ANF has vasodilatory properties and also increases renal sodium and water clearance, NEP inhibition might be a useful treatment both for hypertension and congestive heart failure. However, ANF seems to be most effective in low-renin states. Thus, again, an NEP

inhibitor and an ACE inhibitor in combination might be anticipated to have additive and complementary actions. The NEP/ACE inhibitor is designed such that the NEP-inhibitory action is carried at one end of the molecule, whereas the ACE inhibitory action is carried at the other. Is this a single agent with true dual actions, or is it simply a clever way of bringing together two separate entities as a hybrid structure? Studies to date do not support a greater advantage from omapatrilat use compared to ACE inhibitor therapy.[79]

REFERENCES

1. Ruzicka M, Leenen FHH: Monotherapy versus combination therapy as first-line treatment of uncomplicated arterial hypertension. *Drugs* 61:943, 2001.
2. Moser M, Black HR: The role of combination therapy in the treatment of hypertension. *Am J Hypertens* 11:73S, 1998.
3. Messerli FH, Chander K: Cardiac effects of combination therapy in hypertension. *J Cardiovasc Pharmacol* 35(Suppl 3):S17, 2000.
4. Neutel JM, Smith DHG, Weber MA: Low-dose combination therapy: An important first-line treatment in the management of hypertension. *Am J Hypertens* 14:286, 2001.
4a. Sica DA: Rationale for fixed-dose combinations in the treatment of hypertension: The cycle repeats. *Drugs* 62:443, 2002.
5. Hanson L, Zanchetti A, Carruthers SC, et al: Effects of intensive blood-pressure lowering and low dose aspirin in patients with hypertension: Principal results of the Hypertension Optimal Treatment (HOT) randomized trial. HOT Study Group. *Lancet* 351:1755, 1998.
6. United Kingdom Prospective Diabetes Study Group: Tight blood pressure control and risk of macrovascular and microvascular complications in type 2 diabetes: UKPDS 38. *BMJ* 317:703, 1998.
7. Klahr S, Levey AS, Beck GJ, et al: The effects of dietary protein restriction and blood-pressure control on the progression of chronic renal disease. Modification of Diet in Renal Disease Study Group. *N Engl J Med* 330:877, 1994.
8. Zanchetti A, Hansson L: Introduction: The role of combination therapy in modern antihypertensive therapy. *J Cardiovasc Pharmacol* 35(Suppl 3): S1, 2000.
9. Guidelines Subcommittee 1999 World Health Organization-International Society of Hypertension Guidelines for the management of hypertension. *J Hypertens* 17:151, 1999.
10. Colhoun HM, Dong W, Poulter NR: Blood pressure screening, management and control in England: Results from the Healthy Survey for england 1994. *J Hypertens* 16:747, 1998.
11. Agodoa L, Appel L, Bakris G, et al: Effect of ramipril vs amlodipine on renal outcomes in hypertensive nephrosclerosis. A randomized controlled trial. *JAMA* 285:2719, 2001.
12. Freis ED: Historical development of antihypertensive treatment. In: Laragh JH, Brenner, BM eds. *Hypertension: Pathophysiology, Diagnosis and Management,* 2nd ed. New York: Raven Press, 1995:2741.
13. Laragh JH: Vasoconstriction—volume analysis for understanding and treating hypertension: The use of renin and aldosterone profiles. *Am J Med* 55:261, 1973.
14. Joint National Committee: The Fourth Report of the Joint National Committee on Detection, Evaluation and Treatment of High Blood Pressure (JNC IV). *Arch Intern Med* 148:1023, 1988.
15. Burt VL, Whelton P, Roccella EJ, et al: Prevalence of hypertension in the US adult population. Results from the Third National Health and Nutrition Examination Survey: 1988–1991. *Hypertension* 25:305, 1995.
16. Haria M, Plosker GL, Markham A: Felodipine/metoprolol. A review of the fixed dose controlled release formulation in the management of essential hypertension. *Drugs* 59:141, 2000.
17. Dooley M, Goa KL: Fixed combination verapamil SR/trandolapril. *Drugs* 56:837, 1998.
18. Weir MR: Effects of low dose combination therapy with amlodipine/benazepril on systolic blood pressure. *Cardiovasc Rev Rep* 20:368, 1999.
19. Weber MA, Priest RT, Ricci BA, et al: Low-dose diuretic and a beta-adrenoceptor blocker in essential hypertension. *Clin Pharmacol Ther* 28:149, 1980.

20. Weber MA, Drayer JIM, Laragh JH: The effects of clonidine and propranolol separately and in combination, on blood pressure and plasma renin activity in essential hypertension. *J Clin Pharmacol* 18:233, 1978.

21. Hollifield JW, Sherman K, Slaton P: Age, race and sex as a determinant of successful antihypertensive therapy. *Prev Med* 7:88, 1978.

22. SHEP Investigators: Prevention of stroke by antihypertensive drug treatment in older persons with isolated systolic hypertension: Final results of the Systolic Hypertension in the Elderly Program (SHEP). *JAMA* 265:3255, 1991.

23. Postman CT, Dennesen PJW, deBoo T, Thien T: First dose hypotension after captopril; can it be predicted? A study of 240 patients. *J Hum Hypertens* 6:205, 1992.

24. Saunders E. Weir MR, Kong BW, et al: A comparison of the efficacy and safety of a β-blocker, a calcium channel blocker, and a converting enzyme inhibitor in hypertensive blacks. *Arch Intern Med* 150:1707, 1990.

25. Townsend RR, Holland OB: Combination of converting enzyme inhibitor with diuretic for the treatment of hypertension. *Arch Intern Med* 150:1175, 1990.

26. Andren L, Weiner L, Svensson A, Hansson L: Enalapril with either a "very low" or "low" dose of hydrochlorothiazide is equally effective in essential hypertension. A double-blind trial in 100 hypertensive patients. *J Hypertens* 1:384, 1983.

27. Wyndham RN, Gimenez L, Walker WF, et al: Influence of renin levels on the treatment of essential hypertension with thiazide diuretics. *Arch Intern Med* 147:1021, 1987.

28. Radevski IV, Valtchanova ZP, Candy GP, et al: Antihypertensive effect of low-dose hydrochlorothiazide alone or in combination with quinapril in black patients with mild to moderate hypertension. *J Clin Pharmacol* 40:713, 2000.

29. PROGRESS Collaborative Group: Randomised trial of a perindopril-based blood-pressure-lowering regimen among 6105 individuals with previous stroke or transient ischaemic attack. *Lancet* 358:1033, 2001.

30. Oparil Z, Aurup P, Snavely D, Goldberg A: Efficacy and safety of losartan/hydrochlorothiazide in patients with severe hypertension. *Am J Cardiol* 87:721, 2001.

31. Mackay JH, Arcuri KE, Goldberg Al, et al: Losartan and low dose hydrochlorothiazide in patients with essential hypertension. *Arch Intern Med* 156:278, 1996.

32. Weber MA, Byyny RL, Pratt JH, et al: Blood pressure effects of the angiotensin II receptor blocker losartan. *Arch Intern Med* 155:405, 1995.

32a. Weir MR, Smith DH, Neutel JM, Bedigian MP: Valsartan alone or with a diuretic or ACE inhibitor as treatment for African American hypertensives: Relation to salt intake. *Am J Hypertens* 14:665, 2001.

33. Langtry HD, McClellan KJ: Valsartan/hydrochlorothiazide. *Drugs* 57:751, 1999.

33a. Melian EB, Jarvis B: Candesartan cilexetil plus hydrochlorothiazide combination. *Drugs* 62:787, 2002.

34. Materson BJ, Reda DJ, Cushman WC, et al: A comparison of six antihypertensive agents with placebo. *N Engl J Med* 328:914, 1993.

35. Drayer JI, Keim HJ, Weber MA, et al: Unexpected pressor responses to propranolol in essential hypertension. An interaction between renin, aldosterone and sympathetic activity. *Am J Med* 60:897, 1976.

36. Nicholson JP, Resnick LM, Laragh JH: The antihypertensive effect of verapamil at extremes of dietary sodium intake. *Ann Intern Med* 107:329, 1987.

37. Luft FC, Fineberg NS, Weinberger MH: Long-term effect of nifedipine on blood pressure and sodium homeostasis at varying levels of salt intake in mildly hypertensive patients. *Am J Hypertens* 4:752, 1991.

38. Garthoff B, Bellemann P: Effects of salt loading and nitrendipine on dihydropyridine receptors in hypertensive receptors in hypertensive rats. *J Cardiovasc Pharmacol* 10:S36, 1987.

39. Leenen FHH, Yuan B: Dietary sodium and the antihypertensive effect of nifedipine in spontaneously hypertensive rats. *Am J Hypertens* 5:515, 1992.

40. Weber MA: Prolonged calcium channel blocker therapy of hypertension. *J Cardiovasc Pharmacol* 12(Suppl 4):S16, 1988.

41. Franklin SS, Weir MR, Smith DHG, et al: Combination treatment with sustained release verapamil and indapamide in the treatment of mild-to-moderate hypertension. *Am J Ther* 3:506, 1996.

42. Weir MR, Weber MA, Punzi HA, et al: A dose escalation trial comparing the combination of diltiazem SR with the monotherapies in patients with essential hypertension. *J Hum Hypertens* 6:1, 1992.

43. Thulin T, Hedner T, Gustaffsson S, Olsson S-O: Diltiazem compared with metoprolol as add-on-therapies to diuretics in hypertension. *J Hum Hypertens* 5:107, 1991.

44. Elliott WJ, Polascik TB, Murphy MB: Equivalent antihypertensive effects of combination therapy using diuretic + calcium antagonist compared with diuretic + ACE inhibitor. *J Hum Hypertens* 4:717, 1990.

45. Burris JF, Weir MR, Oparil S, et al: An assessment of diltiazem and hydrochlorothiazide in hypertension. Application of factorial trial design to a multicenter clinical trial of combination therapy. *JAMA* 263:1507, 1990.

46. Weber MA: Clinical pharmacology of centrally active antihypertensive agents. *J Clin Pharmacol* 29:598, 1989.

46a. Sica DA, Gehr TW: Diuretic combinations in refractory oedema states: Pharmacokinetic-pharmaco-dynamic relationships. *Clin Pharmacokin* 30:229, 1996.

47. Hoes AW, Grobbee DE, Lubsen J, et al: Diuretics, β blockers, and the risk for sudden cardiac death in hypertensive patients. *Arch Intern Med* 123:481, 1995.

48. Dahlof B, Hosie J on behalf of the Swedish/UK Study Group: Antihypertensive efficacy and tolerability of a new once-daily felodipine-metoprolol combination compared with each component alone. *Blood Pressure* 2(Suppl 1):22, 1993.

49. Abrahamsson B, Edgar B, Lidman K, Wingstrand K: Design and pharmacokinetics of Logimax, a new extended release combination tablet of felodipine and metoprolol. *Blood Pressure* 2(Suppl):10, 1993.

50. Waeber B, Detry JM, Dahlof B, et al: Felodipine-metoprolol combination tablet: A valuable option to initiate antihypertensive therapy? *Am J Hypertens* 12:915, 1999.

50a. Zannad F, Boivin JM: Ambulatory 24-h blood pressure assessment of the felodipine-metoprolol combination versus amlodipine in mild to moderate hypertension. Lorraine General Hospital Physician Investigators Group. *J Hypertens* 17:1023, 1999.

51. DeQuattro V, Lee D, and the Trandolapril Study Group: Fixed-dose combination therapy with trandolapril and verapamil SR is effective in primary hypertension. *Am J Hypertens* 10(7 Pt 2):138S, 1997.

52. Mancia G, Omboni S, Grassi G: Combination treatment in hypertension: The VeraTran Study. *Am J Hypertens* 10(7 Pt 2):153S, 1997.

53. Elliott WJ, Montoro R, Smith D, et al for the LEVEL (Lexxel vs enalapril) Study Group: Comparison of two strategies for intensifying antihypertensive treatment. Low-dose combination (enalapril + felodipine ER) versus increased dose of monotherapy (enalapril). *Am J Hypertens* 12:691, 1999.

54. Gheinfeld GR, Bakris GL: Benefits of combination angiotensin-converting enzyme inhibitor and calcium antagonist therapy for diabetic patients. *Am J Hypertens* 12:80S, 1999.

55. Messerli FH: Combinations in the treatment of hypertension: ACE inhibitors and calcium antagonists. *Am J Hypertens* 12:86S, 1999.

56. Kuschnir E, Acuna E, Sevilla D, et al: Treatment of patients with essential hypertension: Amlodipine 5 mg/benazepril 20 mg compared with amlodipine 5 mg, benazepril 20 mg and placebo. *Clin Ther* 18:1213, 1996.

56a. Sica DA, Elliott WJ: Angiotensin converting enzyme inhibitors and angiotensin receptor blockers in combination: Theory and practice. *J Clin Hypertens*. 3:383, 2001.

57. Cohn JN, Tognoni G, for the Valsartan Heart failure Trial Investigators: A randomized trial of the angiotensin-receptor blocker valsartan in chronic heart failure. *N Engl J Med* 345:1667, 2001.

58. Hamroff G, Katz SD, Mancini D, et al: Addition of angiotensin II receptor blockade to maximal angiotensin converting enzyme inhibition improves exercise capacity in patients with severe congestive heart failure. *Circulation* 99(8):990–992, 1999.

59. Stergiou GS, Skeva II, Baibas NM, et al: Additive hypotensive effect of angiotensin-converting enzyme inhibition and angiotensin-receptor antagonism in essential hypertension. *J Cardiovasc Pharmacol* 35:937, 2000.

60. Fenichel RR, Lipicky RJ: Combination products as first-line pharmacotherapy. *Arch Intern Med* 54:1429, 1994.

61. Frishman WH, Bryzinski BS, Coulson LR, et al: A multifactorial trial design to assess combination therapy in hypertension: Treatment with bisoprolol and hydrochlorothiazide. *Arch Intern Med* 154:1461, 1994.

62. Neutel JM: Low-dose antihypertensive combination therapy: Its rationale and role in cardiovascular risk management. *Am J Hypertens* 12:73S, 1999.

63. Joint National Committee on Prevention, Detection, Evaluation and Treatment of High Blood Pressure: The Sixth Report of the JNC. *Arch Intern Med* 157:2413, 1997.

64. Prisant LM, Weir MR, Papademetriou V, et al: Low dose drug combination therapy: An alternative first line approach to hypertension treatment. *Am Heart J* 130:359, 1995.

65. Prisant LM, Neutel JM, Papademetriou V, et al: Low-dose combination treatment for hypertension versus single-drug treatment—bisoprolol/hydrochlorothiazide versus amlodipine, enalapril, and placebo: Combined analysis of comparative studies. *Am J Ther* 5:313, 1998.

66. Weinberger, NH: Influence of an angiotensin converting enzyme inhibitor on diuretic-induced metabolic effects in hypertension. *Hypertension* 5(Suppl. 3):132, 1983.

66a. Ciba Geigy: Data on file. Summit, NJ: Geneva Pharmaceuticals.

67. Kaplan NM: Low-dose combination therapy: The rationalization for an ACE inhibitor and a calcium channel blocker in higher risk patients. *Am J Hypertens* 14:8S, 2001.

67a. Messerli FH, Weir MR, Neutel JM: Combination therapy of amlodipine/benazepril versus monotherapy of amlodipine in a practice-based setting. *Am J Hypertens* 15:550, 2002.

68. Cheung DG, Gasster JL, Weber MA: Assessing the duration of the antihypertensive effect with whole-day automated blood pressure monitoring. *Arch Intern Med* 149:2021, 1989.

69. Pfeffer MA, Braunwald E, Moye LA, et al: Effect of captopril on mortality and morbidity in patients with left ventricular dysfunction after myocardial infarction. Results of the Survival and Ventricular Enlargement Trial (SAVE). *N Engl J Med* 327:669, 1992.

70. Cohn JN: The prevention of heart failure: A new agenda. *N Engl J Med* 327:725, 1992.

71. The Heart Outcomes Prevention Evaluation Study Investigators: Effects of an angiotensin-converting-enzyme inhibitor, ramipril, on cardiovascular events and stroke in high-risk patients. *N Engl J Med* 342:145, 2000.

72. Flamenbaum W, Weber MA, McMahon FG, et al: Monotherapy with labetalol compared with propranolol: Differential effects by race. *J Clin Hypertens* 1:56, 1985.

73. Weber MA, Drayer JIM, Kaufman CA: The combined alpha- and beta-adrenergic blocker, labetalol, and propranolol in the treatment of high blood pressure: Similarities and differences. *J Clin Pharmacol* 24:103, 1984.

74. Lessem JN, Weber MA. Antihypertensive treatment with a dual-acting beta-blocker in the elderly. *J Hypertens* 11(Suppl 4):S29, 1993.

75. Frishman WH: Carvedilol. *N Engl J Med* 339:1759, 1998.

76. Packer M, Coats AJS, Fowler MB, et al for the Carvedilol Prospective Randomized Cumulative Survival Study Group: Effect of carvedilol on survival in severe chronic heart failure. *N Engl J Med* 344:1651, 2001.

77. Dargie HJ: Design and methodology of the CAPRICORN trial—a randomised double-blind placebo-controlled study of the impact of carvedilol on morbidity and mortality in patients with left ventricular dysfunction after myocardial infarction. *Eur J Heart Failure* 2:325, 2000.

78. Nawarskas JJ, Anderson JR: Omapatrilat: A unique new agent for the treatment of cardiovascular disease. *Heart Dis* 2:266, 2000.

79. Packer M, Califf RM, Konstam MA, et al: Comparison of omapatrilat and enalapril in patients with chronic heart failure. The Omapatrilat Versus Enalapril Randomized Trial of Utility in Reducing Events (OVERTURE). *Circulation* 106:920, 2002.

CHAPTER 22

Tobacco Smoking, Nicotine, and Nicotine and Non-Nicotine Smoking Cessation Therapies

William H. Frishman

Tom Ky

Anjum Ismail

The history of tobacco smoking can be traced back to pre-Columbian America. When the early Spanish explorers reached the New World, their crew members learned how to use tobacco and later introduced it to Europe. There, Jean Nicot was an early importer and cultivator of a plant he called *Nicotiana tabacum* (after himself). Although known about since the end of the eighteenth century, the substance nicotine was first isolated from tobacco in 1828.[1] Nicotine in cigarette smoke is one of the major factors contributing to the increased cardiovascular risk associated with smoking and is probably the primary cause for tobacco addiction.[2] In this chapter, nicotine from cigarette smoke is discussed as a pharmacologic substance that can have adverse effects in patients with coronary artery disease (CAD). Various nicotine replacement strategies that may be used as therapeutic adjuncts in smoking cessation programs are reviewed as well.

ASSOCIATION OF SMOKING AND HEART DISEASE

The association between cigarette smoking and cardiovascular disease was first proposed in 1934, based on the observation of a sharp rise in the incidence of CAD among cigarette smokers after World War I.[2,3] The first major study strongly correlating smoking with an increased risk of cardiovascular disease was reported in 1958. The investigators described a 70% increase in risk of dying from CAD in smokers compared to nonsmokers.[4,5] Although tobacco smoke could not definitively be shown to be the cause of the increased coronary risk, the evidence was suggestive enough to warrant the first antismoking countermeasures in the 1964 *Surgeon General's Report*.[6] By 1979, that report suggested a definite association between smoking and CAD.[7]

Cigarette and cigar smoking has been shown to accelerate the development of atherosclerotic vascular diseases and can greatly increase the risk of acute coronary events, particularly sudden death.[8–12] Smoking has also been shown to increase the risk of death in patients with left ventricular dysfunction.[12a,12b] Likely mechanisms contributing to the life-threatening effects of smoking are increased sympathetic outflow and heightened activation of the blood coagulation system.[13–17] The blood of cigarette smokers coagulates more readily[18]: platelet aggregability is increased, platelet survival time is decreased, and the bleeding time is shortened.[19,20] The increased risk of platelet thrombus formation with smoking is not prevented by aspirin therapy.[21] Natural fibrinolytic potential is impaired among smokers, as demonstrated by impaired plasminogen activator release.[22] Cigarette smoke can impair endothelium-dependent modulation of vascular tone by inhibiting nitric oxide bioactivity, thereby fostering vasospasm and thrombogenesis.[23,24] Smoking can interfere with the body's own antioxidant defense mechanisms.[25] Cigarette smoking can decrease blood flow in stenosed coronary arteries with or without vasospasm,[26] potentiating endothelial dysfunction in patients with hypercholesterolemia.[27] Quillen and Rossen, using computerized quantitative angiography and intracoronary flow measurements, showed that cigarette smoking constricts both epicardial coronary arteries and myocardial resistance vessels.[28] Almost all cocaine-induced myocardial ischemic events have been seen in cigarette smokers.[29,30] Cigarette smoking can impair the pharmacologic actions of both thyroid hormone[31] and various antianginal drug therapies. Smoking is a major risk factor for coronary vessel restenosis following percutaneous balloon angioplasty, for rethrombosis after thrombolytic therapies,[32–34] and for increased long-term morbidity and mortality after coronary artery bypass surgery.[35] It has also been shown that cigarette smoking is an independent and modifiable determinant of type II diabetes.[36]

It has been shown in North American men and women aged 30 to 74 years that cessation of cigarette smoking increases life expectancy, on average, from 2.6 to 4.4 years in men and from 2.6 to 3.7 years in women.[25] Smoking cessation appears to be a more powerful risk-factor intervention for coronary artery protection than dietary modifications.[37–42]

CHEMICAL COMPOSITION OF TOBACCO

Four thousand compounds can be generated by burning tobacco. Cigarette smoke has two phases: gaseous and particulate. The actual composition of smoke delivered to a smoker depends upon many factors (Table 22-1).

Components of the Gaseous Phase

Carbon monoxide, carbon dioxide, nitrogen oxide, volatile nitrosamines, ammonia, nitrites, volatile sulfur-containing compounds,

TABLE 22-1. Factors Determining Composition of Smoke Delivered to a Smoker

Composition of tobacco
Density of package
Column length of tobacco
Characteristics of paper
Characteristics of filter
Temperature at which tobacco is burned
Velocity of drawing smoke

other nitrogen-containing compounds, alcohols, ketones, aldehydes, and volatile hydrocarbons make up the gaseous phase of tobacco. Some of these substances inhibit ciliary movement in the respiratory tree.

Components of the Particulate Phase

Nicotine, water, and tar make up the particulate phase. Tar consists of polycyclic aromatic hydrocarbons, some of which are potent carcinogens. Tar also contains metallic ions and several radioactive compounds—for example, polonium 210. The actual content of nicotine in tobacco, by weight, can vary from 0.2 to 5%. The most likely life-threatening components of cigarette smoke are carbon monoxide, nicotine, and tar.

PHARMACOKINETICS OF NICOTINE

Nicotine is a major pharmacologically active substance in tobacco, accounting for less than 10% of the dry weight of the plant.[1] It is a tertiary amine composed of both pyridine and pyrrolidine rings and is a volatile base with a pKa of 7.9. On exposure to air, nicotine turns brown and acquires the odor of tobacco. Tobacco alkaloids such as nicotine are synthesized in the plant roots and are transported to the leaves, with the nicotine content highest in the upper stalk. Nicotine content can vary with the type and strain of tobacco and the process used to prepare the tobacco for consumption.[1] Nicotine is very lipophilic and absorbed readily through the buccal membranes, respiratory tract, and skin; however, there is considerable interindividual variability in this absorption. The absorption of nicotine in the stomach is limited because it is a strong base; intestinal absorption is much better. Nicotine must be a salt to be absorbed by the buccal mucosa. The tobacco in cigarettes is acidic, requiring nicotine to be buffered in the lungs and absorbed in the lungs as a salt. The nicotine in cigars and chewing tobacco is a basic salt that can be absorbed in the mouth without being inhaled. About 88% of a systemic nicotine dose can be accounted for by measuring nicotine and its metabolites.[43]

Nicotine is absorbed more slowly from chewing tobacco than from inhalational tobacco; therefore it has a longer duration of effect. Nicotine from chewing tobacco is mainly metabolized in the liver and to some extent in the kidneys and lungs. A significant fraction of inhaled nicotine is metabolized by the lungs.[44,45] Nicotine is metabolized by two major monooxygenases: Cytochrome P450 and flavin-containing monooxygenase (FMO).[46] It undergoes NADPH-dependent oxidation by liver microenzymes. The principal product is nicotine-γ-1′, 5′-immium ion, which is a 5′ carbon atom. In the presence of aldehyde oxidase, it is converted into a γ-lactam derivative, cotinine (Fig. 22-1). The other major product is nicotine N′-oxide.[1,46] The half-life of nicotine administered either by inhalation

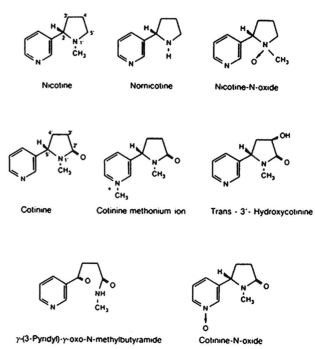

FIGURE 22-1. Chemical structures of nicotine and its major metabolites. (*Reproduced with permission from Benowitz NL, Porchet H, Jacob P III: Pharmacokinetics, metabolism and pharmacodynamics of nicotine. In: Wonnacott S, Russell MAH, Stolerman IP, eds. Nicotine Psychopharmacology: Molecular, Cellular, and Behavioral Aspects. Oxford, UK: Oxford University Press, 1990:112–157.*)

or by the parenteral route is 1 to 2 h. Less than 5% is bound to plasma protein. Both nicotine and its metabolites are rapidly excreted by the kidney[47]; 80 to 90% of a dose of nicotine that is consumed is excreted in the urine as different metabolites.[48] The clearance of nicotine normalized for body weight is significantly slower in smokers than in nonsmokers. A relationship between interindividual differences in nicotine metabolism and CYP26A polymorphism has been shown.[49] The elimination half-life of the metabolite cotinine is similar in nonsmokers and smokers.[50] The half-life of cotinine is 15 h.[51] A steady-state cotinine level for a given degree of nicotine exposure requires 2 days or more of exposure. The amount of cotinine excreted in the urine is about 15%.[52,53] Cotinine levels are used to monitor cigarette smoking in cessation programs.

PHARMACOLOGIC ACTIONS OF NICOTINE

Nicotine has complex central nervous system, behavioral, neuromuscular, endocrine, renal, metabolic, and cardiovascular effects in humans.[54] Nitroso derivatives of nicotine and other nicotine metabolites are carcinogenic.

Nicotine binds stereospecifically to acetylcholine receptors in autonomic ganglia in the adrenal medulla, at neuromuscular junctions, and in the brain.[55] It can produce an increase in alertness and cognitive performance by stimulating the cortex via the locus ceruleus. Its action on the limbic system is called the *reward effect.* At low nicotine doses, a stimulant effect predominates, while at higher doses the reward effect predominates. By activating neurohormonal pathways, nicotine can cause release of acetylcholine, norepinephrine, dopamine, serotonin, vasopressin, beta-endorphin, and growth and adrenocorticotropic hormones.

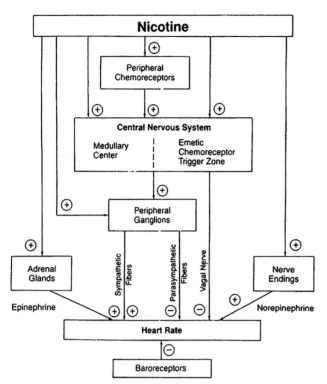

FIGURE 22-2. Cardiovascular effects of nicotine.

Nicotine has both stimulant and depressant phases of action on the cardiovascular system. It can increase heart rate by excitation of the sympathetic or paralysis of parasympathetic nervous system cardiac ganglia and can slow heart rate by an opposing action (Fig. 22-2). Nicotine can also stimulate chemoreceptors of the carotid and aortic bodies and medullary centers, thereby influencing heart rate. Blood pressure can be changed by affecting cardiovascular compensatory reflexes. These effects may be attenuated somewhat in the exercising patient.[56]

NICOTINE ADDICTION

Why do people smoke? Since the mid-1960s, research has been done to examine the motives for cigarette smoking. Smoking motives scales allow the measurement of private events mediated by the proposed neuroregulatory effects of nicotine.[57] Smoking motives questionnaires have been developed based on affect-management models,[58] situations associated with smoking,[59,60] and arousal models.[61] The most commonly found motives are classified as automatic (ATM), addictive (ADD), sedative (SED), stimulatory (STM), psychosocial (SOC), indulgent (IND), and sensorimotor manipulation (SMM).[62] Russell and coworkers in 1974 speculated that social and other nonpharmacologic rewards motivate smoking initially and account for the stronger role of the SOC, IND, and SMM motives early in the smoker's career.[63] Eventually the positive rewards of nicotine, due to its direct and indirect effects on the brain, exert more control as the smoker increasingly uses nicotine to modulate arousal and affective tone, thus accounting for the stronger role of the SED and STM motives as the smoker's addiction progresses.

Shortly after a person smokes a cigarette, the nicotine level in the arterial plasma is approximately double that in the venous plasma, with individual variations.[64] It takes about 7 to 9 s for the drug to reach the brain following absorption in the pulmonary alveoli (Figs. 22-3, 22-4).[65] These findings contribute to the high degree of addictiveness and cardiovascular toxicity of tobacco and smoked forms of other drugs.[66] The average blood cotinine concentration in addicted tobacco smokers is 300 ng/mL. Smokers of <5 cigarettes per day (average 3.9) have average cotinine levels of 54 ng/mL (the cotinine level normalized for cigarette consumption is 14 ng/mL per cigarette). The reasonable cutoff point for the addictive threshold is 50 to 70 ng/mL of cotinine, but in fact there is no sharply demarcated threshold level.[67] In addicted patients, withdrawal from nicotine is characterized by craving, nervousness, restlessness, irritability, anxiety, mood lability, sleep disturbance, drowsiness, impaired concentration, increased appetite, weight gain, blood pressure elevations, and minor somatic complaints.[68,68a] In most smokers, the habit is

FIGURE 22-3. (A) Blood concentrations during and after cigarette smoking for 9 min (1.3 cigarettes), oral snuff (2.5 g), chewing tobacco (7.9 g), and nicotine gum (two 2-mg pieces). Average values for 10 subjects (1 SEM). (B) Nicotine absorption rate profiles, estimated by the point area deconvolution method during and after cigarette smoking, oral snuff, chewing tobacco, and nicotine gum exposure. (*Reproduced with permission from Benowitz NL, Porchet H, Sheiner L, et al: Nicotine absorption and cardiovascular effects with smokeless tobacco use: Comparison with cigarettes and nicotine gum. Clin Pharmacol Ther 44:23–28, 1988.*)

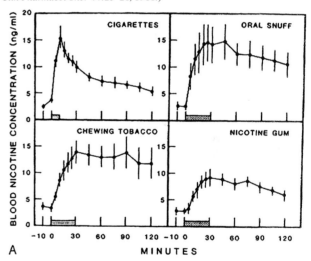

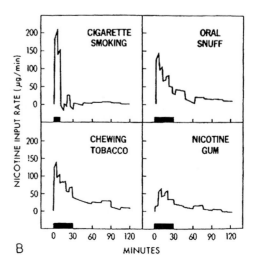

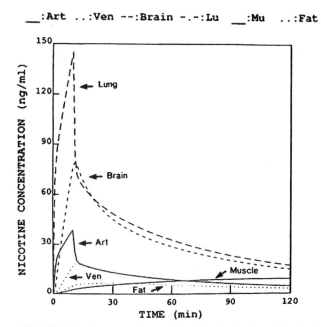

1.5 mg of nicotine in 10 min given I.Pulm.

___:Art ..:Ven --:Brain -.-:Lu ___:Mu ..:Fat

FIGURE 22-4. Perfusion model simulation of the distribution of nicotine in various tissues after infusion of 1.5 mg of nicotine into the lung compartment over 10 min. The dose, route, and dosing regimen were intended to mimic smoking a cigarette. Typical human organ weights and blood flows and partition coefficients from rabbits were used for the simulation.

aggravated by the need to avoid the discomfort of withdrawal. Once an addiction to nicotine develops, it is difficult to break,[69] and more than 90% of smokers who try to quit fail each year.[70] An important component of the policy to reduce tobacco use in the population is to prevent the development of nicotine addiction in the young population.[71,72] It is also important to reduce the effects of secondary smoke, which can be harmful to nonsmokers and may aggravate the nicotine load in current smokers.[73–79]

NICOTINE AS A THERAPEUTIC SUBSTANCE IN SMOKING CESSATION

An increased risk of cancer, cardiovascular disorders, and pulmonary disease with smoking is well established, with blacks being the most susceptible.[80,81] However, instead of trying to quit, 46 million Americans continue to smoke because of nicotine addiction.[82] The pharmacodynamic considerations in the rational treatment of smoking cessation include the following:

1. Setting objectives for treatment—that is, stop smoking completely
2. Setting an appropriate medication and dosing regimen for smoking cessation that is matched to the pathophysiology of the disease—for example, smokeless tobacco, nicotine chewing gum, or a transdermal nicotine delivery system
3. Selecting the optimal dosing regimen
4. Assessing the therapeutic outcome periodically
5. Adjusting therapy as needed to provide optimal benefits with minimal risk[83]

Nicotine replacement therapy is believed to provide benefit by reducing the severity of abstinence symptoms, which are

selective.[66,84–86] Nicotine replacement can contribute to the pathophysiology of acute ischemic events in patients with CAD and to reproductive disturbances during pregnancy.[87,88] However, nicotine replacement appears unlikely to cause more harm than cigarette smoking itself[66]; it may also modify withdrawal symptoms that could aggravate CAD during tobacco withdrawal.[89] In a recent study using the transdermal nicotine patch or placebo, 156 patients with known CAD and a history of smoking more than one pack of cigarettes per day were able to undergo nicotine replacement therapy safely.[90] This observation has been substantiated in others studies.[91] The following types of nicotine replacement therapies are available: smokeless tobacco, nicotine patches (transdermal nicotine replacement system), nicotine polacrilex (nicotine resin complex), nicotine nasal spray, nicotine aerosols and vapors, and other nicotine preparations such as lobeline. There are no notable differences between the nicotine replacement products in their effects on withdrawal, discomfort, perceived helpfulness, or efficacy.[92] Non-nicotine-based therapies are also available.[93,94,94a] They include bupropion, clonidine, nortriptyline, moclobemide and silver acetate, which are discussed below.

Smokeless Tobacco

Smokeless tobacco is associated with far fewer and less serious health problems than cigarette smoking. Smokeless tobacco causes oral cancer at an estimated annual incidence of 26 cases per 100,000. If all American smokers used smokeless tobacco, this would result in 12,000 cases of oral cancer per year. This is 1/20th of all smoking-related cancers, less than 1/10th of smoking-related lung cancers, and less than half the number of oral cancers now attributed to smoking. Cardiovascular disease risks are also decreased.[95] A public health policy that recognizes smokeless tobacco as an alternative to smoking would benefit individuals confronted with the unsatisfactory options of abstinence or continuing to smoke.[96]

Nicotine Patches (Transdermal Nicotine Delivery System)

Nicotine patches were approved by the U.S. Food and Drug Administration (FDA) in 1991 (Fig. 22-5) as an adjunct to concomitant physician support for smoking cessation and were recently approved for over-the-counter use.[37,97–101,101a] Because sufficient nicotine is provided to ameliorate withdrawal symptoms during early abstinence, transdermal nicotine has been shown in multiple studies to improve smoking cessation rates by producing nicotine concentrations less than those resulting from smoking.[102,103] In placebo-controlled trials, the nicotine patch increased quit rates by a factor 2.8 over placebo (Table 22-2).[93] There is evidence suggesting that higher doses of nicotine (44 mg/day) can achieve blood concentrations similar to those produced by smoking, but the benefit of this approach in increasing smoking cessation has not yet been established.[104–106]

Patches should be applied to nonhairy, clean, dry skin of either the upper outer arm or upper body. They should be removed after 24 h and new ones applied. The same skin site should not be used for at least 1 week. The rate of nicotine absorption is maximal between 6 to 12 h, with absolute bioavailability of about 82%.[107] The blood concentration of nicotine plateaus between 16 to 24 h and declines thereafter. About 10% of transdermal nicotine is systemically absorbed after patch removal, showing a reservoir for nicotine

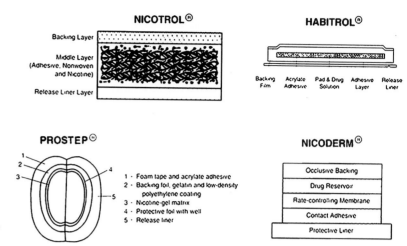

FIGURE 22-5. Design of various transdermal nicotine delivery systems.

in the skin. The fact that bioavailability is not 100% raises the possibility of first-pass metabolism of nicotine by the skin or loss from the skin surface after removal of the patch. The most frequently reported side effects of nicotine patches are local skin irritation and contact sensitization. These reactions have been reported with all 24-h patches, although not with the 16-h patch. Moving the site of patch application daily can reduce the incidence of skin reactions. Sleep disturbances have also been reported with the 24-h patches, and a dose effect has been noted, with the 21-mg patches producing higher rates of sleep disturbance than the 14- or 7-mg patches. Physicians can recommend that patients who have sleep disturbances either use a 16-h patch or remove the 24-h patch before bedtime.[108]

Several different nicotine patch systems are available, some of which are reviewed below. They differ significantly in their pharmacologic kinetics, as described in Table 22-3.

Nicoderm CQ (GlaxoSmithKline Consumer Healthcare, Pittsburgh, PA)

On application, 68% of the nicotine in this patch is absorbed in the circulation and the remainder is lost via evaporation. Plasma concentrations rise rapidly, plateau within 2 to 4 h, then slowly decline. The patch may be worn for 24 h or, to help avoid insomnia,

for 16 h. The recommended treatment duration is for 8 to 12 weeks, as follows: 21 mg daily for first 6 weeks, 14 mg daily for next 2 weeks, then 7 mg daily for 2 weeks. Smaller doses (14 mg) may be started in small individuals, light smokers, and patients with cardiovascular disease. The longer-duration 24-h schedule may be more effective, but this has not been directly tested. On the other hand, the 16-h wearing schedule may produce greater compliance, but this also has not been tested.

Nicotrol (Pharmacia and Upjohn, Peapack, NJ)

Treatment is for 14 to 20 weeks. For the first 12 weeks, 15 mg daily is prescribed, followed by 10 mg daily for 2 weeks, and finally 5 mg daily for 2 weeks.

Safety of Patches

Transdermal nicotine has less effect on platelet activation and catecholamine release than does cigarette smoking; thus its use as a smoking cessation treatment in the patient with CAD is likely to be safer than cigarette smoking.[109] In using any nicotine replacement therapy, patients must stop smoking immediately, be highly motivated, and be supported by their health care provider. The smoking cessation rate reported from various clinics after treatment weaning

TABLE 22-2. Six-Month Quit Rates in Minimal Contact Studies of Nicotine Gum and Patch*

	OTC		Prescription NRT	Risk Ratio for OTC NRT vs. Placebo
	NRT	**Placebo**		
Nicotine gum				
OTC Nicorette data summary, 1995	15	—	18[†]	—
Schneider et al., 1983	13	8	30	1.6
Nicotine patch				
Hays et al., 1997	9	4	—	2.5
Nicoderm data summary, 1996	9	—	7[†]	—
Leischow et al., 1997	5	—	5	—
Nicotrol data summary, 1996	11	—	12	—
Sonderskov et al., 1997	11	4	—	2.8

OTC = over the counter; NRT = nicotine replacement therapy.

*Rates are given in percentages. Due to differences in study design and in data collection, quit rates can be compared within rows but not across rows.

[†]These studies were surveys, not experimental trials. Because so few surveys were returned for carbon monoxide verification, these are self-reported quit rates. With carbon monoxide verification, they are likely to be somewhat lower.

Source: Adapted with permission from Hughes et al.[93] Papers cited within this table are referenced in Hughes et al.[93]

TABLE 22-3. Steady-State Nicotine Pharmacokinetic Parameters for Various Transdermal Nicotine Replacement Systems

Parameters (units)	Dose Absorbed								
	21 mg/day			14 mg/day			7 mg/day		
	Mean	SD	Range	Mean	SD	Range	Mean	SD	Range
Habitrol*									
C_{max} (ng/mL)	17	2	13–19	12	4	6–16	8	2	5–12
C_{avg} (ng/mL)	13	2	9–17	9	3	5–12	6	1	4–10
C_{min} (ng/mL)	9	2	7–14	6	2	3–10	4	1	3–6
T_{max} (h)	6	3	2–9	5	3	0–8	4	4	1–18

	21 mg/day			14 mg/day					
	Mean	SD	Range	Mean	SD	Range			
Nicoderm									
C_{max} (ng/mL)	23	5	13–32	17	3	10–24			
C_{avg} (ng/mL)	17	4	10–26	12	3	8–17			
C_{min} (ng/mL)	11	3	6–17	7	2	4–11			
T_{max} (h)	4	3	1–10	4	3	1–10			

	22 mg/day								
	Mean	SD	Range						
Prostep*									
C_{max} (ng/mL)	16	6	7–31						
C_{avg} (ng/mL)	11	3	6–17						
C_{min} (ng/mL)	5	1	3–9						
T_{max} (h)	9	5	4–24						

	15 mg/day			10 mg/day			5 mg/day		
	Mean	SD	Range	Mean	SD	Range	Mean	SD	Range
Nicotrol									
C_{max} (ng/mL)	13	3	8–18	7	2	5–10	3	1	3–5
C_{avg} (ng/mL)	9	2	5–13	5	1	3–6	3	0.5	2–3
C_{min} (ng/mL)	2	1	1–4	1	0.5	0.5–2	1	0.3	0.3–1
T_{max} (h)	8	3	4–16	9	4	6–16	9	4	3–16

C_{max} = maximum observed plasma concentration; C_{avg} = average plasma concentration; C_{min} = minimum observed plasma concentration; T_{max} = time to maximal plasma concentration; SD = standard deviation.

*Products no longer available but provide examples of previously developed delivery systems.

ranges from 0 to 50%. Special considerations must be noted in using nicotine replacement therapies. If patients continue to smoke with concomitant patch use, they may develop nicotine toxicity, manifest by nausea, abdominal pain, vomiting, diarrhea, diaphoresis, flushing, dizziness, disturbed hearing and vision, confusion, weakness, palpitations, altered respirations, and hypotension. Patients receiving patches may develop nicotine withdrawal with a similar presentation but not to be confused with nicotine toxicity. Nicotine withdrawal in addicted individuals is characterized by craving, nervousness, restlessness, irritability, mood lability, anxiety, drowsiness, sleep disturbances, impaired concentration, increased appetite, and weight gain.

Nicotine patch replacement has therefore been shown to be safe in patients with known CAD; however, it should not be started around the time of acute myocardial infarction or coronary artery surgical procedures. Transient episodes of hypertension have been described with the institution of nicotine replacement therapies.

Smoking and nicotine can increase circulating cortisol and catecholamines. This might influence the pharmacologic effects of various adrenergic blockers and agonists during smoking withdrawal (Table 22-4).

There is strong epidemiologic evidence of a causal and dose-related relationship between cigarette smoking and adverse reproductive outcomes. It is difficult to ascertain how much of this problem is related to nicotine directly. Nicotine replacement therapy may outweigh the risks of cigarette smoking during pregnancy.[88]

Nicotine Gums (Nicotine Polacrilex, Nicotine Resin Complex)

Approved by the FDA in 1984, the dose of these gums varies from 2 to 4 mg, depending on the Fagerstrom Tolerance Questionnaire Score. Highly dependent smokers (>25 cigarettes daily or scoring ≥7) should receive 4 mg (3.4 mg nicotine extracted) initially[110]; others should get the 2-mg (1.4 mg nicotine extracted) strength. An individual cigarette contains, on average, 11 mg of nicotine, of which 0.8 mg is extracted by smoking. The total number of pieces of gum which is recommended daily is 9 to 12, with a maximum of 20 to 30. Even with such use, gum chewers do not match the daily nicotine levels achieved by smoking cigarettes. Each piece should be chewed intermittently for about 30 min. One piece of gum should last 1 to 2 h, with an additional piece being used during the hour if a strong nicotine craving arises. The release of nicotine is related to the speed of chewing. Patients should learn to chew slowly and to self-titrate the nicotine dose. Chewing too quickly leads to excessive production of saliva and the swallowing of nicotine, which can cause gastrointestinal side effects. Advising patients of the "chew and park" method, physicians tell their patient to chew the gum until a

TABLE 22-4. Drugs Requiring Dosage Adjustment During Smoking Cessation

May Require a Decrease in Dose at Cessation of Smoking	Possible Mechanism
Acetaminophen Caffeine Imipramine Oxazepam Pentazocine Propranolol Theophylline	Deinduction of hepatic enzymes on smoking cessation
Insulin	Increase in subcutaneous insulin absorption with smoking cessation
Adrenergic antagonists (e.g., prazosin, labetalol)	Decrease in circulating catecholamines with smoking cessation

May Require an Increase in Dose at Cessation of Smoking	Possible Mechanism
Adrenergic agonists (e.g., isoproterenol, phenylephrine)	Decrease in circulating catecholamines with smoking cessation

Source: Physicians' Desk Reference, 48th ed. Montvale, NJ: Medical Economics Company, 1994:583.

peppery taste emerges and then park it between the cheek and gum until it no longer produces a tingle.

Compliance with nicotine gum is reduced in some people by the demands of oral manipulation, unappealing flavor, jaw fatigue, jaw and mouth soreness, and headaches.[111] Other side effects include hiccups, burping, and nausea, although these effects are generally mild and transient when they occur. Furthermore, acidic beverages (e.g., soda, coffee, beer) have been shown to interfere with buccal absorption of nicotine.[112] Patients should avoid such beverages for 15 min before and during gum chewing. Nicotine gum has been associated with habitual abuse, but it appears to be safe and unrelated to any cardiovascular illnesses or other serious side effects.[113] It was recently approved for over-the-counter sale.

In placebo-controlled trials, nicotine gum increased quit rates by a factor 1.6 over placebo. Recent prospective data indicate that with the use of nicotine gum for as long as 5 years, even with concurrent use of cigarettes, there is no increased risk of cardiovascular or other diseases.[93]

Nicotine Nasal Spray

The nicotine nasal spray (Pharmacia and Upjohn) produces about 50% replacement of nicotine blood concentrations, with a peak concentration being achieved at 5 to 10 min.[114] It delivers nicotine more rapidly than the gum or inhaler but less rapidly than cigarettes.[115] Due to the rapid absorption and need for frequent use, it was thought that the liability and dependence potential of nicotine nasal spray would be high, but recent studies have not found this or other indications of abuse liability.[116,117] Smokers use one to two doses per hour, which may be increased to 40 doses per day for 3 months. The spray was recently approved for clinical use as an aid to smoking cessation and for the relief of nicotine withdrawal symptoms. One dose consists of two squirts, one to each nostril, delivering 0.5 mg of nicotine per squirt. It can be combined with the patch to achieve increased efficacy.[118]

The most common side effects are local irritation of the nose and throat. Other side effects include coughing, sneezing, watery eyes, and runny nose. Reports of moderate to severe nasal and throat irritation usually dissipate or diminish to mild symptoms within a few days of treatment. Long-term nasal complications have not been reported.

Nicotine Inhaler

The nicotine inhaler (Pharmacia and Upjohn) became available as a prescription drug in 1998. It consists of a nicotine cartridge attached to a mouthpiece. Designed to mimic the hand-to-mouth ritual of using a cigarette, the inhaler, unlike cigarettes, actually delivers more nicotine by buccal (36%) than pulmonary (4%) absorption.[108,118a] Like other nicotine replacement therapies, the inhaler consistently doubles quit rates compared with placebo[93] (Table 22-5). The major difference between the inhaler and other nicotine replacement therapies is that it substitutes for the behavioral aspects of cigarette smoking in addition to providing nicotine replacement.[119] Some inhalers require vigorous and frequent inhalation to produce a 30% replacement of nicotine blood concentrations; others produce a higher replacement. Like nicotine gum, success largely depends on the number of doses taken per day. In clinical trials, those smokers who successfully abstained from smoking used between 6 and 16 cartridges per day. A recent study has demonstrated that the combination of the nicotine inhaler and nicotine patch was more effective in achieving smoking cessation than the inhaler alone.[119a]

The inhaler's label states that 80 deep puffs of the inhaler delivers 4 mg of nicotine; however, fewer or shallower puffs may not provide adequate amounts of nicotine. Moreover, the amount of nicotine absorbed from the inhaler is temperature-dependent. Larger amounts of nicotine are delivered at higher temperatures,[120] and bioavailability decreases significantly at temperatures below 10°C.

Common side effects involve local irritation, such as a burning sensation in the throat, coughing, sneezing, and hiccups.[111] Any side effect that decreases compliance may abort effective therapy, since the efficacy of the inhaler relies on heavy use throughout the day.

TABLE 22-5. Six-Month Quit Rates in Specialty Clinic Studies of Nicotine Nasal Spray, Nicotine Inhaler, and Bupropion Hydrochloride

Studies	Abstinence from Smoking, %		
	Active Treatment	Placebo	Risk Ratio
Nasal Spray			
Blondal et al., 1997	29	18	1.6
Hjalmarson et al., 1994	35	15	2.3
Schneider et al., 1995	25	10	2.5
Sutherland et al., 1992	26	10	2.6
Inhaler			
Leischow et al., 1996	21	6	3.5
Mikkelsen et al., 1995	6*	6	1.0
Schneider et al., 1996	17	9	1.8
Tonnesen et al., 1993	17	8	2.1
Bupropion			
Ferry and Burchette, 1994	28	19	1.5
Hurt et al., 1997	27†	16	1.7

*Inhaler alone condition.

†300 mg bupropion hydrochloride condition.

Source: Reproduced with permission from Hughes et al.[93] Papers cited within this table are referenced in Hughes et al.[93]

Nicotine Lozenges

Some smokers prefer oral forms of acute nicotine replacement therapy, but cannot tolerate the chewing of gum. A 2- and 4-mg nicotine lozenge has been tested as a smoking cessation therapy in a placebo-controlled study and was shown to be an effective and safe treatment with an adverse effect rate similar to that seen with nicotine gum.[120a]

Lobeline

This is an alkaloid of *Lobelia inflata* with pharmacologic effects similar to but weaker than those of nicotine. This drug is used as a temporary aid to smoking cessation. Classified as a category III drug, lobeline's safety but not its efficacy has been established by the FDA-OPTC Advisory Panel.[120b,120c] It is available as Bantron, containing 2 mg of lobeline sulfate alkaloid. Because of limited data, no more than 6 weeks of use is recommended.

Nicotine tablets are available for buccal absorption. Nicotine toothpicks have been described, but few data on their efficacy and safety are available.

NON-NICOTINE PREPARATIONS

Bupropion

Bupropion is an atypical antidepressant that has dopaminergic and adrenergic actions.[121] It is available in two sustained-release forms, Wellbutrin and Zyban (Glaxo-Wellcome, Research Triangle Park, NC). Wellbutrin was originally marketed to treat depression, while Zyban was released in 1998 specifically as an aid to smoking cessation.[122,122a] The initial randomized study of placebo versus bupropion with >600 patients showed cessations rates were 19.05, 28.8, 38.6, and 44.2% for placebo and bupropion doses of 100, 150, and 300 mg daily for 7 weeks, respectively.[123] The study excluded

subjects with a history of major depression. Thus, the mechanism of action of bupropion does not rely on the drug's antidepressant effects, as studies have shown bupropion to be equally efficacious in smokers with or without a history of depression.[124] Bupropion, like nicotine replacement therapy, has been shown to consistently double quit rates compared with placebo[93] (Table 22-5). It is a first-line therapy[40,125] (Table 22-6), like the nicotine patch and gum, and should be offered depending on the patient's preference. Bupropion can also be combined with nicotine replacement therapy with greater effects on smoking cessation than either treatment alone.[126]

Using bupropion for smoking cessation does not involve the replacement of nicotine and may be offered to those who dislike or have failed nicotine replacement therapy. Unlike those using nicotine replacement therapy, smokers using bupropion begin treatment 1 week prior to their smoking quit date. The suggested dosage is 300 mg/day and the duration of treatment is 7 to 12 weeks. Patients start bupropion at 150 mg/day for 3 to 5 days and increase to the maximum dose of 300 mg/day, given as 150 mg twice a day. Many smokers state that within 1 week of taking bupropion, their craving for cigarettes is altered and their satisfaction from tobacco use decreased. The decision to stop bupropion depends on an individual's withdrawal phase, which may last 1 month, 3 months, or longer. Treatment can safely be extended, since bupropion was previously used in the treatment of chronic depression for 2 to 3 years. Because bupropion is a non-nicotine-based therapy, there is no rebound phenomenon upon abrupt discontinuation of the drug.

Bupropion can safely be used in combination with the nicotine patch. Combination therapy improves the 1-year quit rate to 25 to 30% compared to a rate of 15 to 20% from monotherapy with counseling.[127] Physicians should consider bupropion and the patch together for patients who have high levels of nicotine dependence, have a history of psychiatric problems, or have failed prior therapy.

Side effects of bupropion include insomnia (30–42%), headache (26%), and dry mouth (10.7%). Insomnia can be managed by taking

TABLE 22-6. Suggestions for the Clinical Use of Pharmacotherapies for Smoking Cessation*

Pharmacotherapy	Precautions/ Contraindications	Adverse Effects	Dosage	Duration
First-line				
Sustained-release bupropion HCl	Hx of seizure Hx eating disorder	Insomnia Dry mouth	150 mg q AM for 3 days then 150 mg bid (begin treatment 1–2 weeks prequit)	7–12 weeks Maintenance up to 6 months
Nicotine gum		Mouth soreness Dyspepsia	1–24 cigarettes per day: 2-mg gum (up to 24 pieces per day); ≥25 cigarettes per day: 4-mg gum (up to 24 pieces per day)	Up to 12 weeks
Nicotine inhaler		Local irritation of mouth and throat	6–16 cartridges/d	Up to 6 months
Nicotine nasal spray		Nasal irritation	8–40 doses/d	3–6 months
Nicotine patch		Local skin reaction; insomnia	21 mg/24 h 14 mg/24 h 7 mg/24 h 15 mg/16 h	4 weeks then 2 weeks then 2 weeks 8 weeks
Second-line				
Clonidine	Rebound hypertension	Dry mouth Drowsiness Dizziness, sedation	0.15–0.75 mg/day	3–10 weeks
Nortriptyline	Risk of arrhythmias	Sedation, dry mouth	75–100 mg/day	12 weeks

*The information in this table is not comprehensive. Please see package insert for additional information. First-line pharmacotherapies have been approved for smoking cessation by the FDA; second-line pharmacotherapies have not.

Source: Reproduced with permission from Ref. 40.

the evening dose more than 4 h before bedtime. Initial studies with higher-dose immediate-release bupropion produced a higher frequency of seizures. More recent data with sustained release preparations at dosages of 300 mg/day or less (as indicated for smoking cessation) has shown the risk of seizures to be no greater than that of typical antidepressants.[128]

Although no seizures were reported in 2400 subjects when screening precautions were used, patients with a history of seizures should not use bupropion. Furthermore, bupropion should not be used in patients with a history of head trauma, heavy alcohol use, or anorexia. Nor should bupropion be used in combination with monoamine oxidase inhibitors or in patients with schizophrenia. Bupropion has been assigned a class B category for pregnancy by the FDA.[128]

Clonidine

Clonidine is an alpha$_2$ agonist marketed as an antihypertensive agent; it has also been recommended for use in the treatment for chronic pain syndromes, menopausal flushing, Tourettes's syndrome, and withdrawal from opiate or alcohol abuse. More recently, studies have investigated clonidine for use as a smoking cessation therapy. The initial study with this drug in 1986 demonstrated that clonidine decreased both craving and nicotine withdrawal symptoms. Randomized trials of up to 4 weeks using 0.15 to 0.4 mg per day showed a doubling of the quit rate compared to placebo.[129] Ten small trials and two large studies have shown a trend for enhanced smoking cessation, but only one trial had efficacy at 6 months.[130]

The recommended dose of clonidine from available studies is 100 μg twice daily, titrated to a maximum of about 400 μg per day as tolerated. Clonidine should be started prior to the quit day to allow time for steady-state plasma concentrations to be achieved before the onset of tobacco withdrawal symptoms. Treatment with clonidine should not be maintained for more than 3 to 4 weeks after smoking cessation, since its efficacy is related to the acute nicotine withdrawal syndrome. Clonidine must be tapered so as to avoid the withdrawal effects of clonidine itself. If clonidine is not tapered, physicians should be wary of the potential of rebound hypertension in hypertensive patients.

The side of effects of clonidine have limited its use in smoking cessation therapy. Sedation, postural hypotension, dizziness, fatigue, and dry mouth are prominent side effects that make it a second-line therapy for smoking cessation. In addition to the failure of nicotine replacement therapy or treatment with bupropion, another consideration for using clonidine may be that, in patients with multiple drug abuse problems, clonidine relieves the withdrawal symptoms of other drugs besides nicotine.

Because its mechanism of action is different from that of nicotine replacement therapy or treatment with bupropion, clonidine may be studied for use in combination with these other treatments. Currently, no studies are available. Future studies will have to demonstrate conclusively that clonidine is effective and has fewer side effects than other treatments before it can be considered as a first-line therapy for smoking cessation.[130a]

Nortriptyline

Nortriptyline is a noradrenergic tricyclic antidepressant drug that has been shown in a randomized controlled trial ($n = 199$) to double the continuous 1-year abstinence rate versus placebo (24 versus 12%).[131] Another randomized controlled study found that at 6 months, 14% of the subjects in the nortriptyline group and 3% of those in the placebo group had remained abstinent.[132] There was significant reduction in withdrawal symptoms of irritability/anger, anxiety/tension, difficulty in concentrating, restlessness, impatience, and insomnia but not for excessive hunger, drowsiness, and increased eating.

Patients receiving nortriptyline experienced more side effects—including dry mouth, dysgeusia, gastrointestinal upset, drowsiness, and sleep disruption. Other adverse reactions include lightheadedness, shaky hands, blurry vision, sedation, serious or lethal toxicity from overdose, and cardiac rhythm disturbances.

More studies are required to assess nortriptyline's efficacy in smoking cessation. Previous studies of nortriptyline have involved intensive counseling (e.g., 12 individual counseling sessions). Participants in the studies, although not depressed, had histories of depression; thus these results cannot be generalized to the general smoking population.[132] Currently, nortriptyline is not approved by the FDA for nicotine dependence and is a second-line intervention for smoking cessation.

Moclobemide

Moclobemide, a monoamine oxidase type A inhibitor, has been used as an aid to smoking cessation after evidence became available that smoking reduced MAO levels in the brain.[132a–c] Adverse effects associated with moclobemide include insomnia and dry mouth.[132c] Its role as a smoking cessation therapy needs to be defined.

Silver Acetate

Silver acetate discourages tobacco use by creating an aversive metallic taste after smoking that is similar to the effect of disulfuram after alcohol use. Initial trials in the 1930s and 1950s with over-the-counter gum, lozenges, and spray did not show efficacy. More recent studies have also failed to show efficacy owing to poor compliance with this regimen. In addition, this method does not address the neurochemical factors of nicotine addiction.[128]

DRUGS UNDER INVESTIGATION

An epilepsy drug called gamma vinyl-GABA has been shown to cause a rise of the transmitter dopamine in the brain's "reward centers" and can stop the craving for nicotine in rats. It is being evaluated as an alternative approach for smoking cessation.[133]

Studies are in progress evaluating the benefits of the selective serotonin reuptake inhibitors doxepin and fluoxetine as smoking cessation therapies. In addition, the opioid antagonists naltrexone and naloxone have been evaluated since endogenous opioids may be involved in the reinforcing properties of nicotine.[133a]

Finally, the non-nicotine medications amfebutamone and the anti-hypertensive mecamylamine have been assessed as part of a smoking cessation therapy along with nicotine replacement.[120c,133b]

CONCLUSION

Cigarette smoking is strongly associated with an increased risk of developing CAD. Smokers with CAD will have significantly lower mortality, fewer ischemic events, and better cardiac function if they stop smoking.[2] Nicotine is one of the substances in cigarette smoke, along with carbon monoxide and tar, that contribute to the mortality risk. Nicotine may be the chemical that contributes most to the addictive quality of cigarette smoke. In various formulations, nicotine can be used as a replacement therapy for cigarette smoking in helping those individuals who wish to break the habit. Nicotine replacement appears to be a safe and effective approach, along with behavioral modification and other pharmacologic treatments[85,133c,134] (see also clonidine discussion in Chap. 16) in patients with known CAD who need to stop smoking. Many new nicotine replacement therapies are available. Nicotine replacement with the nicotine patch and gum are first-line therapies in smoking cessation. Bupropion, a non-nicotine therapy, has joined nicotine replacement therapy as a first-line therapy or as a combination with nicotine replacement therapy. Nicotine in cigarette smoke is indeed a pharmacologic substance and needs to be regulated, as are other drugs.[135]

REFERENCES

1. LeHouezec J, Benowitz NL: Basic and clinical psychopharmacology of nicotine. *Clin Chest Med* 12(4):681, 1991.
2. US Department of Health and Human Services: *The Health Benefits of Smoking Cessation: A Report of the Surgeon General.* Publication CDC 90-8416. Washington DC: DHHS, 1990.
3. US Department of Health and Human Services: *The Health Consequences of Smoking: Cardiovascular Disease. A Report of the Surgeon General's Office on Smoking and Health.* DHHS (PHS) 84-50204.ockville, MD: DHHS, 1983.
4. Hammond EC, Horn D: Smoking and death rates. Report on forty-four months of follow up of 187,783 men: I. Total mortality. *JAMA* 166:1159, 1958.
5. Hammond EC, Horn D: Smoking and death rates. Report on forty-four months of follow up of 187,783 men: II. Death rates by cause. JAMA 166: 1294, 1958.
6. U.S. Public Health Service: *Smoking and Health: Report of the Advisory Committee to the Surgeon General of the Public Health Service Center for Disease Control.* PHS No. 1103. Washington, DC: 1964.
7. U.S. Department of Health, Education and Welfare: *Smoking and Health: A Report of the Surgeon General's Office on Smoking and Health.* DHEW PHS 79-50066. Washington, DC: U, 1979.
8. Matetzky S, Tani S, Kangavari S, et al: Smoking increases tissue factor expression in atherosclerotic plaques. Implications for plaque thrombogenicity. *Circulation* 102:602, 2000.
9. Wang H, Shi H, Zhang L, et al: Nicotine is a potent blocker of the cardiac A-type K+ channels. Effects on cloned Kv4.3 channels and native transient outward current. *Circulation* 102:1165, 2000.
10. Iribarren C, Tekawa IS, Sidney S, Friedman GD: Effect of cigar smoking on the risk of cardiovascular disease. Chronic obstructive pulmonary disease and cancer in men. *N Engl J Med* 340:1773, 1999.
11. Jacobs EJ, Thun MJ, Apicella LF: Cigar smoking and death from coronary heart disease in a prospective study of US men. *Arch Intern Med* 159 2413, 1999.
12. Jee SH, Suh I, Kim IS, Appel LJ: Smoking and atherosclerotic cardiovascular disease in men with low levels of serum cholesterol. The Korea Medical Insurance Corporation Study. *JAMA* 282:2149, 1999.
12a. Suskin N, Sheth T, Negassa A, Yusuf S: Relationship of current and past smoking to mortality and morbidity in patients with left ventricular dysfunction. *J Am Coll Cardiol* 37:1677, 2001.
12b. Lightwood J, Fleischmann KE, Glantz SA: Smoking cessation in heart failure: It is never too late. *J Am Coll Cardiol* 37:1683, 2001.
13. Fitz Gerald GA, Datas JA: Cigarette smoking and hemostatic function. *Am Heart J* 115:267, 1988.
14. Hioki Y, Aoki N, Kawano K, et al: Acute effects of cigarette smoking on platelet-dependent thrombin generation. *Eur Heart J* 22:56, 2001.
15. Fisher SD, Zareba W, Moss AJ, et al for the THROMBO Investigators: Effect of smoking on lipid and thrombogenic factors two months after acute myocardial infarction. *Am J Cardiol* 86:813, 2000.
16. Newby DE, Wright RA, Labinjoh C, et al: Endothelial dysfunction, impaired endogenous fibrinolysis, and cigarette smoking. A mechanism for arterial thrombosis and myocardial infarction. *Circulation* 99:1411, 1999.

17. Narkiewicz K, van de Borne PJH, Hausberg M, et al: Cigarette smoking increases sympathetic outflow in humans. *Circulation* 98:528, 1998.
18. Yarnell JWG, Sweetman PM: Some long term effects of smoking on the hemostatic system: A report from Caerphilly and Speedwell Collaborative Surveys. *J Clin Pathol* 40:909, 1987.
19. Mustard JF, Murphy EA: Effect of smoking on blood coagulation and platelet survival in man. *BMJ* 1:846, 1963.
20. Schmidt KG: Acute platelet activation induced by smoking. *Thromb Haemost* 51:279, 1984.
21. Hung J, Lam JYT, Lacoste L, Letchacovski G: Cigarette smoking acutely increases platelet thrombus formation in patients with coronary artery disease taking aspirin. *Circulation* 92:2432, 1995.
22. Newby DE, McLeod AL, Uren NG, et al: Impaired coronary tissue plasminogen activator release is associated with coronary atherosclerosis and cigarette smoking. Direct link between endothelial dysfunction and atherothrombosis. *Circulation* 103:1936, 2001.
23. Nagy J, Demaster EG, Wittmann I, et al: Induction of endothelial cell injury by cigarette smoke. *Endothelium* 5:251, 1997.
24. Zeiher AM, Schachinger V, Minners J: Long-term cigarette smoking impairs endothelium-dependent coronary arterial vasodilator function. *Circulation* 92:1094, 1995.
25. James RW, Leviev I, Righetti A: Smoking is associated with reduced serum paraoxonase activity and concentration in patients with coronary artery disease. *Circulation* 101:2252, 2000.
26. Zhu B, Parmley WW: Hemodynamic and vascular effects of active and passive smoking. *Am Heart J* 130:1270, 1995.
27. Heitzer T, Yia-Herttuala S, Luoma J, et al: Cigarette smoking potentiates endothelial dysfunction of forearm resistance vessels in patients with hypercholesterolemia: Role of oxidized LDL. *Circulation* 93:1346, 1996.
28. Quillen JE, Rossen JD: Acute effects of cigarette smoking on coronary circulation: Constriction of epicardial and resistance vessels. *J Am Coll Cardiol* 22:642, 1993.
29. Frishman WH, Karpenos A, Molloy TJ: Cocaine-induced coronary artery disease: Recognition and treatment. *Med Clin North Am* 73:475, 1989.
30. Lange RA, Hillis LD: Cardiovascular complications of cocaine use. *N Engl J Med* 345:351, 2001.
31. Muller B, Zulewski H, Huber P, et al: Impaired action of thyroid hormone associated with smoking in women with hypothyroidism. *N Engl J Med* 333:964, 1995.
32. Deanfield J: Cigarette smoking and the treatment of angina with propranolol, atenolol and nifedipine. *N Engl J Med* 310:951, 1984.
33. Sugiishi M, Takatsu F: Cigarette smoking is a major risk factor for coronary spasm. *Circulation* 87:76, 1993.
34. Galan KM, Ubeydullah D, Kern MJ: Increased frequency of restenosis in patients continuing to smoke cigarettes after percutaneous transluminal coronary angioplasty. *Am J Cardiol* 61:260, 1988.
35. Voors AA, van Brussel BL, Plokker T, et al: Smoking and cardiac events after venous coronary bypass surgery: A 1 year follow-up study. *Circulation* 93:42, 1996.
36. Manson JE, Ajani UA, Liu S, et al: A prospective study of cigarette smoking and the incidence of diabetes mellitus among US male physicians. *Am J Med* 109:538, 2000.
37. Grover SA, Gray-Donald K, Joseph L, et al: Life expectancy following dietary modification or smoking cessation: Estimating the benefits of a prudent lifestyle. *Arch Intern Med* 154:1697, 1994.
38. Wagner EH, Curry SJ, Grothaus L, et al: The impact of smoking and quitting on health care use. *Arch Intern Med* 155:1789, 1995.
39. Fichtenberg CM, Glantz SA: Association of the California tobacco control program with declines in cigarette consumption and mortality from heart disease. *N Engl J Med* 343:1772, 2000.
40. The Tobacco Use and Dependence Clinical Practice Guidelines Panel, Staff, and Consortium Representatives: A clinical practice guideline for treating tobacco use and dependence. A US Public Health Service Report. *JAMA* 283:3244, 2000.
41. Wilson K, Gibson N, Willan A, Cook D: Effect of smoking cessation on mortality after myocardial infarction. *Arch Intern Med* 160:939, 2000.
42. Jacobs DR Jr, Adachi H, Mulder I, et al for the Seven Countries Study Group: Cigarette smoking and mortality risk. Twenty-five-year follow-up of the Seven Countries Study. *Arch Intern Med* 159:733, 1999.

43. Benowitz NL: Nicotine metabolic profile in man: Comparison of cigarette smoking and transdermal nicotine. *J Pharmacol Ther* 268:296, 1994.

44. Jacob P III, Benowitz NL: Oxidative metabolism of nicotine in vivo. In: Adikofer F, Thuraus K, eds. *Effects of Nicotine on Biological Systems.* Basel: Birkhauser-Verlag, 1991:35–44.

45. Turner DM, Armitage AK, Briant RH, Dollery CT: Metabolism of nicotine in the isolated perfused dog lung. *Xenobiotica* 5:539, 1975.

46. Cashman JR: Metabolism of nicotine by human liver microsomes stereoselective formation of trans-nicotine N9-oxide. *Clin Res Toxicol* 5:639, 1992.

47. Russell MAH, Feyerabend C: Cigarette smoking: A dependence on high nicotine boli. *Drug Metab* 8:29, 1978.

48. Benowitz NL: Metabolism, pharmacokinetics and pharmacodynamics in man. In: Martin WR, Van Loon GR, Iwamoto ET, Davis L, eds. *Tobacco Smoking and Nicotine: A Neurobiological Approach.* New York: Plenum Press, 1987:357.

49. Nakajima M, Kwon J-T, Tanaka N, et al: Relationship between interindividual differences in nicotine metabolism and CYP2A6 genetic polymorphism in humans. *Clin Pharmacol Ther* 68:72, 2001.

50. Benowitz NL: Nicotine and cotinine elimination pharmacokinetics in smokers and nonsmokers. *Clin Pharmacol Ther* 53:316, 1993.

51. Benowitz NL: Nicotine metabolism in nonsmokers (letter). *Clin Pharmacol Ther* 48:473, 1990.

52. Benowitz NL: Cotinine deposition and effects. *Clin Pharmacol Ther* 34:604, 1983.

53. DeSchepper PJ: Kinetics of cotinine after oral and intravenous administration to man. *Eur J Clin Pharmacol* 31:583, 1987.

54. Benowitz NL: Pharmacological aspects of cigarette smoking and nicotine addiction. *N Engl J Med* 319:1318, 1988.

55. McGehee DS, Heath MJS, Gelber S, et al: Nicotine enhancement of fast excitatory synaptic transmission in CNS by presynaptic receptors. *Science* 269:1692, 1995.

56. Symons JD, Stebbins CL: Hemodynamic and regional blood flow responses to nicotine at rest and during exercise. *Med Sci Sports Exerc* 28:457, 1996.

57. Pomerleau OF, Pomerleau CS: Neuroregulators and the reinforcement of smoking: Towards a biobehavioral explanation. *Neurosci Biobehav Rev* 8:503, 1984.

58. Ikard FF, Green DE, Horn D: A scale to differentiate between types of smoking as related to the management of affect. *Int J Addict* 4:629, 1969.

59. McKennell AC: Smoking motivation factors. *Br J Soc Clin Psychology* 9:8, 1970.

60. Best AJ, Hakstian AR: A situation specific model for smoking behavior. *Addict Behav* 3:79, 1978.

61. Frith CD: Smoking behavior and its relation to the smokers immediate experience. *Br J Soc Clin Psychology* 10:73, 1971.

62. Tate JC: Pharmacological and nonpharmacological smoking motives: A replication and extension. *Addiction* 89(3):321, 1994.

63. Russell MAH, Peto J, Patel UA: The classification of smoking by factorial structure of motives. *J R Statist Soc* 137:313, 1974.

64. Henningfield JE: Higher levels of nicotine in arterial than venous blood after cigarette smoking. *Drug Alcohol Depend* 33(1):23, 1993.

65. Benowitz NL: Clinical pharmacology of inhaled drugs of abuse: Implications in understanding nicotine dependence. *Natl Inst Drug Abuse Res Monogr* 99:12, 1990.

66. Benowitz NL: Nicotine replacement therapy: What has been accomplished. Can we do better? *Drugs* 45(2):157, 1993.

67. Benowitz NL: Establishing nicotine threshold for addiction: The implications for tobacco regulation. *N Engl J Med* 331(2):123, 1994.

68. Flegal KM, Troiano RP, Pamuk ER, et al: The influence of smoking cessation on the prevalence of overweight in the United States. *N Engl J Med* 333:1165, 1995.

68a. Lee D-H, Ha M-H, Kim J-R, Jacobs DR Jr: Effects of smoking cessation on changes in blood pressure and incidence of hypertension. A 4-year follow-up study. *Hypertension* 37:194, 2001.

69. Zellweger J-P: Anti-smoking therapies: Is harm reduction a viable alternative to smoking cessation? *Drugs* 61:1041, 2001.

70. Benowitz NL: Stable isotope studies of nicotine kinetics and bioavailability. *Clin Pharmacol Ther* 49(3):270, 1991.

71. Department of Health and Human Services, Public Health Services: *Preventing Tobacco Use among Young People: A Report of Surgeon General.* Washington, DC: US Government Printing Office, 1994.

72. Johnson J, Ballin S: The power to regulate tobacco. *Circulation* 92:2021, 1995.

73. Otsuka R, Watanabe H, Hirata K, et al: Acute effects of passive smoking on the coronary circulation in healthy young adults. *JAMA* 286:436, 2001.

74. Glantz SA, Parmley WW: Even a little secondhand smoke is dangerous. *JAMA* 286:462, 2001.

75. Liu Y, Zhang J, Watson RR: Environmental tobacco smoke promotes heart disease. *Cardiovasc Rev Rep* 21:589, 2000.

76. Kato M, Roberts-Thomson P, Phillips BG, et al: The effects of short-term passive smoke exposure on endothelium-dependent and independent vasodilation. *J Hypertens* 17:1395, 1999.

77. Hutchison SJ, Sudhir K, Sievers RE, et al: Effects of L-arginine on atherogenesis and endothelial dysfunction due to secondhand smoke. *Hypertension* 34:44, 1999.

78. He J, Vupputuri S, Allen K, et al: Passive smoking and the risk of coronary heart disease—a meta-analysis of epidemiologic studies. *N Engl J Med* 340:920, 1999.

79. Raitakari OT, Adams MR, McCredie RJ, et al: Arterial endothelial dysfunction related to passive smoking is potentially reversible in healthy young adults. *Ann Intern Med* 130:578, 1999.

80. Knight JM, Eliopoulos C, Klein J, et al: Passive smoking in children: Racial differences in systemic exposure to cotinine by hair and urine analysis. *Chest* 109:446, 1996.

81. Sellers EM: Pharmacogenetics and ethnoracial differences in smoking. *JAMA* 280:179, 1998.

82. Centers for Disease Control and Prevention: Cigarette smoking among adults. US 1991. *MMWR* 42:230, 1993.

83. Benowitz NL: Pharmacodynamics of nicotine: Implications for rational treatment of nicotine addiction. *Br J Addict* 86:495, 1991.

84. Henningfield JE: Nicotine medications for smoking cessation. *N Engl J Med* 333:1196, 1995.

85. Law M, Tang JL: An analysis of the effectiveness of interventions intended to help people stop smoking. *Arch Intern Med* 155:1933, 1995.

86. Nicotine replacement for smokers. *Lancet* 357:897, 2001.

87. Benowitz NL: Nicotine and coronary heart disease. *Trends Cardiovasc Med* 1:315, 1991.

88. Benowitz NL: Nicotine replacement therapy during pregnancy. *JAMA* 266:3174, 1991.

89. US Department of Health and Human Services: *The Health Consequences of Smoking: Nicotine Addiction. A Report of the Surgeon General.* Publication CDC 88-8406. Washington, DC: U, 1988.

90. Working Group for the Study of Transdermal Nicotine in Patients with Coronary Artery Disease: Nicotine replacement therapy for patients with coronary artery disease. *Arch Intern Med* 154:989, 1994.

91. Kimmel SE, Berlin JA, Miles C, et al: Risk of acute myocardial infarction and use of nicotine patches in a general population. *J Am Coll Cardiol* 37:1297, 2001.

92. Hajek P, West R, Foulds J, et al: Randomized comparative trial of nicotine polacrilex, a transdermal patch, nasal spray, and an inhaler. *Arch Intern Med* 159:2033, 1999.

93. Hughes JR, Goldstein MG, Hurst RD, Shiffman S: Recent advances in the pharmacotherapy of smoking. *JAMA* 281:72, 1999.

94. Dale LC, Ebbert JO, Hays JT, Hurt RD: Treatment of nicotine dependence. *Mayo Clin Proc* 75:1311, 2000.

94a. Non-nicotine pharmacotherapy may prove useful in smoking cessation. *Drugs Ther Perspect* 17:9, 2001.

95. Rodu B: An alternative approach to smoking control (editorial). *Am J Med Sci* 308(1):32, 1994.

96. Tilashalski K, Rodu B, Cole P: A pilot study of smokeless tobacco in smoking cessation. *Am J Med* 104:456, 1998.

97. Abelin T, Buehler A, Vesanen K, Imhof PR: Controlled trial of transdermal nicotine patch in tobacco withdrawal. *Lancet* 1:7, 1989.

98. Transdermal Nicotine Study Group: Transdermal nicotine for smoking cessation. *JAMA* 266:3133, 1991.

99. Tonneson P, Norregaard J, Simonson K, Sawe U: A double-blind trial of l6 hour transdermal nicotine patch in smoking cessation. *N Engl J Med* 325:311, 1991.

100. Law M, Tang JL: Analysis of the effectiveness of interventions intended to help people stop smoking. *Arch Intern Med* 155:1933, 1995.

101. Fiscella K, Franks P: Cost-effectiveness of the transdermal nicotine patch as an adjunct to physicians smoking cessation counseling. *JAMA* 275:1247, 1996.

101a. Pierce JP, Gilpin EA: Impact of over-the-counter sales on effectiveness of pharmaceutical aids for smoking cessation. *JAMA* 288:1260, 2002.

102. Benowitz NL, Jacob P III, Savanapridi C: Determinants of nicotine intake while chewing nicotine polacrilex gum. *Clin Pharmacol Ther* 45:467, 1987.

103. Gorsline J, Benowitz NL, Rolf CN, et al: Comparison of plasma nicotine concentrations for nicotine transdermal system (NTS), cigarette smoking and nicotine polacrilex (nicotine gum) (abstr). *Clin Pharmacol Ther* 51:129, 1992.

104. Dale LC, Hurt RD, Offord KP, et al: High-dose nicotine patch therapy. Percentage of replacement and smoking cessation. *JAMA* 274:1353, 1995.

105. Jorenby DE, Smith SS, Fiore MC, et al: Varying nicotine patch dose and type of smoking cessation counseling. *JAMA* 274:1347, 1995.

106. Hughes JR: Treatment of nicotine dependence. Is more better? (editorial). *JAMA* 274:1390, 1995.

107. Rigotti NA: Treatment of tobacco use and dependence. *N Engl J Med* 346:506, 2002.

108. Fant RF, Owen LL, Henningfield JE: Tobacco use and cessation. Clinics in Office Practice. *Primary Care* 26:633, 1999.

109. Benowitz NL: Nicotine effects on eicosamoid formation and hemostatic function: Comparison of transdermal nicotine and cigarette smoking. *J Am Coll Cardiol* 22(4):159, 1993.

110. Sachs DPL: Effectiveness of the 4-mg dose of nicotine polacrilex for the initial treatment of high-dependent smokers. *Arch Intern Med* 155:1973, 1995.

111. Medical Economics Company: *Physicians' Desk Reference,* 51st ed. Montvale, NJ: Medical Economics Company, 1997.

112. Henningfield JE, Radzius A, Cooper TM, et al: Drinking coffee and carbonated beverages blocks absorption of nicotine from nicotine polacrilex gum. *JAMA* 264:1560, 1990.

113. Murray RP, Bailey WC, Daniels K, et al: Safety of nicotine polacrilex gum used by 3,094 participants in the lung health study. *Chest* 109:438, 1996.

114. West RJ, Jarvis MJ, Russell MAH, Feyerabend C: Plasma nicotine concentrations from repeated doses of nasal nicotine solution. *Br J Addict* 79:443, 1984.

115. Schneider NG, Lunell E, Olmstead RE, Fagerstrom K-O: Clinical pharmacokinetics of nasal nicotine delivery: A review and comparison to other nicotine systems. *Clin Pharmacokinet* 31: 65, 1996.

116. Hughes JR: Dependence on and abuse of nicotine replace: An update. In: Benowitz NL, ed. *Nicotine Safety and Toxicity.* New York: Oxford University Press, 1998:147–160.

117. Schuh KJ, Schuh LM, Henningfield JE, Stitzer ML: Nicotine nasal spray and vapor inhaler; abuse liability assessment. *Psychopharmacology* 130:352, 1997.

118. Bohadana A, Nilsson F, Rasmussen T, Martinet Y: Nicotine inhaler and nicotine patch as a combination therapy for smoking cessation. A randomized, double-blind, placebo-controlled trial. *Arch Intern Med* 160:3128, 2000.

118a. Schneider NG, Olmstead RE, Franzon MA, Lunell E: The nicotine inhaler: Clinical pharmacokinetics and comparison with other nicotine treatments. *Clin Pharmacokinet* 40:661, 2001.

119. Bollinger C, Zellweger JP, Danielsson T, et al: Smoking reduction with oral nicotine inhalers: Double blind, randomised clinical trial of efficacy and safety. *BMJ* 321:329, 2000.

119a. Blondal T, Gudmundsson LJ, Olafsdottir I, et al: Nicotine nasal spray with nicotine patch for smoking cessation: Randomised trial with six year follow up. *BMJ* 318:285, 1999.

120. Lunell E, Molander L, Andersson SB: Temperature dependency of the release and bioavailability of nicotine from nicotine vapour inhaler: In vitro/in vivo correlation. *Eur J Clin Pharmacol* 52:495, 1997.

120a. Shiffman S, Dresler CM, Hajek P, et al: Efficacy of a nicotine lozenge for smoking cessation. *Arch Intern Med* 162:1267, 2002.

120b. Stead LF, Hughes JR: Lobeline for smoking cessation, *Cochrane Database Syst Rev* CD000124, 2000.

120c. Sutherland G: Current approaches to the management of smoking cessation. *Drugs* 62(Suppl 2):53, 2002.

121. Ascher JA, Cole JO, Colin J, et al: Bupropion: A review of its mechanism of antidepressant activity. *J Clin Psychiatry* 56:395, 1995.

122. Jorenby D: Clinical efficacy of bupropion in the management of smoking cessation. *Drugs* 62(Suppl 2):25, 2002.

122a. Ahluwalia JS, Harris KJ, Catley D, et al: Sustained-release bupropion for smoking cessation in African Americans: A randomized controlled trial. *JAMA* 288:468, 2002.

123. Hurt RD, Sachs DPL, Glover ED, et al: A comparison of sustained release bupropion and placebo for smoking cessation. *N Engl J Med* 337:1195, 1997.

124. Hayford KE, Patten CA, Rummans TA, et al: Efficacy of bupropion for smoking cessation in smokers with a former history of major depression or alcoholism. *Br J Psychiatry.* 174:173, 1999.

125. Sakr A, Andheria M: A comparative multidose pharmacokinetic study of buspirone extended-release tablets with a reference immediate-release product. *J Clin Pharmacol* 41:886, 2001.

126. Jorenby DE, Leischow SJ, Nids MA, et al: A controlled trial of sustained release bupropion, a nicotine patch, or both for smoking cessation. *N Engl J Med* 340:685, 1999.

127. Prochazka A: New developments in smoking cessation. *Chest* 117(4 Suppl 1):169S, 2000.

128. Aubin H-J: Tolerability and safety of sustained-release bupropion in the management of smoking cessation. *Drugs* 62(Suppl 2):45, 2002.

129. Glassman AH, Stetner F, Walsh BT, et al: Heavy smokers, smoking cessation, and clonidine: Results of a double-blind randomized trial. *JAMA* 259:2863, 1988.

130. Covey LS, Glassman AH: A meta-analysis of double-blind placebo controlled trials of clonidine for smoking cessation. *Br J Addict* 86:991, 1991.

130a. Gourlay SG, Stead LF, Benowitz NL: Clonidine for smoking cessation. *Cochrane Data base Syst Rev* CD000058, 2000.

131. Hall SM, Reus VI, Munoz RF, et al: Nortriptyline and cognitive-behavioral therapy in the treatment of cigarette smoking. *Arch Gen Psychiatry* 55:683, 1998.

132. Prochazka AV, Weaver MJ, Keller RT, et al: Treatment: Nortriptyline was associated with an increased rate of 6 month smoking cessation. *Evidenced-based Cardiovasc Med* 3:15, 1999.

132a. Fowler JS, Volkow ND, Wang GJ, et al: Inhibition of monoamine oxidase B in the brain of smokers. *Nature* 379:733, 1996.

132b. Berlin I, Spreux-Varoquaux O, Said S, et al: Effects of past history of major depression on smoking characteristics, monoamine oxidase A and B activities and withdrawal symptoms in dependent smokers. *Drug Alcohol Depend* 45:31, 1997.

132c. Berlin V, Said S, Spreux-Varoquaux O, et al: A reversible monoamine oxidase A inhibitor (moclobemide) facilitates smoking cessation and abstinence in heavy, dependent smokers. *Clin Trial Ther* 8:444, 1995.

133. Wickelgren I: Drug may suppress the craving for nicotine. *Science* 282:1797, 1998.

133a. Covey LS, Sullivan MA, Johnston JA, et al: Advances in non-nicotine therapy for smoking cessation. *Drugs* 59:17, 2000.

133b. Rose JE, Behm FM, Westman EC, et al: Mecamylamine combined with nicotine skin patch facilitates smoking cessation beyond nicotine patch treatment alone. *Clin Trials Ther* 56:86, 1994.

134. Joseph AM, Norman SM, Ferry LH, et al: The safety of transdermal nicotine as an aid to smoking cessation in patients with cardiac disease. *N Engl J Med* 335:1792, 1996.

135. Glantz LH, Annas GJ: Tobacco, the Food and Drug Administration, and Congress. *N Engl J Med* 343:1802, 2000.

Fish Oils, the B Vitamins, and Folic Acid as Cardiovascular Protective Agents

Nathan A. Kruger

William H. Frishman

Jamal Hussain

In recent years, the occurrence of cardiovascular disease has been associated with relative deficiencies of certain food substances in the diet. A form of high-output cardiomyopathy is attributed to thiamine deficiency, which can be treated successfully with vitamin replacement. Most recently, an important risk factor for premature coronary artery disease (CAD) and cerebrovascular disease, homocysteinemia, has been related to nutritional deficiencies of pyridoxine (vitamin B_6), cobalamin (vitamin B_{12}), and folic acid and/or genetic abnormalities in folate metabolism.[1–5] Finally, the omega-3 fatty acids (fish oils), when used as an oral supplement, may prove valuable in primary and secondary prevention of various cardiovascular diseases.

In this chapter, fish oils, the B vitamins (thiamine, pyridoxine, and B_{12}), and folate are discussed as potential drug therapies for the prevention and treatment of cardiovascular disease. The following chapter deals with nutritional antioxidant therapies.

FISH OIL

In the early 1970s, researchers first became interested in the possible role of fish oil in the prevention of atherosclerosis when it was observed that, despite a shorter average life span, Greenland Inuit had a much lower death rate from CAD than western Europeans.[6] The difference in the rate of CAD deaths was attributed to the special Inuit diet—composed mostly of fish and marine animals rich in long-chain polyunsaturated fatty acids (PUFAs). This was in contrast to the Danish diet, which was composed mostly of saturated fats.[7] Although Greenland Inuit consume a high-fat, high-protein diet, their plasma concentrations of total lipids, cholesterol, and triglycerides are significantly lower than those of their Danish counterparts or Inuit living in Denmark.[6] Similarly, a low death rate from coronary heart disease (CHD) was also found in Japanese villages where fish consumption is high.[8,9] The Zutphen study, which followed individuals in the Netherlands for more than 20 years, supported an inverse dose-response relationship between fish consumption and death from CHD.[10] These epidemiologic findings prompted a series of experimental trials investigating the possible role of fish oil in the prevention of atherosclerosis and as a treatment for various cardiovascular disorders (Table 23-1).

Chemistry and Biologic Formation

Fish oil is rich in omega-3 fatty acids. The omega-3 (or n-3) nomenclature denotes the first unsaturated carbon from the methyl end of the molecule and identifies one of two classes of fatty acids, omega-3 and omega-6, that are essential in the diet. This is because mammals lack both delta-12 and delta-15 desaturase enzymes, which are required to create double bonds at the n-6 and n-3 positions, respectively, of an 18-carbon fatty acid precursor. In fish, the two most abundant n-3 fatty acids are eicosapentaenoic acid (EPA, 20:5), a 20-carbon fatty acid with five unsaturated carbon bonds, and docosahexaenoic acid (DHA, 22:6), a 22-carbon fatty acid with six unsaturated carbon bonds (Fig. 23-1). When ingested, EPA accumulates in the membrane phospholipids of platelets, endothelial cells, neutrophils, and erythrocytes.[11–15] EPA can be elongated and desaturated to DHA, but this pathway may not be efficient in humans.[16,17] DHA is incorporated into phospholipids and undergoes retroconversion to EPA within 2 to 4 h after pure DHA ingestion.[18] Recent studies suggest that DHA and EPA are not equivalent when taken as dietary supplements and may have differing pharmacologic effects.[19]

When fatty acids are ingested, they are incorporated into phospholipids and become precursors to biologically active compounds. The metabolic pathway important to n-3 fatty acids is similar to that of eicosanoid metabolism. Arachidonic acid, an n-6 fatty acid derived from plant oil, is the usual substrate of eicosanoid metabolism. When metabolized by cyclooxygenase, arachidonic acid produces the 2-series prostanoids such as thromboxane A_2 (TXA$_2$) and prostacyclin I_2 (PGI$_2$). When n-3 fatty acids are consumed, they replace arachidonic acid and are incorporated into the eicosanoid metabolism pathway, producing 3-series prostanoids and leukotrienes with specific vascular and hemostatic actions (Fig. 23-2). N-3 fatty acids inhibit the synthesis of arachidonic acid from linoleic acid (an 18-carbon n-6 fatty acid).[20] They decrease the plasma and cellular level of arachidonic acid by replacing it at the 2-acyl position in phospholipids[21,22] and compete with arachidonic acid as the substrate for cyclooxygenase and lipoxygenase metabolism.[22,23] TXA$_2$, a product of cyclooxygenase metabolism of arachidonic acid, has potent vasoconstricting and platelet-aggregating effects. However, when n-3 fatty acids are introduced into the platelet membrane by feeding volunteers diets supplemented

TABLE 23-1. Potential Therapeutic Uses of n-3 Fatty Acids in Cardiac Disease

1. Atherosclerosis prevention
2. Decrease in myocardial infarct size
3. Angina pectoris
4. Hyperlipidemia
5. Arrhythmia
6. Prevention of stroke
7. Post PTCA restenosis prevention

with EPA, cyclooxygenase converts EPA into TXA$_3$,[24,25] a structural analog of TXA$_2$ with little platelet-aggregating effect.[26,27] In endothelial cells, EPA is converted by cyclooxygenase to PGI$_3$ and competitively inhibits PGI$_2$ conversion from arachidonic acid. PGI$_3$, unlike the rather inert TXA$_3$, is a potent vasodilator and platelet inhibitor similar to its counterpart, PGI$_2$.[12,14,27] Thus, n-3 fatty acids shift the metabolism of cell-signaling molecules away from thrombosis.

Another class of eicosanoids, the leukotrienes, is also altered by EPA metabolism. Arachidonic acid is metabolized by 5-lipoxygenase to yield the 4-series leukotrienes B$_4$, C$_4$, D$_4$, and E$_4$. Leukotrienes are strong chemoattractants involved in allergic reactions, immune responses, and inflammation. Leukotrienes may also play a part in acute inflammatory responses to myocardial ischemia and vascular injury.[28] When incorporated in neutrophil membrane phospholipids, EPA competitively inhibits the formation of leukotriene B$_4$ from arachidonic acid, and a biologically much less active leukotriene B$_5$ is synthesized that competes against leukotriene B$_4$ for receptor binding.[23] Thus, EPA may have anti-inflammatory actions that could be useful in reducing injury in acute myocardial infarction (MI).

N-3 FATTY ACID STRUCTURES

FIGURE 23-1. The chemical structure of eicosapentaenoic acid and docosahexaenoic acid. Eicosapentaenoic acid consists of 20 carbons (C20) with five double bonds, and the last unsaturated carbon is located third from the methyl end (n-3). Docosahexaenoic acid has 22 carbons (C22) with six double bonds, and also with its last unsaturated carbon located third from the methyl end (n-3).

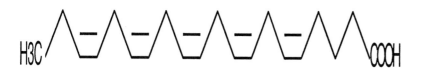

EICOSAPENTAENOIC ACID

(C20:5 n-3)

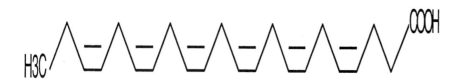

DOCOSAHEXAENOIC ACID

(C22:6 N-3)

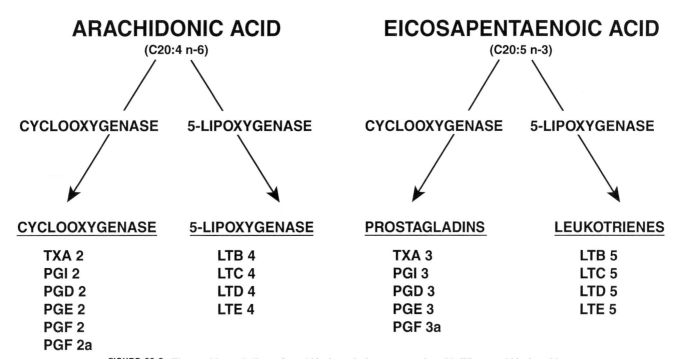

FIGURE 23-2. Eicosanoid metabolism of arachidonic and eicosapentaenoic acid. When arachidonic acid, a n-6 fatty acid, is metabolized by cyclooxygenase, it produces the 2-series prostanoids: thromboxane A_2 (TXA_2), prostaglandin I_2 (PGI_2), prostaglandin D_2 (PGD_2), prostaglandin E_2 (PGE_2), and prostaglandin F_{2a} (PGF_{2a}). When arachidonic acid is metabolized by lipooxygenase, it produces the 4-series leukotrienes: leukotriene B_4 (LTB_4), leukotriene C_4 (LTC_4), leukotriene D_4 (LTD_4), and leukotriene E_4 (LTE_4). As eicosapentaenoic acid replaces arachidonic acid in the phospholipids, it is metabolized by the cyclooxygenase and lipooxygenase to produce the 3-series prostanoids: thromboxane A_3 (TXA_3), prostaglandin I_3 (PGI_3), prostaglandin D_3 (PGD_3), prostaglandin E_3 (PGE_3), and prostaglandin F_{3a} (PGF_{3a}) and the 5-series leukotrienes, leukotriene B_5 (LTB_5), leukotriene C_5 (LTC_5), leukotriene D_5 (LTD_5), and leukotriene E (LTE_5). Dietary consumption of eicosapentaenoic acid leads to decreased synthesis of TXA_2 as well as increased synthesis of TXA_3 and PGI_3, while the synthesis of PGI_2 remains the same.

Pharmacologic Actions

Platelet Function

Repeatedly, n-3 fatty acids have been shown to affect platelet function by prolonging the bleeding time, increasing platelet survival time, decreasing the platelet count and platelet aggregability, and reducing platelet–vessel wall interactions. Dyerberg and Bang demonstrated that the Greenland Inuit have a significantly longer bleeding time than their Danish counterparts, and this "antithrombotic tendency" was thought to result from the dietary n-3 fatty acids consumed by the Inuit. The Inuit demonstrated substantially decreased platelet function, evidenced by the absence of adenosine diphosphate (ADP) and collagen-induced secondary aggregation in half the subjects studied.[11] Human feeding trials with n-3 fatty acid frequently demonstrate increased bleeding times.[29,30] A 40% increase in bleeding time, along with a decreased platelet count, decreased TXA_2 synthesis, and decreased platelet aggregation with ADP and collagen were found in a study involving eight healthy volunteers on a western diet supplemented with cod liver oil.[30] Mortensen et al. also found a similar increase in bleeding time in a double- blind, crossover study of 20 healthy volunteers given fish oil supplements as opposed to vegetable oil supplementation. However, the ADP or collagen-induced platelet aggregation was not altered significantly, even though the threshold concentration for collagen rose by 2% during fish oil supplementation.[31] The increase in bleeding time may be dose-dependent[32,33] and, in some studies,

several weeks elapsed before bleeding times returned to baseline values after supplementation was discontinued.[30,34,35] Prolongation of bleeding time may result from a decreased platelet–vessel wall interaction, as evidenced by decreased platelet aggregation with collagen and ADP. One study gave 6 g/day of EPA for 2 days to eight normal subjects, and showed that fish oil was a potent inhibitor of platelet adhesiveness.[36] Platelet adhesion to fibrinogen and collagen I dropped 60 to 65% after fish oil supplementation. A scanning electron microscopy study of the adherent platelets showed an overall reduction of platelet pseudopodia, which appeared shorter and stubby after fish oil administration.[36]

Fish oil supplementation has been reported to alter other aspects of platelet function. A study by Hay et al. reported a 10% increase in platelet survival time, a 15% fall in platelet count, a 75% fall in the plasma level of platelet factor 4, and a 30% fall in plasma β-thromboglobulin in 13 patients with ischemic heart disease taking 3.5 g/day of EPA supplement for 5 weeks.[37] Platelet factor 4 and β-thromboglobulin are substances released by platelets when interacting with injured blood vessels. Both are chemoattractants for smooth muscle cells and monocytes. Platelet factor 4 may play a role in the hyperplastic response of the injured blood vessel wall.[38] Knapp et al. also found decreased β-thromboglobulin levels and an increased bleeding time in seven normal subjects and in six patients with atherosclerosis taking 10 g/day of EPA for 4 weeks.[39] In this study, the platelet count fell only transiently and the reduction was not significant. The mechanism behind fish oil's possible effect on platelet count has not been elucidated, but the increase in platelet survival suggests a decrease in consumption of platelets that occurs during the platelet–vessel wall interaction. Patients with ischemic heart disease show decreased platelet survival,[15] which may indicate faster turnover of platelets, with a release of growth factors that may encourage the growth of atheromas.[40,41]

Several mechanisms may underlie the modification of platelet function by fish oils. Altered prostacyclin production, rather than thromboxane inhibition, may be the dominant effect, as shown in rat models by Nieuwenhuys et al.[42] Prostacyclin-induced phosphorylation of multiple target proteins may explain the prolonged effects on platelet inhibition. Also, EPA may decrease leukocyte production of platelet activating factor in vitro, and some studies demonstrate decreased thromboxane B_2 (TXB_2) formation in vivo.[43–45] Furthermore, an increased concentration of unsaturated lipid in cell membranes may alter membrane fluidity and thus modify cellular signaling pathways.[46] The change in platelet function after n-3 fatty acid supplementation provides support for an antithrombotic effect of fish oil.

Fibrinolysis and Coagulation Factors

Omega-3 fatty acids influence coagulation pathways and fibrinolysis, but conflicting effects on experimental indices obscure the true clinical relevance of this finding.[47] Plasma fibrinogen level, the best correlate of CHD risk among coagulation markers, is unaltered by amount or type of fat intake. Plasma levels and the activity of factor VII directly correlate with total dietary fat intake and have been shown to increase with fish oil supplementation. However, as demonstrated in type 2 diabetics, this indicator may normalize with an exercise regimen.[47,48] Moreover, fish oils combined with hydroxymethylglutaryl coenzyme A (HMG-CoA) reductase inhibitor therapy may significantly reduce factor VII levels and postprandial hyperlipidemia.[49] Tissue factor pathway inhibitor, in trials by Berrettini, increased after 16 weeks of supplementation but declined in other studies.[47,50] Plasminogen activator inhibitor-1, a potent inhibitor of fibrinolysis, was found to decrease after 4 weeks of treatment in both normal persons and those with CAD.[51] However, subsequent studies have shown both unchanged and even increased activity of plasminogen activator inhibitor-1.[52–54] Recent evidence suggests that omega-3 fatty acids also increase and potentiate protein C.[55,56]

A few reports show that EPA and DHA may have different effects on clotting. In vitro, DHA inhibited clot formation but also inhibited lysis of preexisting clots. EPA enhanced fibrinolysis when added before clot formation but had the opposite effect when added afterwards. A combination supplement enhanced clot formation at low levels but progressively inhibited clotting in higher amounts.[57] Regardless, several double-blind, randomized, controlled studies, including the Coronary Artery Risk Development in Young Adults (CARDIA) study, found no significant changes in coagulation or fibrinolytic markers with fish oil supplementation.[58–60]

Lipids and Lipoproteins

A predominant pharmacologic effect of n-3 fatty acids is in lowering serum triglycerides and VLDL.[61,62] Although this action is well documented in human trials, studies of its mechanism are often performed on other species and must be viewed with due caution. In recent reviews of both human and animal studies, Harris cites effects on other animals that are absent in humans. The metanalyses concluded that species differences as well as experimental designs may account for the discrepancies.[63] Nonetheless, the hypotriglyceridemic effects of fish oils may stem from direct activation of peroxisome-proliferator activated receptor-α (PPAR-α) transcription factors. This mode of action is similar to that of fibrate drugs, which have similar effects on serum lipoproteins. However, whereas mice deficient in PPAR-α do not respond to fibrate drugs, those fed fish oil demonstrate lowered VLDL, triglycerides, and apolipoproteins (apo) A-II and C-III. Still, other effects, such as the lowering of apo A-I, were abolished in the fish oil–fed knockout mice.[64] Further, Anil et al. found indomethacin to suppress the effects of EPA on VLDL and triglyceride production in rat hepatocytes, suggesting a prostaglandin-dependent pathway.[65] These studies suggest that fish oil and fibrate mechanisms may be initially different and provide a molecular rationale for combination treatment.[65,66] Regardless, both therapies result in increased mitochondrial β-oxidation of fatty acids.[67] Also, EPA, but not DHA, increases carnitine acyltransferase mRNA activity and inhibits hepatic lipogenesis, thus reducing the amount of fatty acids available for triglyceride synthesis.[68,69] EPA also directly decreases triacylglycerol formation by inhibiting diacylglycerol acyltransferase in rat hepatocytes.[69]

Fish oil inhibits hepatic VLDL and apoprotein B production in MaxEPA-fed rats, in MaxEPA perfused rat liver, and in humans.[68,70,71] Decreased apo B secretion, not messenger ribonucleic acid (mRNA) translation, may be responsible. Kendrick et al. have shown that EPA causes apo B to be targeted for degradation in the rough endoplasmic reticulum of hamsters.[72,73] Wu et al. have shown in rats that DHA has biphasic effects on apo B and triglyceride levels, initially increasing their secretion; but later it profoundly inhibits secretion of both for at least 8 h.[74] Further, human studies have shown a decrease in apo-B-100 production and have indicated that fish oil supplementation (both 1.8 and 8.5 g/day) may also lower serum Lp(a) levels.[74–76]

In addition to suppressing hepatic lipoprotein production, fish oils may increase lipoprotein catabolism. Human studies have shown hepatic lipase and serum lipoprotein lipase activities to increase after fish oil administration.[77] Omega-3 enrichment may increase VLDL binding to lipoprotein lipase. The increased conversion of VLDL may explain the rise of certain LDL subfractions with fish oil administration.[78] Catabolic augmentation may also explain the increase in clearance and reduced postprandial levels of chylomicrons and chylomicron remnants.[79] Interestingly, increased PPAR-α activity has also been associated in vitro with decreased macrophage production of lipoprotein lipase in the vessel wall.[80]

Atherogenesis and Lipid Peroxidation

Fish oils may attenuate atherosclerotic disease, especially at the early stages of fatty streak formation. This therapeutic potential may stem from interruption of inter- and intracellular signaling processes involved in recruiting atherogenic cells into the vessel wall. De Caterina and coworkers found DHA to inhibit expression of vascular cell adhesion molecule 1 (VCAM-1) in cultures of human saphenous vein epithelium.[81] In proportion to its incorporation into the cell membrane, DHA also inhibited expression of E-selectin, intercellular adhesion molecule 1 (ICAM-1), interleukin-6 (IL-6), and IL-8 in response to IL-1, IL-4, tumor necrosis factor, or bacterial endotoxin (LPS).[81] Decreased macrophage IL-6 production in response to LPS was also observed after 18 weeks of supplementation in healthy human volunteers.[82] Miles and coworkers demonstrated that fish oil decreased the levels of both ICAM-1 and macrophage scavenger receptor-A at the level of the mRNA.[83,84] Further studies by de Caterina et al. revealed that DHA and EPA inhibited activation of the nuclear factor κB (NF-κB) transcription factors, which control expression of adhesion molecules and leukocyte-specific chemoattractants.[85] This effect was shown to be a property of the double bonds in unsaturated fatty acids, was equivalent regardless of position or bond configuration, but was directly proportional to the degree of unsaturation.[86] The doubly bonded fatty acid chain apparently acts as a sink to absorb intracellular hydrogen peroxide production. Intra- and extracellular levels of hydrogen peroxide decrease concomitantly with VCAM-1 mRNA in cells enriched with DHA. Further, polyethylene glycolated catalase, which degrades hydrogen peroxide enzymatically, produces a similar effect when introduced into endothelial cells. Uninhibited, hydrogen peroxide or some other downstream reactive oxygen species induces the NF-κB system and leads to endothelial activation.[85] In accordance with this effect, purified n-3 fatty acids given to hypertriglyceridemic patients for at least 7 months reduced plasma levels of soluble ICAM-1 and E-selectin levels by 9 and 16%, respectively.[87]

Interestingly, the intrinsically greater ability of n-3 fatty acids to be oxidized has led to concern among many investigators that fish oil supplementation may adversely affect atherosclerotic disease. Oxidation of low density lipoprotein (LDL) within vessel walls is a crucial step in atheroma development, and the introduction of n-3 fatty acids should increase the body's aggregate amount of peroxidable substrate. In addition, macrophages with enhanced levels of n-3 fatty acids demonstrate an increased capacity to oxidize LDL in vitro. This occurs via a cyclooxygenase and 15-lipoxygenase–independent mechanism but one that is inhibited by large concentrations of vitamin E.[88]

The majority of recent fish oil trials have included some measurement of LDL oxidation. Methods are varied and include quantifying indices of in vivo oxidation, such as plasma or urinary thiobarbituric acid–reacting substances (TBARS), malondialdehyde, conjugated dienes, or urinary F_2-isoprostanes. Ex vivo indices may report the total peroxidability or oxidation lag time when plasma lipids are exposed to metals such as copper. Unfortunately, the range of results has been as widely varied as the kinds of tests, and little consensus has been reached. For example, McGrath et al. found that patients with type 2 diabetes who were treated with fish oil versus olive oil had increased plasma TBARS. Again, consistent with the hydrogen peroxide mechanism, these patients also demonstrated depleted pools of α-tocopherol (vitamin E).[89] This antioxidant vitamin is known to absorb hydrogen peroxide and other reactive oxygen species but is ultimately consumed in the process. Song and Miyazawa have shown similar elevations in plasma and liver microsomal TBARS as well as decreased α-tocopherol in DHA fed rats.[90] More recently, however, in a double-blinded crossover trial of fish oil versus sunflower oil (oleate) and safflower (linoleate) supplements given to postmenopausal women, overall ex vivo LDL oxidation did not increase.[91] In this and other studies, plasma malondialdehyde and free urinary F_2-isoprostanes decreased with fish oil supplementation despite elevated plasma TBARS.[92–94] In a comparison of fish oil supplementation with and without vitamin E in young women, plasma antioxidant levels were affected in the group given the vitamin, but plasma lipid peroxides were equivalent and unchanged.[95] Ultimately, an aggregate increase of lipid peroxidability with fish oil ingestion may be less clinically relevant than the attenuated leukocyte activity. However, the current evidence is indirect and without consensus.

Tissue Growth Factors and Vessel Wall Inflammation

Fish oils may act at more advanced stages of atherosclerosis, retarding atheroma formation and progression through interactions with several signaling pathways. Omega-3 fatty acids may inhibit monocyte production of IL-1 and tumor necrosis factor,[96,97] substances that are toxic to the endothelium and cause leukocytes to adhere to the endothelium, inducing an inflammatory and procoagulant state.[98,99] Moreover, since IL-1 can stimulate fibroblastic activity with mitogenic effects on smooth muscle cells,[100,101] its inhibition may be important in the prevention of atheroma formation.

Fish oil appears to suppress the production of platelet-derived growth factor (PDGF) from cultured endothelial cells.[102] Also, PDGF-induced migration of human aortic smooth muscle cells is significantly inhibited by n-3 fatty acids in vitro.[103] The work of Asano and others suggests that PDGF fails to induce migration through attenuation of calcium currents and hyperpolarization of resting cell membrane potentials. EPA decreases the intracellular concentration of calcium as well as both the release of calcium from the sarcoplasmic reticulum and calcium entry from the external milieu.[104,105] Attenuation of calcium-mediated stimulation may be important for the atherosclerotic benefits of fish oils but has implications for the antihypertensive and antiarrhythmic properties as well.

Pakala and coworkers demonstrated that EPA and DHA also inhibit vascular smooth muscle cell proliferation in response to thromboxane A_2 as well as to PDGF.[106,107] Serotonin also failed to induce proliferation in EPA- and DHA-pretreated human vascular endothelial cells.[108,109] Proliferation inhibition was optimized with a mixture of EPA and DHA in a ratio similar to that of natural fish oils, but the effect was not produced by other polyunsaturated fatty acids, such as arachidonic, oleic, and γ-linolenic acids.[110] This may be an effect of peroxidation of n-3 fatty acids specifically, which was shown to increase the generation of PGI_2, a known inhibitor of in vitro smooth muscle cell proliferation.[111] EPA-modified expression of transforming growth factor β may also be involved.[112] In vivo, rats and mice fed polyunsaturated fatty acids showed significantly attenuated aortic endothelial migration and smooth muscle proliferation and decreased vessel wall thickness.[113,114] In nonhypercholesterolemic rabbits, Faggin et al. found that dietary fish oil prevented neointima formation after balloon injury of the carotid arteries. This effect was associated with a lower myocyte proliferation index and smaller fibroblasts and smooth muscle cells.[115]

In addition to retarding atheroma formation and progression, evidence suggests that fish oil may induce beneficial vessel wall remodeling. Avula and coworkers attributed higher levels of apoptosis in splenic lymphocytes to n-3 fatty acid–derived lipid peroxides and mediators of apoptosis.[116] Also, moderate levels (15 μg/mL) of EPA kill cloned macrophages through nonapoptotic mechanisms in vitro—apparently by oxidative stress.[117] Moreover, DHA induces apoptosis in vascular smooth muscle cells as a direct PPAR-α ligand in both p38-dependent and p38-independent pathways.[118] The sum of this evidence suggests that n-3 fatty acids may exhibit the therapeutic potential to slow or even reverse atherosclerosis at multiple stages of the disease process.

Endothelial Function

Both human and animal studies show that dietary supplementation of fish oil may increase the release of nitric oxide and restore impaired endothelium-dependent relaxation in hypercholesterolemic subjects.[9,11,120] Endothelial dysfunction is evident by an impaired response to acetylcholine (an endothelium-dependent vasodilator) in subjects with elevated cholesterol levels. This impairment can be reversed by decreasing LDL levels or by dietary supplementation of fish oil in the absence of changes in LDL levels.

Mechanistically oriented studies showed that pretreatment with EPA protects gap junction proteins in human umbilical vein endothelial cells from phosphorylation induced by hypoxia and reoxygenation.[121] This may be due to inhibition of tyrosine kinase activation and parallels the fish oil–induced suppression of protein kinase C seen in renal mesangial cells.[122] Properly functioning gap junctions are regarded as necessary for endothelial cell interactions. Both improved flow-mediated dilation and small artery acetylcholine response have recently been demonstrated in double-blind, randomized, placebo-controlled studies in humans.[123,124] Also, Mori et al. showed that DHA exerts a greater effect than EPA on endothelial relaxation.[125] The improvement in endothelial function and resumption of a normal vasodilatory response in patients with atherosclerosis suggests that fish oil may have beneficial effects in preventing attacks of angina pectoris.

Arrhythmias

Several studies have demonstrated that n-3 fatty acids are possible antiarrhythmic agents. The initial work by McLennan et al. with rats, and later with marmoset monkeys, showed that those fed supplemental fish oil had a decreased incidence and severity of arrhythmias during occlusion and reperfusion of coronary arteries and ventricular fibrillation was prevented.[126,127] Subsequent investigations supported the antiarrhythmic effect of fish oil by demonstrating that PUFAs, especially fish oil, had a protective effect on the appearance of extrasystoles, ventricular tachycardia, and ventricular fibrillation of rat hearts under the conditions of ischemia and reperfusion.[128,129] Billman et al. demonstrated that infusion of free n-3 fatty acids prior to compression of a coronary artery of a prepared dog abolished the expected ischemia and exercise-induced ventricular fibrillation.[130] This suggested that free n-3 fatty acids are the active agents, rather than a change in the composition of myocardial phospholipids. Later studies of cultured rat myocytes supported this assertion.[131] In response, several fish oil supplementation studies showed that about two-thirds of myocardial n-3 fatty acids exist as free, nonesterified fatty acids and in direct proportion to the amount ingested. The remainder are membrane-bound, principally as phosphatidylinositol.[132–134] Leaf et al. further refined the requirements for similarly acting antiarrhythmic molecules. These molecules must consist of a long acyl or hydrocarbon chain, with at least two unsaturated carbon-carbon bonds and a free terminal carboxyl group. Interestingly, these criteria include all-*trans*-retinoic acid, and its antiarrhythmic effects were demonstrated as well.[135]

The antiarrhythmic effects of fish oils may be due to several modifications of cardiac myocyte electrophysiology. As shown by Leaf et al.,[135] n-3 fatty acids cause a slight hyperpolarization of the resting membrane potential as well as prolongation of phase 4 of the cardiac cycle. Also, the threshold voltage for Na^+ channel opening is increased. Thus, a 50% increase of depolarizing stimulus is required to propagate an action potential in isolated myocytes. Subsequent closure of Na^+ channels is shifted to hyperpolarized potentials, requiring that cells return to a relatively hyperpolarized state in order to return the Na^+ channel to an activatable state for subsequent contractions. The prolonged recovery from inactivation should, in theory, counteract the effects of ischemia-induced depolarization.[135–137] However, Kang et al. demonstrated that fish oils, unlike typical type 1 antiarrhythmics, do not cause upregulation of Na channel expression and could even attenuate mexiletine-induced Na channel upregulation.[138]

Inhibition of nitrendipine-sensitive L-type calcium channels by n-3 fatty acids may also be responsible for the antiarrhythmic effect.

Xiao et al. showed that n-3 fatty acids suppressed L-type calcium currents as well as sarcoplasmic reticulum Ca^{2+} release and intracellular Ca^{2+} concentrations in isolated ventricular myocytes.[139] Despite expected negative inotropic effects of fish oils, some evidence suggests that dietary supplementation in rats promotes the efficiency of digitalis and positive inotropy.[140] Further, Kang and Leaf studied the effect of n-3 PUFAs on the contraction of cardiac myocytes in neonatal rats and concluded that at 2 to 10 μM, n-3 PUFAs profoundly reduced the contraction rate without significantly changing the amplitude of the contractions.[141] Also, fish oils appear to prevent the calcium-depleted state caused by nitrendipine and the calcium overload state resulting from ouabain and Bay K8644.[142,143]

Other mechanisms may also account for the antiarrhythmic effects of fish oil. Fish oils may suppress the transient outward flow of potassium.[144] Also, several studies have shown fish oils to inhibit the release of inositol triphosphate, a mechanism that may be responsible for suppressing both ischemia and arrhythmias induced by α-agonists.[145,146] These antiarrhythmic effects may prove beneficial in humans but require further species-specific study.

Anti-Inflammatory Effect

Omega-3 fatty acids inhibit several leukocyte, platelet, and endothelial cell functions, including the generation of inflammatory mediators that may be important in atherogenesis and in the inflammatory response to vascular injury. The pleiotropic effects of fish oil on cellular mediators, many of which are discussed above, are the subjects of recent reviews focusing on inflammation.[16,147] Human trials, as reviewed by Kelley, are plagued by conflicting results, which may be explained by several methodologic inconsistencies. Few studies hold total dietary fat intake constant and include placebo controls, and various amounts of vitamin E intake may further skew results.[148] The preponderance of the evidence suggests that fish oils suppress cytokine production (IL-1 and IL-6 as well as tumor necrosis factor α), and modifies eicosanoid production (decreasing prostaglandin E_2 and leukotriene B_4).[149] Fish oil was also found to blunt the chemotactic responses of both monocytes and neutrophils to leukotriene B_4 and to decrease neutrophil adhesion to the endothelial monolayer treated with leukotriene B_4.[33] Since eicosanoids may be important in the formation of acute inflammation following MI or vascular injury, the alteration in eicosanoid synthesis may be cardioprotective. The anti-inflammatory actions of n-3 fatty acids have also been considered in the treatment of other inflammatory diseases such as asthma, inflammatory bowel disease, IGA nephropathy, lupus, and cancer cachexia.[16,150,151]

Clinical Use

Prevention of Atherosclerosis and Its Complications (Table 23-2)

An epidemiologic study of a Japanese coastal fishing village where the fish consumption is high compared to a farming village where fish consumption is low found an inverse relationship between fish consumption and mortality from CAD.[152] A follow-up study showed a striking five- to eightfold difference in the number of atherosclerotic plaques between the populations and lower incidences of ischemic stroke and angina in the fishing village.[153] The Zutphen study also found an inverse relationship between the amount of fish eaten weekly and the mortality rate from CAD after 20 years of follow-up.[10] In addition, the Chicago Western Electric

TABLE 23-2. Mechanisms by which n-3 Fatty Acids May Prevent Atherosclerosis and Post-PTCA Restenosis

Platelet function
  Decrease platelet factor 4
  Decrease β thromboglobulin
  Increase platelet survival
  Decrease platelet adhesion
  Increase bleeding time
  Decrease platelet count
Cytokines/growth factor
  Decrease IL-1/TNF (monocyte derived)
  Decrease PDGF (endothelium derived)
Inflammatory response
  Decrease LTB_4
  Increase LTB_5
Lipid
  Decrease triglycerides/VLDL
  LDL, HDL, total cholesterol are variable
Coagulation
  Decrease fibrinogen
  Decrease plasminogen activator-1 inhibitor
  Decrease TXA_2
  Increase TXA_3
  Increase PGI_3

TNF = tumor necrosis factor; IL-1 = interleukin-1; VLDL = very low density lipoprotein; LDL = low-density lipoprotein; HDL = high-density lipoprotein; TXA_2 = thromboxane A_2; PGI_3 = prostaglandin I_3; LTB = leukotriene B.

Study showed that fish consumption in men was associated with a decreased long-term risk for death from CAD, especially non–sudden death from MI.[154] These results supported a possible role of fish oil in the prevention of atherosclerosis.

Omega-3 fatty acid supplements, in recent work by von Schacky et al., effectively reduced the progression of human atherosclerotic lesions. In this randomized, double-blind, placebo-controlled study, 223 patients consumed 1.5 g of n-3 fatty acids or placebo daily for 2 years. Angiograms taken before and after the study were compared and showed that the fish oil group had less progression and more regression of atherosclerotic lesions. Quantitative arteriography and clinical events both trended toward benefit but were not significantly different from controls.[155] These results agree with a smaller, earlier study showing a beneficial trend from fish oil but not statistical significance in inhibiting coronary atherosclerosis.[156] Higher consumption of fish and n-3 fatty acids in the Nurses Health Study was associated with a reduced risk of thrombotic cerebral infarctions, particularly in women who did not use aspirin on a regular basis.[157] In the Nurses Study, higher consumption of fish and n-3 fatty acids was also shown to reduce the risk of coronary heart disease, particularly death from coronary heart disease.[157a]

Despite many promising investigations, not all clinical studies have shown benefits. A prospective, 5-year case-control study of male physicians examined the possible relationship between plasma fish oil levels and the incidence of MI.[158] There was no evidence that n-3 fatty acid delayed or prevented the onset of a first heart attack. Plasma levels of n-3 fatty acids were used as biologic markers for fish intake, based on the almost linear relationship with fish or fish oil supplement and plasma levels of EPA and DHA over a range of doses. The effects of a very high level of fish oils were not evaluated in this study.[158] Nonetheless, a reexamination of the U.S. Physicians Health Study correlated fish consumption at least once weekly with decreased risk of sudden cardiac death and decreased total mortality. Other indices of cardiovascular health trended toward benefit,

but not with statistical significance.[159] A recent meta-analysis has provided evidence that dietary and non-dietary intake of n-3 polyunsaturated fatty acids reduced over-all mortality, mortality due to MI, and sudden death in patients with coronary heart disease.[159a]

Other than the possible primary prevention of MI, fish oil may have a role in the secondary prevention of ischemic events. The Diet and Reinfarction Trial (DART) investigators reported that a small increase in dietary fish intake may reduce mortality after MI.[160] A total of 2000 patients were advised to increase their dietary intake of fish or fiber or to decrease their consumption of total fat, with emphasis on using more polyunsaturated vegetable oil. After a 2-year follow-up period, the all-cause mortality was 29% lower for the fish intake group, and this decline was attributed to a 16% decrease in deaths from ischemic heart disease. The survival rate for the group with reduced fat intake was unchanged, while survival for the group emphasizing fiber intake group was worse than that in the other groups. There was no reduction in the rates of nonfatal ischemic heart disease events in any of the three groups. More recently, Singh et al. studied supplementation with n-3 fatty acids for 1 year in 360 patients with suspected acute infarction. In this randomized, double-blind, placebo-controlled trial, the fish oil group had significantly fewer total cardiac events, nonfatal infarctions, and total cardiac deaths. The experimental group also showed a significant reduction in total cardiac arrhythmias, left ventricular enlargement, and angina pectoris compared to controls.[161] In the largest reported clinical trial, the GISSI Prevenzione Investigators (Gruppo Italiano per lo Studio della Sopravvivenza nell'Infarto Miocardico) studied 11,324 recent survivors of MI.[162] In this randomized, open-label, controlled factorial study, patients were administered either 1 g of fish oil per day, 300 mg of vitamin E per day, both, or no treatment starting within 3 months of MI. Over the 3.5 years of the study, the fish oil group showed a 45% decrease in risk of sudden death, a 30% reduction in cardiovascular deaths, and a 20% decrease in all-cause mortality.[162a] Vitamin E supplementation alone conferred no benefit, and the combined treatment was equivalent to fish oil alone.[162]

Noncardiac atherosclerotic vascular diseases may benefit from fish oil as well. The First National Health and Nutrition Examination Survey study group, which involved 5192 persons, found a possible benefit of fish eating more than once a week in lowering stroke incidence in white women aged 45 to 74 years.[163] The age-adjusted risk of stroke incidence in white women who consumed fish more than once a week was about half that of women who never consumed fish. No significant relationship between fish consumption and outcomes was found in white men, but in black men and women combined, there was a significant beneficial association. The possible protective effects of fish oil in the coronary arteries may work in a similar fashion in the cerebral vasculature to protect against ischemic strokes. The results of the Zutphen study and the Japanese fishing village studies supported a positive relationship between fish consumption and decreased incidence of stroke.[153,164] The Physicians' Health Study, involving 21,185 subjects, did not find the same association.[165]

Changes in the parameters of future intervention studies may allow the more subtle benefits of fish oils to be clarified. For example, the Greenland Inuit consume a diet with n-3 fatty acids as the main source of dietary fat over their life span. It is possible that a larger daily dose (i.e., closer to the 10 mg of EPA in the Inuit diet) and a longer follow-up period may be necessary to demonstrate a protective effect of fish oil against the clinical complications of atherosclerosis.

Size of Myocardial Infarct

Dietary fish oils may reduce the size of MI and the incidence of large infarctions. An observational study of 753 patients with acute MI correlated fish oil use prior to infarction with reduced infarction size. Peak levels of creatine kinase and lactate dehydrogenase were significantly less, and the proportion of infarcts classified as smaller was greater in the fish oil group.[166] In animal models, dietary fish oil also favorably affects the size of MI. Culp et al. have demonstrated that chronic dietary supplementation of fish oil for 4 to 6 weeks resulted in smaller infarcts after 24 h of coronary artery occlusion in dogs.[167] Hock et al. found a decreased creatine kinase blood level in fish oil–supplemented rats after 6 h of permanent coronary ligation.[168] Oskarsson et al. fed dogs 0.06 g/kg/day of EPA for 6 weeks and then occluded the left circumflex coronary artery of the dogs for 90 min, followed by 6 h of reperfusion. The dogs who received dietary fish oil had smaller infarctions compared to controls, with no difference in regional coronary perfusion or oxygen consumption.[169] Prospective trials in humans are needed to establish causality and confirm this potential benefit of fish oil ingestion.

Angina Pectoris

Epidemiologic data suggest that fish oil may improve angina symptoms, and several therapeutic investigations examined this issue.[153] In their secondary prevention study, Singh et al. found that fish oil supplementation over a period of 1 year following an acute MI was associated with significantly less angina pectoris.[161] Salachas et al.[170] investigated n-3 fatty acids as a possible treatment for patients with angina pectoris and CAD. Thirty-nine patients were randomized to 1 g of fish oil or olive oil. Weekly anginal attacks, weekly glyceryl trinitrate (GTN) consumption, exercise tolerance time, serum triglycerides, platelet aggregation ratio, and β-thromboglobulin levels were measured at 8 and 12 weeks after initiation of treatment. The group treated with fish oil recorded 41% fewer anginal attacks and concomitantly decreased consumption of GTN. Angina parameters were unchanged in the olive oil–treated group. Exercise tolerance time increased significantly in the fish oil group, whereas the olive oil group experienced a small but insignificant increase in exercise tolerance. Serum triglyceride levels were decreased significantly in the fish oil group and increased slightly in the olive oil group. No difference was found in the platelet aggregation ratio or ß-thromboglobulin levels with either treatment.[170] In a prior study of fish oil in patients with angina, Saynor et al. similarly demonstrated a significant decrease in consumption of GTN and reduction in anginal attack frequency after 2 years of dietary fish oil supplementation.[32] Based on these studies, fish oil appears to have beneficial effects in patients with angina pectoris.

Effects in Percutaneous Transluminal Coronary Angioplasty (PTCA)

Omega-3 fatty acids have been shown to modulate many etiologic factors that are important in postangioplasty restenosis. However, the numerous human clinical trials have shown conflicting results. Explanations for these discrepancies have included variation in the dosage and form of n-3 fatty acids used, the commencement time of supplementation, the definition of restenosis, and the method of evaluating stenosis (stress test versus angiography).[171,172] Most studies involved fewer than 20 subjects.[172] One meta-analysis of seven studies found a small to moderate benefit of fish oil on restenosis but cautioned that a large randomized clinical trial was still needed for confirmation.[171] A second meta-analysis done a year later also suggested a positive result from fish oil, which may be dose-dependent.[172] One large multicenter, randomized, double-blind clinical trial involving 474 subjects receiving either 8 g/day of n-3 fatty acids or corn oil 12 days prior to PTCA and 6 months after PTCA found a 46% restenosis rate in corn oil recipients and 52% restenosis rate in fish oil recipients, based on quantitative angiographic interpretations.[173] Another study, involving 814 patients, that also examined subsequent use of low-molecular-weight heparin failed to show any significant benefit in any group from fish oil administration prior to PTCA.[174] The results of the ESPRIT (Esapent for Prevention of Restenosis Italian Study) showed a small but significant restenosis rate compared to placebo when the fish oil preparation was administered one month before PTCA and maintained for one month there after.[174a]

Most animal studies investigating fish oil's effect on the prevention of postangioplasty restenosis have reported positive results. In a study by Weiner et al., swine were fed a diet high in saturated fats and cholesterol and were given either fish oil supplement or no treatment.[175] Balloon abrasion of coronary arteries was done to stimulate lesion development. After 8 months, the group supplemented with fish oil had less coronary artery encroachment due to intimal hyperplasia than the control group, despite an equivalently elevated cholesterol level.[175] A similar study by Shimokawa et al. demonstrated a decrease in coronary lesion area with fish oil supplementation.[176] Another pig model follow-up study reported both prevention of coronary artery atherosclerosis and regression of existing lesions with fish oil supplementation.[177] Harker et al. found that dietary n-3 fatty acids in large doses eliminated both vascular thrombus formation and vascular lesion formation 6 weeks later at sites of surgical carotid endarterectomy in nonhuman primates.[178] In summary, results of studies done to assess the potential benefit of fish oil in prevention of restenosis after angioplasty have been inconclusive at best.

Hypertension

Several studies suggest a possible blood pressure–lowering effect of fish oil, but the results of both animal and human studies have been conflicting.[179–181] Many of the human clinical trials have been of insufficient size, lacked double-blind randomization, had inadequate run-in periods, and were flawed by methodologic problems.[182–184]

In a meta-analysis that included 17 controlled clinical trials of n-3 fish oil supplementation in humans, Appel et al.[182] found the systolic and diastolic blood pressure change to be -1.0 and -0.5 mm Hg, respectively, in normotensive men, and -5.5 and -3.5 mm Hg, respectively, in untreated hypertensive men. The degree of blood pressure reduction was more significant at higher initial blood pressure levels, but no dose-dependent effect was found. Relatively high doses of n-3 PUFAs of at least 3 g/day can lead to clinically significant reductions in blood pressure in untreated hypertensive subjects.[182] These findings expand upon a prior meta-analysis by Radack and Deck, which found no statistically significant difference between the n-3 PUFA–supplemented group of mostly normotensive subjects. However, only one trial of the four studied involved hypertensive subjects.[185] This single trial showed the greatest reduction in blood pressure. A study evaluating 32 mildly hypertensive men in a randomized, double-blind trial with dietary supplementation of two different doses of fish oil (3 and 15 g/day) demonstrated a significant blood pressure decline only in the high-dose fish oil group, reaching a mean of 5.5/4.5 mm Hg change at the end of 4 weeks of treatment.[183] More recently, Prisco and coworkers found similar results after 2 months, using less than 4 g of fish oils per day, in a randomized controlled trial with 16 normotensive and 16 hypertensive males.[186] Also, a group of 69 overweight hypertensives in a randomized controlled trial showed that dietary fish consumption decreased blood pressure independently and additively with weight reduction.[187] Yosefy and coworkers found similar results in 19 patients who also suffered from diabetes mellitus.[188] In a randomized controlled trial of 45 hypertensive heart transplant recipients, antihypertensive benefit was also observed.[189] In patients with cyclosporine-induced hypertension following cardiac transplantation, a beneficial effect of fish oil was seen on both blood pressure and peripheral vascular resistance.[190] Other evidence is found in obese individuals with markers of insulin resistance; crossover trials showed that 4 weeks of an n-3 fatty acid supplemented diet increased systemic arterial compliance.[191]

In contrast, the Trials of Hypertension Prevention Phase One, a randomized controlled trial of seven interventions in 2182 mildly hypertensive adults, also concluded that moderate amounts of fish oil (i.e., 6 g/day) were unlikely to lower blood pressure in normotensive subjects after either 6 or 18 months.[192,193] Also, a double-blinded, randomized, controlled trial of 4.5 g of daily fish oil in 21 men found no antihypertensive benefit after 8 weeks.[194] These studies illustrate that fish oils do not consistently decrease normal or elevated blood pressure.

Lipid and Lipoprotein Effects

In the original investigation by Bang and Dyerberg, the Greenland Inuit had significantly lower concentrations of total lipids, cholesterol, triglycerides and β-lipoproteins than the Danish controls despite diets that were equally high in fat.[6] The difference in the serum lipid profile was attributed to the Inuit diet, which was high in long-chain PUFAs and low in saturated fat. Key's formula, which describes the serum cholesterol as a function of the fatty acid consumed, was not sufficient to explain the very low serum cholesterol of the Inuit. It was suggested that the long-chain PUFAs, especially timnodonic (C 20:5) and docosahexaenoic (C 22:6) acids from marine mammals in the Inuit diet, had a special metabolic effect leading to lower cholesterol levels. A similar action was believed to have caused lower triglycerides and very low density lipoproteins.[7] Numerous trials have investigated the potential hypolipidemic and cholesterol-lowering effect of fish oil.[195] Described below is a summary of fish oil's effect on the serum lipid profile.

Triglycerides and Very Low Density Lipoprotein (VLDL) Cholesterol

In clinical trials, fish or fish oil supplementation decreases triglycerides in normal and hypertriglyceridemic persons in a dose-dependent manner. Fish oils are among the most powerful triglyceride-lowering agents available and also concomitantly reduce VLDL cholesterol levels.[6,196] Several reviews estimate that n-3 fatty acid supplementation will reduce serum triglycerides by 25 to 30%.[197–199] In hypertriglyceridemic patients, 4 g/day of Omacor was found to have statistically similar lipid and lipoprotein effects as 1200 mg/day of gemfibrozil, including triglyceride- and VLDL cholesterol–reducing effects.[200] Also, fish oil may be used as adjunctive therapy for combined dyslipidemia.[201] Several studies show that adding 900 to 2000 mg/day of fish oil can reduce both serum triglycerides and total cholesterol in hypertriglyceridemic

patients already following regimens similar to those of the Scandinavian Simvastatin Survival Study.[49,202,203] Also, fish oil may increase postprandial triglyceride clearance and reduce postprandial hypertriglyceridemia.[49,204,205]

Low-Density Lipoprotein (LDL) Cholesterol

The plasma LDL level may be affected by fish oil, but the results of numerous studies have included equivocal findings. A meta-analysis by Harris of human trials with less than 7 g/day of supplementation concluded that serum LDL is increased by 5 to 10% by fish oil. Hyperlipidemic subjects experienced greater LDL elevations than normals, but the excursion diminished with time.[199] Subsequent studies suggest that fish oil, especially DHA, may shift the distribution of LDLs to less dense subfractions and reduce the amount of small, dense LDLs. This change, producing more buoyant LDLs, may make them less atherogenic.[19,201,206]

High-Density Lipoprotein (HDL) Cholesterol

The Harris meta-analysis showed that fish oil supplementation increases plasma HDL by 1 to 3%.[199] In phase 1 of the Trials of Hypertension Prevention Study, fish oil was found to increase HDL_2 cholesterol significantly in women but not in men when compared to a control group.[192] Other studies have shown similar increases in HDL_2 and additive effects when combined with a weight-reducing diet.[207] Mori et al. have also suggested that increasing HDL_2 may be a property of DHA but not EPA.[19]

Total Cholesterol

Fish oil did not materially affect the plasma level of total cholesterol in Harris's meta-analysis.[199] However, this study excluded trials utilizing greater than 7 g/day of fish oil; in a few such trials, a significant decrease in serum total cholesterol level was observed.[208] In one study, MaxEPA elicited a dose-dependent response in lowering serum cholesterol.[209] As mentioned previously, fish oil may lower total cholesterol when used as an adjunct to other pharmacologic cholesterol-lowering therapies.

The favorable effect of n-3 fatty acids to lower serum triglycerides is well documented, and their influences over other components of the lipid profile are becoming more so (Table 23-3). Overall, the potential positive influence of fish oil on the lipids may depend on the composition of fat in the diet. Diets containing large amounts of saturated fat may abolish any potential benefit of n-3 fatty acids.

Arrhythmias

Clinical trials on the effects of dietary fish oil on arrhythmias have been limited but encouraging. The Diet and Reinfarction Trial (DART) credited the potential antiarrhythmic effect of fish oil as a possible cause of improved survival after acute MI, but did not measure arrhythmic events directly.[167] Similar improvement in indirect indices of fatal arrhythmias have been subsequently shown

TABLE 23-3. Effects of Fish Oil on Plasma Lipids and Lipoproteins

Total cholesterol	$\leftrightarrow$
Triglyceride	$\downarrow$ 25–30%
Cholesterol	$\leftrightarrow$
HDL cholesterol	$\uparrow$ 1–3%
LDL cholesterol	$\uparrow$ 5–10%
VLDL cholesterol	$\downarrow$ 25%
Lp(a)	$\downarrow$

$\downarrow$ = decrease; $\leftrightarrow$ = unchanged; $\uparrow$ = increased.

by the GISSI investigators.[162] Also, an analysis of the Physicians Health Study correlated fish consumption at least once weekly with a 52% decrease in sudden cardiac deaths, the majority of which involve fatal arrhythmias.[210] This benefit was associated with increased blood levels of long-chain n-3 fatty acids.[210a] Fortunately, a few studies have examined arrhythmias directly. The largest, by Singh et al, found a statistically significant decrease in arrhythmic events and total cardiac deaths when fish oil was administered as secondary prevention post-MI.[161] Earlier, Sellmayer et al. found a reduction of ventricular premature complexes in nearly half of the subjects with frequent premature ventricular arrhythmias given fish oil compared to those patients that received safflower seed oil.[211] A population-based case-control study by Siscovick et al[212] examined 334 cases of primary cardiac arrest and the dietary intake of n-3 PUFA. An intake of 5.5 g of n-3 fatty acids per month, the mean of the third quartile, was associated with a 50% reduction in the risk of primary cardiac arrest. A red blood cell membrane content of n-3 PUFA of 5.0% compared to 3.3% was associated with a 70% reduction in the risk of primary cardiac arrest. Thus, dietary intake of n-3 fatty acids was found to reduce the risk of primary cardiac arrest.[212]

Recently, Christensen et al have provided strong, albeit indirect, evidence of the anti-arrhythmic effects of fish oil in randomized placebo controlled studies.[213] They examined 24-hour heart rate variability, which strongly inversely correlates with arrhythmic events, sudden cardiac death and mortality. This endpoint, as well as the standard deviation of all normal RR intervals, was measured in three different groups: 55 survivors of MI, 29 patients with chronic renal failure at high risk for sudden cardiac death, and 60 healthy volunteers. Significant increases in heart rate variability were found in both groups of diseased patients after 5.2 g/day of fish oil supplementation for 12 weeks. In the healthy subjects, heart rate variability correlated with the granulocytes' content of n-3 fatty acids at baseline. After 12 weeks, a dose-dependent increase in heart rate variability was found with either 2.0 or 6.6 g/day of supplementation in those with low baseline variability.[213] These and other human studies are promising for the potential use of n-3 fatty acids as antiarrhythmic agents.[213a] Ideally, more prospective clinical data are needed to specifically address the issue of antiarrhythmic efficacy, especially in comparison to more established therapies.

Pharmacokinetics

Appropriate dietary intake of n-3 fatty acids can be accomplished directly by consumption of marine foods such as fish, shellfish, or by dietary supplementation with fish oil concentrate. Various types of seafood contain different concentrations of n-3 fatty acids (Table 23-4). Table 23-4 lists the n-3 fatty acid content of several

TABLE 23-4. The n-3 Fatty Acid Content of Various Seafoods

Species	n-3 Fatty Acids (g/100g raw material)
Mackerel	2.5
Trout, lake	1.6
Trout, rainbow	0.5
Herring, Atlantic	1.6
Sardine, canned	1.7
Tuna, albacore	1.3
Tuna, unspecific	0.5
Salmon, chinook	1.4
Salmon, Atlantic	1.2
Blue fish	1.2
Oyster, European	0.5
Crab	0.4
Shrimp	0.4
Cod, Atlantic	0.3
Swordfish	0.2
Lobster	0.2

common marine foods,[214] and Table 23-5 provides a list of EPA and DHA contents in some fish oil concentrates.[215] Omacor, a capsule containing ethyl esters of EPA and DHA, is available in Europe to treat hypertriglyceridemia. The U.S. Food and Drug Administration (FDA) granted it approval only as an orphan drug to treat immunoglobulin A (IgA) nephropathy.

Various fish oil concentrates and seafood, mainly fish, have been used as the source of n-3 fatty acids in various experiments. It appears that n-3 fatty acids are well absorbed after one dose of either fish oil or fish.[216] Although EPA absorption may be more efficient from fish than with concentrates, both provide n-3 fatty acids in a bioavailable form with effects on platelet function.[216]

Various preparations of EPA and DHA are available as triglycerides and as esters of methanol and ethanol. Because of the potential toxic effects of methyl ester, preparations administered to humans are usually are triglyceride or ethyl esters. Both preparations at high doses (27 to 40 g) are equally well absorbed with good absorption of both EPA and DHA.[217] At lower doses (1.0 g EPA), the absorption of the ethyl ester preparation appears less complete than with the triglyceride preparation.[218,219] Different commercially available concentrates can be similar in their form of delivery yet differ in the composition of various n-3 fatty acids. MaxEPA and Amenu were demonstrated to be equivalent in bioavailability.[220] Also, bioavailability was similar between foods fortified with microencapsulated n-3 fatty acids and supplemental capsules.[221] A limited number of studies elucidate potential differences between other preparations in terms of their bioavailability. Aside from the type and form of fatty acid administered, several factors may influence n-3 fatty acid absorption, including the total fat[222] and protein content in the diet.[223]

TABLE 23-5. n-3 Fatty Acid Content of Various Fish Oil Capsules

Product Name	Manufacturer	Milligrams per Capsule	n-3 Fatty Acid Content EPA, mg	n-3 Fatty Acid Content DHA, mg
Promega Pearls Softgels	Parke-Davis	600	600	71
Cardi-Omega 3 capsules	Thompson Medical	1000	180	120
EPA capsules	Nature's Bounty	1000	180	120
MaxEPA capsules	Various: Jones's Medical, Rexall, Moore	1000	180	120
SuperEPA 2000 capsules	Advanced Nutritional	1200	360	240

Source: Adapted with permission from *Drug Facts and Comparisons*.[215]

High amounts of saturated fat may also diminish the potential benefits of EPA and DHA.[224]

A study examining ingestion of Amenu and MaxEPA demonstrated a rapid increase of both EPA and DHA in the plasma at both the 3- and 12-g doses.[220] Other work showed that EPA and DHA ethyl esters in plasma phospholipids exhibit half-lives of about 2 days. Ethyl esters behave biexponentially in plasma triacylglycerols, with initial half-lives of less than 1 day, then slower clearance, with half-lives lasting several days. These results suggest that fish oils may be given every 12 h or less.[225]

Adverse Effects

Fish oil is part of the daily diet and has been consumed in large quantities and over many years in many parts of the world with a low frequency of adverse effects. It is unlikely that fish oil will be toxic when ingested as fish or marine foods. Fish oil concentrates have been used in long-term feeding trials or given in high doses to human subjects without any report of toxicity,[31,173] but more long-term trials are needed to determine a possible toxic dose. The most common side effect reported with the supplementation of large doses of fish oil is gastrointestinal upset, with massive diarrhea and steatorrhea.[226] Less common adverse effects include weight gain, vitamin A and D toxicity, and a foul fish smell. There has been concern regarding possible excessive bleeding and subsequent hemorrhagic stroke from the dietary supplementation of fish oils. However, no clinically significant bleeding was found in one study using fish oil to prevent post-angioplasty restenosis despite invasive surgery and the concomitant use of aspirin.[173]

The seminal fish oil studies, although poorly controlled, prompted the concern that supplementation could impair glycemic control in diabetics. However, in a review of all studies of type 2 diabetics taking fish oil supplements that were published before September 1998, Montori et al. found no statistically significant changes in fasting glucose or HbA_1c levels.[227] An earlier meta-analysis demonstrated no deleterious effects on glycemic control in type 1 or type 2 diabetics from fish oil administration.[228]

Elevation of LDL levels, especially in hyperlipidemic patients given high-dose fish oils, or the possible formation of biologically active oxidation products are other potential concerns.[227] Also, fish oil–induced changes of inflammatory and immune processes are possible adverse effects for persons with preexisting immune suppression but remains with little in vivo human data.

Dose

The appropriate dosage of n-3 fatty acids for optimal cardiovascular benefit in humans is still in question. The optimal dose certainly depends on the effects sought. As little as 1 g/day delivers potent triglyceride-lowering and antiarrhythmic effects, but 3 to 5 g/day has been recommended for therapy of hypertriglyceridemic patients.[197,228] The Greenland Inuit consume approximately 5 to 10 g of n-3 fatty acids a day.[229] Since administration of 6 g of n-3 fatty acids for 7 days inhibited platelet aggregation and this effect did not accelerate with additional supplementation,[230] it was suggested that the optimal dose should be around 3 to 6 g/day.[220] Interestingly the FDA recommends that 3 g/day be the upper limit of total fish oil intake for the general population, because additional intake may adversely alter hemostatic parameters. Such effects may be desired, however. Some authors projected that optimal dosage in high-risk

populations might be as high as 40 to 60 g/day to effect significant reductions in CAD deaths.[221] Further studies are needed to clarify the exact dose of fish oil required to achieve maximal clinical benefits for specific indications.

Conclusion

Based on fish oil's effect on lipids, arrhythmias, platelets, and coagulation factors, fish oil has the potential for use as a cardiovascular medicine. A few secondary prevention studies have shown clinically significant benefits. However, there have not been major prospective primary prevention clinical trials in humans that are able to demonstrate that fish oil supplementation can prevent atherosclerosis and its complications. It is also possible that the antiatherosclerotic beneficial effect of n-3 fatty acids—which is seen in subjects who consume large quantities of fish, such as people living in fishing villages of Japan, the Greenland Inuit, and the subjects in the Zutphen study—is partly related to a decreased consumption of saturated fat. Omega-3 fatty acids may help to prevent the development of atherosclerosis when they are used as a daily supplement to a diet that is low in saturated fat. The potential use of fish oil as a possible triglyceride-lowering agent, antianginal agent or an antiarrhythmic agent is encouraging, but additional study is needed to clarify its effect. Fish oil appears to have limited use in preventing postangioplasty restenosis or lowering blood pressure.

The effects of fish oil supplementation on platelet function appear to be less than those of low-dose aspirin, and the effects on lipids appear to be comparable to those of other therapeutic modalities. Fish oil administration will likely prove to be beneficial in certain high-risk populations and warrants further rigorous study specific to these indications.[231] A recommendation to encourage use of fish oil supplementation in the general population, beyond that of eating more fish, is not appropriate at this time.[232]

VITAMINS B_6 (PYRIDOXINE), B_{12} (COBALAMIN), AND FOLATE

In recent years, vitamins B_6, B_{12}, and folate have gained importance as possible treatments of hyperhomocysteinemia, a potential risk factor for premature atherosclerotic disease and its complications. Fortification of enriched grains with folic acid, a recent requirement in the United States, may impart a significant epidemiologic benefit in the prevention of CHD. In this section, the metabolism of homocysteine is reviewed, along with the published experiences of vitamin therapy for homocysteine elevations.

Homocysteine

The conventional risk factors for cardiovascular disease include smoking, high blood pressure, elevated cholesterol levels, hyperlipidemia, hypertension, diabetes, and a family history of cardiovascular disease. In recent decades, homocysteine has been associated with an increased incidence of cardiovascular disease. In order to understand how homocysteine could be a risk factor for cardiovascular disease, a review of its biochemistry and its related enzymes and vitamins including folate, vitamin B_6 (pyridoxine), and vitamin B_{12} (cobalamin) is required. Both inherited and acquired factors cause hyperhomocysteinemia. Most studies have concluded that an elevated homocysteine level is an independent risk factor for cardiovascular disease and not a proxy for another risk. Ongoing interventional studies—such as the Vitamin Intervention for Stroke Prevention (VISP) trial, the Women's Antioxidant Cardiovascular Disease Study (WACS), and the Heart Outcomes Prevention Evaluation (HOPE-2)—are investigating the efficacy of homocysteine-lowering therapies on cardiovascular disease endpoints. If these trials conclude that a certain therapy efficiently lowers homocysteine levels and that this reduces risk for cardiovascular disease, they will also confirm that homocysteine is an independent risk factor for cardiovascular disease.

Chemistry and Metabolism

Homocysteine is an intermediate sulfhydryl amino acid formed during the conversion of methionine to cysteine.[233] The term *homocysteine* includes the sum of homocysteine, homocystine, and the homocysteine-cysteine mixed disulfide, both free and protein-bound.[234] Methionine is an essential sulfur-containing amino acid supplied from dietary proteins. In its metabolism, methionine is first activated by ATP to make S-adenosylmethionine (SAM). SAM serves as the body's principal methyl donor and then forms S-adenosylhomocysteine, which undergoes hydrolysis to adenosine and homocysteine. Homocysteine can be metabolized through the transsulfuration pathway to form cystathionine or through remethylation pathways to reform methionine. Cystathionine-β-synthase, using pyridoxal phosphate (vitamin B_6) as a cofactor, catalyzes the condensation of homocysteine and serine to form cystathionine. Cystathionine is then converted to cysteine and α-ketobutyrate. In remethylation, homocysteine is metabolized in one of two reaction pathways. In one, 5-methyltetrahydrofolate donates the methyl group and is catalyzed by 5-methyltetrahydrofolate-homocysteine methyltransferase, which uses methylcobalamin as a cofactor. In the second, betaine acts as the methyl donor and the enzyme required is betaine-homocysteine methyltransferase (Fig. 23-3).[235]

Homocysteine metabolism is regulated by dietary intake of methionine, through feedback mechanisms involving SAM and 5-methyltetrahydrofolate.[236] When methionine intake is high, transsulfuration is favored by upregulation of cystathionine-B-synthase and downregulation of the remethylation pathway, and vice versa when methionine supplies are low.[237] Plasma homocysteine is filtered by the kidney and handled there by specific uptake mechanisms and metabolizing enzymes.[238]

Causes of Hyperhomocysteinemia

The concentration of total plasma homocysteine is normally 5 to 15 μmol/L in healthy people.[239] In the absence of renal impairment, elevated plasma homocysteine levels reflect increased cellular export of this potentially toxic metabolite. Intracellular production can be influenced by the concentrations of folate, vitamin B_6, vitamin B_{12}, and in the activity of transsulfuration or remethylation pathway enzymes. Interruption of either the remethylation or transsulfuration pathway produces hyperhomocysteinemia. Moderate, intermediate, and severe hyperhomocysteinemia are defined as total fasting plasma homocysteine of >15 to 30, >30 to 100, and >100 μmol/L, respectively.[240] The diagnosis of hyperhomocysteinemia based on laboratory values should be tempered with knowledge of limitations in measurement. The generally used method with EDTA preserved plasma will artificially elevate homocysteine levels by 10% per hour after about 30 min unless cells are separated out, stabilizing agents are added, or samples are kept on ice and analyzed within 3 h.[241,242]

Prandial status also influences homocysteine levels. Homocysteine elevation after ingestion of a methionine load may indicate vitamin B_6 deficiency or transsulfuration impairment, but otherwise homocysteine levels increase with fasting.[243]

Genetic Causes

Severe hyperhomocysteinemia is usually the result of homozygous cystathionine-B-synthase deficiency. About 1 in 200,000 persons are born homozygous for this disease and develop the classic clinical syndrome of homocystinuria, including premature vascular disease and thrombosis, mental retardation, ectopia lentis, and skeletal abnormalities. The gene for cystathionine-B-synthase can be found on chromosome 21, and, interestingly, patients with trisomy 21 have a very low incidence of cardiovascular disease. Heterozygotes for cystathionine-B-synthase deficiency develop hyperhomocysteinemia to a more moderate degree.

Deficiencies in the remethylation pathway also lead to hyperhomocysteinemia.[233] Kang et al. characterized the symptoms of 5,10-methylene-tetrahydrofolate reductase (MTHFR) deficiency as neurologic abnormalities, atherosclerotic changes, and thromboembolism.[244] They also described a more common thermolabile variant of MHFTR in neurologically normal patients, which is associated with high homocysteine levels and the development of coronary artery disease.[244–246] This variant results from a single nucleotide substitution of thymidine for cytosine at base pair 677 (denoted C677T), corresponding with a substitution of valine for alanine at amino acid 222. This mutated MHFTR has a greater tendency to dissociate into monomers and lose the FAD cofactor, thereby moderately decreasing function.[247] In Europe and North America, an estimated 5 to 15% of the population is homozygous for this mutation, but nearly 40% of French Canadians may be afflicted. Several studies show that affected individuals are more sensitive to dietary folate levels and experience hyperhomocysteinemia only with low folate intake.[248] Other MHFTR polymorphisms, such as A1298C, are much less common and are functionally indistinguishable from the wild-type enzyme. Mutations in methionine synthase, such as A2756G have not been associated with hyperhomocysteinemia alone but correlate with elevated cystathione and are increasingly prevalent in highly hyperhomocysteinemic patients with MHFTR mutations.[249,250] In general, plasma homocysteine levels increase with age and are higher in men.[239]

Acquired

The metabolism of homocysteine requires the presence of folate, vitamin B_6, and vitamin B_{12}. Therefore, a deficiency in any of these vitamins may elevate levels of homocysteine. Deficiencies can result from inadequate intake, poor absorption, or an increase in physiologic demand.[251] Many patients with renal disease exhibit hyperhomocysteinemia and have age-adjusted, cardiovascular-related morbidity and mortality rates twice those of their healthy peers.[252] Plasma homocysteine levels may be influenced by pharmacologic agents such as fenofibrates, methotrexate, or phenytoin. Diseases such as psoriasis, cancer, and hypothyroidism are associated with high levels of homocysteine.[237] Prolonged states of immune activation may deplete tetrahydrofolate by oxidation and result in hyperhomocysteinemia.[253] Interestingly, consumption of coffee has been shown to increase plasma homocysteine; conversely, 6 weeks of abstention by regular consumers reduced total homocysteine by about 1 μmol/L.[254] Any one of the above factors that affect homocysteine levels have the same following result on coronary risk: a total

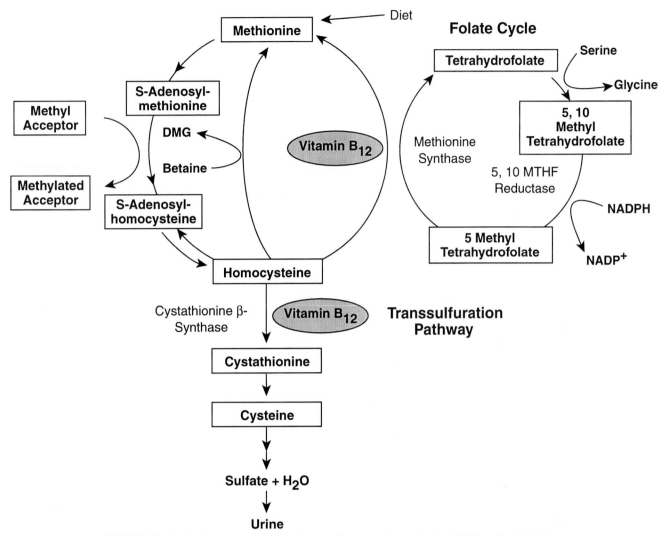

FIGURE 23-3. Methionine cycle: metabolic pathway of homocysteine metabolism. DMG = dimethylglycine; MTHF = methylenetetrahydrofolate; NADP = nicotinamide adenine dinucleotide phosphate (oxidized form); NADPH = nicotinamide adenine dinucleotide phosphate (reduced form). (*From Mayer et al.,*[235] *with permission.*)

homocysteine level increment of 5 μmol/L elevates coronary artery disease risk by as much as an increase in cholesterol of 0.5 mmol/L (Table 23-6).[255]

Pathogenesis of Vascular Disease and Thrombosis

Although the exact mechanisms are controversial and not completely elucidated, homocysteine apparently causes endothelial dysfunction and injury, with platelet activation and coagulation. Sulfhydryl groups per se are reducing agents, but in plasma, homocysteine quickly autooxidizes to form homocysteine, mixed disulfides, and thiolactones. Autooxidation generates superoxide and hydroxyl radicals as well as hydrogen peroxide, which may be responsible for most of the endothelial toxicity.[256] In vitro, cells grown in folate-deficient media drastically increase hydrogen peroxide and homocysteine production and induce the proapoptotic redox-sensitive transcription factor NF-κB.[257] Interestingly, Roth et al. showed that homocysteine exposure of human endothelial cells inhibited NF-κB binding and transcriptional activity, blunting the adhesion molecule expression induced by tumor necrosis

factor.[258] Also through NF-κB induction, homocysteine may alter cell-cycle protein expression and induce proliferation of vascular smooth muscle cells.[259]

Homocysteine cytotoxicity can be modulated by nitric oxide. Homocysteine and nitric oxide react under physiologic conditions to produce S-nitrosohomocysteine, a compound with potent antiplatelet and vasodilatory activity. However, homocysteine can also inhibit production of nitric oxide by endothelial cells, leaving them vulnerable to direct injury and subsequent desquamation via hydrogen peroxide.[260] Stuhlinger et al. showed that homocysteine directly inhibits degradation of asymmetric dimethylarginine by dimethylarginine dimethylaminohydrolase. The subsequently accumulated dimethylarginine is an endogenous inhibitor of nitric oxide synthase.[261] In vivo, fasting hyperhomocysteinemic patients showed blunted endothelium-dependent acetylcholine-induced vasodilation, an effect partially reversed by concomitant administration of the antioxidant vitamin C.[262,263] However, therapeutic trials have shown conflicting results regarding improved vasodilatory responses after homocysteine levels have been lowered.[123,264–268] Also, as a result of decreased nitric oxide production, matrix

TABLE 23-6. Factors Influencing Homocysteine Levels

Genetics
  Transsulfuration abnormalities; diminished or absent cystathionine
    beta-synthase activity (chromosome 21)
  Remethylation abnormalities
    Abnormal methylenetetrahydrofolate reductase (absent or
      thromolabile variant)
    Abnormal methionine synthase
Age/gender
  Homocysteine increases with age
  Homocysteine levels: men > age-matched women
  Postmenopausal women: homocysteine levels increase
Renal function
  Homocysteine increases with increased creatinine
Nutrition
  Vitamin B_6 deficiency
  Vitamin B_{12} deficiency
  Folate deficiency
Disease states
  Severe psoriasis, associated with increased homocysteine levels
    (possibly related to lower folate levels)
  Cancer, acute lymphoblastic leukemia, elevated levels
  Chronic renal failure, increased homocysteine, lowered with dialysis
Medications
  Increase homocysteine
    Methotrexate depletes 5-methyltetrahydrofolate
    Azaribine, a vitamin B_6 antagonist
    Nitric oxide inactivates vitamin B_{12}
    Phenytoin interferes with folate metabolism
    Carbamazepine interferes with folate metabolism
    Estrogen-containing oral contraceptives induce vitamin B_6 deficiency
  Decrease homocysteine
    Penicillamine, a metabolically stable cysteine analogue

Source: Reproduced with permission from Mayer et al.[235]

metalloproteinase activity increases, causing elastinolysis and vascular hypertrophy in rat aortas.[269]

Other mechanisms have been proposed to explain the ability of homocysteine to do harm. Jakubowski proposed both translational and posttranslational pathways for incorporation of homocysteine into proteins, leading to cell damage.[270] Also, homocysteine may interfere with signaling pathways involved with responses to cell stress and hypoxia, as evidenced by concentration-dependent decreases in heme oxygenase-1 expression and extracellular superoxide dismutase secretion.[271,272] Increasing concentrations of extracellular but not intracellular homocysteine decreases endothelin-1 production, apparently via free radical–mediated mechanisms.[273] In mitochondria, homocysteine inhibits gene expression, and plasma homocysteine correlates inversely with mitochondrial DNA content.[274]

Homocysteine can affect coagulation abnormalities by reducing antithrombin III, protein C, and factor VII activities and increasing factor V and prothrombin activities.[256] Hyperhomocysteinemia interacts with factor V Leiden and the prothrombin gene mutation G20210A, significantly increasing the risk of venous thrombosis.[275] In endothelial cell cultures, homocysteine reduces thrombomodulin expression.[276] Products of arachidonic acid peroxidation may cause in vivo platelet activation. Such metabolites are found in higher concentrations in cystathione β-synthase–deficient patients, in direct proportion to homocysteine, but inversely correlating with vitamin E plasma levels.[277] Importantly, autooxidation of homocysteine, through generation of hydroxyl and superoxide radicals, may oxidize LDLs: this is known to lead to the development of atherosclerotic plaques.[240]

Hyperhomocysteinemia and Vascular Disease: Epidemiologic Observations and Studies

Strong prospective and retrospective epidemiologic evidence links elevated homocysteine levels to cardiovascular disease in a graded fashion.[277a–296b,296c] Much effort has been expended to eliminate confounding variables, and most studies agree that hyperhomocysteinemia is an independent risk factor. In the Physicians' Health Study of 14,916 males without known atherosclerosis, those with initial homocysteine levels 12% above normal had a threefold increase in risk of MI compared with normals after an average of 5 years of follow-up.[285] In the study, hyperhomocysteinemia alone was estimated to account for 7% of MIs. In cases of angiographically confirmed atherosclerosis, mortality risk over 4.6 years nearly doubles per every 5 μmol/L over 9 μmol/L on initial measurement of homocysteine.[296] Because the association between homocysteine and cardiovascular disease is shown to exist regardless of the initial metabolic cause, this may represent a cause-and-effect relationship. The fact that many different types of studies agree supports the lack of important biases in most studies investigating homocysteine and cardiovascular disease.[297] The validity of hyperhomocyteinemia as an independent risk factor may be confirmed by ongoing and future prospective interventional trials examining cardiovascular disease and homocysteine-lowering therapy.[298] It has also been shown that an increased plasma homocysteine level is a strong independent risk factor for the development of dementia and Alzheimer's disease.[298a]

Clinical Use

Treatment of homocystinemia and its vascular complications includes lowering plasma homocysteine levels and therapy of thromboembolism. Patients nutritionally deficient in vitamin B_6 exhibit homocystinemia due to diminished transsulfuration. Vitamin B_{12} or folate deficiencies cause homocystinemia by direct impairment of remethylation and inhibition of transsulfation by concomitantly decreased levels of SAM.[236] In either case, supplementation of the deficient vitamin should enable the body to metabolize homocysteine through the affected pathway.[277a] However, even when homocystinemia is not caused by a nutritional deficiency, as in renal impairment, folate significantly decreases homocysteine levels.[1]

Vitamin B_6

The Dietary Reference Intake (DRI; an evolution of Recommended Daily Allowances, and set forth by the National Academy of Sciences in 1997) for vitamin B_6 is approximately 2 mg/day for adults.[299] Because vitamin B_6 is required for amino acid metabolism, physiologic demand is related to protein intake. Dietary vitamin B_6 is converted to its active forms, pyridoxal-5'-phosphate (PLP), and pyridoxamine-5'-phosphate, (PMP) in the liver, red blood cells, and other tissues of humans and animals. The best sources of vitamin B_6 include fish, chicken, organ meats, eggs, and some grains and nuts. Vitamin B_6 deficiency not only leads to homocystinemia but also causes poor growth, anemia, reduced immune response, convulsions, depression and confusion, skin lesions, and kidney stones. A review of the published literature indicates that daily doses of vitamin B_6 under 500 mg for up to 6 months appear safe.[251] However, neurologic symptoms of toxicity begin to appear at intakes greater than 2 g/day.[300]

Vitamin B_{12}

The DRI for vitamin B_{12} is now 2.4 μg/day.[299] The coenzyme forms of cobalamin are 5'deoxyadenosylcobalamin and methylcobalamin. Vitamin B_{12} is synthesized only by microorganisms and is not present in plants. The best sources of vitamin B_{12} include liver, whole milk, eggs, oysters, fresh shrimp, pork, and chicken. In vitamin B_{12} deficiency, N_5-methyltetrahyrofolate, a specific form of tetrahydrofolate, is not efficiently used, which results in the depletion of other active forms of tetrahydrofolate. This situation mimics the signs of megaloblastic anemia with folate deficiency. Vitamin B_{12} deficiency is not normally due to intake problems. Instead, it is due to absorption, as in pernicious anemia, where autoimmune processes destroy the gastric parietal cells responsible for making intrinsic factor needed for B_{12} absorption. Vitamin B_{12}-deficient patients become anemic and may develop late neuropsychiatric symptoms with or without the anemia. Significant amounts of vitamin B_{12} (approximately 4 to 5 g) are stored in the liver; therefore, typically several years of diminished intake elapse before clinical symptoms of B_{12} deficiency develop.

Until recently, it was thought that vitamin B_{12} was not toxic due to its water-solubility, which would allow excess vitamin to be excreted in the urine. However, the Bronx Longitudinal Aging Study, an ongoing prospective study of an ambulatory elderly cohort, showed an increased incidence of mortality and CHD in people with increased blood vitamin B_{12} levels. Each 100 μg increase in B_{12} was associated with a 10% increase in mortality and CHD incidence.[301] Various theories have been proposed to explain the results of this study. Pancharuniti et al.[281] propose that because vitamin B_{12} is found in red meat and eggs, protective benefits derived from the vitamin are outweighed by the high fat and cholesterol content of these foods. Another possibility is that vitamin B_{12} is toxic at high concentrations, because deposits are stored in the liver and may be potentially hepatotoxic and induce liver enzymes.[302] If the Bronx Longitudinal Aging Study's correlation is caused by B_{12} toxicity, it will significantly affect the therapeutic regimen for treating homocystinemia, as described below.

Folate

A vitamin under much scrutiny, folate lowers homocysteine levels in all treated subjects.[286] The DRI for folate is now 400 μg/day.[299] Folic acid is found in green leafy vegetables, liver, lima beans, and whole-grain cereals. Folic acid deficiency leads to growth failure, neural tube defects, and megaloblastic anemia. Deficiency can be due to increases in demand as with pregnancy, decreases in absorption as in alcoholics, certain drugs, and poor intake.

Widespread folic acid supplementation began by January 1998, when the FDA required that all enriched grains contain 140 μg of folic acid per 100 g of product. This was done in an attempt to reduce the risk of neural tube defects, which affect about 4000 pregnancies per year in the United States.[303] Women of childbearing age are also advised to ingest folate supplements even before knowing that they are pregnant because the neural tube closes during the first month of pregnancy.[304] The FDA chose this level of fortification because it was calculated to maximize the probability of attaining adequate (400 μg/day) folate intake by pregnant women while minimizing the chances that the general population would exceed an intake threshold of 1 mg/day. The FDA stated that ingestion of 1 mg/day or more of folic acid should occur only under a physician's supervision and pointed out that such dosages are typically used to treat megaloblastic anemia.[303]

Megaloblastic anemia may result from folic acid or vitamin B_{12} deficiency and is treated with folic acid and vitamin B_{12} together. If treated with folic acid alone, hematologic parameters will normalize in either deficiency, because the added folate bypasses the vitamin B_{12}-dependent metabolic step in hematopoiesis. However, if the anemia was due to vitamin B_{12} deficiency, the primary metabolic insult would continue uncorrected in the nervous system and the patient could develop irreversible neuropsychiatric symptoms. An estimated 500 such cases per year will develop in the U.S., assuming no other changes in health care, because of the current level of folic acid grain enrichment.[305]

Since the onset of folic acid fortification, the Framingham Offspring Study cohort showed a twofold increase in serum folate concentrations, a decrease in mean homocysteine levels from 10.1 to 9.4 μmol/L, and a decrease in the incidence of elevated levels from 18.7 to 9.8%.[306] Tice and coworkers recently calculated that this fortification alone should decrease CHD events by 8% in women and in 13% in men over a 10-year period and conservatively estimate a 1 to 3% reduction in annual CHD mortality. In the same period, adding 1 mg of folic acid and 0.5 mg of cyanocobalamin daily to the diet of all men over age 45 would save more than 300,000 quality-adjusted life years (QALY) and \$2 billion. Providing the same regimen for women over age 55 would save over 140,000 QALYs over the same 10 years.[307] Other authors have also argued for increased levels of folic acid supplementation to cause further lowering of homocysteine,[308] while still others submit that the three major homocysteine-lowering trials currently under way will lose the statistical power needed to prove the benefits of therapy owing to the fortification of grain.[309]

In an intervention therapy study, Ubbink et al. reported that a daily vitamin supplement consisting of 10 mg of pyridoxine, 1 mg of folic acid, and 0.4 mg of cyanocobalamin normalized elevated plasma homocysteine levels within 6 weeks in patients with moderate hyperhomocysteinemia.[310] Administering 1 mg of hydroxycobalamin to B_{12}-deficient patients with hyperhomocysteinemia can normalize homocysteine levels within 2 weeks.[311] Brattstrom et al. reported that a dose of 5 mg of folic acid per day given over a period of 4 weeks could normalize homocysteine levels even in patients with adequate folate intake.[312] Folate therapy can lower homocysteine levels in healthy subjects who had normal folate levels when treated. A recent metanalysis of homocysteine-lowering trials concluded that, from a pretreatment average of 12 mmol/L of plasma homocysteine, between 0.5 and 5 mg/day of folic acid lowers homocysteine by 25%. Adding vitamin B_6 gave no additional benefit, but an additional 7% decrease is afforded by 0.5 mg/day of B_{12}. The absolute and proportional effects were greater at higher pretreatment homocysteine levels.[313] Vitamin therapy may be both cost-effective and efficient in controlling elevated levels of homocysteine (Table 23-7).

Landgren et al. compared plasma homocysteine levels 24 to 36 h after onset of an acute MI with the levels obtained at a 6 weeks' follow-up and with levels in a control group. When the patients were given daily oral folic acid doses of 2.5 mg or 10 mg, homocysteine levels were lowered.[314] Saltzman et al. assessed levels of homocysteine in patients undergoing angioplasty.[315] In this randomized trial, case patients received either 5 mg folic acid or a combination of 1 mg B_{12} with 100 mg B_6. The conclusion of the trial was that elevated homocysteine levels can be treated with folic acid alone, with B_6 combined with B_{12}, or with all three vitamins combined.[315] Recently, Schnyder et al. showed that, if given for 6 months after angioplasty, a combination of 1 mg folic acid, 0.4 mg B_{12}, and 10 mg B_6 daily significantly reduced homocysteine levels and decreased the rate of restenosis (19.6 versus 37.8%) and the need for revascularization (10.8 versus 22.3%), as assessed by quantitative angiography.[316,316a]

TABLE 23-7. Effect of Vitamin Supplementation on Plasma Concentrations of Homocysteine, Cobalamin, Pyridoxal-5′-Phosphate, and Folate

Plasma Index and Group*	0 weeks	2 weeks	Treatment Period 4 weeks	6 weeks	8 weeks
Pyridoxal-5′ phosphate (nmol/L)					
P	44.5±23.6	43.8±19.6	42.2±21.7	41.3±19.4	45.4±26.8
V	39.9±23.0	154.4±62.1[†]	157.0±72.4[†]	157.1±69.0[†]	297.3±114.3[†]
Cobalamin (pmol/L)					
P	215.7±91.3	213.1±110.1	227.8±123.8	241.1±126.5	196.3±77.5
V	220.3±74.4	313.2±99.0[‡]	331.5±110.0[‡]	335.5±111.7[‡]	378.2±133.0[‡]
Folate (nmol/L)					
P	6.2±4.3	5.8±3.4	7.1±5.1	8.3±6.6	6.2±3.1
V	5.6±3.3	20.6±15.6[‡]	27.4±13.8[†]	23.6±14.6[‡]	39.3±21.9[†]
Homocysteine (μmol/L)					
P	24.0±11.3	24.0±12.8	25.2±13.0	22.1±8.5	22.3±9.6
V	28.6±15.2	18.1±9.0	14.1±4.7[‡]	11.5±3.2[†]	10.9±3.0[†]

*Group P received placebo, whereas group V received a vitamin supplement. Vitamin and placebo doses were doubled after 6 weeks.

[†] Significantly different from group P; $P < .001$.

[‡] Significantly different from group P; $P < .05$.

Source: Reproduced with permission from Ubbink et al.[310]

Recent studies have shown that lipid lowering therapy with fibrates may increase plasma homocysteine levels by as much as 40%. Concomitant administration of folic acid and folate with vitamins B_{12} and B_6 has been shown to attenuate these elevations.[317,318]

Studies of genetic defects and epidemiologic data associating high blood homocysteine levels with vascular disease are consistent. Plausible biological mechanisms have been proposed and a safe, inexpensive, and effective therapy is available. Prospective interventional trials are now under way. A public health policy recommendation for widespread screening and intervention for elevated homocysteine levels cannot be made without evidence from randomized clinical trials showing that reduced homocysteine levels can decrease the incidence of cardiovascular disease. Unfortunately, the fortification of grains with folic acid may obscure such results. To optimize the benefits of lowering homocysteine, additional fortification or supplementation may prove appropriate. Folate supplementation might be complemented with 0.4 mg of B_{12} supplements to avoid the undertreatment of pernicious anemia.[319] However, this suggestion does not take into account the latest observation reported from the Bronx Longitudinal Aging Study. If elevated B_{12} levels are shown to cause disease, then supplementation should not be effected without indications of a B_{12} deficiency.[301]

Conclusion

If ongoing and future randomized intervention trials conclude that homocysteine is an independent risk factor and that lowering its levels reduces the risk of cardiovascular disease, then widespread screening for homocysteine levels should be implemented. Screening would be inexpensive and more predictive of risk status than blood pressure. In screening for hyperhomocysteinemia, folate, B_6, and B_{12} levels should be determined. If homocysteine levels are elevated, then the following treatment regimen is suggested: if there is a folate deficiency with normal vitamin levels, administer folate at 5 mg/day for 4 weeks; a B_{12}-deficient state either alone or combined with folate deficiency should be treated with 5 mg/day of folate and 1 mg/day of B_{12} for 4 weeks; a B_6-deficient state either alone or with folate deficiency should be treated with 5 mg/day of folate and 40 mg/day of B_6 for 4 weeks; and a deficiency of all

3 vitamins should be treated with 5 mg/day of folate, 1 mg/day of B_{12}, and 40 mg/day of B_6.[301] If the vitamin levels in the blood are normal and homocysteine remains elevated, this would suggest a genetic defect and lifelong folate therapy alone could be useful in controlling homocysteine levels.

THIAMINE

Thiamine (vitamin B_1), one of the earliest described vitamin substances, plays an essential role in the treatment of "wet beriberi," a dietary thiamine and protein deficiency state characterized by high-output cardiac failure, tachycardia, extensive edema, and depressed ventricular function.[320] Patients with chronic alcoholism or congestive heart failure receiving chronic diuretic therapy may present with thiamine deficiency and experience neurologic as well as cardiovascular effects.[321,322]

Physiologic Function

Thiamine pyrophosphate is the physiologically active form of thiamine and is involved in a series of biochemical reactions involving carbohydrate metabolism. In the citric acid cycle, it serves as a coenzyme in decarboxylation of α-keto acids such as pyruvate and α-ketogluturate. Thiamine is also involved as a cofactor for the enzyme transketolase, which is involved in the hexose monophosphate shunt.[323,324]

Pharmacokinetics

Thiamine is present in most plants and animal tissues, but the most abundant sources of the vitamin are unrefined grain, liver, heart, and kidney. The enrichment of flour and derived food products with the vitamin has contributed to its availability in the western diet.[323]

Dietary thiamine is absorbed in the small intestine by active transport at intakes less than 5 mg/day. At higher doses, passive diffusion becomes important. The portal circulation carries thiamine to the liver where it combines with adenosine triphosphate. The product, thiamine pyrophosphate, is the predominant form in cells and is distributed to all the major organ systems, but free vitamin is found in the plasma. Thiamine is excreted in the urine, depending on how much of the substance is ingested after tissue stores are saturated.[323,324]

Etiology of Thiamine Deficiency

Inadequate intake or increased excretion may cause thiamine deficiency. Inadequate intake is commonly due to consumption of nonenriched grains such as rice and wheat, which are stripped of vitamins by the milling process.[323] Ingestion of raw fish containing microbial thiaminases may destroy the vitamin in the gastrointestinal tract. Chronic alcoholism is associated with low thiamine intake but also with impaired absorption and vitamin storage. Because most chronic alcoholics ingest high carbohydrate diets, the physiologic demand for thiamine is increased. Patients undergoing long-term renal dialysis or intravenous feedings are at high risk of thiamine deficiency.[325] A rare cause of deficiency is thiamine-responsive megaloblastic anemia, a clinical triad of megloblastic anemia with ringed sideroblasts, diabetes mellitus, and progressive sensorineural deafness. The responsible gene, SLC19A2, has recently been mapped and cloned, and its product was determined to normally function as a high-affinity thiamine transmembrane transport protein.[326]

Patients receiving diuretics for long-term management of congestive heart failure may develop thiamine deficiency.[321,322] In healthy volunteers, furosemide was found to increase thiamine excretion in a dose-dependent manner.[327,328] Although the concept of diuretic-induced loss of water-soluble vitamins is generally accepted, some studies fail to show a correlation between furosemide therapy and thiamine pyrophosphate depletion.[329] Hardig et al. noted that thiamine pyrophosphate correlates with hemoglobin concentrations, which are reduced in heart failure patients. After adjusting for this parameter, furosemide-treated patients were found to be deficient in the monophosphate but not the pyrophosphate form of thiamine, suggesting an alteration of thiamine metabolism.[329] Nonetheless, thiamine status in elderly patients, as assessed by erythrocyte transketolase activity, was found to worsen during hospitalization and correlated with the cumulative furosemide dosage as adjusted for the duration of therapy.[330] Also important in congestive heart failure, in cultured heart cells, furosemide and digoxin were found to inhibit thiamine uptake in an additive, dose-related manner.[331] Finally, some evidence suggests that thiamine deficiency may simply be related to age, regardless of concomitant illness.[332]

Clinical Manifestations of Deficiency

Thiamine deficiency will lead to neurologic symptoms and muscle wasting (dry beriberi) as well as cardiac involvement manifest by tachycardia, augmented peripheral vasodilation, and biventricular myocardial failure with extensive accumulation of edema ("wet beriberi").[320,333] In deficiency states, the oxidation of α-ketoacids is dysfunctional, pyruvate will accumulate in the blood, and glucose cannot be utilized anaerobically. Type B lactic acidosis, (or slow lactic acidosis, in contrast to type A or fast lactic acidosis caused by oxygen deprivation) may result from decreased conversion of lactate to glucose. More importantly, however, the central nervous system is deprived of the ATP from the oxidation of ketoacids, and the Wernicke-Korsakoff syndrome results.[334] In peripheral blood

vessels, the decrease in available ATP is believed to cause endothelial swelling, smooth muscle relaxation, and arteriovenous shunting. As resistance vessels become paralyzed, a hyperkinetic state ensues, with increased ventricular filling pressures and decreased peripheral vascular resistance. Pulse pressures may widen and renal and cerebral blood flow decrease in favor of skeletal muscle blood flow, with attendant tachycardia, edema, weakness, dyspnea, and paresthesias of the lower extremities.[320] Cardiac involvement with thiamine deficiency is often related to increased physical exertion and excessive caloric intake, while the polyneuritic form is seen in patients who are relatively inactive or on caloric restriction.[333]

Clinical heart failure may develop explosively in beriberi, with some patients succumbing from their illness within 48 h of symptom onset. Shoshin beriberi is a fulminant form of thiamine deficiency characterized by hypotension, tachycardia, and lactic acidosis, with patients dying of pulmonary edema if not treated.[335,336]

In cardiac catheterization studies in patients with beriberi heart disease, right atrial and pulmonary wedge pressures are elevated, cardiac index is increased, and the arteriovenous oxygen difference is increased.[337,338] These abnormalities may return to normal after treatment with thiamine. Left ventricular ejection fraction may be normal or decreased and may fall further with exercise.[339]

The diagnosis of thiamine deficiency as a cause of heart failure is often made with a recent history of thiamine deficiency for 3 months or longer, an absence of another cause for heart failure, evidence of polyneuritis, and an improvement in clinical symptoms with thiamine replacement. One author cautions that although chronic malnutrition may cause thiamine-induced dilated cardiomyopathy in alcoholics, alcoholism per se may simply predispose the patient to a viral myocarditis, which may cause overlapping symptoms with normal thiamine stores.[340] Clinical presentation alone may thus be highly suggestive of a deficiency but is insufficient for the diagnosis.

Several laboratory modalities provide quantitative assessments of thiamine status. Thiamine pyrophosphate effect (TPPE) measures transketolase enzyme activity when thiamine diphosphate is added to serum. Normal individuals show a TPPE of between zero and 15%; larger effects signify relative deficiency states; and greater than 25% defines severe deficiency.[320] A direct measurement of erythrocyte transketolase levels may be performed on whole blood, and activities that rise from a depressed value after thiamine replacement confirm the diagnosis of a deficiency state.[320,341] High-performance liquid chromatography may even be more precise for identifying a thiamine-deficiency state, as direct measurements of each phosphorylation state of thiamine may be made.[342]

Thiamine deficiency may be present in a significant portion of the elderly population, but the true prevalence is unclear, as most studies thus far have been small. Interestingly, some studies of patients taking loop diuretics failed to show evidence of thiamine deficiency.[328,343] Still, several studies of patients with congestive heart failure or the hospitalized elderly estimate the prevalence of thiamine deficiency to be between 20 and 40%.[344–346]

Replacement of Thiamine

Patients with beriberi heart disease will fail to respond adequately to digitalis and diuretics alone. However, the improvement after the administration of thiamine (up to 100 mg intravenously followed by 25 mg/day orally for 1 to 2 weeks) may be dramatic. A marked diuresis, a decrease in heart size and heart rate, and a clearing of pulmonary congestion may occur within 12 to 48 h.[338] However, the acute reversal of vasodilation induced by correction of the thiamine deficiency may cause the unprepared heart to undergo low-output failure. Therefore, patients with heart failure should receive a glycoside, angiotensin converting enzyme inhibitor, and diuretic therapy along with thiamine replacement treatment.

Thiamine supplements can improve left ventricular function and biochemical evidence of deficiency in some patients with moderate-to-severe congestive heart failure who are receiving long-term furosemide therapy. In a study by Shimon et al.,[325] thiamine replacement for 7 weeks in patients receiving furosemide for 3 months or longer was shown to improve left ventricular ejection fraction by 22%, decrease heart size and heart rate, and increase blood pressure and rate of diuresis. Patients were administered 1 week of intravenous thiamine (200 mg/day) and then 6 weeks of oral thiamine (200 mg/day).

Conclusion

There appears to be no measurable effect of thiamine on the cardiovascular system of humans except in chronic deficiency states.[320] Thiamine replacement therapy may be especially important in alcoholics or patients with refractory chronic congestive heart failure who are receiving diuretics, where an occult vitamin deficiency state may be present.[325]

REFERENCES

1. Morrison HI, Schaubel D, Desmeules M, Wigle DT: Serum folate and risk of fatal coronary heart disease. *JAMA* 275:1893, 1996.
2. Boushey CJ, Beresford SAA, Omenn GS, Motulsky AG: A quantitative assessment of plasma homocysteine as a risk factor for vascular disease. Probable benefits of increasing folic acid intakes. *JAMA* 274:1049, 1995.
3. Jacques PF, Bostom AG, Williams RR, et al: Relation between folate status, a common mutation in methylenetetrahydrofolate reductase, and plasma homocysteine concentrations. *Circulation* 93:7, 1996.
4. Kluijtmans LAJ, van den Heuvel LPWJ, Boers GHJ, et al: Molecular genetic analysis in mild hyperhomocysteinemia: A common mutation in the methylenetetrahydrofolate reductase gene is a genetic risk factor for cardiovascular disease. *Am J Hum Genet* 58:35, 1996.
5. Kang S-S, Wong PWK: Genetic and nongenetic factors for moderate hyperhomocyst(e)inemia. *Atherosclerosis* 119:135, 1996.
6. Bang HO, Dyerberg J: Plasma lipids and lipoproteins in Greenlandic west coast Eskimos. *Acta Med Scand* 192:85, 1972.
7. Bang HO, Dyerberg J Hjoome N: The composition of food consumed by Greenland Eskimos. *Acta Med Scand* 200:69, 1976.
8. Keys A: *Seven Countries: A Multivariate Analysis of Death and Coronary Heart Disease.* Cambridge, MA: Harvard University Press, 1980.
9. Kagawa Y, Nishizawa M, Suzuki M, et al: Eicosapolyenoic acid of serum lipids of Japanese islanders with low incidence of cardiovascular disease. *J Nutr Sci Vitaminol (Tokyo)* 28:441, 1982.
10. Kromhout D, Bosschieter EB, de Lezenne Coulander C: The inverse relation between fish consumption and 20-year mortality from coronary heart disease. *N Engl J Med* 312:1205, 1985.
11. Dyerberg J, Bang HO: Haemostatic function and platelet polyunsaturated fatty acids in Eskimos. *Lancet* 2:433, 1979.
12. Fischer S, Weber PC: Prostaglandin 13 is formed in vivo in man after dietary eicosapentaenoic acid. *Nature* 307:165, 1984.
13. Strasser T, Fischer S, Weber PC: Leukotriene B5 is formed in human neutrophil 5 after dietary supplementation with eicosapentaenoic acid. *Proc Natl Acad Sci U S A* 82:1540, 1985.
14. Bunting S, Gryglewski R, Moncada S, Vane JR: Arterial walls generate from prostaglandin endoperoxides a substance (prostaglandin X) which relaxes strips of mesenteric and coeliac arteries and inhibits platelet aggregation. *Prostaglandins* 12:897, 1976.
15. Steele PP, Weily HS, Davies H, et al: Platelet function studies in coronary artery disease. *Circulation* 48:1194, 1973.
16. Zaloga GP, Marik P: Lipid modulation and systemic inflammation. *Crit Care Clin* 17:25, 2001.
17. Grimsgaard S, Bonaa KH, Hansen JB, Nordoy A: Highly purified eicosapentaenoic acid and docosahexaenoic acid in humans have similar triacylglycerol-lowering effects but divergent effects on serum fatty acids. *Am J Clin Nutr* 66:649, 1997.
18. Fischer S, Vischer A, Preac-Mursic V, Weber PC: Dietary docosahexaenoic acid is retroconverted in men to eicosapentaenoic acid, which can be quickly transformed to prostaglandin 13. *Prostaglandins* 34:367, 1987.
19. Mori TA, Burke V, Reddey IV, et al: Purified eicosapentaenoic acid and docosahexaenoic acid have differential effects on serum lipids and lipoproteins, LDL-particle size, glucose, and insulin, in mildly hyperlipidaemic men. *Am J Clin Nutr* 71:1085, 2000.
20. Holman RT: Nutritional and metabolic interrelationships between fatty acids. *Fed Proc* 23:1062–1067, 1964.
21. Goodnight SH Jr, Harris WS, Connor WE, Illingworth DR: Polyunsaturated fatty acids, hyperlipidemia, and thrombosis. *Arteriosclerosis* 2:87–113, 1982.
22. Siess W, Roth P, Scherer B, et al: Platelet-membrane fatty acids, platelet aggregation, and thromboxane formation during a mackerel diet. *Lancet* 1:441, 1980.
23. Goldman DW, Pickett WC, Goetzl EJ: Human neutrophil chemotactic and degranulating activities of leukotriene B5 (LTB5) derived from eicosapentaenoic acid. *Biochem Biophys Res Commun* 117:282, 1983.
24. Fischer S, Weber PC: Thromboxane A3(TXA3) is formed in human platelet after dietary eicosapentaenoic acid (C20:5 omega-3). *Biochem Biophys Res Commun* 116:1091, 1983.
25. Von Schacky C, Fischer S, Weber PC: Long-term effects of dietary marine omega-3 fatty acids upon plasma and cellular lipids, platelet function and eicosanoid formation in man. *J Clin Invest* 76:1626, 1985.
26. Gryglewski RJ, Salmon JA, Ubatuba FB, et al: Effects of all cis 5, 8, 11, 14, 17 eicosapentaenoic acid and PGH3 on platelet aggregation. *Prostaglandins* 18:453, 1979.
27. Needleman P, Raz A, Minkes MS, et al: Triene prostaglandins: Prostacyclin and thromboxane biosynthesis and unique biological properties. *Proc Natl Acad Sci U S A* 76:944, 1979.
28. Mullane KM, Salmon JA, Kraemer R: Leukocyte derived metabolites of arachidonic acid in ischemia-induced myocardial injury. *Fed Proc* 46:2422, 1987.
29. Thorngren M, Gustafson A: Effects of 11-week increase in dietary eicosapentaenoic acid on bleeding time, lipids, and platelet aggregation. *Lancet* 2:1190, 1981.
30. Lorenz R, Spengler U, Fischer S, et al: Platelet function, thromboxane formation and blood pressure control during supplementation of the western diet with cod liver oil. *Circulation* 67:504, 1983.
31. Mortensen JZ, Schmidt EB, Nielsen AH, Dyerberg J: The effect of N-6 and N-3 polyunsaturated fatty acids on hemostasis, blood lipids and blood pressure. *Haemostasis* 50(2):543, 1983.
32. Saynor R, Verel D, Gillott T: The long-term effect of dietary supplementation with fish lipid concentrate on serum lipids, bleeding time, platelets, and angina. *Atherosclerosis* 50:3, 1984.
33. Schmidt EB, Sorensen PJ, Jersild C, et al: The effect of n-3 polyunsaturated fatty acids on lipids, haemostasis, neutrophil and monocyte chemotaxis in insulin dependent diabetes mellitus. *J Intern Med* 225(Suppl l):201, 1989.
34. Sanders TAB, Naismith DJ, Haines AP, Vickers M: Cod liver oil, platelet fatty acids, and bleeding times. *Lancet* 2:1189, 1980.
35. Sanders TAB, Vickers M, Haines AP: Effect on blood lipids and haemostasis of a supplement of cod liver oil, rich in eicosapentaenoic and docosahexaenoic acids, in healthy young men. *Clin Sci* 61:317, 1981.
36. Li X, Steiner M: Fish oil: A potent inhibitor of platelet adhesiveness. *Blood* 76(5):938, 1990.
37. Hay CRM, Durber AP, Saynor R: Effect of fish oil on platelet kinetics in patients with ischaemic heart disease. *Lancet* 1:1269, 1982.
38. Goldberg ID, Stemerman MB: Vascular permeation of platelet factor 4 after endothelial injury. *Science* 209:611, 1980.
39. Knapp HR, Reilly IAG, Alessandrini P, FitzGerald GA: In vivo indexes of platelet and vascular function during fish oil administration

in patients with atherosclerosis. *N Engl J Med* 314(15):937, 1986.

40. Kaplan DR, Chao FC, Stiles CD, et al: Platelet α granules contain a growth factor for fibroblasts. *Blood* 53:1043, 1979.
41. FitzGerald GA, Smith B, Pedersen AK, Brash AR: Increased prostacyclin biosynthesis in patients with severe atherosclerosis and platelet activation. *N Engl J Med* 310:1065, 1984.
42. Nieuwenhuys CMA, Feijge MAH, Offersmans RFG, et al: Modulation of rat platelet activation by vessel wall-derived prostaglandin and platelet-derived thromboxane: Effects of dietary fish oil on thromboxane-prostaglandin balance. *Atherosclerosis* 154:355, 2001.
43. Martin-Chouly CA, Menier V, Hichami A, et al: Modulation of PAF production by incorporation of arachidonic acid and eicosapentaenoic acid and phospholipid of human leukemic monocyte-like cells THP-1. *Prostaglandins Other Lipid Mediat* 60(4–6):127, 2000.
44. Vericel E, Calzada C, Chapuy P, Lagarde M: The influence of low intake of n-3 fatty acids on platelets in elderly people. *Atherosclerosis* 147(1):187, 1999.
45. Cerbone AM, Cirillo F, Coppola A, et al: Persistent impairment of platelet aggregation following cessation of a short-course dietary supplementation of moderate amounts of n-3 fatty acid ethyl esters. *Thromb Haemost* 82(1):128, 1999.
46. Lund EK, Harvey LJ, Ladha S, et al: Effects of dietary fish oil supplementation on the phospholipid composition and fluidity of cell membranes from human volunteers. *Ann Nutr Metab* 43:290, 1999.
47. Mutanen M, Freese R: Fats, lipids and blood coagulation. *Curr Opin Lipidol* 12:25, 2001.
48. Dunstan DW, Mori TA, Puddey IB, et al: A randomised, controlled study of the effects of aerobic exercise and dietary fish oil on coagulation and fibrinolytic factors in type 2 diabetics. *Thromb Haemost* 81:367, 1999.
49. Nordoy A, Bonaa KH, Sandset, PM, et al: Effect of omega-3 fatty acids and simvastatin on hemostatic risk factors and postprandial hyperlipidemia in patients with combined hyperlipidemia. *Arterioscler Thromb Vasc Biol* 20:259, 2000.
50. Berrettini M, Parise P, Ricotta S, et al: Increased plasma levels of tissue factor pathway inhibitor (TFPI) after n-3 polyunsaturated fatty acids supplementation in patients with chronic atherosclerotic disease. *Thromb Haemost* 75(3):395, 1996.
51. Mehta J, Lawson D, Saldeen T: Reduction in plasminogen activator inhibitor-1 (PAI-1) with omega-3 polyunsaturated fatty acids (PUFA) intake. *Am Heart J* 116:1201, 1988.
52. Hansen J, Grimsgaard S, Nordoy A, Bonaa KH: Dietary supplementation with highly purified eicosapentaenoic acid and docosahexaenoic acid does not influence PAI-1 activity. *Thromb Res* 98(2):123, 2000.
53. Grundt H, Nilsen DW, Hetland O, et al: Atherothrombogenic risk modulation by n-3 fatty acids was not associated with changes in homocysteine in subjects with combined hyperlipidaemia. *Thromb Haemost* 81(4):561, 1999.
54. Toft I, Bonaa KH, Ingebretsen OC, et al: Fibrinolytic function after dietary supplementation with omega 3 polyunsaturated fatty acids. *Arterioscler Thromb Vasc Biol* 17(5):814, 1997.
55. Allman-Farinelli MA, Hall D, Kingham K, et al: Comparison of the effects of two low fat diets with different alpha-linolenic:linoleic acid ratios on coagulation and fibrinolysis. *Atherosclerosis* 142(1):159, 1999.
56. Conquer JA, Cheryk LA, Chan E, et al: Effect of supplementation with dietary seal oil on selected cardiovascular risk factors and hemostatic variables in healthy male subjects. *Thromb Res* 96(3):239, 1999.
57. al-Awadhi AM, Dunn CD: Effects of fish-oil constituents and plasma lipids on fibrinolysis in vitro. *Br J Biomed Sci* 57(4):273, 2000.
58. Archer SL, Green D, Chamberlain M, et al: Association of dietary fish and n-3 fatty acid intake with hemostatic factors in the coronary risk development in young adults (CARDIA) study. *Arterioscler Thromb Vasc Biol* 18(7):1119, 1998.
59. Marckmann P, Bladbjerg EM, Jespersen J: Dietary fish oil (4 g daily) and cardiovascular risk markers in healthy men. *Arterioscler Thromb Vasc Biol* 17(12):3384, 1997.
60. Miller GJ: Effects of diet composition on coagulation pathways. *Am J Clin Nutr* 67(Suppl 3):542S, 1998.

61. Phillipson BE, Rothrock DW, Connor WE, et al: Reduction of plasma lipids, lipoproteins, and apoproteins by dietary fish oils in patients with hypertriglyceridemia. *N Engl J Med* 321:1210, 1985.
62. Borthwick L on behalf of the UK Study Group: The effects of an omega-3 ethyl ester concentrate on blood lipid concentrations in patients with hyperlipidaemia. *Clin Drug Invest* 15:397, 1998.
63. Harris WS: n-3 fatty acids and lipoproteins: Animal studies. *Am J Clin Nutr* 65(Suppl 5):1611S, 1997.
64. Dallongeville J, Bauge E, Tailleux A, et al: Peroxisome proliferator-activated receptor alpha is not rate limiting for the lipoprotein lowering action of fish oil. *J Biol Chem* 276(7):4634, 2001.
65. Anil K, Jayadeep A, Sudhakaran PR: Effect of n-3 fatty acids on VLDL production by hepatocytes is mediated through prostaglandins. *Biochem Mol Biol Int* 43(5):1071, 1997.
66. Froyland L, Madsen L, Vaagenes H, et al: Mitochondrion is the principal target for nutritional and pharmacological control of triglyceride metabolism. *J Lipid Res* 38(9):1851, 1997.
67. Madsen L, Rustan AC, Vaagenes H, et al: Eicosapentaenoic and docosahexaenoic acid affect mitochondrial and peroxisomal fatty acid oxidation in relation to substrate preference. *Lipids* 35(9):951, 1999.
68. Wong SH, Nestel PJ, Trimble RP, et al: The adaptive effects of dietary fish and safflower oil on lipid and lipoprotein metabolism in perfused rat liver. *Biochim Biophys Acta* 792:103, 1984.
69. Berge RK, Madsen L, Vaagenes H, et al: In contrast with docosahexaenoic acid, eicosapentaenoic acid and hypolipidaemic derivatives decrease hepatic synthesis and secretion of triacylglycerol by decreased diacylglycerol acyltransferase activity and stimulation of fatty acid oxidation. *Biochem J* 343(1):191, 1999.
70. Nestel PJ, Connor WE, Reardon MF, et al: Suppression by diets rich in fish oil of very low density lipoprotein production in man. *J Clin Invest* 74:82, 1984.
71. Harris WS, Connor WE, Illingworth DR, et al: Effects of fish oil on VLDL triglyceride kinetics in humans. *J Lipid Res* 31(9):1549, 1990.
72. Kendrick JS, Higgins JA: Dietary fish oils inhibit early events in the assembly of very low density lipoproteins and target apoB for degradation within the rough endoplasmic reticulum of hamster hepatocytes. *J Lipid Res* 40(3):504, 1999.
73. Kendrick JS, Wilkinson J, Cartwright IJ, et al: Regulation of the assembly and secretion of very low density lipoproteins by the liver. *Biol Chem* 379(8–9):1033, 1998.
74. Wu X, Shang A, Jiang H, Ginsberg HN: Demonstration of biphasic effects of docosahexaenoic acid on apolipoprotein B secretion in HepG2 cells. *Arterioscler Thromb Vasc Biol* 17:3347, 1997.
75. Herrmann W, Biermann J, Kostner GM: Comparison of effects of n-3 to n-6 fatty acids on serum level of lipoprotein(a) in patients with coronary artery disease. *Am J Cardiol* 76:459, 1995.
76. Shinozaki K, Kambayashi J, Kawasaki T, et al: The long term effect of eicosapentaenoic acid on serum levels of lipoprotein (a) and lipids in patients with vascular disease. *J Atheroscler Thromb* 2(2):107, 1996.
77. Harris WS, Lu G, Rambjor GS, et al: Influence of n-3 fatty acid supplementation on the endogenous activities of plasma lipases. *Am J Clin Nutr* 66(2):254, 1997.
78. Lu G, Windsor SL, Harris WS: Omega-3 fatty acids alter lipoprotein subfraction distributions and the invitro conversion of very low density lipoproteins to low density lipoproteins. *J Nutr Biochem* 10:151, 1999.
79. Harris WS, Hustvedt BE, Hagen E, et al: N-3 fatty acids and chylomicron metabolism in the rat. *J Lipid Res* 38:503, 1997.
80. Michaud SE, Renier G: Direct regulatory effect of fatty acids on macrophage lipoprotein lipase: Potential role of PPARs. *Diabetes* 50(3):660, 2001.
81. De Caterina R, Libby P: Control of endothelial leukocyte adhesion molecules by fatty acids. *Lipids* 31:57S, 1996.
82. Abbate R, Gori AM, Martini F, et al: n-3 PUFA supplementation, monocyte PCA expression and interleukin-6 production. *Prostaglandins Leukot Essent Fatty Acids* 54(6):439, 1996.
83. Miles EA, Wallace FA, Calder PC: Dietary fish oil reduces intercellular adhesion molecule 1 and scavenger receptor expression on murine macrophages. *Atherosclerosis* 152:43, 2000.
84. Miles EA, Wallace FA, Calder PC: Reduction of scavenger receptor expression and function by dietary fish oil is accompanied by a reduction in scavenger receptor mRNA. *Lipids* 34S:215S, 1999.

85. De Caterina, Spiecker M, Solaini G, et al: The inhibition of endothelial activation by unsaturated fatty acids. *Lipids* 34S:191S, 1999.

86. Massaro M, Carluccio MA, Bonfrate C, et al: The double bond in unsaturated fatty acids is the necessary and sufficient requirement for the inhibition of expression of endothelial leukocyte adhesion molecules through interference with nuclear factor κB activation. *Lipids* 34S:213S, 1999.

87. Abe Y, El-Masri B, Kimball KT, et al: Soluble cell adhesion molecules in hypertriglyceridemia and potential significance on monocyte adhesion. *Arterioscler Thromb Vasc Biol* 18(5):723, 1998.

88. Suzukawa M, Abbey M, Clifton P, Nestel P: Enhanced capacity of n-3 fatty acid-enriched macrophages to oxidize low density lipoprotein mechanisms and effects of antioxidant vitamins. *Atherosclerosis* 124:157, 1996.

89. McGrath LT, Brennan GM, Donnelly JP, et al: Effect of dietary fish oil supplementation on peroxidation of serum lipids in patients with non-insulin dependent diabetes mellitus. *Atherosclerosis* 121:275, 1996.

90. Song JH, Miyazawa T: Enhanced level of n-3 fatty acid in membrane phospholipids induces lipid peroxidation in rats fed dietary docosahexaenoic acid oil. *Atherosclerosis* 155:9, 2001.

91. Higdon JV, Du SH, Lee YS, et al: Supplementation of postmenopausal women with fish oil does not increase overall oxidation of LDL ex vivo compared to dietary oils rich in oleate and linoleate. *J Lipid Res* 42(3):407, 2001.

92. Higdon JV, Liu J, Du SH, et al: Supplementation of postmenopausal women with fish oil rich in eicosapentaenoic acid and docosahexaenoic acid is not associated with greater in vivo lipid peroxidation compared with oils rich in oleate and linoleate by plasma malondialdehyde and F(2)-isoprostanes. *Am J Clin Nutr* 72(3):714, 2000.

93. Mori TA, Dunstan DW, Burke V, et al: Effects of dietary fish and exercise training on urinary F2-isoprostane excretion in non-insulin dependent diabetic patients. *Metabolism* 48:1402, 1999.

94. Mori TA, Puddey IB, Burke V, et al: Effect of omega-3 fatty acids on oxidative stress in humans: GCMS measurement of urinary F2-isoprostane excretion. *Redox Rep* 5:45, 2000.

95. Turley E, Wallace JM, Gilmore WS, Strain JJ: Fish oil supplementation with and without added vitamin E differentially modulates plasma antioxidant concentrations in healthy women. *Lipids* 33(12):1163, 1998.

96. Endres S, Ghorbani R, Kelly VE, et al: The effect of dietary supplementation with n-3 polyunsaturated fatty acids on the synthesis of interleukin-1 and tumor necrosis factor by mononuclear cells. *N Engl J Med* 320:265, 1989.

97. Endres S, von Schacky C: n-3 Polyunsaturated fatty acids and human cytokine synthesis. *Curr Opin Lipidol* 7:48, 1996.

98. Dinarrello CA, Mier JW: Current concepts: Lymphokines. *N Engl J Med* 317:940, 1987.

99. Beutler B, Cerami A: Cachectin: More than a tumor necrosis factor. *N Engl J Med* 316:379, 1987.

100. Libby P, Warner SJC, Friedman GB: Interleukin-1: A mitogen for human vascular smooth muscle cells that induces the release of growth inhibiting prostanoids. *J Clin Invest* 81:487, 1988.

101. Elias JA, Gustilo K, Baeder W, Freundlich B: Synergistic stimulation of fibroblast prostaglandin production by recombinant interleukin-1 and tumor necrosis factor. *Immunol* 138:3812, 1987.

102. Fox PL, DiCorleto PE: Regulation of production of a platelet-derived growth factor-like protein by cultured bovine aortic endothelial cells. *J Cell Physiol* 121:298, 1987.

103. Mizutani M, Asano M, Roy S, et al: Omega-3 polyunsaturated fatty acids inhibit migration of human vascular smooth muscle cells in vitro. *Life Sci* 61(19):PL269, 1997.

104. Asano M, Nakajima T, Hazama H, et al: Influence of cellular incorporation of n-3 eicosapentaenoic acid on intracellular Ca^{2+} concentration and membrane potential in vascular smooth muscle cells. *Atherosclerosis* 138:117, 1998.

105. Hirafuji M, Ebihara T, Kawahara F, et al: Effect of docosahexaenoic acid on intracellular calcium dynamics in vascular smooth muscle cells from normotensive and genetically hypertensive rats. *Res Commun Mol Pathol Pharmacol* 102(1):29, 1998.

106. Pakala R, Pakala R, Sheng WL, Benedict CR: Vascular smooth muscle cells preloaded with eicosapentaenoic acid and docosahexaenoic acid fail to respond to serotonin stimulation. *Atherosclerosis* 153:47, 2000.

107. Pakala R, Pakala R, Benedict CR: Thromboxane A_2 fails to induce proliferation of smooth muscle cells enriched with eicosapentaenoic acid and docosahexaenoic acid. *Prostaglandin Leukot Essent Fatty Acids* 60(4):275, 1999.

108. Pakala R, Pakala R, Benedict CR: Eicosapentaenoic acid and docosahexaenoic acid block serotonin-induced smooth muscle cell proliferation. *Arterioscler Thromb Vasc Biol* 19(10):3316, 1999.

109. Pakala R, Pakala R, Sheng WL, Benedict CR: Serotonin fails to induce proliferation of endothelial cells preloaded with eicosapentaenoic acid and docosahexaenoic acid. *Atherosclerosis* 145:137, 1999.

110. Pakala R, Pakala R, Radcliffe JD, Benedict CR: Serotonin-induced endothelial cell proliferation is blocked by omega-3 fatty acids. *Prostagland Leukot Essent Fatty Acids* 60(2):115, 1999.

111. Saito J, Terano T, Hirai A, et al: Mechanisms of enhanced production of PGI_2 in cultured rat vascular smooth muscle cells enriched with eicosapentaenoic acid. *Atherosclerosis* 131:219, 1997.

112. Nakayama M, Fukuda N, Watanabe Y, et al: Low dose of eicosapentaenoic acid inhibits the exaggerated growth of vascular smooth muscle cells from spontaneously hypertensive rats through suppression of transforming growth factor-beta. *J Hypertens* 17(10):1421, 1999.

113. Nobukata H, Ishikawa T, Obata M, Shibutani Y: Long-term administration of highly purified eicosapentaenoic acid ethyl ester improves the dysfunction of vascular endothelial and smooth muscle cells in male WBN/Kob rats. *Metabolism* 49(12):1588, 2000.

114. Fan YY, Ramos KS, Chapkin RS: Dietary gamma-linolenic acid suppresses aortic smooth muscle cell proliferation and modifies atherosclerotic lesions in apolipoprotein E knockout mice. *J Nutr* 131(6):1675, 2001.

115. Faggin E, Puato M, Chiavegato A, et al: Fish oil supplementation prevents neointima formation in nonhypercholesterolemic balloon-injured rabbit carotid artery by reducing medial and adventitial cell activation. *Arterioscler Thromb Vasc Biol* 20(1):152, 2000.

116. Avula CP, Zaman AK, Lawrence R, Fernandes G: Induction of apoptosis and apoptotic mediators in Balb/C splenic lymphocytes by dietary n-3 and n-6 fatty acids. *Lipids* 34:921, 1999.

117. Fyfe DJ, Abbey M: Effects of n-3 fatty acids on growth and survival of J774 macrophages. *Prostaglandins Leukot Essent Fatty Acids* 62(3):201, 2000.

118. Diep QN, Touyz RM, Schiffrin EL: Docosahexaenoic acid, a peroxisome proliferator-activated receptor-alpha ligand, induces apoptosis in vascular smooth muscle cells by stimulation of p38 mitogen-activated protein kinase. *Hypertension* 36(5):851, 2000.

119. Goode GK, Garcia S, Heagerty AM: Dietary supplementation with marine fish oil improves in vitro small artery endothelial function in hypercholesterolemic patients. A double-blind placebo-controlled study. *Circulation* 96:2802, 1997.

120. Tagawa H, Shimokawa H, Tagawa T, et al: Long-term treatment with eicosapentaenoic acid augments both nitric oxide-mediated and non-nitric oxide-mediated endothelium-dependent forearm vasodilatation in patients with coronary artery disease. *J Cardiovasc Pharmacol* 33: 633, 1999.

121. Zhang YW, Morita I, Yao XS, Murota S: Pretreatment with eicosapentaenoic acid prevented hypoxia/reoxygenation-induced abnormality in endothelial gap junction intercellular communication through inhibiting the tyrosine kinase activity. *Prostaglandins Leukot Essent Fatty Acids* 61(1):33, 1999.

122. McCarty MF: A central role for protein kinase C overactivity in diabetic glomerulosclerosis: Implications for prevention with antioxidants, fish oil, and ACE inhibitors. Med Hypoth 50(2):155, 1998.

123. Goodfellow J, Bellamy MF, Ramsey MW, et al: Dietary supplementation with marine omega-3 fatty acids improve systemic large endothelial function in subjects with hypercholesterolemia. *J Am Coll Cardiol* 35(2):265, 2000.

124. Goode GK, Garcia S, Heagerty AM: Dietary supplementation with marine fish oil improves in vitro small artery endothelial function in hypercholesterolemic patients: A double-blind placebo-controlled study. *Circulation* 96(9):2802, 1997.

125. Mori TA, Watts GF, Burke V, et al: Differential effects of eicosapentaenoic acid and docosahexaenoic acid on forearm vascular reactivity of the microcirculation in hyperlipidaemic, overweight men. *Circulation* 102:1264, 2000.

126. McLennan PL, Abeywardena MY, Charnock JS: Dietary fish oil prevents ventricular fibrillation following coronary artery occlusion and reperfusion. *Am Heart J* 116(3):709, 1988.

127. McLennan PL, Bridle TM, Abeywardena MY, Charnock JS: Comparative efficacy of n-3 and n-6 polyunsaturated fatty acids in modulating ventricular fibrillation threshold in marmoset monkeys. *Am J Clin Nutr* 58(5):6669, 1993.

128. Isenssee H, Jacob R: Differential effects of various oil diets on the risk of cardiac arrhythmias in rats. *J Cardiovasc Risk* 1(4):353, 1994.

129. Al Makdessi S, Brandle M, Ehrt M, et al: Myocardial protection by ischemic preconditioning: the influence of the composition of myocardial phospholipids. *Molec Cell Biochem* 145(1):69, 1995.

130. Billman GE, Kang JX, Leaf A: Prevention of sudden cardiac death by dietary pure ω-3 polyunsaturated fatty acids in dogs. *Circulation* 99:2452, 1999.

131. Weylandt KH, Kang JX, Leaf A: Polyunsaturated fatty acids exert antiarrhythmic actions as free acids rather than in phospholipids. *Lipids* 31(9):977, 1996.

132. Conquer JA, Holub BJ: Effect of supplementation with different doses of DHA on the levels of circulating DHA as non-esterified fatty acid in subjects of Asian Indian background. *J Lipid Res* 39(2):286, 1998.

133. Nair SS, Leitch J, Garg ML: Specific modifications of phosphatidylinositol and nonesterified fatty acid fractions in cultured porcine cardiomyocytes supplemented with n-3 polyunsaturated fatty acids. *Lipids* 34(7):697, 1999.

134. Nair SS, Leitch J, Falconer J, Garg ML: Cardiac (n-3) non-esterified fatty acids are selectively increased in fish oil-fed pigs following myocardial ischemia. *J Nutr* 129(8):1518, 1999.

135. Leaf A, Kang JX, Xiao YF, Billman GE: N-3 fatty acids in the prevention of cardiac arrhythmias. *Lipids* 34S:S187, 1999.

136. Xiao YF, Wright SN, Wang GK, et al: Fatty acids suppress voltage-gated Na$^+$ currents in HEK293t cells transfected with the alpha-subunit of the human cardiac Na$^+$ channel. *Proc Natl Acad Sci U S A* 95(5):2680, 1998.

137. Kang JX, Xiao YF, Leaf A: Free, long-chain, polyunsaturated fatty acids reduce membrane electrical excitability in neonatal rat cardiac myocytes. *Proc Natl Acad Sci U S A* 92(9):3997, 1995.

138. Kang JX, Li Y, Leaf A: Regulation of sodium channel gene expression by class I antiarrhythmic drugs and n-3 polyunsaturated fatty acids in cultured neonatal rat cardiac myocytes. *Proc Natl Acad Sci U S A* 94(6):2724, 1997.

139. Xiao YF, Gomez AM, Morgan JP, et al: Suppression of voltage-gated L-type Ca^{2+} currents by polyunsaturated fatty acids in adult and neonatal rat ventricular myocytes. *Proc Natl Acad Sci U S A* 94(8):4182, 1997.

140. Bernard M, Gerbi A, Barbey O, et al: Dietary fish oil promotes positive inotropy and efficiency of digitalis. *Lipids* 34S:S195, 1999.

141. Kang JX, Leaf A: Effects of long-chain polyunsaturated fatty acids on the contraction of neonatal rat cardiac myocytes. *Proc Natl Acad Sci U S A* 91(21):9886, 1994.

142. Pepe S, Bogdanov K, Hallaq H, et al: Omega 3 polyunsaturated fatty acid modulates dihydropyridine effects on L-type Ca^{2+} channels, Ca^{2+}, and contraction in adult rat cardiac myocytes. *Proc Natl Acad Sci U S A* 91(19):8832, 1994.

143. Hallaq H, Smith TW, Leaf A: Modulation of dihydropyridine sensitive calcium channels in heart cells by fish oil fatty acids. *Proc Natl Acad Sci U S A* 89(5):1760, 1992.

144. Singleton CB, Valenzuela SM, Walker BD, et al: Blockade by n-3 polyunsaturated fatty acid of the Kv4.3 current stably expressed in Chinese hamster ovary cells. *Br J Pharmacol* 127(4):941, 1999.

145. Anderson KE, Du XJ, Sinclair AJ, et al: Dietary fish oil prevents reperfusion Ins(1,4,5)P3 release in rat heart: possible antiarrhythmic mechanism. *Am J Physiol* 271:H1483, 1996.

146. Nair SS, Leich J, Garg ML: Suppression of inositol phosphate release by cardiac myocytes isolated from fish oil-fed pigs. *Mol Cell Biochem* 215(1–2):57, 2000.

147. Kelley DS: Modulation of human immune and inflammatory responses by dietary fatty acids. *Nutrition* 17:669, 2001.

148. Meydani SN, Lichtenstein AH, Cornwall S, et al: Immunologic effects of national cholesterol education panel step-2 diets with and without fish-derived N-3 fatty acid enrichment. *J Clin Invest* 92(1):105, 1993.

149. Kelley DS, Taylor PC, Nelson GJ, et al: Docosahexaenoic acid ingestion inhibits natural killer cell activity and production of inflammatory mediators in young healthy men. *Lipids* 34:317, 1999.

150. Stenson WF, Cort D, Rodgers J, et al: Dietary supplementation with fish oil in ulcerative colitis. *Ann Intern Med* 116(8):609–614, 1992.

151. Robinson DR: Alleviation of autoimmune disease by dietary lipids containing omega-3 fatty acids. *Rheum Dis Clin North Am* 17(2):213, 1991.

152. Hirai A, Terano T, Saito H, et al: Eicosapentaenoic acid and platelet function in Japanese. In: Lovenburg W, Yamori Y, eds. *Nutritional Prevention of Cardiovascular Disease.* New York: Academic Press, 1984:231–239.

153. Yamada T, Strong JP, Ishii T: Atherosclerosis and omega-3 fatty acids in the populations of a fishing village and a farming village in Japan. *Atherosclerosis* 153:469, 2000.

154. Daviglus ML, Stamler J, Orencia AJ, et al: Fish consumption and the 30-year risk of fatal myocardial infarction. *N Engl J Med* 336:1046, 1997.

155. Von Schacky C, Angerer P, Kothny W, et al: The effect of dietary omega-3 fatty acids on coronary atherosclerosis: A randomized, double-blind, placebo-controlled trial. *Ann Intern Med* 130:554, 1999.

156. Sacks FM, Stone PH, Gibson CM, et al: Controlled trial of fish oil for regression of human coronary atherosclerosis: Harp Research Group. *J Am Coll Cardiol* 24(7):1492, 1995.

157. Iso H, Rexrose KM, Stampfer MJ, et al: Intake of fish and omega-3 fatty acids and risk of stroke in women. *JAMA* 285:304, 2001.

157a. Hu FB, Bronner L, Willett WC, et al: Fish and omega-3 fatty acid intake and risk of coronary heart disease in women. *JAMA* 287:1815, 2002.

158. Guallar E, Hennekens CH, Sacks F, et al: A prospective study of plasma fish oil levels and incidence of myocardial infarction in US male physicians. *J Am Coll Cardiol* 25:387, 1995.

159. Albert CM, Hennekens CH, O'Donnell CJ, et al: Fish consumption and risk of sudden cardiac death. *JAMA* 279(1):23, 1998.

159a. Bucher HC, Hengstler P, Schindler C, Meier G: N-3 polyunsaturated fatty acids in coronary heart disease: A meta-analysis of randomized controlled trials. *Am J Med* 112:298, 2002.

160. Burr ML, Fehily AM, Gilbert JF, et al: Effects of changes in fat, fish, and fibre intakes on death and myocardial reinfarction: Diet and reinfarction trial (DART). *Lancet* 2:757, 1989.

161. Singh RB, Niaz MA, Sharma JP, et al: Randomized, double-blind, placebo-controlled trial of fish oil and mustard oil in patients with suspected acute myocardial infarction: the Indian Experiment of Infarct Survival—4. *Cardiovasc Drugs Ther* 11(3):485, 1997.

162. GISSI-Prevenzione Investigators: Dietary supplementation with n-3 polyunsaturated fatty acids and vitamin E after myocardial infarction: Results of the GISSI-prevenzione Trial: Gruppo Italiano per lo Studio della Sopravvivenza nell'Infarto Miocardico. *Lancet* 354:447, 1999.

162a. Marchioli R, Barzi F, Bomba E, et al: Early protection against sudden death by n-3 polyunsaturated fatty acids after myocardial infarction: Time course analysis of the results of the Gruppo Italiano per lo Studio della Sopravvivenza nell'Infarto Miocardico (GISSI) Prevenzione. *Circulation* 105:1897, 2002.

163. Gillum RF, Mussolino ME, Madans JH: The relationship between fish consumption and stroke incidence. *Arch Intern Med* 156:537, 1996.

164. Keli SO, Feskens EJM, Kromhout D: Fish consumption and risk of stroke: The Zutphen study. *Stroke* 25:328, 1994.

165. Morris MC, Manson JE, Rosner B, et al: Fish consumption and cardiovascular disease in the Physicians' Health Study: A prospective study. *Am J Epidemiol* 142:166, 1995.

166. Landmark K, Abdelnoor M, Urdal P, et al: Use of fish oils appears to reduce infarct size as estimated from peak creatine kinase and lactate dehydrogenase activities. *Cardiology* 89(2):94, 1998.

167. Culp BR, Lands WEM, Lucchesi BR, Pitt B, Romson J: The effect of dietary supplementation of fish oil on experimental myocardial infarction. *Prostaglandins* 20:1021, 1980.

168. Hock CE, Holahan MA, Reibel DK: Effect of dietary fish oil on myocardial phospholipids and myocardial ischemic damage. *Am J Physiol* 252:554, 1987.

169. Oskarsson HJ, Godwin J, Gunnar RM, Thomas JX: Dietary fish oil supplementation reduces myocardial infarct size in a canine model of ischemia and reperfusion. *J Am Coll Cardiol* 2(5):1280, 1993.

170. Salachas A, Papadopoulos C, Sakadamis G, et al: Effect of a low-dose fish oil concentrate on angina, exercise tolerance time, serum triglycerides, and platelet function. *Angiology* 45(12):1023, 1994.

171. O'Connor GT, Malenka DJ, Olmstead EM, et al: A meta-analysis of randomized trials of fish oil in prevention of restenosis following coronary angioplasty. *Am J Prev Med* 8:186, 1992.

172. Gapinski JP, VanRuiswyk JV, Heudebert GR, Schectman GS: Preventing restenosis with fish oils following coronary angioplasty. *Arch Intern Med* 153:1595, 1993.

173. Leaf A, Jorgensen MB, Jacobs AK et al: Do fish oils prevent restenosis after coronary angioplasty (Fish Oil Restenosis Trial). *Circulation* 90(5):2248, 1994.

174. Cairns JA, Gill J, Morton B, et al: Fish oils and low-molecular-weight heparin for the reduction of restenosis after percutaneous transluminal coronary angioplasty: The EMPAR Study. *Circulation* 94(7):1553, 1996.

174a. Maresta A, Balduccelli M, Varani E, et al: Prevention of postcoronary angioplasty restenosis by omega-3 fatty acids: Main results of the Esapent for Prevention of Restenosis Italian Study (ESPRIT). (On-line article) *Am Heart J* 143:e5, 2002.

175. Weiner BH, Ockene IS, Levine PH, et al: Inhibition of atherosclerosis by cod-liver oil in a hyperlipidemic swine model. *N Engl J Med* 315:841, 1986.

176. Shimokawa H, Vanhoutte PM: Dietary cod-liver oil improves endothelium dependent responses in hypercholesterolemic and atherosclerotic porcine coronary arteries. *Circulation* 78:1421, 1989.

177. Sassen LMA, Hartog JM, Lamers JMJ, et al: Mackerel oil and atherosclerosis in pigs. *Eur Heart J* 10:838, 1989.

178. Harker LA, Kelly AB, et al: Interruption of vascular thrombus formation and vascular lesion formation by dietary n-3 fatty acids in fish oil in nonhuman primates. *Circulation* 87(3):1017, 1993.

179. Kowe PR, Lungershausen YK, Rogers PF, et al: Effects of dietary sodium and fish oil on blood pressure development in stroke-prone spontaneous hypertensive rats. *J Hypertens* 9(7):639, 1991.

180. Howe PR, Rogers PF, Lungershausen Y: Blood pressure reduction by fish oil in adult rats with established hypertension-dependence on sodium intake. *Prostagland Leukot Essent Fatty Acids* 44(2): 113, 1991.

181. Croft KD, Beilin LJ, Vandongen R, Mathews SE: Dietary modification of fatty acid and prostaglandin synthesis in the rat. *Biochim Biophys Acta* 795:196, 1984.

182. Appel LT, Miller ER III, Seidler AJ, Wheiton PK: Does supplementation of diet with "fish oil" reduce blood pressure? A meta-analysis of controlled clinical trials. *Arch Intern Med* 153(12):1429, 1993.

183. Knapp HR: n-3 Fatty acids and human hypertension. *Curr Opin Lipidol* 7:30, 1996.

184. Herold PM, Kinsella MS and EK: Fish oil consumption and decreased risk of cardiovascular disease: A comparison of findings from animal and human feeding trials. *Am J Clin Nutr* 43:566, 1986.

185. Radack K, Deck C: The effect of omega-3 polyunsaturated fatty acids on blood pressure: A methodologic analysis of the evidence. *J Am Coll Nutr* 8(5):376, 1989.

186. Prisco D, Paniccia R, Bandinelli B, et al: Effect of medium term supplementation with a moderate dose of n-3 polyunsaturated fatty acids on blood pressure in mild hypertensive patients. *Thromb Res* 91(3):105, 1998.

187. Bao DQ, Mori TA, Burke V: Effects of dietary fish and weight reduction on ambulatory blood pressure in overweight hypertensives. *Hypertension* 32(4):710, 1998.

188. Yosefy C, Viskoper JR, Laszt A, et al: The effect of fish oil on hypertension, plasma lipids and hemostasis in hypertensive, obese, dyslipidemic patients with and without diabetes mellitus. *Prost Leukot Essent Fatty Acids* 61(2):83, 1999.

189. Holm T, Andreassen AK, Aukrust P, et al: Omega-3 fatty acids improve blood pressure control and preserve renal function in hypertensive heart transplant recipients. *Eur Heart J* 22(5):428, 2001.

190. Ventura H, Milani T, Lavie CJ, et al: Cyclosporine-induced hypertension: efficacy of omega-3 fatty acids in patients after cardiac transplantation. *Circulation* 88:281, 1993.

191. Nestel PJ, Pomeroy SE, Sasahara T, et al: Arterial compliance in obese subjects is improved with dietary plant n-3 fatty acid from flaxseed oil despite increased LDL oxidizability. *Arterioscler Thromb Vasc Biol* 17(6):1163, 1997.

192. Sacks FM, Hebert P, Appel LJ, et al: The effect of fish oil on blood pressure and high-density lipoprotein cholesterol levels in phase 1 of the Trials of Hypertension Prevention. *J Hypertens* (Suppl) 12(7):S23, 1994.

193. Whelton PK, Kumanyika SK, Cook NR, et al: Efficacy of nonpharmacologic interventions in adults with high-normal blood pressure: Results from phase 1 of Trials of Hypertension Prevention. Trials of Hypertension Prevention Collaborative Research Group. *Am J Clin Nutr* 65(2 Suppl):652S, 1997.

194. Gray DR, Gozzip CG, Eastham JH, Kashyap ML: Fish oil as an adjuvant in the treatment of hypertension. *Pharmacotherapy* 16(2): 295, 1996.

195. Harris WS: Dietary fish oil and blood lipids. *Curr Opin Lipidol* 7:3, 1996.

196. Schmidt EB, Varming K, Svaneborg N, Dyerberg J: N-3 polyunsaturated fatty acid supplementation (Pikasol) in men with moderate and severe hypertriglyceridaemia: A dose response study. *Ann Nutr Metab* 36(5–6):283, 1992.

197. Weber P, Raederstorff D: Triglyceride-lowering effect of omega-3 LC-polyunsaturated fatty acids—a review. *Nutr Metab Cardiovasc Dis* 10(1):28, 2000.

198. Harris WS: n-3 Fatty acids and lipoproteins: comparison of results from human and animal studies. *Lipids* 31:243, 1996.

199. Harris WS: n-3 fatty acids and serum lipoproteins: Human studies. *Am J Clin Nutr* 65(5Suppl):164S, 1997.

200. Stalenhoef AFH, de Graaf J, Wittekoek ME, et al: The effect of concentrated n-3 fatty acids versus gemfibrozil on plasma lipoproteins, low density lipoprotein heterogeneity and oxidizability in patients with hypertriglyceridemia. *Atherosclerosis* 153:129, 2000.

201. Alaswad K, O'Keefe JH Jr, Moe RM: Combination drug therapy for dyslipidemia. *Curr Atheroscler Rep* 1(1):44, 1999.

202. Nakamura N, Hamazaki T, Ohta M, et al: Joint effects of HMG-CoA reductase inhibitors and eicosapentaenoic acids on serum lipid profile and plasma fatty acid concentrations in patients with hyperlipidemia. *Int J Clin Lab Res* 29(1):22, 1999.

203. Durrington, PN, Bhatnagar D, Mackness MI, et al: An omega-3 polyunsaturated fatty acid concentrate administered for one year decreased triglycerides in simvastatin treated patients with coronary heart disease and persisting hypertriglyceridemia. *Heart* 85(5):544, 2001.

204. Emken EA, Adlof RO, Duval SM, Nelson GJ: Effect of dietary docosahexaenoic acid on desaturation and uptake in vivo of isotope-labeled oleic, linoleic, and linolenic acids by male subjects. *Lipids* 34:785, 1999.

205. Harris WS, Connor WE, Alam N, Illingworth DR: Reduction of postprandial triglyceridemia in humans by dietary n-3 fatty acids. *J Lipid Res* 29:1451, 1988.

206. Calabresi L, Donati D, Pazzucconi F, et al: Omacor in familial combined hyperlipidemia: Effects on lipids and low density lipoprotein subclasses. *Atherosclerosis* 148:387, 2000.

207. Mori TA, Bao DQ, Burke V, et al: Dietary fish as a major component of a weight reducing diet: Impact on serum lipids, glucose and insulin metabolism in overweight hypertensive subjects. *Am J Clin Nutr* 70:817, 1999.

208. Herold PM, Kinsella MS, Kinsella JE: Fish oil consumption and decreased risk of cardiovascular disease: A comparison of findings from animal and human feeding trials. *Am J Clin Nutr* 43:566, 1986.

209. Sanders TAB, Roshanai F: The influence of different types of W-3 polyunsaturated fatty acid on blood lipids and platelet function in healthy volunteers. *Clin Sci* 64:91, 1983.

210. Albert CM, Campos H, Stampfer MJ, et al: Blood levels of long-chain n-3 fatty acids and the risk of sudden death. *N Engl J Med* 346:1113, 2002.

211. Sellmayer A, Witzgall H, Lorenz RL, Weber PC: Effects of dietary fish oil on ventricular premature complexes. *Am J Cardiol* 76:974, 1995.

212. Siscovick DS, Raghunathan TE, King I, et al: Dietary intake and cell membrane levels of long-chain n-3 polyunsaturated fatty acids and the risk of primary cardiac arrest. *JAMA* 274(17):1363, 1995.

213. Christensen JH, Dyerberg J, Schmidt EB: N-3 Fatty acids and risk of sudden cardiac death assessed by 24-hour heart rate variability. *Lipids* 34S:S197, 1999.

213a. Christensen JH, Schmidt EB: Fish oil and the risk of sudden cardiac death. *Cardiovasc Rev Rep* 23:435, 2002.

214. Hepburn FN, Exler J, Weihrauch JL: Provisional tables on the content of omega-3 fatty acids and other fat components of selected foods. *J Am Diet Assoc* 86:788, 1986.

215. *Drug Facts and Comparisons by Facts and Comparisons.* 50th ed. St. Louis, Mo: Wolters Kluwer Company, 1996:l92.

216. Silverman DI, Ware JA, Sacks FM, Pasternak RC: Comparison of the absorption and effect on platelet function of a single dose of n-3 fatty acids given as fish or fish oil. *Am J Clin Nutr* 53:65, 1991.

217. Nordoy A, Barstad L, Connor WE, Hatcher L: Absorption of the n-3 eicosapentaenoic and docosahexaenoic acids as ethyl esters and triglycerides by humans. *Am J Clin Nutr* 53:1185, 1991.

218. Lawson LD, Hughes BG: Human absorption of fish oil fatty acids as triglycerides, free fatty acids or ethyl esters. *Biochem Biophys Res Commun* 152:328, 1988.

219. El Boustani S, Coletta C, Monnier L, et al: Enteral absorption in man of eicosapentaenoic acid in different chemical forms. *Lipids* 22:711, 1987.

220. Marsen TA, Pollok M, Oette K, Baldamus CA: Pharmacokinetics of omega-3 fatty acids during ingestion of fish oil preparations. *Prostagland Leukot Essent Fatty Acids* 46:191, 1992.

221. Wallace JM, McCabe AJ, Robson PJ, et al: Bioavailability of n-3 polyunsaturated fatty acids (PUFA) in foods enriched with microencapsulated fish oil. *Ann Nutr Metab* 44(4):157, 2000.

222. Suchy N, Sullivan JF: Endogenous fatty acids in alimentary triglycerides in normolipidemic young males. *Am J Clin Nutr* 28:36, 1975.

223. Meyer JH, Stevenson EA, Watts HD: The potential role of protein in the absorption of fat. *Gastroenterology* 70:232, 1976.

224. Nordoy A, Hatcher L, Goodnight S, et al: Effects of dietary fat content, saturated fatty acids, and fish oil on eicosanoid production and hemostatic parameters in normal men. *J Lab Clin Med* 123(6):914, 1994.

225. Zuijdgeest-van Leeuwen SD, Dagnelie PC, Rietveld T, et al: Incorporation and washout of orally administered n-3 fatty acid ethyl esters different plasma lipid fractions. *Br J Nutr* 82(6):481, 1999.

226. Koehler HU, Luley C: Hypertriglyceridemia and omega-3 fatty acids. *Adv Exp Med Biol* 243:339, 1988.

227. Montori VM, Farmer A, Wollan PC, Dineen SF: Fish oil supplementation in type 2 diabetes: A quantitative systematic review. *Diabetes Care* 23:1407, 2000.

228. Friedberg CE, Heine RJ, Janssen MJFM, Grobbee DE: Fish oil and glycemic control in diabetes: A meta-analysis. *Diabetes Care* 21:494, 1998.

229. Dyerberg J, Bang HO, Hjorne N: Fatty acid composition of the plasma lipids in Greenland Eskimos. *Am J Clin Nutr* 28:958, 1975.

230. Von Schacky C, Weber PC: Metabolism and effects of platelet function of the purified eicosapentaenoic and eicosahexaenoic acids in humans. *J Clin Invest* 76:2446, 1985.

231. Colquhoun DM: Nutraceuticals: Vitamins and other nutrients in coronary heart disease. *Curr Opin Lipidol* 12:639, 2001.

232. Mori TA, Beilin LJ: Long-chain omega-3 fatty acids, blood lipids and cardiovascular risk reduction. *Curr Opin Lipidol* 12:11, 2001.

233. Rees MM, Rodgers GM: Homocystinemia: Association of a metabolic disorder with vascular disease and thrombosis. *Thromb Res* 71:337, 1993.

234. Fortin LJ, Genest J Jr: Measurement of homocysteine in the prediction of arteriosclerosis. *Clin Biochem* 28:155, 1995.

235. Mayer EL, Jacobsen DW, Robinson K: Homocysteine and coronary atherosclerosis. *J Am Coll Cardiol* 27:517, 1996.

236. Selhub J: Homocysteine metabolism. *Annu Rev Nutr* 19:217, 1999.

237. Mayer EL, Jacobsen DW, Robinson K: Homocysteine and coronary atherosclerosis. *J Am Coll Cardiol* 27:517, 1996.

238. Friedman, AN, Bostom AG, Selhub J, et al: The kidney and homocysteine metabolism. *J Am Soc Nephrol* 12(10):2181, 2001.

239. Nygard O, Vollset SE, Refsum H, et al: Total plasma homocysteine and cardiovascular risk profile: The Hordaland Homocysteine Study. *JAMA* 274:1526, 1995.

240. Kang SS, Wong PWK, Malinow MR: Hyperhomocysteinemia as a risk factor for occlusive vascular disease. *Annu Rev Nutr* 12:279, 1992.

241. Korzun WJ, Ho QV: Stability of plasma total homocysteine concentrations in EDTA-whole blood kept on ice. *Clin Lab Sci* 13(4):196, 2000.

242. Nauck M, Bisse E, Nauck M, Wieland H: Pre-analytical conditions affecting the determination of the plasma. *Clin Chem Lab Med* 39(8):675, 2001.

243. Nurk E, Tell GS, Nygard O, et al: Plasma total homocysteine is influenced by prandial status in humans: The Hordaland Homocysteine Study 1. *J Nutr* 131:1214, 2001.

244. Kang SS, Wong PWK, Susmano A, et al: Thermolabile methylenetetrahydrofolate reductase: An inherited risk factor for coronary artery disease. *Am J Hum Genet* 48:536, 1991.

245. Morimoto K, Haneda T, Okamoto K, et al: Methylenetetrahydrofolate reductase gene polymorphism, hyperhomocysteinemia, and cardiovascular diseases in chronic hemodialysis patients. *Nephron* 90(1):43, 2002.

246. Lievers KJ, Boers GH, Verhoef P, et al: A second common variant in the methylenetetrahydrofolate reductase (MTHFR) gene and its relationship to MTHFR enzyme activity, homocysteine and cardiovascular disease risk. *J Mol Med* 79(9):522, 2001.

247. Yamada K, Chen Z, Rozen R, Mathews RG: Effects of common polymorphisms on the properties of recombinant human methylenetetrahydrofolate reductase. *Proc Natl Acad Sci U S A* 98:14853, 2001.

248. Cortese C, Motti C: MTHFR gene polymorphism, homocysteine and cardiovascular disease. *Public Health Nutr* 4(2B):493, 2001.

249. Feix A, Fritsche-Polanz R, Kletzmayr J, et al: Increased prevalence of combined MTR and MTHFR genotypes in individuals with severely elevated total homocysteine plasma levels. *Am J Kidney Dis* 38(5):956, 2001.

250. Geisel J, Zimbelmann I, Schorr H, et al: Genetic Defects as important factors for moderate hyperhomocysteinemia. *Clin Chem Lab Med* 39(8):698, 2001.

251. Gaby SK, Bendich A, Singh VN, Machlin LJ, eds. *Vitamin Intake and Health.* New York: Marcel Dekker, 1991.

252. Friedman JA, Dwyer JT: Hyperhomocysteinemia as a risk factor for cardiovascular disease in patients undergoing hemodialysis. *Nutr Rev* 53:197, 1995.

253. Fuchs D, Jaeger M, Widner B, et al: Is hyperhomocysteinemia due to the oxidative depletion of folate rather than to insufficient dietary intake? *Clin Chem Lab Med* 39(8):691, 2001.

254. Christensen B, Mosdol A, Retterstol L, et al: Abstention from filtered coffee reduces the concentration of plasma homocysteine and serum cholesterol—a randomized controlled trial. *Am J Clin Nutr* 74(3):302, 2001.

255. Boushey CJ, Beresford SAA, Omenn GS, Motulsky AG: A quantitative assessment of plasma homocysteine as a risk factor for vascular disease. *JAMA* 274:1049, 1995.

256. Welch GN, Loscalzo J: Homocysteine and atherothrombosis. *N Engl J Med* 338:1042, 1998.

257. Chern CL, Huang RF, Chen YH, et al: Folate deficiency-induced oxidative stress and apoptosis are mediated via homocysteine-dependent overproduction of hydrogen peroxide and enhanced activation of NF-kappaB in human Hep G2 cells. *Biomed Pharmacother* 55(8):434, 2001.

258. Roth J, Goebeler M, Ludwig S, et al: Homocysteine inhibits tumor necrosis factor-induced activation of endothelium via modulation of nuclear factor-kappa β activity. *Biochem Biophys Acta* 1540(2):154, 2001.

259. Tsai JC, Wang H, Perrella MA, et al: Induction of cyclin A gene expression by homocysteine in vascular smooth muscle cells. *J Clin Invest* 97:146, 1996.

260. Wu LL, Wu J, Hunt SC, et al: Plasma homocysteine as a risk factor for early familial coronary artery disease. *Clin Chem* 40:552, 1994.

261. Stuhlinger MC, Tsao PS, Her JH, et al: Homocysteine impairs the nitric oxide synthase pathway: Role of asymmetric dimethyl arginine. *Circulation* 104(21):2569, 2001.

262. Virdis A, Ghiadoni L, Cardinal H, et al: Mechanisms responsible for endothelial dysfunction induced by fasting hyperhomocystinemia in normotensive subjects and patients with essential hypertension. *J Am Coll Cardiol* 38(4):1106, 2001.

263. Nappo F, DeRosa N, Marfella R, et al: Impairment of endothelial functions by acute hyper-homocysteinemia and reversal by antioxidant vitamins. *JAMA* 281:2113, 1999.

264. van Dijk RA, Rauwerda JA, Steyn M, et al: Long-term homocysteine-lowering treatment with folic acid plus pyridoxine is associated with decreased blood pressure but not with improved brachial artery endothelium-dependent vasodilation or carotid artery stiffness: A 2-year, randomized, placebo-controlled trial. *Arterioscler Thromb Vasc Biol* 21(12):207, 2001.

265. Pullin CH, Ashield-Watt PA, Burr, et al: Optimization of dietary folate or low-dose folic acid supplements lower homocysteine but do not enhance endothelial function in healthy adults, irrespective of the methylenetetrahydrofolate reductase (C677T) genotype. *J Am Coll Cardiol* 38(7):1799, 2001.

266. Chambers JC, Ueland PM, Obeid OA, et al: Improved vascular endothelial function after oral B vitamins. An effect mediated through reduced concentrations of free plasma homocysteine. *Circulation* 102:2479, 2000.

267. Title LM, Cummings PM, Giddens K, et al: Effect of folic acid and antioxidant vitamins on endothelial dysfunction in patients with coronary artery disease. *J Am Coll Cardiol* 36:758, 2000.

268. Lentz SR, Piegors DJ, Malinow R, Heistad DD: Supplementation of atherogenic diet with B vitamins does not prevent atherosclerosis or vascular dysfunction in monkeys. *Circulation* 103:1006, 2001.

269. Mujumdar VS, Aru GM, Tyagi SC: Induction of oxidative stress by homocysteine impairs endothelial function. *J Cell Biochem* 82(3):491, 2001.

270. Jakubowski H: Protein N-homocysteinylation: Implications for atherosclerosis. *Biomed Pharmacother* 55(8):443, 2001.

271. Sawle P, Foresti R, Green CJ, Motterlini R: Homocysteine attenuates endothelial haem oxygenase-1 induction. *FEBS Lett* 508(3):403, 2001.

272. Drunat S, Moatti N, Paul JL, et al: Homocysteine-induced decrease in endothelin-1 production is initiated at the extracellular level and involves oxidative products. *Eur J Biochem* 268(20):5287, 2001.

273. Nonaka H, Tsujino T, Watari Y, et al: Taurine prevents the decrease in expression and secretion of extracellular superoxide dismutase induced by homocysteine: amelioration of homocysteine-induced endoplasmic reticulum stress by taurine. *Circulation* 104(10):1165, 2001.

274. Lim S, Kim MS, Park KS, et al: Correlation of plasma homocysteine and mitochondrial DNA content in peripheral blood in healthy women. *Atherosclerosis* 158(2):399, 2001.

275. Seligsohn U, Lubetsky A: Genetic susceptibility to venous thrombosis. *N Engl J Med* 344:1222, 2001.

276. Zhang G, Zhao H, Zhang L: Effects of homocysteine on human vascular endothelial cells, platelet aggregation, and heparin cofactor activity. *Zhonghua Xue Ye Xue Za Zhi* 20(9):471, 2001.

277. Davi G, Di Minno G, Coppola A, et al: Oxidative stress and platelet activation in homozygous homocysteinuria. *Circulation* 104(10):1124, 2001.

277a. Malinow MR, Stampfer MJ: Role of plasma homocysteine in arterial occlusive diseases. *Clin Chem* 40:857, 1994.

278. Malinow MR, Nieto FJ, Szklo M, et al: Carotid artery intimal-medial wall thickening and plasma homocysteine in asymptomatic adults: The Atherosclerosis Risk in Communities Study. *Circulation* 87:1107, 1993.

279. Selhub J, Jacques PF, Bostom AG, et al: Association between plasma homocysteine concentrations and extracranial carotid artery stenosis. *N Engl J Med* 332:286, 1995.

280. Dalery K, Lussier-Cacan S, Selhub J, et al: Homocysteine and coronary artery disease in french canadian subjects: Relation with vitamins B12, B6, pyridoxal phosphate, and folate. *Am J Cardiol* 75:1107, 1995.

281. Pancharuniti N, Lewis CA, Sauberlich HE, et al: Plasma homocysteine, folate, and vitamin B12 concentrations and risk for early-onset coronary artery disease. *Am J Clin Nutr* 59:940, 1994.

282. den Heijer M, Keijzer MB: Hyperhomocysteinemia as a risk factor for venous thrombosis. *Clin Chem Lab Med* 39(8):710, 2001.

283. Clarke R, Daly L, Robinson K, et al: Hyperhomocysteinemia: An independent risk factor for vascular disease. *N Engl J Med* 324:1149, 1991.

284. Verhoef P, Stampfer MJ: Prospective studies of homocysteine and cardiovascular disease. *Nutr Rev* 53:283, 1995.

285. Stampfer MJ, Malinow MR, Willett WC, et al: A prospective study of plasma homocysteine and risk of myocardial infarction in United States physicians. *JAMA* 268:877, 1992.

286. Arnesen E, Refsum H, Bonaa KH, et al: Serum total homocysteine and coronary heart disease. *Int J Epidemiol* 24:704, 1995.

287. Alfthan G, Pekkanen J, Jauhiainen M, et al: Relation of serum homocysteine and lipoprotein(a) concentrations to atherosclerotic disease in a prospective Finnish population based study. *Atherosclerosis* 106:9, 1994.

288. Taylor LM Jr, DeFrang RD, Harris EJ, et al: The association of elevated homocysteine with progression of symptomatic peripheral arterial disease. *Vasc Surg* 13:128, 1991.

289. Cattaneo M, Lombardi R, Lecchi A, et al: Low levels of vitamin B(6) are independently associated with a heightened risk of deep-vein thrombosis. *Circulation* 104(20):2442, 2001.

290. Evans RW, Shaten BJ, Hempel JD, et al: Homocyst(e)ine and risk of cardiovascular disease in the Multiple Risk Factor Intervention Trial. *Arterioscler Thromb Vasc Biol* 17:1947, 1997.

291. Bostom AG, Shemin D, Verhoef P, et al: Elevated fasting total plasma homocysteine levels and cardiovascular disease outcomes in maintenance dialysis patients: A prospective study. *Arterioscler Thromb Vasc Biol* 17:2554, 1998.

292. Folsom AR, Nieto FJ, McGovern PG, et al: Prospective study of coronary heart disease incidence in relation to fasting total homocysteine, related genetic polymorphisms, and B vitamin: The Atherosclerosis Risk in Communities (ARIC) study. *Circulation* 98:204, 1998.

293. Moustapha A, Naso A, Nahlawi M, et al: Prospective study of hyperhomocystinemia as an adverse cardiovascular risk factor in end-stage renal disease. *Circulation* 97:138, 1998.

294. Stehouwer CD, Weijenberg MP, van den Berg M, et al: Serum homocysteine and risk of coronary heart disease and cerebrovascular disease in elderly men: A 10-year follow-up. *Arterioscler Thromb Vasc Biol* 18:1895, 1998.

295. Wald NJ, Watt HC, Law MR, et al: Homocysteine and ischemic heart disease: Results of a prospective study with implications regarding prevention. *Arch Intern Med* 158:862, 1998.

296. Nygard O, Nordrehaug JE, Refsum H, et al: Plasma homocysteine levels and mortality in patients with coronary artery disease. *N Engl J Med* 337:230, 1997.

296a. Fairfield KM, Fletcher RH: Vitamins for chronic disease prevention in adults. Scientific review. *JAMA* 287:3116, 2002.

296b. Ford ES, Smith SJ, Stroup DF, et al: Homocyst(e)ine and cardiovascular disease: A systematic review of the evidence with special emphasis on case-control studies and nested case-control studies. *Intl J Epidemiol* 31:59, 2002.

296c. Nurk E, Tell GS, Vollset SE, et al: Plasma total homocysteine and hospitalizations for cardiovascular disease. The Hordaland Homocysteine Study. *Arch Intern Med* 162:1374, 2002.

297. Fermo I, Vigano D'Angelo S, Paroni R, et al: Prevalence of moderate hyperhomocysteinemia in patients with early-onset venous and arterial occlusive disease. *Ann Intern Med* 123:747, 1995.

298. Stampfer MJ, Rimm EB: Folate and cardiovascular disease. Why we need a trial now. *JAMA* 275:1929, 1996.

298a. Seshadri S, Beiser A, Selhub J, et al: Plasma homocysteine as a risk factor for dementia and Alzheimer's disease. *N Engl J Med* 346:476, 2002.

299. Morrison G, Hark L: *Medical Nutrition and Disease*. 2nd ed. Malden, MA: Blackwell Science, 1999:37.

300. Tucker KL, Mahnken B, Wilson PWF, et al: Folic acid fortification of the food supply. Potential benefits and risks for the elderly population. *JAMA* 276:1879, 1996.

301. Zeitlin A, Frishman WH, Chang CJ: The association of vitamin B12 and folate blood levels with mortality and cardiovascular morbidity incidence in the old: The Bronx Longitudinal Aging Study. *Am J Ther* 4(7-8):275, 1997.

302. McLaren DS: The luxus vitamins A and B12. *Am J Clin Nutr* 34:1611, 1981.

303. Bentley JR, Ferrini RL, Hill LL: American College of Preventive Medicine public policy statement: Folic acid fortification of grain products in the United States to prevent neural tube defects. *Am J Prev Med* 16:264, 1999.

304. Mills JL: Fortification of foods with folic acid—how much is enough? *N Engl J Med* 342:1442, 2000.

305. Romano PS, Waitzman NJ, Scheffler RM, Pi RD: Folic acid fortification of grain: an economic analysis. *Am J Public Health* 85(5):667, 1995.

306. Jacques PF, Selhub J, Bostom AG, et al: The effect of folic acid fortification on plasma folate and total homocysteine concentrations. *N Engl J Med* 340:1449, 1999.

307. Tice JA, Ross E, Coxson PG, et al: Cost effectiveness of vitamin therapy to lower plasma homocysteine levels for the prevention of coronary heart disease: Effects of grain fortification and beyond. *JAMA* 286:936, 2001.

308. Malinow MR, Duell PB, Hess DL, et al: Reduction of plasma homocyst(e)ine levels by breakfast cereal fortified with folic acid in patients with coronary heart disease. *N Engl J Med* 338:1009, 1998.

309. Bostom AG, Selhub J, Jacques PF, Rosenberg IH: Power shortage: Clinical trials testing the "homocysteine hypothesis" against a background of folic acid-fortified cereal grain flour. *Ann Intern Med* 135(2):133, 2001.

310. Ubbink JB, Vermaak WJH, Merwe A, et al: Vitamin B12, vitamin B6, and folate nutritional status in men with hyperhomocysteinemia. *Am J Clin Nutr* 57:47, 1993.

311. Brattstrom LE, Israelsson B, Lindgarde F, et al: Higher total plasma homocysteine in vitamin B12 deficiency than heterozygosity for homocystinuria due to cystathionine-B-synthase deficiency. *Metabolism* 34:1073, 1985.

312. Brattstrom LE, Israelsson B, Jeppson JO, et al: Folic acid-an innocuous means to reduce plasma homocysteine. *Scand J Clin Invest* 48:215, 1988.

313. Homocysteine Lowering Trialists' Collaboration: Lowering blood homocysteine with folic acid based supplements: Meta-analysis of randomised trials. *BMJ* 316:894, 1998.

314. Landgren F, Israelsson B, Lindgren A, et al: Plasma homocysteine in acute myocardial infarction: Homocysteine-lowering effect of folic acid. *J Intern Med* 237:381, 1995.

315. Saltzman E, Mason JB, Jacques PF, et al: B vitamin supplementation lowers homocysteine levels in heart disease (abstr). *Clin Res* 42:172A, 1994.

316. Schnyder G, Roffi M, Pin R, et al: Decreased rate of coronary restenosis after lowering of plasma homocysteine levels. *N Engl J Med* 345:1593, 2001.

316a. Schnyder G, Roffi M, Flammer Y, et al: Effect of homocysteine-lowering therapy with folic acid, vitamin B$_{12}$, and vitamin B$_6$ on clinical outcome after percutaneous coronary intervention: The Swiss Heart Study: A randomized controlled trial. *JAMA* 288:973, 2002.

317. Dierkes J, Westphal S, Kunstmann S, et al: Vitamin supplementation can markedly reduce the homocysteine elevation induced by fenofibrate. *Atherosclerosis* 158(1):161, 2001.

318. Stule T, Melenovsky V, Grauova B, et al: Folate supplementation prevents plasma homocysteine increase after fenofibrate therapy. *Nutrition* 17(9):721, 2001.

319. Oakley GP Jr, Adams MJ, Dickinson CM: More folic acid for everyone, now. *J Nutr* 126:751S, 1996.

320. Leslie D, Gheorghiade M: Is there a role for thiamine supplementation in the management of heart failure? *Am Heart J* 131:1248, 1996.

321. Yui Y, Itokawa Y, Kawai C: Furosemide-induced thiamine deficiency. *Cardiovasc Res* 14:537, 1980.

322. Seligmann H, Halkin H, Rauchfleisch S, et al: Thiamine deficiency in patients with congestive heart failure receiving long-term furosemide therapy: A pilot study. *Am J Med* 91:151, 1991.

323. Statius Van Eps LW, Schouten H: Water and electrolyte metabolism in thiamine deficiency. *Neth J Med* 28:408, 1985.

324. Marcus R, Coulston AM: Water soluble vitamins. In: Hardman G, Limbird LE, eds. *Goodman & Gilman's The Pharmacological Basis of Therapeutics.* 10th ed. New York: McGraw Hill, 2001: 1753–1771.

325. Shimon I, Almog S, Vered Z, et al: Improved left ventricular function after thiamine supplementation in patients with congestive heart failure receiving long-term furosemide therapy. *Am J Med* 98:485, 1995.

326. Neufeld EJ, Fleming JC, Tartaglini E, Steinkamp MP: Thiamine-responsive megaloblastic anemia syndrome: A disorder of high-affinity thiamine transport. *Blood Cells Mol Dis* 27(1):135, 2001.

327. Rieck J, Halkin H, Almog S, et al: Urinary loss of thiamine is increased by low doses of furosemide in healthy volunteers. *J Lab Clin Med* 134(3):238, 1999.

328. Yue QY, Beermann B, Lindstrom B, Nyquist O: No difference in blood thiamine diphosphate levels between Swedish Caucasian patients with congestive hear failure treated with furosemide and patients without heart failure. *J Intern Med* 242(6):491, 1997.

329. Hardig L, Daae C, Dellborg M, et al: Reduced thiamine phosphate, but not thiamine diphosphate, in erythrocytes in elderly patients with congestive heart failure treated with furosemide. *J Intern Med* 247(5):597, 2000.

330. Suter PM, Haller J, Hany A, Vetter W: Diuretic use: A risk for subclinical thiamine deficiency in elderly patients. *J Nutr Health Aging* 4(2)69, 2000.

331. Zangen A, Botzer D, Zangen R, Shainberg A: Furosemide and digoxin inhibit thiamine uptake in cardiac cells. *Eur J Pharmacol* 361(1):151, 1998.

332. Wilkinson TJ, Hanger HC, George PM, Sainsbury R: Is thiamine deficiency in elderly people related to age or co-morbidity? *Age Aging* 29(2):111, 2000.

333. Rodeheffer RJ, Gersh BJ, Kannel AJ: Myocarditis, dilated cardiomyopathy, and specific myocardial disease. In: Giuliani ER, Fuster V, Gersh B, McGoon MD, eds. *Cardiology: Fundaments and Practice,* 2nd ed. St. Louis: Mosby, 1991:1827.

334. Luft FC: Lactic acidosis update for critical care clinicians. *J Am Soc Nephrol* 12:S17, 2001.

335. Blankenhorn MA: Effect of vitamin deficiency on the heart and circulation. *Circulation* 11:288, 1995.

336. Naidoo DP, Rawat R, Dyer RB, et al: Cardiac beriberi: A report of four cases. *S Afr Med J* 72:283, 1987.

337. Burwell CS: Beriberi heart disease. *Trans Assoc Am Phys* 60:59, 1947.

338. Akbarian M: Hemodynamic studies in beriberi heart disease. *Am J Med* 41:197, 1966.

339. Webster MWI, Ikram H: Myocardial function in alcoholic cardiac beriberi. *Int J Cardiol* 17:213, 1987.

340. Constant J: The alcoholic cardiomyopathies—genuine and pseudo. *Cardiology* 91(2):92, 1999.

341. Kawai C, Wakabayashi A, Matsumura T, Yui Y: Reappearance of beriberi heart disease in Japan. *Am J Med* 69:383, 1980.

342. Talwar D, Davidson H, Cooney J, et al: VitaminB(1) status assessed by direct measurement of thiamin pyrophosphate in erythrocytes of whole blood by HPLC: Comparison with erythrocyte transketolase activation assay. *Clin Chem* 46(5):704, 2000.

343. Levy WC, Soine LA, Huth MM, Fishbein DP: Thiamine deficiency in congestive heart failure. *Am J Med* 93:705, 1992.

344. Brady JA, Rock CL, Horneffer MR: Thiamine status, diuretic medications, and the management of congestive heart failure. *J Am Diet Assoc* 95(5):541, 1995.

345. Pepersack T, Garbusinski J, Robberrecht J, et al: Clinical relevance of thiamine status amongst hospitalized elderly patients. *Gerontology* 45(2):96, 1999.

346. Lee DC, Chu J, Satz W, et al: Low plasma thiamine levels in patients admitted through the emergency department. *Acad Emerg Med* 7(10):1156, 2000.

Antioxidant Vitamins and Enzymatic and Synthetic Oxygen-Derived Free-Radical Scavengers in the Prevention and Treatment of Cardiovascular Disease

William H. Frishman

Nathan A. Kruger

Devraj U. Nayak

Babak A. Vakili

Coronary artery disease (CAD) is currently the leading cause of death in the United States, accounting for one out of three deaths. Free radicals play a key role in the pathogenesis and progression of this disease. The potential role of antioxidants in therapeutic protection against free radical–induced tissue damage has been the subject of great controversy in recent years. If antioxidants serve a protective role through combating the harmful effects of free radicals, it is foreseeable that long-term antioxidant therapy may play a major part in reducing both the prevalence of CAD and the incidence of its complications.

In this chapter, the pathogenesis of free-radical production and cell injury is discussed, and drug treatments to alter the generation of free radicals and their pathologic consequences are reviewed with respect to atherosclerosis and myocardial ischemic injury.

FREE RADICALS

In the structure of atoms, electrons occupy regions of space surrounding the nucleus called orbitals, and each orbital can hold a maximum of two electrons. A free radical is a molecule containing one or more electrons that are spinning alone in an orbital in the outer valence shell. These are known as unpaired electrons. Because the lone electron exists in a relatively a high-energy state, free radicals are extremely reactive, with a very short life span measured in microseconds. They can be generated in humans by three separate chemical reactions: homolytic cleavage and loss or addition of electrons to molecules. Once formed, a free radical may react with second molecules, itself becoming nonradical while transforming the second into a free radical. Alternatively, free radicals can combine their unimpaired electrons with other molecules and form covalent bonds or accept an electron from other molecules to form a pair of electrons. These latter reactions terminate the chain of free-radical reactions and are the basic mechanism of action of antioxidants and free-radical scavengers.

In vivo, the majority of free-radical formation is thought to occur as electrons move down the mitochondrial respiratory chain, where oxygen (O_2) is enzymatically reduced to water through the addition of four electrons and two protons. It has been shown that 1 to 2% of electrons can leak from the mitochondrion during this process.[1] These electrons can lead to the nonenzymatic reduction of the surrounding O_2 molecules and subsequent formation of free radicals.[2–4]

Free radical–induced injury has been implicated in the etiology of numerous human diseases including neurodegenerative diseases, various lung diseases, hepatitis, renal injury, muscular dystrophies, diabetes mellitus, retinopathy of prematurity, CAD, and certain types of cancers.[5–14a] Oxygen-derived free radicals are capable of damaging various biological substances, such as proteins, carbohydrates, lipids, vitamins, DNA, RNA, and many micronutrients.[15] Apart from causing cellular and tissue damage, free radicals also play a beneficial role in numerous biological systems. They are produced by phagocytes to exert a bactericidal effect, play a role in modulating vascular tone, provide a defense mechanism against tumor growth (nitric oxide), and also serve to catalyze certain enzymatic reactions.[16,17] Free radicals also activate transcription factors that participate in different stages of cellular growth, wound healing, and fibrosis.

The direct measurement of free radicals in vivo is an extremely difficult task, mainly because they are very reactive and unstable and consequently short-lived. Hence, it is nearly impossible to measure free radicals chemically directly from blood or urine samples. Most assessments are therefore done indirectly through measuring end products of reactions between free radicals and biological molecules such as lipids, proteins, and DNA or conversely through measurement of antioxidant levels in serum or tissues.[18,19] Electron spin resonance spectrometry has been used to detect free radicals directly; however, its use is limited mainly to tissues ex vivo. The technical difficulties encountered in the direct measurement of free radicals in vivo pose a great limitation on our ability to detect the source and site of free-radical production. At this point most assays are semiquantitative, and more sensitive and specific methods for detection of free radicals in vivo are needed.

Reaction #1: $O_2 + e^- \longrightarrow O_2^{-\bullet}$

Reaction #2: $Fe^{2+} + O_2 \longrightarrow Fe^{3+} + O_2^{-\bullet}$

Reaction #3: $Cu^+ + O_2 \longrightarrow Cu^{2+} + O_2^{-\bullet}$

Reaction #4: $2O_2^{-\bullet} + 2H^+ \xrightarrow{\text{SOD}^\bullet} H_2O_2 + O_2$

Reaction #5: $O_2 + 2e^- + 2H^+ \longrightarrow H_2O_2$

Reaction #6: $O_2^{-\bullet} + H_2O_2 \longrightarrow {}^\bullet OH + OH^- + O_2$

Reaction #7: $H_2O_2 + Fe^{2+} \longrightarrow {}^\bullet OH + OH^- + Fe^{3+}$

Reaction #8: ${}^\bullet OH + O_2^{-\bullet} + H^+ \longrightarrow {}^1O_2 + H_2O$

FIGURE 24-1. Various chemical reactions leading to the generation of free radicals.

Oxygen-Derived Free Radicals (Fig. 24-1)

Superoxide Anion (O_2^{-*})

This radical is generated by the addition of a single electron to O_2 (reaction #1) or through autoxidation of reduced transitional metals in the presence of oxygen (reactions #2 and 3). As seen in reaction #4, the superoxide anion also serves as a substrate in the production of hydrogen peroxide (H_2O_2). It also participates in the reduction of transitional metal ions, which play an important role in the production of free radicals. The superoxide anion is not deemed to have a substantial damaging effect by itself. However, at low pH, it can form a perhydroxyl radical (HO_2), a more reactive and potent oxygen radical, that is capable of causing significant cellular damage.[3] In addition to the above-mentioned mechanisms, the superoxide anion can also be generated through many endogenous biochemical reactions, such as those mediated by nicotinamide adenine dinucleotide phosphate (NADPH) oxidase and the cytochrome P450 systems.[20,21]

Hydroxyl Radical (${}^\bullet OH$)

The hydroxyl radical is formed through the Haber Weiss reaction between H_2O_2 and superoxide anion (reaction #6), or by the direct breakdown of H_2O_2 in the presence of transitional metal ions (reaction #7). The hydroxyl radical is considered the most potent and reactive of all oxygen species,[11] and it can react with virtually any molecule. Therefore, it exerts most of its cellular damage at or very close to its site of production.[2,3]

Hydrogen Peroxide (H_2O_2)

Hydrogen peroxide is produced when two superoxide anions react together in the presence of the enzyme superoxide dismutase (SOD, reaction #4), or by the two-electron reduction of oxygen (reaction #5). H_2O_2 is not regarded as a free radical; in fact, it belongs to a group of molecules collectively known as reactive oxygen species (ROS). This group includes all molecules that are somehow involved in the production of free-radical species. H_2O_2 is relatively less reactive and mainly serves as a source for the production of the hydroxyl radical.[2,3]

Singlet Oxygen (${}^1O_2$)

Like H_2O_2, singlet oxygen is considered to be a reactive oxygen species. It can be formed through a free-radical reaction (reaction #8) or generated from ground-state triplet oxygen in the presence of light. Singlet oxygen plays an important role in free radical–induced damage in tissues such as the eye and skin.[2]

Oxygen-derived free radicals are the most abundant form of free radicals produced in vivo; however, they are not the only forms. Other less common free radicals include a variety of carbon-centered radicals (peroxyl and alkoxyl radicals), sulfur radicals, and a number of toxic compounds including carbon tetrachloride.[3,22,23] The former can be generated through the process of lipid peroxidation.

Lipid Peroxidation

Lipid peroxidation, and more specifically the oxidative modification of low-density lipoproteins (LDL) into oxidized LDL (oLDL), has been implicated in the enhanced atherogenicity of LDL and the development of CAD.[13,15] Lipid peroxidation is a chain reaction initiated and continued by the production of free radicals. The process starts by the oxidation of a polyunsaturated fatty acid (PUFA:H) in the presence of a free radical (R$^\bullet$), such as hydroxyl radical. A fatty acid radical (PUFA$^\bullet$) is generated in this manner and quickly reacts with an oxygen molecule to form a fatty acid peroxyl radical (PUFAOO$^\bullet$). The latter can further oxidize another PUFA, forming a lipid hydroperoxide (PUFAOOH) and a fatty acid radical (PUFA$^\bullet$), hence propagating the radical chain reaction[24,25]:

$$PUFA:H + R^\bullet \to PUFA^\bullet + RH$$

$$PUFA^\bullet + O_2 \to PUFAOO^\bullet$$

$$PUFAOO^\bullet + PUFA:H \to PUFAOOH + PUFA^\bullet$$

In the presence of transitional metal ion catalysts (M^{n+}), lipid hydroperoxides are further broken down into a number of free radicals including alkoxyl radicals (PUFAO$^\bullet$), fatty acid peroxyl radical (PUFAOO$^\bullet$), and aldehydes. Therefore, a single initiating reaction driven by a free-radical species is capable of causing extensive cellular damage in a self-perpetuating chain reaction. Unlike free radicals, aldehydes are more stable compounds and are capable of diffusing into and injuring tissues located far away from their original site of production[26]:

$$PUFAOOH + M^{n+} \to PUFAO^\bullet + OH^- + M^{(n+1)+}$$

$$PUFAOOH + M^{(n+1)+} \to PUFAOO^\bullet + H^+ + M^{n+}$$

OXIDIZED LDL AND ATHEROGENESIS

LDL is a spherical molecule with a central core containing cholesteryl esters and triglyceride molecules. It is surrounded by an outer layer of free cholesterol, fatty acids, and phospholipids. About half of all fatty acids in LDL are polyunsaturated fatty acids (PUFAs), which are highly vulnerable to the process of lipid peroxidation. Apolipoprotein B (apo B), the signal protein recognized by normal LDL receptors, is embedded in this outer layer. During the oxidative modification of LDL into oLDL, apo B is chemically modified so that it can no longer bind to the normal LDL receptor. Instead, it is picked up by acetyl (scavenger) LDL receptors on monocytes, macrophages, and endothelial cells. These receptors are not subject to the same regulatory mechanisms that control the presence of normal LDL receptors on cell membranes.[27,28] In other words, these receptors are not downregulated in the presence of high intracellular cholesterol levels. Hence, macrophages continue to accumulate LDL until they are converted to lipid-laden foam cells. When foam cells necrose, their toxic contents (oLDL, aldehydes,

FIGURE 24-2. Schematic outline of the oxidative modification hypothesis, showing the several ways in which oxidized LDL is potentially more atherogenic than native LDL. Monocytes, the major precursors for foam cells in the fatty streak, are shown adhering to the endothelium and then penetrating to the subendothelial space. Oxidized LDL can directly stimulate this by virtue of its lysolecithin content, and lightly oxidized LDL (MM-LDL) can stimulate it indirectly by increasing the release of MCP-1 from endothelial cells. Oxidized LDL is a ligand for the scavenger receptor that is expressed as the monocyte differentiates to a tissue macrophage, and this leads to the accumulation of lipids in the developing foam cells. This monocyte/macrophage differentiation can be facilitated by the release of macrophage-colony stimulating factor (M-CSF) from endothelial cells under the influence of MM-LDL. Finally, oxidized LDL can induce endothelial damage and thus facilitate the atherogenic process by allowing entry of elements from the blood and adherence of platelets. Additional properties of oxidized LDL not shown here that may make it more atherogenic are the facts that it is immunogenic and that it interferes with response of arteries to endothelial-derived relaxation factor (EDRF). (*Reproduced with permission from Steinberg.*[28])

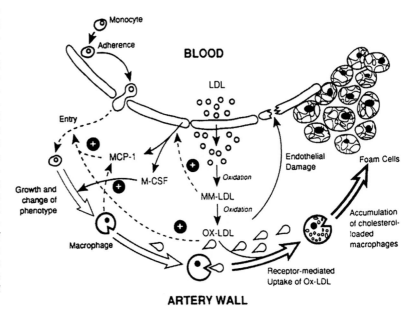

and free radicals) are spilled into the intimal space, stimulating an inflammatory process whereby more neutrophils and macrophages are recruited (Fig. 24-2).

Oxidized LDL damages the integrity of endothelial cells and also stimulates them to release cytokines and chemotactic factors while inducing the formation of endothelial leukocyte adhesion molecules (ELAMs), leading to the migration of macrophages into the subendothelial space.[11,29] Also, the actions of endothelium-derived relaxing factor are inhibited by oLDL.[30] Through induction of the gene responsible for coding the A chain of endothelium-derived growth factor, oLDL stimulates the proliferation of smooth muscle cells. Oxidized LDL induces the formation of autoantibodies against itself[31,32] and provokes an immune response within the atherosclerotic plaque by activating T cells.[33,34]

Prevention of LDL oxidation may play a significant role both in delaying and arresting the development of atherosclerotic plaques, thereby reducing the risk of CAD. To prevent the autooxidation of PUFAs, a number of antioxidants exist within the LDL particle. These include retinoids, beta carotenes, alpha carotenes, gamma tocopherol, and alpha tocopherol.[12]

DEFENSE AGAINST OXIDATIVE DAMAGE

Several natural mechanisms involving antioxidants have evolved to protect the lipids and other biomolecules of cellular components from free radical–mediated oxidation. When the capacity of the antioxidant defense system is exceeded by free-radical load, damage to cells and tissues may occur. The defense mechanisms against tissue damage induced by free-radical and reactive oxygen species (ROS) can be divided into two general categories. The first comprises preventive measures that are closely involved with the site of free-radical generation. These mechanisms decrease electron leakage (through compartmentalization) and reduce the availability of certain catalysts needed for the generation of free radicals. Examples of such microenvironments include mitochondrions, lysosomes, and peroxisomes. Peroxisomes serve as structures in which H_2O_2-generating enzymes are sequestered. Transitional metal ions,

such as Fe^{2+}, serve to enhance many oxidation reactions. Their sequestration by chelating agents (transferrin, ferritin, carnosine, ceruloplasmin, and homocarnosine) help to prevent them from participating in and catalyzing free-radical reactions.[3,5,35,36]

The second category of defense is made up of intercepting or scavenging antioxidants. They are composed of enzymatic and nonenzymatic substances and are found in both the lipid and aqueous compartments of cells. These scavengers act to decompose formed free radicals and ROSs. Intracellular enzymatic scavengers include catalase, SOD, and glutathione peroxidase; they play an important part in the breakdown of hydroperoxides (Fig. 24-3). Catalase is predominantly found in peroxisomes and acts on H_2O_2. Glutathione peroxidase is found in the cytosol and acts on both H_2O_2 and free-fatty acid hydroperoxides.[3] Glutathione peroxidase is a selenium-dependent enzyme; in some studies, selenium levels have been found to correlate inversely with the risk of CAD. SOD catalyzes the dismutation of superoxide anion to hydrogen peroxide, which is subsequently broken down by either catalase or glutathione peroxidase.[37] Three different types of superoxide dismutase enzymes exist. Two of these contain copper and magnesium and are found in the cytosol and bound to vascular endothelium, respectively. The third contains magnesium and is found in the mitochondrial matrix. Magnesium deficiency has been associated with increased cell death and peroxidation following exposure to free radicals, presumably secondary to a decrease in cellular antiperoxidative properties.[2,38] Table 24-1 contains a more complete list of enzymatic antioxidants, along with their main action.

Nonenzymatic antioxidants can be divided into two groups: lipophilic (vitamin E and beta carotene) and hydrophilic (vitamin C)

FIGURE 24-3. Chemical reactions involving hydrogen peroxide and free-radical development.

$$2\ H_2O_2 \xrightarrow{\text{Catalase}} O_2 + 2H_2O$$

$$2GSH + H_2O_2 \xrightarrow{\text{GP°}} GssG + 2H_2O$$

$$O_2^{-\bullet} + O_2^{-\bullet} + 2H^+ \xrightarrow{\text{Super Oxide Dismutase}} H_2O_2 + O_2$$

TABLE 24-1. Enzymatic Antioxidants and Their Action

Enzyme	Target of Action
Catalase	Hydrogen peroxide
Glutathione	Hydrogen peroxide
Peroxidase	Hydrogen peroxide
Superoxide dismutase	Superoxide anion
Cytochrome oxidase system	Detoxifies 95–99% of oxygen in cells

antioxidants.[2,39] The former are mostly present in cell membranes, while the latter reside in the cell cytoplasm, plasma, and other intra/extracellular fluids (Table 24-2 and Fig. 24-4).

NUTRITIVE ANTIOXIDANTS (VITAMINS AND MINERALS)

Alpha Tocopherol (Vitamin E) (Fig. 24-5)

Alpha tocopherol, the most active form of vitamin E, is a lipid-soluble antioxidant and is the major form of antioxidant present in lipid layers such as cell membranes, mitochondrial membranes, and LDL.[40,41] Its dietary source is mostly animal tissues, vegetable oils, seeds, and grains. Alpha tocopherol provides the main antioxidant defense in the LDL particle and is the most plentiful of all lipophilic antioxidants in humans (1 per every 2000 phospholipid molecules or about 5–10 tocopherols per LDL particle).[42] Despite its relative scarcity compared with other lipid moieties, alpha tocopherol is a highly effective antioxidant. It preferentially donates the hydrogen (H^+) from the hydroxyl group on its ring structure to free radicals because of highly favorable reaction kinetics. Upon accepting the hydrogen ion, the radical species is quenched and the lipid peroxidation reaction chain may be broken.[12,39] By donating a hydrogen ion, vitamin E (A-OH) becomes a free radical (A-O·) with the unpaired electron delocalized into the aromatic ring structure (reaction 1).

1. $A\text{-}OH + R^\cdot \rightarrow A\text{-}O^\cdot + RH$

2. $A\text{-}O^\cdot + R^\cdot \rightarrow A\text{-}OH + R$

3. $A\text{-}O^\cdot + PUFA \rightarrow A\text{-}OH + PUFA^\cdot + O_2 \rightarrow PUFAOO^\cdot$

4. $A\text{-}O^\cdot + QH_2 \rightarrow A\text{-}OH + QH^\cdot \rightarrow$ nonradical products

The ensuing fate of the tocopherol radical is determined by a number of factors. In the presence of a highly reactive oxidant of

TABLE 24-2. Naturally Occurring Lipid-Soluble and Water-Soluble Antioxidant Substances

Lipid-Soluble	Water-Soluble
Alpha tocopherol	Ascorbic acid
Gamma tocopherol	Glutathione
Hydrogen beta carotene	Uric acid
Alpha carotene	Cysteine
Lutein	Bilirubin
Cryptoxanthine	Albumin
Cantaxanthine	
Zeaxanthin	
Phytofluene	
Lycopene	
Ubiquinol	
2-Hydroxyesterone	
2-Hydroxyestradiol	

sufficient abundance, a radical-radical reaction is likely, creating nonradical products (reaction 2). In the presence of a less reactive or less abundant radical, however, reaction kinetics favor interactions with a polyunsaturated lipid moiety in the LDL particle and generation of a fatty acid radical, which quickly undergoes peroxidation (reaction 3).[43] This tocopherol-mediated peroxidation appears to be permissive of oxidation, and the extent of its action depends on reaction conditions; it should be noted that vitamin E has not been demonstrated to increase oxidation of phospholipids in vivo. Alternatively, in the presence of a coantioxidant, a strong reducing agent—such as ascorbate, ubiquinol-10, or hydroquinone—the tocopherol radical efficiently reacts to regenerate tocopherol and a coantioxidant radical (reaction 4). Importantly, coantioxidant radicals terminate the process by virtue of their instability, by movement into an aqueous environment, and/or recycling through other cellular processes.[44]

Nonredox activities of vitamin E may also confer antiatherosclerotic properties. As proposed by Neuzil et al., by destabilizing membranous structures, vitamin E may cause activation of caspase-3 and caspase-6, proapoptotic proteases that cleave the p65 subunit of the redox-dependent transcription factor NF-κB.[44] Through inhibition of NF-κB, vitamin E has been shown to inhibit cytokine stimulation of monocytes and expression of adhesion molecules.[45] Similar inhibition of the expression of adhesion molecules was shown when oLDL was used to stimulate vitamin E-treated endothelial cells.[46] Vitamin E may also modify cellular signaling and cytokine release through inhibition of protein kinase C. Apparently, alpha tocopherol stimulates protein phosphatase 2A, which downregulates the protein kinase Cα isotype by dephosphorylation.[47] The gamma-tocopherol moiety has also been suggested as a scavenger of radical nitrogen species, causing decreased activation of cyclooxygenase.[48] In turn, vitamin E has been shown to inhibit platelet aggregation.[49] Gene transcription may be regulated through the newly discovered alpha tocopherol–associated protein. Alpha tocopherol has been shown to downregulate transcription of class A scavenger receptors in macrophages and the CD 36 scavenger receptor in smooth muscle cells.[50,51] Finally, vitamin E may also cause increased degradation of hydroxymethylglutaryl coenzyme A (HMG-CoA) in hepatocytes, suppressing cholesterol synthesis.[52]

Clinical trials have not shown any cardiovascular benefit from an intake of vitamin E.[52a,52b] Most observational studies tend to correlate vitamin E intake or blood levels with decreasing risk of cardiovascular disease. However, most prospective therapeutic studies have failed to show significant benefits. Also, only a small proportion of the animal models that utilize doses similar to those taken by humans showed decreases in atherosclerosis or beneficial effects on lipids.[44] For example, vitamin E has been shown to protect the endothelium against various insults in cholesterol-fed guinea pigs and to reduce postischemic dysfunction in dogs after transient coronary artery occlusion.[53,54] Ubiquinol-10 and vitamin E in combination have also shown a promising antiatherogenic effect in mice.[55] In humans, lower levels of serum tocopherol have been found in subjects with abdominal obesity[56] and in patients experiencing variant angina.[57] Gey et al. found an inverse relation between the rate of heart disease and plasma levels of vitamin E and C in European men.[58] Tissue levels of vitamins C and E have been shown to be significantly lower and lipid peroxidation products higher in smokers than in nonsmokers.[59] Vitamin E supplementation has been found to suppress leukocyte production of oxygen-free radicals in patients with myocardial infarction (MI).[60] Daily supplementation with alpha tocopherol increases plasma LDL alpha tocopherol levels as

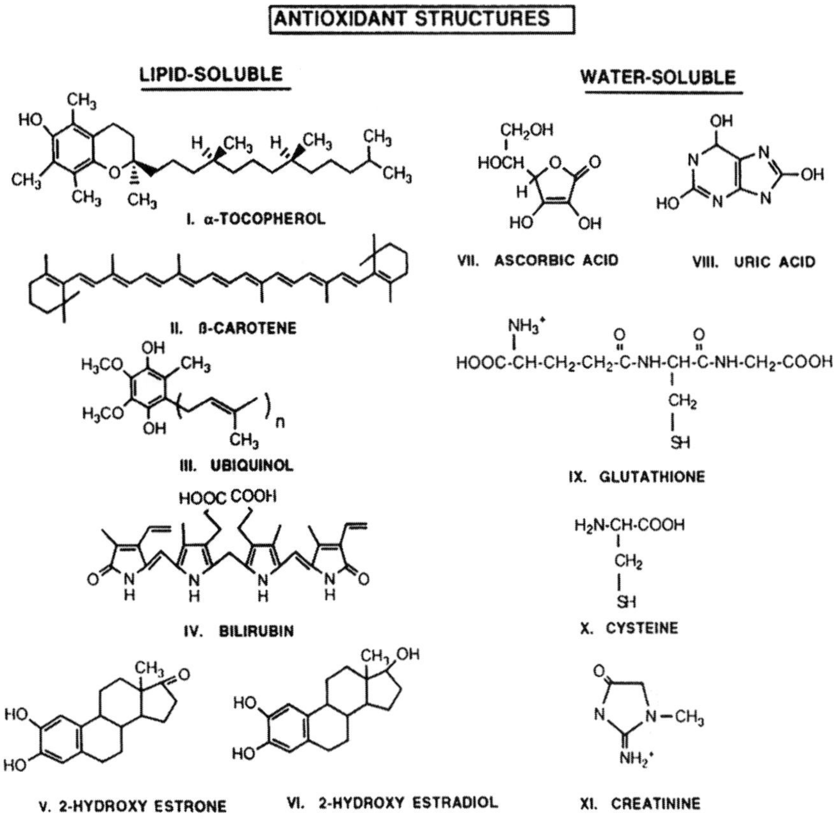

ANTIOXIDANT STRUCTURES

LIPID-SOLUBLE   **WATER-SOLUBLE**

I. α-TOCOPHEROL

II. ß-CAROTENE

III. UBIQUINOL

IV. BILIRUBIN

V. 2-HYDROXY ESTRONE

VI. 2-HYDROXY ESTRADIOL

VII. ASCORBIC ACID

VIII. URIC ACID

IX. GLUTATHIONE

X. CYSTEINE

XI. CREATININE

FIGURE 24-4. Structures of common lipid- and water-soluble antioxidants. (*Reproduced with permission from Krinsky*[39])

well as the oxidation resistance of LDL.[61] The oxidation resistance of LDL is defined as the length of time (lag phase) before the onset of lipid peroxidation.[62] However, this method has been disputed as inappropriate because of direct interactions of the transitional metal reagents and vitamin E.[44,62] More recently, three urinary indices of lipid peroxidation were analyzed by gas chromatography/mass spectrometry by Meagher et al., but no significant changes were found after 8 weeks of vitamin E supplementation at various levels.[63] On serial coronary angiography, vitamin E supplementation was associ-

ated with a reduction in the progression of coronary artery lesions for mild/moderate lesions.[64] Among over 22,000 Finnish male smokers without CAD, there was a modest risk reduction in the incidence of angina pectoris with daily vitamin E supplementation.[65] Also, a combination of vitamins E and C was correlated with less progression of carotid atherosclerosis after 3 years, but only in men.[66] On the contrary, the Perth Carotid Ultrasound Disease Assessment Study recently showed only a minimal association between vitamin E intake or plasma levels and atherosclerosis.[67] Other work has

FIGURE 24-5. The vitamin E cycle: synergistic action of water- and lipid-soluble antioxidants. Nonenzymatic and enzymatic mechanisms for the regeneration of chromanoxyl radicals.

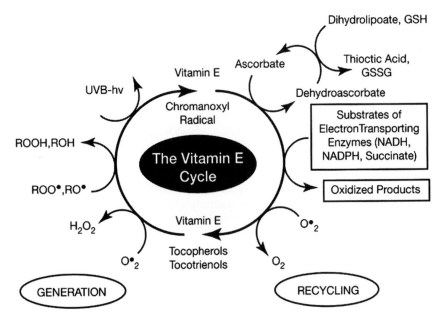

TABLE 24-3. Trials of Antioxidant Vitamins in Cardiovascular Disease Involving More than 1000 Middle-Aged Patients

Trial Name	Study Participants	Antioxidant and Daily Dose	Primary Cardiovascular Endpoint	Results
WHS	40,000 postmenopausal U.S. nurses	Vitamin E 600 IU/day β-carotene 50 mg qod (3 × 2 factorial with aspirin)	MI, stroke and death from cardiovascular disease	
HPS	20,536 persons with previous angina, stroke, claudication, or diabetes	Vitamin E 600 mg/day + β-carotene 20 mg/day + Vitamin C 250 mg/day	Total mortality	No benefit
HOPE	9000 persons with previous MI, stroke or PVD, and diabetes	Vitamin E 400 IU/day	MI, stroke, and death from cardiovascular disease	No benefit
WACS	8000 female nurses with previous cardiovascular disease	Vitamin C 1 g/day or Vitamin E 400 IU/day or β-carotene 20 mg/day (2 × 2 × 2 factorial)	MI, stroke, coronary revascularization, and death from cardiovascular disease	
GISSI Prevention	12,000 persons with recent MI (<3 months)	Vitamin E 300 mg/day	Total mortality	No benefit

MI = myocardial infarction; PVD = peripheral vascular disease; WHS = Women's Health Study; HPS = Heart Protection Study; HOPE = Heart Outcomes Prevention Evaluation; WACS = Women's Atherosclerosis Cardiovascular Study; GISSI = Gruppo Italiano per lo Studio della Sopravvivenza nell-Infarto Miocardico Acuto.

Source: Adapted from Jha P, Flather M, Lonn E: The antioxidant vitamins and cardiovascular disease. A critical review of epidemiologic and clinical trial data. *Ann Intern Med* 123:860, 1995, with permission.

shown that the concentration of vitamin E in erythrocytes, rather than plasma, better correlates with atherosclerotic disease.[68]

Large observational studies provide the strongest support for the utility of vitamin E. In the Nurses' Health Study, both vitamin E and beta carotene were shown to have protective effects against the risk of major coronary heart disease in 90,000 women in the two highest intake categories.[69] The findings of the Health Professionals' Follow-up Study were very similar to those of the Nurses' Health Study, again showing a reduction in risk of coronary artery events in those men with higher intakes of vitamin E (50,000 men participated in the study).[42] Among 34,000 postmenopausal women without known CAD, mortality due to coronary heart disease was lower among those whose initial dietary reports indicated a high intake of vitamin E from food.[70] In comparing the highest and lowest quintiles of vitamin E intake, the relative risk of mortality was 0.38. The Established Populations for Epidemiologic Studies of the Elderly Trial and other studies have also correlated vitamin E intake with decreased risk of heart disease and mortality.[71-73] Many authors criticize the fact that vitamin supplements may simply serve as a proxy for lifestyle or good dietary habits in observational studies; other such studies have failed to shown any benefit to vitamin E intake.[74,75]

Two major prospective clinical trials clearly show a reduction in nonfatal MI and cardiovascular death with vitamin E. In the Cambridge Heart Antioxidant Study, 2002 patients with angiographically-proven coronary atherosclerosis were randomized to receive daily vitamin E supplementation or placebo.[76] The vitamin E group had a significantly reduced risk of non-fatal MI and cardiovascular death (relative risk 0.53 for combined endpoints and 0.23 for non-fatal MI alone). The Secondary Prevention with Antioxidants of Cardiovascular Disease in Endstage Renal Disease trial also showed a 70% reduction in the total MI rate and a 54% reduction in the primary endpoints of MI, ischemic stroke, peripheral vascular disease, and unstable angina.[77] In contrast, in the Alpha Tocopherol–Beta Carotene Cancer Prevention Study, supplementation with alpha tocopherol was found not to be associated with a decreased risk of CAD in Finnish male smokers, nor did it affect the risk for large abdominal aortic aneurysms.[78,79] The Heart Outcomes Prevention Evaluation (HOPE) study showed no beneficial effect from vitamin E (400 IU/day) on total mortality or cardiovascular deaths in high-risk patients.[80] Using carotid ultrasound measurements, vitamin E was shown to have no effect on the progression of atherosclerosis.[81] Similarly, the GISSI III study showed no significant benefit of vitamin E therapy[82] (Table 24-3).

Recently the HDL–Atherosclerosis Treatment Study found no significant benefits from an antioxidant regimen of 1000 mg of vitamin C, 25 mg of natural beta carotene, and 100 μg of selenium and 800 IU of alpha tocopherol given for 3 years to CAD patients with low HDL. The study also showed that the antioxidants lowered HDL-2 levels, both alone and in combination with simvastatin and niacin.[83] No benefits of vitamin E were shown in the Primary Prevention Project, but it was stopped prematurely at 3.8 years.[84] Proponents of vitamin E have levied several criticisms against existing large-scale trials, including the failure to measure total dietary antioxidant intake or antioxidant status and the use of vitamin E in advanced stages of atherosclerosis, when the disease may have progressed too far to be mitigated by antioxidants.[44,85,86]

In addition, water-soluble analogues of vitamin E have been developed (Trolox, MDL 74,405), which appear to be useful in reducing free radical–induced injury in experimental myocardial ischemia.[87] Clinical studies with these compounds remain to be done.

Beta Carotene

Beta carotene, like alpha tocopherol, is a lipid-soluble antioxidant. It is a precursor of vitamin A and is found in fruits and vegetables.[88] Verlangieri et al. reported on an inverse relationship between the decline of heart disease and increased vegetable consumption in the United States.[89] Beta carotene is a free-radical scavenger that has been shown to protect against oxidative damage of LDL in vitro and that also provides effective antioxidant action mainly against singlet oxygen species.[90,91] The scavenging activity of beta carotene is thought to occur only at low oxygen tensions.[92] At higher O_2 tensions, beta carotene has been postulated to exert a prooxidant effect through the formation of peroxyl radicals, which in turn keeps the lipid peroxidation cycle moving. Beta carotene may also play a role in preventing damage to the endothelial cells by decreasing the uptake of oLDL.[93] Some evidence supports a cardiovascular benefit from vitamin A. The Massachusetts Elderly Cohort Study showed that those taking high levels of beta carotene had a lower risk of cardiovascular mortality.[94] In The Basel Prospective Study, high levels of beta carotene were associated with protection against ischemic heart disease.[95] The European Community Multicenter Study, which measured levels of vitamin E and beta carotene in adipose tissue, showed that those in the lowest quintile of beta carotene had a higher risk of MI.[96] The follow-up study of The Lipid Research Clinics Coronary Primary Prevention Trial further supported data that higher serum carotenoid levels are associated with a decreased risk of coronary heart disease.[97]

Many studies have found no significant benefits from vitamin A. In the Physicians' Health Study, 22,000 male physicians took beta carotene or placebo for 12 years; the rate of MI and death was identical in both groups.[98] Daily supplementation with beta carotene did not decrease the risk of developing angina in 22,000 Finnish male smokers without known coronary disease who were followed up for 5 years.[65] In a skin cancer prevention trial, there was no reduction in overall risk of death or cardiovascular mortality between those men and women taking daily beta-carotene supplements versus placebo.[99] In this study, however, those with the highest initial plasma carotene levels had a lower risk of all-cause and cardiovascular death. In 34,000 postmenopausal women without known coronary heart disease, the intake of carotenoids (from supplement or food) was not associated with a decrease in death from coronary heart disease when other risk factors were accounted for.[78] Most recently, the HDL–Atherosclerosis Treatment Study found no significant benefit from an antioxidant regimen that included 25 mg/day of beta carotene given for 3 years to patients with coronary disease and low HDL. Rather, the antioxidants were found to lower levels of HDL-2.[83] The bulk of the available data to date would suggest that supplementation with beta carotene has no role to play in reducing the risk of atherosclerotic heart disease.

Some recent studies even point to severe adverse effects of vitamin A intake. In the Alpha Tocopherol Beta Carotene Cancer Prevention Study, beta-carotene supplementation was found to be associated with a higher risk of CAD.[78] In this study, the mortality rate was higher in the beta-carotene group from both ischemic heart disease and cancer. The study investigators also reported no improvement in the risk of abdominal aortic aneurysm with beta carotene.[79] Furthermore, a trial comparing placebo and a combination of beta carotene plus vitamin A in 18,000 smokers and workers exposed to asbestos was stopped prematurely after a significantly increased relative risk of lung cancer was discovered in the active treatment group.[100] In a recent analysis of the Nurses' Health Study, which followed 72,377 postmenopausal women for over 18 years, ingestion of high amounts of vitamin A (as retinol but not beta carotene) significantly increased the risk of osteoporotic hip fracture.[101] The bulk of the available data suggest that beta carotene or vitamin A supplementation has no role to play in reducing the risk of atherosclerotic heart disease and may otherwise adversely affect health in certain populations.

Other lipid-soluble antioxidants are present in much lower quantities than alpha tocopherol and beta carotene, and their mechanisms of action and significance in preventing oxidative damage have not been clearly elucidated to date. They are listed in Table 24-2.

Ascorbic Acid (Vitamin C)

Ascorbic acid has a number of well-defined biological actions, including participation in the formation of collagen and the synthesis of bile, catecholamines, carnitine, and cholesterol.[101a] Ascorbic acid is also an effective free-radical scavenger that exerts most of its action in aqueous solutions, both within the cellular cytoplasm and in plasma.[102] Vitamin C is thought to act as the main line of antioxidant defense in plasma and other aqueous solutions. In vitro, it has been shown to regenerate alpha tocopherol from tocopheroxyl radical (Fig. 24-5), which is the reduced form of alpha tocopherol.[103] Ascorbic acid has been shown to prevent LDL oxidation; to increase LDL's resistance to transitional metal ion-, hypochlorous acid- and chloramine-induced oxidation; and to act synergistically along with alpha tocopherol in preventing LDL oxidation in vitro.[104–107] In experiments using human plasma in vitro, free-radical initiation and accumulation was demonstrated only after vitamin C had been mostly consumed.[2] Vitamin C has been shown to prevent the initiation of transitional metal ion and the propagation of lipid peroxidation in human LDL.[108] Vitamin C also has beneficial effects on plasma lipids. There seems to be a negative correlation between total cholesterol, triglycerides, and LDL and serum vitamin C levels; high-density lipoproteins correlated positively with vitamin C levels.[109]

Like other antioxidants, vitamin C may improve endothelial function by protecting nitric oxide from oxidation.[110,111] Vitamin C may also reduce venous tone by activating vascular smooth muscle channels.[112] Attenuated endothelium-dependent vasodilation has been shown in patients with a variety of cardiac diagnoses— but, interestingly, not in one study involving healthy elderly subjects.[113–115] Vitamin C supplementation has been shown to reverse endothelial vasomotor dysfunction in patients with CAD, including the vasomotor abnormalities seen in chronic cigarette smokers.[116–118] Smokers demonstrate decreased levels of vitamin C and require up to 60 mg more of this vitamin than nonsmokers. A single 3-g dose of vitamin C has been shown to reduce the increase in oxidative indices caused by brief (1.5 h to several days) episodes of passive smoking by nonsmokers.[119] Vitamin C appears to protect against the free-radical formation produced by cigarette smoke and can reduce neutrophil and monocyte adhesion to the vascular endothelium.[120]

Gey et al. suggested that men in countries with higher rates of mortality from heart disease had, on average, levels of vitamin C in plasma that bordered on being deficient.[121] In the follow-up of the first National Health and Nutrition Survey, men reporting an intake of 50 mg or more of vitamin C per day had a standardized mortality ratio of 0.58 for all cardiovascular disease.[122] In the Basel Prospective Study, low levels of vitamin C in plasma were associated with higher mortality from ischemic heart disease.[95] In the Nurses' Health Study, however, there was no statistically significant relationship between vitamin C intake and CAD.[69] Riemersma et al. made the same observation in patients with MI.[123] In men and women over 55 years of age, an inverse relationship was found between vitamin C intake and average thickness of arterial walls.[124] Vitamin C levels have been found to be lower in patients with intermittent claudication.[125]

In summary, although some epidemiologic evidence correlates vitamin C intake with a reduced rate of cardiovascular disease, the few existing clinical trials have not shown significant benefits.

Flavonoids

Since the discovery of the "French paradox"—i.e., that certain Mediterranean populations enjoy a lower rate of mortality due

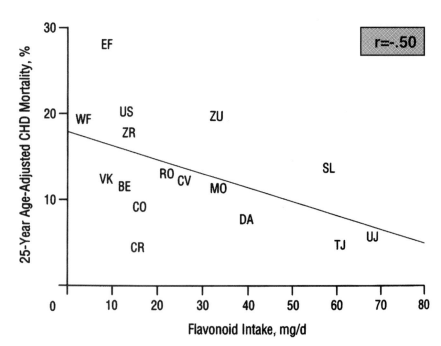

FIGURE 24-6. Average flavonoid intake and age-adjusted mortality from coronary heart disease (CHD) afer 25 years of follow-up (The Seven Countries Study). BE = Belgrade, Serbia; CO = Corfu, Greece; CR = Crete, Greece; CV = Crevalcore, Italy; DA = Dalmatia, Croatia; EF = East Finland; MO = Montegiorgio, Italy; RO = Rome, Italy; SL = Slavonia, Croatia; TJ = Tanushimaru, Japan; US = US Railroad; UJ = Ushibuka, Japan; VK = Velika Krsna, Serbia; WF = West Finland; ZR = Zrenjanin, Serbia; ZU = Zutphen, the Netherlands. (*Reproduced with permission from Keli SO, et al: Dietary flavonoids, antioxidant vitamins, and incidence of stroke. The Zutphen Study. Arch Intern Med 154:637, 1996.*)

to cardiovascular disease despite a diet high in saturated fat and red wine—interest in flavonoids has increased. Flavonoids first attracted the interest of pharmacologists when their vitamin-like properties were described in the 1930s. A heterogeneous group of diphenylpropane derivatives with strong antioxidant and free radical–scavenging properties, they are found in tea, onions, red wine, apples, and other fruits and vegetables.[126] The color of most fruits and vegetables is imparted by flavonoids, and the astringency of red wine and tea is largely a product of flavonoid tannins. There are five major flavonoids, which include the flavonols quercetin, kaempferol, and myricetin and the flavones aplgenin and luteolin; the average dietary intake of these substances is approximately 25 mg daily.[127] Discovery of their antioxidant and weak estrogenic properties have sparked recent interest in isoflavones, coumestans, and lignans, which are nonsteroidal flavones commonly called phytoestrogens (see Chap. 36).[128–130]

Three epidemiologic studies have suggested the benefits of diets high in flavonoids (black tea, apples, onions) as being protective against coronary heart disease (Fig. 24-6) and stroke (see Chap. 47).[131–133] Various mechanisms of flavonoid action have resulted from in vitro and animal studies; however, few human data, especially from prospective trials, exist.

Antioxidant properties appear to confer the majority of benefits of flavonoids.[134] In experimental studies, flavonoids have been shown to scavenge free radicals such as superoxide anions and lipid peroxy radicals.[135,136] The molecules quercetin and silibin have been shown to reduce ischemia-reperfusion injury, putatively through scavenging nitric oxide–derived free radicals or nitric oxide directly.[137,138] Flavonoids appear to inhibit the oxidative modification of LDL by macrophages, and like vitamin C, to serve as coantioxidants of vitamin E.[139,140] They do not, however, delay LDL oxidation once vitamin E in LDL is consumed.[134] A study by da Silva et al. suggests that flavonoids may be more potent inhibitors of LDL oxidation than vitamins C and E.[141] Flavonoids have also been shown to inhibit LDL modifications by glucose autooxidation, implying a mechanism of reducing complications of diabetes.[142] In apo E–deficient mice, flavonoids from green teat were shown to attenuate the development of atherosclerosis.[143] Red wine, which

contains 10 to 20 mg/L of different flavonoids, has been shown to provide antioxidant activity for 4 h in human volunteers.[144] Nonalcoholic red wine extract and quercetin have also been shown to inhibit LDL oxidation when ingested by humans.[145]

In addition, flavonoids, through their antioxidant action, appear in vitro and in vivo to reduce platelet aggregation while causing disaggregation of preformed platelet thrombi.[146] Cyclooxygenase, lipoxygenase, and xanthine oxidase may also be inhibited by some flavonoids.[147,148] Flavonoids have been shown in experimental studies to inhibit endothelial expression of leukocyte adhesion molecules in vitro[149] and may reduce the extent of MI by this mechanism.[150] Flavonoids have been shown in vitro to inhibit the hypertrophy of vascular smooth muscle that is induced by angiotensin.[151] The flavonoids have been used as protective agents against doxorubicin-induced cardiomyopathy.[152] Finally, some flavonoids have been shown to have calcium-entry blocking activity.

Data on the absorption and metabolism of flavonoids are lacking. Natural flavonoids are glycosylated, which plays an uncertain role in influencing absorption. Once absorbed, glucuronide conjugation commonly occurs, but at varying sites, which may affect the biological activity of the compounds.[138] It is not known if all flavonoids are beneficial, with evidence to suggest that some may increase cholesterol uptake in LDL. Furthermore, as would be expected in a heterogeneous group of compounds, both antitumor and mutagenic properties have been described, and concerns have been raised that excess intake may be toxic.[128] As such, the optimal amount of flavonoids in the diet, form or method of supplementation, and dose are uncertain.[153] Nonetheless, many flavonoids are available as food supplements in doses as high as 500 and 1000 mg, an amount that may be 10 to 20 times the daily intake in a typical vegetarian diet.[128] A recent epidemiologic report from the Physician's Health Study did not show a strong inverse association between intake of flavonoids and total CAD.[154] Until these issues are resolved in prospective controlled studies, patients may be encouraged to consume a diet that includes tea, apples, and onions in generous amounts. Current research does not support the benefits of supplemental flavonoid intake, but further research is needed.

Selenium

The metabolic relationships between the mineral selenium and vitamin E are very close.[155] Selenium is a cofactor of the enzyme glutathione peroxidase, which serves as an antioxidant and is found in the platelets and the arterial walls.[156] In contrast to vitamin E, which prevents formation of lipid hydroperoxides in cell membranes and LDL by acting as a biological free-radical trap, selenium and glutathione peroxidase help destroy lipid hydroperoxides already formed by peroxidation of polyunsaturated fatty acids.[157] Selenium thereby defends against the free-radical oxidative stress that escapes the protection of vitamin E.

Selenium is an essential mineral in the diet with a requirement for adults of 50 μg/day. Since selenium supplementation can increase the enzyme activity of glutathione reductase,[158] it has been suggested that this approach might reduce the risk of atherosclerotic heart disease by preventing the formation of oLDL.

Low plasma selenium levels have been associated with increased platelet aggregability, higher production of thromboxane A_2, and decreased production of prostacyclin.[159,160] Patients with low levels of selenium in plasma demonstrate a higher rate of MI in some cohort studies, although other studies show no such relationship.[161–166] One review concluded that the epidemiologic evidence for selenium in humans is equivocal.[167] Nonetheless, selenium has been shown to improve APACHE scores in critically ill patients and to reduce the need for dialysis.[168]

A recent substudy report from the Physician's Health Study showed no relationship between selenium blood levels and the risk of MI in well-nourished subjects.[166] However, these findings do not rule out the possibility of an increased risk of MI in severe selenium deficiency. Also, questions have been raised about the reliability of plasma selenium levels, and other methods to obtain accurate body measurement have been proposed.[164]

Conclusion

Free-radical formation is associated with a number of pathologic processes, including CAD. Nutritional antioxidants offer a line of defense against the generation and propagation of free radical species and the oxidative damage they cause. Data available from clinical trials and observational studies seem to point toward the beneficial effect of certain antioxidants on coronary heart disease and its complications. However, due to the difficulty of measuring levels of free radicals in tissues in vivo and the observational nature of most data, it may be difficult to identify more direct and convincing evidence for the role of free radicals and antioxidants in CAD.[168a] There are many unaccountable confounding factors that perturb some of the study results, such as the dietary habits and lifestyles of the participants, and these in part account for some of the confusion surrounding the use of antioxidants. More clinical trials are in progress that examine the role of nutritional antioxidants in heart disease. Meanwhile, physicians are faced with a number of patients who are either self-prescribed or are interested in taking antioxidant supplementation as a means of primary or secondary prevention for coronary heart disease. In many cases a physician must make individual decisions regarding long-term antioxidant supplementation based on the existing data. For those patients, it seems that vitamin E at doses around 400 IU/day has no protective role in decreasing the risk of heart disease. Similarly, Vitamin A cannot be recommended as a dietary supplement, as most clinical trials have shown no benefit in terms of coronary heart disease prevention and,

in fact, this vitamin may increase cancer risk and osteoporosis. Data on vitamin C and flavonoids are not as extensive and more trials are needed. Vitamin C at doses between 250 and 500 mg per day seems to saturate all vitamin C receptors and may have some potential benefit both in terms of preventing heart disease and infections, especially in cigarette smokers. Coantioxidant combinations of vitamins E and C may be necessary to test the oxidation hypothesis. A recent placebo-controlled study with combinations of Vitamin E, Vitamin C and B-carotene showed no protective benefit.[168b] Needless to say, ongoing clinical trials should shed some new light on our current knowledge on antioxidant therapy, and additional basic research studies are needed. However, only with this increased knowledge can we begin to make more intelligent and directed recommendations as to the use of antioxidants.

REPERFUSION INJURY AND FREE RADICALS

In the previous sections, the effects of antioxidant therapy on the atherosclerotic process were reviewed. Free-radical generation also plays an important role in reperfusion injury and subsequent myocardial damage during an ischemic injury to the heart.[37,169] During myocardial ischemia, free radicals are generated by injured myocardial cells, neutrophils that have migrated to the injured area, platelets, and endothelial cells.[37] The myocardial and endothelial cells are targets of free-radical damage. Similarly, the reintroduction of oxygen to the ischemic myocardium can increase cellular injury by increasing the production of free radicals. This promotes lipid peroxidation and additional substrate for the xanthine oxidase system (see below). A rise in intracellular calcium during myocardial ischemia and reperfusion can increase the activity of cellular adenosine triphosphatases (ATPases), proteases, and phospholipases, which generate additional free radicals, causing additional cell injury.[37] In the heart, oxygen radicals may be generated by several mechanisms, such as mitochondrial respiration, activated neutrophils, and (in some species) xanthine oxidase activity. Activity of these mechanisms can be greatly enhanced in postischemic hearts. For instance, ischemia alters the redox state of the mitochondrial respiratory chain and promotes the accumulation of xanthine (through ATP hydrolysis). Both events may prepare the heart for a subsequent burst of oxygen free-radical formation upon resumption of mitochondrial respiration and stimulation of xanthine oxidase activity, when oxygen is reintroduced at reflow. Furthermore, following reperfusion, neutrophils accumulate within the previously ischemic area.[170] Activated neutrophils may then release oxygen radicals in large amounts. Finally, in addition to this enhanced potential for oxygen radical production, postischemic hearts may also exhibit a decrease in tissue concentrations of various "scavengers,"—for example, enzymes or chemicals that inactivate oxygen radicals.[171]

No-Reflow Phenomenon

When reperfusion occurs after prolonged ischemia, it may not be sufficient to relieve the previously occluded epicardial coronary artery to ensure adequate and uniform myocardial perfusion, because significant impairment to flow may occur at the microvascular level. This phenomenon has been termed "no-reflow."[170] The main determinant of no-reflow is activation of neutrophils in the microvasculature. Postischemic reperfusion is accompanied by release of proinflammatory cytokines, such as tumor necrosis factor alpha and interleukins 1 and 6.[172] These cytokines, in turn, induce exposure of adhesion molecules on the surface of endothelium, neutrophils, and myocytes and stimulate release of interleukin 8, a cytokine with marked proinflammatory and neutrophil-activating properties. In addition, other factors may promote neutrophil activation and adhesion to the vessel wall in postischemic tissues, such as reduced nitric oxide concentrations and increased release of activating mediators.[172,173] Activated neutrophils adhere tightly to capillary endothelium, thus mechanically blocking flow. At the same time, the vasodilator reserve is impaired in postischemic vessels, secondary to a reduced generation of nitric oxide and prostacyclin, whereas enhanced endothelin formation and damage to vascular beta-adrenergic receptors increase vasoconstriction[172,173]; in addition, activated neutrophils release vasoconstricting mediators. The prevalence of vasoconstriction in postischemic vessels reduces the pressure gradient in the capillaries, thus favoring further neutrophil accumulation.

Treatment of Reperfusion Injury

A therapeutic approach to maximize the salvage of viable myocardium during an acute MI would be to combine thrombolysis with therapy designed to minimize free-radical damage and thrombogenicity in both the ischemic and reperfusion phases.[37] Because of the multiple sources of free-radical generation during these phases, therapy can be aimed at various sites (Table 24-4). The most direct means of limiting production of free radicals is by limiting production of the principal oxygen metabolites: superoxide anion, hydrogen peroxide, and the hydroxyl radical.

The use of allopurinol, superoxide dismutase, catalase, *N*-acetylcysteine, magnesium, mannitol, and adenosine as antioxidants and free-radical scavengers for the treatment of myocardial injury are reviewed.

Allopurinol

Both the cardiac myocyte and the vascular endothelial cell are targets of free-radical damage during myocardial ischemia and reperfusion. Rosen and Freeman,[174] utilizing spin-trapping techniques, have detected production of the superoxide anion by cultured endothelial cells and the subsequent generation of free radicals by lipid peroxidation. Endothelial cells contain the enzymes cyclooxygenase and lipoxygenase[175,176] and, as such, are vulnerable to the toxic byproducts of arachidonic acid metabolism. In addition, the endothelial cell

TABLE 24-4. Therapeutic Options to Minimize Free Radical Damage during Myocardial Ischemia and Reperfusion

Xanthine oxidase inhibitor (allopurinol)

Enzymatic free radical scavengers and antioxidants [superoxide dismutase (h-SOD), catalase, glutathione, alpha-tocopherol, peroxidase, coenzyme Q_{10}]

Synthetic antioxidants [iron chelators (deferoxamine), mannitol, dimethylsulfoxide]

Inhibitors of arachidonic acid metabolism [anti-inflammatory agents (aspirin, indomethacin)]

Antiplatelet and antineutrophil agents, inhibitors of platelet aggregation, inhibitors of neutrophil chemotaxis and adherence

Antilipolytic agents (nicotinic acid)

Phospholipase inhibitors (mepacrine)

Calcium-entry blockers

β-Adrenergic blockers

Adenosine

possesses the enzyme xanthine oxidase, which generates the superoxide anion during its conversion of either xanthine or hypoxanthine to uric acid:

$$\text{Xanthine} + H_2O + 2O_2 \text{ xanthine oxidase} \rightarrow$$
$$\text{Uric acid} + 2\,O_2^{\cdot-} + 2H^+$$

In normal tissue, the enzyme functions as xanthine dehydrogenase, which reduces NAD+ but does not form free-radical metabolites. As demonstrated by McCord et al.[177] in the rat heart, however, during ischemia, xanthine dehydrogenase rapidly converts to the oxidase form. This conversion is catalyzed by a protease whose activity is controlled by an increase in calcium ions in the cytosol. As discussed, this increase in calcium is itself facilitated by free-radical damage. Hypoxia also promotes the degradation of adenine nucleotides with a resultant increase in hypoxanthine,[178] which provides increased substrate for xanthine oxidase. This free radical-generating system becomes increasingly important during the stage of reperfusion. With the reintroduction of oxygen, xanthine oxidase acts on the substrate accumulated during the ischemic phase to generate a burst of free radicals.

The production of superoxide anion could be inhibited by the use of the xanthine oxidase inhibitor allopurinol. Several laboratories have reported a beneficial effect of pretreatment with allopurinol on the extent of myocardial injury. Chambers and colleagues[179] reported a decrease in infarct size in dogs pretreated with allopurinol and subjected to 1 h of ischemia followed by 4 h of reperfusion. This was confirmed by Werns et al.,[180] also in a canine model, after a 90-min occlusion and 6 h of reperfusion. Kingma et al. were able to demonstrate a reduced infarct size in closed-chest dogs pretreated with allopurinol and then subjected to 24 h of occlusion.[181] Other investigators have also been able to show decreased myocardial injury in canine models pretreated with allopurinol.[182,183]

In addition to the decreased infarct sizes with the administration of allopurinol, some investigators have reported fewer arrhythmias and decreased release of creatine kinase.[184,185] Myers et al. reported that administration of allopurinol during hypoxia reduced creatine kinase upon reoxygenation in isolated buffer-perfused hearts.[185]

In contrast, Reimer and Jennings[186] found no significant decrease in infarct size with the use of allopurinol in dogs subjected to 40 min of ischemia followed by 4 days of reperfusion. Downey and coworkers[187] examined the effect of allopurinol on infarct size in the rabbit heart, which is more similar to the human heart in that it contains only small quantities of xanthine oxidase.[188] After 45 min of occlusion followed by 3 h of reperfusion, there was no significant difference in infarct size in rabbits pretreated with allopurinol versus controls. Despite this finding and the low xanthine oxidase activity in human hearts, allopurinol appears to be effective against ischemia/reperfusion injury in some human trials. Allopurinol has been reported to reduce the mortality[189] and morbidity[190] of patients undergoing cardiac surgery. Several clinical studies in patients undergoing cardiac surgery demonstrated that pretreatment with allopurinol resulted in decreased release of myocardial enzymes,[190] improved postoperative cardiac performance measured by cardiac index, reduced need for inotropic support,[189,191] and reduced incidence of cardiac complications such as arrhythmias, heart failure, and infarctions.[189–193] Using direct spin-trapping measurements, pretreatment with allopurinol was also shown to reduce the amount of free radicals generated during the first minute of reperfusion during coronary bypass surgery.[194] Also, allopurinol treatment has been associated with significant improvement in granulocyte counts, cardiac enzymes, and malondialdehyde levels (an index of lipid peroxidation) in cardiopulmonary bypass patients and in ex vivo models.[195] However, in a prospective, randomized trial study by Taggart et al., allopurinol was not shown to have cardioprotective effects during coronary artery surgery.[196] As suggested by these authors, their results might have been due to an insufficient dose of allopurinol (although it was similar to the dose used in other clinical studies) or the possibility that free radicals are not important determinants of myocardial injury in cardiac surgery.

The cardioprotective mechanism of action of allopurinol has not been fully elucidated in the mammalian heart. It has been postulated that allopurinol and its metabolite, oxypurinol, are free-radical scavengers.[197,198] Perhaps the beneficial effects of allopurinol seen in species with low myocardial xanthine oxidoreductase activity—such as rabbits, pigs, and humans—may thus be attributed to the free radical scavenging effects rather than the inhibition of xanthine oxidoreductase.[188,199] Other possible mechanisms of benefit with allopurinol may include the preservation of the adenine nucleotide pool[200] or effects on the endothelium. The endothelial cell is a source of xanthine oxidase, and most studies have not addressed the effect of xanthine oxidase–derived free radicals on endothelial cell injury. Allopurinol may prove to be particularly beneficial in preventing endothelial cell damage, vascular injury, and thrombogenicity.[201] Additional studies in humans to confirm these hypotheses still need to be done. In related work, allopurinol has shown benefits in treating idiopathic dilated cardiomyopathy. Cappola et al. showed that intracoronary infusion of various amounts of allopurinol, in addition to standard therapy, improved cardiac efficiency after 15 min.[202] In a dog model of heart failure, allopurinol increased contractility and responsiveness to dopamine.[203] In humans, however, allopurinol showed no significant effect on resting autonomic tone, as indicated by time domain heart rate variability, or on dysrhythmia count in stable heart failure patients.[204] As of now, there is no strong evidence to recommend allopurinol treatment to prevent myocardial reperfusion injury.

Enzymatic Free-Radical Scavengers and Antioxidants

The production of free radicals can be limited by the use of endogenous enzymes that function as natural cellular defense mechanisms or by the use of synthetic substance having similar properties.[205] By preventing the accumulation of the principal free radicals, these substances decrease the ability of radicals to form additional toxic metabolites.

The use of endogenous intracellular scavengers of the superoxide anion, hydrogen peroxide, and the hydroxyl radical in the animal model has been encouraging in minimizing reperfusion injury of the myocardium. However, despite experimental evidence of the cytotoxic oxygen free–radical production during ischemia and mainly reperfusion, controversy exists on the role of these radicals in myocardial stunning, reperfusion arrhythmias, and irreversible reperfusion injury (myocardial infarct).[206] In this regard, many studies have been undertaken to examine the capacity of these anti–free radical therapies to limit MI size.

Superoxide Dismutase (SOD)

Superoxide radicals may react with various molecules, resulting in either direct damage or potentially harmful products. They also react avidly with nitric oxide—which is constantly produced by the endothelium and maintains basal vascular tone—to form peroxynitrite,

a potent oxidant.[207–209] An abundance of peroxynitrite, as identified by nitrotyrosine protein adducts, has been demonstrated in atherosclerotic lesions, and overproduction of peroxynitrite has been implicated in atherogenesis.[209–211] The protective scavenging function against superoxide is provided mainly by SOD present in the extracellular space and within cells of the vascular wall.[212,213] There are three isoenzymes of SOD: the secreted extracellular SOD (EC-SOD), cytosolic CU/Zn-SOD, and mitochondrial Mn-SOD.[212,213] In mouse cardiomyocytes, expression of Mn-SOD was shown to be upregulated by signal transduction by an activator of transcription-3. This pathway conferred protection against ischemia/reperfusion injury and was suggested as a target of therapy,[214] EC-SOD has a high affinity for heparin sulfate proteoglycan, which appears to be the most important physiologic ligand of EC-SOD.[215,216] An Arg213→Gly mutation at the heparin-binding domain has been identified in a small proportion of the healthy population.[217,218] The mutation is associated with very high plasma EC-SOD levels[217,218] and impairs the affinity for heparin at the endothelial cell surface.[218,219] Wang et al., in their study of 590 white Australian patients with angiographically documented CAD, showed that the mean plasma EC-SOD in female patients was significantly higher than that in male patients, and there was also a positive correlation with age.[220] Plasma EC-SOD in current smokers was much lower than that in nonsmokers, and ex-smokers had intermediate levels. Levels were significantly lower in patients with a history of MI than in those without such a history, and low plasma EC-SOD was independently associated with an increased likelihood of a history of MI and CAD.[221] Thus, higher levels of EC-SOD also tend to be associated with delayed onset of MI.[220] Interestingly, expression of SOD and other antioxidant enzymes has been found to be inducible in patients with congestive heart failure by exercise training.[222]

In experimental studies, SOD has been shown to preserve left ventricular function after reperfusion. However, the existing data suggest that this phenomenon depends on the duration of ischemia. The experimental results published to date have generally concluded that antioxidant therapy enhances the recovery of mechanical function after 15 min of coronary occlusion.[223] Myers et al.[224] found that pretreatment with SOD and catalase could improve the recovery of myocardial function, as measured by systolic wall thickening, after 15 min of occlusion followed by reperfusion. However, a study by Ambrosio et al. demonstrated that recovery of myocardial function in rabbit hearts was possible after 30 min of global ischemia.[225] Conversely, it has been demonstrated that when the duration of ischemia is prolonged to 2 h to produce subendocardial infarction, SOD given with catalase at the time of reperfusion does not alleviate the postischemic contractile dysfunction.[226] Several experimental studies[226–228] have failed to show a beneficial effect of SOD on recovery of contractile function after 60 to 120 min of ischemia.

On the basis of the positive results obtained from human recombinant SOD in experimental models, two clinical studies were completed. In a pilot study of 23 patients with acute MI successfully reperfused with tissue plasminogen activator or urokinase, Murohara et al. found that SOD failed to improve left ventricular function but did reduce the number of reperfusion arrhythmias.[229] Similarly, in a large multicenter, randomized placebo-controlled clinical trial, Flaherty et al. found that administration of SOD at the time of reperfusion failed to improve recovery of left ventricular function in patients who underwent successful percutaneous transluminal coronary angioplasty for acute MI.[230] As suggested by the authors, these results may be explained by varying durations of ischemia;

irreversible injury may have occurred in prolonged ischemia. The doses of SOD may have been too high, which has been shown to be ineffective and can even increase infarct size.[231,232] Another plausible mechanism to be considered is insufficient delivery of SOD due to the lack of adequate blood flow to the area.[228] Perhaps the rate of generation of hydrogen peroxide from SOD may exceed the capability of endogenous catalase and/or glutathione peroxidase to detoxify hydrogen peroxide, which could potentially generate more reactive hydroxyl radicals by the Haber-Weiss and Fenton reactions.[233,234]

In contrast, the use of free-radical scavengers for the treatment of reperfusion arrhythmias has provided favorable results.[235] Free-radical scavengers, such as SOD, have reduced the occurrence of reperfusion arrhythmias, whereas perfusion of hearts with free-radical generating systems increased the incidence of reperfusion arrhythmias.[236] Riva et al. found the effect of SOD on reperfusion arrhythmias to be dose-dependent in the anesthetized rat. Dose-response curves showed 10 mg/kg of SOD to have the most antiarrhythmic activity, while higher doses did not provide additional benefit.[237] In a study by Nejima et al., SOD reduced reperfusion arrhythmias but failed to reduce infarct size.[238] However, both groups of animals were treated with prophylactic lidocaine, which has been shown to impair the formation of oxygen free radicals. Similarly, in a recent pilot study of 23 patients, Murohara et al. reported that intravenous administration of SOD after acute MI had beneficial effects on reperfusion arrhythmias but not on left ventricular function.[229]

Several studies have suggested that free-radical scavengers may be used to protect the mitochondria from injury. Otani and coworkers[239] studied the effect of SOD and catalase on ischemic/reperfused isolated rabbit heart mitochondria. They measured subsequent hydroxyl radical production by electron spin resonance spectroscopy and followed coenzyme Q10 levels and ATP production to determine the extent of free radical production and mitochondrial injury. SOD plus catalase prevented the increase in hydroxyl radical, the decrease in coenzyme Q10 levels, and the decrease in ATP generation that were observed after reperfusion in untreated hearts. Other free radical scavengers such as dimethylsulfoxide (DMSO) have also been shown to preserve mitochondrial oxidative phosphorylating activity in globally ischemic rabbit hearts.[240]

At this juncture, SOD is being used in clinical trials to enhance graft survival in renal transplantation and as an adjunctive treatment for patients with severe head injury.[241,242] In experimental studies, SOD has been shown to prolong life span by its antioxidative actions.[243] Strategies have also been developed to prolong the half-life of SOD either by conjugating the enzyme to polyethylene glycol or by using liposomal encapsulation to both prolong SOD activity and target its effects to specific organs.[244] Recently, lecithinized Cu/Zn-SOD, which sustains high tissue concentrations longer than unconjugated SOD, was found to attenuate infarct size in a rat model to a greater extent than unmodified or polyethylene glycol–conjugated SOD.[245,246] In other studies, polyethylene glycol–conjugated SOD was shown to inhibit infarct extension during early reperfusion in a canine model.[247] The clinical studies to date remain inconclusive on the beneficial effects of h-SOD in reperfusion injury. Additional clinical trials are needed to confirm the favorable results of SOD in experimental studies.

Catalase

Catalase, a free-radical scavenger of hydrogen peroxide, is another enzyme that has been investigated for its role in minimizing ischemia and reperfusion injury of the myocardium. With increased oxidative stress in humans, there is a specific upregulation of catalase gene expression.[248] Hydrogen peroxide has been shown in several studies to be cytotoxic, either by direct effect[249] or through the superoxide-mediated generation of more reactive hydroxyl radicals by the Haber-Weiss and Fenton reactions.[233,234] Many investigators have examined the effects of catalase on limiting myocardial reperfusion injury. However, since the majority of the previous studies have examined the effects of catalase given in conjunction with SOD,[224,249,250] there have been only a few studies that have investigated the role of catalase alone in its ability to limit myocardial reperfusion injury.[251–253]

The results of the studies involving catalase have been conflicting. Several studies have demonstrated beneficial effects on the recovery of contractile function or reduction of myocardial infarct size using combination of SOD and catalase.[249,250,254] However, it is uncertain whether the beneficial effects are attributed to the independent effects of SOD, catalase, or both.

Studies in which catalase was examined alone have in general yielded negative results. In a study by Werns et al. in 1985, SOD treatment reduced infarct size in anesthetized dogs, but catalase treatment after 90 min of regional ischemia did not.[255] In another study by Gallagher et al., where conscious dogs were used, catalase also failed to alter the size of infarction after 3 h of coronary occlusion and 45 min of reperfusion.[251] Perhaps in this study, the damage produced by 3 h of ischemia was not amenable to reduction by drug intervention.[251] In a separate study that examined the effect of catalase on myocardial stunning in dogs subjected to 15 min of ischemia and then 4 h of reperfusion, Jeroudi et al. studied the effects of various doses of catalase given alone or in combination with superoxide.[252] The authors found that recovery of the myocardium was significantly improved by the combination of SOD and catalase but not by SOD or catalase alone.[253] These authors suggested that both superoxide anion and hydrogen peroxide contributed significantly to the pathogenesis of myocardial stunning after regional ischemia. In contrast, Myers et al. were able to demonstrate favorable effects of catalase in two separate studies.[184,253] In one study, catalase alone was found to attenuate postischemic dysfunction after 2 h of hypothermic cardioplegia in rabbit hearts.[253] The authors speculated that catalase was effective due to its ability to reduce the extracellular concentration of hydrogen peroxide. In another study by Myers et al., catalase was demonstrated to reduce the release of creatine kinase upon reoxygenation.[184]

N-Acetylcysteine

Some recent clinical studies have demonstrated that the intravenous infusion of N-acetylcysteine during thrombolysis was associated with a decrease in infarct size and better preservation of left ventricular function, probably due to the antioxidant and free radical scavenger properties of N-acetylcysteine. In short- and long-term studies of patients with unstable angina and a threat of infarct, the intravenous or oral administration of N-acetylcysteine in association with nitroglycerin is highly effective in decreasing the risk of acute MI.[256]

Magnesium

Clinical studies suggest that magnesium has beneficial effects in patients with acute MI by preserving left ventricular ejection fraction, decreasing infarct size, and limiting mortality (see Chap. 12).[257] This has been postulated to occur through the effect of magnesium as a physiologic calcium-channel blocker.[258] Garcia et al. demonstrated for the first time that magnesium also reduces free-radical formation during an occlusion-reperfusion sequence in a canine model.[259] Magnesium may attenuate free-radical production in one of two ways: it may directly inhibit free-radical production or may facilitate the scavenging of free radicals.[259] One study showed that magnesium inhibits reduced nicotinamide-adenine dinucleotide phosphate oxidase, an enzyme that produces superoxide radical.[260] This study also found that although magnesium does facilitate free radical scavenging, it does so at only a minimal level compared with other scavengers, such as the transition metal manganese. Thus, the mechanism for magnesium's attenuation of free radicals may be through inhibition of free-radical production upon reperfusion and not by direct scavenging of radicals already present. Dickens et al.[261] showed that, compared with magnesium-rich cells, magnesium deficiency within endothelial cells increased cytotoxicity from oxyradicals beginning at a relatively short 15 min of exposure to the free radicals. Thus, magnesium may also protect the endothelial cell from oxygen free radical injury. This action may explain the recent results of Rukshin et al., who showed that magnesium may attenuate coronary stent thrombosis in swine.[262] Magnesium may also confer benefit during occlusion-reperfusion sequences by its action as a physiologic calcium channel blocker.[258,260,263] Magnesium inhibits calcium overload during initial phases of reperfusion through inhibition of calcium transport across most calcium channels.[258]

Shibata et al.[264] recently studied the effects of magnesium pretreatment of patients with acute MI on the incidence of reperfusion injuries. Thirty-eight patients were treated with either intravenous magnesium or placebo along with coronary reperfusion therapy within 6 h of onset. The incidence of reperfusion arrhythmia was significantly lower in the magnesium group and, at the postreperfusion stage, there was a tendency for the degree of ST-segment reelevation in the magnesium group to be lower.[264] In stark contrast, in the Fourth International Study of Infarct Survival (ISIS-4), comprising 58,050 patients, magnesium therapy did not reduce 5-week mortality, either in the general population (7.64 versus 7.24%) or in specific subgroups.[265] Although this study aroused considerable controversy over its methodology, subsequent studies have corroborated its findings. A later study confirmed that intravenous magnesium delivered before, during, and after reperfusion did not decrease myocardial damage and did not improve the short-term clinical outcome in patients with acute MI treated with direct angioplasty.[266] In isolated cardiomyocytes, magnesium was also shown not to protect from hypoxic injury.[267] Notwithstanding the controversy surrounding the ISIS-4 study, magnesium has not been clearly shown to confer significant clinical benefit in reperfusion injuries as an antioxidant, and much conflicting evidence exists.

Mannitol (Synthetic Antioxidant)

Some investigators have suggested that the major danger of superoxide anion radical and hydrogen peroxide accumulation is due to the production of hydroxyl radicals.[268] Furthermore, the formation of hydroxyl radicals has been implicated as the actual mechanism of free-radical damage, which is attributed to its high reactivity and the fact that there are no host enzyme systems to scavenge hydroxyl radicals once formed.[268]

Mannitol is an oxygen free–radical scavenger of the hydroxyl radical (OH·) by forming a mannitol radical through the reaction $(MH_2 + OH^{\cdot} \rightarrow MH^{\cdot} + H_2O)$. The mannitol radical then undergoes dimerization or disproportionation.[269] Experimental studies report that mannitol limits injury to the myocardium after ischemia and reperfusion.[270–272] However, several mechanisms could account for the observed beneficial effects of mannitol: (1) the hyperosmotic properties of mannitol could help reduce myocardial cell swelling[271,273]; (2) mannitol could decrease blood viscosity and thus reduce sludging within the coronary arteries[270]; and (3) as a scavenger of hydroxyl radicals, mannitol may reduce myocardial injury by inhibiting the production of free radicals.[274]

A few studies report that mannitol may reduce MI size.[270–272] In dogs, Kloner et al. showed that mannitol pretreatment resulted in a 50% reduction in the amount of myocardial necrosis in the posterior papillary muscles after the dogs were subjected to 40 min of coronary occlusion and 48 h of reperfusion.[270] However, there was no significant difference in the extent of electrocardiographic (ECG) ST-segment elevation or mortality from control. Similarly, Powell et al. demonstrated that mannitol may reduce the mean percentage of necrotic cells.[273] Both of these studies selected the posterior papillary muscle as being representative of the myocardium at risk. In a more recent study by Justicz et al., mannitol administered during coronary occlusion was also found to increase salvage of the ischemic myocardium after 75 min of left anterior descending artery (LAD) occlusion followed by 45 min of reperfusion.[272] The areas of infarct and areas at risk were determined by planimetric analysis. In contrast, Harada et al. were not able to show a reduction in myocardial infarct size in a different animal model.[275] In this study, mannitol was infused in anesthetized baboons at 105 min post-coronary occlusion until reperfusion was allowed at 2 h. No significant difference was noted in the mean summated ST-segment elevations between the control and treated groups. The authors attributed the differences to the poor collateral circulation in the baboon, short duration of the treatment, and negation of the beneficial effects of mannitol by the adverse effects of volume overload, which consequently led to an increase in myocardial wall stress.[275]

Cardiac effects of mannitol have also been examined in the clinical setting. In early work by Willerson et al., mannitol was administered to 20 patients undergoing cardiac catheterization; the investigators found that mannitol increased coronary blood flow by 39%.[276] In a study by Ferreira et al.,[277] mannitol was shown to reduce reperfusion during coronary artery bypass surgery. This prospective trial of 40 patients showed that the addition of mannitol to a cardioplegic solution significantly reduced the number of atrial arrhythmias. Furthermore, myocardial biopsies performed before ischemia and at the time of reperfusion showed no significant differences in the group that received mannitol. The authors suggested the beneficial effects of mannitol were more likely due to free-radical scavenging properties because the standard cardioplegic solution had higher osmolarity than the mannitol solution.[277] In a study by Laskowski et al., 84 consecutive patients with acute MI were given streptokinase therapy.[278] Half of these patients randomly received mannitol infusion in conjunction with ascorbic acid infusion, whereas the controls received only the standard fibrinolytic therapy. The authors found that the administration of mannitol with ascorbic acid decreased the number of complications, such as left ventricular insufficiency and ventricular ectopic beats. However, it is unclear whether these benefits could be attributed to the antioxidant effects of ascorbic acid, mannitol, or both drugs. Future randomized studies are necessary to establish the role of mannitol as a therapeutic agent in limiting myocardial ischemia and reperfusion injury.

Adenosine

Adenosine has unique properties for myocardial protection during reperfusion therapy (see Chap. 32) and is believed to play an important role as a natural mediator of the adverse effects from ischemia.[279] Its ubiquitous nature, multiple effects, and multiple receptor types and locations make the exact mechanism of action in myocardial protection difficult to pinpoint. However, a number of its properties provide possible antioxidant protection.[280] Adenosine replenishes high-energy phosphate stores in endothelial cells and myocytes.[281] It is a potent vasodilator, modulates cardiac adrenergic responses,[282] and inhibits neutrophil function and the generation of free radicals via adenosine A_2 receptor stimulation[279,283,284]; it also inhibits neutrophil-mediated endothelial damage.[285] In animal reperfusion models,[286–288] adenosine was consistently found to reduce infarct size after 24 to 72 h, whether by intracoronary or intravenous administration, after 40 to 90 min (but not after 180 min) of coronary occlusion, with adenosine infused for 60 to 150 min. The reduction in infarct size was accompanied by improved regional left ventricular function, improved coronary blood flow, less capillary plugging and neutrophil accumulation, and improved microscopic endothelial and microvascular integrity. Data concerning the use of adenosine following acute MI in humans are limited. Garratt et al.[289,290] used acute and follow-up technetium-99m sestamibi single-photon emission computed tomography (SPECT) scanning to measure infarct size in a group of patients with acute MI treated with direct angioplasty with intravenous adenosine 70 μg/kg/min continued for 1 h after coronary patency was restored. Lidocaine was also administered. There was 55% early salvage of the original ischemic area, and minimal evidence of infarct by SPECT at 6 weeks. The infarct size was significantly smaller than that in historical controls, although the historical controls had infarct size determined at the time of hospital discharge. Marzilli et al.[291] studied coronary flow with and without intracoronary adenosine in a group of 40 consecutive patients undergoing direct angioplasty. Twenty patients were treated with 4 mg of intracoronary adenosine for more than 4 min, and 20 controls were treated with saline solution. Residual coronary stenosis was similar, but coronary flow was brisker in adenosine-treated patients; no-reflow was less common (0 versus 30%). These are the first data suggesting a treatment to improve tissue perfusion despite adequate epicardial coronary flow—a property viewed as lacking in current reperfusion strategies.[292] Two phase II clinical trials evaluated the effects of adenosine in acute MI. The Acute Myocardial Infarction Study of Adenosine (AMISTAD) trial randomized approximately 300 patients to a 3-h intravenous infusion of 70 μg/kg/min adenosine versus open-label control, in conjunction with thrombolytic therapy, for acute MI within 6 h of symptom. The primary endpoint was SPECT sestamibi–determined infarct size at 5 to 7 days. The results of the study showed a possible benefit of adenosine, but the trial was under-powered to assess mortality.[292a] A follow-up study in 2,118 patients with acute MI (AMISTAD-II) also showed a benefit of adenosine therapy in combination with thrombolysis.[292b] A sister trial, the Adenosine Lidocaine Infarct Zone Viability Enhancement Trial (ALIVE) evaluated adenosine in conjunction with direct angioplasty, with a sample size of approximately 220 and a primary endpoint of myocardial salvage based on acute and follow-up SPECT sestamibi imaging.[293] These trials suggest a basis for further evaluation of adenosine as a myocardial protective agent for acute MI.

N-2 Mercaptoproprionyl Glycine (MPG)

MPG is a safe and well-tolerated drug that is used clinically to reduce radiation-induced tissue injury.[294,295] It appears to work by reacting directly with free-radical species, promoting the resynthesis of glutathione, or acting as an alternative substrate for glutathione peroxidase, thereby limiting the cytotoxic effects of H_2O_2 and lipid peroxides. This compound has been shown to significantly reduce MI size both in the early moments[296,297] and for as long as 48 h[14a,298] after reperfusion. It has also been shown to significantly reduce the oxidative damage of doxorubicin (adriamycin) in rats.[299]

Gene Therapy

In experimental animals, it has recently been demonstrated that targeted mutation of the P66[shc] gene induces resistance to oxidative stress and can prolong the life span.[300] Whether genetic manipulation of P66[shc] can provide greater protection against reactive oxygen species than that of catalase and SOD needs to be determined. Also, adenoviral vectors have been used to transfect Mn-SOD into rat hearts and were shown to be protective against ischemia-reperfusion injury.[301] In addition, rabbits have been transfected with adenovirus expressing EC-SOD in their livers. Liberation of the overexpressed enzyme with heparin prior to and during myocardial ischemia reduced infarct size by 25% in the experimental group.[302] Transgenic mice that overexpress human Cu/Zn-SOD have also been found to have relative resistance to cardiac ischemia.[303]

CONCLUSION

Enzymatic and nonenzymatic approaches to reversing the toxicity of free radical formation in myocardial ischemia and reperfusion have shown promise in experimental studies but have yet to be of proven value in humans.

REFERENCES

1. Boveris A, Oshino N, Chance B: The cellular production of hydrogen peroxide. *Biochem J* 128:617, 1972.
2. Balz F: Reactive oxygen species and antioxidant vitamins: Mechanisms of action. *Am J Med* 97:3A5s, 1994.
3. Cheeseman KH, Slater TF: An introduction to free radical biochemistry. *Br Med Bull* 49(3):481, 1993.
4. McCord JM: The evolution of free radicals and oxidative stress. *Am J Med* 108:652, 2000.
5. Evans PH: Free radicals in brain metabolism and pathology. *Br Med Bull* 49(3):577, 1993.
6. Ryrfeldt A, Bannenberg G, Moldeus P: Free radicals and lung disease. *Br Med Bull* 49(3):588, 1993.
7. Poli G: Liver damage due to free radicals. *Br Med Bull* 49(3):604, 1993.
8. Baud L, Ardaillou R: Involvement of reactive oxygen species in kidney damage. *Br Med Bull* 49(3):621, 1993.
9. Jackson MJ, O'Farrell S: Free radicals and muscle damage. *Br Med Bull* 49(3):630, 1993.
10. Wolff SP: Diabetes mellitus and free radicals. *Br Med Bull* 49(3):642, 1993.
11. Lubec G: The hydroxyl radical: From chemistry to human disease. *J Invest Med* 44:324, 1996.
12. Esterbauer H, Wag G, Puhl H: Lipid peroxidation and its role in atherosclerosis. *Br Med Bull* 49(3):566, 1993.

13. Ames BN: Dietary carcinogens and anticarcinogens: Oxygen radicals and degenerative diseases. *Science* 221:1256, 1983.
14. Andreoli TE: Free radicals and oxidative stress. *Am J Med* 108:650, 2000.
14a. Lefer DJ, Granger DN: Oxidative stress and cardiac disease. *Am J Med* 109:315, 2000.
15. Gey KF: Prospects for the prevention of free radical disease, regarding cancer and cardiovascular disease. *Br Med Bull* 49(3):679, 1993.
16. Moncada S, Palmer RMJ, Higgs EA: Nitric oxide: Physiology, pathophysiology and pharmacology. *Pharmacol Rev* 43:109, 1991.
17. Winrow VR, PG Winyard, CJ Morris, Blake DR: Free radicals in inflammation: Second messengers and mediators of tissue destruction. *Br Med Bull* 49(3):506, 1993.
18. Pryor WA, Godber SS: Non-invasive measures of oxidative stress status in humans. *Free Radic Biol Med* 10:177, 1991.
19. Slater TF: Overview of methods used for detecting lipid peroxidation. *Methods Enzmol* 105:283, 1984.
20. Kehrer JP, Smith CV: Free radicals in biology: Sources reactivities and roles in the etiology of human diseases. In: Frei B, ed. *Natural Antioxidants in Human Health and Disease.* Orlando, FL: Academic Press, 1994:25.
21. Ames BN, Shigenaga MK, Hagen TM: Oxidants, antioxidants and the degenerative disease of aging. *Proc Natl Acad Sci USA* 90:7915, 1993.
22. Slater TF: Necrogenic action of carbon tetrachloride in the rat: A speculative mechanism based on activation. *Nature* 209:36, 1966.
23. Cheeseman KH, Albano E, Tomasi A: Biochemical studies on the metabolic activation of haloalkanes. *Environ Health Perspect* 64:85, 1985.
24. Porter N: Autoxidation of polyunsaturated fatty acids: Initiation, propagation and product distribution (basic chemistry). In: Vigo-Pelfrey C, ed. *Membrane Lipid Oxidation.* Boca Raton, FL: CRC Press, 1990:33.
25. Esterbauer H, Zollner H, Schaur R: Aldehydes formed by lipid peroxidation: Mechanisms of formation, occurrence and determination. In: Vigo-Pelfrey C, ed. *Membrane Lipid Peroxidation.* Boca-Raton, FL: CRC Press, 1990:239.
26. Borg D: Oxygen free radicals and tissue injury. In: Tarr M, Samson F, eds. *Oxygen Free Radicals in Tissue Damage.* Boston: Birkhauser, 1993:12.
27. Steinberg D, Parthasarathy S, Carew T, et al: Beyond cholesterol. Modifications of low density lipoprotein that increases its atherogenicity. *N Engl J Med* 320:915, 1989.
28. Steinberg D: Antioxidants and antiatherosclerosis. A current assessment. *Circulation* 84:1420, 1991.
29. Rajavashisth T, Andalibi A, Territo M, et al: Induction of endothelial cell expression of granulocyte and macrophage colony stimulating factors by modified low density lipoproteins. *Nature* 344:254, 1990.
30. Schmidt K, Graier W, Kostner G, et al: Activation of soluble guanylate cyclase by nitrovasodilators is inhibited by oxidized low density lipoprotein. *Biochem Biophys Res Commun* 172:614, 1990.
31. Bui MN, Sack MN, Moutsatsos G, et al: Autoantibody titers to oxidized low-density lipoprotein in patients with coronary atherosclerosis. *Am Heart J* 131:663, 1996.
32. Bergmark C, Wu R, deFaire U, et al: Patients with early-onset peripheral vascular disease have increased levels of autoantibodies against oxidized LDL. *Arterioscler Thromb Vasc Biol* 15:441, 1995.
33. Wood K, Cadogan M, Ramshaw A, et al: The distribution of adhesion molecules in human atherosclerosis. *Histopathology* 22(5):437, 1993.
34. Parmus D, Brown D, Mitchinson M: Serum antibodies to oxidized LDL and ceroid in chronic periaortitis. *Arch Pathol Lab Med* 114:383, 1990.
35. Esterbauer H, Dieber-Rothender M, Waeg G, et al: Biochemical, structural and functional properties of oxidized low density lipoprotein. *Chem Res Toxicol* 3:77, 1990.
36. Rangan U, Bulkley G: Prospects for treatment of free radical mediated tissue injury. *Br Med Bull* 49(3):700, 1993.
37. Maza S, Frishman W: Therapeutic options to minimize free radical damage and thrombogenicity in ischemic/reperfused myocardium. *Med Clinics North Am* 172(1):227, 1988.
38. Dickens B, Weglicki W, Li Y, et al: Magnesium deficiency in vitro enhances free radical induced intracellular oxidation and cytotoxicity in endothelial cells. *FEBS Lett* 311:187, 1992.
39. Krinsky N: Mechanism of action of biological antioxidants. *Soc Exper Biol Med* 200:248, 1992.

40. Ferrari R, Visioli O, Caldarera C: Vitamin E and the heart: Possible role as antioxidants. *Acta Vitamin Enzymol* 5:11, 1982.
41. Ferrari R, Cargoni A, Ceconi C, et al: Role of oxygen in myocardial ischemic and reperfusion damage: Protective effects of vitamin E. In: Hayaishi O, Mino M, eds. *Clinical and Nutritional Aspects of Vitamin E.* New York: Elsevier, 1987:209.
42. Rimm E, Stampfer M, Ascherio A, et al: Vitamin E supplementation and risk of coronary heart disease among men. *N Engl J Med* 328:1450, 1993.
43. Upston JM, Terentis AC, Stocker R: Tocopherol-mediated peroxidation of lipoproteins: Implications for vitamin E as a potential antiatherogenic supplement. *FASEB J* 13:977, 1999.
44. Neuzil J, Weber C, Kontush A: The role of vitamin E in atherogenesis: Linking the chemical, biological and clinical aspects of the disease. *Atherosclerosis* 157:257, 2001.
45. Erl W, Weber C, Wardemann C, Weber PC: Alpha-tocopheryl succinate inhibits monocytic cell adhesion to endothelial cells by suppressing NF-κB activation. *Am J Physiol* 273:H634, 1997.
46. Yoshida N, Manabe H, Terasawa Y, et al: Inhibitory effects of vitamin E on endothelial-dependent adhesive interactions with leukocytes induced by oxidized low density lipoprotein. *Biofactors* 13(1-4):279, 2000.
47. Ricciarelli R, Tasinato A, Clement S, et al: Tocopherol specifically inactivates cellular protein kinase Cα by changing its phosphorylation state. *Biochem J* 334:243, 1998.
48. Wu D, Hayek MG, Meydani NS: Vitamin E and macrophage cyclooxygenase regulation in the aged. *J Nutr* 131:382S, 2001.
49. Freedman JE, Kearney JF: Vitamin E inhibition of platelet aggregation is independent of antioxidant activity. *J Nutr* 131:374S, 2001.
50. Assi A, Breyer I, Feher M: Nonantioxidant functions of alpha-tocopherol in smooth muscle cells. *J Nutr* 131:378S, 2001.
51. Ricciarelli R, Zingg J-M, Azzi A: Vitamin E reduces the uptake of oxidized LDL by inhibiting CD36 scavenger receptor expression in cultured aortic smooth muscle cells. *Circulation* 102:82, 2000.
52. Packer L, Weber SU, Rimbach G: Molecular aspects of α-tocotrienol antioxidant action and cell signalling. *J Nutr* 131:369S, 2001.
52a. Fairfield KM, Fletcher RH: Vitamins for chronic disease prevention in adults. Scientific review. *JAMA* 287:3116, 2002.
52b. Fletcher RM, Fairfield KM: Vitamins for chronic disease prevention in adults. Clinical applications. *JAMA* 287:3127, 2002.
53. Qiao Y, Yokomaya M, Kameyama K, Asano G: Effect of vitamin E on vascular integrity in cholesterol fed guinea pigs. *Arterioscler Thromb* 13:1885, 1993.
54. Zughaib M, Tang X, Schleman M, et al: Beneficial effects of MDL 74,405, a cardioselective water soluble alpha tocopherol analogue, on recovery of function of stunned myocardium in intact dogs. *Cardiovasc Res* 28:235, 1994.
55. Thomas SR, Leichtweis SB, Pettersson K, et al: Dietary cosupplementation with vitamin E and coenzyme Q(10) inhibits atherosclerosis in apolipoprotein E gene knockout mice. *Arterioscler Thromb Vasc Biol* 21(4):585, 2001.
56. Ohrvall M, Tengblad S, Vessby B: Lower tocopherol serum levels in subjects with abdominal obesity. *J Intern Med* 234:53, 1993.
57. Miwa K, Miyagi Y, Igawa A, et al: Vitamin E deficiency in variant angina. *Circulation* 94:14, 1996.
58. Gey K, Puska P: Plasma vitamin E and A inversely correlated to mortality from ischemic heart disease in cross cultural epidemiology. *Ann NY Sci* 570:254, 1989.
59. Mezzetti A, Lapenna D, Pierdomenico S, et al: Vitamins E, C and lipid peroxidation in plasma and arterial tissue of smokers and nonsmokers. *Atherosclerosis* 112(1):91, 1995.
60. Herbaczynska-Cedro K, Klosiewicz-Wasek B, Cedro K, et al: Supplementation with vitamins C and E suppresses leukocyte oxygen free radical production in patients with myocardial infarction. *Eur Heart J* 16:1044, 1995.
61. Dieber-Rotheneder M, Puhl H, Waeg G, et al: Effect of oral supplementation with d-alpha tocopherol on the vitamin E content of human low density lipoprotein and resistance to oxidation. *J Lipid Res* 32:1325, 1991.
62. Jialal I, Fuller CJ, Huet BA: The effect of α-tocopherol supplementation on LDL oxidation. A dose-response study. *Arterioscler Thromb Vasc Biol* 15:190, 1995.

63. Meagher EA, Barry OP, Lawson JA, et al: Effects of vitamin E on lipid peroxidation in healthy persons. *JAMA* 285:1178, 2001.

64. Hodis H, Mack W, LaBree L, et al: Serial coronary angiographic evidence that antioxidant vitamin intake reduces progression of coronary artery atherosclerosis. *JAMA* 273(23):1849, 1995.

65. Rapola J, Virtamo J, Haukka J, et al: Effect of vitamin E and beta carotene on the incidence of angina pectoris: A randomized, double blind, controlled trial. *JAMA* 275:693, 1996.

66. Salonen JT, Nyyssonen K, Salonen R, et al: Antioxidant supplementation in atherosclerosis Prevention (ASAP) study: A randomized trial of the effect of vitamin E and C on 3–year progression of carotid atherosclerosis. *J Intern Med* 248(5):377, 2000.

67. McQuillan BM, Hung J, Beilby JP, et al: Antioxidant vitamins and the risk of carotid atherosclerosis. The Perth Carotid Ultrasound Disease Assessment Study (CUDAS). *J Am Coll Cardiol* 38(7):1788, 2001.

68. Simon E, Gariepy J, Cogny A, et al: Erythrocyte, but not plasma, vitamin E concentration is associated with carotid intima-media thickening in asymptomatic men at risk for cardiovascular disease. *Atherosclerosis* 159(1):193, 2001.

69. Stampfer MJ, Hennekens CH, Manson JE, et al: Vitamin E consumption and the risk of coronary disease in women. *N Engl J Med* 328:1444, 1993.

70. Kushi LH, Folsom AR, Prineas RJ, et al: Dietary antioxidant vitamins and death from coronary heart disease in postmenopausal women. *N Engl J Med* 334:1156, 1996.

71. Losonczy KG, Harris TB, Havlik RJ: Vitamin E and vitamin C supplement use and risk of all-cause and coronary heart disease mortality in older persons: The Established Populations for Epidemiologic Studies of the Elderly. *Am J Clin Nutr* 64:190, 1996.

72. Meyer F, Bairati I, Dagenais GR: Lower ischemic heart disease incidence and mortality among vitamin supplement users. *Can J Cardiol* 12:930, 1996.

73. Knekt P, Reunanen A, Jarvinen R, et al: Antioxidant vitamin intake and coronary mortality in a longitudinal population study. *Am J Epidemiol* 139:1180, 1994.

74. Kromhout D, Bloemberg BP, Feskens EJ, et al: Alcohol, fish, fibre and antioxidant vitamins intake do not explain population differences in coronary heart disease mortality. *Int J Epidemiol* 25:753, 1996.

75. Sahyoun NR, Jacques PF, Russell RM: Carotenoids, vitamins C and E, and mortality in an elderly population. *Am J Epidemiol* 144:501, 1996.

76. Stephens NG, Parsons A, Schofield PM, et al: Randomized control trial of vitamin E in patients with coronary disease: Cambridge Heart Antioxidant Study. *Lancet* 347:781, 1996.

77. Boaz M, Smetana S, Weinstein T, et al: Secondary prevention with antioxidants of cardiovascular disease in end-stage renal disease (SPACE): Randomized placebo controlled trial. *Lancet* 356:1213, 2000.

78. The Alpha-Tocopherol Beta Carotene Cancer Prevention Study Group: The effect of vitamin E and beta carotene on the incidence of lung cancer and other cancers in male smokers. *N Engl J Med* 330:1029, 1994.

79. Tornwall ME, Virtamo J, Haukka JK, et al: Alpha-tocopherol (vitamin E) and beta-carotene supplementation does not affect the risk for large abdominal aortic aneurysm in a controlled trial. *Atherosclerosis* 157(1):167, 2001.

80. The Heart Outcomes Prevention Evaluation Study Investigators: Effects of an angiotensin converting enzyme inhibitor, ramipril, on cardiovascular events and stroke in high-risk patients. *N Engl J Med* 342:145, 2000.

81. Lonn EM, Yusuf S, Dzavik V, et al for the SECURE Investigators: Effects of ramipril and vitamin E on atherosclerosis. The Study to Evaluate Carotid Ultrasound Changes in Patients Treated with Ramipril and Vitamin E (SECURE). *Circulation* 103:919, 2001.

82. Latini R, Santoro E, Masson S, et al for the GISSI-3 Investigators: Aspirin does not interact with ACE inhibitors when both are given early after acute myocardial infarction: Results of the GISSI-3 trial. *Heart Dis* 2:185, 2000.

83. Brown BG, Zhao XQ, Chait A, et al: Simvastatin and niacin, antioxidant vitamins, or the combination for the prevention of coronary disease. *N Engl J Med* 345:1583, 2001.

84. de Gaetano G, Collaborative Group of the Primary Prevention Project: Low-dose aspirin and vitamin E in people at cardiovascular risk: A randomised trial in general practice. *Lancet* 357:89, 2001.

85. Jialal I, Traber M, Devaraj S: Is there a vitamin E paradox? *Curr Opin Lipidol* 12:49, 2001.

86. Steinberg D: Is there a potential therapeutic role for vitamin E or other antioxidants in atherosclerosis? *Curr Opin Lipidol* 11:603, 2000.

87. Tang X-L, Kaur H, Sun J-Z, et al: Effect of the hydrophilic α-tocopherol analog MDL 74,405 on detection of hydroxyl radicals in stunned myocardium in dogs. *Am Heart J* 130:940, 1995.

88. Harris W: The prevention of atherosclerosis with antioxidants. *Clin Cardiol* 15:636, 1992.

89. Verlangieri A, Kapeghian J, El-Dean S, et al: Fruits and vegetable consumption and cardiovascular disease mortality. *Med Hypoth* 16: 7, 1985.

90. Burton G, Ingold K: Beta-carotene: An unusual type of antioxidant. *Science* 224:569, 1984.

91. Sies H, Stahl W: Vitamins E and C, beta-carotene, and other carotenoids as antioxidants. *Am J Clin Nutr* 62(Suppl):1315S, 1995.

92. Liebler D: Antioxidant reactions of carotenoids. *Ann NY Acad Sci* 691:20, 1993.

93. Keaney J, Gaziano J, Xu A, et al: Dietary antioxidants preserve endothelium dependent vessel relaxation in cholesterol fed rabbits. *Proc Natl Acad Sci U S A* 90:11880, 1993.

94. Gaziano JM, Manson JE, Branch LG, et al: A prospective study of consumption of carotenoids in fruits and vegetables and decreased cardiovascular mortality in the elderly. *Ann Epidemiol* 5:255, 1995.

95. Gey K, Stahelin H, Eicholzer M: Poor plasma status of carotene and vitamin C is associated with higher mortality from ischemic heart disease and stroke: Basel Prospective Study. *Clin Invest* 342:1379, 1993.

96. Kardinaal AF, Kok, FJ, Ringstad J, et al: Antioxidants in adipose tissue and risk of myocardial infarction: The EURAMIC study. *Lancet* 342:1379, 1993.

97. Morris D, Kritchevsky S, Davis C: Serum carotenoids and coronary heart disease. *JAMA* 272:1439, 1994.

98. Hennekens C, Buring J, Manson J, et al: Lack of effect of long-term supplementation with beta carotene on the incidence of malignant neoplasms and cardiovascular disease. *N Engl J Med* 334:1145, 1996.

99. Greenberg ER, Baron JA, Karagas MR, et al: Mortality associated with low plasma concentration of beta carotene and the effect of oral supplementation. *JAMA* 275:699, 1996.

100. Omenn GS, Goodman GE, Thornquist MD, et al: Effects of a combination of beta carotene and vitamin A on lung cancer and cardiovascular disease. *N Engl J Med* 334:1150, 1996.

101. Feskanich D, Singh V, Willet WC, Colditz GA: Vitamin A intake and hip fractures among postmenopausal women. *JAMA* 287:47, 2002.

101a. Libby P, Aikawa M: Vitamin C, collagen, and cracks in the plaque. *Circulation* 105:1396, 2002.

102. Stocker R, Frei B: Endogenous antioxidant defenses in human blood plasma. In: Sies H, eds. *Oxidative Stress: Oxidants and Antioxidants.* London: Academic Press, 1991:213.

103. Weber C, Erl W, Weber K, Weber PC: Increased adhesiveness of isolated monocytes to endothelium prevented by vitamin C intake in smokers. *Circulation* 93:1488, 1996.

104. Jialal I, Grundy S: Preservation of the endogenous antioxidants in low density lipoprotein by ascorbate but not probucol during oxidative modification. *J Clin Invest* 87:597, 1991.

105. Retsky K, Freeman M, Frei B: Ascorbic acid oxidation product(s) protect low density lipoprotein against atherogenic modification. Anti rather than pro-oxidant activity of vitamin C in the presence of transitional metal ions. *J Biol Chem* 268:1304, 1993.

106. Jessup W, Rankin S, deWhalley CV, et al: Alpha tocopherol consumption during low density lipoprotein oxidation. *Biochem J* 265:399, 1990.

107. Carr AC, Tijerina T, Frei B: Vitamin C protects against and reverses specific hypochlorous acid- and chloramine-dependent modifications of low-density lipoprotein. *Biochem J* 346(2):491, 2000.

108. Retsky K, Frei B: Vitamin C prevents metal ion dependent initiation and propagation of lipid peroxidation in human low density lipoproteins. *Biochim Biophys Acta* 1257(3):279, 1995.

109. Howard P, Meyers D: Effect of vitamin C on lipids. *Ann Pharmacother* 29(11):1129, 1995.

110. Hamabe A, Takase B, Uehata A, et al: Impaired endothelium-dependent vasodilation in the brachial artery in variant angina pectoris and the effect of intravenous administration of vitamin C. *Am J Cardiol* 87:1154, 2001.

111. Ting HH, Timimi FK, Haley EA, et al: Vitamin C improves endothelium-dependent vasodilation in forearm resistance vessels of humans with hypercholesterolemia. *Circulation* 95:2617, 1997.

112. Grossmann M, Dobrev D, Himmel HM, et al: Ascorbic acid-induced modulation of venous tone in humans. *Hypertension* 37:949, 2001.

113. Price KD, Price CSC, Reynolds RD: Hyperglycemia-induced ascorbic acid deficiency promotes endothelial dysfunction and the development of atherosclerosis. *Atherosclerosis* 158:1, 2001.

114. Singh N, Graves JE, MacAllister RJ, Singer DRJ: Vitamin C does not alter endothelium-dependent dilatation in the forearm of elderly humans. *Br J Pharmacol* 126:96, 1999.

115. Chambers JC, McGregor A, Jean-Marie J, et al: Demonstration of rapid onset vascular endothelial dysfunction after hyperhomocysteinemia. An effect reversible with vitamin C therapy. *Circulation* 99:1156, 1999.

116. Heitzer T, Just H, Munzel T: Antioxidant vitamin C improves endothelial dysfunction in chronic smokers. *Circulation* 94:6, 1996.

117. Gokce N, Keaney JF Jr, Frei B, et al: Long-term ascorbic acid administration reverses endothelial vasomotor dysfunction in patients with coronary artery disease. *Circulation* 99:3234, 1999.

118. Hirashima O, Kawano H, Motoyama T, et al: Improvement of endothelial function and insulin sensitivity with vitamin C in patients with coronary spastic angina. *J Am Coll Cardiol* 35:1860, 2000.

119. Valkonen MM, Kuusi T: Vitamin C prevents the acute atherogenic effects of passive smoking. *Free Radic Biol Med* 28(3):428, 2000.

120. Weber C, Erl W, Weber K, Weber PC: Increased adhesiveness of isolated monocytes to endothelium is prevented by vitamin C intake in smokers. *Circulation* 93:1488, 1996.

121. Gey K, Brubacher G, Stahelin H: Plasma levels of antioxidant vitamins in relation to ischemic heart disease and cancer. *Am J Nutr* 45:1368, 1987.

122. Enstrom J, Kanim L, Klein M: Vitamin C intake and mortality among a sample of the United States population. *Epidemiology* 3:194, 1992.

123. Riemersma RA, Carruthers KF, Elton FA, Fox KAA: Vitamin C and the risk of acute myocardial infarction. *Am J Clin Nutr* 71:1181, 2000.

124. Kritchevsky S, Shimakawa T, Tell G, et al: Dietary antioxidants and carotid artery wall thickness. The ARIC Study. Atherosclerosis Risk in Communities. *Circulation* 92:2142, 1995.

125. Langlois M, Duprez D, Delanghe J, et al: Serum vitamin C concentration is low in peripheral arterial disease and is associated with inflammation and severity of atherosclerosis. *Circulation* 103:1863, 2001.

126. Hertog MGL, Hollman PCH, Katan MB, Kromhout D: Estimation of daily intake of potentially anticarcinogenic flavonoids and their determinants in adults in The Netherlands. *Nutr Cancer* 20:21, 1993.

127. Willaman JJ: Some biological effects of flavonoids. *J Am Pharm Assoc* 44:404, 1995.

128. Skibola CF, Smith, MT: Potential health impacts of excessive flavonoid intake. *Free Radic Biol Med* 29(3–4):375, 2000.

129. Hwang J, Sevanian A, Hodis HN, Ursini F: Synergistic inhibition of LDL oxidation by phytoestrogens and ascorbic acid. *Free Radic Biol Med* 29(1):79, 2000.

130. Hwang J, Hodis HN, Sevanian A: Soy and alfalfa phytoestrogen extracts become potent low-density lipoprotein antioxidants in the presence of acerola cherry extract. *J Agric Food Chem* 49(1):308, 2001.

131. Hertog MG, Feskens EJM, Hollman PCH, et al: Dietary antioxidant flavonoids and risk of coronary heart disease: The Zutphen Elderly Study. *Lancet* 342:1007, 1993.

132. Knekt P, Jarvinen R, Reunanen A, Maatela J: Flavonoid intake and coronary mortality in Finland: a cohort study. *BMJ* 312:478, 1996.

133. Hertog MGL, Kromhout D, Aravanis C, et al: Flavonoid intake and long-term risk of coronary heart disease and cancer in the Seven Countries Study. *Arch Intern Med* 155:381, 1995.

134. Viana M, Barbas C, Bonet B, et al: In vitro effects of flavonoid-rich extract on LDL oxidation. *Atherosclerosis* 123:83, 1996.

135. Robak J, Gryglewski RJ: Flavonoids are scavengers of superoxide anions. *Biochem Pharmacol* 37:837, 1988.

136. Husain SR, Cillard J, Cillard P: Hydroxy radical scavenging activity of flavonoids. *Phytochem* 26:2489, 1987.

137. Shoskes DA: Effect of bioflavonoids quercetin and curcumin on ischemic renal injury: A new class of renoprotective agents. *Transplantation* 66:147, 1998.

138. Nijveldt RJ, van Nood E, van Hoorn DEC, et al: Flavonoids: A review of probable mechanisms of action and potential applications. *Am J Clin Nutr* 74(4):418, 2001.

139. DeWhalley CV, Rankin SM, Hoult JRS, et al: Flavonoids inhibit the oxidative modification of low density lipoproteins. *Biochem Pharmacol* 39:1743, 1990.

140. Negre-Salvayre A, Salvayre R: Quercetin prevents the cytotoxicity of oxidized LDL by macrophages. *Free Radic Biol Med* 12:101, 1992.

141. da Silva EL, Abdalla DS, Terao J: Inhibitory effects of flavonoids on low-density lipoprotein peroxidation catalyzed by mammalian 15–lipoxygenase. *IUBMB Life* 49(4):289, 2000.

142. Exner M, Hermann M, Hofbauer R, et al: Genistein prevents the glucose autoxidation mediated atherogenic modification of low-density lipoprotein. *Free Radic Res* 34(1):101, 2001.

143. Miura Y, Chiba T, Tomita I, et al: Tea catechins prevent the development of atherosclerosis in apoprotein E–deficient mice. *J Nutr* 131(1):27, 2001.

144. Maxwell S: Red wine and antioxidant activity in serum (letter). *Lancet* 344:193, 1994.

145. Chopra M, Fitzsimons PE, Strain JJ, et al: Nonalcoholic red wine extract and quercetin inhibit LDL oxidation without affecting plasma antioxidant vitamin and carotenoid concentrations. *Clin Chem* 46(8 Pt 1):1162, 2000.

146. Osman HE, Maalej N, Shanmuganayagam D, Folts JD: Grape juice but not orange or grapefruit juice inhibits platelet activity in dogs and monkeys. *J Nutr* 128:2307, 1998.

147. Laughton MJ, Evans PJ, Moroney MA, et al: Inhibition of mammalian 5–lipoxygenase and cyclo-oxygenase by flavonoids and phenolic dietary additives. Relationship to antioxidant activity and to iron ion-reducing ability. *Biochem Pharmacol* 42:1673, 1991.

148. Cos P, Ying L, Calomme M, et al: Structure-activity relationship and classification of flavonoids as inhibitors of xanthine oxidase and superoxide scavengers. *J Nat Prod* 61:71, 1998.

149. Gerritsen ME, Carley WW, Ranges GE, et al: Flavonoids inhibit cytokine-induced endothelial cell adhesion protein gene expression. *Am J Pathol* 147:278, 1995.

150. Carrea FP, Lesnefsky EJ, Kaiser DG, Horwitz LD: The lazaroid U74006F, a 21-amino steroid inhibitor of lipid peroxidation, attenuates myocardial injury from ischemia and reperfusion. *J Cardiovasc Pharmacol* 20:230, 1992.

151. Natarajan R, Gonzales N, Lanting L: Role of the lipoxygenase pathway in angiotensin II–induced smooth muscle cell hypertrophy. *Hypertension* 23:I142, 1994.

152. Van Acker SABE, Kramer K, Grimbergen JA, et al: Monohydroxyethylrutoside as protector against chronic doxorubicin-induced cardiotoxicity. *Br J Pharmacol* 115:1260, 1995.

153. Rice-Evans E. Flavonoid antioxidants. *Curr Med Chem* 8(7):797, 2001.

154. Rimm EB, Katan MB, Ascherio A, et al: Relation between intake of flavonoids and risk for coronary heart disease in male health professionals. *Ann Intern Med* 125:384, 1996.

155. Levander OA: Selenium and sulfur in antioxidant protective systems: Relationships with vitamin E and malaria. *Proc Soc Exp Biol Med* 200:255, 1992.

156. Rotruck JT, Pope AL, Ganther ME, et al: Selenium, biochemical role as a component of glutathione peroxidase. *Science* 179:588, 1973.

157. Hoekstra WG: Biochemical function of selenium and its relation to vitamin E. *Fed Proc* 34:2083, 1975.

158. Salonen JT: Selenium in ischaemic heart disease. *Intl J Epidemol* 16:323, 1987.

159. Salonen JT, Salonen R, Seppanen K, et al: Relationship of serum selenium and antioxidants to plasma lipoproteins, platelet aggregability and prevalent ischaemic heart disease in Eastern Finnish men. *Atherosclerosis* 70:155, 1988.

160. Hampel G, Watanabe K, Weksler B, Jaffe EA: Selenium deficiency inhibits prostacyclin release and enhances production of platelet activating factor by human endothelial cells. *Biochim Biophys Acta* 1006:151, 1989.

161. Salonen JT, Salonen R, Penttila I, et al: Serum fatty acids, apolipoproteins, selenium and vitamin antioxidants and the risk of death from coronary artery disease. *Am J Cardiol* 56:226, 1985.

162. Virtamo J, Valkeila E, Alfthan G, et al: Serum selenium and the risk of coronary heart disease and stroke. *Am J Epidemiol* 122:276, 1985.

163. Ringstad J, Jacobsen BK, Thomassen Y, Thelle DS: The Tromso Heart Study: Serum selenium and risk of myocardial infarction. A nested case-control study. *J Epidemiol Commun Health* 41:329, 1987.

164. Kok FJ, Hofman A, Witteman JCM, et al: Decreased selenium levels in acute myocardial infarction. *JAMA* 261:1161, 1989.

165. Suadicani P, Hein HO, Gyntelberg F: Serum selenium concentration and risk of ischemic heart disease in a prospective cohort study of 3000 males. *Atherosclerosis* 96:33, 1992.

166. Salvini S, Hennekens CH, Morris JS, et al: Plasma levels of the antioxidant selenium and risk of myocardial infarction among US physicians. *Am J Cardiol* 76:1218, 1995.

167. Kwiterovich PO: The effect of dietary fat, antioxidants, and prooxidants on blood lipids, lipoproteins, and atherosclerosis. *J Am Diet Assoc* 97(7 Suppl):S31, 1997.

168. Angstwurm MW, Schottdorf J, Schopohl J, et al: Selenium replacement in patients with severe systemic inflammatory response syndrome improves clinical outcome. *Crit Care Med* 27:1807, 1999.

168a. Steinberg D, Witztum JL: Is the oxidative modification hypothesis relevant to human atherosclerosis? Do the antioxidant trials conducted to date refute the hypothesis? *Circulation* 105:2107, 2002.

168b. Heart Protection Study Collaborative Group: MRC/BHF Heart Protection Study of antioxidant vitamin supplementation in 20536 high-risk individuals: A randomised placebo-controlled trial. *Lancet* 360:23, 2002.

169. Buffon A, Santini SA, Ramazzotti V, et al: Large, sustained cardiac lipid peroxidation and reduced antioxidant capacity in the coronary circulation after brief episodes of myocardial ischemia. *J Am Coll Cardiol* 35:633, 2000.

170. Ambrosio G, Weisman HF, Mannisi JA, Becker LC: Progressive impairment of regional myocardial perfusion after initial restoration of postischemic blood flow. *Circulation* 80:1846, 1989.

171. Ferrari R, Ceconi C, Curello S, et al: Oxygen mediated myocardial damage during ischemia and reperfusion: Role of the cellular defenses against oxygen toxicity. *J Mol Cell Cardiology* 17:937, 1985.

172. Entman ML, Smith WC: Postreperfusion inflammation: A model for reaction to injury in cardiovascular disease. *Cardiovasc Res* 28:1301, 1994.

173. Hansen PR: Role of neutrophils in myocardial ishemia and reperfusion. *Circulation* 91:1872, 1995.

174. Rosen GM, Freeman BA: Detection of superoxide generated by endothelial cells. *Proc Natl Acad Sci U S A* 81:7269, 1984.

175. Johnson AR, Revtyak G, Campbell WB: Arachidonic acid metabolites and endothelial injury: Studies with cultures of human endothelial cells. *Fed Proc* 44:19, 1985.

176. Kuhn H, Ponicke K, Halle W, et al: Evidence for the presence of lipoxygenase pathway in cultured endothelial cells. *Biomed Biochim Acta* 42:K1, 1983.

177. McCord JM, Roy RS, Schaffer SW: Free radicals and myocardial ischemia: The role of xanthine oxidase. In: Harris P, Poole-Wilson PA, eds. *Advances in Myocardiology*. Vol. 5. New York: Elsevier Science, 1985:183.

178. McCord JM: Oxygen-derived free radicals in post-ischemic tissue injury. *N Engl J Med* 312:159, 1985.

179. Chambers DE, Parks DA, Patterson G, et al: Xanthine oxidase as a source of free radical damage in myocardial ischemia. *J Mol Cell Cardiol* 17:145, 1985.

180. Werns SW, Shea MJ, Mitsos SE, et al: Reduction of the size of the infarction by allopurinol in the ischemic-reperfused canine heart. *Circulation* 73:518, 1986.

181. Kingma JG Jr, Denniss AR, Hearse DJ, et al: Limitation of infarct size for 24 hours by combined treatment with allopurinol plus verapamil during acute myocardial infarction in the dog. *Circulation* 75:V25, 1987.

182. Bando K, Tago M, Teramoto S: Prevention of free radical–induced myocardial injury by allopurinol. Experimental study in cardiac preservation and transplantation. *J Thorac Cardiovasc Surg* 95:465, 1988.

183. Stewart JR, Crute SL, Loughlin V, et al: Prevention of free radical–induced myocardial reperfusion injury with allopurinol. *J Thorac Cardiovasc Surg* 90:68, 1985.

184. Myers CL, Weiss SJ, Kirsh MH, Shlafer M: Involvement of hydrogen peroxide and hydroxyl radical in the oxygen paradox: Reduction of creatine kinase release by catalase, allopurinol, or deferoxamine but not by superoxide dismutase. *J Mol Cell Cardiol* 17:675, 1985.

185. Manning AS, Coltart DJ, Hearse DJ: Ischemia and reperfusion induced arrhythmias in the rat. Effects of xanthine oxidase inhibition with allopurinol. *Circ Res* 55:545, 1984.

186. Reimer KA, Jennings RB: Failure of the xanthine oxidase inhibitor allopurinol to limit infarct size after ischemia and reperfusion in dogs. *Circulation* 71:1069, 1985.

187. Downey JM, Miura T, Eddy LJ, et al: Xanthine oxidase is not a source of free radicals in the ischemic rabbit heart. *J Mol Cell Cardiol* 19:1053, 1987.

188. Morgan EJ: The distribution of xanthine oxidase. *Biochem J* 20:1282, 1926.

189. Johnson WD, Kayser KL, Brenowitz JB, Saedi SF: A randomized controlled trial of allopurinol in coronary bypass surgery. *Am Heart J* 121:20, 1991.

190. Tabayashi K, Suzuki Y, Nagamine S, et al: A clinical trial of allopurinol (Zyloric) for myocardial protection. *J Thorac Cardiovasc Surg* 101:713, 1991.

191. Coghlan JG, Flitter WD, Clutton SM, et al: Allopurinol pretreatment improves postoperative recovery and reduces lipid peroxidation in patients undergoing coronary artery bypass grafting. *J Thorac Cardiovasc Surg* 107:248, 1994.

192. Movahed A, Nair KG, Ashavaid TF, Kumar P: Free radical generation and the role of allopurinol as a cardioselective agent during coronary artery bypass grafting surgery. *Canad J Cardiol* 12:138, 1996.

193. Clancy RR, McGaurn SA, Goin JE: Allopurinol neurocardiac protection trial in infants undergoing heart surgery using deep hypothermic circulatory arrest. *Pediatrics* 108:61, 2001.

194. Tarkka MR, Vuolle M, Kaukinen S: Effect of allopurinol on myocardial oxygen free radical production in coronary bypass surgery. *Scand Cardiovasc J* 34(6):593, 2000.

195. Belboul A, Roberts D, Borjesson R, Johnsson J: Oxygen free radical generation in healthy blood donors and cardiac patients: The protective effect of allopurinol. *Perfusion* 16(1):59, 2001.

196. Taggart DP, Young V, Hooper J: Lack of cardioprotective efficacy of allopurinol in coronary artery surgery. *Br Heart J* 71:177, 1994.

197. Hoey BM, Butler J, Halliwell B: On the specificity of allopurinol and oxypurinol as inhibitors of xanthine oxidase. A pulse radiolysis determination of rate constants for reaction of allopurinol and oxypurinol with hydroxyl radicals. *Free Radic Res Commun* 4:259, 1988.

198. Das DK, Engleman RM, Clement R, et al: Role of xanthine oxidase inhibitor as free radical scavenger: A novel mechanism of action of allopurinol and oxypurinol in myocardial salvage. *Biochem Biophys Res Commun* 148:314, 1987.

199. Janssen M, Van der Meer P, De Jong JW: Antioxidant defences in rat, pig, guinea pig, and human hearts: Comparison with xanthine oxidoreductase activity. *Cardiovasc Res* 27:2052, 1993.

200. Khatib SY, Farah H, El-Migdadi F: Allopurinol enhances adenine nucleotide levels and improves myocardial function in isolated hypoxic rat heart. *Biochemistry* 66:328, 2001.

201. Maza SR, Frishman WH: Therapeutic options to minimize free radical damage and thrombogenicity in ischemic/reperfused myocardium. *Am Heart J* 114:1206, 1987.

202. Cappola TP, Kass DA, Nelson GS: Allopurinol improves myocardial efficiency in patients with idiopathic dilated cardiomyopathy. *Circulation* 104(20):2407, 2001.

203. Ukai T, Cheng CP, Tachibana H, et al: Allopurinol enhances the contractile response to dobutamine and exercise in dogs with pacing-induced heart failure. *Circulation* 103(5):750, 2001.

204. Shehab AM, Butler R, MacFadyen RJ, Struthers AD: A placebo-controlled study examining the effect of allopurinol on heart rate variability and dysrhythmia counts in chronic heart failure. *Br J Clin Pharmacol* 51(4):329, 2001.

205. Torok B, Roth E, Bar V, et al: Effects of antioxidant therapy in experimentally induced heart infarcts. *Basic Res Cardiol* 81:167, 1986.

206. Kloner RA, Przyklenk K, Whittaker P: Deleterious effects of oxygen radicals in ischemia/ reperfusion: Resolved and unresolved issues. *Circulation* 80:1115, 1989.

207. Beckman JS, Koppenol WH: Nitric oxide, superoxide, and peroxynitrite: the good, the bad, and the ugly. *Am J Physiol* 271:C1424, 1996.

208. Kroncke K-D, Fehsel K, Kolb-Bachofen V: Nitric oxide: Cytotoxicity versus cytoprotection: how, why, when and where? *Nitric Oxide Biol Chem* 1:107, 1997.

209. Beckman JS, Beckman TW, Chen J, et al: Apparent hydroxyl radical formation by peroxynitrite: Implications for endothelial injury

from nitric oxide and superoxide. *Proc Natl Acad Sci U S A* 86:1620, 1990.

210. Beckman JS, Ye YZ, Anderson PG, et al: Extensive nitration of protein tyrosines in human atherosclerosis detected by immunohistochemistry. *Biol Chem Hoppe Seyler* 5:81, 1994;.

211. Buttery LDK, Springall DR, Chester AH, et al: Inducible nitric oxide synthase is present within human atherosclerotic lesions and promotes the formation and activity of peroxynitrite. *Lab Invest* 75:77, 1996.

212. Stralin P, Karlsson K, Johansson BO, Marklund SL: The interstitium of the human arterial wall contains very large amounts of extracellular superoxide dismutase. *Arterioscler Thromb Vasc Biol* 15:2032, 1995.

213. Weisger RA, Fridovich I: Mitochondrial superoxide dismutase: site of synthesis and intramitochondrial localization. *J Biol Chem* 248:4793, 1973.

214. Negoro S, Kunisada K, Fujio Y: Activation of signal transducer and activator of transcription 3 protects cardiomyocytes from hypoxia/reoxygenation-induced oxidative stress through the upregulation of manganese superoxide dismutase. *Circulation* 28;104(9):979, 2001.

215. Abrahamsson T, Brandt U, Marklund SL, Sjoqvist PO: Vascular bound recombinant extracellular superoxide dismutase type C protects against the detrimental effects of superoxide radicals on endothelium-dependent arterial relaxation. *Circ Res* 70:264, 1992.

216. Karlsson K, Marklund SL: Heparin induced release of extracellular superoxide dismutase to human blood plasma. *Biochem J* 242:55, 1987.

217. Yamada H, Yamada Y, Adachi T, et al: Molecular analysis of extracellular superoxide dismutase gene associated with high levels in serum. *Jpn J Hum Genet* 40:177, 1995.

218. Sandstorm J, Nilsson P, Karlsson K, Marklund SL: 10-fold increase in human plasma extracellular superoxide dismutase content caused by a mutation in heparin-binding domain. *J Biol Chem* 269:19163, 1994.

219. Adachi T, Yamada H, Yamada Y, et al: Substitution of glycine for arginine-213 in extracellular-superoxide dismutase impairs affinity for heparin and endothelial cell surface. *Biochem J* 313:235, 1996.

220. Wang XL, Adachi T, Sim AS, Wilcken DEL: Plasma extracellular superoxide dismutase levels in an Australian population with coronary artery disease. *Arterioscler Thromb Vasc Biol* 12:1915, 1998.

221. Landmesser U, Merten R, Spiekermann S, et al: Vascular extracellular superoxide dismutase activity in patients with coronary artery disease. Relation to endothelium-dependent vasodilation. *Circulation* 101:2264, 2000.

222. Ennezat PV, Malendowicz SL, Testa M: Physical training in patients with chronic heart failure enhances the expression of genes encoding antioxidative enzymes. *J Am Coll Cardiol* 38(1):194, 2001.

223. Bolli R: Mechanism of myocardial "stunning." *Circulation* 82:723, 1990.

224. Myers ML, Bolli R, Lekich RF, et al: Enhancement of recovery of myocardial function by oxygen free radical scavengers after reversible regional ischemia. *Circulation* 72:915, 1985.

225. Ambrosio G, Weisfeldt ML, Jacobus WE, Flaherty JT: Evidence for a reversible oxygen radical-mediated component of reperfusion injury: Reduction by recombinant human superoxide dismutase administered at the time of reflow. *Circulation* 75:282, 1987.

226. Przyklenk K, Kloner RA: "Reperfusion injury" by oxygen-derived free radicals? Effect of superoxide dismutase plus catalase, given at the time of reperfusion, on myocardial infarct size, contractile function, coronary microvasculature, and regional myocardial blood flow. *Circ Res* 64:86, 1989.

227. Asinger RW, Peterson DA, Elsperger KJ, et al: Long-term recovery of LV wall thickening after one hour of ischemia is not affected when superoxide dismutase and catalase are administered during the first 45 min of reperfusion (abstr). *J Am Coll Cardiol* 11:163A, 1988.

228. Patel BS, Jeroudi MO, O'Neill PG, et al: Effect of human recombinant superoxide dismutase on canine myocardial infarction. *Am J Physiol* 258:H369, 1990.

229. Murohara Y, Yui Y, Hattori R, Kawai C: Effects of superoxide dismutase on reperfusion arrhythmias and left ventricular function in patients undergoing thrombolysis for anterior wall acute myocardial infarction. *Am J Cardiol* 67:765, 1991.

230. Flaherty JT, Pitt B, Gruber JW, et al: Recombinant human superoxide dismutase (h-SOD) fails to improve recovery of ventricular function in patients undergoing coronary angioplasty for acute myocardial infarction. *Circulation* 89:1982, 1994.

231. Omar BA, Gad NM, Jordan MC, et al: Cardioprotection by Cu, Zn-superoxide dismutase is lost at high doses in the reoxygenated heart. *Free Radic Biol Med* 9:465, 1990.

232. Omar BA, McCord JM: The cardioprotective effect of Mn-superoxide dismutase is lost at high doses in the postischemic isolated rabbit heart. *Free Radic Biol Med* 9:473, 1990.

233. Starke PE, Farber JL: Ferric iron and superoxide ions are required for the killing of cultured hepatocytes by hydrogen peroxide: Evidence for the participation of hydroxyl radicals formed by an iron-catalyzed Haber-Weiss reaction. *J Biol Chem* 260:10099, 1985.

234. Halliwell B: Superoxide-dependent formation of hydroxyl radicals in the presence of iron salts is a feasible source of hydroxyl radicals in vivo (letter). *Biochem J* 205:461, 1982.

235. Manning AS, Hearse DJ: Reperfusion-induced arrhythmias: mechanisms and prevention. *J Mol Cell Cardiol* 16:497, 1984.

236. Bernier M, Hearse DJ, Manning AS: Reperfusion-induced arrhythmias and oxygen-derived free radicals: Studies with "anti-free radical" interventions and a free radical–generating system in the isolated perfused rat heart. *Circ Re*s 58:331, 1986.

237. Riva E, Manning AS, Hearse DJ: Superoxide dismutase and the reduction of reperfusion-induced arrhythmias: In vivo dose-response studies in the rat. *Cardiovasc Drugs Ther* 1:133, 1987.

238. Nejima J, Knight DR, Fallon JT, et al: Superoxide dismutase reduces reperfusion arrhythmias but fails to salvage regional function or myocardium at risk in conscious dogs. *Circulation* 79:143, 1989.

239. Otani H, Tanaka H, Inoue T, et al: In vitro study on contribution of oxidative metabolism of isolated rabbit heart mitochondria to myocardial reperfusion injury. *Circ Res* 55:168, 1984.

240. Shlafer M, Kane PF, Kirsch MM: Effects of dimethylsulfoxide on the globally ischemic heart: Possible general relevance to hypothermic organ preservation. *Cryobiology* 19:61, 1982.

241. Land W, Schneeberger H, Schleibner S, et al: The beneficial effect of human recombinant superoxide dismutase on acute and chronic rejection events in recipients of cadaveric renal transplants. *Transplantation* 57:211, 1994.

242. Stein J: PEG-SOD offers new hope for patients with severe head injury. *Inpharma* 899:15, 1993.

243. Melov S, Ravenscroft J, Malik S, et al: Extension of life-span with superoxide dismutase/catalase mimetics. *Science* 289:1567, 2000.

244. Jadot G, Vaille A, Maldonado J, Vanelle P: Clinical pharmacokinetics and delivery of bovine superoxide dismutase. *Clin Pharmacokinet* 28:17, 1995.

245. Nakajima H, Hangaishi M, Ishizaka N, et al: Lecithinized copper, zinc-superoxide dismutase ameliorates ischemia-induced myocardial damage. *Life Sci* 69(8):935, 2001.

246. Hangaishi M, Nakajima H, Taguchi J: Lecithinized Cu, Zn-superoxide dismutase limits the infarct size following ischemia-reperfusion injury in rat hearts in vivo. *Biochem Biophys Res Commun* 285(5):1220, 2001.

247. Kanamasa K, Ishida N, Ishikawa K: Protective effect of PEG-SOD against early coronary reperfusion injury assessed in reperfused and non-reperfused ischaemic areas of the same heart. *Acta Cardiol* 56(3):181, 2001.

248. Rubin R, Farber JL: Mechanisms of the killing of cultured hepatocytes by hydrogen peroxide. *Arch Biochem Biophys* 228:450, 1984.

249. Przyklenk K, Kloner RA: Superoxide dismutase plus catalase improve contractile function in the canine model of the "stunned myocardium." *Circ Res* 58:148, 1986.

250. Greenfield DT, Greenfield LJ, Hess ML: Enhancement of crystalloid cardioplegic protection against global normothermic ischemia by superoxide dismutase plus catalase but not diltiazem in the isolated, working rat heart. *J Thorac Cardiovasc Surg* 95:799, 1988.

251. Gallagher KP, Buda AJ, Pace D, et al: Failure of superoxide dismutase and catalase to alter size of infarction in conscious dogs after 3 h of occlusion followed by reperfusion. *Circulation* 73:1065, 1986.

252. Jeroudi MO, Triana FJ, Patel BS, Bolli R: Effect of superoxide dismutase and catalase, given separately, on myocardial "stunning." *Am J Physiol* 259:H889, 1990.

253. Myers CL, Weiss SJ, Kirsh MM, et al: Effects of supplementing hypothermic crystalloid cardioplegic solution with catalase, superoxide dismutase, allopurinol, or deferoxamine on functional recovery of globally ischemic and reperfused isolated hearts. *J Thorac Cardiovasc Surg* 91:281, 1986.

254. Jolly SR, Kane WJ, Bailie MB, et al: Canine myocardial reperfusion injury. Its reduction by the combined administration of superoxide dismutase and catalase. *Circ Res* 54:277, 1984.

255. Werns SW, Shea MJ, Driscoll EM, et al: The independent effects of oxygen radical scavengers on canine infarct size. Reduction by superoxide dismutase but not catalase. *Circ Res* 56:895, 1985.

256. Marchetti G, Lodola E, Licciardello L, Colombo A: Use of N-acetylcysteine in the management of coronary artery diseases. *Cardiologia* 44(7):633, 1999.

257. Woods KL, Fletcher S: Long term outcome after intravenous magnesium sulphate in suspected acute myocardial infarction: The second Leicester Intravenous Magnesium Intervention Trial (LIMIT-2). *Lancet* 343:816, 1994.

258. Woods KL: Possible pharmacological actions of magnesium in acute myocardial infarction. *Br J Clin Pharmacol* 32:3, 1991.

259. Garcia LA, Dejong SC, Martin SM, et al: Magnesium reduces free radicals in an in vivo coronary occlusion reperfusion model. *J Am Coll Cardiol* 32:536, 1998.

260. Afanas'ev IB, Suslova TB, Cheremisina ZP, et al: Study of antioxidant properties of metal aspartates. *Analyst* 1995;120:859, 1998.

261. Dickens BF, Weglicki WB, Li YS, Mak IT: Magnesium deficiency in vitro enhances free radical-induced intracellular oxidation and cytotoxicity in endothelial cells. *FEBS Lett* 311:187, 1992.

262. Rukshin V, Azarbal B, Shah PK, et al: Intravenous magnesium in experimental stent thrombosis in swine. *Arterioscler Thromb Vasc Biol* 21(9):1544, 2001.

263. Shechter M, Kaplinsky E, Rabinowitz B: The rationale of magnesium supplementation in acute MI: A review of the literature. *Arch Intern Med* 152:2189, 1992.

264. Shibata M, Ueshima K, Harada M, et al: Effect of Mg pretreatment and significance of matrix metalloproteinase-1 and interleukin-6 levels in coronary reperfusion therapy for patients with acute myocardial infarction. *Angiology* 50(7):573, 1999.

265. ISIS-4 (Fourth International Study of Infarct Survival) Collaborative Group: ISIS-4: A randomised factorial trial assessing early oral captopril, oral mononitrate, and intravenous magnesium sulphate in 58,050 patients with suspected acute myocardial infarction. *Lancet* 345(8951):669, 1995.

266. Santoro GM, Antoniucci D, Bolognese L, et al: A randomized study of intravenous magnesium in acute myocardial infarction treated with direct coronary angioplasty. *Am Heart J* 140(6):891, 2000.

267. Gallagher MM, Allshire AP: Failure of magnesium to protect isolated cardiomyocytes from effects of hypoxia or metabolic poisoning. *Clin Cardiol* 23(7):530, 2000.

268. Hammond B, Hess ML: The oxygen free radical system: Potential mediator of myocardial injury. *J Am Coll Cardiol* 6:215, 1985.

269. Ouriel K, Ginsburg ME, Patti CS, et al: Preservation of myocardial function with mannitol reperfusate. *Circulation* 72(Suppl 2):II254, 1985.

270. Kloner RA, Reimer KA, Willerson JT, Jennings RB: Reduction of experimental myocardial infarct size with hyperosmolar mannitol. *Proc Soc Exp Biol Med* 151:677, 1976.

271. Powell Jr WJ, DiBora DR, Flores J, Leaf A: The protective effect of hyperosmotic mannitol in myocardial ischemia and necrosis. *Circulation* 54:603, 1976.

272. Justicz AG, Farnsworth WV, Soberman MS, et al: Reduction of myocardial infarct size by poloxamer 188 and mannitol in a canine model. *Am Heart J* 122:671, 1991.

273. Powell WJ Jr, DiBona DR, Flores J, et al: Effects of hyperosmotic mannitol in reducing ischemic cell swelling and minimizing myocardial necrosis. *Circulation* 53(Suppl 3):I45, 1976.

274. Del Maestro RF, Thau HH, Bjork J, et al: Free radicals as mediators of tissue injury. *Acta Physiol Scand* 492(Suppl 1):43, 1980.

275. Harada RN, Limm W, Piette LH, McNamara JJ: Failure of mannitol to reduce myocardial infarct size in the baboon. *Cardiovasc Res* 26:893, 1992.

276. Willerson JT, Curry GC, Atkins JM, et al: Influence of hypertonic mannitol on ventricular performance and coronary blood flow in patients. *Circulation* 51:1095, 1975.

277. Ferreira R, Burgos M, Llesuy S, et al: Reduction of reperfusion injury with mannitol cardioplegia. *Ann Thorac Surg* 48:77, 1989.

278. Laskowski H, Minczykowski A, Wysocki H: Mortality and clinical course of patients with acute myocardial infarction treated with streptokinase and antioxidants: mannitol and ascorbic acid. *Int J Cardiol* 48:235, 1995.

279. Ely SW, Berne RM: Protective effects of adenosine in myocardial ischemia. *Circulation* 85:893, 1992.

280. Forman MB, Velasco CE, Jackson EK: Adenosine attenuates reperfusion injury following regional myocardial ischemia. *Cardiovasc Res* 27:9, 1993.

281. Mauser M, Hoffmeister HM, Nienaber C, Schaper W: Influence of ribose, adenosine, and "AICAR" on the rate of myocardial adenosine triphosphate synthesis during reperfusion after coronary artery occlusion in the dog. *Circ Res* 56:220, 1985.

282. Richardt G, Wass W, Kranzhofer R, et al: Adenosine inhibits exocytotic release of endogenous noradrenaline in rat heart: A protective mechanism in early myocardial ischemia. *Circ Res* 61:117, 1987.

283. Cronstein BN, Kramer SB, Weissman G, Hirschhorn R: Adenosine: A physiologic modulator of superoxide anion generation by human neutrophils. *J Exp Med* 158:1160, 1983.

284. Jordan JE, Zhao Z, Sato H, et al: Adenosine A2–receptor activation attenuates reperfusion injury by inhibiting neutrophil accumulation, superoxide generation and coronary endothelial adherence. *J Pharmacol Exp Ther* 280:301, 1997.

285. Cronstein BN, Levin RI, Belanoff J, et al: Adenosine: An endogenous inhibitor of neutrophil-mediated injury to endothelial cells. *J Clin Invest* 78:760, 1986.

286. Babbitt DG, Bermani R, Forman MB: Intracoronary adenosine administered after reperfusion limits vascular injury after prolonged ischemia in the canine model. *Circulation* 80:1388, 1989.

287. Babbitt DG, Virmani R, Vildibill HD, et al: Intracoronary adenosine administration during reperfusion following 3 hours of ischemia: Effects on infarct size, ventricular function, and regional myocardial blood flow. *Am Heart J* 120:808, 1990.

288. Pitarys CJ, Virmani R, Vildibill HD, et al: Reduction of myocardial reperfusion injury by intravenous adenosine administered during the early reperfusion period. *Circulation* 83:237, 1991.

289. Garratt KN, Gibbons RJ, Reeder GS, et al: Intravenous adenosine and lidocaine to limit reperfusion injury during acute myocardial infarction: preliminary data. *J Am Coll Cardiol* 25(suppl):104A, 1995.

290. Garratt KN, Holmes DR Jr, Molina-Viamonte V, et al: Intravenous adenosine and lidocaine in patients with acute myocardial infarction. *Am Heart J* 136(2):196, 1998.

291. Marzilli M, Marraccini P, Gliozheni E, et al: Intracoronary adenosine as an adjunct to combined use of primary angioplasty in acute MI: Beneficial effects on angiographically assessed no-reflow (abstr). *J Am Coll Cardiol* 28(suppl):406A, 1996.

292. Lincoff AM, Topol EJ: Illusion of reperfusion. Does anyone achieve optimal reperfusion during acute myocardial infarction? *Circulation* 88:1361, 1993.

292a. Mahaffey KW, Puma JA, Barbagelata A, et al for the AMISTAD Investigators: Adenosine as an adjunct to thrombolytic therapy for acute myocardial infarction. *J Am Coll Card* 34:1711, 1999.

292b. Williams ES, Miller JM: Results from late-breaking clinical trials Sessions at the American College of Cardiology 51st Annual Scientific Session. *J Am Coll Cardiol* 40:1, 2002.

293. Gibbons RJ, Christian TF, Hopfenspirger M, et al: Myocardium at risk and infarct size after thrombolytic therapy for acute MI: Implications for the design of randomized trials of acute myocardial intervention. *J Am Coll Cardiol* 24:616, 1994.

294. Suguhara T, Horikawa M, Hikita M, et al: Studies on a sulfhydryl radioprotector of low toxicity. *Experientia* 27:53, 1977.

295. Devi P: Chemical radiation protection by alpha-mercapto-propionyl glycine. *J Nucl Med Allied Sci* 27:327, 1983.

296. Mitsos SE, Fantone JC, Gallagher KP, et al: Canine myocardial reperfusion injury: protection by a free radical scavenger, N-2 mercaptopropionyl glycine. *J Cardiovasc Pharmacol* 8:978, 1986.

297. Mitsos SE, Askew TE, Fantone JC, et al: Protective effects of N-3-mercapto-propionyl glycine against myocardial reperfusion injury after neutrophil depletion in the dog: evidence for the role of intracellular-derived free radicals. *Circulation* 73:1077, 1986.

298. Horwitz LD, Fennessey PV, Shikes RH, et al: Marked reduction in myocardial infarct size due to prolonged infusion of an antioxidant during reperfusion. *Circulation* 89:1792, 1994.

299. el-Missiry MA, Othman AI, Amer MA, Abd el-Aziz MA: Attenuation of the acute Adriamycin-induced cardiac and hepatic oxidative toxicity by N-(2-mercaptopropionyl) glycine in rats. *Free Radic Res* 35(5):575, 2001.

300. Migliaccio E, Giorgia M, Mele S, et al: The p66[shc] adaptor protein controls oxidative stress response and life span in mammals. *Nature* 402:309, 1999.

301. Abunasra HJ, Smolenski RT, Morrison K, et al: Efficacy of adenoviral gene transfer with manganese superoxide dismutase and endothelial nitric oxide synthase in reducing ischemia and reperfusion injury. *Eur J Cardiothorac Surg* 20(1):153, 2001.

302. Li Q, Bolli R, Qiu Y, et al: Gene therapy with extracellular superoxide dismutase protects conscious rabbits against myocardial infarction. *Circulation* 103(14):1893, 2001.

303. Chen Z, Oberley TD, Ho Y, et al: Overexpression of CuZnSOD in coronary vascular cells attenuates myocardial ischemia/reperfusion injury. *Free Radic Biol Med* 29(7):589, 2000.

CHAPTER 25

Use of Prostacyclin and Its Analogues in the Treatment of Pulmonary Hypertension and Other Cardiovascular Diseases

William H. Frishman

Masoud Azizad

Yogesh Agarwal

Daniel W. Kang

The prostaglandin and prostacyclin (PGI$_2$) story begins in 1933, when von Euler discovered a lipophilic substance in the seminal fluid. Erroneously thinking that this substance was produced predominantly in the prostate, he called it prostaglandin.[1] Many years later, prostacyclin was isolated and synthesized by Moncada et al.,[2] and that same year its chemical structure was described by Whittaker et al.[3] (Fig. 25-1). Prostacyclin is now commercially available for intravenous administration as epoprostenol (Flolan), and many stable analogues, including some for oral and inhalational use, are undergoing investigation.

Prostacyclin is found in all tissues and body fluids and is the major metabolite of arachidonic acid in the vasculature.[4] Arachidonic acid is metabolized by cyclooxygenase to PGG$_2$ and then by PG hydroperoxidase into PGH$_2$. These compounds are converted into prostacyclin by PGI$_2$ synthetase[5,6] (Fig. 25-2). Prostacyclin is produced predominantly in the endothelium and also by smooth muscle[4,5,7,8] and has interesting physiologic activity in relation to the cardiovascular system. It is the most potent vasodilator known and affects both the pulmonary and the systemic circulation.[9] Relaxation of the blood vessels is caused by increases in intracellular cAMP of vascular smooth muscle. Prostacyclin has also been noted to prevent smooth muscle proliferation. Platelet aggregation and adhesion are inhibited by the increase of intracellular cAMP induced by prostacyclin.[10,11] An interesting note is that platelet aggregation is inhibited before adhesion.[12]

These features have made it a very attractive substance for the treatment of many different cardiovascular diseases. Patients with primary pulmonary hypertension (PPH), congestive heart failure (CHF), myocardial ischemia, Raynaud's phenomenon, and peripheral vascular disease have all been treated with epoprostenol and its more stable analogues.

EPOPROSTENOL

Epoprostenol is the first synthetic prostacyclin to become commercially available and is currently approved for use in patients with PPH. It has the same structure as prostacyclin and is a very unstable molecule; its in vitro half-life at physiologic pH is approximately 6 min and is noted to be longer in alkaline solutions.[13] It is also degraded by light. The product must be freeze-dried and stored at temperatures between 15 and 25°C. The drug must be reconstituted just prior to administration in a glycine buffer with a pH of 10.5 and must be protected from exposure to light during reconstitution and infusion. At room temperature, a single infusion should be completed within 8 h after the medication is reconstituted. Epoprostenol must be administered intravenously, since it is degraded by the gastrointestinal tract before it can be absorbed.

Epoprostenol's in vivo half-life in humans is not measurable. In animal models, the half-life of epoprostenol is 2.7 min. It is hydrolyzed to 6-ketoprostaglandin F1$_\alpha$ in vitro,[5] but in vivo, PGI$_2$ undergoes catalyzed oxidation to 15-*keto*-PGI$_2$.[14] It has been noted that apolipoprotein (apo A-I), a molecule associated with high-density lipoproteins (HDL), can prolong the half-life of prostacyclin.[15]

Clinical Use

Studies done with epoprostenol have usually initiated the infusion rate at a dose ranging from 1 to 2 ng/kg/min with increases in the infusion rate at 5- to 15-min increments of 1 to 2 ng/kg/min until the appearance of side effects or the desired long-term infusion dose is obtained.[16–22] The manufacturer of the drug recommends initiating the infusion with epoprostenol at 2 ng/kg/min and increasing it at increments of 2 ng/kg/min every 15 min. The drug is titrated until the appearance of side effects, including systemic hypotension, or until the desired long-term infusion dose is obtained. The infusion rate can be easily lowered to a dose at which there are no side effects, and if severe systemic hypotension develops, the infusion can be stopped, with the patient returning to baseline hemodynamic status quickly.[23] This method can be used in both acute hemodynamic testing and long-term infusion. With long-term infusion, the dosage can easily be readjusted to meet the patient's changing needs. Tolerance to prostacyclin has been observed, but the dose can be downtitrated while preserving its therapeutic activity, especially if a high cardiac output state is observed.[24]

Several side effects are noted with the drug, most commonly flushing, headache, nausea and vomiting, anxiety, and systemic hypotension. Other less common side effects are chest pain, dizziness,

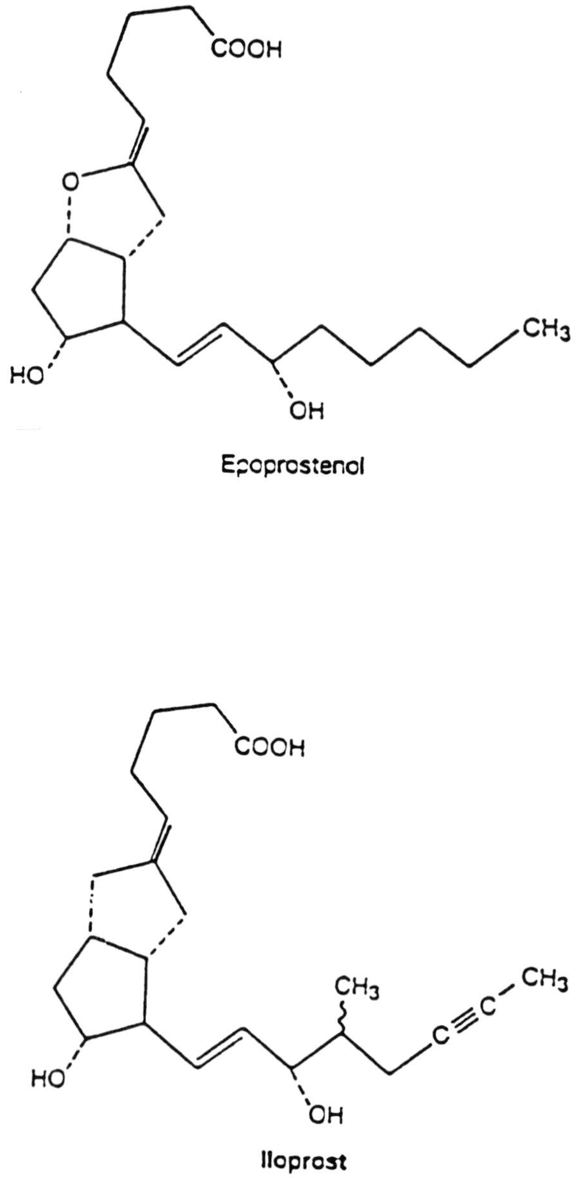

FIGURE 25-1. Chemical structures of epoprostenol (prostacyclin, PGI_2) and iloprost.

bradycardia, abdominal pain, sweating, dyspepsia, hyperesthesia, paresthesia, tachycardia, headache, diarrhea, flulike symptoms, and jaw pain (Table 25-1). These unwanted effects are easily reversed by discontinuing the medication.[23]

Most problems with long-term administration of the drug are related to the need for continuous intravenous delivery. These conditions include sepsis, line occlusion secondary to thrombosis, and pump failure—problems that can result in fatalities. Long-term studies have shown that most patients are able to reconstitute and properly administer their medication safely at home.[16–22]

Primary Pulmonary Hypertension

PPH is an idiopathic disease that is divided into three groups based on pathology: plexogenic arteriopathy, venoocclusive disease, and capillary hemangiomatosis. All three conditions can also be complicated by thrombosis in situ.[25,25a] Plexogenic arteriopathy is the most common form and is characterized by abnormalities

in the intima and media of precapillary vessels, which can range from mild neointimal proliferation to intimal fibrosis, plexiform lesions, and necrotizing arteritis.[26] Pulmonary venoocclusive disease is less common and is characterized by fibrosis of the endovascular walls of small- and medium-sized veins.[25] The least common form, pulmonary capillary hemangiomatosis, is characterized by proliferation of the capillary network, leading to changes in the arterial bed.[25–27]

Although the mechanisms behind the disease are not completely elucidated, it does appear that there are definite features of the disease process.[28] There is an imbalance of endothelial mediators of vascular tone characterized by an unfavorable balance between thromboxane A and prostacyclin, predisposing the vasculature to thrombosis and constriction.[29] There is also an increase in the production of endothelin by the pulmonary vasculature,[30] a decrease in endothelial clearance, and an increase in circulating endothelin levels in patients with PPH,[31] which causes further vasoconstriction. In addition, plasma serotonin concentrations are raised in PPH patients.[32] It also seems that there is a cycle involving vascular injury from an unknown cause in susceptible individuals,[26] which leads to smooth muscle invasion of the endothelium and a further disruption of the normal balance of vascular tone and coagulation mediators, further predisposing the endothelium to thrombosis and obstruction.[25] A defect in K^+ channels in the smooth muscle cells of the pulmonary artery may add to vasoconstriction. Intracellular calcium is an important regulator of smooth muscle contraction and proliferation, and the voltage-gated K^+ channels that determine cytoplasmic concentrations of free Ca^{+2} may be defective in patients with PPH.[33] Presenting symptoms of the disease are dyspnea on exertion, syncope, and chest pain pain.[27,34]

The estimated annual incidence of PPH is one to two cases per million people per year, and the mean age at diagnosis is 36 years.[28] The disease has a poor prognosis. The results of a national registry of patients with PPH published in 1991[35] found that patients had a mean survival of 2.8 years after diagnostic catheterization was performed. In this study, the survival rate at 1 year was 68%; at 3 years, 48%; and at 5 years, 34%. In this registry, 39% of the patients had been diagnosed with PPH before being entered into the registry, but there was no significant difference between their survival rates and the survival rates of those who had not been previously diagnosed.

Traditionally, this disease has been treated with strong arterial vasodilators, such as calcium-channel blockers,[36] anticoagulants,[37] and supplemental oxygen when needed.[37a] Nitrates have also been used as a treatment, and rarely cardiac glycosides and diuretics are used, but only with extreme caution.[38–40] Recently, the orally active endothelin antagonist bosentan was approved for clinical use in patients with PPH (see Chap. 31).[40a] There are always a number of patients who fail to respond to medical treatment. Heart and lung transplantation[41] and lung transplantation[42,43] have been employed successfully in patients with PPH.

Epoprostenol was approved by the U.S. Food and Drug Administration (FDA) for use in patients with PPH and seems to be useful in two ways. First, epoprostenol use appears to provide a safe method to screen patients with PPH for responsiveness to drug therapy. Second, epoprostenol has been shown to prolong survival in patients with New York Heart Association (NYHA) class III and IV heart failure secondary to PPH.

There are well-defined goals for screening responsiveness to drug therapy in PPH. Not all patients respond to medication, and some have an unfavorable response. An ideal response to administration of medication in patients with PPH would be a 20% decrease

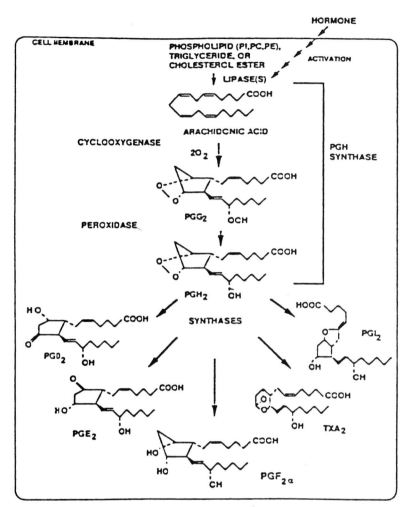

FIGURE 25-2. Hormone-activated prostanoid biosynthesis in a model cell. Although all products of "cyclooxygenase pathway" are shown, usually only one prostanoid is formed as a major product by a given cell type. PGH = prostaglandin endoperoxide; PI, PC, and PE = phosphatidylinositol, phosphatidylcholine, and phosphatidylethanolamine, respectively; PGG_2, PGD_2, PGE_2, and PGF_{2a} = prostaglandin G_2, D_2, E_2, and F_{2a}, respectively; PGI_2 = prostacyclin; TXA_2 = thromboxane A_2. (*Reproduced with permission from Smith WL: Prostanoid biosynthesis and mechanism of action. Am J Physiol 263:F181–F191, 1992.*)

in pulmonary vascular resistance (PVR) or a decrease in PVR with a 20% decrease in pulmonary artery pressure (PAP) with or without an increase in cardiac output. An unfavorable response would be the development of symptomatic systemic hypotension or an observed decrease in cardiac output. A nonresponder to therapy would be a person who did not show any significant change in PVR or PAP without the development of adverse side affects.[44]

Epoprostenol seems to be an ideal screening agent for identifying responsiveness to medical therapy in patients with PPH.[38] Advantages of this medication are its easy titratability, its potency, and its short half-life.[38] Other medications used for screening responsiveness to therapy in patients with PPH are acetylcholine,[45] adenosine,[46] nitric oxide,[47] and sublingual nifedipine.[48] Epoprostenol is more potent than acetylcholine, giving it an advantage in this respect.[49] Adenosine causes a decrease in pulmonary pressure, but it is suggested that this result is secondary to its actions on cardiac output and not because of its effects on the pulmonary vasculature.[50,51] Nitric oxide seems to be comparable to epoprostenol in many of its hemodynamic actions. It has a short half-life and causes a decrease in PVR. In a comparative study, Jolliet et al. compared the effects of sequentially administered nitric oxide, PGI_2, and nifedipine in 10 patients with precapillary pulmonary hypertension for screening patient responsiveness to vasodilators.[52] They concluded that nitric oxide inhalation had a predictive ability at least as good or perhaps better than PGI_2 without the associated decrease in systemic vascular resistance (SVR), systemic mean

arterial pressure, and consequent increase in heart rate and cardiac index. Nitric oxide also does not cause systemic hypotension. However, it is not clear at this time whether nitric oxide will replace epoprostenol as a screening agent for assessing responsiveness to medical treatment in PPH.[53] Sublingual nifedipine has also been shown to have effects on the pulmonary and systemic circulations similar to those of epoprostenol. However, the utility of nifedipine is limited by its longer half-life.[48]

If the patient has a favorable drop in PVR with epoprostenol without experiencing systemic hypotension, it is a good indication that the patient will have a favorable response to longer-acting vasodilators such as nifedipine.

The other use for prostacyclin is in severely ill PPH patients who do not seem to be responding to other medical therapy. Recent studies have shown that long-term infusion of epoprostenol can improve survival in patients with PPH.

In 1990, Rubin et al.[16] published the result of a small randomized trial looking at the effect of epoprostenol in patients with PPH who had not responded to traditional therapy or had adverse reactions to therapy. They studied 24 patients with PPH with NYHA classes III and IV heart failure for 8 weeks and found that patients who received epoprostenol improved symptomatically and had improved hemodynamic function. Acutely, epoprostenol caused no change in PAP, decreased PVR from 27 to 32%, decreased systemic blood pressure, and increased cardiac output by 40%. At 2 months, there were no statistically significant changes in the hemodynamics of

TABLE 25-1. Adverse Events with Epoprostenol Infusion

Adverse Events in ≥1% of Patients	Epoprostenol (% Pts, $n = 391$)*
During Acute Dose Ranging†	
Flushing	58
Headache	49
Nausea/vomiting	32
Hypotension	16
Anxiety, nervousness, agitation	11
Chest pain	11
Dizziness	8
Bradycardia	5
Abdominal pain	5
Musculoskeletal pain	3
Dyspnea	2
Back pain	2
Sweating	1
Dyspepsia	1
Hypesthesia/parestheia	1
Tachycardia	1

Adverse Events in ≥1% of Patients	Epoprostenol (% Pts, $n = 52$)	Standard Therapy (% Pts, $n = 54$)
Occurrence More Common with Epoprostenol		
General		
Chills, fever, sepsis, flu-like symptoms	25	11
Cardiovascular		
Tachycardia	35	24
Flushing	42	2
Gastrointestinal		
Diarrhea	37	6
Nausea/vomiting	67	48
Musculoskeletal		
Jaw pain	54	0
Myalgia	44	31
Nonspecific musculoskeletal pain	35	15
Neurologic		
Anxiety/nervousness, tremor	21	9
Dizziness	83	70
Headache	83	33
Hypesthesia, hyperesthesia, paresthesia	12	2
Occurrence More Common with Standard Therapy		
Cardiovascular		
Heart failure	31	52
Syncope	13	24
Shock	0	13
Respiratory		
Hypoxia	25	37

*Thrombocytopenia has been reported during uncontrolled clinical trials in patients receiving epoprostenol.

†Interpretation of adverse events is complicated by the clinical features of primary pulmonary hypertension, which are similar to some of the pharmacologic effects of epoprostenol (dizziness, syncope). Adverse events probably related to the underlying disease include dyspnea, fatigue, chest pain, right ventricular failure, and pallor. Several adverse events, on the other hand, can clearly be attributed to epoprostenol, including headache, jaw pain, flushing, diarrhea, nausea and vomiting, flu-like symptoms, and anxiety/nervousness. In an effort to separate the adverse effects of the drug from those of the underlying disease, the following lists adverse events that occurred at a rate at least 10% different in the two groups in controlled trials.

Source: Reproduced from package insert for Flolan.

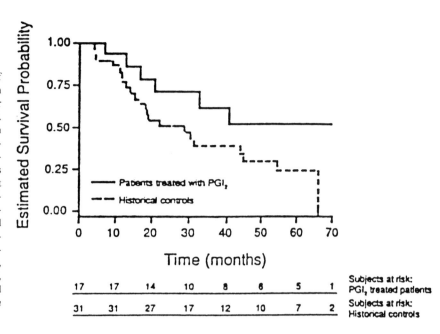

FIGURE 25-3. In patients with PPH, a comparison of survival probabilities between patients treated with prostacyclin and historical controls. Kaplan-Meier observed survival probability curves for NYHA class III and IV patients treated with prostacyclin ($n = 17$) and historical controls from the NIH Registry [NYHA class III and IV patients receiving standard therapy including anticoagulant agents ($n = 31$)]. Survival function was calculated at 6-month intervals for 5 years. Survival was significantly improved in the patients treated with prostacyclin ($P = .045$). The 1-, 2-, and 3-year predicted survival rates estimated by the NIH Primary Pulmonary Hypertension Registry equation for the patients treated with prostacyclin were 63.2, 50.4, and 41.1% respectively; for the historical controls, the predicted survival rates were 65.2, 52.1, and 42.4%, respectively. (*Reproduced with permission from Barst et al.*[17])

either group as compared with the beginning of therapy; however, there was a decrease in PVR from 21.6 to 13.9 U in the epoprostenol group, which approached statistical significance. Perhaps more interesting is that all the epoprostenol patients had an improvement in their NYHA functional class, compared with two patients receiving conventional therapy. Both groups also had improvement in the distance walked during a 6-min walk test, with the epoprosentol group showing a larger increase in distance walked.

Seventeen of these patients were followed from 37 to 69 months in an open, uncontrolled trial.[17] When compared with historical controls, this group showed a decrease in mortality, with a 3-year survival rate of 63.3%, compared with 40.6% in the control group (Fig. 25-3). These patients also had an improvement of approximately 100 m in a 6-min walk test after 6 and 18 months of treatment with epoprostenol, and they showed some improvement in their hemodynamic variables (Table 25-2).

Barst et al.[18] published the results of the largest epoprostenol trial in patients with PPH. In this study, 81 patients were randomized to receive epoprostenol or standard therapy for 12 weeks. Again, there was a dramatic improvement in exercise capacity and

a decrease in mortality with epoprostenol. Patients who received epoprostenol were able to walk farther during a 6-min walk test after 12 weeks of epoprostenol infusion. The control group showed a 29-m decrease in the distance walked in 6 min. Functional class improved in 40% of the epoprostenol group in this study. While 48% did not have any change in functional class, 13% worsened. In the control group, 3% improved in functional class, whereas 87% remained unchanged and 10% worsened. It should be noted that only survivors who did not undergo transplant were included in the above figures and that there were no deaths in the epoprostenol group and eight among the controls. Cardiac parameters also improved with epoprostenol treatment (Table 25-3). Patients treated with epoprostenol also reported improvement using the Nottingham Health Profile.

Hinderliter et al.[19] later expanded on this trial by describing the echocardiographic changes associated with long-term epoprostenol therapy. The echocardiographic results showed that patients treated with continuous infusion of epoprostenol for 12 weeks had a lower maximal tricuspid regurgitant jet velocity, less right ventricular dilatation, an improved curvature of the intraventricular septum

TABLE 25-2. Hemodynamic Effects of Continuous Epoprostenol Infusion in Patients with Primary Pulmonary Hypertension after 6 Months and 12 Months of Follow-Up (Mean ± SD)

	Baseline ($n = 18$)	6 Months ($n = 16$)	12 Months ($n = 14$)
Mean right atrial pressure (mm Hg)	11 ± 7	7 ± 5	8 ± 6
Mean pulmonary arterial pressure (mm Hg)	61 ± 15	55 ± 11	54 ± 16
Mean systemic arterial pressure (mm Hg)	91 ± 13	90 ± 14	84 ± 11
Cardiac index (L/min/m^2)	1.9 ± 0.6	2.3 ± 0.6	2.5 ± 0.8
Heart rate (bpm)	81 ± 13	81 ± 13	89 ± 13
Mixed venous saturation (%)	59 ± 12	67 ± 7	64 ± 12
Arterial oxygen saturation (%)	93 ± 6	93 ± 6	92 ± 10
Stroke volume (mL per beat)	41 ± 18	53 ± 18	51 ± 23
Total pulmonary resistance (U)	22 ± 11	15 ± 6	14 ± 6
Total systemic resistance (U)	31 ± 11	25 ± 11	22 ± 10

Source: Reproduced with permission from Barst et al.[17]

TABLE 25-3. Hemodynamic Effects of Epoprostenol (E) and Conventional Therapy (CT) in Patients with Primary Pulmonary Hypertension after 12 Weeks of Follow-Up

Variable	Change from Baseline*		Difference between Treatments	95% CI
	E	**CT**		
Mean pulmonary artery pressure (mm Hg)	-4.8 ± 1.3	1.9 ± 1.6	-6.7	-10.7 to -2.6
Mean right atrial pressure (mm Hg)	-2.2 ± 1.1	0.1 ± 0.9	-2.3	-5.2 to 0.7
Mean systemic artery pressure (mm Hg)	-4.8 ± 1.2	-0.9 ± 1.7	-3.9	-9.6 to 1.7
Mean pulmonary capillary wedge pressure (mm Hg)	0.4 ± 1.2	-1.0 ± 1.6	1.4	-2.5 to 5.3
Cardiac index (L/min/M^2)	0.3 ± 0.1	-0.2 ± 0.2	0.5	0.2 to 0.9
Heart rate (bpm)	-0.9 ± 2.5	-1.8 ± 1.5	0.9	-5.2 to 7.2
Systemic arterial oxygen saturation (%)	2.0 ± 1.6	-0.6 ± 1.4	2.6	-1.8 to 7.1
Mixed venous oxygen saturation (%)	1.2 ± 1.8	-2.6 ± 2.0	3.8	-1.6 to 9.2
Stroke volume (mL/beat)	6.6 ± 2.2	-3.5 ± 3.3	10.1	2.5 to 17.8
Pulmonary vascular resistance (mmHg/L/min)	-3.4 ± 0.7	1.5 ± 1.2	-4.9	-7.6 to -2.3
Systemic vascular resistance (mmHg/L/min)	-4.00 ± 1.0	2.1 ± 1.4	-6.1	-9.5 to -2.8

*$\pm$ values are the mean ($\pm$SE) changes from baseline. 95% confidence intervals (CI) are for comparisons between treatment groups. A CI that does not contain 0 indicates statistical significance.

Source: Reproduced with permission from Barst et al.[18]

(during diastole and systole), and also a trend toward less tricuspid regurgitation when compared with patients randomized to conventional therapy.

Shapiro et al. studied the long-term effects of continuous epoprostenol therapy (>330 days in 18 patients and 90–190 days in 25 patients).[54] They demonstrated improved survival over 1, 2, and 3 years of 80% ($n = 36$), 75% ($n = 17$), and 49% ($n = 6$), respectively, compared with the historical control subjects at 10, 20, and 30 months of 88% ($n = 31$), 56% ($n = 27$), and 47% ($n = 17$), respectively. They also described a method for noninvasive long-term follow-up of patients with PPH (see Fig. 25-3).

In a recent publication, McLaughlin et al.[20] suggested that the effects of prostacyclin treatment in PPH go beyond those of immediate vasodilation. After establishing baseline hemodynamic variables in 27 patients with severe PPH, the investigators then evaluated their response to the administration of adenosine, a vasodilator, and long-term therapy with epoprostenol. When the hemodynamic responses to the two treatments were compared, it was found that epoprostenol therapy caused a long-term reduction in PVR that exceeded the short-term reduction achieved with adenosine. Furthermore, long-term epoprostenol therapy also reduced PVR in patients who showed no short-term response to adenosine.

It has also been observed that continuous prostacyclin therapy can also reduce endothelial cell injury, an etiologic factor in the development of PPH. Prostacyclin infusion in patients favorably reduces the plasma levels of P-selectin while increasing thrombomodulin levels, markers of endothelial injury, and altered hemostasis.[55] The drug can also improve the balance between endothelin clearance and release, an abnormality seen in patients with PPH.[56]

Although epoprostenol does not constitute a cure for PPH, it provides a substantial improvement as a palliative treatment for the disease.[56a] Higenbottam et al.[21] have studied patients with PPH in England since the early 1980s, looking at the effect of epoprostenol use on heart and lung transplantation. His group studied 44 patients, 25 of whom received epoprostenol, and measured the time to transplantation and its success. In this study, they noted that epoprostenol doubled the time on the waiting list for transplant or until death. They also noted that epoprostenol was the one factor that influenced longevity the most. However, it should be noted that a total of only 10 patients were transplanted, and that 7 of these patients received epoprostenol.[21]

Secondary Pulmonary Hypertension

Although prostacyclin infusions have been found to be successful in treating patients with PPH, the role of this drug in treating secondary pulmonary hypertension has not been well studied. In an uncontrolled, compassionate-use clinical experience with prostacyclin in 33 patients with secondary pulmonary hypertension associated with congenital heart disease, collagen vascular disease, and peripheral thromboembolic and portopulmonary hypertension, the drug was shown to be of benefit.[57] The drug was also shown to benefit patients with pulmonary hypertension and associated congenital heart defects.[58]

Congestive Heart Failure (CHF)

Epoprostenol has also been studied extensively in patients with CHF. Initially, the data were very encouraging about the potential benefit of epoprostenol infusion in patients with NYHA classes III and IV CHF. Short-term studies showed that the drug could be safely administered,[59,60] and one small, long-term study by Sueta et al.[22] showed that classes III and IV CHF patients improved with epoprostenol. In this study, they examined 33 patients with classes III and IV CHF who were not responding to conventional therapy. These patients were randomized to receive conventional therapy or were given a continuous infusion of epoprostenol in addition to conventional therapy for 12 weeks. Patients underwent an initial dosing trial to determine the maximum tolerated dose of epoprostenol.

Long-term infusion was initiated at a rate of 4 ng/kg/min below this dose and subsequently increased to achieve maximal benefit. The patients who received epoprostenol had improvements in cardiac output, walking distance during a 6-min walk test, and functional class.

However, a large-scale study, the Flolan International Randomized Survival Trial (FIRST),[61] was terminated early when the investigators noticed an increase in mortality among the epoprostenol group. In this study, patients were randomized to receive epoprostenol and conventional therapy. Patients who received epoprostenol underwent an initial dosing trial and were started on an infusion rate 40% below the maximally tolerated dose. During the trial, there were 171 deaths, 105 among those receiving epoprostenol—an amount deemed to be excessive. There were also no reported symptomatic benefits to receiving therapy. There was no increase in exercise capacity, and there were no reported improvements in quality of life using the Nottingham Health Profile.

In a recent publication, Montalescot et al.[62] found that epoprostenol was effective in improving pulmonary vascular tone and right ventricular afterload in patients with pulmonary hypertension secondary to end-stage heart failure. It was also demonstrated that epoprostenol has a significant positive inotropic effect in patients with severe heart failure,[24] which may relate to the disappointing results observed in the FIRST trial.[62a] In contrast to its effects with long-term administration, the acute administration of prostacyclin remains of particular interest as a pharmacologic test in evaluating the reversibility of vascular resistance before orthotopic heart transplantation. It appears that prostacyclin may also be used in more unstable patients awaiting heart transplantation or in patients with acute right ventricular dysfunction of the donor heart after transplantation.

Other Uses

Epoprostenol has been studied in patients with myocardial ischemia. Patients with angina actually experienced an increase in the frequency of their symptoms while receiving epoprostenol.[63] This appears to be secondary to a coronary steal effect.[64] The drug has also been studied in patients undergoing percutaneous transluminal coronary angioplasty to see whether it helps to prevent reocclusion. However, there is no observed benefit to adding epoprostenol to heparin during the 36-h time period following angioplasty when compared with the addition of placebo.[65]

Epoprostenol has also been used in acute myocardial infarction. In animal models, epoprostenol has been shown to reduce infarct size,[66-68] decrease oxygen demand,[68] and prevent arrhythmia.[69] Studies have shown that epoprostenol can be administered safely to patients during acute myocardial infarction; however, epoprostenol infusion does not appear to promote recanalization of occluded arteries[70,71] and has not yet been shown to reduce infarct size.[72] Initial studies in humans also showed that epoprostenol could be administered safely in combination with thrombolytics.[73,74] However, it is still not clear whether the addition of epoprostenol enhances thrombolytic therapy.[75]

Another area in which epoprostenol has been used is in peripheral vascular disease. It should be noted that with this disease, epoprostenol is not required on a long-term basis; rather, it is given for a few days with sustained benefits. Studies have shown a benefit with epoprostenol infusion in terms of wound healing and the postponement of amputation in patients with severe ischemic disease. Patients also show a reduction in rest pain that can last for several months after the initial infusion.[76-79]

Intermittent infusion of epoprostenol can benefit patients with intractable Raynaud's phenomenon. Two studies showed that such patients who were treated with epoprostenol had a decrease in the number of painful episodes and the severity of these episodes when compared with placebo. Likewise, these studies also showed some improvement in the temperature of the fingertips. These benefits were still seen after 2 months of follow-up.[80,81] A later study that used epoprostenol in treating Raynaud's phenomenon did not observe any long-term benefits in terms of blood flow and finger temperature.[82] This study also failed to adequately assess the patient's subjective response to therapy. Therefore, although the investigations did show that there was no physiologically measurable difference between epoprostenol and placebo after 6 weeks, they also did not produce any data to suggest epoprostenol affects the number and severity of painful attacks.[82]

There have also been studies that have examined the potential benefit of using epoprostenol to control hypertensive crises in pregnant women near full term. These studies showed that epoprostenol had the same effects as hydralazine in reducing blood pressure.[83] The authors speculate that epoprostenol may have a potential use in pregnant women with severe hypertension who need rapid control to undergo delivery or a procedure. In a small study involving 4 women with PPH, prostacyclin and nifedipine contributed to 3 out of 4 successful pregnancies. Delay of diagnosis contributed in the case of the woman who did not have a successful outcome.[84] However, more studies need to be done to see whether acute blood pressure lowering in pregnancy will be a potential indication for the use of epoprostenol.

Epoprostenol has also been used in procedures that require extracorporeal circulation, such as dialysis[85,86] and cardiopulmonary bypass.[87] One study in patients with a history of type II heparin-induced thrombocytopenia undergoing cardiopulmonary bypass procedures showed that thrombocyte counts were higher when epoprostenol was added to heparin as compared to the use of heparin alone.[88] The favorable risk/benefit ratio associated with epoprostenol relates to easier protamine reversal and decreased postoperative blood loss. A similar study, attempted by DiSesa et al.,[89] showed that systemic hypotension remained a problem in using epoprostenol, DiSesa's group also noticed that patients who received epoprostenol had a decreased oxygen tension after the procedure, although none of these patients had end-organ damage as a result. Furthermore, the investigators noticed that patients who received epoprostenol also required more blood transfusions. Therefore, the benefit of epoprostenol in these procedures is still unclear.

ILOPROST

Iloprost is a more stable analogue of epoprostenol and has a similar structure, with some minor modifications (see Fig. 25-1). It has similar effects on platelet aggregability[90-92] and vasodilation.[93,94] Iloprost is two to seven times more potent as an inhibitor of platelet aggregation than as a vasodilator.[92,95] Because of its structural modifications, iloprost has a half-life of 13 min[96] and is not degraded by light. It is metabolized by beta oxidation.[97] Drug elimination is substantially reduced in patients with renal failure[98] and severe hepatic disease.[99] This drug is reconstituted in a solution with physiologic pH and has been administered intravenously, by inhalation, and orally. When taken orally, less than 20% of the medication reaches the systemic circulation.[97]

TABLE 25-4. Comparison of the Acute Hemodynamic Effect of Epoprostenol and Iloprost in Patients with Primary Pulmonary Hypertension*

	HR (bpm)	CI (L/min/m²)	SI (mL/m²)	MPAP (mm Hg)	SVO₂ (%)	PVR (mm Hg/min/L)	SVR (mm Hg/min/L)
First baseline	89.3 (15.2)	1.9 (0.7)	21.4 (8.5)	67.6 (13.8)	57.1 (8.1)	17.1 (8.5)	24.0 (8.1)
Iloprost max	89.5 (15.4)	2.5 (0.7)	29.6 (11.8)	63.0 (13.9)	66.5 (4.8)	13.2 (6.0)	18.9 (7.9)
Second baseline	89.7 (15.1)	1.9 (0.6)	22.4 (7.2)	69.4 (13.2)	59.1 (7.2)	16.5 (8.2)	22.6 (8.1)
Prostacyclin max	89.4 (16.4)	2.8 (0.7)	31.6 (9.8)	63.8 (18.0)	63.3 (7.2)	12.5 (6.0)	17.7 (8.6)
Third baseline	90.4 (14.9)	2.0 (0.4)	22.5 (10.2)	68.9 (19.2)	56.3 (9.1)	16.4 (8.5)	23.5 (8.4)
	NS	$P < .05$	$P < .05$	$P < .05$	NS	$P < .05$	$P < .05$

HR = heart rate; CI = cardiac index; SI = stroke index; MPAP = mean pulmonary artery pressure; SVO₂ = venous/arterial oxygenation; PVR = pulmonary vascular resistance; SVR = systemic vascular resistance; NS = not significant.

*Patients were given alternating intravenous infusions of iloprost or epoprostenol; infusion was then discontinued for 15 min. After the patient returned to baseline hemodynamic status, infusion of the other drug was started. The initial infusion was randomly assigned, and both medications were titrated to maximally tolerated doses.

Source: Reproduced with permission from Fink AN, Frishman WH, Ahmad A: Uses of prostaglandins and prostacyclin in cardiovascular disease. In: Frishman WH, Sonnenblick EH, eds. *Cardiovascular Pharmacotherapeutics*. New York: McGraw Hill, 1997; 557–570.

When administered acutely, iloprost is similar to epoprostenol in its effects in patients with PPH. Scott et al.[100] noted that there were no significant differences between these drugs and their effects on heart rate, cardiac index, PVR, PAP, and SVR (Table 25-4). A long-term study with iloprost has also been done in patients with pulmonary hypertension secondary to systemic sclerosis.[101] In this study, aerosolized iloprost caused marked pulmonary vasodilation, with maintenance of gas exchange and systemic arterial pressure. Iloprost therapy may be life-saving in decompensated right heart failure from pulmonary hypertension secondary to lung fibrosis. This is especially true for patients who cannot tolerate systemic vasodilator therapy because of the associated shunting and drop in systemic arterial pressure. A long-term study with iloprost has also been done in patients with pulmonary hypertension secondary to systemic sclerosis and primary antiphospholipid syndrome.[102] In this study, there was improvement in patients' NYHA class and some improvement in PVR. However, this study included only five patients. Nonetheless, it did show that iloprost could be administered safely for long periods in patients with pulmonary hypertension.[102]

Aerosolization of prostacyclin or iloprost has been shown to cause selective pulmonary vasodilation, an increase in cardiac output, and improved venous and arterial oxygenation in patients with severe PPH.[103,104,140a] Iloprost inhalation has also been shown to cause a rapid decrease in levels of atrial natriuretic peptide and cyclic GMP in parallel with pulmonary vasodilation and hemodynamic improvement.[105]

In 2000, Hoeper et al. demonstrated that aerosolized iloprost may be a potential alternative for the treatment of PPH.[106] While continuous intravenous infusion of epoprostenol is an effective treatment for PPH, this approach requires the insertion of a permanent central venous catheter, with the associated risk of serious complications. These investigators evaluated 24 patients with PPH who received aerosolized iloprost for at least 1 year. These patients had significant increases in walking distance and cardiac output, while mean pulmonary arterial pressure and pulmonary vascular resistance showed statistically significant declines (Table 25-5). Olschewski et al. found similar results regarding the efficacy of inhaled iloprost to treat PPH.[107] The addition of oral sildenafil to an inhaled iloprost

TABLE 25-5. Hemodynamic Variables and Exercise Capacity in 24 Patients with Primary Pulmonary Hypertension Treated with Inhaled Iloprost*

Measurement	Baseline Preinhalation	Baseline Postinhalation	3 Months Preinhalation	3 Months Postinhalation	12 Months Preinhalation	12 Months Postinhalation
Heart rate (bpm)	84 ± 13	84 ± 13	82 ± 15	79 ± 13	82 ± 10	80 ± 10
Mean systemic arterial pressure (mm Hg)	98 ± 14	100 ± 14	93 ± 10†	92 ± 12	90 ± 13†	89 ± 13
Mean pulmonary arterial pressure (mm Hg)	59 ± 10	50 ± 13	52 ± 11†	44 ± 12	52 ± 15†	43 ± 16
Mean right atrial pressure (mm Hg)	8 ± 7	7 ± 6	5 ± 4†	4 ± 4	5 ± 4†	4 ± 4
Cardiac output (L/min)	3.8 ± 1.4	4.5 ± 1.4	4.0 ± 1.2	4.5 ± 1.2	4.4 ± 1.3†	4.8 ± 1.4
Pulmonary vascular resistance (dyn-s-cm⁻⁵)	1205 ± 467	866 ± 415	1001 ± 437†	728 ± 330	925 ± 469†	704 ± 440
Systemic vascular resistance (dyn-s-cm⁻⁵)	2088 ± 712	1791 ± 508	1884 ± 506†	1646 ± 397	1660 ± 494†‡	1534 ± 467
Stroke volume (mL per beat)	46 ± 16	55 ± 16	50 ± 16†	57 ± 15	55 ± 16†‡	61 ± 19
Mixed venous oxygen saturation (%)	62 ± 8	68 ± 8	65 ± 7†	70 ± 7	67 ± 8†	70 ± 7
6-min walk distance (m)	278 ± 96	ND	353 ± 69†	ND	363 ± 135†	ND

*Values are means ±SD. "Preinhalation" and "postinhalation" denote before and immediately after inhalation of iloprost; ND = not done.

† $P < .05$ for the comparison of preinhalation variables at 3 months or 12 months with preinhalation variables at baseline.

‡ $P < .05$ for the comparison of preinhalation variables at 12 months with preinhalation variables at 3 months.

Source: Reproduced with permission from Hoeper et al.[106]

regimen has also been shown to provide greater benefit than iloprost alone.[108,108a]

Although inhaled iloprost appears to benefit patients with mild to moderate forms of PPH, it is less likely to be of benefit in treating patients with severe forms of PPH. Schenk et al. posed that while iloprost demonstrated short-term hemodynamic benefits, it could not be utilized as an alternative chronic treatment in patients with severe pulmonary hypertension.[109] In a small, uncontrolled trial, aerosolized iloprost reduced PAP and increased cardiac output by significant amounts. The effect of iloprost lasted for 20 min and was similar at different doses of intravenous epoprostenol. However, a persistent treatment change to inhaled iloprost could not be achieved because all patients developed signs of right heart failure. After termination of iloprost inhalation, return to standard epoprostenol therapy led to a restoration of clinical and hemodynamic benefit. Other studies have also demonstrated the limitation of inhaled iloprost in treating severe forms of PPH.[110,110a]

The one condition in which iloprost has been extensively studied has been inoperable peripheral vascular disease. Iloprost causes a significant improvement in symptoms when compared with placebo and also extends the amount of time to amputation. Dormandy[111] found that 51% of iloprost-treated patients experienced improvement in terms of ulcer healing and a decrease in pain. The United Kingdom Severe Limb Ischemia Study[112] showed that at 6 months, 32% of patients treated with iloprost had to undergo amputation, compared with 47% in the control group.

Iloprost has also been used on patients with thromboangiitis obliterans.[113] Of patients treated with iloprost, 63% had relief of rest pain, compared with 28% in the placebo group, and there was complete healing of trophic lesions in 35% of patients treated with iloprost, compared to a lower rate of healing with placebo. At 5 months of follow-up, 88% of the iloprost patients reported improvement in their condition, compared with 21% in an aspirin control group.[113]

In a multicenter, double-blind study of patients with thromboangiitis obliterans, those receiving iloprost had significantly better pain relief as compared to their placebo counterparts (63% versus 49% respectively; $P = .02$). However, in this study, iloprost was no more effective than placebo at healing these patients' ulcer lesions.[114,114a]

Iloprost has also been shown to benefit patients with Raynaud's phenomenon. Two retrospective studies showed that slightly more than half of the patients who received iloprost benefited.[115,116] There is also one prospective study showing that iloprost treatment had an equivalent benefit when compared with nifedipine therapy in these patients.[117]

Oral iloprost has also been used in patients with Raynaud's syndrome that is unresponsive to conventional therapy. Belch et al.[118] found that patients treated with oral iloprost had a decrease in the frequency and severity of their attacks when compared with a group receiving placebo. However, differences never reached statistical significance because of the number studied and the high rate of improvement in the placebo group. However, it should be noted that a 60% change would have been required to reach statistical significance in this particular study.

Studies with iloprost in patients with angina showed similar results to epoprostenol—namely, increases in the amount of nitroglycerin consumed by patients, in chest pain, and in ST-segment depression on electrocardiography (ECG).[119,120]

Iloprost has been studied as an adjuvant therapy to thrombolysis in acute myocardial infarction. Topol et al.[121] studied 50 patients who were randomized to receive recombinant tissue-type plasminogen activator (rtPA) alone, or in combination with iloprost; they found no benefit with the addition of iloprost in terms of coronary artery patency. They also observed that patients who received iloprost had diminished recovery of ejection fraction and infarct zone wall motion.

Iloprost has been looked at in procedures requiring extracorporeal circulation. There is no clear indication that intravenous iloprost has any benefit during cardiopulmonary bypass. Martin et al.[122] showed that there may be slight improvement in thrombocyte counts for the 24 h after surgery, and Massonnet-Castel et al.[123] did not find any difference between iloprost and heparin. Likewise, there is no demonstrable benefit to using iloprost during hemodialysis.[86]

In an experimental model of endotoxemia, the administration of iloprost was shown to attenuate leukocyte adherence and to improve intestinal microvascular blood flow, suggesting a potential for its use in the treatment of endotoxin-induced intestinal injury.[124]

Although iloprost is not available in the United States at the current time, it may one day be approved for the treatment of intractable Raynaud's phenomenon and PPH.

OTHER AGENTS

Prostaglandin E_1 (PGE$_1$) has pharmacologic actions similar to those of prostacyclin (PGI$_2$), although it is not as potent. It has both vasodilatory and antithrombotic effects. Because the discovery of PGE$_1$ preceded that of PGI$_2$ and its more stable analogues, it was initially studied in many of the same situations for which these newer agents are now being used. Preliminary studies were performed to evaluate the efficacy and safety of PGE$_1$ in acute myocardial infarction,[125,126] CHF,[127] Raynaud's phenmenon,[128] peripheral vascular disease,[129] and open-heart surgery in children.[130] However, more definitive investigations were not conducted, possibly since more potent and stable agents have been discovered.

Taprostene is a stable analogue of prostacyclin. It has similar physiologic effects, namely, inhibition of platelet aggregation and vasodilation, albeit it is not as potent an agent.[131] There is limited experience using taprostene in patients with peripheral vascular disease.[132,133] Taprostene has also been tested in a small group of patients with stable angina, where it did not cause any ECG ST-segment depressions when compared with placebo.[134]

Taprostene has also been used in combination with thrombolytics in acute myocardial infraction. In the Seruplase Taprostene Acute Reocclusion Trial (START),[135] taprostene was compared with placebo for improved arterial patency following the use of seruplase. In this study, no advantage or disadvantage was seen in the taprostene group in obtaining arterial patency. However, it should be noted that this was a relatively small trial and that there were a significant number of patients who did not have a follow-up angiogram. Although taprostene may be shown to be effective in coronary angioplasty, it must still be studied prospectively in a larger trial.

Ciprostene is another stable analogue of prostacyclin. This agent has been used in patients with severe peripheral vascular disease without much improvement in symptomatology.[136,137] One quantitative study looked at the effect of ciprostene on coronary artery reocclusion after percutaneous transluminal coronary angioplasty and found that the addition of ciprostene may have a long-term benefit in reducing the degree of long-term stenosis. Ciprostene-treated patients had decreased angiographic restenosis (41 to 53%; $P = .058$) compared to the placebo group.[138]

There is limited experience with another stable prostacyclin analogue, treprostinil (UT-15, formerly known as 15AU81). Its pharmacologic profile is similar to that of epoprostenol but has a significantly longer half-life. This agent has been used safely in one trial in patients with severe CHF.[139] A phase II study compared the hemodynamic effects of UT-15 when administered intravenously and subcutaneously and found that both acute intravenous and subcutaneous administration increased cardiac output and decreased total PVR and mean PAP in patients with PPH. Although this agent, with its long half-life, shows promise, more studies are needed to determine whether UT-15 will one day be useful for treating patients with severe CHF. More recently the effect of UT-15 on peripheral blood flow of the limbs was studied in 8 patients with severe intermittent claudication. Ultrasonography measurements revealed a 29% ($P = .003$) increase in blood flow in the common femoral artery.[140] Treprostinil has also been used subcutaneously in patients with PPH and was found to improve exercise tolerance. Based on this experience, the FDA has approved treprostinil for use in pulmonary hypertension.

Cicaprost and beraprost are two stable prostacyclin analogues that can be used in oral form.[141,141a] Two pilot studies on the effect of cicaprost in patients with Raynaud's phenomenon have shown that there is minimal improvement if any. However, the appropriate dosage of cicaprost and proper treatment regimen are still unknown, and more studies are needed to see whether cicaprost will be a useful therapy for patients with Raynaud's phenomenon.[142,143,143a] Beraprost, with both vasodilating and antiplatelet properties, has been shown with intermittent claudication in a placebo-controlled pilot study to improve walking distance in patients with intermittent claudication.[144] In a study of PPH patients, the drug was shown to enhance survival.[145] In another study, beraprost was shown to improve exercise capacity and symptoms in patients with pulmonary artery hypertension, in particular, those with PPH.[145a] Beraprost has also been shown to enhance pulmonary vasodilation in children with pulmonary hypertension when used simultaneously with inhaled nitric oxide. This combination may offer an alternative mode of treatment for patients with postoperative pulmonary hypertension and PPH who do not respond to inhaled nitric oxide alone or conventional therapy.[146]

A pilot study by Okano et al.[147] evaluated the efficacy of beraprost sodium in 12 patients with severe PPH unresponsive to

calcium-channel blockers and inhaled nitric oxide. An acute response was evaluated after one dose of beraprost sodium (2 μg/kg) in 6 patients. Chronic response with a daily dose of 80 to 180 μg in 10 patients over an average of 2 months was assessed. Only 1 patient responded acutely, 3 showed no response, while 8 showed improvement in functional class and were still alive with the same dose of beraprost sodium during a mean of 5 months of follow-up. One patient died suddenly at 18 months. Beraprost sodium may be the first treatment option in patients with severe symptoms of PPH before resorting to intravenous PGI$_2$, with its inherent risks and increased medical costs. However, before such treatment can be recommended, further multicenter clinical trials are needed to investigate the long-term effects of the drug.[145a]

Recent studies have demonstrated the efficacy of beraprost in relieving symptoms in patients having PPH, intermittent claudication, and digital necrosis in systemic sclerosis. Nagaya et al. showed the possible benefits of beraprost in improving mean survival for patients with mild forms of PPH as compared to patients receiving conventional therapy (i.e., with anticoagulants and calcium-channel blockers).[145] Kaplan-Meier survival curves demonstrated that the 1-, 2-, and 3-year survival rates for the beraprost group were 96, 86, and 76%, respectively, as compared with 77, 47, and 44%, respectively, in the conventional treatment group ($P < .05$). However, the study was limited for the following reasons: it was retrospective, and it studied patients with mainly mild PPH who naturally might have longer survival rates than those with severe PPH. Lievre et al., in a multicenter trial, studied the efficacy of beraprost in 549 patients with intermittent claudication.[148] After a 4-week placebo run-in phase, patients were randomized to receive either beraprost ($n = 209$) or placebo ($n = 213$) in a double-blind manner for 6 months. Success was defined as an improvement of >50% in pain-free walking distance at 6 months in the absence of severe cardiovascular events. The beraprost group had better success (43.5%) than the placebo group (33.3%, $P = .036$). Pain-free walking distances increased by 81.5 and 52.5%, respectively, in the beraprost and placebo groups ($P = .001$) and maximum walking distances by 60.1 and 35.0%, respectively ($P = .004$) (Fig. 25-4). In a third study, Vayssairat et al. found encouraging results with beraprost in patients with systemic sclerosis.[149] Patients ($n = 107$) with systemic sclerosis were randomized in a double-blind fashion. Although the incidence of digital ulcerations in the beraprost group was found

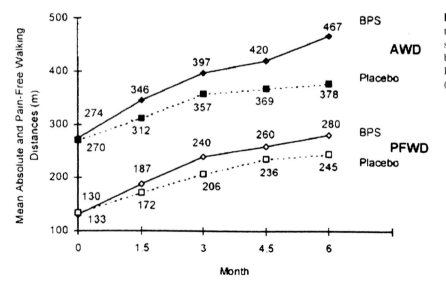

FIGURE 25-4. Pain-free and absolute walking distances. Comparison of mean absolute (AWD, solid symbols) and mean pain-free (PFWD, open symbols) walking distances for beraprost (BPS) (solid lines) and placebo (dashed lines) groups, in meters. *(Reproduced with permission from Lievre et al.[148])*

to be statistically less than that in the placebo group (48.1 versus 58.8%, $P = .325$), the beneficial effects of active treatment were observed in the following study end points: the overall well-being of the beraprost group was significantly better than that of the placebo counterparts ($P = .047$), the onset of digital ulceration was markedly delayed in the beraprost group compared to the placebo group ($P = .057$), and the level of von Willebrand factor decreased significantly more in the beraprost group ($P = .0001$). Finally, the study showed that beraprost benefited those patients with distal systemic sclerosis.

CONCLUSION

Epoprostenol is now available in the United States and is approved for use in patients with PPH. Although this agent has been used with limited success in other areas, there is a great amount of work to be done with its more stable analogues.[150,151] Recently, trepostinil, a prostacyclin analogue was approved for subcutaneous use in PPH. Perhaps one of these other agents will provide an oral therapy for PPH, a valuable treatment for severe CHF, a palliative treatment for inoperable peripheral vascular disease or intractable Raynaud's phenomenon, or as a useful adjunct to standard therapy of acute myocardial infarction.

REFERENCES

1. von Euler US: Zur Kenntnis der pharmakologischen Wirkungen von Nativsekreten und Extrakten mannlicher accessorisher Geschlectsdrussen. *Arch Exp Pathol Pharmacol* 75:78, 1934.
2. Moncada S, Gryglewski R, Bunting S, Vane JR: An enzyme isolated from the arteries transforms prostoglandin endoperoxides to an unstable substance that inhibits platelet aggregation. *Nature* 263:663, 1976.
3. Whittaker N, Bunting S, Salmon J, et al: The chemical structure of prostaglandin X (prostacyclin). *Prostaglandins* 12:915, 1976.
4. Bunting S, Gryglewski R, Moncada S, Vane JR: Arterial walls generate from prostaglandin endoperoxides a substance (prostaglandin X) which relaxes strips of mesenteric and coeliac arteries and inhibits platelet aggregation. *Prostaglandins* 12:897, 1976.
5. Moncada S, Herman AG, Higgs EA, Vane JR: Differential formation of prostacyclin (PGX or PGI$_2$) by layers of the arterial wall: An explanation for the antithrombotic properties of vascular endothelium. *Thromb Res* 11:323, 1977.
6. Marcus AJ, Weksler BB, Jaffe EA: Enzymatic conversion of prostaglandin endoperoxide H$_2$ and arachidonic acid to PGI$_2$ by cultured human endothelial cells. *Biol Chem* 253:7138, 1978.
7. Weksler BB, Marcus AJ, Jaffe EA: Synthesis of prostaglandin I$_2$ (prostacyclin) by cultured human bovine endothelial cells. *Proc Natl Acad Sci USA* 74:3922, 1977.
8. MacIntyre DE, Pearson JD, Gordon JL: Localization and stimulation of prostacyclin production in vascular cells. *Nature* 271:549, 1978.
9. Moncada S, Vane JR: Pharmacology and endogenous roles of prostaglandin endoperoxides, thromboxane A2, and prostacyclin. *Pharmacol Rev* 30:293, 1979.
10. Nakagawa O, Tanaka I, Usui T, et al: Molecular cloning of human prostacyclin receptor cDNA and its gene expression in the cardiovascular system. *Circulation* 90:1643, 1994.
11. Tateson JE, Moncada S, Vane JR: Effects of proctacyclin (PGX) on cyclic AMP concentrations in human platelets. *Prostagandins* 13:389, 1977.
12. Higgs EA, Moncada S, Vane JR, et al: Effects of prostacyclin (PGI$_2$) on platelet adhesion to rabbit arterial subendothelium. *Prostaglandins* 16:17, 1978.
13. Cho MJ, Allen MA: Chemical stability of PGI$_2$ in aqueous solutions. *Prostaglandins* 15:943, 1978.
14. Wong PY, Sun FF, McGiff JC: Metabolism of prostacyclin in blood vessels. *J Biol Chem* 253:5555, 1978.
15. Yui Y, Aoyama T, Morishita H, et al: Serum prostacyclin stabilizing factor is identical to apoprotein A-I (apo-I): A novel function of apo A-I. *J Clin Invest* 82:803, 1988.
16. Rubin LJ, Mendoza J, Hood M, et al: Treatment of primary pulmonary hypertension with continuous intravenous prostacyclin (epoprostenol): Results of a randomized trial. *Ann Intern Med* 112:485, 1990.
17. Barst RJ, Rubin LJ, McGoon MD, et al: Survival in primary pulmonary hypertension with long term continuous intravenous prostacyclin. *Ann Intern Med* 121:409, 1994.
18. Barst RJ, Rubin LJ, Long WA, et al: A comparison of continuous epoprostenol (prostacyclin) with conventional therapy for primary pulmonary hypertension. *N Engl J Med* 334:296, 1996.
19. Hinderliter AL, Park WW, Barst RJ, et al: Effects of long-term infusion of prostacyclin (epoprostenol) on echocardiographic measures of right ventricular structure and function in primary pulmonary hypertension. *Circulation* 95:1479, 1997.
20. McLaughlin VV, Genthner DE, Panella MM, Rich S: Reduction in pulmonary vascular resistance with long-term epoprostenol (prostacyclin) therapy in primary pulmonary hypertension. *N Engl J Med* 338:273, 1998.
21. Higenbottam TW, Spiegelhalter D, Scott JP, et al: Prostacyclin (epoprostenol) and heart-lung transplantation as treatments for severe pulmonary hypertension. *Br Heart J* 70:366, 1993.
22. Sueta CA, Gheorghiade M, Adams KF, et al: Safety and efficacy of epoprostenol in patients with severe congestive heart failure. *Am J Cardiol* 75:34A, 1995.
23. Cremona G, Higenbottam T: Role of prostacyclin in the treatment of primary pulmonary hypertension. *Am J Cardiol* 75:67A, 1995.
24. Rich S, McLaughlin VV: The effects of chronic prostacyclin therapy on cardiac output and symptoms in primary pulmonary hypertension. *J Am Coll Cardiol* 34:1184, 1999.
25. Rubin LJ: Pathology and pathophysiology of primary pulmonary hypertension. *Am J Cardiol* 75:51A, 1995.
25a. Lehrman S, Romano P, Frishman W, et al: Primary pulmonary hypertension and cor pulmonate. *Cardiol in Rev* 2002: in press.
26. Rubin LJ, Barst RJ, Kaiser LR, et al: Primary pulmonary hypertension: ACCP Consensus Statement. *Chest* 104:236, 1993.
27. Pietra GG, Edwards WD, Kay JM, Rich S: Histopathology of primary pulmonary hypertension: A qualitative study of pulmonary blood vessels from 58 patients in the National Heart, Lung and Blood Institute primary pulmonary hypertension registry. *Circulation* 80:1198, 1989.
28. Gaine S, Lewis R: Primary pulmonary hypertension. *Lancet* 353:719, 1998.
29. Christman BW, McPherson CD, Newman JH, et al: An imbalance between the excretion of thromboxane and prostacyclin metabolites in pulmonary hypertension. *N Engl J Med* 327:70, 1992.
30. Giaid A, Yanagisawa M, Langleben D, et al: Expression of endothelin-1 in the lungs of patients with pulmonary hypertension. *N Engl J Med* 328:173, 1993.
31. Stewart DJ, Levy RD, Cernacek P, Langleben D: Increased plasma endothelin-1 in the lungs of patients with pulmonary hypertension. *N Engl J Med* 114:467, 1991.
32. Herve P, Launay JM, Scrobohaci ML, et al: Increased plasma serotonin in primary pulmonary hypertension. *Am J Med* 99:249, 1995.
33. Yuan X-J, Wang J, Juhaszova M, et al: Attenuated K+ channel gene transcription in primary pulmonary hypertension. *Lancet* 352:726, 1998.
34. Rich S, Dantzker DR, Ayres SM, et al: Primary pulmonary hypertension: a national prospective study. *Ann Intern Med* 107:236, 1987.
35. D'Alonzo GE, Barst RJ, Ayres SM, et al: Survival in patients with primary pulmonary hypertension: Results from a national prospective registry. *Ann Intern Med* 115:343, 1991.
36. Rubin LJ: Calcium channel blockers in primary pulmonary hypertension. *Chest* 88:257S, 1985.
37. Fuster V, Steele PM, Edwards WD, et al: Primary pulmonary hypertension: natural history and the importance of thrombosis. *Circulation* 70:580, 1984.
37a. Dobkin J, Reichel J: Drug treatment of primary pulmonary hypertension. In: Frishman WH, Sonnenblick EH (eds). *Cardiovascular Pharmacotherapeutics*. New York: McGraw-Hill, 1997:1173–1183.

38. Rubin LJ: Primary pulmonary hypertension: Practical therapeutic recommendations. *Drugs* 43:37, 1992.

39. Rich S: Medical treatment of primary pulmonary hypertension: A bridge to transplantation? *Am J Cardiol* 75:63A, 1995.

40. Alpert MA, Pressly TA, Mukerji V, et al: Acute and long-term effects of nifedipine on pulmonary hypertension associated with diffuse systemic sclerosis, the CREST syndrome and mixed connective tissue diseases. *Am J Cardiol* 68:1687, 1991.

40a. Rubin LJ, Badesch DB, Barst RJ, et al: Bosentan therapy for pulmonary arterial hypertension. *N Engl J Med* 346:896, 2002.

41. Reitz BA, Wallwork JL, Hunt SA, et al: Heart-lung transplantation: Successful therapy for patients with pulmonary vascular disease. *N Engl J Med* 306:557, 1982.

42. Pasque MK, Trulock EP, Kaiser LD, Cooper JD: Single lung transplantation for pulmonary hypertension: Three months hemodynamic follow-up. *Circulation* 84:2275, 1991.

43. Doud JR, McCabe MM, Montoya A, Garrity ER: The Loyola University lung transplant experience. *Arch Intern Med* 153:2769, 1993.

44. Galie N, Ussi G, Passarelli P, et al: Role of pharmacologic tests in the treatment of primary pulmonary hypertension. *Am J Cardiol* 75:55A, 1995.

45. Marshall RJ, Helmholz HF, Shepherd JT: Effect of acetylcholine on pulmonary vascular resistance in a patient with idiopathic pulmonary hypertension. *Circulation* 20:391, 1959.

46. Morgan MJ, McCormack DG, Griffiths MJD, et al: Adenosine as a vasodilator in primary pulmonary hypertension. *Circulation* 84:1145, 1991.

47. Frostell C, Fratacci MD, Wain JC, et al: Inhaled nitric oxide: A selective pulmonary vasodilator reversing hypoxic pulmonary vasoconstriction. *Circulation* 83:2038, 1991.

48. Rozkovec A, Stradling JR, Shepherd G, et al: Prediction of favorable responses to long term vasodilator treatment of pulmonary hypertension by short term administration of epoprostenol (prostacyclin) or nifedipine. *Br Heart J* 59:696, 1988.

49. Palewsky HI, Long W, Crow J, Fishman AP: Prostacyclin and acetylcholine as screening agents for acute pulmonary vasodilator responsiveness in primary pulmonary hypertension. *Circulation* 82:2018, 1990.

50. Scrader BJ, Inbar S, Kaufman L, et al: Comparison of the effects of adenosine and nifedipine in pulmonary hypertension. *J Am Coll Cardiol* 19:1060, 1992.

51. Inbar S, Schrader BJ, Kaufmann E, et al: Effects of adenosine in combination with calcium channel blockers in patients with primary pulmonary hypertension. *J Am Coll Cardiol* 21:413, 1993.

52. Jolliet P, Bulpa P, Thorens JB, et al: Nitric oxide and prostacyclin as test agents of vasoreactivity in severe precapillary pulmonary hypertension: Predictive ability and consequences on haemodynamics and gas exchange. *Thorax* 52:369, 1997.

53. Sitbon O, Brenot F, Denjean A, et al: Inhaled nitric oxide as a screening vasodilator agent in primary pulmonary hypertension: A dose-response study and comparison with prostacyclin. *Am J Respir Crit Care Med* 151:384, 1995.

54. Shapiro SM, Oudiz RJ, Cao T, et al: Primary pulmonary hypertension: Improved long-term effects and survival with continuous intravenous epoprostenol infusion. *J Am Coll Cardiol* 30:343, 1997.

55. Sakamaki F, Kyotani S, Nagaya N, et al: Increased plasma P-selectin and decrease thrombo-modulin in pulmonary arterial hypertension were improved by continuous prostacyclin therapy. *Circulation* 102:2720, 2000.

56. Langleben D, Barst RJ, Badesch D, et al: Continuous infusion of epoprostenol improves the net balance between pulmonary endothelin-1 clearance and release in primary pulmonary hypertension. *Circulation* 99:3266, 1999.

56a. Sitbon O, Humbert M, Nunes H, et al: Long-term intravenous epoprostenol infusion in primary pulmonary hypertension. *J Am Coll Cardiol* 40:780, 2002.

57. McLaughlin VV, Genthner DE, Panella MM, et al: Compassionate use of continuous prostacyclin in the management of secondary pulmonary hypertension: A case series. *Ann Intern Med* 130:740, 1999.

58. Berman Rosenzweig E, Kerstein D, Barst RJ: Long-term prostacyclin for pulmonary hypertension with associated congenital heart defects. *Circulation* 99:1858, 1999.

59. Yui Y, Nakajima H, Kawai C, Murakami T: Prostacyclin therapy in patients with refractory congestive heart failure. *Am J Cardiol* 50:320, 1982.

60. Auinger C, Virgolini I, Weissel M, et al: Prostacyclin (PGI$_2$) increases left ventricular ejection fraction (LVEF). *Prostaglandins Leukot Essent Fatty Acids* 36:149, 1989.

61. Califf RM, Adams KF, McKenna WJ, et al: A randomized controlled trial of epoprostenol therapy for severe congestive heart failure: The Flolan International Randomized Survival Trial (FIRST). *Am Heart J* 134:44, 1997.

62. Montalescot G, Drobinski G, Meurin P, et al: Effects of prostacyclin on the pulmonary vascular tone and cardiac contractility of patients with pulmonary hypertension secondary to end-stage heart failure. *Am J Cardiol* 82:749, 1998.

62a. Shah MR, Stinnett SS, McNulty SE, et al: Hemodynamics as surrogate end points for survival in advanced heart failure: An analysis from FIRST. *Am Heart J* 141:908, 2001.

63. Bugiardini R, Galvani M, Ferrini D, et al: Myocardial ischemia induced by prostacyclin and iloprost. *Clin Pharmacol Ther* 38:101, 1985.

64. Bugiardini R, Galvani M, Ferrini D, et al: Myocardial ischemia during intravenous prostacyclin administration: Hemodynamic findings and precautionary measures. *Am Heart J* 113:234, 1987.

65. Gershlick AH, Spriggins D, Davies SW, et al: Failure of epoprostenol to inhibit platelet aggregation and to prevent restenosis after coronary angioplasty: Results of a randomized placebo controlled trial. *Br Heart J* 71:7, 1994.

66. Jugdutt BJ, Hutchins GM, Bulkley BH, Becker LC: Dissimilar effect of prostacyclin, prostaglandin E$_1$ and prostaglandin E$_2$ on myocardial infarct size after coronary occlusion in conscious dogs. *Circ Res* 49:685, 1981.

67. Ogletree Ml, Lefer AM, Smith JB, Nicolaou KC: Studies on the protective effect of prostacyclin in acute myocardial ischemia. *Eur J Pharmacol* 56:95, 1979.

68. Ribeiro L, Brandon T, Hopkins D, et al: Prostacyclin in experimental myocardial ischemia: Effect on hemodynamics, regional myocardial blood flow, infarct size and mortality. *Am J Cardiol* 47:835, 1981.

69. Starnes VA, Primm RK, Woosley RL, et al: Administration of prostacyclin prevents ventricular fibrillation following coronary occlusion in conscious dogs. *J Cardiovasc Pharmacol* 4:765, 1982.

70. Kiernan FJ, Kluger J, Regnier J, et al: Epoprostenol sodium (prostacyclin) infusion in acute myocardial infarction. *Br Heart J* 56:428, 1986.

71. Henriksson P, Edhag O, Wennmalm A: Prostacyclin offers protection against early extension of acute myocardial infarction. *Adv Prostaglandins Thromboxane Leukot Res* 17:435, 1987.

72. Armstrong PW, Langevin LM, Watts DG: Randomized trial of prostacyclin infusion in acute myocardial infarction. *Am J Cardiol* 61:455, 1988.

73. Blasko G, Berentey E, Harsanyi A, Sas G: Intracoronarily administered prostacyclin and streptokinase for treatment of myocardial infarction. *Adv Prostaglandins Thromboxane Leukot Res* 11:385, 1983.

74. Uchida Y, Hanai T, Hasegawa K, et al: Recanalization of obstructed coronary artery by intracoronary administration of prostacyclin in patients with acute myocardial infarction. *Adv Prostaglandins Thromboxane Leukot Res* 11:377, 1983.

75. Hackett D, Davies G, Attilio M: Effect of prostacyclin on coronary occlusion in acute myocardial infarction. *Int J Cardiol* 26:53, 1990.

76. Hossman V, Heinen A, Anel H, Fitzgerald GA: A randomized, placebo controlled trial of prostacyclin (PGI$_2$) in peripheral arterial disease. *Thromb Res* 22:481, 1981.

77. Pardy BJ, Lewis JD, Eastcott HHG: Preliminary experience with prostaglandin E$_1$ and I$_2$ in peripheral vascular disease. *Surgery* 88:826, 1981.

78. Vermylen J, Chamore DAF, Machin SJ, et al: Prostacyclin in inoperable ischemic rest pain. *Acta Ther* 6:33, 1980.

79. Belch JJF, McArdle B, Pollock JG, et al: Epoprostenol (prostacyclin) and severe arterial disease: A double-blind trial. *Lancet* 1(8320):315, 1983.

80. Belch JJF, Newman P, Drury JK, et al: Intermittent epoprostenol (prostacyclin) infusion in patients with Raynaud's syndrome: A double-blind control trial. *Lancet* 1(8320):313, 1983.

81. Dowd PM, Martin MFR, Cooke ED, et al: Treatment of Raynaud's phenomenon by intravenous infusion of prostacyclin (PGI_2). *Br J Dermatol* 106:81, 1982.

82. Kingma K, Wollersheim H, Thein T: Double-blind, placebo-controlled study on hemodynamics in severe Raynaud's phenomenon: The acute vasodilatory effect is not sustained. *J Cardiovasc Pharmacol* 26:388, 1995.

83. Moodley J, Gouws E: A comparative study of the use of epoprostenol and dihydralazine in severe hypertension in pregnancy. *Br J Gynecol* 99:727, 1992.

84. Easterling T, Ralph D, Schmucker B: Pulmonary hypertension in pregnancy: Treatment with pulmonary vasodilators. *Obstet Gynecol* 93:494, 1999.

85. Caruana RJ, Smith MC, Clyne D, et al: Controlled study of heparin verses epoprostenol sodiun (prostacyclin) as the sole anticoagulant for chronic hemodialysis. *Blood Purif* 9:296, 1991.

86. Dibble JB, Kalra PA, Orchard MA, et al: Prostacyclin and iloprost do not effect action of standard dose heparin on hemostatic function during hemodialysis. *Thromb Res* 49:385, 1988.

87. Aren C, Feddersen K, Radegran K: Effects of prostacyclin infusion on platelet activation and postoperative blood loss in coronary bypass. *Ann Thorac Surg* 36:49, 1983.

88. Aouifi A, Blanc P, Piriou V: Cardiac surgery with cardiopulmonary bypass in patients with type II heparin-induced thrombocytopenia. *Ann Thorac Surg* 71:678, 2001.

89. DiSesa VJ, Huval W, Lelcuk S, et al: Disadvantages of prostacyclin infusion during cardiopulmonary bypass: A double-blind study of 50 patients having coronary revascularization. *Ann Thorac Surg* 38:514, 1984.

90. Fisher CA, Kappa JR, Sinha AK, et al: Comparison of equimolar concentrations of iloprost, prostacyclin, and prostaglandin E_1 on human platelet function. *J Lab Clin Med* 109:184, 1987.

91. Saniabadi AR, Belch JJF, Lowe GDO, et al: Comparison of inhibitory actions of prostacyclin and a new prostacyclin analogue on the aggregations of human platelet in whole blood. *Hemostasis* 17:147, 1987.

92. Schror K, Darius H, Matzky R, Ohlendorf R: The antiplatelet and cardiovascular action of a new carbacyclin derivative (ZK 36 374)-equipotent to PGI_2 in vitro. *Naunyn Schmiedebergs Arch Pharmacol* 316:252, 1981.

93. Parsons AA, Whalley ET: Effects of prostanoids on human and rabbit basilar arteries precontracted in vitro. *Cephalalgia* 9:165, 1989.

94. Schroder G, Beckman R, Schillinger E: Studies on vasorelaxant effects and mechanisms of iloprost in isolated preparations. In: Gryglewski RJ, Stock G, eds. *Prostacyclin and Its Stable Analogue Iloprost.* Berlin: Springer Verlag, 1987:129.

95. Belch JJ, Greer I, McLaren M, et al: The effects of intravenous ZK 36-374, a stable prostacyclin analogue, on normal volunteers. *Prostaglandins* 28:67, 1984.

96. Kaukinen S, Ylitalo P, Pessi T, Vapaatalo H: Hemodynamic effects of iloprost, a prostacyclin analog. *Clin Pharmacol Ther* 36:464, 1984.

97. Krause W, Humpel M, Hoyer GA: Biotransformation of the stable prostacyclin analogue, iloprost, in the rat. *Drug Metab* 12:645, 1984.

98. Hildebrand M, Krause W, Fabian H, et al: Pharmacokinetics of iloprost in patients with chronic renal failure and maintenance hemodialysis. *Int J Clin Pharmacol Res* 10:285, 1990.

99. Hildebrand M, Krause W, Angeli P, et al: Pharmacokinetics of iloprost in patients with hepatic dysfunction. *Int J Clin Pharmacol Ther Toxicol* 28:430, 1990.

100. Scott JP, Higenbottam T, Wallwork J: The acute effect of the synthetic prostacyclin analogue iloprost in primary pulmonary hypertension. *Br J Clin Pract* 44:231, 1990.

101. Olschewski H, Ghofrani H, Walmrath D, et al: Inhaled prostacyclin and iloprost in severe pulmonary hypertension secondary to lung fibrosis. *Am J Respir Crit Care Med* 160:600, 1999.

102. De La Mata J, Gomez-Sanchez MA, Aranzana M, Gomez-Reino JJ: Long-term iloprost infusion therapy for severe pulmonary hypertension in patients with connective tissue diseases. *Arthritis Rheum* 37:1528, 1994.

103. Olschewski H, Walmrath D, Schermuly R, et al: Aerosolized prostacyclin and iloprost in severe pulmonary hypertension. *Ann Intern Med* 124:820, 1996.

104. Mikhail G, Gibbs J, Richardson M, et al: An evaluation of nebulized prostacyclin in patients with primary and secondary pulmonary hypertension. *Eur Heart J* 18:1499, 1997.

104a. Olschewski S, Simonneau G, Galié N, et al: Inhaled iloprost for severe pulmonary hypertension. *N Engl J Med* 347:322, 2002.

105. Wiedemann R, Ardeschir Ghofrani H, Weissmann N, et al: Atrial natriuretic peptide in severe primary and nonprimary pulmonary hypertension: response to iloprost inhalation. *J Am Coll Cardiol* 38:1130, 2001.

106. Hoeper M, Schwarze M, Ehlerding S, et al: Long-term treatment of primary pulmonary hypertension with aerosolized iloprost, a prostacyclin analogue. *N Engl J Med* 342:1866, 2000.

107. Olschewski H, Ardeschir H, Schmehl T, et al: Inhaled iloprost to treat severe pulmonary hypertension. *Ann Intern Med* 132:435, 2000.

108. Wilkens H, Guth A, König J, et al: Effect of inhaled iloprost plus oral sildenafil in patients with primary pulmonary hypertension. *Circulation* 104:1218, 2001.

108a. Ghofrani HA, Wiedemann R, Rose F, et al: Combination therapy with oral sildenafil and inhaled iloprost for severe pulmonary hypertension. *Ann Intern Med* 136:515, 2002.

109. Schenk P, Petkov V, Madl C, et al: Aerosolized iloprost therapy could not replace long-term intravenous epoprostenol (prostacyclin) administration in severe pulmonary hypertension. *Chest* 119:296, 2000.

110. Ewert R, Wensel R, Opitz CF: Aerosolized iloprost for primary pulmonary hypertension (correspondence). *N Engl J Med* 343:1421, 2000.

110a. Machherndl S, Kneussl M, Baumgartner H, et al: Long-term treatment of pulmonary hypertension with aerosolized iloprost. *Eur Respir J* 17:8, 2001.

111. Dormandy J: Use of the prostacyclin analogue iloprost in the treatment of patients with critical limb ischemia. *Therapie* 46:319, 1991.

112. UK Severe Limb Ischemia Study Group: Treatment of limb threatening ischemia with intravenous iloprost: A ramdomized double-blind placebo-controlled study. *Eur J Vasc Surg* 5:511, 1991.

113. Fiessinger JN, Schafer M: Trial of iloprost versus aspirin treatment for critical limb ischemia of thromboangiitis obliterans. *Lancet* 335:555, 1990.

114. Anonymous: Oral iloprost in the treatment of thromboangiitis obliterans (Buerger's disease): A double-blind, randomized, placebo-controlled trial. *Eur J Vasc Endovasc Surg* 15: 300, 1998.

114a. Scorza R, Caronni M, Mascagni B, et al: Effects of long-term cyclic iloprost therapy in systemic sclerosis with Raynaud's phenomenon. A randomized, controlled study. *Clin Exp Rheumatol* 19:503, 2001.

115. Watson HR, Belcher G: Retrospective comparison of iloprost with other treatments for secondary Raynaud's phenomenon. *Ann Rheum Dis* 50:359, 1991.

116. Darton K, Tanner SB, Watson HR, et al: Long term follow-up of iloprost infusion in patients with connective tissue disease using infra-red thermography (abstr). *Br J Rheum* 30 (Suppl 2):76, 1991.

117. Rademaker M, Cooke ED, Almond NE, et al: Comparison of intravenous infusion of iloprost and oral nifedipine in treatment of Raynaud's phenomenon in patients with systemic sclerosis: A double blind randomized study. *Br Med J* 298:561, 1989.

118. Belch JJF, Capell HA, Cooke ED, et al: Oral iloprost as a treatment for Raynaud's syndrome: A double blind multicenter placebo controlled study. *Ann Rheum Dis* 54:197, 1995.

119. De Caterina R, Pelosi G, Carpeggiani C, et al: Iloprost in Prinzmetal's angina. *Am J Cardiol* 58:553, 1986.

120. Bugiardini R, Galvani M, Ferrini D, et al: Myocardial ischemia during intravenous prostacyclin administration: Hemodynamic findings and precautionary measures. *Am Heart J* 113:234, 1987.

121. Topol EJ, Ellis SG, Califf RM, et al: Combined tissue-type plasminogen activator and prostacyclin therapy for acute myocardial infarction. *J Am Coll Cardiol* 14:877, 1989.

122. Martin W, Spyt T, Thomas I, et al: Quantification of extracorporeal platelet deposition in cardiopulmonary bypass: Effects of ZK 36374, a prostacyclin analogue. *Eur J Nucl Med* 15:128, 1989.

123. Massonnet-Castel S, Farge D, Tournay D, et al: Utilisation d'une prostacyclin de synthese en circulation extracorporelle. *Presse Med* 25:113, 1992.

124. Lehmann C, König J-P, Dettmann J, et al: Effects of iloprost, a stable prostacyclin analog, on intestinal leukocyte adherence and microvascular blood flow in rat experimental endotoxemia. *Crit Care Med* 29:1412, 2001.

125. Popat KD, Pitt B: Hemodynamic effects of prostaglandin E_1 infusion in patients with acute myocardial infarction and left ventricular failure. *Am Heart J* 103:485, 1982.

126. Sharma B, Wyeth RP, Gimenez HJ, Franciosa JA: Intercoronary prostaglandin E_1 plus streptokinase in acute myocardial infarction. *Am J Cardiol* 58:1161, 1986.

127. Awan NA, Evenson MK, Needham KE, et al: Cardiocirculation and myocardial energetic effects of prostaglandin E_1 in severe left ventricular failure due to chronic coronary heart disease. *Am Heart J* 102:703, 1981.

128. Lucas GS, Simms MH, Caldwell NM, et al: Hemorrheological effects of prostaglandin E_1 infusion in Raynaud's syndrome. *J Clin Pathol* 37:870, 1984.

129. Pardy BJ, Lewis JD, Eastcott HH: Preliminary experience with prostaglandins E_1 and I_2 in peripheral vascular disease. *Surgery* 88:826, 1980.

130. Rubis LJ, Stephenson LW, Johnston MR, et al: Comparison of effects of prostaglandin E_1 and nitroprusside on pulmonary vascular resistance in children after open-heart surgery. *Ann Thorac Surg* 32:563, 1981.

131. Barth H, Lintz W, Michel G, et al: Inhibition of platelet aggregation by intravenous administration of the biochemically stable prostacyclin analogue CG 4203 in man. *Naunyn Schmiedebergs Arch Pharmacol* 324(Suppl):R60, 1983.

132. Darius H, Kopp H, Mulfinger A, et al: Pilot study of the effects of taprostene (CG 4203) in patients with advanced peripheral arterial disease. *Prog Clin Biol Res* 301:417, 1989.

133. Virgolini I, Fitscha P, O'Grady J, et al: Effects of taprostene, a chemically stable prostacyclin analogue, in patients with ischemic peripheral vascular disease: A placebo controlled double-blind trial. *Prostaglandins Leukot Essent Fatty Acids* 38:31, 1989.

134. Hopf R, Schofl E, Frings M, Sohngen W: Einfluss des prostacyclin analogons taprostene auf die ischamische ST-streckensenkung im belastungs-EKG koronarkranker. *Zeit Kardiol* 83:258, 1994.

135. Bar FW, Meyer J, Michels R, et al: The effect of taprostene in patients with acute myocardial infarction treated with thrombolytic therapy: Results of the START study. *Eur Heart J* 14:1118, 1993.

136. Linet OI, Luderer JR, Froeschke M, et al: Ciprostene in patients with peripheral vascular disease: An open-labeled, tolerance trial. *Prostaglandins Leukot Essent Fatty Acids* 34:9, 1988.

137. The Ciprostene Study Group: The effect of ciprostene in patients with peripheral vascular disease (PAD) characterized by ischemic ulcers. *J Clin Pharmacol* 31:81, 1991.

138. Raizner AE, Hollman J, Abukhalil J, et al: Ciprostene for restenosis revisited: Quantitative analysis of angiograms (abstr). *J Am Coll Cardiol* 21:321A, 1993.

139. Patterson JH, Adams KF, Gheorghiade M, et al: Acute hemodynamic effects of the prostacyclin analog 15AU81 in severe congestive heart failure. *Am J Cardiol* 75:26A, 1995.

140. Moller ER III, Klugherz B: Trial of a novel prostacyclin analog, UT-15, in patients with severe intermittent claudication. *Vasc Med* 5:231, 2000.

141. Hildebrand M, Staks T, Nieuweboer B: Pharmacokinetics and pharmacodynamics of cicaprost in healthy volunteers after oral administration of 5 to 20 micrograms. *Eur J Clin Pharmacol* 39:149, 1990.

141a. Melian EB, Goa KL: Beraprost: A review of its pharmacology and therapeutic efficacy in the treatment of peripheral arterial disease and pulmonary arterial hypertension. *Drugs* 62:107, 2002.

142. Lau CS, McLaren M, Saniabadi A, et al: The pharmacological effects of cicaprost, an oral prostacyclin analogue, in patients with Raynaud's syndrome secondary to systemic sclerosis: A preliminary study. *Clin Exp Rheumatol* 9:271, 1991.

143. Lau CS, Belch JJ, Madhok R, et al: A randomized, double-blind study of cicaprost, an oral prostacyclin analogue, in the treatment of Raynaud's phenomenon secondary to systemic sclerosis. *Clin Exp Rheumatol* 11:35, 1993.

143a. Pope J, Fenlon D, Thompson A, et al: Iloprost and cisaprost for Raynaud's phenomenon in progressive systemic sclerosis. *Cochrane Database Syst Rev* 2:CD000953, 2000.

144. Lievre M, Azoulay S, Lion L, et al: A dose-effect study of beraprost sodium in intermittent claudication. *J Cardiovasc Pharmacol* 27:788, 1996.

145. Nagaya N, Uematsu M, Okano Y, et al: Effect of orally active prostacyclin analogue on survival of outpatients with primary pulmonary hypertension. *J Am Coll Cardiol* 34:1188, 1999.

145a. Galié N, Humbert M, Vachiéry J-L, et al: Effects of beraprost sodium, an oral prostacyclin analogue, in patients with pulmonary arterial hypertension: A randomized, placebo-controlled, double-blind trial. *J Am Coll Cardiol* 30:1496, 2002.

146. Ichida F, Uese K, Tsubata S, et al: Additive effect of beroprost on pulmonary vasodilation by inhaled nitric oxide in children with pulmonary hypertension. *Am J Cardiol* 80:662, 1997.

147. Okano Y, Hoshioka T, Shimouchi A, et al: Orally active prostacyclin analogue in primary pulmonary hypertension (letter). *Lancet* 349:1365, 1997.

148. Lievre M, Morand S, Besse B, et al: Oral beraprost sodium, a prostaglandin I2 analogue, for intermittent claudication. *Circulation* 102:426, 2000.

149. Vayssairat M: Preventive effect of an oral prostacyclin analog, beraprost sodium, on digital necrosis in systemic sclerosis. *J Rhematol* 26:2173, 1999.

150. Fink AN, Frishman WH, Azizad M, Agarwal Y: Use of prostacyclin and its analogues in the treatment of cardiovascular disease. *Heart Dis* 1:29, 1999.

151. Saji T, Nakayama T, Ishikita T, Matsuura H: Current status and future prospect of prostacyclin therapy for pulmonary hypertension—intravenous, subcutaneous, inhaled, and oral PGI_2 derivatives. *Nippon Rinsho* 59:1132, 2001.

CHAPTER 26

Selective and Nonselective Dopamine-Receptor Agonists

William H. Frishman

Hilary Hotchkiss

Dopamine, the endogenous precursor of both norepinephrine and epinephrine, is used predominantly in intensive care unit settings as an intravenous pharmacotherapy for patients with ventricular dysfunction and various forms of shock. Dopamine acts at low doses by stimulating specific peripheral dopaminergic receptors, which are classified into two major subtypes (Fig. 26-1): D_{A1} receptors, which, when stimulated, mediate arterial vasodilation in the coronary, renal, cerebral, and mesenteric arteries as well as natriuresis and diuresis; and D_{A2} receptors, which are located in presynaptic areas and, when stimulated, mediate the inhibition of norepinephrine release.[1-3] At increasingly higher doses, dopamine, in addition, selectively activates the beta$_1$-adrenergic receptors, leading to both a positive inotropic and a chronotropic effect on the heart (see Chap. 13). Next, the alpha$_1$- and alpha$_2$-adrenergic receptors are activated, leading to an increase in systemic vascular resistance and blood pressure due to vasoconstriction (Table 26-1).

For a number of years, there has been interest in newer pharmacologic agents that share some of the qualities of dopamine but have their own unique advantages. Each is an agonist at one or both of the peripheral dopaminergic receptors (Table 26-2). The first of these agents, fenoldopam, is specific for the D_{A1} receptor, and in contrast to dopamine may have weak alpha-antagonist activity.[4-6] Fenoldopam has been shown to have no significant activity at the D_{A2} or beta receptors.[6a] Although available in an oral formulation, fenoldopam has rapid metabolism and poor bioavailability via the oral route; thus the focus has been on its intravenous use. Over the past 10 years, an increasing database has accumulated in support of fenoldopam for hypertensive emergencies. Some have considered it a first-line agent secondary to a predictable vasodilatory mediated decrease in blood pressure, with minimal hypotensive overshoot, combined with a natriuretic and diuretic response. In December 1997, fenoldopam was approved by the U.S. Food and Drug Administration (FDA) for short-term use (48 h) as a parenteral antihypertensive agent for use in hypertensive emergencies. A second dopamine agonist, ibopamine, is an orally active prodrug that activates D_{A1}, D_{A2}, beta receptors, and alpha receptors, with a dose response similar to that of to dopamine. The drug was developed due to its orally available formulation with thoughts that it would be useful in the long-term treatment of congestive heart failure (CHF). Ibopamine was used in Europe; however, in 1996, a large-scale clinical trial, the Prospective Randomized study of Ibopamine on Mortality and Efficacy (PRIME II) was stopped early owing to increased mortality.[7] It has been hypothesized that the increase in mortality with ibopamine was due to its increasing adrenergic agonist activity. Further clinical investigation of this agent has therefore

been halted. Dopexamine, another intravenous dopamine-receptor agonist, is being evaluated particularly in patients with CHF who require major abdominal surgery. Dopexamine predominantly acts at the D_{A1} and beta$_2$-adrenergic receptors; thus interest has focused on those properties that would increase cardiac output as well as both intestinal and renal blood flow. Finally, specific D_{A2}-selective agonists such as bromocriptine are being used in clinical trials to treat systemic hypertension. The mechanism of pharmacologic action is the presynaptic inhibition of norepinephrine release. In this chapter, the clinical pharmacology of the dopaminergic agonists is reviewed, following a discussion of the peripheral dopaminergic receptors.

DOPAMINE RECEPTORS

Molecular pharmacologists have divided the dopaminergic receptors into various subtypes. The peripheral dopaminergic receptors, D_{A1} and D_{A2}, have been the target of various cardiovascular pharmacotherapies that do not cross the blood-brain barrier and therefore do not affect the central nervous system's dopaminergic receptors. A number of distinct dopamine receptors in the central nervous system have been found. They have been broken down into two groups: D_1-like and D_2-like. The D_1-like group includes the specific receptors D_{1A}, D_{1B}, and D_5. These are G protein–linked receptors that stimulate adenylate cyclase, causing an increase in intracellular cAMP. The D_2-like group includes D_2, D_3, and D_4. These are also G protein–linked receptors, but they inhibit adenylate cyclase and thus also the formation of cAMP. The D_1- and D_2-like receptors are all distinct; however, they are currently grouped on the basis of their similarities. The peripheral dopamine receptors have a different nomenclature and are classified into two distinct families—D_{A1} and D_{A2} receptors.[7,8] Recent studies have found the D_{A1} receptors to be similar to the D_1-like central receptors and the D_{A2} receptors to be similar to the D_2-like central receptors. However, additional study is required before a firm conclusion can be made regarding the significance of these similarities. The remainder of this chapter concentrates solely on the peripheral dopamine receptors and their activation.

D_{A1} receptors are located postsynaptically on the smooth muscle of the renal, coronary, cerebral, and mesenteric arteries (Table 26-3). Their activation results in vasodilation through an increase in cyclic adenosine monophosphate (cAMP)–dependent protein kinase A activity. This causes relaxation of smooth muscle.[1,7] This vasodilatory effect tends to be strongest in the renal arteries,

AUTONOMIC
GANGLION

PREJUNCTIONAL
SYMPATHETIC NERVE TERMINAL

POSTJUNCTIONAL
VASCULAR EFFECTOR CELL

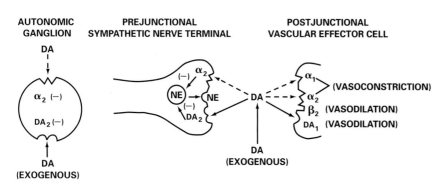

FIGURE 26-1. Receptors a2 and D_2 are located on the autonomic ganglion and prejunctional sympathetic nerve terminal to inhibit release of norepinephrine. Receptors a1 and a2 are located on the postjunctional vascular effector cell to cause vasoconstriction. D_1 receptors and b2 adrenoreceptors are also located on the postjunctional vascular effector cell and induce vasodilation. When dopamine is injected exogenously, it acts on D_1 and D_2 receptors at lower doses and on a1 and a2 adrenoreceptors at higher doses. Dopamine has little or no effect on b2 adrenoreceptors. Dopamine also acts on b1 adrenoreceptors on myocardial cells to increase cardiac contractility. (*From Goldberg LI, Murphy MB: Dopamine. In: Messerli FH, ed. Cardiovascular Drug Therapy. Philadelphia: Saunders, 1990:1083–1089.*)

where blood flow can be increased up to 35% in normal arteries and up to 77% in patients with unilateral renal disease (dopamine doses were 1 mg/kg/min).[9,10] Recent evidence points to additional D_{A1} receptors located in the tubule of the kidney, which seem to be directly responsible for the natriuresis that is also seen with dopamine administration.[10] Although their exact role in renal tubular physiology has not been established, the receptors have been shown to regulate both the Na^+/K^+-ATPase pump and the Na^+/H^+ exchanger.[11-15] Bertorello and Aperia have demonstrated that dopamine agonists inhibit the Na^+/K^+-ATPase pump[11]; however, Lee has recently pointed out the difficulty of dissecting the natriuretic response due to increased blood flow from the natriuretic response secondary to Na^+/K^+-ATPase inhibition.[10] While the exact mechanism of D_{A1}-receptor activation in the kidney remains uncertain, natriuresis associated with dopamine infusion is quite clear. Abnormalities in the renal D_{A1} receptors may, in fact, contribute to the etiology of some cases of systemic hypertension.[16] Based on the combined effects of activated D_{A1} receptors, research on selective D_{A1} agonists has focused on their use as a treatment for systemic hypertension and for hypertensive crises, particularly in patients with impaired renal function. The advantage of this pharmacologic approach over currently available antihypertensive medications would be the maintenance of renal perfusion combined with natriuretic and diuretic effects. In addition, some research on D_1 agonists has

focused on the possibility of increased myocardial blood flow with this treatment.[17] Since currently available vasodilators often exhibit coronary steal, a D_{A1} agonist might correct this problem. Finally, the potential use of D_{A1} agonists for CHF is attractive based on the reduction in afterload caused by their selective vasodilatory ability.

Peripheral D_{A2} receptors are located on presynaptic adrenergic nerve terminals and on sympathetic ganglia; when activated, they inhibit norepinephrine release.[18] They are located on the adrenal cortex, where they inhibit angiotensin II–mediated aldosterone secretion.[19,20] D_{A2} receptors are also located in the pituitary gland; when stimulated, they can inhibit prolactin release. The D_{A2} receptors in the emetic center of the medulla, when stimulated, can induce nausea and vomiting.[18] D_{A2} receptors are thought to be present in the kidney, although their function is unknown.[21] The consequence of D_2-receptor activation has been experimentally shown to be a reduction in cAMP.[8] The combined effects of inhibiting both norepinephrine-induced vasoconstriction and aldosterone release with selective D_{A2} agonists is an attractive approach for the treatment of both hypertension and CHF. A large number of D_{A2} agonists have recently been used to treat hypertension and are discussed below. Haeusler et al. wrote that presynaptically acting agents are among the few types of drugs that have not been thoroughly researched for the treatment of hypertension.[22] With respect to their use in heart failure, D_{A2} agonists would treat the associated edema by

TABLE 26-1. Adrenergic and Dopaminergic Receptors: Locations, Roles, and Agonists

Receptors	Location	Roles	Agonists
α_1	Postsynaptic	↑ Vascular contraction and cardiac inotropism	PE, NE, E, EP, DA
α_2	Presynaptic	↑ Vascular (vein) contraction	E, NE, EP, DA
	Postsynaptic	↓ NE & renin release	
		↓ H_2O, Na^+ reabsorption	
β_1	Postsynaptic	↑ Cardiac inotropism and chronotropism	I, NE, EP, DA
		↑ Lipolysis	
β_2	Presynaptic	↑ Vasodilation (artery)	I, EP
	Postsynaptic	↑ NE and renin release	
		↑ Cardiac chronotropism and inotropism	
D_{A1}	Postsynaptic	↑ Vasodilation	Fenoldopam, EP, DA
		↓ H_2O, Na^+ reabsorption	
D_{A2}	Presynaptic	↓ Ganglionic transmission	Bromocriptine, EP, DA
		↓ NE and aldosterone release	

PE = phenylephrine; NE = norepinephrine; E = epinephrine; EP = epinine; DA = dopamine; I = isoproterenol; ↑ = increase; ↓ = decrease.

Source: Reproduced from Itoh H: Clinical pharmacology of ibopamine. *Am J Med* 90(Suppl 5B): 36s, 1991.

TABLE 26-2. Actions of Dopaminergic Agonists and Their Oral Availability

	Dopamine	Ibopamine	Fenoldopam	Dopexamine	Bromocriptine
D_{A1} (vasodilation)	+++	+++	+++	+++	−
D_{A2} (vasodilation, emesis, inhibits prolactin)	+++	+++	−	+	+++
α (vasoconstriction)	++	+	−	−	−
β_1 (inotropic, chronotropic)	+++	++	−	−	−
β_2 (vasodilation)	+	++	−	++	−
Oral availability	−	yes	minimal	−	yes

+++ = major action; ++ = moderate action; + = minimal action; − = no action.

inhibiting aldosterone secretion and could reduce afterload through the inhibition of norepinephrine release.

DOPAMINE-RECEPTOR AGONISTS

Dopamine

Dopamine, the parent agonist, is given intravenously at varying doses to achieve different hemodynamic effects. In the low-dose range (2 to 5 μ/kg/min), dopamine activates only D_{A1} and D_{A2} receptors.[23] It is used at this dose to improve renal perfusion during acute low-cardiac-output situations such as cardiogenic, septic, and hypovolemic shock (Table 26-4). Diuresis and natriuresis are also observed at this dose.[23] At a somewhat higher dose (5 to 10 μg/kg/min), dopamine also activates beta$_1$ receptors for a chronotropic and inotropic effect.[23] Heart rate may actually increase, decrease, or stay the same, depending on the balance of beta$_1$ or D_{A2} receptors found in a particular person.[18] A higher number of beta$_1$ receptors causes an increase in heart rate, while a higher number of D_{A2} receptors causes a decrease in heart rate because of the inhibition of norepinephrine release. At this dose level, dopamine has been used to treat heart failure, often in combination with vasodilators such as nitroprusside or nitroglycerin.[23] In addition, if used with dobutamine, a beta$_1$ agonist, the increase in cardiac output can be magnified.[18] Side effects with this dose of dopamine may include arrhythmia and/or tachycardia.[18] At the highest levels of dopamine infusion (10 to 20 μg/kg/min), both alpha$_1$ and alpha$_2$ vasoconstrictive receptors are activated. Blood pressure may now increase, along with systemic vascular resistance. Because these peripheral effects occur at highly variable doses in different individuals, renal perfusion and blood pressure must be carefully watched during any dopamine infusion. In addition, potential adverse effects of dopamine may occur at these high doses and can include the occurrence of arrhythmias, myocardial ischemia, and a reduction in blood flow to the limbs.[23] Although these effects are rare, high-dose dopamine must be used with caution and in closely monitored situations.

The use of low-dose dopamine as a renal protective agent during acute conditions that place patients at risk of impaired renal function is nearly standard practice, despite the lack of strong clinical evidence. During recent years, a number of investigators have questioned the use of "renal dose" dopamine, suggesting that low-dose dopamine does not have the renoprotective effects previously thought. In a multicenter, randomized, double-blind, placebo-controlled trial of 328 critically ill patients, Bellomo et al.[24] looked at the effects of low-dose dopamine on renal function. Outcome measures included increase in serum creatinine from baseline, the need for dialysis, duration of stay in hospital and/or an intensive care unit, and death. These investigators found no significant protection from renal dysfunction conferred by dopamine. In another double-blind randomized controlled trial of 126 patients, Lassnigg et al.[25] looked at the renoprotective effects of low-dose dopamine after cardiac surgery. They found no significant difference in the concentration of serum creatinine or the need for dialysis between the groups that received low-dose dopamine or placebo. Whether physicians should continue to use low-dose dopamine in these situations remains to be seen.[25a]

Fenoldopam

Fenoldopam is well known as a potent selective D_{A1} agonist. There is also weak evidence that fenoldopam has mild alpha-antagonist activity at the alpha$_2$ receptor site.[4-6a] Unlike dopamine, fenoldopam has no significant effects on alpha$_1$, beta-adrenergic, or D_{A2} receptors. It acts as a vasodilator, being up to six to nine times as potent as dopamine itself, particularly in the renal bed (Fig. 26-2). It is poorly soluble in lipids, thus does not penetrate the blood-brain barrier and has no central nervous system effects. Fenoldopam is available

TABLE 26-3. Dopamine Receptors Outside the Blood-Brain Barrier

Receptor Type	Location	Physiologic Response
D_1	Kidney	Renal vasodilation, diuresis, natriuresis, direct inhibition of renin secretion
	Select arterial blood vessels	Vasodilation
D_2	Peripheral adrenergic nerve terminals	Inhibition of norepinephrine
	Sympathetic ganglia	Inhibition of transmission
	Adrenal cortex	Inhibition of aldosterone secretion
	Pituitary gland	Inhibition of prolactin release
	Area postrema of the CNS	Emesis
	Kidney	Unknown

Source: Adapted with permission from Carey.[21]

TABLE 26-4. Cardiovascular Indications for Dopaminergic-Receptor Agonists

Agent	Peripheral Dopaminergic Receptor Action	Indication
Dopamine*	Nonselective	Shock, acute treatment of CHF
Ibopamine	Nonselective	Chronic treatment of CHF
Fenoldopam*	D_1 selective	Acute treatment of hypertensive emergencies
Dopexamine	D_1 selective	Acute treatment of CHF; low cardiac output, post–cardiac surgery
Bromocriptine,	D_2 selective	Chronic treatment of hypertension
Carmoxirole	D_2 selective	Low cardiac output

*Denotes that the drug is currently available for this use.

in an oral formulation; however, its bioavailability is inconsistent (10–35%) and poor when it is taken with food. Metabolism is rapid (half-life of about 10 min); thus, frequent administration is required for sustained effect.[26–28] For these reasons, fenoldopam is primarily used via the intravenous route and has been investigated most widely in the treatment of both hypertensive emergencies and urgencies.

Hypertensive emergency is a condition that affects 2.4 to 5.2% of hypertensive patients in the United States.[28a,28b] This condition—defined as a diastolic blood pressure >115 mm Hg and/or end-organ damage such as encephalopathy, intracranial hemorrhage, pulmonary edema, dissecting aortic aneurysm or acute myocardial infarction—requires immediate care. Historically, sodium nitroprusside has been the preferred agent to treat these patients.[29] It is a potent venous and arterial dilator, with a rapid onset of action, a short half-life, a low incidence of tolerance, and a high predictability of response. However, sodium nitroprusside has some disadvantages, including thiocyanate toxicity, a possible deterioration in renal function, and a possible coronary steal due to its potent vasodilation of both arteries and veins. Alternative intravenous

FIGURE 26-2. Chemical structure of the dopamine-receptor agonist fenoldopam compared with that of dopamine.

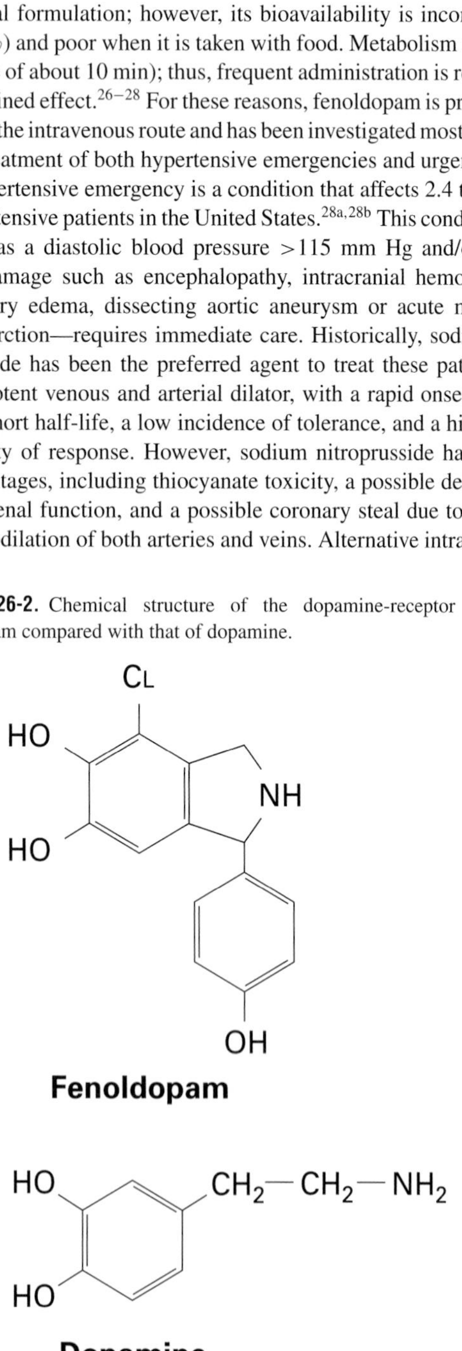

Fenoldopam

Dopamine

agents have also been used to treat hypertensive emergency, including labetalol, esmolol, nicardipine, and nitroglycerin. Intravenous fenoldopam therapy offers an alternative with potentially fewer side effects and the potential additional advantage of renal protection.[30]

Fenoldopam has been investigated and its effects reported on in the literature for more than 20 years. Among the reported clinical trials, there are data from over 1000 patients who have been treated with fenoldopam for hypertension. Some of these studies have been noncomparative. Of those that are comparative, most compare fenoldopam to sodium nitroprusside. Investigations of fenoldopam in hypertensive adults have demonstrated a clear dose-response relationship in lowering both systolic and diastolic blood pressure, along with a dose-related reflex tachycardia.[26,31–34] Significantly, at doses that reduce the blood pressure into target ranges, little overshoot hypotension is observed.

Tumlin et al., in a recent study as part of the Fenoldopam Study Group,[34] enrolled 107 patients in a randomized double-blinded study evaluating four different fixed doses of fenoldopam for 24 h in patients with hypertensive emergency, defined as diastolic blood pressure >120 mm Hg and/or target-organ damage including new renal dysfunction, hematuria, acute CHF, myocardial ischemia, or grade III–IV retinopathy. Of these patients, 94 received 0.01, 0.03, 0.1, or 0.3 μg/kg/min of fenoldopam for 24 h. The mean time to achieve a 20-mm Hg reduction in diastolic blood pressure was 132.8±15.1, 125±17.0, 89.3±12.6, and 55.2±12.8 min respectively, illustrating a dose-dependent effect in lowering of blood pressure. At the highest dose (0.3 μg/kg/min), heart rate increased by an average of 11 beats per minute. It was reported that two patients in the study developed hypotension, although the dose in these two patients was not specified.

In comparison with nitroprusside, fenoldopam has been shown to have equal efficacy in reducing blood pressure and to produce fewer side effects. In a randomized prospective trial of fenoldopam versus sodium nitroprusside in hypertensive adults with diastolic blood pressure >120 mm Hg, Panecek et al. enrolled 183 patients.[32] The dose of each medication was titrated to achieve a diastolic blood pressure of 95 to 110 mm Hg, or a maximum reduction of 40 mm Hg, and patients remained in the study for at least 6 h. Results of the study showed equivalent antihypertensive efficacy with similar adverse events. Ten patients were withdrawn from the study in the fenoldopam group, five for hypotension, and five others for flushing, hypokalemia, tachycardia, and a gastrointestinal bleed. Eleven patients were withdrawn from the nitroprusside group; ten secondary to hypotension and one with palpitations and dizziness.[32] In a smaller study of 33 patients, Pilmer et al. found similar results: equal efficacy for the treatment of severe systemic hypertension with fenoldopam and sodium nitroprusside, with no difference in rate or severity of adverse events.[26] A number of other studies have been similar. There were no studies comparing efficacy or safety of fenoldopam to agents other than nitroprusside for the treatment of hypertension.

The natriuretic and diuretic effects of fenoldopam in hypertensive patients have been studied in smaller trials, including both noncomparative and comparative studies with sodium nitroprusside. Murphy et al., in a study of 10 patients with hypertension, found that intravenous fenoldopam was associated with a 46% increase in urinary flow rate and a 202% increase in sodium excretion.[35] GFR increased by 6%. Shusterman et al., in a study of 22 patients, 11 on fenoldopam and 11 on nitroprusside, showed, in addition to natriuresis and diuresis, a significant increase in creatinine clearance in the fenoldopam group.[36] These studies point to additional effects of fenoldopam and also illustrate the advantage of fenoldopam over nitroprusside in treating hypertension in patients with chronic renal insufficiency or CHF who would benefit from natriuresis and diuresis.

The adverse-effect profile of fenoldopam is similar to that of nitroprusside, including reflex tachycardia and a more moderate risk of hypotension. Elliot et al. point out that intraocular pressure increases with fenoldopam but not with nitroprusside; thus it is important to be aware that fenoldopam is contraindicated in patients with glaucoma.[37,38]

While the majority of clinical trials with fenoldopam have focused on its use for hypertensive crisis, some researchers are looking at the potential use of fenoldopam for other indications.[39,40] Kini et al.[40] and Tumlin et al.[41] have suggested that fenoldopam may be a useful adjunct in preventing radiocontrast nephropathy in patients with chronic renal insufficiency who are undergoing cardiac catheterization. Investigators have evaluated the use of fenoldopam in elderly patients undergoing repair of an abdominal aortic aneurysm.[39]

Ibopamine

Ibopamine is an orally active diisobutyric ester of epinine (*N*-methyldopamine) with a bioavailability of 75%.[42] When ingested, ibopamine is a prodrug converted by intestinal and hepatic plasma esterases to epinine, the active compound having properties very similar to those of dopamine. Epinine has a plasma half-life of 1.5 to 3 h in normal men and 4.5 h in patients with CHF.[43,44] It is excreted through the kidneys after sulfate conjugation or oxidation in the liver. Using doses of 100 to 200 mg three times daily, epinine activates both the D_1 and D_2 receptors equally. At increasingly higher doses, epinine activates beta$_1$ and beta$_2$ receptors, and eventually epinine acts as an agonist, although to a lesser extent than dopamine.[45] Extensive clinical investigation has been done using ibopamine as an agent to treat CHF. Although, for some time, ibopamine had seemed to be an agent with promise in the treatment of CHF, a large-scale clinical trial in Europe led to startling conclusions. The second Prospective Randomized Study of Ibopamine on Mortality and Efficacy in Heart Failure (PRIME-2) was a European multicenter, randomized, placebo controlled study looking at patients with class III or IV heart failure, on optimum management, who were then assigned to receive ibopamine or placebo. After 1906 patients were enrolled, preliminary results of the study found an increase in the mortality in the ibopamine group (25 versus 20% in the placebo group). Thus the trial was terminated early.[7]

The reasons for increased mortality with ibopamine are unclear. The authors pointed out that the use of an antiarrhythmic drug at baseline was a predictor for an adverse effect in ibopamine-treated patients; however, ibopamine is not thought to be proarrhythmic. Others have suggested that the stimulation of catecholamine receptors may be the more important variable in the increase in mortality.

Dopexamine

Dopexamine is a novel drug that most strongly activates beta$_2$-adrenergic receptors, but it also activates D_{A1} receptors. It differs from dopamine in that it does not activate beta$_1$- or alpha-adrenergic receptors. It is also reported to inhibit neuronal reuptake of norepinephrine. Like dopamine, dopexamine is available only in intravenous form; thus its use has focused on acute treatment rather than chronic therapy.[46] Thus far, dopexamine has been used only experimentally in humans and in small numbers of patients. It has been used in human studies at infusion rates of 1 to 6 μg/kg/min for the treatment of CHF.[46,47] Dopexamine has often been compared with both dopamine and dobutamine with respect to their hemodynamic and inotropic effects in patients with CHF.[48] Compared with dobutamine, dopexamine offers the advantage of mild inotropy, which stimulates beta$_1$ receptors directly, causing a larger inotropic effect. Dopexamine also lacks the important stimulation of alpha receptors, which causes vasoconstriction in patients treated with dopamine. It is also being studied as a treatment for postoperative low cardiac output, particularly following coronary artery bypass grafting. These studies illustrate effects of dopexamine, which include vasodilation, natriuresis, diuresis, and inotropy. The basis for the inotropic effect of dopexamine remains unclear. One explanation points to the rise in plasma norepinephrine due to the inhibition of norepinephrine reuptake as the cause for this effect.[48,49] Another study points to the activation of beta$_2$ adrenoceptors as the cause, although beta$_1$, not beta$_2$, receptors have traditionally been associated with an increase in contractility.[50]

Recent studies have investigated the use of dopexamine during major abdominal surgeries.[51–53] The thought is that under stressful conditions, the nonspecific response of endogenous catecholamines includes generalized vasoconstriction with preserved blood flow to the brain and heart. During major abdominal surgeries, endogenous catecholamines in combination with local vasoactive substances often cause gut ischemia, particularly in patients with CHF. A drug that might promote increased intestinal blood flow in this situation would be beneficial. In a study of 18 adult patients, Muller et al. looked at splanchnic oxygenation during major abdominal surgery.[52] They found that dopexamine improves oxygenation at the serosal side of the gut. Suojaranta-Ylinen et al., however, found no improvement in regional tissue oxygenation in patients treated with dopexamine who were undergoing major abdominal surgery.[53] A third study looked at hepatoprotective effects of dopexamine during hemihepatectomy surgery and found no beneficial effects.[51] Thus, combined results appear inconclusive concerning this theme.

Bromocriptine and Other D$_2$-Selective Agonists

Selective D_{A2}-receptor agonists represent another class of drugs that have been experimented with for the treatment of hypertension. Traditionally, patients with hypertension are characterized by a relative excess of plasma norepinephrine. Thus, a D_{A2}-selective agonist would reduce plasma norepinephrine and consequently vasodilate peripheral arteries and reduce blood pressure. Included in this class of drugs are, among others, bromocriptine, carmoxirole, ropinirole, quinpirole, co-dergocrine, and cabergoline. In general, these drugs have also been investigated for use in treating Parkinson's disease and are known to cross the blood-brain barrier. As a result, while the majority of drugs in this class may have beneficial effects in hypertension, they may also be associated with severe side effects from the activation of central dopaminergic receptors. Quinn et al. found that bromocriptine lowers blood pressure in normal and hypertensive individuals.[54] Walden et al., using similar doses to those in the Quinn study, however, found that bromocriptine was not effective in lowering blood pressure in hypertensive patients.[55] Lahlou et al. found that bromocriptine induced tachycardia via central D_2 stimulation.[56] Other studies reported associations between bromocriptine and loss of vision and between bromocriptine and angiopathy. One report found that bromocriptine, used at low dose to suppress lactation, induced myocardial infarction.[57]

A number of studies found that both the D_2-receptor agonists carmoxirole and ropinirole have potent antihypertensive effects; however, inadequate numbers of studies prevent conclusions from being drawn regarding their safety and efficacy.[57a] These drugs also cross the blood-brain barrier to an extent. However, they can stimulate two central areas that lie outside the blood-brain barrier, the pituitary gland and the chemoreceptor trigger zone in the area postrema, inducing prolactin release and nausea and vomiting.

In summary, D_2 selective agonists represent a class of drugs with potential as antihypertensive agents. These agents cross the blood-brain barrier, thereby additional research is needed to find peripheral D_2 agonists that do not have central nervous system effects.

Other Compounds

Other dopamine-receptor agonists that are in early development include the D_1-selective agonist YM-435,[51] the dopexamine-like compound FPL63012AR,[58] and the dopaminergic prodrugs gluDOPA[53] and docarbomine, which are converted to dopamine in the proximal tubule of the kidney to provide a hypotensive and natriuretic effect.[59] Docarpamine, an orally active dopamine prodrug, has been found in early studies to have some benefit in the treatment of refractory ascites secondary to cirrhosis.[60,61]

CONCLUSION

Nonselective and selective dopaminergic agonists are available for the treatment of hypertensive crisis and possibly CHF. In addition to intravenous dopamine, a nonselective agonist used for treatment of ventricular dysfunction and for the preservation of renal blood flow in low-output states, newer agents have and continue to be evaluated in clinical trials.

Fenoldopam is a selective D_1 agonist that is used to treat patients with hypertensive emergency. Because of bioavailability problems with the oral formulation, only the intravenous form is in use. Fenoldopam was FDA approved for the treatment of hypertensive emergency and has promise as a first-line agent for this condition. Ibopamine, which is an orally active derivative of dopamine, has dopaminergic D_1 and D_2 activity, alpha$_1$, alpha$_2$, beta$_1$, and beta$_2$ activity. This drug was extensively evaluated in the 1980s and 1990s, however, a large clinical trial revealed increased mortality, thus this drug is no longer in use. Dopexamine is an intravenous beta$_2$ and D_{A1} receptor agonist that is being studied in patients with CHF

and low cardiac output states, particularly in the context of major abdominal surgery. Selective D_2 agonists are available that can inhibit the release of norepinephrine from sympathetic nerve terminals, thereby resulting in the reduction of systemic blood pressure. However, many of these drugs cross the blood-brain barrier and affect the nigrostriatal and mesolimbic central dopaminergic systems. Carmoxirole and ropinirole appear to have less central nervous system activity and may ultimately become useful drugs for treating systemic hypertension.

REFERENCES

1. Goldberg LI, Volkman PH, Kohli JD: A comparison of the vascular dopamine receptor with other dopamine receptors. *Annu Rev Pharmacol Toxicol* 18:57, 1978.
2. Goldberg LI, Kohli JD: Peripheral pre- and post-synaptic dopamine receptors: Are they different from dopamine receptors in the central nervous system? *Commun Psychopharmacol* 3:447, 1979.
3. Goldberg LI, Kohli JD: Identification and characterization of dopamine receptors in the cardiovascular system. *Cardiologia* 32:1603, 1987.
4. Kohli JD, Glock D, Goldberg LI: Relative D_{A1}-dopamine-receptor agonist and alpha-adrenoceptor antagonist activity of fenoldopam in the anesthetized dog. *J Cardiovasc Pharmacol* 11:123, 1988.
5. Nakamura S, Kohli JD, Rajfer SI: Alpha-adrenoceptor blocking activity of fenoldopam (SK&F 82526), a selective D_{A1} agonist. *J Pharm Pharmacol* 38:113, 1986.
6. Ohlstein EH, Zabko-Potapovich B, Berkowitz BA: The D_{A1} receptor agonist fenoldopam (SK&F 82526) is also an alpha 2-adrenoceptor antagonist. *Eur J Pharmacol* 118:321, 1985.
6a. Murphy MB, Murray C, Shorten GD: Fenoldopam: A selective peripheral dopamine receptor agonist. *N Engl J Med* 345:1548, 2001.
7. Hampton JR, van Veldhuisen DJ, Kleber FX, et al: Randomised study of effect of ibopamine on survival in patients with advanced severe heart failure. Second Prospective Randomised Study of Ibopamine on Mortality and Efficacy (PRIME II) Investigators. *Lancet* 349:971, 1997.
8. Francis GS: Receptor systems involved in norepinephrine release in heart failure: focus on dopaminergic systems. *Clin Cardiol* 18:I13, 1995.
9. Lee MR: Dopamine and the kidney. *Clin Sci (Colch)* 62:439, 1982.
10. Lee MR: Dopamine and the kidney: Ten years on. *Clin Sci (Colch)* 84:357, 1993.
11. Bertorello A, Aperia A: Regulation of Na$^+$,K$^+$-ATPase activity in kidney proximal tubules: Involvement of GTP binding proteins. *Am J Physiol* 256:F57, 1989.
12. Felder CC, Campbell T, Albrecht F, Jose PA: Dopamine inhibits Na($+$)-H$+$ exchanger activity in renal BBMV by stimulation of adenylate cyclase. *Am J Physiol* 259:F297, 1990.
13. Felder CC, Albrecht FE, Campbell T, et al: cAMP-independent, G protein-linked inhibition of Na+/H+ exchange in renal brush border by D1 dopamine agonists. *Am J Physiol* 264:F1032, 1993.
14. Gesek FA, Schoolwerth AC: Hormonal interactions with the proximal Na($+$)-H$+$ exchanger. *Am J Physiol* 258:F514, 1990.
15. Carey RM: Renal dopamine system. Paracrine regulator of sodium homeostasis and blood pressure. *Hypertension* 38:297, 2001.
16. Jose PA, Eisner GM, Felder RA: Role of dopamine in the pathogenesis of hypertension. *Clin Exp Pharmacol Physiol Suppl* 26:S10, 1999.
17. Shi Y, Zalewski A, Bravette B, et al: Selective dopamine-1 receptor agonist augments regional myocardial blood flow: Comparison of fenoldopam and dopamine. *Am Heart J* 124:418, 1992.
18. Murphy MB, Vaughn CJ: Dopamine. In: Messerli FH (ed). *Cardiovascular Drug Therapy.* Philadelphia: WB Saunders, 1996:1162–1166.
19. Lokhandwala MF, Barrett RJ: Cardiovascular dopamine receptors: Physiological, pharmacological and therapeutic implications. *J Auton Pharmacol* 2:189, 1982.
20. Lokhandwala MF, Hegde SS: Cardiovascular pharmacology of adrenergic and dopaminergic receptors: Therapeutic significance in congestive heart failure. *Am J Med* 90:2S, 1991.
21. Carey RM: Dopamine, hypertension and the potential for agonist therapy. In: Laragh JG, Brenner BB, eds. *Hypertension: Pathophysiology,*

Diagnosis and Management, 2nd ed. New York: Raven Press, 1995: 2937–2952.

22. Haeusler G, Lues I, Minck KO, et al: Pharmacological basis for antihypertensive therapy with a novel dopamine agonist. *Eur Heart J* 13(Suppl D):129, 1992.

23. van Veldhuisen DJ, Girbes AR, de Graeff PA, Lie KI: Effects of dopaminergic agents on cardiac and renal function in normal man and in patients with congestive heart failure. *Int J Cardiol* 37:293, 1992.

24. Bellomo R, Chapman M, Finfer S, et al: Low dose dopamine in patients with early renal dysunction: A placebo-controlled randomized trial. Australian and New Zealand Intensive Care Society (ANZICS) Clinical Trials Group. *Lancet* 356:2139, 2000.

25. Lassnigg A, Donner E, Grubhofer G, et al: Lack of renoprotective effects of dopamine and furosemide during cardiac surgery. *J Am Soc Nephrol* 11(1):97, 2000.

25a. Kellum JA, Decker JM: Use of dopamine in acute renal failure: A meta-analysis. *Crit Care Med* 29:1526, 2001.

26. Pilmer BL, Green JA, Panacek EA, et al: Fenoldopam mesylate versus sodium nitroprusside in the acute management of severe systemic hypertension. *J Clin Pharmacol* 33:549, 1993.

27. Blanchett DG, Green JA, Nara A, et al: The effect of food on pharmacokinetics and pharmacodynamics of fenoldopam in class III heart failure. *Clin Pharmacol Ther* 49:449, 1991.

28. Clancy A, Locke-Haydon J, Cregeen RJ, et al: Effect of concomitant food intake on absorption kinetics of fenoldopam (SK&F 82526) in healthy volunteers. *Eur J Clin Pharmacol* 32:103, 1987.

28a. Mansoor GA, Frishman WH: Comprehensive management of hypertensive emergencies and urgencies. *Heart Disease* 4:2002, in press.

28b. Phillips RA, Greenblatt J, Krakoff LR: Hypertensive emergencies: Diagnosis and management. *Prog Cardiovasc Dis* 45:33, 2002.

29. Abdelwahab W, Frishman W, Landau A: Management of hypertensive urgencies and emergencies. *J Clin Pharmacol* 35:747, 1995.

30. Oparil S, Aronson S, Deeb GM, et al: Fenoldopam: A new parenteral antihypertensive. Consensus round table on the management of perioperative hypertension and hypertensive crises. *Am J Hypertens* 12:653, 1999.

31. Munger MA, Rutherford WF, Anderson L, et al: Assessment of intravenous fenoldopam mesylate in the management of severe systemic hypertension. *Crit Care Med* 18:502, 1990.

32. Panacek EA, Bednarczyk EM, Dunbar LM, et al: Randomized, prospective trial of fenoldopam vs sodium nitroprusside in the treatment of acute severe hypertension. Fenoldopam Study Group. *Acad Emerg Med* 2:959, 1995.

33. Post JB, Frishman WH: Fenoldopam: a new dopamine agonist for the treatment of hypertensive urgencies and emergencies. *J Clin Pharmacol* 38:2, 1998.

34. Tumlin JA, Dunbar LM, Oparil S, et al: Fenoldopam, a dopamine agonist, for hypertensive emergency: A multicenter randomized trial. Fenoldopam Study Group. *Acad Emerg Med* 7:653, 2000.

35. Murphy MB, McCoy CE, Weber RR, et al: Augmentation of renal blood flow and sodium excretion in hypertensive patients during blood pressure reduction by intravenous administration of the dopamine-1 agonist fenoldopam. *Circulation* 76:1312, 1987.

36. Shusterman NH, Elliott WJ, White WB: Fenoldopam, but not nitroprusside, improves renal function in severely hypertensive patients with impaired renal function. *Am J Med* 95:161, 1993.

37. Elliott WJ, Karnezis TA, Silverman RA, et al: Intraocular pressure increases with fenoldopam, but not nitroprusside, in hypertensive humans. *Clin Pharmacol Ther* 49:285, 1991.

38. Everitt DE, Boike SC, Piltz-Seymour JR, et al: Effect of intravenous fenoldopam on intraocular pressure in ocular hypertension. *J Clin Pharmacol* 37:312, 1997.

39. Gilbert TB, Hasnain JU, Flinn WR, et al: Fenoldopam infusion associated with preserving renal function after aortic cross-clamping for aneurysm repair. *J Cardiovasc Pharmacol Ther* 6:31, 2001.

40. Kini A, Mitre C, Kamran M, et al: Changing trends in incidence and predictors of radiographic contrast nephropathy after percutaneous coronary intervention with use of fenoldopam. *Am J Cardiol* 89:999, 2002.

41. Tumlin JA, Wang A, Murray PT, Mathur VS: Fenoldopam mesylate blocks reductions in renal plasma flow after radiocontrast dye infusion: A pilot trial in the prevention of contrast nephropathy. *Am Heart J* 143:894, 2002.

42. Ventresca GP, Lodola E: Clinical pharmacokinetics of ibopamine on different diseases and conditions. *Arzneimittelforschung* 38:1175, 1988.

43. Girbes AR, Milner AR, McCloskey BV, et al: Oral ibopamine substitution in patients with intravenous dopamine dependence. *Cardiology* 86:391, 1995.

44. Metra M, Dei CL: Clinical efficacy of ibopamine in patients with chronic heart failure. *Clin Cardiol* 18:I22, 1995.

45. Pouleur H: Neurohormonal and hemodynamic effects of ibopamine. *Clin Cardiol* 18:I17, 1995.

46. Gollub SB, Elkayam U, Young JB, et al: Efficacy and safety of a short-term (6–h) intravenous infusion of dopexamine in patients with severe congestive heart failure: A randomized, double-blind, parallel, placebo-controlled multicenter study. *J Am Coll Cardiol* 18:383, 1991.

47. Asanoi H, Sasayama S, Sakurai T, et al: Intravenous dopamine in the treatment of acute congestive heart failure: Results of a multicenter, double-blind, placebo-controlled withdrawal study. *Cardiovasc Drugs Ther* 9:791, 1995.

48. Tan LB, Littler WA, Murray RG: Comparison of the haemodynamic effects of dopexamine and dobutamine in patients with severe congestive heart failure. *Int J Cardiol* 30:203, 1991.

49. Tan LB, Littler WA, Murray RG: Beneficial haemodynamic effects of intravenous dopexamine in patients with low-output heart failure. *J Cardiovasc Pharmacol* 10:280, 1987.

50. Napoleone P, Ricci A, Ferrante F, Amenta F: Dopexamine hydrochloride in the human heart: Receptor binding and effects on cAMP generation. *Eur Heart J* 13:1709, 1992.

51. Marx G, Leuwer M, Holtje M, et al: Low-dose dopexamine in patients undergoing hemihepatectomy: An evaluation of effects on reduction of hepatic dysfunction and ischaemic liver injury. *Acta Anaesthesiol Scand* 44:410, 2000.

52. Muller M, Boldt J, Schindler E, et al: Effects of low-dose dopexamine on splanchnic oxygenation during major abdominal surgery. *Crit Care Med* 27:2389, 1999.

53. Suojaranta-Ylinen RT, Ruokonen ET, Takala JA: The effect of dopexamine on regional tissue oxygenation, systemic inflammation and amino acid exchange in major abdominal surgery. *Acta Anaesthesiol Scand* 44:564, 2000.

54. Quinn N, Illas A, Lhermitte F, Agid Y: Bromocriptine in Parkinson's disease: A study of cardiovascular effects. *J Neurol Neurosurg Psychiatry* 44:426, 1981.

55. Walden RJ, Hernandez J, Bhattacharjee P, et al: Bromocriptine in the treatment of hypertension. *Eur J Clin Pharmacol* 30:141, 1986.

56. Lahlou S, Duarte GP, Demenge P: Central dopaminergic origin of bromocriptine induced tachycardia in normotensive rats. *Cardiovasc Res* 27:2022, 1993.

57. Eickman FM: Recurrent myocardial infarction in a postpartum patient receiving bromocriptine. *Clin Cardiol* 15:781, 1992.

57a. Carmoxirole. In: Messerli FH, ed. *Cardiovascular Drug Therapy,* 2nd ed. Philadelphia: Saunders, 1996:1189.

58. Smith GW, Farmer JB, Ince F, et al: FPL 63012AR: A potent D_1-receptor agonist. *Br J Pharmacol* 100:295, 1990.

59. Lee MR: Five years' experience with gamma-L-glutamyl-L-dopa: A relatively renally specific dopaminergic prodrug in man. *J Auton Pharmacol* 10(Suppl 1):s103, 1990.

60. Funasaki T, Tsutsumi M, Takase S, et al: Effects of a new orally active prodrug, docarpamine, on refractory ascites: A pilot study. *Am J Gastroenterol* 94:2475, 1999.

61. Doggrell SA: The therapeutic potential of dopamine modulators on the cardiovascular and renal systems. *Expert Opin Invest Drugs* 11:631, 2002.

Natriuretic and Other Vasoactive Peptides

William H. Frishman

Domenic A. Sica

Judy W.M. Cheng

Youngsoo Cho

Bradley G. Somer

In 1981, de Bold et al[1] infused a homogenized rat extract that triggered a potent natriuresis and diuresis, as well as a small kaliuresis, supporting prior theories that suggested the heart was more than merely a mechanical pump.[2,3] This paved the way for the notion that the heart was also an endocrine organ. Subsequent fractionation and bioassay of rat atrial homogenates confirmed that this natriuretic bioactivity resided in the atrial granules.[4] On the heels of these original observations, several groups isolated atrial natriuretic peptide (ANP) in a pure form and determined its amino acid sequence. Shortly thereafter, a series of related peptides were isolated, further suggesting the endocrine capabilities of the heart. In 1988, Sudoh et al. discovered a peptide in porcine brain with structural homology and biological properties similar to ANP.[5] Although subsequent studies showed it to be secreted predominantly by ventricular tissue,[6,7] the peptide retained the name brain natriuretic peptide (BNP). Soon after the discovery of BNP, C-type natriuretic peptide (CNP) was also isolated from porcine brain.[8] Although CNP production occurs mostly in the central nervous system (CNS)[9] and vascular endothelium,[10] its structural homology and similarities in metabolism with the other natriuretic peptides led to its inclusion in the same family of peptide hormones. As a result of these findings, there developed an explosive interest in cardiac peptide research, which has led to the heart being recognized as a true endocrine organ.[11]

This chapter reviews the molecular biology, physiology, and pathophysiology of the natriuretic peptides, and uses the discussion as a foundation for exploring the peptides' therapeutic application. In this review, the quantification of doses used in the cited pharmacologic studies, as well as the methods and durations of peptide administration, are usually omitted. This was done because one objective of the chapter is to highlight the results of studies done with the pharmacologic manipulation of the natriuretic peptides, and not necessarily to describe the individual study. The reader is referred to the cited articles for additional information in this regard.

NATRIURETIC PEPTIDES

Molecular Biology, Synthesis, and Release

There are many similarities in structure, gene regulation and synthesis of the various members of the natriuretic peptide family. Each of the three major natriuretic peptides (ANP, BNP, and CNP) has a 17-amino-acid ring structure in which a number of the amino acid residues are conserved across the members of the family (Fig. 27-1).[12] The pathways for synthesis of ANP, BNP, and CNP are depicted in Figs. 27-2, 27-3, and 27-4, and the biologic characteristics are compared in Table 27-1.[13]

Atrial Natriuretic Peptide

The circulating and biologically active form of human ANP comprises a 28-amino-acid peptide with a 17-amino-acid ring closed by a disulfide bond between two cysteine residues (Fig. 27-1). Its synthesis begins with transcription of its gene from the short arm of chromosome 1 (Fig. 27-2).[14] The messenger RNA is processed,[14,15] translated into the 151-amino-acid prepro-ANP,[16] and subsequently cleaved, producing the 126 amino acid pro-ANP,[17] a biologically inactive polypeptide, which is stored in myocyte granules.[18,19] After cleavage by a membrane-bound protease, the 28-amino-acid ANP that is the carboxy-terminal fragment, biologically active, and major circulating form is released, along with an N-terminal pro-ANP (N-ANP) consisting of 98 amino acids.[19–21] In an effort to maintain stores of preformed ANP within myocyte granules, 1 to 3% of total atrial transcription is devoted to synthesis of ANP.[22] Interestingly, the amino acid sequence of ANP has been highly preserved across species.[23,24]

Although the nomenclature uses many terms to describe ANP, including atriopeptin, cardionatrin, auriculin, and atrin, for the purposes of this review, the term *ANP* will be used to describe the biologically active 28-amino-acid atrial-derived polypeptide that is the major circulating form in humans.[20] The term *N-ANP* will be used to describe the 98-amino-acid N-terminal pro-ANP. ANP possesses a disulfide bond that is required for its biologic activity.[25] Its plasma half-life is short, ranging from 1 to 3 min.[26] The normal range for plasma ANP is approximately 10 to 100 pg/mL.[27]

The atria are the primary sites of ANP synthesis with the synthetic capacity of right atrial myocytes exceeding that of left atrial cells.[28] ANP gains circulatory access via the coronary sinus emptying into the right atrium,[29] although some may be released via Thebesian veins into the left atrium and ventricles.[30] ANP release occurs in direct proportion to atrial mechanical load, with increased right atrial pressure[31,32] and distention[33] the major stimuli for release. Transmural, rather than intramural, atrial pressure is required

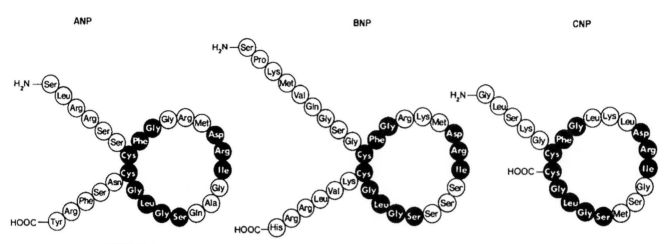

FIGURE 27-1. Mature forms of peptides belonging to the human atrial natriuretic peptide (ANP), brain natriuretic peptide (BNP), and C-type natriuretic peptide (CNP) families. Filled circles are amino acids, that are common to the three members of the human natriuretic peptide family. The mature forms shown are ANP, BNP-32, and CNP-22. (*Modified with permission from Nakao K, et al: Molecular biology and biochemistry of the natriuretic peptide system. I: Natriuretic peptides. J Hypertens 10:907–912, 1992.*)

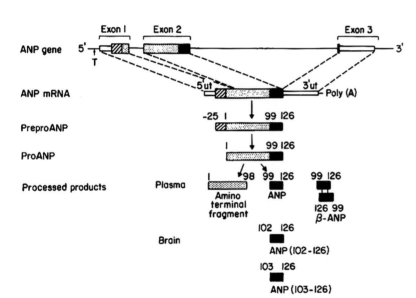

FIGURE 27-2. Structure of the human ANP gene and subsequent steps through to the mature (processed) products found in human plasma or forms found in the brain. Solid black sections are those that ultimately constitute the mature ANP peptide. Stippled areas are those from which the amino terminal fragment is derived. Diagonal striped sections represent the region coding for the signal peptide or the signal peptide itself. (*Modified with permission from Nakao K, et al: Molecular biology and biochemistry of the natriuretic peptide system. I: Natriuretic peptides. J Hypertens 10:907–912, 1992.*)

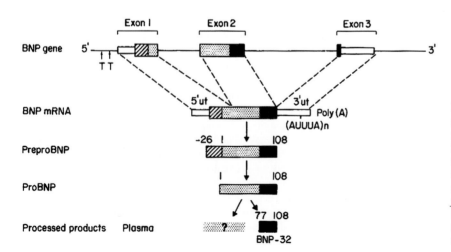

FIGURE 27-3. Structure of the human BNP gene and subsequent steps to the mature processed product (BNP-32). Solid black sections are those that encode for and ultimately become the mature BNP-32 peptide. Stippled area are those that code for or constitute the remainder of the pro-BNP molecule. It is not known whether this portion is secreted. (*Modified with permission from Nakao K, et al: Molecular biology and biochemistry of the natriuretic peptide system. I: Natriuretic peptides. J Hypertens 10:907–912, 1992.*)

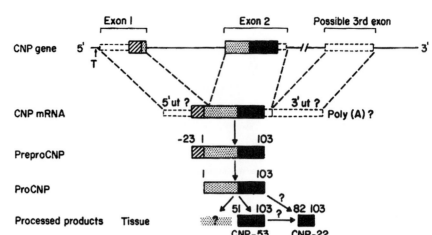

FIGURE 27-4. Structure of the human CNP gene and steps through to the mature CNP-53 or CNP-22 products. Solid black regions are those that code for and become CNP-53 (or CNP-22). Stippled areas code for the remainder of the pro-CNP molecule. It is not known whether the latter portion of pro-CNP is secreted. The uncertain regions in the gene structure are outlined with dashed lines. (*Modified with permission from Nakao K, et al: Molecular biology and biochemistry of the natriuretic peptide system. I: Natriuretic peptides. J Hypertens 10:907–912, 1992.*)

to stimulate ANP release because experimental cardiac tamponade inhibits volume expansion-induced release of ANP.[33] Additionally, evidence suggests that in normal cardiac function subjects, levels of ANP and BNP are pulsatile with an interval of 36 min (range, 21 to 77 min) for ANP and a pulse interval for BNP of 48 min (range, 24 to 77 min).[34] The significance of this phenomenon remains unknown.

A number of endogenous factors including endothelin, arginine vasopressin, and catecholamines, directly stimulate the atrial secretion of ANP.[35–39] Interestingly, ventricular expression of the ANP gene is much greater in fetal life and decreases shortly after birth.[40] Although adult ventricular ANP gene expression is about 1 to 2% that of the atria,[14,40] various stimuli can upregulate ventricular synthesis of ANP. They include either acute or chronic volume loading,[41] acute heart failure, coarctation of the abdominal aorta, hypertrophic heart disease,[42] and left ventricular aneurysm.[43] It has been suggested that hypoxia is an independent stimulus for ventricular natriuretic peptide release,[44] although these data have not been consistently demonstrated.[45] ANP transcripts are also present in noncardiac tissues such as the brain, anterior pituitary, eye, lung, thymus, vascular tissue, kidney, gastrointestinal tract, and adrenal medulla. The ANP produced by extracardiac sources behaves mainly as an autocrine/paracrine hormone and its function is not fully established. Moreover, the kidneys show a different pro-

cessing of the precursor peptide, so that urodilatin, a mature peptide of 32 amino acids (instead of 28), is produced.[46]

Brain Natriuretic Peptide

BNP retains the 17-amino-acid ring structure of the natriuretic peptide family, and in humans, BNP-32 is the major form of the hormone in atrial tissue (Fig. 27-1).[47] Alternatively, human plasma has been reported to contain either BNP-32 alone[48] or both BNP-32 and a high-molecular-weight BNP component (probably pro-BNP),[49–51] which has been detected in the peripheral blood of patients with CHF.[50,52] Its biosynthesis is directed from the distal short arm of human chromosome 1 (Fig. 27-3).[53] BNP arises from a single precursor prepro-BNP molecule translated from the BNP messenger RNA (mRNA). In humans, for instance, by removal of a hydrophobic 26-amino-acid signal peptide, the 135-amino-acid prepro-BNP is reduced to a 109-amino-acid peptide, pro-BNP.[54] This peptide is further processed to the C-terminal 32-amino-acid human BNP, the principal storage form in the human heart. In contrast to ANP, there is much variability in the length and structure of BNP across species, and the predominant forms differ considerably resulting in considerable cross-species variation in actions.[55] For further discussion, the term *BNP* will be used to describe BNP-32.

TABLE 27-1. Human Natriuretic Peptides

	ANP	BNP	CNP
Major sites of synthesis	Cardiac atrium	Cardiac ventricle	Brain, vascular, endothelium, kidney tubules
Major stimulus synthesis	Atrial transmural	Ventricular wall tension	? Cytokines,? other natriuretic peptides
Major plasma forms	ANP$_{99-126}$	BNP$_{77-108}$ (BNP-32) and pro-BNP	? (Very low levels)
Plasma half-life	3 min	21 min	2.6 min
Baroreceptor type	NPR-A	NPR-A, ?other	NPR-B
C-receptor affinity	High	Lower than ANP/CNP	High
Affinity for EPA	High	Lower than ANP/CNP	High
Major actions	Natriuresis vasodepression, antimitogenesis	Natriuresis, vasodepression, inhibition of aldosterone, ?antimitogenesis	?Vasodepression, antimitogenesis

ANP = atrial natriuretic peptide; BNP = brain natriuretic peptide; CNP = C-type natriuretic peptide; EPA = endopeptidase EC.24.11; NPR-A = natriuretic peptide receptor subtype A; NPR-B = natriuretic peptide receptor subtype B; R.

Source: Modified with permission from Espiner EA, Richards AM, et al. Natriuretic hormones. *Endocr Metab Clin North Am* 24:481–509, 1995.

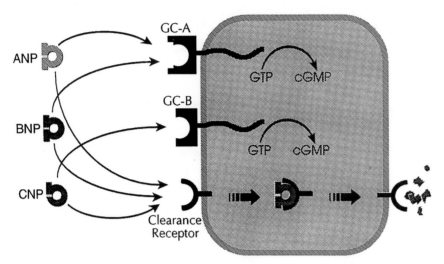

FIGURE 27-5. Binding of the natriuretic peptides to the biologic (guanylyl cyclase) and clearance (C-ANP) receptors. The binding specificity of the natriuretic peptides ANP and BNP bound to the GC-A receptor, and of CNP bound to the GC-B receptor, combined with the unique tissue distribution between the GC-A and GC-B receptors, is consistent with the possibility of fundamentally distinct biologic activity of ANP and BNP as compared to that of CNP. All three of the natriuretic peptides bind to the clearance receptor with high affinity. (*Modified with permission from Lewicki JA, Protter AA: Physiologic studies of the natriuretic peptide family. In: Laragh JH, Brenner BM, eds. Hypertension: Pathophysiology, Diagnosis and Management, 2nd ed. New York: Raven, 1995:1029–1053.*)

BNP is found in significantly lower concentrations than ANP in human plasma. In healthy controls, the plasma BNP concentration is 0.90 umol/mL, which is less than one-sixth that of the plasma ANP concentration.[56,57] Despite this, BNP has a comparatively long plasma half-life (approximately 22 min), due, presumably, to a greater volume of distribution,[58] a reduced affinity for clearance receptors,[59] and a slower rate of hydrolysis.[60]

Unlike ANP, which is produced primarily in the cardiac atria, BNP is made primarily by cardiac ventricles and released constitutively into the blood.[7] This was proven during isolated heart perfusion experiments with approximately 60% of the BNP secretory rate being maintained after atrial removal, with atrial removal reducing ANP secretory rate to less than 5% in these experiments.[61] BNP is also released into the coronary sinus. BNP is greatly increased in states of ventricular overload,[62,63] as well as in states of hypertrophic cardiomyopathy (even in the absence of increases in intraventricular pressure from volume overload).[57,64] As noted already with ANP secretion, it is probable that BNP secretion occurs in response to increased ventricular wall tension, and that its secretion increases in proportion to the severity of left ventricular dysfunction.[63,65] This response, however, is not sustained, presumably because the storage capacity of BNP in ventricular tissue, like that of ANP, is limited.[66,67]

Although the mechanisms for increased secretion of ANP and BNP appear to be similarly based on myocardial wall tension, a recent study suggests that the physiologic regulation of ANP and BNP differs in normal subjects. ANP secretion was shown to be modulated primarily by volume loading and salt intake, whereas BNP responded primarily to physical exercise.[68,69] In contrast to ANP, in which ventricular expression decreases soon after birth, plasma BNP concentrations in healthy subjects show a marked, rapid, and preferential increase immediately after birth, which suggests that BNP has a physiologic role distinct from that of ANP in the perinatal circulatory changes from fetus to neonate.[70]

Although BNP is primarily produced in the ventricles, it is also produced in smaller amounts by the atria.[71] Some atrial granules contain both BNP and ANP,[72] which may explain the observation that ANP and BNP are co-secreted in some experimental settings, as was most recently described in the equine atrium.[73] Extracardiac BNP synthesis has been reported in the human adrenal medulla, CNS, lung, thyroid, kidney, spleen, uterus, and muscle.[74,75] The presence of local synthesis of ANP, as mentioned earlier, and of BNP

in peripheral organs suggest paracrine and/or autocrine functions for these natriuretic peptides.[75]

C-Natriuretic Peptide

CNP was isolated and determined to consist of two forms, 22 and 53 amino acids in length, respectively; 11 of the 17 amino acids within the core of each are identical for ANP and BNP (Fig. 27-1).[8] Analysis of the amino acid sequence inferred from DNA clones encoding CNP indicate that the initial translation product, prepro-CNP, is 126 amino acids in length, and its processing to mature forms involves at least two proteolytic cleavage steps: initial removal of a 23-amino-acid signal sequence yielding a 103-amino-acid prohormone (pro-CNP103) and subsequent proteolytic processing to yield one of two mature peptide forms, CNP53 or CNP22 (Fig. 27-4).[76] Unlike BNP, the precursor forms of CNP are probably the most highly conserved of the natriuretic peptide family.[77]

Compared to other members of the natriuretic peptide family, the role and regulation of CNP is just now beginning to be understood. Production occurs primarily in brain tissue, especially the cerebellum and spinal cord,[78] where its concentration far exceeds those of ANP and BNP.[9] CNP is also produced in appreciable amounts in endothelial and vascular smooth-muscle tissues, where ANP and BNP can stimulate its production.[79,80] CNP was not originally thought to be synthesized by human cardiac tissue;[81] more recent investigative work, however, has provided evidence of CNP mRNA gene expression in the atria and ventricles of rats.[82]

In contrast to ANP and BNP, no changes in plasma immunoreactive CNP are observed in subjects with either mild CHF[83] or severe CHF, a state characterized by increased myocardial wall tension.[84] CNP is thought to be either a neuropeptide or a vascular peptide, and is usually undetectable in cardiac tissue.[85,86] For this reason, CNP is only described briefly in the upcoming discussion, and only as it compares with the other natriuretic peptides.[87]

Physiologic Actions

Atrial Natriuretic Peptide

ANP appears to act in four principal ways to oppose the activity of the renin-angiotensin-aldosterone (RAA) axis: it (a) causes vasorelaxation, (b) blocks aldosterone secretion by the adrenal cortex, (c) inhibits kidney renin secretion, and (d) opposes the sodium

TABLE 27-2. Reported Effects of ANP in Humans

Vascular effects
Vasodilatation
Hemoconcentration
Hormonal effects
   Decrease in plasma renin activity
   Decrease in aldosterone, cortisol, ACTH, TSH, and prolactin
   Inhibition of vasopressin secretion and/or effects
   Induction of pancreatic secretion
   Modulation of insulin secretion and/or metabolism
   May be endogenous antagonist to angiotensin II
Renal effects
   Natriuresis, diuresis with no concomitant kaliuresis
   Increase in GFR
   Decrease in effective renal plasma flow
   Increase in filtration fraction
   Increase in renovascular resistance
   Increase in urinary volume and electrolytes
Central nervous system effects
   Modulation of sympathetic activity
   Increase in heart rate
   Increase in lipolysis
   Effects on blood pressure/volume regulatory regions in the brain
Cardiac effects
   Coronary vasodilatation
   Left-ventricular performance enhancement
   Cardiac output reduction
   Coronary blood flow (varied effects)
Pulmonary effects
   Relaxation of vascular smooth-muscle cells
   Relaxation of the trachea
Adrenal effects
   Blocks release of aldosterone
Pituitary effects
   Posterior pituitary: inhibition of ADH production and release
   Anterior pituitary: inhibition of ACTH, TSH, and prolactin
Intestinal effects
   Effect on fluid movement across intestinal membrane
Growth regulatory effects
   Inhibits growth and cell proliferation

ACTH = adrenocorticoatrophic hormone; ADH = antidiuretic hormone; ANP = atrial natriuretic peptide; GFR = glomerular filtration rate; TSH = thyroid-stimulating hormone.

Source: Modified from DeZeeuw, et al: Atrial natriuretic factor: Its (patho) physiological significance in humans. *Kidney Int* 41:1115–1133, 1992.

(Na^+)-retaining action of aldosterone.[27] In addition, CNS effects, such as its inhibiting antidiuretic hormone (ADH) secretion,[88] and/or reducing salt appetite and water drinking[89,90] reinforce the ability of ANP to reduce plasma volume (Fig. 27-5) (Table 27-2).

Vascular Effects

ANP has two predominant vascular actions: first, it causes vasodilatation and second it redistributes plasma volume to the extravascular space.[91] ANP effects vasodilatation by decreasing intracellular Ca^{2+} concentrations.[92] The vasodilatory effect seems to be mediated by the second messenger, cyclic GMP (guanosine $3',5'$-monophosphate).[93,94] In one study, the forearm intra-arterial infusion of ANP produced a dose-dependent vasodilatation to about 60% of that produced by sodium nitroprusside.[95] ANP can also modulate the vasopressor effect of norepinephrine.[96] ANP also appears to reset the baroreflex control of heart rate in a way that favors bradycardia and opposes cardioacceleration. These effects may be related, at least in part, to an interaction between ANP and angiotensin-II.[97]

Renal Effects

ANP receptor binding in the kidney leads to a rise in urinary cyclic GMP excretion.[98] ANP produces both a natriuresis and a diuresis due to both renal hemodynamic and direct tubular actions.[99] The increase in renal blood flow (RBF) produced by ANP does not last as long as the natriuretic effect, suggesting two separate and distinct processes. ANP also inhibits renin release.[100] ANP promotes natriuresis and diuresis via a series of mechanisms,[101] which are not mutually exclusive one of the other, including: (a) an increase in glomerular filtration rate (GFR), which occurs as a consequence of afferent arteriolar vasodilation and efferent arteriolar vasoconstriction,[102,103] and enhanced Na^+ delivery to the medullary collecting duct;[104,105] (b) inhibition of Na^+ reabsorption by medullary collecting ducts secondary to reduction in the effects of aldosterone and/or angiotensin-II;[101,105] (c) redistribution of blood flow to deeper nephrons with less Na^+ reabsorptive capacity;[102] and (d) decreased secretion and/or effect of ADH.[88,89] On a more primary level ANP may be an endogenous antagonist to angiotensin-II[103] as their binding sites overlap in the brain, kidney and adrenal cortex.[106] An additional intriguing action of ANP is its ability to induce a natriuresis without a concomitant kaliuresis.[107] When increased potassium (K^+) excretion occurs, it seems to correlate with an enhanced tubular flow rate.[27] ANP inhibits renin release by secondary effects at the macular densa or, less likely, via a direct effect on the juxtaglomerular cells.[100]

Adrenal Effects

The zona glomerulosa cells contain specific ANP binding sites[108] and ANP both inhibits aldosterone synthesis and blocks the release of aldosterone that typically follows angiotensin-II infusions.[109,110] The inhibitory effect on aldosterone production can be overcome in a dose-dependent fashion by secretagogues such as angiotensin-II and corticotropin.[111] In addition, ANP may be an endogenous antagonist to angiotensin II.[103,106]

Cardiac Effects

Although ANP does not appear to have a direct negative or positive inotropic effect,[112] by decreasing blood volume, and thereby venous return, ANP can have a negative impact on cardiac output.[113] In experimental studies, ANP has been shown to depress myocardial contractility in normal myocytes, whereas there is no effect on contractility in hypertrophied myocytes.[114] ANP may increase,[115] decrease,[113] or have no effect on coronary blood flow.[116] ANP can act as a modulator of baroreflex function. It appears to reset the baroreflex control of heart rate in a manner that favors bradycardia and opposes cardioacceleration.[97]

CNS Effects

Although plasma ANP and BNP do not cross the blood-brain barrier, they access sites outside this barrier—such as the subfornical organ and the area postrema. As in the periphery, a pattern has emerged in which ANP opposes many of the central actions of angiotensin-II.[117] Thus, ANP's primary actions in the CNS oppose the conservation of Na^+ and water and thereby aid in regulating fluid volume and cardiovascular-renal (CVR) homeostasis. ANP also acts in the brain stem to decrease sympathetic tone.[118] In rodents with genetic forms of hypertension, inhibiting the actions of endogenous ANP in the nucleus tractus solitarii further elevates BP, suggesting a tonic role for ANP in central BP regulatory mechanisms.

Pituitary

Pharmacologic levels of ANP inhibit ADH production and release from the posterior pituitary.[119] Its effect on the anterior pituitary includes attenuation of basal secretion of adrenocorticotropin hormone and a decrease in plasma cortisol concentration. Pharmacologic levels of ANP also have been shown to reduce both thyroid releasing hormone induced-thyrotropin secretion as well as the release of prolactin in women.[120]

Other Effects

Intestine   Studies have found that ANP infusion may affect fluid movement across the intestinal membrane in rats.[121]

Cell Growth Regulation   There is evidence that ANP has growth regulatory properties in a variety of tissues such as the adrenal gland, kidney, vascular smooth muscle, brain, bone, myocytes, red blood cell precursors, and endothelial cells. For example, ANP inhibits growth in the zona glomerulosa, to behave in an antimitogenic and antiproliferative fashion in cultured glomerular mesangial cells, and to inhibit cell proliferation in vascular smooth-muscle cells.[122] ANP also inhibits endothelin release from cultured cells and the intact aorta.[123] Recent studies also show that ANP, as well as the other natriuretic peptides, can inhibit DNA synthesis in cardiac fibroblasts during cardiac hypertrophy.[124]

Brain Natriuretic Peptide

BNP has pharmacologic actions that are qualitatively similar to those of ANP. Thus, the spectrum of actions ascribed to ANP, including effects on the kidney (natriuresis and diuresis), the vasculature (hypotension and decreased intravascular fluid volume), and hormone balance (decreased plasma renin and aldosterone) have all been demonstrated with BNP administration in both experimental animals and humans.[58] BNP, though, may elicit quantitatively different effects from ANP, particularly in pathophysiologic settings.[76] The more prominent renal effects of BNP could potentially be related to its decreased avidity for the two principle metabolic pathways, and, hence, its longer half-life. Despite this, in a recent study ANP and BNP were shown to have similar efficacy in blunting the systemic pressor response to angiotensin-II and norepinephrine.[125,126] However, ANP was significantly more potent, on a molar basis, than BNP in terms of attenuating the aldosterone response to angiotensin-II. Interestingly, BNP has been recently shown to have a vasodilator effect on the coronary artery system[127] and to be a more potent vasodilator of the placental vasculature than is ANP.[128]

Considering that cross species homology amongst BNP is as highly variable as it is, interpretations of animal studies must be undertaken with caution.

C-Natriuretic Peptide

The physiologic effects of CNP differ from those of ANP and BNP. Administration of CNP has been reported to produce a hypotensive response in association with a decrease in cardiac output.[129] Renal effects, such as diuresis and/or natriuresis, appear not to occur with CNP. It has been speculated that CNP decreases arterial pressure and cardiac output by decreasing venous return, an effect consistent with the observation that CNP relaxes preconstricted canine veins.[79] Infusions of CNP-22 in normal humans did not affect BP or Na+ excretion, but are associated with significant, but small, increases in plasma cyclic guanosine monophosphate (GMP) and ANP (unpublished observations). These increases may be attributable to CNP's effect on ANP metabolism and degradation by competing for binding to EC24.11 and/or NPR-C receptors. In the dog, CNP has been shown to have positive chronotropic and inotropic effects.[130]

A possible paracrine function for CNP is receiving increasing interest following reports of its antiproliferative effects; for example, inhibition of thymidine uptake[131] or inhibition of vascular smooth-muscle cell growth.[132] CNP inhibits DNA synthesis induced by a number of vascular smooth-muscle mitogens and is twentyfold more potent than ANP as an antimitogen.[131] CNP may also play a key pathophysiologic role in regulating vascular tissue organization and vascular tone. In rats, infusions of CNP-22 have significantly reduced luminal restenosis after injury to the arterial vessel wall.[133]

Few studies have dealt with the central actions of CNP. In sheep, intracerebroventricular infusions of CNP induced a rapid fall in mean arterial BP, suggesting a role for this hormone in the central regulation of BP.[134,135]

Role of the Natriuretic Peptides in Fluid and Electrolyte Balance

Atrial Natriuretic Peptide

ANP is importantly linked to the regulation of fluid and electrolyte balance.[121] A true physiologic antagonism exists between ANP and the RAA system that can allow the body to finely tune both systemic BP and volume status.[136] In addition, the presence of secretory-like morphologic characteristics in the heart-muscle cells of many species and the fact that ANP has been highly preserved across species,[23,24] suggest both an evolutionary strategy to maintain water and electrolyte balance and a possible physiologic mechanism to offset pathologic conditions.[137] In addition, the fact that ANP can be found in areas of the brain involved in thirst[89] and cardiovascular function,[138] as well as in the adrenal medulla, lung, aortic arch, renal distal collecting duct cells, and spinal ganglion,[139] lends support to the notion of its having an important physiologic role. Despite these observations, some believe that ANP may exert only a trivial effect on renal Na+ excretion during normal living conditions, and with adequate dietary Na+ intake ANP may not be important at all.[140,141] However, it has been suggested that ANP may defend against massive and acute volume expansion.[139]

Urodilatin

ANP gene is expressed in many noncardiac tissues including the kidney. In the kidney, alternate processing of the precursor protein of ANP produces a 32-amino-acid peptide (ANP 95-126) originally isolated from human urine called urodilatin.[142] Urodilatin may act as a paracrine hormone and may be involved in the local regulation of Na+ and water processing in the kidney. Interestingly, the dose of urodilatin necessary to initiate a diuresis and natriuresis is less than the dose of ANP required to produce the same effect.[143] Urodilatin also appears to be much more resistant than ANP to endopeptidase inactivation.[144]

Brain Natriuretic Peptide

As detailed elsewhere, BNP binds to the same receptor (NPR-A) as ANP, is found in similar locations, and has similar physiologic actions. Both peptides antagonize the RAA system, although in this regard, ANP is more potent on a molar basis. Despite the fact that the species homology amongst BNP forms so far identified is much less striking than ANP, they perform similar roles, perhaps acting synergistically, in fluid and electrolyte balance.

C-Natriuretic Peptide

As mentioned previously, CNP exhibits little renal activity, even when administered in high doses directly into the renal artery.[110] The lack of natriuretic and diuretic response by the kidney to CNP supports the notion that the effects of CNP are fundamentally distinct from those of ANP and BNP.[76]

Natriuretic Peptide Receptors

Three natriuretic peptide receptors have been identified in humans, mapping to three different chromosomes.[145] Two of these receptor subtypes, NPR-A and NPR-B, are unique in containing an intracellular guanylate cyclase catalytic domain, which mediates most of the biologic actions of natriuretic peptides through the production of the second messenger, cyclic GMP.[146] A second intracellular region, termed the *kinase homology domain* because of its structural homology with known tyrosine kinase proteins, is believed to contain an ATP binding site, and studies suggest that in the absence of ligand binding, this region inhibits the activity of the guanylyl cyclase domain (Fig. 27-5).[76] The third receptor, NPR-C (also termed *clearance receptor*) is not thought to be associated with any known intracellular mediator and may function chiefly in the uptake, internalization and intracellular lysosomal degradation of hormone (Fig. 27-5).[147] Some studies indicate that occupancy of this receptor activates the phosphoinositol pathway, inhibits cyclic ANP production, and mediates some of the actions of ANP and other natriuretic peptides on cell proliferation, as well as mediating their neuromodulatory action within the nervous system.[148]

The selectivity of these different receptors for each of the three natriuretic peptides has been assessed in cell preparations,[149] and in cell cultures expressing the cloned human receptors,[150] by measuring binding affinities and production of cyclic GMP. These studies show that CNP has a minimal effect on cyclic GMP production by the NPR-A receptor,[150] which is selective for both ANP and BNP, having the rank order of selectivity ANP > BNP > CNP.[149] In contrast, the NPR-B receptor is selective for CNP[149,150] with a rank order of selectivity of CNP > ANP > BNP.[149] In keeping with its role as a clearance receptor, the NPR-C receptor has a broad specificity, and, not surprisingly, this receptor binds all three natriuretic peptides, the order of binding affinity being ANP > CNP > BNP, which may be one of the factors behind the longer half-life of BNP.[149]

There have been many studies undertaken to localize and to draw distinctions between these receptors by assessing receptor mRNA expression in different tissues. Across species mRNA, the encoding NPR-A receptor has been found in the kidney, glomerular cells, adrenal gland, pituitary, brain, heart, liver, lung, and aorta.[151–153] NPR-B has more variation in its distribution in some species, and in others, it is primarily confined to the adrenal, pituitary, and brain (monkey).[151] These findings are consistent with the dominant functional role of ANP and BNP, with the exclusion of CNP at the levels of the glomerular and inner medullary collecting duct of the kidney.[151] As expected NPR-C was found to be the most abundant receptor in most tissues, and is widely distributed.

There have been recent reports about the possible role of defective ANP receptors as a cause for systemic hypertension.[154] There have also been recent studies undertaken to determine if ANP autoregulates its own receptor function by suppressing the transcription of its guanylyl cyclase-linked receptor.[155] The reproducibility of these observations, as well as their physiologic import, remains unclear at this time.

Metabolism of Natriuretic Peptides

Removal of the natriuretic peptides from the circulation is affected mainly by binding to clearance receptors and enzymatic degradation, and, to a lesser extent, by elimination through the kidney (Fig. 27-5).

Enzymatic Degradation

ANP is metabolized by neutral endopeptidase EC 3.4.24.11, neutral endopeptidase 24.11,[156] enkephalinase, atriopeptidase, and neutral metalloendopeptidase 24.11, a Zn-dependent glycoprotein metallopeptidase that cleaves a variety of other active peptides, including enkephalins and substance P.[157] The rate-limiting step is the cleavage by neutral endopeptidase of the disulfide ring to produce a ring-open metabolite, which has markedly diminished in vitro biologic activity and receptor-binding affinity.[158] While the role of this enzyme has been most extensively characterized with respect to the metabolism of ANP, BNP and CNP are also presumably affected the same way. Of the three natriuretic peptides, CNP is the preferred substrate for the enzyme, followed by ANP and BNP, for which the enzyme has the lowest affinity.[159]

These findings are consistent with the patterns of plasma natriuretic peptide response to acute enzyme inhibition observed in vivo. Neutral endopeptidase has been found in the kidney, intestine, lungs, CNS, lymph nodes, male genital tract, neutrophils, fibroblasts, endothelium, adrenal capsule, and in the blood.[160–163] Within the CNS, neutral endopeptidase inactivates opioid peptides.[164] In the kidney, neutral endopeptidase is located mainly in the glomerulus and at the proximal tubule,[165] and it is interesting to note that neutral endopeptidase and angiotensin-converting enzyme (ACE) share some common renal site localization, as well as substrate similarities.[166] This raises the question of whether or not and to what degree ACE-neutral endopeptidase and ANP interact.[167]

Removal Mediated by Clearance Receptors

The clearance receptors (NPR-C) have affinity for all three natriuretic peptides. These receptors show structural homology to the biologic receptors (NPR-A, NPR-B) in their extracellular domain, but are unique in having a relatively short intracellular region with no guanylyl cyclase domain (Fig. 27-5).[168] These receptors function as a clearance site for the natriuretic peptides, removing excess peptides by eliminating their intracellular stores and/or, slowly releasing them into the circulation. These receptors may deliver the natriuretic peptides to intracellular lysosomal peptidase[169] and protect the body from excess surges of the natriuretic peptides and overproduction of cyclic GMP.[170,171] The disappearance rate of BNP is much longer than that of ANP or CNP, presumably due to the relatively decreased affinity for the NPR-C receptor (ANP > CNP > BNP).[172]

The most important site for peptide clearance from the circulation was once believed to be the kidney.[173] However, it is now believed that the kidney plays a less-significant role in peptide metabolism.[174] Important clearance sites probably include the lung or a combination of the lung, kidney, liver/splanchnic vascular bed, and the large-muscle beds.[175,176] Some studies suggest that clearance receptors have greater capacity for clearing circulating natriuretic peptides than other peptide elimination pathways.[22] Comparative studies in rats, however, show that both pathways (enzymatic and NPR-C) contribute nearly equally to ANP clearance. Together the two pathways account for >70% of ANP total body clearance.[177] The remainder is accounted for by renal elimination (<15%) and other unspecified degradative enzymes.

Natriuretic Peptides in Disease

Conditions with Increased Blood Levels of Natriuretic Peptides

Atrial Natriuretic Peptide

Increased atrial pressure and atrial distention, as mentioned above, are immediate stimuli for increased ANP production (Fig. 27-6). There are several conditions associated with an increased ANP blood level. These conditions include CHF;[178] supraventricular tachycardia;[104,179] an increased heart rate or pacing frequency;[180,181] valvular heart disease;[182] idiopathic cardiomyopathies;[182] coronary artery disease;[183] hypertension;[184] chronic renal failure (CRF);[185] exercise;[186] secretion of antidiuretic hormone;[183] pregnancy;[187] secretion of mineralocorticoids and glucocorticoids;[188] viral

myocarditis;[189] cardiac amyloidosis;[190] cirrhosis;[191] salt feeding;[192] head-down tilt;[192] water immersion;[193] radiotherapy myocardial damage;[193a] and increasing age.[194] Prostaglandins[195] and thyroid hormone[196] also affect ANP blood levels.

Brain Natriuretic Peptide

BNP secretion occurs in response to increased ventricular wall tension and cardiac overload. Studies in humans indicate that plasma BNP is elevated in a number of pathophysiologic conditions, similar to what is observed with ANP.

For example, BNP, like ANP, is increased in CHF;[62,64,197,197a] myocardial infarction (MI);[198,198a] idiopathic cardiomyopathy;[57,63] hypertension;[199] CRF;[48] high Na+ diets;[200] supraventricular tachycardia;[201] pregnancy;[197] cirrhosis;[202] and increasing age.[203] However, both the degree and the time course of these increases in ANP and BNP differ between various pathologic conditions.

Despite the close correlation of ANP and BNP in volume-expanded states, studies in humans show that these two hormones differ in their release characteristics to an acute stimulation. For example, supine posture,[204] acute exercise,[205] acute intravenous saline loading,[206] and pressor angiotensin-II infusions[207] all promptly increase ANP, but the effect on BNP is small or insignificant. This may be due to the response of atrial tissue, which contains little readily releasable BNP, in contrast to the abundant stores of preformed ANP. Additionally, in response to acute ventricular or atrial pacing, BNP levels do not show any increase, in contrast to a marked increase in

FIGURE 27-6. Diagram showing the regulation and actions of natriuretic peptides. Aldo = aldosterone; BP = blood pressure; FF = filtration fraction. (*Modified with permission from Espiner EA: Physiology of natriuretic peptides. J Intern Med 235:527, 1994*).

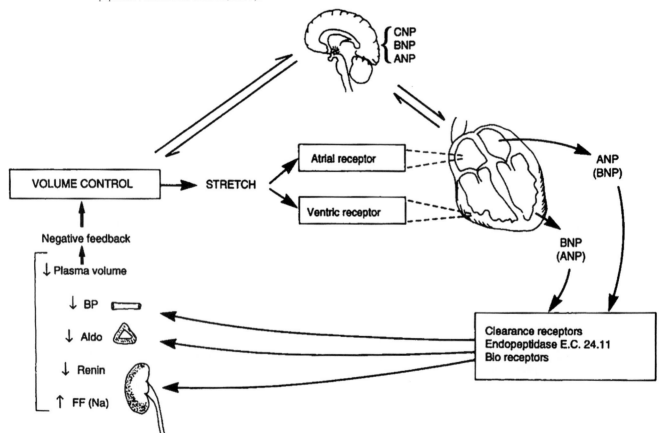

ANP levels.[208] Predictably, the responses of ANP and BNP differ according to the distribution of increased pressure within the separate chambers of the heart; for example, ANP would be substantially more elevated than BNP in mitral stenosis. These results suggest that the regulatory mechanisms and pathophysiologic significance of BNP differs from those of ANP.

C-Natriuretic Peptide

High concentrations of CNP are found in the CNS, and CNP concentrations in cardiac tissue are very low or undetectable. Thus, the pathophysiologic roles of CNP seem to be different from those of ANP and BNP. Plasma CNP levels are not increased in hypertension[209] and congestive heart failure (CHF).[76,84] Although plasma levels of CNP are not increased, Wei et al reported that CNP was increased threefold in ventricular myocardium of severe CHF patients.[84] This, coupled with the fact that plasma levels of CNP are increased in septic shock,[210] may reflect cytokine-stimulated CNP secretion from the vascular endothelium. These findings may suggest that CNP may be involved in vascular remodeling, as occurs after injury.[13] Recent studies additionally show that CNP is elevated in patients with CRF.[85] It has been suggested that CNP, a vasodilator, protects against overhydration and vasoconstriction in patients with CRF.[76] Thus, CNP may participate in the regulation of cardiovascular and body fluid homeostasis together with, but in a manner different than, ANP and BNP.

Congestive Heart Failure

Atrial Natriuretic Peptide

ANP plasma levels are increased in CHF[211] approximately 3 to 13 times normal, and levels of ANP have been shown to correlate directly with the severity of myocardial disease, clinical prognosis, right atrial and pulmonary capillary wedge pressures, and inversely with cardiac index, stroke volume, and BP.[212] In chronic CHF, hypersecretion of ANP by the ventricles also occurs.[41] Over 3 to 4 weeks, even a small increase in ANP may account for an increased excretion of 2 to 3 L of isotonic saline. Therefore, increased ANP in CHF, although not adequately compensating for the fluid retention seen in this disease, may help to prevent further episodes of decompensation.[140] Interestingly, studies show that even with severe CHF, with ANP levels 10 times the normal amount, the atrium still maintains its sensitivity to atrial stretch. This was indicated by the finding of significantly decreased plasma ANP levels directly related to reduced atrial pressure induced by various CHF drug therapies.[213]

The increase in ANP may also occur to counteract opposing pressor mechanisms and to reduce ventricular preload and afterload. Because ANP helps to redistribute fluid to the extravascular space, edema formation in CHF and other conditions may be partly attributable to ANP.[214] When animals with CHF are given anti-ANP monoclonal antibodies, the hemodynamic profile worsens and Na+ excretion falls,[215] which again underscores the importance of ANP in modifying CHF. Studies using synthetic ANP infusions report blunting of the natriuretic response in compensated and decompensated stages of CHF.[216] The fact that both norepinephrine and angiotensin-II can overcome the effects of ANP in advanced stages of CHF supports the notion that a diminished renal responsiveness to ANP may result from overactivity of the RAA and sympathetic nervous systems.[104] This may explain why in patients with CHF, despite high endogenous ANP levels, there remains an elevated peripheral vascular resistance with inadequate urine output.[179,211,212]

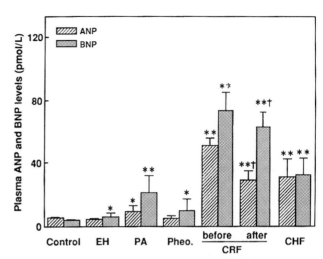

FIGURE 27-7. Bar graph shows plasma levels of atrial natriuretic peptide (ANP) and brain natriuretic peptide (BNP) in patients with various cardiovascular diseases. Valves are mean + SEM. After = after hemodialysis; before = before hemodialysis; CHF = chronic heart failure (n = 11); CRF = chronic renal failure (n = 61); EH = essential hypertension (n = 32); PA = primary aldosteronism (n = 20); Pheo = pheochromocytoma (n = 4). (*Modified with permission from Naruse M, et al: Atrial and brain natriuretic peptides in cardiovascular diseases. Hypertension 23(Suppl 1):1231–1235, 1994.*)

This phenomenon is compounded by the fact that, in CHF, a point is reached where the atrial myocytes are synthesizing and releasing ANP at a maximum capacity: thus, at progressive stages of CHF, there is a relative ANP tissue deficiency.[217] This suggests an approach aimed at augmenting the activity of ANP as a potential form of therapy.

Brain Natriuretic Peptide

Plasma BNP concentrations are remarkably elevated in patients with CHF in proportion to its severity (as much as a 300-fold increase as compared with the control), and exceeds plasma ANP concentrations in severe cases (New York Heart Association class III/IV) (Figs. 27-7 and 27-8).[6,218–228f] Other studies have used the ANP/BNP ratio in CHF as a prognostic indicator with conflicting opinions as to its significance.[6] As with ANP, BNP levels are elevated in cor-pulmonale[229] and primary pulmonary hypertension,[230] suggesting that the right ventricle can contribute considerably to circulating BNP levels. Secretion of BNP in CHF is mainly from the ventricles,[231] but the atria also contribute.[84] Significant quantities of both BNP and pro-BNP are observed in the plasma of CHF patients.[63,64,67] Plasma BNP correlates strongly with increases in both end-diastolic volume and left ventricular end-diastolic pressures, in contrast to ANP levels that correlate mainly with the level of pulmonary capillary wedge pressure (PCWP). Because BNP is predominately secreted by the ventricular myocardium and has a prolonged plasma half-life (~22 min), it has been speculated that it would be a more sensitive and specific indicator of abnormal ventricular function than ANP.[66]

C-Natriuretic Peptide

In contrast to ANP and BNP, circulating CNP levels are not elevated in patients with CHF, although atrial and ventricular CNP content is increased.[84]

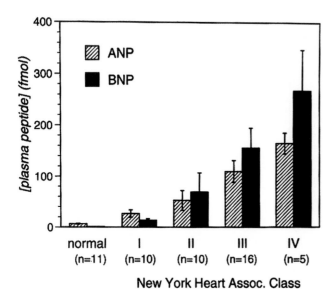

FIGURE 27-8. Elevated levels of plasma ANP and BNP in patients with congestive heart failure compared with normal subjects. Patients are grouped by severity of disease according to the New York Heart Association guidelines. (*Modified with permission from Lewicki JA, Protter AA: Physiologic studies of the natriuretic peptide family. In: Laragh JH, Brenner BM, eds. Hypertension: Pathophysiology, Diagnosis and Management. 2d ed. New York: Raven, 1995:1029–1053.*)

Hypertension

Atrial Natriuretic Peptide

ANP levels are increased in patients with systemic hypertension.[232] ANP levels correlate with left-atrial size in hypertension, and ANP levels are higher than those of normal controls in patients with untreated mild systemic hypertension and are even higher in patients with treated but uncontrolled essential hypertension.[232] ANP levels may be elevated in hypertension in an attempt to reduce the workload on the heart,[233] and the peptide may actually participate as a physiologic compensatory mechanism against hypertension and its consequences.[234] For example, studies show that the elevated ANP levels found in hypertension may provide a peripheral vasodilatory effect,[95,235] which might be the mechanism for a concurrent hypotensive effect. Others believe that elevated ANP levels may cause an extravascular fluid shift and natriuresis with a resultant reduction in cardiac venous return, lower ventricular filling pressures, a fall in cardiac output, and a hypotensive effect.[236]

Interestingly, the importance of ANP in the control of hypertension, as well as its compensatory effects, are highlighted by recent studies, which showed that a mutation in the ANP gene[237] or receptor[238] can increase the susceptibility to essential hypertension. Additionally, inappropriately low basal plasma ANP concentrations may be related to the development of essential hypertension in offspring of hypertensive families.[239] The clinical and pharmacologic implications of these studies remain to be defined.

Brain Natriuretic Peptide

In hypertensive patients, plasma BNP concentrations are significantly higher than in borderline hypertensives or normotensive controls.[46] Patients with left ventricular hypertrophy (LVH) had higher plasma BNP concentrations than did those patients without LVH, and there has been a suggestion of a positive correlation

between BNP levels and the echocardiographic left ventricular mass index.[66,239a] The increases in plasma BNP concentration in patients are much more prominent than those in plasma ANP concentration, due mainly to augmented secretion from the ventricle and the longer half-life of BNP.[6] In hypertensive rat models, ventricular BNP expression increases with progression of the hypertension,[240] and a positive correlation is observed between plasma BNP concentrations and systolic BP.[241] Furthermore, BNP ventricular gene expression is already induced at the onset of the hypertensive state and is preferentially responsive to the development of hypertension as compared with ANP.[240] These findings support the concept that BNP represents a sensitive marker of cardiac changes associated with hypertension.

C-Natriuretic Peptide

CNP levels do not correlate significantly with either systolic or diastolic BP and are not raised in hypertension.[209]

Acute Myocardial Infarction

The levels of both plasma ANP and BNP rise soon after an acute MI.[198] In patients with acute MI, the plasma BNP concentration is remarkably elevated on admission (approximately twentyfold as high as the control), whereas the plasma ANP concentration is only slightly elevated (by only threefold).[198] In contrast to ANP levels, which decrease in a short period of time, BNP levels continue to rise and peak at 16 h. Both ANP and BNP levels and their sustained increases correlate with hemodynamic outcomes (filling pressures, left ventricular ejection fraction, CHF, anterior infarction, etc).[198] In this regard, the plasma ANP and BNP concentrations should represent a good indicator of prognosis in patients with acute MI. BNP may be a more sensitive marker due to its earlier and more prominent increase, and the fact that in most patients it is correlated well with the serum levels of creatine kinase and cardiac myosin light chain I.[208]

Therapeutic Applications

Changes in plasma levels of ANP and BNP in normal individuals can induce a natriuresis, suppress the RAA system, and significantly decrease systemic BP.[242,243] Because of these various physiologic actions of the natriuretic peptides, manipulation of ANP or BNP levels continues to hold promise in the treatment of various CVR and renal disorders.[244,245] Multiple therapeutic strategies have involved attempts to either augment plasma levels and/or effects of endogenous natriuretic peptides or to provide exogenous ANP or BNP. These strategies include the use of ANP and BNP infusion, neutral endopeptidase (NEP) inhibitors, and clearance-receptor ligands. Much research has focused on ANP and BNP infusion, as well as on NEP inhibitor use, in the context of CHF and hypertension, and is discussed here. In addition, the use of ANP in the realm of renal disorders is considered. Finally, the measurement of plasma levels of peptides as potential markers for ventricular dysfunction, as well as their use in diagnosing cardiac function and structural abnormalities, are discussed.

ANP Administration

Congestive Heart Failure

The intravenous administration of exogenous ANP in various doses seems to have a beneficial effect in patients with CHF. For example, patients with CHF who receive ANP demonstrate an increase in stroke index, a decrease in PCWP,[246] and an increase in cardiac index, with no change in either BP or heart rate.[246] Large bolus doses of ANP in patients with CHF have produced an acute fall in cardiac preload, afterload, and peripheral vascular resistance. The effects are accompanied by natriuresis, diuresis, and suppression of plasma aldosterone.[191,247] Such results, however, are not always reproducible.[248] Despite some clinical successes, many investigators stress caution and point to a dissociation between levels of ANP and the degree of natriuresis in CHF, and the ANP blunting effect discussed below.[212,249] This diminished target-organ responsiveness in CHF suggests that abnormalities in the ANP pathway may contribute to abnormal Na^+ and water retention in this condition.[249] Nevertheless, the ability of ANP to produce natriuresis, diuresis, and suppression of plasma aldosterone concentrations,[215,247] inhibit aldosterone synthesis, block the release of aldosterone associated with angiotensin-II infusion,[109,110] produce falls in both cardiac preload and afterload, and decrease peripheral vascular resistance,[247] suggests that augmenting the effects of ANP may be useful in the treatment of CHF.

Infusion of synthetic ANP in healthy subjects causes natriuresis, diuresis, suppression of the RAA axis, a hemoconcentrating effect, and a reduction of the PCWP.[249] In one normal volunteer study, a synthetic ANP lowered systolic arterial and left ventricular filling pressures and raised the hematocrit, suggesting a contraction of plasma volume, while not changing other hemodynamic variables. However, in patients with CHF, PCWP and systemic vascular resistance fell significantly, cardiac index rose, and BP remained unchanged. The contraction of plasma volume seen in normal subjects did not occur in the heart-failure patients. Plasma aldosterone concentrations fell in both normal and patient groups. The pronounced natriuretic effect in normal subjects was markedly attenuated in patients with CHF[212] and abnormalities of the ANP pathway may have contributed to abnormal Na^+ and water retention in these patients.[249] Despite this effect, hemodynamic improvement in patients with CHF receiving an ANP analogue can occur.[212,250] For example, when anaritide, a synthetic analogue of ANP, was given to patients with CHF, peripheral vascular resistance and filling pressure were reduced, cardiac output, diuresis, and natriuresis increased, and no adverse effects occurred on the coronary circulation.[250]

Despite the favorable hemodynamic effects of ANP, enthusiasm has waned for the use of this peptide to treat CHF and other edematous states.[76] This lack of enthusiasm arises, in large part, from observations that the renal actions of ANP are blunted substantially in these clinical settings,[251,252] and that ANP has a very short half-life.[6,26] One explanation put forth by Abraham et al[253] is that diminished delivery of Na^+ to the distal renal tubular site of natriuretic peptide action leads to relative resistance to the renal effects of natriuretic peptides. Support for the hypothesis comes from studies which show that maneuvers that increase distal renal tubular Na^+ delivery, such as angiotensin-II receptor antagonism, furosemide, low-dose mannitol, and renal denervation, reverse natriuretic peptide resistance in experimental models and in humans.[254–257]

The paracrine hormone urodilatin (ANP 95-126), a natriuretic peptide of renal origin, has shown greater efficacy than ANP when infused over a prolonged period of time. It is effective because it is not subject to tolerance and it does not facilitate neurohumoral activation.[258] Urodilatin's higher potency than ANP and its resistance to endopeptidase inactivation may make it advantageous over ANP as a therapeutic agent.[144] Another recent study suggested that increased levels of angiotensin-II are responsible for the development of Na^+ retention and of the blunted renal response to ANP

in CHF. The investigators suggest that losartan, an angiotensin-II-receptor blocker, could be used to improve the natriuretic response to ANP.[257] The effectiveness of this approach to counteract the blunting of ANP activity remains to be clinically proven.

Hypertension

ANP infusion reduces systemic BP in hypertensive animals and in hypertensive subjects.[259,260] The infusion of ANP into patients with hypertension causes a greater decrease in BP than in normotensives, and the effect has persisted for more than 2 h.[261] Natriuresis due to ANP is significantly greater in hypertensives than that observed in normal subjects.[262] The decrease in BP with ANP occurs concomitantly with suppression of renin, aldosterone, and catecholamine, and with an increase in hematocrit, Na^+ excretion, and plasma and urinary cyclic GMP concentrations.[107,259] Long-term infusions of ANP, lasting up to several days, reduce BP even at plasma ANP levels in the upper physiologic range.[107,259,263] The long-term infusions are also more effective in BP reduction in hypertensives than in normotensives, and persist even after ANP or cyclic GMP has disappeared.[261,263] Some research studies, however, show less-favorable results. In one study, a bolus of ANP followed by a 45-minute infusion enhanced natriuresis and increased GFR, norepinephrine, and plasma renin activity, while not affecting aldosterone, and causing no greater hypotensive effect than in normotensives.[264] The available evidence does suggest that in hypertensive patients the natriuretic effect of ANP is enhanced, but the vasodepressor effects may be attenuated.[262,264] Anaritide, a synthetic form of ANP, can produce a diuresis and natriuresis indicating that synthetic ANP may have a beneficial effect as a partial treatment for hypertension.[250]

In spite of these promising studies, the clinical development of synthetic ANP as a potential antihypertensive agent has been inhibited by its lack of oral bioavailability.[76]

Recently, studies have shown that the somatic delivery of the human ANP gene could induce a sustained reduction of systemic BP in young hypertensive rats.[265] This raises the question of the feasibility of using ANP gene therapy for the treatment of human hypertension in the future.

Renal Disease

ANP has also been used to test its role in the treatment of renal disorders. In a recent study, Allgren et al[245] performed a multicenter, randomized, double-blind, placebo-controlled clinical trial of anaritide (a synthetic form of ANP) in 504 critically ill patients with acute tubular necrosis. The patients received a 24-h infusion of anaritide or placebo. Anaritide did not improve the overall rate of dialysis-free survival; in fact, it may worsen dialysis-free survival in patients without oliguria. The investigators did find that anaritide may improve dialysis-free survival in patients with oliguria. In another study, synthetic ANP was shown to improve renal function in the immediate postischemic period in a model of acute renal failure.[266]

BNP Administration

Congestive Heart Failure

With enthusiasm for ANP use fading, a next logical step was to attempt clinical trials using BNP infusion, because BNP's half-life was much longer than ANP and initial trials had not shown any renal attenuation of effect with BNP use.[267,268] Some of the first infusions of BNP were first performed in normal men. These studies showed BNP infusion led to either suppression of the RAA system or to increased urine Na$^+$ excretion.[58,269,270] Encouraged by the findings in normal men, experiments began with administration of BNP for various durations to patients with CHF.

Nesiritide is the first human BNP made by recombinant DNA technology available for human use. The hemodynamic effects of nesiritide are characterized by venous and arterial dilation, resulting in decreased preload and afterload. A dose of 0.015 μg/kg/min reduces PCWP by an average of 6 mm Hg, right atrial pressure (RAP) by an average of 3 mm Hg, mean pulmonary pressure by an average of 5.5 mm Hg, and systemic vascular resistance (SVR) by an average of 150 dyn·sec·cm^{-5}. Although nesiritide has no direct positive inotropic effect, cardiac index (CI) also increases by an average of 0.2 L/min/m^2 secondary to a dose-dependent afterload reduction.[271,272] Following discontinuation of nesiritide, PCWP returns to within 10% of baseline in 2 h, but no rebound increase to levels above baseline state is observed.[272]

In addition to hemodynamic effects, administration of nesiritide has been demonstrated to reduce plasma aldosterone and norepinephrine levels.[273,274] This effect persists 4 h after discontinuation of drug administration. Nesiritide also demonstrates diuretic effect in clinical trials.[273,275] The renal hemodynamic effects of nesiritide appear to be that of reducing efferent arteriolar vasoconstriction, which would tend to augment glomerular filtration rate and filtration fraction in the setting of decreasing renal perfusion. Additionally, both proximal and distal sodium reabsorption are reduced, which results in an increase in sodium excretion.

In patients with CHF, nesiritide administered intravenously demonstrated a biphasic disposition from the plasma. The mean terminal half-life of nesiritide is approximately 18 min and mean volume of distribution at steady state is estimated to be 0.19 L/kg (Scios Inc., data on file). At steady state, plasma B-type natriuretic peptide levels increase from baseline endogenous levels by approximately three- to sixfold, with nesiritide infusion doses ranging from 0.01 to 0.03 μg/kg/min.

Human BNP is cleared mainly via binding to cell-surface clearance receptors with subsequent cellular internalization and lysosomal proteolysis. Some are also cleared by proteolytic cleavage of the peptide by endopeptidases or by renal filtration (Scios Inc., data on file). The average total body clearance is approximately 9.2 mL/min/kg. Clearance of nesiritide is not affected by age, gender, race/ethnicity, baseline endogenous BNP level, severity of heart failure (HF), or concomitant administration of angiotensin-converting enzyme inhibitor (ACEI).

With the recommended dose of nesiritide of 2 μg/kg intravenous bolus followed by 0.01 μg/kg/min infusion, 60% of the 3-h effect (dose of nesiritide is titrated every 3 h; see dose and administration) on PCWP reduction is achieved within 15 min after the bolus and reaches 95% of the 3-h effect within an hour. Approximately 70% of the 3-h effect on systolic blood pressure (SBP) reduction is reached within 15 min. The pharmacodynamic half-life of the onset and offset of the hemodynamic effect of nesiritide is longer than what the pharmacokinetic half-life would predict (Scios Inc., data on file).

Colucci and colleagues studied the clinical efficacy and compared the effects of nesiritide to conventional treatment in patients who were admitted with decompensated HF.[271] Patients hospitalized were enrolled to either the efficacy trial or to the comparative trial. In the efficacy trial, 127 patients were randomized into either 6-h infusions of placebo or 1 of 2 doses of nesiritide (0.015 or 0.03 μg/kg/min) preceded by bolus doses of 0.3 and 0.6 μg/kg, respectively. Subsequently, the blind was broken and patients were

maintained on open-label treatment for up to 7 days. The majority of patients had New York Heart Association (NYHA) class III or IV HF and a mean left ventricular ejection fraction of 22%, a mean of PCWP of 28 mm Hg, and a CI of 1.9 L/min/m^2. Nesiritide caused dose-dependent reduction in PCWP (6 to 9.6 mm Hg) resulted in 60% and 67% improvement in global clinical status as compared with 14% of those receiving placebo ($P < .001$). It also reduced dyspnea in approximately 55% of patients compared with 12% in those receiving placebo ($P < .001$). Hypotension resulted in discontinuation of study drug in only one patient who was receiving the 0.03 μg/kg/min dose. In the comparative trial, 305 patients were randomized to open-label treatment with standard care intravenous agents or double-blind treatment with one of two dose levels of nesiritide (0.015 μg/kg/min infusion preceded by a 0.3 μg/kg bolus or 0.03 μg/kg/min infusion preceded by a 0.6 μg/kg bolus). The duration of therapy was based on usual clinical criteria and ranged up to 7 days. A majority of patients in the trial were in NYHA class III HF. Among the 102 patients randomized to standard therapy, 57% were treated with dobutamine, 19% with milrinone, 18% with nitroglycerin, 6% with dopamine, and 1% with amrinone. End-points such as global clinical status and dyspnea were assessed as in the efficacy trials. They were similar to those observed with standard intravenous therapy. The most common adverse event with nesiritide was hypotension, which was symptomatic in 11% and 17% of patients treated with the 0.015 μg/kg/min and 0.03 μg/kg/min dose, respectively, as compared to 4% in patients receiving standard therapy. Other adverse events were similar in frequency in the nesiritide and standard treatment groups, except for the frequency of nonsustained ventricular tachycardia, which decreased with the 0.03 μg/kg/min dose of nesiritide (1% in the 0.03 μg/kg/min vs 10% in 0.015 μg/kg/min dose group vs 8% in standard treatment group, $P < .02$).[271]

The Vasodilation in the Management of Acute Congestive Heart Failure (VMAC) trial was a multicenter, randomized, double-blind, placebo-controlled study looking at the hemodynamic and clinical effects of nesiritide compared with nitroglycerin therapy for symptomatic decompensated HF.[272] Four hundred and ninety-eight patients with dyspnea at rest from HF were randomized to a 3-h placebo-controlled period, during which they received nitroglycerin, placebo, fixed-dose nesiritide, or adjustable-dose nesiritide. At the end of this period, the placebo group was crossed over to a prespecified treatment with either nitroglycerin or fixed-dose nesiritide. Duration of treatment after crossover was at the discretion of the investigators. Patients receiving adjustable-dose nesiritide continued on this same regimen. For 3 h, nesiritide was administered as a 2 μg/kg intravenous bolus followed by an infusion of 0.01 μg/kg/min in both the fixed-dose and the adjustable-dose groups. After the first 3 h, the adjustable-dose group could have the nesiritide dose increased by administering a 1 μg/kg intravenous bolus followed by an increase of 0.005 μg/kg/min over the previous infusion rate. The maximum allowable infusion rate was 0.03 μg/kg/min. The primary end-points were change in PCWP and dyspnea at the end of the 3 h. Both nesiritide treatment groups (i.e., fixed dose and adjusted dose) were pooled for study analysis. At the 3-h time point, nesiritide significantly decreased PCWP as compared with either placebo ($P < .001$) or nitroglycerin ($P < .027$) added to standard care. At 24 h the reduction in PCWP was greater in the nesiritide group than in the nitroglycerin group, but patients reported no significant differences in dyspnea and only modest improvement in global clinical status. The most common adverse effect was headache, which occurred less often in nesiritide-treated patients

(8%) than in the nitroglycerin-treated patients (20%) ($P = .003$). Symptomatic hypotension was uncommon and similar in frequency in both groups (5%).[272]

The Prospective, Randomized Evaluation of Cardiac Ectopy with Dobutamine or Natrecor Therapy (PRECEDENT) trial examined the proarrhythmic effects of nesiritide and dobutamine.[276,277] Two hundred and forty-six patients with NYHA class III or class IV HF were randomized to one or two doses of nesiritide (0.015 or 0.03 μg/kg/min) or dobutamine (minimum dose of 5 μg/kg/min) and underwent Holter monitoring for 24 h before and during treatment. When compared with either dose of nesiritide, dobutamine was associated with significant increases in premature ventricular beats (PVC) (average change in hourly total PVC as compared with baseline: dobutamine +69; nesiritide 0.015 μg/kg/min: −13; and nesiritide 0.03 μg/kg/min: −5; $P < .002$).

A post-hoc analysis combining the long-term mortality results from the Comparative Trial by Colucci and the PRECEDENT trials (reflecting a total of 507 patients) demonstrated that when compared with treatment with dobutamine, treatment with nesiritide 0.015 μg/kg/min was associated with a reduction in cumulative 6-month mortality by 37% (15.8% vs 25%, $P = .03$).[278] This observed mortality difference could not be explained by differences in baseline demographics, severity or etiology of congestive HF, or other comorbid conditions. However, further trials are required to confirm this effect and to establish the optimal dose to maximize the effect.

A recent pharmacoeconomic study has demonstrated an advantage of nesiritide over dobutamine in the treatment of decompensated CHF.[279]

The safety profile of nesiritide was obtained by compiling data from the different randomized clinical trials within the dose range of 0.01 to 0.03 μg/kg/min.[271,274,276,278] The studied patient population is representative of a compromised chronic HF population, including comorbidities such as significant atrial and ventricular arrhythmias, diabetes, hypertension, significant renal insufficiency, and acute coronary syndromes. The most common side effect of nesiritide was dose-related hypotension (11 to 35%), by which approximately half of the side effects were symptomatic. Incidence of other side effects was similar to the controlled groups. Nesiritide may affect renal function in patients with severe heart failure whose renal function may depend on the activity of the renin-angiotensin-aldosterone system. In the VMAC study, when nesiritide was initiated at doses higher than 0.01 μg/kg/min, there was an increased rate of elevated serum creatinine over baseline as compared with standard therapies, although the rate of acute renal failure and need for dialysis was not increased.[272]

No trial specifically examined potential drug interactions with nesiritide. There is also no long-term study that evaluates carcinogenic potential of nesiritide (Scios Inc., data on file).

The recommended dose of nesiritide is an intravenous bolus of 2 μg/kg followed by a continuous infusion at a dose of 0.01 μg/kg/min. Nesiritide should not be initiated at a dose that is above the recommended dose to prevent excessive hypotension or worsening of renal function. Dose of nesiritide can be adjusted 0.005 μg/kg/min (preceded by a bolus of 1 μg/kg) every 3 h up to a maximum of 0.03 μg/kg/min.[272] There is limited experience with administering nesiritide for longer then 72 h. However, in the VMAC study, duration of treatment was not specified.[272] The longest infusion was 161 days in a NYHA class IV patient who was poorly responsive to other intravenous therapies while awaiting a cardiac transplant.[76] The patient responded well clinically and tolerated therapy for 161 days. No tolerance or tachyphylaxis was observed.[280] BNP is also being evaluated in a subcutaneous injectable form.[281]

Nesiritide is physically and chemically incompatible with injectable formulations of heparin, insulin, ethacrynate sodium, bumetanide, enalaprilat, hydralazine, and furosemide. These drugs should not be coadministered with nesiritide through the same intravenous catheter. Injectable drugs that contain sodium metabisulfite as a preservative are also incompatible with nesiritide.[76]

Hypertension

In recent studies, BNP infusion was shown in hypertensive patients to progressively reduce left ventricular end-diastolic and -systolic volume, whereas stroke volume did not show any significant change.[282] Additionally, it induced a significant increase in urinary Na^+ excretion, GFR, and urine flow rate with a concomitant decrease in aldosterone.[283] Cardiac output, arterial pressure, and peripheral vascular resistance did not change significantly.[282] The lack of effects on systemic hemodynamics was probably due to a compensatory activation of the sympathetic nervous system.[282] The results of these studies indicate that BNP influences CVR homeostasis by reducing cardiac preload through its natriuretic effects.[282,283] Similar to ANP, the natriuretic response to BNP appears to be enhanced by hypertension.[76] The clinical use of BNP as a potential antihypertensive agent still requires clarification.

Neutral Endopeptidase (Vasopeptidase) Inhibitors

Natriuretic peptides have the potential to be of therapeutic value in cardiovascular disorders such as hypertension and heart failure. A barrier for their widespread pharmacologic application relates to their large peptide structure, and their need to be given parenterally. This problem was overcome by several pharmaceutical companies who developed orally active NEP inhibitors. These substances inhibit the breakdown of endogenous natriuretic peptides, and it was hoped that by so doing, the therapeutic potential of the natriuretic peptides could be harnessed by prolonging their activity.[284] However, NEP degrades many other endogenous peptides, including angiotensin-II, bradykinin, and substance P. Inhibitors of NEP were initially designed to block the degradation of enkephalins and were assessed for their analgesic properties.[66]

Several classes of NEP inhibitors have been developed, and are discussed in Chap. 44. The main classes include mercaptoalkyl inhibitors, carboxyalkyl inhibitors, phosphoramidite inhibitors, and dual-metalloprotease inhibitors. Recently the FDA Cardiorenal Advisory Panel rejected the application of omapatrilat, a dual-metalloproteinase inhibitor, for use in systemic hypertension.

Clearance-Receptor Blockade

Atrial Natriuretic Peptide

Another approach in the pharmacologic manipulation of ANP includes use of clearance-receptor blockade with a ligand often derived from ANP. ANP-derived peptides lacking biologic activity are able to bind to clearance receptors and give ANP some protection from breakdown.[171] Research in this area has combined such receptor blockade with NEP inhibition. In one study, clearance-ANP, an ANP analogue that binds to the clearance receptor with high affinity, but has little, if any, biologic activity, and SCH 39,370, a potent and specific inhibitor of NEP, were used to block the nonenzymatic and enzymatic pathways of ANP removal, respectively.[285] While clearance-ANP alone is known to cause a decrease in elimination of

ANP via blockade of the clearance-receptor mechanism of degradation, and SCH 39,370 alone potentiates ANP effects, both produced a fifteenfold increase in the area under the ANP plasma concentration curve.[285]

Other work in this area has demonstrated diuresis and natriuresis after clearance-receptor ligand administration,[286] as well as a vasodepressor response.[287] Interestingly, in the latter study, no significant alteration in plasma ANP levels occurred when the ligand was given alone, but when SQ 28,603 was given concomitantly, ANP concentrations rose and the depressor activity was additive.[287] More recent studies have shown that coadministration of sinorphan (ecadotril) and AP811 (an ANP-C receptor ligand) had greater effects on endocrine and renal parameters than the administration of either substance alone.[287] Unfortunately, the long-term studies do not suggest that such combined therapy has sustained hypotensive effects.[288]

Brain Natriuretic Peptide

The effects of clearance-receptor blockade and its effect on BNP have not been evaluated to date.

Other Potential Uses

Natriuretic peptides are used in other disease states, such as various Na^+-retaining states such as nephrotic syndrome or cirrhotic ascites;[289] MI, in which the natriuretic and minimal kaliuretic effects may be useful in the water and sodium retention of acute myocardial infarction;[290] analgesia, as inhibition of neutral endopeptidase produces opioid-like effects by raising the extracellular level of endogenous enkephalins;[291] and chronic hypoxic pulmonary hypertension, because ANP decreases pulmonary artery pressure when infused into the right atrium.[292]

Adverse Effects of Natriuretic Peptide Usage

Complications with manipulation of ANP have been reported. Hypotension and bradycardia can occur with ANP, urodilatin, or synthetic ANP infusions.[260,293,294] It appears that doses greater than 10 pmol/kg/min and duration of infusion in excess of 2 h may predispose to this side effect. Diminished venous return, leading to a fall in filling pressure, may contribute to these side effects.[295] High doses of ANP frequently caused hypotensive and bradycardic episodes in both normal and hypertensive subjects at the beginning of, during, or immediately after infusion, and last for several hours. This hypotension is associated with a compensatory increase in plasma catecholamines, renin activity, and aldosterone levels.

The use of a synthetic ANP in CHF produces marked drops in pulmonary capillary wedge and arterial blood pressures requiring intravenous saline treatment.[246] For example, in one study, 17% of patients with CHF who were given anaritide experienced side effects that were usually related to hypotension.[250] Sinus tachycardia and bradycardia have also been described with ANP analogue use. These arrhythmias did cease without harmful effects minutes after the infusion was stopped. However, because of these side effects, there is some question regarding the usefulness and safety of ANP analogues in CHF treatment.[296]

Resistance to ANP in pathologic states may also limit its therapeutic effectiveness.[212] This is evident from the fact that although there are highly elevated ANP levels in CHF, peripheral vascular resistance remains high and there is still inadequate urine output. This

can be explained by the possibilities of ANP receptor downregulation or uncoupling of ANP and cyclic monophosphate production under chronic conditions of ANP increase seen with severe CHF[297] and essential hypertension.[298,299] This pharmacologic tolerance to ANP has also limited the long-term therapeutic effectiveness of the various forms of ANP enhancement, such as the NEP inhibitors.[157] Urodilatin[258] and BNP[300] both show less resistance than ANP in pathologic states and appear to be more promising long-term therapeutic approaches.

Conclusion

The two decades of active natriuretic peptide research has produced tremendous insight into the molecular biology, physiology, and pathophysiology of these hormones, establishing the principle that the heart is a pump as well as a true endocrine organ. In addition, several approaches toward the pharmacologic manipulation of natriuretic peptides in vivo have been developed.

The natriuretic peptides play a fundamental role in the regulation of vascular hemodynamics. They play a crucial role in maintaining vascular fluid homeostasis, and act to counterbalance the RAA system, endothelin, vasopressin and various actions of the sympathetic nervous system. In their role as such, these peptides are part of the human body's natural system of checks and balances. They perform important protective functions in many acute situations and have proved useful in altering hemodynamics in many studies on congestive heart failure. BNP may be more beneficial than ANP in the treatment of CHF due to a longer half-life and an apparent lack of renal attenuation.[300a] A recombinant form of BNP is approved for clinical use in decompensated heart failure.[301] Another area where the natriuretic peptides may be of use is in the treatment of renal disorders such as acute renal failure.

A promising use of these peptides may be as markers for disease. In the near future, routine immunoassay of ANP and BNP may provide a preliminary test of ventricular function, or other abnormalities, and may permit physicians to more carefully select patients for further investigation and treatment.[228f] The natriuretic peptide field is still in its infancy and further investigation of the natriuretic peptide family promises to add new insights into their mechanism of action, and improved potential clinical uses in the future.

OTHER VASODILATOR PEPTIDES

Recently three new vasodilator peptides, which may be important substances in cardiovascular regulation, have been described in humans: adrenomedullin, calcitonin gene-related peptide, and vasoactive intestinal peptide.

Adrenomedullin

Structure, Biosynthesis, and Molecular Biology

Adrenomedullin (ADM) is a polypeptide that contains 52 amino acids and one intramolecular disulfide bond. The C-terminal amino acid, tyrosine, is amidated, a characteristic of other biologically active peptides (Fig. 27-9).[302] ADM shares some structural similarity to human calcitonin gene-related peptide (CGRP). They both have a C-terminal amide, a G-residue ring structure, and a terminal amide substitution, which are important for biologic activity.[302]

The cDNA encoding the precursors of human porcine and rat ADM have been successfully cloned.[303,304] The biosynthesis of

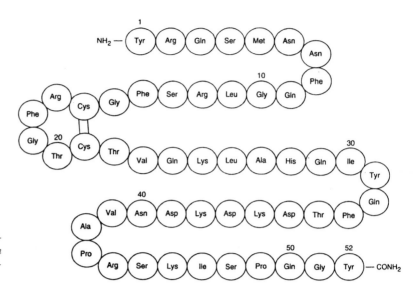

FIGURE 27-9. Complete amino acid sequence of human adrenomedullin. (*Reproduced with permission from Kitamura K, et al: Adrenomedullin: Implications for hypertension research. Drugs 49:485–95, 1995.*)

ADM is similar to that of other active peptide substances in that it has a precursor polypeptide (proadrenomedullin), which is sequentially cleaved by the enzyme peptidylglycine C-amidating monooxygenase to generate the active molecule.[302] The gene for human ADM was isolated from a human genomic library and is found on a single locus of chromosome 11.[305] The ADM gene has three introns and four exons. The 5′ flanking region contains several *cis*-acting elements that may be important in the regulation of ADM gene expression. Consensus sites for AP-1 and AP-2 binding have been identified in addition to cyclic AMP-regulated enhancer sites. Pathways involving induction of cyclic AMP and protein kinase A are thought to result in AP-2-mediated transcriptional activation. Because ADM itself can induce cyclic AMP formation, it may exert feedback controls on its own production.

There is also another vasodilatory peptide, referred to as proadrenomedullin N-20 terminal peptide (PAMP), which is produced from the same preprohormone as ADM.[306,307] This peptide is also quite potent in its vasodilatory actions, but there is less known about this substance as compared with ADM.

Distribution

ADM is found in picomolar concentrations in the human plasma and has also been found in the adrenal medulla, brain, GI organs, lungs, heart, and kidneys.[308] The clearance of ADM appears to be via the kidney, as suggested by the increase in plasma concentration seen in patients with renal failure.[309] Active production of ADM has been demonstrated in endothelial cells.[310] Studies to identify the sites of production and clearance of ADM in humans have been performed. These studies showed no significant differences in concentrations of ADM at various sampling sites in the right-sided circulation. In addition, increases in ADM levels were noted in the coronary sinus. The level of ADM found in the aorta was slightly lower than that measured in the pulmonary artery, suggesting that the pulmonary circulation may be one of the sites for ADM clearance.[311] The rate of secretion of ADM from endothelial cells was found to be comparable to that of endothelin-1. Endothelial cells are assumed to be one of the major sources of plasma ADM.[312] The presence of ADM-specific receptors on vascular smooth-muscle cells (VSMC)[313,314] raises interesting possibilities, because ADM and endothelin are physiologically antagonistic to each other. In addition, both rat and

bovine VSMC produce ADM, suggesting a possible autoregulation role.[315] The production of ADM from cultured VSMC in rats is about one-sixth that of the production of ADM from rat endothelial cells.[315] The low level of ADM content in VSMC suggests that ADM produced by VSMC is being secreted for its local effects.

Enhanced ADM production from cultured arterial VSMC was demonstrated in response to many extracellular signals. Based on these results, it has been proposed that a physiologic level of hydrocortisone may be sufficient to regulate ADM production in VSMC in vivo. These data suggest that the increased production of ADM in VSMC is mainly due to the activation of ADM gene transcription as demonstrated by the increase in the ADM mRNA levels.[316] The concentration of ADM in the aorta, heart ventricle, kidney, and lung is less than 3% of that in adrenal medulla, yet high levels of ADM mRNA were found in the other tissues.[316] This raises the possibility that ADM biosynthesized in these tissues is rapidly and constitutively secreted into blood or may function as an autocrine or paracrine regulator. In contrast, adrenal ADM is thought to be stored in granules and secreted through a regulatory pathway.

Stimulation of adrenal medullary cells via nicotinic receptors caused the release of ADM along with catecholamines by exocytosis involving calcium ions.[312] The molar ratio of ADM to catecholamines secreted into the medium after nicotinic receptor stimulation was found to be quite similar to the ratio stored in adrenal medullary cells. Because catecholamines are stored exclusively in chromaffin granules, it is possible that ADM may also be stored in the same or similar location.[302]

Table 27-3 lists factors that stimulate ADM production. Lipopolysaccharide is a major component of bacterial endotoxin,

TABLE 27-3. Factors Influencing Adrenomedullin Production

Interleukin-1	Aldosterone
Interleukin-1α	Hydrocortisone
Interleukin-1β	Retinoic acid
Tumor necrosis factor-α	Thyroid hormone
Tumor necrosis factor-α	Dexamethasone
Lipopolysaccharide	

Source: Reproduced from Frishman WH, et al: Natriuretic peptides, and other vasoactive peptides: Implications for future drug therapy. In: Frishman WH, Sonnenblick EH, eds. *Cardiovascular Pharmacotherapeutics*. New York: McGraw-Hill, 1997:595.

whereas tumor necrosis factor-alpha (TNFα) and interleukin (IL)-1β are major inflammatory cytokines involved in the development of endotoxic shock. In the 5′ upstream region of the ADM gene, the conventional sites required for the activation of gene regulation by TNFα, IL-1β, and lipopolysaccharide are not found. Instead, in these regions, several homologous sequences are found.[317,318] It is hypothesized that these proinflammatory cytokines may still play a part in the hypotension of sepsis, which might be caused by excessive ADM in the vasculature.[319] However, the regulation of the ADM gene may occur via other unknown mechanisms that may utilize the homologous sequences.[317,318]

Mechanism of Action

ADM produces a dose-dependent increase in intracellular cyclic AMP levels. It is postulated that the effect on vasodilatation is due to stimulation of cyclic AMP production in VSMC.[320] The vasodilatory effect is similar to the mechanism of vasodilation induced by CGRP.[302] This is in contrast to the vasodilatory effects of ANP and nitroglycerin, which activate guanylyl cyclase, thereby increasing cyclic GMP. The hypotensive effects of ADM are comparable with that of CGRP, which has already been established as one of the most potent vasodilators.[321] Adrenomedullin also has an antimigration action on SMCs,[322] as well as capabilities to inhibit endothelin production from both VSMC and glomerular mesangial cells.[323,324] It can suppress mitogenesis in mesangial cells,[325] while having sympatholytic properties.[326] The vasodilatory effect of adrenomedullin is not blocked by the prior administration of propranolol or atropine, suggesting that this action is not mediated through the adrenergic or cholinergic systems. However, recent studies have demonstrated that the infusion of a CGRP-receptor antagonist (hCGRP$_{8-37}$) prior to administration of ADM resulted in the subsequent blocking of its vasodilatory activity. In isolated rat hearts, preinfusion of hCGRP$_{8-37}$ markedly attenuated the vasodilatory response. This effect has also been demonstrated in the mesenteric circulation.[327] Therefore, it is thought that ADM may exert its effects via CGRP receptors. However, in bovine aortic endothelial cells, it was found that ADM does not share the same receptor site with CGRP based on binding studies.[328] Furthermore, there is speculation that ADM acts on different receptors besides CGRP, depending on different end organs.[329] In contrast, in human neuroblastoma cell lines, ADM demonstrated a potent competition with hCGRP for binding sites. Both substances were demonstrated to cause an increase in cyclic AMP.[327]

ADM also increased intracellular calcium in a dose-dependent manner in a process mediated by phospholipase C activation and inositol triphosphate formation. This increase in calcium is biphasic, with the initial transient increase reflecting release from intracellular storage sites, whereas the prolonged increase is secondary to influx of extracellular calcium through ion channels in the plasma membrane. The increase in intracellular calcium seemed to result in activation of nitric oxide synthase by monitoring cyclic GMP activation.[328] Thus, the vasodilatory responses of ADM seem to be mediated by at least two mechanisms involving direct action on VSMC by increasing cyclic AMP, which probably inactivates myosin light-chain kinase, and an action on endothelial cells to cause release of nitric oxide, which is, in itself, a potent vasodilator.[328] Studies have demonstrated that administration of N$_2$-nitro-L-arginine methyl ester (L-NAME), which is an inhibitor of the nitric oxide systems in some vascular preparations, inhibited the systemic vasodepressor responses to ADM without any effect

on the action of CGRP.[330] A similar infusion of the cyclooxygenase inhibitor, meclofenamate, had no effect on the response to ADM or CGRP. In bovine aortic endothelial cells, intracellular cyclic GMP levels were significantly increased by ADM, with the effect being blocked in the presence of inhibitors of nitric oxide synthase. An increase in intracellular calcium should result in enhanced muscle contraction. However, ADM was not shown to cause an increase in intracellular calcium in smooth-muscle cells, unlike the findings in endothelial cells, suggesting that signal transduction systems may be different depending on the cell lines.

Like ADM, PAMP also has vasodilatory effects. However, its signals are different than those of ADM. PAMP does not act via nitric oxide nor via cyclic AMP; it acts via potassium ion channels, which eventually exert a presynaptic inhibition of sympathetic nerves innervating blood vessels.[306]

Hemodynamic Actions

In a study done in rats, the intravenous administration of ADM caused a potent hypotensive effect without any changes seen in the heart rate. This blood-pressure-lowering action was accompanied by an increase in stroke volume and cardiac index.[331] These results suggest that the hypotensive effect of ADM occurs as a result of peripheral vasodilatation. The decrease in mean blood pressure was closely correlated with a decrease in the total peripheral vascular resistance. In addition, the increase in cardiac stroke volume and cardiac index might have been due to a direct positive inotropic action on the heart.[331] Because cyclic AMP is the effector molecule for the positive inotropic actions of β agonists, it may be possible that ADM has the same action in the heart. Another action common to both ADM and PAMP is an inhibitory action on angiotensin-II and aldosterone secretion.[307]

The lack of tachycardia in response to systemic hypotensive effects is unique to ADM. There is some controversy regarding the effects of ADM on the heart, with the lack of tachycardia being attributed to a negative chronotropic effect.[331] It appears that ADM interferes with the baroreceptor reflex arc by an unknown mechanism. CGRP, while producing potent vasodilatation, also causes marked increases in cardiac output and possesses positive inotropic activity.

Studies in humans show that plasma adrenomedullin levels rapidly increase with orthostatic challenges in a stimuli-dependent manner and swiftly return to baseline levels after the subject resumes the supine position.[332]

Studies have demonstrated that ADM centrally injected in the brain induced a long-lasting vasopressor effect and that these effects were blocked by prior administration of the hCGRP antagonist (hCGRP$_{8-37}$). However, unlike CGRP, ADM is barely detectable in the brain under normal situations.[331,333] These findings suggest that ADM receptors may exist in the brain, and that both ADM and CGRP may share the same receptors. It has also been found that both ADM and PAMP act to inhibit adrenocorticotropin hormone (ACTH) secretion.[334,335] However, a recent study found that the infusion of ADM into healthy volunteers showed an increase in plasma prolactin, the only pituitary hormone to show any significant changes, suggesting that the proposed role for ACTH control may still need further study.[336] In addition, ADM acts to inhibit thirst and salt appetite by direct effects on the brain.[337–339]

ADM also has potent renal vasodilatory effects along with diuretic actions. Intrarenal infusion of ADM causes a marked increase in natriuresis and diuresis. These effects are presumably due to an increase in both the glomerular filtration rate and the

TABLE 27-4. Conditions Associated with High Adrenomedullin Activity

Congestive heart failure
Acute myocardial infarction
Pheochromocytoma
Primary aldosteronism
Essential hypertension

Source: Reproduced from Frishman WH, et al: Natriuretic peptides, and other vasoactive peptides: Implications for future drug therapy. In: Frishman WH, Sonnenblick EH, eds. *Cardiovascular Pharmacotherapeutics*. New York: McGraw Hill, 1997:596.

fractional excretion of sodium with a decrease in distal tubular sodium reabsorption.[340] With a high dose of ADM into the renal artery, a kaliuresis can also be induced. No concomitant changes were noted in plasma renin, aldosterone, cyclic GMP, or atrial natriuretic peptide levels from experiments done on dogs. However, in an experiment performed on rats, it was observed that aldosterone release in response to angiotensin-II and potassium was inhibited by ADM.[341] The potency of ADM to cause diuresis in dogs was comparable with that of atrial natriuretic peptide. The presence of a plateau of natriuretic actions at higher concentrations suggests that specific ADM receptors may be involved in this action. Human studies have also shown that the threshold for biologic activity of ADM is lower for a change in the arterial pressures than it is for urinary electrolyte effects.[342] Unlike ADM, PAMP has not been seen to have any role within the renal system.

Adrenomedullin as a Biologic Marker for Cardiovascular Diseases and Potential Therapeutic Roles

Recent studies show that immunoreactive ADM levels are significantly higher in patients with severe hypertension as compared with normotensives (Table 27-4). The augmentation of ADM levels in patients with hypertension appears to be progressive and proportional to the severity of hypertension.[302] Ventricular ADM levels have also been observed to correlate with the extent of cardiac hypertrophy in rats,[343] and the presence of coronary vasospasm.[344]

When compared with those seen in normotensives, plasma ADM levels were increased 26% in hypertensive patients without end-organ damage, and 45% in those with organ damage. In addition, the elevation in ADM levels was more prominent in renal failure than in those patients with hypertension alone.[345] Moreover, ADM levels correlate with norepinephrine, ANP, and cyclic AMP levels in plasma, suggesting that plasma ADM levels increase in association with changes in sympathetic nervous system activity and body fluid volume in hypertension and renal failure. As described earlier, plasma ANP levels also increase in response to expanded plasma volume either acutely or chronically,[346] and it is possible that a similar response to expanded plasma volume is shown by ADM. However, plasma ADM levels were not found to be elevated either at rest or during hypertensive crisis in patients with pheochromocytoma, even though epinephrine and norepinephrine levels were markedly elevated.[311] Similarly, plasma ADM levels did not correlate with epinephrine levels. Recently, ADM was described to be elevated in patients with primary aldosteronism, suggesting that ADM may counteract vasopressor influences in the body.[347]

Due to the detection of ADM in the pulmonary circulation, a study was performed on rats with pulmonary hypertension. Chronic infusion of rat ADM significantly lessened the increase in right ventricular systolic pressure and the ratio of right ventricular weight-to-body weight seen after the treatment. ADM also attenuated the medial thickening of the pulmonary artery.[348,349] Whether or not ADM may have the same kind of results in human pulmonary hypertension requires further study.

A preliminary report in humans described an ADM infusion with beneficial effects in patients with pulmonary hypertension.[350] Another recent study was completed in humans to assess the biologic effects of ADM administration on systemic hemodynamics. Administration of low doses (2 and 8 ng/min/kg) of ADM reduced mean arterial pressure, systolic arterial pressure, and diastolic arterial pressure in the absence of compensatory responses in sympathetic activity or renin release (Fig. 27-10).[340] However, more studies are needed to assess whether there is a dose-response relationship at a higher dose of ADM in order to evaluate a possible therapeutic role.

Plasma ADM has been found to be elevated in patients with CHF and acute myocardial infarction, with the levels increasing even more with higher grades of failure, as classified by the New York Heart Association.[351-355] ADM immunoreactivity was more intense in the atria in both normal and failing hearts. In contrast, significant increases in ventricular immunoreactivity were noted in the failing heart as compared with normal ventricular tissue.[356] Increases in plasma ADM have also been observed in patients undergoing cardiac surgery,[357,358] in patients with septic shock,[359] pulmonary hypertension,[360] and mitral stenosis.[361]

ADM is an important factor in regulating local and systemic vascular tone by its activity as an autocrine/paracrine and circulating hormone. In the setting of CHF, it has been postulated that ADM acts as a counteracting mechanism to reduce elevated cardiac afterload. It is also known that nitric oxide production in the peripheral vasculature is invariably impaired within CHF patients, as demonstrated by ADM measurements done on the forearm and skin in human volunteers (Figs. 27-11 and 27-12). Thus, the speculation is that if nitric oxide is involved in ADM-induced vascular effects, the vasodilatory potency of ADM may be severely blunted in this disorder.[362] However, ADM plays a role in important paracrine effects in regulating other cardiovascular functions as well as renal function.[363] In lieu of these actions, it is hypothesized that ADM may have an important therapeutic role in patients with CHF.

In a clinical study it was demonstrated that the intravenous infusion of ADM resulted in beneficial hemodynamic and renal effects in patients with CHF.[364]

Calcitonin Gene-Related Peptide

Calcitonin gene-related peptide is a vasoregulatory substance that is released by peptidergic sensory nerve endings, including those found in the heart.[365,366] CGRP has positive chronotropic and inotropic actions and is a potent vasodilator.[365,367,368]

Similar to adrenomedullin and the natriuretic peptides, marked elevations in plasma CGRP concentrations are found in patients with congestive heart failure,[369] septic shock,[370] and acute myocardial infarction.[371]

CGRP appears to be involved in a negative feedback loop in the heart.[372] Bradykinin stimulates cardiac sensory C fibers which release CGRP. In turn, CGRP causes the release of histamine from cardiac mast cells, which inhibits further release of CGRP from the sensory nerves.

CGRP has been found to be useful as a treatment for Raynaud's phenomenon. This is of interest because CGRP receptors are decreased in the digital vessels of patients with this condition.[373,374]

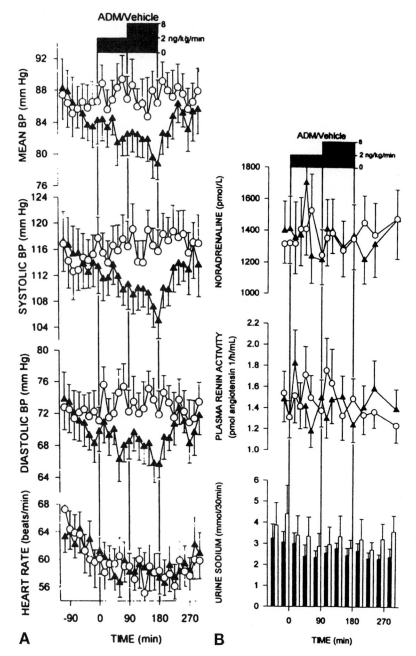

A

B

FIGURE 27-10. Arterial pressure and heart rate recordings in eight healthy subjects who received intravenous adrenomedullin (ADM) (▲) and time-matched vehicle infusions (O). Data are shown as means + SEM. Differences between ADM and vehicle were statistically significant for systolic pressure from the start of infusion to completion of the study ($P = .04$) and for mean pressure over the first 90 min of infusion ($P = .04$). The decline in mean arterial pressure over the entire 180-minute period of ADM administration and the fall in diastolic pressure for the first 90 min of ADM infusion were of marginal statistical significance ($P = .05$). Heart rate was not different on the two study days. BP = blood pressure. (*Reproduced with permission from Lainchbury JG, et al: Adrenomedullin: A hypotensive hormone in man. Clin Sci (London) 92:467–472, 1997, with permission from Biochemical Society of the Medical Research Society.*)

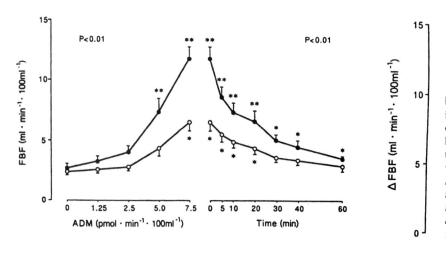

FIGURE 27-11. Forearm blood flow (FBF) response induced by local infusion of ADM and decay curves of FBF after cessation of ADM administration in 10 healthy subjects (●) and 18 patients with congestive heart failure (CHF) (O). *$P < .05$; **$P < .01$ versus baseline. (*Reproduced with permission from Nakamura M, et al: Potent and long-lasting vasodilatory effects of adrenomedullin in humans: Comparisons between normal subjects and patients with chronic heart failure. Circulation 95:1214–1221, 1997.*)

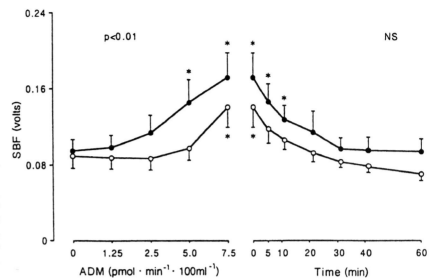

FIGURE 27-12. Skin blood flow (SBF) induced by local infusion of ADM and decay curves of SBF after cessation of ADM administration in 10 healthy subjects (●) and 18 patients with congestive heart failure (CHF) (O). *$P < .05$ versus baseline. (*Reproduced with permission from Nakamura M, et al: Potent and long-lasting vasodilatory effects of adrenomedullin in humans: Comparisons between normal subjects and patients with chronic heart failure. Circulation 95:1214–1221, 1997.*)

Vasoactive Intestinal Peptide

Vasoactive intestinal peptide (VIP) is a neuropeptide found throughout the central and peripheral nervous systems.[375] It is stored in the parasympathetic nerve terminals and has been found to have positive inotropic and chronotropic effects, as well as powerful vasodilator and natriuretic actions.[376]

Similar to other vasoactive peptides, VIP is thought to counteract harmful effects of the vasoconstrictor influences of an activated sympathetic and renin-angiotensin system.[377] VIP plasma levels are elevated in acute myocardial infarction, and it may serve as a prognostic marker,[378] as well as a potential pharmacologic agent, in managing patients with hemodynamic compromise.

CONCLUSION

ADM, CGRP, and VIP are among a growing list of biologic vasodepressor substances that may have importance in normal hemodynamic regulation and in the pathophysiology of various cardiovascular diseases. ADM has been thought to serve as a normal counterbalance to vasoconstricting substances produced by the body such as endothelin and norepinephrine. It may also serve to counter extreme vasoconstrictor influences in congestive heart failure, myocardial infarction, and hypertension.

Similar to ANP and BNP, ADM, CGRP, and VIP appear to be markers of disease severity in congestive heart failure. They could also be infused as drugs in patients to produce vasodilatory and diuretic actions. In the future, orally active drugs could be produced that might enhance either the production or the release of these vasoactive peptides in the body and inhibit their metabolism. Such an approach might provide an innovative treatment for patients with hypertension and congestive heart failure.[379]

REFERENCES

1. de Bold AJ, Borenstein HB, Veress AT, Sonnenberg H: A rapid and potent natriuretic response to intravenous injection of atrial myocardial extract in rats. *Life Sci* 28:89, 1981.
2. de Bold AJ, Raymond JJ, Bencosme SA: Atrial specific granules of the rat heart: Light microscopic staining and histochemical reactions. *Histochem Cytochem* 26:1094, 1978.
3. Luria MH, Adelson EI, Lochaya S: Paroxysmal tachycardia and polyuria. *Ann Intern Med* 65:461, 1966.
4. Garcia R, Cantin M, Thibault G, et al: Relationship of specific granules to the natriuretic and diuretic activity of rat atria. *Experientia* 38:1071, 1982.
5. Sudoh T, Kangawa K, Minamino N, Matsuo H: A new natriuretic peptide in porcine brain. *Nature* 332:78, 1988.
6. Mukoyama M, Nakao K, Hosoda K, et al: Brain natriuretic peptide as a novel cardiac hormone in humans. *J Clin Invest* 87:1402, 1991.
7. Hosoda K, Nakao K, Mukoyama M, et al: Expression of brain natriuretic peptide gene in human heart: Production in the ventricle. *Hypertension* 17:1152, 1991.
8. Sudoh I, Minamino N, Kangawa K, Matsuo H: C-type natriuretic peptide (NP): A new member of natriuretic peptide family identified in porcine brain. *Biochem Biophys Res Commun* 168:863, 1990.
9. Minamino N, Makino Y, Tateyama H, et al: Characterization of immunoreactive human C-type natriuretic peptide in brain and heart. *Biochem Biophys Res Commun* 179:535, 1991.
10. Suga S, Nakao K, Itoh H, et al: Endothelial production of C-type natriuretic peptide and its marked augmentation by transforming growth factor-beta. *J Clin Invest* 90:1145, 1992.
11. Currie MG, Geller DM, Cole BR, et al: Bioactive cardiac substances: Potent vasorelaxant activity in mammalian atria. *Science* 221:71, 1983.
12. Yandle TG: Biochemistry of natriuretic peptide. *J Intern Med* 235:561, 1994.
13. Espiner EA, Richards AM, Yandle TG, Nicholls MG: Natriuretic hormones. *Endocr Metab Clinics North Am* 24:481, 1995.
14. Seidman CE, Bloch KD: Molecular approaches to the study of atrial natriuretic factor. *Am J Med Sci* 294:144, 1987.
15. Oikawa S, Imai M, Ueno A, et al: Cloning and sequence analysis of cDNA encoding a precursor for human atrial natriuretic polypeptide. *Nature* 309:724, 1984.
16. Seidman CE, Duby AD, Choi E, et al: The structure of rat preproatrial natriuretic factor as defined by a complementary DNA clone. *Science* 225:324, 1984.
17. Zisfein JB, Matsueda GR, Fallon JT, et al: Atrial natriuretic factor: Assessment of its structure in atria and regulation of its biosynthesis with volume depletion. *J Mol Cell Cardiol* 18:917, 1986.
18. Thibault G, Cartier F, Garcia R, et al: The human atrial natriuretic factor (hANF): Purification and primary structure. *Clin Invest Med* 7(Suppl 2):59, 1984.
19. Kangawa K, Fukuda A, Matsuo H: Structural identification of β- and γ-human atrial natriuretic polypeptides. *Nature* 313:397, 1985.
20. Sugawara A, Nakao K, Morii N, et al: Significance of a-human atrial natriuretic polypeptide as a hormone in humans. *Hypertension* 8(Suppl I):I151, 1986.

21. Gutkowska J, Bourassa M, Roy D, et al: Immunoreactive atrial natriuretic factor (IR-ANF) in human plasma. *Biochem Biophys Res Commun* 128:1350, 1985.

22. Wilkins MR, Needleman P: Effect of pharmacological manipulation of endogenous atriopeptin activity on renal function. *Am J Physiol* 262:F161, 1992.

23. Seidman CE, Bloch CE, Klein KA, et al: Nucleotide sequences of the human and moose atrial natriuretic factor. *Science* 226:1206, 1984.

24. Kangawa K, Fukuda A, Kubot I, et al: Identification in rat atrial tissue of multiple forms of natriuretic polypeptides of about 3,000 daltons. *Biochem Biophys Res Commun* 121:585, 1984.

25. Chartier L, Schiffrin E, Thibault G: Effect of atrial natriuretic factor (ANF) related peptides on aldosterone secretion by adrenal glomerulosa cells: Critical role of the intramolecular disulphide bond. *Biochem Biophys Res Commun* 122:171, 1984.

26. Gnadinger MP, Lang RE, Hasler L, et al: Plasma kinetics of synthetic alpha-human atrial natriuretic peptide in man. *Miner Electrolyte Metab* 12:371, 1986.

27. Birney MH, Penney DG: Atrial natriuretic peptide: A hormone with implications for clinical practice. *Heart Lung* 19:174, 1990.

28. Baxter JD, Lewicki JA, Gardner DG: Atrial natriuretic peptide. *Biotech* 6:529, 1988.

29. Genest J, Cantin M: Atrial natriuretic factor. *Circulation* 75(Suppl I): I118, 1987.

30. Obata K, Yasue H, Okumura K, et al: Atrial natriuretic poly-peptide is removed by the lungs and released into the left atrium as well as the right atrium in humans. *J Am Coll Cardiol* 15:1537, 1990.

31. Katsube ND, Schwartz D, Needleman P: Release of atriopeptin in the rat by vasoconstrictors or water immersion correlates with changes in right atrial pressure. *Biochem Biophys Res Commun* 133:937, 1985.

32. Metzler CH, Lee ME, Thrasher TN, Ramsay DJ: Increased right or left atrial pressure stimulates release of atrial natriuretic peptide in conscious dogs. *Endocrinology* 119:2396, 1986.

33. Edwards BS, Zimmerman RS, Schwab TR, et al: Atrial stretch, not pressure, is the principal determinant controlling the acute release of atrial natriuretic factor. *Circ Res* 62:191, 1988.

34. Pedersen EB, Pedersen HB, Jensen KT: Pulsatile secretion of atrial natriuretic peptide and brain natriuretic peptide in healthy humans. *Clin Sci (London)* 97:201, 1999.

35. Sonnenberg H, Veress AT: Cellular mechanism of release of atrial natriuretic factor. *Biochem Biophys Res Commun* 124:443, 1984.

36. Petterson A, Rickstein SE, Towle AC, et al: Effect of blood volume expansion and sympathetic denervation on plasma levels of atrial natriuretic factor in rat. *Acta Physiol Scand* 124:309, 1985.

37. Levin ER, Isackson PJ, Hu R-M: Endothelin increases atrial natriuretic peptide production in cultured rat diencephalic neurons. *Endocrinology* 128:2925, 1991.

38. Levin ER, Hu R-M, Rossi M, Pickart M: Arginine vasopressin stimulates atrial natriuretic peptide gene expression and secretion from rat diencephalic neurons. *Endocrinology* 131:1417, 1992.

39. Huang W, Lee D, Yang Z, et al: Norepinephrine stimulates immunoreactive (IR) atrial natriuretic peptide (ANP) secretion and pro-ANP mRNA expression from rat hypothalamic neurons in culture: Effect of alpha$_2$-adrenoceptors. *Endocrinology* 130:2426, 1992.

40. Bloch KD, Seidman JG, Naftilan JD, et al: Neonatal atria and ventricles secrete atrial natriuretic factor via tissue-specific secretory pathways. *Cell* 457:695, 1986.

41. Lattion AL, Michel JB, Arnauld E, et al: Myocardial recruitment during ANF mRNA increase with volume overload in the rat. *Am J Physiol* 251:H890, 1986.

42. Takemura G, Fujiwara H, Mukoyama M, et al: Expression and distribution of atrial natriuretic peptide in human hypertrophic ventricle of hypertensive hearts and hearts with hypertrophic cardiomyopathy. *Circulation* 83(1):181, 1991.

43. Saito Y, Nakao K, Arai H, et al: Relationship between ventricular expression of atrial natriuretic polypeptide gene and hemodynamic parameter in old myocardial infarction. *J Cardiovasc Pharmacol* 13(Suppl 6):S1, 1989.

44. Toth M, Vuorinen KH, Vuolteenaho O, et al: Hypoxia stimulates release of ANP and BNP from perfused rat heart ventricular myocardium. *Am J Physiol* 266:H1572, 1994.

45. Klinger JR, Pietras L, Warburton R, Hill NS: Reduced oxygen tension increases atrial natriuretic peptide release from atrial cardiocytes. *Exp Biol Med* 226:847, 2001.

46. Schulz-Knappe P, Forssmann K, Herbst F, et al: Isolation and structural analysis of "urodilatin," a new peptide of the cardiodilatin-(ANP)-family, extracted from human urine. *Klin Wochenschr* 66:752, 1988.

47. Tateyama H, Himo J, Minamino N, et al: Characterization of immunoreactive brain natriuretic peptide in human cardiac atrium. *Biochem Biophys Res Commun* 166:1080, 1990.

48. Kohno M, Horio T, Yokokawa K, et al: Brain natriuretic peptide as a cardiac hormone in essential hypertension. *Am J Med* 92:29, 1992.

49. Tateyama H, Hino J, Minamino N, et al: Concentrations and molecular forms of human brain natriuretic peptide in plasma. *Biochem Biophys Res Commun* 185:760, 1992.

50. Yandle TG, Richards AM, Gilbert A, et al: Assay of brain natriuretic peptide (BNP) in human plasma evidence for high molecular weight BNP as a major plasma component in heart failure. *J Clin Endocrinol Metab* 76:832, 1993.

51. Morita E, Yasue H, Yoshimura M, et al: Increased plasma levels of brain natriuretic peptide in patients with acute myocardial infarction. *Circulation* 88:82, 1993.

52. Richards AM, Doughty R, Nicholls MG, et al: Plasma N-terminal pro-brain natriuretic peptide and adrenomedullin: Prognostic utility and prediction of benefit from carvedilol in chronic ischemic left ventricular dysfunction. Australia-New Zealand Heart Failure Group. *J Am Coll Cardiol* 37:1781, 2001.

53. Tamura N, Ogawa Y, Yasoda A, et al: ANP, BNP in tandem in rat, human and man: Two cardiac natriuretic peptide genes are organised in tandem in the mouse and human genomes. *Cell Cardiol* 28:1811, 1996.

54. Seilhamer JJ, Arfsten A, Miller JA, et al: Human and canine gene homologs of porcine brain natriuretic peptide. *Biochem Biophys Res Commun* 165:650, 1989.

55. Kambayashi Y, Nakao K, Kimura H, et al: Biological characterization of human brain natriuretic peptide (BNP) and rat BNP: Species-specific actions of BNP. *Biochem Biophys Res Commun* 173:599, 1990.

56. Mukoyama M, Nakao K, Saito Y, et al: Increased human brain natriuretic peptide in congestive heart failure. *N Engl J Med* 323:757, 1990.

57. Luchner A, Burnett JC Jr, Jougasaki M, et al: Evaluation of brain natriuretic peptide as marker of left ventricular dysfunction and hypertrophy in the population. *J Hypertens* 18:1121, 2000.

58. Holmes SJ, Espiner EA, Richards AM, et al: Renal, endocrine, and hemodynamic effects of human brain natriuretic peptide in normal man. *J Clin Endocrinol Metab* 76:91, 1993.

59. Mukoyama M, Nakao K, Hosoda K, et al: Brain natriuretic peptide as a novel cardiac hormone in humans. Evidence for an exquisite dual natriuretic peptide system, ANP and NP. *J Clin Invest* 87:1402, 1991.

60. Kenny AJ, Bourne A, Ingram J: Hydrolysis of human and pig natriuretic peptides, urodilatin. C-type natriuretic peptide and some C-receptor ligands by endopeptidase-24.11. *Biochem J* 291:83, 1993.

61. Ogawa Y, Nakao K, Mukoyama M, et al: Natriuretic peptides as cardiac hormones in normotensive and spontaneously hypertensive rats: The ventricle as the major site of synthesis and secretion of brain natriuretic peptide. *Circ Res* 69:491, 1991.

62. Yoshimura M, Yasue H, Okumura K, et al: Different secretion patterns of atrial natriuretic peptide and brain natriuretic peptide in patients with congestive heart failure. *Circulation* 87:464, 1993.

63. Koglin J, Pehlivanli S, Schwaiblmair M, et al: Role of brain natriuretic peptide in risk stratification of patients with congestive heart failure. *J Am Coll Cardiol* 38:1934, 2001.

64. Yoshibayashi M, Kamiya T, Saito Y, Matsuo H: Increased plasma levels of brain natriuretic peptide in hypertrophic cardiomyopathy. *N Engl J Med* 329:433, 1993.

65. Kinnunen P, Vuolteenaho O, Ruskoaho H: Mechanisms of atrial and brain natriuretic peptide release from rat ventricular myocardium: Effect of stretching. *Endocrinology* 132:1961, 1993.

66. Espiner EA: Physiology of natriuretic peptides. *J Intern Med* 235:527, 1994.

67. Moe GW, Grima EA, Wong NL, et al: Plasma and cardiac tissue atrial and brain natriuretic peptides in experimental heart failure. *J Am Coll Cardiol* 27:720, 1996.

68. Wambach G, Koch J: BNP plasma levels during acute volume expansion and chronic sodium loading in normal men. *Clin Exp Hypertens* 17:619, 1995.

69. Nishikimi T, Morimoto A, Ishikawa K, et al: Different secretion patterns of adrenomedullin, brain natriuretic peptide, and atrial natriuretic peptide during exercise in hypertensive and normotensive subjects. *Clin Exp Hypertens* 19:503, 1997.

70. Yoshibayashi M, Kamiya T, Saito Y, et al: Plasma brain natriuretic peptide concentrations in healthy children from birth to adolescence: Marked and rapid increase after birth. *Eur J Endocrin* 133:207, 1995.

71. Doyama K, Fukumoto M, Takemura G, et al: Expression and distribution of brain natriuretic peptide in human right atria. *J Am Coll Cardiol* 32:1832, 1998.

72. Nakamura S, Naruse M, Naruse K, et al: Atrial natriuretic peptide and brain natriuretic peptide coexist in the secretory granules of human cardiac myocytes. *Am J Hypertens* 4:909, 1991.

73. Mifune H, Richter R, Forssmann WG: Detection of immunoreactive atrial and brain natriuretic peptides in the equine atrium. *Anat Embryol* 192:117, 1995.

74. Lee YJ, Lin SR, Shin SJ, et al: Brain natriuretic peptide is synthesized in the human adrenal medulla and its messenger ribonucleic acid expression along with that of atrial natriuretic peptide are enhanced in patients with primary aldosteronism. *J Clin Endo Metab* 79:1476, 1994.

75. Gerbes AL, Dagnino L, Nguyen T, Nemer M: Transcription of brain natriuretic peptide and atrial natriuretic peptide genes in human tissues. *J Clin Endocrinol Metab* 78:1307, 1994.

76. Lewicki JA, Protter AA: Physiologic studies of the natriuretic peptide family. In: Laragh JH, Brenner BM, eds. *Hypertension: Pathophysiology, Diagnosis, and Management,* 2d ed. New York: Raven Press, 1995:1029.

77. Ogawa Y, Nakao K, Nakagawa H, et al: Human C-type natriuretic peptide. Characterization of the gene and peptide. *Hypertension* 19:809, 1992.

78. Minamino N, Aburaya M, Kojima M, et al: Distribution of C-type natriuretic peptide and its messenger RNA in rat central nervous system and peripheral tissue. *Biochem Biophys Res Commun* 197:326, 1993.

79. Wei C, Aarhus LL, Miller VM, et al: Action of C-type natriuretic peptide in isolated canine arteries and veins. *Am J Physiol* 264:H71, 1993.

80. Woodard GE, Rosado JA, Brown J: Expression and control of C-type natriuretic peptide in rat vascular smooth muscle cells. *Am J Physiol Regul Integr Comp Physiol* 282:R156, 2002.

81. Takahashi T, Allen PD, Izumo S: Expression of A-, B-, and C-type natriuretic peptide genes in failing and developing human ventricles. *Circ Res* 71:9, 1992.

82. Vollmar AM, Gerbes A, Nemer, Schulz R: Detection of C-type natriuretic peptide (CNP) transcript in the rat heart and immune organs. *Endocrinology* 132:1872, 1993.

83. Daggubati S, Parks JR, Overton RM, et al: Adrenomedullin, endothelin, neuropeptide Y, atrial, brain, and C-natriuretic prohormone peptides compared as early heart failure indicators. *Cardiovasc Res* 36:246, 1997.

84. Wei C, Heublein D, Perrela M, et al: Natriuretic peptide system in human heart failure. *Circulation* 88:1004, 1993.

85. Totsune K, Takahashi K, Murakama O, et al: Elevated plasma C-type natriuretic peptide concentrations in patients with chronic renal failure. *Clin Sci (London)* 87:319, 1994.

86. Clerico A, Iervasi G, Pilo A: Turnover studies on cardiac natriuretic peptides: Methodological, pathophysiological and therapeutical considerations. *Curr Drug Metab* 1:85, 2000.

87. Kalra PR, Anker SD, Struthers AD, Coats AJ: The role of C-type natriuretic peptide in cardiovascular medicine. *Eur Heart J* 22:997, 2001.

88. Samson WK: Recent advances in ANF research. *Trends Endocrinol Metab* 3:86, 1992.

89. Burrell LM, Lambert HJ, Baylis PH: Effect of ANP on thirst and arginine-vasopressin release in humans. *Am J Physiol* 260:R475, 1991.

90. Blackburn RE, Samson WK, Fulton RJ, et al: Central oxytocin and ANP receptors mediate osmotic inhibition of salt appetite in rats. *Am J Physiol* 269:R245, 1995.

91. Ishihara T, Aisaka K, Hattori K, et al: Vasodilatory and diuretic actions of alpha-human atrial natriuretic polypeptide. *Life Sci* 36:1205, 1985.

92. Takeuchi K, Abe K, Yasujima M, et al: Difference between the effects of atrial natriuretic peptide and calcium antagonist on cytosolic free calcium in cultured vascular smooth muscle cells. *J Cardiovasc Pharmacol* 13(Suppl 6):S13, 1989.

93. Cornwell TL, Lincoln TM: Regulation of intracellular Ca^{2+} levels in cultured vascular smooth muscle cells: reduction of Ca^{2+} by atriopeptin and 8-bromo-cyclic GMP is mediated by cyclic GMP-dependent protein kinase. *J Biol Chem* 264:1146, 1989.

94. Sarcevic B, Brookes V, Martin TJ, et al: Atrial natriuretic peptide-dependent phosphorylation of smooth muscle cell particulate fraction proteins is mediated by cyclic GMP-dependent protein kinase. *J Biol Chem* 264:20648, 1989.

95. Bolli P, Muller FB, Linder L, et al: The vasodilating effect of atrial natriuretic peptide in normotensive and hypertensive humans. *J Cardiovasc Pharmacol* 13(Suppl 6):S75, 1989.

96. Yasujima M, Abe K, Kohzuki M, et al: Atrial natriuretic factor inhibits the hypertension induced by chronic infusion of norepinephrine in conscious rats. *Circ Res* 57:470, 1985.

97. Volpe M: Atrial natriuretic peptide and baroreflex control of circulation. *Am J Hypertens* 5:488, 1992.

98. Ishikawa S, Saito T, Okada K, et al: Atrial natriuretic factor increases cyclic GMP and inhibits cyclic AMP in rat renal papillary collecting tubule cells in culture. *Biochem Biophys Res Commun* 130:1147, 1985.

99. Dunn BR, Troy JL, Ichikawa I, Brenner BR: Effect of atrial natriuretic peptide (ANP) on hydraulic pressures in the rat renal papilla. In: Brenner BM, Laragh JH, eds. *Biologically Active Atrial Peptides.* Proceedings of the First World Congress. New York: Raven Press, 1987: 416.

100. Kurtz A, Della Bruna R, Pfeilschifter J, et al: Atrial natriuretic peptide inhibits renin release from juxtaglomerular cells by a cyclic GMP-mediated process. *Proc Natl Acad Sci U S A* 83:4769, 1986.

101. Needleman P, Greenwald JE: Atriopeptin: A cardiac hormone intimately involved in fluid, electrolyte and blood pressure homeostasis. *N Engl J Med* 314:828, 1986.

102. Buckalew VM, Morris M, Hamilton RW: Atrial natriuretic factors. *Adv Intern Med* 32:1, 1987.

103. Harris PJ, Thomas D, Morgan TO: Atrial natriuretic peptide inhibits angiotensin-stimulated proximal tubular sodium and water reabsorption. *Nature* 326:697, 1987.

104. Huang CL, Lewicki J, Johnson LK, Cogan MG: Renal mechanism of action of rat atrial natriuretic factor. *J Clin Invest* 75:769, 1985.

105. Atlas SA, Laragh JH: Atrial natriuretic peptide: A new factor in hormonal control of blood pressure and electrolyte homeostasis. *Ann Rev Med* 37:397, 1986.

106. Mendelsohn FAO, Allen AM, Chai SY, et al: Overlapping distributions of receptors for atrial natriuretic peptide and angiotensin II visualized by in vitro autoradiography: Morphological basis of physiological antagonism. *Can J Physiol Pharmacol* 65:1517, 1987.

107. Richards AM, Espiner EA, Ikram H, Yandle TG: Atrial natriuretic factor in hypertension: Bioactivity at normal plasma levels. *Hypertension* 14:261, 1989.

108. Mantyh CR, Kruger L, Brecha NC, Mantyh PW: Localization of specific binding sites for atrial natriuretic factor in peripheral tissues of the guinea pig, rat and human. *Hypertension* 8:712, 1986.

109. Franco-Saenz R, Atarashi K, Takagi M, et al: Effect of atrial natriuretic factor on renin and aldosterone. *J Cardiovasc Pharmacol* 13(Suppl 6):S31, 1989.

110. Campbell WB, Currie MG, Needleman P: Inhibition of aldosterone biosynthesis by atriopeptins in rat adrenal cells. *Circ Res* 57:113, 1985.

111. Cuneo RC, Espiner EA, Nicholls MG, et al: Effect of physiological levels of atrial natriuretic peptide on hormone secretion: Inhibition of angiotensin-induced aldosterone secretion and renin release in normal man. *J Clin Endocrinol Metab* 65:765, 1987.

112. Lainchbury JG, Burnett JC Jr, Meyer D, Redfield MM: Effects of natriuretic peptides on load and myocardial function in normal and heart failure dogs. *Am J Physiol Heart Circ Physiol* 278:H33, 2000.

113. Pegram BL, Kardon MB, Tippodo NC, et al: Atrial extract: Hemodynamics in Wistar-Kyoto and spontaneously hypertensive rats. *Am J Physiol* 249:H265, 1985.

114. Tajima M, Bartunek J, Weinberg EO, et al: Atrial natriuretic peptide has different effects on contractility and intracellular pH in normal and

hypertrophied myocytes from pressure-overloaded hearts. *Circulation* 98:2760, 1998.

115. Bauman RP, Rembert JC, Himmelstein SI, et al: Effects of atrial natriuretic factor on transmural myocardial blood flow distribution in the dog. *Circulation* 76:705, 1987.

116. Burnett JC Jr, Rubanyi GM, Edwards BS, et al: Atrial natriuretic peptide decreases cardiac output independent of coronary vasoconstriction. *Proc Soc Exp Biol Med* 186:313, 1987.

117. Samson WK: Atrial natriuretic factor inhibits dehydration and hemorrhage-induced vasopressin release. *Neuroendocrinology* 40:277, 1985.

118. Schulz HD, Gardner DG, Deschepper CF, et al: Vagal C-fiber blockade abolishes sympathetic inhibition by atrial natriuretic factor. *Am J Physiol* 155:R6, 1988.

119. Obana K, Naruse M, Inagami T, et al: Atrial natriuretic factor inhibits vasopressin secretion from rat posterior pituitary. *Biochem Biophys Res Commun* 132:1088, 1985.

120. Kentsch M, Lawrenz R, Ball P, et al: Effects of atrial natriuretic factor on anterior pituitary hormone secretion in normal man. *Clin Invest* 70:549, 1992.

121. Reddy S, Kelly D, Cochineas C, Gyory AZ: Additive and synergistic interaction of atrial natriuretic peptide and volume expansion. *Am J Physiol* 255:F66, 1988.

122. Appel RG: Growth-regulatory properties of atrial natriuretic factor. *Am J Physiol* 262:F911, 1992.

123. Kohno M, Horio T, Ikeda M, et al: Angiotensin II stimulates endothelin-1 secretion in cultured rat mesangial cells. *Kidney Int* 42:860, 1992.

124. Cao L, Gardner OG. Natriuretic peptides inhibit DNA synthesis in cardiac fibroblasts. *Hypertension* 25:227, 1995.

125. Cargill RI, Struthers AD, Lipworth BJ: Comparative effects of atrial natriuretic peptide and brain natriuretic peptide on the aldosterone and pressor responses to angiotensin II in man. *Clin Sci* 88:81, 1995.

126. Clemens LE, Almirez RG, Baudouin KA, et al: Human brain natriuretic peptide reduces blood pressure in normotensive and acute norepinephrine-induced hypertensive rats. *Am J Hypertens* 10:654, 1997.

127. Okumura K, Yasue H, Fujii H, et al: Effects of brain natriuretic peptide on coronary artery diameter and coronary hemodynamic variables in humans: Comparison with effects on systemic hemodynamic variables. *J Am Coll Cardiol* 25:342, 1995.

128. Holeberg G, Kossenjans W, Brewer A, et al: The action of two natriuretic peptides (ANP and BNP) in the human placental vasculature. *Am J Obstet Gynec* 172:71, 1995.

129. Clavell AL, Stingo AJ, Wei CM, et al: C-type natriuretic peptide: A selective cardiovascular peptide. *Am J Physiol* 264:R290, 1993.

130. Beaulieu P, Cardinal R, Pagé P, et al: Positive chronotropic and inotropic effects of C-type natriuretic peptide in dogs. *Am J Physiol* 273:H1933, 1997.

131. Porter JG, Catalano R, McEnroe G: C-type natriuretic peptide inhibits growth factor-dependent DNA synthesis in smooth muscle cells. *Am J Physiol* 263:C1001, 1992.

132. Furuya M, Yoshida M, Hayashi Y, et al: C-type natriuretic peptide is a growth inhibitor of rat vascular smooth muscle cells. *Biochem Biophys Res Commun* 177:927, 1991.

133. Furuya M, Aisaka K, Miyazaki T, et al: C-type natriuretic peptide inhibits intimal thickening after vascular injury. *Biochem Biophys Res Commun* 193:248, 1993.

134. Charles CJ, Richards AM, Espiner EA: Central C-type natriuretic peptide but not atrial natriuretic factor lowers blood pressure and adrenocortical secretion in normal conscious sheep. *Endocrinology* 131:1721, 1992.

135. Sakamoto M, Nishimura M, Takahashi H: Brain atrial natriuretic peptide family abolishes cardiovascular haemodynamic alterations caused by hypertonic saline in rats. *Clin Exp Pharmacol Physiol* 26:684, 1999.

136. Johnston CI, Hodsman PG, Kohzuki M, et al: Interaction between atrial natriuretic peptide and the renin angiotensin aldosterone system. Endogenous antagonists. *Am J Med* 87(Suppl 6B):24S, 1989.

137. de Bold AJ: Atrial natriuretic factor: A hormone produced by the heart. *Science* 230:767, 1985.

138. Inagami T, Tanaka I, McKenzie JC, et al: Discovery of atrial natriuretic factor in the brain: Its characterization and cardiovascular implication. *Cell Mol Neurobiol* 9:75, 1989.

139. Flynn TG, Davies PL: The biochemistry and molecular biology of atrial natriuretic factor. *Biochem J* 232:313, 1985.

140. Schrier RW: Pathogenesis of sodium and water retention in high-output and low-output cardiac failure, nephrotic syndrome, cirrhosis and pregnancy. *N Engl J Med* 319:1065, 1988.

141. Weil J, Strom TM, Heim JM, et al: Influence of diurnal rhythm, posture and right atrial size on plasma atrial natriuretic peptide levels. *Z Kardiol* 77(Suppl 2):36, 1988.

142. Feller SM, Gagelmann M, Forssmann WG: Urodilatin: A newly described member of the ANP family. *Trends Pharmacol Sci* 10:93, 1989.

143. Saxenhofer H, Raseli A, Weidmann P, et al: Urodilatin, a natriuretic factor from kidneys, can modify renal and cardiovascular function in men. *Am J Physiol* 259:F832, 1990.

144. Gagelmann M, Hock D, Forssmann WG: Urodilatin (CDD/ANP-95-126) is not biologically inactivated by a peptidase from dog kidney cortex membranes in contrast to atrial natriuretic peptide/cardiodilatin (alpha-hANP/CDD-99-126). *FEBS Lett* 233:249, 1988.

145. Lowe DG, Klisak I, Sparkes RS, et al: Chromosomal distribution of three members of the human natriuretic peptide receptor/guanylyl cyclase gene family. *Genomics* 8:304, 1990.

146. Mantymaa P, Vuolteenaho O, Marttila M, Ruskoaho H: Atrial stretch induces rapid increase in brain natriuretic peptide but not in atrial natriuretic peptide gene expression in vitro. *Endocrinology* 133;1470, 1993.

147. Maack T, Okolicany J, Koh GY, Price DA: Functional properties of atrial natriuretic factor receptors. *Semin Nephrol* 13:50, 1993.

148. Levin ER: Natriuretic peptide C-receptor: More than a clearance receptor. *Am J Physiol* 264:E483, 1993.

149. Suga SI, Nakao K, Hosoda K, et al: Receptor selectivity of natriuretic peptide family, atrial natriuretic peptide, brain natriuretic peptide, and C-type natriuretic peptide. *Endocrinology* 130:229, 1993.

150. Koller KJ, Lowe DG, Bennett GL, et al: Selective activation of the B-natriuretic peptide receptor by C-type natriuretic peptide (CNP). *Science* 252:120, 1991.

151. Wilcox JN, Augustine A, Goeddel DV, Lowe DG: Differential regional expression of three natriuretic peptide genes within primate tissues. *Mol Cell Biol* 11:3454, 1991.

152. Tallerico-Melnyk T, Yip CC, Watt VM: Widespread co-localization of messenger RNAs encoding the guanylate cyclase-coupled natriuretic peptide receptors in rat tissues. *Biochem Biophys Res* 189:610, 1992.

153. Nunez DJR, Dickson MC, Brown MJ: Natriuretic peptide receptor messenger RNAs in the rat and human heart. *J Clin Invest* 90:1966, 1992.

154. Marcil J, Anand-Srivastava MB: Defective ANF-R2/ANP-C receptor-mediated signaling in hypertension. *Mol Cell Biochem* 149-150:223, 1995.

155. Cao L, Wu J, Gardner DG: Atrial natriuretic peptide suppresses the transcription of its guanylyl cyclase-linked receptor. *J Biol Chem* 270:24871, 1995.

156. Seymour AA, Norman JA, Asaad MM, et al: Possible regulation of atrial natriuretic factor by neutral endopeptidase 24.11 and clearance receptors. *J Pharmacol Exp Ther* 256:1002, 1991.

157. Achilihu G, Frishman WH, Landau A: Neutral endopeptidase inhibitors and atrial natriuretic peptide. *J Clin Pharmacol* 31:758, 1991.

158. Seymour AA, Swerdel JN, Fennell SA, Delaney NG: Atrial natriuretic peptides cleaved by endopeptidase are inactive in conscious spontaneously hypertensive rats. *Life Sci* 43:2265, 1988.

159. Kenny AJ, Bourne A, Ingram J: Hydrolysis of human and pig brain natriuretic peptides, urodilatin, C-type natriuretic peptide and some C-receptor ligands by endopeptidase-24.11. *Biochem J* 291:83, 1993.

160. Gee NS, Bowes MA, Buck P, Kenny AJ: An immunoradiometric assay for endopeptidase 24.11 shows it to be a widely distributed enzyme in pig tissues. *Biochem J* 228:119, 1985.

161. Erdos EG, Schulz WW, Gafford JT, Defendiri R: Neutral metalloendopeptidase in human male genital tract: Comparison to angiotensin I converting enzyme. *Lab Invest* 52:437, 1985.

162. Johnson AR, Ashton J, Schulz WW, Erdos EG: Neutral metalloendopeptidase in human lung tissue and cultured cells. *Am Rev Resp Dis* 132:564, 1985.

163. Schiebinger RJ, Pratt JH, Kem DC: The adrenal capsule alters the response of zona glomerulosa cells to atrial natriuretic peptide. *Endocrinology* 123:492, 1988.

164. Erdos EG, Skidgel RA: Neutral endopeptidase 24.11 (enkephalinase) and related regulators or peptide hormones. *FASEB J* 3:145, 1989.

165. Shima M, Seino Y, Torikai S, Imai M: Intrarenal localization of degradation of atrial natriuretic peptide in isolated glomeruli and cortical nephron segments. *Life Sci* 43:357, 1988.

166. Schulz WW, Hagler K, Buja L, Erdos G: Ultrastructural localization of angiotensin I converting enzyme (EC 3.4.15.1) and neutral metalloendopeptidase (EC 3.4.24.11) in the proximal tubule of the human kidney. *Lab Invest* 59:789, 1988.

167. Richards AM, Rao G, Espiner EA, Yandle T: Interaction of angiotensin-converting enzyme inhibition and atrial natriuretic factor. *Hypertension* 13:193, 1989.

168. Almeida FA, Suzuki M, Scarborough RM, et al: Clearance function of type C receptors of atrial natriuretic factor in rats. *Am J Physiol* 256:R469, 1989.

169. Murthy KK, Thibault G, Cantin M: Binding and intracellular degradation of atrial natriuretic factor by cultured vascular smooth muscle cells. *Mol Cell Endocrinol* 67:195, 1989.

170. Porter JG, Wang Y, Schwartz K, et al: Characterization of the atrial natriuretic peptide clearance receptor using a vaccinia virus expression vector. *J Biol Chem* 263:18827, 1988.

171. Maack T, Suzuki M, Almeida FA, et al: Physiological role of silent receptors of atrial natriuretic factor. *Science* 238:675, 1987.

172. Maack T: Receptors of atrial natriuretic factor. *Annu Rev Physiol* 54:11, 1992.

173. Sybertz EJ, Chiu PJS, Vemulapalli S, et al: SCH 39370, a neutral metalloendopeptidase inhibitor, potentiates biological responses to atrial natriuretic factor and lowers blood pressure in desoxycorticosterone acetate-sodium hypertensive rats. *J Pharmacol Exp Ther* 250:624, 1989.

174. Barclay PL, Bennet JA, Samuels GMR, Shepperson NB: The atriopeptidase inhibitor (±) candoxatrilat reduces the clearance of atrial natriuretic factor in both intact and nephrectomized rats: Evidence for an extrarenal site of action. *J Pharmacol Biochem* 41:841, 1991.

175. Hollister AS, Rodeheffer RJ, White FJ, et al: Clearance of atrial natriuretic factor by lung, liver and kidney human subjects and the dog. *J Clin Invest* 83:623, 1989.

176. Hollister AS, Inagami T: Atrial natriuretic factor and hypertension. *Am J Hypertens* 4:850, 1991.

177. Yandle TG: Biochemistry of natriuretic peptides. *J Intern Med* 235:561, 1994.

178. Nakaoka H, Imataka K, Amano M, et al: Plasma levels of atrial natriuretic factor in patients with congestive heart failure. *N Engl J Med* 313:892, 1985.

179. Tikkanen I, Metsarinne K, Fyhrquist F, Leidenius R: Plasma atrial natriuretic peptide in cardiac disease and during infusion in healthy volunteers. *Lancet* 2:66, 1985.

180. Bilder GE, Siegl PKS, Schofield TL, Friedman PA: Chronotropic stimulation: A primary effector for release of atrial natriuretic factor. *Circ Res* 64:799, 1989.

181. Rankin AJ, Courneya CA, Wison N, Ledsom JR: Tachycardia releases atrial natriuretic peptide in the anesthetized rabbit. *Life Sci* 38:1951, 1986.

182. Cantin M, Genest J: The heart as an endocrine gland. *Hypertension* 10(Suppl I):I118, 1997.

183. Manning PT, Schwartz D, Katsube NC, et al: Vasopressin-stimulated release of atriopeptin: Endocrine antagonists in fluid homeostasis. *Science* 229:395, 1985.

184. Singer DRJ, Sagnella GA, Markandu ND, et al: Atrial natriuretic peptide, blood pressure and age. *Lancet* 2:1394, 1987.

185. Trippodo NC: An update on the physiology of atrial natriuretic factor. *Hypertension* 10(Suppl I):I122, 1987.

186. Somers VK, Anderson JV, Conway J, et al: Atrial natriuretic peptide is released by dynamic exercise in man. *Horm Metab Res* 18:871, 1986.

187. Cusson JR, Gutkowska J, Rey E, et al: Plasma concentration of atrial natriuretic factor in normal pregnancy. *N Engl J Med* 313:1230, 1985.

188. Weidman P, Matter DR, Matter EE, et al: Glucocorticoid and mineralocorticoid stimulation of atrial natriuretic peptide release in man. *J Clin Endocrinol Metab* 66:1233, 1988.

189. Morii N, Makao K, Matsumori A, et al: Increased synthesis and secretion of atrial natriuretic polypeptide during viral myocarditis. *J Cardiovasc Pharmacol* 13(Suppl 6):S5, 1989.

190. Takemura G, Takatsu Y, Doyama K, et al: Expression of atrial and brain natriuretic peptides and their genes in hearts of patients with cardiac amyloidosis. *J Am Coll Cardiol* 31:254, 1998.

191. Tang J, Xie CW, Xu CB, et al: Therapeutic actions of alpha-human atrial natriuretic polypeptide in 16 clinical cases. *Life Sci* 40:2077, 1987.

192. Hollister AS, Tanaka I, Imada T, et al: Sodium loading and posture modulate human atrial natriuretic factor plasma levels. *Hypertension* 8(Suppl II):II106, 1986.

193. Ogihara T, Shima J, Hara H, et al: Significant increase in plasma immunoreactive atrial natriuretic polypeptide concentration during water immersion. *Life Sci* 38:2413, 1986.

193a. Wondergem J, Strootman EG, Frölich M, et al: Circulating atrial natriuretic peptide plasma levels as a marker for cardiac damage after radiotherapy. *Radiother Oncol* 58:295, 2001.

194. Cappuccio FP, MacGregor G, Strazzullo P, et al: Characteristics of the distribution of plasma atrial natriuretic peptides in a cross-sectional study of middle-aged untreated male workers. *J Cardiovasc Pharmacol* 13(Suppl 6):S51, 1989.

195. Gardner DG, Schultz HD: Prostaglandins regulate the synthesis and secretion of the atrial natriuretic peptide. *J Clin Invest* 86:52, 1990.

196. Vesely DL, Winters CJ, Sallman AL: Prohormone atrial natriuretic peptides 1-30 and 31-67 increase in hyperthyroidism and decrease in hypothyroidism. *Am J Med Sci* 297:209, 1989.

197. Saito Y, Nakao K, Itoh H, et al: Brain natriuretic peptide is a novel cardiac hormone. *Biochem Biophys Res Commun* 158:360, 1989.

197a. Yoshimura M, Mizuno Y, Nakayama M, et al: B-type natriuretic peptide as a marker of the effects of enalapril in patients with heart failure. *Am J Med* 112:716, 2002.

198. Morita E, Yasue H, Yoshimura M, et al: Increased plasma levels of brain natriuretic peptide in patients with acute myocardial infarction. *Circulation* 88:82, 1993.

198a. DeLemos JA, Morrow DA, Bentley JH, et al: The prognostic value of B-type natriuretic peptide in patients with acute coronary syndromes. *N Engl J Med* 345:1014, 2001.

199. Richards AM: The natriuretic peptides and hypertension. *J Intern Med* 235:543, 1994.

200. Lang CC, Coutie WJ, Khong TK, et al: Dietary sodium loading increases plasma brain natriuretic peptide levels in man. *J Hypertens* 9:779, 1991.

201. Kohno M, Horio T, Toda I, et al: Cosecretion of atrial and brain natriuretic peptides during supraventricular tachyarrhythmias. *Am Heart J* 123:1382, 1992.

202. La Villa G. Romanelli RG, Casini-Raggi V, et al: Plasma levels of brain natriuretic peptide in patients with cirrhosis. *Hepatology* 16:156, 1992.

203. Richards AM, Crozier IG, Yandle TG, et al: Brain natriuretic factor: Regional plasma concentrations and correlations with haemodynamic state in cardiac disease. *Br Heart J* 69:414, 1993.

204. Wilkins MA, Su XL, Palaye MD, et al: The effects of posture change and continuous positive airway pressure on cardiac natriuretic peptides in congestive heart failure. *Chest* 107:909, 1995.

205. Tomiyama H, Kushiro T, Imai S, et al: Changes in the E/A ratio induced by handgrip-exercise are related to plasma ANP level, but not to changes in BNP in mild essential hypertension. *Jpn Circ J* 59:617, 1995.

206. Espiner EA: Hormones of the cardiovascular system. In: DeGroot LJ, ed. *Endocrinology.* 3rd ed. Philadelphia: WB Saunders, 1995:2895.

207. Richards AM, Crozier IG, Espiner EA, et al: Plasma brain natriuretic peptide and endopeptidase 24.11 inhibition in hypertension. *Hypertension* 22:231, 1993.

208. Naruse M, Takeyama Y, Tanabe A, et al: Atrial and brain natriuretic peptides in cardiovascular diseases. *Hypertension* 23(Suppl I):I231, 1994.

209. Cheung BM, Brown MJ: Plasma brain natriuretic peptide and C-type natriuretic peptide in essential hypertension. *J Hypertens* 12:449, 1994.

210. Hama N, Itoh H, Shirakami G, et al: Detection of C-type natriuretic peptide in human circulation and marked increase of plasma CNP level in septic shock patients. *Biochem Biophys Res Commun* 198:1177, 1994.

211. Dickstein K, Abrahamsen S, Aarsland T: Plasma N-terminal atrial natriuretic peptide predicts hospitalization in patients with heart failure. *Scand Cardiovasc J* 32:361, 1998.

212. Cody RJ, Atlas SA, Laragh JH, et al: Atrial natriuretic factor in normal subjects and heart failure patients: Plasma level, renal hormonal, and hemodynamic responses to peptide infusion. *J Clin Invest* 78:1362, 1986.

213. Lewis BS, Makhoul N, Dakak N, et al: Atrial natriuretic peptide in severe heart failure: Response to controlled changes in atrial pressures during intravenous nitroglycerin therapy. *Am Heart J* 124:1009, 1992.

214. Munzel T, Drexler H, Holtz J, et al: Mechanisms involved in the response to prolonged infusion of atrial natriuretic factor in patients with chronic heart failure. *Circulation* 83:191, 1991.

215. Lee ME, Miller WL, Edwards BS, Burnett JC Jr: Role of endogenous atrial natriuretic factor in acute congestive heart failure. *J Clin Invest* 84:1962, 1989.

216. Hoffman A, Burnett JC, Haramati A, Winaver J: Effects of atrial natriuretic factor in rats with experimental high output heart failure. *Kidney Inter* 33:656, 1988.

217. Perrella MA, Marulies KB, Burnett JC Jr: Pathophysiology of congestive heart failure: role of atrial natriuretic factor and therapeutic implications. *Can J Physiol Pharmacol* 69:1576, 1991.

218. Dao Q, Krishnaswamy P, Kazanegra R, et al: Utility of B-type natriuretic peptide in the diagnosis of congestive heart failure in an urgent-care setting. *J Am Coll Cardiol* 37:379, 2001.

219. Cheng V, Kazanagra R, Garcia A, et al: A rapid bedside test for B-type peptide predicts treatment outcomes in patients admitted for decompensated heart failure: A pilot study. *J Am Coll Cardiol* 37:386, 2001.

220. Maisel AS, Koon J, Krishnaswamy P, et al: Utility of B-natriuretic peptide as a rapid, point-of-care test for screening patients undergoing echocardiography to determine left ventricular dysfunction. *Am Heart J* 141:367, 2001.

221. McDonagh TA, Cunningham AD, Morrison CE, et al: Left ventricular dysfunction, natriuretic peptides, and mortality in an urban population. *Heart* 86:21, 2001.

222. Maeda K, Tsutamoto T, Wada A, et al: High levels of plasma brain natriuretic peptide and interleukin-6 after optimized treatment for heart failure are independent risk factors for morbidity and mortality in patients with congestive heart failure. *J Am Coll Cardiol* 36:1587, 2000.

223. Knight EL, Fish LC, Kiely DK, et al: Atrial natriuretic peptide and the development of congestive heart failure in the oldest old: A seven-year prospective study. *J Am Geriatr Soc* 47:407, 1999.

224. Yamamoto K, Burnett JC Jr, Bermudez EA, et al: Clinical criteria and biochemical markers for the detection of systolic dysfunction. *J Cardiac Fail* 6:194, 2000.

225. Troughton RW, Frampton CM, Yandle TG, et al: Treatment of heart failure guided by plasma aminoterminal brain natriuretic peptide (N-BNP) concentrations. *Lancet* 355:1126, 2000.

226. Andersson B, Hall C: N-terminal proatrial natriuretic peptide and prognosis in patients with heart failure and preserved systolic function. *J Cardiac Fail* 6:208, 2000.

227. Fruhwald FM, Fahrleitner A, Watzinger N, et al: Natriuretic peptides in patients with diastolic dysfunction due to idiopathic dilated cardiomyopathy. *Eur Heart J* 20:1415, 1999.

228. Morrison LK, Harrison A, Krishnaswamy P, et al: Utility of B-natriuretic peptide assay in differentiating congestive heart failure from lung disease in patients presenting with dyspnea. *J Am Coll Cardiol* 39:202, 2000.

228a. Cowie MR, Mendez GF: BNP and congestive heart failure. *Prog Cardiovasc Dis* 44:293, 2002.

228b. McCullough PA, Nowak RM, McCord J, et al: B-type natriuretic peptide and clinical judgment in emergency diagnosis of heart failure. Analysis from Breathing Not Properly (BNP) Multinational Study. *Circulation* 106:416, 2002.

228c. Bettencourt P, Ferreira S, Azevedo A, Ferreira A: Preliminary data on the potential usefulness of B-type natriuretic peptide levels in predicting outcome after hospital discharge in patients with heart failure. *Am J Med* 113:215, 2002.

228d. Ribeiro ALP, dos Reis AM, Barros MVL, et al: Brain natriuretic peptide and left ventricular dysfunction in Chagas' disease. *Lancet* 360:461, 2002.

228e. Krüger S, Graf J, Kunz D, et al: Brain natriuretic peptide levels predict functional capacity in patients with chronic heart failure. *J Am Coll Cardiol* 40:718, 2002.

228f. Maisel AS, Krishnaswamy P, Nowak RM, et al: Rapid measurement of B-type natriuretic peptide in the emergency diagnosis of heart failure. *N Engl J Med* 347:161, 2002.

229. Lang CC, Coutie WJ, Struthers AD, et al: Elevated levels of brain natriuretic peptide in acute hypoxaemic chronic obstructive pulmonary disease. *Clin Sci (Colch)* 83:529, 1992.

230. Nagaya N, Nishikimi T, Uematsu M, et al: Plasma brain natriuretic peptide as a prognostic indicator in patients with primary pulmonary hypertension. *Circulation* 102:865, 2000.

231. Nakamura M, Kawata Y, Yoshida H, et al: Relationship between plasma atrial and brain natriuretic peptide concentration and hemodynamic parameters during percutaneous transvenous mitral valvulotomy in patients with mitral stenosis. *Am Heart J* 124:1283, 1992.

232. Santucci A, Ferri C, Cammarella I, et al: Plasma atrial natriuretic peptide in young normotensive subjects with a family history of hypertension and in young hypertensive patients. *Am J Hypertens* 3:782, 1990.

233. Goetz KL: Physiology and pathophysiology of atrial peptides. *Am J Physiol* 254:E1, 1998.

234. Itoh H, Nakao K, Mukoyama M, et al: Chronic blockade of endogenous atrial natriuretic polypeptide (ANP) by monoclonal antibody against ANP accelerates the development of hypertension in spontaneously hypertensive and deoxycorticosterone acetate-salt-hypertensive rats. *J Clin Invest* 84:145, 1989.

235. Winquist RJ: The relaxant effects of atrial natriuretic factor on vascular smooth muscle. *Life Sci* 37:1081, 1985.

236. Ebert TJ, Skelton MM, Cowley AW: Dynamic cardiovascular responses to infusions of atrial natriuretic factor in humans. *Hypertension* 11:537, 1988.

237. Rutledge DR, Sun Y, Ross EA: Polymorphisms within the atrial natriuretic peptide gene in essential hypertension. *J Hypertens* 13:953, 1995.

238. Lopez MJ, Wong Sk, Kishimoto I, et al: Salt-resistant hypertension in mice lacking the guanylyl cyclase-A receptor for atrial natriuretic peptide. *Nature* 378:65, 1995.

239. Mo R, Myking OL, Lund Johansen P, Omvick P: The Bergen Blood Pressure Study: Inappropriately low levels of circulating atrial natriuretic peptide in offspring of hypertensive families. *Blood Pressure* 3:223, 1994.

239a. Vasan RS, Benjamin EJ, Larson MG, et al: Plasma natriuretic peptides for community screening for left ventricular hypertrophy and systolic dysfunction. The Framingham Heart Study. *JAMA* 288:1252, 2002.

240. Dagnino L, Lavigne JP, Nemer M: Increased transcripts for B-type natriuretic peptide in spontaneously hypertensive rats: Quantitative polymerase chain reaction for atrial and brain natriuretic peptide transcripts. *Hypertension* 20:690, 1992.

241. Yokota N, Aburaya M, Yamamoto Y, et al: Increased plasma brain natriuretic peptide levels in DOCA-salt hypertensive rats: Relation to blood pressure and cardiac concentration. *Biochem Biophys Res Commun* 173:632, 1990.

242. Cheung B, Dickerson J, Ashby M, et al: Effects of physiological increments in human alpha-atrial natriuretic peptide and human brain natriuretic peptide in normal male subjects. *Clin Sci (Colch)* 86:723, 1994.

243. Anderson J, Struthers A, Christofides N, Bloom S: Atrial natriuretic peptide: An endogenous factor enhancing sodium excretion in man. *Clin Sci (Colch)* 70:327, 1986.

244. Jardine AG, Northridge DB, Connell JMC: Harnessing therapeutic potential of atrial natriuretic peptide. *Klin Wochenschr* 67:902, 1989.

245. Allgren RL, Marbury TC, Noor R et al: Anaritide in acute tubular necrosis. *N Engl J Med* 336:828, 1997.

246. Goy JJ, Waeber B, Nussberger J, et al: Infusion of atrial natriuretic peptide to patients with congestive heart failure. *J Cardiovasc Pharmacol* 12:562, 1988.

247. Riegger AJG, Kromer EP, Koshsiek K: Der natriuretische vorhoffaktor bei schwerer kongestiver herzinsuffizienz. *Deutsch Med Wochenschr* 110:1607, 1985.

248. Firth BG, Perna R, Bellomo JF, Toto RD: Cardiorenal effects of atrial natriuretic factor administration in congestive heart failure: Natriuresis and diuresis without hemodynamic alterations. *Am J Med Sci* 297:203, 1989.

249. Kohzuki M, Hodsman GP, Harrison RW, et al: Atrial natriuretic peptide infusion in chronic heart failure in the rat. *J Cardiovasc Pharmacol* 13(Suppl 6):S43, 1989.

250. Fifer MA, Molina CR, Quiroz AC, et al: Hemodynamic and renal effects of atrial natriuretic peptide in congestive heart failure. *Am J Cardiol* 65:211, 1990.

251. Saito Y, Nakao K, Nishimura K, et al: Clinical application of atrial natriuretic polypeptide in patients with congestive heart failure: Beneficial effects on left ventricular function. *Circulation* 76:115, 1987.

252. Eiskjaer H, Bagger JP, Danielsen H, et al: Attenuated renal excretory response to ANP in congestive heart failure in man. *Int J Cardiol* 33:61, 1991.

253. Abraham WT, Lowes BD, Ferguson DA, et al: Systemic hemodynamic, neurohormonal, and renal effects of a steady-state infusion of human brain natriuretic peptide in patients with hemodynamically decompensated heart failure. *J Cardiac Failure* 4:37, 1998.

254. Abraham WT, Lauwaars ME, Kim JK, et al: Reversal of atrial natriuretic peptide resistance by increasing distal tubular sodium delivery in patients with decompensated cirrhosis. *Hepatology* 22:737, 1995.

255. Connelly TP, Francis GS, Williams KJ, et al: Interactions of intravenous atrial natriuretic factor with furosemide in patients with heart failure. *Am Heart J* 127:392, 1994.

256. Koepke JP, DiBona GF: Blunted natriuresis to atrial natriuretic peptide in chronic sodium-retaining disorders. *Am J Physiol* 252:F865, 1987.

257. Abassi ZA, Kelly G, Golomb E, et al: Losartan improves the natriuretic response to ANP in rats with high-output heart failure. *J Pharm Exper Ther* 268:224, 1994.

258. Elsner D, Muders F, Muntze A, et al: Efficacy of prolonged infusion of urodilatin (ANP-95-126) in patients with congestive heart failure. *Am Heart J* 129:766, 1995.

259. Cusson JR, Thibault G, Cantin M, Larochelle P: Prolonged low-dose infusion of atrial natriuretic factor in essential hypertension. *Clin Exp Hypertens* A12:111, 1990.

260. Franco-Saenz R, Somani P, Mulrow PJ: Effect of atrial natriuretic peptide (8-33-Met ANP) in patients with hypertension. *Am J Hypertens* 5:266, 1992.

261. Tonolo G, Richards AM, Manunta P, et al: Low-dose infusion of atrial natriuretic factor in mild essential hypertension. *Circulation* 80:893, 1989.

262. Richards AM, Nicholls MG, Espiner EA, et al: Effects of α-human atrial natriuretic peptide in essential hypertension. *Hypertension* 7:812, 1985.

263. Hamet P, Testaert E, Palmour R, et al: Effect of prolonged infusion of ANF in normotensive and hypertensive monkeys. *Am J Physiol* 257:690, 1989.

264. Weidmann P, Gnadinger MP, Ziswiler HR, et al: Cardiovascular, endocrine and renal effects of atrial natriuretic peptide in essential hypertension. *J Hypertens* 4(Suppl 2):S71, 1986.

265. Lin KF, Chao J, Chao L: Human atrial natriuretic peptide gene delivery reduces blood pressure in hypertensive rats. *Hypertension* 26:847, 1995.

266. Pollock DM, Opgenorth TJ: Beneficial effect of the atrial natriuretic factor analog A68828 in postischemic acute renal failure. *J Pharmacol Exp Ther* 255:1166, 1990.

267. Boland DG, Abraham WT: Natriuretic peptides in heart failure. *Cong Heart Fail* Mar/Apr:23, 1998.

268. Grantham JA, Borgeson DD, Burnett JC Jr: BNP: Pathophysiological and potential therapeutic roles in acute congestive heart failure. *Am J Physiol* 272:R1077, 1997.

269. La Villa G, Fronzaroli C, Lazzeri C, et al: Cardiovascular and renal effects of low-dose brain natriuretic peptide infusion in man. *J Clin Endocrinol Metab* 78:1166, 1994.

270. McGregor A, Richards M, Espiner E, et al: Brain natriuretic peptide administered to man: Ations and metabolism. *J Clin Endocrinol Metab* 70:1103, 1990.

271. Colucci WS, Elkayam U, Horton DP, et al: Intravenous nesiritide, a natriuretic peptide, in the treatment of decompensated congestive heart failure. Nesiritide Study Group. *N Engl J Med* 343:246, 2000.

272. Publication Committee for the VMAC Investigators: Intravenous nesiritide vs nitroglycerin for treatment of decompensated congestive heart failure. A randomized controlled trial. *JAMA* 287:1531, 2002.

273. Abraham WT, Lowes BD, Ferguson DA, et al: Systemic hemodynamic, neurohormonal, and renal effects of a steady-state infusion of human brain natriuretic peptide in patients with hemo-dynamically decompensated heart failure. *J Cardiac Fail* 4:37, 1998.

274. Brunner-LaRocca HP, Kaye DM, Woods RL, et al: Effects of intravenous brain natriuretic peptide on regional sympathetic activity in

patients with chronic heart failure as compared with healthy control subjects. *J Am Coll Cardiol* 37:1221, 2001.

275. Marcus LS, Hart D, Packer M, et al: Hemodynamic and renal excretory effects of human brain natriuretic peptide infusion in patients with congestive heart failure: A double-blind, placebo-controlled, randomized crossover trial. *Circulation* 94:3184, 1996.

276. Burger AJ, Horton DP, Elkayam U, et al: Nesiritide is not associated with proarrhythmic effects of dobutamine in the treatment of decompensated CHF: The PRECEDENT Study. *J Cardiac Fail* 5(Suppl 1):49, 1999.

277. Burger AJ, Horton DP, Elkayam U, et al: Evidence of ventricular ectopy at baseline is not predictive of the proarrhythmic effects of dobutamine in the treatment of decompensated CHF: The PRECEDENT Study. *J Cardiac Fail* 6(Suppl 2):46, 2000.

278. Elkayam U, Silver MA, Burger AJ, Horton DP: The effect of short-term therapy with nesiritide (B-type natriuretic peptide) or dobutamine on long-term survival. *J Cardiac Fail* 6(Suppl 2):45, 2000.

279. Silver MA, Horton DP, Ghali JK, Elkayam U: Effect of nesiritide versus dobutamine on short-term outcomes in the treatment of patients with acutely decompensated heart failure. *J Am Coll Cardiol* 39:798, 2002.

280. Elkayam U, Silver MA, Burger AJ, et al: Limitations of commonly used titrated doses of intravenous nitroglycerin in patients with acute decompensated heart failure. *J Card Fail* 7(Suppl 2):12, 2001.

281. Chen HH, Grantham JA, Schirger JA, et al: Subcutaneous administration of brain natriuretic peptide in experimental heart failure. *J Am Coll Cardiol* 36:1706, 2000.

282. LaVilla G, Bisi G, Lazzeri C, et al: Cardiovascular effects of brain natriuretic peptide in essential hypertension. *Hypertension* 25:1053, 1995.

283. Lazzeri C, Franchi F, Porciani C, et al: Systemic hemodynamics and renal function during brain natriuretic peptide infusion in patients with essential hypertension. *Am J Hypertens* 8:799, 1995.

284. Wilkins MR, Unwin RJ, Kenny AJ: Endopeptidase 24.11 and its inhibitors: Potential therapeutic agents for edematous disorders and hypertension. *Kidney Int* 43:273, 1993.

285. Chiu PJS, Tetzloff G, Romano MT, et al: Influence of c-ANP receptor and neutral endopeptidase on pharmacokinetics of ANF in rats. *Am J Physiol* 260:R208, 1991.

286. Vemulapalli S, Chiu PJS, Brown A, et al: The blood pressure and renal responses to SCH 24826, a neutral metallo-endopeptidase inhibitor, and C-ANF (4-23) in DOCA-salt hypertensive rats. *Life Sci* 49:383, 1991.

287. Wegner M, Stasch JP, Hirth-Dietrich C, et al: Interaction of a neutral endopeptidase inhibitor with an ANP-C receptor ligand in anesthetized dogs. *Clin Exp Hypertens* 17:861, 1995.

288. Koepke JP, Tyler LD, Blehm DJ, et al: Chronic atriopeptin regulation of arterial pressure in conscious hypertensive rats. *Hypertension* 16:642, 1990.

289. Schwartz JC, Malfroy B, De La Baume S: Biological inactivation of enkephalins and the role of enkephalin-dipeptidyl-carboxypeptidase (enkephalinase) as neuropeptidase. *Life Sci* 29:1715, 1981.

290. Nakamura A, Arakawa N, Kato M: Renal, hormonal and hemodynamic effects of low-dose infusion of atrial natriuretic factor in acute myocardial infarction. *Am Heart J* 120:1078, 1990.

291. Ronco P, Pollard H, Galceran M, et al: Distribution of enkephalinase (membrane metalloendopeptidase EC 3.4.24.11) in rat organs: Detection using a monoclonal antibody. *Lab Invest* 58:210, 1988.

292. Liu L, Cheng H, Chin W, et al: Atrial natriuretic peptide lowers pulmonary arterial pressure in patients with high-altitude disease. *Am J Med Sci* 298:397, 1989.

293. Janssen WMT, de Jong PE, van der Hem GK, de Zeeux D: Effect of human atrial natriuretic peptide on blood pressure after sodium depletion in essential hypertension. *Br Med J* 293:351, 1986.

294. Kentsch M, Drummer C, Gerzer R, Muller-Esch G: Severe hypotension and bradycardia after continuous intravenous infusion of urodilatin (ANP 95-126) in a patient with congestive heart failure. *Eur J Clin Invest* 25:281, 1995.

295. Cheung BM, Dickerson JE, Ashley MJ, et al: Effects of physiological increments in human atrial natriuretic peptide and human brain natriuretic peptide in normal male subjects. *Clin Sci (Colch)* 86:723, 1994.

296. Anand IS, Kalra GS, Ferrari R, et al: Hemodynamic, hormonal and renal effects of atrial natriuretic peptide in untreated congestive cardiac failure. *Am Heart J* 118:500, 1989.

297. Tsutamoto T, Kanamori T, Wada A, Kinoshita M: Uncoupling of atrial natriuretic peptide extraction and cyclic guanosine mono-phosphate production in the pulmonary circulation in patients with severe heart failure. *J Am Coll Cardiol* 20:541, 1992.

298. Weidman P, Ferrari P, Allemann Y, et al: Developing essential hypertension: a syndrome involving ANF deficiency? *Can J Physiol Pharmacol* 69:1582, 1991.

299. Mittal CK: Decreased atrial natriuretic peptide receptors in the adrenal gland of genetically hypertensive rats. *Am J Hypertens* 6:431, 1993.

300. Yoshimura M, Yasue H, Morita E, et al: Hemodynamic, renal and hormonal responses to brain natriuretic peptide infusion in patients with congestive heart failure. *Circulation* 84:1581, 1991.

300a. McMurray J, Pfeffer MA: New therapeutic options in congestive heart failure. Part I. *Circulation* 105:2099, 2002.

301. Cheng JWM: Nesiritide: Review of clinical pharmacology and role in heart failure management. *Heart Dis* 4:199, 2002.

302. Kitamura K, Kangawa K, Matsuo H, Eto T: Adrenomedullin: Implications for hypertension research. *Drugs* 49:485, 1995.

303. Kitamura K, Sakata J, Kangawa K, et al: Cloning and characterization of cDNA encoding a precursor for human adrenomedullin. *Biochem Biophys Res Commun* 194:720, 1993.

304. Kitamura K, Kangawa K, Kojima M, et al: Complete amino acid sequence of porcine adrenomedullin and cloning of cDNA encoding its precursor. *FEBS Letter* 338(3):306, 1994.

305. Ishimitsu T, Kojima M, Kangawa K, et al: Genomic structure of human adrenomedullin gene. *Biochem Biophys Res Commun* 203:631, 1994.

306. Samson WK, Murphy TC, Resch ZT: Proadrenomedullin N-terminal 20 peptide inhibits adrenocorticotropin secretion from cultured pituitary cells, possibly via activation of a potassium channel. *Endocrine* 9(3):269, 1998.

307. Samson WK: Adrenomedullin and the control of fluid and electrolyte homeostasis. *Annu Rev Physiol* 61:363, 1999.

308. Samson WK, Bode AM, Murphy TC, Resch ZT: Antisense oligonucleotide treatment reveals a physiologically relevant role for adrenomedullin gene products in sodium intake. *Brain Res* 818:164, 1999.

309. Sato K, Hirata Y, Imai T, Iwashita M, Mariuo F: Characterization of immunoreactive ADM in human plasma and urine. *Life Sci* 57:189, 1995.

310. Sugo S, Minamino N, Kangawa K, et al: Endothelial cells actively synthesize and secrete adrenomedullin. *Biochem Biophys Res Commun* 201:1160, 1994.

311. Nishikimi T, Kitamura K, Saito Y, et al: Clinical studies on the sites for circulating adrenomedullin in human subjects. *Hypertension* 24:600, 1994.

312. Katoh F, Niina H, Kitamura K, et al: Ca^{2+} dependent cosecretion of adrenomedullin and catecholamines mediated by nicotinic receptors in bovine cultured adrenal medullary cells. *FEBS Lett* 348:61, 1994.

313. Ishizaka Y, Tanaka M, Kitamura K, et al: Adrenomedullin stimulates cyclic AMP formation in rat vascular smooth muscle cells. *Biochem Biophys Res Commun* 200:642, 1994.

314. Eguchi S, Hirata Y, Kano H, et al: Specific receptors for adrenomedullin in cultured rat vascular smooth muscle cells. *FEBS Lett* 340:226, 1994.

315. Sugo S, Minamino N, Shoji H, et al: Production and secretion of adrenomedullin from vascular smooth-muscle cells: Augmented production by tumor necrosis factor. *Biochem Biophys Res Commun* 203:719, 1994.

316. Minamino, N, Shoji H, Sugo S, et al: Adrenocortical steroids, thyroid hormones and retinoic acid augment the production of adrenomedullin in vascular smooth muscle cells. *Biochem Biophys Res Commun* 211:686, 1995.

317. Leitman DC, Ribeiro RC, Mackow ER, et al: Identification of a tumor necrosis factor-responsive element in the tumor necrosis factor alpha gene. *J Biol Chem* 266:9343, 1991.

318. Shin HS, Drysdale BE, Shin ML, et al: Definition of a lipopolysaccharide-responsive element in the 5′-flanking regions of MuRantes and Crg-2. *Mol Cell Biol* 14:2914, 1994.

319. Ueda S, Nishio K, Minamino N, et al: Increased plasma levels of ADM in patients with systemic inflammatory response syndrome. *Am J Respir Crit Care Med* 160(1):132, 1999.

320. Brain S, Williams TJ, Tippins JR, et al: Calcitonin gene related peptide is a potent vasodilator. *Nature* 313:54, 1985.

321. Barber DA, Park YS, Burnett JC Jr, Miller VM: Adrenomedullin-mediated relaxations in veins are endothelium-dependent and distinct from arteries. *J Cardiovasc Pharmacol* 30:695, 1997.

322. Horio T, Kohno M, Kano H, et al: Adrenomedullin as a novel antimigration factor of vascular smooth muscle cells. *Circ Res* 77(4):660, 1995.

323. Kohno M, Kano H, Horio T, et al: Inhibition of endothelin production by adrenomedullin in vascular smooth muscle cells. *Hypertension* 25(6):1185, 1995.

324. Kohno M, Yasunari K, Yokokawa K, et al: Interaction of adrenomedullin and platelet-derived growth factor on rat mesangial cell production of endothelin. *Hypertension* 27:663, 1996.

325. Chini EN, Choi E, Grande JP, et al: Adrenomedullin suppresses mitogenesis in rat mesangial cells via cyclic AMP pathway. *Biochem Biophys Res Commun* 215:868, 1995.

326. Matsumura K, Abe I, Tsuchihashi T, Fujishima M: Central adrenomedullin augments the baroreceptor reflex in conscious rabbits. *Hypertension* 33:992, 1999.

327. Entzeroth M, Doods HN, Wieland HA, Wiene W: Adrenomedullin mediates vasodilation via CGRP1 receptors. *Life Sci* 56:PL19, 1995.

328. Shimekake Y, Nagata K, Ohta S, et al: Adrenomedullin stimulates two signal transduction pathways, cyclic AMP accumulation and Ca^{2+} mobilization in bovine aortic endothelial cells. *J Biol Chem* 270:4412, 1995.

329. Samson WK, Murphy TC, Resch ZT: Central mechanisms for the hypertensive effects of preproadrenomedullin-derived peptides in conscious rats. *Am J Physiol* 274:R1505, 1998.

330. Feng CJ, Kang B, Kaye AD, et al: L-NAME modulates responses to adrenomedullin in the hindquarters vascular bed of the rat. *Life Sci* 55:PL433, 1994.

331. Ishiyama Y, Kitamura K, Ichiki Y, et al: Hemodynamic effects of a novel hypotensive peptide, human adrenomedullin, in rats. *Eur J Pharmacol* 241:271, 1993.

332. Rössler A, László Z, Haditsch B, et al: Orthostatic stimuli rapidly change plasma adrenomedullin in humans. *Hypertension* 34:1147, 1999.

333. Sakata J, Shimokubo T, Kitamura K, et al: Molecular cloning and biological activities of rat adrenomedullin, a hypotensive peptide. *Biochem Biophys Res Commun* 195:921, 1993.

334. Parkes DG, May CN: ACTH-suppressive and vasodilator actions of adrenomedullin in conscious sheep. *J Neuroendocrinol* 7:923, 1995.

335. Samson WK, Murphy T, Schell DA: A novel vasoactive peptide, adrenomedullin, inhibits pituitary adrenocorticotropin release. *Endocrinology* 136:2349, 1995.

336. Meeran K, O'Shea D, Upton PD, et al: Circulating adrenomedullin does not regulate systemic blood pressure but increases plasma prolactin after intravenous infusion in humans: A pharmacokinetic study. *J Clin Endocrinol Metab* 82:95, 1997.

337. Charles CJ, Lainchbury JG, Lewis LK, et al: The role of adrenomedullin. *Am J Hypertens* 12:166, 1999.

338. Jougasaki M, Wei C, Aarhus LL, et al: Renal localization and actions of adrenomedullin: A natriuretic peptide. *Am J Physiol* 268:F657, 1995.

339. Samson WK, Murphy TC: Adrenomedullin inhibits salt appetite. *Endocrinology* 138:613, 1997.

340. Lainchbury JG, Cooper GJS, Coy DH, et al: Adrenomedullin: A hypotensive hormone in man. *Clin Sci (Colch)* 92:467, 1997.

341. Yamaguchi T, Baba K, Doi Y, Yano K: Effect of adrenomedullin on aldosterone secretion by dispersed rat adrenal zona glomerulosa cells. *Life Sci* 56:379, 1995.

342. Ishimitsu T, Nishikimi T, Saito Y, et al: Plasma levels of adrenomedullin, a newly identified hypotensive peptide in patients with hypertension and renal failure. *J Clin Invest* 94:2158, 1994.

343. Morimoto A, Nishikimi T, Yoshihara F, et al: Ventricular adrenomedullin levels correlate with the extent of cardiac hypertrophy in rats. *Hypertension* 33:1146, 1999.

344. Kamiya H, Okumura K, Sone T, et al: Plasma adrenomedullin levels in the coronary circulation in vasospastic angina pectoris. *Am J Cardiol* 85:656, 2000.

345. Yamaji T, Ishibashi M, Takaku F: Atrial natriuretic factor in human blood. *J Clin Invest* 76:1705, 1985.

346. Hirata Y, Ishii M, Fukui K, et al: A possible physiological role of atrial natriuretic factor in body fluid volume regulation. *J Cardiovasc Pharmacol* 13(Suppl 1):S63, 1989.

347. Kato J, Kitamura K, Kuwasako K, et al: Plasma adrenomedullin patients with primary aldosteronism. *Am J Hypertens* 8:997, 1995.

348. Yoshihara F, Nishikimi T, Horio T, et al: Chronic infusion of adrenomedullin reduces pulmonary hypertension and lessens right ventricular hypertrophy in rats administered monocrotaline. *Eur J Pharmacol* 355:33, 1998.

349. Yang BC, Lippton H, Gumusel B, et al: Adrenomedullin dilates rat pulmonary artery rings during hypoxia: Role of nitric oxide and vasodilator prostaglandins. *J Cardiovasc Pharmacol* 28:458, 1996.

350. Nagaya N, Nishikimi T, Kyotani S, et al: Pulmonary vasodilator responses to adrenomedullin in patients with pulmonary hypertension. *Circulation* 100(Suppl I):I240, 1999.

351. Jougasaki M, Wei CM, McKinley LJ, Burnett JC Jr: Elevation of circulating and ventricular adrenomedullin in human congestive heart failure. *Circulation* 92:286, 1995.

352. Richards AM, Doughty R, Nicholls MG, et al: Plasma N-terminal pro-brain natriuretic peptide and adrenomedullin. Prognostic utility and prediction of benefit from carvedilol in chronic ischemic left ventricular dysfunction. *J Am Coll Cardiol* 37:1781, 2001.

353. Jougasaki M, Rodeheffer R, Redfield M, et al: Cardiac secretion of adrenomedullin in human heart failure. *J Clin Invest* 97:2370, 1996.

354. Kobayashi K, Kitamura K, Hirayama N, et al: Increased plasma adrenomedullin in acute myocardial infarction. *Am Heart J* 131: 676, 1996.

355. Øie E, Vinge LE, Yndestad A, et al: Induction of a myocardial adrenomedullin signaling system during ischemic heart failure in rats. *Circulation* 101:415, 2000.

356. Lainchbury JG, Nicholls MG, Espiner EA, et al: Bioactivity and interactions of adrenomedullin and brain natriuretic peptide in patients with heart failure. *Hypertension* 34:70, 1999.

357. Nishikimi T, Hayashi Y, Iribu G, et al: Increased plasma adrenomedullin concentrations during cardiac surgery. *Clin Sci (Colch)* 94:585, 1998.

358. Amado JA, Fidalgo I, García-Unzueta MT, et al: Patients with poor preoperative ejection fraction have a higher plasma response of adrenomedullin in response to open heart surgery. *Acta Anaesthesiol Scand* 43:829, 1999.

359. Nishio K, Akai Y, Murao Y, et al: Increased plasma concentrations of adrenomedullin correlate with relaxation of vascular tone in patients with septic shock. *Crit Care Med* 25:953, 1997.

360. Yoshibayashi M, Kamiya T, Kitamura K, et al: Plasma levels of adrenomedullin in primary and secondary pulmonary hypertension in patients <20 years of age. *Am J Cardiol* 79:1556, 1997.

361. Yamamoto K, Ikeda U, Sekiguchi H, Shimada K: Plasma levels of adrenomedullin in patients with mitral stenosis. *Am Heart J* 135:542, 1998.

362. Nakamura M, Yoshida H, Makita S, et al: Potent and long-lasting vasodilatory effects of adrenomedullin in humans: Comparisons between normal subjects and patients with chronic heart failure. *Circulation* 95:1214, 1997.

363. Nagaya N, Nishikimi T, Horio T, et al: Cardiovascular and renal effects of adrenomedullin in rats with heart failure. *Am J Physiol* 276:R213–R218, 1999.

364. Nagaya N, Satoh T, Nishikimi T, et al: Hemodynamic, renal, and hormonal effects of adrenomedullin infusion in patients with congestive heart failure. *Circulation* 101:498, 2000.

365. Franco-Cereceda A: Calcitonin gene-related peptide and tachykinins in relation to local sensory control of cardiac contractility and coronary vascular tone. *Acta Physiol Scand* 569(Suppl):1, 1988.

366. Maggi CA: Tachykinins and calcitonin gene-related peptide (CGRP) as co-transmitters released from peripheral endings of sensory nerves. *Prog Neurobiol* 45:1, 1995.

367. Poyne DR: Calcitonin gene-related peptide: Multiple actions, multiple receptors. *Pharmacol Ther* 56:23, 1992.

368. Tan KKC, Brown MJ, Hargreaves RJ, et al: Calcitonin gene-related peptides as an endogenous vasodilator: Immunoblockade studies in vivo with an anti-calcitonin gene-related peptide monoclonal antibody and its Fab fragment. *Clin Sci (Colch)* 89:565, 1995.

369. Anand IS, Gurden J, Wander GS, et al: Cardiovascular and hormonal effects of calcitonin gene-related peptide in congestive heart failure. *J Am Coll Cardiol* 17:208, 1991.

370. Griffin EC, Aiyar N, Slivjak MJ, et al: Effect of endotoxicosis on plasma and tissue levels of calcitonin gene-related peptide. *Circ Shock* 38:50, 1992.

371. Mair J, Lechlenner P, Langle T, et al: Plasma CGRP in acute myocardial infarction. *Lancet* 335:168, 1990.

372. Imamura M, Smith N, Garbarg M, Levi R: Histamine H3-receptor-mediated inhibition of calcitonin gene-related peptide release from cardiac C fibers. *Circ Res* 78:863, 1996.

373. Shawket S, Dickerson C, Hazelman B, et al: Prolonged effect of CGRP in Raynaud's patients: A double-blind, randomised comparison with prostacyclin. *Br J Clin Pharmacol* 32:209, 1991.

374. Bunker CB, Terenghi G, Springall DR, et al: Deficiency of calcitonin gene-related peptide in Raynaud's phenomenon. *Lancet* 336:1530, 1990.

375. Lundberg JM: Evidence for a coexistence of vasoactive intestinal peptide (VIP) and acetyl-choline in neurons of cat exocrine glands: Morphological, biochemical and functional studies. *Acta Physiol Scand* 496:1, 1981.

376. Frase LL, Gaffney FA, Lane LD, et al: Cardiovascular effects of vasoactive intestinal peptide in healthy subjects. *Am J Cardiol* 60:1356, 1987.

377. McAlpine HM, Morton JJ, Leckie B, et al: Neuroendocrine activation after acute myocardial infarction. *Br Heart J* 60:117, 1988.

378. Lucia P, Caiola S, Coppola A, Maroccia E, et al: Effect of age and relation to mortality on serial changes of vasoactive intestinal peptide in acute myocardial infarction. *Am J Cardiol* 77:644, 1996.

379. Shimosawa T, Shibagaki Y, Ishibashi K, et al: Adrenomedullin, an endogenous peptide, counteracts cardiovascular damage. *Circulation* 105:106, 2002.

PART III

New Drug Classes in Development

Potassium-Channel Openers and Sodium/Hydrogen–Channel Effectors

William H. Frishman

Benjamin Y. Lee

Isaac Galandauer

Alex Huanphong Phan

In this chapter, two classes of drugs that work on cell membrane ion channels are discussed: the potassium-channel openers and the sodium hydrogen–channel effectors. Agents from both drug classes are being evaluated for use in the treatment of various cardiovascular disorders.

POTASSIUM-ION CHANNEL

The potassium channels are a diverse group of transmembrane proteins that allow for the selective permeability of potassium ions.[1] These channels play an important role in maintaining the resting potential of cell membranes and helping to control cell excitability.[2] In vascular smooth muscle, they help to modulate vasomotion; for this reason, the potassium channel is considered to be an important pharmacologic target in the treatment of cardiac and vascular disease.

Various drugs that open the potassium channel are in clinical development and some have already been used in clinical practice (e.g., diazoxide, minoxidil, pinacidil, and nicorandil).

Potassium Channels and Channel-Mediated Effects on Vascular Smooth Muscle

Cloning techniques have helped identify a large, heterogeneous number of potassium channels (Table 28-1): voltage-sensitive channels, calcium ion–activated channels, receptor-coupled channels, the adenosine 5'-triphosphate (ATP)-sensitive channels, and the sodium ion–activated potassium channel.[2] These channels are found all over the body and help to modulate various physiologic functions.

The calcium-activated and ATP-sensitive potassium channels help to modulate vascular tone.[3] When the potassium channels are closed, there is an increase in intracellular potassium concentration and a smaller membrane potential. This depolarization action causes an opening of voltage-sensitive calcium-ion channels and an increased intracellular calcium-ion influx. This calcium influx causes an increase in vascular smooth muscle contraction. When the potassium channel is opened, there is an opposite effect on smooth muscle contraction: the cell membrane is hyperpolarized and the voltage-sensitive calcium-ion channels close with a decreased intracellular calcium-ion influx, causing a subsequent relaxation effect on vascular smooth muscle (Fig. 28-1).[4]

It has been shown that even small pertubations in membrane potential by the opening and closing of potassium channels can have important effects on the contractile function of myocardial tissue and vascular smooth muscle.[3] However, the arteries in the body can vary in their sensitivity to potassium-channel opening and closing, showing that vasomotion in various blood vessels may be influenced by many other factors (e.g., local metabolites, catecholamines, and angiotensin).[3,4]

The Adenosine Triphosphate (ATP)–Sensitive Potassium (KATP) Channel

The KATP channel has been studied most extensively because of the availability of multiple pharmacologic agents that can either activate or inhibit the channel. Noma in 1983 first demonstrated that cardiac KATP channels played an important role in mediating an endogenous self-defense mechanism in ischemic hearts.[5] Subsequently, these KATP channels have been found to exist in the pancreas,[6] smooth muscle,[7] skeletal muscle,[8] brain,[9,10] and kidney.[11]

KATP channels are composed of a sulfonylurea receptor (SUR) subunit and an inward-rectifying K^+ channel subunit that belongs to the Kir6.0 subfamily (Kir6.x: Kir6.2 or Kir6.1) (Fig. 28-2A and B).[13] Kir6.x serves as the pore-forming subunit, and SUR is an important regulatory subunit.[14] Three isoforms of SUR have been cloned and are designated as SUR1 (pancreatic type), SUR2A (cardiac type), and SUR2B [vascular smooth muscle (VSM) type].[15] Tetrameric assembly of the SUR/Kir6.x complex (Fig. 28-2C) forms a functional KATP channel identical to the native one. That is, the SUR1/Kir6.2, SUR2A/Kir6.2, and SUR2B/Kir6.1 channels are thought to be KATP channels in pancreatic beta cells, cardiac myocytes, and VSM cells, respectively.[16,17]

These KATP channels are regulated via several established and controversial mechanisms. The primary inhibitory effect of ATP occurs at the Kir6.x pore subunit[18] and does not involve

TABLE 28-1. Classification of Potassium-Ion Channels

Voltage-sensitive channels
    Delayed (outward) rectifier (I_{KV})
    Anomalous (inward) rectifier (IR/I_{K1})
    Transient outward A-current (I_A)
Calcium (Ca^{2+})-activated channels (IK(Ca))
    High conductance (K_L)
    Intermediate conductance (K_M)
    Low conductance (Ks)
Receptor-coupled channels
    Protein kinase C–activated (close channel)
    Acetylcholine- and adenosine-activated (open channel)
Others
    ATP-sensitive channel (KATP, KG)—ATP reduces opening
    Sodium-activated (KNa)

hydrolysis. This site does not distinguish between ATP-bound to magnesium (Mg) or free ATP[19] and is inhibited by both. ATP also appears to exert a hydrolysis-dependent stimulation/maintenance action at the SUR regulatory subunit,[12] although the exact mechanism remains unclear.[18] The SUR subunit also modulates several other interactions, including: inhibition by sulfonylurea compounds, stimulation by Mg-bound nucleotide diphosphates (MgNDPs), and stimulation by KATP channel openers.[12] The nucleotide-binding domains (NBDs) of SUR are indispensable for the last two actions.[20] The KATP channel can also be influenced by acetylcholine, catecholamines, angiotensin II, A_1-adenosine receptors through G-protein coupling during myocardial ischemia, and by cyclic AMP–dependent protein kinase A or protein kinase C.[4]

In endocrine organs, KATP channels regulate the release of insulin, prolactin, and growth hormone, linking bioenergetic metabolism to membrane excitability.[6] As discussed earlier, membrane KATP channels affect voltage-sensitive calcium channels and can cause vessels to either dilate or contract. In cardiac myocytes, the KATP channel is predominantly closed at physiologic concentrations of intracellular ATP.[5,21] However, these channels respond differently under physiologic versus stressed conditions.[22,23] Sensitivity to sulfonylureas is drastically reduced in metabolically stressed cardiac cells,[24,25] and ATP-inhibitory or channel-closing capacity is decreased with an acidic intracellular pH (which occurs during ischemia or anoxia).

KATP CHANNEL–OPENING DRUGS

The KATP-channel openers are a heterogeneous group of organic compounds (Table 28-2, Fig. 28-3). The distinction between the vasodilation produced by the KATP-channel openers (Fig. 28-1) and other vasodilator compounds is demonstrated by the "potassium paradox." Vasodilation produced by the KATP-channel openers in vitro is almost completely inhibited by exogenous potassium used in high concentrations.[26]

Although KATP-channel openers are now believed to act on the SUR regulatory subunit,[20] the exact mechanism of this interaction is still under investigation. Also, how the SUR subunit interacts with the Kir6.x pore subunit is unknown. As a consequence, much of the activity in new drug discovery has resulted in compounds structurally related to cromakalim and pinacidil (Fig. 28-3).

Understanding the mechanism of action of KATP-channel openers has been aided by the discovery of KATP channel–inhibiting (channel closing) agents such as the sulfonyloreas tolbutamide and glibenclamide.[2,27]

KATP-channel openers seem to stimulate KATP channels by binding to the same sites as MgNDPs on the SUR subunit[20] (Fig. 28-4). By allowing the channel to open, the cascade of events illustrated in Fig. 28-1 will occur, leading to smooth muscle relaxation. In addition, the KATP-channel openers may inhibit the release of calcium ions from the sarcoplasmic reticulum,[28] cause an increase in calcium ion extrusion from the cell, and reduce the calcium sensitivity of the contractile proteins.[2]

Use in Systemic Hypertension

Abnormalities of the KATP channel have been suggested as a possible etiologic factor in systemic hypertension.[3] Recent data suggest that impairment of hyperpolarization by potassium efflux through KATP channels may contribute to elevated renovascular resistance.[29] Initial efforts focused on the use of KATP-channel openers as antihypertensive agents; however, clinical studies have revealed no clear advantages over other commonly used antihypertensive drugs.[26] As vasodilators, some of the KATP channel–opening agents can cause reflex tachycardia, edema, headache, and flushing, which have also limited their clinical use.[2]

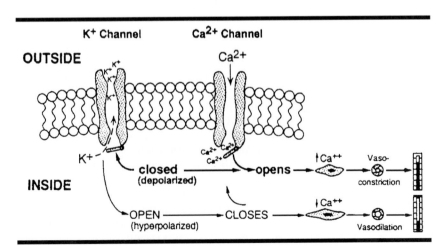

FIGURE 28-1. Schematic depiction of interactions between potassium and calcium channels and their effects on blood pressure. Closed potassium channels lower membrane potential and open voltage-sensitive calcium channels. These effects increase the contractility of vascular smooth muscle and elevate blood pressure. Open potassium channels raise membrane potential and close calcium channels sensitive to voltage. These effects decrease the contractility of vascular smooth muscle and lower blood pressure. (*Reproduced with permission from Furspan.*[4])

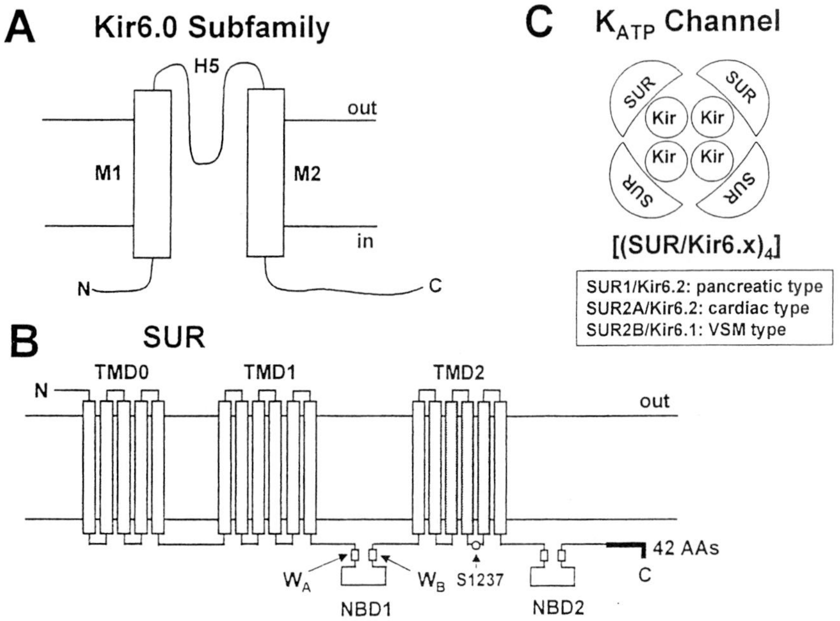

FIGURE 28-2. Structure of the K_{ATP} channel as a complex of SUR and Kir6.x channel subunits. *Panel A:* Membrane topology of Kir 6.0 subfamily. The Kir6.x (Kir6.2 or Kir6.1) channel subunit has a minimal structure, with only a "pore" region (H5) and two flanking transmembrane TM segments, M1 and M2. *Panel B:* Membrane topology of SUR. SUR has two nucleotide-binding domains (NBDs) and 17 TM segments arranged in three groups (TMD0, TMD1, and TMD2) of 5, 6, and 6 TM segments. The TM segments 14 to 16 are filled with light gray. TMD = transmembrane domain; W_A = Walker-A motif; W_B = Walker-B motif; Aas = amino acids. *Panel C:* Proposed structure of K_{ATP} channel. (*Reproduced with permission from Yokoshiki et al.*[13])

Minoxidil (Fig. 28-3) is available for clinical use in the United States as a treatment for refractory hypertension that is not responsive to other antihypertensive treatments. However, it can cause pronounced reflex sympathetic stimulation, often requiring concomitant beta- blocker therapy.

Diazoxide (Fig. 28-3) is a parenteral drug used to treat hypertensive urgencies and emergencies. This drug is a powerful arteriolar dilator with no effect on venous capacitance.[30] Its use is primarily limited to hypertensive urgencies in which nitroprusside is the preferred drug but intensive care monitoring is not possible. It has also been used in obstetric hypertensive emergencies refractory to hydralazine.[31] Diazoxide opens KATP channels that regulate membrane potential in vascular smooth muscle. This effect, in turn, decreases calcium entry into the myocytes via voltage-dependent calcium channels (Fig. 28-1).[32]

In the past, pinacidil (Fig. 28-3) has been used as an oral therapy in clinical trials for mild to moderate hypertension, with[33] and

TABLE 28-2. Chemical Classes of Potassium-Channel Openers

Benzopyrans
　Cromakalim (BRL 34915)
　Levo-cromakalim (BRL 38227)
　Bimakalim (EMD 52692; SR 44866)
　Celikalim (WAY 120491)
Pyridines
　Pinacidil
　Nicorandil
　Apricalim
Pyrimidines
　Minoxidil sulfate
Benzothiadiazines
　Diazoxide
Thioformamides
　RP 52891
　RP 49356
Endotoxin derivatives
　Monophosphoryl lipid A (MLA)

without[34] a diuretic. As in the case of minoxidil, when pinacidil as used as a direct peripheral arterial dilator, reflex tachycardia was often encountered, requiring treatment with a beta blocker. Pinacidil also caused headache, flushing, palpitations, edema, weight gain, dizziness, hypertrichosis, and, on electrocardiography (ECG), T-wave abnormalities.[35] This drug is no longer being evaluated for the treatment of hypertension.

There is little information available regarding the KATP-channel openers cromakalim,[36] levo-cromakalim,[37] and bimakalim[38] as antihypertensive drugs. Nicorandil was shown to have a transient effect on blood pressure in clinical studies and appears to be more effective as an antianginal agent[38a] (see Chap. 37).

The drug KRN 4884, a novel long-acting potassium-channel opener, has been shown to be an effective antihypertensive agent in preliminary studies and is undergoing additional investigation.[39] The drug activates cardiac KATP channels by decreasing the affinity of the channels to ATP and by a mechanism independent of intracellular ATP.[40]

Other KATP-channel openers with the potential for use in systemic hypertension have recently become available. The benzopyran Y-27152[41,42] is reported to have a prolonged antihypertensive effect with less associated tachycardia than equally hypotensive doses of nifedipine and lemarkalim. As with all other KATP-channel openers, pharmacologic tolerance was not observed after 8 h of therapy. Tissue-specific KATP channel openers may allow for greater use of these drugs in the future to treat hypertension.

Use in Angina Pectoris

The KATP-channel openers used in various experiments have been shown to relax coronary smooth muscle and are known coronary artery dilators.[2,43] Thus far, most research exploring antianginal effects has centered around the nicotinamide derivative nicorandil, a KATP-channel opener that also has nitrovasodilatory actions[38a] (see Chaps. 33 and 37). The activation of KATP channels leads to the dilation of arterial resistance vessels, whereas the nitrate-like

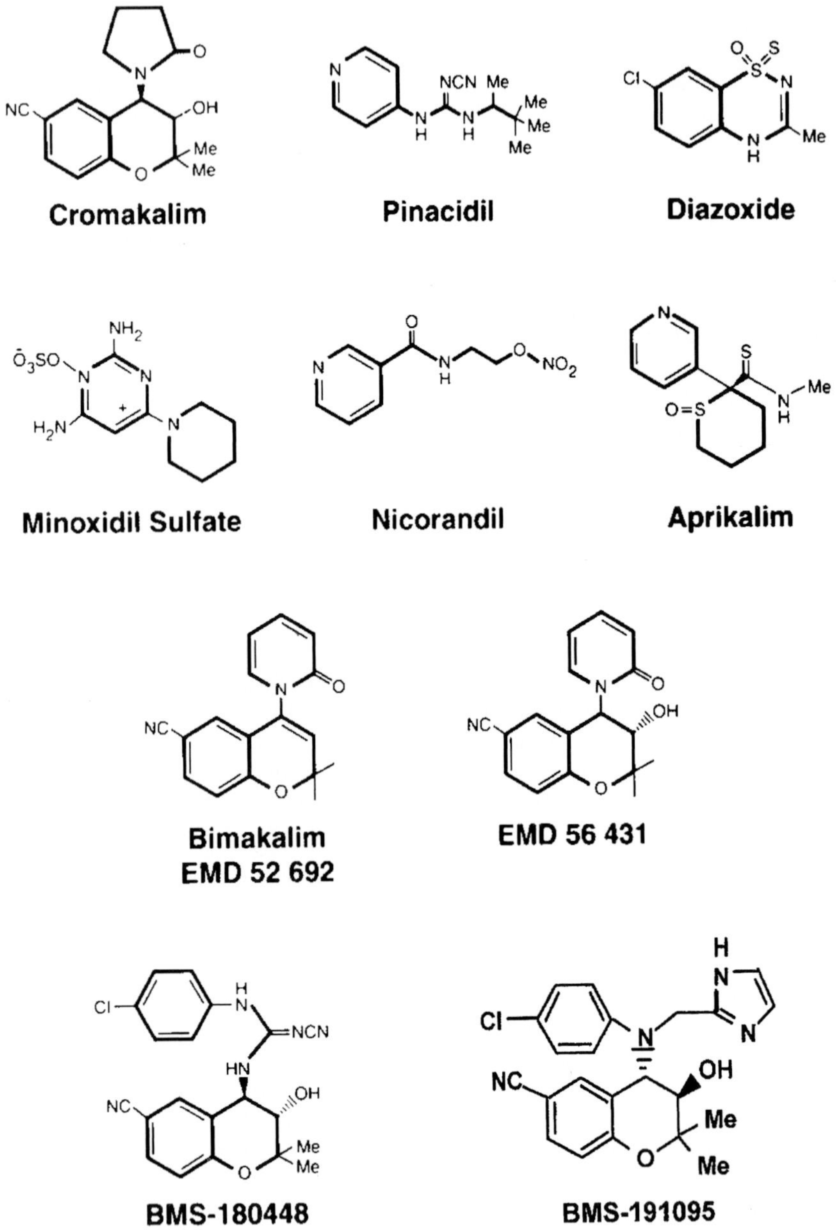

FIGURE 28-3. Chemical structures of nicorandil, bimakalim, EMD 56,431, cromakalim, pinacidil, diazoxide, minoxidil sulfate, aprikalim, BMS 180448, BMS 191095, monophosphoryl lipid A.

properties dilate venous capacitance vessels.[44] Thus, this drug acts as a balanced coronary and peripheral vasodilator.

Nicorandil has been used as an antianginal agent and in clinical studies has been shown to be as potent a drug as isosorbide dinitrate without causing tolerance.[45] Reflex tachycardia is not seen with nicorandil, since the doses used for antianginal treatment are lower than those needed to reduce blood pressure.[46,47] In active control comparisons, Nicorandil was shown to be as effective as beta blockers[48] and calcium-channel blockers[49] in relieving symptoms in both effort-related and vasospastic anginal syndromes. Nicorandil was also demonstrated to have an antioxidant effect on free-radical production and an anti-inflammatory action not observed with nitroglycerin.[50,51]

Due to the multifaceted hemodynamic effects of nicorandil, the issue of drug tolerance, seen with nitrates, has remained controversial. Despite the favorable effects of nicorandil described above, a recent placebo-controlled study in patients with angina pectoris could not demonstrate an improvement in exercise tolerance compared to placebo.[52] However, although the anti-ischemic effects appeared to decline, the hemodynamic effects at rest were not affected. Also, data from studies in healthy volunteers indicate that cross-tolerance between nicorandil and nitroglycerin does not develop.[53] Another recent study concluded that although nicorandil was effective in treating stable angina, isosorbide dinitrate proved to be superior, with a greater decrease in the frequency of angina attacks.[45] The recently completed IONA study (Impact of Nicorandil in Angina) showed that the drug caused a significant improvement in major coronary events in patients with stable angina.[54] Nicorandil may need to be used in a long-acting sustained-release formulation to show benefit.

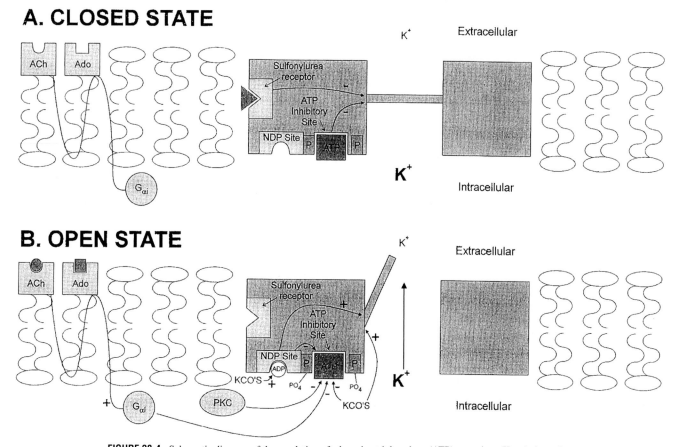

FIGURE 28-4. Schematic diagram of the regulation of adenosine triphosphate (ATP) potassium (K_{ATP}) channels. K_{ATP} channel is closed (A) in response to increases in intracellular ATP concentration. Channel opening is inhibited by binding of ATP to the ATP inhibitory site. Drug binding to the sulfonylurea receptor also decreases the open state probability of the channel. In contrast, nucleotide diphosphates (NDPs) such as adenosine diphosphate (ADP) antagonize ATP-induced inhibition of channel opening, an action that requires occupation of a phosphorylation site (P) by inorganic phosphate (PO_4) and causes opening of the K_{ATP} channel (B). Acetylcholine (ACh) and adenosine (Ado) enhance channel opening via stimulation of membrane receptors coupled to inhibitory G ($G_{\alpha i}$) proteins. Activated $G_{\alpha i}$ and protein kinase C (PKC) antagonize ATP inhibitory gating of the channel. Potassium channel openers (KCOs) enhance opening of the K_{ATP} channel through a direction action on the channel, by augmenting the stimulatory effects of NDPs on channel opening or by antagonizing the inhibitory effect of ATP on the channel. (*Reproduced with permission from Kersten JR, Gross GJ, Pagel PS, Warltier DC; Activation of adenosine-triphosphate-regulated potassium channels mediation of cellular and organ protection. Anesthesiology 88:497, 1998.*)

KATP Channels in Myocardial Ischemia Preconditioning

In addition to their roles in endocrine organs and vascular smooth muscle, KATP channels are believed to be involved in the cardio-protective action seen with ischemic preconditioning[55–61b] (also described in Chap. 32).

Murry was the first to describe the phenomenon known as ischemic preconditioning,[62] the most powerful self-defense mechanisms against ischemia-reperfusion–induced myocardial necrosis known. With brief periods of ischemia followed by reperfusion, the heart, by a mechanism that is still being studied, becomes resistant to subsequent insults. In 1992, Gross and Auchampach were among the first to implicate the role of the cardiac KATP channel in the ischemic preconditioning phenomenon.[63] In their studies, dogs were preconditioned with 10 min of left anterior descending artery (LAD) occlusion, followed by 60 min of LAD occlusion and a 4-h reperfu-

sion period. They found that preconditioned dogs showed a decrease in infarct size, an effect that was abolished by the potassium-channel blocker glibenclamide administered 10 min before or immediately after preconditioning. Administering glibenclamide to dogs that had not been preconditioned did not result in a decrease in infarct size.

Since a KATP-channel blocker can abolish the beneficial effect of preconditioning, many researchers believe that the KATP channel is actively involved in ischemic preconditioning. Indeed, pre-treatment in experimental models with intravenous aprikalim (another KATP-channel opener) resulted in reduced infarct size from what was seen in control animals.[63] Gross and Auchampach[63] concluded from their studies that KATP-channel opening is involved in both triggering preconditioning and sustaining the protective effect where there is a prolonged ischemic insult. This explains why glibenclamide, when given before or shortly after preconditioning, abolished the protective effect of KATP-channel opening. To make sure that this effect is due to its KATP-channel blocking activity and not a glucose metabolizing effect, Auchampach et al. compared the effect of glibenclamide and sodium 5-hydroxydecanoate (5-HD), a nonsulfonylurea KATP-channel blocker, in preconditioned and control dogs.[64] Preconditioning was blocked by both compounds independently of the changes in plasma glucose level, a result duplicated in studies by Grover et al.[65] Neither compound had an effect on nonpreconditioned dogs. The finding that the protective effect of preconditioning is related to KATP-channel activation has been confirmed by other investigations in pig,[66] rabbit,[67] and dog[68] models.

Originally it was believed that during ischemia, the ensuing decrease in ATP would lead to opening of KATP channels in cardiac myocytes and shortening of the action potential duration, thereby reducing calcium overload and myocardial damage.[69] However, recent studies have shown that the beneficial effects of ischemic preconditioning or KATP-channel openers are not dependent on a shortened action potential,[70] and attention has shifted to the role of the mitochondrial KATP channel (see "New Drugs and Selectivity," below).

Adenosine and the KATP Channel in Myocardial Protection

Adenosine is also found to be protective against myocardial ischemic damage (see Chap. 32). In the isolated blood-perfused rabbit heart, Liu et a. found that intracoronary infusion of adenosine, which is released during ischemia, is as effective as preconditioning in reducing infarct size.[71,72] This effect was abolished with an adenosine antagonist.[73] Using different animal models, Tsuchida et al. (in anesthetized rabbits),[74] Downey et al. (in rats),[75] Yao and Gross (in dogs),[76] and Schwarz et al. (in pigs)[77] showed that alpha$_1$-receptor antagonists abolished the protective effect of adenosine. Li and Kloner, however, failed to reproduce the cardioprotective effect of adenosine in rats.[78] Moreover, Auchampach and Gross found no mimicry of preconditioning when 50 or 400 μg/min of adenosine or 2 μg/kg/min of dipyridamole (an adenosine uptake inhibitor) were infused for 5 min separately before the 60-min occlusion.[79] Miura et al.[80] suggested that dipyridamole, as an adenosine uptake inhibitor, increases the relative availability of adenosine to cardiac myocytes, which explains why Auchampach and Gross were able to reduce infarct size by combining adenosine and dipyridamole.[79] However, in an experiment by Yao and Gross,[76] infusion of adenosine for 10 min before a 10-min occlusion decreased infarct size to the same extent as preconditioning.

Yao and Gross showed that, at doses too low to affect infarct size, glibenclamide and 5-HD abolished the protective effect of adenosine.[76] Also, Van Winkle et al.[81] showed that 5-HD also blocked the anti-infarct effect of R-PIA (a selective A$_1$-receptor agonist) in pigs. This suggests that adenosine mediates its cardioprotective effect via the KATP channel.[82] While an earlier study implicated a G protein as a possible mediator between the A$_1$ receptor and the KATP channel,[83] a recent study has shown that protein kinase C (PKC) acts downstream from the A$_1$ receptor to stimulate KATP channels.[84] PKC activation enhanced the cardioprotective effect of adenosine, and all beneficial effects were abolished when a KATP-channel antagonist was added. Studies involving delayed cardioprotection (24 to 72 h), which is less understood than classic acute preconditioning, have also pointed to PKC as an important mediator between the A$_1$ receptor and the KATP channel.[85,86]

It seems that in the initial ischemic insult, the opening capacity of the KATP channel is either primed or increased such that,

with subsequent insults, the channel will be able to open rapidly or to a greater extent. Increased PKC activity due to increased levels of adenosine, via A$_1$-receptor activation, may be the priming agent.[84,87] The cardiac myocytes may then be more responsive to the protective action of adenosine during the subsequent prolonged ischemia. Although it has been shown that the cardioprotective effect of KATP-channel opening is independent of vasodilation, it is not known whether the cardioprotective effect of adenosine is also independent of its coronary vasodilatory effect. Furthermore, although there are many studies confirming that the cardioprotective effect of adenosine is as effective as that of KATP-channel openers, no study has proven that the effects of adenosine and KATP-channel openers are additive.

Acetylcholine and the KATP Channel in Myocardial Protection

Liu and Downey,[72] in trying to provide further evidence for Gi protein coupling in ischemic preconditioning, found that acetylcholine mimics preconditioning in rabbits. Yao and Gross[76] found that this mimicry can also occur in dogs. In addition, it was shown that the threshold for ventricular fibrillation was significantly raised in preconditioned and acetylcholine-treated animals compared with those receiving saline or glibenclamide.[72] Shiki and Hearse[88] also agreed that a short period of regional ischemia decreased the chance of premature ventricular contractions (PVCs), tachycardia, and fibrillation in anesthetized rats. These data suggest that acetylcholine has an antifibrillatory effect.

The mechanism of preconditioning in the various models that appear to mimic it is unclear at present; what is clear is that the effect is unlikely to be due to an increase in coronary blood flow. Yao and Gross[76] showed no changes in systemic hemodynamics, risk area, or collateral blood flow in the acetylcholine group. Although the acetylcholine group had an increase in LAD flow, this returned to baseline before the occlusion period.

5-HD and glibenclamide abolish the protective effect of acetylcholine, implying that the protective mechanism is via the cardiac KATP channel. Acetylcholine opens potassium channels in myocytes via the activation of M2 muscarinic receptors.[81] The stimulation of M2 receptors increases KATP-channel activity via the Gi protein.[65] Liu and Downey[72] and Thornton et al.,[89] using isolated perfused rabbit hearts, also support the hypothesis that acetylcholine mediates its protective effect via the M2 receptor, Gi activation, and regulation of the KATP channel.

Cardioprotective Effect and KATP-Channel Openers

By now, the involvement of KATP channels in ischemic preconditioning and the cardioprotective effects of KATP-channel openers are widely accepted. However, the precise details and mechanisms of these effects are still being uncovered and investigated. Earlier studies established the consistent ability of KATP-channel openers to mimic ischemic preconditioning.

Nicorandil was shown to possess a clear advantage over calcium-channel blockers in that it could protect the ischemic myocardium at a concentration that caused very little cardiodepression.[90] Nicorandil enhanced recovery of regional systolic shortening during reperfusion after a 10- to 15-min coronary artery occlusion. This effect was not found when using sodium nitroprusside (nitrovasodilator), but it was mimicked by another potassium opener, bimakalim (EMD 52692).[90] Bimakalim decreased infarct size to the same degree as nicorandil, and like nicorandil, the drug improved the recovery of isovolumic left ventricular minute work during myocardial reperfusion when compared with control. This improvement was accompanied by a preservation of total adenine nucleotide concentrations at 30 min of reperfusion. Also, Grover et al.[91] found that the protective effect of nicorandil was exerted directly on the myocardium and was independent of its peripheral or coronary dilator activities.

In a separate study, Grover et al.[92] showed, in an isolated rat heart model of ischemia and reperfusion, that both pinacidil and cromakalim enhanced postischemic recovery of contractile function, reduced reperfusion contracture, and reduced LDH release. Galinances,[93] Cohen et al.,[94] Ohta,[95] and Tosaki and Hellegouarch,[96] by studying structurally dissimilar cardiac KATP-channel openers at different concentrations, showed that the anti-ischemic potency of most potassium-channel openers is similar at 1 to 10 μM. It is evident that the cardioprotective effect is related to KATP-channel activation. Also, in all the studies mentioned above, all cardioprotective effects were completely abolished by KATP-channel antagonists (either glibenclamide or sodium 5-HD).

However, KATP channels are not solely responsible for ischemic preconditioning, since KATP-channel openers cannot confer the same level of cardioprotection as classic ischemic preconditioning.[55] A continuous infusion of aprikalim[63] or bimakalim[97–99] reduced infarct size (31–63%) to a lesser degree than classic ischemic preconditioning (79–85%). Also, Yao and Gross noticed that the memory of protection is shorter with KATP-channel openers than with classic ischemic preconditioning.[100] When bimakalim was infused for 5 min followed by a 60-min washout to imitate the 5-min coronary artery occlusion and 60-min reperfusion protocol, bimakalim-induced protection had disappeared, while the protection by ischemic preconditioning was still present. Interestingly, when adenosine and bimakalim administration were combined, the memory for protection could be extended to more than 60 min.

Besides the evidence suggesting that elements other than KATP channels have a role in cardioprotection, several recent studies have shown that the sarcolemmal KATP channel may not actually be responsible for preconditioning. As early as 1994, Yao et al. demonstrated that doses of bimakalim that had no effect on action potential duration still had the ability to limit infarct size.[101] In the same study, dofetilide, a class III antiarrhythmic agent that does not have an effect on KATP channels, abolished the action potential duration by ischemia but had no effect of the protection by ischemic preconditioning. Current studies point to the mitochondrial KATP channel as the nonsarcolemmal element that may be responsible for cardioprotection (see "New Drugs and Selectivity," below).

In fact, a study by Pomerantz et al., using the mitochondrial specific KATP-channel opener diazoxide, showed that infarct size was decreased to the same extent as with adenosine.[102] There are numerous studies showing the effects of mitochondrial KATP channels; however, their exact role in cardioprotection is still up for debate.

New Drugs and Selectivity

Monophosphoryl Lipid A (MLA)

A new compound that has shown significant promise as a cardioprotective agent is monophosphoryl lipid A (MLA), an endotoxin derivative (Table 28-2, Fig. 28-3).

In rabbits, within the narrow dose range of 5 to 10 μg/kg, endotoxin has been shown to reduce infarct size when administered 24 h before ischemia.[103] Similar results have been seen in the rat.[104] In spite of these intriguing reports, the narrow therapeutic index of endotoxin and its potentially severe side effects (diffuse intravascular coagulation, neutrophil activation, multiorgan failure) preclude its consideration as a cardioprotective compound. MLA is an amphipathic polyesterified diglucosamine monophosphate derivative of lipid A (the minimal substructural pharmacophore of endotoxin)[105] and appears to be devoid of endotoxin's undesirable effect.

In situ experiments in rabbits have shown that intravenous bolus dosing with MLA can reduce infarct size following 3 or 48 h of reperfusion.[106,107] In these studies, investigators saw a biphasic profile of cardioprotective activity with ischemic tolerance observed at 10 to 20 min after dosing and with protection reappearing 6 to 36 h following administration of a single 35-μg/kg dose of MLA (with a peak at 24 h). This observation of an acute and delayed window of protection with MLA is similar to that reported following classic ischemic preconditioning[108] or administration of an adenosine A_1-receptor agonist.[109] Interestingly, both the acute[110] and delayed[111–113] windows of ischemic tolerance induced by MLA are abolished by glibenclamide and sodium 5-HD (KATP-channel antagonists) in both dogs and rabbits. This strongly implies a role for KATP channels in the cardioprotective effects seen with MLA.[113]

In contrast to the more traditional KATP-channel openers (i.e., cromakalim, pinacidil, diazoxide), research involving MLA has revealed more about delayed cardioprotection than the acute window. The delayed ischemic tolerance induced by MLA is related to the upregulation of inducible nitric oxide synthase (iNOS).[114] In both rat and porcine models, a dose-responsive increase in iNOS mRNA as detected by Northern blot analysis was observed 4 to 8 h after administration of cardioprotective doses of MLA.[115,116] Zhao and Elliott theorize that ischemic challenges following the administration of MLA may result in tyrosine kinase-dependent phosphorylation and activation of this MLA-induced iNOS pool, leading to nitric oxide-dependent activation of the myocardial KATP channels.[114,117]

While the upregulation of iNOS cannot explain the acute cardioprotection (10 to 20 min) with MLA, the ability of KATP-channel antagonists to block this effect suggests that KATP channels are somehow involved.[110] While work is still ongoing to elucidate the exact mechanism of acute protection, it has been proposed MLA's known ability to activate kinases may lead to activation of protein kinase C, a purported mediator between the adenosine A_1 receptor and the KATP channel. Alternatively, MLA may cause acute ischemic tolerance via phosphorylation of constitutive pools of iNOS, as has been reported for endotoxin,[117] ultimately resulting in nitric oxide-mediated KATP channel activation.[110]

While clinical investigation of MLA as a potential cardioprotective agent has only recently begun, early studies show that doses of up to at least 20 μg/kg may be safely given to humans.[118] Future results may show a superior or synergistic role for MLA when compared to more traditional KATP-channel openers in developing ischemic tolerance.

Tissue Selectivity

Most systemic KATP-channel openers are nonselective with hemodynamic actions such as tachycardia. Most are more potent as vasodilators than as cardioprotectants[119] with the exception of aprikalim,[26] which is cardioprotective without major hemodynamic effects. Yet aprikalim's small therapeutic window makes it difficult to use clinically. To solve these problems, BMS 182264[26] was developed as a more selective KATP-channel opener. BMS 182264 combines the structural features of cromakalim and pinacidil. It also exhibits the same vascular effects, namely, smooth muscle–relaxing and antihypertensive activities. There is good correlation between vasorelaxation and ^{86}Rb+ efflux caused by BMS 182264, suggesting that potassium-channel opening is partly responsible for the vasorelaxation effect. Radioligand-binding studies using rat aortic smooth muscle cells have indicated that cromakalim, 3[H]P-1075 (an analog of pinacidil), and BMS 182264 show a good correlation between their smooth muscle–relaxant potencies and binding affinities to potassium channels.[120–122] BMS 182264 also displaced 3[H]P-1075 from its binding site in a competitive manner, suggesting that the drugs bind to a similar receptor site or sites.

Steinberg et al.[123] have shown that the smooth muscle–relaxing effect of cromakalim, nicorandil, and pinacidil all correlate with their effect on action potential shortening in Purkinje fiber and ventricular tissue. This indicates a common mechanism of action of these drugs in cardiac and smooth muscle. KATP-channel openers that have antianginal effects without causing systemic hemodynamic disturbances are needed.

Unlike cromakalim and pinacidil, BMS 182264 has no effect on the action potential in guinea pig papillary muscle. Cromakalim and pinacidil shortened action potential duration in a concentration-dependent manner, with cromakalim causing 80% shortening of APD at 100 μmol/L. Although BMS 182264 has a similar vasorelaxant potency to cromakalim, it has no effect on action potential duration (APD) at up to 100-μmol/L concentrations.[124] This suggest that cardiac action potential and smooth muscle relaxation with BMS 182264 may occur by different mechanisms or with different receptors.[125] In addition, it suggests that BMS 182264 is more selective for smooth muscle than pinacidil or cromakalim.[126] It offers the hope that modification of existing KATP-channel openers can achieve selectivity. BMS 182264 is now undergoing clinical trials in patients with angina.

An analog of cyanoguanidine called BMS 180448 racemic causes an increased time to contracture after ischemia with a potency similar to that of cromakalim.[26] However, it is 40 to 50 times less potent than cromakalim as a vasorelaxing agent and 30 to 40 times less potent than cromakalim as a coronary dilator. It has been shown that BMS 180448 is efficacious in several models of myocardial ischemia without affecting hemodynamic variables.[127] It has been demonstrated that the cardioprotective effect of BMS 180448 racemic is via its role as a potassium-channel opener; the effect is abolished when there is pretreatment of the heart with potassium blocker glyburide or sodium 5-HD.[128] It has also been shown that the 3S,4R enantiomer of BMS 180447 (that is, BMS 180448) is a more active anti-ischemic agent than its 3R,4S enantiomer, BMS 180449. The facts that both 180448 and 180449 have similar vasorelaxing activities and 180448 is the more anti-ischemic agent suggest that the vasorelaxant effect is not stereoselective. The vasorelaxant and anti-ischemic effects may occur via different mechanisms. The exact mechanism of this dissociation is not known. Also, the facts that bimakalim and BMS 180448 shorten APD less than cromakalim but are as effective as cromakalim as antianginal agents with little hemodynamic effect suggest a possible separation between APD shortening and cardioprotection.[26]

The lack of correlation between anti-ischemia and smooth muscle–relaxing potencies for a variety of KATP-channel openers has led to the clinical development of BMS 180448. Like cromakalim, BMS 180448 has anti-ischemic activity. Unlike cromakalim, BMS 180448 is only 1/100 as effective as a smooth mus-

cle relaxant, which allows BMS 180448 to remain a glyburide-reversible antianginal agent without affecting hemodynamics.[26] This clearly is an improvement from the older KATP-channel openers, which lack selectivity. It is postulated that the existence of receptor subtypes in different tissues could be responsible for the selectivity of BMS 180448.

Presently there are potassium-channel opener agents that are more selective as coronary dilators, which are undergoing investigation. It is generally agreed that the cardioprotective effect of KATP-channel openers is independent of their coronary dilating activity. However, KATP-channel openers with potent coronary dilating activity can still be useful antianginal agents for correcting the imbalance between myocardial oxygen delivery and utilization.

RWJ 26629[129] has been reported to be more potent than cromakalim and calcium blockers both in its antihypertensive and coronary vasodilatory properties. It increases coronary blood flow with greater potency and duration than cromakalim or nifedipine without affecting contractile force. However, RWJ 26629 still has the side effect of reflex tachycardia, suggesting that an even greater selectivity for the coronary artery is needed.

Another drug under investigation is TCV 295. Its glibenclamide-reversible antihypertensive effect is longer than with levocromakalim and nisoldipine, and with oral dosing, TCV 295 causes less reflex tachycardia at the same hypotensive potency. However, TCV 295 given intravenously can cause a rapid increase in heart rate. Its selectivity for coronary dilatation, long duration of action, lack of tolerance, and lack of rebound hypertension makes it a promising antihypertensive and antianginal agent.[130]

Cell Selectivity—Mitochondrial KATP Channels

While most early studies in the development of KATP-channel openers implicated sarcolemmal KATP channels as the site of action, more current research has suggested that that this may not be the case.[131] Many studies have demonstrated the role of mitochondrial KATP channels as the actual site of action in myocardial preconditioning.[132–136]

In 1994, Yao and Gross published a study showing that low doses of the KATP-channel opener bimakalim, which did not enhance APD shortening, produced a cardioprotective effect equal to that of two higher doses that did enhance APD shortening.[101] Since APD shortening is a result of sarcolemmal KATP-channel activation, the results of this study implicated an alternative site of action for KATP-channel openers. In addition, Grover et al. showed that administration of dofetilide, a class III antiarrhythmic drug hat prevented APD shortening, did not antagonize the cardioprotective effects of ischemic preconditioning.[137] Based on these and similar findings, many researchers proposed an intracellular site of action for KATP channel openers.

The first mitochondrial KATP (mito-KATP) channel was identified in 1991 by Inoue et al. in the inner mitochondrial membrane of rat hepatocytes.[138] In contrast to sarcolemmal KATP channels, which seem to affect electrical activity, the mito-KATP channels appear to be involved in the regulation of mitochondrial matrix volume.[139] Opening of mito-KATP channels leads to inner membrane depolarization, matrix swelling, slowing of ATP synthesis, and accelerated respiration.[140]

Evidence that the mito-KATP channel might play a role in cardioprotection was first presented by Garlid et al. in 1997.[141] In this study, it was shown that diazoxide is a selective opener of mito-KATP channels. In reconstituted bovine heart mitochondria, diazoxide opened mito-KATP channels with a $K_{1/2}$ (the concentration at which 50% of the maximal effect on mito-KATP channels is observed) of 0.8 μmol/L, while opening the sarcolemmal KATP channels at only 800 μmol/L.[141] In addition, these authors observed that diazoxide, at concentrations that would not open sarcolemmal KATP channels (5–20 μmol/L), produced cardioprotective effects equal to those of cromakalim, a nonselective KATP-channel opener, at similar concentrations. Beneficial effects of both drugs were blocked by the KATP-channel antagonists glibenclamide and 5-HD.

Further support for diazoxide being a selective mito-KATP–channel opener has been provided in studies by Liu et al.,[142] Wang et al.,[143] and Sato et al.[144] In these studies, concentrations of diazoxide that were too low to open sarcolemmal KATP channels were still able to mimic the cardioprotective effects of ischemic preconditioning. These authors also found evidence suggesting that 5-HD may be a selective mito-KATP–channel antagonist.[143] Sato et al.[144] also suggested that protein kinase C, a postulated intermediate in the signaling pathway responsible for ischemic preconditioning,[145] could modulate mito-KATP–channel activity.

Since arrhythmogenesis seen with KATP-channel openers have mainly been associated with agents that are not mito-KATP–selective, such as pinacidil, mito-KATP–channel openers may be able avoid such problematic side effects.[131] Indeed, nicorandil and BMS-180448, two agents believed to be mito-KATP–selective, seem to possess cardioprotective properties without any proarrhythmic or hypotensive effects.[146] Conversely, HMR-1883, a selective sarcolemmal KATP-channel antagonist, has been shown to be a potent antifibrillatory agent in a canine model of myocardial ischemia.[147]

Problems with the Development of Potassium-Channel Openers

Arrhythmogenesis

As pointed out in the earlier discussion of hypertension, one problem investigators encountered with KATP-channel openers was reflex sympathetic activity and tachycardia. Another problem raised was the possibility of arrhythmogenesis due to APD shortening by KATP-channel openers.[148–151]

Several early studies have demonstrated the potential for KATP-channel openers to induce arrhythmia. In vivo experiments with dogs showed that the KATP-channel opener causes shortening of the refractory period in cardiac tissue. However, the shortening was more pronounced in the atrium than the ventricle. In addition, a statistically significant shortening of the refractory period was produced only at doses that decreased the blood pressure by 30 to 40% or more.[152,153] This finding, that a high dose of KATP channel opener is needed for arrhythmogenesis, is also supported by a study of pinacidil in isolated guinea pig hearts.[154] Another study showed that pinacidil injected into the LAD of canine hearts induced action potential shortening and ST-segment elevation. However, the 50% reduction in the activation recovery interval suggests that supratherapeutic concentrations of the drug may have been used.

The study by Chi et al.[155] is often cited as evidence that pinacidil is proarrhythmic; however, critics argue that the heart rate was not controlled and infarct size was not determined in the pinacidil-treated dogs used in the study. Since the treated animals had a decrease in blood pressure and an increase in heart rate, the increase in sympathetic activity (increase in heart rate) may have led to the development of larger infarcts and the higher incidence of arrhythmia. For the same reason, critics have also dismissed the results

of another study[156] where pinacidil was found to cause irreversible ventricular fibrillation.

D'Alonzo and Grover[157] feel that a proarrhythmic effect may be peculiar to pinacidil and not a class effect. However, Spinelli and Colatsky[158] argue that this effect has also been seen in cromakalim and its active enantiomer lemakalim and that it may therefore be a general property of this drug class. Studies using more cardioselective KATP-channel openers—such as BMS 180448[159] and BMS 191095[160]—will help to resolve this controversy by eliminating hypotension and tachycardia as confounding factors.

It is important to note that the majority of evidence supporting an arrhythmogenic quality in KATP-channel openers comes only from animal models. Depending on the experimental conditions—i.e. conscious versus anesthetized animal, global versus regional ischemia, and the species used—potassium-channel openers can be proarrhythmic or antiarrhythmic. Remme and Wilde[161] proposed that the problem of proarrhythmogeneity with KATP-channel openers might be overestimated. In fact, Patel et al. recently showed that nicorandil, as an antianginal agent, significantly reduced the incidence of nonsustained ventricular tachycardia compared to placebo.[162] Similar effects have been seen with nicorandil in patients with idiopathic ventricular tachycardia.[163] Also, studies with MLA pretreatment have shown a decrease in incidence of ventricular fibrillation and ventricular tachycardia related to ischemia.[116,164] Thus far, no clinical trials involving KATP-channel openers have shown an increase in the occurrence of arrhythmias, although transient T-wave inversion or T-wave flattening may be seen on electrocardiogram.[165]

It is an issue of risk versus benefit: potassium-channel openers antagonize triggered arrhythmia but induce reentry arrhythmia.[166,167] However, it is unclear which arrhythmia predominates in the human ischemic heart. It is argued that the cardioprotective effect of KATP-channel openers negates its questionable proarrhythmic activity. Also, the emerging role of specific mitochondrial KATP-channel openers, which have minimal arrhythmogenic potential, may allow this discussion to become a nonissue.

Conclusion

It has now been 20 years since the discovery of the cardiac KATP channel by Noma, and the subsequent development of a new group of organic drugs that modulate the KATP channel has ushered in a new branch of cardiovascular pharmacology.

The various available KATP-channel openers appear to be potent vasodilators with antihypertensive, anti-ischemic, and myocardial protective actions. They may not cause drug tolerance—a problem seen with other vasodilators such as the nitrates.

Various potassium-channel openers have been used in the treatment of hypertension, and their use as antianginal agents, myocardial protectants, and drugs for the treatment of peripheral vascular disease is being investigated. In addition, recent pharmacologic discoveries have led to the introduction of KATP channel openers that are both specific in their cardioprotective effects and potentially more favorable in their adverse effect profiles.

SODIUM/HYDROGEN-CHANNEL EFFECTORS

The plasma membrane sodium/hydrogen exchanger (NHE) may play a key role in the pathophysiology of cardiac ischemia and reperfusion injury of the heart,[168] since it is directly involved in

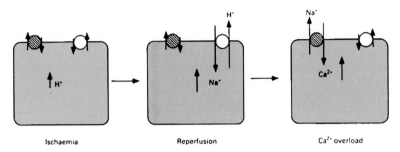

Ischaemia   Reperfusion   Ca²⁺ overload

FIGURE 28-5. Putative series of events illustrating how intracellular acidosis can lead to Ca^{2+} overload. Excess intracellular protons, resulting from ischemia, lead to decreased intracellular pH. During reperfusion, the resulting acid load activates the Na^+/H^+ exchanger, resulting in increased intracellular Na^+. Subsequently, the increased intracellular Na^+ results in increased intracellular Ca^{2+} through the actions of the Na^+/CA^{2+} exchanger. Excess intracellular Ca^{2+} is known to have a variety of detrimental effects, resulting in cell damage and possibly in the generation of arrhythmias. (*Reproduced with permission from Fliegel and Frohlich.*[190])

the maintenance of cellular homeostasis. There are three interdependent effects that play a role in the impairment of both ischemic and reperfused myocardial tissue. These effects are decreased intracellular pH, and intracellular sodium and calcium overload.[169]

During the first few minutes of ischemia and reperfusion, an excessive activation of the exchanger seems to cause intracellular sodium overload (Figs. 28-5 and 28-6). As long as there is sufficient ATP available, the excessive levels of intracellular sodium can be removed to the extracellular space by the sodium/potassium ATPase channel, which extracts the sodium against its gradient[169]. However, as ATP is lost from the system, sodium again begins to accumulate in the intracellular space. Sodium and calcium transports are linked by a 3-sodium-calcium exchange, therefore, raised intracellular sodium levels result in calcium overload, which can endanger the tissue. At the same time, intracellular acidosis, which may reduce the harmful effects of the raised intracellular calcium, is counteracted by the active NHE, thus further increasing the intracellular sodium. The consequences of these events are the potentiation of malignant cardiac arrhythmias, myocardial contracture, and necrosis.[168]

It is the excessive activity of the sodium/hydrogen pump that supports these pathophysiologic events. Therefore it could be assumed that these harmful events might be ameliorated through the use of NHE inhibitors (Fig. 28-7). The prototypes associated with this activity are amiloride and its analogues. At low doses, amiloride

is a potassium-sparing diuretic, which was shown to be a potent NHE blocker in the distal convoluted tubules of the kidney. However, it is only a weak nonspecific NHE inhibitor in the heart, requiring higher doses to achieve this effect. As NHE inhibitors in the heart, amiloride derivatives are more effective than the parent compound itself, since they are more specific for this activity.[168] Despite the ability of these agents to inhibit NHE, various nonspecific actions and relatively low potency have restricted their eventual therapeutic development.[170] This has led to the development of the novel benzoylguanidine compounds HOE 642 (cariporide) and EMD 96785 (eniporide) (Fig. 28-8). These new drugs have been involved in recent and ongoing clinical trials and have been proven to be safer and more specific and potent than earlier compounds.

Sodium-Hydrogen Exchange

The NHE exchanges intracellular hydrogen for extracellular sodium. This antiporter runs on the concentration gradients of sodium and hydrogen and is involved in the maintenance of pH, volume homeostasis, and cell growth in both polar and nonpolar cells. While the exchanger is mainly affected by intracellular pH, autocrine and paracrine factors may also influence channel activity.[170,171]

There are six isoforms of the NHE transporter: NHE1 to NHE6. They represent distinct gene products and exhibit differences in their

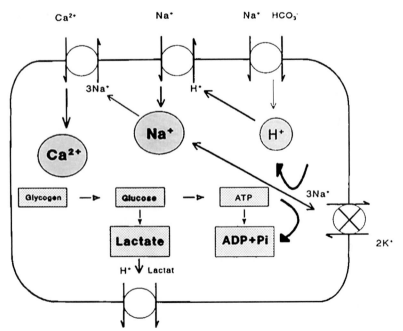

FIGURE 28-6. Active Na^+/H^+ exchange in ischemic cardiac myocytes. Elevated intracellular Na^+ concentrations cause an intracellular Ca^{2+} overload. Anaerobic metabolism is driven by high intracellular Ca^{2+} and the excretion of H^+. (*Reproduced with permission from Scholz and Albus.*[168])

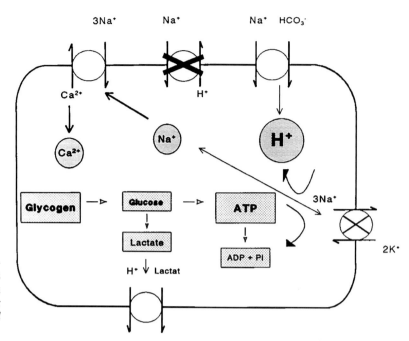

FIGURE 28-7. Inhibited Na^+/H^+ exchange in ischemic cardiac myocytes. Reduced intracellular Na^+ concentrations prevent intracellular Ca^{2+} overload. Anaerobic metabolism is inhibited by reduced intracellular Na^+ and intracellular acidification. (*Reproduced with permission from Scholz and Albus.*[168])

primary structures, patterns of tissue expression, membrane localization, functional properties, and physiologic roles.[172,173] NHE1 to NHE5 share 34 to 60% amino acid homology, whereas NHE6 shares only 20% homology with other isoforms.[170] While NHE1 is expressed in almost all mammalian cells, NHE2 to NHE5 are more restricted in their patterns of expression. NHE6 is localized intracellularly and may play a role in regulating intramitochondrial Na^+ and H^+ levels as well as mitochondrial Ca^{2+} levels.[174,175] The various isoforms also show differences in their sensitivities to inhi-

FIGURE 28-8. Chemical structures of cariporide (HOE-642) and eniporide (EMD-96785).

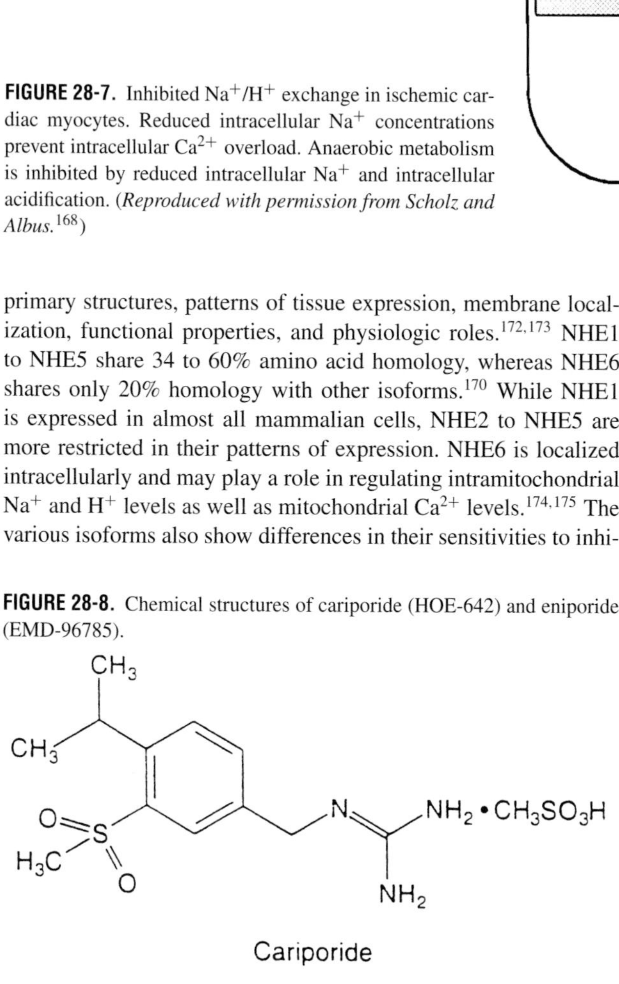

Cariporide

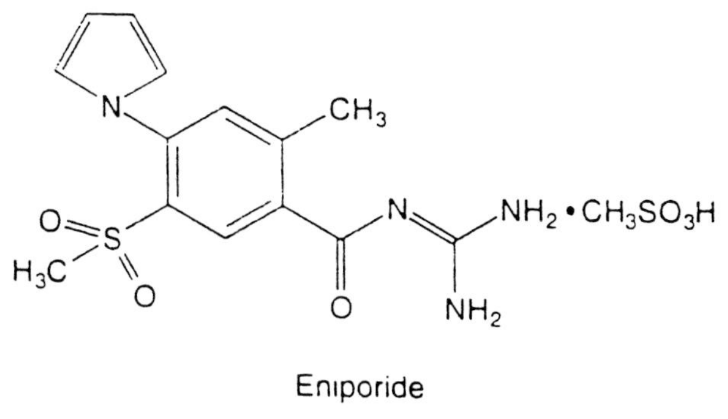

Eniporide

bition by amiloride and its derivatives, which are the prototypical NHE inhibitors and are generally not specific for NHE subtypes.[176] All studies to date indicate that NHE1 is the predominant isoform present in mammalian myocardium (Fig. 28–9).[177] Cardiac cells lack NHE2 to NHE5, and further research is necessary to uncover the potential role of NHE6 in the heart either under normal or pathologic conditions.

NHE1 contains 815 amino acids and consists of two separate functional domains. The N-terminal domain is a 500–amino acid transmembrane domain with 12 transmembrane-spanning segments, and the C-terminal domain is a 315–amino acid hydrophilic cytoplasmic domain.[172,173] The transmembrane domain is mainly responsible for proton extrusion,[178] and the cytoplasmic domain is responsible for modulation of NHE1 activity, mainly by phosphorylation-dependent reactions.[179] Recent studies have shown that NHE1 is predominantly located at the intercalated disk region of atrial and ventricular myocytes near gap junction proteins and also along the transverse tubular system.[180] Since both of these elements are highly sensitive to intracellular pH, it is hypothesized that, under normal conditions, NHE1 influences cell-to-cell ion-dependent communication and also intracellular Ca^{2+} levels.[180]

The predominant factor that influences NHE1 activity is intracellular pH.[181]. Within the normal range of intracellular pH, 7.1 to 7.3, NHE1 activity is negligible; but as intracellular pH decreases, the exchanger rapidly becomes activated.[170] Increasing H^+ concentration is detected by an H^+ sensor on the cytoplasmic surface of the exchanger and accounts for the sensitivity of NHE1 to intracellular pH. Although the exact mechanism of this process is poorly understood, it is believed that the binding of H^+ to the cytoplasmic sensor causes a conformational change resulting in exchanger activation.[178] Besides intracellular pH, several extrinsic factors can modulate NHE1 activity by increasing its sensitivity of the H^+ sensor to intracellular H^+ ions. Such factors include endothelin-1,[182] angiotensin II,[183] alpha$_1$-adrenergic agonists,[184] thrombin,[185] and growth factors.[186–188] These factors most likely increase the sensitivity of the NHE1 H^+ sensor via phosphorylation reactions involving the C-terminal domain.[179,186]

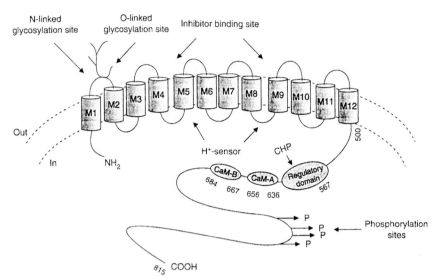

FIGURE 28-9. Putative topologic model of the 815–amino acid Na$^+$/H$^+$ exchange (NHE) isoform NHE1, showing 12 transmembrane-spanning segments and the hydrophilic carboxyl terminus with indications of proposed regulatory sites. The transmembrane domain represents the site of functional ion exchange, whereas the cytoplasmic region represents the major site for regulation via phosphorylation-dependent and -independent reactions. The regulatory domain is the major determinant of the set point of the exchanger and involves regulation by growth factors as well as osmotic stress; it is possibly regulated by calcineurin homologous protein (CHP). Both high- (CaM-A) and low- (CaM-B) affinity calmodulin binding sites on the C-terminal domain of NHE1 have been identified; these are linked to NHE1 activation. Stimulation of these binding sites is thought to represent the basis for the reversal of the autoinhibitory state of the antiporter, which normally exists under unstimulated conditions when intracellular calcium levels are low. (*Reproduced with permission from Karmazyn et al.*[170])

Sodium/Hydrogen Exchange in Ischemia

In myocardial ischemia there are at least three discrete phases. The first phase extends until the myocardium ceases to contract, the second is the period of ischemic arrhythmias, and the third is characterized by a lack of mechanical and electrical activity.[169] In the beginning of the ischemic insult, myocardial cells are subject to changes in their metabolism and ion-transport activity. Due to the limited quantity of oxygen present, the cells rely on anaerobic glycolysis for their energy needs.[189] However, the energy demands of the system remain, in that the Na$^+$K$^+$-ATPase system is still active. The degradation of ATP produces protons that, under normal physiologic conditions, are degraded in the mitochondria. However, since the mitochondrial activity ceases in the first seconds of ischemia, these protons accumulate and decrease the intracellular pH.[169] Several defense mechanisms present in the cell aim to decrease the effects of the decreased pH. One of these is through the activation of NHE1.

The NHE is the dominant mechanism against decreased intracellular pH.[168] It is usually not active under normal physiologic conditions, as evidenced by its unresponsiveness to amiloride or other inhibitors during normal physiologic events.[190] It is responsible for most of the sodium influx associated with pH recovery and reperfusion,[169] although some of the sodium that enters comes from the sodium hydrocarbon transporter.[168] With this increase in Na$^+$, there is an increase in the activity of the Na$^+$K$^+$-ATPase. As stated, the degradation of ATP generates more protons, enhancing anaerobic glycolysis and the formation of lactate. All this creates a cycle by which there is further enhancement of NHE1 antiporter activity.[169]

The decrease in intracellular pH is soon followed by a decrease in extracellular pH, also occurring in the first stage of ischemia.[168] While NHE1 drives protons out of the cell, they are not washed away from the extracellular space surrounding the cells. Thus, the external pH begins to decrease. With this, there are no longer hydrogen, HCO$_3^-$, or lactate gradients to allow for NHE1 to work efficiently. There is, therefore, no proton extrusion from the cell allowing both the intracellular and extracellular environments to acidify.[169] NHE1 is totally quiescent at an approximate pH$_e$ (extracellular pH) of 6.3,[168] which is usually achieved after 10 to 15 min of ischemia.

This is a change from the resting pH of 7.2.[190] The decrease in pH also inhibits the function of anaerobic glycolysis, which, at best, produces only 50% of the ATP produced with aerobic glycolysis. These events ultimately result in a decrease in contractility by affecting a number of steps involved in the excitation-contraction coupling and a decrease in the calcium binding to contractile elements.[190]

With the loss of ATP and the inefficient anaerobic glycolysis, the Na$^+$K$^+$-ATPase begins to falter, which leads to additional increases in intracellular sodium. This problem is confounded by the finding that cardiotoxic ischemic metabolites, such as hydrogen peroxide[191] and lysophosphatidylcholine (LPC),[192] can also stimulate NHE1 activity and further increase sodium influx. The increases in sodium are followed by increases in the internal Ca^{2+} levels, for the calcium is regulated by the 3Na$^+$/Ca^{2+} exchanger. Transgenic mice that overexpress this 3Na$^+$/Ca^{2+} exchanger show an increased sensitivity to ischemic injury.[193] This exchanger is driven by sodium and calcium gradients under physiologic conditions. With excessive sodium, the system fails to extrude the calcium from the cell and may actually reverse to extrude excess sodium for calcium, further increasing the intracellular calcium levels. This excess calcium is what is actually deleterious to the cell, since it can cause overexcitability and electrical instability.[169] The calcium also uncouples mitochondrial function and causes cellular hypercontraction and arrhythmias, thus impeding the function of the heart and aggravating the ischemic state.[190]

During ischemia, there is another occurrence that derails normal metabolic functioning. Adrenergic nerve endings are involved in the uptake of norepinephrine from the extracellular space, using a sodium-driven mechanism. The norepinephrine is transported into vesicles in the cells and exchanged for protons there. In ischemia, there is derangement of metabolism and ion homeostasis. Due to the high levels of intracellular Na$^+$, there is a decrease in the activity of norepinephrine uptake, which can lead to the development of cardiac arrhythmias.[169]

Reperfusion is sometimes used in the rescue of ischemic tissue. Initially, this causes a washout of the acidic extracellular fluid, which is in the ischemic area. However, this creates a huge pH gradient between the intra- and extracellular environments. This gradient reactivates all the pH-regulated systems to a maximum level, which will cause the intracellular Na^+ to increase through NHE1 as well as through the action of the sodium-dependent hydrocarbon transport.[169] This all causes cell alkalization,[194] which aims to return the intracellular pH to normal levels.

However, the increase in sodium cannot be properly extruded by the Na^+K^+-ATPase, as there is a lack of ATP present. There is a further sodium overload and a secondary rise in calcium, which leads to calcium overload through the sodium/calcium exchanger. The exchanger will either stop removing calcium or reverse to remove excess sodium and deposit calcium.[168] With depressed pH, the deleterious effects of excess calcium are usually stifled. In reperfusion, the pH is returned to its average of 7.2, allowing the excess calcium to take its effect, which results in arrhythmias, myocardial stunning, and necrosis.[169] In nerve endings, sodium overload as well as ATP depletion result in norepinephrine overflow, perpetuating arrhythmias and enhancing the myocardial damage due to excessive intracellular calcium.[169]

The true adverse effects of reperfusion occur in the initial 2 min. It is in this short time that there is pH imbalance, resulting in damage to myocardial cells. If NHE1 is inhibited in the first 2 min, much of the damage caused by the ischemia and reperfusion can be avoided, since after the first 2 min of reperfusion there is enough regenerated ATP to deal with the excess sodium through the Na^+K^+-ATPase system.

Finally, while ischemia-enhanced NHE1 activity has been well documented, less information is available on the ability of ischemia to regulate NHE1 expression. In fact, a recent study has shown that myocardial ischemia or the direct administration of cardiotoxic compounds, such as LPC and hydrogen peroxide, can increase tissue levels of NHE1 mRNA.[195] This suggests that both increased activity as well as increased expression may stimulate the NHE1 exchanger.

NHE Inhibition

With inhibition of the sodium/hydrogen antiporter, there is a decrease in sodium influx into myocardial cells. With a decrease in the influx, there is a reduction in the amount of sodium that must be extruded by the Na^+K^+-ATPase; thus, less ATP is required by the body's myocardial cells. This could potentially delay or avoid all the harmful effects associated with sodium and the subsequent calcium overload.[169]

In ischemic tissue, the decrease in intracellular pH is accentuated by NHE1 inhibition. This would enhance the inhibition of anaerobic glycolysis and decrease the degradation of ATP (Fig. 28-7). Due to the decrease in ATP degradation, there would also be fewer protons released. The diminution of lactate efflux from the cardiac tissue and the decrease in the lactate content imply that there is a decrease in lactate production. There are also increases in glycogen stores. The inhibition of NHE1 would also potentially prevent the overflow of norepinephrine, which, as stated, is frequently seen with ischemia and reperfusion injuries.[169] The reduction in norepinephrine contributes also to the reduction in calcium overload, which means that there would be potential for a lower incidence of arrhythmias. Furthermore, a reduction in calcium levels indicates that there would be less myocardial necrosis, since it is the abundance of calcium on the cell that accelerates this process.[190]

The inhibition of NHE also affects myocardial reperfusion. Damage during reperfusion is associated with the acidic extracellular environment being washed away and subsequent NHE1 reactivation causing a sodium overload. A decrease in NHE1 activity

would prevent the sudden surge of intracellular sodium, avoiding cellular injury. Again, there would be a decrease in the amount of ATP expended, and the retarded levels of intracellular sodium would also prevent the rampant increases in intracellular calcium.[168]

Amiloride and Analogues

Amiloride and its analogues are the prototypical sodium inhibitors, inhibiting the sodium/hydrogen antiporter, as well as effecting the sodium/calcium exchanger and the Na^+K^+-ATPase. Analogues of amiloride, specifically those with hydrophobic substitutions on the 5-amino nitrogen, are known to be more potent than their parent compound.[196] Likewise, analogues with two substitutions are usually more effective than those with only one substitution. However, the only residue that must remain unsubstituted is the guanidine group, because it is important for the activity of the molecule and the inhibition of sodium channels.[197] Some of the more potent analogues are 5(*N*-methyl-*N* isopropyl), 5(*N*-methyl-*N*-isobutyl), 5(ethyl-*N*-isopropyl), 5(*N*,*N* hexamethylene), and 5(*N*,*N* dimethyl). These compounds are 10 to 500 times more potent than the unsubstituted amiloride.[196]

High concentrations of an NHE inhibitor can inhibit protein synthesis in cells and in cell-free systems. Under these circumstances, amiloride is quite toxic. Amiloride competes with sodium for the external site of the NHE; thus, to compete successfully, a high concentration of amiloride, in excess of 10^{-4}, is required. This can also inhibit the paracellular cation permeability in epithelia and ATPase. Since amiloride is also a weak base, it also can alter the pH.[198] The analogues are superior, for they are more than 100 times as potent. Therefore low doses are effective too, avoiding the toxicity associated with elevated amiloride levels in the blood.[198]

Other than being studied as a diuretic, amiloride has been the focus of very few amiloride trials in humans. However, one clinical study did show the antiarrhythmic properties of amiloride.[199] In this investigation, 6 of 31 patients with inducible ventricular tachycardia had an antiarrhythmic response to amiloride, with 5 responding to a dose of 20 mg/day and 1 patient responding to a dose of 10 mg/day. Another 6 patients had partial antiarrhythmic effects recorded. To prove that K^+ values were not significant, a potassium resin–binding agent was added to lower the slightly elevated potassium levels to the normal range. Even when these levels were lowered, antiarrhythmic activity was still associated with amiloride. In another part of the study, it was noticed that of 15 patients who had greater than 20 premature ventricular complexes per hour, amiloride was able to suppress arrhythmia in 8.

The 12 patients who responded favorably to the drug responded better than they would have on other antiarrhythmic drugs, for amiloride was seen to be 4.5 times more effective than the others. Although 5 patients did experience some spontaneous nonsustained arrhythmias, exacerbation of arrhythmia was not apparent. Random variability does not explain these results.[199]

The antiarrhythmic and cardioprotective effects of amiloride have also been established in many animal models. In rats, amiloride decreased the heart rate in a dose-dependent manner, an effect apparently based on proton retention.[200] During the first minutes of reperfusion, NHE inhibition by amiloride caused a decrease in intracellular sodium and prevented a rise in calcium.

Monensin is a drug that can block the effects of amiloride; when it was added in the trial, the NHE was reactivated. Furthermore, maneuvers to decrease the sodium transsarcolemmal gradients, by decreasing the external sodium concentrations or applying NH_4Cl, exhibited the same positive effects as the addition of amiloride. During reperfusion, it was also noticed that there was an increase in sarcolemmal peroxidation; amiloride was able to reduce some of this free radical formation. As stated, amiloride was able to prevent, in a dose-dependent fashion, the ventricular tachycardia or fibrillation associated with reperfusion.[200]

Studies in dogs have also shown the ability of amiloride to suppress arrhythmia,[201] decrease infarct size,[201] and prevent contractile dysfunction related to postischemic "stunned" myocardium.[202] Interestingly, the ability to prevent contractile dysfunction was thought to be related to an inhibition of the Na^+/Ca^+ exchanger and not the NHE.[202]

After these early studies established the efficacy of amiloride in inhibiting the NHE, researchers proved that the amiloride analogues had similar effects at much lower concentrations. DMA [5(N,N dimethyl)amiloride] is a more selective NHE1 inhibitor and 10 times more potent than amiloride. In studies performed in animals, the analogue restored contractile function and reduced myocardial injury after ischemic reperfusion. In one such study, DMA (10 μmol/L) caused a significant improvement in ATP decay and a decrease in myocardial wall tension.[203] Another analogue, HMA [5(N,N hexamethylene)amiloride], also acts as an NHE inhibitor, with a potency that is 4 times that of DMA or 40 times that of amiloride. In an experiment performed on rats using a myocardial reperfusion model, HMA 2.5 μmol/L improved the recovery of developed myocardial tension and protected against a rise in resting tension.[203] This analogue in another trial also worked quite rapidly.[204] There was a 97 + 8.1% chance that with the use of HMA, a return to normal levels of sodium would occur within 1 min. It was only after 5 min that amiloride was able to achieve this normal level of intracellular sodium concentration. EIPA [5(N-ethyl-N-isopropyl) amiloride] is even more potent than HMA. At 1 μmol/L, EIPA significantly improved the recovery of developed tension after myocardial reperfusion and depressed the increase in resting tension exhibited in untreated cardiac muscle.[203] In a related study, 1 μmol/L was effective in mildly depressing active tension, while a dose of 5 to 10 μmol/L depressed active tension fully.[203]

In these amiloride analogue studies, it has been suggested that an inhibitor of the Na^+/Ca^{2+} exchanger might be beneficial in myocardial ischemia and reperfusion.[202] However, in these same experiments as those described above, verapamil, a calcium-channel blocker, did not show similar effects in the recovery of generated tension or in the rate of relaxation. Also, verapamil had no beneficial effect on postischemic recovery of the heart. This is because for calcium-channel blockers to be effective, they must be employed prior to the development of ischemia.[203] The calcium-channel blockers may not be effective alone in reperfusion, for there is a sodium-hydrogen-calcium system that needs to be considered.

Benzoylguanidine NHE Inhibitors

Despite the ability of amiloride and its analogues to inhibit NHE, their eventual clinical use has been limited by various nonspecific actions, lack of selectivity against NHE1, and relatively low potency. This has led to the development of novel benzoylguanidine compounds targeted specifically against NHE1, increasing the potential for treatment in patients with coronary artery disease (CAD). Recent clinical trials have tested this new class of NHE1-specific inhibitors in human subjects.[204–212]

The prototype for this group of compounds is HOE-694 (3-methylsulphonyl-4-piperidinobenzoyl-guanidine methanesulfonate).[170] However, recent clinical development has largely centered around two newer benzoylguanidine compounds, cariporide (HOE-642) and eniporide (EMD-96785) (Fig. 28-8). Both of these drugs are promising because they appear to be selective inhibitors of the cardiac specific NHE1 isoform.[170,212,212a]

While the mechanism of action of NHE1 inhibitors is not completely understood, their effects on the antiporter involve binding to sites on the lipophilic transmembrane region. By constructing a variety of chimeric NHE constructs, Orlowski and Kandasam demonstrated potential sites on a number of transmembrane units to which these drugs can bind.[176] Using site-directed mutagenesis, Wang et al. have shown that the histidine 349 residue may be of particular importance for interaction of NHE1 with inhibitors, at least of the amiloride series.[213] It is not known whether this can be extended to the more recently developed benzoylguanidine compounds.

Clinical development and testing of NHE1-specific benzoylguanidine compounds in cardiac disease has been very rapid, reflecting the consistent and excellent protection with these agents demonstrated in animal studies. The first such study, termed the GUARDIAN (Guard During Ischemia Against Necrosis) trial, was an ambitious combined phase II/phase III double-blind, randomized, placebo-controlled study of 11,590 patients to assess different doses of cariporide in individuals with acute coronary syndromes with outcomes evaluation at 36 days.[214,215] The population of patients included those with unstable angina pectoris/non-Q-wave myocardial infarction (MI) as well as patients undergoing high-risk percutaneous transluminal coronary angioplasty coronary artery bypass grafting (CABG).

The GUARDIAN trial revealed that cariporide is well tolerated, although it failed to demonstrate an overall significant attenuation (10%) of the two primary events, mortality and incidence of MI. However, favorable effects among the three major subgroups were observed, especially a significant reduction in the event rate in patients undergoing CABG receiving the highest dose of 120 mg of cariporide intravenously every 8 h. This dose appeared to be effective in reducing the overall incidence of Q-wave MI by about 40%.

This suggests that, perhaps, optimal dosages and plasma therapeutic levels were not achieved in this study. It is possible that future studies using higher doses of cariporide may show a significant decrease in cardiac events in high-risk patients. In fact, results from a relatively small clinical trial with 100 patients demonstrated improved left ventricular function when cariporide was administered prior to balloon angioplasty in patients with acute MI.[216]

A larger (approximately 1300 patients) clinical evaluation for patients with acute MI has been completed in which the NHE1-selective inhibitor eniporide was assessed as an adjunct therapy to early reperfusion in a phase II placebo-controlled multicenter European trial, the ESCAMI (Evaluation of the Safety and the Cardioprotective effects of Eniporide in Acute Myocardial Infarction) study. In this study, eniporide was administered prior to angioplasty or thrombolytic therapy in an attempt to minimize reperfusion injury. The final results showed no beneficial effects of eniporide on infarct size or clinical outcomes.[217]

While initial results of clinical trials with benzoylguanidine compounds have been less than overwhelming, there continues to be significant promise for use of these drugs in the treatment of cardiac disease.[217a] Based on mechanism of action, their use would be most beneficial if they were administered prior to or early after the onset of ischemia.[218] Other NHE inhibitors under development include zoniporide[219] and SM-20550.[220]

NHE Inhibition versus Ischemic Preconditioning

While the first half of this chapter focused on KATP channels and their role in the phenomenon of ischemic preconditioning, the question exists as to whether cardioprotective effects of NHE1 inhibition occur via a similar mechanism.[221–223] Studies to date indicate that benefits of NHE inhibition occur by different physiologic pathways when compared to ischemic preconditioning. In fact, NHE1 inhibition offers added protection when administered to preconditioned hearts.[224]

Protection by ischemic preconditioning has generally been considered the most effective known cardioprotective strategy. This has recently been challenged in a study that demonstrated comparable protection by NHE1 inhibition in terms of infarct size reduction in dogs subjected to coronary artery ligation for 60 min.[225] However, when the period of occlusion was extended to 90 min, preconditioning failed to exert salutary effects, although NHE1 inhibition reduced infarct size by 70%.[226] This indicates that NHE1 inhibition may confer superior protection to ischemic preconditioning under certain circumstances.

CONCLUSION

The sodium-hydrogen exchanger is markedly active in ischemia and reperfusion. Inhibition of this exchanger definitely decreases intracellular Na^+ and subsequently decreases intracellular Ca^{2+} overload. Inhibitors also decrease the rate of ATP depletion during ischemia and reperfusion. Such action reduces the chance that malignant arrhythmias and/or myocardial necrosis will develop.[227,228] Amiloride and analogues have been proven to be potent NHE inhibitors. However, amiloride alone is nonspecific; in order for it to be effective, it must be taken at excessively high levels. This can prove to be toxic. In contrast, new benzoylguanidine compounds, such as cariporide and eniporide, are more potent and NHE1-selective, accomplishing the same desired results of less specific NHE inhibitors while not requiring excessive doses to be effective.

The most promising situation for the use of NHE1 inhibitors in humans is in a typical ischemia/reperfusion situation, when the inhibitor can be present at all times, as during cardiac surgery. It could also be beneficial in cardiac transplantation and percutaneous coronary angioplasty, where coronary blood flow is transiently stopped. Use of the inhibitors may also be effective in patients with unstable angina pectoris and myocardial infarction, when there is risk of myocardial contractile abnormalities and arrhythmias.[168] It is very likely and hopeful that new therapeutic strategies will emerge, based on both the clinical trials that have been or are currently being undertaken as well as the obviously rapid development of a large number of new NHE1-selective inhibitors.

REFERENCES

1. Ashford MLJ, Bond CT, Blair TA, Adelman JP: Cloning and functional expression of a rat heart KATP channel. *Nature* 370:456, 1994.
2. Lenz T, Wagner G: Potential role of potassium channel openers for treatment of cardiovascular disease. In: Laragh JH, Brenner BM, eds. *Hypertension, Pathophysiology, Diagnosis and Management,* 2nd ed. New York: Raven Press, 1995: 2953–2968.
3. Yuan JX, Blaustein MP: Cellular potassium transport. In: Izzo L Jr, Black HR, eds. *Hypertension Primer,* 2nd ed. Dallas: American Heart Association, 1999:56, 388.
4. Furspan PB: Potassium channels. In: Izzo L Jr, Black HR, eds. *Hypertension Primer.* Dallas: American Heart Association, 1993:38.
5. Noma A: ATP regulated potassium channels in cardiac muscle. *Nature* 305:147, 1983.
6. Petersen OH, Findlay I: Electrophysiology of the pancreas. *Physiol Rev* 67:1054, 1983.
7. Standen NB, Quayle JM, Davies NW, et al: Hyperpolarizing vasodilators activate ATP sensitive potassium channels in arterial smooth muscle. *Science* 245:177, 1989.
8. Spruce AE, Standen NB, Stanfield PR: Voltage dependent ATP sensitive potassium channels of skeletal muscle membrane. *Nature* 316:736, 1985.
9. Treherne JM, Ashford MLJ: The regional distribution of sulfonylurea binding sites in rat brain. *Neuroscience* 40:523, 1991.
10. Takano M, Noma A: The ATP sensitive potassium channel. *Prog Neurobiol* 41:21, 1993.
11. Quast U: ATP-sensitive K^+ channels in the kidney. *Naunyn Schmiedebergs Arch Pharmacol* 354:213, 1996.
12. Yokoshiki H, Sunagawa M, Seki T, Sperelakis N: ATP-sensitive K^+ channels in pancreatic, cardiac, and vascular smooth muscle cells. *Am J Physiol* 274:C25, 1998.
13. Yokoshiki H, Kohya T, Tomita F, et al: Pharmacological regulators of ATP-sensitive K^+ channels. In: Kanno M, Hattori Y, eds. Current Aspects of Cellular And Subcellular Mechanism of Drug Actions. Sapporo, Japan: Hokkaido University School of Medicine, 2000:65–77.
14. Inagaki N, Gonoi T, Clement JP IV, et al: Reconstitution of IK_{ATP}: An inward rectifier subunit plus the sulfonylurea receptor. *Science* 270:1166, 1995.
15. Inagaki N, Seino S: ATP-sensitive potassium channels: Structures, functions, and pathophysiology. *Jpn J Physiol* 48:397, 1998.
16. Seino S: ATP-sensitive potassium channels: A model of heteromultimeric potassium channel/receptor assemblies. *Annu Rev Physiol* 61:337, 1999.
17. Aguilar-Bryan L, Clement JP IV, Gonzalez G, et al: Toward understanding the assembly and structure of KATP channels. *Physiol Rev* 78:227, 1998.
18. Tucker SJ, Gribble FM, Zhao C, et al: Truncation of Kir6.2 produces ATP-sensitive K^+ channels in the absence of the sulfonylurea receptor. *Nature* 387:179, 1997.
19. Nakashima H, Kakei M, Tanaka H: Activation of the ATP sensitive K channel by decavanadate in guinea pig ventricular myocytes. *Eur J Pharmacol* 233:219, 1993.
20. Shyng S, Ferrigni T, Nichols CG: Regulation of KATP channel activity by diazoxide and MgADP: Distinct functions of the two nucleotide binding folds of the sulfonylurea receptor. *J Gen Physiol* 110:643, 1997.
21. Ashcroft SJH, Ashcroft FM: Properties and functions of ATP sensitive K channels. *Cell Signals* 2:197, 1990.
22. Furukawa T, Kimura S, Furukawa N, et al: Role of cardiac ATP regulated potassium channels in differential responses of endocardial and epicardial cells to ischemia. *Circ Res* 68:1693, 1991.
23. Cameron JS, Kimura S, Jackson-Burns DA, et al: ATP sensitive K^+ channels are altered in hypertrophied ventricular myocytes. *Am J Physiol* 255:H1254, 1988.
24. Findlay I: Sulphonylurea drugs no longer inhibit ATP sensitive K^+ channels during metabolic stress in cardiac muscle. *J Pharmacol Exp Ther* 266:456, 1993.
25. Venkatesh N, Lamp ST, Weiss JN: Sulfonylureas, ATP sensitive K^+ channels, and cellular K loss during hypoxia, ischemia, and metabolic inhibition in mammalian ventricle. *Circ Res* 69:623, 1991.
26. Atwal KS: Pharmacology and structure activity relationships for KATP modulators: Tissue selective KATP openers. *J Cardiovasc Pharmacol* 24:S12, 1994.
27. Tung RT, Kurachi Y: On the mechanism of nucleoside diphosphate activation of the ATP sensitive K^+ channels in ventricular cells of guinea pig. *J Physiol (London)* 437:239, 1991.
28. Quast U, Cook NS: Moving together: K^+-channel openers and ATP-sensitive K^+-channels. *Trends Pharmacol Sci* 10:431, 1989.

29. Mimuro T, Kawata T, Onuki T, et al: The attenuated effect of ATP-sensitive K$^+$ channel opener pinacidil on renal haemodynamics in spontaneously hypertensive rats. *Eur J Pharmacol* 358 (2):153, 1998.

30. Huysmans FT, Thien T, Koene RA: Acute treatment of hypertension with slow infusion of diazoxide. *Arch Intern Med* 143:882, 1983.

31. Hanson AS, Linas SL: Refractory and malignant hypertension. In: Bennett WM, McCarron DA, eds. Pharmacology and Management of Hypertension. New York: Churchill Livingstone, 1994:166.

32. Quayle JM, Nelson MT, Standen NB: ATP-sensitive and inwardly rectifying potassium channels in smooth muscle. *Physiol Rev* 77(4):1165, 1997.

33. Goldberg MR, Offen WW: Pinacidil with and without hydrochlorothiazide. Dose response relationships from results of a 4x3 factorial design study. *Drugs* 36(Suppl 7):83, 1988.

34. Goldberg MR: Clinical pharmacology of pinacidil, a prototype for drugs that affect potassium channels. *J Cardiovasc Pharmacol* 12(Suppl 2):S41, 1988.

35. Friedel HA, Brodgen RN: Pinacidil: A review of its pharmacodynamic and pharmacokinetic properties, and therapeutic potential in the treatment of hypertension. *Drugs* 39:929, 1990.

36. Singer DR, Markandu ND, Miller MA, et al: Potassium channel stimulation in normal subjects and in patients with essential hypertension: An acute study with cromakalim (BRL 34915). *J Hypertens* 7(Suppl 6):S294, 1989.

37. Grover GJ: Protective effects of ATP sensitive potassium channel openers in experimental myocardial ischemia. *J Cardiovasc Pharmacol* 24(Suppl 2):S18, 1994.

38. Senior R, Buchner-Moell D, Raftery E, Lahiri A: Potent hemodynamic effects of bimakalim, a new potassium channel opener, in man. *J Cardiovasc Pharmacol* 2:717, 1993.

38a. Gomma AH, Purcell HJ, Fox KM: Potassium channel openers in myocardial ischaemia. Therapeutic potential of nicorandil. *Drugs* 61:1705, 2001.

39. Kawahara J-i, Kashiwabara T, Ogawa N, et al: Antihypertensive properties of KRN4884, a novel long-lasting potassium channel opener. *J Cardiovasc Pharmacol* 33:292, 1999.

40. Shinbo A, Ono K, Iijima T: Activation of cardiac ATP-sensitive K$^+$ channels by KRN4884, a novel K$^+$ channel opener. *J Pharmacol Exp Ther* 283:770, 1997.

41. Nakajima T, Shinohara T, Yaoka O, et al: Y-27152, a long-acting K$^+$ channel opener with less tachycardia: Antihypertensive effects in hypertensive rats and dogs in conscious state. *J Pharmacol Exp Ther* 261:730, 1992.

42. Uematsu T, Kosuge K, Hirosawa S, et al: Pharmacokinetics and safety of a novel long-acting prodrug-type potassium channel opener Y-27152, in healthy volunteers. *J Clin Pharmacol* 36:439, 1996.

43. O'Rourke ST: Effects of potassium channel blockers on resting tone in isolated coronary arteries. *J Cardiovasc Pharmacol* 27:636, 1996.

44. Knight C, Purcell H, Fox K: Potassium channel openers: Clinical applications in ischemic heart disease—overview of clinical efficacy of nicorandil. *Cardiovasc Drugs Ther* 9(Suppl 2):229, 1995.

45. Ciampricotti R, Schotborgh CE, de Kam PJ, van Herwaarden RH: A comparison of nicorandil with isosorbide mononitrate in elderly patients with stable coronary heart disease: the SNAPE study. *Am Heart J* 139(5):939, 2000.

46. Goldschmidt M, Landzberg BR, Frishman WH: Nicorandil. A potassium channel opening drug for the treatment of ischemic heart disease. *J Clin Pharmacol* 36:559, 1996.

47. Doring G: Anti-anginal and anti-ischemic efficacy of nicorandil in comparison with isosorbide 5-mononitrate and isosorbide dinitrate: Results from two multi-center, double-blind, randomized studies with stable coronary heart disease patients. *J Cardiovasc Pharmacol* 20(Suppl 3):S74, 1992.

48. Raftery EB, Lahiri A, Hughes LO, Rose EL: A double blind comparison of a beta-blocker and a potassium channel opener in exercise induced angina. *Eur Heart J* 14(Suppl B):35, 1993.

49. SWAN Study Group: Comparison of the anti-ischaemic and anti-anginal effects of nicorandil and amlodipine in patients with symptomatic stable angina pectoris: The SWAN study. *J Clin Basic Cardiol* 2:213, 1999.

50. Naito A, Aniya Y, Sakanashi M: Antioxidative action of the nitrovasodilator nicorandil: Inhibition of oxidative activation of liver microsomal glutathione S-transferase and lipid peroxidation. *Jpn J Pharmacol* 65:209, 1994.

51. Jaraki O, Strauss WE, Francis S, Stamler JS: Antiplatelet effects of a novel antianginal agent, nicorandil. *J Cardiovasc Pharmacol* 23:24, 1994.

52. Rajaratnam R, Brieger DB, Hawkins R, Freedman SB: Attenuation of anti-ischemic efficacy during chronic therapy with nicorandil in patients with stable angina pectoris. *Am J Cardiol* 83(7):1120, 1999.

53. Tabone X, Funck-Brentano C, Billon N, Jaillon P: Comparison of tolerance to intravenous nitroglycerin during nicorandil and intermittent nitroglycerin patch in healthy volunteers. *Clin Pharmacol Ther* 56(6 Pt 1):672, 1994.

54. The IONA Study group: Effect of nicorandil on coronary events in patients with stable angina: The Impact Of Nicorandil in Angina (IONA) randomised trial. *Lancet* 359:1269, 2002.

55. Duncker DJ, Verdouw PD: Role of K$^+$ ATP channels in ischemic preconditioning and cardioprotection. *Cardiovasc Drugs Ther* 14:7, 2000.

56. Haruna T, Horie M, Kouchi I, et al: Coordinate interaction between ATP-sensitive K$+$ channel and Na$^+$,K$^+$-ATPase modulates ischemic preconditioning. *Circulation* 98:2905, 1998.

57. Baker JE, Holman P, Gross GJ: Preconditioning in immature rabbit hearts. Role of K$_{ATP}$ channels. *Circulation* 99:1249, 1999.

58. Gross GJ: Recombinant cardiac ATP-sensitive potassium channels and cardioprotection. *Circulation* 98:1479, 1998.

59. Kevelaitis E, Peynet J, Mouas C, et al: Opening of potassium channels. The common cardio-protective link between preconditioning and natural hibernation? *Circulation* 99:3079, 1999.

60. Tomai F, Crea F, Chiariello L, Gioffrè PA: Ischemic preconditioning in humans. Models, mediators and clinical relevance. *Circulation* 100:559, 1999.

61. Gomma AH, Purcell HJ, Fox KM: Potassium channel openers in myocardial ischaemia. Therapeutic potential of nicorandil. *Drugs* 61:1705, 2001.

61a. Kloner RA, Jennings RB: Consequences of brief ischemia: Stunning, preconditioning and their clinical implications. Part 2. *Circulation* 104:3158, 2001.

61b. Suzuki M, Sasaki N, Miki T, et al: Role of sarcolemmal K$_{ATP}$ channels in cardioprotection against ischemia/reperfusion injury in mice. *J Clin Invest* 109:509, 2002.

62. Murry CE, Jennings RB, Reimer KA: Preconditioning with ischemia: A delay of lethal cell injury in ischemic myocardium. *Circulation* 74:1124, 1986.

63. Gross GJ, Auchampach JA: Blockade of ATP sensitive potassium channels prevents myocardial preconditioning in dogs. *Circ Res* 70:223, 1992.

64. Auchampach JA, Grover GJ, Gross GJ: Blockade of ischemic preconditioning in dogs by the novel ATP dependent K$^+$ channel antagonist sodium 5-hydroxydecanoate. *Cardiovasc Res* 26:1054, 1992.

65. Grover GJ, Sleph PG, Dzwonczyk S: Role of myocardial ATP sensitive K$^+$ channels in mediating preconditioning in the dog heart and their possible interaction with adenosine A1 receptor. *Circulation* 86:1310, 1992.

66. Rohmann S, Weygandt H, Schelling P, et al: Effect of bimakalim (EMD 52692), an opener of ATP-sensitive potassium channel, on infarct size, coronary blood flow, regional wall function, and oxygen consumption in swine. *Cardiovasc Res* 28:858, 1994.

67. Toombs CF, Norman NR, Groppi VE, et al: Limitation of myocardial injury with the K$^+$ channel opener cromakalim and the nonvasoactive analog U-89,232: Vascular versus cardiac action in vitro and in vivo. *J Pharmacol Exp Ther* 263:1261, 1992.

68. Grover GJ, Dzwonczyk S, Parham CS, Sleph PG: The protective effects of cromakalim and pinacidil on reperfusion function and infarct size in isolated perfused rat hearts and anesthetized dogs. *Cardiovasc Drug Ther* 4:465, 1990.

69. Wilde AA, Escande D, Schumacher CA, et al: Potassium accumulation in the globally ischemic mammalian heart. A role for the ATP-sensitive potassium channel. *Circ Res* 67:835, 1990.

70. Szewczyk A, Marban E: Mitochondria: a new target for K$^+$ channel openers? *Trends Pharmacol Sci* 20(2):157, 1999.

71. Liu GS, Thornton J, Van Winnie DM, et al: Protection against infarction afforded by preconditioning is mediated by A$_1$ adenosine receptors in rabbit hearts. *Circulation* 84:350, 1991.

72. Liu GS, Downey JM: Acetylcholine preconditions rabbit heart: Further evidence for Gi protein coupling in preconditioning (abstr). *Circulation* 86(Suppl):I-174, 1992.

73. Fossett M, DeWeille JR, Green RD, et al: Antidiabetic sulfonylureas control action potential properties in heart cells via high affinity receptors that are linked to ATP-dependent K$^+$ channels. *J Biol Chem* 263:7933, 1988.

74. Tsuchida A, Miura T, Imura O: Role of adenosine receptor activation in infarct size limitation by preconditioning in the heart (abstr). *Circulation* 84(Suppl II):II-191, 1991.

75. Downey JM, Liu GS Thornton JD: Adenosine and the anti-infarct effects of preconditioning. *Cardiovasc Res* 27:3, 1993.

76. Yao Z, Gross GJ: A comparison of adenosine-induced cardioprotection and ischemic preconditioning in dogs: Efficacy, time course of KATP channels. *Circulation* 89:1229, 1994.

77. Schwarz ER, Mohri M, Sack S, Arras M: The role of adenosine and its A$_1$ receptor in ischemic preconditioning (abstr). *Circulation* 84(Suppl II):II-191, 1991.

78. Li Y, Kloner RA: The cardioprotective effects of ischemic "preconditioning" are not mediated by adenosine receptors in rat hearts. *Circulation* 87:1642, 1993.

79. Auchampach JA, Gross GJ: Adenosine A$_1$ receptors, KATP channels and ischemic preconditioning in dogs: Efficacy, time course, and role of KATP channels. *Am J Physiol* 264:H1327, 1993.

80. Miura T, Yellon DM, Hearse DJ, Downey JM: Determinants of infarct size during permanent occlusion of a coronary artery in the closed chest dog. *J Am Coll Cardiol* 9:647, 1987.

81. Van Winkle DM, Chien GL, Wolff RA, et al: Intra-coronary infusion of R phenyl isoprophyl adenosine prior to ischemia reperfusion reduces myocardial infarct size in swine (abstr). *Circulation* 8(Suppl IV):I-213, 1992.

82. Toombs CF, McGee DS, Johnston WE, Vinten-Johansen J: Protection from ischemic reperfusion injury with adenosine pretreatment is reversed by inhibition of ATP sensitive potassium channels. *Cardiovasc Res* 27:623, 1993.

83. Kirsch GE, Codina J, Birnbaumer L, Brown AM: Coupling of ATP-sensitive K$^+$ channels to A$_1$ receptors by G proteins in rat ventricular myocytes. *Am J Physiol* 259:H820, 1990.

84. Liang BT: Protein kinase C-dependent activation of KATP channel enhances adenosine-induced cardioprotection. *Biochem J* 336(Pt 2):337, 1998.

85. Baxter GF, Marber MS, Patel VC, Yellon DM: Adenosine receptor involvement in a delayed phase of myocardial protection 24 h after ischemic preconditioning. *Circulation* 90:2993, 1994.

86. Baxter GF, Goma FM, Yellon DM: Involvement of protein kinase C in the delayed cytoprotection following sublethal ischaemia in rabbit myocardium. *Br J Pharmacol* 115: 222, 1995.

87. Sato T, Sasaki N, O'Rourke B, Marbán E: Adenosine primes the opening of mitochondrial ATP-sensitive potassium channels. A key step in ischemic preconditioning? *Circulation* 102:800, 2000.

88. Shiki K, Hearse DJ: Preconditioning of ischemic myocardium: Reperfusion induced arrhythmias. *Am J Physiol* 253:H1470, 1987.

89. Thornton JD, Liu GS, Downey JM: Pretreatment with pertussis toxin blocks the protective effect of preconditioning: Evidence for Gi protein mechanism. *J Mol Cell Cardiol* 25:311, 1993.

90. Gross JA, Auchampach JA, Maruyama M, et al: Cardioprotective effects of nicorandil. *J Cardiovasc Pharmacol* 20:S22, 1992.

91. Grover GJ, Newburger J, Sleph PG, et al: Cardioprotective effects of the potassium channel opener cromakalim: Stereo-selectivity and effects on myocardial adenine nucleotides. *J Pharmacol Exp Ther* 257:156, 1991.

92. Grover GJ, McCullough JR, Henry DE, et al: Anti-ischemic effects of the potassium channel activators pinacidil and cromakalim and the reversal of these effects with the K$^+$ channel blocker glyburide. *J Pharmacol Exp Ther* 251:98, 1989.

93. Galinances M, Shattock MJ, Hearse DJ: Effects of potassium channel modulation during global ischemia in isolated rat heart with and without cardioplegia. *Cardiovasc Res* 26:1063, 1992.

94. Cohen NM, Wise RM, Wechsler AS, Damiano RJ: Elective cardiac arrest with a hyperpolarizing adenosine triphosphate sensitive potassium channel opener. *J Thorac Cardiovasc Surg* 106:317, 1993.

95. Ohta H, Jinno Y, Harada K, et al: Cardioprotective effects of KRN 2391 and nicorandil on ischemic dysfunction in perfused rat heart. *Eur J Pharmacol* 204:171, 1991.

96. Tosaki A, Hellegouarch A: Adenosine triphosphate sensitive potassium channel blocking agent ameliorates, but the opening agent aggravates, ischemia reperfusion induced injury. *J Am Coll Cardiol* 23:487, 1994.

97. Picard S, Criniti A, Iwashiro K, et al: Protection of human myocardium in vitro by K$_{ATP}$ activation with low concentrations of bimakalim. *J Cardiovasc Pharmacol* 34:162, 1999.

98. Auchampach JA, Gross GJ: Reduction in myocardial infarct size by the new potassium channel opener bimakalim. *J Cardiovasc Pharmacol* 23:554, 1994.

99. Rohmann S, Weygandt H, Schelling P, et al: Effect of bimakalim (EMD 52692), an opener of ATP sensitive potassium channels, on infarct size, coronary blood flow, regional wall function, and oxygen consumption in swine. *Cardiovasc Res* 28:858, 1994.

100. Yao Z, Mizumura T, Mei DA, Gross GJ: KATP channels and memory of ischemic preconditioning in dogs: Synergism between adenosine and KATP channels. *Am J Physiol* 272:H334, 1997.

101. Yao Z, Gross GJ: Effects of the KATP channel opener bimakalim on coronary blood flow, monophasic action potential duration, and infarct size in dogs. *Circulation* 89:1769, 1994.

102. Pomerantz BJ, Robinson TN, Morrell TD, et al: Selective mitochondrial adenosine triphosphate-sensitive potassium channel activation is sufficient to precondition human myocardium. *J Thorac Cardiovasc Surg* 120:387, 2000.

103. Rowland RT, Cleveland JC, Meng X, et al: A single endotoxin challenge induces delayed myocardial protection against infarction. *J Surg Res* 63(1):193, 1996.

104. Maulik N, Watanabe M, Engelman D, et al: Myocardial adaptation to ischemia by oxidative stress induced by endotoxin. *Am J Physiol* 269:C907, 1995.

105. Ribi E: Beneficial modification of the endotoxin molecule. *J Biol Resp Mod* 3:1, 1984.

106. Weber P, Smart M, Comerford M, et al: Monophosphoryl lipid A mimics both first and second window of ischemic preconditioning and preserves myocardial sarcoplasmic reticular calcium pump. *J Mol Cell Cardiol* 29(6):A233, 1997.

107. Cluff C, Heindel M, Elliott GT: Protection from cardiac ischemia/reperfusion injury after treatment of rabbits with monophosphoryl lipid A is durable. *J Mol Cell Cardiol* 30(6):A80, 1998.

108. Marber MS, Latchman DS, Walker JM, Yellon DM: Cardiac stress protein elevation 24 hours after brief ischemia or heat stress is associated with resistance to myocardial infarction. *Circulation* 88:1264, 1993.

109. Baxter GF, Yellon DM: Time course of delayed myocardial protection after transient adenosine A$_1$-receptor activation in the rabbit. *J Cardiovasc Pharmacol* 29(5):631, 1997.

110. Weber P, Comerford M, Smith J, Elliott GT: Monophosphoryl lipid A (MLA) induces "first window" preconditioning which is blocked by glibenclamide. *J Mol Cell Cardiol* 30(6):A18, 1998.

111. Mei DA, Elliott GT, Gross GJ: KATP channels mediate late preconditioning against infarction produced by monophosphoryl lipid A. *Am J Physiol* 271(40):H2723, 1996.

112. Elliott GT, Comerford ML, Smith JR, Zhao L: Myocardial ischemia/reperfusion protection using monophosphoryl lipid A is abrogated by the ATP-sensitive potassium channel blocker glibenclamide. *Cardiovasc Res* 32:1071, 1996.

113. Janin Y, Qian Y-Z, Hoag JB, et al: Pharmacologic preconditioning with monophosphoryl lipid A is abolished by 5-hydroxydecanoate, a specific inhibitor of the K$_{ATP}$ channel. *Cardiovasc Res* 32(3):337, 1998.

114. Zhao L, Elliott GT: Pharmacologic enhancement of tolerance to ischemic cardiac stress using monophosphoryl lipid A: A comparison with antecedent ischemia. *Ann NY Acad Sci* 874:229, 1999.

115. Yoshida T, Rousou JA, Flack JEI, et al: Induction of iNOS expression by monophosphoryl lipid A: A pharmacological approach of ischemic preconditioning of swine hearts undergoing open heart surgery. *Circulation* 96(8):I620, 1997.

116. Tosaki A, Maulik N, Elliott GT, et al: Preconditioning of rat heart with monophosphoryl lipid A: A role for nitric oxide. *J Pharmacol Exp Ther* 285(3):1274, 1998.

117. Pan J, Burgher KL, Szczepanik AM, Ringheim GE: Tyrosine phosphorylation of inducible nitric oxide synthase: Implications for potential post-translational regulation. *Biochem J* 314(Pt 3):889, 1996.

118. Elliott GT: Monophosphoryl lipid A: A novel agent for inducing pharmacologic myocardial preconditioning. *J Thromb Thrombolysis* 3(3):225, 1996.

119. Gross GJ: Letter to the editor. *Cardiovasc Res* 28:139, 1994.

120. Bray KM, Quast U: A specific binding site for K$^+$ channel openers in rat aorta. *J Biol Chem* 267:1169, 1992.

121. Manley PW, Quast U, Andres H, Bray K: Synthesis and radioligand binding studies with a titrated pinacidil analoT: Receptor interactions of structurally different classes of potassium channel openers and blockers. *J Med Chem* 36:2004, 1993.

122. Dickinson KEJ, Cohen RB, Bryson CC, et al: Characterization of KATP channels in smooth muscle cells and cardiac myocytes with [3H]P-1075. *FASEB J* 7:A354, 1993.

123. Steinberg MI, Ertel P, Smallwood JK, et al: The relation between vascular relaxant and cardiac electrophysiological effects of pinacidil. *J Cardiovasc Pharmacol* 12(Suppl 2):S30, 1988.

124. Conder ML, Normandin DE, Atwal KS, McCullough JR: Evidence for vascular selectivity of the K channel opener BMS 182264. *Biophys J* 61:A250, 1992.

125. Veldkamp MW, VanGinneken ACG, Opthof T, Bouman LN: Action potential shortening in metabolically inhibited ventricular myocytes occurs before the opening of ATP regulated K channels. *Circulation* 88(4 Pt 2):I-293, 1993.

126. Atwal KS, Grover GJ, Ahmed S, et al: Cardioselective anti-ischemic ATP sensitive potassium channel openers. *J Med Chem* 36:3971, 1993.

127. Grover GJ, Parham CS: Protective effects of a cardioselective ATP sensitive potassium channel opener BMS 180448 in 2 stunned myocardium models. *J Am Coll Cardiol* 23:42A, 1994.

128. Grover GJ, Sargent CS, McCullough JR, Atwal KS: In vitro anti-ischemic profile of activity of a novel cardioselective KATP opener, BMS 180448. *Pharmacologist* 35:178, 1993.

129. Katx LB, Giardino EC, Salata JJ, et al: RW 26629, a new potassium channel opener and vascular smooth muscle relaxant: A potential antihypertensive and antianginal agent. *J Pharmacol Exp Ther* 267:648, 1993.

130. Kusumoto K, Awane Y, Kitayoshi T, et al: Antihypertensive and cardiovascular effects of a new potassium channel opener, TCV 295, in rats and dogs. *J Cardiovasc Pharmacol* 24:929, 1994.

131. Gross GJ, Fryer RM: Sarcolemmal versus mitochondrial ATP-sensitive K$^+$ channels and myocardial preconditioning. *Circ Res* 84(9):973, 1999.

132. Miura T, Liu Y, Goto M, et al: Mitochondrial ATP-sensitive K$^+$ channels play a role in cardioprotection by Na$^+$-H$^+$ exchange inhibition against ischemia/reperfusion injury. *J Am Coll Cardiol* 37:957, 2001.

133. Kevelaitis E, Oubénaïssa A, Peynet J, et al: Preconditioning by mitochondrial ATP-sensitive potassium channel openers. An effective approach for improving the preservation of heart transplants. *Circulation* 100(Suppl 9):II-345, 1999.

134. Wang L, Cherednichenko G, Hernandez L, et al: Preconditioning limits mitochondrial Ca^{2+} during ischemia in rat hearts: Role of K$_{ATP}$ channels. *Am J Physiol* 280:H2321, 2001.

135. Sanada S, Kitakaze M, Asanuma H, et al: Role of mitochondrial and sarcolemmal K$_{ATP}$ channels in ischemic preconditioning of the canine heart. *Am J Physiol* 280:H256, 2001.

136. Kowaltowski AJ, Seetharaman S, Paucek P, Garlid KD: Bioenergetic consequences of opening the ATP-sensitive K$^+$ channel of heart mitochondria. *Am J Physiol* 280:H649, 2001.

137. Grover GS, D'Alonso AJ, Parham CS, Darbenzio RB: Cardioprotection with the KATP channel opener cromakalim is not correlated with ischemic myocardial action potential duration. *J Cardiovasc Pharmacol* 26:145, 1995.

138. Inoue I, Nagase H, Kishi K, Higuti T: ATP-sensitive K$^+$ channel in the mitochondrial inner membrane. *Nature* 352:244, 1991.

139. Paucek P, Mironova G, Mahdi F, et al: Reconstitution and partial purification of the glibenclamide-sensitive ATP-dependent K$^+$ channel from rat liver and beef heart mitochondria. *J Biol Chem* 267:26062, 1992.

140. Holmuhamedov EL, Jovanovic S, Dzeja PP, et al: Mitochondrial ATP-sensitive K$^+$ channels modulate cardiac mitochondrial function. *Am J Physiol* 275:H1567, 1998.

141. Garlid K, Paucek P, Yarov-Yarovoy V, et al: Cardioprotective effect of diazoxide and its interaction with mitochondrial ATP-sensitive K$^+$ channels: Possible mechanism of cardioprotection. *Circ Res* 81:1072, 1997.

142. Liu Y, Sato T, O'Rourke B, Marban E: Mitochondrial ATP-dependent potassium channels: Novel effectors of cardioprotection? *Circulation* 97:2463, 1998.

143. Wang S, Cone J, Liu Y: Dual roles of mitochondrial K$_{ATP}$ channels in diazoxide-mediated protection in isolated rabbit hearts. *Am J Physiol* 280:H246, 2001.

144. Sato T, O'Rourke B, Marban E: Modulation of mitochondrial ATP-dependent K$^+$ channels by protein kinase C. *Circ Res* 83:110, 1998.

145. Liu Y, Ytrehus K, Downey J: Evidence that translocation of protein kinase C is a key event during ischemic preconditioning of rabbit myocardium. *J Mol Cell Cardiol* 26:661, 1994.

146. Sato T, Sasaki N, O'Rourke B, Marbán E: Nicorandil, a potent cardioprotective agent, acts by opening mitochondrial ATP-dependent potassium channels. *J Am Coll Cardiol* 35:514, 2000.

147. Billman GE, Englert HC, Scholkens BA: HMR 1883, a novel cardioselective inhibitor of the ATP-sensitive potassium channel. Part II: Effects on susceptibility to ventricular fibrillation induced by myocardial ischemia in conscious dogs. *J Pharmacol Exp Ther* 286:1465, 1998.

148. Colatsky TJ, Follmer CH, Starmer CF: Channel specificity in antiarrhythmic drug action. Mechanism of potassium channel block and its role in suppressing and aggravating cardiac arrhythmias. *Circulation* 82:2235, 1990.

149. Lynch JJ Jr, Sanguinetti MC, Kimura S, Bassett AL: Therapeutic potential of modulating K currents in the diseased myocardium. *FASEB J* 6:2952, 1992.

150. Antzelevitch C, DiDiego JM: Role of K channel activators in cardiac electrophysiology and arrhythmias. *Circulation* 85:1627, 1992.

151. Wilde AAM: Role of ATP sensitive K$^+$ channel current in ischemic arrhythmias. *Cardiovasc Drug Ther* 7 (Suppl 3):521, 1993.

152. de la Coussaye JE, Eledjam JJ, Bruelle P, et al: Electrophysiologic and arrhythmogenic effects of the K$^+$ channel agonist BRL 38227 in anesthetized dogs. *J Cardiovasc Pharmacol* 22:722, 1993.

153. Spinelli W, Follmer C, Parsons R, Colatsky T: Effects of cromakalim, pinacidil and nicorandil on cardiac refractoriness and arterial pressure in open chest dogs. *Eur J Pharmacol* 179:243, 1990.

154. Padrini R, Bova S, Cargnelli G, et al: Effects of pinacidil on guinea pig isolated perfused heart with particular reference to the proarrhythmic effect. *Br J Pharmacol* 105:715, 1992.

155. Chi L, Uprichard ACG, Lucchesi BR: Profibrillatory actions of pinacidil in a conscious canine model of sudden coronary death. *J Cardiovasc Pharmacol* 15:452, 1990.

156. Lu H, Remeysen P, DeClerck F: The protection by ischemic preconditioning against myocardial ischemia and reperfusion induced arrhythmias is not mediated by ATP sensitive K channels in rats. *Coron Artery Dis* 4:649, 1993.

157. D'Alonzo AJ, Grover GJ: Potassium channel openers are unlikely to be proarrhythmic in the diseased human heart. *Cardiovasc Res* 28:924, 1994.

158. Spinelli W, Colatsky TJ: Proarrhythmic potential of the potassium channel openers. *Cardiovasc Res* 28:926, 1994.

159. D'Alonzo AJ, Grover GJ, Darbenzio RB, et al: Hemodynamic and cardiac effects of BMS-180448, a novel K$^+$ATP opener, in anesthetized dogs and isolated rat hearts. *Pharmacology* 52(2):101, 1996.

160. Grover GJ, D'Alonzo AJ, Garlid KD, et al: Pharmacologic characterization of BMS-191095, a mitochondrial K(ATP) with no peripheral vasodilator or cardiac action potential shortening activity. *J Pharmacol Exp Ther* 297(3):1184, 2001.

161. Remme CA, Wilde AA: KATP channel openers, myocardial ischemia, and arrhythmias—should the electrophysiologist worry? *Cardiovasc Drugs Ther* 14(1):21, 2000.

162. Patel DJ, Purcell HJ, Fox KM: Cardioprotection by opening of the KATP channel in unstable angina. *Eur Heart J* 20:51, 1999.

163. Kobayashi Y, Miyata A, Tanno K, et al: Effects of nicorandil, a potassium channel opener, on idiopathic ventricular tachycardia. *J Am Coll Cardiol* 32:1377, 1998.

164. Yamashita N, Hoshida S, Otsu K, et al: Monophosphoryl lipid A provides biphasic cardioprotection against ischemia-reperfusion injury in rat hearts. *Br J Pharmacol* 128(2): 412, 1999.

165. Goldberg MR: Clinical pharmacology of pinacidil, a prototype for drugs that affect potassium channels. *J Cardiovasc Pharmacol* 12(Suppl. 2):S41, 1988.

166. Robert E, Delye B, Aya G, et al: Comparison of proarrhythmogenic effects of two potassium channel openers, levcromakalim (BRL 38227) and nicorandil (RP 46417): A high-resolution mapping study on rabbit heart. *J Cardiovasc Pharmacol* 29(1):109, 1997.

167. Coetzee WA, Wells T, Avkiran M: Anti-arrhythmic effects of levcromakalim in the ischaemic rat heart: A dual mechanism of action? *Eur J Pharmacol* 402(3):263, 2000.

168. Scholz W, Albus U: Potential of selective sodium-hydrogen exchange inhibitors in cardiovascular therapy. *Cardiovasc Res* 29:184, 1995.

169. Scholz W, Albus U: Na$^+$/H$^+$ exchange and its inhibition in cardiac ischemia and reperfusion. *Basic Res Cardiol* 88:443, 1993.

170. Karmazyn M, Sostaric JV, Gan XT: The myocardial Na$^+$/H$^+$ exchanger: A potential therapeutic target for the prevention of myocardial ischaemic and reperfusion injury and attenuation of postinfarction heart failure. *Drugs* 61(3):375, 2001.

171. Buhagiar KA, Hansen PS, Bewick N, Rasmussen HH: Protein kinase C epsilon contributes to regulation of the sarcolemmal Na$^+$-K$^+$ pump. *Am J Physiol* 50:C1059, 2001.

172. Wakabayashi S, Shigekawa M, Pouyssegur J: Molecular physiology of vertebrate Na$^+$/H$^+$ exchangers. *Physiol Rev* 77:51, 1997.

173. Orlowski J, Grinstein S: Na$^+$/H$^+$ exchangers of mammalian cells. *J Biol Chem* 272:22373, 1997.

174. Numata M, Petrecca K, Lake N, Orlowski J: Identification of a mitochondrial Na$^+$/H$^+$ exchanger. *J Biol Chem* 273:6951, 1998.

175. Nass R, Rao R: Novel localization of a Na$^+$/H$^+$ exchanger in a late endosomal compartment of yeast. Implications for vacuole biogenesis. *J Biol Chem* 273:21054, 1998.

176. Orlowski J, Kandasamy RA: Delineation of transmembrane domains of the Na$^+$/H$^+$ exchanger that confer sensitivity to pharmacological antagonists. *J Biol Chem* 271:19922, 1996.

177. Orlowski J, Kandasamy RA, Shull GE: Molecular cloning of putative members of the Na/H exchanger gene family. cDNA cloning, deduced amino acid sequence, and mRNA tissue expression of the rat Na/H exchanger NHE-1 and 2 structurally related proteins. *J Biol Chem* 267:9331, 1992.

178. Kinsella JL, Heller P, Froehlich JP: Na$^+$/H$^+$ exchanger: proton modifier site regulation of activity. *Biochem Cell Biol* 76:753, 1998.

179. Bianchini L, Pouyssegus J: Regulation of the Na$^+$/H$^+$ exchanger isoform NHE1: role of phosphorylation. *Kidney Int* 49:1038, 1996.

180. Petrecca K, Atanasiu R, Grinstein S, et al: Subcellular localization of the Na$^+$/H$^+$ exchanger NHE1 in rat myocardium. *Am J Physiol* 276:H709, 1999.

181. Wu ML, Vaughan-Jones RD: Interaction between Na$^+$ and H$^+$ ions on Na-H exchange in sheep cardiac Purkinje fibers. *J Mol Cell Cardiol* 29:1131, 1997.

182. Woo SH, Lee CO: Effects of endothelin-1 on Ca^{2+} signaling in guinea pig ventricular myocytes: Role of protein kinase C. *J Mol Cell Cardiol* 31:631, 1999.

183. Gunasegaram S, Haworth RS, Hearse DJ, Avkiran M: Regulation of sarcolemmal Na$^+$/H$^+$ exchanger activity by angiotensin II in adult rat ventricular myocytes: Opposing actions via AT$_1$ versus AT$_2$ receptors. *Circ Res* 85:919, 1999.

184. Yokoyama H, Yasutake M, Avkiran M: α_1-Adrenergic stimulation of sarcolemmal Na$^+$-H$^+$ exchanger activity in rat ventricular myocytes: Evidence for selective mediation by the α_{1A}-adreno receptor subtype. *Circ Res* 82:1078, 1998.

185. Yasutake M, Haworth RS, King A, Avkiran M: Thrombin activates the sarcolemmal Na$^+$-H$^+$ exchanger: Evidence for a receptor-mediated mechanism involving protein kinase C. *Circ Res* 79:705, 1996.

186. Wakabayashi S, Fafournoux P, Sardet C, Pouyssegur J: The Na$^+$/H$^+$ antiporter cytoplasmic domain mediates growth factor signals and controls "H($^+$)-sensing". *Proc Natl Acad Sci U S A* 89:2424, 1992.

187. Bianchini L, L'Allemain G, Pouyssegur J: The p42/p44 mitogen-activated protein kinase cascade is determinant in mediating activation of the Na$^+$/H$^+$ exchanger (NHE1 isoform) in response to growth factors. *J Biol Chem* 272:271, 1996.

188. Counillon L, Pouyssegur J: Structure-function studies and molecular regulation of the growth factor activatable sodium-hydrogen exchanger (NHE-1). *Cardiovasc Res* 29:147, 1995.

189. Allen DG, Orchard CH: Myocardial contractile function during ischemia and hypoxia. *Circ Res* 60:153, 1987.

190. Fliegel L, Frohlich O: The Na\H exchanger: An update on structure, regulation and cardiac physiology. *Biochem J* 296:273, 1993.

191. Sabri A, Byron KL, Samarel AM, et al: Hydrogen peroxide activates mitogen-activated protein kinases and Na$^+$-H$^+$ exchange in neonatal rat cardiac myocytes. *Circ Res* 82:1053, 1998.

192. Hoque ANE, Haist JV, Karmazyn M: Na$^+$-H$^+$ exchange inhibition protects against mechanical, ultrastructural, and biochemical impair-

ment induced by low concentrations of lysophospha-tidylcholine in isolated rat hearts. *Circ Res* 80:95, 1997.

193. Cross HR, Lu L, Steenbergen C, et al: Overexpression of the cardiac Na$^+$/Ca^{2+} exchanger increases susceptibility to ischemia/reperfusion injury in male, but not female, transgenic mice. *Circ Res* 83:1215, 1998.

194. Soleimani M, Singh G: Physiologic and molecular aspects of the Na$^+$/H$^+$ exchangers in health and disease processes. *J Invest Med* 43(5):419, 1995.

195. Gan XT, Chakrabarti S, Karmazyn M: Modulation of Na$^+$/H$^+$ exchange isoform 1 mRNA expression in isolated rat hearts. *Am J Physiol* 277:H993, 1999.

196. Kleyman TR, Cragoe EJ: Amiloride and its analogs as tools in the study of ion transport. *J Membr Biol* 105:1, 1988.

197. Vigne P, Frelin C, Cragoe EJ, Lazdunski M: Structure activity relationships of amiloride and certain of its analogues in relation to the blockade of the Na/H exchange system. *Mol Pharmacol* 25:131, 1983.

198. Mahnensmith RL, Aronson PS: The plasma membrane sodium-hydrogen exchanger and its role in physiological and pathophysiological processes. *Circ Res* 56:773, 1985.

199. Duff HJ, Mitchell LB, Kavanagh KM, et al: Amiloride: Antiarrhythmic and electrophysiologic actions in patients with inducible sustained ventricular tachycardia. *Circulation* 79(6):1257, 1989.

200. Yano K, Maruyama T, Makino N, et al: Effects of amiloride on the mechanical, electrical and biochemical aspects of ischemic-reperfusion injury. *Mol Cell Biochem* 121:75, 1993.

201. Duff HJ, Lester NM, Rohmberg M: Amiloride. Antiarrhythmic and electrophysiological activity in the dog. *Circulation* 78:1469, 1988.

202. Smart SC, LoCurto A, Schultz JE, et al: Intra-coronary amiloride prevents contractile dysfunction of postischemic "stunned" myocardium. Role of hemodynamic alterations and inhibition of Na$^+$/H$^+$ exchange and L-type Ca^{2+} channels. *J Am Coll Cardiol* 26:1365, 1995.

203. Meng HP, Maddaford TG, Pierce GN: Effect of amiloride and selected analogues on postischemic recovery of cardiac contractile function. *Am J Physiol* 264:H1831, 1993.

204. Karmazyn M, Ray M, Haist JV: Comparative effects of Na$^+$/H$^+$ exchange against cardiac injury produced by ischemia/reperfusion, hypoxia/regeneration and the calcium paradox. *J Cardiovasc Pharmacol* 21:172, 1993.

205. Kovar A, Peters T, Beier N, Derendorf H: Pharmacokinetic/ pharmacodynamic evaluation of the NHE inhibitor eniporide. *J Clin Pharmacol* 41:139, 2001.

206. Kusumoto K, Haist JV, Karmazyn M: Na$^+$/H$^+$ exchange inhibition reduces hypertrophy and heart failure after myocardial infarction in rats. *Am J Physiol* 280:H738, 2001.

207. Schäfer C, Ladilov YV, Schäfer M, Piper HM: Inhibition of NHE protects reoxygenated cardiomyocytes independently of anoxic Ca^{2+} overload and acidosis. *Am J Physiol* 279:H2143, 2000.

208. Fukuhiro Y, Wowk M, Ou R, et al: Cardioplegic strategies for calcium control. Low Ca^{2+}, high Mg^{2+}, citrate, or Na$^+$/H$^+$ exchange inhibitor HOE-642. *Circulation* 102(Suppl III):III-319, 2000.

209. Humphreys RA, Haist JV, Chakrabarti S, et al: Orally administered NHE1 inhibitor cariporide reduces acute responses to coronary occlusion and reperfusion. *Am J Physiol* 276:H749, 1999.

210. Symons JD, Correa SD, Schaefer S: Na$^+$/H$^+$ exchange inhibition with cariporide limits functional impairment caused by repetitive ischemia. *J Cardiovasc Pharmacol* 32:853, 1998.

211. Kim Y-IL, Herijgers P, Laycock SK, et al: Na$^+$/H$^+$ exchange inhibition improves long-term myocardial preservation. *Ann Thorac Surg* 66:436, 1998.

212. Strömer H, deGroot MC, Horn M, et al: Na$^+$/H$^+$ exchange inhibition with HOE 642 improves postischemic recovery due to attenuation of Ca^{2+} overload and prolonged acidosis on reperfusion. *Circulation* 101:2749, 2000.

212a. Loennechen JP, Wisloff U, Falck G, et al: Effects of cariporide and losartan on hypertrophy, calcium transients, contractility, and gene expression in congestive heart failure. *Circulation* 105:1380, 2002.

213. Wang D, Balkovetz DF, Warnock DG: Mutational analysis of transmembrane histidines in the amiloride-sensitive Na$^+$/H$^+$ exchanger. *Am J Physiol* 269:C392, 1995.

214. Theroux P, Chaitman BR, Danchin N, et al: Inhibition of the sodium-hydrogen exchanger with cariporide to prevent myocardial infarction

in high-risk ischemic situations: main results of the GUARDIAN trial. *Circulation* 102:3032, 2000.

215. Yellon DM, Baxter GF: Sodium-hydrogen exchange in myocardial reperfusion injury (commentary). *Lancet* 356:522, 2000.

216. Rupprecht HJ, vom Dahl J, Terres W, et al: Cardioprotective effects of the Na$^+$/H$^+$ exchange inhibitor cariporide in patients with acute anterior myocardial infarction undergoing direct PTCA. *Circulation* 101:2902, 2000.

217. Zeymer U, Suryapranata H, Monassier JP, et al for the ESCAMI Investigators: The Na$^+$/H$^+$ exchange inhibitor eniporide as an adjunct to early reperfusion therapy for acute myocardial infarction. Results of the Evaluation of the Safety and Cardioprotective Effects of Eniporide in Acute Myocardial Infarction (ESCAMI) Trial. *J Am Coll Cardiol* 38:1644, 2001.

217a. Avkiran M, Marber MS: Na$^+$/H$^+$ exchange inhibitors for cardioprotective therapy: Progress, problems, and prospect. *J Am Coll Card* 39:747, 2002.

218. Menown IB, Adgey AAJ: Cardioprotective therapy and sodium-hydrogen exchange inhibition: current concepts and future goals (editorial comment). *J Am Coll Cardiol* 38:1651, 2001.

219. Knight DR, Smith AH, Flynn DM, et al: A novel sodium-hydrogen exchanger isoform-1 inhibitor, zoniporide, reduces ischemic myocardial injury in vitro and in vivo. *J Pharmacol Exp Ther* 297:254, 2001.

220. Yamamoto S, Matsui K, Kitano M, Ohashi N: SM-20550, a new Na$^+$/H$^+$ exchange inhibitor and its cardioprotective effect in ischemic/reperfused isolated rat hearts by preventing Ca^{2+} overload. *J Cardiovasc Pharmacol* 35:855, 2000.

221. Karmazyn M: The role of the myocardial sodium-hydrogen exchanger in mediating ischemic and reperfusion injury. From amiloride to cariporide. *Ann NY Acad Sci* 874: 326, 1999.

222. Gumina RJ, Beier N, Schelling P, Gross GJ: Inhibitors of ischemic preconditioning do not attenuate Na$^+$/H$^+$ exchange inhibitor mediated cardioprotection. *J Cardiovasc Pharmacol* 35:949, 2000.

223. Avkiran M: Protection of the myocardium during ischemia and reperfusion. Na$^+$/H$^+$ exchange inhibition versus ischemic preconditioning. *Circulation* 100:2469, 1999.

224. Shipolini AR, Yokoyama H, Galinanes M, et al: Na$^+$/H$^+$ exchanger activity does not contribute to protection by ischemic preconditioning in the isolated rat heart. *Circulation* 96:3617, 1997.

225. Gumina RJ, Mizumura T, Beier N, et al: A new sodium/hydrogen exchange inhibitor, EMD 85131, limits infarct size in dogs when administered before or after coronary artery occlusion. *J Pharmacol Exp Ther* 286:175, 1998.

226. Gumina RJ, Buerger E, Eickmeier C, et al: Inhibition of Na$^+$/H$^+$ exchanger confers greater cardioprotection against 90 minutes of myocardial ischemia than ischemic preconditioning in dogs. *Circulation* 100:2519, 1999.

227. Duff HJ, Brown E, Cragoe EJ, Rohmberg M: Antiarrhythmic activity of amiloride: mechanisms. *J Cardiol Pharmacol* 17:879, 1991.

228. Harper IS, Bond JM, Chacon E, et al: Inhibition of NHE preserves viability, restores mechanical function and prevents the pH paradox in reperfusion injury to rat neonatal myocytes. *Basic Res Cardiol* 88:430, 1993.

CHAPTER 29

Serotonin and Its Antagonists in Cardiovascular Disease

William J. Elliott

William H. Frishman

Various circulating substances are involved in blood pressure control in human beings, and among these the effects of serotonin are now well recognized. Its importance in human hypertension and other cardiovascular disorders was not appreciated initially, as serotonin antagonism induced by various chemical substances affected blood pressure in conflicting ways. The recent discovery of serotonin receptor subtypes has rekindled interest in examining serotonin antagonism as a pharmacologic approach for treating cardiovascular disease.[1]

In this chapter the cardiovascular effects of serotonin are reviewed, and potential pharmacologic therapies involving serotonin antagonism are discussed.

SEROTONIN RECEPTOR SUBTYPES AND CLASSIFICATION SCHEMES

Serotonin (5-hydroxytryptamine, often abbreviated "5-HT") is a naturally occurring monoamine with many different cardiovascular effects, even when administered at an identical dose within the same arterial segment. As with dopamine, the direct effects of serotonin and its agonists in the cardiovascular system can be most easily explained by their actions on different receptors.[2] Unlike dopamine, which activates, in sequence with increasing doses, dopamine-1, dopamine-2, and then other receptors, specific serotonin receptors exist in many different subtypes that are activated by serotonin and few other natural agonists.[3] Serotonin receptors have been classified in several distinct schemes.[4] The most comprehensive (see Table 29-1) attempts to integrate operational pharmacology (using experimental results with various agonists and antagonists) and molecular biology (especially cloning studies). Some authors[5,6] prefer using the prefix "S" rather than "5-HT" to identify and subgroup serotonin receptors, but the terminology is otherwise interchangeable.[1] This classification scheme has special relevance for the central nervous system (CNS), in which serotonin serves as a major neurotransmitter and has many important effects, many of which are amenable to pharmacologic manipulation.[7] An older system that characterized receptors by their affinity for classic pharmacologic antagonists[8] ("D" = Dibenzyline or phenoxybenzamine, "M" = morphine) has been largely replaced; "D" receptors are classified in the 5-HT$_{2A}$ family and "M" receptors belong to the 5-HT$_3$ family.

The diverse effects of serotonin and its several agonists and antagonists are perhaps best understood by reference to the seven known subfamilies of 5-HT-receptors. In the cardiovascular system, the various subtypes of the 5-HT$_1$- and 5HT$_2$-receptors are the most important (Table 29-1). The 5-HT$_3$ and 5-HT$_4$ subfamilies also have defined pharmacologic functions in the CNS and especially in the gastrointestinal system. Recent work with ondansetron and several analogues have made these the drugs of choice for preventing chemotherapy-induced nausea and vomiting. The 5-HT$_5$ through 5-HT$_7$ receptor subfamilies have been cloned, but their physiologic and pharmacologic roles are still unclear, since no agonists or antagonists have yet been identified. More such subfamilies are likely to be discovered as the Human Genome Project nears completion.

The 5-HT$_1$-receptors have five subtypes, of which the 1A and 1D are the most important in cardiovascular medicine. The synthesis and release of dilating substances from vascular endothelium is increased through the 5-HT$_1$ receptor, which eventually leads to local vasodilation. In addition, stimulation of the 5-HT$_1$ receptor inhibits adrenergic neurotransmission, leading to decreased norepinephrine transmission and eventually vasodilation. When vascular smooth muscle is exposed to serotonin, the 5-HT$_1$ receptor mediates at least some of the direct vasodilation that results. In the cerebral circulation, stimulation of 5-HT$_{1D}$ receptors results in vasoconstriction, and is the reported mechanism by which 5HT$_1$ agonists (eletriptan, rizatriptan, almotriptan frovatriptan, naratriptan, sumatriptan, zolmitriptan) relieve migraine headache.[9,10]

The cardiovascular responses of the 5-HT$_2$ receptors have been much more elegantly and thoroughly characterized, primarily because more specific and more powerful antagonists and agonists exist for this receptor subtype. The primary direct effect of serotonin involving the 5-HT$_{2A}$ receptors is vasoconstriction. In addition, platelet aggregation is enhanced when 5-HT$_{2A}$ receptors are activated, leading to an increase in thrombus formation from both platelet clumps and narrowed blood vessels. Somewhat later than either of these two effects, other vasoconstricting agents are also produced, probably also through stimulation of the 5-HT$_{2A}$ receptor; so far, prostaglandin F$_{2a}$, norepinephrine, angiotensin II, histamine, and thromboxanes have all been found to increase locally after stimulation of the 5-HT$_{2A}$ receptor.

CARDIOVASCULAR EFFECTS OF SEROTONIN

The classic, immediate response of many large blood vessels to most concentrations of serotonin is vasoconstriction. These effects are most obvious in the splanchnic, renal, pulmonary, and especially cerebral arteries as well as in some precapillary vessels. In many arterioles and large veins, however, there is often vasodilation due

TABLE 29-1. Subtypes of Serotonin [5-Hydroxytryptamine ("5-HT")] Receptors

Serotonin Receptor Subtype	Intron?	Second Messenger	Tissue of Interest	Function	Agonist	Antagonist
1A (5-HT$_{1A}$)	No	↓ Adenylate cyclase	Raphe nucleus, hippocampus	Autoreceptor	8-OH-DPAT, Flesinoxan	WAY 100135, Sprioxatrine
1B* (5-HT$_{1B}$)	No	↓ Adenylate cyclase	Subiculum, substantia nigra	Autoreceptor	CP 93129	None
1D (5-HT$_{1D}$)	No	↓ Adenylate cyclase	Cerebral blood vessels	Vasoconstriction	Sumatriptan and analogues	None
1E (5-HT$_{1E}$)	No	↓ Adenylate cyclase	Cortex, striatum	Unknown	None	None
1F† (5-HT$_{1F}$)	No	↓ Adenylate cyclase	Brain and peripheral nervous system	Unknown	None	None
2A (5-HT$_{2A}$)	Yes	↑ Phospholipase C	Platelets, vascular and other smooth muscle(s)	Aggregation, contraction	α-Methyl-5-HT, DOI	Ketanserin, Ritanserin, LY53857, MDL 100,907
2B (5-HT$_{2B}$)	Yes	↑ Phospholipase C	Gastric fundus	Contraction	α-Methyl-5-HT, DOI	LY53857
2C (5-HT$_{2C}$)	Yes	↑ Phospholipase C	Choroidal plexus	Unknown	α-Methyl-5-HT, DOI	LY53857, Mesulergine
3 (5-HT$_3$)	Yes	Ligand-sensitive ion channel	Peripheral nerves, area postrema	Neuronal excitation	2-Methyl-5-HT	Ondansetron and analogues
4 (5-HT$_4$)	Yes	↑ Adenylate cyclase	Hippocampus, gastrointestinal tract	Neuronal excitation	Renzapride; 5-methoxytryptamine	GR 113808
5A (5-HT$_{5A}$)	Yes	Unknown	Hippocampus	Unknown	None	None
5B (5-HT$_{5B}$)	Yes	Unknown	Unknown	Unknown	None	None
6 (5-HT$_6$)	Yes	↑ Adenylate cyclase	Striatum	Unknown	None	None
7 (5-HT$_7$)	Yes	↑ Adenylate cyclase	Hypothalamus, intestines	Unknown	None	None

8-OH-DPAT = 8-hydroxy-(2-N,N-dipropylamine)-tetralin; DOI = 1-(2,5-dimethoxy-4-iodophenyl)isopropylamine. Other abbreviations refer to proprietary compounds currently in development.

Source: Adapted and updated with permission from Sanders-Bush.[3]

to locally-produced nitric oxide (and possibly other endothelium-derived relaxing factors[11]) and blockade of norepinephrine release from sympathetic nerves. A few seconds later, the same vessels sometimes contract, in response to the local increase in vasoconstrictor substances listed above.

The effects of serotonin on the contracting heart and its innervation are also complex. Usually, serotonin has positive inotropic and chronotropic effects on intact hearts, resulting in increased pulse rate, stroke volume, and cardiac output. These findings have recently been seen in both normotensive and hypertensive humans.[12] These effects, however, may be moderated or even obviated by simultaneous stimulation of afferent nerves from baroreceptors and chemoreceptors. Extreme bradycardia and hypotension after serotonin administration has been attributed to its effects on the vagus nerve (the "Bezold-Jarisch reflex"). Thus the final result of serotonin's effects on the cardiovascular system is often difficult to predict, as there is a delicate balance between direct cardiac effects of serotonin and the combined effects of autonomic and reflex responses to it.

Effects of Serotonin in Hypertension and Atherosclerosis

Apart from serotonin's effects on platelets that increase thrombus formation, much work in both laboratory animals and humans

has implicated serotonin in the altered vascular responses seen in hypertension, atherosclerosis, and more diseased blood vessels.[13,14] After atherosclerotic deposits in blood vessels reduce flow, many organs develop collateral circulation to overcome the relative ischemia. These collateral vessels are often exquisitely sensitive to the vasoconstrictive effects of serotonin.[15] Enhanced vasoconstriction to serotonin is also a characteristic of atherosclerotic vessels from monkeys, humans, and rats; some authorities believe this is an integral part of the endothelial dysfunction seen during "vascular remodeling" and repair of sick vessels.[16] In coronary heart disease, increased frequency of vasospastic angina has been correlated with increased serum levels of serotonin[17]; impairment of serotonin-mediated release of nitric oxide is thus implicated in the pathophysiology of angina pectoris. Altered reactivity to serotonin has also been seen in the infarct-related arteries of patients with recent myocardial infarction.[18]

Perhaps analogous to these observations, altered sensitivity of blood vessels to serotonin has also been seen in hypertensive patients. Both hypertensive and elderly patients have a more exuberant constrictive response to exogenous serotonin and appear to have lost some of the vasodilatory response seen in normotensive or younger individuals. Although the mechanism is unclear, the loss of the intact endothelial lining containing 5-HT$_1$ receptors and the enzymatic machinery that produces nitric oxide may be part of the explanation. Hypertensive patients also have diminished platelet levels of serotonin, suggesting increased release of serotonin in the peripheral circulation, which would lead to further local vasoconstriction and platelet aggregation.[19] Peripheral monoamine oxidase also appears to be somewhat less efficient in hypertensive patients compared to normotensive controls, leading to impaired clearance of free serotonin from blood in hypertensives.[20] Last, serotonin stimulates aldosterone production in both rats and humans,[21] which may further exacerbate salt and water retention in hypertensives.[22]

Many of the better-known effects of serotonin occur in the CNS, which may also be true in hypertension. Careful studies in rats have identified serotoninergic neurons in the raphe nucleus that probably contain 5-HT$_{1A}$ receptors. When very small amounts of serotonin or a 5-HT$_{1A}$ agonist are injected into these areas, neuronal uptake is quickly followed by major increases in blood pressure, which can be blocked by methylsergide, as well as tachycardia and increased renal sympathetic nerve activity.[23] Elaborate studies in rats have suggested that some of the actions of centrally acting antihypertensive drugs (e.g., clonidine, methyldopa) may be mediated through serotonin-related pathways.

Although the pathophysiology is probably complex, serotonin has been linked both epidemiologically and genetically to hypertension, atherosclerosis, and coronary heart disease events. In a study of 121 consecutive male patients undergoing cardiac catheterization, high serotonin levels ($\geq$1000 nmol/L) were associated not only with angiographically proven coronary disease (odds ratio: 3.4, 95% confidence interval 1.2–9.8, $P = .024$), even after adjustment for traditional risk factors, but also with the incidence rate of cardiac events (death, myocardial infarction, or unstable angina).[24] Whether this is related somehow to an insertion/deletion polymorphism of the promoter region of the serotonin transporter gene (HTT,SLC6A4) is unclear, but that genotype has been linked to higher cholesterol levels and heart disease in several groups of older people.[25]

SPECIFIC SEROTONIN ANTAGONISTS

Ketanserin

Ketanserin (Sufrexal, Janssen Pharmaceutica, Beerse, Belgium) has served as the focal point for much of the recent research exploring the use of serotonin antagonists in hypertension and other diseases. It was the first serotonin antagonist to be developed for use in humans and has been approved for hypertension in several European countries, Argentina, the Philippines, and Thailand. One long-term clinical trial assessing vascular events using ketanserin has been completed,[26] but the interpretation of the results is controversial.

Ketanserin has complex pharmacologic properties. It is a very potent antagonist at 5-HT$_{2A}$ receptors; is somewhat less potent at blocking 5-HT$_{2C}$ receptors; and has little (if any) activity at the various 5-HT$_1$, 5-HT$_3$, or 5-HT$_4$ receptors. In addition, it has high affinity for alpha$_1$-adrenergic receptors and for histamine H$_1$-receptors.[27] Although controversial, some believe that some, if not much, of its acute efficacy in otherwise normal hypertensive humans is due to its effect as an alpha blocker. The simplest evidence comes from a study of 30 hypertensive patients who received 10 mg of intravenous ketanserin, which lowered their mean arterial pressure by 22%. After pretreatment with the alpha$_1$-adrenergic blocker prazosin (12 mg/day), the blood pressure–lowering effect was blunted.[28] In sheep, pretreatment with prazosin abolished the hypotensive response to ketanserin.[29] On the other hand, ketanserin had a significant hypotensive effect in four normotensive patients with autonomic insufficiency due to an efferent sympathetic

lesion who were otherwise unresponsive to phentolamine (20 mg intravenously).[28]

The CNS effects of ketanserin on blood pressure are also complex and may also involve alpha-adrenergic receptors. The primary reasons to invoke a central effect of ketanserin on blood pressure are the lack of reflex tachycardia (which would be expected with any peripheral vasodilator) and the frequent side effects of fatigue, sedation, and sleep disturbance (usually attributed to CNS penetration of any drug). Ketanserin and clonidine share the ability to alter electroencephalograms (EEGs), suggesting a similar central mechanism.[30] In cats, both ketanserin and prazosin produced similar inhibition of sympathetic nerve discharge (measured from the inferior cardiac nerve), and pretreatment with one prevented a further change after administration of the other.[31] In elegant radioactive ligand–binding studies, competition experiments in pig and human brain tissues between ketanserin and compounds that selectively label alpha$_1$-adrenoreceptors was essentially complete, suggesting a limited role for central 5-HT$_2$ receptors as a part of ketanserin's mechanism of action.

Ketanserin has many pharmacokinetic properties that are desirable for a chronic antihypertensive agent. Its onset of action is gradual, and its plasma elimination half-life is 12 to 25 h. Most of the chronic treatment studies, however, have used twice-daily dosing, perhaps because the drug was initially developed in the early 1980s, when once-daily dosing was not as important a consideration. It is about 50% bioavailable after oral administration and is primarily cleared by hepatic metabolism.

Ketanserin for Systemic Hypertension

The antihypertensive efficacy of ketanserin is now well researched, with more than 5000 patients in placebo-controlled studies.[32] At equivalent doses, it has little antihypertensive effect in normotensive individuals. It is effective both orally (in typical doses of 20 to 80 mg twice daily) and intravenously (typically in a 10-mg loading dose followed by 2 to 4 mg/h). It appears to be more effective in the elderly than in younger patients but may lower diastolic more than systolic pressure. In direct comparative studies, ketanserin 40 mg twice daily had a blood pressure–lowering effect similar to that of metoprolol 200 mg/day, propranolol 160 mg/day, captopril 100 mg/day, enalapril 20 mg/day, or hydrochlorothiazide 50 mg/day. At 20 to 40 mg twice daily, ketanserin may be less effective as monotherapy than nifedipine 20 mg twice daily[33] but more effective than methyldopa 250 to 500 twice daily.[34] Like other antihypertensive agents, ketanserin reduces left ventricular hypertrophy during long-term effective antihypertensive treatment. Ketanserin has no significant effect on plasma lipid levels or carbohydrate metabolism, even in patients with diabetes mellitus. Although it manifests little hypokalemia by itself, the potential for cardiac dysrhythmias when taken with potassium-depleting diuretics may be a problem (see below). This phenomenon has been linked to ketanserin's minor but potentially important prolongation of the QT interval on the electrocardiogram in a dose-dependent fashion, which may increase the risk for torsades de pointes. This dysrhythmia has not yet been seen with ketanserin alone. The adverse effects of ketanserin are otherwise similar in frequency to those of other commonly used antihypertensive drugs. The most frequent symptomatic side effects are dizziness, fatigue, sleep disturbances, somnolence, dry mouth, edema, and weight gain; most are dose-dependent.

Most of the initial studies with ketanserin were intended to provide data on 3 months of exposure to the drug. Several of the longer-term studies have shown no diminution in antihypertensive efficacy with longer treatment periods, but weight gain, edema, and other adverse effects may limit enthusiasm for its long-term use. The combination of ketanserin with either beta blockers or angiotensin converting enzyme (ACE) inhibitors appears to be both effective and safe. Although a diuretic would appear both to be effective and to militate against weight gain and pedal edema, there are concerns about the adverse cardiac effects of hypokalemia that may occur with this combination.

Intravenous ketanserin has been used for hypertensive emergencies and urgencies. Several open-label studies and comparative trials have shown a consistent effect of intravenously administered ketanserin, with only a mild reflex tachycardia. These studies are consistent with the idea that the acute mechanism of action of ketanserin given intravenously is primarily vasodilatation. Several studies in postoperative patients (post–coronary bypass,[35,36] postcraniotomy[37]) have shown impressive hypotensive effects without untoward changes in either cardiac, renal, or intracranial function.

Ketanserin for Pregnancy-Induced Hypertension

Preeclampsia is a disease of pregnancy characterized by hypertension, platelet activation, endothelial dysfunction, reduced vasodilator prostaglandin production, and increased plasma levels of the vasoconstrictors thromboxane A_2 and serotonin. Since ketanserin is not known to be teratogenic, it was a good candidate for several hypertensive syndromes that occur in pregnancy, including the prevention of eclampsia.[6]

The simplest and most direct experience with ketanserin in pregnancy is its use in the management of established severe hypertension and preeclampsia. A case report of the successful use of intravenous ketanserin in reducing elevated blood pressure in a woman with an intrauterine death was published in 1984 and was followed by two double-blind, placebo-controlled crossover studies with similar results. First intravenous and then oral ketanserin was found to be moderately effective in reducing blood pressure in preeclamptic women with viable fetuses. Several comparative studies—first after and then against, hydralazine—were then completed; 162 women were enrolled, and the efficacy of ketanserin or hydralazine in controlling blood pressure was found to be similar. In the largest study, ketanserin was better tolerated, but neonatal and maternal outcomes were similar.[6]

Chronic hypertension of pregnancy has also been treated successfully in several studies using oral ketanserin. In the comparative study against methyldopa, there were similar reductions in blood pressure, but the group receiving ketanserin had slightly higher blood pressures toward the end of pregnancy. Neither group had any untoward complications.[6]

In a study of a series of 15 patients with the HELLP (hemolysis, elevated liver enzymes, and low platelets) syndrome[38] who received ketanserin, it was also concluded that it successfully prolonged pregnancy for 1 to 22 days, with a significant decrease in blood pressure overall and a decrease in platelet count in 11 patients.[39]

A large, randomized trial was organized to investigate the potential role of ketanserin in preventing preeclampsia in 138 women with diastolic blood pressure higher than 80 mm Hg before 20 weeks of gestation. Although both groups received aspirin, half were randomized to ketanserin 40 mg/day and half received matching placebo. Doses could be doubled if diastolic blood pressure exceeded 90 mm Hg. During the pregnancy, ketanserin was associated (Fig. 29-1) with fewer cases of preeclampsia (2 versus 13, $P = .006$), severe hypertension (6 versus 17, $P = .02$), and a trend to fewer perinatal deaths (1 versus 6, $P = .28$). Rates of abruptio placentae were lower and mean birth weight was higher in the ketanserin group. Although few obstetricians now recommend aspirin for preventing preeclampsia, the authors concluded that ketanserin prevented many of the undesired outcomes commonly seen among pregnant women with mild to moderate midtrimester hypertension,[40] but there are concerns about the generalizability of this conclusion to clinical practice, where aspirin is seldom recommended during pregnancy.

Ketanserin for Pulmonary Hypertension

Many associated diseases involving serotonin manifest as pulmonary hypertension.[41] Because the pulmonary circulation is especially well supplied with serotonin receptors and pulmonary neuroendocrine cells produce large amounts of serotonin, several 5-HT$_2$ antagonists have been studied in various models of these diseases. Most of these studies in rats or dogs have shown an improvement, especially acutely, after administration of 5-HT$_2$ antagonists.

In human primary pulmonary hypertension, there have been at least two studies using intravenous ketanserin. One involved 10 patients and resulted in a mean 18% drop in pulmonary vascular resistance.[42] A further study of 20 patients, 8 of whom had not responded to any other vasodilator, showed a similar and significant improvement, and there was a clinically important response in three others.[43] Many other studies of patients with pulmonary hypertension due to other causes have also generally shown an improvement in pulmonary vascular resistance and few adverse effects.[41] Since the development of stable prostaglandin analogues and the withdrawal from the market of appetite suppressants and other drugs thought to cause pulmonary hypertension,[44] the effects of ketanserin in pulmonary hypertension have not been as intensively studied.

Pulmonary hypertension is sometimes observed as part of progressive systemic sclerosis (scleroderma). One study of 14 such patients has noted a significant reduction in pulmonary arterial pressures at right heart catheterization after intravenous ketanserin, but 3 patients had a paradoxical increase; in 2, both pulmonary pressures and vascular resistance normalized.[45] The number of patients who responded acutely to ketanserin was greater than with nifedipine (3 of 6), captopril (3 of 5), and isosorbide dinitrate (2 of 4). Long-term administration of serotonin antagonists has not yet been studied in this condition.

Ketanserin for Portal Hypertension

The portal circulation is another that should be amenable to treatment with serotonin antagonists, given the large number of receptors present there and the propensity to hypertension, especially in advanced liver disease. Several rat studies, both with[46] and without[47,48] a beta-blocker, showed that acute administration of ketanserin and even ritanserin[46] reduced portal pressures. Similar studies have been carried out in humans. Acute dosing studies have shown an effect of ketanserin,[49] with or without propranolol,[50] in reducing several measures of portal pressure or splanchnic blood flow[51] without reducing hepatic blood flow. A longer-term study of 16 patients who were given oral ketanserin for about a month also reduced hepatic venous pressure gradient by about 15% over the long term, but about half developed side effects, and 3 developed encephalopathy, thought to be due to the worsening of their severe liver disease.[52] A similar study was done with propranolol and ritanserin in 10 patients; the 5 who lowered their suprahepatic venous pressure gradient more than 3 mm Hg were successfully treated for more than 100 days.[53] After discontinuation of ritanserin, the values returned to baseline.

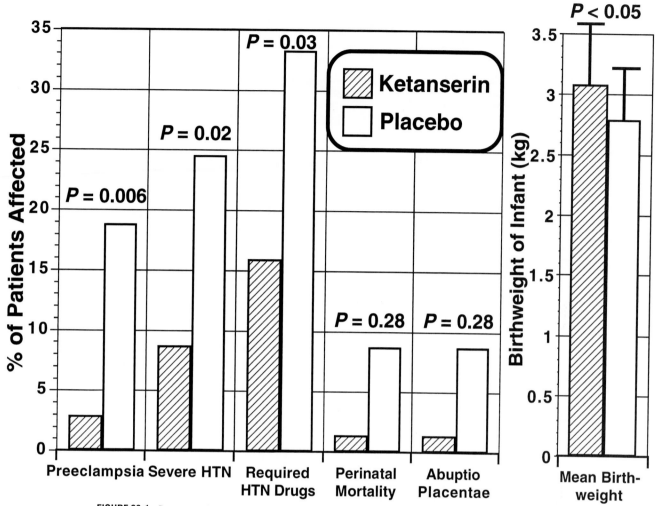

FIGURE 29-1. Summary of the results of a randomized, placebo-controlled clinical trial of intravenous ketanserin versus placebo in the prevention of preeclampsia and other adverse consequences of pregnancy-associated hypertension.[40] The primary outcome measure was preeclampsia, shown on the left. Mean birth weights (and standard deviation) are shown (in kilograms) on the right.

Ketanserin for Peripheral Arterial Disease

Ketanserin has also been studied extensively in conditions other than hypertension. Perhaps the disease of greatest interest was peripheral vascular disease (see Chap. 50), since the vasodilatory effects of a serotonin antagonist on atherosclerotic arteries should be beneficial. Several small studies were done, many of which showed improvement in walking times in patients with intermittent claudication. In a pooled analysis of 13 randomized, placebo-controlled studies, there was a slight, nonsignificant improvement in treadmill times (65 versus 25%) but a significant difference in deterioration (23 versus 35%) and a significant difference in the incidence of major cardiovascular events (9 versus 0) among those randomized to ketanserin.[54]

The first potentially definitive long-term clinical trial with "hard endpoints" using a serotonin antagonist was performed with ketanserin. The primary objective was to see whether the drug prevented complications of peripheral vascular disease, including vascular death, myocardial infarction, stroke, abdominal ischemia requiring surgery, and/or above-knee amputation. Although less than half of the enrolled 3899 patients were hypertensive, they all had documented intermittent claudication and a unilateral ankle-arm

index ≤0.85. All subjects were allowed to take other antihypertensive drugs if needed. After a 1-month single-blind placebo-control period, subjects were randomized to either ketanserin (20 mg thrice daily, increasing to 40 mg thrice daily after 1 month) or placebo. After an average of 5 months of treatment, 6 subjects were discontinued by the Data Safety and Monitoring Board (DSMB) because of a QT_c >500 ms, 4 of whom had been randomized to ketanserin. Four months later, all patients taking a diuretic were discontinued because of an excess risk of death (35 of 167 on ketanserin versus 15 of 144 on placebo). After slightly more than 1 year of average follow-up, the study was concluded, but the results remain controversial. In the intent-to-treat cohort that included all randomized patients, there was no significant difference across treatments in the primary outcome (bottom panel of Fig. 29-2). Because the DSMB noted harm to one treatment group's subjects taking potassium-losing diuretics or antidysrhythmic drugs (without knowing which specific treatment group was affected), a secondary analysis was performed. This analysis excluded all patients who were either taking a potassium-losing diuretic (a stratification apparently not made by the DSMB) or antidysrhythmic agents and found a nonsignificant 23% reduction compared to placebo in the number of primary endpoints

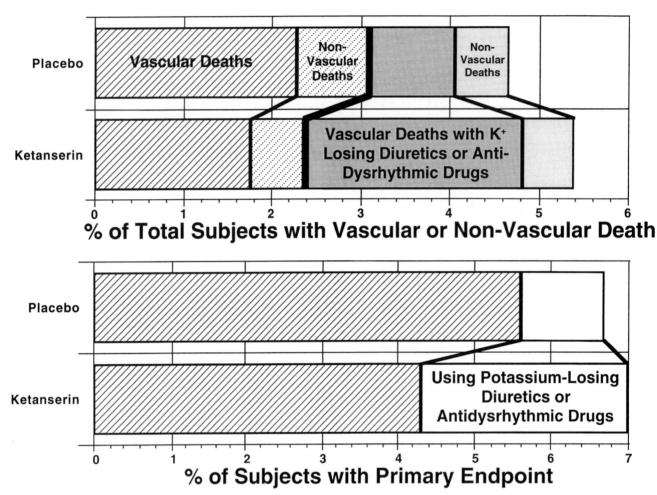

FIGURE 29-2. Summary of the results of a randomized, placebo-controlled clinical trial of oral ketanserin versus placebo in prevention of complications of peripheral vascular disease, the PACK (Prevention of Atherosclerotic Complications with Ketanserin) Trial.[26] The primary outcome measure was first myocardial infarction, stroke, above-knee amputation, operation for abdominal ischemia, or vascular death, shown in the bottom panel, stratified according to whether the patients did not (cross-hatched bars) or did (open bars) take potassium-losing diuretics or antidysrhythmic drugs. If the latter patients are excluded from the analysis, there was a nonsignificant 23% lower risk of the primary event with ketanserin versus placebo. Ketanserin was associated with a significantly higher number of vascular deaths (top panel) in the group receiving the above-noted drugs; but if these patients are excluded, there was, overall, a slight and barely significant reduction in the ketanserin group in patients having either a primary or secondary endpoint.

among those randomized to ketanserin ($P = .11$ by Fisher's exact test).[26]

There still remains controversy about the PACK trial results, primarily because of the excluded subjects.[55] One analysis focuses only on the subgroup of patients receiving potassium-losing diuretics and/or antidysrhythmic drugs, for whom ketanserin would now be considered contraindicated. In this subgroup, there were 71 patients with primary endpoints among the 416 patients randomized to ketanserin, compared to only 45 of the 412 assigned to placebo ($P = .012$ by Fisher's exact test). This corresponds to a 56% (95% CI: 10–121%) increase in risk for the primary endpoint. The vascular and all-cause mortality data from this subgroup are even more compelling: ketanserin was associated with 47 vascular and 11 non-vascular deaths (see Fig. 29-2, top panel), whereas placebo had only 19 and 12, respectively. For ketanserin, this corresponds to a relative risk of vascular death of 2.44 (95% CI: 1.46–4.10, $P = .0004$). The corresponding relative risk for all-cause mortality was 1.85 (95%

CI: 1.22–2.80, $P = .003$). These data are reasonably compelling arguments against using ketanserin in patients taking potassium-losing diuretics and were presumably the reason why the DSMB's decision was never criticized.

The controversy about the PACK trial's interpretation derives from how the remaining data are analyzed. If analyses are restricted to the subgroup of patients who did not take potassium-losing diuretics or antidysrhythmic drugs, the differences in neither primary endpoints nor deaths (either vascular or all-cause) reach traditional levels of statistical significance. All these trends, however, are in favor of ketanserin (Fig. 29-2), and the overall analysis (any primary or secondary endpoint) was significantly in favor of ketanserin (196 versus 249, relative risk reduction 20%, 95% CI: 4–32%, $P = .03$ by Fisher's exact test). The DSMB, who were never aware of which set of results pertained to the placebo group, began the process resulting in the discontinuation of study drug in patients who were at risk. Some therefore feel that the drug should be evaluated *only* for those patients for whom it would not in the future be contraindicated[56] and that the secondary analyses should be considered more important, perhaps even more so than the preplanned analyses. Others believe more strongly in rigorous enforcement of the "intent-to-treat" principle, which would *not* condone any analysis that excluded any of the randomized subjects. In the case of the PACK trial, their point of view is probably easier to advocate. There were no significant differences between treatment groups in the other preplanned endpoints in substudies, including either the absolute value or change in pain-free walking time on the treadmill or change in the ankle blood pressure at the end of 1 year.[57] The significant improvement in the ankle-arm index in the ketanserin group was presumably due to ketanserin's antihypertensive effect. The ketanserin group did have lessened platelet aggregation responses to serotonin, but most other comparisons of platelet function across all randomized patients were not significant.[58]

Ketanserin for Raynaud's Phenomenon in Scleroderma

The only clinical use for ketanserin that merits a separate entry in the Cochrane Database of Systematic Reviews is Raynaud's phenomenon in progressive systemic sclerosis.[59] Unfortunately, only 3 of 18 reviewed trials included sufficient objective detail to be incorporated into the meta-analysis. The conclusion was that "ketanserin is not an outstanding drug for treatment of Raynaud's phenomenon in scleroderma." The major limitation was that the small doses of ketanserin (40 mg/day) typically used in these studies are not significantly more efficacious than placebo, and the placebo response rate was inordinately high.

Ketanserin for Angina Pectoris

Although ketanserin has a strong theoretical basis for being an effective antianginal agent,[1] one study of 10 patients during ketanserin infusion showed no change in cardiac lactate extraction despite a small but significant drop in cardiac oxygen consumption.[60] The only clinical trial to test the antianginal effect of ketanserin using traditional treadmill tests showed no improvement with single 20- or 40-mg doses in 10 patients with chronic stable angina who were also treated with beta-adrenergic blockers.[61] The authors concluded that ketanserin is unlikely to increase exercise times by more than 20%, and such experiments have not been repeated.

Ketanserin for Vasospastic Angina Pectoris

Coronary spasm is also a clinical problem that should theoretically be amenable to prevention and treatment with a serotonin antagonist. Unfortunately, the results of clinical tests appear to differ from the expected result, as well as those of tests done on hanging strips of coronary arteries. Although serotonin infusion was followed by occlusive spasm in both stable angina and variant angina patients in two separate studies, ketanserin failed to prevent vasospasm in variant angina as well as in distal segments in patients with stable angina.[62] In a different study of 7 patients with stable coronary disease, ketanserin blunted serotonin-induced coronary vasospasm.[63] In a third study, 10 patients with coronary disease treated with 10 mg of ketanserin intravenously showed no significant changes in arterial diameter but did have reduced blood pressures.[64] These apparently contradictory observations have led to complex discussions of the relative importance of the various 5-HT receptors involved in coronary spasm, but no clinical utility for ketanserin for Prinzmetal's angina or coronary spasm was seen during coronary catheterization.

Ketanserin for Preventing Restenosis after Angioplasty

The process of restenosis after coronary angioplasty might benefit from serotonin antagonists, by either reduction of platelet aggregation or coronary vasodilation. Results from several small series of patients given ketanserin immediately before angioplasty suggested a reduction in early restenosis, but only one small study did long-term follow-up. A large clinical trial was therefore organized that included either placebo or a 40-mg oral loading dose of ketanserin before the angioplasty and chronic dosing thereafter (40 mg twice daily). The primary endpoint was death, myocardial infarction, or revascularization during 6 months after the angioplasty. A total of 658 patients were enrolled, but there were no significant differences between groups after 6 months in either the number of subjects reaching the primary endpoint or from the results of quantitative angiography (Fig. 29-3).[65]

Ketanserin for Preventing Vascular Complications of Cardiac Surgery

There are two types of postsurgical situations in which the coronary vessels often develop problems. Because of handling and other trauma, many veins and even internal mammary arteries used in coronary artery bypass grafting develop intra- and postoperative spasm, reducing flow to the already ischemic grafted area. This is a situation in which the potential vasodilatory and the antiplatelet effects of ketanserin might be useful. Ketanserin has been extensively used in the treatment of perioperative hypertension seen with cardiac surgery, and 18 papers have generally agreed that such treatment is effective in reducing blood pressure. There has, however, so far been no reinvestigation of the patients to see if such treatment prevents any vascular complications, either in the immediate postop period or in the longer term.

Another common problem after transplantation of the heart or other arterial segments is accelerated atherosclerosis in the transplanted arteries. Although some have attributed this to hypertension, dyslipidemia, and the high doses of immunosuppressant drugs used, ketanserin may also be useful.[66] So far, this has been investigated only in aortic transplantation in two strains of rats. Although one strain showed an impressive reduction of intimal thickening in the transplanted hearts after chronic, high-dose (10 mg/kg/day) ketanserin, this was not seen in a second rat strain.[67]

Ketanserin for Heart Failure

A vasodilating drug that does not increase heart rate would be expected to be beneficial in heart failure due to systolic dysfunction. Ketanserin has been given, both acutely[68–70] and chronically,[71] to heart failure patients, and some improvement was seen in hemodynamics,[68–71] circulating[69] and other catecholamine levels,[72] and platelet response to serotonin.[69] The study with the longest duration of treatment was 1 year and included only five patients.[71] Since ACE inhibitors have proven to be so beneficial for heart failure, enthusiasm for using ketanserin in this disease has diminished.

Ketanserin for Pulmonary Embolism

Because pulmonary embolism involves both platelet aggregation and a vasoconstrictor response in an artery plentifully supplied with serotonin receptors, ketanserin seemed an obvious potential therapy. A series of four studies in dogs, either pretreated with ketanserin or treated with intravenous ketanserin just after iatrogenic pulmonary embolization, showed improved hemodynamics,[73–76]

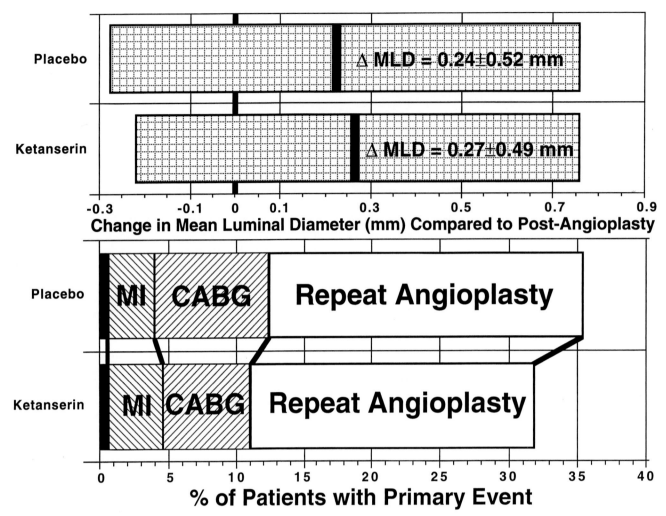

FIGURE 29-3. Summary of the results of a randomized, multicenter, placebo-controlled clinical trial of oral ketanserin versus placebo in the prevention of cardiovascular sequelae and restenosis after coronary angioplasty, the PARK (Post-Angioplasty Restenosis with Ketanserin) Trial.[65] On the bottom panel are displayed the components of the primary endpoint: death (dark bars at left), myocardial infarction (diagonally cross-hatched bars at left), coronary artery bypass grafting (CABG; diagonally cross-hatched bars at right), or repeat angioplasty (open bars). The overall difference between treatments was not significantly different ($P = .38$). The first secondary endpoint was the overall change in mean luminal diameter (MLD) of the angioplastied coronary artery, compared to the postangioplasty diameter (top panel); shown are the mean values for each group (dark vertical lines) and one standard deviation in each direction (hatched box). The difference between treatments was not statistically significant ($P = .50$).

oxygen delivery,[73–75] and platelet responses,[73] although not usually into the normal ranges. It is noteworthy that these dog studies used a much higher dose (mg/kg) than is usually given to humans. Only one human series has so far been reported; 10 patients significantly improved both their pulmonary arterial pressures and their oxygenation after intravenous ketanserin.[77] Since the introduction of thrombolytic agents, enthusiasm for ketanserin to treat pulmonary embolism has waned.

Ritanserin and Congeners

Ritanserin is a fascinating analogue of ketanserin that was developed partly in an attempt to dissect the alpha-blocking effects of ketanserin from its serotonin-blocking properties. There is less information available about ritanserin (1069 citations in MEDLINE through July 2002, compared to 3855 for ketanserin). Although ritanserin has now been shown in binding studies and in classic

pharmacologic experiments in laboratory animals to be completely without alpha-blocking properties, it has subsequently been shown to block not only 5-HT$_{2A}$ receptors (which would presumably be useful in cardiovascular disease) but also 5-HT$_{2C}$ receptors. These receptors are involved in many centrally mediated phenomena, including neurotransmission, especially in the limbic and choroid areas. As a result, ritanserin has been most intensively studied in psychiatric illnesses, including schizophrenia and addictions to alcohol or cocaine. In the largest study of 80 patients with cocaine addiction, ritanserin was not any better than placebo, over and above outpatient psychosocial therapy.[78] Similarly, in a study of 423 detoxified alcohol-dependent individuals, two doses of ritanserin were not significantly different than placebo in behavioral or reported alcohol-seeking behavior, but there was a dose-related increase in the QT$_c$ interval in those randomized to ritanserin.[79] In a three-dose study of ritanserin in Germany comprising 493 subjects, there were no significant benefits over placebo on several measures of symptoms and social functioning.[80] Ritanserin has also been subjected to a placebo-controlled clinical trial in 51 women with fibromyalgia. Although "feeling refreshed in the morning" and headache were significantly improved in the ritanserin group, there were no objective differences in serum markers between ritanserin and placebo.[81]

There are a few studies in laboratory animals suggesting a potential for ritanserin in cardiovascular disease. Ritanserin has been found to reduce collar-induced hypersensitivity to serotonin in rabbit carotids,[82] increase blood flow in middle cerebral artery occlusion in rats,[83] produce no change in local blood flow after scalding in dogs' femoral areas,[84] and diminish potassium-induced contractions in rat aortic strips.[85] A computer-based molecular modeling study also showed some major similarities between ketanserin's and ritanserin's binding to the putative 5-HT$_{2C}$ receptors.[86]

Early in the development of ritanserin for human use, however, it was found to have essentially no activity in treating systemic hypertension,[87,88] even when compared directly to ketanserin,[89,90] and further efforts to develop it for cardiovascular uses have largely been abandoned. Perhaps an exception would be in centrally mediated hypertension; a small study of 11 patients with Cushing's disease found no significant differences between ritanserin and ketanserin in several measures of corticotropin production.[91] One study of 24 normotensive volunteers who underwent forearm plethysmography showed little effect of ritanserin to infused norepinephrine or angiotensin II.[92]

Cinanserin shares many of the pharmacologic properties of ritanserin but has not been as extensively studied (311 citations in MEDLINE through July 2002). Again, most of the research with this compound pertains to its effects in the CNS, but some potential cardiovascular applications exist. Studies in dogs[93] or rats[94] subjected to pacing-induced myocardial ischemia showed that cinanserin could protect the heart from ST-segment elevations better than saline.

Flesinoxan is a serotoninergic drug with a different pharmacologic mechanism, acting primarily by stimulating the 5-HT$_{1A}$ receptor centrally.[95] It has apparently not been administered to human hypertensive patients, probably because it also failed to lower blood pressure in experimental animals.[96] It has been extensively studied, however (180 citations in MEDLINE through June 2001), mostly as a pharmacologic probe for the 5-HT$_{1A}$ receptor.[97]

Naftidrofuryl (also known as nafronyl, Gevatran, or Praxilene, Lipha Pharmaceuticals, Lyon, France) is a 5-HT$_2$-receptor antagonist that has been used for intermittent claudication since 1968 and is licensed for this use and/or for acute stroke therapy in several European countries.[98,99] Naftidrofuryl is thought both to enhance tissue oxygenation by inhibiting succinodehydrogenase[100] and to cause peripheral vasodilation, in addition to its possible rheological effects on platelets and erythrocytes.[101] The Cochrane Review of intravenous naftidrofuryl versus placebo for critical limb ischemia included seven trials and 229 subjects.[102] The conclusion was that naftidrofuryl produced nonsignificant improvements in the reduction of pain or skin necrosis as well as ankle systolic blood pressure. The intravenous formulation was withdrawn from the European market in 1985 due to excessive side effects.[103] The effects of naftidrofuryl either for intermittent claudication[104] or to prevent dementia[105] are currently being collected by the Cochrane Collaborative and are expected to result in meta-analyses shortly. A prior meta-analysis summarized the effects of 600 mg/day of naftidrofuryl against placebo in five clinical trials in 880 patients.[106] Naftidrofuryl had significant benefits on subjective "success/failure" decisions and change in pain-free walking distance on a treadmill ($P \leq .003$). Limited clinical trial evidence to date with naftidrofuryl in acute stroke indicates no survival benefit and a mild beneficial response in limiting disability.[107] Comparative trials in acute stroke against other vasodilators (e.g., nimodipine) or thrombolytic agents are lacking.

Sarpogrelate (MCI-9042, Anplag, Mitsubishi-Tokyo Pharmaceutical Co. Ltd., Tokyo, Japan), a selective 5-HT$_{2a}$ receptor blocker, has been shown to inhibit serotonin-induced coronary spasm in a porcine model.[108] The drug has also been shown to inhibit serotonin-induced proliferation of porcine coronary smooth muscle cells, suggesting a potential for use in improving the patency of coronary artery bypass grafts.[109] In addition, the drug has been shown to improve the exercise capacity of patients with angina pectoris by augmenting the coronary circulation, possibly by an antiplatelet action.[110,110a]

AT-1015 (Ajinomoto Co., Shiga, Japan) is a novel 5-HT$_{2a}$-receptor blocker that has a high affinity for 5-HT$_{2a}$ and 5-HT$_{2c}$; unlike ketanserin, it does not prolong the electrocardiographic QT interval.[111] In an animal model, the drug was shown to block both vascular and platelet 5-HT$_{2a}$ receptors and to prevent experimentally induced peripheral vascular lesions.[111]

Urapidil

Urapidil (Eupressyl in France, Ebrantyl in Italy, Ebrantil in Israel, Mediatensyl and others in other countries) is another pharmacologically complex agent, with inhibitory activity at peripheral postsynaptic alpha$_1$-adrenoreceptors and partial agonist activity at central serotonin 5-HT$_{1A}$ receptors.[112] At higher doses, it can block alpha$_2$- and beta$_1$-adrenoreceptors. There remains debate about the importance of its antagonism of central serotonin receptors as a part of its usual antihypertensive and other cardiovascular uses. Its chemical structure differs greatly from those of prazosin, terazosin, and doxazosin. Like other alpha$_1$-blockers, though urapidil reduces blood pressure by decreasing peripheral resistance and without reflex tachycardia.

As an antihypertensive drug, oral urapidil has been thoroughly studied, both in placebo-controlled and comparative studies against other traditional antihypertensive agents. MEDLINE (through July 2002) lists 571 citations for urapidil. It may be particularly beneficial in older hypertensives, more than 5000 of whom have now been studied in clinical trials.[113] It has few metabolic side effects and can be used in dyslipidemic or diabetic patients without significant effect on the concomitant disease.[114] Urapidil can be combined with a diuretic, beta-blocker, calcium antagonist, or ACE inhibitor, and the combination produces a further reduction in blood pressure. Adverse effects are typically mild, and include dizziness, headache, nausea, fatigue, stomach irritation, orthostatic hypotension, palpitations, and skin rash. It is eliminated both by renal and hepatic excretion, and has a relatively short serum elimination half-life of 3 h; the disadvantage of this short half-life has been overcome by a recently introduced sustained-release preparation.[114]

Most of the recent work with urapidil has involved the intravenous formulation, which has been extensively studied in many types of hypertensive emergencies.[115,116] It has been studied in patients post–coronary artery bypass[117] and in others with pulmonary edema[118] and preeclampsia.[119] In comparative studies (especially against intravenous ketanserin[117]), it was similarly effective and reasonably well tolerated in the short term.[112]

The only long-term clinical experience with urapidil derives from an open-label study of 3216 hypertensive patients with a previous cardiovascular event. These individuals received 3 years of treatment with urapidil, which lowered both systolic and diastolic blood pressures by 14.4 and 15%, respectively.[120] There was no change in mean heart rate, either supine or standing, and no significant change in other disease parameters was noted among the diabetic or dyslipidemic subjects. Opinions of the treatment were improved in both physicians and patients.[121]

Other Agents in Development

Several serotonin antagonists are currently being studied, either in laboratory animals and/or tissue culture or in clinical trials. Perhaps the most interesting, in terms of being very specific for a particular serotonin receptor, is MDL 100,907, which binds very tightly to the 5-HT_{2A} receptor. There is hope that this molecule may help unravel some of the effects of ketanserin that may not be due to such a specific effect on this receptor. Of the 127 citations found in MEDLINE (through July 2002), none are relevant to hypertension or cardiovascular medicine.

A somewhat less selective serotonin antagonist, LY 53857, binds to each of the subtypes of 5-HT_2 receptors. This compound has been extensively tested (173 citations in MEDLINE through July 2002), but has no antihypertensive effect in spontaneously hypertensive rats.[122] This experiment has cast doubt on a major role of central 5-HT receptors in blood pressure regulation.[123]

Other 5-HT_2 receptor antagonists that are still being evaluated include MDL 28,133A,[124] DV-7028,[125] and LY-272015.[126] There are also several 5-HT_1 receptor antagonists that are currently being tested, including A-74283.[127]

NON-CARDIOVASCULAR CONDITIONS FOR WHICH SEROTONIN ANTAGONISTS MAY BE HELPFUL

Despite the extensive work with serotoninergic receptor antagonists and agonists in hypertension and other cardiovascular conditions, only a few widely used drugs have evolved for clinical use. There remain, however, many potential uses for drugs with this mechanism of action in noncardiovascular areas of medicine. These are summarized briefly in Table 29-2.

CONCLUSION

After a role for serotonin was first proposed in cardiovascular medicine by Irvine Page in 1956, many chemicals have been synthesized and many experiments done to elaborate the complex system of receptors for serotonin that exist today. The compound that is most advanced in treating cardiovascular disease is ketanserin, which has been tested in two major clinical trials. Despite conflicting interpretations of the PACK trial, ketanserin clearly has the potential for increasing mortality (ascribed to the prolongation of the QT_c interval) when coadministered with potassium-losing diuretics. There is, however, little doubt that the many interesting serotonin agonists and antagonists studied in multiple laboratories and clinics have improved our understanding of this complex system and hold promise for future progress in both cardiovascular and noncardiovascular medicine.

TABLE 29-2. Noncardiovascular Therapeutic Areas of Interest for Serotoninergic Drugs

Carcinoid syndrome
Familial platelet storage pool diseases
Platelet cell membrane disorders (e.g., paroxysmal nocturnal hemoglobinuria, antiphospholipid syndrome)
Thrombocytopenia in persistent pulmonary hypertension in the newborn
Acute respiratory failure
Airway obstruction (perhaps including asthma)
Neurogenic bladder
Collagen disorders
Radiation pneumonitis

REFERENCES

1. Slassi A: Recent advances in 5-HT1B/1D receptor antagonists and agonists and their potential therapeutic applications. *Curr Top Med Chem* 2:559, 2002.
2. Hindle AT: Recent developments in the physiology and pharmacology of 5-hydroxytryptamine. *Br J Anaesth* 73:395, 1994.
3. Sanders-Bush E, Mayer SE: 5-Hydroxytryptamine (serotonin) receptor agonists and antagonists. In: Hardman JG, Limbird LE, Molinoff PB, et al, eds: *Goodman & Gilman's The Pharmacological Basis of Therapeutics.* New York: McGraw-Hill, 1996, 249.
4. Hoyer D, Clarke DE, Fozard JR, et al: VII International Union of Pharmacology classification of receptors for 5-hydroxytryptamine. *Pharmacol Rev* 46:157, 1994.
5. Frishman WH, Okin S, Huberfield S: Serotonin antagonism in the treatment of systemic hypertension: The role of ketanserin. *Med Clin North Am* 72:501, 1988.
6. Steyn DW, Odendaal HJ: Serotonin antagonism and serotonin antagonists in pregnancy: Role of ketanserin *Obstet Gynecol Surv* 55:582, 2000.
7. Kosten TR, Markou A, Koob GF: Depression and stimulant dependence: Neurobiology and pharmacotherapy. *J Nerv Ment Dis* 186:737, 1998.
8. Gaddum JH, Picarelli ZP: Two kinds of tryptamine receptors. *Br J Pharmacol* 12:323, 1957.
9. Burkiewicz JS, Chan JD, Alldredge BK: Eletriptan. Serotonin 5-HT1B/1D receptor agonist for the acute treatment of migraine. *Formulary* 35:129, 2000.
10. Ferrari MD, Roon KI, Lipton RB, Goadsby PJ: Oral triptans (serotonin 5-HT1B/1D agonists) in acute migraine treatment: A meta-analysis of 53 trials. *Lancet* 358:1668, 2001.
11. Yokota Y, Imaizumi Y, Asano M, et al: Endothelium-derived relaxing factor released by 5-HT: Distinct from nitric oxide in basilar arteries of normotensive and hypertensive rats. *Br J Pharmacol* 113:324, 1994.
12. Missouris CG, Cappuccio FP, Varsamis E, et al: Serotonin and heart rate in hypertensive and normotensive subjects. *Am Heart J* 135:838, 1998.
13. Koba S, Pakala R, Watanabe T, et al: Vascular smooth muscle proliferation. Synergistic interaction between serotonin and low density lipoproteins. *J Am Coll Cardiol* 34:1644, 1999.
14. Ito T, Ikeda U, Shimpo M, et al: Serotonin increases interleukin-6 synthesis in human vascular smooth muscle cells. *Circulation* 102:2522, 2000.
15. Wright L, Homans D, Laxson D, et al: Effects of serotonin and thromboxane A2 on blood flow through moderately well developed coronary artery vessels. *J Am Coll Cardiol* 19:687, 1992.
16. Heistad DD, Armstrong ML, Baumbach GL, Faraci FM: Sick vessel syndrome. Recovery of atherosclerotic and hypertensive vessels. *Hypertension* 26:509, 1995.
17. Shimada T, Murakami Y, Hashimoto M, et al: Impairment of serotonin-mediated nitric oxide release across the coronary bed in patients with coronary spastic angina. *Am J Cardiol* 83:953, 1999.
18. Mongiardo R, Finocchiaro ML, Beltrame J, et al: Low incidence of serotonin-induced occlusive coronary artery spasm in patients with recent myocardial infarction. *Am J Cardiol* 78:84, 1996.
19. Baudouin-Legros M, Le Quan-Bui K, Guicheney P, et al: Platelet serotonin in essential hypertension and in mental depression. *J Cardiovasc Pharmacol* 7(Suppl 7):S12, 1985.

20. Vanhoutte P, Luscher T: Serotonin and the blood vessel wall. *J Hypertens* 4(Suppl 1):S29, 1986.

21. Watts SW: The development of enhanced arterial serotonergic hyperresponsiveness in mineralocorticoid hypertension. *J Hypertens* 16: 811, 1998.

22. Mantero F, Rooco S, Opocher G, et al: Effect of ketanserin in primary hyperaldosteronism. *J Cardiovasc Pharmacol* 7(Suppl 7):S172, 1985.

23. McCall RB, Clement ME: Role of serotonin-1A and serotonin-2 receptors in the central regulation of the cardiovascular system. *Pharmacol Rev* 46:231, 1994.

24. Vikenes K, Farstad M, Nordrehaug JE: Serotonin is associated with coronary artery disease and cardiac events. *Circulation* 100:483, 1999.

25. Comings DE, MacMurray JP, Gonzalez N, et al: Association of the serotonin transporter gene with serum cholesterol levels and heart disease. *Mol Genet Metab* 67:248, 1999.

26. Prevention of atherosclerotic complications: Controlled trial of ketanserin. Prevention of Atherosclerotic Complications with Ketanserin Trial Group. *BMJ* 298:424, 1989.

27. Janssen PAJ: 5-HT2 receptor blockade to study serotonin-induced pathology. *Trends Pharmacol Sci* 4:198, 1983.

28. Weiting GJ, Woitticz AJ, Man in't Veld AJ, Schalekamp MA: 5-HT, alpha-adrenoreceptors, and blood pressure. Effects of ketanserin in essential hypertension and autonomic insufficiency. *Hypertension* 6: 100, 1984.

29. Nelson MA, Coghlan JP, Denton DA, et al: Serotonergic mechanisms and blood pressure in sheep. *J Cardiovasc Pharmacol* 7(Suppl 7): S117, 1985.

30. Reimann I, Ziegler G, Ludwig L, Frolich J: Central and autonomic nervous system side-effects of ketanserin. *Arzneimittelforschung* 36:1681, 1986.

31. McCall RB, Harris LT: Characterization of the central sympathoinhibitory action of ketanserin. *J Pharmacol Exp Ther* 241:736, 1987.

32. Brogden RN, Sorkin EM: Ketanserin—a review of its pharmacodynamic and pharmacokinetic properties, and therapeutic potential in hypertension and peripheral vascular disease. *Drugs* 40:903, 1990.

33. Hannedouche T, Fillastre JP, Mimran A, et al: Ketanserin versus nifedipine in the treatment of essential hypertension in patients over 50 years old: An international multicenter trial. *J Cardiovasc Pharmacol* 10(Suppl 3):S107, 1987.

34. Zin C, Copertari P, Landi E, et al: Evaluation of a new antihypertensive agent ketanserin versus methyldopa in the treatment of essential hypertension in older patients: An international multicenter trial. *J Cardiovasc Pharmacol* 10(Suppl 3):S113, 1987.

35. Petry A, Wulf H, Baumgartel M: The influence of ketanserin or urapidil on haemodynamics, stress response, and kidney function during operations for myocardial revascularisation. *Anaesthesia* 50:312, 1995.

36. van der Stroom JG, van Wezel HB, Langemeijer JJ, et al: A randomized multicenter double-blind comparison of urapidil and ketanserin in hypertensive patients after coronary artery surgery. *J Cardiothor Vasc Anesth* 11:726, 1997.

37. Felding M, Cold GE, Jacobsen CJ, et al: The effect of ketanserin upon postoperative blood pressure, cerebral blood flow and oxygen metabolism in patients subjected to craniotomy for cerebral tumours. *Acta Anaesthesiol Scand* 39:582, 1995.

38. Egerman RS, Sibai BM: HELLP syndrome. *Clin Obstet Gynecol* 42:381, 1999.

39. Spitz B, Witters K, Hanssens M, et al: Ketanserin, a 5-HTA2 serotonergic receptor antagonist, could be useful in the HELLP syndrome. *Hypertens Pregnancy* 12:183, 1993.

40. Steyn DW, Odendaal HJ: Randomised controlled trial of ketanserin and aspirin in prevention of pre-eclampsia. *Lancet* 350:1267, 1997.

41. Egermayer P, Town GI, Peacock AJ: Role of serotonin in the pathogenesis of acute and chronic pulmonary hypertension. *Thorax* 54:161, 1999.

42. McGoon MD, Vliestra RE: Vasodilator therapy for primary pulmonary hypertension. *Mayo Clin Proc* 59:672, 1984.

43. McGoon MD, Vliestra RE: Acute hemodynamic response to the S2-serotonergic receptor antagonist, ketanserin, in patients with primary pulmonary hypertension. *Int J Cardiol* 14:303, 1987.

44. Naeije R, Wauthy P, Maggiorini M, et al: Effects of dexfenfluramine on hypoxic pulmonary vasoconstriction and embolic pulmonary hypertension in dogs. *Am J Respir Crit Care Med* 151:692, 1995.

45. Seibold JR, Molony RR, Turkevich D, et al: Acute hemodynamic effects of ketanserin in pulmonary hypertension secondary to systemic sclerosis. *J Rheumatol* 14:519, 1987.

46. Pomier-Layrargues G, Giroux L, et al: Combined treatment of portal hypertension with ritanserin and propranolol in conscious and unrestrained cirrhotic rats. *Hepatology* 15:878, 1992.

47. Cummings SA, Groszmann RJ, Kaumann AJ: Hypersensitivity of mesenteric veins to 5-HT and ketanserin-induced reduction of portal pressure in portal hypertensive rats. *Br J Pharmacol* 89:501, 1986.

48. Cummings SA, Kaumann AJ, Groszmann RJ: Comparison of the hemodynamic responses to ketanserin and prazosin in portal hypertensive rats. *Hepatology* 8:1112, 1988.

49. Hadengue A, Lee SS, Moreau R, et al: Beneficial hemodynamic effects of ketanserin in patients with cirrhosis: Possible role of serotonergic mechanisms in portal hypertension. *Hepatology* 7:644, 1987.

50. Hadengue A, Moreau R, Cerini R, et al: Combination of ketanserin and verapamil or propranolol in patients with alcoholic cirrhosis: Search for an additive effect. *Hepatology* 9:83, 1989.

51. Gibson PR, Gibson RN, Donlan JD, et al: A comparison of Doppler flowmetry with conventional assessment of acute changes in hepatic blood flow. *J Gastroenterol Hepatol* 11:14, 1996.

52. Vorobioff J, Garcia-Tsao G, Groszmann R, et al: Long-term hemodynamic effects of ketanserin, a 5-hydroxytryptamine blocker, in portal hypertensive patients. *Hepatology* 9:88, 1989.

53. Ladero Quesada JM, Diez Ordonez S, et al: [Addition of ritanserin to the treatment with propranolol in cirrhotic patients: Effects on portal pressure] (in Spanish). *Anales Med Interna* 11:162, 1994.

54. Clement DL, Duprez D: Effect of ketanserin in the treatment of patients with intermittent claudication: Results from 13 placebo-controlled parallel group studies. *J Cardiovasc Pharmacol* 10(Suppl 3):S89, 1987.

55. DeMets DL, Pocock SJ, Julian DG: The agonising negative trend in monitoring of clinical trials. *Lancet* 354:1983, 1999.

56. Chalmers TC, Murray GD: Retrospective analyses for hypothesis generation. A commentary of the PACK trial (Prevention of Atherosclerotic Complications with Ketanserin). *Clin Exp Hypertens* 11:1117, 1989.

57. Verstraete M: The PACK trial: Morbidity and mortality effects of ketanserin. Prevention of atherosclerotic complications. *Vasc Med* 1:135, 1996.

58. The PACK Trial Group. Platelet function during long-term treatment with ketanserin of claudicating patients with peripheral atherosclerosis. A multi-center, double-blind, placebo-controlled trial. *Thromb Res* 55:13, 1989.

59. Pope J, Fenlon D, Thompson A, et al: Ketanserin for Raynaud's phenomenon in progressive systemic sclerosis (*Cochrane Review*). In: *The Cochrane Library*. Oxford, UK: Update Software, 2001.

60. Walker JM, Wilmshurst PT, Juul SM, Coltart DJ: Acute effects of ketanserin on left ventricular function, metabolism, and coronary blood flow. *Br J Clin Pharmacol* 17:301, 1984.

61. Cameron HA, Cameron CM, Ramsay LE: Comparison of single doses of ketanserin and placebo in chronic stable angina. *Br J Clin Pharmacol* 22:114, 1986.

62. McFadden EP, Bauters C, Lablanche JM, et al: Effect of ketanserin on proximal and distal coronary constrictor responses to intracoronary infusion of serotonin in patients with stable angina, patients with variant angina, and control patients. *Circulation* 82:187, 1992.

63. Golino P, Piscione F, Willerson J, et al: Divergent effects of serotonin on coronary artery dimension and blood flow in patients with coronary atherosclerosis and control patients. *N Engl J Med* 1991;324:641, 1992.

64. Hood S, Birnie D, Nasser A, Hillis WS: Effect of ketanserin on central haemodynamics and coronary circulation. *J Cardiovasc Pharmacol* 32:983, 1998.

65. Serruys PW, Klein W, Tijssen JP, et al: Evaluation of ketanserin in the prevention of restenosis after percutaneous transluminal coronary angioplasty. A multicenter randomized double-blind placebo-controlled trial. *Circulation* 88:1588, 1993.

66. Ishida T, Kawashima S, Hirata K, et al: Serotonin-induced hypercontraction through 5-hydroxytryptamine 1B receptors in atherosclerotic rabbit coronary arteries. *Circulation* 103:1289, 2001.

67. Geerling RA, De Bruin RWF, Scheringa M, et al: Ketanserin reduces graft atherosclerosis after aorta transplantation in rats. *J Cardiovasc Pharmacol* 27:307, 1996.

68. Demoulin JC, Bertholet M, Soumagne D, et al: 5-HT2-receptor block-ade in the treatment of heart failure. A preliminary study. *Lancet* 1:1186, 1981.

69. Grobecker H, Gessler I, Delius W, et al: Effect of ketanserin on hemodynamics, plasma-catecholamine concentrations, and serotonin uptake by platelets in volunteers and patients with congestive heart failure. *J Cardiovasc Pharmacol* 7(Suppl 7):S102, 1985.

70. Majid PA, Morris WM, Sole MJ: Hemodynamic and neurohumoral effects of ketanserin, a 5-HT2 receptor antagonist in patients with congestive heart failure. *Can J Cardiol* 3:70, 1987.

71. Brune S, Schmidt T, Tebbe U, Kreuzer H: Influence of long-term treat-ment with ketanserin on blood pressure, pulmonary artery pressure, and cardiac output in patients with heart failure. *Cardiovasc Drugs Ther* 4(Suppl 1):85, 1990.

72. Majid PA, Sole MJ: Effect of 5-hydroxytryptamine blockade with ketanserin on myocardial uptake of epinephrine and norepinephrine in patients with congestive heart failure. *J Clin Pharmacol* 27:661, 1987.

73. Huval WV, Mathieson MA, Stemp LI, et al: Therapeutic benefits of 5-hydroxytryptamine inhibition following pulmonary embolism. *Ann Surg* 197:220, 1983.

74. Thompson JA, Millen JE, Glauser FL, Hess ML: Role of 5-HT2 receptor inhibition in pulmonary embolism. *Circ Shock* 20:299, 1986.

75. Breuer J, Meschig R, Breuer HW, Arnold G: Effects of serotonin on the cardiopulmonary circulatory system with and without 5-HT2-receptor blockade by ketanserin. *J Cardiovasc Pharmacol* 7(Suppl 7): S64, 1985.

76. Fitzpatrick JM, Grant BJ: Effects of pulmonary vascular obstruc-tion on right ventricular afterload. *Am Rev Respir Dis* 141:944, 1990.

77. Huet Y, Brun-Buisson C, Lemaire F, et al: Cardiopulmonary effects of ketanserin infusion in human pulmonary embolism. *Am Rev Respir Dis* 135:114, 1987.

78. Cornish JW, Maany I, Fudala PJ, et al: A randomized, double-blind, placebo-controlled study of ritanserin pharmacotherapy for cocaine dependence. *Drug Alcohol Depend* 61:183, 2001.

79. Johnson BA, Jasinski DR, Galloway GP, et al: Ritanserin in the treat-ment of alcohol dependence–a multi-center clinical trial. Ritansin Study Group. *Psychopharmacology* 128:206, 1996.

80. Wiesbeck GA, Weijers HG, Chick J, Boening J: The effects of ri-tanserin on mood, sleep, vigilance, clinical impression, and social functioning in alcohol-dependent individuals. Ritanserin in Alco-holism Work Group. *Alcohol Alcohol* 35:384, 2000.

81. Olin R, Klein R, Berg PA: A randomised double-blind 16-week study of ritanserin in fibromyalgia syndrome: Clinical outcome and analysis of autoantibodies to serotonin, gangliosides and phospholipids. *Clin Rheumatol* 17:89, 1998.

82. Geerts IS, Matthys KE, Herman AG, Bult H: Involvement of 5-HT1B receptors in collar-induced hypersensitivity to 5-hydroxytryptamine of the rabbit carotid artery. *Br J Pharmacol* 127:1327, 1999.

83. Back T, Prado R, Zhao W, et al: Ritanserin, a 5-HT2 receptor an-tagonist, increases subcortical blood flow following photothrom-botic middle cerebral artery occlusion in rats. *Neurol Res* 20:643, 1998.

84. Taheri PA, Lippton HL, Force SD, et al: Analysis of regional hemo-dynamic regulation in response to scald injury. *J Clin Invest* 93:147, 1994.

85. Okoro EO, Marwood JF: Effects of 5HT2 receptor antagonists to potassium depolarization in rat isolated aorta. *Clin Exp Pharmacol Physiol* 24:34, 1997.

86. Kristiansen K, Dahl SG: Molecular modeling of serotonin, ketanserin, ritanserin and their 5-HT2C receptor interactions. *Eur J Pharmacol* 306:195, 1996.

87. Hedner T, Pettersson A, Persson B: Chronic 5-HT2-receptor blockade by ritanserin does not reduce blood pressure in patients with essential hypertension. *Acta Med Scand* 222:307, 1987.

88. Stott DJ, Saniabadi AR, Hosie J, et al: The effects of the 5-HT2 an-tagonist ritanserin on blood pressure and serotonin-induced platelet aggregation in patients with untreated essential hypertension. *Eur J Clin Pharmacol* 35:123, 1988.

89. Hosie J, Stott DJ, Robertson JIS, Ball SG: Does acute serotonergic type-2 antagonism reduce blood pressure? Comparative effects of single doses of ritanserin and ketanserin in essential hypertension. *J Cardiovasc Pharmacol* 10(Suppl 3):S86, 1987.

90. Chau NP, Pithois-Merli I, Levenson J, Simon AC: Comparative haemodynamic effects of ketanserin and ritanserin in the proximal and distal upper limb circulations of hypertensive patients. *Eur J Clin Pharmacol* 37:215, 1989.

91. Sonino N, Fava GA, Fallo F, et al: Effect of the serotonin antago-nists ritanserin and ketanserin in Cushing's disease. *Pituitary* 3:55, 2000.

92. Bruning TA, Change PC, Blauw GJ, et al: Interactions between sero-tonin and endogenous and exogenous noradrenaline in the human forearm. *Blood Press* 3:309, 1994.

93. Grover GJ, Parham CS, Youssef S, Ogletree ML: Protective effect of the serotonin receptor antagonist cinaserin in two canine mod-els of pacing-induced myocardial ischemia. *Pharmacology* 50:286, 1995.

94. Grover GJ, Sargent CA, Dzwonczyk S, et al: Protective effect of serotonin (5-HT2) receptor antagonists in ischemic rat hearts. *J Car-diovasc Pharmacol* 22:664, 1993.

95. Chamienia AL, Johns EJ: The cardiovascular and renal functional responses to the 5-HT1A receptor agonist flesinoxan in two rat models of hypertension. *Br J Pharmacol* 118:1891, 1996.

96. Dabire H, Chamiot-Clerc P, Chaouche-Teyara K, et al: Acute and chronic sympathoinhibition on carotid artery diameter of sponta-neously hypertensive rats: Effects of clonidine and flesinoxan. *Clin Exp Pharmacol Physiol* 27:715, 2000.

97. van Zwieten PA, Blauw GJ, van Brummelen P: The role of 5-hydroxytryptamine and 5-hydroxytryptaminergic mechanisms in hypertension. *Br J Clin Pharmacol* 30(Suppl 1):69S, 1990.

98. Naftidrofuryl (Praxilene). *Drug Ther Bull* 26:25, 1988.

99. Barradell LB, Brogden RN: Oral naftidrofuryl. A review of its phar-macology and therapeutic use in the management of peripheral oc-clusive arterial disease. *Drugs Aging* 8:299, 1996.

100. Wiernsperger NF: Serotonin, 5-HT2 receptors, and their blockade by naftidrofuryl: A targeted therapy of vascular diseases. *J Cardiovasc Pharmacol* 23(Suppl 3):S37, 1994.

101. Hiatt WR: New treatment options in intermittent claudication: The US experience. *Int J Clin Pract* (Suppl 119):20, 2001.

102. Smith FB, Bradbury AW, Fowkes FGR: *Intravenous Naftidrofuryl for Critical Limb Ischaemia. Cochrane Database Syst Rev* 2000; CD 002070.

103. Smith P, Loy C, Wong M: *Naftidrofuryl (Nafronyl, Praxilene) for Cognitive Impairment [Protocol]*. Oxford, UK: Update Software, 2001.

104. Ausejo M, Saenz A, Hoold S, et al: *Naftidrofuryl for Intermittent Claudication [Protocol]*. Oxford, UK: Update Software, 2001.

105. Gold M: The efficacy of naftidrofuryl in patients with vascular or mixed dementia. *Clin Ther* 22:1251, 2000.

106. Lehert P, Comte S, Gamand S, Brown TM: Naftidrofuryl in intermit-tent claudication: A retrospective analysis. *J Cardiovasc Pharmacol* 23(Suppl 3):S48, 1994.

107. Steiner TJ: Naftidrofuryl after acute stroke: A review and a hypothesis. *J Cardiovasc Pharmacol* 16(Suppl 3):S58, 1990.

108. Miyata K, Shimokawa H, Higo T, et al: Sarpogrelate, a selective 5-HT2A serotonergic receptor antagonist, inhibits serotonin-induced coronary artery spasm in a porcine model. *J Cardiovasc Pharmacol* 35:294, 2000.

109. Sharma SK, Del Rizzo DF, Zahradka P, et al: Sarpogrelate inhibits serotonin-induced proliferation of porcine coronary artery smooth muscle cells: Implications for long-term graft patency. *Ann Thorac Surg* 71:1856, 2001.

110. Tanaka T, Fujita M, Nakae I, et al: Improvement of exercise capac-ity by sarpogrelate as a result of augmented collateral circulation in patients with effort angina. *J Am Coll Cardiol* 32:1982, 1998.

110a. Kinugawa T, Fujita M, Lee J-D, et al: Effectiveness of a novel sero-tonin blocker, for patients with angina pectoris. *Am Heart J* 144; e1, 2002 (online article).

111. Kihara H, Hirose K, Koganei H, et al: AT-1015, a novel serotonin (5-HT)2 receptor antagonist, blocks vascular and platelet 5-HT2A re-ceptors and prevents the laurate-induced peripheral vascular lesion in rats. *J Cardiovasc Pharmacol* 35:523, 2000.

112. Dooley M, Goa KL: Urapidil. A reappraisal of its use in the manage-ment of hypertension. *Drugs* 56:929, 1998.

113. Hansson L, Petitet A: Review of studies with urapidil in elderly hy-pertensives. *Blood Press* 3(Suppl):21, 1995.

114. Oren S, Turkot S, Paran E, et al: Efficacy and tolerability of slow-release urapidil (Ebrantil) in hypertensive patients with non-insulin

dependent diabetes mellitus (NIDDM). *J Hum Hypertens* 10:123, 1996.

115. Hirschl MM, Binder M, Bur A, et al: Safety and efficacy of urapidil and sodium nitroprusside in the treatment of hypertensive emergencies. *Intens Care Med* 23:885, 1997.

116. Alijotas-Reig J, Bove-Farre I, de Cabo-Frances F, Angles-Coll R: Effectiveness and safety of prehospital urapidil for hypertensive emergencies. *Am J Emerg Med* 19:130, 2001.

117. van der Stroom JG, van Wezel HB, Langemeijer JJ, et al: A randomized multicenter double-blind comparison of urapidil and ketanserin in hypertensive patients after coronary artery surgery. *J Cardiothorac Vasc Anesth* 11:729, 1997.

118. Schreiber W, Woisetschlager C, Binder M, et al: The Nitura Study–effect of nitroglycerin or urapidil on hemodynamic, metabolic, and respiratory parameters in hypertensive patients with pulmonary edema. *Intens Care Med* 24:557, 1998.

119. Wacker J, Werner P, Walter-Sack I, Bastert G: Treatment of hypertension in patients with pre-eclampsia: A prospective parallel-group study comparing dihydralazine with urapidil. *Nephrol Dialysis Transplant* 13:318, 1998.

120. Godeau P, Allaert FA, Barrier J, et al: [Course of ischemic risk in treated atheromatous hypertensive patients. The PRIHAM study (Prognosis of Ischemic Risk in Atheromatous Patients under Mediatensyl)] (in French). *Ann Med Interne (Paris)* 147:403, 1996.

121. Godeau P, Allaert FA, Barrier J, et al: [Course of ischemic risk in treated atheromatous hypertensive patients. The PRIHAM Study] (in French). *Ann Med Interne (Paris)* 146:530, 1995.

122. Cohen ML, Fuller RW, Kurz KD: LY 53857, a selective and potent serotonergic (5-HT2) receptor antagonist, does not lower blood pressure in the spontaneously hypertensive rat. *J Pharmacol Exp Ther* 227:327, 1983.

123. Dabire H: Central 5-hydroxytryptamine (5-HT) receptors in blood pressure regulation. *Therapie* 46:421, 1991.

124. Hseih CP, Sakai K, Bruns GC, Dage RC: Effects of MDL 28,133A, a 5-HT2 receptor antagonist, on platelet aggregation and coronary thrombosis in dogs. *J Cardiovasc Pharmacol* 24:761, 1994.

125. Pawlak D, Adamkiewicz M, Malyszko J, et al: Vascular and cardiac effects of DV-7028, a selective, 5-HT2-receptor antagonist in rats. *J Cardiovasc Pharmacol* 32:266, 1998.

126. Watts SW, Fink GD: 5-HT2B-receptor antagonist LY-272015 is antihypertensive in DOCA-salt-hypertensive rats. *Am J Physiol* 276:H944, 1999.

127. Lee JY, Hancock AA, Warner RB, et al: Cardiovascular activity of A-74283, a 5-hydroxytryptamine 1A agent, in the spontaneously hypertensive rat. *Pharmacology* 56:17, 1998.

128. Herve P, Drouet L, Dosquet C, et al: Primary pulmonary hypertension in a patient with familial platelet storage pool disease: Role of serotonin. *Am J Med* 89:117, 1990.

Imidazoline-Receptor Agonist Drugs for the Treatment of Systemic Hypertension and Congestive Heart Failure

William H. Frishman

Sameet A. Palkhiwala

Austin Yu

Fay Rim

The role of the central nervous system (CNS) in regulating vasomotor tone and control of blood pressure has been well described in both experiments and clinical trials using central-acting antihypertensive drugs, such as alpha-methyldopa and clonidine.[1] The central regulation of cardiovascular tone and blood pressure is based on the response of the autonomic nervous system in the medulla oblongata to variations in the activity of the carotid sinus and the aortic arch baroreceptors. Afferent fibers from the carotid and aortic baroreceptors form the tractus solitarius and terminate in the nucleus tractus solitarius. From here, axons project to the ventromedial area (depressor) and rostral-ventrolateral (pressor) areas of the medulla. Any changes in blood pressure will cause changes in firing of the carotid and aortic baroreceptors, which will then result in an increase or decrease in both sympathetic outflow and vagal impulses in order to maintain arterial pressure. If the autonomic nervous system has an abnormality anywhere in these pathways, it could result in systemic hypertension.[2,3]

At this time, diuretics, beta-adrenergic blockers, calcium-channel blockers, angiotensin-II receptor blockers and angiotensin converting enzyme (ACE) inhibitors are considered first-line agents in treating patients with hypertension. Central-acting antihypertensive agents, such as alpha methyldopa and clonidine, have been limited to second- and third-line use due to associated adverse drug effects such as dry mouth, sedation, impotence, and sympathetic overactivity upon sudden withdrawal of the medications.

Rilmenidine and moxonidine are representatives of a new class of central-acting antihypertensive drugs, the imidazoline receptor agonists (Fig. 30-1). Rilmenidine was first registered in France in 1987 and is the first oxazoline-derived agent of its kind.[1] It was originally thought that rilmenidine, like clonidine and alpha methyldopa, mediated its antihypertensive actions by decreasing sympathetic outflow via activation of alpha$_2$-adrenergic receptors in brain medullary structures,[4–8] but more recently it has been found that the drug acts centrally through a newly discovered class of receptors, the nonadrenergic imidazoline receptors.[9–13] This chapter discusses what is known about these receptors and the clinical pharmacology of rilmenidine and moxonidine, the first orally active imidazoline-receptor agonists.

THE IMIDAZOLINE RECEPTORS

At this time, two subtypes of imidazoline receptors have actually been isolated; they have been designated as I-1 and I-2.[13a–18] Both receptors bind to idazoxan, a nonspecific alpha$_2$-adrenergic and imidazoline antagonist, but the I-1 imidazoline receptor has a greater affinity for clonidine, its congener *para*-amonoclonidine, and rilmenidine.[11,14,16,18a] These imidazoline receptors are insensitive to catecholamines, and the distribution in the brain of I-1 and I-2 receptors differs. The I-1 receptor has a more restricted distribution involving the rostral ventrolateral medulla,[19] particularly the C1 area of the rostral ventrolateral reticular nucleus.[20] The I-1 receptor is also found in the hippocampus, hypothalamus, and striatum but not in the frontal cortex.[19] These receptors are assumed to be on the plasma membranes of neurons[19] and are thought to be linked to G proteins (Fig. 30-2).[21] It is the activation of the I-1 receptor that is thought to be responsible for the antihypertensive actions of both rilmenidine and moxonidine.[18]

The I-2 receptor has been implicated in natural neuroprotective processes in the setting of ischemic infarction.[13a,22,23] The I-2 receptor has a much wider area of distribution than the I-1 receptor, having been found in liver,[24] platelets,[25,26] adipocytes,[27] kidney,[28,29] stomach,[30] glial cells,[31] cardiac myocytes,[32] vascular smooth muscle,[32] and chromaffin cells of the adrenal medulla.[14] The distribution of the I-2 receptor is also more widespread in the brain and includes the cerebral cortex.[33] The I-2 receptor also differs from the I-1 receptor in that it is almost exclusively expressed on the mitochondrial membrane[34] in cells that contain this receptor, including chromaffin cells[14] and astrocytes.[35] The I-2 receptor is not found on the plasma membrane of neurons,[36] as is the case with the I-1 receptor.[19]

The imidazoline receptor protein has been found to have a molecular weight of 70 kDa,[37] but the amino acid sequence of the receptor has not yet been elucidated. The isolated receptor protein has been found to have binding sites exclusively for imidazolines and not for alpha$_2$ agonists or antagonists.[6,37] The 70-kDa protein was purified from adrenal chromaffin cells. Efforts to identify the imidazoline binding site have also demonstrated a 43-kDa protein purified from human brainstem, which has been shown

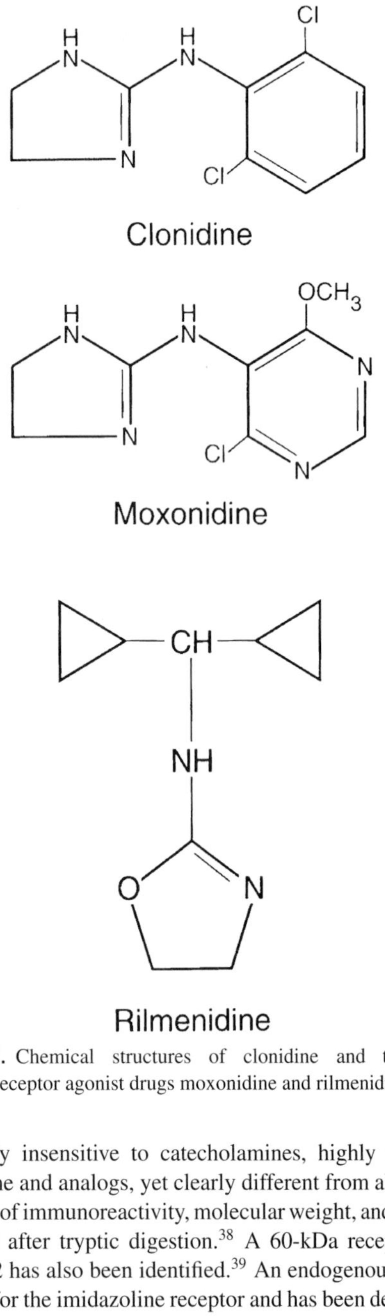

FIGURE 30-1. Chemical structures of clonidine and the selective imidazoline- receptor agonist drugs moxonidine and rilmenidine.

to be largely insensitive to catecholamines, highly sensitive to [3H]clonidine and analogs, yet clearly different from alpha$_2$ receptors in terms of immunoreactivity, molecular weight, and amino acid composition after tryptic digestion.[38] A 60-kDa receptor protein most like I-2 has also been identified.[39] An endogenous ligand has been found for the imidazoline receptor and has been described as a low-molecular-weight, heat-resistant, acid-stable substance identified in rat brains.[40,41] This endogenous ligand has been referred to as clonidine-displacing substance. It has been shown to bind selectively to the imidazoline I-1 receptor in the rostral ventrolateral medulla of rats, and microinjection of clonidine-displacing substance into the rostral ventrolateral medulla results in a reduction in arterial blood pressure.[42] In terms of the signaling transduction mechanism, many questions remain. In PC12 pheochromocytoma cells, stimulation of I-1 receptors elicited the release of prostaglandin E[43] and arachidonic acid.[44] It has also been shown that the I-1 receptor is coupled to phosphatidylcholine-selective phospholipid, leading to the generation of diacylglyceride.[45] Activation of the I-1 receptor–coupled phosphatidylcholine-specific phospholipase C may also result in downstream activation of mitogen-activated protein kinase[46] (Fig. 30-3). I-1 cellular responses also include inhibition of sodium-hydrogen exchange across the cell membrane

and induction of catecholamine synthetic enzymes.[38] In addition, it is hypothesized that signaling may be related to interleukins.[47] Radioligand-binding studies have identified the presence of imidazoline receptors in the rostral ventrolateral medulla along with the paucity of alpha$_2$ adrenoceptors in this same area of distribution.[18a] In contrast, alpha$_2$ adrenoceptors have been found in abundance in areas shown to be responsible for sedation, such as the nucleus tractus solitarius, locus ceruleus, and frontal cortex, while imidazoline receptors were not found in these areas.[48] This difference in affinity for the two receptor types is how rilmenidine and moxonidine differ from clonidine. These imidazoline receptor agonists are more selective for the imidazoline receptors in the ventrolateral region of the medulla oblongata, whereas clonidine is more selective for the alpha$_2$-adrenergic receptor in the locus ceruleus (Fig. 30-4).[9] Rilmenidine has a 2.5 times greater selectivity for imidazoline receptors than for alpha$_2$-adrenergic receptors.[49]

Studies have shown that rilmenidine exerts its antihypertensive effect at the same CNS sites as clonidine, and has a similar mechanism of action in bringing about its antihypertensive effects.[11,12] Originally, it was thought that clonidine's actions were achieved through its agonistic activity at the alpha$_2$-adrenergic receptor resulting in decreased pre- and postganglionic discharge in sympathetic nerves[50,51] to the heart and blood vessels, and a facilitation of the vagal baroreceptor reflex,[52] resulting in hypotension and bradycardia. However, experiments in rats and rabbits have shown that drugs having an imidazoline structure, such as clonidine, rilmenidine, and moxonidine, are hypotensive when injected in minute quantities into the rostral ventrolateral medulla, while alpha methylnorepinephrine, an alpha$_2$ agonist lacking an imidazoline structure, is inactive in this area of the brain.[10,11,53,54] Hypotension was achieved with alpha methylnorepinephrine when injected into the nucleus tractus solitarius, while clonidine, which has an imidazoline structure with alpha$_2$-agonist activity, had no effect on blood pressure at this site except in very high concentrations.[10] These results have led to the conclusion that imidazoline receptors in the rostral ventrolateral medulla are responsible for the antihypertensive activity of clonidine, but recent studies have found evidence to suggest that some of clonidine's hypotensive activities may still be mediated through the alpha$_2$ adrenoreceptors.[55]

RILMENIDINE

Animal Studies

Studies in the spontaneously hypertensive rat (SHR) and the rabbit have demonstrated the interaction between imidazoline receptors and rilmenidine.[55] Idazoxan, a nonspecific alpha-adrenoreceptor blocker and imidazoline receptor blocker, and 2-methoxyidazoxan, a highly specific alpha$_2$-adrenoceptor blocker, were used to determine their effect on the antihypertensive qualities of rilmenidine and clonidine. In the SHR, the antihypertensive effect of rilmenidine was completely reversed with idazoxan and only partially (36%) reversed with 2-methoxyidazoxan.[55] These same studies also revealed that rilmenidine-induced bradycardia was reversed by both antagonists, 87 and 81% respectively.[55] These results agree with previous studies showing that the bradycardia produced by rilmenidine and clonidine is due to agonist activity at the alpha$_2$ adrenoreceptor, and that this bradycardia is reversed with selective alpha$_2$-adrenoreceptor antagonism.[56,57] Similar results were found in normotensive rabbits.[55] In these studies, the

CDS and its putative imidazoline receptor

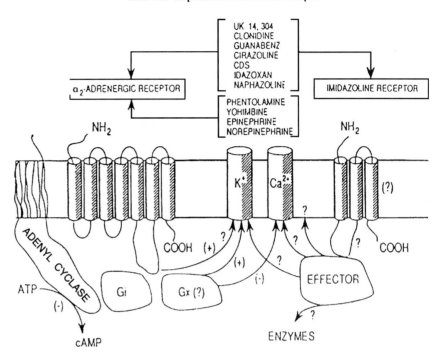

FIGURE 30-2. Schematic representation of alpha$_2$-adrenoreceptors, an imaginary imidazoline site, and their postulated sites of action in the cell. [*Reproduced with permission from Atlas D: Clonidine displacing substance (CDS) and its putative imidazoline receptors. New leads for further divergence of α_2-adrenergic receptor activity. Biochem Pharmacol 1991; 41: 1541–1549.*]

hypotensive effects of rilmenidine were also reversed by idazoxan but not by 2-methoxyidazoxan. However, both idazoxan and 2-methoxyidazoxan reversed the antihypertensive effects of clonidine by similar degrees. The bradycardia induced by both rilmenidine and clonidine was also reversed by 2-methoxyidazoxan. Another study demonstrated that clonidine, rilmenidine, and moxonidine decrease blood pressure and heart rate in a time-dependent manner in stroke-prone SHR.[58] A study in rabbits showed rilmenidine to potentially have antiarrhythmic effects mediated by blunted sympathetic outflow to the heart and vascular beds.[59]

Under normal physiologic conditions, salt and water balance, along with mean arterial pressure, are maintained by the kidney with modulations from local, neural, and hormonal inputs. Hypertension can result when the mean arterial pressure and the hormonal

and neural inputs to the kidney are not able to adequately maintain of sodium and water balance. Rilmenidine has been shown to increase sodium excretion, osmolar clearance, and urine flow rates in one kidney (1K)-sham normotensive rats when infused directly into the renal artery.[60] In 1K-1C (1 clamp) hypertensive rats, the increase in sodium excretion, osmolar clearance, and urine flow rate were not seen to the same extent as in 1K-sham rats, suggesting that the renal effects of rilmenidine are diminished in 1K-1C hypertensive rats.[60] These findings indicate that 1K-1C rats have a decrease in the activity or a blunted response from the imidazoline receptor when stimulated, resulting in sodium and fluid retention and ultimately, hypertension.[60] Other studies with rilmenidine revealed that intravenous administration of rilmenidine did not have a direct natriuretic effect on the kidneys but did increase total and fractional

FIGURE 30-3. Signaling pathways coupled to I-1 imidazoline receptors. (*Reproduced with permission from Ernsberger.*[113])

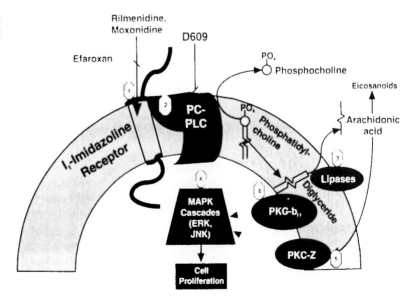

Sites of Action of Centrally Acting Antihypertensive Drugs

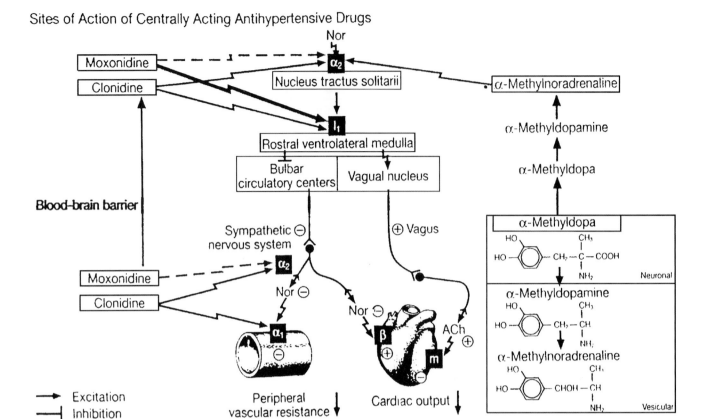

FIGURE 30-4. Sites of action of centrally acting antihypertensive agents. (*Reproduced with permission from Palm D, Hellenbrecht D, Quiring K: Pharmakologie noradrenerger und adrenerger Systeme. In: Forth W, Henschler D, Rummel W, Starke K, eds. Allgemeine und Spezielle Pharmacologie und Toxikologie. Mannheim, Germany:BI Wissenschaftsverlag, 1992:148–199.*)

excretion of sodium and osmoles from innervated kidneys of Wistar rats, while surgically denervated kidneys showed no change in natriuresis.[61] Direct recording of renal sympathetic nerve activity after infusion of rilmenidine showed a profound decrease in sympathetic activity.[61] These data indicate that the increase in sodium excretion and osmolar clearance with rilmenidine is brought about through central inhibition of renal sympathetic nerve activity. Additional studies in SHR demonstrate that the decrease in arterial pressure seen with rilmenidine is accompanied by a decrease in salt appetite and a restoration of the blood pressure–natriuresis relationship, resulting in a resetting of long-term blood pressure control.[62] In humans, rilmenidine has been shown to decrease the glomerular filtration rate and filtration fraction while causing an increase in sodium reabsorption.[63] In a study that compared rilmenidine and alpha methylnoradrenaline and their influence on central inhibition of renal sympathetic nerve activity, it was shown that both drugs lowered mean arterial pressure.[64] However, there were differences in effects on burst frequency and amplitude and baroreflex curves suggesting a difference in mechanism. The study also showed that 2-MI (methoxyidazoxan) to some extent reversed the actions of alpha methylnoradrenaline and rilmenidine. From these data it was proposed that alpha$_2$-adrenoreceptor hypotension may be involved in the rabbit renal sympathetic baroreflex and that rilmenidine may activate alpha$_2$ adrenoreceptors through activation of imidazoline receptors. A study of rilmenidine in Holtzman rats investigated the role of the imidazoline receptor of the paraventricular nucleus in the hypothalamus on the pressor effects of angiotensin II at the subfornical organ.[65] It was shown that rilmenidine decreased the pressor

effects of angiotensin II and, unlike captopril, rilmenidine did not impair the autoregulation of renal blood flow while modulating its hypotensive effect.[66] The study also established that the paraventricular nucleus interacts with the subfornical organ via imidazoline receptors in control of arterial blood pressure.

Neuroprotection in Ischemic Infarction with Rilmenidine

There has been recent evidence from animal studies to suggest that agents that interact with imidazoline receptors may reduce the size of focal ischemic infarctions.[22,67,68] This neuroprotection is thought to be mediated through the I-2 subclass of imidazoline receptors.[13a] As stated above, the I-2 receptor is found throughout the cerebral cortex on the mitochondrial membrane of astrocytes.[69] These I-2 receptors have not been found to be coupled to G protein–linked second messenger systems, since the levels of cyclic adenosine monophosphate, cyclic gunaosine monophosphate, or phosphoinositiol are not increased with activation of the I-2 receptor.[70] There have been experiments with kidney cells suggesting that the I-2 receptor may be coupled to Na$^+$ and H$^+$ ion channels.[71] Agents that interact with the imidazoline receptor, such as rilmenidine and clonidine, increase the influx of $^{45}Ca^{2+}$ into adrenal chromaffin cells.[70] Studies have found that agents which are agonistic and antagonistic at the imidazoline receptor are neuroprotective in the setting of cerebral ischemia. This association was first discovered with idazoxan,[67,68] an alpha$_2$-adrenergic receptor and imidazoline receptor antagonist. The neuroprotection was initially thought to come about by antagonistic activity at the alpha$_2$-adrenergic receptor; but with the isolation of the imidazoline receptor, it is now thought that neuroprotection is actually due to some interaction with the imidazoline receptor.[22] Maiese et al. have compared the effect of rilmenidine, idazoxan, and SKF-86466 (a specific alpha$_2$-adrenergic receptor antagonist) on the extent of cerebral infarction following occlusion of the middle cerebral artery in the rat.[22] These same authors found that rilmenidine elicited a significant dose-dependent protective effect on neuronal tissue to 33% of control, while idazoxan produced a significant reduction in cerebral infarction size by 22%. SKF-86466, on the other hand, did not result in reduction in the size of ischemic infarction. The experiments also went on to examine whether the neuroprotection was due to changes in local cerebral blood flow by increasing cerebral blood flow to 200% of control. There was no increased preservation of ischemic tissue despite doubling of blood flow. The authors concluded that the mechanism of neuroprotection for rilmenidine and idazoxan does not appear to be secondary to interaction at the alpha$_2$-adrenergic receptor or an elevation of local cerebral blood flow, because these factors did not lead to a reduction in the volume of infarction after occlusion of the middle cerebral artery (Fig. 30-5). The results suggest that the neuroprotective effects of rilmenidine and idazoxan occur through an interaction with the imidazoline receptor, but the exact nature of the interaction is unclear because rilmenidine is an agonist while idazoxan is an antagonist.

The specific cause of cell death in the setting of cerebral ischemia is unclear and probably multifactorial, but it is thought that the progression to cell death starts with the inactivation of energy-dependent ion and neurotransmitter uptake pumps on the neuronal membranes and astrocytes secondary to hypoxia.[72] This results in an excessive release of the neurotransmitter L-glutamate, which stimulates a subclass of glutamate receptors, N-methyl-D-aspartate (NMDA) and α-amino-3-hydroxy-5-methyl-4-isoxazole proprionic acid, leading to an accumulation of intracellular Ca^2 and Na$^+$.[72] The elevated levels of intracellular Ca^{2+} activates Ca^{2+}-dependent lipolytic and proteolytic enzymes, which generates nitric oxide, and eventually superoxides, which ultimately result in cell death.[72] The elevated levels of Na$^+$ intracellularly also result in cell death by leading to cellular swelling and eventually lysis. A number of agents appear to interfere with the cascade of events discussed above, including superoxide dismutase,[73,74] which destroys oxygen-free radicals; calcium-channel antagonists,[75,76] which block the entry of Ca^{2+}; and MK-801[77,78] which interferes with the stimulation of the NMDA receptors while causing antagonism of Ca^{2+} entry. In addition, barbiturates[35,79] and hypothermia[80] have been found to be neuroprotective by decreasing cellular metabolism.

Studies with rilmenidine in the setting of cerebral ischemia suggest that its site of action in the ischemic penumbra is mediated through the I-2 receptor on the mitochondrial membrane[34] in the

FIGURE 30-5. Proposed mechanism to account for salvage in focal ischemia by rilmenidine (RIL). (*A*) Neuron and astrocyte with I-2 receptors (I-2R) localized to astrocytic mitochondria. (*B*) Effects of focal ischemia in releasing glutamate (GLU) from afferent glutamatergic terminal, thereby increasing Ca^{2+} entry into neurons, leading to toxic levels of the ion. (*C*) Proposed action of rilmenidine to increase Ca^{2+} entry only into cortical astrocytes, since cortical neurons do not harbor IRs. (*D*) The action of rilmenidine on ischemia, in which stimulation of Ca^{2+} entry into astrocytes reduces the amounts available to entry into neurons, thus acting to limit damage in neurons in the penumbra. NMDA = N-methyl-D-aspartate. (*Reproduced with permission from Reis et al.*[13a])

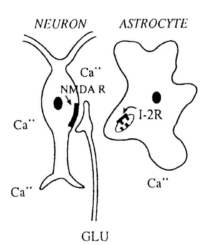

A. CONTROL

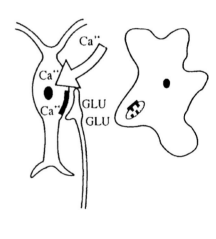

B. ISCHEMIA

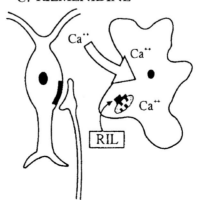

C. RILMENIDINE

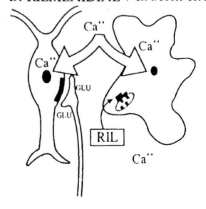

D. RILMENIDINE + ISCHEMIA

astrocytes[69] of the cerebral cortex.[33] This conclusion is based upon experiments which found that I-1 receptors are not found in the cerebral cortex,[81] while almost all I-2 receptors in the brain are found on the mitochondrial membranes in astrocytes.[34] The exact cellular mechanism responsible for neuroprotection elicited by rilmenidine is still unclear, but one theory—based on the Ca^{2+} hypothesis of ischemic cell death, along with the findings of Ca^{2+} influx in bovine adrenal chomaffin cells with stimulation of the imidazoline receptors[70]—has the astrocytes acting as an extracellular sink for Ca^{2+},[13a] thus diverting some of the Ca^{2+} from the neurons into the astrocytes, which are the only cells in the frontal cortex with I-2 receptors.[37] Rilmenidine evokes a release of Ca^{2+} from intracellular stores in astrocytes, which may trigger the influx of extracellular Ca^{2+} into these cells.[82] This theory is further reinforced by results showing that reductions in extracellular Ca^{2+} can provide some degree of neuroprotection in cerebral ischemia.[83,84]

Clinical Trials in Hypertension

The results of clinical trials have demonstrated the efficacy and safety of rilmenidine in the treatment of systemic hypertension.[85–89] Similar results have been obtained in hypertensive subpopulations having diabetes mellitus,[90,91] syndrome X,[92] renal insufficiency,[93,94] and left ventricular hypertrophy,[95] as well as in the elderly.[96,97] The efficacy of rilmenidine has been found to be comparable to that of first-line antihypertensive drugs such as atenolol[98] and hydrochlorothiazide[95,99] and to second-line central acting agents such as alpha methyldopa[100] and clonidine[85]; in addition, the drug is as well tolerated as atenolol[98] and hydrochlorothiazide.[97] There is also no evidence of the "clonidine withdrawal syndrome" with sudden termination of rilmenidine.[100] Long-term hypertension treatment with rilmenidine has produced a reduction in left ventricular mass[31] comparable to that of nifedipine.[101]

In the elderly population, rilmenidine has been found to be well tolerated[96,97] and as efficacious as hydrochlorothiazide[97] in lowering both systolic and diastolic blood pressure. There were no cases of orthostatic hypotension observed, and no clonidine withdrawal syndrome was seen with the sudden termination of rilmenidine.[96] The lack of orthostatic hypotension with rilmenidine treatment may be due to an increase in baroreflex sensitivity.[102] Pelemans et al. found that rilmenidine did not induce changes in blood chemistries, in contrast to hydrochlorothiazide.[97] The hydrochlorothiazide group demonstrated a significant decrease in both potassium and chloride serum levels, while uric acid levels were increased. There were no significant differences in serum lipids between rilmenidine- and hydrochlorothiazide-treated patients. The hydrochlorothiazide group had a significant decrease in weight of 1 kg, while the rilmenidine group had no change in weight. It was concluded that rilmenidine is both well tolerated and as efficacious as hydrochlorothiazide in lowering blood pressure in the elderly, without the associated serum chemistry changes commonly seen with hydrochlorothiazide.

Pharmacokinetics and Use in Patients with Renal Insufficiency

Rilmenidine is rapidly and almost completely absorbed regardless of food intake. A peak plasma drug concentration is reached in 1.5 to 2 h, and the drug's elimination half-life is approximately 8 h. Rilmenidine's hypotensive properties are maintained well beyond its plasma half-life. Rilmenidine has a volume of distribution of 4.2 L/kg, and less than 10% of drug is bound to plasma proteins. The main route of elimination of rilmenidine is by the kidneys, with 65% of the dose being excreted as unchanged drug with only traces of metabolites from oxazoline ring hydrolysis or oxidation. Renal clearance is 300 mL/min, and total clearance is 450 mL/min.[8] There is no drug accumulation with repeated dosing,[87] and steady state is reached by the third day of dosing.[8] Hypertension does not influence the absorption, distribution, or elimination of rilmenidine.[8] In the elderly, drug absorption is delayed and the elimination half-life is prolonged to 13 h, probably secondary in older subjects to a 12% decrease in the drug's volume of distribution and a 50% decrease in apparent total clearance.[8] The pharmacokinetic/pharmacodynamic relationship is also not influenced by rate of infusion. In comparing the effect profile of different intravenous infusion rates of rilmenidine by saccadic eye movements, electroencephalogram, blood pressure, and heart rate, there was no significant difference between a fast and slow infusion used to achieve a target concentration.[103]

The pharmacokinetics of rilmenidine are altered in the setting of renal insufficiency and renal failure, as would be expected, since the main route for drug elimination is renal. In patients with a creatinine clearance of 30 mL/min/1.73 m^2, elimination half-life is extended to 29 h; and in patients with severe renal impairment, the elimination half-life of drug is prolonged to 42 h.[94] These results have led to the following proposals for dosage changes in patients with renal impairment. In hypertensive patients with a creatinine clearance of 15 to 30 mL/min/1.73 m^2, rilmenidine 1 mg every other day should be given.[94] In patients with more severe renal impairment, the drug can be given every 3 days as necessary. Hypertensive patients undergoing hemodialysis do not require an additional dose of rilmenidine after a standard 4-h dialysis session because the drug is poorly dialyzable.[94]

MOXONIDINE

Moxonidine is also a selective imidazoline I-1 receptor agonist with 40 to 70 times greater affinity for I-1 imidazoline receptors than for alpha$_2$ receptors in the bovine rostral ventrolateral medulla oblongata.[54] When it was compared against rilmenidine, moxonidine had a threefold greater affinity for the I-1 imidazoline receptor in the ventrolateral medulla, which correlates with the threefold higher dose of rilmenidine required in order to attain a similar level of antihypertensive efficacy. The affinity for the alpha$_2$-adrenergic receptor is nearly the same for the two agents when I-1 receptors are masked. Moxonidine was also found to be more selective for the I-1 imidazoline receptor than both rilmenidine and clonidine. Clonidine was found to be twice as potent as moxonidine at the I-1 receptor, but moxonidine was considerably more selective at this receptor when compared to clonidine. Moxonidine also had the highest agonist activity at the I-1 versus the I-2 imidazoline receptor, with efaroxan being the most selective antagonist. Moxonidine was determined to be more selective and more potent than rilmenidine. Moxonidine, like rilmenidine, has been found to elicit a dose-dependent decrease in arterial blood pressure when injected into the rostral ventrolateral medulla of SHR.[104]

In addition to moxonidine's antihypertensive effects, animal studies have shown that moxonidine reduces free fatty acids[105] and urine protein excretion,[106] improves insulin secretion[105] and glucose tolerance,[107] and increases urine flow rate via augmented sodium excretion.[108] The drug has also been shown to improve corticocerebral blood flow in both normal and ischemic conditions and may be beneficial in the management of cerebral ischemia.[109]

Clinical Experience

The hypotensive properties of moxonidine are due to a reduction in peripheral vascular resistance secondary to a centrally mediated decrease in adrenergic tone.[110–117] There is also a 26 and 33.5% reduction in serum norepinephrine, and a 23 and 35.5% reduction in plasma renin activity in hypertensive patients 4 to 6 h after single oral doses of moxonidine 0.25 and 0.4 mg respectively.[111,112] Epinephrine levels were not significantly reduced in 4 to 6 h but were significantly lower 6 to 9 h following a single 0.25-mg dose.[112] Moxonidine has also been shown to stimulate plasma atrial natriuretic peptide (ANP) and increase urinary guanosine monophosphate (GMP) excretion.[118]

Cardiac hemodynamics—such as cardiac output, stroke volume and pulmonary artery pressure—are unaffected by moxonidine.[111,119] In a study by Huting et al.,[119] there was no change in left ventricular ejection fraction but there was a fall in left ventricular end-systolic volume from 75 to 64 mL and end-diastolic volume from 164 to 151 mL in 12 hypertensive patients taking moxonidine 0.2 mg twice daily. In patients with left ventricular hypertrophy, a 6-month course of moxonidine has been associated with a significant reduction in ventricular septal thickness.[120] In hypertensive patients with microalbuminuria, moxonidine was shown to significantly reduce urine albumin excretion.[121] Unlike other antihypertensive drugs, such as beta-blockers, moxonidine does not seem to affect either the plasma lipid profile or lipoprotein composition.[122]

In comparative studies, moxonidine has shown comparable hypotensive effectiveness and tolerability when compared against agents from each major class of antihypertensive medication currently being used. In comparison with clonidine at equivalent hypotensive doses,[123,124] the incidence of dry mouth was 20% with moxonidine versus 46% with clonidine, while the incidence of tiredness was 13% versus 17% respectively. Similarly, moxonidine was found to be comparable in antihypertensive effectiveness to atenolol,[125] immediate-release nifedipine,[126] sustained-release nifedipine,[119,127] captopril,[128,129] enalapril,[130] prazosin,[131] and hydrochlorothiazide.[132] In the prazosin-moxonidine comparisons, the number of adverse effects was similar with both drugs. However, there were significantly fewer episodes of orthostatic hypotension in the moxonidine group compared to the prazosin group (1 versus 13, respectively), but the reverse was true for dry mouth, with 16 patients in the moxonidine group versus 2 in the prazosin group.

Recent data suggest that the activation of imidazoline pathway may be beneficial in the treatment of glaucoma by reducing intraocular pressure.[133,133a] Retinal microvessel disease can also be targeted with moxonidine by causing potent vasoconstriction.[134]

Pharmacokinetics of Moxonidine

A study by Weinmann and Rudolph[135] with [^{14}C] radiolabeled moxonidine showed the drug is 89% absorbed orally and has a bioavailability of 88% regardless of food intake. The T_{max} for moxonidine is about 1 h, with a C_{max} of 1.5 ng/mL 15 to 30 min after an oral dose of 0.2 mg. The volume of distribution for moxonidine is 1.83 L/kg. Similar to rilmenidine, the antihypertensive activity of moxonidine

is longer than would be expected given its half-life of 2 h with essentially complete excretion of drug by 24 h. Moxonidine is excreted almost entirely via the renal route. Renal excretion accounts for 90–96% of the total drug elimination with less than 2% of the drug being excreted in the feces. Repeated dosing does not cause drug accumulation. The apparent total plasma clearance in 12 healthy males was 830 mL/min, and the renal clearance was 530 mL/min, suggesting that the drug is secreted into the renal tubule.

The pharmacokinetics of moxonidine are unchanged in the hypertensive and the elderly patient, with no need to adjust dosing in these populations. There does not appear to be any drug-drug interaction between moxonidine and hydrochlorothiazide, glibenclamide or digoxin over a 5-day treatment course. In patients with renal insufficiency, there is a statistically significant increase in the half-life and C_{max}, and a decrease in the apparent total clearance with increasing renal insufficiency. Though plasma concentrations of moxonidine in patients with glomerular filtration rates <30 mL/min were unchanged after repeated dosing, titration of dosage to effect may be required.[135,136,136a]

USE OF CLONIDINE AND IMIDAZOLINE-RECEPTOR AGONISTS IN THE TREATMENT OF CONGESTIVE HEART FAILURE

Symptomatic congestive heart failure (CHF) is characterized by sympathetic neurohormonal activation and pathologically elevated peripheral vascular resistance.[137] The increase in cardiac sympathetic activity has been shown to be a strong predictor of clinical outcome,[138] and high levels of neurohormones are considered to be a marker of poor prognosis.[139,140] This activation would be intended to restore circulatory pressure and volume by stimulating myocardial contractility, constriction of peripheral arteries, and sodium and fluid retention. Though initially effective, in the long run, the increased sympathetic activity results in increased preload and afterload, myocardial dysfunction, and further decompensation.

Therapy for chronic CHF has been aimed at specific mechanisms including suppression of the renin-angiotensin-aldosterone axis and sympathetic blockade with peripheral alpha- and beta-adrenergic-receptor blockers. The efficacy of beta-adrenergic-receptor blockers provides evidence that the inhibition of sympathetic activity is beneficial in patients with CHF. While beta-blockers inhibit beta-adrenergic receptors in the neuroeffector junction, they may not reduce efferent sympathetic outflow[141] or antagonize other compounds released at the adrenergic nerve terminals, such as dopamine and neuropeptide Y.[142] With the above in mind, investigators have begun to evaluate the role of central sympathetic inhibition as an adjunct therapeutic modality in CHF.[143]

Studies have been undertaken to examine the effects of clonidine on cardiac sympathetic activity in patients with CHF. A pilot study demonstrated the effects of sympathetic suppression with clonidine after 2 to 3 h and after 1 week of follow-up in 20 patients with CHF. They found that clonidine reduced preload, heart rate, and arterial pressure—all indices of myocardial energy demand.[144] Specifically, the following was reported: decreases of 8% in mean arterial pressure, 23% in right arterial pressure, 19% in mean pulmonary artery pressure, and 12% in heart rate; increase of 17% in stroke volume; and no significant changes in cardiac output or systemic vascular resistance.[144] A drop in plasma norepinephrine of 28% after the initial dose and 68% after 1 week of therapy was also reported.[144] Another study of clonidine in 9 CHF patients concluded that clonidine caused a marked reduction in sympathetic activity directed at the heart, and the negative inotropic effects appear to be secondary to the reduction in sympathetic drive.[143] An intravenous dose of 150 μg of clonidine produced a 59% reduction in cardiac norepinephrine spillover.[143]

There has recently been some experience with moxonidine and the sustained-release formulation of the drug showing that the increased sympathetic activation in CHF can be reduced.[145,146] A study evaluated the acute neurohormonal and hemodynamic effects of a single oral dose of moxonidine (0.4 or 0.6 mg) in a double-blind randomized study of 32 CHF patients. Moxonidine produced a dose-dependent vasodilator response and was well tolerated. After 6 h, the 0.6-mg dose of moxonidine produced significant reductions in mean systemic arterial pressure, mean pulmonary arterial pressure, systemic vascular resistance, heart rate, and plasma norepinephrine. Stroke volume was unchanged.[147]

Despite these potentially beneficial features, the results of a recent placebo-controlled survival trial using moxonidine in patients with class II to IV CHF [MOXCON (Moxonidine for Congestive Heart Failure)] showed an increased mortality rate with the drug.[148] Deaths in the active-treatment group appeared to be sudden and were found at all doses (0.25 mg twice daily to 1.5 mg twice daily). An excess of acute myocardial infarctions were also seen in the moxonidine group compared to the placebo group: 17 versus 6. As expected, plasma norepinephrine levels fell in moxonidine-treated patients, raising questions regarding the hypothesis that excess sympathetic nervous activation is harmful and should be inhibited in patients with heart failure. Survival studies using clonidine or rilmenidine have not been reported.

ANTIARRHYTHMIC ACTIONS

The involvement of the sympathetic nervous system in the genesis of ventricular dysrhythmias is well documented. In animal studies, restoration of sympathovagal balance by centrally acting drugs, such as the imidazoline selective drugs, has been shown to prevent these dysrhythmias.[149,150] However, in heart failure patients, the drugs have been associated with an increased risk of sudden death. Clinical trials need to be done to confirm this finding in humans.

CONCLUSION

In summary, rilmenidine, and moxonidine are representatives of a new class of centrally active antihypertensive agents having a greater selectivity for the imidazoline receptor relative to the alpha$_2$-adrenergic receptor.[151] This receptor selectivity allows these second-generation agents to have central antihypertensive properties, while being associated with fewer central adverse effects (such as dry mouth, sedation, and tiredness) compared to older agents such as clonidine and methyldopa. These imidazoline receptor agonists appear to lower blood pressure by decreasing central sympathetic outflow and decreasing plasma catecholamine and renin levels without affecting serum blood uric acid, electrolytes, or the lipid profile.

Although they are not yet approved for clinical use in the United States, the safety and efficacy of these agents have been well demonstrated in multiple clinical trials in hypertensive patients, including patients with concurrent illnesses.[152–154] Left ventricular hypertrophy has been shown to regress during treatment with both rilmenidine and moxonidine. The efficacy of these agents has been shown to be comparable to that of first-line antihypertensive agents, including atenolol and hydrochlorothiazide, and moxonidine has also been shown to be comparable in its blood pressure–lowering action to nifedipine, captopril, and prazosin. Both rilmenidine and moxonidine were tolerated as well as the antihypertensive medications to which they were compared in these trials. Rilmenidine has also been shown to be neuroprotective in the setting of focal cerebral ischemia in animal studies. These agents also provide the convenience of once-daily dosing for the treatment of hypertension.

As for the role of imidazoline receptor agonists in the treatment of CHF, the outlook is less clear. Though these agents may blunt the neurohormonal excesses seen in heart failure, survival trials to date have not shown any benefit, with the potential for an increased mortality risk.

REFERENCES

1. Safar ME, Laurent S: Rilmenidine. In: Messerli R, ed. *Cardiovascular Drug Therapy, 2nd ed.* Philadelphia: Saunders, 1996:633.
2. Esler M: The sympathetic system and hypertension. *Am J Hypertens* 13(Suppl):99S, 2000.
3. Brook RD, Julius S: Autonomic imbalance, hypertension, and cardiovascular risk. *Am J Hypertens* 13(Suppl):112S, 2000.
4. Van Zwieter P: Pharmacology of alpha$_2$-adrenoceptor agonist rilmenidine. *Am J Cardiol* 61:6D, 1988.
5. Koenig-Berard E, Tierney C, Beau B, et al: Cardiovascular and central nervous system effects of rilmenidine (S-3341) in rats. *Am J Cardiol* 61:22D, 1988.
6. Velasco M, Luchsinger A: Central acting antihypertensive drugs: Past, present, and future. *Am J Ther* 2:255, 1995.
7. Timmermans PBMWM, Van Zwieter PA: Postsynaptic alpha$_1$- and alpha$_2$-adrenoreceptors in the circulatory system of pithed rats: Selective stimulation of the alpha$_2$ type by B-HT 933. *Eur J Pharmacol* 63:199, 1980.
8. Singlas E, Ehrhardt JD, Zech P, et al: Pharmacokinetics of rilmenidine. *Am J Cardiol* 61:54D, 1988.
9. Dontenwill M, Tibirica E, Greney G, et al: Role of imidazoline receptors in cardiovascular regulation. *Am J Cardiol* 74:3A, 1994.
10. Bousquet P, Feldman J, Schwartz J: Central cardiovascular effects of alpha-adrenergic drugs: Difference between catecholamines and imidazolines. *J Pharmacol Exp Ther* 230:230, 1984.
11. Feldman F, Tibirica E, Brica G, et al: Evidence for the involvement of imidazoline receptor in the central hypotensive effect of rilmenidine in the rabbit. *Br J Pharmacol* 100:600, 1990.
12. Head GA, Burke SL: I$_1$ imidazoline receptors in cardiovascular regulation: The place of rilmenidine. *Am J Hypertens* 13(Suppl):89S, 2000.
13. Sy GY, Bruban V, Bousquet P, Feldman J: Nitric oxide and central antihypertensive drugs. One more difference between catecholamines and imidazolines. *Hypertension* 37:246, 2001.
13a. Reis D, Regunathan S, Golanov G, Feinstein D: Protection of focal ischemic infarction by rilmenidine in the animal: Evidence that interactions with central imidazoline receptors may be neuro-protective. *Am J Cardiol* 74:25A, 1994.
14. Regunthan S, Meeley MP, Reis DJ: Expression on nonadrenergic imidazoline sites in chromaffin cell and mitochondrial membranes of bovine adrenal medulla. *Biochem Pharmacol* 45:1667, 1993.
15. Ernsberger P, Damon TH, Graf LM, et al: Moxonidine, a central acting antihypertensive agent, is selective for I-1 imidazoline sites. *J Pharmacol Exp Ther* 264:172, 1993.
16. Gomez RO, Ernsberger P, Feinland G, Reis DJ: Rilmenidine lowers arterial pressure via imidazoline receptors in the brainstem C1 area. *Eur J Pharmacol* 195:181, 1991.
17. Bousquet P: Identification and characterization of I$_1$ imidazoline receptors: Their role in blood pressure regulation. *Am J Hypertens* 13(Suppl):84S, 2000.

18. Bousquet P, Dontenwill M, Greney H, Feldman J: Imidazoline receptors in cardiovascular and metabolic diseases. *J Cardiovasc Pharmacol* 35(Suppl 4):S21, 2000.

18a. Ernsberger P, Meeley MP, Mann JJ, Reis DJ: Clonidine binds to imidazoline binding sites as well as alpha$_2$-adrenoreceptors in the ventrolateral medulla. *Eur J Pharmacol* 134:1, 1987.

19. Kamisaki Y, Ishikawa T, Takao Y, et al: Binding of [^{3}H]p-aminoclonidine to two sites, α_2-adrenoceptors and imidazoline binding sites: Distribution of imidazoline binding sites in rat brain. *Brain Res* 514:15, 1990.

20. Reis DJ, Ruggiero DA, Morrison SJ: The C1 area of the rostral ventrolateral medulla: A critical brainstem region for control of resting and reflex integration of arterial pressure. *Am J Hypertens* 291:2363S, 1989.

21. Ernsberger P, Graves ME, Graff L, et al: I1-imidazoline receptors. Definition, characterization, distribution, and transmembrane signaling. *Ann NY Acad Sci* 763:22, 1995.

22. Maiese K, Pek L, Berger SB, Reis DJ: Reduction in focal cerebral ischemia by agents acting at imidazole receptors. *J Cereb Blood Flow Metab* 12(1):53, 1992.

23. Yamamato S, Golanov EV, Berger SB, Reis DJ: Inhibition of nitric oxide synthesis increases focal ischemic infarction in rat. *J Cereb Blood Flow Metab* 12(5):717, 1992.

24. Zonnenschein R, Diamant S, Atlas D: Imidazoline receptor in rat hepatocytes: A subtype of α_2-adrenergic receptor or a new receptor? *Eur J Pharmacol* 183:853, 1990.

25. Petrusewicz J, Kaliszan R: Human blood platelet alpha adrenoceptor in view of the effects of various imidazol(in)e drugs on aggregation. *Gen Pharmacol* 22(5):819, 1991.

26. Piletz JE, Sletten K: Nonadrenergic imidazoline binding sites on human platelets. *J Pharmacol Exp Ther* 267(3):1493, 1993.

27. Diamant S, Eldar-Geva T, Atlas D: Imidazoline binding sites in human placenta: Evidence for heterogeneity and a search for physiological function. *Br J Pharmacol* 106:1019, 1992.

28. Coupry I, Atlas D, Pedevin RA, et al: Imidazoline-guanidinium receptive sites in renal proximal tubule: Asymmetric distribution, regulation by cations and interaction with an endogenous clonidine displacing substance. *J Pharmacol Exp Ther* 252:293, 1989.

29. Ernsberger P, Feinland G, Meeley MP, Reis DJ: Characterization and visualization of clonidine-sensitive imidazoline sites in rat kidney which recognize clonidine-displacing substance. *Am J Hypertens* 3:90, 1990.

30. Molderings GJ, Donecker K, Burian M, et al: Characterization of I2 imidazoline and sigma binding sites in the rat and human stomach. *J Pharmacol Exp Ther* 285(1):170, 1998.

31. Van Zwieten PA: Central imidazoline (I1) receptors as targets of centrally acting antihypertensives: moxonidine and rilmenidine. *J Hypertens* 15(2):117, 1997.

32. Molderings GJ, Gothert M: Imidazoline binding sites and receptors in cardiovascular tissue. *Gen Pharmacol* 1999; 32(1):17, 1997.

33. Mallard NJ, Hudson AL, Nutt DJ: Characterization and autoradiographical localization of non-adrenoreceptor idazoxan binding sites in the rat brain. *Br J Pharmacol* 106:1019, 1992.

34. Meeley MP, Regunathan S, Roberts S, et al: Distinct sub-cellular localization of imidazoline and α_2-adrenergic receptors in bovine cerebral cortex. *Soc Neurosci Abstr* 18:59l, 1992.

35. Michenfelder JD, Milde JH, Sundt TM Jr: Cerebral protection by barbiturate anesthesia. Use after middle cerebral artery occlusion in Java monkeys. *Arch Neurol* 33:345, 1976.

36. Regunathan S, Feinstein DL, Reis DJ: Expression of non-adrenergic sites in rat cerebral cortical astrocytes. *J Neurosci Res* 1993; 34:6811, 1976.

37. Wang WH, Regunathan S, McGowan D, et al: An antiserum to idazoxan recognizes an immunoreactive substance in human serum and cerebral spinal fluid, which is not agmatine. *Neurochem Int* 30:85, 1997.

38. Ernsberger P: The I-1 imidazoline receptor and its cellular signaling pathways. *Ann NY Acad Sci* 881:35, 1999.

39. Limon I, Coupry I, Lanier SM, Parini A: Purification and characterization of mitochondrial imidazoline-guanidium receptive site from rabbit kidney. *J Biol Chem* 267:21645, 1992.

40. Atlas D, Burstein Y: Isolation of an endogenous clonidine-displacing substance from rat brain. *FEBS Lett* 170:387, 1984.

41. Atlas D, Burstein Y: Isolation and partial purification of a clonidine-displacing endogenous brain substance. *Eur J Biochem* 144:287, 1984.

42. Meeley MP, Ernsberge PR, Granata AR, Reis DJ: An endogenous clonidine-displacing substance from bovine brain: Receptor binding and hypotensive actions in the ventrolateral medulla. *Life Sci* 38:1119, 1986.

43. Ernsberger P, Graves ME, Graff LM: I-1 imidazoline receptors: Definition, characterization, distribution, and transmembrane signaling. *Ann NY Acad Sci* 763:22, 1995.

44. Ernsberger P: Arachadonic acid release from PC12 pheochromocytoma cells is regulated by I-1 imidazoline receptors. *J Auton Nerv Syst* 72:147, 1998.

45. Separovic D, Kester M, Ernsberger P: Coupling of I-1 imidazoline receptors to diacylglyceride accumulation in PC12 rat pheochromocytoma cells. *Mol Pharmacol* 49:668, 1996.

46. Zhang J, El-mas MM, Abdel-Rahman AA: Imidazoline I-1 receptor induced activation of phosphatidylcholine-specific phospholipase C elicits mitogen-activated protein kinase phosphorylation in PC12 cells. *Eur J Pharmacol* 415(2-3):117, 2001.

47. Musgave IF: Novel targets and techniques in imidazoline receptor research. *Ann NY Acad Sci* 881:301, 1999.

48. Bricca G, Zhang J, Greney H, et al: Relevance of the use of [^{3}H]-clonidine to identify imidazoline receptors in the rabbit brainstem. *Br J Pharmacol* 110:1537, 1993.

49. Bricca G, Dontenwill M, Molines A, et al: Rilmenidine selectivity for imidazoline receptors in human brain. *Eur J Pharmacol* 163: 373, 1989.

50. Guyenet PG, Cabot JC: Inhibition of sympathetic preganglionic neurons by catecholamines and clonidine: Mediation by an α-adrenergic receptor. *J Neurosci* 1: 908, 1981.

51. Sun MK, Guyenet PG: Effect of clonidine and gamma-aminobutyric acid on the discharges of medullo-spinal sympathoexcitatory neurons in the rat. *Brain Res* 368:1, 1986.

52. Gillis R, Gatti PJ, Quest JA: Mechanism of the antihypertensive effect of α_2-agonists. *J Cardiovasc Pharmacol* 8(Suppl 8):S38, 1986.

53. Ernsberger P, Guiliano R, Willette RN, Reis DJ: Role of imidazoline receptors in the vasodepressor response to clonidine analogs in the rostral ventrolateral medulla. *J Pharmacol Exp Ther* 253:408, 1990.

54. Ernsberger P, Westbrooks L, Christen O, Schafer SG: A second generation of centrally acting antihypertensive agents act on putative I1-imidazoline receptors. *J Cardiovasc Pharmacol* 1992; 20:S1, 1990.

55. Sannajust F, Head G: Involvement of imidazoline-preferring receptors in regulation of sympathetic tone. *Am J Cardiol* 74:7A, 1994.

56. Deckert V, Lachaud V, Parini A, Elghozi JL: Contribution of alpha-2-adrenoceptors to the central cardiovascular effects of clonidine and S8350 in anaesthetized rats. *Clin Exp Pharmacol Physiol* 18:401, 1991.

57. Dabire H, Mouille P, Fournier B, Schmitt H: Pre- and post-synaptic α_2-adrenoreceptor blockade by (imidazolinyl-2-)-2-benzodioxane 1-4 (170150): Antagonistic action on central effects of clonidine. *Arch Int Pharmacodyn Ther* 254:262, 1981.

58. Medvedev OS, Kunduzova OR, Murashev AN, Medvedeva NA: Chronopharmacological dependence of antihypertensive effects of the imidazoline-like drugs in stroke-prone spontaneously hypertensive rats. *J Auton Nerv Syst* 72(2-3):170, 1998.

59. Roegel JC, Yannoulis N, De Jong W, et al: Preventive effect of rilmenidine on the occurrence of neurogenic ventricular arrhythmias in rabbits. *J Hypertens Suppl* 16(3):S39, 1998.

60. Li P, Penner SB, Smyth DD: Attenuated renal response to moxonidine and rilmenidine on kidney one-clip hypertensive rats. *Br J Pharmacol* 112:200, 1994.

61. Kline R, van der Mark J, Cechetteo D: Natriuretic effect of rilmenidine in anesthetized rats. *Am J Cardiol* 74:20A, 1994.

62. Cechetto DF, Kline RL: Complementary antihypertensive action of rilmenidine on the pressure-natriuresis relationship and sodium preference in spontaneously hypertensive rats. *J Hypertens Suppl* 16(3):S13, 1998.

63. Fauvel JP, Najem R, Ryon B, et al: Effects of rilmenidine on stress-induced peak blood pressure and renal function. *J Cardiovasc Pharmacol* 34:41, 1999.

64. Head GA: Comparison of renal sympathetic baroreflex effects of rilmenidine and alpha-methylnoradrenaline in the ventrolateral medulla of the rabbit. *J Hypertens* 18:1263, 2000.

65. Saad WA, Camargo LA, Silveira JE, et al: Imidazoline receptors of the paraventricular nucleus on the pressor response induced by stimulation of the subfornical organ. *J Physiol Paris* 92(1):25, 1998.

66. Bauduceau B, Mayaudon H, Dupuy O: Rilmenidine in the hypertensive type-2 diabetic: A controlled pilot study versus captopril. *J Cardiovasc Risk* 7(1):57, 2000.

67. Gustafson I, Miyauchi Y, Wieloch T: Postischemic administration of idazoxan, an α_2-adrenergic receptor antagonist, decreases neuronal damage in the rat brain. *J Cereb Blood Flow Metab* 9:171, 1989.

68. Gustafson I, Weterberg E, Wieloch T: Protection against ischemic-induced neuronal damage by the α_2-adrenergic receptor antagonist idazoxan: Influence of time of administration and possible mechanisms of action. *J Cerebr Blood Flow Metab* 10:885, 1989.

69. Ruggiero DA, Milner TA, Wang H, et al: Imidazoline receptor-associated binding protein in the central nervous system. *Soc Neurosci Abstr* 18:591, 1992.

70. Regunathan S, Evinger MJ, Meeley MP, Reis DJ: Effect of clonidine and other imidazole-receptor binding agents on second messenger systems and calcium influx in bovine adrenal chromaffin cells. *Biochem Pharmacol* 1991; 42:2011, 1992.

71. Bidet M, Poujeol P, Parini A: Effect of imidazolines on Na^+ transport and intracellular pH in renal proximal tubule cells. *Biochem Biophys Acta* l024:l73, 1990.

72. Siesjo BK: Pathophysiology and treatment of focal cerebral ischemia. Part 1: Pathophysiology. *J Neurosurg* 77:167, 1992.

73. Imaizumi S, Woolworth V, Fichman RA, Chan PH: Liposome-entrapped superoxide dismutase reduces cerebral infarction in cerebral ischemia in rats. *Stroke* 21:1312, 1990.

74. Liu TH, Beckman JS, Freeman BA, et al: Polyethylene glycol-conjugated superoxide dismutase and catalase reduce ischemic brain injury. *Am J Physiol* 256:H589, 1989.

75. Kucharzyk J, Chew W, Derugin J, et al: Nicardipine reduces ischemic brain injury. Magnetic resonance imaging/spectroscopy study in cats. *Stroke* 20:268, 1989.

76. Jacewicz M, Brint S, Tanabe J, et al: Nimodipine pretreatment improves cerebral blood flow and reduces brain edema in conscious rats subjected to focal cerebral ischemia. *J Cereb Blood Flow Metab* 1990; 10:903, 1989.

77. Park CK, Nehis DG, Teasdale GM, McCulloch J: Focal ischemia of the rat brain: Autoradiographic determination of cerebral glucose utilization, glucose content, and blood flow. *J Cerebr Blood Flow Metab* 9:617, 1986.

78. Ozyurt E, Graham DI, Woodruff GN, McCulloch J: Protective effect of the glutamate antagonist, MK-801, in focal cerebral ischemia in the cat. *J Cereb Blood Flow Metab* 8:138, 1988.

79. Smith A, Hoff J, Nielsen S, Larson C: Barbiturate protection in acute focal cerebral ischemia. *Stroke* 5:1, 1974.

80. Onesti ST, Baker CJ, Sun PP, Solomon RA: Transient hypothermia reduces focal ischemic brain injury in the rat. *Neurosurgery* 29:369, 1991.

81. Wikber JE, Uhlen S: Further characterization of the guinea pig cerebral cortex idazoxan receptor solubilization, distinction from the imidazole site, and demonstration of cirazoline as an idazoxan receptor selective drug. *J Neurochem* 55:192, 1990.

82. Ozog MA, Wilson JX, Dixon SJ, Cechetto DF: Rilmenidine elevates cytosolic free calcium concentration in suspended cerebral astrocytes. *J Neurochem* 71(4):1429, 1998.

83. Raley-Susman KM, Lipton P: In vitro ischemia and protein synthesis in the rat hippocampal slice: The role of calcium and NMDA receptor activation. *Brain Res* 515:27, 1990.

84. Amagasa M, Ogawa A, Yoshimoto T: Effect of calcium and calcium antagonists against deprivation of glucose and oxygen in guinea pig hippocampal slices. *Brain Res* 526:1, 1990.

85. Fillastre JP, Letac B, Galinier F, et al: A multicenter double-blind comparative study of rilmenidine and clonidine in 333 hypertensive patients. *Am J Cardiol* 61(Suppl):81D, 1988.

86. Ostermann G, Brisgand B, Schmitt J, Fillastre JP: Efficacy and acceptability of rilmenidine for mild to moderate systemic hypertension. *Am J Cardiol* 1988; 61:76D, 1988.

87. Beau B, Mahieux F, Paraire M, et al: Efficacy and safety of rilmenidine for arterial hypertension. *Am J Cardiol* 61:95D, 1988.

88. Pillion G, Fevier B, Codis P, Schutz D: Long-term control of blood pressure by rilmenidine in high-risk populations. *Am J Cardiol* 74:58A, 1994.

89. Reid JL: Rilmenidine: A clinical overview. *Am J Hypertens* 13(Suppl):106S, 2000.

90. Mpoy M, Vandeleene B, Ketelslegers JM, Lambert A: Treatment of systemic hypertension in insulin-treated diabetes mellitus with rilmenidine. *Am J Cardiol* 61:91D, 1988.

91. Dupuy O, Bauduceau B, Mayaudon H: Efficacy of rilmenidine: A selective I_1 imidazoline receptor binding agent in diabetic hypertensive patients. *Am J Hypertens* 13(Suppl):123S, 2000.

92. De Luca N, Izzo R, Fontana D, et al: Haemodynamic and metabolic effects of rilmenidine in hypertensive patients with metabolic syndrome X. A double-blind parallel study versus amlodipine. *J Hypertens* 18(10):1515, 2000.

93. Lins R, Daelemans R, Dratwa M, et al: Acceptability of rilmenidine and long-term surveillance of plasma concentration in hypertensive patients with renal insufficiency. *Am J Med* 87(Suppl 3C):41S, 1989.

94. Aparicio M, Dratwa M, El Esper N, et al: Pharmacokinetics of rilmenidine in patients with chronic renal insufficiency and in hemodialysis patients. *Am J Cardiol* 74:43A, 1994.

95. Trimarco B, Rosiello G, Sarno D, et al: Effects of one-year treatment with rilmenidine on systemic hypertension-induced left ventricular hypertrophy in hypertensive patients. *Am J Cardiol* 74:36A, 1994.

96. Galley P, Manciet G, Hessel JL, Michel JP: Antihypertensive efficacy and acceptability of rilmenidine in elderly hypertensive patients. *Am J Cardiol* 61:86D, 1988.

97. Pelemans W, Verhaeghe J, Creytens G, et al: Efficacy and safety of rilmenidine in elderly patients: A double blind comparison with hydrochloro-thiazide. *Am J Cardiol* 74:51A, 1994.

98. Dallocchio M, Gosse P, Grollier G, et al: La rilmenidine, un nouvel antihypertenseur dans le traitement de premiere intention de L'hypertension arterielle essentielle. Etude multicentrique en double aveugle contre atenolol. *Presse Med* 20:1265, 1991.

99. Fiorentini C, Guillet C, Guzaai M: Etude multicentrique en double aveugle comparant la rilmenidine 1 mg et l-hydrochlorothia-zide 25 mg chez 244 patients. *Arch Mal Coeur* 82(V):39, 1989.

100. UK Working Party on Rilmenidine: Rilmenidine in mild to moderate essential hypertension—a double blind, randomized, parallel group, multicenter comparison with methyldopa in 157 patients. *Clin Ther Res* 47:194, 1990.

101. Sadowski Z, Szwed H, Kuch-Wocial A, et al: Regression of left ventricular hypertrophy in hypertensive patients after 1 year of treatment with rilmenidine: A double-blind, randomized, controlled (versus nifedipine) study. *J Hypertens Suppl* 16(3):S55, 1998.

102. Harron DWG: Antihypertensive drugs and baroreflex sensitivity. *N Engl J Med* 321:952, 1989.

103. De Visser SJ, van Gerven JM, Schoemaker RC, Cohen AF: Concentration-effect relationships of two infusion rates of the imidazoline antihypertensive agent rilmenidine for blood pressure and development of side-effects in healthy subjects. *Br J Clin Pharmacol* 51(5):423, 2001.

104. Haxhiu MA, Dreshaj I, Erokwu B, et al: Vasodepression elicited in hypertensive rats by the selective I_1-imidazoline agonist moxonidine administered into the rostral ventrolateral medulla. *J Cardiovasc Pharmacol* 20(Suppl 4):S11, 1992.

105. Ernsberger P, Ishizuka T, Liu S, et al: Mechanisms of antihyperglycemic effects of moxonidine in the obese spontaneously hypertensive Koletsky rat (SHROB). *J Pharmacol Exp Ther* 288(1):139, 1999.

106. Yakubu Madus FE, Johnson WT, Zimmerman KM, et al: Metabolic and hemodynamic effects of moxonidine in the Zucker diabetic fatty rat model of type 2 diabetes. *Diabetes* 48(5):1093, 1999.

107. Henriksen EJ, Jacob S, Fogt DL, et al: Antihypertensive agent moxonidine enhances muscle glucose transport in insulin-resistant rats. *Hypertension* 30(6):1560, 1997.

108. Smyth DD, Penner SB: Imidazoline receptor mediated natriuresis: Central and/or peripheral effect? *J Auton Nerv Syst* 72(2-3):155, 1998.

109. Csete K, Papp JG: Effects of moxonidine on corticocerebral blood flow under normal and ischemic conditions in conscious rabbits. *J Cardiovasc Pharmacol* 35(3):417, 2000.

110. MacPhee GJA, Howie CA, et al: A comparison of the haemodynamic and behavioural effects of moxonidine and clonidine in normotensive subjects. *Br J Clin Pharmacol* 33:261, 1992.

111. Mitrovic V, Patyna W, Huting J, Schepper M: Hemodynamic and neurohumoral effects of moxonidine in patients with essential hypertension. *Cardiovasc Drugs Ther* 1991; 5:967, 1992.

112. Kirch H, Hutt H-J, Planitz N: Pharmacodynamic action and pharmacokinetics of moxonidine after single oral administration in hypertensive patients. *J Clin Pharmacol* 30:1088, 1990.

113. Ernsberger P: Pharmacology of moxonidine: An I_1-imidazoline receptor agonist. *J Cardiovasc Pharmacol* 35(Suppl 4):S27, 2000.

114. Messerli F: Moxonidine: A new and versatile antihypertensive. *J Cardiovasc Pharmacol* 35(Suppl 4):S53, 2000.

115. Schacter M, Luszick J, Jager B, et al: Safety and tolerability of moxonidine in the treatment of hypertension. *Drug Saf* 19:191, 1998.

116. Moxonidine a better tolerated centrally acting antihypertensive? *Drugs Ther Perspect* 14:12, 1999.

117. Greenwood JP, Scott EM, Stoker JB, Mary DA: Chronic I_1-imidazoline agonism. Sympathetic mechanisms in hypertension. *Hypertension* 35:1264, 2000.

118. Mukaddam-Daher S, Gutkowska J: Atrial natriuretic peptide is involved in renal actions of moxonidine. *Hypertension* 35:1215, 2000.

119. Huting J, Mitrovic V, Behavar J, Schlepper M: Vergleich der Wirkungen von Moxonidin und Nifedipin auf die linksventrikulare Function bei Monotherapie der essentiellen Hypertonie. *Jerz/Kreislauf* 24:132, 1992.

120. Eichstadt G, Gatz G, Schroder R, Kreuz D: Linksventrikulare Hypertrophieregression unter einer Therapie mit Moxonidin. *J Pharmacol Ther* 1:12, 1991.

121. Krespi PG, Makris TK, Hatzizacharias AN, et al: Moxonidine effect on microalbuminuria, thrombomodulin, and plasminogen activator inhibitor-1 levels in patients with essential hypertension. *Cardiovasc Drugs Ther* 12(5):463, 1998.

122. Elisaf MS, Petris C, Bairaktari E, et al: The effects of moxonidine on plasma lipid profile and on LDL subclass distribution. *J Hum Hypertens* 13(11):781, 1999.

123. Planitz V: Comparison of moxonidine and clonidine HCl in treating patients with hypertension. *J Clin Pharmacol* 27:46, 1987.

124. Planitz V: Crossover comparison of moxonidine and clonidine in mild to moderate hypertension. *Eur J Clin Pharmacol* 27:147, 1984.

125. Prichard BNC, Simmons R, Rooks MJ, et al: A double-blind comparison of moxonidine and atenolol in the management of patients with mild to moderate hypertension. *J Cardiovasc Pharmacol* 20(Suppl 4):S45, 1992.

126. Wolf R: The treatment of hypertensive patients with a calcium antagonist or moxonidine. A comparison. *J Cardiovasc Pharmacol* 20(Suppl 4):S42, 1992.

127. Mangiameli S, Privitera A, Jonte G, Low-Kroger A: Moxonidine versus nifedipine retard in the treatment of mild to moderate hypertension. *Zeitschr Allgemeinmed* 68:862, 1992.

128. Ollivier JP, Christen MO, Schafer SG: Moxonidine: A second generation of centrally acting drugs. An appraisal of clinical experience. *J Cardiovasc Pharmacol* 20(Suppl 4):S31, 1992.

129. Chrisp P, Faulds D: Moxonidine: A review of its pharmacology and therapeutic use in essential hypertension. *Drugs* 44:993, 1992.

130. Kuppers HE, Jager BA, Luszick JH, et al: Placebo-controlled comparison of the efficacy and tolerability of once-daily moxonidine and enalapril in mild-to-moderate essential hypertension. *J Hypertens* 15(1):93, 1997.

131. Planitz V: Intra-individual comparison of moxonidine and prazosin in hypertensive patients. *Eur J Clin Pharmacol* 229:645, l986.

132. Moxonidine for hypertension. *Drug Ther Bull* 35(5):33, 1997.

133. Chu TC: Potential mechanisms of moxonidine-induced ocular hypotension: Role of norepinephrine. *J Ocul Pharmacol Ther* 13(6):489, 1997.

133a. Ogidigben MJ, Potter DE: Central imidazoline (I[1]) receptors modulate aqueous hydrodynamics. *Curr Eye Res* 22:358, 2001.

134. Spada CS, Nieves AL, Burke JA, et al: Differential effects of alpha-adrenoceptor agonists on human retinal microvessel diameter. *J Ocul Pharmacol Ther* 17(3):255, 2001.

135. Weinmann H-J, Rudolph M: Clinical pharmacokinetics of moxonidine. *J Cardiovasc Pharmacol* 20(Suppl 4):S37, 1992.

136. Dominiak P, Keogh JP, Prichard BNC: Moxonidine. In: Messerli F, ed. *Cardiovascular Drug Therapy,* 2nd ed. Philadelphia: Saunders 1996:651.

136a. Kirch W, Hutt HJ, Planitz V: The influence of renal function on clinical pharmacokinetics of moxonidine. *Clin Pharmacokinet* 15:245, 1988.

137. Cohn JN, Levine TB, Olivari MT, et al: Plasma norepinephrine as a guide to prognosis in patients with chronic congestive heart failure. *N Engl J Med* 311:819, 1984.

138. Kaye DM, Lefkovits J, Jennings GL, et al: Adverse consequences of high sympathetic nervous activity in the failing human heart. *J Am Coll Cardiol* 26:1257, 1995.

139. Rector TS, Olivari MT, Levine TB, et al: Predicting survival for an individual with congestive heart failure using the plasma norepinephrine concentration. *Am Heart J* 114:148, 1987.

140. Keogh AM, Baron DW, Hickie JB: Prognostic guides in patients with idiopathic or ischemic dilated cardiomyopathy assessed for cardiac transplantation. *Am J Cardiol* 65:903, 1990.

141. Newton GE, Parker JD: Acute effects of $beta_1$-selective and nonselective beta-adrenergic receptor blockade on cardiac sympathetic activity in congestive heart failure. *Circulation* 94:353, 1996.

142. Kaye DM, Lambert GW, Lefkovits J, et al: Neurochemical evidence of cardiac sympathetic and increased central nervous system norepinephrine turnover in severe congestive heart failure. *J Am Coll Cardiol* 23:570, 1994.

143. Azevedo ER, Newton MD, Parker JD: Cardiac and sypathetic activity in response to clonidine in human heart failure. *J Am Coll Cardiol* 33:186, 1999.

144. Manolis AJ, Olympios C, Sifaki M, et al: Suppressing sympathetic activation in congestive heart failure. *Hypertension* 26:719, 1995.

145. Swedberg K, Bergh C-H, Dickstein K, et al for the Moxonidine Investigators: The effects of moxonidine, a novel imidazoline, on plasma norepinephrine in patients with congestive heart failure. *J Am Coll Cardiol* 35:398, 2000.

146. Swedberg K, Bristow MR, Cohn JN, et al. Effects of sustained-release moxonidine, an imidazoline agonist, on plasma norepinephrine in patients with chronic heart failure. *Circulation* 105:179, 2002.

147. Dickstein K, Manhenke C, Aarsland T, et al: Acute hemodynamic and neurohormonal effects of moxonidine in congestive heart failure secondary to ischemic or idiopathic dilated cardiomyopathy. *Am J Cardiol* 83:1638, 1999.

148. Dogrell SA: Moxonidine: Some controversy. *Expert Opin Pharmacother* 2(2):337, 2001.

149. Poisson D, Christen M-O, Sannajust F: Protective effects of I_1-antihypertensive agent moxonidine against neurogenic cardiac arrhythmias in halothane-anesthetized rabbits. *J Pharmacol Exper Ther* 293:929, 2000.

150. Bousquet P, Feldman J: Drugs acting on imidazoine receptors. A review of their pharmacology, their use in blood pressure control and their potential interest in cardioprotection. *Drugs* 58:799, 1999.

151. Dubar M, Pillion G: I, agents: A new approach to the treatment of hypertension. *Ann NY Acad Sci* 763:642, 1995.

152. Yu A, Frishman WH: Imidazoline receptor agonist drugs: A new approach to the treatment of systemic hypertension. *J Clin Pharm* 36:98, 1996.

153. Szabo B: Imidazoline antihypertensive drugs: A critical review on their mechanism of action. *Pharmacol Ther* 93:1, 2002.

154. Greenblatt JP, Coplan NL, Phillips RA: New drugs in hypertension management. *Cardiovasc Rev Rep* 23:458, 2002.

Endothelin as a Therapeutic Target in the Treatment of Cardiovascular Disease

William H. Frishman

Sukhdeep Kaur

Inderpal Singh

Praveen Tamirisa

Endothelin is a naturally occurring polypeptide substance with potent vasoconstrictor actions. It was originally described as endotensin or endothelial contracting factor in 1985 by Hickey et al.,[1] who reported on their finding of a potent, stable vasoconstricting substance produced by cultured endothelial cells. Subsequently, Yanagisawa et al.[2] isolated and purified the substance from the supernatant of cultured porcine aortic and endothelial cells and then went on to prepare its cDNA. This substance was subsequently renamed endothelin.

Endothelins are the most potent vasoconstrictors known to date. Their chemical structure is closely related to that of certain neurotoxins (sarafotoxins) produced by scorpions and the burrowing asp (*Atractapsis engaddensin*).[3] Endothelins have now been isolated in various cell lines from multiple organisms. They are considered autocoids/cytokines[4] given their wide distribution, their expression during ontogeny and adult life, their primary role as intracellular factors, and the complexity of their biologic effects.

This chapter reviews the biologic effects of endothelin, its receptors, the possible role of endothelin in various pathophysiologic states and as a disease marker, as well as the experimental and clinical experiences with endothelin receptor blockers in the treatment of various systemic illnesses.

STRUCTURE

Endothelin is a polypeptide consisting of 21 amino acids. There are three closely related isoforms: endothelin-1, 2, and 3 (ET1, ET2, and ET3, respectively) that differ in a few of the amino acid constituents (Fig. 31-1). The endothelin molecules have several conserved amino acids, including the last six-carboxyl (C)-terminal amino acids and four cysteine residues that form two intrachain disulfide bonds between residues 1 to 15 and 3 to 11. These residues might have biologic implications particularly in relation to three-dimensional structure and function. The main differences in the endothelin isopeptides reside in their N-terminal segments. ET1, the peptide originally identified by Yanagisawa and the major isoform generated in blood vessels, is the most potent vasoconstrictor and appears to be of greatest significance in cardiovascular regulation.[5,6]

PRODUCTION

The genes for the various endothelin isoforms have been sequenced and are found to be scattered in different chromosomes.[7] Current evidence suggests that they arose from a common ancestor by exon duplication followed by gene duplication with subsequent dispersion of the different genes. ET1 is located on chromosome 6. Regulation of endothelin synthesis takes place primarily at the level of transcription. Factors known to enhance the release of endothelin are shown in Table 31-1.[8] These include various vasoactive hormones, growth factors, mediators of inflammation, and lipoproteins as well as physicochemical factors like hypoxia and vascular shear. In contrast, other factors—like endothelin-derived nitric oxide, natriuretic peptides, heparin, and some dilator prostanoids—inhibit the generation of ET1 by promoting the production of cyclic guanosine monophosphate (cGMP).[9] In the 5' gene flanking sequence, there are binding sites for activating protein 1 (AP1),[6] GATA2 protein, and the nuclear factor binding element[10] through which angiotensin II and transforming growth factor beta act to induce the expression of ET1. Cytokines such as interleukin-2 can turn on the production of endothelin. Plasma cytokines are elevated in several conditions, including shock, congestive heart failure, and hypercholesterolemia and may contribute to the increased levels of endothelin that are observed in these conditions.[11]

Endothelin has been demonstrated to be produced from endothelial as well as nonendothelial cells. The synthesis of endothelin's parallels that of the various peptide hormones in that a precursor polypeptide is sequentially cleaved to generate the active form. Initially, preproendothelin, a 212–amino acid peptide is produced[12] (Fig. 31-2). It is then converted into proET1 after removal of a secretory sequence and cleavage by a furin-like enzyme. This big ET1 thus produced is converted into additional ET1 by one of several endothelin converting enzymes.[13] Endothelin-converting enzymes are a family of metalloproteinases with different tissue distributions, biologic activities and selectivity toward endothelin isoforms under various conditions.[14,15] Some amount of big ET1 is secreted in conjunction with ET1 into the circulation, where it may be converted into additional ET1 by extracellular mechanisms. The fully formed endothelin molecule is then broken down into inactive peptides by

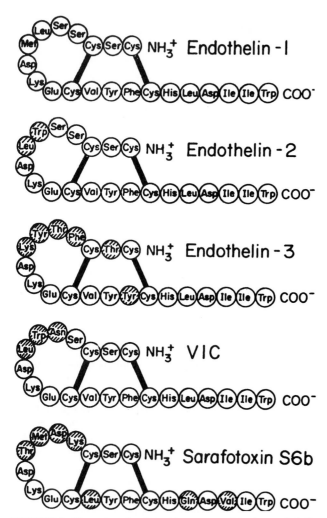

FIGURE 31-1. Illustration of amino acid sequences of the three endothelin isoforms: ET1, ET2, and ET3. (*Reproduced with permission from Kramer et al.*[4])

as yet uncharacterized proteases. Some of the candidates are the lysosomal protective protein (deamidase) and enkephalinase (neutral endopeptidase EC 24.11).[16–18] A majority of plasma ET1 (about 90%) is cleared during the first passage through the lungs.[19] Pulmonary clearance of radiolabeled ET1 may be receptor mediated as it can be blocked by pretreatment with a large dose of unlabelled ET1.[20] Since circulating ET1 is rapidly cleared from the circulation, circulating concentration of big ET1 and the inactive C-terminal fragment of big ET1 formed by cleavage of big ET1 may

TABLE 31-1. Factors Known to Release Endothelin

Thrombin	Cyclosporine
TGFβ	Insulin-like growth factor
Arginine vasopressin	Bombesin
Hypoxia	Cortisol
Phorbol ester	LDL-cholesterol
Glucose	Hypercholesterolemia
Angiotensin II	Changes in shear stress on vascular wall
Interleukin-1	Epidermal growth factor
Fibroblast growth factor	

Source: Tamirisa P, Frishman WH, Kumar A: Endothelin and endothelin antagonists. Roles in cardiovascular health and disease. *Am Heart J* 130:601–610, 1995, with permission.

be more accurate reflectors of endothelin generation than endothelin levels.[21]

The secretion of endothelin occurs within minutes after exposure to inducing stimuli. The plasma half-life of ET1 is between 4 to 7 min, while that of its mRNA is about 15 to 20 min.[5] Vascular cells can therefore rapidly adjust endothelin production for the regulation of vascular tone.[22] Recently, intracellular vesicles containing both mature endothelin and endothelin-converting enzyme have been identified in endothelial cells.[23] However, it remains unclear whether intracellular stored peptide represents an important pool available for rapid release.

ENDOTHELIN RECEPTORS

The receptors for endothelin have been isolated and their genes cloned.[24–26] The receptors are classified on the basis of their affinity for the various endothelin isoforms (Table 31-2). So far two receptors, ETA and ETB, are well characterized. The ETA receptor has 10 times more binding affinity for ET1 than ET3. The ETB receptor has nearly identical affinity for all three isopeptides. In humans, ETA and ETB receptors exhibit significant sequence similarity, having about 63% amino acid identity and a high degree of sequence conservation across mammalian species (about 90%).[27] Functional data point to the presence of possible subtypes of the endothelin receptors on the basis of responses to various agonists and antagonists; but to date, molecular studies have not been able to support this subclassification.[8,28]

The endothelin receptors belong to the rhodopsin superfamily, which contains other members like the beta₁-adrenergic, beta₂-adrenergic, serotonin₁, serotonin₂, and vasopressin₁ and vasopressin₂ receptors. Members of this family are characterized by the presence of seven hydrophobic transmembrane segments in the receptor that span the membrane, with their action mediated by G proteins. The receptors appear to be glycoproteins, with the sugar moiety being a possible constituent for ligand interaction.[25] The ETA receptors probably recognize the tertiary structure of both the N- and C-terminal segments, while the ETB receptors recognize predominantly the C-terminal parts, explaining the differences in affinities of the two receptors for the isoforms.[29]

The differential distribution of the endothelin receptors in various tissues is responsible for the multiplicity of actions attributed to endothelin. The mRNA for the ETA receptor is expressed in the heart, aorta, and blood vessels of the brain but not in the endothelial cells, suggesting that vascular expression of this receptor occurs selectively in vascular smooth muscle cells.[30] On the other hand, mRNA for the ETB receptor is most highly expressed in cultured endothelial cells, where receptor activation leads to the production of vasodilator substances including nitric oxide. ETB receptors may also be found in vascular smooth muscle, where they can mediate vasoconstriction. The overall hemodynamic effect of endothelin in a given organ depends on the receptor type being stimulated, its location, and its relative abundance.

ETA receptors are dynamic entities and can be upregulated by hypoxia, various tissue growth factors, cyclic adenosine monophosphate (cAMP), and estrogens, whereas ETB receptors can be upregulated by C-type natriuretic factor and angiotensin II.[22] ETA receptors can be down-regulated by endothelins, angiotensin II and certain tissue growth factors, and ETB receptors are down-regulated by cAMP and catecholamines.[22]

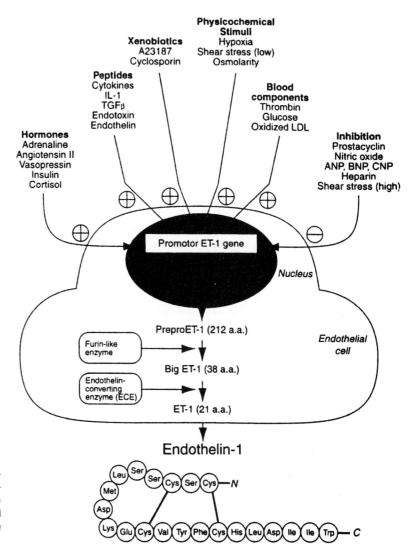

FIGURE 31-2. Factors that alter the synthesis of endothelin-1 (ET1 and the pathway for its generation. IL-1 = interleukin; TGFβ = transforming growth factor beta; LDL = low-density lipoprotein; ANP, BNP, CNP = atrial, brain, and c-type natriuretic peptides, respectively. (*Reproduced with permission from Webb and Strachan.*[8])

MECHANISM OF ACTION

Circulating concentrations of ET1 are in the picomolar range, much lower than the concentrations required to cause vascular contraction, both in vitro and in vivo. Also, about two-thirds of endothelin produced by endothelial cells is directionally released toward the adjacent smooth muscle cells, where it exerts local paracrine and autocrine effects.[31] The binding of endothelin to its receptor is very tight, with relatively slow dissociation, which might result in prolonged action. An important factor to consider is that some of the effects seen in vitro may not be biologically relevant to what transpires in vivo.[32] The binding of endothelin to its receptor leads to multiple effects (Fig. 31-3). Activation of phospholipase C by means of a G protein causes consequent hydrolysis of phosphatidylinositol, forming cytosolic inositol 1,4,5 trisphosphate (IP3) and membrane-bound diacylglycerol. The newly formed IP3 causes release of calcium from storage sites in the sarcoplasmic reticulum. It also facilitates the entry of extracellular calcium via Dhp-sensitive

TABLE 31-2. Endothelin Receptors and Their Antagonists

Receptor Type	ETA	ETB
Affinity	ET1 > ET2 ≫ ET3	ET1 = ET2 = ET3
Location	VSMC	EC, VSMC
Action	Vasoconstriction	Vasodilation, vasoconstriction
Upregulators	Hypoxia, cAMP	Angiotensin II
Downregulators	Endothelins, angiotensin II	cAMP
Selective agonist	—	Endothelin-3
Selective antagonist	BQ-123	BQ-788

VSMC = vascular smooth muscle cells; EC = endothelial cells; ET = endothelin; cAMP = cyclic adenosine monophosphate.

Source: Kaur S, Frishman WH, Singh I, et al: Endothelin as a therapeutic target in the treatment of cardiovascular disease. *Heart Disease* 3:176, 2001, with permission.

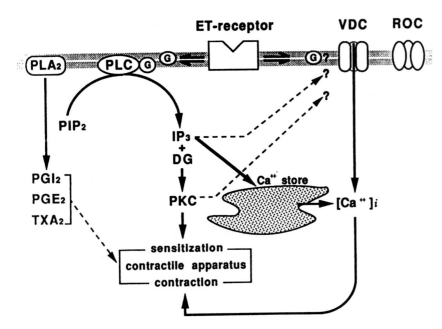

FIGURE 31-3. Intracellular signal transduction pathways activated by endothelins (ETs). Activated endothelin receptor stimulates phospholipase C (PLC) and phospholipase A2 (PLA2). Activated endothelin receptor also stimulates voltage-dependent calcium channels (VDC) and probably receptor-operated calcium channel (ROC). Inositol triphosphate (IP3) elicits release of calcium ion from caffeine-sensitive calcium store. Protein kinase C (PKC) activated by diacylglycerol (DG) sensitizes contractile apparatus. Elevated intracellular free calcium ion induces contraction. Cyclooxygenase products [prostacyclin (PGI2), prostaglandin E (PGE2 thromboxane A2 (TXA2)] modify the contraction. IP2 = inositol biphosphate. [*Reproduced with permission from Masaki T, Kimura S, Yanagisawa M, Goto K: Molecular and cellular mechanism of endothelin regulation: Implications for vascular function. Circulation 84(4):1457–1468, 1991.*]

voltage channels. The total intracellular free calcium increases, with the initial increase reflecting the release from cellular stores while the latter increase reflects net inward calcium entry across the cell membrane.[33-36] The greater concentration of intracellular calcium often associates with calmodulin and modulates diverse processes such as neurotransmitter release, secretion, activation of enzymes like myosin light chain kinases (which activate cellular contractile machinery), etc.[37] Nifedipine and other calcium-channel blockers can inhibit the influx of extracellular calcium, thereby antagonizing some of the actions of endothelin.[38-40]

The sustained release of diacylglycerol causes prolonged activation of protein kinase C, which, by causing phosphorylation of various proteins, could result in either activation or inactivation of proteins and the regulation of gene expression.[41] Endothelin has also been noted to cause increase in intracellular pH, perhaps by stimulating the sarcolemmal sodium-hydrogen antiporter. This increased intracellular pH can enhance the sensitivity of the myofilaments to calcium, thereby augmenting contraction even without changing the calcium concentration.[42,43] It has also been noted that the increase in intracellular pH can, by itself, stimulate hypertrophic and mitogenic responses in different cells.[44,45]

The binding of endothelin to its receptor might also alter ion-channel permeability (such as the voltage-dependent L-type calcium channels via G proteins) and cause activation of other secondary messengers (e.g., production of prostanoids by activating phospholipase A) or release of nitric oxide.[19,46-48] Nitric oxide has been shown to antagonize some of the effects of endothelin on vascular smooth muscle contraction, perhaps by decreasing release of endothelin from endothelial cells.[49] In addition, experiments have revealed a competitive inhibition of ET1 binding to its receptors in cardiac membranes of rats by potassium channel–opening agents. These agents have been shown to exert cardioprotective action after experimental myocardial infarction in rats by suppressing cardiac arrhythmias that may be due, in part, to inhibition of the proarrhythmic effects of cardiac endothelin. It has been suggested that ET1 may close adenosine 5'-triphosphate (ATP)-sensitive potassium channels,[50-52] thereby preventing efflux of potassium from the cell, resulting in depolarization of membranes and contraction of muscle.

THE ENDOTHELIN ANTAGONISTS

Much of our knowledge about the role of endothelin in various pathophysiologic states as well as the effects of exogenous endothelin has come from the research with endothelin antagonists. Several antagonists to endothelin have been discovered in recent years (Table 31-3). The original receptor antagonist was isolated from the cultured broth of *Streptomyces misakiensis*, but this had low potency in binding and functional assays. In the subsequent years, an array of peptide and endothelin-receptor antagonists have been developed. While some of the agents are receptor-specific for either the ETA or ETB subtypes, others are nonspecific. However, these compounds are hydrolyzed by peptidase in the systemic circulation and the gastrointestinal tract.[53] Recently, research has been focused on the development of orally active

TABLE 31-3. Some Peptide and Nonpeptide Endothelin-Receptor Antagonists

Endothelin receptor selectivity		
ET$_A$	ET$_B$	ET$_A$ET$_B$
Peptide molecules		
BQ 123	BQ 788	PD 142893
BQ 485	IRL 1038	PD 145065
BQ 610	A-192621.1	
FR 139317		
Nonpeptide molecules		
PD 155080		Bosentan (RO 470203)
PD 156707		RD 46-2005
PD 180988		TAK-044
BMS 182874		L-751281
BMS 193884		SB 209670
A-127722		SB 217242 (enrasentan)
LU 135252 (darusentan)		CP 170687
L 754141		J-104132
2D 1611		Tezosentan
TA 0115		
Sitaxsentan		

Source: Adapted with permission from Benigni and Remuzzi.[53]

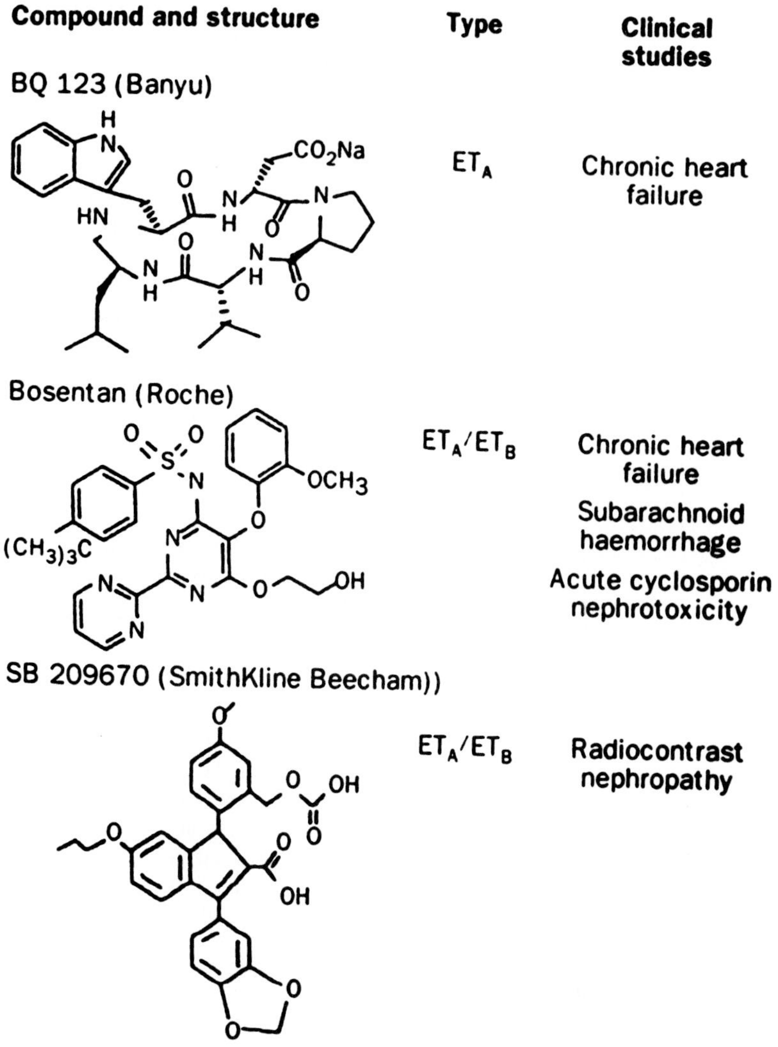

Compound and structure | **Type** | **Clinical studies**

BQ 123 (Banyu)

ET$_A$ — Chronic heart failure

Bosentan (Roche)

ET$_A$/ET$_B$ — Chronic heart failure; Subarachnoid haemorrhage; Acute cyclosporin nephrotoxicity

SB 209670 (SmithKline Beecham))

ET$_A$/ET$_B$ — Radiocontrast nephropathy

FIGURE 31-4. Some endothelin-receptor antagonists under clinical development. (*Reproduced with permission from Benigni and Remuzzi.*[53])

nonpeptide antagonists (Fig. 31-4). There are also other classes of drugs (Table 31-4) that either interfere with endothelin release or modify its metabolism.

The use of endothelin antagonists, which can be administered either intravenously or orally, not only helps elucidate the mechanisms by which endothelin mediates its effects but may also be of potential benefit in the treatment of patients with systemic hypertension, myocardial ischemia, restenosis following angioplasty, congestive heart failure, subarachnoid hemorrhage, renal failure, asthma, pulmonary hypertension, allograft rejection, and sepsis.[53a]

TABLE 31-4. Nonspecific Endothelin Antagonists*

Endothelin-converting enzyme inhibitors
Angiotensin-converting enzyme inhibitors
Angiotensin II-receptor blockers
Calcium-entry blockers
Potassium-channel openers
Adenosine
Nitroglycerin
Nitric oxide

*These antagonists interfere with the release or modify the actions of endothelin.

Source: Reproduced with permission from Tamirisa P, Frishman WH, Kumar A: Endothelins and endothelin antagonism: In: Frishman WH, Sonnenblick EH, eds. *Cardiovascular Pharmacotherapeutics.* New York: McGraw Hill, 1997, p. 697.

Clinical trials are now in progress using endothelin antagonists for many of these conditions, with some promising results (Table 31-5). However, hepatotoxicity has been observed with several of the compounds used, suggesting that long-term safety data are needed.

PATHOPHYSIOLOGIC ROLES OF ENDOTHELIN: EFFECTS OF ENDOTHELIN ANTAGONISM

Regulation of Vascular Tone and Systemic Hypertension

Endothelin is the most potent vasoconstrictor known today and has an exceptionally long duration of physiologic action[19,53b] (Fig. 31-5). Intravenous injections of endothelin in animals cause a transient fall in systolic blood pressure (ETB) followed by a prolonged pressor response (ETA).[2,6] The vasoconstrictor action of endothelin is mediated by ETA receptors in the vascular smooth muscle, while the vasodilation effect is mediated via the ETB receptors on the endothelial cells, which cause release of prostacyclin and nitric oxide.[53a] There is evidence for the presence of endothelin-dependent vascular tone in healthy humans. Infusion of BQ-123, an ETA receptor antagonist, into the forearm of healthy subjects, as well as systemic administration of TAK-044, a mixed ETA/ETB antagonist,

TABLE 31-5. Partial List of Endothelin Antagonists Under Clinical Testing

Substance	Receptor Selectivity	Disease
BQ-123	A	Transplantation, HF, MI, subarachnoid hemorrhage, renal ischemia
BQ-788	B	HF
BMS 193884	A	HF
J-10432	A	Hypertension
L-754142	A	Renal ischemia
LU 135252 (darusentan)	A	HF, pulmonary hypertension, atherosclerosis, progressive nephropathies
PD-142893	A/B	Progressive nephropathies
PD-145065	A/B	Subarachnoid hemorrhage
PD-156707	A	HF
RO 47-0203 (bosentan)	A/B	Transplantation, HF, MI, atherosclerosis, pulmonary hypertension, subarachnoid hemorrhage, renal ischemia, progressive nephropathies
RO 61-1790	A	Subarachnoid hemorrhage
SB-209670	A/B	Radiocontrast nephropathy
TA-0115	A	HF
TAK-044	A/B	Atherosclerosis, subarachnoid hemorrhage, renal transplant rejection
ZD 1611	A	Obstructive lung disease, pulmonary hypertension

HF = heart failure; MI = myocardial infarction.

Source: Reproduced with permission from Spieker et al.[72b]

resulted in vasodilatation with an increase in forearm blood flow.[54,55] The overall hemodynamic effect of endothelin depends on the balance between ETA-mediated vasoconstriction and ETB-mediated vasodilatation and natriuresis. ETB receptor-mediated generation of nitric oxide appears to oppose the vasoconstrictor effects of endogenous ET1 in healthy humans. In hypercholesterolemic animals, endothelial dysfunction is associated with an ETA receptor–mediated increase in coronary tone.[56]

The definitive role of endothelin in maintaining normal blood pressure, as well as its role in the etiology of systemic hypertension, remains unclear.[56a,b] Endothelin levels are increased in some salt-sensitive models of hypertension, such as the deoxycorticosterone acetate (DOCA) salt hypertensive rat and DOCA salt–treated spontaneously hypertensive rat (SHR).[57,58] The direct mitogenic effects of endothelin result in the hypertrophy of vascular smooth muscle seen in these animals, contributing to the hypertension-induced hypertrophy.[59] Normalization or lowering of blood pressure in experimental animals by ETA- or ETA/ETB-receptor blockade sug-

gests that endothelin may participate in the pathophysiology of hypertension. Also, endothelin antagonism results in the blunting of hypertrophic vascular remodeling.[57–59] However, in contrast to the benefit derived from treatment with an endothelin antagonist in the hypertensive models that overexpress ET1, the hypertensive models that do not overexpress ET1 did not exhibit any regression of vascular hypertrophy.[60] The concentration of ET1 in animal models of hypertension is raised in accelerated hypertension and is positively correlated with serum levels of creatinine, probably reflecting a decrease in the clearance of endothelin.[61]

Conflicting results have also been reported in humans regarding the role of endothelin in the etiology of systemic hypertension. In a report on two patients with hemangioendothelioma, increased levels of endothelin were found to coexist with high blood pressure levels, which resolved with successful resection of the tumor. With recurrence of the tumor in one patient, an increase in blood pressure was reported.[62] However, endothelin levels are usually found to be normal in human hypertensives; hypertensive patients with

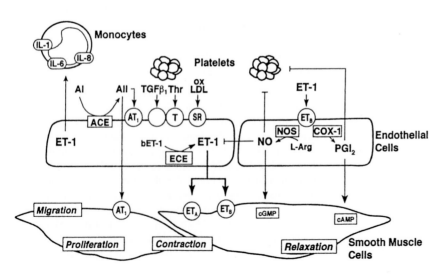

FIGURE 31-5. Endothelin-1 (ET1) exerts vasoconstriction and proliferation via ET_A receptors on smooth muscle cells. Endothelial ET_B receptors mediate vasodilation via release of nitric oxide (NO) and prostacyclin. ETB receptors in the lung clear ET1 from plasma. AI/II = angiotensin I/II; AT = angiotensin receptor; cAMP = cyclic adenosine monophosphate; cGMP = cyclic guanosine monophosphate; COX = cyclooxygenase; ECE = endothelin-converting enzyme; IL = interleukin; L-Arg = L-arginine; NOS = nitric oxide synthase; oxLDL = oxidized low-density lipoprotein; PGI_2 = prostacyclin; SR = scavenger receptor; T = thrombin receptor; TGF = transforming growth factor; Thr = thrombin. (*Reproduced with permission from Spieker et al.[72b]*)

preserved renal function have been shown to have concentrations of endothelin similar to those of normotensives.[63] The plasma levels of endothelin tend to increase with age and are higher in males than in females in both normotensive and hypertensive subjects.[64] Hypertensive African Americans, in whom hypertension is often severe and salt-sensitive, have much higher concentrations of endothelin than Caucasians, indicating possible racial differences in the production of endothelin.[65,65a] In a recent study, TAK-044, an ETA/ETB antagonist, caused a greater degree of vasodilation in the forearm vessels of atients with essential hypertension than in normotensive subjects despite similar plasma circulating endothelin concentrations in the two groups, suggesting a possible role for ET1 in the pathogenesis of hypertension.[66] Normotensive offspring of hypertensive parents have also been shown to have enhanced plasma endothelin responses to mental stress, suggesting the presence of a genetically determined endothelial dysfunctional state at an early stage preceding the development of hypertension.[67]

A close and complex interaction between ET1 and the renin angiotensin system has been seen. Angiotensin II has been found to increase endothelin levels in vitro from endothelial cells, suggesting one possible mechanism by which angiotensin-converting enzyme (ACE) inhibition could be functional in vivo.[68] ACE inhibitors can also indirectly interfere with endothelin as increased levels of bradykinin decrease release of endothelin. ACE inhibitors can cause regression of intimal hyperplasia, unlike other antihypertensive drugs that are ineffective in this regard, suggesting that they might be blocking the mitogenic actions of endothelin.[69] In rats infused with angiotensin II, a known stimulant of ET1 expression, endothelin antagonists lowered blood pressure and reduced myocardial fibrosis and hypertrophic remodeling in cardiac and small arteries.[70,70a] Interestingly, an additive reduction in blood pressure was seen when ETA/ETB inhibition with bosentan was added to ACE inhibition in hypertensive dogs.[71]

The role of endothelin antagonists in hypertension is being studied extensively, and clinical studies are ongoing.[66] In a recent randomized, placebo-controlled trial, it was shown that administration of the ETA/ETB antagonist bosentan at a dose of 1000 mg twice a day for 4 weeks decreased 24-h ambulatory diastolic pressure in patients with essential hypertension by about 10 mm Hg.[72] The selective ETA receptor antagonist, darusentan, has also shown clinical efficacy as an antihypertensive drug.[72a] Numerous well-tolerated drugs already exist that can be used to control hypertension effectively. Nevertheless, the potential additional benefits of endothelin antagonists on atherogenesis, cardiac hypertrophy, and renal function make these agents important drugs to pursue developmentally.[72b]

Endothelin has been implicated as a possible cause for secondary hypertension in various conditions. The use of cyclosporine therapy is frequently complicated by the development of hypertension, which was initially thought to be due to increased levels of circulating endothelin. However, after the development of new, specific, and sensitive assays for endothelin, it was shown that there were no significant differences in the endothelin levels of normal and hypertensive patients.[73] Also, in healthy human subjects, the concentration of immunoreactive endothelin does not increase with cyclosporine therapy,[74] In animal models, endothelin receptor blockade using BQ-123 and the nonselective receptor blocker bosentan has resulted in the amelioration of cyclosporine-induced hypertension.[75,76] It is postulated that such beneficial effects may be seen despite normal concentrations of endothelin, since Endothelins are essentially a paracrine system rather than a circulating hormone,

thus making the significance of a change or the lack of change in plasma endothelin levels unclear.

Higher levels of plasma endothelin have been seen in preeclamptic patients than in nonhypertensive pregnant females.[77] Magnesium sulfate has been shown to be clinically beneficial in the treatment of high blood pressure in preeclampsia, possibly by decreasing plasma concentrations of ET1.[78] Apart from the vasoactive effects of ET1, an interesting study has demonstrated the mitogenic effects of ET1 on proliferation and invasion of trophoblastic cells, thereby implying a possible role in the etiology of preeclampsia.[79] In addition, endothelin has been implicated in the hypertensive states associated with chronic renal failure,[80] erythropoietin use,[81] and pheochromocytoma.[82]

Atherosclerosis

Hypercholesterolemia leads to profound alterations in the regulation of vascular tone. In this condition, low-density liprotein (LDL)-cholesterol accumulates in vascular walls. Experimental studies have shown that oxidatively modified LDL induces the production of ET1 by human macrophages and can increase both endothelin formation and its release from endothelial cells.[83,84] High plasma levels of endothelin have been described in patients with atherosclerosis[85] and hypercholesterolemia.[85a]

One of the early mechanisms for atherosclerosis includes the migration of monocytes into the intimal layer of blood vessels where they become activated and stimulate the release of multiple factors. It has been demonstrated in vitro that endothelin can serve as a chemotactic agent for monocytes, therefore its role as an initiator of the atherosclerotic process has been strengthened.[86,87] Endothelin could also stimulate the migration and proliferation of vascular smooth muscle cells, thereby sustaining the atherosclerotic process.[40,88] Calcium-channel blockers have been shown to reduce the chemotactic movements of monocytes, perhaps by interfering with calcium ion fluxes. The vasoconstrictor effects of endothelin may be more significant in atherosclerotic vessels, in which the opposing biological effects of nitric oxide are lost.[89,90]

The stimulation of ET1 production and the enhancement of its mitogenic action on smooth muscle by insulin may contribute to the accelerated vascular disease processes that are associated with both hyperinsulinemia and diabetes mellitus.[91] It was recently demonstrated that the use of chronic endopeptidase inhibition therapy could modulate the activity of endothelin-converting enzyme in experimental atherosclerosis.[92] Moreover, mixed ETA/ETB-receptor blockade noticeably improves renal artery vascular function in rats with streptozotocin-induced diabetes.[93]

ETA and ETB receptors are present in medial smooth muscle segments of femoral arteries obtained from patients with peripheral vascular disease, indicating a potential role of endothelin in this condition.[94]

Myocardial Ischemia

Myocardial ischemia can enhance the release of endothelin by cardiomyocytes and increase its vasoactive effects in rats. Infusion of ET1 directly into the coronary circulation of animals results in the development of myocardial infarction, with impaired ventricular functioning and the development of arrhythmias.[95] Endothelin is clearly shown to be a powerful coronary artery constrictor in various experimental models.[96,97] Intravenous infusions of ET1 reduce coronary blood flow by >90%. A substantial increase in endothelin levels distal to the ligation site has been demonstrated in experimental models.[98] Endothelin has also been shown to lower the threshold for ventricular fibrillation in dogs.[99] An increase in ET1 has been observed in cardiac tissue after experimental myocardial infarction in rats, while pretreatment with an anti-endothelin gamma globulin in this model can reduce infarct size by as much as 40%.[100]

Plasma endothelin levels and urinary endothelin excretion are increased in patients with myocardial infarction as well as in vasospastic, stable, unstable, and postinfarction angina.[88,100–102a] Patients who undergo successful thrombolysis with early reperfusion have lower endothelin levels than those subjects who do not have early reperfusion. On the other hand, in animal models, the concentration of ET1 was greatly increased during reperfusion, implying a role for ET1 in reperfusion injuries.[103] Plasma endothelin levels can also predict hemodynamic complications in patients with myocardial infarction.[104] Those patients with the highest plasma endothelin levels after myocardial infarction had the highest creatinine phosphokinase (CPK) and CPK-MB levels and the lowest angiographically determined ejection fractions.[105] Plasma levels of ET1 measured 3 days after infarction have been shown to be a predictor of 1-year mortality.[101] Thus, it has been suggested that endothelin levels may have a role in risk stratification after acute myocardial infarction.[106] Infusion of ETA-receptor antagonist drugs prior to an ischemic insult can also reduce infarct size in animals[107] through a possible myocardial energy–preserving action.[108] In rats with myocardial infarction, chronic endothelin-receptor blockade leads to attenuation of progressive ventricular dilatation and improvement of ventricular function, suggesting that endothelin may have a role in ventricular remodeling.[109,110] Endothelin has also been shown to reduce ischemia-reperfusion injury in dogs.[110a]

It is also suggested that the time course of endothelin-receptor antagonism may be important, since its early use after myocardial infarction has been seen to be detrimental.[111] In a recent randomized, double-blind control trial, bosentan was shown, under acute conditions, to cause vasodilatation of the coronary arteries in patients with stable coronary artery disease.[112] Since endothelin also has vasoproliferative properties, chronic therapy with endothelin antagonists might be beneficial for reversing structural changes in diseased coronary arteries, in addition to causing vasodilatation. Long-term studies are needed to determine the therapeutic potential of endothelin antagonists in patients with coronary artery disease.

Left Ventricular Function and Congestive Heart Failure

Congestive heart failure (CHF) is associated with stimulation of compensatory neurohormonal reflexes associated with activation of the renin-angiotensin and sympathetic nervous systems, setting up a vicious cycle of deteriorating cardiac function. High-affinity receptors for endothelin have been demonstrated in both the atria and ventricles.[113,113a] Intravenous administration of ET1 produces a delayed prolonged augmentation of left ventricular performance in addition to its biphasic vasoactive effects of an initial transient vasodilation followed by a sustained vasoconstriction.[114] The actions of endothelin on isolated hearts, cardiac muscle, and instrumented intact animals are all consistent with the hemodynamics found in CHF (Figure 31-6).[72b,115,116]

Endothelin is also a potent secretagogue of atrial natriuretic factor, a naturally occurring antagonist of endothelin that acts by

inhibiting its release.[117] The ETA receptor appears to mediate Endothelin's actions of vasoconstriction and stimulation of atrial natriuretic peptide secretion, and the ETB receptor mediates endothelin-induced vasodilation and activation of the renin-angiotensin-aldosterone system.[118,119] Urinary water excretion is mediated through both receptors, but sodium excretion is mediated through the ETA receptor.

Increased levels of endothelin have been described in animal models as well as patients with CHF and are found to correlate with increases in left ventricular end-diastolic volume, left atrial pressure, and pulmonary artery pressures.[106,109,120–123d] These raised levels of endothelin are due to increased production, since levels of the precursor "big" endothelin is also increased.[124] Increased endothelin production may play a direct and contributory role in the progression of CHF,[121] and in the increased pulmonary artery pressures seen in patients with chronic heart failure.[125] Increased levels of endothelin have also been observed in endothelial cells infected with *Trypanosoma cruzi* in experimental Chagas' cardiomyopathy[126] and in a murine model of viral myocarditis.[127]

It has been suggested that increased levels of endothelin may be playing an important role in the increased systemic vascular resistance observed in CHF.[128] In animal models of heart failure, treatment with endothelin antagonists is associated with reduced systemic vascular resistance, improved hemodynamics, improved endothelial function, a reduced progression of left ventricular dysfunction, an attenuation of left ventricular chamber remodeling, and increased survival.[120–122,129,129a] Also available are clinical data suggesting that treatment with endothelin-receptor antagonists can favorably influence the course of human heart failure.[72a,125] In the early clinical trials of endothelin antagonists in heart failure, patients were taken off ACE inhibitors. Treatment with bosentan resulted in an improvement in both systemic and pulmonary hemodynamics without inducing reflex tachycardia or increasing concentrations of angiotensin II or norepinephrine.[130] These beneficial effects were similar to those seen with ACE inhibitors. The question was then whether endothelin antagonists would be of benefit to patients receiving ACE inhibitors. However, there is now evidence that the addition of an endothelin-converting enzyme inhibitor (phosphoramidon), an ETA-receptor antagonist (BQ-123), or an endothelin-receptor blocker (bosentan) combined with an ACE inhibitor or A–II-receptor blocker can result in additional vasodilatation and improved hemodynamics.[131–134a] ACE inhibitors, in turn, benefit patients with heart failure because of their anti-endothelin actions.[106]

Although selective ETA-receptor blockers as well as nonselective endothelin antagonists have been studied in CHF,[125,134b,c] the optimal agent class remains a subject of discussion and ongoing research (Table 31-5) This is the case because of the possible adverse effects of blockade of ETB receptor–induced vasodilatation.[135–136d]

A clinical trial (Research on Endothelin Antagonists in Chronic Heart Failure; REACH-1) investigated the long-term effects of bosentan on clinical events in CHF and showed an improvement in symptoms.[136a] However, the trial had to be stopped prematurely because of elevated liver enzymes with active therapy. Bosentan can interact with bile excretion in larger oral doses. Lower dosages of bosentan were evaluated in the Endothelin Antagonist Bosentan for Lowering Cardiac Events in Heart Failure (ENABLE) trials. ENABLE 1 and ENABLE 2 were conducted concurrently with the first trial, enrolling U.S. patients and patients from Europe and Australia, respectively. In these placebo-controlled, double-blind trials, patients assigned to bosentan were given an initial dose of 6.25 mg twice daily for 4 weeks, followed by 12.5 mg twice daily for the

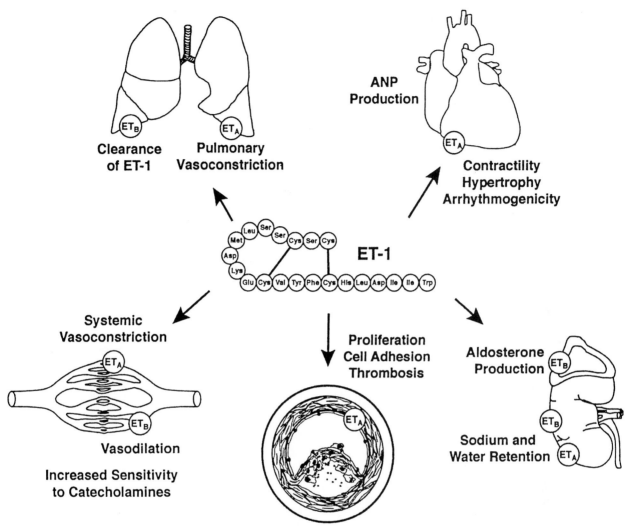

FIGURE 31-6. Pathophysiologic role of endothelin-1 (ET1) in congestive heart failure. In the heart, ET1 contributes to contractility. In addition to its vasoconstrictive effects in the systemic and pulmonary circulation, ET1 leads to hypertrophy of myocardial and smooth muscle cells. The pulmonary circulation is an important source of ET1 but is also involved in the clearance of ET1. In the kidney, ET1 regulates sodium and water excretion. ANP = atrial natriuretic peptide.

duration of follow up. The trials were designed to determine if bosentan would have an effect on the primary outcome of death and heart failure hospitalizations or the second outcome of all-cause death. Enrolled patients had severe heart failure (NYHA) class III, IV) and a mean left ventricular ejection fraction of 25%. In these trials, bosentan failed to reduce mortality or hospitalizations, and may have contributed to higher rates of adverse effects.[136e] The orally active selective ETA blockers darusentan (LU 135252) and BMS-192884 are also being evaluated in patients with heart failure.[136a] Tezosentan, the first intravenous ETA/ETB antagonist, has also been evaluated as treatment in acute and chronic heart failure, with no benefit seen.[136c]

Enrasentan was also shown to be of no clinical benefit (ENCORE trial) in patients already receiving heart failure therapies including diuretics, ACE inhibitors, digoxin, and beta-blockers.

ET1 levels decrease with heart failure therapy, and it appears that ET1 is an independent, noninvasive predictor of the functional and hemodynamic response to beta-blocker therapy with carvedilol in patients with CHF.[137] In another study, the level of big ET1 in plasma in patients with advanced heart failure was found to be strongly related to survival and was a better predictor of outcome than existing markers.[106]

Ventricular and Vascular Hypertrophy

Endothelin increases DNA synthesis in vascular smooth muscle cells, cardiomyocytes, fibroblasts, glial cells, mesangial cells, etc., and causes protooncogene expression, cell proliferation, and hypertrophy.[40,138–140] It acts in synergy with various factors such as transforming growth factor, epidermal growth factor, plateletderived growth factor, basic fibroblast growth factor, and insulin to potentiate cellular transformation or replication.[140a] Endothelin, per se, may not be a direct mediator of angiogenesis but may function as a comitogenic factor.[40,141] The locally produced ET1 that acts as an autocrine and/or paracrine factor may be more important than the circulating endothelin.[140] Increased protein synthesis induced by endothelin may play a role in myocardial hypertrophy.[142,143] Marked increase in prepro ET1 mRNA and mature ET1 was found in the ventricles of rats, where concentric hypertrophy was induced experimentally.[144] The inhibitory effect of the ET1 antagonist BQ-123 and the ETA antagonist LU 127043 on hypertrophy has been observed in both in vitro and in vivo studies using animal models.[145–147a] Bosentan exerts an inhibitory action on cardiac hypertrophy in rats with salt-induced hypertension. As the inhibitory action of bosentan on cardiac hypertrophy was relatively stronger than antihypertensive effects, a direct action of this drug on the effects of locally produced endothelin has been suggested.[148]

Neointima Formation Following Trauma to the Vascular Wall

The efficacy of coronary angioplasty is limited by the high incidence of restenosis. ET1 induces the proliferation of vascular smooth muscle in culture via activation of the ETA-receptor subtype—a response normally attenuated by an intact, functional endothelium. In addition, ET1 also induces the expression and release of several protooncogenes/growth factors that modulate the migration and proliferation of smooth muscle as well as and matrix formation. In addition to inhibiting smooth muscle proliferation in vitro, endothelin-receptor antagonism with SB 209670 or DMS 182874 ameliorates the degree of neointima formation observed following carotid artery angioplasty in the rat.[149,150] Recently, bosentan was shown to prevent graft arteriosclerosis in rat cardiac allografts.[151] Such observations raise the possibility that ET1 antagonists might serve as novel therapeutic agents in the control of postangioplasty restenosis and in post–cardiac bypass allograft disease.[152–152b]

Cardiac Arrhythmias

Intrapericardial endothelin infusion causes severe, dose-dependent ventricular arrhythmias via its action on ETA receptors. This is thought to be a direct arrhythmogenic effect of endothelin, independent of its vasoconstrictive action. Both selective ETA receptor blocker (LU 135.252) and bosentan inhibit endothelin-induced arrhythmogenesis.[153,154]

Pulmonary Hypertension

Pulmonary hypertension is characterized by endothelial injury, smooth muscle proliferation, and pulmonary vasoconstriction. ET1 has been implicated in the pathophysiology of both primary and secondary pulmonary hypertension in view of its vasoconstrictor and mitogenic properties. The plasma concentration as well as the immunoreactivity and expression of m-RNA for ET1 in the endothelial cells of hypertrophied pulmonary vessels are increased in both primary and secondary pulmonary hypertension.[155,156,156a] In the rat

model of pulmonary hypertension induced by exposure to a hypoxic environment, pulmonary ET1- and ETA- and ETB-receptor gene expression is upregulated.[157] The clearance of ET1 was thought to be decreased in patients with primary pulmonary hypertension as compared to controls.[158] However, a recent study in which blood was sampled directly from the pulmonary artery has suggested an absence of a transpulmonary gradient for ET1.[159] Endothelin has been implicated as a plausible contributor in the pathophysiology of pulmonary hypertension seen in patients with varied conditions such as Takayasu's arteritis, fenfluramine use, scleroderma, high-altitude pulmonary edema, and congenital heart disease as well as those who have had cardiopulmonary bypass surgery.[160–163a]

In experimental animals, the orally active ETA- and ETB-receptor blocker bosentan, as well as such selective ETA-receptor blockers as TA-0201 and CI-1020, have been shown to prevent both hypoxia-induced pulmonary hypertension and pulmonary artery remodeling.[164–166] In another study in rats, combined treatment with an oral ETA antagonist and an oral prostacyclin analog was more effective in ameliorating pulmonary hypertension and right ventricular hypertrophy than either drug alone.[167] The selective ETA antagonist LU 135252 and nonselective antagonist BSF 420627 were both shown to reduce monocrotaline-induced pulmonary hypertension in rats.[167a] Clinical studies using endothelin antagonists in patients with pulmonary hypertension have been carried out and some are ongoing (Tables 31-5 and 31-6). In a recent study, it was shown that short-term ETA-receptor antagonism significantly improves hemodynamics in patients with severe chronic pulmonary artery hypertension.[168a]

The FDA has approved bosentan (Tracleer) as the first oral drug for the treatment of pulmonary hypertension. The efficacy of bosentan was based on 2 placebo-controlled studies with symptomatic, severe (WHO class III-IV) primary pulmonary hypertension or pulmonary hypertension due to scleroderma or other connective tissue diseases or autoimmune diseases. Bosentan was added to current therapy that included vasodilators, anti-coagulants, diuretics, digoxin, or supplemental oxygen. The drug was shown to improve exercise ability and decrease the rate of clinical worsening. The starting dose was 62.5 mg twice daily for 4 weeks and then increased to 125 mg twice daily. Higher doses are not recommended due to the potential for liver toxicity. Dose adjustment is not required in patients with renal impairment.[168b] The drug is not available in pharmacies; it is dispensed via a direct distribution program by the manufacturer.

Asthma

Increased endothelin concentrations have been demonstrated in the bronchoalveolar lavage and bronchial epithelial cells from

TABLE 31-6. Clinical Trials with Endothelin Antagonists in CHF and Pulmonary Hypertension

Study	Compound	Patients	Primary Endpoint
HEAT	Darusentan	HF	Chronic hemodynamic efficacy
ET-005	Darusentan	HF	LV mass and function, symptoms
ENABLE	Bosentan	HF	Combined morbidity and mortality
BREATHE-1	Bosentan	Pulmonary hypertension	Change in 6-min walk test
	Tezosentan	Acute HF	Hemodynamics
	BMS 193884	HF	Hemodynamics

ENABLE = Endothelin Antagonist Bosentan for Lowering Cardiac Events in Heart Failure; CHF = congestive heart failure; ET = endothelin; HEAT = Heart Failure ET(A) Receptor Blockade Trial; = HF = heart failure; LV = left ventricular

Source: Reproduced with permission from Spieker et al.[72b]

endobronchial biopsies in asthmatic patients. Endothelin has been shown to be a potent bronchoconstrictor via production of thromboxane, and its level has been shown to correlate with the degree of resting airflow obstruction. This action is opposed by the local nitric oxide production that it stimulates, with an end result probably depending on the balance between these two opposing forces as well as other factors. Since endothelin also stimulates fibroblast proliferation and collagen deposition, it may play a significant role in causing irreversible airway wall thickening in chronic bronchial hyperresponsiveness.[169]

Immunoreactive endothelin has been shown to be increased in subjects with asthma receiving treatment only with beta$_2$ agonists but not in subjects with asthma also receiving corticosteroid therapy.[170] The increase in levels of cytokine-stimulated release of endothelin has been shown to be reduced or even normalized in patients treated with dexamethasone. It has been proposed that the beneficial effects of steroids in asthma may be related to the inhibition of endothelin synthesis.[171] Moreover, the endothelin receptor antagonists BQ-123 and SB-209670 have been shown to decrease both the number of eosinophils in the bronchoalveolar lavage fluid of mice with antigen-induced lung inflammation as well as the neutrophilic infiltration in the lungs, thereby highlighting the potential role of endothelin antagonists in the treatment of asthma.[172] Endothelin release has also been shown to be increased in the initial phase of airway inflammation as well as in the lungs of mice with experimentally induced respiratory viral infection.[173,174]

The ETA antagonist 2D 1611 is now being evaluated as a treatment modality in patients with chronic obstructive pulmonary disease and pulmonary hypertension.

Growth and Development

Endothelin is essential for normal embryonic development. Mice homozygous for ET1 mutations have severe cardiovascular malformations affecting the aorta and the ventricular septum.[175] ETA knockout mice develop lesions that mimic those seen in the velocardiofacial and CATCH-22 (cardiac anomaly, abnormal face, thymic hypoplasia, cleft palate, hypocalcemia, chromosome 22 deletions) syndromes in humans.[176] The disruption of ET3 or ETB receptors produced mice with an aganglionic megacolon due to the absence of neural crest–derived melanocytes and enteric neurons. This pathologic finding is thought to correspond to that seen in Hirschsprung's disease, in which a missense mutation of the ETB-receptor gene has been identified in some patients.[177,178]

Cerebrovascular Disease

The production of endothelin does not appear to contribute to basal tone in the cerebral circulation.[179] However, ET1 produces a potent and long-lasting contraction of the cerebral vessels in both in vitro and in vivo studies predominantly by activation of ETA receptors.[180] Laboratory and clinical investigations suggest that endothelin may play a role in the pathogenesis of delayed cerebral vasospasm in patients with subarachnoid hemorrhage and ischemic stroke, since high levels of endothelin have been demonstrated in the cerebrospinal fluid of these patients.[181] Endothelin-receptor inhibitors have been suggested as potential treatment agents for patients with subarachnoid hemorrhage in order to influence cerebral vasoconstriction and delay neuronal death[182]; trials are in progress with some of the selective and nonselective agents (Table 31-5).

ETA or ETA/ETB antagonists have been shown to be protective in animal models of stroke.[183–185]

Renal Function, Acute Renal Failure, and Nephrotoxicity

Endothelin can cause increased renal vascular resistance, decreased renal blood flow, and decreased glomerular filtration—effects resembling those seen in renal failure. Studies with endothelin antagonists in animal models of renal failure provide evidence for a role of endothelin in the pathophysiology of acute renal failure. Endothelin antagonists prevented renal failure in dogs after ischemic injury.[186] In transplant models, BQ-123 prevented ischemia-reperfusion damage in rat kidneys.[187] There is indirect evidence for a role of endothelin in other forms of renal disease, such as experimental models of membranous nephropathy, lupus, and diabetes.[53] In an interesting study of diabetic animals with overt proteinuria, chronic use of the nonselective endothelin antagonist PD-142893 was as effective as an ACE inhibitor for improving blood pressure and proteinuria.[188] Increased expression of ET1 in the glomerulus and endothelium of vessels from the kidney in DOCA salt–hypertensive rats indicates a pathophysiologic role of endothelin in renal dysfunction in hypertension.[189] Indeed, the administration of endothelin antagonists to DOCA salt–treated spontaneously hypertensive rats, which develop malignant hypertension and vascular and glomerular fibrinoid necrosis, resulted in the amelioration of the renal lesions.[190] In addition, treatment with an endothelin antagonist normalizes expression of the collagen I gene and leads to regression of renal vascular fibrosis in NG-nitro-L-arginine methyl ester (L-NAME)–induced hypertension.[191] There is some evidence regarding the role of endothelin in radiocontrast-induced renal failure, but conclusive evidence for a protective role of endothelin antagonism is still lacking.[192]

Clinical studies are now in progress evaluating various endothelin antagonists as treatment for patients with progressive nephropathy, renal ischemia, renal transplant rejection, and radiocontrast nephropathy (Table 31-5).

Inflammation and Pain

Endothelin has been suggested to have a potential role as an inflammatory mediator.[192a] Pain, tissue swelling, and infiltration by inflammatory cells appear to involve activation of the ETB receptor.[193] There may be a potential role for ETB-receptor antagonists as therapeutic agents in inflammatory disorders.

SIDE EFFECTS

Bosentan was the first dual ET$_{A/B}$ receptor antagonist to undergo phase II/III testing for indications that require long-term administration, such as systemic pulmonary hypertension and heart failure.[53] In these studies, a number of cases of asymptomatic transaminase elevation were observed to occur—a process that appeared to be dose-dependent.[72,136a,194] These findings suggested that bosentan administration could cause liver injury. No liver biopsies were performed in these patients and the transaminase elevations resolved shortly after the discontinuation of bosentan. Subsequent studies have shown that bosentan induces liver injury through inhibition of the canalicular bile salt export pump, and that the cholestatic potency of bosentan is increased by the concomitant administration of glyburide, a known inhibitor of the bile salt export pump.[194,195] Inhibition of this pump causes intracellular accumulation of cytotoxic bile salts and bile salt–induced liver cell damage.

Additionally, the ENABLE trials showed an increased rate of fluid retention in patients receiving bosentan for the treatment of heart failure.[136e]

CONCLUSION

Endothelin, a potent vasoconstrictor and mitogenic agent, plays a role in multiple disease entities involving various organ systems in both experimental animals and human beings. In the few years since endothelin's discovery, much progress has been made in the development of specific receptor antagonists. Endothelin antagonists have helped to elucidate the role of endothelin in normal physiologic processes and in the pathogenetic mechanisms of several conditions; in addition, these agents offer great promise as a new therapeutic intervention. Peptide and, lately, orally active nonpeptide endothelin antagonists are under clinical investigation. Bosentan is now approved for use in pulmonary hypertension. Efforts are now under way to customize more specific antagonists and, by utilizing the known structure of endothelin, to modify key amino acids and thus create novel agents. Another innovative approach is to control endothelin action by interfering with the endothelin-converting enzyme essential for the production of the active compounds. There are still ongoing questions regarding the efficacy and safety of selective versus nonselective receptor blockers. Hepatotoxicity has been observed with some compounds. Additional research should help resolve safety issues so as to ultimately optimize the clinical benefits of endothelin antagonism.

REFERENCES

1. Hickey KA, Rubanyi GM, Paul RJ, Highsmith RF: Characterization of a coronary vasoconstrictor produced by cultured endothelial cells. *Am J Physiol* 248:550, 1985.
2. Yanagisawa M, Kurihara H, Kimura S, et al: A novel potent vasoconstrictor peptide produced by vascular endothelial cells. *Nature* 332:411, 1988.
3. Kloog Y, Ambar I, Sokolovsky M, et al: Sarafotoxin, a novel vasoconstrictor peptide: Phosphoinositide hydrolysis in rat heart and brain. *Science* 242:268, 1988.
4. Kramer BK, Nishida M, Kelly RA, Smith TW: Endothelins: Myocardial actions of a new class of cytokines. *Circulation* 85:350, 1992.
5. Inoue A, Yanagisawa M, Takuwa Y, et al: The human preproendothelin-1 gene. *J Biol Chem* 264:14954, 1989.
6. Inoue A, Yanagisawa M, Kimura S, et al: The human endothelin family: Three structurally and pharmacologically distinct isopeptides predicted by three separate genes. *Proc Natl Acad Sci U S A* 86:2863, 1989.
7. Yanagisawa M, Masaki T: Molecular biology and biochemistry of the endothelins. *Trends Pharmacol Sci* 10:374, 1989.
8. Webb DJ, Strachan FE: Clinical experience with endothelin antagonists. *Am J Hypertens* 11(4 Pt 3):71S, 1998.
9. Gray G, Webb D: The endothelin system and its potential as a therapeutic target in cardiovascular disease. *Pharmacol Ther* 72:109, 1996.
10. Miyauchi T, Yanagisawa M, Tomizawa T, et al: Increased plasma concentration of endothelin-1 and big endothelin-1 in acute myocardial infarction. *Lancet* 2:53, 1989.
11. Warner TD, Klemm P: What turns on the endothelins? *Inflamm Res* 45:51, 1996.
12. Saida K, Kometani N, Masuda H, et al: Structure of mouse preproendothelin-3 and phylogenetic analysis of the endothelins. *J Cardiovasc Pharmacol* 36(Suppl 1):S1, 2000.

13. Shimada K, Matsushita Y, Wakabayashi K, et al: Cloning and functional expression of human endothelin converting enzyme CDNA. *Biochem Biophy Res Commun* 207:807, 1995.
14. Webb DJ, Monge JC, Rabelink TJ, Yanagisawa M. Endothelin: New discoveries and rapid progress in the clinic. *Trends Pharmacol Sci* 19: 5, 1998.
15. Brown CD, Barnes K, Turner AJ: Functional significance of the isoforms of endothelin-converting enzyme-1. *J Cardiovasc Pharmacol* 36(Suppl 1):S26, 2000.
16. Jackman HL, Morris PW, Rabito SF, et al: Inactivation of endothelin 1 by an enzyme of the vascular endothelial cells. *Hypertension* 21:925, 1993.
17. Sokolovsky M, Galron R, Kloog Y, et al: Endothelins are more sensitive than sarafotoxins to neutral endoproteinase: Possible physiological significance. *Proc Natl Acad Sci U S A* 87:4702, 1990.
18. Vijayaraghavan J, Scicli AG, Carretero OA, et al: The hydrolysis of endothelins by neutral endopeptidase 24.11 (enkephalinase). *J Biol Chem* 265:14150, 1990.
19. DeNucci G, Thomas R, D'Orleans-Juste P, et al: Pressor effects of circulating endothelin are limited by its removal in the pulmonary circulation and by the release of prostacyclin and endothelin derived relaxing factor. *Proc Natl Acad Sci U S A* 85:9797, 1988.
20. Sirvio ML, Metsarinne K, Saijonmaa, Fyhrquist F. Tissue distribution and half-life of 125I-endothelin in the rats: Importance of pulmonary clearance. *Biochem Biophys Res Commun* 167:1191, 1990.
21. Plumpton C, Ferro CJ, Haynes WG, et al: The increase in human plasma immunoreactive endothelin but not big endothelin-1 or its C-terminal fragment induced by systemic administration of the endothelin antagonist TAK-044. *Br J Pharmacol* 119:311, 1996.
22. Levin ER: Mechanisms of disease: Endothelin. *N Engl J Med* 333: 356, 1995.
23. Turner AJ, Murphy LJ: Molecular pharmacology of endothelin converting enzymes. *Biochem Pharmacol* 51(2):91, 1996.
24. Arai H, Hori S, Aramori I, et al: Cloning and expression of a cDNA encoding an endothelial receptor. *Nature* 348:730, 1990.
25. Lin HY, Kaji EH, Winkel GK, et al: Cloning and functional expression of a vascular smooth muscle endothelin 1 receptor. *Proc Natl Acad Sci U S A* 88:3185, 1991.
26. Sakurai T, Yanagisawa M, Masaki T: Molecular characterisation of the endothelin receptors. *Trends Pharmacol Sci* 13:103, 1992.
27. Sakamoto A, Yanagisawa M, Sakurai T, et al: Cloning and functional expression of human cDNA for the ETB endothelin receptor. *Biochem Biophys Res Commun* 178:656, 1991.
28. Bax WA, Saxena PR: The current endothelin receptor classification: Time for reconsideration? *Trends Pharmacol Sci* 15(10):379, 1994.
29. Sakurai T, Goto K: Endothelins: Vascular actions and clinical implications. *Drugs* 46(5):795, 1993.
30. Hosoda K, Nakao K, Hiroshi-Arai, et al: Cloning and expression of human endothelin-1 receptor cDNA. *FEBS Lett* 287(1–2):23, 1991.
31. Yoshimoto S, Ishizaki Y, Sasaki T, Murota SI: Effect of carbon dioxide and oxygen on endothelin production by cultured porcine cerebral endothelial cells. *Stroke* 22:378, 1991.
32. Nathan C, Sporn M: Cytokines in context. *J Cell Biol* 113:981, 1991.
33. Chan J, Greenberg DA: Endothelin and calcium signaling in NG 108-15 neuroblastoma X glioma cells. *J Pharmacol Exp Ther* 258:524, 1991.
34. Ohnishi A, Yamaguchi K, Kusuhara M, et al: Mobilization of intracellular calcium by endothelin in Swiss 3T3 cells. *Biochem Biophys Res Commun* 161:489, 1989.
35. Takuwa N, Takuwa Y, Yanagisawa M, et al: A novel vasoactive peptide stimulates mitogenesis through inositol lipid turnover in Swiss 3T3 fibroblasts. *J Biol Chem* 264:7856, 1989.
36. Takuwa Y, Masaki T, Yamashita K: The effects of the endothelin family peptides on cultured osteoblastic cells from rat calvariae. *Biochem Biophy Res Commun* 170:998, 1990.
37. Miller RC, Pelton JT, Huggins JP: Endothelins—from receptors to medicine. *Trends Pharmacol Sci* 14(2):54, 1993.
38. Nakaki T, Nakayama M, Yamamoto S, Kato R: Endothelin-mediated stimulation of DNA synthesis in vascular smooth muscle cells. *Biochem Biophys Res Commun* 158:880, 1989.
39. Nilsson J, Sjolund M, Palmberg L, et al: The calcium antagonist nifedipine inhibits arterial smooth muscle proliferation. *Atherosclerosis* 58:109, 1985.

40. Battistini B, Chailler P, D'Orleans-Juste P, et al: Growth regulatory properties of endothelins. *Peptides* l4:385, 1993.

41. Brown KD, Littlewood CJ: Endothelin stimulates DNA synthesis in Swiss 3T3 cells, synergy with polypeptide growth factors. *Biochem J* 263:977, 1989.

42. Fabiato A, Fabiato F: Effects of pH on the myofilaments and the sarcoplasmic reticulum of skinned cells from cardiac and skeletal muscles. *J Physiol* 276:233, 1978.

43. Allen DG, Orchard CH: The effects of changes of pH on intracellular calcium transits in mammalian cardiac muscle. *J Physiol* 335:555, 1983.

44. Komuro I, Kurihara H, Sugiyama T, et al: Endothelin stimulates c-fos and c-myc expression and proliferation of vascular smooth muscle cells. *FEBS Lett* 238:249, 1988.

45. Simonson MS, Wann S, Mene P, et al: Endothelin stimulates phospholipase C, Na^+/H^+ exchange, c-fos expression, and mitogenesis in rat mesangial cells. *J Clin Invest* 83:708, 1989.

46. Chakravarthy U, Archer DB: Endothelin—a new vasoactive ocular peptide. *Br J Ophthalmol* 76:l07, 1992.

47. Nakami A, Hirata Y, Ishikawa M, et al: ET-1 and ET-3 induce vasorelaxation via common generation of endothelium derived nitric oxide. *Life Sci* 50:677, 1992.

48. Nakamuta M, Takayanagi R, Sakai Y, et al: Cloning and sequence analysis of cDNA encoding human non-selective type of endothelin receptor. *Biochem Biophys Res Commun* l77:34, 1991.

49. Vincent R, Hogie M, Clozel M, Thuillez C: In vivo evidence of an endothelin-induced vasopressor tone after inhibition of nitric oxide synthesis in rats (abstr). *Circulation* 90(4 Pt 2):1, 1994.

50. Haynes WG, Waugh CJ, Dockrell MEC, et al: Modulators of calcium and potassium channels: their effects on endothelin-1 binding to cardiac membranes. *J Cardiovasc Pharmacol* 22(Suppl):S154, 1993.

51. Grover GJ, Dzwonczyk S, Parham CS, Sleph PG: The protective effects of cromakalim and pinacidil on reperfusion function and infarct size in anaesthetised dogs. *Cardiovasc Drugs Ther* 4:465, 1990.

52. Kerr MJ, Wilson R, Shanks RG: Suppression of ventricular arrhythmias after coronary artery ligation by pinacidil, a vasodilator drug. *J Cardiovasc Pharmacol* 7:875, 1985.

53. Benigni A, Remuzzi G: Endothelin antagonists. *Lancet* 353(9147):133, 1999.

53a. Lüscher TF, Barton M: Endothelins and endothelin receptor antagonists. Therapeutic considerations for a novel class of cardiovascular drugs. *Circulation* 102:2434, 2000.

53b. MacCarthy PA, Pegge NC, Prendergast BD, et al: The physiological role of endogenous endothelin in the regulation of human coronary vasomotor tone. *J Am Coll Cardiol* 37:137, 2001.

54. Haynes WG, Webb DJ: Contribution of endogenous generation of endothelin-1 to basal vascular tone. *Lancet* 344:852, 1994.

55. Haynes WG, Ferro CJ, O'Kane KP, et al: Systemic endothelin receptor blockade decreases peripheral vascular resistance and blood pressure in humans. *Circulation* 93(10):1860, 1996.

56. Stangl K, Dschietzig T, Laule M, et al: Pulmonary big endothelin affects coronary tone and leads to enhanced, ET(A)-mediated coronary constriction in early endothelial dysfunction. *Circulation* 96(9):3192, 1997.

56a. Schiffrin EL: Role of endothelin-1 in hypertension. *Hypertension* 34(Pt 2):876, 1999.

56b. Cardillo C, Kilcoyne CM, Waclawiw M, et al: Role of endothelin in the increased vascular tone of patients with essential hypertension. *Hypertension* 33:753, 1999.

57. Li JS, Lariviere R, Schiffrin EL: Effect of a nonselective endothelin antagonist on vascular remodeling in deoxycorticosterone acetate-salt hypertensive rats. Evidence for a role of endothelin in vascular hypertrophy. *Hypertension* 24(2):183, 1994.

58. Doucet J, Gonzalez W, Michel JB: Endothelin antagonists in salt-dependent hypertension associated with renal insufficiency. *J Cardiovasc Pharmacol* 27(5):643, 1996.

59. Schiffrin EL, Lariviere R, Li JS, Sventek P: Enhanced expression of the endothelin-1 gene in blood vessels of DOCA-salt hypertensive rats: Correlation with vascular structure. *J Vasc Res* 33(3):235, 1996.

60. Schiffrin EL: Endothelin and endothelin antagonists in hypertension. *J Hypertens* 16(12 Pt 2):1891, 1998.

61. Kohno M, Murakawa K, Horio T, et al: Plasma immunoreactive endothelin-1 in experimental malignant hypertension. *Hypertension* 18(1):93, 1991.

62. Yokokawa K, Tahara H, Kohno M, et al: Hypertension associated with endothelin-secreting malignant hemangioendothelioma. *Ann Intern Med* 114(3):213, 1991.

63. Schiffrin EL, Thibault G: Plasma endothelin in human essential hypertension. *Am J Hypertens* 4(4 Pt 1):303, 1991.

64. Tomobe Y, Miyauchi T, Saito A, et al: Effects of endothelin on the renal artery from spontaneously hypertensive and Wistar Kyoto rats. *Eur J Pharmacol* l52:373, 1988.

65. Ergul S, Parish DC, Puett D, Ergul A: Racial differences in plasma endothelin-1 concentrations in individuals with essential hypertension. *Hypertension* 28(4):652, 1996.

65a. Ergul S: Hypertension in black patients. An emerging role of the endothelin system in salt-sensitive hypertension. *Hypertension* 36:62, 2000.

66. Taddei S, Virdis A, Ghiadoni L, et al: Vasoconstriction to endogenous endothelin-1 is increased in the peripheral circulation of patients with essential hypertension. *Circulation* 100:1680, 2000.

67. Noll G, Wenzel RR, Schneider M, et al: Increased activation of sympathetic nervous system and endothelin by mental stress in normotensive offspring of hypertensive parents. *Circulation* 93:866, 1996.

68. Ciafre SA, D'Armiento FP, DiGregorio F, et al: Angiotensin II stimulates endothelin-1 release from human endothelial cells. *Recenti Progr Med* 84(4):248, 1993.

69. Powell JS, Clozel JP, Muller RK, et al: Inhibitors of angiotensin converting enzyme prevent myointimal proliferation after vascular injury. *Science* 245:186, 1989.

70. Moreau P, d'Uscio LV, Shaw S, et al: Angiotensin II increases tissue endothelin and induces vascular hypertrophy: Reversal by ET(A)-receptor antagonist. *Circulation* 96(5):1593, 1997.

70a. Ammarguellat F, Larouche I, Schiffrin EL: Myocardial fibrosis in DOCA-salt hypertensive rats. Effect of endothelin ET_A receptor antagonism. *Circulation* 103:319, 2001.

71. Donckier JE, Massart PE, Hodeige D, et al: Additional hypotensive effect of endothelin-1 receptor antagonism in hypertensive dogs under angiotensin-converting enzyme inhibition. *Circulation* 96(4):1250, 1997.

72. Krum H, Viskoper RJ, Lacourciere Y, et al—Bosentan Hypertension Investigators: The effect of an endothelin-receptor antagonist, bosentan, on blood pressure in patients with essential hypertension. *N Engl J Med* 338(12):784, 1998.

72a. Nakov R, Pfarr E, Eberle S, on behalf of the HEAT Investigators: Darusentan: An effective endothelin-receptor antagonist for treatment of hypertension. *Am J Hypertens* 15:583, 2002.

72b. Spieker LE, Noll G, Ruschitzka FT, Lüscher TF: Endothelin receptor antagonists in congestive heart failure: A new therapeutic principle for the future? *J Am Coll Cardiol* 37:493, 2001.

73. Miyauchi T, Yanagisawa M, Iida K, et al: Age and sex related variation of plasma endothelin-1 concentration in normal and hypertensive subjects. *Am Heart J* 123(4 Pt 1):1092, 1992.

74. Sturrock ND, Lang CC, MacFarlane LJ, et al: Serial changes in blood pressure, renal function, endothelin and lipoprotein (a) during the first 9 days of cyclosporin therapy in males. *J Hypertens* 13(6):667, 1995.

75. Phillips PA, Rolls KA, Burrell LM, et al: Vascular endothelin responsiveness and receptor characteristics in vitro and effects of endothelin receptor blockade in vivo in cyclosporin hypertension. *Clin Exp Pharmacol Physiol* 21:223, 1994.

76. Bartholomeusz B, Hardy KJ, Nelson AS, Phillips PA: Bosentan ameliorates cyclosporin A–induced hypertension in rats and primates. *Hypertension* 27(6):1341, 1996.

77. Sudo N, Kamoi K, Ishibashi M, Yamaji T: Plasma endothelin-1 and big endothelin-1 levels in women with pre-eclampsia. *Acta Endocrinol (Copenh)* 129(2):114, 1993.

78. Mastrogiannis DS, O'Brien WF, Krammer J, Benoit R: Potential role of endothelin-1 in normal and hypertensive pregnancies. *Am J Obstet Gynecol* 165(6 Pt 1):1711, 1991.

79. Cervar M, Puerstner P, Kainer F, Desoye G: Endothelin-1 stimulates the proliferation and invasion of first trimester trophoblastic cells in vitro—a possible role in the etiology of preeclampsia? *J Invest Med* 44(8):447, 1996.

80. Takahashi K, Totsune K, Mori T: Endothelin in chronic renal failure. *Nephron* 66(4):373, 1994.

81. Carlini R, Obialo CI, Rothstein M: Intravenous erythropoietin (rHuEPO) administration increases plasma endothelin and blood pressure in hemodialysis patients. *Am J Hypertens* (6):103, 1993.

82. Oishi S, Sasaki M, Sato T: Elevated immunoreactive endothelin levels in patients with pheochromocytoma. *Am J Hypertens* 7(8):717, 1994.

83. Boulanger CM, Tanner FC, Bea ML, et al: Oxidized low density lipoprotein induces mRNA expression and release of endothelin from human and porcine endothelium. *Circ Res* 70:1191, 1992.

84. Martin-Nizard F, Houssaini HS, Lestavel-Delattre S, et al: Modified low density lipoproteins activates macrophages to secrete ir-ET. *FEBS Lett* 293:127, 1991.

85. Lerman A, Edwards BS, Hallett JW, et al: Circulating and tissue endothelin immunoreactivity in advanced atherosclerosis: *N Engl J Med* 325:997, 1991.

85a. Cardillo C, Kilcoyne CM, Cannon RO, Panza JA: Increased activity of endogenous endothelin in patients with hypercholesterolemia. *J Am Coll Cardiol* 36:1483, 2000.

86. Dagassan PH, Breu V, Clozel M, et al: Up-regulation of endothelin B receptors in atherosclerotic human coronary arteries. *J Cardiovasc Pharmacol* 27:147, 1996.

87. Lerman A, Holmes Jr. DR, Bell MR, et al: Endothelin in coronary endothelial dysfunction and early atherosclerosis in humans. *Circulation* 92:2426, 1995.

88. Haynes WG, Webb DJ: The endothelin family: Local hormones with diverse roles in health and disease? *Clin Sci* 84:485, 1993.

89. Lopez JA, Armstrong ML, Piegos DJ, Hepstad DD: Vascular responses to endothelin-1 in atherosclerotic primates. *Arteriosclerosis* 10:1113, 1990.

90. Miki S, Takeda K, Kiyama M, et al: Modulation of endothelin-1 coronary vasoconstriction in spontaneously hypertensive rats by the nitric oxide system. *Am J Hypertens* 13:83, 2000.

91. Frank HJL, Levin ER, Hu R-M, Pedram A: Insulin stimulates endothelin binding and action on cultured vascular smooth muscle cells. *Endocrinology* 133:1092, 1993.

92. Grantham JA, Schirger JA, Wennberg PW, et al: Modulation of functionally active endothelin-converting enzyme by chronic neutral endopeptidase inhibition in experimental atherosclerosis. *Circulation* 101:1976, 2000.

93. Arikawa E, Verma S, Dumont AS, McNeill JH: Chronic bosentan treatment improves renal artery vascular function in diabetes. *J Hypertens* 19:803, 2001.

94. Dashwood MR, Jagroop IA, Gorog DA, Bagger JP: A potential role for endothelin-1 in peripheral vascular disease. *J Cardiovasc Pharmacol* 36(Suppl 1):S93, 2000.

95. Karwatowska-Prokopezuk E, Wennmalm A: Effects of endothelin on coronary flow, mechanical performance, oxygen uptake and formation of purines and on outflow of prostacyclin in the isolated rabbit heart. *Circ Res* 66:46, 1990.

96. Traverse JH, Judd D, Bache RJ: Dose-dependent effect of endothelin-1 on blood flow to normal and collateral-dependent myocardium. *Circulation* 93:558, 1996.

97. Cannan CR, Burnett JC Jr, Brandt RR, Lerman A: Endothelin at pathophysiological concentrations mediates coronary vasoconstriction via the endothelin-A receptor. *Circulation* 92:3312, 1995.

98. Kurihara H, Yamaoki K, Nahai R: Endothelins: A potent vasoconstrictor associated with coronary vasospasm. *Life Sci* 44:1937, 1989.

99. Salvati P, Chierchia S, Dho L, et al: Proarrhythmic activity of intracoronary endothelin in dogs: Relation to the site of administration and to changes in regional flow. *J Cardiovasc Pharmacol* 17:1007, 1991.

100. Watanabe T, Suzuki N, Shimamoto N, et al: Contribution of endogenous endothelins to the extension of myocardial infarct size in rats. *Circ Res* 69:370, 1991.

101. Omland T, Lie RT, Aakvaag A, et al: Plasma endothelin determination as a prognostic indicator of 1 year mortality after acute myocardial infarction. *Circulation* 89:1573, 1994.

102. Salomone OA, Elliott PM, Calvino R, et al: Plasma immunoreactive endothelin concentration correlates with severity of coronary artery disease in patients with stable angina pectoris and normal ventricular function. *J Am Coll Cardiol* 28:14, 1996.

102a. Ruschitzka F, Moehrlen U, Quaschning T, et al: Tissue endothelin-converting enzyme activity correlates with cardiovascular risk factors in coronary artery disease. *Circulation* 102:1086, 2000.

103. Brunner F, Dutoit EF, Opie LH: Endothelin release during ischemia and reperfusion of isolated perfused rat hearts. *J Mol Cell Cardiol* 24:1291, 1992.

104. Lechleitner P, Genser N, Mair J, et al: Endothelin-1 in patients with complicated and uncomplicated myocardial infarction. *Clin Invest* 70(12):1070, 1992.

105. Lechleitner P, Genser N, Mair J, et al: Plasma immunoreactive endothelin in the acute and subacute phases of myocardial infarction in patients undergoing fibrinolysis. *Clin Chem* 39(6):955, 1993.

106. Pacher R, Stanek B, Hulsmann M, et al: Prognostic impact of big endothelin-1 plasma concentrations compared with invasive hemodynamic evaluation in severe heart failure. *J Am Coll Cardiol* 27:633, 1996.

107. Grover GJ, Dzwonczyk S, Parham CS: The endothelin-1 receptor antagonist BQ-123 reduces infarct size in a canine model of coronary occlusion and reperfusion. *Cardiovasc Res* 27(9):1613, 1993.

108. Iimuro M, Kaneko M, Matsumoto Y, et al: Effects of an endothelin receptor antagonist TAK-044 on myocardial energy metabolism in ischemia/reperfused rat hearts. *J Cardiovasc Pharmacol* 35:403, 2000.

109. Mulder P, Richard V, Derumeaux G, et al: Role of endogenous endothelin in chronic heart failure: Effect of long-term treatment with an endothelin antagonist on survival, hemodynamics, and cardiac remodeling. *Circulation* 96(6):1976, 1997.

110. Fraccarollo D, Hu K, Galuppo P, et al: Chronic endothelin receptor blockade attenuates progressive ventricular dilation and improves cardiac function in rats with myocardial infarction: Possible involvement of myocardial endothelin system in ventricular remodeling. *Circulation* 96(11):3963, 1997.

110a. Galiuto L, DeMaria AN, del Balzo U, et al: Ischemia-reperfusion injury at the microvascular level. Treatment by endothelin A–selective antagonist and evaluation by myocardial contrast echocardiography. *Circulation* 102:3111, 2000.

111. Nguyen QT, Cernacek P, Calderoni A, et al: Endothelin A receptor blockade causes adverse left ventricular remodeling but improves pulmonary artery pressure after infarction in the rat. *Circulation* 98(21):2323, 1998.

112. Wenzel RR, Fleisch M, Shaw S, et al: Hemodynamic and coronary effects of the endothelin antagonist bosentan in patients with coronary artery disease. *Circulation* 98(21):2235, 1998.

113. Hirata Y: Endothelin-1 receptors in cultured vascular smooth muscle cells and cardiocytes of rats. *J Cardiovasc Pharmacol* 13:S157, 1989.

113a. Dhein S, Giesslere C, Wangemann T, et al: Differential pattern of endothelin-1 induced inotropic effects in right atria and left ventricles of the human heart. *J Cardiovasc Pharmacol* 36:564, 2000.

114. Ohno M, Li W, Cheng C-P: Effects of endothelin-1 on left ventricular performance in conscious dogs: Assessment by pressure-volume analysis (abstr) *Circulation* 90(4 Pt 2):I, 1994.

115. MacCarthy PA, Grocott-Mason R, Prendergast BD, Shah AM: Contrasting inotropic effects of endogenous enodthelin in the normal and failing human heart. Studies with an intracoronary ET$_A$ receptor antagonist. *Circulation* 101:142, 2000.

116. Burrell KM, Molenaar P, Dawson PJ, Kaumann AJ: Contractile and arrhythmic effects of endothelin receptor agonists in human heart in vitro: blockade with SB 209670. *J Pharmacol Exp Ther* 292:449, 2000.

117. Moe GW, Ferrazzi S, Naik G, Howard RJ: Endothelin in heart failure: Temporal evolution, source of production and interaction with atrial natriuretic peptide (abstr) *Circulation* 90(4 Pt 2):I, 1994.

118. Baertschi AJ, Pedrazzini T, Aubert J-F, et al: Role of endothelin receptor subtypes in volume-stimulated ANF secretion. *Am J Physiol Heart Circ Physiol* 278:H493, 2000.

119. Sütsch G, Bertel O, Rickenbacher P, et al: Regulation of aldosterone secretion in patients with chronic congestive heart failure by endothelins. *Am J Cardiol* 85:973, 2000.

120. Sakai S, Miyauchi T, Kobayashi M, et al: Inhibition of myocardial endothelin pathway improves long-term survival in heart failure. *Nature* 384(6607):353, 1996.

121. Spinale FG, Walker JD, Mukherjee R, et al: Concomitant endothelin receptor subtype-A blockade during the progression of pacing-induced congestive heart failure in rabbits. Beneficial effects on left ventricular and myocyte function. *Circulation* 95(7):1918, 1997.

122. Mishima T, Tanimura M, Suzuki G, et al: Effects of long-term therapy with bosentan on the progression of left ventricular dysfunction and remodeling in dogs with heart failure. *J Am Coll Cardiol* 35:222, 2000.

123. Rodeheffer RJ, Lerman A, Heublein DM, Burnett JC Jr: Increased plasma concentrations of endothelin in congestive heart failure in humans. *Mayo Clin Proc* 67(8):719, 1992.

123a. Zolk O, Quattek J, Sitzler G, et al: Expression of endothelin-1, endothelin-converting enzyme, and endothelin receptors in chronic heart failure. *Circulation* 99:2118, 1999.

123b. Yamauchi-Kohno R, Miyauchi T, Hoshino T, et al: Role of endothelin in deterioration of heart failure due to cardiomyopathy in hamsters. Increase in endothelin-1 production in the heart and beneficial effect of endothelin-A receptor antagonist on survival and cardiac function. *Circulation* 99:2171, 1999.

123c. Pieske B, Beyermann B, Breu V, et al: Functional effects of endothelin and regulation of endothelin receptors in isolated human nonfailing and failing myocardium. *Circulation* 99:1802, 1999.

123d. Selvais PL, Robert A, Ahn S, et al: Direct comparison between endothelin-1, N-terminal proatrial natriuretic factor, and brain natriuretic peptide as prognostic markers of survival in congestive heart failure. *J Cardiac Failure* 6:201, 2000.

124. Erbas T, Erbas B, Kabakci G, et al: Plasma big-endothelin levels, cardiac autonomic neuropathy, and cardiac functions in patients with insulin-dependent diabetes mellitus. *Clin Cardiol* 23:259, 2000.

125. Givertz MM, Colucci WS, LeJemtel TH, et al: Acute endothelin A receptor blockade causes selective pulmonary vasodilation in patients with chronic heart failure. *Circulation* 101:2922, 2000.

126. Wittner M, Morris SA, Christ GJ, et al: Infection of cultured human endothelial cells increases endothelin levels (abstr). *Circulation* 90(4 Pt 2):I, 1994.

127. Ono K, Matsumori A, Shioi T, et al: Contribution of endothelin-1 to myocardial injury in a murine model of myocarditis. Acute effects of bosentan, and endothelin receptor antagonist. *Circulation* 100:1823, 1999.

128. Webb DJ: Evidence for endothelin-1-mediated vasoconstriction in severe chronic heart failure. Endothelin antagonism in heart failure. *Circulation* 92:3372, 1995.

129. Berger R, Stanek B, Hülsmann M, et al: Effects of endothelin A receptor blockade on endothelial function in patients with chronic heart failure. *Circulation* 103:981, 2001.

129a. Takeuchi Y, Kihara Y, Inagaki K: Endothelin-1 has a unique oxygen-saving effect by increasing contractile efficiency in the isolated rat heart. *Circulation* 103:1557, 2001.

130. Kiowski W, Sutsch G, Hunziker P, et al: Evidence for endothelin-1-mediated vasoconstriction in severe chronic heart failure. *Lancet* 346(8977):732, 1995.

131. Haynes WG, Webb DJ: Endothelin as a regulator of cardiovascular function in health and disease. *J Hypertens* 16(8):1081, 1998.

132. Love MP, Haynes WG, Gray GA, et al: Vasodilator effects of endothelin-converting enzyme inhibition and endothelin ETA receptor blockade in chronic heart failure patients treated with ACE inhibitors. *Circulation* 94(9):2131, 1996.

133. Sutsch G, Kiowski W, Yan XW, et al: Short-term oral endothelin-receptor antagonist therapy in conventionally treated patients with symptomatic severe chronic heart failure. *Circulation* 98(21):2262, 1998.

134. Fraccarollo D, Bauersachs J, Galuppo P, et al: Effects of combined endothelin A receptor blockade plus ACE inhibition in rats with chronic heart failure (abstr). *J Am Coll Cardiol* 37(Suppl A):151A, 2001.

134a. New RB, Sampson AC, King MK, et al: Effects of combined angiotensin II and endothelin receptor blockade with developing heart failure. Effects on left ventricular performance. *Circulation* 102:1447, 2000.

134b. Sakai S, Miyauchi T, Yamaguchi I: Long-term endothelin receptor antagonist administration improves alterations in expression of various cardiac genes in failing myocardium of rats with heart failure. *Circulation* 101:2849, 2000.

134c. Wada A, Tsutamoto T, Ohnishi M, et al: Effects of a specific endothelin-converting enzyme inhibitor on cardiac, renal, and neurohumoral functions in congestive heart failure. Comparison of effects with those of endothelin A receptor antagonism. *Circulation* 99:570, 1999.

135. Wada A, Tsutamoto T, Fukai D, et al: Comparison of the effects of selective endothelin ETA and ETB receptor antagonists in congestive heart failure. *J Am Coll Cardiol* 30(5):1385, 1997.

136. Love MP, Ferro CJ, Haynes WG, et al: Selective or non-selective endothelin receptor blockade in chronic heart failure? *Circulation* 94(suppl 1):2899, 1996.

136a. Packer M, Caspi A, Charlon V, et al: Multicenter, double-blind, placebo-controlled study of long-term endothelin blockade with bosentan in chronic heart failure—results of the REACH-1 trial. *Circulation* 98 (Suppl S):12, 1998.

136b. Ruschitzka F, Noll G, Mitrovic V, et al: Clinical and hemodynamic effects of chronic selective ETA-receptor blockade in congestive heart failure (HEAT, Heart Failure ETA Receptor Blockade Trial). *Eur Heart J* 71(Suppl S):705, 2000.

136c. Torre-Amione G, Young JB, Durand J-B, et al: Hemodynamic effects of tezosentan, an intravenous dual endothelin receptor antagonist, in patients with class III to IV congestive heart failure. *Circulation* 103:973, 2001.

136d. Ellahham SH, Charlon V, Abassi Z, et al: Bosentan and endothelin system in congestive heart failure. *Clin Cardiol* 23:803, 2000.

136e. Moore J: ENABLE 1, 2: Bosentan did not improve HF symptoms. *Today Cardiol* 5:8, 2002.

137. Krum H, Gu A, Wilshire Clement M, et al: Changes in plasma endothelin-1 levels reflect clinical response to beta blockade in chronic heart failure. *Am Heart J* 131:337, 1996.

138. Hassoun PM, Thappa V, Landman MJ, Fanburg BL: Endothelin-1: Mitogenic activity on pulmonary artery smooth muscle cells and release from hypoxic endothelial cells. *Proc Soc Exp Biol Med* 199:165, 1992.

139. Ito H, Hirata Y, Hiroe M, et al: ET-1 induces hypertrophy with enhanced expression of muscle specific genes in cultured neonatal rat cardiomyocytes. *Circ Res* 69:209, 1991.

140. Ito H: Endothelins and cardiac hypertrophy. *Life Sci* 61(6):585, 1997.

140a. Yang Z, Krasnici N, Lüscher TF: Endothelin-2 potentiates human smooth muscle cell growth to PDGF. Effects of ETA and ETB receptor blockade. *Circulation* 100:5, 1999.

141. Bek EL, McMillen MA: Endothelins are angiogenic. *J Cardiovasc Pharmacol* 36(Suppl 1):S135, 2000.

142. Chua BH, Kreba CJ, Chua CC, Diglio CA: Endothelin stimulates protein synthesis in smooth muscle cells. *Am J Physiol* 262:E412, 1992.

143. Stash J-P, Hirth-Dietrich C, Frobel K, Wegner M: Prolonged endothelin blockade prevents hypertension and cardiac hypertrophy in stroke-prone spontaneously hypertensive rats. *Am J Hypertens* 8:1128, 1995.

144. Yorikane R, Sakai S, Miyauchi T, et al: Possible involvement of endothelin-1 in cardiac hypertrophy. *Arzneim Forsch* 44(3A):412, 1994.

145. Ito H, Hirata Y, Adachi S, et al: Endothelin-1 is an autocrine/paracrine factor in the mechanism of angiotensin II-induced hypertrophy in cultured rat cardiomyocytes. *J Clin Invest* 92(1):398, 1993.

146. Ito H, Adachi S, Tamamori M, et al: Mild hypoxia induces hypertrophy of cultured neonatal rat cardiomyocytes: A possible endogenous endothelin-1-mediated mechanism. *J Mol Cell Cardiol* 28(6):1271, 1996.

147. Ito H, Hiroe M, Hirata Y, et al: Endothelin ETA receptor antagonist blocks cardiac hypertrophy provoked by hemodynamic overload. *Circulation* 89(5):2198, 1994.

147a. Ehmke H, Faulhaber J, Münter K, et al: Chronic ETA receptor blockade attenuates cardiac hypertrophy independently of blood pressure effects in renovascular hypertensive rats. *Hypertension* 33:954, 1999.

148. Karam H, Heudes D, Hess P, et al: Respective role of humoral factors and blood pressure in cardiac remodeling of DOCA hypertensive rats. *Cardiovasc Res* 31(2):287, 1996.

149. Douglas SA, Louden C, Vickery-Clark LM: A role for endogenous endothelin-1 in neointimal formation after rat carotid artery balloon angioplasty: Protective effects of the novel nonpeptide endothelin receptor antagonist SB 209670. *Circ Res* 75:190, 1994.

150. Ferrer P, Valentine M, Jenkins-West T, et al: Orally active endothelin receptor antagonist BMS-182874 suppresses neointimal development in balloon-injured rat carotid arteries. *J Cardiovasc Pharmacol* 26:908, 1995.

151. Okada K, Nishida Y, Murakami H: Role of endogenous endothelin in the development of graft arteriosclerosis in rat cardiac allografts: Antiproliferative effects of bosentan, a nonselective endothelin receptor antagonist. *Circulation* 97(23):2346, 1998.

152. Kyriakides ZS, Kremastinos DT, Georgiades M, et al: Endothelin A receptor antagonism may prevent in-stent restenosis in humans (abstr). *J Am Coll Cardiol* 37(Suppl A):14A, 2001.

152a. Huckle WR, Drag MD, Acker WR, et al: Effects of L-749,329, an ET$_A$/ET$_B$ endothelin receptor antagonist, in a porcine coronary artery injury model of vascular restenosis. *Circulation* 103:1899, 2001.

152b. Kyriakides ZS, Kremastinos DH, Kolettis TM, et al: Acute endothelin-A receptor antagonism prevents normal reduction of myocardial ischemia on repeated balloon inflations during angioplasty. *Circulation* 102:1937, 2000.

153. Merkely B, Szabó, Gellér L, et al: The selective endothelin-A-receptor antagonist LU 135.252 inhibits the direct arrhythmogenic action of endothelin-1. *J Cardiovasc Pharmacol* 36(Suppl 1):S314, 2000.

154. Horkay F, Gellér L, Kiss O, et al: Bosentan the mixed endothelin-A-and B-receptor antagonist suppresses intrapericardial endothelin-1-induced ventricular arrhythmias. *J Cardiovasc Pharmacol* 36(Suppl 1):S320, 2000.

155. Stewart DJ, Levy RD, Cernacek P, Langleben D: Increased plasma endothelin-1 in pulmonary hypertension: Marker or mediator of disease? *Ann Intern Med* 114:464, 1991.

156. Giaid A, Yanagisawa M, Langleben D, et al: Expression of endothelin-1 in the lungs of patients with pulmonary hypertension. *N Engl J Med* 328:1732, 1993.

156a. Snopek G, Pogorzelska H, Rywik TM, et al: Usefulness of endothelin-1 concentration in capillary blood in patients with mitral stenosis as a predictor of regression of pulmonary hypertension after mitral valve replacement or valvuloplasty. *Am J Cardiol* 90:188, 2002.

157. Li H, Chen SJ, Chen YF, et al: Enhanced endothelin-1 and endothelin receptor gene expression in chronic hypoxia. *J Appl Physiol* 77(3):1451, 1994.

158. Dupuis J, Cernacek P, Tardif JC, et al: Reduced pulmonary clearance of endothelin-1 in pulmonary hypertension. *Am Heart J* 135(4):614, 1998.

159. Mikhail G, Chester AH, Gibbs JS, et al: Role of vasoactive mediators in primary and secondary pulmonary hypertension. *Am J Cardiol* 82(2):254, 1998.

160. Barman SA, Isales CM: Fenfluramine potentiates canine pulmonary vasoreactivity to endothelin-1. *Pulm Pharmacol Ther* 11(2–3):183, 1998.

161. Reddy VM, Hendricks-Munoz KD, Rajasinghe HA, et al: Postcardiopulmonary bypass pulmonary hypertension in lambs with increased pulmonary blood flow. A role for endothelin 1. *Circulation* 95(4):1054, 1997.

162. Akazawa H, Ikeda U, Kuroda T, Shimada K: Plasma endothelin-1 levels in Takayasu's arteritis. *Cardiology* 87(4):303, 1996.

163. Lutz J, Gorenflo M, Habighorst M, et al: Endothelin-1- and endothelin-receptors in lung biopsies of patients with pulmonary hypertension due to congenital heart disease. *Clin Chem Lab Med* 37(4):423, 1999.

163a. Sartori C, Vollenweider L, Löffler B-M, et al: Exaggerated endothelin release in high-altitude pulmonary edema. *Circulation* 99:2665, 1999.

164. Chen SJ, Chen YF, Meng QC, et al: Endothelin-receptor antagonist bosentan prevents and reverses hypoxic pulmonary hypertension in rats. *J Appl Physiol* 79(6):2122, 1995.

165. Itoh H, Yokochi A, Yamauchi-Kohno R, Maruyama K: Effects of the endothelin ET(A) receptor antagonist, TA-0201, on pulmonary arteries isolated from hypoxic rats. *Eur J Pharmacol* 376(3):233, 1999.

166. Sheedy W, Haleen S, Morice AH: The effect of the ETA receptor antagonist (CI-1020) in rats with established hypoxic pulmonary hypertension. *Pulm Pharmacol Ther* 11(2–3):173, 1998.

167. Ueno M, Miyauchi T, Sakai S, Goto K: The combined treatment of oral endothelin (ET)-A receptor antagonist and oral prostacyclin (PGI2) analog is more greatly effective in ameliorating pulmonary hypertension (PH) and right ventricular (RV) hypertrophy than each drug alone in rats (abstr). *Circulation* 100 (Suppl 1):I, 1999.

167a. Jasmin J-F, Lucas M, Cernacek P, Dupuis J: Effectiveness of a nonselective ET$_{A/B}$ and a selective ET$_A$ antagonist in rats with monocrotaline-induced pulmonary hypertension. *Circulation* 103:314, 2001.

168. Apostolopoulou SC, Kyriakides Z, Webb DJ, et al: Endothelin A receptor antagonism improves pulmonary and systemic hemodynamics in patients with severe pulmonary hypertension (abstr). *Circulation* 100(Suppl 1):I, 1999.

168a. Barst RJ, Rich S, Widlitz A, et al: Clinical efficacy of sitaxsentan, an endothelin-A receptor antagonist, in patients with pulmonary arterial hypertension. Open-label pilot study. *Chest* 121:1860, 2002.

168b. Elliott WT, Chan J: Bosentan tablets (Tracleer-Actelion). *Intern Med Alert* 4:13, 2002.

169. Howarth PH, Redington AE, Springall DR, et al: Epithelially derived endothelin and nitric oxide in asthma. *Int Arch Allergy Immunol* 107(1–3):228, 1995.

170. Redington AE, Springall DR, Meng Q, et al. Immunoreactive endothelin in bronchial biopsy specimens: Increased expression in asthma and modulation by corticosteroid therapy. *J Allergy Clin Immunol* 100:544, 1997.

171. Yang Q, Laporte J, Battistini B, Sirois P: Effects of dexamethasone on the basal and cytokine-stimulated release of endothelin-1 from guinea-pig cultured tracheal epithelial cells. *Can J Physiol Pharmacol* 75:576, 1997.

172. Fujitani Y, Trifilieff A,Tsuyuki S, et al: Endothelin receptor antagonists inhibit antigen-induced lung inflammation in mice. *Am J Respir Crit Care Med* 155:1890, 1997.

173. Finsnes F, Christensen G, Lyberg T, et al: Increased synthesis and release of endothelin-1 during the initial phase of airway inflammation. *Am J Respir Crit Care Med* 158:1600, 1998.

174. Carr MJ, Spalding LJ, Goldie RG, Henry PJ: Distribution of immunoreactive endothelin in the lungs of mice during respiratory viral infection. *Eur Respir J* 11:79, 1998.

175. Kurihara Y, Kurihara H, Oda H, et al: Aortic arch malformations and ventricular septal defect in mice deficient in endothelin-1. *J Clin Invest* 96(1):293, 1995.

176. Clouthier DE, Hosoda K, Richardson JA, et al: Cranial and cardiac neural crest defects in endothelin-A receptor-deficient mice. *Development* 125(5):813, 1998.

177. Hosoda K, Hammer RE, Richardson JA, et al: Targeted and natural (piebald-lethal) mutations of endothelin-B receptor gene produce megacolon associated with spotted coat color in mice. *Cell* 79(7):1267, 1994.

178. Puffenberger EG, Hosoda K, Washington SS, et al: A missense mutation of the endothelin B receptor gene in multigenic Hirschsprung's disease. *Cell* 79:1257, 1994.

179. Faraci FM, Heistad DD. Regulation of the cerebral circulation: Role of endothelium and potassium channels. *Physiol Rev* 78(1):53, 1998.

180. Pierre LN, Davenport AP, Katusic ZS: Blockade and reversal of endothelin-induced constriction in pial arteries from human brain. *Stroke* 30(3):638, 1999.

181. Suzuki H, Sata S, Suzuki Y, et al: Increased endothelin concentration in CSF from patients with subarachnoid hemorrhage. *Acta Neurol Scand* 81:553, 1990.

182. Kikkawa K, Saito A, Iwasaki H, et al: Prevention of cerebral vasospasm by a novel endothelin receptor antagonist, TA-0201. *J Cardiovasc Pharmacol* 34:666, 1999.

183. Willette RN, Zhang H, Mitchell MP, et al: Nonpeptide endothelin antagonist. Cerebrovascular characterization and effects on delayed cerebral vasospasm. *Stroke* 25(12):2450, 1994.

184. Tatlisumak T, Carano RA, Takano K, et al: A novel endothelin antagonist, A-127722, attenuates ischemic lesion size in rats with temporary middle cerebral artery occlusion: a diffusion and perfusion MRI study. *Stroke* 29(4):850, 1998.

185. Lambert G, Lambert E, Fassot C, et al: Subarachnoid haemorrhage-induced sympatho-excitation in rats is reversed by bosentan or sodium nitroprusside. *Clin Exp Pharmacol Physiol* 28:200, 2001.

186. Brooks DP, dePalma PD, Gellai M, et al: Nonpeptide endothelin receptor antagonists. III. Effect of SB 209670 and BQ123 on acute renal failure in anesthetized dogs. *J Pharmacol Exp Ther* 271(2):769, 1994.

187. Buyukgebiz O, Aktan AO, Haklar G, et al: BQ-123, a specific endothelin (ETA) receptor antagonist, prevents ischemia-reperfusion injury in kidney transplantation. *Transplant Int* 9(3):201, 1996.

188. Benigni A, Colosio V, Brena C, et al: Unselective inhibition of endothelin receptors reduces renal dysfunction in experimental diabetes. *Diabetes* 47(3):450, 1998.

189. Deng LY, Day R, Schiffrin EL: Localization of sites of enhanced expression of endothelin-1 in the kidney of DOCA-salt hypertensive rats. *J Am Soc Nephrol* 7(8):1158, 1996.

190. Li JS, Schurch W, Schiffrin EL: Renal and vascular effects of chronic endothelin receptor antagonism in malignant hypertensive rats. *Am J Hypertens* 9(8):803, 1996.

191. Boffa JJ, Tharaux PL, Dussaule JC, Chatziantoniou C: Regression of renal vascular fibrosis by endothelin receptor antagonism. *Hypertension* 37(2 Pt 2):490, 2001.

192. Sung JM, Shu GH, Tsai JC, Huang JJ: Radiocontrast media induced endothelin-1 mRNA expression and peptide release in porcine aortic endothelial cells. *J Formosa Med Assoc* 94(3):77, 1995.

192a. Tschaikowsky K, Sagner S, Lehnert N, et al: Endothelin in septic patients: Effects on cardiovascular and renal function and its relationship to proinflammatory cytokines. *Crit Care Med* 28:1854, 2000.

193. Griswold DE, Douglas SA, Martin LD, et al: Targeted disruption of the endothelin-B-receptor gene attenuates inflammatory nociception and cutaneous inflammation in mice. *J Cardiovasc Pharmacol* 36(Suppl 1):S78, 2000.

194. Fattinger K, Funk C, Pantze M, et al: The endothelin export pump: A potential mechanism for hepatic adverse reactions. *Clin Pharmacol Ther* 69:223, 2001.

195. Stieger B, Fattinger K, Madon J, et al: Drug- and estrogen-induced cholestasis through inhibition of the hepatocellular bile salt export pump of rat liver. *Gastroenterology* 118:422, 2000.

CHAPTER 32

Adenosine-Receptor Agonism and Antagonism in Cardiovascular Disease

William H. Frishman

Eugenia Gianos

Jay Lee

Bradley G. Somer

Adenosine, a purine nucleoside, is present in all cells and released under a variety of different physiologic and pathophysiologic circumstances to affect various bodily actions. The effects of adenosine are mediated by the stimulation of three distinct receptors, A_1, A_2, and A_3. The main cardiovascular effects of adenosine-receptor (AR) stimulation are vasodilation, which includes the coronary vasculature; inhibition of platelet aggregation; and atrioventricular (AV) conduction blockade. Adenosine is currently being used for the treatment of some supraventricular arrhythmias and as a diagnostic agent in radionucleotide perfusion studies. There is also evidence suggesting its potential use in ischemic preconditioning, as a treatment for angina pectoris, as therapy for heart failure, and in the prevention of reperfusion injury. Also of note is its potential clinical application in systemic hypertension and hyperlipidemia. There are also promising data to support a role for AR manipulation in a variety of noncardiovascular conditions. The study of adenosine's pharmacology, which is reviewed in this chapter, has provided important new information regarding the regulation of body homeostasis and has suggested a promising and innovative approach for the future prevention and treatment of a variety of cardiovascular disorders.

ADENOSINE SYNTHESIS, RELEASE, AND CLEARANCE

Adenosine (Fig. 32-1) is synthesized extracellularly through the metabolic degradation of adenine nucleotides such as adenosine monophosphate (AMP) and adenosine triphosphate (ATP) by the enzyme 5′-nucleotidase, which is found bound to cell membranes. This enzyme also accounts for one of the two intracellular mechanisms of adenosine synthesis. This multimodal synthesis allows for adenosine to be produced both intra- and extracellularly; thus cells that release adenine nucleotides (e.g., ATP) into the extracellular space are potential sources for adenosine. The main cells which account for this release are the platelets and endothelial cells.[1] Also of note is that with any event leading to ischemia or hypoxia where oxygen demand outweighs supply and where large amounts of ATP are metabolized completely, adenosine becomes a by-product.[2] The other major mode of adenosine synthesis is

through the intracellular metabolism of S-adenosylhomocysteine by S-adenosylhomocysteine hydrolase, resulting in the release of both adenosine and homocysteine.[3] This mechanism predominates during periods of normoxia.[3]

Adenosine exerts its action by binding to specific receptors, resulting in the activation and manipulation of a second messenger with resultant alteration of cellular functions. The half-life of adenosine in human blood is less than 1 s.[4] Such a short half-life is determined by rapid adenosine transport and clearance into cells, via an energy-dependent nucleotide transport system,[5] as part of a salvage pathway to maintain intracellular ATP. This system can be overwhelmed when there is hypoxia leading to adenosine accumulation in several tissues.[6] Once in the cell, adenosine is either metabolized by phosphorylation with adenosine kinase to AMP through the salvage pathway or deaminated by adenosine deaminase to inosine, which is degraded into hypoxanthine, xanthine, and eventually uric acid, which is excreted in the urine. Figure 32-1 provides an overview of adenosine synthesis and clearance.

RECEPTORS MEDIATING BIOLOGIC ACTIVITY OF ADENOSINE: CLASSIFICATION, MOLECULAR BIOLOGY, STRUCTURE, AND FUNCTION

The receptors for adenosine that mediate biologic activity are found on cardiomyocytes in both the atria and ventricles, in the sinus node and atrioventricular (AV) nodes, and on ventricular pacemaker cells. ARs are also found on coronary vascular endothelial and smooth muscle cells. Besides the heart, biologically active AR exist in the central nervous system (CNS),[7–9] kidney,[10,11] skeletal muscles,[12] blood cells,[13] adipose tissue,[14] spermatozoa,[15] bronchotracheal tree,[16] pancreas,[17] liver, and endocrine glands.[18]

ARs are grouped as purinergic (P1)-type receptors, which are sensitive to adenosine and its analogs. This is in contrast to P2 receptors, which respond more to adenine nucleotides such as ATP.[19] Among the P1 (adenosine) receptors there are intracellular P-site receptors that require an intact purine ring for activation and are of little physiologic importance. There are also the more important R-site receptors, found on cell membranes, that require the

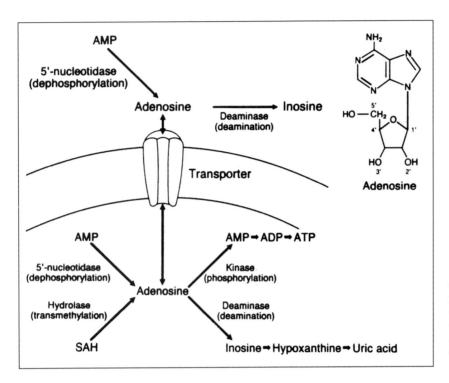

FIGURE 32-1. Adenosine molecular structure, production and metabolism. ADP = adenosine diphosphate; AMP = adenosine monophosphate; ATP = adenosine triphosphate; SAH = S-adenosyl homocystine. (*Reproduced with permission from Shen W-K, Kurachi Y: Mechanisms of adenosine-mediated actions on cellular and clinical cardiac electrophysiology. Mayo Clinic Proc 70:275, 1995.*)

ribose moiety for activation. There are currently various subtypes of adenosine cell surface R-type receptors, classified on the basis of the different mechanisms of action that they mediate and their different tissue distributions. The classification of receptor subtype was originally determined by the different mechanism of surface receptor–mediated signal transduction, although other criteria such as agonist/antagonist rank-order potency data were also used to determine AR subtype. The A_1 receptors were originally determined to be those which, when stimulated at the receptor R-site, caused adenylate cyclase to be inhibited (originally termed Ri receptors), leading to decreased intracellular cyclic AMP. A_2 receptors, when stimulated, activate adenylate cyclase (originally termed Ra receptors), leading to potentiation of intracellular cAMP. Two subtypes of A_2 ARs have been identified: A_{2a} and A_{2b}. More recently, studies have suggested that there also is an A_3 receptor subtype, which is activated by adenosine via a mechanism more typical of A_1 receptors;

however, this receptor is not blocked by typical AR antagonists. This receptor also has a unique distribution and physiologic function, discussed further on.[20]

In general, all of the ARs are from the family of receptors known as cell surface receptors of the G protein–coupled type, similar to the muscarinic[21] and adrenergic[22] receptor systems. The architecture of the receptors comprises the typical seven stretches of hydrophobic helical regions, each composed of 22 to 26 amino acids that traverse the cell membrane.[23] Figure 32-2 displays the typical AR structure. The cytoplasmic domain of the receptor, including the three intracellular loops and the carboxy-terminal tail, interacts with subunits of the unique G protein, which then alters its structure and binds GTP, resulting in further signal transduction. This results in either the activation or inactivation of adenylate cyclase, depending on whether the receptor was A_2 or A_1 and A_3 respectively.

FIGURE 32-2. The typical adenosine receptor structure. (*Reproduced with permission from Schott et al.[190]*)

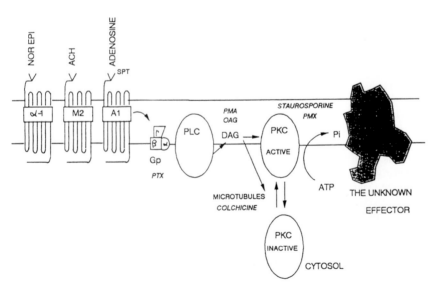

A_1 ARs have been cloned from rat,[24,25] rabbit,[26] bovine,[27,28] and human[29–32] cDNA libraries. The gene has been localized to chromosome 1q32.1.[33] The various clones encode a protein of 326 amino acids with a corresponding molecular mass of about 36 kd. The expressed products of the isolated clones bind to the AR agonist with the potency order of (-)-N6-(R-phenylisopropyl) adenosine(R-PIA)>5 =-N-ethylcarboxamidoadenosine(NECA)> (+)-N6 phenylisopropyladenosine (S-PIA)—the configuration conventionally used to define the A_1 AR.[25,30,32] Bovine A_1 AR is a little different in that it is a 328–amino acid protein and the rank-order potency is R-PIA>S-PIA>NECA.[27,28] The trend is that the A_1 AR subtype usually has a higher affinity to N6-substituted adenosine analogues than to the 5'-substituted analogue. Analysis of tissue mRNA by Northern blotting and in situ hybridization show that A_1 ARs are expressed in detectable amounts in the brain, spinal cord, fat, testis, heart,[24,25,28] and medullary and papillary collecting ducts of the kidney.[34] In the heart, A_1 ARs are mostly distributed in myocardial cells.[35–39]

The A_1 ARs, when bound to a ligand agonist, cause adenylate cyclase to be inhibited[40,41] through activation of a Gi protein. The resulting decrease in cAMP results in an alteration of the activity of cAMP-activated protein kinase and a resultant alteration in cell function. Other potential effects resulting from A_1 AR stimulation have subsequently been discovered. These include stimulation of K^+ conductance,[42] inhibition of calcium (Ca^{2+}) conductance,[43] stimulation of phospholipase C, and generation of a Ca^{2+} second messenger and protein kinase C signal.[44,45] In the heart, the A_1 ARs are located on the cardiomyocytes and on coronary smooth muscle.[46] The proposed role for A_1 ARs in the heart is mediated through two pathways. When the receptor is stimulated by adenosine, there is a direct action on potassium (K^+) channels, with a resultant hyperpolarizing K^+ efflux mediated by a Gk protein. This accounts for functions that slow automaticity. The other mechanism of action is indirect and entails the inhibition of adenylate cyclase through a Gi protein. This antagonizes the action of the beta-adrenergic system, which acts by stimulating adenylate cyclase via G_s protein, thereby increasing cAMP concentration and leading to the activation of several ionic channels, including Ca^{2+} channels and pacemaker function currents. A_1 AR activation inhibits this beta-adrenergic activity through the inhibition of cAMP.

A_2 ARs are subtyped into the A_{2a} and A_{2b} ARs. When stimulated, both receptor subtypes activate adenylate cyclase, thus triggering the production of the cAMP second messenger. This defines the A_2 AR. Another proposed mechanism for the action of the A_2 AR, is the activation of the ATP sensitive potassium channel, resulting in a hyperpolarized cell and decreased effector action.[47] The A_{2a} AR differs from the A_{2b} AR in that the A_{2a} AR has a high-affinity adenosine-sensitive site and A_{2b} ARs have a low-affinity site.[48] CGS 21680 has been shown to bind selectively to A_{2a} ARs.[49] Other selective A_{2a} AR agonists have since been identified.[50] The rank-order potencies in functional studies utilizing agonists and antagonists are very different. The other major difference between these receptor subtypes is found in their predominant anatomic locations in the brain—A_{2a} AR is found mostly in the striatum, and A_{2b} AR is distributed diffusely in the brain.[48,51] In the heart, A_2 receptors are largely distributed in coronary vascular smooth muscle and endothelial cells.[35–39]

The A_{2a} AR has been cloned from rat,[52] canine,[53] and human[54] cDNA libraries. The various clones encode a protein of 410 to 412 amino acids, with a corresponding molecular weight of about 45 kd. The additional amino acids that make A_{2a} ARs so much larger than

A_1 ARs are due to a long carboxy-terminal tail of undetermined significance. Analysis of tissue mRNA by Northern blotting shows that transcript is present in the striatum, heart, kidney, and lung. Pharmacologic studies have observed the presence of A_{2a} ARs in platelets,[55] on coronary endothelial cells,[56] and in the liver.[57]

The A_{2b} AR has been cloned from rat[58,59] and human[60] cDNA libraries. The clones encode a protein of about 330 amino acids, structurally more similar to A_1 AR than to A_{2a} AR. The A_{2b} ARs are relatively more difficult to study since they have very low affinity to their agonists; also, less is known about them functionally.[60a] They are studied more typically by their increased affinity to certain antagonists, since the affinity of the A_{2b} ARs to these antagonists is greater than that of the A_{2a} ARs.[59] Analysis of tissue mRNA by Northern blotting demonstrated presence of a large amount of transcript in cecum, large intestine, and bladder, with lesser amounts present in the lungs, brain, and spinal cord.[58]

A_3 ARs have been cloned from rat,[61,62] sheep,[63] mouse,[64] and human[65] cDNA libraries. The gene encodes a receptor that is 317 to 320 amino acids long, similar in size to the A_1 AR. Pharmacologic functional studies have been done on this receptor. The properties of the rat A_3 AR differ somewhat from those of the human in that studies on the rat A_3 AR demonstrate that several xanthine derivatives—which normally inhibit ARs nonselectively—will display little binding at this receptor.[62] In humans, however, A_3 ARs do bind certain xanthine antagonists with relatively moderate affinity.[65] This can be explained by the fact that human A_3 ARs display only a 72% overall amino acid identity to rat A_3 ARs. The tissue distribution of A_3 AR mRNA in the human is reported as lung = liver > brain = aorta > testis > heart.[4]

For A_3 ARs, the mechanisms of signal transduction and the resultant effector responses are not well characterized. Pharmacologic studies are somewhat limited, as selective high-affinity agonists and antagonists are still required for further investigation. However, different mechanisms of signal transduction and effector activity have been speculated. Some believe that the mechanism is similar to that of A_1 AR, whereby adenylate cyclase is inhibited and cAMP levels are subsequently decreased. This is based on a study showing a G protein–coupled receptor that binds both to [^{3}H] NECA and the A_1-selective agonist [^{125}] [N_6-(4-aminophenyl)-ethyladenosine, or APNEA] but not the A_1-selective antagonists [^{3}H] DPCPX, [^{3}H] xanthine amine congener (XAC), or the A_{2a}-selective agonist [^{3}H] CGS21680, which inhibits adenylate cyclase.[62] This yields indirect evidence for the existence of another receptor subtype that inhibits cAMP production yet does not bind to A_1 AR antagonists. Other mechanisms have been proposed for the enhanced antigen-induced secretion from mast cells due to adenosine antagonists. It has been reported that activation of A_3 ARs results in elevation of inositol phosphate levels, leading to increased intracellular calcium.[66,67] This response was sensitive to both cholera and pertussis toxins.[66] Another proposed mechanism is the activation of potassium ion efflux, resulting in membrane repolarization and promoting enhancement of antigen-stimulated calcium influx.[68]

Functionally, investigators have reported that A_3 AR stimulation can cause both mast cell degranulation[67] and a hypotensive response.[69] A_3 AR stimulation may also play a role in ischemic preconditioning.[70] A_3 receptors also appear to play a role in the human lung in mediating inhibition of eosinophil chemotaxis. These receptors may be useful in the treatment of diseases such as asthma and rhinitis, which are largely eosinophil-dependent diseases.[71]

PHYSIOLOGIC ACTIONS OF ADENOSINE

Adenosine accumulates in various tissue interstitia when there is a period of localized ischemia or hypoxia. AR activation can then result in various physiologic effects in different tissues. Many of these adenosine actions are well described; however, others are only just beginning to be understood. For an overview of the physiologic effects of adenosine, see Table 32-1.

Cardiovascular Effects

Adenosine has multiple effects on the cardiovascular system, including electrophysiologic actions, hemodynamic alterations, and effects on blood pressure, cholesterol, thrombogenesis, and angiogenesis. For an overview of the cardiovascular effects of adenosine, see Table 32-2.

Electrophysiologic Effects

Adenosine has negative chronotropic, dromotropic, and inotropic actions. The proposed mechanism for adenosine's inhibitory action on nodal cell tissue entails the direct activation of a dis-

TABLE 32-1. Adenosine Receptor Subtypes Mediating Biologic Effects

Biologic Effects of Adenosine	Receptor Subtype
CNS effects	
Decreased transmitter release	A_1
Sedation	A_1
Decreased locomotor activity	A_{2a}
Anticonvulant	A_1
Chemoreceptor stimulation	A_2
Hyperalgesia	?
Cardiovascular effects	
Vasodilation	A_{2a}, A_{2b}, A_3
Vasoconstriction	A_1
Bradycardia	A_1
Platelet inhibition	A_{2a}
Negative cardiac inotropy and dromotropy	A_1
Angiogenesis	?
Renal effects	
Decreased GFR*	A_1
Mesangial cell contraction	A_1
Antidiuresis	A_1
Inhibition of renin release	A_1
Respiratory effects	
Bronchodilator	A_2
Bronchoconstrictor	A_1
Mucus secretion	?
Respiratory depression	A_2
Immunologic effects	
Immunosuppression	A_2
Neutrophil chemotaxis	A_1
Neutrophil superoide generation (inhibition)	A_{2a}
Mast-cell degranulation	A_2
Metabolic effects	
Inhibition of lipolysis	A_1
Stimulation of glucose uptake	?
Increase of insulin sensitivity	A_1
Stimulation of gluconeogenesis	A_2

*GFR = glomerular filtration rate.

Source: Adapted with permission from Collis MG, Hourani SMO: Adenosine receptor subtypes. *Trends Pharmacol Sci* 14:360, 1993.

tinct subtype of cell membrane potassium channel by an activated A_1-receptor-ligand complex, resulting in a hyperpolarizing outward current.[72] This results in both slowing of the sinus rate and slowing of AV-nodal conduction. This same mechanism occurring in atrial myocytes results in both shortening of the atrial action potential duration and negative inotropy.[73] Supraventricular tissue also contains A_1 receptors, which, when ligand-bound, inhibit beta receptor–stimulated adenylyl cyclase.[74] Both of these mechanisms of action in supraventricular tissue with adenosine are identical to those activated by the stimulation of the cholinergic M_2 receptors. There is recent evidence to suggest that these ARs may be subject to agonist-induced desensitization/downregulation, with a resultant decrease in the hyperpolarizing potassium ion current with prolonged exposure.[75]

On the ventricular myocytes, receptor-ligand binding leads to adenylate cyclase inhibition and ultimately a decreased Ca^{2+} influx when initiated by beta-receptor activation. There is also less of a response of the sarcoplasmic reticulum and subsequent Ca^{2+} release. Activation of $I_{k(Ach)}$ channels is not the mechanism for this activity. These actions of adenosine account for an antagonism of the positive inotropic and chronotropic effects and the arrhythmogenic activity induced by adrenergic receptor activation.[76]

Vascular Effects

The vascular effects of adenosine vary in the type of response depending on which receptor is stimulated, which is, in turn, dependent on the vascular bed and on the species. Even within the coronary circulation itself, adenosine has a more potent effect on the small coronary arteries than on the large ones, which tend to vasodilate more in response to ATP through activation of P_2 receptors.[77] In the coronary circulation, it is believed that the A_2 ARs play an important role, and their activation results in vasodilation.[78] It is likely that both vascular smooth muscle and endothelial cell receptors are activated in this response.[79] Smooth muscle cells respond to adenosine agonists by increasing cAMP production, resulting in cAMP-dependent kinase activation and phosphorylation of myosin light chain kinase, leading to less effective myosin light chain phosphorylation and consequently a poor actin-myosin interaction. This results in decreased smooth muscle contraction[80] and vasodilation. Other studies show that low concentrations of adenosine relax vascular smooth muscle cells primarily by decreasing intracellular Ca^{2+} levels by decreasing sarcolemmal permeability to Ca^{2+} and thus decreasing influx[81] or by enhanced Ca^{2+} sequestration.[82,83] Some studies have shown that adenosine-induced vasodilation also involves the activation of ATP-sensitive K^+ channels, as glibenclamide, a K^+-channel antagonist, attenuates vasodilation both in the isolated heart[84] and in vivo.[85–87] A_2 B receptors have been shown to mediate relaxation in human small coronary arteries through K^+-sensitive receptors.[88] There also appears to be a role for adenosine stimulation of nitric oxide via A_2 receptors, which may independently stimulate vasodilation.[89,90] These findings correspond to other studies showing that K^+-ATP channels are not involved in adenosine-induced coronary vasodilation.[91] Each of these mechanisms may in fact contribute to adenosine's vasodilatory effects, either as separate activators of vasodilation or as part of a cascade of events.

Endothelial cells are also important in helping to mediate the vasodilator action of adenosine.[92] There is experimental evidence for this concept from the infusion of adenosine linked to a macromolecule, which can limit advancement of the molecule from the lumen across the endothelium into the smooth muscle. Yet vasodilation can still be induced.[93] Also, the vasodilatory effect of adenosine

TABLE 32-2. Cardiovascular Effects of Adenosine

Organ	Action	Receptor Type	Effect on Blood Pressure
Vascular smooth muscle endothelium	Vasodilation*	A_{2a}/A_{2b}	↓
Sinoatrial and atrioventricular node	Sinus slowing, AV prolongation	A_1	↓
Kidney	↓ Renin release	A_1	↓
Vasculature	↑ Renin release	A_2	↑
Sympathetic efferent nerves	↓ Norepinephine release	A_1	↓
Brainstem (nucleus tractus solitarii)	↓ Sympathetic activity	A_{2a}	↓
Renal afferents	↑ Sympathetic activity	?	↑
Arterial chemoreceptors	↑ Sympathetic activity	A_2	↑
Myocardial efferents	↑ Sympathetic activity	A_1	↑
Skeletal muscle afferents	↑ Sympathetic activity	?	↑

*Adenosine can produce vasoconstriction in certain vascular beds.

Source: Adapted with permission from Biaggioni and Mosqueda-Garcia.[140]

was attenuated by removal of the endothelium in the isolated dog coronary artery, and the effect was greater when adenosine was then applied to the luminal side of the artery rather than to the adventitial side.[94] Data from these studies suggest that there might be a different mechanism involved in endothelium-induced vasodilation from that observed in smooth muscle–induced vasodilation. Some studies have shown that vasodilation does not occur from adenylate cyclase activation by the stimulation of endothelial A_2 receptors.[95] It is proposed, however, that adenosine activates guanylate cyclase and increases the intracellular cyclic guanosine monophosphate (cGMP). This action is attenuated by theophylline, suggesting that ARs are the mediators of this response. The rank order potency for the elevation of cGMP with various ligands suggests a pattern similar to that of the A_1 receptors.[96] Adenine nucleotides may enhance the production and release of endothelium-derived relaxing factor (EDRF) from endothelial cells.[97] It is possible that this factor consists of nitric oxide,[98,99] prostanoids, or other endothelium-dependent factors not yet characterized.[100,101] There are also reports of adenosine-induced vasorelaxation of the guinea pig aorta mediated by an intracellular "P-site" AR-induced mechanism.[102]

There are precipitating vascular insults that induce adenosine release and the resultant vasodilation action. This serves a protective role against the potential harm from these vascular insults. To be specific, adenosine is released from the heart during any event in which O_2 demand is greater than supply, such as ischemia,[103] enhanced O_2 consumption,[104,105] and hypoxia.[106] Adenosine is also released in the brain in response to similar conditions,[107] suggesting an important role of adenosine in the local regulation of blood flow. Evidence for this is based on a few experimental observations. First, studies show that adenosine results in vasodilation even at extremely low concentrations,[108] at doses even lower than believed to occur physiologically. Furthermore, correlations between the amounts of endogenous adenosine released and the extent of the increase in blood flow have been observed in brain[107] and cardiac muscle.[108] Other studies show that both AR antagonists[109] and adenosine deaminase–induced blockade of endogenous adenosine[110] can attenuate the vasodilatory response. These factors being considered, adenosine has long been proposed to be a mediator of reactive hyperemia; during ischemic conditions, adenosine does seem to contribute to the reactive hyperemia in skeletal muscle[111,112] and the heart.[113]

Other studies that investigated the role of adenosine in alteration of coronary hemodynamics suggest that the substance plays an important role in coronary autoregulation,[108,114–116] so that if cardiac perfusion pressure is altered within the nonischemic range,

adenosine may be responsible for maintenance of constant flow. Other studies have suggested, however, that adenosine may not be the active mediator.[117,118]

During ischemic conditions, adenosine release from the ischemic myocardium was markedly reduced when the alpha$_1$-adrenergic receptor antagonist prazosin was added.[119] It was hypothesized that stimulation of this receptor activates protein kinase C,[120] which, under hypoxic conditions, may affect the enzymes responsible for alterations in adenosine levels. It has also been shown that stimulation of alpha$_2$-adrenergic receptors with the alpha agonist clonidine could enhance coronary vasodilation.[121,122] Thus, during ischemia, there is also an increase in the coronary vascular sensitivity to adenosine. Although other mechanisms—including the activation of ATP-sensitive K^+ channels,[123] nitric oxide,[98] prostaglandins,[124] the kallikrein-kinin system,[125] histamine,[126] and increased potassium ions[127]—might be involved in coronary vasodilation and limitation of ischemic changes, adenosine's role is well documented, with supporting evidence to suggest potential therapeutic application with the substance.

Adenosine plays a role in the vascular response in a wide variety of other tissues. It has been shown to inhibit collagen and total protein synthesis in vascular smooth muscle cells and by this effect to protect against vascular hypertrophy.[128] In the pulmonary circulation, adenosine was shown to induce vasodilation by activation of A_{2b} ARs via a K^+ channel–dependent mechanism.[129] Also, dipyridamole caused pulmonary vasodilatation in the ovine fetus, yet it is believed that this response is not mediated primarily by adenosine, but rather by a cGMP elevation secondary to phosphodiesterase blockade.[130] Other studies have shown that in the pulmonary circulation, adenosine mediates an initial phasic contraction in guinea pigs via activation of the A_1 ARs, followed by a tonic contraction and a slow relaxation.[131] This transient pulmonary vasoconstriction has also been observed in sheep[132] and cats[133] but not yet in humans.[134]

There are also reports of transient vasoconstriction in other tissues, including the kidney,[135] with transient decreases in renal blood flow[136]; in the rat hepatic circulation[137]; in primate coronary artery strips[138]; and in certain other vascular beds.[139] The mechanisms, receptor type, cell type responsible, and physiologic importance of these actions have not been elucidated.

Effect on Blood Pressure

It is clear that adenosine has a vasodilatory effect and therefore affects blood pressure as well.[139a] The effects of adenosine on blood pressure may also be the result of actions on both the renin-angiotensin and autonomic nervous systems (Table 32-2).[140]

Adenosine is known to inhibit renin release via A_1-receptor stimulation.[136,141,142] There is in vitro evidence that A_2 receptors are present in the kidney, which could potentiate renin release[143]; however from studies of nonselective AR antagonists, it is evident that the A_1 receptor/renin inhibition is the predominant in vivo response.[144] Also, the specific A_1 AR antagonist 1,3-dipropryl-8-sulfophenylxanthine (DPSPX), increases plasma renin activity in rats,[145] and selective AR inhibition has been shown to potentiate the same response in humans,[146] suggesting that an endogenous physiologic tonic inhibition of renin is mediated by these receptors.[140] This tubuloglomerular feedback, whereby adenosine controls renin secretion and glomerular filtration rate (GFR), may indicate a role for adenosine in coupling energy metabolism or ATP reserves with tubular sodium transport.[147] Also, angiotensin II has been shown to increase release of adenosine from rat lung,[148] thus probably inhibiting further release of renin with an attenuation of the renin-angiotensin system and suggesting that adenosine may be involved in a negative feedback process.[140] There is also evidence to show that intrabrachial infusion of adenosine can result in the release of angiotensin II from both the coronary bed[149] and the forearm,[150] an effect inhibited by intraarterial theophylline. This effect could be blocked by captopril, yet vasodilation was not even enhanced,[150] suggesting that the release of AII was not significant enough to oppose adenosine-induced vasodilation. However, losartan-induced AT_1-receptor blockade has been shown to enhance vasodilation induced by A_2 AR agonism.[151]

Continuous infusion of adenosine can reduce the glomerular filtration rate by afferent arteriolar vasoconstriction, with efferent arteriolar vasodilation, leading to a reduction in renal blood flow and a decreased urine output. All of these effects return to normal with discontinuation of the infusion.[152] Studies with specific AR_1 and AR_2 antagonists in the rabbit kidney showed that these receptors mediated opposite effects on the afferent arteriole. Adenosine constricted afferent arterioles via A_1 receptors and dilated preconstricted afferent arterioles via A_2 receptors when A_1 receptors were blocked,[153] which may be associated with the differing effects of these receptors on renin secretion.

It has also been shown in patients with congestive heart failure (CHF) that stimulation of ARs decreased overall renal blood flow, but with no corresponding change in renal artery cross-sectional area. This suggested that adenosine may effect intrarenal resistance blood vessels rather than large conductance vessels.[154]

As far as the adenosine effect on the autonomic nervous system is concerned, the substance has been shown to inhibit presynaptic release of almost all neurotransmitters in both the brain and the periphery,[155,156] including norepinephrine.[157] It is likely that endogenous adenosine inhibits adrenergic neurotransmission in humans. Adenosine also inhibits presynaptic acetylcholine release and blocks the postsynaptic calcium ion current in the superior cervical sympathetic ganglia of the rat.[158] However, adenosine has also been shown to increase the pressor effects of nicotine in rats, suggesting stimulation of sympathetic ganglia.[159] These studies suggest that adenosine may contribute somewhat to blood pressure homeostasis by peripheral neuromodulation. However, adenosine may play a more important role in central cardiovascular regulation.

These studies have shown that the intracerebroventricular administration of adenosine can produce a dose-dependent reduction in blood pressure and heart rate, with the effect being antagonized by caffeine,[160,161] suggesting that adenosine may play a role in the central decrease in sympathetic tone.[162] This central control of systemic blood pressure may be mediated by A_3 receptors, since activation of these receptors brought about a decrease in blood pressure that was independent of heart rate.[163] The nucleus tractus solitarius has been the most studied structure for adenosine activity, since it is here that ARs are found in the highest density[164,165] and also because this region is of great importance in reflex cardiovascular control. Microinjection of adenosine in this region has shown a dose-related decrease in blood pressure, heart rate,[166—168] and renal sympathetic tone,[169] all actions being blocked by adenosine antagonists. Based on studies with selective agonists, these effects are believed to be mediated by A_{2a} ARs.[170] However, some studies have shown that activation of A_3 ARs present in the CNS induces a decrease in blood pressure with no change of heart rate.[163] Given that these effects are mediated by glutamate release in the nucleus tractus solitarius (NTS),[171] it is likely that adenosine uncharacteristically acts as a neurostimulant in this region. This is supported by the observation that kynurenic acid, a glutamate-receptor antagonist, could inhibit the effect of both glutamate and adenosine.[166] NTS interstitial glutamate levels were increased with the microinjection of adenosine, correlating with a decrease in blood pressure.[166] When intra-NTS injection of adenosine was studied in spontaneously hypertensive rats (SHR) compared with Wistar rats, SHRs had a reduced hypotensive effect,[172] suggesting a potential role for ARs in altered blood pressure homeostasis and the development of hypertension. The regulation of blood pressure in the NTS may be mediated by a combination of both nitric oxide (NO) and adenosine, since these were individually shown to decrease blood pressure and this effect could be blocked by antagonists specific for each.[173]

The area postrema region of the brain, a region lacking the blood-brain barrier, is also likely involved in cardiovascular control, as microinjection of adenosine into this region evokes decreased blood pressure, bradycardia,[168] and decreased renal sympathetic nerve activity.[169] Neuronal cell groups in the spinal cord at levels T8–T10 have also been shown to mediate cardiovascular control in microinjection studies.[174,175] Many other regions of the brain have been studied for the possibility of adenosine-mediated activity, but these studies have not resulted in any definitive findings. Thus, it is likely that this adenosine activity is linked predominantly to specific regions of the brain. Although it is likely that adenosine plays a role in central blood pressure homeostasis, the degree to which AR modulation contributes to the development of systemic hypertension is not well understood. Adenosine typically behaves as a neuroinhibitor for efferent nerves; however, for afferent nerves, adenosine typically behaves as a neurostimulant.[176,177] It has been shown that adenosine excites chemoreceptors in carotid bodies and the aortic arch.[176] Intracarotid injections of adenosine in rats[178] and cats[176] increase carotid sinus nerve activity, an effect that is blocked by 8-phenyltheophylline and therefore likely to be mediated by A_2 ARs.[179] Adenosine administration has been shown to increase both minute ventilation and blood pressure if injected into the aortic arch, proximal to the site of origin of the carotid arteries, but it has no effect if infused into the descending aorta.[180,181] These effects are inhibited with adenosine antagonists[182,183] and are potentiated with dipyridamole.[184] The pressor effects are not seen in patients with autonomic dysfunction, implying that sympathetic activation is likely the mechanism of this action.[181] Also, intracoronary infusion of adenosine reflexively increases systemic blood pressure,[185] but only if autonomic function is intact, implying that adenosine stimulates myocardial afferent nerves, resulting in sympathetic activation. Although this was found to clearly be the case in animals, most likely by activation of A_1,[186,187] these results would be difficult to confirm in humans.[188]

It can be seen that there is a physiologic interplay between the vasorelaxant effects of AR activation and its effects on the renin-angiotensin system, the afferent and efferent autonomic nervous system, and the central cardiovascular regulatory center. In combination, activation of these receptors may act to control blood pressure homeostasis, and if the system is altered, it might contribute to the pathophysiology of hypertension, suggesting that AR manipulation may have therapeutic benefit.

Ischemic Preconditioning, Myocardial Stunning, and Reperfusion Injury

AR activation is one of the mechanisms proposed to explain the phenomenon of ischemic preconditioning, whereby, with antecedent brief periods of either regional or global sublethal ischemia (and reperfusion) induced by complete or partial occlusion or by rapid ventricular pacing, the myocardium is protected from subsequent periods of more prolonged ischemia. For example adenosine has been shown to decrease the predicted infarct size in animals by 75%.[189] Preconditioning dramatically increases the tolerance of the myocardium at risk to an otherwise lethal ischemic event. This phenomenon can be reproduced in a wide variety of animal models.[190–196] Preconditioning is also believed to suppress ischemia and reperfusion-induced life-threatening arrhythmias—which typically occur minutes after coronary artery occlusion and after reperfusion[197]—and to enhance recovery of myocardial contractile function during reperfusion following an ischemic period (myocardial stunning). Two types of preconditioning are described: classic preconditioning, which provides protection to the myocardium within minutes of initiation of the preconditioning stimulus, and a so-called second window of protection, which can provide protection to the myocardium for a day. This type of preconditioning in humans, during percutaneous transluminal coronary angioplasty (PTCA), has been observed to reduce anginal symptoms and ST-segment changes, which occur less frequently in subsequent balloon inflations than with the first inflation.[198,199]

There are many proposed mechanisms for this endogenous protection, but by far the most popular involves the release of adenosine and the activation of ARs.[200] Both A_1 and A_3 receptors appear to be involved in the preconditioning effect, with studies showing that stimulation of these receptors in the human atrium mimics the effects of preconditioning.[201] Further evidence for the role of A_3 receptors in preconditioning lies in the fact that increased expression of the A_3 receptor in cardiac myocytes has cardioprotective effects in the face of ischemia.[202]

The mechanism of action downstream from the AR has been found to involve both the phosphorylation of protein kinase C and the activation of mitochondrial K^+-ATP channels.[203,204] This hypothesized sequence of events, with the AR upstream from protein kinase C, was confirmed by studies where the combination of protein kinase C activation and AR blockade was protective, while that of AR activation and protein kinase C blockade was not.[205]

A_1 AR activation with R(-)N6-(2-phenyl-isopropyl) adenosine (R-PIA) or 2-chloro-N6-cyclopentyl-adenosine (CCPA) produces protection from ischemic injury in a manner similar to that of ischemic preconditioning.[206,207] This effect is attenuated by adenosine antagonists.[193,194,198] It is also proposed that ARs play a role in a delayed phase of myocardial protection, the "second window

of protection," which occurs 24 h after the antecedent ischemic event.[208] It has been suggested that the mechanism of A_1 AR activation and protection might be via the potentiation of KATP channels,[203,204,209] since the administration of a KATP–channel blocker resulted in the loss of the protective effect that is produced by adenosine agonists.[210] Downey et al.[211] reproduced the induction of ischemic preconditioning using adenosine analogues specific for the A_1 AR and the attenuation of this effect with adenosine antagonists. These investigators propose that adenosine's action is mediated through the activation of protein kinase C by a mechanism of translocation of the protein kinase C molecule after first exposure into the cell membrane for a short time, rendering it more susceptible to subsequent activation. Thus a mechanism for the memory component in ischemic preconditioning is hypothesized.[212] Yet it is unknown which consequent protein phosphorylation results in this protective effect. Figure 32-2 summarizes this hypothesis. Increased collateral blood flow is unlikely to be the mechanism[211]; prostaglandins also are not the mediators, as cyclooxygenase inhibition did not block the protective effect of ischemic preconditioning.[213,214] Another study shows that this outcome is unlikely due to antioxidant effects,[215] Thus, the exact mechanism for ischemic preconditioning is as yet unknown.

Another proposed mechanism for the myocardial protection afforded by ischemic preconditioning involves the activation of A_3 ARs.[215a] This was first proposed when it was shown that a selective A_3 AR antagonist attenuated the preconditioning-induced reduction in infarct size seen in rabbit hearts.[216] A proposed mechanism of this action involves A_3 AR–induced mast cell and macrophage activation when adenosine is released during ischemia. This results in the release of cytokines and chemotactic factors, lending itself to the recruitment of neutrophils and eosinophils. The theory continues that with preconditioning, there is minor release of cytokines and histamines from the mast cells with A_3-receptor stimulation. During transient ischemia, there would be no damage, as there is not enough of an inflammatory response. During subsequent stimulation due to ischemia, the mast cells would be relatively depleted and then there would be a relatively small inflammatory response.[70] Figure 32-3 summarizes this hypothesis. These are the proposed mechanisms of ischemic preconditioning. The rest of this section discusses the resultant protection afforded by preconditioning. In general, preconditioning can reduce infarct size with subsequent coronary occlusion. It has also been shown to protect the heart from reperfusion arrhythmias and to improve recovery from myocardial stunning.

There have been reports that the preconditioned isolated perfused rat and rabbit heart display improved postischemic recovery of contractile function of the ventricles.[217,218] The stunned myocardium is characterized by metabolic and functional dysfunction occurring after ischemia, which may persist for hours to days, as manifest by contractile dysfunction, decreased myocardial cell volume, and ionic alterations.[219–222] It is important to determine the mechanisms of action of myocardial stunning, as it has broad medical implications for understanding myocardial preservant interventions such as thrombolysis, angioplasty of stenotic/occluded coronary arteries, reduction of infarct size in the setting of acute MI with subsequent preservation of myocardial function, cardioplegic arrest during cardiothoracic surgery, and organ preservation techniques in cardiac transplantation.

One proposal is that the cell, after being exposed to ischemia, experiences a fall in tissue P_{O_2}, with a resultant rapid mitochondrial ATPase-mediated hydrolysis of ATP. Thus, ATP levels fall

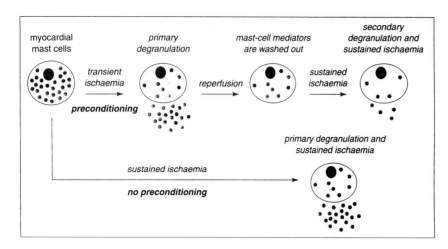

FIGURE 32-3. The hypothetical involvement of mast cells and adenosine A_3 receptors in myocardial preconditioning. Mast cells degranulate and hence release histamines, leukotrienes, and other substances that accentuate myocardial injury when this release occurs in conjunction with sustained myocardial hypoxia. (*Reproduced with permission from Walker.*[71])

dramatically. There is also reduced substrate to form AMP and ADP.[223–227] It has also been proposed that, in the stunned myocardium, there is microvascular injury caused by inadequate perfusion, probably due to myocardial cell swelling, microvascular thrombosis, vascular smooth muscle dysfunction, and leukocyte plugging.[228–230] Another likely contributor to this phenomenon is the formation of oxygen-derived free radicals from activated neutrophils and from the endothelium, leading to cellular oxidative stress and damage.[231–233] There also may be an effect on calcium availability, cell sensitivity to calcium, and calcium overload.[234]

It has also been proposed that the improvement of cardiac function in the stunned myocardium occurs via adenosine and ARs.[235,236] This effect was enhanced with administration of adenosine or its analogues.[237] The effect was also potentiated by increased endogenous adenosine levels with adenosine deaminase[238,239] and by inhibition of nucleoside transport into endothelial cells.[240] Adenosine enhances the recovery of stunned myocardium by stimulating glycolysis and improving energy balance during ischemia, inhibiting calcium (Ca^{2+}) influx through L-type Ca^{2+} channels, blocking norepinephrine release, and attenuating contractile response to beta$_1$-adrenoceptor stimulation.[241] Other studies have shown that preconditioning induced by A_1 activation does not account for improved functional recovery after global ischemia in the isolated rabbit heart.[242] It is also likely that ARs do not play a role in the mechanism of suppression of reperfusion arrhythmias by ischemic preconditioning.[243]

Nevertheless, adenosine has been shown to limit infarct size in a canine model of occlusion of the left anterior descending artery with 72-h reperfusion.[244] Also, both regional and global indices of ventricular function were substantially improved in the adenosine-treated group versus control. Adenosine also reduced the degree of neutrophil infiltration and capillary plugging and enhanced endothelial preservation.[245] This protective effect was observed with 90- and 120-min coronary artery occlusions but was lost with a 180-min occlusion.[246] These results were reproduced with a 90-min occlusion followed by a 72-h reperfusion. Infarct size was reduced by adenosine from 35 to 17% in the area at risk. There was also enhanced regional ventricular function, reduced capillary plugging, and preservation of endothelial cell structure in the adenosine-treated group.[247] Studies using adenosine antagonists have supported its role in protection against reperfusion injury.[248] AR antagonism increases infarct size when the antagonist is administered during ischemia,

but this also occurs when the antagonist is administered solely at reperfusion, suggesting that adenosine plays a clear role in reperfusion injury.[249] Thus, it is likely that adenosine administration can significantly lower infarct size if the occlusion is less than 3 h in duration.

In addition, adenosine is involved in the second window of protection. This is associated with the induction of stress proteins and/or A_3 AR–mediated release of antioxidants in the heart, which probably mediate the limitation of infarct size.[250] This late response is also blocked by AR antagonism and induced by an exogenous adenosine agonist.[251] Contrary to the short-lived, more time-specific early preconditioned response, the late phase can persist for 72 h from the event[252]; thus noninvasive treatment interventions inducing pharmacologic ischemic preconditioning might be more appropriate for this phase of protection. However, this concept is relatively new and not well studied. Nevertheless, it is clear that adenosine plays a central role in the two types of ischemic preconditioning; thus, there is the potential for a pharmacologic manipulation of adenosine and its receptors, with therapeutic benefit in this area.

ADENOSINE IN THE TREATMENT OF DISEASE

Pharmacologic Manipulation of Adenosine

Adenosine's pharmacologic actions can be manipulated in a variety of ways, including administration of synthetic adenosine and synthetic analogues acting as agonists or AR antagonists as well as by the potentiation of adenosine via the inhibition of adenosine deaminase of active nucleotide transport.

Endogenous Adenosine Potentiation via Transport and Deaminase Inhibitors

As mentioned previously, adenosine is cleared by cellular uptake via an active nucleoside carrier system. Several agents inhibit the nucleoside transporter and thus theoretically cause elevation of adenosine levels. These agents include dipyridamole, dilazep, hexobendine, mioflazine, lidoflazine, soluflazine, nitrobenzylmercaptopurine (NBMPR), and draflazine[253] (Table 32-3). Dipyridamole is a potent uptake inhibitor, with a Ki in the range of 10 to 300 nm in humans.[254–256] It is believed that dipyridamole

TABLE 32-3. Comparative Data on Some Adenosine Transport Inhibitors

Parameter	Dilazep	Dipyridamole	Mioflazine	Draflazine
Potency				
In vitro	A	B	B	A
In vivo	A	D	D	A
Specificity	B	D	B	A
Duration of action	D	C	A	A
Oral bioavailability	D	D	C	A

A = excellent; B = good; C = moderate; D = poor.

Source: Adapted with permission from van Belle.[72]

potentiates the cardiovascular actions of endogenous adenosine approximately fourfold in humans.[184]

Multiple theories are used to explain both the mode of action and the therapeutic role of dipyridamole[257,258]; however, the most accepted explanation is that dipyridamole works via adenosine potentiation secondary to the inhibition of nucleoside transport.[254,255] This appears to be conclusive, as the actions of dipyridamole are blocked by adenosine antagonists.[259,260] Consequently, the physiologic actions of dipyridamole are very similar to those of adenosine itself. The therapeutic effects of this action are discussed later in this chapter.

The clear advantage of dipyridamole is that it potentiates an endogenous substance, adenosine, in a site-specific and temporally specific fashion; that is, adenosine is released for doing a job and is able to be more efficient performing the physiologic or metabolic task. Also, adenosine would act only where it is produced, thereby also offering a benefit by alleviating the potential side effects that would be seen from systemic administration of adenosine.[261]

Another class of adenosine potentiators are the adenosine deaminase inhibitors, which inhibit the breakdown of adenosine into inosine and hyoxanthine.[262] Examples are 2-deoxycoformycin and EHNA. These drugs enhance tissue and interstitial adenosine in the setting of myocardial ischemia and reperfusion and promote the restoration of ATP while also improving postischemic ventricular function,[263,264] probably by enhanced purine salvage and reduced free radical–induced injury.[265]

Therapeutic Application of Adenosine's Pharmacologic Manipulation

Arrhythmias

Conduction delay or AV block produced by adenosine is a result of activation of the A_1 AR[266]; this has been shown to occur in the pig and human AV node as well.[267–269] Adenosine is therefore used clinically to block AV nodal conduction transiently in supraventricular tachycardia, in which the AV node is part of the reentrant pathway.[267] Also, by producing AV block and decreasing the heart rate, the oxygen demand in the heart is reduced, thus protecting the myocardium from oxygen deprivation. The SA node is depressed with high doses of adenosine, similar to what is observed in severe ischemia.[267] Other pacemaker cells, such as the His bundle and the Purkinjie fiber, are also depressed by adenosine.[266,270] These effects are also discussed in Chap. 17. ATP has also been used to terminate supraventricular tachycardia, although its effect is probably related to its breakdown to adenosine.

Cardioprotection: Myocardial Ischemia, Ischemic Preconditioning, Reperfusion Injury and Myocardial Stunning, Infarct Size Limitation

Many pharmacologic effects of adenosine agonists are potentially useful in the treatment of ischemic heart disease. In fact, stimulation of the AR subtypes plays some role in this protective action. Activation of the A_2 receptor inhibits both platelet[271] and neutrophil activation[272] and thus probably plays a role in protection from myocardial stunning and reperfusion injury[273] from microvascular injury. Activation of A_1 ARs induces the profound cardioprotective effects of ischemic preconditioning and is thought to limit ischemic injury.[273] More recently, A_3 receptors have been implicated in the role of ischemic preconditioning as well.[273]

Ischemic preconditioning has been shown to occur with adenosine, adenosine agonists, and adenosine potentiation mechanisms, including transport inhibitors and adenosine deaminase (ADA) inhibitors. The importance of developing a clinically useful drug for ischemic preconditioning, reperfusion injury and arrhythmias, and myocardial stunning is clear. It would also be important to use this pharmacologic approach in the setting of an acute myocardial infarction (MI) as an adjunct to thrombolysis for protecting the myocardium at risk. It may be useful to precondition the myocardium pharmacologically for higher-risk coronary angioplasties and coronary artery bypass grafts (CABGs).

The use of adenosine as a preconditioning agent during coronary revascularization procedures that expose the myocardium to periods of ischemia has recently been evaluated in a number of clinical trials. The preliminary results of one clinical trial using adenosine in patients undergoing CABG showed that the agent is safe and well tolerated and can improve postoperative hemodynamic function.[274] Patients in the adenosine arm of the study required less postoperative inotropic agents and their morbidity and mortality rates were decreased. In a separate study, administration of dipyridamole caused a decrease in the number of adverse cardiovascular events up to 48 h after balloon angioplasty.[275] The role of adenosine in PTCA has also been studied with the intracoronary administration of either exogenous adenosine or an adenosine-enhancing agent. This study also showed an increased myocardial tolerance to ischemia, as evidenced by the improved balloon inflation times, reduction in electrocardiographic signs of ischemia, and anginal discomfort, with even more protection offered by the liberation of endogenous adenosine.[276] In addition, adenosine, as an adjunct to primary PTCA in acute MI was shown to ameliorate coronary blood flow, prevent the no-reflow phenomenon, and improve ventricular function; it was associated with a more favorable clinical course.[277] It appears, from the results of these individual clinical trials, that adenosine can be an effective agent for cardioprotection in high-risk angioplasty procedures.

Many different adenosine analogues have been prepared, but they are of limited use clinically because of the associated systemic side effects. This is a problem with adenosine-related therapy in general; thus tissue-specific preparations are of utmost importance if therapeutic utility is to be established. The pharmacologic agent that has been studied most extensively in surgical ischemia and reperfusion is acadesine (AICA riboside). This is a weak inhibitor of ADA and adenosine kinase, and its special usefulness is that it can increase endogenous adenosine selectively in the ischemic tissue but is pharmacologically silent in nonischemic tissues. This is so because it requires ATP for its catabolism. When acadesine was evaluated in elective CABG patients, there was a decreased incidence of adverse ischemic events in the active drug study arm.[278,279] Acadesine prevents injury induced by ischemia and reperfusion of isolated cardiomyocytes[280] and in in vivo preparations.[281,282] Acadesine's effects are abolished by AR antagonists.[280–282] BN-063, an A_1 AR agonist, has also been shown to attenuate myocardial reperfusion injury in rats, displaying infarct size reduction and an antiarryhthmic effect during myocardial occlusion followed by reperfusion.[283] Future research will likely focus on site-specific potentiation of endogenous adenosine, for the reasons previously mentioned.

Much of the explanation for adenosine-mediated cardioprotection has been previously discussed, including the mechanisms, as much as they are known for ischemic preconditioning, for protection in reperfusion injury and myocardial stunning, and for its effect on infarct size reduction. There are a few more mechanisms responsible for adenosine-induced cardioprotection.

Adenosine plays a protective role in ischemia by mediating the formation of collateral circulation, resulting in an increased supply/demand ratio. It has been shown that adenosine is also involved in angiogenesis.[284] Molecular biology data show that in a hypoxic milieu, increased interstitial adenosine causes heightened proliferation of endothelial cells in culture, and the stimulation of A_1 and A_2 ARs induced the production of vascular endothelial growth factor, leading to angiogenesis.[285] Morphologic data indicate that chronic, intermittent dipyridamole administration, which elevates adenosine levels, increases the length density of endomyocardial capillaries by 33% in hypertensive and 11% in normotensive rabbits.[285] Experimental data suggest that chronic treatment with dipyridamole increases collateral flow and decreases exercise-induced left ventricular dysfunction in the myocardial region dependent upon a critical coronary stenosis.[285] Also, dipyridamole can increase the formation of new capillaries in rat heart.[286] Prospective, properly designed trials are needed to assess convincingly the efficacy of the drug used over a long period of time.[285]

In recent studies of retinal angiogenesis in both canine and human cell lines, it was shown that oxygen deprivation led to increased release of adenosine and increased synthesis of vascular endothelial growth factor (VEGF). Peak adenosine levels correlated with increased cell proliferation and active vasculogenesis. These studies concur that it is the A_2 AR that is responsible for adenosine's role in angiogenesis; however, they differ on the type of A_2 receptor responsible for this action. In studies of human cell lines, the A_{2b} receptor was found to increase neovascularization, possibly through increased angiogenic growth factor, whereas in dogs it was the A_{2A} receptor that increased vascular development.[287–290] In other studies, dipyridamole, an inhibitor of adenosine breakdown, was found to increase the formation of new capillaries in the rat heart.[286] It also increased endomyocardial capillary length density and collateral flow and decreased exercise-induced left ventricular dysfunction in the rabbit heart. These studies and clinical data from human trials illustrate the potential benefits of the drug in the treatment of angina.[285,286]

Another possible protective effect of adenosine in coronary disease is the inhibition of platelet aggregation and adhesion and the prevention of neutrophil activation, all of which have been associated with the formation of thromboemboli and reperfusion injury.[291] It appears that adenosine, through the activation of both A_1 and A_2 receptors, acts to prevent platelet adhesion and loss of myocardial function.[292] This may be due to adenosine's ability to inhibit the thrombin-induced expression of P-selectins on platelets and neutrophil-platelet adhesion.[293] Studies have also shown that adenosine inhibits neutrophil function by suppressing the release of arachidonic acid and the synthesis of leukotrienes.[294,295] Through

A_2 receptor–mediated inhibition of superoxide generation and the adherence of polymorphonuclear neutrophils (PMNs) to coronary artery endothelium, adenosine reduces PMN-induced coronary endothelial injury.[296] These effects of adenosine on platelets and neutrophils illustrate a role for adenosine in the prevention of ischemic heart disease and protection against reperfusion-induced microvascular disease.

Some of the well-known cardioprotective effects of adenosine administration have also been noted with the administration of volatile anesthetic agents such as isoflurane and sevoflurane.[297] The cardioprotective effects of these volatile agents were blocked in rabbits and dogs by adenosine antagonists and also by the administration of glibencamide, a KATP–channel inhibitor. These findings lead to the conclusion that the cellular mechanism involves activation of ARs and opening of KATP channels.[298,299] Separate studies in rabbits have shown that inhibitors of protein kinase C blocked these protective effects.[300] In canine studies, pertussis toxin pretreatment together with the administration of isoflurane also blocked these effects, showing the involvement of Gi proteins in the cascade of events.[301] From the accumulation of these data, it appears that the effects of these volatile agents may be mediated by a series of events similar to those involved in ischemic preconditioning, namely, activation of ARs, activation of a Gi protein, phosphorylation of protein kinase C, and activation of K^+-ATP channels. The protective effect of isoflurane has also been shown to persist for at least 15 min beyond its withdrawal, which could explain its ability to minimize ischemia intraoperatively.[298]

Another possible protective effect in coronary disease with AR stimulation is interfering with both platelet aggregation and platelet adhesion.[291] Activation of A_2 ARs results in the inhibition of platelets.[271] This action may prevent the progression of ischemic heart disease and may also provide some protection against reperfusion-induced microvascular disease, which could result in contractile dysfunction. Thus, from all of the available evidence, adenosine appears to potentially be a powerful cardioprotective agent.

To test whether adenosine could provide additional benefit to thrombolysis regarding cardioprotection in a human reperfusion study of patients with MI, a randomized study was carried out comparing intravenous adenosine (70 μg/kg/min for 3 h) versus placebo [the Acute Myocardial Infarction Study of Adenosine (AMISTAD)].[302] Final infarct size was assessed 6 days later in 83% of patients and was found to be smaller in those treated with adenosine compared to those on placebo; the difference was entirely due to benefit in anterior compared with nonanterior infarcts. In patients with both acute and follow up imaging (26%), the myocardial salvage index (defined as the percent of myocardium at risk that was viable on final imaging) was higher in patients with anterior MI. There were no significant differences in clinical outcomes between treatment groups, but the overall number of events was small. This study supports the evidence for adenosine as a cardioprotective agent. The small sample size, the use of a surrogate endpoint (infarct size), and an insignificant increase in clinical events with adenosine highlights the need for a large, randomized trial to assess clinical outcomes of this therapy.

Hypertension

For reasons already mentioned, it would seem that adenosine could be a good antihypertensive agent. It is a vasodilator, an inhibitor of norepinephrine and renin release as well as sinus node activity, and it has central antihypertensive effects. Adenosine can prevent cardiac remodeling associated with hypertension.[303] Intravenous adenosine has been shown to have a hypotensive effect in most animals without the reflex sympathetic activity characteristic of other vasodilators. Intravenous adenosine is also a potent hypotensive agent in anesthetized humans.[304] Intravenous dipyridamole has also been shown to have a hypotensive effect by reducing systemic vascular resistance while producing near maximal coronary vasodilation. Systolic blood pressure is reported to either decrease,[305] remain the same,[306] or increase,[307] whereas diastolic blood pressure decreases.[305,306]

Unfortunately adenosine's potential utility as an oral antihypertensive agent is somewhat limited. The main problems are its very short duration of action, acid-lability, and its side-effect profile. Its renal side effects, as mentioned, include decreased renal blood flow, decreased GFR, and oliguria, all of which are reversible. Adenosine also produces significant coronary vasodilation at doses that have a minute effect on blood pressure.[308] This may be beneficial in some patients; however, when CABG patients were given adenosine to control blood pressure postoperatively, many developed ST-segment depression on the electrocardiogram, whereas they did not with nitroprusside.[309] This effect is most likely due to a coronary steal phenomenon, which is clearly documented with dipyridamole use.[310] In order to limit the systemic side effects, great efforts has been made to develop selective adenosine analogues.

A_1-selective agonists are potent antihypertensive agents in both normotensive and spontaneously hypertensive rats (SHRs).[311,312] Since it is believed that A_1 agonists have no peripheral vasodilating activity in rats,[311] other mechanisms must be responsible. A_1-selective agonists decrease renin release[311,313] and can cause bradycardia[311–313] in rats, resulting in decreased cardiac output with a hypotensive effect. This bradycardia is probably the limiting factor in the therapeutic use of these agents.

A_2-selective agonists can decrease blood pressure due to vasodilation.[314] In contrast, in A_2 AR activation, there is tachycardia and an increase in cardiac output, with a reported increase in plasma renin activity.[311,313] These effects are explained by a reflexive enhancement of sympathetic activity in response to the vasodilation, as they can be nullified by beta-blockade.[311,314] Y-341 is an A_2 AR-selective agonist that has been studied in animal models. It is an acid-stable oral agent with a prolonged duration of action. The drug has been shown to cause a sustained hypotensive effect over 5 days with a single dose in SHRs, with no significant change in heart rate.[315] However, there are species differences in the cardiovascular effects of adenosine, thus calling into question the reliability of extrapolating the results of rat studies in evaluating the therapeutic effects of adenosine in humans.[140]

Intravenous adenosine lowers blood pressure in virtually all animal models. However, in conscious humans, intravenous adenosine increases systolic blood pressure, heart rate, and sympathetic efferent nerve activity[316] as well as catecholamines.[184] This is believed to be due entirely to an enhanced sympathetic response to adenosine, as the opposite effect occurs in patients with degeneration of the autonomic nervous system.[181] It is believed that this effect is not entirely because of a vasodilator-induced baroreflex but is probably also due to a direct sympathetic stimulation of chemoreceptors at the aortic arch.[180,181] This sympathetic discharge certainly limits its therapeutic effectiveness of adenosine, and which receptor subtype is responsible is really unknown. A_2 ARs can mediate arterial chemoreceptor activation,[317] and they are also involved in neuroexcitation in the nucleus of the tractus solitarius and other CNS nuclei.[318] It remains clear that in order to use the manipulation

of AR-receptors as a new therapeutic option in hypertension, more must be learned about the function of ARs and their physiologic effect on blood pressure control in humans.

Heart Failure

Endogenous adenosine accumulation by ultra-low-dose dipyridamole infusion in patients with chronic heart failure has been shown to improve the hemodynamic profile of patients by decreasing pulmonary and, to a minor degree, systemic vascular resistance while increasing the cardiac index.[319]

Adenosine has also been implicated as a cause for the poor renal function associated with heart failure. The effects of the A_1 AR receptor antagonist, CVT-124 (BG-9719) have been evaluated in patients with heart failure with the demonstration of increased sodium excretion without decreasing glomerular function.[319a]

OTHER POTENTIAL THERAPEUTIC ACTIONS

Adenosine potentiation will likely prove to be a promising cardiovascular intervention in the future. There are, however, other organ systems where adenosine may provide some therapeutic benefit. In the CNS, adenosine is a neuroprotectant. Regulation of adenosine levels could play a role in the therapy of stroke and epilepsy and in pain control.[320] In a phase I clinical trial, intrathecal adenosine administration, showed an attenuation of different types of experimental pain.[321] Other CNS studies in monkey models have shown that adenosine A_{2A} receptor antagonists have antiparkinsonian effects, with a reduced propensity to elicit dyskinesias.[322] They might therefore be useful agents in the treatment of Parkinson's disease. Adenosine obviously may play a role in the ischemic preconditioning of skeletal muscle as well as in situations such as vascular and musculoskeletal reconstructive surgery as well as in limb procurement for transplantation in the future.[323] There is also promise for the use of adenosine agonists as anti-inflammatory drugs, since adenosine appears to be a potent anti-inflammatory agent. In fact, the anti-inflammatory effect of methotrexate is believed to stem from local adenosine release.[324] The combination of anti-inflammatory and matrix metalloproteinase-regulating properties of adenosine or adenosine-regulating agents suggests that treatment with such agents might be useful in rheumatoid arthritis.[325]

Adenosine is also used as an aid in diagnostic studies. It is an endogenous vasodilator that is used in conjunction with perfusion scintigraphy[326] and echocardiography[327–329] for the diagnosis of coronary artery disease.[330] An adenosine A_{2A} agonist, CGS-21680, has been evaluated in myocardial perfusion imaging and appears to have coronary dilator actions comparable to those of adenosine.[331]

ADENOSINE ANTAGONISM

Adenosine antagonists are widely used drugs in the form of caffeine and theophylline. Caffeine is a commonly used neurostimulant and can produce antiepileptic and neuroprotective changes.[332] Caffeine, a nonselective antagonist, blocks A_1, A_{2a}, A_{2b}, and A_3 ARs.[333] A description of the therapeutic use of caffeine is beyond the scope of this chapter.

Theophylline, a potent AR antagonist and phosphodiesterase inhibitor, is a powerful drug used in the treatment of asthma and acts both as a bronchodilator and an anti-inflammatory agent. Theophylline nonselectively blocks A_1, A_{2a}, and A_{2b} but not A_3 ARs in the rat.[334] Using several types of knockout mice, investigators have shown that adenosine induces increased vascular permeability by binding to the A_3 AR on mast cells, with resultant mast cell activation and mediator release.[335] This action appears to be independent of mast cell activation through its receptor for immunoglobulin E (IgE). These findings are of particular relevance because of the long interest in the possible role of adenosine in the pathogenesis of asthma.[335] Studies with theophylline and other adenosine antagonist in guinea pigs have shown possible therapeutic benefits in the management of bronchial asthma.[336] Since studies with adenosine are still inconclusive, the action of theophylline in the lungs is believed to be due to its phosphodiesterase inhibitory action.[337]

Theophylline has had a resurgence of use as a cardiovascular agent since it was found to have antiadenosine effects. The drug has coronary dilator, positive inotropic, chronotropic, and diuretic effects. Theophylline has beneficial effects on exercise-induced angina[338] and intermittent claudication,[339] perhaps by reducing vascular steal. Theophylline can prevent adenosine-induced chest pain.[340] Theophylline can reverse heart blocks, seen with acute MI, that may be adenosine-induced. Its use as a myocardial stimulant probably relates to its phosphodiesterase inhibitory effect.

There is also evidence of clinical utility in using AR antagonists for the treatment of contrast media–induced acute renal failure,[341,342] in cisplatin-induced renal failure,[343] as an adjunct to furosemide in congestive heart failure,[344] and as a diuretic in puromycin aminonucleoside–induced nephrotic rats.[345]

The use of theophylline in cardiovascular medicine is limited by its potential to induce convulsions and arrhythmias. Adenosine antagonists devoid of these effects could allow for a wider therapeutic use of these compounds in cardiovascular medicine.

THERAPEUTIC PITFALLS

Each apparent action of AR activation, when first examined, appears to be of possible therapeutic benefit; however, there are many associated side effects from treatment that limit the use of this form of treatment.

During intravenous bolus injection of adenosine for the diagnosis of arrhythmia, there are dose-dependent side effects both in frequency and in severity, including diaphoresis, light-headedness, chest pain, dyspnea,[346,347] nausea, vomiting, headache, and anxiety. If adenosine is inhaled, it may produce bronchoconstriction in patients with asthma.[348] Most of these symptoms are tolerated and are very brief. If the patient has prolonged adenosine-induced chest pain, administration of theophylline should alleviate the symptoms. Also of note is that a bolus administration of adenosine can elicit a proarrhythmic response[346,347] with premature atrial and ventricular contractions being the most common arrhythmias seen. Frequently, episodes of transient asystole and heart block are observed, but they are short-lived and reverse rapidly without intervention.

Other limiting side effects include a significant decrease in renal blood flow, a decrease in GFR, and oliguria. Also, the adenosine transport inhibitors will decrease coronary and systemic vascular resistance, increase coronary blood flow, and decrease blood pressures.[349] This effect is utilized in the dipyridamole stress test to induce an area of relative ischemia where there is coronary stenosis, and a cardiac steal is produced by nonselective global coronary dilation. Another side effect of adenosine is profound bradycardia.

The major side effects of ADA inhibitors include a compromise in immune function. The other hesitancy in using them is that genetic deficiencies in ADA are associated with premature mortality,[350] neurologic abnormalities, and hepatic dysfunction.[351] The combination of ADA and transport inhibitors produces systemic side effects, including therapy-limiting hypotension.[352]

In addition to all of these side effects, there are multiple limitations to the use of adenosine. Some of these can be escaped by pharmacologic manipulation, whereas other limitations will be more difficult to bypass. At present, the most limiting issue in AR research is the fact that systemic side effects must be controlled. It was initially believed that by utilizing agonists specific for the AR subtype, the side effects would be reduced. This has proved not to be the case. The further challenge for adenosine will be to target specific cells involved in the underlying pathophysiologic process, such as those cells being exposed to ischemia, thus avoiding the deleterious systemic effects. Other problems with adenosine are its short duration of action and its acid-lability. Oral adenosine agents are now available; however, these preparations are just beginning to be examined in clinical trials.

Another major limiting factor with the use of adenosine that will be difficult to overcome is the issue of receptor desensitization and tachyphylaxis. This problem underlies all of the possible uses of adenosine except for its transient use during arrhythmias. In a study to determine whether unstable anginal episodes can cause ischemic preconditioning in preparation for an MI, it was shown that the induced protection waned after multiple 5-min coronary occlusions but reappeared after a 180-min ischemia-free period,[353] suggesting that a patient with just one episode of angina would be more protected than one with multiple attacks. The same holds true in therapy. With adenosine, it has been shown that the functional desensitization is associated with a decrease in membrane A_1 AR expression and impaired G-protein coupling.[354,355] Some studies have shown that G protein–coupled receptor kinases (GRKs) may be important in mediating the agonist-induced phosphorylation and consequent desensitization of G protein–coupled receptors responses such that in cells that express high levels of GRK_2, low agonist concentrations may be sufficient to trigger GRK-mediated desensitization.[356] While another study showed that phosphorylation of the C-terminal 14 amino acids of the rat A_3 AR is crucial for rapid desensitization to occur, the identity of the critical phosphorylation sites has remained unknown.[357] Studies demonstrated that the simultaneous mutation of three threonine residues to alanine residues dramatically reduces agonist-stimulated phosphorylation and rapid desensitization of the rat A_3 AR.[357] In order to escape this limitation, much more needs to be learned about the mechanism of this pharmacologic tolerance.

Another limiting factor with the clinical use of adenosine is that most of the studies have been done with animals. Since AR tissue specificity, receptor affinity, and receptor subtype distribution vary from animal to humans, one cannot extrapolate from animal to human studies.

CONCLUSION

Our understanding of adenosine and ARs is still in its infancy. Adenosine has current clinical use in the diagnosis and treatment of supraventricular tachycardias; dipyridamole, which affects adenosine, is used as a study aid for the noninvasive diagnosis of coronary disease and as an agent to decrease platelet aggregation. There is growing clinical evidence that adenosine potentiation in a site-specific manner may be useful for reperfusion injury and as a cardioprotectant approach to be used prior to invasive coronary artery studies that require intermittent coronary occlusion. With ongoing drug development, there will come more useful antagonist and agonist preparations that will be easier to use in clinical investigations. More needs to be learned about the physiology of ARs in humans, as most of the previous work has been done in rats. Whether the manipulation of adenosine will make it clinically useful in the management of hypertension is unlikely at this stage. It seems, however, that the future clinical work on adenosine will focus more on its cardioprotective aspects in myocardial ischemia. There is much work to be done in adenosine drug development regarding drug delivery, new clinical uses of adenosine, limiting AR desensitization, and eliminating systemic side effects of the drug's analogues.

REFERENCES

1. Pearson JD, Hellewell PG, Gordon JL: Adenosine uptake and adenine nucleotide metabolism by vascular endothelium. In: Berne RM, Rall TW, Rubio R, eds. *Regulatory Function of Adenosine.* Boston: Martinus Nijhoff, 1983:333.

2. Deussen A, Borst M, Schrader J: Formation S-adenosylhomocysteine in the heart: I. An index of free intracellular adenosine. *Circ Res* 63:240, 1988.

3. Achterberg PW, de Tombe PP, Harmsen E, de Jong JW: Myocardial s-adenylhomocysteine hydrolase is important for adenosine production during normoxia. *Biochem Biophy Acta* 840:393, 1985.

4. Moser GH, Schrader J, Deussen A: Turnover of adenosine in plasma of human and dog blood. *Am J Physiol* 26:C799, 1989.

5. Jarvis SM: Nitrobenzylthioinosine-sensitive nucleoside transport system. Mechanism of inhibition by dipyridamole. *Mol Pharmacol* 30:659, 1986.

6. Bockman EL, McKenzie JE: Tissue adenosine content in active soleus and gracilis muscles of cats. *Am J Physiol* 244:H552, 1983.

7. Phillis JW, Wu PH: The role of adenosine in central neurotransmission. In: Berne PM, Rall TW, Rubio R, eds. *Regulatory Function of Adenosine.* Boston: Martinus Nijhoff, 1983:133, 419.

8. McBean DE, Harper M, Rudolph KA: Effects of adenosine and its analogues on porcine basilar arteries: Are only A_2 receptor involved? *J Cereb Flow Metab* 8:40, 1988.

9. Rivkees SA, Price SL, Zhou FC: Immunohistochemical detection of A_1 adenosine receptors in rat brain with emphasis on localization in the hippocampal formation, cerebral cortex, cerebellum and basal ganglia. *Brain Res* 677:193, 1995.

10. Stefanovic V, Valhovic P: A_2 adenosine receptors in human glomerular mesangial cells. *Experientia* 51:360, 1995.

11. Arend LJ, Thompson CI, Spielman WS: Dipyridamole decreases glomerular filtration in the sodium-depleted dog: Evidence for mediation by intrarenal adenosine. *Circ Res* 56:242, 1985.

12. Bockman EL, Berne RM, Rubio R: Adenosine and active hyperaemia in dog skeletal muscle. *Am J Physiol* 230:1531, 1976.

13. Cronstein BN, Kramer SB, Rosenstein ED, et al: Adenosine modulates the generation of superoxide anion by stimulated human neutrophils via interaction with a specific cell surface receptor. *Ann NY Acad Sci* 451:291, 1985.

14. Szillat D, Bukowieki LJ: Control of brown adipose tissue lipolysis and respiration by adenosine. *Am J Physiol* 245:E555, 1983.

15. Minelli A, Miscetti P, Allegrucci C, Mezzasoma I: Evidence of A_1 adenosine receptor on epidydimal bovine spermatozoa. *Arch Biochem Biophys* 322:272, 1995.

16. Merten MD, Kammouni W, Figarella C: Evidence for, and characterization of a lipopolysaccharide-inducible adenosine A_2 receptor in human tracheal gland serous cells. *FEBS Lett* 369:202, 1995.

17. Rodriguez-Nodal F, San Roman JI, Lopez-Novoa JM, Calvo JJ: Effect of adenosine and adenosine agonists on amylase release from rat pancreatic lobules. *Life Sci* 57:PL253, 1995.

18. Budohoshki L, Challiss RAJ, McManus B, Newsholme EA: Effects of analogues of adenosine and methylanthines on insulin sensitivity in the soleus muscle of the rat. *FEBS Lett* 167:1, 1984.

19. Burnstock G: A basis for distinguishing two types of purinergic receptors. In: Bolis L, Straub RW, eds. *Cell Membrane Receptors for Drugs and Hormones: A Multidisciplinary Approach.* New York: Raven Press, 1978:107.

20. Zhou QY, Chuanyu L, Olah ME, et al: Molecular cloning and characterization of an adenosine receptor: The adenosine A_3 receptor. *Proc Natl Acad Sci U S A* 89:7432, 1992.

21. Hulme EC, Birdsall NJM, Bockley NJ: Muscarinic receptor subtypes. *Annu Rev Pharmacol Toxicol* 30:633, 1990.

22. Ostrowski J, Kjelsberg MA, Caron MG, Lefkowitz RJ: Mutagenesis of the α2 adrenergic receptor. How structure elucidates function. *Ann Rev Pharmacol Toxicol* l32:167, 1992.

23. Henderson R, Baldwin JM, Ceska T, et al: Model for the structure of bacteriorhodopsin based on high-resolution electron cryomicroscopy. *J Mol Biol* 213:899, 1990.

24. Reppert SM, Weaver DR, Stehle JH, Rivkee SA: Molecular cloning and characterization of a rat A_1 adenosine receptor that is widely expressed in brain and spinal cord. *Mol Endocrinol* 5:1037, 1991.

25. Mahan LC, McVittie LD, Smyk-Randall EM, et al: Cloning and expression of an A_1 adenosine receptor from a rat brain. *Mol Pharmacol* 40:1, 1991.

26. Bhattacharya S, Dewitt DL, Burnatowska-Hledin M, et al: Cloning of an adenosine A_1 receptor-encoding gene from rabbit. *Gene* 128:285, 1993.

27. Tucker AL, Linden J, Robeva AS, et al: Cloning and expression of a bovine adenosine A_2 receptor cDNA. *FEBS Lett* 297:107, 1992.

28. Olah ME, Ren H, Ostrowski J, et al: Cloning, expression, and characterization of the unique bovine A_1 adenosine receptor: Studies on the ligand binding site by site-directed mutagenesis. *J Biol Chem* 267:10764, 1992.

29. Linden J, Tucker AL, Robeva AS, et al: Properties of recombinant adenosine receptors. *Drug Dev Res* 28:232, 1993.

30. Ren H, Stiles GL: Characterization of the human A_1 adenosine receptor gene: Evidence for alternative splicing. *J Biol Chem* 269:3104, 1994.

31. Townsend-Nicholson A, Shine J: Molecular cloning and characterization of a human brain A_1 adenosine receptor cDNA. *Mol Brain Res* 16:36, 1992.

32. Libert F, Van Sande L, Lefort A, et al: Cloning and functional characterization of a human A_1 adenosine receptor. *Biochem Biophys Res Commun* 187:919, 1992.

33. Townsend-Nicholson A, Baker E, Schofield PR, Sutherland GR: Localization of the adenosine A_1 receptor subtype gene (ADORA1) to chromosome 1q32.1. *Genomics* 26:423, 1995.

34. Weaver DR, Reppert SM: Adenosine receptor gene expression in rat kidney. *Am J Physiol* 263:F991, 1992.

35. Belardinelli L, Linden J, Berne RM: The cardiac effects of adenosine. *Prog Cardiovasc Dis* 32:73, 1989.

36. Hori M, Kitakaze M: Adenosine, the heart, and coronary circulation. *Hypertension* 18:565, 1991.

37. Ely SW, Berne RM: Protective effects of adenosine in myocardial ischemia. *Circulation* 85:893, 1992.

38. Londos C, Wolff J: Two distinct adenosine-sensitive sites on adenylate cyclase. *Proc Natl Acad Sci U S A* 74:5482, 1977.

39. Kusachi SJ, Thompson RD, Olsson RA: Ligand selectivity of dog coronary adenosine receptor resembles that of adenylate cyclase stimulatory (Ra) receptors. *J Pharmacol Exp Ther* 227:316, 1983.

40. Londos C, Cooper DMF, Wolf J: Subclasses of eternal adenosine receptors. *Proc Natl Acad Sci U S A* 77:2551, 1980.

41. Van Calker D, Muller M, Hamprecht B: Adenosine inhibits the accumulation of cyclic AMP in the cultured brain cells. *Nature* 276:839, 1978.

42. Trussel LO, Jackson MS: Adenosine-activated potassium conductance in cultured striatal neurons. *Proc Natl Acad Sci U S A* 82:4857, 1985.

43. Scholz KP, Miller RJ: Analysis of adenosine actions on Ca^{2+} currents and synaptic transmission in cultured rat hippocampal pyramidal neurons. *J Physiol* 435:373, 1991.

44. Gerwins P, Fredholm BB: ATP and its metabolite adenosine act synergistically to mobilize intracellular calcium via the formation of inositol 1,4,5-triphosphate in a smooth muscle cell line. *J Biol Chem* 267:16081, 1992.

45. Marala RB, Mustafa SJ: Adenosine analogues prevent phorbol ester-induced PKC depletion in porcine coronary artery via A_1 receptor. *Am J Physiol* 268:H271, 1995.

46. Hussain T, Mustafa SJ: Binding of A1 adenosine receptor ligand [3H]8-cyclopentyl-1,3-dipropylxanthine in coronary smooth muscle. *Circ Res* 77:194, 1995.

47. Akatsuka Y, Egashira K, Katsuda Y, et al: ATP sensitive potassium channels are involved in adenosine A_2 receptor mediated coronary vasodilatation in the dog. *Cardiovasc Res* 28:906, 1994.

48. Daly JW, Butts-Lamb P, Padgett W: Subclasses of adenosine receptors in the central nervous system: Interaction with caffeine and related methylxanthines. *Cell Mol Neurobiol* 3:69, 1983.

49. Jarvis MF, Schulz R, Hutchison AJ, et al: [3H]CSG 21680, a selective A_2 adenosine receptor agonist directly labels A_2 receptors in rat brain. *J Pharmacol Exp Ther* 251:888, 1989.

50. Monopoli A, Conti A, Zocchi C, et al: Pharmacology of the new selective A_2 adenosine receptor agonist 2-hexynyl-5'-N-ethylcarbox-amidoadenosine. *Arzneim Forsch/Drug Res* 44:1296, 1994.

51. Bruns RF, Lu GH, Pugsley TA: Characterization of the A_2 adenosine receptor labeled by [3H]NECA in rat striatal membranes. *Mol Pharmacol* 29:331, 1986.

52. Fink JS, Weaver DR, Rivkees SA, et al: Molecular cloning of the rat A_2 adenosine receptor: Selective co-expression with D2 dopamine receptors in rat striatum. *Mol Brain Res* 14:186, 1992.

53. Maenhaut C, VanSande J, Libert F, et al: RDC8 codes for an adenosine receptor with physiological constitutive activity. *Biochem Biophy Res Commun* 173:1169, 1990.

54. Furlong TJ, Pierce KD, Selbie LA, Shine J: Molecular characterization of human adenosine A_2 receptor. *Mol Brain Res* 15:62, 1992.

55. Huttemann E, Ukena D, Lenschow W, Schwabe U: Ra adenosine receptors in human platelets: Characterization by 5-N-ethylcarbox-amido[3H]-adenosine binding in relation to adenylate cyclase activity. *Naunyn Schmiedebergs Arch Pharmacol* 325:226, 1984.

56. Schiele JO, Schwabe U: Characterization of the adenosine receptor in microvascular coronary endothelial cells. *Eur J Pharmacol* 269:51, 1994.

57. Johnson RA: Mn2+ does not uncouple adenosine "Ra" receptors from the liver adenylate cyclase. *Biochem Biophys Res Commun* 105:347, 1982.

58. Stehle JH, Rivkees SA, Lee JJ, et al: Molecular cloning and expression of the cDNA for a novel A_2 adenosine receptor subtype. *Mol Endocrinol* 6:384, 1992.

59. Rivkees SA, Reppert SM: RFL9 encodes an A_{2B}-adenosine receptor. *Mol Endocrinol* 6:1598, 1992.

60. Pierce KD, Furlong TJ, Selbie LA, Shine J: Molecular cloning and expression of an adenosine A_{2B} receptor from the human brain. *Biochem Biophys Res Commun* 187:86, 1992.

60a. Morrison RR, Talukder MAH, Ledent C, Mustafa SJ: Cardiac effects of adenosine in A_{2A} receptor knockout hearts: Uncovering A_{2B} receptors. *Am J Physiol* 282:H437, 2002.

61. Meyerhof W, Muller-Brechlin R, Richter D: Molecular cloning of a novel putative G-protein coupled receptor expressed during rat spermatogenesis. *FEBS Lett* 284:155, 1991.

62. Zhou Q-Y, Olah ME, Johnson RA, et al: Molecular cloning and characterization of an adenosine receptor: the A_3 adenosine receptor. *Proc Natl Acad Sci U S A* 89:7432, 1992.

63. Linden J, Taylor HE, Robeva AS, et al: Molecular cloning and functional expression of a sheep A_2 adenosine receptor with widespread tissue distribution. *Mol Pharmacol* 44:524, 1993.

64. Zhao Z, Francis C, Ravid K: Characterization of the mouse A_3 adenosine receptor gene: Exon/intron organization and promoter activity. *Genomics* 57:152, 1999.

65. Salvatore CA, Jacobson MA, Taylor HE, et al: Molecular cloning and characterization of the A_3 adenosine receptor. *Proc Natl Acad Sci U S A* 90:10365, 1993.

66. Ali H, Cunha-Melo JR, Saul WF, Beaven MA: Activation of phospholipase C via adenosine receptors provides synergistic signals for secretion in antigen-stimulated RBL-2H3 cells: Evidence for a novel adenosine receptor. *J Biol Chem* 265:745, 1990.

67. Ramkumar V, Stiles GL, Beaven MA, Ali H: The A_3 adenosine receptor is the unique adenosine receptor which facilitates release of allergic mediators in mast cells. *J Biol Chem* 268:16667, 1993.

68. Qian Y-X, McCloskey MA: Activation of mast cell K^+ channels through multiple G protein-linked receptors. *Proc Natl Acad Sci U S A* 90:7844, 1993.

69. Fozzard JR, Carruthers AM: Adenosine A_3 receptors mediate hypotension in the angiotensin II-supported circulation in the pithed rat. *Br J Pharmacol* 109:3, 1993.

70. Linden J: Cloned adenosine A_3 receptors: Pharmacological properties, species differences and receptor functions. *Trends Pharmacol Sci* 15:298, 1994.

71. Walker BA, Jacobson MA, Knight DA, et al: Adenosine A_3 receptor expression and function in eosinophils. *Am J Respir Cell Mol Biol* 16:531, 1997.

72. van Belle H: Specific metabolically active anti-ischemic agents. In: Singh BN, Dzau VJ, Vanhoutte PM, Woosley RL, eds: *Cardiovascular Pharmacology and Therapeutics.* New York: Churchill Livingstone, 1994:217.

73. Tawfik-Schlieper H, Klotz KN, Kreye VAW, Schwabe U: Characterization of the K^+ channel-coupled adenosine receptor in guinea pig atria. *Naunyn Schmiedebergs Arch Pharmacol* 340:684, 1989.

74. Wilken A, Tawfik-Schlieper H, Klotz KN, Schwabe U: Pharmacological characterization of the adenylate cyclase-coupled adenosine receptor in isolated guinea pig atrial myocytes. *Mol Pharmacol* 37:916, 1990.

75. Bunemann M, Pott L: Down regulation of A_1 adenosine receptors coupled to muscarinic K^+ current in cultured guinea pig atrial myocytes. *J Physiol* 482:81, 1995.

76. Dobson JG Jr, Ordway RW, Fenton RA: Endogenous adenosine inhibits catecholamine contractile responses in normoxic hearts. *Am J Physiol* 251:H455, 1986.

77. White TD, Angus JA: Relaxant effects of ATP and adenosine on canine large and small coronary arteries in vitro. *Eur J Pharmacol* 143:119, 1987.

78. Bertolet BD, Belardinelli L, et al: Selective attenuation by N-0861 (N^6-endonorboran-2-yl-9-methyladenine) of cardiac A_1 adenosine receptor-mediated effects in humans. *Circulation* 93:1871, 1996.

79. Abebe W, Mukujina SR, Mustafa SJ: Adenosine receptor-mediated relaxation of porcine coronary artery in presence and absence of endothelium. *Am J Physiol* 266:H2018, 1994.

80. Herlihy JT, Bockman EL, Berne RM, Rubio R: Adenosine relaxation of isolated vascular smooth muscle. *Am J Physiol* 230:1239, 1976.

81. Harder DR, Belardinelli L, Sperelakis N, et al: Differential effects of adenosine and nitroglycerin on the action potential of large and small coronary arteries. *Circ Res* 44:176, 1979.

82. Fenton RA, Rubio BR, Berne RM: Effect of adenosine on calcium uptake by intact and cultured vascular smooth muscle. *Am J Physiol* 242:H797, 1982.

83. Ramagopal MV, Mustafa SJ: Effect of adenosine and its analogues on calcium influx in coronary artery. *Am J Physiol* 255:H1492, 1988.

84. Daut J, Maier-Rudolph W, von Beckerath N, et al: Hypoxic dilation of coronary arteries is mediated by ATP-sensitive potassium channels. *Science* 247:1341, 1990.

85. Belloni FL, Hintze T: Glibenclamide attenuates adenosine-induced bradycardia and coronary vasodilatation. *Am J Physiol* 261:H720, 1991.

86. Akatsuka Y, Egashira K, Katsuda Y, et al: ATP sensitive potassium channels are involved in adenosine A_2 receptor mediated coronary vasodilatation in the dog. *Cardiovasc Rev* 28: 06, 1994.

87. He HM, Wang H, Xiao WB: Relationship between adenosine-induced vascular effects and ATP-sensitive K^+ channels. *Zhongguo Yao Li Xue Bao* 20(3):257, 1999.

88. Kemp BK, Cocus TM: Adenosine mediates relaxation of human small resistance-like coronary arteries via A_{2B} receptors. *Br J Pharmacol* 126:1796, 1999.

89. Ikeda U, Kurosaki K, Shimpo M, et al: Adenosine stimulates nitric oxide synthesis in rat cardiac myocytes. *Am J Physiol* 273(1 Pt 2):H59, 1997.

90. Carpenter LB, Baker RS, Greenberg S, Clark KE: The role of nitric oxide in mediating adenosine-induced increases in uterine blood flow in the oophorectomized nonpregnant sheep. *Am J Obstet Gynecol* 183:46, 2000.

91. Makujina SR, Olanrewaju HA, Mustafa SJ: Evidence against KATP channel involvement in adenosine receptor-mediated dilation of epicardial vessels. *Am J Physiol* 267:H716, 1994.

92. Nees S, Herzog Z, Becker BF, et al: The coronary endothelium: A highly active metabolic barrier for adenosine. *Basic Res Cardiol* 80:515, 1985.

93. Olsson RA, Davis CC, Khouri EM: Coronary vasoactivity of adenosine covalently linked to polylysine. *Life Sci* 21:1343, 1977.

94. Matsuda H, Imai S: Effects of adenosine and adenine nucleotides on the diameter of the isolated perfused pig coronary artery (abstr). *Jpn J Pharmacol* 52(Suppl II):116, 1990.

95. Newman WH, Becker BF, Heier M, Gerlach E: Endothelium-mediated coronary dilatation by adenosine does not depend on endothelial adenylate cyclase activation: Studies in isolated guinea pig hearts. *Pflugers Arch* 413:1, 1988.

96. Kurtz A: Adenosine stimulates guanylate cyclase activity in vascular smooth muscle cells. *J Biol Chem* 262:6296, 1987.

97. Rubanyi GM, Romero JC, Vanhoutte PM: Flow-induced release of endothelium derived relaxing factor. *Am J Physiol* 250:H1145, 1986.

98. Abebe W, Hussain T, Olanrewaju H, Mustafa SJ: Role of nitric oxide in adenosine receptor-mediated relaxation of porcine coronary artery. *Am J Physiol* 269:H1672, 1995.

99. Zhao T, Xi L, Chelliah J: Inducible nitric oxide synthase mediates delayed myocardial protection induced by activation of adenosine A_1 receptors. Evidence from gene-knockout mice. *Circulation* 102:902, 2000.

100. Headrick JP, Berne RM: Endothelium-dependent and independent relaxations to adenosine in guinea pig aorta. *Am J Physiol* 259:H62, 1990.

101. Furchgott RF: Role of endothelium in the responses of vascular smooth muscle to drugs. *Annu Rev Pharmacol Toxicol* 24:175, 1984.

102. Collis MG, Brown VM: Adenosine relaxes the aorta by interacting with an A_2 receptor and an intracellular site. *Eur J Pharmacol* 96:61, 1983.

103. Bardenheuer H, Schrader J: Supply-to-demand ratio for oxygen determines formation of adenosine by the heart. *Am J Physiol* 250:H173, 1986.

104. McKensie JE, McCoy FP, Bockman EL: Myocardial adenosine and coronary resistance during increased cardiac performance. *Am J Physiol* 239:H509, 1980.

105. Watkinson WP, Foley DH, Rubio R, Berne RM: Myocardial adenosine formation with increased cardiac performance in the dog. *Am J Physiol* 96:H13, 1979.

106. Berne RM: Cardiac nucleotides in hypoxia: Possible role in regulation of coronary blood flow. *Am J Physiol* 204:317, 1963.

107. Berne RM, Rubio R, Curnish RR: Release of adenosine from ischemic brain: Effect on cerebral vascular resistance and incorporation into cerebral adenine nucleotides. *Circ Res* 35:262, 1974.

108. Schrader J, Haddy FJ, Gerlach E: Release of adenosine, inosine and hypoxanthine from isolated guinea pig heart during hypoxia, flow-autoregulation and reactive hyperemia. *Pflugers Arch* 369:1, 1977.

109. Mohrman DE, Heller LJ: Effect of aminophylline on adenosine and exercise dilatation of rat creamaster arterioles. *Am J Physiol* 246:H195, 1984.

110. Proctor KG; Reduction of contraction-induced arteriolar vasodilatation by adenosine deaminase on theophylline. *Am J Phsyiol* 247:H195, 1984.

111. Dobson JG Jr, Rubio R, Berne RM: Role of adenosine nucleotides, adenosine and inorganic phosphate in the regulation of skeletal muscle blood flow. *Circ Res* 29:375, 1971.

112. Schwartz LM, McKenzie JE: Adenosine and active hyperemia in soleus and gracilis muscle of cats. *Am J Physiol* 258:H1295, 1990.

113. Berne RM: The role of adenosine in the regulation of coronary blood flow. *Circ Res* 47:807, 1980.

114. Shryock JC, Snowdy S, Baraldi PG, et al: A_{2A}-adenosine receptor reserve for coronary vasodilation. *Circulation* 98:711, 1998.

115. Yada T, Richmond KN, van Bibber R, et al: Role of adenosine in local metabolic coronary vasodilation. *Am J Physiol* 276:H1425, 1999.

116. Belardinelli L, Shryock JC, Snowdy S, et al: The A_{2A} adenosine receptor mediates coronary vasodilation. *J Pharmacol Exp Ther* 284:1066, 1998.

117. Dole WP, Yamada N, Bishop VS, Olsson RA: Role of adenosine in coronary blood flow regulation after reductions in perfusion pressure. *Circ Res* 56:517, 1985.

118. Hanley FL, Grattan MT, Stevens MB, Hoffman JIE: Role of adenosine in coronary autoregulation. *Am J Physiol* 251:H558, 1986.

119. Kitakaze M, Hori M, Tamai J, et al: α1-Adrenoceptor activity regulates release of adenosine from the ischemic myocardium in dogs. *Circ Res* 60:631, 1987.

120. Kitakaze M, Hori M, Iwakura K, et al: Protein kinase C regulates production of adenosine in hypoxic myocytes of rats (abstr). *Circulation* 80(Suppl II):II-498, 1989.

121. Kitakaze M, Hori M, Gotoh K, et al: Beneficial effects of α2-adrenoceptor activity on ischemic myocardium during coronary hypoperfusion in dogs. *Circ Res* 65:1632, 1989.

122. Hori M, Kitakaze M, Tamai J, et al: α2-Adrenoceptor stimulation can augment coronary vasodilation maximally induced by adenosine in dogs. *Am J Physiol* 257:H132, 1989.

123. Frishman WH, Wang S, Gurell D, Yashar P: Potassium channel openers and sodium-hydrogen channel effectors. In: Frishman WH, Sonnenblick EH, eds: *Cardiovascular Pharmacotherapeutics*. New York: McGraw-Hill. 1997:619.

124. Blass KE, Forster W, Zehl U: Coronary vasodilation: Interactions between prostacyclin and adenosine. *Br J Pharmacol* 69:555, 1980.

125. Lochner W, Parratt JR: A comparison of the effects of locally and systemically administered kinins on coronary blood flow and myocardial metabolism. *Br J Pharmacol* 26:17, 1966.

126. Trzeciakowski JP, Levi R: Cardiac histamine: A mediator in search of function. *Trends Pharmacol Sci* 2:14, 1981.

127. Hirche H, Franz C, Bos L, et al: Myocardial extracellular K+ and H+ increase in noradrenaline release as possible cause of early arrhythmias following acute coronary artery occlusion in pigs. *J Mol Cell Cardiol* 12:579, 1980.

128. Dubey RK, Gillespie DG, Jackson EK: Adenosine inhibits collagen and total protein synthesis in vascular smooth muscle cells. *Hypertension* 33(Pt II):190, 1999.

129. Haynes J Jr, Obiako B, Thompson WJ, Downey J: Adenosine-induced vasodilation: Receptor characterization in pulmonary circulation. *Am J Physiol* 268:H1862, 1995.

130. Abman SH: Dipyridamole, a cGMP phosphodiesterase inhibitor, causes pulmonary vasodilation in the ovine fetus. *Am J Physiol* 269:H473, 1995.

131. Szentmiklosi AJ, Ujfalusi A, Cseppento A, et al: Adenosine receptors mediate both contractile and relaxant effects in the main pulmonary artery of guinea pigs. *Naunyn Schmiedebergs Arch Pharmacol* 351:417, 1995.

132. Biaggioni I, King LS, Enayat N, et al: Adenosine produces pulmonary vasoconstriction in sheep. Evidence for thromboxane A_2/prostaglandin endoperoxide receptor activation. *Circ Res* 65:1516, 1989.

133. Neely CF, Haile DM, Cahill BE, Kadowitz PJ: Adenosine and ATP produce vasoconstriction in the feline pulmonary vascular bed by different mechanisms. *J Pharmacol Exp Ther* 258:753, 1991.

134. Edlund A, Sollevi A, Linde B: Haemodynamic and metabolic effects of infused adenosine in man. *Clin Sci* 79:131, 1990.

135. Osswald H: Renal effects of adenosine and their inhibition by theophylline in dogs. *Naunyn Schmiedebergs Arch Pharmacol* 288:79, 1975.

136. Osswald H: The role of adenosine in the regulation of glomerular filtration rate and renin secretion. *Trends Pharmacol Sci* 5:94, 1984.

137. Vom Dahl S, Wettsetin M, Gerok W, Haussinger D: Stimulation of release of prostaglandin D2 and thromboxane B2 from perfused rat liver by extracellular adenosine. *Biochem J* 270:39, 1990.

138. Nakane T, Chiba S: Adenosine constricts the isolated and perfused monkey coronary artery. *Heart Vessels* 5:71, 1990.

139. Biaggioni I: Contrasting excitatory and inhibitory effects of adenosine in blood pressure regulation. *Hypertension* 20:457, 1992.

139a. Saadjian AY, Levy S, Franceschi F, et al: Role of endogenous adenosine as a modulator of syncope induced during tilt testing. *Circulation* 106:569, 2002.

140. Biaggioni I, Mosqueda-Garcia R: Adenosine in cardiovascular homeostasis and the pharmacologic control of its activity. In: Laragh JH, Brenner BM, eds. *Hypertension: Pathophysiology, Diagnosis and Management*, 2nd ed. New York: Raven Press, 1995:1125.

141. Tagawa H, Vander AJ: Effects of adenosine compounds on renal function and renin secretion in dogs. *Circ Res* 26:327, 1970.

142. Jackson EK: Adenosine: A physiological brake on renin release. *Annu Rev Pharmacol Toxicol* 31:1, 1991.

143. Churchill PC, Churchill MC: A_1 and A_2 adenosine receptor activation inhibits and stimulates renin secretion of rat cortical slices. *J Pharmacol Exp Ther* 232:589, 1985.

144. Kuan C-J, Wells JN, Jackson EK: Endogenous adenosine restrains renin release during sodium restriction. *J Pharmacol Exp Ther* 249:110, 1989.

145. Kuan C-J, Wells JN, Jackson EK: Endogenous adenosine restrains renin release in conscious rats. *Circ Res* 66:637, 1990.

146. van Buren M, Bijlsma JA, Boer P, et al: Natriuretic and hypotensive effects of adenosine-1 blockade in essential hypertension. *Hypertension* 22:728, 1993.

147. Osswald H. Adenosine and tubuloglomerular feedback. *Blood Purif* 15(4–6):243, 1997.

148. Bottiglieri DF, Kost CK Jr, Jackson EK: Angiotensin II-induced [3H]adenosine release from in situ rat lung. *J Cardiovasc Pharmacol* 16:101, 1990.

149. Taddei S, Salvetti A: Vascular tissue renin-angiotensin system in hypertensive humans. *J Hypertens* 10(Suppl 7):S165, 1992.

150. Taddei S, Virdis A, Favilla S, Salvetti A: Adenosine activates a vascular renin-angiotensin system in hypertensive subjects. *Hypertension* 19:672, 1992.

151. Smits GJ, Kitzen JM, Perrone MH, Cox BF: Angiotensin subtype 1 blockade selectively potentiates adenosine subtype 2-mediated vasodilation. *Hypertension* 22:221, 1993.

152. Zall S, Milocco I, Ricksten SE: Effects of adenosine on renal function and central hemodynamics after coronary artery bypass surgery. *Anesth Analg* 76:493, 1993.

153. Yaoita H: Effect of adenosine on isolated afferent arterioles. *Nippon Jinzo Gakkai Shi* 41 (7):697, 1999.

154. Elkayam U: Renal circulatory effects of adenosine in patients with chronic heart failure. *J Am Coll Cardiol* 32(1):211, 1998.

155. Dunwiddie TV: The physiological role of adenosine in the central nervous system. *Int Rev Neurobiol* 27:63, 1985.

156. White TD: Role of adenosine compounds in autonomic neurotransmission. *Pharmacol Ther* 38:129, 1988.

157. Wakade AR, Wakade TD: Inhibition of noradrenaline release by adenosine. *J Physiol* 282:35, 1978.

158. Henon BK, McAfee DA: The ionic basis of adenosine receptor actions on postganglionic neurones in the rat. *J Physiol* 336:601, 1983.

159. von Borstel RW, Evoniuk GE, Wurtman RJ: Adenosine potentiates sympathomimetic effects of nicotinic agonists in vivo. *J Pharmacol Exp Ther* 236:344, 1986.

160. Hedner T, Hedner J, Wessberg P, Jonasson T: Regulation of breathing in the rat: Indications for a role of central adenosine mechanisms. *Neurosci Lett* 33:147, 1982.

161. Barraco RA, Phillis JW, Campbell WR, et al: The effects of central injections of adenosine analogs on blood pressure and heart rate in the rat. *Neuropharmacology* 25:675, 1986.

162. Laborit H, Manzo-Fay G, Baron C, Hasni H: Changes in plasma catecholamine levels after the intraperitoneal and intracerebroventricular administration of the adenosine analogues and of clonidine in conscious rats. *Res Commun Chem Pathol Pharmacol* 68:307, 1990.

163. Stella L, de Novellis V, Marabese I, et al: The role of A_3 adenosine receptors in central regulation of arterial blood pressure. *Br J Pharmacol* 125(3):437, 1998.

164. Deckert J, Bsserbe JC, Klein E, Marangos PJ: Adenosine uptake sites in the brain: Regional distribution of putative subtypes in relationship to adenosine A_1 receptors. *J Neurosci* 8:2338, 1988.

165. Marangos PJ, Patel J, Clark-Rosenberg R, Martino AM: D[3H] nitrobenzylthioinosine binding as a probe for the study of adenosine uptake sites in brain. *J Neurochem* 39:184, 1982.

166. Mosqueda-Garcia R, Tseng CJ, Appalsamy M, et al: Cardiovascular excitatory effects of adenosine in the nucleus of the solitary tract. *Hypertension* 18:494, 1991.

167. Barraco RA, Janusz CJ, Polasek PM, et al: Cardiovascular effects of microinjection of adenosine into the nucleus tractus solitarius. *Brain Res Bull* 20:129, 1988.

168. Tseng CJ, Biaggioni I, Appalsamy M, Robertson D: Purinergic receptors in the brainstem mediate hypotension and bradycardia. *Hypertension* 11:191, 1988.

169. Mosqueda-Garcia R, Appalsamy M, Robertson D: Mechanisms of the central cardiovascular effects of adenosine interaction with brain L-glutamate. *Neuroscience* 15(2): 1178, 1989.

170. Barraco RA, El-Ridi MR, Ergene E, Phillis JW: Adenosine receptor subtypes in the brainstem mediate distinct cardiovascular response patterns. *Brain Res Bull* 26:59, 1991.

171. Talman WT: Kynurenic acid microinjected into the nucleus tractus solitarius of rat blocks the arterial baroreflex but not responses to glutamate. *Neurosci Lett* 102:247, 1989.

172. Mosqueda-Garcia R, Tseng CJ, Appalsamy M, et al: Cardiovascular excitatory effects of adenosine in the nucleus of the solitary tract. *Hypertension* 18:494, 1991.

173. Lo WC: Cardiovascular effects of nitric oxide and adenosine in the nucleus tractus solitarii of rats. *Hypertension* 32(6):1034, 1998.

174. Mosqueda-Garcia R, Tseng CJ, Beck C, et al: Adenosine in central cardiovascular control. In: Kunos G, Ciriello J, eds. *Central Neural Mechanisms in Cardiovascular Regulation.* New York: Springer-Verlag 1991:165.

175. Galosy RA, Clarke LK, Vasko MR, Crawford IL: Neurophysiology and neuropharmacology of cardiovascular regulation and stress. *Neurosci Behav Rev* 5:137, 1981.

176. McQueen DS, Ribeiro JA: Effect of adenosine on carotid chemoreceptor activity in the cat. *Br J Pharmacol* 74:129, 1981.

177. Katholi RE, Hageman GR, Whitlow PL, Woods WT: Hemodynamic and afferent renal nerve responses to intrarenal adenosine in the dog. *Hypertension* 5(Suppl I):I-149, 1983.

178. Monteiro EC, Ribeiro JA: Ventilatory effects of adenosine mediated by carotid body chemoreceptors in the rat. *Naunyn Schmiedebergs Arch Pharmacol* 335:143, 1987.

179. McQueens DS, Ribeiro JA: Pharmacological characterization of the receptor involved in chemoexcitation induced by adenosine. *Br J Pharmacol* 88:615, 1986.

180. Watt AH, Reid PG, Stephens MR, Routledge PA: Adenosine induced respiratory stimulation in man depends on site of infusion. Evidence for an action on the carotid body? *Br J Clin Pharmacol* 23:486, 1987.

181. Biaggioni I, Olafsson B, Robertson RM, et al: Cardiovascular and respiratory effects of adenosine in conscious man. Evidence for chemoreceptor activation. *Circ Res* 61:779, 1987.

182. Biaggioni I, Paul S, Puckett A, Arzubiaga C: Caffeine and theophylline as adenosine receptor antagonists in humans. *J Pharmacol Exp Ther* 258:588, 1991.

183. Smits P, Lenders JWM, Thien T: Caffeine and theophylline attenuate adenosine-induced vasodilation in humans. *J Clin Pharmacol Ther* 48:410, 1990.

184. Biaggioni I, Onrot J, Hollister AS, Robertson D: Cardiovascular effects of adenosine infusion in man and their modulation by dipyridamole. *Life Sci* 39:2229, 1986.

185. Cox DA, Vita JA, Treasure CB, et al: Reflex increase in blood pressure during the intracoronary administration of adenosine in man. *J Clin Invest* 84:592, 1989.

186. Montano N, Lombardi F, Ruscone TG, et al: The excitatory effect of adenosine on the discharge activity of the afferent cardiac sympathetic fibers. *Cardiologia* 36:953, 1991.

187. Dibner-Dunlap ME, Kinugawa T, Thames MD: Activation of cardiac sympathetic afferents: Effects of exogenous adenosine and adenosine analogues. *Am J Physiol* 265:H395, 1993.

188. Crea F, Pupita G, Galassi AR, et al: Role of adenosine in pathogenesis of anginal pain. *Circulation* 81:164, 1990.

189. Murry CE, Jennings RB, Reimer KA: Preconditioning with ischemia: A delay of lethal cell injury in ischemic myocardium. *Circulation* 74:1124, 1986.

190. Schott RJ, Rohmann S, Braun ER, Schaper W: Ischemic preconditioning reduces infarct size in swine myocardium. *Circ Res* 66:1133, 1990.

191. Tsuchida A, Miura T, Miki T, et al: Role of adenosine receptor activation in myocardial infarct size limitation by ischemic preconditioning. *Cardiovasc Res* 26:456, 1992.

192. Velasco CE, Turner M, Cobb MA, et al: Myocardial reperfusion injury in the canine model after 40 minutes of ischemia: Effects on intracoronary adenosine. *Am Heart J* 122:1561, 1991.

193. Liu GS, Thornton J, Van Winkle DM, et al: Promotion against infarction afforded by preconditioning is mediated by A_1 adenosine receptors. *Naunyn Schmiedebergs Arch Pharmacol* 337:687, 1988.

194. Gross GJ, Auchampach JA: Blockade of ATP-sensitive potassium channels prevents myocardial preconditioning in dogs. *Circ Res* 70:223, 1992.

195. Murry CE, Richard VJ, Reimer KA, Jennings RB: Ischemic preconditioning slows energy metabolism and delays ultrastructural damage during a sustained ischemic episode. *Circ Res* 66:913, 1990.

196. Yellon DM, Baxter GF, Marber MS: Angina reassessed: Pain or protector? *Lancet* 347:1059, 1996.

197. Parratt JR, Vegh A: Pronounced antiarrhythmic effects of ischemic preconditioning. *Cardioscience* 5:9, 1994.

198. Deutsch E, Berger M, Kussmaul WG, et al: Adaptation to ischemia during PTCA. *Circulation* 82:2044, 1990.

199. Jain A, Gettes LS: Patterns of ST segment change during acute no flow myocardial ischemia produced by balloon occlusion during angioplasty of the left anterior descending coronary artery. *Am J Cardiol* 67:305, 1991.

200. McCully JD, Toyoda Y, Uematsu M, et al: Adenosine-enhanced ischemic preconditioning: Adenosine receptor involvement during ischemia and reperfusion. *Am J Physiol* 280:H591, 2001.

201. Carr CS: Evidence for the role for both the adenosine A_1 and A_3 receptors in protection of isolated human atrial muscle against simulated ischaemia. *Cardiovasc Res* 36: 52, 1997.

202. Dougherty C: Cardiac myocytes rendered ischemia resistant by expressing the human adenosine A_1 or A_3 receptor. *FASEB J* 12:1785, 1998.

203. Sato T: Adenosine primes the opening of mitochondrial ATP-sensitive potassium channels: A key step in ischemic preconditioning? *Circulation* 102:800, 2000.

204. Miura T: Role of mitochondrial ATP-sensitive K^+ channels and PKC in anti-infarct tolerance afforded by adenosine A_1 receptor activation. *J Am Coll Cardiol* 35:238, 2000.

205. Iliodromitis EK: The PKC activator PMA preconditioning rabbit heart in the presence of adenosine receptor blockade: Is 5'-nucleotidase important? *J Mol Cell Cardiol* 30:2201, 1998.

206. Thornton JD, Liu GS, Olsson RA, Downey JM: Intravenous pretreatment with A_1 selective adenosine analogues protects the heart against infarction. *Circulation* 85:659, 1992.

207. Liu GS, Thornton JD, Van Winkle DM, et al: Protection against infarction afforded by preconditioning is mediated by A_1 adenosine receptors in rabbit heart. *Circulation* 84:350, 1991.

208. Bater GF, Marber MS, Patel VC, Yellon DM: Adenosine receptor involvement in a delayed phase of myocardial protection 24 hours after ischemic preconditioning. *Circulation* 90:2993, 1994.

209. Bernardo NL, Okubo S, Maaieh MM: Delayed preconditioning with adenosine is mediated by opening of ATP-sensitive K^+ channels in rabbit heart. *Am J Physiol* 277:H128, 1999.

210. Van Winkle DM, Chien GL, Davis RF: Myocardial ischemic preconditioning. *Adv Pharmacol* 31:99, 1994.

211. Downey JM, Cohen MV, Ytrehus K, Liu Y: Cellular mechanisms in ischemic preconditioning: the role of adenosine and protein kinase C. *Ann NY Acad Sci* 723:82, 1994.

212. Strasser RH, Braun-Dullaeus R, Walendzik H, Marquetant R: Alpha 1-receptor-independent activation of protein kinase C in acute myocardial ischemia. Mechanisms for sensitization of the adenyl cyclase system. *Circ Res* 70:1303, 1992.

213. Li Y, Kloner R: Cardioprotective effects of ischaemic preconditioning are not mediated by prostanoids. *Cardiovasc Res* 26:226, 1992.

214. Liu GS, Stanley AHS, Downey JM: Cyclooxygenase products are not involved in the protection against myocardial infarction afforded by preconditioning in rabbit. Cyclooxygenase pathways involvement in preconditioning. *Am J Cardiovasc Pathol* 4:157, 1992.

215. Turrens JF, Thornton J, Barnard ML, et al: Protection from reperfusion injury by preconditioning hearts does not involve increased antioxidant defenses. *Am J Physiol* 262:H585, 1992.

215a. Peart J, Flood A, Linden J, et al: Adenosine-mediated cardioprotection in ischemic-reperfused mouse heart. *J Cardiovasc Pharmacol* 39:117, 2002.

216. Liu GS, Richards SC, Olsson RA, et al: Evidence that the adenosine A_3 receptor may mediate the protection afforded by preconditioning in the isolated rabbit heart. *Cardiovasc Res* 28:1057, 1994.

217. Cave AC, Collis CS, Downey JM, Hearse DJ: Improved functional recovery by ischaemic preconditioning is not mediated by adenosine in the globally ischaemic isolated rat heart. *Cardiovasc Res* 27:663, 1993.

218. Omar BA, Hanson A, Bose S, McCord J: Reperfusion with pyruvate eliminates ischemic preconditioning: An apparent role for enhanced glycolysis (abst). *FASEB J* 5:A1257, 1991.

219. Ellis SG, Henschke CI, Sandor T, et al: Time course of function and biochemical recovery of myocardium salvaged by reperfusion. *J Am Coll Cardiol* 1:1047, 1983.

220. Braunwald E, Kloner RA: The stunned myocardium: Prolonged ischemic ventricular dysfunction. *Circulation* 66:1146, 1982.

221. Patel B, Kloner RA, Przyklenk K, Braunwald E: Post-ischemic myocardial "stunning": A clinically relevant phenomenon. *Ann Intern Med* 108:626, 1988.

222. Tennant R, Wiggers CJ: The effect of coronary occlusion on myocardial contraction. *Am J Physiol* 112:351, 1935.

223. Reimer KA, Hill ML, Jennings RB: Prolonged depletion of ATP and the adenine nucleotide pool due to delayed resynthesis of adenine nucleotide following reversible ischemic injury in dogs. *J Mol Cell Cardiol* 13:229, 1981.

224. Swain JL, Sabina RL, McHale PA, et al: Prolonged myocardial adenine nucleotide depletion after brief ischemia in the open chest dog. *Am J Physiol* 242:H818, 1982.

225. DeBoer FWV, Ingwall JS, Kloner RA, Braunwald E: Prolonged derangements of canine myocardial purine metabolism after a brief coronary artery occlusion not associated with anatomic evidence of necrosis. *Proc Natl Acad Sci U S A* 77:5471, 1980.

226. Thourani VH, Ronson RS, Van Wylen DGL, et al: Adenosine-supplemented blood cardioplegia attenuates postischemic dysfunction after severe regional ischemia. *Circulation* 100(Suppl II):II-376, 1999.

227. Ward HB, Kriett JB, Einzig S, et al: Adenine nucleotides and cardiac function following global myocardial ischemia. *Surg Forum* 34:264, 1983.

228. Heyndrickx GR, Baig H, Nellens P, et al: Depression of regional blood flow and wall thickening after brief coronary artery occlusions. *Am J Physiol* 234:H653, 1978.

229. Stahl LD, Weiss HR, Becker LC: Myocardial oxygen consumption, oxygen supply/demand heterogeneity, and microvascular patency in regionally stunned myocardium. *Circulation* 77:865, 1988.

230. Bolli R, Triana JF, Jeroudi MO: Prolonged impairment of coronary vasodilation after reversible ischemia: Evidence for microvascular stunning. *Circ Res* 67:332, 1990.

231. Garlick PB, Davies MJ, Hearse DJ, Slater TF: Direct detection of free radicals in the reperfused rat heart using electron-spin resonance spectroscopy. *Circ Res* 61:757, 1987.

232. Zweier JL, Flaherty JT, Weisfeldt ML: Direct measurement of free radical generation following reperfusion of ischemic myocardium. *Proc Natl Acad Sci U S A* 84:1404, 1987.

233. Bolli R, Jeroudi MO, Patel BS, et al: Direct evidence that oxygen-derived free radicals contribute to post-ischemic myocardial dysfunction in the intact dog. *Proc Natl Acad Sci U S A* 86:4695, 1989.

234. Bolli R: Mechanism of myocardial stunning. *Circulation* 82:723, 1990.

235. Toyoda Y, DiGregorio V, Parker FA, et al: Anti-stunning and anti-infarct effects of adenosine-enhanced ischemic preconditioning. *Circulation* 102(Suppl III):III-326, 2000.

236. Lasley RD, Jahania MS, Mentzer RM Jr: Beneficial effects of adenosine A_{2A} agonist CGS-21680 in infarcted and stunned porcine myocardium. *Am J Physiol* 280:H1660, 2001.

237. Lasley RD, Rhee JW, Van Wylen DGL, Mentzer RM Jr: Adenosine A1 receptor mediated protection of the globally ischemic isolated rat heart. *J Mol Cell Cardiol* 22:39, 1990.

238. Dorheim TA, Hoffman A, Van Wylen DGL, Mentzer RM: Enhanced interstitial fluid adenosine attenuates myocardial stunning. *Surgery* 110:136, 1991.

239. Zhu G-Y, Chen S-G, Zou C-M: Protective effect of an adenosine deaminase inhibitor on ischemia-reperfusion injury in isolated perfused rat heart. *Am J Physiol* 259:H835, 1990.

240. Masuda M, Demeulemeester A, Chen C-C, et al: Cardioprotective effects of nucleoside transport inhibition in rabbit hearts. *Ann Thorac Surg* 52:1300, 1991.

241. Kersten J, Orth K, Pagel P, et al: Role of adenosine in isoflurane-induced cardioprotection. *Anesthesiology* 86:1128, 1997.

242. Hendrikx M, Toshima Y, Mubagwa K, Flameng W: Improved functional recovery after ischemic preconditioning in the globally ischemic rabbit heart is not mediated by adenosine A_1 receptor activation. *Basic Res Cardiol* 88:576, 1993.

243. Miura T, Ishimoto R, Sakamoto J, et al: Suppression of reperfusion arrhythmia by ischemic preconditioning in the rat: Is it mediated by the adenosine receptor, prostaglandin, or bradykinin receptor? *Basic Res Cardiol* 90:240, 1995.

244. Olafsson B, Foreman MB, Puett DW, et al: Reduction of reperfusion injury in the canine prepartion by intracoronary adenosine: Importance of the endothelium and the no-reflux phenomenon. *Circulation* 76:1135, 1987.

245. Babbitt DG, Virmani R, Forman MB: Intracoronary adenosine administered after reperfusion limits vascular injury after prolonged ischemia in the canine model. *Circulation* 80:1388, 1989.

246. Babbitt DG, Virmani R, Vildibill HD, et al: Intracoronary adenosine administration during reperfusion following 3 hours of ischemia: Effects on infarct size, ventricular function, and regional myocardial blood flow. *Am Heart J* 120:808, 1990.

247. Ptarys CJ, Virmani R, Vildibill HD, et al: Reduction of myocardial reperfusion injury by intravenous adenosine administered during the early reperfusion period. *Circulation* 83:237, 1991.

248. Rynning SE, Hexeberg E, Birkeland S, et al: Blockade of adenosine receptors during ischemia increases systolic dysfunction but does not affect diastolic creep in stunned myocardium. *Eur Heart J* 15:1705, 1994.

249. Zhao AQ, Nakanishi K, McGee DS, et al: A$_1$ receptor mediated myocardial infarct size reduction by endogenous adenosine is exerted primarily during ischemia. *Cardiovasc Res* 28:270, 1994.

250. Yellon DM, Baxter GF: A second window of protection or delayed preconditioning phenomenon: Future horizons for myocardial protection. *J Mol Cell Cardiol* 27:1023, 1995.

251. Baxter GF, Marber MS, Patel VC, Yellon DM: Adenosine receptor involvement in a delayed phase of myocardial protection 24 hours after ischemic preconditioning. *Circulation* 90:2993, 1994.

252. Baxter GF, Marber MS, Patel VC, Yellon DM: Adenosine receptor involvement in a delayed phase of myocardial protection 24 hours after ischemic preconditioning. *Circulation* 90:2993, 1994.

253. Rongen GA, Smits P, Ver Donck K, et al: Hemodynamic and neurohumoral effects of various grades of selective adenosine transport inhibition in humans. *J Clin Invest* 95:658, 1995.

254. Kubler W, Spieckerman PG, Bretschneider HJ: Influence of dipyridamole (Persantin) on myocardial adenosine metabolism. *J Mol Cell Cardiol* 1:23, 1970.

255. Van Belle H: Uptake and deamination of adenosine by blood: Species differences, effects on pH, ions, temperature, and metabolic inhibitors. *Biochem Biophys Acta* 192:124, 1969.

256. Newby AC: How does dipyridamole elevate extracellular adenosine concentration? Predictions from a three-compartment model of adenosine formation and activation. *Biochem J* 237:845, 1986.

257. Weishaar RE, Burrows SD, Kobylarz DC, et al: Multiple molecular forms of cyclic nucleotide phosphodiesterase in cardiac and smooth muscle and in platelets. Isolation, characterization and effects of various reference phosphodiesterase inhibitors and cardiotonic agents. *Biochem Pharmacol* 3:787, 1986.

258. Fitzgerald GA: Dipyridamole (review). *N Engl J Med* 316:1247, 1987.

259. Sollevi A, Ostergren J, Fagrell B, Hjemdahl P: Theophylline antagonizes cardiovascular responses to dipyridamole in man without affecting increases in plasma adenosine. *Acta Physiol Scand* 121:165, 1984.

260. Smits P, Straatman C, Pijpers E, Thien T: Dose-dependent inhibition of the hemodynamic response to dipyridamole by caffeine. *Clin Pharmacol Ther* 50:529, 1991.

261. Van Belle H: Nucleoside transport inhibition: A therapeutic approach to cardioprotection via adenosine? *Cardiovasc Res* 27:68, 1993.

262. Achterberg PW, deJong JW: Adenosine deaminase inhibition and myocardial adenosine metabolism during ischemia. *Adv Myocardiol* 6:465, 1985.

263. Zhu Q, Chen S, Zou C: Protective effects of an adenosine deaminase inhibition on ischemia-reperfusion injury in isolated perfused rat heart. *Am J Physiol* 259:H835, 1990.

264. Dorheim TA, Van Wylen DGL, Mentzer RM: Effect of adenosine deaminase inhibition on cardiac interstitial fluid purine metabolites during myocardial ischemia and reperfusion. *Surg Forum* 41:243, 1990.

265. Abd-Elfattah A, Jessen ME, Lekven J, et al: Pharmacologic intervention for the prevention of reperfusion injury using specific inhibitors of adenosine nucleoside transport and adenosine deaminase. *Cardiovasc Drug Ther* 1:210, 1987.

266. Belardinelli L, Linden J, Berne RM: The cardiac effects of adenosine. *Prog Cardiovasc Dis* 32:73, 1989.

267. DiMarco JP, Sellers TD, Berne RM, et al: Adenosine: Electrophysiologic effects and therapeutic use for terminating paroxysmal supraventricular tachycardia. *Circulation* 68:1253, 1983.

268. Wu L, Belardinelli L, Zablocki JA, et al: A partial agonist of the A$_1$-adenosine receptor selectively slows AV conduction in guinea pig hearts. *Am J Physiol* 280:H334, 2001.

269. Glatter KA, Cheng J, Dorostkar P, et al: Electrophysiologic effects of adenosine in patients with supraventricular tachycardia. *Circulation* 99:1034, 1999.

270. Shen W-K, Kurachi Y: Mechanisms of adenosine-mediated actions on cellular and clinical cardiac electrophysiology. *Mayo Clinic Proc* 70:274, 1995.

271. Hourani SMO, Cusack NJ: Pharmacologic receptors on blood platelets. *Pharmacol Rev* 43:243, 1991.

272. Firestein GS, Bullough DA, Erion MD, et al: Inhibition of neutrophil adhesion by adenosine and an adenosine kinase inhibitor: The role of selectins. *J Immunol* 154:326, 1995.

273. Forman MB, Velasco CE, Jackson EK: Adenosine attenuates reperfusion injury following regional myocardial ischemia. *Cardiovasc Res* 27:9, 1993.

274. Mentzer R, Birjiniuk V, Khuri S, et al: Adenosine myocardial protection: Preliminary results of a phase II clinical trial. *Ann Surg* 229:643, 1999.

275. Heidland UE: Adjunctive intracoronary dipyridamole in the interventional treatment of small coronary arteries: A prospectively randomized trial. *Am Heart J* 139(6):1039, 2000.

276. Heidland UE: Preconditioning during percutaneous transluminal coronary angioplasty by endogenous and exogenous adenosine. *Am Heart J* 140(5):813, 2000.

277. Frishman WH, Chiu R, Landzberg BR, Weiss M: Medical therapies for the prevention of restenosis following percutaneous coronary interventions. *Curr Prob Cardiol* 23:533, 1998.

278. Mangano DT: Effects of acadesine on myocardial infarction, stroke, and death following surgery. A meta-analysis of the 5 international randomized trials. The Multicenter Study of Perioperative Ischemia (McSPI) Research Group. *JAMA* 277:325, 1997.

279. Leung JM, Stanley T, Mathew J, et al: An initial multicenter, randomized control trial on the safety and efficacy of acadesine in patients undergoing coronary artery bypass graft surgery. *Anesth Analg* 778:420, 1994.

280. Gruver EJ, Toupin D, Smith TW, Marsh JD: Acadesine improves tolerance to ischemic injury in rat cardiomyocytes. *J Mol Cell Cardiol* 26:1187, 1994.

281. Hori M, Kitakaze M, Takashima S, et al: AICA riboside improves myocardial ischemia in coronary microembolization in dogs. *Am J Physiol* 267:H1483, 1994.

282. Tsuchida A, Yang S, Burckhartt B, et al: Acadesine extends the window of protection afforded by ischemic preconditioning. *Cardiovasc Res* 28:379, 1994.

283. Lee YM, Sheu JR, Yen MH: BN-063, a newly synthesized adenosine A$_1$ receptor agonist, attenuates myocardial reperfusion injury in rats. *Eur J Pharmacol* 278:251, 1995.

284. Adair TH, Gay WJ, Montani J-P: Growth regulation of the vascular system: Evidence for a metabolic hypothesis. *Am J Physiol* 259:R393, 1990.

285. Picano E, Michelassi C: Chronic oral dipyridamole as a "novel" antianginal drug: The collateral hypothesis. *Cardiovasc Res* 33(3):666, 1997.

286. Mattfeldt T, Mall G: Dipyridamole-induced capillary endothelial cell proliferation in the rat heart: A morphometric investigation. *Cardiovasc Res* 17:229, 1983.

287. Lutty GA: 5′ nucleotidase and adenosine during retinal vasculogenesis and oxygen-induced retinopathy. *Invest Ophthalmol Vis Sci* 41(1):218, 2000.

288. Benoit H: Effect of NO, vasodilator prostaglandins, and adenosine on skeletal muscle angiogenic growth factor gene expression. *J Appl Physiol* 86(5):1513, 1999.

289. Taomoto M: Localization of adenosine A$_{2a}$ receptor in retinal development and oxygen-induced retinopathy. *Invest Ophthalmol Vis Sci* 41(1):230, 2000.

290. Grant MB: Adenosine receptor activation induces vascular endothelial growth factor in human retinal endothelial cells. *Circ Res* 85(8):699, 1999.

291. Kitakaze M, Hori M, Sato H, et al: Endogenous adenosine inhibits platelet aggregation during myocardial ischemia in dogs. *Circ Res* 69:1402, 1991.

292. Seligmann C: Adenosine endogenously released during early reperfusion mitigates postischemic myocardial dysfunction by inhibiting platelet adhesion. *J Cardiovasc Pharmacol* 32(1):156, 1998.

293. Minamoto T: Endogenous adenosine inhibits P-selectin-dependent formation of coronary thromboemboli during hypoperfusion in dogs. *J Clin Invest* 101(8):1643, 1998.

294. Krump E: Adenosine. An endogenous inhibitor of arachidonic acid release and leukotriene biosynthesis in human neutrophils. *Adv Exp Med Biol* 447:107, 1999.

295. Jordan JE: Adenosine A$_2$ receptor activation attenuates reperfusion injury by inhibiting neutrophil accumulation, superoxide generation and coronary endothelial adherence. *J Pharmacol Exp Ther* 280(1): 301, 1997.

296. Zhao ZQ: Adenosine A$_2$-receptor activation inhibits neutrophil-mediated injury to coronary endothelium. *Am J Physiol* 271(4 Pt 2): H1456-, 1996.

297. Haessler R, Kuzume K, Chein GL, et al: Anaesthetics alter the magnitude of infarct limitation by ischaemic preconditioning. *Cardiovasc Res* 28:1574, 1994.

298. Roscoe AK: Isoflurane, but not halothane, induces protection of human myocardium via adenosine A$_1$ receptors and adenosine triphosphate-sensitive potassium channels. *Anesthesiology* 92(6):1692, 2000.

299. Ismaeil MS: Mechanisms of isoflurane-induced myocardial preconditioning in rabbits. *Anesthesiology* 90(3):812, 1999.

300. Cope DK: Volatile anesthetics protect the ischemic rabbit myocardium from infarction. *Anesthesiology* 86(3):699, 1997.

301. Toller WG: Isoflurane preconditions myocardium against infarction via activation of inhibitory guanine nucleotide binding proteins. *Anesthesiology* 92(5):1400, 2000.

302. Mahaffey KW, Puma JA, Barbagelata A, et al for the AMISTAD Investigators: Adenosine as an adjunct to thrombolytic therapy for acute myocardial infarction. *J Am Coll Cardiol* 34:1711, 1999.

303. Dubey RK, Gillespie DG, Zacharia LC, et al: A$_{2B}$ receptors mediate the antimitogenic effects of adenosine in cardiac fibroblasts. *Hypertension* 37(Pt. 2):716, 2001.

304. Sollevi A, Lagerkranser M, Irestedt L, et al: Controlled hypotension with adenosine in cerebral aneurysm surgery. *Anesthesia* 61:400, 1984.

305. Brown BG, Josephson MA, Petersen RB, et al: Intravenous dipyridamole combined with isometric handgrip for near maximal acute increase in coronary flow in patients with coronary artery disease. *Am J Cardiol* 48:1077, 1981.

306. Sollevi A, Ostergren J, Fagrell B, Hjemdahl P: Theophylline antagonizes cardiovascular responses to dipyridamole in man without affecting increases in plasma adenosine. *Acta Physiol Scand* 121:165, 1984.

307. Smits P, Straatman C, Pijpers E, Thien T: Dose-dependent inhibition of the hemodynamic response to dipyridamole by caffeine. *Clin Pharmacol Ther* 50:529, 1991.

308. Owall A, Ehrenberg J, Brodin LA, et al: Effects of low-dose adenosine on myocardial performance after coronary artery bypass surgery. *Acta Anaesthesiol Scand* 37:140, 1993.

309. Zall S, Kirno K, Milocco I, Richsten S-E: Vasodilation with adenosine or sodium nitroprusside after coronary artery bypass surgery: A comparative study on myocardial blood flow and metabolism. *Anesth Analg* 76:498, 1993.

310. Picano E, Simonetti I, Masini M, et al: Transient myocardial dysfunction during pharmacologic vasodilatation as an index of reduced coronary reserve: A coronary hemodynamic and echocardiographic study. *J Am Coll Cardiol* 8:84, 1986.

311. Webb RL, McNeal RB Jr., Barclay BW, Yasay GD: Hemodynamic effects of adenosine agonists in the conscious spontaneously hypertensive rat. *J Pharmacol Exp Ther* 254:1090, 1990.

312. Francis JE, Webb RL, Ghai GR, et al: Highly selective adenosine A$_2$ receptor agonists in a series of N-alkylated 2-aminoadenosines. *J Med Chem* 34:2570, 1991.

313. Gerencer RZ, Finegan BA, Clanachan AS: Cardiovascular selectivity of adenosine receptor agonists in anesthetized dogs. *Br J Pharmacol* 107:1048, 1992.

314. Webb RL, Barclay BW, Graybill SC: Cardiovascular effects of adenosine A$_2$ agonists in the conscious spontaneously hypertensive rat: A comparative study of three structurally distinct ligands. *J Pharmacol Exp Ther* 259:1203, 1991.

315. Yagil Y, Miyamoto M: The hypotensive effect of an oral adenosine analog with selectivity for the A$_2$ receptor in the spontaneously hypertensive rat. *Am J Hypertens* 8:509, 1995.

316. Biaggioni I, Killian TJ, Mosqueda-Garcia R, et al: Adenosine increases sympathetic nerve traffic in humans. *Circulation* 83:1668, 1991.

317. McQueens DS, Ribeiro JA: Pharmacological characterization of the receptor involved in chemoexcitation induced by adenosine. *Br J Pharmacol* 8:615, 1986.

318. Barraco RA, El-Ridi MR, Ergene E, Phillis JW: Adenosine receptor subtypes in the brainstem mediate distinct cardiovascular response patterns. *Brain Res Bull* 26:59, 1991.

319. Cortigiani L, Baroni M, Picano E, et al: Acute hemodynamic effects of endogenous adenosine in patients with chronic heart failure. *Am Heart J* 136:37, 1998.

319a. Gottlieb SS: Renal effects of adenosine A$_1$-receptor antagonists in congestive heart failure. *Drugs* 61:1387, 2001.

320. Foster AC, Miller LP, Weisner JB: Regulation of endogenous adenosine levels in the CNS: Potential for therapy in stroke, epilepsy and pain. *Adv Exp Med Biol* 370:427, 1994.

321. Rane K, Segerdahl M, Goiny M, Sollevi A: Intrathecal adenosine administration—a phase 1 clinical safety study in healthy volunteers, with additional evaluation of its influence on sensory thresholds and experimental pain. *Anesthesiology* 89:1108, 1998.

322. Grondin R, Bedard P, Hadj A, et al: Antiparkinsonian effect of a new selective adenosine A$_{2A}$ receptor antagonist in MPTP-treated monkeys. *Neurology* 52:1673, 1999.

323. Pang CY, Forrest CR: Acute pharmacologic preconditioning as a new concept and alternative approach for prevention of skeletal muscle ischemic necrosis. *Biochem Pharmacol* 49:1023, 1995.

324. Cronstein BN: Adenosine, an endogenous anti-inflammatory agent. *J Appl Physiol* 76:5, 1994.

325. Boyle D, Sajjadi F, Firestein G: Inhibition of synoviocyte collagenase gene expression by adenosine receptor stimulation. *Arthritis Rheum* 39:924, 1996.

326. Verani MS, Mahmarian JJ, Hixson JB, et al: Diagnosis of coronary artery disease by controlled coronary vasodilation with adenosine and thallium-201 scintigraphy in patients unable to exercise. *Circulation* 82:80, 1990.

327. Zoghbi W: Use of adenosine echocardiography for diagnosis of coronary artery disease. *Am Heart J* 122: 285, 1991.

328. Marwick T, Willemart B, D'Hondt AM, et al: Selection of the optimal nonexercise stress for the evaluation of ischemic regional myocardial dysfunction and malperfusion: Comparison of dobutamine and adenosine using echocardiography and ^{99m}Tc-MIBI single photon emission computed tomography. *Circulation* 87:345, 1993.

329. Tawa CB, Baker WB, Kleiman NS, et al. Comparison of adenosine echocardiography, with and without isometric handgrip, to exercise echocardiography in the detection of ischemia in patients with coronary artery disease. *J Am Soc Echo* 9:33, 1996.

330. Nagueh S, Kopelen H, Zoghbi W: Effects of adenosine on left ventricular filling dynamics in patients with and without coronary artery disease: A Doppler echocardiographic study. *Am Heart J* 135:647, 1998.

331. He Z-X, Cwajg E, Hwang W, et al: Myocardial blood flow and myocardial update of ^{201}Tl and ^{99m}Tc-sestamibi during coronary vasodilation induced by CGS-21680, a selective adenosine A$_{2A}$ receptor agonist. *Circulation* 102:438, 2000.

332. Fredholm BB: Astra Award Lecture. Adenosine, adenosine receptors and the action of caffeine. *Pharmacol Toxicol* 76:93, 1995.

333. Varani K, Portaluppi F, Gessi S, et al: Dose and time effects of caffeine intake on human platelet adenosine A$_{2A}$ receptors. Functional and biochemical aspects. *Circulation* 102:285, 2000.

334. Ji XD, Gallo-Rodriguez C, Jacobson KA: A selective agonist affinity label for A$_3$ adenosine receptors. *Biochem Biophys Res Commun* 203:570, 1994.

335. Tilley SL, Wagoner VA, Salvatore CA, et al: Adenosine and inosine increase cutaneous vasopermeability by activating A(3) receptors on mast cells. *J Clin Invest* 105:361, 2000.

336. Kanazawa H, Fujiwara H, Shoji S, et al: Adenosine modulates endothelin-induced bronchoconstriction in guinea pig airway. *Int Arch Allergy Immunol* 112(1):83, 1997.

337. Weinberger M, Hendeles L: Drug therapy: Theophylline in asthma. *N Engl J Med* 334:1380, 1996.

338. Crea F, Pupita G, Galassi AR, et al: Comparative effects of theophylline and isosorbide dinitrate on exercise capacity in stable angina pectoris and their mechanism of action. *Am J Cardiol* 64:1098, 1989.

339. Picano E, Testa R, Pogliani M, et al: Increase in walking capacity after aminophylline administration in intermittent claudication. *Angiology* 4:1035, 1989.

340. Sylven C, Beerman B, Jonzon B, et al: Angina pectoris-like pain provoked by adenosine in healthy volunteers. *Br Med J* 293:227, 1986.

341. Osswald H, Gleiter C, Muhlbauer B: Therapeutic use of theophylline to antagonize renal effects of adenosine. *Clin Nephrol* 43:S33, 1995.

342. Pflueger A, Larson TS, Nath KA, et al: Role of adenosine in contrast media–induced acute renal failure in diabetes mellitus. *Mayo Clin Proc* 75:1275, 2000.

343. Nagashima K, Kusaka H, Karasawa A: Protective effects of KW-3902, an adenosine A1-receptor antagonist, against cisplatin-induced acute renal failure in rats. *Jpn J Pharmacol* 67(4):349, 1995.

344. Gottlieb SS, Skettino SL, Wolff A, et al: Effects of BG9719 (CVT-124), an A_1-adenosine receptor antagonist, and furosemide on glomerular filtration rate and natriuresis in patients with congestive heart failure. *J Am Coll Cardiol* 35:56, 2000.

345. Kusaka H, Nagashima K, Karasawa A: Effects of KW-3902, an adenosine A1-receptor antagonist, on ascites volume in puromycin aminonucleoside (PAN)-induced nephrotic rats. *Jpn J Pharmacol* 68:213, 1995.

346. Rankin AC, Oldroyd KG, Chong E, et al: Value and limitations of adenosine in the diagnosis and treatment of narrow and broad complex tachycardia. *Br Heart J* 62:195, 1989.

347. DiMarco JP, Sellers TD, Lerman BB, et al: Diagnostic and therapeutic use of adenosine in patients with supraventricular tachyarrhythmias. *J Am Coll Cardiol* 6:417, 1985.

348. Cushley MJ, Tattersfield AE, Holgate ST: Adenosine-induced bronchoconstriction in asthma: Antagonism by inhaled theophylline. *Am Rev Respir Dis* 129:380, 1984.

349. Galinanes M, Qiu Y, Van Belle H, Hearse DJ: Metabolic and functional effects of the nucleoside transporter inhibitor R75231 in ischemic and blood reperfused rabbit heart. *Cardiovasc Res* 27:90, 1993.

350. Seegmiller JE: Diseases of purine and pyrimidine metabolism. In: Bondy PK, Rosenberg LE, eds. *Metabolic Control and Disease,* 8th ed. Philadelphia: Saunders, 1980:777.

351. Bollinger ME, Arredondo-Vega FX, Santisteban I, et al: Hepatic dysfunction as a complication of adenosine deaminase deficiency. *N Engl J Med* 334:1367, 1996.

352. Zughaib ME, Abd-Elfattah AS, Jeroudi MO, et al: Augmentation of endogenous adenosine attenuates myocardial stunning independently of coronary flow or hemodynamic effects. *Circulation* 88:2369, 1993.

353. Cohen MV, Yang X, Downey JM: Conscious rabbits became tolerant to multiple episodes of ischemic preconditioning. *Circ Res* 74:998, 1994.

354. Lee HT, Thompson CI, Hernandez A, et al: Cardiac desensitization to adenosine analogs after prolonged R-PIA infusion in vivo. *Am J Physiol* 265:H1916, 1993.

355. Olah ME, Stiles GL: Adenosine receptor subtypes: Characterization and therapeutic regulation. *Annu Rev Pharmacol Toxicol* 35:581, 1995.

356. Mundell S, Luty J, Willets J, et al: Enhanced expression of G protein–coupled receptor kinase 2 selectively increases the sensitivity of A_{2A} adenosine receptors to agonist-induced desensitization. *Br J Pharmacol* 125:347, 1998.

357. Palmer T, Stiles GL: Identification of threonine residues controlling the agonist-dependent phosphorylation and desensitization of the rat A(3) adenosine receptor. *Mol Pharmacol* 57:539, 2000.

Nitric Oxide Donor Drugs in the Treatment of Cardiovascular Diseases

William H. Frishman

Armin Helisch

Nauman Naseer

Jason Lyons

Richard M. Hays

For years the vasculature was viewed as a static network of resistance vessels responsible for the maintenance of arterial pressure. However, the discovery of nitric oxide (NO), an endogenous vasodilator molecule that is synthesized by the vascular endothelium, among many other cells, has allowed a new biologic understanding of the dynamic features of the vasculature.[1] It is now thought that many cardiovascular and pulmonary diseases are characterized by endothelial dysfunction with consequent subphysiologic concentrations of NO.[2]

As a result, interest has arisen in a class of drugs loosely termed *NO donors,* which are organic nitrates that in physiologic conditions release NO. In addition, administration of NO gas by inhalation and of dietary L-arginine has been studied. It is believed that these agents may allow the replacement of NO and the amelioration of some cardiac and pulmonary-vascular diseases. This chapter reviews the discovery and biology of nitric oxide, some of its functions in the human body, its role in the pathogenesis of cardiovascular and pulmonary diseases, and the potential utility of NO donors, NO synthase (NOS) modulators, L-arginine, and inhaled NO as therapeutic agents. The organic nitrates, which are donors of exogenous NO, and sodium nitroprusside are discussed in Chap. 14, and the use of NO in children is discussed in Chap. 49.

BIOLOGIC FEATURES OF NITRIC OXIDE

In 1980, Furchgott and Zawadzki,[3] during their studies of vascular biology, noted that acetylcholine (ACh) induced vasodilation in vivo; however, in experiments conducted in vitro with isolated blood vessels, ACh was inconsistent in its vasodilatory properties and at times caused vasoconstriction. Evaluating this discrepancy, they found that inadvertent removal of the intimal surface of the blood vessels before the experiments resulted in the vessels' inability to dilate when exposed to ACh. Furthermore, subsequent experiments demonstrated that careful handling of the vessels to preserve an intact endothelium allowed the blood vessels to retain their vasodilatory properties. It was then postulated that ACh-stimulated

endothelium released a substance causing the relaxation of smooth muscle; this later became known as endothelium-derived relaxing factor (EDRF).

Subsequently it was recognized that EDRF was an unstable humoral agent released by the endothelium and resulting in smooth muscle relaxation. It also was appreciated that some vasodilating drugs, the mechanism of action of which is the release of NO, mimicked the effect of EDRF (Fig. 33-1), leading to the suggestion that EDRF is NO.[4,5] Following this line of reasoning, two groups of researchers in 1987 demonstrated that EDRF and NO are identical: they possess the same biologic activity, stability, and susceptibility to an inhibitor and to a potentiator.[6,7]

It was also shown that hemoglobin has an important transport and buffer function for NO. Heme iron has a very strong affinity for NO and acts like an NO scavenger. The β-chains of hemoglobin have highly reactive cysteine residues (Cysβ93) which are S-nitrosylated in the lung when red blood cells are oxygenated. The NO groups are released during arterial-venous transit, bound to glutathione and other small molecular erythrocytic thiols, and are transferred to vascular endothelial receptors.[8] This is explained by the reactivity of the Cysβ93 residues, which is high in the oxy- (or R structure) and low in the deoxy-conformation (or T structure) of hemoglobin. Within the R structure, the formation of methemoglobin (FE_{III}), which occurs after NO scavenging by the metal center of hemoglobin, facilitates NO group release from the Cysβ93 residues.[8] This allosteric control of NO delivery may be an important element of efficient O_2 utilization as NO suppresses mitochondrial respiration.[9]

NO is synthesized by the vascular endothelial cells in response to any of many stimuli: ACh, adenine nucleotides, thrombin, substance P, A23187 (a calcium ionophore), bradykinin, hypoxia, vasoactive hormones, and shear stress from blood flow.[10–12] In two experiments it was shown that NO is produced from the amino acid L-arginine. In one experiment, cultured endothelial cells deprived of L-arginine were not able to produce NO; however, supplementation of L-arginine restored the NO-producing ability in this cell line.[13] In a more definitive experiment, use of radiolabeled L-arginine and mass spectrometry analysis revealed that labeled

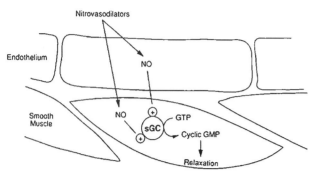

FIGURE 33-1. Nitrovasodilators such as sodium nitroprusside and nitroglycerin release NO spontaneously or through enzymatic reaction. Liberated NO stimulates soluble guanylate cyclase (sGC) in vascular smooth-muscle cell, resulting in enhanced synthesis of cyclic guanosine monophosphate (cGMP) from guanosine triphosphate (GTP); increased concentrations of cGMP in smooth muscle cells leads to their relaxation. (*Reproduced with permission from Moncada and Higgs.*[30])

NO was produced from the terminal guanidino nitrogen atoms of L-arginine.[13] L-Arginine is catabolized into NO and citrulline by NOS (Fig. 33-2),[14,15] of which there are three main classes (Table 33-1).

One is a constitutive enzyme class with one type (eNOS or Nos III) present in the vascular endothelium, cardiac myocytes, platelets, megakaryocytes; the second (nNOS or Nos I) is in neuronal cells, skeletal muscle, neutrophils, pancreatic islets, endometrium and respiratory and gastrointestinal epithelia. These enzymes are dependent on a calcium transient in the host cell to sustain binding of calmodulin and are involved in homeostatic processes such as moment-to-moment blood pressure regulation, neurotransmission, and peristalsis.[16–21]

The third main class is an inducible enzyme (iNOS or Nos II), which is found in macrophages, platelets, myocardium, megakaryocytes, respiratory epithelia, and many other cells. It has a tightly bound calmodulin subunit, requires only very low levels of Ca^{2+} for activation, and has a much higher maximal enzymatic activity than the constitutive enzymes.[17,19–21] Expression of iNOS is mainly reserved for infection or inflammation, and it is induced by a wide range of cytokines, microbes, microbial cell products, and some tumor cells. Excess production of NO by iNOS may be involved in the pathogenesis of septic shock.[22]

NO-induced vasorelaxation is mainly mediated by cyclic guanosine monophosphate (cGMP). A study by Rapaport and Murad in 1983[23] demonstrated that in the rat aorta, vasorelaxation was

TABLE 33-1. Characteristics of NOS Isoforms

	Type I	Type II	Type III
Other designation	nNOS	iNOS	eNOS
Expression	Constitutive	Inducible	Constitutive
Intracellular location	Cytosolic	Cytosolic	Membrane
Calcium activation	+	−	+
Nitric oxide output	Low	High	Low

NOS = nitric oxide synthase; nNOS = neuronal NOS; iNOS = inducible NOS; eNOS = endothelial NOS.

Source: Hart CM: Nitric oxide in adult lung disease. *Chest* 111:1409, 1999, with permission.

associated with increased concentrations of cGMP in a time- and concentration-dependent manner. A more recent study has shown that NO increases the intracellular concentration of calcium, leading to the activation of soluble guanylate cyclase in vascular smooth muscle. Activated soluble guanylate cyclase leads to phosphorylation of intracellular proteins by activation of a specific cGMP-dependent protein kinase, resulting in vasorelaxation (Fig. 33-2).[24] Other mechanisms may contribute to NO-induced vasodilation, like direct activation of calcium-dependent potassium channels.[25]

Other biologic effects of NO are related to its interaction with reactive oxygen species molecules.[26–28] Vascular endothelial cells, monocytes, and smooth muscle cells all have been shown to produce superoxide (O_2^-), which apparently antagonizes the action of EDRF (NO). O_2^- and NO react to form peroxynitrite ($ONOO^-$), which can cause lipid peroxidation and vascular endothelial dysfunction. However, NO is also a very effective peroxyl radical scavenger and a much more effective antioxidant than, for example, α-tocopherol (vitamin E).[26] The NO/O_2^- balance appears to be an important determinant of many physiologic and pathophysiologic processes, including atherosclerosis and ischemia-reperfusion injury. Figure 33-3 shows a simplified summary of the physiologic chemistry of NO.

BIOLOGIC FUNCTIONS OF NO RELATIVE TO CARDIOVASCULAR DISEASE

NO was first discovered in the vascular system. However, in the past 10 years, scientists have discovered that it is a ubiquitous molecule, utilized throughout the human body. Figure 33-4 summarizes the main biologic effects of NO.

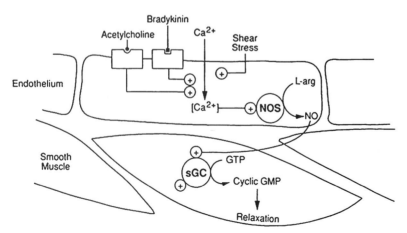

FIGURE 33-2. Shear stress or receptor activation of vascular endothelium by bradykinin or acetylcholine results in influx of calcium. Consequent increase in intracellular calcium stimulates constitutive NO synthase (NOS). NO formed from L-arginine (L-arg) by this enzyme diffuses to nearby smooth muscle cells, in which it stimulates soluble guanylate cyclase (sGC), resulting in the relaxation of these cells. GTP = guanosine triphosphate. (*Reproduced with permission from Moncada and Higgs.*[30])

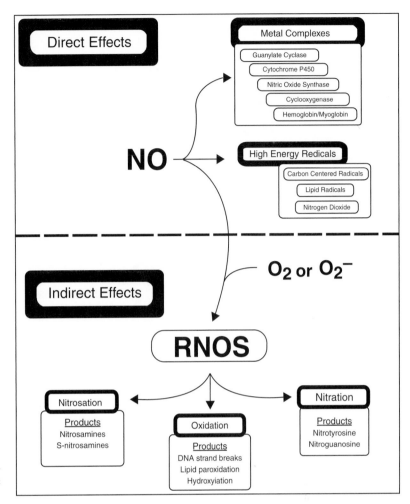

FIGURE 33-3. Physiologic chemistry of NO. RNOS = reactive nitric oxygen species. (*Reproduced with permission from Grisham et al.*[53])

Vascular Tone

As discussed earlier, NO is an endogenous vasodilator. This property is demonstrated by intravascular infusion of a competitive inhibitor of NO synthase, N^G-monomethyl-L-arginine (L-NMMA), which results in potent vasoconstriction (Fig. 33-5).[29] L-NMMA itself has no intrinsic constrictor activity; rather its hypertensive mechanism is the inhibition of the body's endogenous vasodilator mechanism. Hence, it is now understood that vascular tone is maintained in part by balance of the body's endogenous vasodilating mechanism against constrictor stimuli.[30] In blood vessels, endothelium-derived NO activates guanylate cyclase to generate cGMP from guanosine triphosphate (GTP) in smooth muscle cells, elevates cellular cGMP concentrations, and causes smooth muscle relaxation.[31] NO also inhibits the release of endothelin-1 (a vasoconstrictor) from endothelial cells[31-33] and the release of thromboxane A2 from the platelets.[34,35] Thus, NO plays an essential role in regulating vascular tone and hemodynamics.[36-38]

Hemostasis

NO acts as an endogenous inhibitor of platelet aggregation and adhesion.[39,40] NO, when released into the vascular lumen, diffuses into platelets, causing an increase in cGMP. This response begins a cascade of cGMP-dependent phosphorylation that results in the reduction of the intracellular calcium concentration. Platelet activation requires a sudden increase in intracellular calcium, so reduced intra-

cellular concentrations inhibit platelet aggregation.[41] As a result of this effect, NO inhibits platelet adhesion to the vessel wall, inhibiting initial thrombus formation by inhibiting aggregation[42] and hence the autocrine stimulation and recruitment of adjacent platelets.[43]

Inflammation

NO plays an important role in the body's inflammatory process. Its exact function is unclear: some studies have shown it to be proinflammatory, and others have shown it to be anti-inflammatory. In rats with acute inflammation, NO synthase inhibitors have been shown to reduce the degree of inflammation.[30] However, in a recent study,[44] it was found that NOS inhibitors, administered locally, exacerbated inflammation and prolonged its resolution as a result of an increase in the proinflammatory mediators, histamine, leukotriene B_4 (LTB$_4$), O_2^-, and cytokine-induced neutrophil chemoattractant (CINC), suggesting that the local production of NO is protective. By contrast, administering NOS inhibitors systemically ameliorated inflammation, thereby showing differential anti-inflammatory properties of NOS inhibitors depending on their route of administration. Endogenously formed NO is thought to promote a number of chronic inflammatory diseases, such as rheumatoid arthritis, hepatitis, inflammatory bowel disease, septic and hemorrhagic shock, and certain autoimmune disorders.[44-48]

However, a study of NO synthase inhibitors has shown that inhibition of NO production increases leukocyte adherence 15-fold,

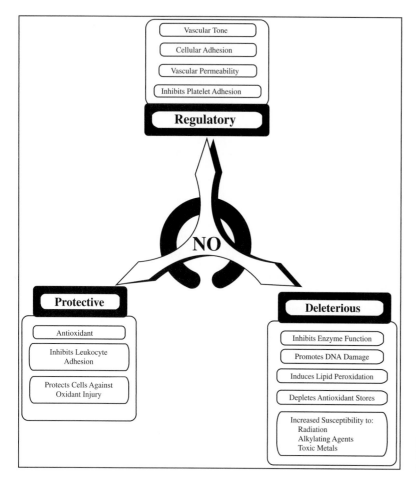

FIGURE 33-4. Regulatory, protective and deleterious biologic effects of nitric oxide (NO). (*Reproduced with permission from Grisham et al.*[53])

whereas supplementation with L-arginine, a precursor to NO, attenuates this increased adhesion. This result suggests that NO may be an endogenous modulator of leukocyte adhesion and that acute inflammation may be caused by reduced concentrations of NO.[49,50] Indeed, it is well established that exogenous NO donors are very effective at inhibiting polymorphonuclear adhesion in vivo.[45,51] In addition, a 1992 study examining the effect of NO on superoxide anion production found that NO inhibits neutrophilic superoxide anion generation by direct action on an as yet unidentified membrane component of the nicotinamide-adenine dinucleotide phosphate (NADPH) oxidase. This inhibition may provide an endothelial cell defense mechanism against neutrophil-mediated inflammation and injury.[52] Consideration of the timing, location, and rates of production of NO and reactive nitrogen oxide species may help identify which of the many NO-dependent reactions are important in modulating the inflammatory response.[53]

Smooth Muscle Proliferation

NO has been shown to have inhibitory effects on smooth muscle proliferation and migration.[31,32,54] In rat models, NO was shown to decrease neointimal proliferation after balloon-induced arterial injury.[55,56]

Apoptosis

NO has been shown to induce apoptosis via stimulation of soluble guanylate cyclase both in cardiac and vascular smooth muscle cells in vitro.[57,58] NO also inhibits apoptosis in endothelial cells, possibly through two mechanisms: (1) increasing cGMP generation, which interrupts apoptotic signaling, and (2) direct inhibition of cysteine protease (caspase) activity. The decision for a cell to undergo apoptosis is the result of a shift in the balance between the antiapoptotic and proapoptotic forces within a cell. NO contributes to this balance by suppressing the apoptotic pathway at multiple levels and by several mechanisms (Fig. 33-6). Inhibition of caspase activity by S-nitrosylation is the best-characterized mechanism for the inhibition of apoptosis by NO and is likely to be effective in cells that can efficiently carry out S-nitrosylation. Higher rates of NO production overwhelm cellular protective mechanisms and shift the balance toward apoptotic death in some cell types. The presence of superoxide (O_2^-) may also divert NO to a toxic pathway by leading to the formation of peroxynitrite. Additional studies should ultimately elucidate the many factors that determine whether NO promotes or inhibits apoptosis.[59,59a]

Angiogenesis and Wound Healing

NO stimulates endothelial cell proliferation and angiogenesis, thereby playing an important role in wound healing and in the microcirculation.[57,60] It was demonstrated that eNOS-deficient knockout mice manifest impaired wound healing and angiogenesis.[60] Diseases in which a deficit in vascular endothelial growth factor (VEGF) expression has been identified, such as diabetes,[61] may benefit from a therapeutic increase in eNOS activity or even local delivery of NO to promote wound healing. Recent work

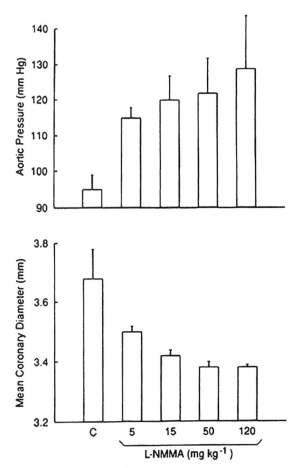

FIGURE 33-5. Infusion of N^G = monomethyl-L-arginine (L-NMMA) (5–120 mg/kg) causes dose-dependent increase in aortic pressure and vasoconstriction of coronary arteries. C = control value prior to treatment. (*Reproduced with permission from Chu et al.[29]*)

by Kullo et al.[62] has demonstrated that successful transfection of vascular tissues with adenoviral vectors encoding eNOS (AdeNOS). AdeNOS gene transfer in the setting of impaired wound healing

could potentially increase eNOS activity in wounds and thereby allow normal wound repair to occur.

CARDIOVASCULAR AND PULMONARY DISEASES CHARACTERIZED BY REDUCED CONCENTRATIONS OF NO

Many cardiovascular diseases are characterized by endothelial dysfunction, with concomitant subphysiologic levels of NO. Though usually not the primary cause of the disease, the relative lack of NO can contribute to further physiologic derangements and may potentiate the natural course of the disease.

Systemic Hypertension

As expected, there is ample evidence that essential hypertension is characterized in part by endothelial dysfunction with subphysiologic levels or impaired vascular response to NO.[63] In 1992 it was accepted on the basis of animal studies that acute blockade of NO synthesis resulted in increases in systemic blood pressure. It was not known if chronic blockade of NO synthesis, consistent with endothelial dysfunction, would produce hypertension. Rats were exposed to an NO synthase inhibitor for 2 months; compared with control animals, the rats undergoing long-term exposure manifested systemic hypertension.[64] In a corroborating study, rats that were exposed to 4 to 6 weeks of NO blockade demonstrated an increase in systemic blood pressure.[65]

In 1990, Panza et al. observed in patients with hypertension that the response of forearm vasculature to ACh (an endothelium-dependent vasodilator) was diminished (Fig. 33-7), yet the vasculature maintained a normal response to nitroprusside (an endothelium-independent vasodilator) (Fig. 33-8).[66] A recent review by Kojda and Harrison suggested that the impaired endothelium-dependent vasodilation is due to an increase in superoxide formation, resulting in a decrease in NO concentrations.[67] A decrease in NOS activity has also been suggested, including genetic variants of eNOS.[68] While there is little dispute that NO levels are decreased in hypertension, the role or responsibility of these decreased NO levels

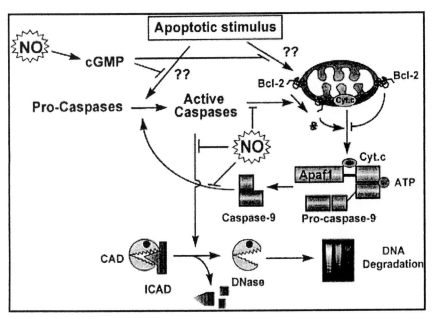

FIGURE 33-6. NO suppresses apoptosis by two mechanisms: (1) through the activation of soluble guanylyl cyclase, NO can increase cGMP levels. Cyclic guanosine monophosphate (cGMP) interrupts apoptotic signaling in some cell types, including hepatocytes, splenocytes, and PC12 cells. (2) NO also directly inhibits caspase activity in many cells. Through these mechanisms, NO can prevent the degradation of Bcl-2 family members and cytochrome C (Cyt.c) release from mitochondria. This prevents the activation of downstream caspases and the terminal events in apoptosis, such as the cleavage of the inhibitor of caspase-dependent activated DNase (ICAD) and the activation of caspase-dependent activated DNase (CAD). (*Reproduced with permission from Kim et al.[59]*)

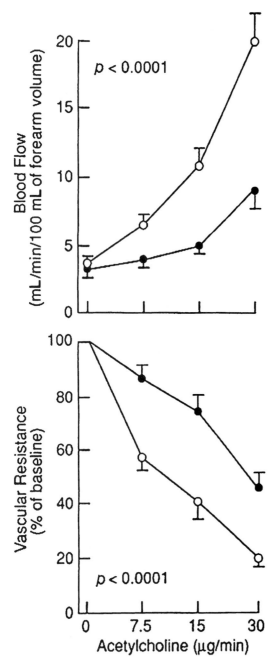

FIGURE 33-7. Reduced response of forearm blood flow and vascular resistance to acetylcholine (endothelium-dependent vasodilator) in 18 patients with hypertension (solid circles) compared with 18 patients with normal blood pressure (open circles). (*Reproduced with permission from Panza et al.*[66])

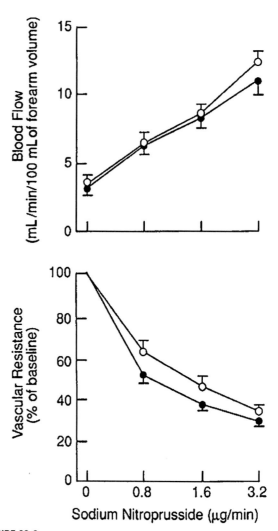

FIGURE 33-8. Normal response of forearm blood flow and vascular resistance to sodium nitroprusside (endothelium-independent vasodilator) in 18 patients with hypertension (solid circles) and in 18 patients with normal blood pressure (open circles). (*Reproduced with permission from Panza et al.*[66])

Myocardial Ischemia and Reperfusion

Coronary artery occlusion may result in myocardial cell death. Reperfusion can salvage ischemic tissue but may also contribute to myocardial cellular injury by allowing polymorphonuclear neutrophil leukocytes (PMNs) to infiltrate the site of injury. Reperfusion injury can be explained by endothelial dysfunction. In experiments by Tsao et al.,[71] coronary arteries did not lose their NO-producing ability while ischemic, but on reperfusion, they became dysfunctional within 2.5 min; and after 20 min, they were nearly maximally dysfunctional. This dysfunction could be prevented by providing superoxide dismutase before reperfusion. In addition, significant myocardial cell damage did not occur until hours after reperfusion, suggesting that endothelial dysfunction occurs on reperfusion. This dysfunction may be caused by oxygen-derived free radicals,[45,72] and endothelial dysfunction occurs before myocardial cell necrosis. A recent study confirmed the finding of decreased NO levels after reperfusion. In addition, it was shown that the adherence of PMNs to endothelial cells is increased when NO concentrations decrease with reperfusion and that this could be prevented with the addition of

in the pathogenesis of hypertension in humans is yet to be elucidated. Arnal et al. state that the decreased NO bioavailability seen with hypertension could be due to numerous secondary causes and not primarily responsible for hypertension.[69] Therefore, hypertension is characterized by decreased NO bioavailability, but the role it plays in the pathogenesis and maintenance of hypertension is still an important question that needs to be answered. Indirectly increased NO production has been shown to occur with various antihypertensive drugs, and could, in part, explain their mechanisms of action.[70]

L-arginine, a precursor of NO.[73,74] In contrast to these earlier findings, ischemia has now been shown to stimulate increased local NO production, which may decrease the coronary vascular resistance of the vessels perfusing ischemic myocardium, thereby potentially improving myocardial contractility and metabolic function.[75] However, in a review, Zweier et al. suggest that in postischemic tissues, NOS-independent NO generation can result in cellular injury, with a loss of organ function.[76,77] In myocardial ischemia/reperfusion, increased NO production by circulating neutrophils was demonstrated, which was further enhanced by aspirin. This results in significant platelet inhibition unrelated to the known inhibitory effect of aspirin on thromboxane A_2 production.[78] These more recent observations suggest that decreased local NO production related to endothelial injury occurs somewhat later in the development of reperfusion injury. Ischemic preconditioning appears to protect not only against reperfusion-related myocardial dysfunction but also against reperfusion-related coronary endothelial dysfunction.[79] A review by Bolli states that the late effects of preconditioning can be pharmacologically reproduced with NO donors, adenosine receptor agonists, endotoxin derivatives, or opioid receptor agonists.[80]

In patients with angina secondary to coronary vasospasm and without angiographic stenosing coronary artery disease, a deficiency of endothelial NO activity in the spasm arteries was recently demonstrated. This resulted in increased local sensitivity to the vasodilating effect of nitroglycerin and to the vasoconstrictive effect of ACh.[81]

Splanchnic Ischemia and Reperfusion

Mesenteric ischemia and reperfusion can result in lethal circulatory shock as a result of endothelial dysfunction. In one study in cats, splanchnic artery occlusion for 90 min followed by reperfusion resulted in hypotension and death. Examination of the mesenteric vasculature revealed that these animals had impaired ability to vasodilate in response to endothelium-dependent vasodilators yet responded normally to endothelium-independent vasodilators. In addition, the infusion of superoxide dismutase before reperfusion markedly reduced the amount of endothelial dysfunction, improved arterial blood pressure, and improved survival.[82] The role of peroxynitrite, formed from the interaction of superoxide molecules and NO, is under question. Cuzzocrea et al. showed that an increase in peroxynitrite (seen 90 min following reperfusion) is produced from eNOS rather than iNOS and suggests that the increased peroxynitrite contributes to the reperfusion injury.[83] However, Lefer et al. demonstrated that peroxynitrite inhibited leukocyte rolling and adhesion within mesenteric venules.[82] The protection of endothelial function may therefore be crucial to the prevention of circulatory shock resulting from splanchnic ischemia and reperfusion.

Atherosclerosis

The activities of everyday life require that the coronary arteries have the ability to dilate. Angiographic studies have shown that normal coronary arteries dilate in response to exercise and exposure to low temperatures, yet mildly atherosclerotic vessels vasoconstrict in response to these stimuli,[84–86] predisposing patients with atherosclerosis to myocardial ischemia.

In one study of the mechanism for atherosclerotic impairment of endothelium-dependent vasodilation, patients with angiographically smooth left anterior descending (LAD) coronary arteries were compared with patients with irregular LAD arteries consistent with mild atherosclerosis. The comparison involved the arteries' ability to dilate when exposed to increases in blood flow, a known stimulus for endothelium-dependent vasodilation. The arteries' ability to dilate in response to an endothelium-independent vasodilator (nitroglycerin) was also evaluated.

All of the arteries responded normally to nitroglycerin, and whereas the angiographically normal arteries dilated in response to increases in blood flow, the ability of the atherosclerotic vessels to dilate was impaired. Because the arteries maintained a normal response to endothelium-independent vasodilators, the failure of the atherosclerotic vessels to dilate in response to endothelium-dependent stimuli is consistent with endothelial dysfunction with probable decreased NO production.[87] Reviews by Tentolouris et al.[88] and Wever et al.[89] state that there are numerous benefits of L-arginine administration with respects to coronary atherosclerosis. Tentolouris et al. also conclude that stimulation of endogenous NO production could inhibit atherogenesis.[88] Similar evidence for endothelial dysfunction has been found in patients with hypercholesterolemia and diabetes mellitus.[27,90–93] The underlying mechanisms may be related to (1) a decreased synthesis or release of NO[21]; (2) increased inactivation of NO (e.g., by superoxide)[27,89]; (3) a reduced degradation of asymmetric-dimethyl-L-arginine (ADMA), an endogenous inhibitor of NO synthase[94]; (4) theoretically also a decreased responsiveness of the vascular smooth muscle cell NO–guanylate cyclase pathway; and/or (5) increased release of vasoconstricting agonists, such as prostanoids.[91] Oxidized LDL, probably the most important factor in the pathophysiology of early atherosclerosis, not only inactivates EDRF directly but also impairs the expression of NO synthase in endothelial cells[92,95,96] and inhibits NO synthesis in platelets, thereby stimulating platelet activity.[21,27] Recent studies are suggesting the importance of a proper balance of NO, with its antioxidant capabilities, versus peroxynitrite, a byproduct of NO with superoxide molecules.[89,97] Wever et al.[89] propose that NOS III has a dual role in the pathogenesis of atherosclerosis by increasing oxidative stress in a hyperlipidemic and atherosclerotic environment. However, Dusting et al. propose that NOS II is increased in atherosclerosis.[98] Clearly, the role of NO and NOS in atherosclerosis is still unclear.

Recently an endogenous NO inhibitor, ADMA, was found in plasma and noted to be evaluated in patients with risk factors for atherosclerosis.[99] Statins have also been shown to enhance NO production; this may explain some of the protective benefit of statins in patients with atherosclerotic heart disease.[100,101]

Congestive Heart Failure

Patients with advanced congestive heart failure (CHF) exhibit systemic vasoconstriction produced by neural, hormonal, and local vascular factors. In addition, in these patients the vascular responses to physiologic stimuli are abnormal, as the ability to vasodilate peripheral vessels in response to ischemia or exercise may be lost.

Studies in animals and human beings have shown that the basal release of NO in chronic CHF is normal or possibly enhanced and may function in a compensatory role as an antagonist to neurohormonal vasoconstricting forces. Other studies suggest that in patients with heart failure, there is a decrease in the basal release of nitric oxide in the coronary circulation.[102] However, these studies also have shown that endothelium-mediated dilation is depressed, presumably because of an impaired ability of the endothelium to release NO on stimulation. More recent studies have also concluded that a change in expression or regulation of eNOS or an increase in plasma concentration of inhibitors of eNOS may be responsible for a relative decrease in NO.[103,104] This depression probably accounts for the abnormal vascular responses seen in these patients.[105–109] It has also been shown that NO is produced by the heart (endothelium, vascular smooth muscle cells, cardiac myocytes, and neurons) and that it attenuates the positive inotropic and chronotropic response to the stimulation of beta-adrenergic receptors.[109a] Basal NO production by cNOS[18] appears to have only a mild moderating effect on the latter; however, excessive NO production by iNOS may be one of the reasons for the myocardial depression and the beta-adrenergic hyporesponsiveness associated with sepsis, myocarditis, cardiac transplant rejection, and dilated cardiomyopathy.[19,22,110–111a] These findings were substantiated in a study by Drexler et al., in which they found that N^G-monomethyl-L-arginine (L-NMMA) (an inhibitor of NOS) enhanced the positive inotropic response to beta stimulation in failing hearts.[112] In addition to peripheral endothelial dysfunction in chronic CHF, the coronary vasculature's ability to dilate is impaired. Treasure et al.[113] found that in response to ACh, coronary blood flow increased greatly in control patients, whereas coronary blood flow in patients with CHF exhibited no significant increase.

Pulmonary Vascular Disease

NOS inhibitors caused pulmonary vasoconstriction when administered to normal volunteers, demonstrating that the tonic or constitutive production of NO by the pulmonary vasculature regulates pulmonary vascular tone and resistance under normal conditions.[114] NOS inhibitors also enhanced hypoxia-induced increases in pulmonary vascular resistance,[115] whereas inhaled NO prevented hypoxia-induced pulmonary vasoconstriction in normal volunteers,[116] suggesting that NO can also regulate the response to vasoconstrictive stimuli in the lung.

In addition to its effects on vascular tone, the continuous production of NO in the pulmonary vasculature may also play an important role in vascular homeostasis through its ability to inhibit such proinflammatory events as platelet activation and aggregation[117] and leukocyte adhesion.[118] NO produced by inflammatory cells participates in host defense against specific microorganisms,[119] and NO produced by inhibitory nonadrenergic noncholinergic (NANC) neurons modulates bronchomotor tone. Thus, current evidence indicates that NO plays an important role in the regulation of vascular, airway, and inflammatory events in the lung. Pulmonary vascular resistance is regulated in part by continuous local production of NO.[120,121] Pulmonary hypertension and right heart failure are known results of hypoxemia and pulmonary hypertension induced by chronic obstructive pulmonary disease (COPD). A study in rats with chronic hypoxic pulmonary hypertension has demonstrated endothelial dysfunction with a loss in pulmonary endothelium-dependent relaxation.[122]

A 1991 study examined pulmonary arteries obtained from patients with COPD for their ability to dilate when exposed to known vasodilatory pharmacologic agents. The COPD arteries at maximum dilation achieved only 50% of the control arteries' maximum dilation capacity. However the experimental and control arteries showed equivalent dilation in response to sodium nitroprusside (an endothelium-independent vasodilator). Thus the COPD arteries lost some of their endothelium-dependent vasodilating ability.[123]

The cause of the endothelial dysfunction may be related to chronic hypoxemia; the ability of the vessels to vasodilate (an in-

dicator of endothelial function) was related directly to the partial pressure of arterial oxygen immediately before experimentation.[123] Furthermore, bovine pulmonary endothelial cells when made hypoxic have an impaired ability to release NO on stimulation.[124] It is possible that hypoxemia results in endothelial dysfunction and decreased NO production, leading to pulmonary hypertension and its sequelae. Giaid and Saleh[121] elegantly demonstrated a significantly diminished expression of NO synthase in the vascular endothelium of pulmonary arteries of patients with primary or secondary pulmonary hypertension and severe morphologic abnormalities. It is unclear whether this is a cause or an effect of pulmonary hypertension. However, this finding, combined with our knowledge about the inhibitory effects of NO on vascular tone and smooth muscle cell proliferation,[125] strongly suggest a role of the decrease of NO production in the initiation and/or progression of pulmonary hypertension.[121,126]

Additional studies will be required to determine whether altered pulmonary vascular endothelial NO production plays a pathogenetic role in the vascular remodeling of patients with obstructive airway disease. Low concentrations of inhaled NO prevented hypoxia-induced pulmonary hypertension in rats.[127]

Summary

Endothelial dysfunction is present in numerous cardiovascular and pulmonary disease states; as a result, NO and NO donors hold great promise for the treatment of these diseases. The remainder of this chapter reviews the pharmacologic features of NO donors and the most recent applications of NO, NO donors, and L-arginine as therapeutic agents in cardiovascular and pulmonary diseases.

PHARMACOLOGIC ASPECTS OF NO DONORS

A wide variety of NO donors are available. They differ in structure, and in the enzymatic and/or chemical mechanisms by which they are made biologically active. Table 33-2 lists the major classes of NO donors, along with mechanisms of NO generation. NO donor compounds can be classified into six categories, based on the atom to which the NO-releasing moiety is attached. These categories are O-NO donors, transition metal NO complexes, heterocyclic NO donors, S-NO donors, N-NO donors, and C-NO donors.[128]

NO Donor Compounds

O-NO Donors

Organic Nitrates
Nitroglycerin's ability to produce NO is dependent on the donation of three electrons, probably from the thiol group of cysteine.[129] Tolerance to nitroglycerin may occur partly because of its required biotransformation to generate NO, even though the hypothesis of thiol group depletion has not been supported by more recent observations.[130,131] Nitrate tolerance appears to be partly related to an increased endothelial superoxide anion generation, leading to degradation of NO and to increased endothelin-1 levels that sensitize the vessel to the vasoconstricting effects of angiotensin II and catecholamines.[131] Neurohumoral activation leads to intravascular fluid accumulation/ retention and may contribute to the development of nitrate tolerance.[131]

TABLE 33-2. General Characteristics of NO Donors

Chemical Class	General Structure	Examples	Mechanisms of NO Generation
Organic nitrates	$R_3C\text{-}ONO_2$	Nitroglycerin, isosorbide dinitrate	Mostly enzymatic
Organic nitrites	$R_3C\text{-}ONO$	Isoamyl nitrite, isobutyl nitrite	Enzymatic and chemical hydrolysis
Ferrous nitro complexes	$[(CN)_5Fe^{2+}]NO$	Sodium nitroprusside	Chemical reduction and enzymatic
Sydnonimines	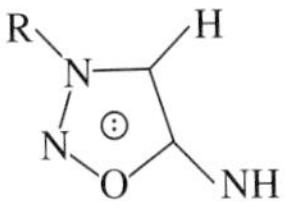	Molsidomine, pirsidomine, linsidomine (SIN-1)	Ring removal through hepatic metabolism (not for SIN-1), then chemical hydrolysis
Furoxans	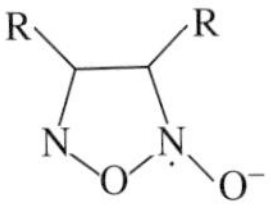	Multiple investigational agents	Chemical
S-Nitrosothiols	$R_3C\text{-}S\text{-}NO$	S-Nitrosocysteine, S-nitroso-N-acetylpenicillamine, S-nitrosocaptopril	Chemical hydrolysis and enzymatic
Nucleophile adducts	$R_2N\text{-}[N(O)NO]^-$	Diethylamine-NO, spermine-NO	Chemical

Source: Bauer et al.,[132] with permission.

Organic Nitrites

Spontaneous release and enzymatic catalysis have been described as the NO-generating mechanisms for these agents.[132] Their hydrolytic stability is much lower than that of respective organic nitrates, which limits their usability.[133] The enzyme involved in the generation of NO appears to be different from that involved in the metabolism of organic nitrates.[132]

Transition Metal NO Complexes

It is believed that NO binding to protein metal complexes such as hemoglobin may play a key role in the function of NO within the body. Transition metal NO complexes act as NO^+, NO^-, and $NO^\bullet$ donors. Sodium nitroprusside is the only clinically used chemical in the group (Fig. 33-9).

Sodium nitroprusside requires chemical reduction for NO release, with the obligate generation of cyanide as a by-product.[134,135] Because cyanide inhibits NO action, higher doses of sodium nitroprusside may be required.[134,136] However, the marked activation of soluble guanylate cyclase and vasodilation caused by this agent does not appear to be exclusively related to generation of NO.[133] Nitroprusside is used clinically to treat hypertensive emergencies and acute heart failure.

Dinitrosyl-iron complexes are mononuclear iron-NO complexes. Low-molecular-weight thiols, amino acids, peptides and proteins can function as coordinating ligands. However, their physiologic significance is unclear. Compound 28 and Roussin's salts are nitrosyl complexes of iron-sulfur clusters that can also release NO; however, the mechanism is unclear.[128]

Heterocyclic NO Donors

Sydnonimines

Linsidomine (SIN-1) arises from hepatic cleavage of the prodrug molsidomine which has been used clinically in Europe and Japan for several years (Fig. 33-10) and does not require any cofactors for the generation of NO (Fig. 33-11).[133,137] The formation of superoxide anions[133] is a potential drawback of these drugs.

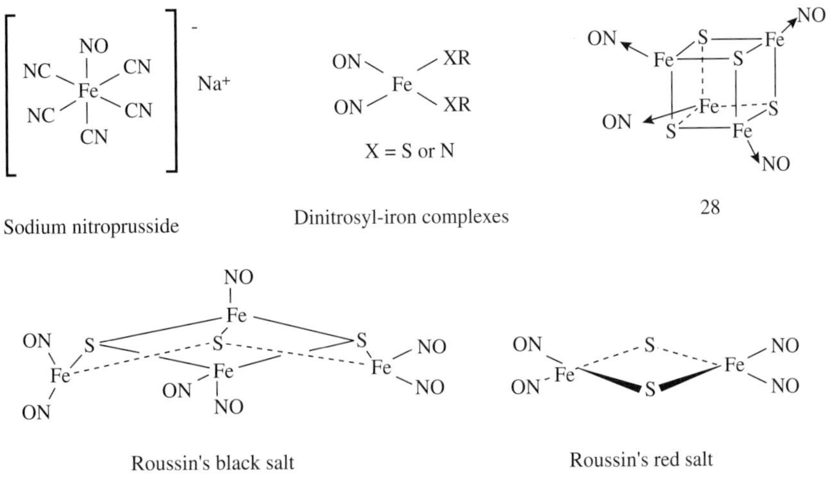

FIGURE 33-9. Some common transition metal NO complexes. (*Reproduced with permission from Hou et al.*[128])

Sodium nitroprusside

Dinitrosyl-iron complexes

X = S or N

28

Roussin's black salt

Roussin's red salt

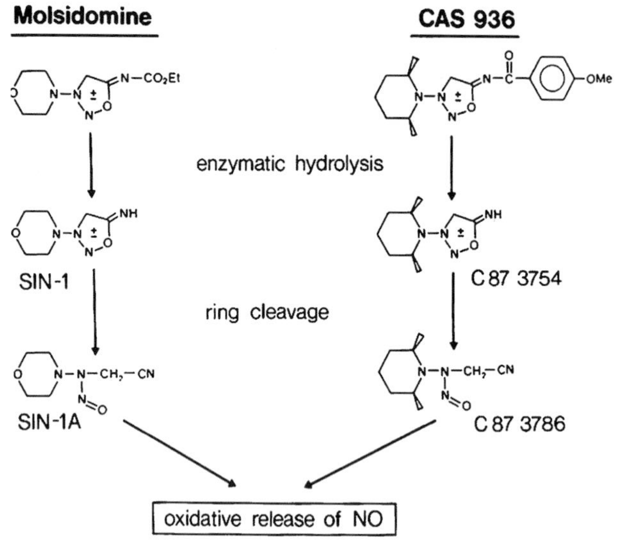

Molsidomine

CAS 936

enzymatic hydrolysis

ring cleavage

oxidative release of NO

FIGURE 33-10. First steps in in vivo metabolism of molsidomine leading to release of NO (left) and the respective process suggested for persidomine (CAS 936) (right). (*From Bohn H, Beyerle R, Martorana PA, Schönafinger X: CAS936, a novel sydnonimine with direct vasodilating and nitric-oxide donating properties: Effects on isolated blood vessels. J Cardiovasc Pharmacol 18:522, 1991.*)

Pirsidomine, a highly active NO donor, is metabolized in an analogous way, and is believed to have biologic properties similar to those of isosorbide dinitrate (Fig. 33-10).[136] Unlike organic nitrates, the sydnonimines do not induce tolerance.[138]

Furoxans

These are another group of heterocyclic compounds that have been shown to activate guanylate cyclase via NO liberation. Their capacity to release NO and to dilate vessels is related to the substitutions at the heterocyclic ring,[139] and in some of the more recently developed agents does not seem to be dependent on the presence of thiols.[140] A lack of physiologic tolerance makes this type of NO donor attractive in the treatment of cardiovascular disease. However, the mutagenicity of this type of compound is a further drawback for its future drug development.

Oxatriazole Derivatives

GEA 5024 was found to inhibit PMN activation and endothelial cell–mediated oxidation of LDL.[139,141] These effects are believed to result from NO formation. This compound may have 10-fold greater potency than SIN-1 or S-nitroso-N-acetyl pencillamine (SNAP).[128]

S-NO Donors (S-Nitrosothiols)

Many of these substances occur physiologically, being derived from protein and low-molecular-weight thiols; they appear to mediate nitric oxide–like bioactivity in addition to effects related to NO group transfer involving either NO^+ or NO^-.[142,143] The recently discovered biologic importance of S-nitrosylation of hemoglobin was previously described.[8] Numerous biologic functions of RSNOs continue to be uncovered to date. For example, it has recently been reported that blood flow is regulated by nitrosohemoglobin via the release of NO. Additionally, S-nitrosylation of certain thiol groups on the calcium release channel may regulate the channel.[144] Synthetic agents of interest include S-nitrosocaptopril.[143] It can influence vital systems that control arterial pressure and vasodilatation. It accomplishes this through inhibition of the angiotensin converting enzyme (ACE) and activation of soluble guanylate cyclase (SGC).[145]

N-NO Donors

According to their chemical structures, N-NO donor compounds can be further classified as diazeniumdiolates, N-nitrosamines, N-hydroxy-N-nitrosamines, and N-nitrosoamides.

Diazeniumdiolates (Previously Called Nucleophile NO Adducts, NONOates)

A promising type of NO donor now in development is the NO-nucleophile, also known as NONOates. Morley and Keefer[146] have shown that these compounds have the ability to generate NO spontaneously in vitro and in vivo. They are produced by exposing solutions of nucleophile compounds to a few atmospheres of NO gas, with the resulting chemical reaction $X^- + 2NO \rightarrow X-[N(O)-NO]^-$. The resulting compound is stable as a solid and highly soluble in aqueous media. Decomposition yields 2 mol of NO per mol of donor: $X-[N(O)NO] \rightarrow X^- + 2 NO$. The rate of decomposition is dependent on pH, temperature, and identity of the molecule X. Therefore the rate of NO generation can be chemically predicted and adjusted.[146] A study of the vasoactivity of these compounds has demonstrated that there is linear correlation among the NONOates as to their ability to release NO and their vasodilating properties.[146]

Their mechanism of NO production confers on the NONOates a unique advantage: unlike other nitrovasodilators, they generate NO spontaneously, without any requirements for electron transfer, cofactors, metabolic activation, or oxidation-reduction activation.[146] Because the NONOates are stable as solids yet highly soluble, have chemically predictable reactions, spontaneously generate NO, and show a high correlation between NO release and vasodilation. They hold great promise as therapeutic agents.

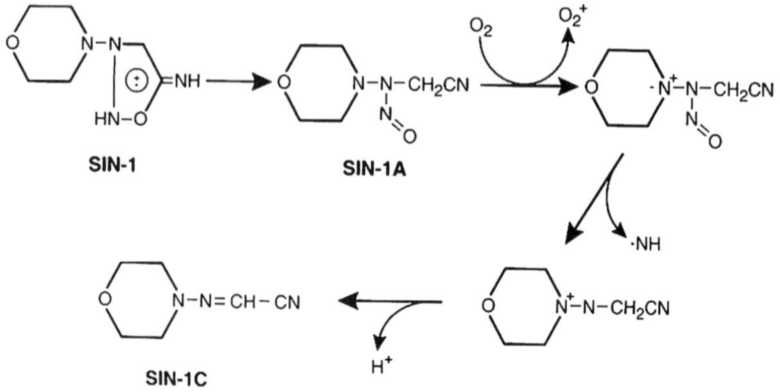

SIN-1 **SIN-1A**

SIN-1C

FIGURE 33-11. Pathway of NO formation for SIN-1, In the first step, SIN-1 undergoes hydrolytic opening to the nitrosamine SIN-1A. This compound then is attached by molecular oxygen and converted to a radical cation while oxygen is reduced to superoxide. The highly unstable radical compound is stabilized by NO splitoff and deprotonation. (*Reproduced with permission from Feelisch.[133]*)

N-Hydroxy-N-Nitrosamines

Cupferron, widely employed as a metal chelating agent and a polymerization inhibitor, generates NO by enzymatic oxidation as well as in electrochemical and chemical reactions. The antineoplastic drug alanosine and antihypertensive agent dopastin are believed to generate NO via biotransformation.[147]

N-Nitrosoamide

Streptozotocin, an *N*-nitrosoamide, is an anticancer drug. Like many NO donors, it can release NO upon ultraviolet irradiation. The effects noted are accumulation of nitrite, vasodilatation of aortic tissue, and SGC stimulation.[128]

C-NO Donors

This class consists of nitro- and nitrosocompounds, guanidine-related compounds, and oxime-related compounds. These compounds have been shown to manifest pharmacologic aspects associated with NO. These effects include activation of SGC, relaxation of isolated vascular smooth muscle, and inhibition of platelet-aggregation in vivo. In addition, these compounds show hypotensive, antithrombotic, and antianginal effects in vivo.

Other Pharmacologic Sources of NO

L-arginine has been used to treat cardiovascular conditions that include angina pectoris, congestive heart failure, syndrome X, and hypertension.

L-Arginine Supplementation

Many investigators have conducted clinical trials evaluating L-arginine, the substrate for NO synthase to increase NO production.[148–159] In cases of L-arginine depletion, the rationale for this approach is obvious.[160] In other cases, the rationale for this approach has been questioned, as the intracellular L-arginine concentration is generally much higher than that required for the very efficient NOS.[161] Intracellular L-arginine concentrations are approximately 1 to 2 mmol/L in freshly isolated endothelial cells or endothelial cells in the presence of 0.2 to 0.4 mmol/L-arginine, but the K_m value of purified endothelial NO synthase for arginine is only 2.9 μmol/L.[162] These observations imply that eNOS may be saturated with intracellular arginine and that endothelial NO synthesis may not respond to alterations in extracellular arginine concentrations. However, increasing extracellular arginine concentrations from 0.1 to 10 mmol/L in a dose-dependent manner increases NO production by cultured endothelial cells, and elevating plasma arginine levels enhance systemic and vascular NO production.[34,163] A number of theories have been proposed to explain this Arg paradox, including colocalization of the arginine transporter (CAT-1) and eNOS in membrane-associated caveolae, intracellular compartmentation of arginine, an interaction between arginine and glutamine, alterations in eNOS dimerization, and the competitive inhibition of eNOS by endogenous inhibitors (e.g., ADMA).[34,163] Other potential explanations for the efficacy of L-arginine supplementation include the possibility of intracellular compartmentalization of L-arginine and the reversal of the inhibitory effect of substances like L-glutamine on NO release.[161] There may be other endogenous inhibitors of NO synthesis as well. N^G-monomethyl-L-arginine (L-NMMA), an inhibitor of NO synthesis, is present in the plasma of patients with renal failure, for example.[164] L-arginine is also known to be the substrate for other processes, including arginine decarboxylase, which catalyzes the synthesis of agmantine. The latter is an endogenous noncatecholamine alpha$_2$ agonist that decreases peripheral sympathetic outflow by an effect in the nucleus tractus soli-

tarius and therefore might be involved in the antihypertensive effect of L-arginine.[149,157] Whatever the mechanism, L-arginine supplementation has been reported to be effective in some clinical settings (see below).

Inhaled Nitric Oxide

There has been increasing interest in the use of inhaled nitric oxide for the diagnosis and treatment of a variety of cardiothoracic diseases and in cardiothoracic surgery.[165–168] Fullerton and McIntyre[169] have recently reviewed the biochemistry, toxicity, experimental studies, and therapeutic applications of inhaled NO; therapeutic applications are discussed in a later section.

One of the major advantages of the administration of NO by inhalation is the concentration of its therapeutic effect on the pulmonary circulation, without producing general systemic vasodilation. NO crosses the alveolar-capillary membrane and improves gas exchange and relaxes the pulmonary vascular smooth muscle.[170] Careful control of the level of inhaled NO is critical, to avoid toxicity not only from high levels of methemoglobin but also from nitrogen dioxide, the oxidation product of NO.[169] Some investigators have reported a rebound phenomenon with rapid hemodynamic and gas-exchange deterioration after discontinuing inhaled nitric oxide is abruptly discontinued.[171,172]

Additional Approaches for Manipulating NO Production and Bioavailability

The goal of therapy should be to have NO donors that are target-specific, with low tolerance and toxicity, and development of hybrid molecules utilizing the biologic function of NO with other pharmaceutical moieties. The addition of alkyl moieties has been exploited to prevent the spontaneous release of NO and to increase the delivery to the liver, where hepatic enzymes stimulate the release of NO. This organ-specific NO delivery strategy effectively reduced experimentally induced liver damage in an animal model.[173] Gene therapy that increases the expression of NOS at localized sites is also under exploration as a strategy to enhance the local rate of NO production in specific vascular beds.[174,175] A new class of drugs (NO-nonsteroidal anti-inflammatory drugs, or NO-NSAIDs) have been shown to have comparable or superior anti-inflammatory and analgesic activity to standard NSAIDs while sparing the gastrointestinal tract and kidney of injury.[176,177]

Glutathione, a reduced thiol that modulates redox states and forms adducts of NO, has been evaluated in patients with decreased endothelial function and has been shown to improve endothelial function selectively by enhancing NO activity.[178]

Attempts have also been made to interfere with NO production in shock and myocardial infarction. L-NMMA administration in cardiogenic shock was shown to be safe and had favorable clinical and hemodynamic effects.[179] L-NMMA is a potent vasoconstrictor and may have a role in septic shock, large myocardial infarctions, and congestive heart failure where enhanced NO activity is present.[180]

NO DONORS IN THE TREATMENT OF CARDIOVASCULAR AND PULMONARY DISEASES

Coronary Artery Disease

Recent research studies have focused on understanding the role of NO and NO donors in the development and prevention of atherosclerosis and subsequent coronary artery disease. Moreover, with the increased use of invasive treatments for coronary artery disease, NO and NO donors are also being investigated for their role in preventing unwanted sequelae from procedures like percutaneous transluminal coronary angioplasty (PTCA) and stenting.

NO Donors

Nitrates have long been the standard treatment for myocardial ischemia–induced angina pectoris. These agents cause epicardial artery dilation and dilation of compliant stenoses in order to redistribute coronary flow toward jeopardized myocardium.[136] The limitation of nitrate therapy is the development of tolerance to the agent (tachyphylaxis) with long-term administration.[181] There are multiple possible mechanisms for the development of nitrate tolerance. It was hoped that the newer NO donors, releasing NO spontaneously, would not be subject to antianginal tolerance.

Wagner and coworkers[182] compared slow-release preparations of molsidomine (8 mg PO tid) with isosorbide dinitrate (40 mg PO tid). A significant attenuation of the anti-ischemic effects of both drugs after 4 days was observed without any significant difference between them. On the other hand, Unger et al.[183] reported on a group of patients with ischemic cardiomyopathy who were randomized to receive intravenous isosorbide dinitrate, molsidomine, or placebo for 24 h. All three groups received enalapril to inhibit renin-angiotensin activation. In the molsidomine (+enalapril) group, a sustained decrease of the pulmonary capillary wedge pressure was achieved without evidence of tolerance. In a study of C87-3754, a derivative of the syndonimine pirsidomine, which is metabolized to C87-3786 (Fig. 33-10), a maximal coronary artery dilation of $9.8 \pm 1.3\%$ was found on day 1 of continuous infusion in dogs.[184] By the end of day 1, the diameters diminished to 60% of the maximally achieved diameters and then remained constant throughout the 5-day infusion period. The right atrial pressure remained decreased during the infusion period, and the heart rate remained increased by 25% without changes in mean arterial pressure. These results differ markedly from those of a similar study of nitroglycerin, in which no dilation was evident 2 days after the beginning of the infusion.[185] The situation becomes more complicated by the fact that some of the novel NO donors, like pirsidomine (CAS 936), which is metabolized to C87-3754 and C87-3786 (Fig. 33-10), may have vasodilating properties unrelated to their metabolites and unrelated to the release of NO.[141] A study comparing ACh, nitroglycerin, and CAS 754 (an active metabolite of pirsidomine) revealed vasodilatory properties unique to CAS 754: this agent selectively dilated the large epicardial arteries and had an extremely long-lasting effect compared with the effects of nitroglycerin and ACh.[186]

In addition to the beneficial effects with endothelial dysfunction and platelet activation, NO and NO donors have been shown to inhibit the proliferation[187,188] and migration[189] of vascular smooth muscle cells, leukocyte recruitment,[190] and microvascular permeability elicited by mast cell activation.[191] Furthermore, studies have shown inhibitory effects on monocyte chemotaxis and superoxide inactivation.[27,47]

In a study of rabbits treated with molsidomine, an increase of fatty streak development was seen in the treated group.[192] This was thought to be related to the corelease of superoxide anion from the sydnonimine and stresses the need for care in selecting the NO donor to be used.[133] In addition, Bult et al.[192] noted a downregulation of endothelial NO production in the rabbits on molsidomine.

In reference to the syndnonimines, the NO donors releasing NO spontaneously, there still is no conclusive evidence that they are impervious to tachyphylaxis, as initially hoped. Unger et al. in 1994,[183]

addressed whether molsidomine was as susceptible to tolerance as isosorbide dinitrate. At 24 h, they found that the only the patients treated with molsidomine had significantly decreased pulmonary capillary wedge pressures. The authors suggested that due to the difference in mechanism of the two drugs, an impaired biotransformation of nitrates is involved in tolerance induced by high doses of isosorbide dinitrate in congestive heart failure. Sutsch et al.[193] examined whether subjects pretreated with nitroglycerine (NTG) would be susceptible to the vasodilating effects of molsidimine. In this study, 33 healthy subjects were randomly divided into two groups. One group received 1 week of NTG administration whereas the other group received placebo. The vascular responses to linsidomine were assessed before and 7 days after initiation of the study. These authors concluded that the short-term administration of sydnonimines can overcome the loss of vascular relaxation associated with long-term NTG therapy. Lehmann et al. examined molsidomine, a sydnonimine, versus IS5MN for the development and underlying mechanism of tachyphlyaxis.[194] They concluded that molsidomine had longer-lasting effects even while producing a more prominent fluid shift. However, they also concluded that the fluid shift has no essential role in nitrate tolerance development. A recent study by Messin et al.[195] compared the efficacy of molsidomine retard 8 mg bid, and molsidomine 4 mg tid in 90 patients with stable angina. They used clinical outcome for their comparison and showed that after 6 weeks of treatment, there was still a significant improvement in the patients' clinical outcome with both forms of therapy. However, they concluded that the molsidomine retard reduces myocardial ischemia more efficiently at the submaximal exercise level, has a more prolonged effect on exercise tolerance, and maintains its benefit at a somewhat higher level after 6 weeks of treatment.

L-Arginine

Intracoronary infusion of L-arginine has been shown to normalize the defective acetylcholine-induced vasodilation of coronary microvessels in patients with hypercholesterolemia[90] and in those with microvascular angina pectoris.[196] In patients with coronary artery disease and hypertension, no such effect was observed.[197] Unlike the coronary dilation seen with nitrates, no significant beneficial effect of L-arginine on the large epicardial arteries has been observed.[87,186,198]

Thirteen weeks of oral administration of L-arginine was shown to result in an increased generation of vascular NO, a reduced endothelial release of superoxide anions, and regression of intimal atherosclerotic lesions in rats on a high-cholesterol diet.[199] Another group, however, supplemented rabbits on a high-cholesterol diet for 7 to 14 weeks with oral L-arginine and found a significant effect on the extent of atherosclerotic lesions limited to the descending aorta of males but no effect in the ascending aorta or in females.[200] In this study, plasma L-arginine levels remained only transiently elevated in the supplemented group of animals; also, effects on acetylcholine-induced hindlimb conductance were transient, raising questions on the long-term benefit of dietary L-arginine in the prevention of atherosclerosis.

Previous studies have demonstrated that an intracoronary infusion of L-arginine normalizes the defective acetylcholine-induced vasodilation of coronary microvessels in patients with hypercholesterolemia[90] and in patients with microvascular angina pectoris[196] as well in those with atherosclerosis.[201] A later study by Lerman et al., in 1997,[154] examined the effects of 6 months of oral L-arginine supplementation (3 g tid). They demonstrated that the chronic oral L-arginine supplementation improved coronary small vessel endothelial function in association with a significant improvement in symptoms and a decrease in plasma endothelin concentrations. However, in a study by Blum et al.,[159] 30 patients with coronary artery disease on appropriate medical therapy were orally supplemented with 9 g/day for 1 month of L-arginine. This study concluded that chronic oral L-arginine supplementation does not improve NO bioavailability in this population of patients. Loscalzo and Walsh[47] comment on the discrepancy of Blum's study with previous studies showing beneficial effects of oral L-arginine (e.g., Lerman et al). Possible explanations, according to Loscalzo and Walsh, include limited cellular uptake, competitive inhibition of eNOS, or limited cofactor availability for eNOS.

Quyyumi recently examined the topic of stereospecificity and concluded that parenteral arginine produces non-stereospecific peripheral vasodilation and improves endothelium-dependent vasodilation in patients with stable coronary artery disease.[202]

Angiography and Stenting

With the increasing use of surgical intervention to treat coronary artery disease (PTCA, stenting, bypass), NO and NO donors have been investigated to evaluate their potential use in improving the immediate and long-term benefits of these procedures.

Inhaled NO—80 ppm continuously for 2 weeks—and FK 409, a new orally active NO donor [(±)-(E)-4-ethyl-2-hydroxyimino-5-nitro-3-hexenamide], have both been shown to decrease neointima proliferation following balloon injury of the rat carotid artery.[188,203] This effect is probably mediated by the inhibitory effects of NO on the proliferation[187,188,203,204] and migration[189] of vascular smooth muscle. Von der Leyen et al[204a] successfully employed an in vivo gene transfer method to transfect rat carotid arteries after balloon injury and found a 70% reduction of neointima formation 14 days after balloon injury.

The ACCORD study was a prospective, multicenter, randomized trial involving 700 stable patients with coronary artery disease who were scheduled for angioplasty. They were randomized to receive direct NO donors or diltiazem prior to and 6 months following the procedure. The study concluded that treatment with intravenous linsidomine followed by oral molsidomine (direct NO donors) was associated with a modest improvement on the long-term angiographic results after angioplasty but had no effect on clinical outcome.[205] The improvement in long-term angiographic result was due to a better immediate angiographic result that was not associated with an increase in periprocedural complications or more extensive late loss in luminal diameter. As for the ability for the NO donors to be effective in preventing restenosis, the restenosis rate seen was 38% in the NO donor group versus 46.5% in the diltiazem group ($P = .026$), which is not reduced compared to previous trials, where the restenosis rates ranged from 30 to 70%.

Mandinov et al. looked into the relationship of NO and coronary vasoconstriction seen in the distal vessel segment following PTCA.[206] They concluded that in patients with acute ischemia, the epicardial coronary arteries show an enhanced vasoconstriction after PTCA. Since the response to NTG is maintained, Mandinov et al. suggest that endothelial dysfunction rather than structural factors is likely to be the etiology of the vasoconstriction. However, Uren et al., in a small study of 10 patients, concluded that a reduced production or release of NO in the coronary circulation does not seem to be responsible for the impaired vasodilator response after angioplasty.[207] While the methods of these studies differed, it would seem that further investigation is warranted to determine whether NO and NO donors can play a beneficial effect in PTCA by reducing its adverse sequelae.

The most recent studies looking at NO and vascular smooth muscle proliferation are focusing on NO modulating expression of cell cycle regulatory proteins.[208–210] Most recently, Bohl and West described a polymeric biomaterial they developed that is capable of providing localized and sustained production of NO for the prevention of thrombosis and restenosis in vitro. By covalently incorporating NO donors into the biomaterial, they describe hours to months of NO production.[211] Whether this technology will have clinical benefits will have to be assessed in future clinical trials.

Myocardial Ischemia and Reperfusion Injury

Most studies agree on the role oxygen free radicals and cytokines play in contributing to myocardial ischemia and reperfusion injury (MIR). However, there is an ongoing debate over whether NO is beneficial or detrimental when used for MIR injury. Numerous experiments have shown that NO and NO donors are beneficial in decreasing MIR injury.[212–215]

Johnson et al.[216] studied the effect of direct NO supplementation on MIR. An intravenous solution of NO was infused after coronary occlusion and was continued during reperfusion. It was found that the area of myocardial necrosis was significantly reduced in the NO-treated cats and that these cats had fewer neutrophils in their necrotic areas than did the control animals. This study suggests that direct supplementation with NO may have a therapeutic role in MIR. However, authentic NO is difficult to use and can even be toxic in large doses[217]; consequently NO donors may be useful for NO supplementation.

Lefer et al.[218] tested this hypothesis with the use of SPM-5185, a cysteine-containing NO donor. It was found that NO supplementation reduced myocardial necrosis by 70% in areas of regional MIR (Fig. 33-12) and that the necrotic core of the control animals had 2.4 times more neutrophils per unit area than did that of the treated animals. SPM-5185 also was tested in experiments involving global MIR. After global ischemia and reperfusion, the experimental animals exhibited 95% recovery of contractile ability, whereas the control animals retained only approximately 40% of their previous contractile ability (Fig. 33-13). As with the regional MIR experiment, the NO-treated animals had a significant reduction in neutrophil activity.[218] The pirsidomine derivative C87-3754 has been used in the study of MIR. Compared to control, it was found that the same amount of myocardium was jeopardized in C873754-treated animals, yet less than half of the amount of necrotic injury that was seen in the control animals developed. In addition, in the experimental animals, neutrophil activity was significantly reduced.[90] Similar results were found by Masini et al. in a murine model. They report significant myocardial protection from ischemia/reperfusion (I/R) injury and histamine release with endogenous NO production as well as with NO donors (sodium nitroprusside, SIN-1, glyceryl trinitrate).[214] Furthermore, they report additional beneficial effects with infusion of superoxide dismutase (SOD) as well as an attenuation of histamine and LDH release with administration of L-arginine following NOS inhibitor infusion. More recently, Langford et al.[219] demonstrated persistent platelet activation in patients with acute myocardial infarction and unstable angina, which occurred in spite of treatment with aspirin, but platelet function was inhibited by intravenous glyceryl dinitrate and S-nitroso-glutathione, both NO donors and the latter possibly more platelet-specific.

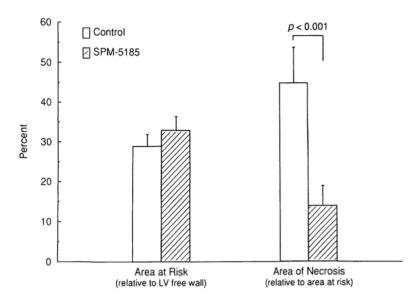

FIGURE 33-12. Myocardial area at risk and area of necrosis with use of NO donor SPM-5185 compared with placebo. Area at risk was approximately equivalent yet NO supplementation greatly reduced area of necrosis. LV = left ventricular. (*Reproduced with permission from Lefer at al.*[218])

The European Study for the Prevention of Infarct with Molsidomine (ESPRIM)[220] randomized 4017 patients with suspected acute myocardial infarction to intravenous linsidomine for 48 h followed by oral molsidomine for 12 days versus placebo in addition to conventional treatment including thrombolytic therapy. Unfortunately no reduction of all-cause 35-day mortality was found; also, long-term mortality (mean follow-up 13 months), major and minor adverse effects were similar in both groups. Randomization occurred on average 8 h after onset of symptoms, and 30% of all patients had received nitrates before, which, together with a lower than expected overall mortality rate, could have diluted any possible beneficial effect. Another speculative disadvantage may have been the above-mentioned superoxide anion cogeneration by sydnonimines,[133] which may antagonize NO and its effects.[27,221]

Grisham et al.[45] looked into the generation of superoxide anions with respect to simultaneous NO formation. Their review suggests that it is the concentrations of NO and O_2^- relative to each other that will determine whether there will be attenuation or enhancement of MIR injury. It is typically thought that the basal concentration of NO is high and has protective qualities, whereas, during an ischemic event, there is an increase in superoxide anions and free radicals, which increases the radical:NO ratio and results in a decrease in the protective qualities inherent to NO.

Therefore it is not surprising to find recent studies indicating that increased NO concentrations can contribute to MIR rather than inhibit it.[222–224] Hill et al.[223] examined the relation of NO concentrations and "overproduction" of NO seen with an increase in certain cytokines. They recognized the beneficial effects of NO in basal states but suggested that with the increases in TNF-alpha, IL-1, and endotoxin seen with cardiopulmonary bypass, there is an activation of iNOS, causing release of large amounts of NO, which may cause tissue injury.

Congestive Heart Failure

NO release has been shown to decrease tissue oxygen consumption in the failing myocardium.[224a] In addition, the ability of NO donors or activation of a local kinin system by amlodipine and ACE inhibitors, or a neutral endopeptidase inhibitor to release NO to lower myocardial oxygen demand suggests an additional cardioprotective

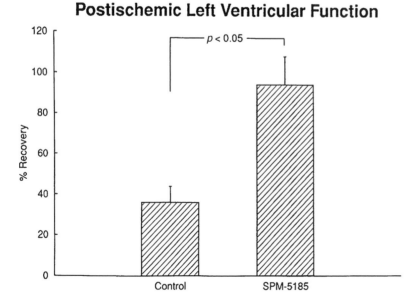

FIGURE 33-13. Postischemic global left ventricular function with use of NO donor SPM-5185 compared with placebo. (*Reproduced with permission from Lefer et al.*[218])

mechanism of NO, which may contribute to the beneficial effects currently used in the treatment of heart failure.

The use of inhaled NO (80 ppm) may not be advisable in patients with congestive heart failure due to left ventricular dysfunction, as it lowers pulmonary vascular resistance effectively and thereby increases the left ventricular filling pressure.[225] On the other hand, oral nitric oxide donors like the sydnonimines are known to decrease preload much as organic nitrates do.[183,226]

Concomitant ACE inhibitor therapy might be advisable to decrease activation of the renin-angiotensin system during long-term NO therapy.[131,183] In a recent nonrandomized, uncontrolled study, intravenous infusion of 20 g of L-arginine over 1 h in patients with congestive heart failure increased endogenous NO synthesis and appeared to transiently increase stroke volume and cardiac output without any change in heart rate, but with a decreased mean arterial pressure and systemic vascular resistance.[227] A randomized, double-blind, placebo-controlled crossover study of 6 weeks' oral supplementation with 5.6 to 12.6 g/day L-arginine in 15 patients with moderate to severe heart failure was quite encouraging.[228] The patients on L-arginine had a significantly increased forearm blood flow during forearm exercise but not in the basal state, an improved arterial compliance as assessed by pulse contour analysis, a significant fall of circulating plasma endothelin levels, some increased distances during a 6-min walk test, and better scores on a quality-of-life questionnaire.

Possible mechanisms for the beneficial effects of L-arginine supplementation are now under investigation. Recent studies have concluded that there may be a benefit to L-arginine supplementation in heart failure because of the existence of a variety of mechanisms by which L-arginine, NO, or NOS activity is decreased. These mechanisms include a decrease of in vitro and in vivo L-arginine transport,[229] decreased synthesis via a change in regulation or expression of eNOS, or a possible increase in plasma inhibitors of eNOS.[103]

However, in another double-blind study of 20 patients with class III to IV heart failure (and 7 healthy controls), 4 weeks of supplementation with 20 g/day of L-arginine versus placebo did not show any significant improvement of ACh-induced forearm blood flow and vascular resistance relative to basal blood flow and vascular resistance.[230] The increased distance on a 6-min walk test in this study did not achieve statistical significance. Prior et al. also demonstrated only a transient improvement to ACh-induced vasodilation with oral L-arginine.[231]

Further research and a larger study will be needed to assess the practical benefits and the mechanisms of L-arginine in patients with congestive heart failure.

Recently it was demonstrated that inhaled NO could improve gas exchange in patients with CHF, in contrast to other vasodilators, which can worsen oxygenation by creating ventilation/perfusion ($\dot{V}/\dot{Q}$) mismatches.[232] It has also been shown in patients with severe pressure-overload hypertrophy that intracoronary administration of NO donors exerts a marked decrease in left ventricular end-diastolic pressure without affecting left ventricular systolic pump function. Thus it appears that the hypertrophied myocardium is susceptible to NO donors with a marked improvement in diastolic function.

Splanchnic Ischemia and Reperfusion

As in the case of MIR, the splanchnic vasculature exhibits profound damage and subsequent systemic morbidity on reperfusion, in part because of low concentrations of NO. Madesh et al. demonstrated

that there is a component of splanchnic ischemia-reperfusion where structural and functional alterations of mitochondria are present. He additionally found that with the use of a NO donor these alterations may be attenuated.[233]

Lefer et al.[217] showed that cats without NO supplementation demonstrated a decrease in mean arterial pressure (MAP) and were dead after <2 h of reperfusion. However cats that received NO supplementation had a transient decrease in MAP with subsequent return of MAP to normal levels and increased survival. These observations were confirmed in a study by Schleiffer et al.[234] In addition, the biochemical markers of shock (plasma cathepsin D activity and plasma myocardial depressant factor) were increased with reperfusion; however, NO supplementation significantly attenuated the release of these molecules. Results of similar studies[235–238] correlate with the findings of Lefer et al.[217] In experimental animals, splanchnic ischemia and reperfusion without NO caused the animals to die after <60 min. However, NO infusion improved the survival time of the animals and attenuated the plasma activity of cathepsin D and myocardial depressant factor.[235]

Ischemic Arrhythmia

As discussed earlier, NO has a role in MIR injuries; NO supplementation reduces the damage associated with myocardial ischemia. NO supplementation might therefore reduce the incidence of arrhythmia caused by ischemia. Furthermore, the vasodilator and antiplatelet aggregatory properties of NO are very similar to properties of prostacyclin and adenosine, and these agents have demonstrated antiarrhythmic effects.[239,240] A 1983 study found that molsidomine (an NO donor) protects against ventricular fibrillation caused by MIR.[241] More recently, Gyorgi et al. demonstrated an increase in survival and a decrease in ectopic beats, ventricular tachycardia and ventricular fibrillation in dogs that received intracoronary nitrates before and during coronary artery occlusion.[242]

Wainwright and Martorana[243] recently studied the effect of pirsidomine on the incidence of ventricular arrhythmia and electrocardiographic changes. The animals treated with pirsidomine had a later onset of ectopic ventricular arrhythmia and a reduced total number of arrhythmias (Fig. 33-14). In addition, although ventricular fibrillation developed in all animals, pirsidomine delayed its onset. With initiation of ischemia, all animals demonstrated ST-segment depression. Pirsidomine had a normalizing effect on the ST segments, which showed a return to baseline; in the control animals, ST-segment depression was sustained.[240]

As with the other areas of investigation concerning NO, there is an increasing interest in the ability of L-arginine supplementation to reproduce the effects of NO or NO donors. Fei et al. examined the effects of intrapericardial delivery of L-arginine in dogs undergoing acute coronary occlusion with concomitant sympathetic stimulation.[244] They found that L-arginine supplementation was able to decrease the severity of ischemic ventricular arrhythmias. Tosaki et al. also demonstrated that MLA (monophosphoryl lipid A) is an inducer of iNOS.[245] They infused MLA into rats and found that, at a dosage of 450 μg, there was a decrease in ventricular fibrillation and ventricular tachycardia.

Pulmonary Hypertension

Because NO is the body's endogenous vasodilator, it could be supposed that NO supplementation would ameliorate pulmonary artery hypertension. However, systemic infusion of NO does not affect the pulmonary vasculature, since NO is inactivated by hemoglobin.

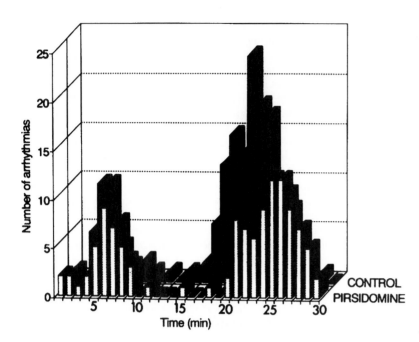

FIGURE 33-14. Distribution of arrhythmias during 30-min occlusion (open bars, control; solid bars, pirsidomine supplementation). Number of arrhythmias is decreased and onset is later with pirsidomine. (*Reproduced with permission from Wainwright and Martorana.*[243])

Inhalational NO on the other hand, offers an effective mode of NO delivery in this disease state.

Initial studies by Pepke-Zaba et al.[246] showed that in patients with pulmonary hypertension, inhalation of NO reduced pulmonary vascular resistance by approximately 30% from baseline values without affecting systemic vascular resistance. There is now evidence that in newborns with persistent pulmonary hypertension,[152,247–249] patients undergoing surgical correction of congenital heart disease,[154,250,251] patients experiencing pulmonary hypertension and hypoxemia following lung transplantation,[252–256] and in other settings in which pulmonary hypertension is present,[153] inhaled NO lowers pulmonary vascular resistance and may be of clinical benefit. In addition, NO inhalation immediately after mitral valve replacement has been shown to cause pulmonary artery vasodilation and hemodynamic improvement in patients with mild chronic pulmonary artery hypertension caused by mitral stenosis.[151,257] One promising use appears to be in the assessment of pulmonary vascular reactivity in patients with pulmonary hypertension.[170] Inhaled NO (10 to 40 ppm) was compared with prostacyclin in patients with primary pulmonary hypertension.[258] Inhaled NO has also demonstrated its usefulness in the assessment of reversibility of pulmonary hypertension in patients with chronic congestive heart failure.[259] Isolated reports have suggested that inhaled nitric oxide has also provided benefits in the management of end-stage primary pulmonary hypertension[260] and end-stage idiopathic pulmonary fibrosis.[261] Inhaled NO has also been shown to increase endothelin-1 levels, a potential cause of rebound pulmonary hypertension.[261a]

Several studies led to the conclusion that inhaled NO exerts the greatest benefit to gas exchange in the lung, from which the pathophysiology stems, primarily from intrapulmonary shunt [e.g., adult respiratory distress syndrome (ARDS)] rather than $\dot{V}/\dot{Q}$ mismatching, which occurs in COPD.[262,263] Because ARDS characteristically causes hypertension, pulmonary vasodilation from NO inhalation may improve gas exchange. It is postulated that blood flow to those regions with decreased ventilation produces areas of low $\dot{V}/\dot{Q}$ ratios. Admixture of blood perfusing low $\dot{V}/\dot{Q}$ regions with blood from areas with more normal $\dot{V}/\dot{Q}$ ratio creates hypoxemia.

The inhaled NO distributes preferentially to those areas with greater ventilation, stimulating localized vasodilation and enhanced blood flow to the well-ventilated lung units while simultaneously stealing perfusion from more poorly ventilated areas. In human trials, more than 30 studies have now reported the application of inhaled NO to patients with ARDS.[264] In general, however, these studies suggest that in the absence of sepsis, 60 to 80% of ARDS patients will respond to inhaled NO at doses of <20 ppm, exhibiting at least 20% increases in the ratio of PaO_2 to the fraction of inspired oxygen and 10 to 20% reductions in intrapulmonary right-to-left shunt or pulmonary artery pressure. Response rates in patients with septic ARDS have been variable, probably due to the concomitant administration of vasopressors that antagonize the vasodilatory effects of NO.[265,266] The duration of response to inhaled NO is controversial. Some studies have shown that prolonged inhalation of NO (>7 days) provided persistent improvements in oxygenation and pulmonary hemodynamics without evidence of tachyphylaxis,[267,268] although a recent randomized controlled trial demonstrated that such an effect was transient (<24 h).[269] Several multicenter trials have been initiated; these have shown no improvement in mortality in patients with ARDS receiving NO.[270–273] Some studies have looked at pulmonary vasoconstrictors,[274,275] phosphodiesterase inhibitors,[276,277] the use of PEEP,[278] prone position,[279] and permissive hypercapnia[280] to enhance the effects of inhaled NO in reducing pulmonary hypertension in patients with ARDS, emphasizing the fact that inhaled NO should be looked upon as a combined-modality treatment strategy in ARDS and not as a single agent. The inhaled NO may also contribute in ARDS through its anti-inflammatory[281,282] antiplatelet,[283] and antioxidant effects[284] and by decreasing capillary leak and improving the barrier function of the alveolar-capillary membrane.[285] Whether all the beneficial effects of nitric oxide will translate into improved patient outcomes will require carefully designed studies with rigorously selected patient populations.

In high-altitude pulmonary edema, nitric oxide inhalation (40 ppm for 15 min) has been shown to decrease the elevated pulmonary artery pressures and improve arterial oxygenation associated with a shift of blood flow from edematous to nonedematous lung segments.[286] Recent studies in murine models have shown that NO may have a role in therapy of massive pulmonary embolism.[287-289]

POTENTIAL ADVERSE EFFECTS OF NO

Under normal conditions, NO produced in low concentrations acts as a physiologic messenger and cytoprotective (antioxidant) factor through direct interactions with transition metals and other free radicals. Alternatively, when substantial amounts of NO are produced, the chemistry of NO will lead to the formation of dinitrogen trioxide and peroxynitrite. These reactive nitrogen molecules will, in turn, mediate both oxidative and nitrosative stresses, which are the pathologic basis for the cytoxicity attributed to NO in circulatory shock and ischemia-reperfusion injury.[290] In these conditions, the pharmacologic thrust has been to use inhibitors of both NO and the NOS.

CONCLUSION

NO has been shown to be a biologic substance important to normal physiologic functioning. It appears to be an endogenous vasodilator and is involved in hemostasis, inflammation, smooth muscle proliferation, apoptosis, angiogenesis, and wound healing. Endothelial cell dysfunction often leads to diminished NO production; this reduction in NO concentrations may be an etiologic factor in systemic hypertension, myocardial and splanchnic ischemia, atherosclerosis, CHF, and pulmonary vascular disease. The ongoing development of novel NO donors represents a prospective trend in the search for effective drugs. Future clinical studies will probably define additional strategies for manipulating the NO pathway in vivo because basic investigation continues to refine our understanding of nitric oxide biology.

REFERENCES

1. Alexander RW, Dzau VJ: Vascular biology. The past 50 years. *Circulation* 102:IV-112, 2000.
2. Culotta E, Koshland DE Jr: NO news is good news. *Science* 258:1862, 1992.
3. Furchgott RF, Zawadzki JV: The obligatory role of endothelial cells in the relaxation of arterial smooth muscle by acetylcholine. *Nature* 288:373, 1980.
4. Furchgott RF: Studies on relaxation of rabbit aorta by sodium nitrite: The basis for the proposal that acid-activatable inhibitory factor from bovine retractor penis is inorganic nitrite and the endothelium-derived relaxing factor. In: Vanhoutte P, ed. *Vasodilatation: Vascular Smooth Muscle, Peptides, Autonomic Nerves and Endothelium.* New York: Raven Press, 1988:401.
5. Ignarro LJ, Byrns RE, Buga GM, Wood KS: Endothelium-derived relaxing factor from pulmonary artery and vein possesses pharmacological and chemical properties identical to those of nitric oxide radical. *Circ Res* 61:866, 1987.
6. Palmer RMJ, Ferrige AG, Moncada S: Nitric oxide release accounts for the biological activity of endothelium derived relaxing factor. *Nature* 327:524, 1987.
7. Ignarro LJ, Buga GM, Woods KS, et al: Endothelium derived relaxation factor produced and released from artery and vein is nitric oxide. *Proc Natl Acad Sci U S A* 84:9265, 1987.
8. Jia L, Bonaventura J, Stamler JS: S-nitroshemoglobin: A dynamic activity of blood involved in vascular control. *Nature* 380:221, 1996.
9. Shen W, Hintze TH, Wolin MS: Nitric oxide. An important signaling mechanism between vascular endothelium and parenchymal cells in the regulation of oxygen consumption. *Circulation* 92:3505, 1995.

10. Moncada S, Palmer RMJ, Higgs EA: Nitric oxide: Physiology, pathophysiology, and pharmacology. *Pharmacol Rev* 43:109, 1991.
11. Schena M, Mulatero P, Schiavone D, et al: Vasoactive hormones induce nitric oxide synthase mRNA expression and nitric oxide production in human endothelial cells and monocytes. *Am J Hypertens* 12:388, 1999.
12. Tousoulis D, Tentolouris C, Crake T, et al: Effects of L- and D-arginine on the basal tone of human diseased coronary arteries and their responses to substance P. *Heart* 81:505, 1999.
13. Palmer RMJ, Ashton DS, Moncada S: Vascular endothelial cells synthesize nitric oxide from L-arginine. *Nature* 333:664, 1988.
14. Marletta MA : Nitric oxide: Biosynthesis and biological significance. *Trends Biochem Sci* 14:488, 1989.
15. Bredt DS, Snyder SH: Isolation of nitric oxide synthetase, a calmodulin-requiring enzyme. *Proc Natl Acad Sci U S A* 87:682, 1990.
16. Förstermann U, Nakane M, Tracey WR, Pollock JS: Isoforms of nitric oxide synthase: Functions in the cardiovascular system. *Eur Heart J* 14(Suppl 1):10, 1993.
17. Nathan C, Xie QW: Nitric oxide synthases: Roles, tolls, and controls. *Cell* 78:915, 1994.
18. Hattler BG, Oddis CV, Zeevi A, et al: Regulation of constitutive nitric oxide synthase activity by the human heart. *Am J Cardiol* 76:957, 1995.
19. Hare JM, Loh E, Creager MA, Colucci WS: Nitric oxide inhibits the positive inotropic response to β-adrenergic stimulation in humans with left ventricular dysfunction. *Circulation* 92:2198, 1995.
20. Mehta JL, Chen LY, Kone BC, et al: Identification of constitutive and inducible forms of nitric oxide synthase in human platelets. *J Lab Clin Med* 125:370, 1995.
21. Chen LY, Mehta P, Mehta JL: Oxidized LDL decreases L-arginine uptake and nitric oxide synthase protein expression in human platelets. *Circulation* 93:1740, 1996.
22. Cobb JP, Danner RL: Nitric oxide and septic shock. *JAMA* 275:1192, 1996.
23. Rapaport RM, Murad F: Agonist induced endothelium dependent relaxation in rat thoracic aorta may be mediated through cGMP. *Circ Res* 52:352, 1983.
24. Waldman SA, Murad F: Biochemical mechanisms underlying vascular smooth muscle relaxation: The guanylate cyclase cyclic GMP system. *J Cardiovasc Pharmacol* 12(suppl 5):S115, 1988.
25. Bolotina VM, Najibi S, Palacino JJ, et al: Nitric oxide directly activates calcium-dependent potassium channels in vascular smooth muscle. *Nature* 368:850, 1994.
26. Darley-Usmar V, Wiseman H, Halliwell B: Nitric oxide and oxygen radicals: A question of balance. *FEBS Lett* 369:131, 1995.
27. Keaney JF, Vita JA: Atherosclerosis, oxidative stress, and antioxidant protection in endothelium-derived relaxing factor action. *Prog Cardiovasc Dis* 38:129, 1995.
28. Rajagopalan S, Harrison DG: Reversing endothelial dysfunction with ACE inhibitors. A new trend? (editorial). *Circulation* 94:240, 1996.
29. Chu A, Chambers DE, Lin CC, et al: Effects of inhibition of nitric oxide formation on basal vasomotion and endothelium-dependent responses of the coronary arteries in awake dogs. *Clin Invest* 87:1964, 1991.
30. Moncada S, Higgs A: The L-arginine-nitric oxide pathway. *N Engl J Med* 329:2002, 1993.
31. Ignarro L J, Cirino G, Casini A, Napoli C: Nitric oxide as a signaling molecule in the vascular system: An overview. *J Cardiovasc Pharmacol* 34:879, 1999.
32. Maxwell A J, Cooke JP: Cardiovascular effects of L-arginine. *Curr Opin Nephrol Hypertens* 7:63, 1998.
33. Christou H, Adatia I, Van Marten LJ, et al: Effect of inhaled nitric oxide on endothelin-1 and cyclic guanosine 5′-monophosphate plasma concentrations in newborn infants with persistent pulmonary hypertension. *J Pediatr* 130:603, 1997.
34. Dellipizzi A, Nasjletti A: Involvement of nitric oxide and potassium channels in the reduction of basal tone produced by blockade of thromboxane A2/prostaglandin H2 receptors in aortic rings of hypertensive rats. *Clin Exp Hypertens* 20(8):903, 1998.
35. Wade ML, Fitzpatrick FA: Nitric oxide modulates the activity of the hemoproteins prostaglandin I2 synthase and thromboxane A2 synthase. *Arch Biochem Biophys* 347(2):174, 1997.

36. Chowdhary S, Vaile JC, Fletcher J, et al: Nitric oxide and cardiac autonomic control in humans. *Hypertension* 36:264, 2000.

37. Blackman DJ, Morris-Thurgood JA, Atherton JJ, et al: Endothelium-derived nitric oxide contributes to the regulation of venous tone in humans. *Circulation* 101:165, 2000.

38. Wilkinson IB, Qasem A, McEniery CM, et al: Nitric oxide regulates local arterial distensibility in vivo. *Circulation* 105:213, 2002.

39. Andrews NP, Husain M, Dakak N, Quyyumi AA: Platelet inhibitory effect of nitric oxide in the human coronary circulation: Impact of endothelial dysfunction. *J Am Coll Cardiol* 37:510, 2001.

40. Wang GR, Zhu Y, Halushka PV, et al: Mechanism of platelet inhibition by nitric oxide: In vivo phosphorylation of thromboxane receptor by cyclic GMP-dependent protein kinase. *Proc Natl Acad Sci U S A* 95(9):4888, 1998.

41. Bassenge E: Antiplatelet effects of endothelium derived relaxing factor and nitric oxide donors. *Eur Heart J* 12(Suppl E):5, 1991.

42. Radomski MW, Moncada S: The biological and pharmacological role of nitric oxide in platelet function. *Adv Exp Med Biol* 344:251, 1993.

43. Freedman JE, Loscalzo J, Barnard MR, et al: Nitric oxide released from activated platelets inhibits platelet recruitment. *J Clin Invest* 100:350, 1997.

44. Paul-Clark MJ, Gilroy DW, Willis D, et al: Nitric oxide synthase inhibitors have opposite effects on acute inflammation depending on their route of administration. *J Immunol* 166:1169, 2001.

45. Grisham MB, Granger DN, Neil D, Lefer DJ: Modulation of leukocyte-endothelial interactions by reactive metabolites of oxygen and nitrogen: Relevance to ischemic heart disease. *Free Radic Biol Med* 25:404, 1998.

46. Hierholzer C, Harbrecht B, Menezes JM, et al: Essential role of induced nitric oxide in the initiation of the inflammatory response after hemorrhagic shock. *J Exp Med* 187:917, 1998.

47. Loscalzo J, Walsh G: Nitric oxide and its role in the cardiovascular system. *Prog Cardiovasc Dis* 38:87, 1995.

48. Palombella VJ, Conner EM, Fuseler JW, et al: Role of the proteasome and NF-kB in streptococcal cell wall-induced polyarthritis. *Proc Natl Acad Sci U S A.* 95:15671, 1998.

49. Kubes P, Suzuki M, Granger DN: Nitric oxide an endogenous modulator of leukocyte adhesion. *Proc Natl Acad Sci USA* 88:4651, 1991.

50. Hickey MJ, Kubes P: Role of nitric oxide in regulation of leukocyte-endothelial cell interactions. *Exp Physiol* 82:339, 1997.

51. Granger DN, Kubes P: Nitric oxide as anti-inflammatory agent. *Methods Enzymol* 269:434, 1996.

52. Clancy RM, Leszczynska-Piziak J, Abramsom SB: Nitric oxide, an endothelial cell relaxation factor, inhibits neutrophil superoxide anion production via a direct action on the NADPH oxidase. *J Clin Invest* 90:1116, 1992.

53. Grisham MB, Jourd'Heuil D, Wink DA: Physiological chemistry of nitric oxide and its metabolites: Implications in inflammation. *Am J Physiol Gastrointest Liver Physiol* 276:G315, 1999.

54. Mooradian DL, Hutsell TC, Keefer LK: Nitric oxide (NO) donor molecules: Effect of NO release rate on vascular smooth muscle cell proliferation in vitro. *J Cardiovasc Pharmacol* 25:674, 1995.

55. Seki J, Nishio M, Kato Y, et al: FK 409, a new nitric-oxide donor, suppresses smooth muscle proliferation in the rat model of balloon angioplasty. *Atherosclerosis* 117:97, 1995.

56. Lee JS, Adrie C, Jacob HJ, et al: Chronic inhalation of nitric oxide inhibits neointimal formation after balloon-induced arterial injury. *Circ Res* 78:337, 1996.

57. Lincoln TM, Cornwell TL, Komalavilas P, Boerth N: Cyclic GMP-dependent protein kinase in nitric oxide signaling. *Methods Enzymol* 269:149, 1996.

58. Pinsky DJ, Aji W, Szabolcs M, et al: Nitric oxide triggers programmed cell death (apoptosis) of adult rat ventricular myocytes in culture. *Am J Physiol* 277:H1189, 1999.

59. Kim Y-M, Bombeck CA, Billiar TR: Nitric oxide as a bifunctional regulator of apoptosis. *Circ Res* 84:253, 1999.

59a. Gao F, Gao E, Yue T-L, et al: Nitric oxide mediates the antiapoptotic effect of insulin in myocardial ischemia-reperfusion. The roles of PI-3 kinase and endothelial nitric oxide synthase phosphorylation. *Circulation* 105:1497, 2002.

60. Lee PC, Salyapongse AN, Bragdon GA, et al: Impaired wound healing and angiogenesis in eNOS-deficient mice. *Am J Physiol* 277:H1600, 1999.

61. Frank S, Hubner G, Breier G, et al: Regulation of vascular endothelial growth factor expression in cultured keratinocytes. Implications for normal and impaired wound healing. *J Biol Chem* 270:12607, 1995.

62. Kullo IJ, Mozes G, Schwartz RS, et al: Enhanced endothelium-dependent relaxation after gene transfer of recombinant endothelial nitric oxide synthase to rabbit carotid arteries. *Hypertension* 30:314, 1997.

63. Thomas GD, Zhang W, Victor RG: Nitric oxide deficiency as a cause of clinical hypertension. Promising new drug targets for refractory hypertension. *JAMA* 285:2055, 2001.

64. Baylis C, Mitruka B, Deng A: Chronic blockade of nitric oxide synthesis in the rat produces systemic hypertension and glomerular damage. *J Clin Invest* 90:278, 1992.

65. Ribiero MO, Antunes E, Nucci GD, et al: Chronic inhibition of nitric oxide synthesis: A new model of arterial hypertension. *Hypertension* 20:298, 1992.

66. Panza JA, Quyyumi AA, Brush JE, Epstein SE: Abnormal endothelium dependent vascular relaxation in patients with essential hypertension. *N Engl J Med* 323:22, 1990.

67. Kojda G, Harrison D: Interactions between NO and reactive oxygen species: Pathophysiological importance in atherosclerosis, hypertension, diabetes and heart failure. *Cardiovasc Res* 43:562, 1999.

68. Kato N, Sugiyama T, Morita H, et al: Lack of evidence for association between the endothelial nitric oxide synthase gene and hypertension. *Hypertension* 33:933, 1999.

69. Arnal JF, Dinh-Xuan AT, Pueyo M, et al: Endothelium-derived nitric oxide and vascular physiology and pathology. *Cell Mol Life Sci* 55(8-9):1078, 1999.

70. Frishman WH: β-adrenergic blockers. In: Izzo JL Jr, Black HR (eds): *Hypertension Primer.* 3rd ed. Dallas: American Heart Association, in press.

71. Tsao S, Aoki N, Lefer DJ, et al: Time course of endothelial dysfunction and myocardial injury during myocardial ischemia and reperfusion in the cat. *Circulation* 82:1402, 1990.

72. Ambrosio G, Tritto I: Reperfusion injury: Experimental evidence and clinical implications. *Am Heart J* 138(2 Pt 2):S69, 1999.

73. Ma X, Weyrich AS, Lefer DJ, Lefer AM: Diminished basal nitric oxide release after myocardial ischemia and reperfusion promotes neutrophil adherence to coronary endothelium. *Circ Res* 72:403, 1993.

74. Vinten-Johansen J, Zhao ZQ, Nakamura M, et al: Nitric oxide and the vascular endothelium in myocardial ischemia-reperfusion injury. *Ann NY Acad Sci* 874(2 Pt 2): 354, 1999.

75. Kitakaze M, Node K, Minamino T, et al: Role of nitric oxide in regulation of coronary blood flow during myocardial ischemia in dogs. *J Am Coll Card* 27:1804, 1996.

76. Zweier JL, Samouilov A, Kuppusamy P: Non-enzymatic nitric oxide synthesis in biological systems. *Biochim Biophys Acta* 1411(2-3): 250, 1999.

77. Csonka C, Szilvassy Z, Fulop F, et al: Classic preconditioning decreases the harmful accumulation of nitric oxide during ischemia and reperfusion in rat hearts. *Circulation* 100:2260, 1999.

78. López-Farré A, Riesco A, Digiuni E, et al: Aspirin-stimulated nitric oxide production by neutrophils after acute myocardial ischemia in rabbits. *Circulation* 94:83, 1996.

79. Richard V, Kaeffer N, Tron C, Thuillez C: Ischemic preconditioning protects against coronary endothelial dysfunction induced by ischemia and reperfusion. *Circulation* 89:1254, 1994.

80. Bolli R: The late phase of preconditioning. *Circ Res* 87:972, 2000.

81. Kugiyama K, Yasue H, Okumura K, et al: Nitric oxide activity is deficient in spasm arteries of patients with coronary spastic angina. *Circulation* 94:266, 1996.

82. Ma XL, Johnson G 3rd, Lefer AM: Mechanisms of inhibition of nitric oxide production in a murine model of splanchnic artery occlusion shock. *Arch Intern Pharmacodyn Ther* 311:89, 1991.

83. Cuzzocrea S, Zingarelli B, Caputi AP: Role of constitutive nitric oxide synthase and peroxynitrite production in a rat model of splanchnic artery occlusion shock. *Life Sci* 63:789, 1998.

84. Nabel EG, Ganz P, Gordon JB, et al: Dilation of normal and constriction of atherosclerotic coronary arteries caused by the cold pressor test. *Circulation* 77:43, 1988.

85. Gage JE, Hess OM, Murakami T, et al: Vasoconstriction of stenotic coronary arteries during dynamic exercise in patients with classic angina pectoris: Reversibility by nitroglycerin. *Circulation* 73:865, 1986.

86. Gordon JB, Zebede J, Wayne RR, et al: Coronary constriction with exercise: Possible role for endothelial dysfunction and alpha tone (abstr). *Circulation* 74(Suppl 2):481, 1986.

87. Cox DA, Vita JA, Treasure CB, et al: Atherosclerosis impairs flow mediated dilation of coronary arteries in humans. *Circulation* 87:458, 1989.

88. Tentolouris C, Tousoulis D, Goumas G, et al: L-Arginine in coronary atherosclerosis. *Int J Cardiol* 75(2-3):123, 2000.

89. Wever R, Luscher T, Cosentino F, et al: Atherosclerosis and two faces of endothelial nitric oxide synthase. *Circulation* 97:108, 1998.

90. Drexler H, Zeiher AM, Meinzer K, Just H: Correction of endothelial dysfunction in coronary microcirculation of hypercholesterolemic patients by L-arginine. *Lancet* 338:1546, 1991.

91. Williams SB, Cusco JA, Roddy MA, et al: Impaired nitric oxide-mediated vasodilation in patients with non-insulin-dependent diabetes mellitus. *J Am Coll Cardiol* 27:567, 1996.

92. Vergnani L, Hatrik S, Ricci F, et al: Effect of native and oxidized low-density lipoprotein on endothelial nitric oxide and superoxide production. Key role of L-arginine availability. *Circulation* 101:1261, 2000.

93. Napoli C, Lerman LO: Involvement of oxidation-sensitive mechanisms in the cardiovascular effects of hypercholesterolemia. *Mayo Clin Proc* 76:619, 2001.

94. Ito A, Tsao PS, Adimoolam S, et al: Novel mechanism for endothelial dysfunction. Dysregulation of dimethylarginine dimethylaminohydrolase. *Circulation* 99:3092, 1999.

95. Liao JK, Shin WS, Lee WY, Clark SL: Oxidized low-density lipoprotein decreases the expression of endothelial nitric oxide synthase. *J Biol Chem* 270:319, 1995.

96. Jessup W: Oxidized lipoproteins and nitric oxide. *Curr Opin Lipidol* 7:274, 1996.

97. Patel R, Levonen A, Crawford J, et al: Mechanisms of the pro- and antioxidant actions of nitric oxide in atherosclerosis. *Cardiovasc Res* 47:465, 2000.

98. Dusting GJ, Fennessy P, Yin ZL, et al: Nitric oxide in atherosclerosis: Vascular protector or villain? *Clin Exp Pharmacol Physiol Suppl* 25:S34, 1998.

99. Miyazaki H, Matsuoka H, Cooke JP, et al: Endogenous nitric oxide synthase inhibitor. A novel marker of atherosclerosis. *Circulation* 99:1141, 1999.

100. Mital S, Zhang X, Zhao G, et al: Simvastatin upregulates coronary vascular endothelial nitric oxide production in conscious dogs. *Am J Physiol* 279:H2649, 2000.

101. Laufs U, Endres M, Custodis F, et al: Suppression of endothelial nitric oxide production after withdrawal of statin treatment is mediated by negative feedback regulation of Rho GTPase gene transcription. *Circulation* 102:3104, 2000.

102. Mohri M, Egashira K, Tagawa T, et al: Basal release of nitric oxide is decreased in the coronary circulation in patients with congestive heart failure. *Hypertension* 30:50, 1997.

103. Katz SD, Khan T, Zeballos GA, et al: Decreased activity of the L-arginine nitric oxide metabolic pathway in patients with congestive heart failure. *Circulation* 99:2113, 1999.

104. Drexler H: Nitric oxide synthases in the failing human heart. A double-edged sword? *Circulation* 99:2972, 1999.

105. Drexler H, Hayoz D, Münzel T, et al: Endothelial function in chronic congestive heart failure. *Am J Cardiol* 69:1596, 1992.

106. Kaiser L, Spickard RC, Olivier NB: Heart failure depresses endothelium dependent responses in canine femoral artery. *Am J Physiol* 256:H962, 1989.

107. Drexler H, Lu W: Endothelial dysfunction of hindquarter resistance vessels in experimental heart failure. *Am J Physiol* 262:H1640, 1992.

108. Habib F, Dutka D, Crossman D, et al: Enhanced basal nitric oxide production in heart failure: Another failed counter-regulatory vasodilator mechanism? *Lancet* 344:371, 1994.

109. Winlaw DS, Smythe GA, Keogh AM, et al: Increased nitric oxide production in heart failure. *Lancet* 345:390, 1994.

109a. Node K, Kitakaze M, Yoshihara F, et al: Increased cardiac levels of nitric oxide in patients with chronic heart failure. *Am J Cardiol* 86:474, 2000.

110. Haywood GA, Tsao PS, von der Leyen H, et al: Expression of inducible nitric oxide synthase in human heart failure. *Circulation* 93:1087, 1996.

111. Lewis NP, Tsao PS, Rickenbacher PR, et al: Induction of nitric oxide synthase in the human cardiac allograft is associated with contractile dysfunction of the left ventricle. *Circulation* 93:720, 1996.

111a. Gealekman O, Abassi Z, Rubinstein I, et al: Role of myocardial inducible nitric oxide synthase in contractile dysfunction and β-adrenergic hyporesponsiveness in rats with experimental volume-overload heart failure. *Circulation* 105:236, 2002.

112. Drexler H, Kastner S, Strobel A, et al: Expression, activity and functional significance of inducible nitric oxide synthase in the failing human heart. *J Am Coll Cardiol* 32:955, 1998.

113. Treasure CB, Vita JA, Cox DA, et al: Endothelium dependent dilation of the coronary microvasculature is impaired in dilated cardiomyopathy. *Circulation* 81:772, 1990.

114. Stamler JS, Loh E, Roddy MA, et al: Nitric oxide regulates basal systemic and pulmonary vascular resistance in healthy humans. *Circulation* 89:2035, 1994.

115. Blitzer M, Loh E, Roddy MA, et al: Endothelium-derived nitric oxide regulates systemic and pulmonary vascular resistance during acute hypoxia in humans. *J Am Coll Cardiol* 28:91, 1996.

116. Frostell C, Blomqvist H, Hedenstierna G, et al: Inhaled nitric oxide selectively reverses human hypoxic pulmonary vasoconstriction without causing systemic vasodilation. *Anesthesiology* 78:427, 1993.

117. Cheung PY, Salas E, Schulz R, et al: Nitric oxide and platelet function: Implications for neonatology. *Semin Perinatol* 21:409, 1997.

118. Hickey MJ, Kubes P: Role of nitric oxide in regulation of leukocyte-endothelial cell interactions. *Exp Physiol* 82:339, 1997.

119. Gaston B, Drazen J, Loscalzo J, et al: State of the art: The biology of nitrogen oxides in the airways. *Am J Respir Crit Care Med* 149:538, 1994.

120. Cooper CJ, Landzberg MJ, Anderson TJ, et al: Role of nitric oxide in the local regulation of pulmonary vascular resistance in humans. *Circulation* 93:266, 1996.

121. Giaid A, Saleh D: Reduced expression of endothelial nitric oxide synthase in the lungs of patients with pulmonary hypertension. *N Engl J Med* 333:214, 1995.

122. Adnot S, Ruffestin B, Eddahibi S, et al: Loss of endothelium relaxant activity in the pulmonary circulation of rats exposed to chronic hypoxemia. *J Clin Invest* 87:155, 1991.

123. Dihn-Xuan AT, Higenbottam TW, Clelland CA, et al: Impairment of endothelium dependent pulmonary artery relaxation in chronic obstructive lung disease. *N Engl J Med* 324:1539, 1991.

124. Warren JB, Maltby NH, MacCormack D, Barnes DJ: Pulmonary endothelium derived relaxing factor is impaired in hypoxia. *Clin Sci (Colch)* 77:671, 1989.

125. Mooradian DL, Hutsell TC, Keefer LK: Nitric oxide (NO) donor molecules: Effect of NO release rate on vascular smooth muscle cell proliferation in vitro. *J Cardiovasc Pharmacol* 25:674, 1995.

126. Ozaki M, Kawashima S, Yamashita T, et al: Reduced hypoxic pulmonary vascular remodeling by nitric oxide from the endothelium. *Hypertension* 37:322, 2001.

127. Horstman DJ, Frank DU, Rich GF: Prolonged inhaled NO attenuates hypoxic, but not monocrotaline-induced, pulmonary vascular remodeling in rats. *Anesth Analg* 86:74, 1998.

128. Hou YC, Janczuk A, Wang PG: Current trends in the development of nitric oxide donors. *Curr Pharm Des* 5:417, 1999.

129. Ignarro LJ, Gruetter CA: Requirements of thiol for activation of coronary arterial guanylate cyclase by glyceryl trinitrate and sodium nitrite: Possible involvement of s-nitrosothiols. *Biochim Biophys Acta* 631:221, 1980.

130. Boesgaard S, Aldershvile J, Poulsen HE, et al: Nitrate tolerance in vivo is not associated with depletion of arterial or venous thiol levels. *Circ Res* 74:115, 1994.

131. Münzel T, Kurz S, Heitzer T, Harrison DG: New insights into mechanisms underlying nitrate tolerance. *Am J Cardiol* 77:24C, 1996.

132. Bauer JA, Booth BP, Fung H-L: Nitric oxide donors: Biochemical pharmacology and therapeutics. In: Ignarro L, Murad F, eds. *Nitric Oxide: Biochemistry, Molecular Biology, and Therapeutic Implications.* New York: Academic Press, 1995:361.

133. Feelisch M: The biochemical pathways of nitric oxide formation from nitrovasodilators: Appropriate choice of exogenous NO donors and

aspects of preparation and handling of aqueous NO solutions. *J Cardiovasc Pharmacol* 17(suppl 3):S25, 1991.

134. Bate JN, Bake MT, Guerra R Jr, Harrison DG: Nitric oxide generation from nitroprusside by vascular tissue: Evidence that reduction of the nitroprusside anion and cyanide loss are required. *Biochem Pharmacol* 42:S157, 1991.

135. Michenfelder JD, Tinker JH: Cyanide toxicity and thiosulfate production during chronic administration of sodium nitroprusside in the dog: Correlation with a human case. *Anesthesiology* 47:441, 1977.

136. Brown GB, Bolson E, Petersen RB, et al: The mechanism of nitroglycerin action: Stenosis vasodilatation as a major component of drug response. *Circulation* 64:1089, 1981.

137. Belhassen L, Carville C, Pelle G, et al: Molsidomine improves flow-dependent vasodilation in brachial arteries of patients with coronary artery disease. *J Cardiovasc Pharmacol* 35:560, 2000.

138. Bohn H, Martorana PA, Schonafinger K: Cardiovascular events of the new NO donor, persidomine. Hemodynamic profile and tolerance studies in anesthetized and conscious dogs. *Eur J Pharmacol* 220:71, 1992.

139. Ferioli R, Folco GC, Ferretti C, et al: A new class of furoxan derivatives as NO donors: Mechanism of action and biological activity. *Br J Pharmacol* 114:816, 1995.

140. Hecker M, Vorhoff W, Bara AT, et al: Characterization of furoxans as a new class of tolerance-resistant nitrovasodilators. *Naunyn-Schmiedebergs Arch Pharmacol* 351:426, 1995.

141. Bohn H, Beyerle R, Martorana PA, Schonafinger X: CAS 936, a novel sydnonimine with direct vasodilating and nitric oxide-donating properties: Effects on isolated blood vessels. *J Cardiovasc Pharmacol* 18:522, 1991.

142. Stamler JS: S-nitrosothiols and the bioregulatory actions of nitrogen oxides through reactions with thiol groups. *Curr Top Microbiol Immunol* 196:16, 1995.

143. Arnelle DR, Stamler JS: NO^+, $NO^\bullet$, and NO^- donation by S-nitrosothiols: Implications for regulation of physiological functions by S-nitrosylation and acceleration of disulfide formation. *Arch Biochem Biophys* 318:279, 1995.

144. Xu I, Eu JP, Meissner G, Stamler JS: Activation of the cardiac calcium release channel (ryanodine receptor) by poly-S-nitrosylation. *Science* 279:234, 1998.

145. Loscalzo J, Smick D, Andon N, Cooke J: S-nitrosocaptopril. I. Molecular characterization and effects on the vasculature and/or platelets. *J Pharmacol Exp Ther* 249:726, 1989.

146. Morley D, Keefer LK: Nitric oxide/nucleophile complexes: A unique class of nitric oxide-based vasodilators. *J Cardiovasc Pharmacol* 22(Suppl 7):S3, 1993.

147. Vega JM, Garrett RH: Siroheme: A prosthetic group of the Neurospora crassa assimilatory nitrite reductase. *J Biol Chem* 250:7980, 1975.

148. Castillo L, DeRojas, TC, Chapman TE, et al: Splanchnic metabolism of dietary arginine in relation to nitric oxide synthesis in normal adult man. *Proc Natl Acad Sci U S A* 90:193, 1993.

149. Cannon RO III: Oral L-arginine (another active ingredient) for ischemic heart disease? *J Am Coll Cardiol* 39:46, 2002.

150. Blum A, Hathaway L, Mincemoyer R, et al: Effects of oral L-arginine on endothelium-dependent vasodilation and markers of inflammation in healthy postmenopausal women. *J Am Coll Cardiol* 35:271, 2000.

151. Bøttcher M, Bøtker HE, Sonne H, et al: Endothelium-dependent and -independent perfusion reserve and the effects of L-arginine on myocardial perfusion in patients with syndrome X. *Circulation* 99:1795, 1999.

152. Berkenboom G, Crasset V, Unger P, et al: Absence of L-arginine effect on coronary hypersensitivity to serotonin in cardiac transplant recipients. *Am J Cardiol* 84:1882, 1999.

153. Bode-Böger SM, Böger RH, Löffler M, et al: L-arginine stimulates NO-dependent vasodilation in healthy humans—effect of somatostatin pretreatment. *J Invest Med* 47:43, 1999.

154. Lerman A, Burnett JC Jr, Higano ST, et al: Long-term L-arginine supplementation improves small-vessel coronary endothelial function in humans. *Circulation* 97:2123, 1998.

155. Blum A, Porat R, Rosenschein U, et al: Clinical and inflammatory effects of dietary L-arginine in patients with intractable angina pectoris. *Am J Cardiol* 83:1488, 1999.

156. Campisi R, Czernin J, Schöder H, et al: L-arginine normalizes coronary vasomotion in long-term smokers. *Circulation* 99:491, 1999.

157. Siani A, Pagano E, Iacone R, et al: Blood pressure and metabolic changes during dietary L-arginine supplementation in humans. *Am J Hypertens* 13:547, 2000.

158. Kaposzta Z, Baskerville PA, Madge D, et al: L-arginine and S-nitroso-glutathione reduce embolization in humans. *Circulation* 103:2371, 2001.

159. Blum A, Hathaway L, Mincemoyer R, et al: Oral L-arginine in patients with coronary artery disease on medical management. *Circulation* 101:2160, 2000.

160. Gold, ME, Bush PA, Ignarro LJ: Depletion of arterial L-arginine causes reversible tolerance to endothelium dependent relaxation. *Biochem Biophys Res Commun* 164:714, 1989.

161. Arnal J-F, Münzel T, Venema RC, et al: Interactions between L-arginine and L-glutamine change endothelial NO production. *J Clin Invest* 95:2565, 1995.

162. Harrison DG: Cellular and molecular mechanisms of endothelial cell dysfunction. *J Clin Invest* 100:2153, 1997.

163. Wu G, Flynn NE, Flynn SP, et al: Dietary protein or arginine deficiency impairs constitutive and inducible nitric oxide synthesis by young rats. *J Nutr* 129:1347, 1999.

164. Ribiero AS, Roberts NB, Lane C, et al: Accumulation of the endogenous L-arginine analogue N^G-monomethyl-L-arginine in human end-stage renal failure patients on regular hemodialysis. *Exp Physiol* 81:475, 1996.

165. Mahoney PD, Loh E, Blitz LR, Herrmann HC: Hemodynamic effects of inhaled nitric oxide in women with mitral stenosis and pulmonary hypertension. *Am J Cardiol* 87:188, 2001.

166. Hoehn T, Krause MF: Response to inhaled nitric oxide in premature and term neonates. *Drugs* 61:27, 2001.

167. Krasuski RA, Warner JJ, Wang A, et al: Inhaled nitric oxide selectively dilates pulmonary vasculature in adult patients with pulmonary hypertension, irrespective of etiology. *J Am Coll Cardiol* 36:2204, 2000.

168. Miller OI, Tang SF, Keech A, et al: Inhaled nitric oxide and prevention of pulmonary hypertension after congenital heart surgery: A randomised double-blind study. *Lancet* 356:1464, 2000.

169. Fullerton DA, McIntyre RC Jr: Inhaled nitric oxide: Therapeutic applications in cardiothoracic surgery. *Ann Thorac Surg* 61:1856, 1996.

170. Atz AM, Adatia I, Lock JE, Wessel DL: Combined effects of nitric oxide and oxygen during acute pulmonary vasodilatory testing. *J Am Coll Cardiol* 33:813, 1999.

171. Gerlach H, Pappert D, Lewandowski K, et al: Long-term inhalation with evaluated low doses of nitric oxide for selective improvement of oxygenation in patients with adult respiratory syndrome. *Intens Care Med* 19:443, 1993.

172. Lavoie A, Hall J, Olson D, et al: Life-threatening effects of discontinuing inhaled nitric oxide in severe respiratory failure. *Am J Respir Crit Care Med* 153:1985, 1996.

173. Saavedra JE, Billiar TR, Williams DL, et al: Targeting nitric oxide delivery in vivo: Design of a liver selective NO donor prodrug that blocks tumor necrosis factor-α-induced apoptosis and toxicity in the liver. *J Med Chem* 40:1947, 1997.

174. Tzeng E, Shears LL, Robbins PD, et al: Vascular gene transfer of the human inducible nitric oxide synthase: Characterization of activity and effects on myointimal hyperplasia. *Mol Med* 2:211, 1996.

175. von der Leyen HE, Dzau VJ: Therapeutic potential of nitric oxide synthase gene manipulation. *Circulation* 103:2760, 2001.

176. Wallace JL, Elliott SN, Del Soldato P, et al: Gastrointestinal sparing anti-inflammatory drugs: The development of nitric oxide-releasing NSAIDs. *Drug Dev Res* 42:144, 1998.

177. Wallace JL, Reuter B, Cicala C, et al: Novel nonsteroidal anti-inflammatory drug derivatives with markedly reduced ulcerogenic properties in the rat. *Gastroenterology* 107:173, 1994.

178. Prasad A, Andrews NP, Padder FA, et al: Glutathione reverses endothelial dysfunction and improves nitric oxide bioavailability. *J Am Coll Cardiol* 34:507, 1999.

179. Cotter G, Kaluski E, Blatt A, et al: L-NMMA (a nitric oxide synthase inhibitor) is effective in the treatment of cardiogenic shock. *Circulation* 101:1358, 2000.

180. Wang D, Yang X-P, Liu Y-H, et al: Reduction of myocardial infarct size by inhibition of inducible nitric oxide synthase. *Am J Hypertens* 12:174, 1999.

181. Abrams J: Tolerance to organic nitrates. *Circulation* 74:1181, 1986.

182. Wagner F, Gohlke-Bärwolf C, Trenk D, et al: Differences in the antiischemic effects of molsidomine and isosorbide dinitrate (ISDN) during acute and short-term administration in stable angina pectoris. *Eur Heart J* 12:994, 1991.

183. Unger P, Vachiery J, de Cannière D, et al: Comparison of the hemodynamic responses to molsidomine and isosorbide dinitrate in congestive heart failure. *Am Heart J* 128:557, 1994.

184. Bassenge E, Zanzinger J: Effectiveness of an NO releasing pirsidomine derivative on coronary conductance during long term administration. *J Cardiovasc Pharmacol* 22(suppl 7):S22, 1993.

185. Stewart DJ, Holtz J, Bassenge E: Long-term nitroglycerin treatment: Effect on direct and endothelium-mediated large coronary artery dilation in conscious dogs. *Circulation* 75:847, 1987.

186. Drieu La Rochelle C, Dubois-Raude JC, Richard V, Hittinger L, et al: The role of NO release in the control of large and small coronary artery tone in conscious dogs. *J Cardiovasc Pharmacol* 22(Suppl 7):S17, 1993.

187. Mooradian DL, Hutsell TC, Keefer LK: Nitric oxide (NO) donor molecules: Effect of NO release rate on vascular smooth muscle cell proliferation in vitro. *J Cardiovasc Pharmacol* 25:674, 1995.

188. Seki J, Nishio M, Kato Y, et al: FK 409, a new nitric-oxide donor, suppresses smooth muscle proliferation in the rat model of balloon angioplasty. *Atherosclerosis* 117:97, 1995.

189. Sarkar R, Meinberg EG, Stanley JC, et al: Nitric oxide reversibly inhibits the migration of cultured vascular smooth muscle cells. *Circ Res* 78:225, 1996.

190. Neviere R, Guery B, Mordon S, et al: Inhaled NO reduces leukocyte-endothelial cell interactions and myocardial dysfunction in endotoxemic rats. *Am J Physiol* 278: H1783, 2000.

191. Gaboury JP, Niu X, Kubes P: Nitric oxide inhibits numerous features of mast cell-induced inflammation. *Circulation* 93:318, 1996.

192. Bult J, De Meyer GRY, Herman AG: Influence of chronic treatment with a nitric oxide donor on fatty streak development and reactivity of the rabbit aorta. *Br J Pharmacol* 114:1371, 1995.

193. Sutsch G, Kim JH, Bracht C, Kiowski W: Lack of cross-tolerance to short-term linsidomine in forearm resistance vessels and dorsal hand veins in subjects with nitroglycerin tolerance. *Clin Pharmacol Ther* 62(5):538, 1997.

194. Lehmann G, Hahnel I, Reiniger G, et al: Infusions with molsidomine and isosorbide-5-mononitrate in congestive heart failure: Mechanisms underlying attenuation of effects. *J Cardiovasc Pharmacol* 31:212, 1998.

195. Messin R, Karpov Y, Baikova N, et al: Short- and long-term effects of molsidomine retard and molsidomine non-retard on exercise capacity and clinical status in patients with stable angina: A multicenter randomized double-blind crossover placebo-controlled trial. *J Cardiovasc Pharmacol* 31:271, 1998.

196. Egashira K, Hirooka Y, Kuga T, et al: Effects of L-arginine supplementation on endothelium-dependent coronary vasodilation in patients with angina pectoris and normal coronary angiograms. *Circulation* 94:130, 1996.

197. Hirooka Y, Egashira K, Imaizumi T, et al: Effect of L-arginine on acetylcholine-induced endothelium-dependent vasodilation differs between the coronary and forearm vasculatures in humans. *J Am Coll Cardiol* 24:948, 1994.

198. Stewart DJ, Holtz J, Bassenge E: Long-term nitroglycerin treatment: Effect on direct and endothelium-mediated large coronary artery dilation in conscious dogs. *Circulation* 75:847, 1987.

199. Candipan RC, Wang B, Buitrago R, et al: Regression or progression. Dependency on vascular nitric oxide. *Arteriothromb Vasc Biol* 16:44, 1996.

200. Jeremy RW, McCarron J, Sullivan D: Effects of dietary L-arginine on atherosclerosis and endothelium-dependent vasodilation in the hypercholesterolemic rabbit. *Circulation* 94:498, 1996.

201. Quyyumi A, Dakak N, Diodati J, et al: Effect of L-arginine on human coronary endothelium-dependent and physiologic vasodilation. *J Am Coll Cardiol* 30(5):1220, 1997.

202. Quyyumi A: Does acute improvement of endothelial dysfunction in coronary artery disease improve myocardial ischemia? A double-blind comparison of parenteral D- and L-arginine. *J Am Coll Cardiol* 32(4):904, 1998.

203. Lee JS, Adrie C, Jacob HJ, et al: Chronic inhalation of nitric oxide inhibits neointimal formation after balloon-induced arterial injury. *Circ Res* 78:337, 1996.

204. LeTourneau T, Van Belle E, Corseaux D, et al: Role of nitric oxide in restenosis after experimental balloon angioplasty in the hypercholesterolemic rabbit: Effects on neointimal hyperplasia and vascular remodeling. *J Am Coll Cardiol* 33:876, 1999.

204a. Von der Leyen HE, Gibbons GH, Morishita R, et al: Gene therapy inhibiting neointimal vascular lesion: In vivo transfer of endothelial cell nitric oxide synthase gene. *Proc Natl Acad Sci U S A* 92:1137, 1995.

205. Lablanche J, Grollier G, Lusson J, et al: Effect of the direct nitric oxide donors linsidomine and molsidomine on angiographic restenosis after coronary balloon angioplasty. The ACCORD Study. *Circulation* 95(1):83, 1997.

206. Mandinov L, Kaufmann P, Eberli F, Hess OM: Enhanced coroncary vasoconstriction after PTCA in patients with ischemia. *Basic Res Cardiol* 93(Suppl 3):44, 1998.

207. Uren N, Crake T, Lefroy D, et al: Altered resistive vessel function after coronary angioplasty is not due to reduced production of nitric oxide. *Cardiovasc Res* 32:1108, 1996.

208. Sandirasegarane L, Charles R, Bourbon N, Kester M: NO regulates PDGF-induced activation of PKB but not ERK in A7r5 cells: Implication for vascular growth arrest. *Am J Physiol Cell Physiol* 279(1):C225, 2000.

209. Kibbe MR, Li J, Nie S, et al: Inducible nitric oxide synthase (iNOS) expression upregulates p21 and inhibits vascular smooth muscle cell proliferation through p42/44 mitogen-activated protein kinase activation and independent of p53 and cyclic guanosine monophosphate. *J Vasc Surg* 31(6):1214, 2000.

210. Tanner FC, Meier P, Greutert H, et al: Nitric oxide modulates expression of cell cycle regulatory proteins: A cytostatic strategy for inhibition of human vascular smooth muscle cell proliferation. *Circulation* 101(16):1982, 2000.

211. Bohl KS, West JL: Nitric oxide-generating polymers reduce platelet adhesion and smooth muscle cell proliferation. *Biomaterials* 21(22):2273, 2000.

212. Jordan JE, Zhao Z-Q, Vinten-Johansen J: The role of neutrophils in myocardial ischemia-reperfusion injury. *Cardiovasc Res* 43(4):860, 1999.

213. Vinten-Johnsen J, Zhao ZQ, Nakamura M, et al: Nitric oxide and the vascular endothelium in myocardial ischemia-reperfusion injury. *Ann NY Acad Sci* 874:354, 1999.

214. Masini E, Salvemini D, Ndisang JF, et al: Cardioprotective activity of endogenous and exogenous nitric oxide on ischaemia reperfusion injury in isolated guinea pig hearts. *Inflamm Res* 48:561-568, 1999.

215. Massoudy P, Zahler S, Barankay A, et al: Sodium nitroprusside during coronary artery bypass grafting: Evidence for an antiinflammatory action. *Ann Thorac Surg* 67(4):1059, 1999.

216. Johnson G III, Tsao PS, Lefer AM: Cardioprotective effects of authentic nitric oxide in myocardial ischemia with reperfusion. *Crit Care Med* 19:244, 1991.

217. Lefer AM, Siegfried MR, Ma XL: Protection of ischemia-reperfusion injury by sydnonimine NO donors via inhibition of neutrophil-endothelium interaction. *J Cardiovasc Pharmacol* 22(suppl 7):S27, 1993.

218. Lefer DJ, Nakanishi K, Vinten-Johansen J: Endothelial and myocardial cell protection by a cysteine-containing nitric oxide donor after myocardial ischemia and reperfusion. *J Cardiovasc Pharmacol* 22(suppl 7):S34, 1993.

219. Langford EJ, Wainwright RJ, Martin JF: Platelet activation in acute myocardial infarction and unstable angina is inhibited by nitric oxide donors. *Arterioscler Thromb Vasc Biol* 16:51, 1996.

220. European Study of Prevention of Infarct with Molsidomine (ESPRIM) group: The ESPRIM trial: Short-term treatment of acute myocardial infarction with molsidomine. *Lancet* 344:91, 1994.

221. Darley-Usmar V, Wiseman H, Halliwell B: Nitric oxide and oxygen radicals: A question of balance. *FEBS Lett* 369:131, 1995.

222. Ambrosio G, Tritto I: Reperfusion injury: Experimental evidence and clinical implications. *Am Heart J* 138(2 Pt 2):S69, 1999.

223. Hill GE: Cardiopulmonary bypass-induced inflammation: Is it important? *J Cardiothorac Vasc Anesth* 12(2 Suppl 1):21, 1998.

224. Ferrari R, Agnoletti L, Comini L, et al: Oxidative stress during myocardial ischaemia and heart failure. *Eur Heart J* 19(Suppl B):B2, 1998.

224a. Loke KE, Laycock SK, Mital S, et al: Nitric oxide modulates mitochondrial respiration in failing human heart. *Circulation* 100:1291, 1999.

225. Loh E, Stamler JS, Hare JM, et al: Cardiovascular effects of inhaled nitric oxide in patients with left ventricular dysfunction. *Circulation* 90:2780, 1994.

226. Stengele E, Ruf G, Jähnchen E, et al: Short-term hemodynamic and antianginal effects of pirsidomine, a new sydnonimine. *Am J Cardiol* 77:937, 1996.

227. Koifman B, Wollman Y, Bogomolny N, et al: Improvement of cardiac performance by intravenous infusion of L-arginine in patients with moderate congestive heart failure. *J Am Coll Cardiol* 26:1251, 1995.

228. Rector TS, Bank AJ, Mullen KA, et al: Randomized, double-blind, placebo-controlled study of supplemental oral L-arginine in patients with heart failure. *Circulation* 93:2135, 1996.

229. Kaye DM, Ahlers BA, Autelitano DJ, et al: In vivo and in vitro evidence for impaired arginine transport in human heart failure. *Circulation* 102:2707, 2000.

230. Chin-Dusting JPF, Kaye DM, Lefkovits J, et al: Dietary supplementation with L-arginine fails to restore endothelial function in forearm resistance arteries with severe heart failure. *J Am Coll Cardiol* 27:1207, 1996.

231. Prior DL, Jennings GLR, Chin-Dusting JP: Transient improvement of acetylcholine responses after short-term oral L-arginine in forearms of human heart failure. *J Cardiovasc Pharmacol* 36(1):31, 2000.

232. Matsumoto A, Momomura S, Sugiura S, et al: Effect of inhaled nitric oxide on gas exchange in patients with congestive heart failure. A randomized, controlled trial. *Ann Intern Med* 130:40, 1999.

233. Madesh M, Ramachandran A, Pulimood A, Vadranam M: Attenuation of intestinal ischemia/reperfusion injury with sodium nitroprusside: Studies on mitochondrial function and lipid changes. *Biochim Biophys Acta* 1500(2):204, 2000.

234. Schleiffer R, Raul F: Prophylactic administration of L-arginine improves the intestinal barrier function after mesenteric ischaemia. *Gut* 39(2):194, 1996.

235. Aoki N, Johnson G III, Lefer AM: Beneficial effects of two forms of NO administration in feline splanchnic artery occlusion shock. *Am J Physiol* 258:G275, 1990.

236. Haklar G, Ulukaya-Durakbasa C, Yuksel M, et al: Oxygen radicals and nitric oxide in rat mesenteric ischaemia-reperfusion: Modulation by L-arginine and NG-nitro-L-arginine methyl ester. *Clin Exp Pharmacol Physiol* 25(11):908, 1998.

237. Kubes P, Sihota E, Hickey MJ: Endogenous but not exogenous nitric oxide decreases TNF-alpha-induced leukocyte rolling. *Am J Physiol* 273(3 Pt 1):G628, 1997.

238. Lefer AM, Lefer DJ: The role of nitric oxide and cell adhesion molecules on the microcirculation in ischaemia-reperfusion. *Cardiovasc Res* 32(4):743, 1996.

239. Coker SJ, Parratt JR: Prostacyclin: Antiarrhythmic or arrhythmogenic? Comparison of the effects of intravenous and intracoronary prostacyclin and ZK36374 during coronary artery occlusion and reperfusion in anaesthetized greyhounds. *J Cardiovasc Pharmacol* 5:557, 1983.

240. Wainwright CL, Parrat JR: An antiarrhythmic effect of adenosine during myocardial ischemia and reperfusion. *Eur J Pharmacol* 146:183, 1988.

241. Martorana PA, Mogilev AM, Kettenbach B, Nitz R-E: Effect of molsidomine on spontaneous ventricular fibrillation following myocardial ischemia and reperfusion in the dog. *Adv Myocardiol* 4:606, 1983.

242. Gyorgy K, Vegh A, Rastegar MA, et al: Isosorbide-2-mononitrate reduces the consequences of myocardial ischaemia, including arrhythmia severity: Implications for preconditioning. *Cardiovasc Drugs Ther* 14(5):481, 2000.

243. Wainwright CL, Martorana PA: Pirsidomine, a novel nitric oxide donor, suppresses ischemic arrhythmias in anesthetized pigs. *J Cardiovasc Pharmacol* 22(suppl 7):S44, 1993.

244. Fei L, Baron AD, Henry DP, Zipes DP: Intrapericardial delivery of L-arginine reduces the increased severity of ventricular arrhythmias during sympathetic stimulation in dogs with acute coronary occlusion: Nitric oxide modulates sympathetic effects on ventricular electrophysiological properties. *Circulation* 96(11):4044, 1997.

245. Tosaki A, Maulik N, Elliott GT, et al: Preconditioning of rat heart with monophosphoryl lipid A: A role for nitric oxide. *J Pharmacol Exp Ther* 285(3):1274, 1998.

246. Pepke-Zaba J, Higenbottam TW, Dinh-Xuan AT, et al: Inhaled nitric oxide as a cause of selective pulmonary vasodilation in pulmonary hypertension. *Lancet* 338:1173, 1991.

247. Kinsella JP, Neish SR, Shaffer E, Abman SH: Low-dose inhalational nitric oxide in persistent pulmonary hypertension of the newborn. *Lancet* 340:819, 1992.

248. Betit P, Thompson J: Inhaled nitric oxide in the management of cardiopulmonary disorders in infants and children. *Respir Care Clin North Am* 3:459, 1997.

249. Upanemunda RH: Current status of inhaled nitric oxide therapy in the perinatal period. *Early Hum Dev* 47:247, 1997.

250. Robert JD Jr, Lang P, Bigatello LM, et al: Inhaled nitric oxide in congenital heart disease. *Circulation* 87:447, 1993.

251. Tworetzky W, Bristow J, Moore P, et al: Inhaled nitric oxide in neonates with persistent pulmonary hypertension. *Lancet* 357:118, 2001.

252. Adatia I, Lillehei C, Arnold JH, et al: Inhaled nitric oxide in the treatment of postoperative graft dysfunction after lung transplantation. *Ann Thorac Surg* 57:1311, 1994.

253. Fugino S, Nagahiro I, Triantafillou AN, et al: Inhaled nitric oxide at the time of harvest improves early lung allograft function. *Ann Thorac Surg* 63:1383, 1997.

254. Bhabra MS, Hopkinson DN, Shaw TE, et al: Low-dose nitric oxide inhalation during initial reperfusion enhances rat lung graft function. *Ann Thorac Surg* 63:339, 1997.

255. Date H, Triantafillou AN, Trulock EP, et al: Inhaled nitric oxide reduces human lung allograft dysfunction. *J Thorac Cardiovasc Surg* 111:913, 1996.

256. Meyer KC, Love RB, Zimmerman JJ: The therapeutic potential of nitric oxide in lung transplantation. *Chest* 113:1360, 1998.

257. Girard C, Lehot JJ, Pannetier JC, et al: Inhaled nitric oxide after mitral valve replacement in patients with chronic pulmonary artery hypertension. *Anesthesiology* 77:880, 1992.

258. Inhaled nitric oxide as a screening agent in primary pulmonary hypertension: A dose-response study and comparison with prostacyclin. *Am J Respir Crit Care Med* 151:384, 1995.

259. Semigran M, Cockrill B, Kacmarek R, et al: Hemodynamic effects of inhaled nitric oxide in heart failure. *J Am Coll Cardiol* 24:982, 1994.

260. Snell G, Salmonsen R, Bergin P, et al: Inhaled nitric oxide used as a bridge to heart-lung transplantation in a patient with end-stage pulmonary hypertension. *Am J Respir Crit Care Med* 151:1263, 1995.

261. Channick R, Hoch R, Newhart J, et al: Improvement in pulmonary hypertension and hypoxemia during nitric oxide inhalation in a patient with end-stage pulmonary fibrosis. *Am J Respir Crit Care Med* 149:811, 1994.

261a. Pearl JM, Nelson DP, Raake JL, et al: Inhaled nitric oxide increases endothelin-1 levels: A potential cause of rebound pulmonary hypertension *Crit Care Med* 30:89, 2002.

262. Sanna A, Kurtansky, A, Veriter C, et al: Bronchodilator effect of inhaled nitric oxide in healthy men. *Am J Respir Crit Care Med* 150:1702, 1994.

263. Barbera JA, Roger N, Roca J, et al: Worsening of pulmonary gas exchange with nitric oxide inhalation in chronic obstructive pulmonary disease. *Lancet* 347:436, 1996.

264. Troncy E, Francoeur M, Blaise G: Inhaled nitric oxide: Clinical applications, indications, and toxicology. *Can J Anaesth* 44:973, 1997.

265. Krafft P, Fridrich P, Fitzgerald RD, et al: Effectiveness of nitric oxide inhalation in septic ARDS. *Chest* 109:486, 1996.

266. Manktelow C, Bigatello LM, Hess D, et al: Physiological determinants of the response to inhaled nitric oxide in patients with acute respiratory distress syndrome. *Anesthesiology* 87:297, 1997.

267. Bigatello LM, Hurford WE, Kacmarek RM, et al: Prolonged inhalation of low concentrations of nitric oxide in patients with severe adult respiratory distress syndrome: Effects on pulmonary hemodynamics and oxygenation. *Anesthesiology* 80:761, 1994.

268. Rossaint R, Falke KJ, Lopez F, et al: Inhaled NO for the adult respiratory distress syndrome. *N Engl J Med* 328:399, 1993.

269. Michael JR, Barton RG, Saffl, JR, et al: Inhaled nitric oxide versus conventional therapy: Effect on oxygenation in ARDS. *Am J Respir Crit Care Med* 157:1372, 1998.

270. Dellinger RP, Zimmerman JL, Taylor RW, et al: Effects of inhaled nitric oxide in patients with acute respiratory distress syndrome: Results of a randomized phase II trial. *Crit Care Med* 26:15, 1998.

271. Groupe d'etude sur le NO inhale' au cours de l'ARDS. Inhaled NO in ARDS: Presentation of a double blind randomized multicentric study (abstr). *Am J Respir Crit Care Med* 153:A590, 1996.

272. Lundin S, Mang H, Smithies M, et al: Inhalation of nitric oxide in acute lung injury: Preliminary results of a European multicenter study (abstr). *Intens Care Med* 23(Suppl 1):S2, 1997.

273. Schwebel C, Beure, P Perdrix JP, et al: Early nitric oxide inhalation in acute lung injury: Results of a double-blind randomized study. (abstr) *Intens Care Med* 23(Suppl 1):S2, 1997.

274. Lu Q, Mourgeon E, Law-Koune J, et al: Dose-response curves of inhaled nitric oxide with and without intravenous almitrine in nitric oxide responding patients with acute respiratory distress syndrome. *Anesthesiology* 83:929, 1995.

275. Wysocki M, Delclaux C, Roupie E, et al: Additive effect on gas exchange of inhaled nitric oxide and intravenous almitrine bismesylate in the adult respiratory distress syndrome. *Int Crit Care Med* 20:2254, 1994.

276. Kinsella JP, Torielli F, Ziegler JW, et al: Dipyridamole augmentation of response to nitric oxide. *Lancet* 346:647, 1995.

277. Ichinose F, Adrie C, Hurford WE, et al: Prolonged pulmonary vasodilator action of inhaled nitric oxide by zaprinast in awake lambs. *J Appl Physiol* 78:1288, 1995.

278. Puybasset L, Rouby J, Mourgeon E, et al: Factors influencing the cardiopulmonary effects of inhaled nitric oxide in acute respiratory failure. *Am J Respir Crit Care Med* 152:318, 1995.

279. Papazian L, Bregeon F, Gaillat F, et al: Respective and combined effects of prone position and inhaled nitric oxide in patients with acute respiratory distress syndrome. *Am J Respir Crit Care Med* 157:580, 1998.

280. Puybasset L, Stewart T, Rouby J, et al: Inhaled nitric oxide reverses the increase in pulmonary vascular resistance induced by permissive hypercapnia in patients with ARDS. *Anesthesiology* 80:1254, 1994.

281. Bloomfield GL, Holloway S, Ridings PC, et al: Pretreatment with inhaled nitric oxide inhibits neutrophil migration and oxidative activity resulting in attenuated sepsis-induced acute lung injury. *Crit Care Med* 25:584, 1997.

282. Chollet-Martin S, Gatacel C, Kermarrec N, et al: Alveolar neutrophil functions and cytokine levels in patients with adult respiratory distress syndrome during nitric oxide inhalation. *Am J Respir Crit Care Med* 153:985, 1996.

283. Samama CM, Diaby M, Fellahi JL, et al: Inhibition of platelet aggregation by inhaled nitric oxide in patients with acute respiratory distress syndrome. *Anesthesiology* 83:56, 1995.

284. Rubbo H, Darley-Usmar V, Freeman BA: Nitric oxide regulation of tissue free radical injury. *Chem Res Toxicol* 9:809, 1996.

285. Benzing A, Brautigam P, Geiger K, et al: Inhaled nitric oxide reduces pulmonary transvascular albumin flux in patients with acute lung injury. *Anesthesiology* 83:1153, 1995.

286. Scherrer U, Vollenweider L, Delabays A, et al: Inhaled nitric oxide for high-altitude pulmonary edema. *N Engl J Med* 334:624, 1996.

287. Tanus-Santos JE, Moreno H Jr, Moreno RA, et al: Inhaled nitric oxide improves hemodynamics during a venous air infusion (VAI) in dogs. *Intens Care Med* 25:983, 1999.

288. Dschietzig T, Laule M, Alexiou K, et al: Coronary constriction and consequent cardiodepression in pulmonary embolism are mediated by pulmonary big endothelin and enhanced in early endothelial dysfunction. *Crit Care Med* 26:510, 1998.

289. Tanus-Santos JE, Gordo WM, Udelsmann A, et al: Nonselective endothelin-receptor antagonism attenuates hemodynamic changes after massive pulmonary air embolism in dogs. *Chest* 118:175, 2000.

290. Liaudet L, Garcia Soriano F, Szabo C: Biology of nitric oxide signaling. *Crit Care Med* 28(Suppl):N37, 2000.

Specific Inhibitors of Renin in Cardiac Therapy

William H. Frishman

Michael H. Shanik

Cherry Lin

The renin-angiotensin system (RAS) functions as a primary regulator in the physiologic control of blood pressure and fluid volume. Angiotensin converting enzyme (ACE) inhibitors (see Chap. 10) have been successfully studied and utilized effectively in treating systemic hypertension and congestive heart failure.[1] Recent studies have shown that ACE inhibitors are effective in reducing the risk of cardiovascular death, myocardial infarction, and stroke in patients at high risk for cardiovascular events but without left ventricular dysfunction or heart failure.[2] However, long-term treatment with ACE inhibitors does not completely suppress the circulatory RAS, as plasma angiotensin II (A-II) and aldosterone levels tend to return toward pretreatment levels. Theories have evolved in an attempt to explain the higher than expected levels of A-II and aldosterone despite continued ACE inhibitor treatment. It has been suggested that A-II is produced via pathways that do not employ ACE. Studies have demonstrated that there are other enzymes involved in the formation of A-II. Urata et al.[3] identified a chymostatin-sensitive pathway for conversion of A-I to A-II in the human heart. Other studies have also demonstrated alternate pathways of A-II formation. Okunishi et al.[4] found that a unique enzyme known as CAGE (chymostatin-sensitive A-II generating enzyme) was responsible for converting A-I to A-II. A series of studies in healthy human patients measured the change in renal blood flow in response to three ACE inhibitors at maximum doses, three angiotensin receptor blockers (ARBs), or two renin inhibitors. A meta-analysis demonstrated that the ARBs and renin inhibitors had comparable renal vascular responses that were substantially greater than the response from ACE inhibitors[5] (Fig. 34-1). This significant observation demonstrates a renin-dependent but ACE-independent pathway for A-II generation. Renin inhibitor peptide was found to be more effective than ACE inhibition in blocking A-II formation,[6] thus supporting this idea. The implications for therapeutics are important; if it is the A-II that is responsible for tissue destruction, renin inhibition might provide greater efficacy than ACE inhibition. Furthermore, the protussive agent bradykinin and the vasoconstricting agent substance P, which are normally degraded by ACE, accumulate when the enzyme is inhibited. This may be related to the side effects observed with all ACE inhibitors, which include the occasional case of angioneurotic edema and the more frequent occurrence of cough. This chapter reviews the development of a more specific form of therapy for cardiovascular disease—renin inhibition.

THE RENIN-ANGIOTENSIN SYSTEM

Synthesis of renin begins with the formation of preprorenin, which is cleaved during translation to prorenin by removal of a 23–amino acid signal peptide.[7,8] A 43–amino acid prosegment is removed from prorenin to produce renin, which is packed for storage and release. Some prorenin is directly released into the circulation. Prorenin and renin are stored in granules in the juxtaglomerular cells in the macula densa, located in the nephron's distal tubules. Both prorenin and renin are released from the storage granules in response to a reduction in glomerular afferent arteriolar blood pressure, sympathetic nerve stimulation, or a reduced rate of sodium ion delivery to the distal tubules. There might not be a direct active translocation of renin storage granules but rather a swelling of the granules lying alongside the plasma membrane.[9] The swelling or shrinking of the granules might be a result of potassium and chloride movement into or out of the granules. Studies have demonstrated that nonselective inhibitors of cyclooxygenase (COX) activity prevent stimulation of renin secretion by a reduction in luminal NaCl concentration in the macula densa.[10] COX-2 was found to be involved in the macula densa control of renin secretion, indicating that COX-2 expressing epithelial cells in the tubuloglomerular contact area are a likely source of prostaglandins. The prostaglandins then are involved in the signaling pathway between the macula densa and renin-producing granular cells. The contraction of the actin-myosin network might also play a significant role (Fig. 34-2).

Renin is a single-chain aspartyl protease that is formed from prorenin by removal of a 43–amino acid prosegment followed by release of a Lys^{65}-Arg^{66} dipeptide.[11,12] From three-dimensional x-ray crystallography studies of aspartyl proteases, these proteins were revealed to be bilobal with a pronounced cleft between the two lobes, where the two aspartyl residues of the catalytic sites are located close together, one on each side of the cleft.[13] Prorenin and renin are released into the circulation in a ratio of 10 prorenin for every renin molecule.[14] Renin differs from other aspartyl proteases in its action at a neutral pH, and its specificity for only one known substrate, angiotensinogen. This high specificity of renin for angiotensinogen makes it an ideal target for pharmacologic intervention (as discussed later in the chapter).

Angiotensinogen is a 14–amino acid α_2-globulin of hepatic origin with a molecular weight of 55 to 65 kDa, which varies with the

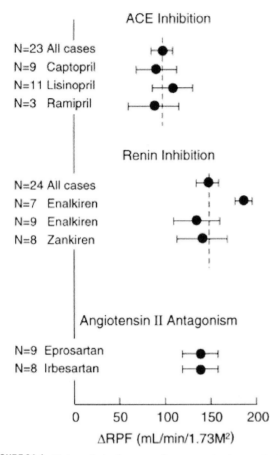

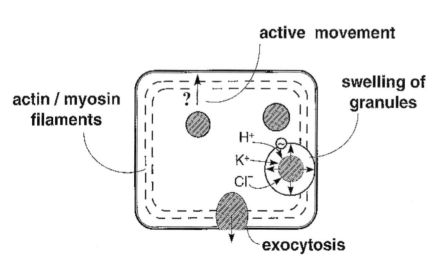

FIGURE 34-1. Meta-analysis of renovascular response to pharmacologic interruption of the renin system in healthy young men who were in balance on a 10-mEq sodium intake. Each agent was studied at the top of its dose–renovascular response relationship. The virtual identity of the responses to renin inhibition and A-II antagonists makes it exceedingly likely that this represents the contribution of endogenous renin-dependent A-II formation triggered by the low-salt diet. From the ratio of the flow increase induced by ACE inhibition and the alternative blockers, one can calculate that approximately two-thirds of A-II formation under these conditions is ACE-dependent and one-third is generated by alternative, non-ACE pathways. *(Reproduced with permission from Hollenberg NK, Fisher ND, Price DA: Pathways for angiotensin II generation in intact human tissue. Hypertension 32: 387, 1998.)*

degree of glycosylation.[15] Human angiotensinogen differs from rat or hog angiotensinogen by the presence of a Leu[10]-Val[11] cleavage site instead of a Leu[10]-Leu[11] bond and also by the nature of the residues that immediately follow on the C-terminal side of the scissile bond.[16,17] This explains the high specificity of human renin for human angiotensinogen, the necessity of modeling renin inhibitors on the human angiotensinogen sequence and the need to do clinical testing in primates.

Enzymatic cleavage of angiotensinogen by renin is the rate-limiting step in the intrinsic series of RAS (Fig. 34-3). When renin interacts with angiotensinogen, the two aspartic acids of the active site hydrolyze the relatively fragile C-N bond by the water molecule buried in the active site. One strategy in making renin inhibitors is to replace this fragile transition state tetrahedral C-N bond with a virtually uncleavable bond such as a C-C bond (transition state analogue). The minimal substrate recognized and cleaved by renin is an octapeptide (His[6]-Tyr[13]) including the cleavage site.[18] Angiotensin-I (A-I), a 10–amino acid fragment, is removed from angiotensinogen after the interaction with renin.[19] The released A-I circulates in the bloodstream until it comes into contact with ACE in the lungs. When A-I interacts with ACE, two amino acids from its carboxy-terminal dipeptide are cleaved, producing A-II, an octapeptide. This angiotensin converting activity is highly dependent on the presence of chloride anions as a cofactor.[20] ACE is not specific for A-I; it also interacts with bradykinin, enkephalins, substance P, neurotensin, and luteinizing hormone-releasing hormones.

A-II exerts numerous hemodynamic effects. In addition to increasing blood pressure by promoting the local release of endothelin to cause vasoconstriction,[21] A-II has several other direct and indirect effects that lead to increased intravascular volume, sodium retention, and blood pressure. A-II has a direct effect on the kidney to increase absorption of salt and water as well as an indirect effect through stimulation of aldosterone release from the adrenal gland. Aldosterone acts at the distal tubules and cortical collecting ducts of the kidney to stimulate sodium and water retention and potassium secretion. Another way A-II increases intravascular volume is to act centrally to stimulate thirst and enhance antidiuretic hormone release. Also through its effect on the central nervous system, A-II can directly augment myocardial contractility and enhance sympathetic nervous tone, causing additional release of renin.[22] Cardiomyocytes bind and activate native human prorenin.[22a] Data to support the inotropic effect of A-II come from studies using the renin inhibitor

FIGURE 34-2. Intracellular events regulating the exocytosis of renin from renal (JGE) cells. Although an active movement of renin storage granules toward the plasma membrane for induction of exocytosis is less likely, a swelling of the storage granules by KCL influx driven by the activity of a proton pump appears to be relevant. Also, the action-myosin filaments could play a role for renin secretion by influencing the access of the storage vesicles to the plasma membrane. *(Reproduced with permission from Kurtz and Wagner.[9])*

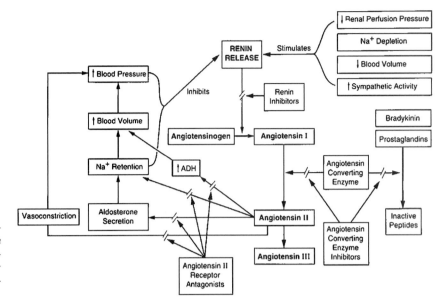

FIGURE 34-3. Schematic representation of the renin-angiotensin-aldosterone system. (*Reproduced with permission from Foote EF, Halstenson CE: New therapeutic agents in the management of hypertension: Angiotensin II-receptor antagonists and renin inhibitors. Ann Pharmacother 27:1495, 1993.*)

remikiren. By comparing intravenous to intracardiac infusion of remikiren, it was found that myocardial contractility is increased by renin-dependent A-II formation in the heart.[23] Further studies have demonstrated that A-II also contributes to cell proliferation, left ventricular hypertrophy, vascular media hypertrophy, neointima formation in atherosclerosis, and nephrosclerosis by stimulation of the AT_1 receptor.[24] It has also been proposed that A-II plays an integral role in the pathogenesis of hypertension-induced end-organ damage. In a recent study, A-II was found to cause monocyte recruitment and a vascular inflammatory response in the kidney.[25] Finally, A-II can promote its own release through a positive feedback effect on the liver's production of angiotensinogen.[26] Thus, A-II can exert a wide variety of actions to elevate systemic blood pressure, and the control of A-II production or activity could provide effective control of elevated blood pressure and other cardiovascular disorders.

THE DEVELOPMENT OF RENIN INHIBITORS

The history of renin inhibitor development has involved the development of four classes of compounds (Table 34-1). The first approach to renin inhibition was the development of specific renin antibodies directed against the enzyme.[27,28] Initially, the antibodies were generated against unpurified crude renal extracts, which had questionable specificity.[29] Antibodies with a high degree of specificity have been generated from pure renin abstracts. Administration of antirenin antisera,[30] Fab fragment, and monoclonal antibodies[31,32] lower both the blood pressure and plasma renin activity (PRA). Although shown to be effective, this immunologic approach is limited because the antibodies are orally inactive due to their inability to be absorbed intact from the gastrointestinal tract, and with repeated intravenous administration the antibodies can induce antigenic reactions. The

TABLE 34-1. Classes of Renin Inhibitors

Renin antibodies (antisera, monoclonal antibodies, Fab fragments)
Synthetic derivatives of the prosegment of renin precursor
Pepstatin analogues
Angiotensinogen analogues

second class of renin inhibitor drug is a synthetic derivative of a prosegment of renin precursor, which can inhibit human renin activity but with low potency.[33,34]

The next development in the evolution of renin inhibitors was based on structure-activity relationships. The peptide sequence of angiotensinogen was modified to produce an inhibitor that would bind tightly to renin and would not be cleaved by renin or other proteases. The modification of angiotensinogen was based on the transition state configuration which has the greatest stability and binding of the enzyme to the substrate. Inhibitors that mimic the transitional structure of the hydrolysis of the Leu-Val amide bond should form a strong interaction with the enzyme, greater than the substrate analogues (Fig. 34-4).

Based on this principle, the third class of drugs was modeled on the activity of pepstatin, a natural pentapeptide isolated from actinomyces culture[35] that universally inhibits aspartyl protease enzymes with a high inhibitory potency for pepsin and a low inhibitory activity for renin.[36,37] Pepstatin contains two statin residues, the central one of which determines the binding affinity of renin for pepstatin by acting as a mimic of the transition state for the scissile peptide bond cleaved by renin.[38] Pepstatin analogues have been synthesized, corresponding to the general formula: A-X-Y-Sta-Ala-Sta-R,[39] in which various changes in the nature of the A, X, and Y groups are made to improve the inhibitory potency against human renin. The analogues having a Phe in place of Val in the X position and His or an amino acid with an aliphatic side chain in the Y position show the highest inhibition of human plasma renin activity. 3-Methyl statin derivatives of pepstatin[40] have been synthesized and their renin inhibitory activity evaluated. However, pepstatin analogues unfortunately exhibit poor specificity and affinity for human renin, and this has limited their experimental and potential clinical use.

The fourth class of renin inhibitors, the angiotensinogen (substrate) analogues (Fig. 34-5) hold the greatest promise. The early substrate analogue inhibitors of renin were derivatives of the tetrapeptide sequence Leu^{10}-Leu-Val-Tyr^{13}, found in equine angiotensinogen.[41] Later, the use of an octapeptide substrate, which competes for renin activity to form an inactive product several amino acids shorter than A-I, was shown to be effective in renin inhibition.[42] Attempts were also made to evaluate the inhibitory effect of several other modified fragments of angiotensinogen. One

transition state for amide bond hydrolysis

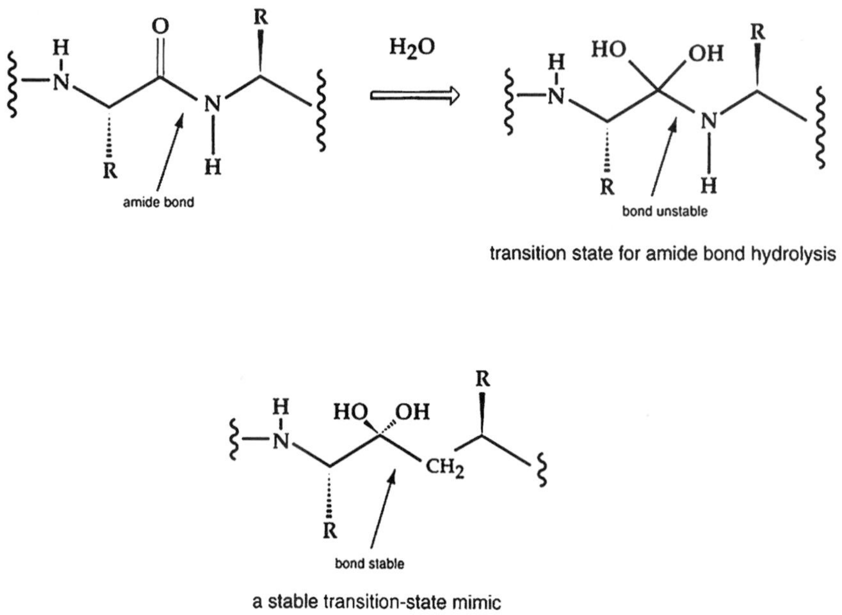

a stable transition-state mimic

FIGURE 34-4. A transition-state structure for amide bond hydrolysis and a stable transition-state mimic. (*Reproduced with permission from Kleinert HD, Baker WR, Stein HH: Renin inhibitors. Adv Pharmacol 22:207, 1991.*)

alteration includes substitution of the D-enantiomer D-Leu for the Leu[10] or Leu[11] of the scissile peptide bond, which is not cleaved by renin in the substrate.[42] This change results in a significant increase in the inhibitory potency of this angiotensinogen fragment. Replacement of the Leu[10]-Leu[11] scissile bond with a hydrophobic dipeptide (Phe-Phe) yields the renin inhibitor peptide (RIP) Pro[1]-His-Pro-Phe-His-Phe-Phe-Val-Tyr-Lys.[43] RIP was the first compound to demonstrate that stabilization of the scissile bond of a renin substrate would produce in vivo pharmacologic effects.[44] Szelke et al.[45] prepared a series of angiotensinogen analogues in which potent renin inhibition was achieved by reducing the scissile peptide bond (-CO-NH-) to form a reduced isostere (CH$_2$-NH-), which renders the scissile bond uncleavable by renin. Several of these initial analogue inhibitors were found to exhibit μmol/L potency.[41,43]

The synthesis of more specific and more potent inhibitors of renin was accomplished by replacing the Leu[10]-Leu[11] scissile bond of human angiotensinogen with a statin residue mimicking the central statin residue of pepstatin. In this case, the ability of the statin residue to act as an analogue of the transition state[38] enables it to achieve a very high binding affinity and specificity for renin. Extensive studies have been made of the interaction of the active sites and subsites of renin with angiotensinogen analogues incorporating statine[46–48] as well as other transition-state analogues—such as norstatine,[49,50] difluorostatine,[51,52] cyclohexylalanyl congeners of statine,[53–55] cyclostatine,[56] dihydroxyethylene,[57,58] dehydrohydroxyethylene,[59] and phosphinic derivatives[60]—replaced at various substrate analogue subsites. The presence of a phenylalanine (Phe) residue or an aromatic group at P$_3$ and a histidine (or histidine analogue) at P$_2$ positions of the substrate analogue gives a high affinity for the inhibitor, whereas the P$_2'$ and P$_3'$ positions are not crucial in determining inhibitory activity.[61–63]

The application of the concept of transition-state mimetics has revolutionized the organic chemistry of renin inhibition. In fact, potent and specific lower-molecular-weight substrate analogue inhibitors have been synthesized as tetrapeptides,[48,64] tripeptides,[46,47] dipeptides,[20,41,65] pseudopeptides,[65a] and even nonpeptidic compounds.[66,67] Moreover, conformationally constrained cyclic renin inhibitors[68] have been produced, and these preparations

exhibit a high binding affinity for human renin as well as increased metabolic stability.

CLINICAL PHARMACOLOGY

The clinical significance of renin inhibition relates directly to preventing the initiation of biochemical reactions in the RAS described. Renin inhibitors block the renin-catalyzed hydrolytic cleavage of angiotensinogen by competitively binding to the active site and subsites of renin and remaining bound but noncleavable by the enzyme. The generation of A-I required for formation of A-II by action of the ACE is inhibited and consequently A-II becomes unavailable to maintain its vasopressor and volume regulatory effects on the circulation. Consequently, renin inhibitors decrease PRA, systemic vascular resistance, and systemic blood pressure.

A number of significant pharmacologic responses to various renin inhibitors have been observed. The first in a series of transition state inhibitors to be tested in humans was H-142. This decapeptide produced clear reduction in diastolic blood pressure in salt depleted, normotensive subjects, only slight reduction in systolic blood pressure, and a significant increase in heart rate.[69] Intravenous infusion of statine-containing renin inhibitor (SCRIP)[70] to conscious, sodium-deficient dogs decreased mean arterial pressure (MAP) and caused suppression of PRA. Chronic intraperitoneal infusion of CGP-29287 to sodium-depleted, normotensive marmosets decreased PRA and reduced blood pressure.[71] In conscious, chronically instrumented, sodium-replete *Macaca* species, perfusion of SR-43845 decreased blood pressure with a notable inhibitory effect on PRA.[72] Infusion of two different doses (0.125 and 0.25 mg/kg) of CGP-38560A induced a modest but significant hypotensive response in 12 hypertensive patients.[73] In 18 patients with essential hypertension, intravenous administration of enalkiren (A-64662)[74] resulted in both a sustained dose-dependent decrease in blood pressure and PRA in sodium-repleted and sodium-depleted conditions. Thus, the dependency of blood pressure on the RAS during basal conditions in hypertensive patients has been demonstrated.

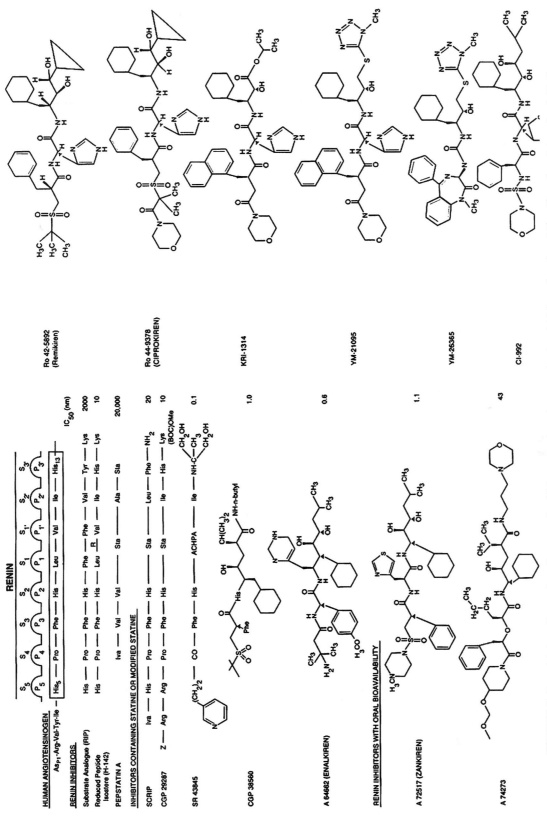

FIGURE 34-5. Potential sites of interaction of human renin with human angiotensinogen and various inhibitors. S_1 to S_5 and S_1' to S_5' are the subsites of renin binding to the corresponding amino acids, P_1 to P_5 and P_1' to P_5', located on the left and right of the Leu^{10}- Val^{11} cleavage site, respectively. NH_2-terminal amino acid sequence of human angiotensinogen and the minimal octapeptide substrate (His^6-His^{13} in box) cleaved by renin are indicated. Structures of various renin inhibitors with their IC_{50} (nM) are indicated. From top to bottom: RIP = renin inhibitor peptide, first substrate analogue synthesized; R = substrate analogue synthesized in which CO-NH bond to be cleaved is replaced by CH_2-NH or CH(OH)-CH; pepstatin A; SCRIP = statin-containing renin inhibitor peptide and other pseudopeptides containing an analogue of the central statine (sta) acting as the intermediary for the transitional state of enzyme hydrolysis; CGP 29287, SR 43845, CGP 38560, A 64662, A 72517, A 74273, Ro 42-5892, Ro 44-9375, KRI 1314, YM21095, YM26365, CI-992.

593

One of the drugs that has been studied extensively in both normotensive and hypertensive patients is enalkiren. Enalkiren is a potent dipeptide renin inhibitor.[75] The drug's volume of distribution includes a V_C of 4.8 L and a V_B of 18.57 L due to its high binding to plasma protein (94%) and its limited ability to cross cellular barriers.[76] After intravenous administration, enalkiren exhibits a biphasic elimination with a distribution and elimination half-life of 15±6 min and 1.6±0.43 h, respectively.[77–79] Oral experiments in rats have shown that it is poorly absorbed: however, while exhibiting moderate portal drug levels, enalkiren was subjected to high liver extraction.[80] Despite the relatively short elimination half-life, enalkiren has been shown to produce prolonged (>6 h) dose-related suppression of PRA and significant lowering of blood pressure.[81] Both systolic and diastolic blood pressure are decreased in a dose-dependent manner, with no effect on heart rate. The reduction in blood pressure is enhanced by salt depletion[74] and pretreatment or concomitant diuretic treatment.[74,82–84] Enalkiren infusion leads to a progressive fall in blood pressure, PRA, A-II, and plasma aldosterone with no change in cardiac output or pulse rate.[78,85] PRA remained significantly suppressed for as long as 24 h after enalkiren; however, A-II and aldosterone returned to approximate baseline levels. Boger et al.[86] conducted a study to evaluate the effects of chronic administration (1 week) of enalkiren in humans. This study showed that the drug was well tolerated and that a prolonged, pronounced blood pressure reduction was achieved, the magnitude of which increased with repeated dosing. No evidence of pharmacologic tolerance or tachyphylaxis was demonstrated. The finding that enalkiren has a sustained effect in lowering blood pressure was also demonstrated by Fisher et al.[87] The study demonstrated that although the plasma concentration and activity of enalkiren waned after discontinuation of intravenous infusion, the influence of the agent on renal plasma flow was sustained. The study suggested that in the face of rising plasma A-II concentration, enalkiren exerted its main influence outside the plasma compartment (perhaps enalkiren-induced interruption of local, intrarenal formation of A-II). This local intrarenal formation of A-II has been demonstrated.[88] Although enalkiren is an effective antihypertensive drug, its clinical usefulness is limited because of its poor bioavailability.[89]

Although a wide variety of effective renin inhibitors have been developed, the impediment of grossly limited oral bioavailability has stemmed movement toward clinical application of this new family of drugs. An orally active renin inhibitor must be predictably absorbed from the gastrointestinal tract and must elicit a dose-related lowering of blood pressure when given orally. Newer and orally active renin inhibitors are emerging that achieve these pharmacologic goals.

Zankiren (A-72517) has significant oral bioavailability in several animal species.[90] This peptide is modeled on the structure of the intravenously effective renin inhibitor enalkiren, having undergone several structural changes resulting in its enhanced oral bioavailability.[91,92] These changes include enhanced lipophilicity and reduced ability to form conjugates through the removal of the P_2 histidine and the NH_2 terminal β-alanine of enalkiren. The enhanced lipophilicity of the drug improves oral absorption and the reduced conjugate formation limits hepatic elimination. In several species in which the drug was evaluated, the predominant obstacle to oral bioavailability was hepatic elimination. The bioavailabilities included 8, 24, 32, and 53% in the monkey, rat, ferret and dog, respectively, after 10-mg/kg doses of A-72517.[90] The IC_{50} of zankiren measured at pH 7.4 is 1.1, 0.24, 9.4, 110, and 1400 nmol/L in the plasma of humans, monkey, guinea pig, dog, and rat, respectively.[90] Various doses of intravenous A-72517 cause dose-dependent

decreases in MAP, PRA, and left ventricular end-diastolic pressure in sodium-depleted dogs.[92] No significant change in the rate of increase of left ventricular pressure during the hypotensive responses occurred, but dose-related increases in contractility compared with baseline were noted, indicating the possible involvement of a local RAS within the heart, as mentioned previously.[23] When zankiren (250 mg PO) was administered to healthy male volunteers pretreated with furosemide, a maximal reduction in blood pressure of 10.0±3.7 mm Hg was observed at peak effect between 1 to 2 h after intake.[93] Statistically significant reduction in MAP was observed throughout the 6 h postdosing observation, with no effect at 24 h. In another study, zankiren was administered to healthy men, and plasma renin activity and renal plasma flow were measured.[94] Plasma renin activity decreased with the smallest dose (5 mg), and the effect was sustained. The increase in renal plasma flow was dose-related.

A-74273 is another nonpeptide-based renin inhibitor with a molecular weight of 787 kDa.[95] This compound has significant oral bioavailability in several animal species as well as an inhibitory concentration of 43 nmol/L for dog renin.[95] Oral bioavailability is 1.9±1.5, 26±15, 31±15, and 54±13% in the monkey, rat, ferret, and dog, respectively, after 10-mg/kg doses. In addition, A-74273 is broken down into two metabolites known as A-78030 and A-78242, and these retain 50% of the potency of their parent compound. In salt-depleted dogs, oral A-74273 reveals dose-dependent reductions in MAP, PRA, and blood pressure. The maximum decrease in MAP was 44±3 mm Hg, with a maximal PRA suppression of 98±1% and blood pressure decreased over time with an area under the curve of 61±13% mm Hg/h, all seen with 30-mg/kg oral dosing.[95] At 3 h after dosing in sodium-repleted dogs, using 30 and 60 mg/kg doses of A-74273, decreases in MAP occurred: 67±5 and 68±5 mm Hg, respectively.[96] No difference in bioavailability between doses was noted, but significantly increased drug concentrations were observed for the 60-mg/kg dose.[96] Thus, it was concluded from this study that higher doses tend to prolong rather than increase the maximal response to A-74273.

Remikiren (Ro 42-5892) is a nonpeptide orally active renin inhibitor.[97] This inhibitor has a high systemic plasma clearance, a high volume of distribution and a long terminal half-life (7 h).[98] The in vitro IC_{50} of remikiren is 0.5 ng/mL[97,99]; in vivo, it is 1.7 ng/mL.[98] Whole-body autoradiography was used to determine the distribution of remikiren in laboratory animals.[100] The kidney consistently showed the highest concentrations of drug-related material. The majority of retained material was intact remikiren, even 24 h after administration (after both intravenous and oral dosing). It appears as if the kidney acts as a reservoir for the drug despite the high plasma clearance of the drug. Data on the renal effects of continued treatment with remikiren, however, were not available until van Paassen[101] studied the effect of 8 days of remikiren treatment at 600 mg once daily. Remikiren induced a significant peak fall in MAP of 11.2 +/−0.8%, which was more pronounced in patients with impaired renal function. Glomerular filtration rate remained stable, whereas effective renal plasma flow increased. Filtration fraction and renal vascular resistance fell. Remikiren induced a cumulative sodium loss of −82+/−22 mmol and a positive potassium balance of 49+/−9 mmol. Proteinuria also fell by 27% in patients with overt proteinuria at onset. No side effects were observed. These data suggest a renoprotective role of renin inhibition. Remikiren causes oral dose-related declines in A-II and PRA in normotensive men given different oral doses of this drug.[102] However, no changes in blood pressure, heart rate, inactive renin, or plasma aldosterone are seen in these normotensive men. Remikiren was given in a short-term study in patients with essential hypertension, either as monotherapy or with hydrochlorothiazide.[103] Its antihypertensive effect during short-term administration was not significant, but when it was combined with a diuretic, a marked potentiation occurred. The study demonstrated that remikiren is orally active and well tolerated in patients. Remikiren (1 mg/kg IV or 10 mg/kg PO) was shown to be markedly more effective than CGP 38560A or enalkiren in reducing arterial pressure in sodium-depleted normotensive squirrel monkeys and was as effective as cilazapril, a long-acting ACE inhibitor.[104] In an 8-day study of 24 hypertensive men with initial diastolic pressures ranging from 95 to 115 mm Hg, significant blood pressure responses were seen, with a maximum reduction of 9.8 mm Hg recorded relative to placebo.[105] This response was maintained 24 h after the first dose, with a net average decrease of 8.6 mm Hg. This study also revealed that a 600-mg dose is at the top of the dose-response curve for this drug. With both oral (600 mg) and intravenous (100 μg/kg or 1 mg/kg) administration, PRA and A-II fell to undetectable levels within 10 min and returned to baseline in a dose-dependent manner by 24 h.[106] The onset of blood pressure decline occurred within 20 min of drug administration and remained depressed for 24 h with both oral and intravenous administration. The blood pressure changes were not accompanied by reflex tachycardia. To demonstrate the optimal mode of remikiren delivery, a slow intravenous infusion was compared with a bolus infusion with respective PRA AUC (area under the curve) results of 1.7 ± 6 and 4.9 ± 2.5 ng AI/mL/h^2.[107] This would indicate an advantage in using a sustained-release or transcutaneous formulation for the delivery of this drug. The bioavailability of the drug has been determined to be less than 1%, mainly attributable to high first-pass effect rather than poor absorption.[98] After oral administration in animal studies, the major elimination pathway is extensive liver metabolism followed directly by biliary excretion of both the metabolite and unchanged compound, with minor urinary elimination of the unchanged compound. However, potency is considered high, as peak antihypertensive effect is seen at a point in which drug levels are not detectable in the bloodstream of patients.[105] These studies also demonstrate that the drug is clinically effective only in those patients who necessitate a therapeutic effect (hypertensive effect), and this may, in turn, reveal an inherent safeguard against potential overdose with this treatment.

Another transition-state renin inhibitor, ciprokiren (Ro 44-9375), has been shown to lower blood pressure after long-term oral administration of very low doses or transdermal application. The extent of blood pressure reduction with these low doses is equal to that after high oral doses given acutely. In vitro, at a pH of 7.4, this compound inhibited renin with an IC$_{50}$ of 0.65, 1.0, 65, 29, and 780 nmol/L in human, squirrel monkey, guinea pig, dog, and rat, respectively.[108] It is hypothesized that ciprokiren inhibited renin located in the extraplasmic site. With 0.1 mg/kg ciprokiren, arterial blood pressure was reduced with no change in PRA, demonstrating the dissociation between hemodynamic effects and inhibition of plasma renin.[109] There was marked peripheral vasodilation, which was not increased by additional ACE inhibition. After intravenous administration of 0.1 mg/kg of ciprokiren, mean arterial blood pressure decreased by 20 to 30 mm Hg, without change in heart rate, and the effect lasted for more than 8 h.[108] Ciprokiren also was shown to have potent oral activity with maximal blood pressure lowering of 40 mm Hg, with 3 mg/kg in normotensive monkeys and with 0.3 mg/kg in the hypertensive monkey.[108] The same blood pressure drop was obtained at a dose that is 10-fold lower than remikiren. Chronic (7 days) daily oral treatment with 1 μg/kg showed a pro-

gressive blood pressure decrease with a maximal response reached after 1 week. This drug was also applied transdermally with similar hemodynamic effects. A norstatine-containing inhibitor, KRI-1314, selectively inhibits human and monkey renin. When given to sodium-depleted Japanese monkeys, it lowered the blood pressure and PRA without affecting heart rate.[110] The absorption of KRI-1314 from the gastrointestinal tract occurs in a relatively low, slow, and continuous manner, as with constant blood levels for at least 7 h after oral administration.[110]

The inhibitor YM-21095, after both intravenous and oral administration to primates, produced a reduction in blood pressure and an inhibition of PRA in a dose-dependent manner.[111] The bioavailability determined in dogs was low, $0.16\pm0.04\%$.[112] To improve this low bioavailability, YM-26365, a smaller nonpeptide molecule with no peptide bonds and a replacement of the C-terminal portion (P$_2$ and P$_3$), was synthesized. The systemic bioavailability of 9.6% was calculated by comparing the AUC after a 3-mg/kg intravenous infusion of YM-26365 to that of 30 mg/kg orally in rats.[113] YM-26365 inhibited human plasma renin with an IC$_{50}$ value of 2.9 nmol/L but did not affect plasma renin in dogs, rabbits, and rats.[113] In addition to inhibiting renin, YM-26365 also had inhibitory effects on cathepsin D and ACE. Due to its resistance to proteolytic degradation and low molecular weight, this inhibitor does not appear to be subject to an extensive first-pass effect.

When compared to captopril, the renin inhibitor ES-8891, which appeared to inhibit renin secretion from the kidney, produced a significant reduction in MAP and PRA after short-term oral administration.[114] In another study that compared captopril to a renin inhibitor,[115] it was observed that the effect of acute intravenous administration of the renin inhibitor CP80794 was comparable to that of the ACE inhibitor. This comparative study evaluated left ventricular, systemic, and peripheral blood flow effects in conscious dogs with advanced heart failure. Both drugs had similar effects on left ventricular systemic hemodynamics, but CP80794 caused a significantly greater increase in renal blood flow compared to the ACE inhibitor. Other studies have demonstrated that renin inhibitors had greater effects than ACE inhibitors on renal plasma flow[5] (Fig. 34-1) and that they are more effective than ACE inhibition in blocking systemic A-II formation.[6] One speculation is that renin inhibitors, which are highly lipophilic, have access to crucial pools of intrarenal renin, differentiating their tissue distribution within the kidney from that of ACE inhibitors.[116]

Another oral renin inhibitor is CI-992, which reduces MAP in hypertensive and renal hypertensive monkeys and does not appear to produce tolerance in the MAP or PRA reduction effects after 5 days of oral dosing.[117] However, in contrast to observations following intravenous administration, a trend for decreasing mean arterial blood pressure with increasing plasma CI-992 was not apparent following oral CI-992 administration in monkeys.[118] The human renin inhibitors EMD 58265 and U71038 (long-acting orally active agents with high water-solubility) were compared to the ACE inhibitor enalaprilat.[119] Both renin inhibitors exerted a greater blood pressure–lowering effect than the ACE inhibitor in rabbits.

A renin inhibitor has yet to be approved for use in humans. Typically the renin inhibitors have been large and peptidic, which have limited their oral bioavailability. While the search for new peptide inhibitors of renin has led to the development of new, lower-molecular-weight agents,[120–122] some focus has recently been on nonpeptide inhibitors. A similar approach led to the development of losartan, which is a small nonpeptidic A-II antagonist. CGP 60536B is the first completely nonpeptide low-molecular-weight renin inhibitor.[123]

Aliskiren (SPP100) is a new orally active nonpeptide renin inhibitor that has been shown to be an effective once-daily antihypertensive agent causing a significant and sustained decrease in PRA, A-I, and A-II plasma levels.[123a] Other groups have attempted to synthesize similar small, highly potent renin inhibitors.[124] These new inhibitors used angiotensinogen as a template; the focus was on the P_2-P_3-P_4 segment of the inhibitors while maintaining a known transition state analogue at P_1-P_1'. These have demonstrated good oral bioavailability in monkeys, and the structure of renin inhibitors has been simplified. They have been studied in the human renin infused rat,[125] demonstrating high potency, dose dependence, and bioavailability following oral administration. Similar small, nonpeptidic inhibitors have been designed with limited potency and water solubility.[126] A recent attempt to utilize crystal structure analysis of renin-inhibitor complexes combined with computational methods was used to develop novel nonpeptide orally active inhibitors of renin.[127] The results are promising; the compounds demonstrated high in vitro affinity and specificity for renin, favorable bioavailability, and excellent oral efficacy in lowering blood pressure in primates. Future studies with these new inhibitors are indicated to establish their efficacy in human subjects.

A recent development has been the class of agents that has substituted piperidines.[128-130] By high-throughput screening of the Roche compound library, a simple 3,4-disubstituted piperidine lead compound was identified.[128] Two representatives of this new class were complexed with recombinant human renin, and an unexpected induced-fit adaptation of the enzyme was discovered.[128] The observed induced-fit adaptations of the renin active site suggest that there is latent conformational flexibility.[128] This might therefore represent a novel paradigm for inhibition of renin. The most active substituted piperidines showed activities in the picomolar range and, when compared to previously developed renin inhibitors, are of much higher potency.[129]

Finally, another technique that has been suggested is covalently linking renin inhibitors to the red cell surface.[131] Red blood cells were labeled with an antirenin pharmacophore, and the inhibitory activity specific to the extracellular surface of red cells was measured. Renin inhibition by labeled cells varied according to the concentrations of labeling agent. This demonstrates the feasibility of exploiting covalently bound pharmacophores for drug targeting. Advantages of red blood cell-anchored drugs over free drugs include longer half-life and an intravascular volume of distribution.[132] This would be particularly useful for renin inhibitors, which have been troubled by metabolic instability and/or excretion in the bile. By attaching the drugs to red cells, the bile and urinary excretion would be circumvented. In addition, a red cell–linked moiety would be more difficult to modify than the free drug because of the red cell surface.

A dissociation between suppression of PRA and the blood pressure–lowering response induced by renin inhibitors has been observed, as well as a phenomenon of recruitment of dose-related blood pressure decrement despite complete suppression of PRA.[70,71,75] The explanation for these observations is still a matter of debate.

The consideration of a tissue-based RAS system outside of the intravascular space has been suggested as being important.[88,133] Price et al.[134] have proposed that an activated intrarenal renin system is involved in diabetic nephropathy, despite the low-renin state. However, an additional non-renin-mediated mechanism of action for renin inhibitors in nephropathic states may be a possibility and requires further investigation. Renin inhibitors do not have any direct chronotropic effects on the heart, and like ACE inhibitors, their hypotensive effects do not cause reflex tachycardia.[86,135-137] Administration of these inhibitors usually is followed by a dose-dependent increase in renin secretion,[138] thereby necessitating a high dose of the inhibitor for effective in vivo renin inhibition; however, tachyphylaxis or tolerance has not yet been observed with chronic administration of these agents.[86]

CLINICAL APPLICATION

Renin has a specific action in the RAS, and as a result, the use of specific renin inhibitors in clinical investigations will help to better delineate the role of RAS in the pathogenesis of essential hypertension. Animal models of hypertension will also contribute to our understanding of the RAS. Renal hypertension was induced by ligation of the left caudal renal artery and right nephrectomy to create a novel renal hypertensive guinea pig,[139] which could be a useful model for comparing and contrasting different RAS inhibitors. Another animal model is the human renin infused rat.[125]

Three pharmacologic targets within the RAS have been renin inhibition, ACE inhibitors, and angiotensin antagonists. The latter two have garnered much success, but renin inhibitor development has lagged behind. Although the therapeutic potential is clear, there are several reasons why renin inhibition has not developed as a successful class of drugs. The cost of synthesis, continuing problems with oral bioavailability, and the remarkable success of the competitor class—the A-II antagonists, have impeded progress.[140] Because of the greater specificity of action for renin inhibitors (compared to ACE inhibitors), a more limited side effect profile with these drugs is expected, and their availability for clinical use will create more opportunity for better selection and tailoring of suitable antihypertensive pharmacotherapy according to individual patient characteristics. Synergistic effects resulting in a more efficacious antihypertensive regimen would be expected from combination therapy of a renin inhibitor with an ACE inhibitor, a finding that has been confirmed.[141-143]

Renin inhibition has potential therapeutic efficacy in the treatment of renovascular hypertension[144,145] and congestive heart failure.[146-148] However, renin inhibition may also demonstrate clinical utility in a number of other clinical scenarios. Conditions such as stroke, myocardial infarction, scleroderma,[149] renal trauma, and acute closure of renal artery grafts[150] are all associated with high levels of plasma renin.[151] Corneal application of the inhibitor enalkiren decreases intraocular pressure in unanesthetized rabbits and anesthesized monkey,[152] thus suggesting a possible functional role of RAS in modulation of intraocular pressure and the potential clinical utility of renin inhibitors as ocular pressure–lowering agents. Further study is needed in this regard. Finally, renin may have a direct vasculotoxic effect unrelated to its hypertensive consequences.[151]

POTENTIAL ADVERSE REACTIONS

Although significant adverse reactions have not yet been observed with renin inhibitors, several may be considered. By blocking the RAS-mediated increase in aldosterone secretion, renin inhibitors would be expected to potentiate hyponatremic and hyperkalemic states. In addition, long-term renin inhibition therapy may induce pharmacologic tolerance with renin hypersecretion, as well as the phenomenon of rebound hypertension after abrupt cessation of chronic therapy. This hypersecretion also would result in an increased release of prorenin, which might have unknown effects on local tissue RAS. Finally, excessive levels of prorenin, with its localized vasodilatory potential, also may predispose to hypoperfusion injury in various tissues in patients with diabetes mellitus or toxemia of pregnancy.[151]

Minor adverse effects of enalkiren include malaise,[78] rash,[153] palpitations,[153] nocturia,[153] dizziness,[74] and an excessive decline in blood pressure.[74,84] Remikiren is very well tolerated, having the minor adverse effect of diarrhea after a very high dose.[98]

OBSTACLES

Renin inhibitors have been extensively studied for over 30 years. Several areas remain problematic; among them, the assay for evaluation of potency of a renin inhibitor, the source of renin activity, the choice and source of substrate, the pH of the test system, the measurements of the product of enzymatic reaction and A-I, high cost, and poor oral bioavailabilty.

One of the most interesting problems is that of the species-specific nature of the available substrate inhibitor. Primate renin cleaves all mammalian angiotensinogen to A-I, but nonprimate renin will not cleave primate angiotensinogen.[154] KRI-1314 strongly inhibited PRA in humans and monkeys, but acted weakly on PRA in dogs, rabbits, guinea pigs, and rats.[111] This species-specificity is secondary to the location of the scissile bond in the primate substrate in between Leu and Val, whereas it is between Leu and Leu in nonprimate angiotensinogen.[155] The species-specificity may be due to differences in the three-dimensional structures of individual renins. Thus, this species-specificity has limited our ability to adequately test renin inhibitors in various animal models, but useful animal models have been developed in recent years.[125,139]

In addition, the route of elimination of the renin inhibitors remains unclear. Since renin is eliminated primarily by the liver and to a lesser extent by the kidney, administration of a renin inhibitor immediately leads to a dose-dependent[72] increase in renin secretion.[138] To inhibit the newly released renin, renin inhibitors must remain at a high concentration for a long period of time. Most of the renin is cleaved or rapidly metabolized and blood pressure recovers within minutes after stopping intravenous drug administration. The elimination of renin inhibitors is unclear; it is not known if the inhibitors are removed independently or complexed with renin. It is also unclear whether the elimination pattern of renin influences the route and speed of renin inhibitor clearance from the circulation.

CONCLUSION

The RAS is exceedingly intricate and of great physiologic significance. Moreover, there has been great progress over recent years in the development of orally active renin inhibitor agents that have important clinical potential, both as effective antihypertensive drugs and as treatment for other cardiovascular conditions. However, many of the development programs have been curtailed because of the success of A-II antagonists in the management of hypertension. The implications of successful renin blockade are as broad and far-reaching as the complexity of the RAS itself.

REFERENCES

1. Weber MA, Laragh JH: Hypertension: Steps forward and steps backward: The Joint National Committee, Fifth Report. *Arch Intern Med* 13:154, 1993.
2. Yusuf S, Sleight P, Pogue J, et al: Effects of an angiotensin-converting-enzyme inhibitor, ramipril, on cardiovascular events in high-risk patients. *N Engl J Med* 342:145, 2000.
3. Urata H, Healy B, Stewart R, et al: Angiotensin II forming pathways in normal and failing human hearts. *Circ Res* 66:883, 1990.
4. Okunishi H, Oka Y, Shiota N, et al: Marked species-difference in the vascular angiotensin II-forming pathways: Humans versus rodents. *Jpn J Pharmacol* 62:207, 1993.
5. Hollenberg NK, Pharmacologic interruption of the renin-angiotensin system and the kidney: Differential responses to angiotensin-converting enzyme and renin inhibition. *J Am Soc Nephrol* 10(Suppl 11): S239, 1999.
6. Allan DR, Hui KY, Coletti C, Hollenberg NK: Renin vs angiotensin-converting enzyme inhibition in the rat: Consequences for plasma and renal tissue angiotensin. *J Pharmacol Exp Ther* 283:661, 1997.
7. Dzau VJ, Burt DW, Pratt RE: Molecular biology of the renin angiotensin system. *Am J Physiol* 255:F563, 1988.
8. Baxter JD, James MN, Chu WN, et al: The molecular biology of human renin and its gene. *Yale J Biol Med* 62:493, 1989.
9. Kurtz A, Wagner C: Regulation of renin secretion by angiotensin II-ATI receptors. *J Am Soc Nephrol* 10(Suppl 11):S162, 1999.
10. Traynor TR, Smart A, Briggs JP, et al: Inhibition of macula densa–stimulated renin secretion by pharmacological blockade of cyclooxygenase-2. *Am J Physiol* 277:F706, 1999.
11. Pratt RE, Ouellete AJ, Dzau VJ: Biosynthesis of renin: Multiplicity of active and intermediate forms. *Proc Natl Acad Sci U S A* 80:6809, 1983.
12. Galen FX, Devaux C, Houot AM, et al: Renin biosynthesis by human tumoral juxtaglomerular cells. Evidence for a renin precursor. *J Clin Invest* 73:1144, 1984.
13. Corvol P, Chauveau D, Jeunemaitre X, Menard J: Human renin inhibitor peptides. *Hypertension* 16:1, 1990.
14. Derkx FHM, Wenting GJ, Man In't Veld AJ, et al: Control of enzymatically inactive renin in man under various pathologic conditions: Implications for the interpretation of renin measurements in peripheral and renal venous plasma. *Clin Sci Mol Med* 54:529, 1978.
15. Clauser E, Gaillard I, Wei L, Corvol P: Regulation of angiotensinogen gene. *Am J Hypertens* 2:403, 1989.
16. Tewksbury DA, Dart RA, Travis J: The amino terminal amino acid sequence of human angiotensinogen. *Biochem Biophys Res Commun* 99:1311, 1981.
17. Kageyama R, Ohkubo M, Nakanishi S: Primary structure of human preangiotensinogen deduced from the cloned cDNA sequence. *Biochemistry* 23:3603, 1984.
18. Skeggs LT, Lentz KE, Kahn JR, Hochstrasser H: Kinetics of the reaction of renin with nine synthetic peptide substrates. *J Exp Med* 128:13, 1968.
19. Hilgers KF, Veelken R, Müller DN, et al: Renin uptake by the endothelium mediates vascular angiotensin formation. *Hypertension* 38:243, 2001.
20. Cushman DW, Ondetti MA: Inhibitors of angiotensin converting enzyme. In: Ellis GP, West GB, eds. *Progress in Medicinal Chemistry.* Amsterdam: Elsevier/North Holland Biomedical Press, 1980:42–104.
21. Hahn AWA, Resnik TJ, Scott-Burden T, et al: Stimulation of endothelin mRNA and secretion in rat vascular smooth muscle cells: A novel autocrine function. *Cell Reg* 1:649, 1990.
22. Ferrario CM: The renin angiotensin system: Importance in physiology and pathology. *J Cardiovasc Pharmacol* 15(Suppl 3):S1, 1990.
22a. Saris JJ, Derkx FHM, Lamers JMJ, et al: Cardiomyocytes bind and activate native human prorenin. Role of soluble mannose 6-phosphate receptors. *Hypertension* 37(Pt 2):710, 2001.
23. van Kats JP, Sassen LM, Danser AH, et al: Assessment of the role of the renin-angiotensin system in cardiac contractility utilizing the renin inhibitor remikiren. *Br J Pharmacol* 117:891, 1996.
24. Unger T: Neurohormonal modulation in cardiovascular disease. *Am Heart J* 139:S2, 2000.
25. Mervaala EMA, Muller DN, Park JK, et al: Monocyte infiltration and adhesion molecules in a rat model of high human renin hypertension. *Hypertension* 33:389, 1999.

26. Tewksbury DA: Angiotensinogen: Biochemistry and molecular biology. In: Laragh JH, Brenner BM, eds. *Hypertension: Pathophysiology, Diagnosis and Management.* New York: Raven Press, 1990, pp 1197–1216.

27. Johnson CA, Wakerlin GE: Antiserum for renin. *Proc Soc Exp Biol Med* 44:277, 1940.

28. Deodhar SD, Haas E, Goldblatt H: Production of antirenin to homologus renin and its effect on experimental renal hypertension. *J Exp Med* 119:425, 1964.

29. Helmer OM: Studies on renin antibodies. *Circulation* 17:648, 1958.

30. Dzau VJ, Kopelman RI, Barger AC, Haber E: Renin-specific antibody for study of cardiovascular homeostasis. *Science* 207:1091, 1980.

31. Wood JM, Baum HP, Bews JPA, et al: Effects of chronic administration of a monoclonal antibody against human renin in the marmoset. *Clin Exp Hypertens Part A* A9:1467, 1987.

32. Wood JM, Heusser C, Gulati N, et al: Monoclonal antibodies against human renin. Blood pressure effects in the marmoset. *Hypertension* 8:600, 1986.

33. Evin G, Devin J, Castro B, et al: Synthesis of peptides related to the prosegment of mouse submaxillary gland renin precursor: An approach to renin inhibitors. *Proc Natl Acad Sci U S A* 81:48, 1984.

34. Cumin F, Evin G, Fehrentz JA, et al: Inhibition of human renin by synthetic peptides derived from its prosegment. *J Biol Chem* 260:9154, 1985.

35. Aoyagi T, Kunimoto S, Morishima H, et al: Effect of peptstatin on acid proteases. *J Antibotic (Tokyo)* 24:687, 1971.

36. Gross F, Lazar J, Orth H: Inhibition of renin-angiotensinogen reaction by pepstatin. *Science* 175:656, 1972.

37. Miller RP, Poper CH, Wilson CW, Devito E: Renin inhibition by pepstatin. *Biochem Pharmacol* 21:2941, 1972.

38. Boger J, Lohr NS, Ulm EH, et al: Novel renin inhibitors containing the amino acid statine. *Nature* 303:81, 1983.

39. Guegan R, Diaz J, Cazaubon C, et al: Pepstatin analogues as novel renin inhibitors. *J Med Chem* 29:1152, 1986.

40. Rich DH, Bernatowicz MS, Agarwal NS, et al: Inhibition of aspartic protease by pepstatin and 3–methyl statine derivatives of pepstatin. Evidence for collected substrate enzyme inhibition. *Biochemistry* 24:3165, 1985.

41. Kokubu T, Ueda E, Fujimoto S: Peptide inhibitor of the renin angiotensin system. *Nature* 217:46, 1968.

42. Poulsen K, Burton J, Haber E: Competitive inhibitors of renin. *Biochemistry* 12:3877, 1973.

43. Burton J, Cody RJ, Herd AJ, Haber E: Specific inhibition of renin by an angiotensinogen analogue: Studies in sodium depletion and renin-dependent hypertension. *Proc Natl Acad Sci U S A* 77:5476, 1980.

44. Zusman RM, Burton J, Christensen D, et al: Hemodynamic effects of a competitive renin inhibitory peptide in humans: Evidence for multiple mechanisms of action. *Trans Am Assoc Physicians* 96:365, 1983.

45. Szelke M, Leckie BJ, Hallett A, et al: Potent new inhibitors of human renin. *Nature* 299:555, 1982.

46. Kokubu T, Hiwada K, Nagae A, et al: Statine-containing dipeptide and tripeptide inhibitors of human renin. *Hypertension* 8(Suppl II):II-1, 1986.

47. Kokubu T, Hiwada K, Murakami E, Muneta S: In vitro inhibition of human renin by statine-containing tripeptide renin inhibitor (ES 1005). *J Cardiovasc Pharmacol* 10(Suppl 7):S88, 1987.

48. Bock MG, Diapardo RM, Evans BE, Rittle KE: Renin inhibitors. Statine-containing tetrapeptides with varied hydrophobic carboxy terminal. *J Med Chem* 30:1853, 1987.

49. Iizuka J, Kamijo T, Kubota T, et al: New human renin inhibitors containing an unnatural amino acid, norstatine. *J Med Chem* 31:701, 1988.

50. Toda N, Miyazoki M, Etoh Y, et al: Human renin inhibiting dipeptide. *Eur J Pharmacol* 129:393, 1986.

51. Thaisrivongs S, Pals DT, Kati WM, et al: Difluorostatine and difluorostatone containing peptides as potent and specific renin inhibitors. *J Med Chem* 28:1553, 1985.

52. Thaisrivongs S, Pals DT, Kati WM, et al: Design and synthesis of potent and specific renin inhibitors containing difluorostatine, difluorostatone and related analogues. *J Med Chem* 29:2080, 1986.

53. Boger J, Payen LS, Perlow DS, et al: Renin inhibitors: Syntheses of subnanomolar competitive transition-state analogue inhibitors containing a novel analogue of statine. *J Med Chem* 28:1779, 1985.

54. Dellaria JF, Maki RG, Bopp BA, et al: Optimization and in vivo evaluations of a series of small potent and specific renin inhibitors containing a novel Leu-Val replacement. *J Med Chem* 30:2137, 1987.

55. Hui KY, Holtzman EJ, Quinones MA, et al: Design of rat renin inhibitory peptides. *J Med Chem* 31:1679, 1988.

56. Hiwada K, Kokubu T, Murakami K, et al: A highly potent and long-acting oral inhibitor of human renin. *Hypertension* 11:708, 1988.

57. Luly JR, BaMaung N, Soderquist J, et al: Renin inhibitors. Dipeptide analogues of angiotensinogen, utilizing a dihydroxyethylene transition-state mimic at the scissile bond to impart greater inhibitory potency. *J Med Chem* 31:2264, 1988.

58. Kleinert HD, Luly JR, Marcotte PA, et al: Renin inhibitors: Improvements in the stability and biological activity of small peptides containing novel Leu-Val replacements. *FEBS Lett* 230(1–2):38, 1988.

59. Kempf DJ, Delara E, Stein HH, et al: Renin inhibitors based on novel dipeptide analogues. Incorporation of the dihydroxyethylene isostere at the scissile bond. *J Med Chem* 30:1978, 1987.

60. Allen MC, Fuhrer W, Tuck B, et al: Renin inhibitors. Synthesis of transition state analogue inhibitors containing phosphorus acid derivatives at the scissile bond. *J Med Chem* 32:1652, 1989.

61. Evin G, Devin J, Castro B, et al: New potent inhibitors of human renin.In: Hruby VJ, Rich DH, eds. *Peptides: Structure and Function. Proceedings of the 8th American Peptide Symposium.* IL: Piere Chemical Co, 1984:583–590.

62. Sawyer TK, Pals DT, Mao B, et al: Design, structure-activity, and molecular modeling studies of potent renin inhibitory peptides having N-terminal Nin-For-Trp (Ftr): Angiotensinogen congeners modified by P_1-$P_1$1 Phe-Phe, Sta, Leu Psi [CH(OH)CH$_2$] Val or Lew Psi [CH$_2$BG] Val substitutions. *J Med Chem* 31:18, 1988.

63. Haber E, Hui KY, Carlson WD, Bernatowicz MS: Renin inhibitors: A search or principles of design. *J Cardiovasc Pharmacol* 10(Suppl 7):S54, 1987.

64. Bock MG, Dipardo RM, Evans BE, et al: Renin inhibitors containing hydrophilic groups: Tetrapeptides with enhanced aqueous solubility and nanomolar potency. *J Med Chem* 31:1918, 1988.

65. Glassman HN, Kleinert HD, Boger RS, et al: Clinical pharmacology of enalkiren, a novel dipeptide renin inhibitor. *J Cardiovasc Pharmacol* 16(Suppl 40):S76, 1990.

65a. Paruszewski R, Jaworski P, Winiecka I, et al: New renin inhibitors with pseudodipeptidic units in p(1)-p(1′) and p(2′)-p(3′) positions. *Chem Pharm Bull* 50:850, 2002.

66. DeGasparo M, Cumin F, Nussberger J, et al: Pharmacological investigation of a new renin inhibitor in normal sodium-unrestricted volunteers. *Br J Clin Pharmacol* 27:587, 1989.

67. Boyd SA, Fung AKL, Baker WR, et al: C-terminal modifications of nonpeptide renin inhibitors: Improved oral bioavailability via modification of physiochemical properties. *J Med Chem* 35:1735, 1992.

68. Sham HL, Bolis G, Stein HH, et al: Renin inhibitors. Design and synthesis of a new class of conformationally restricted analogues of angiotensinogen. *J Med Chem* 31:284, 1988.

69. Webb DJ, Manhem PJ, Ball SG, et al: A study of the renin inhibitor H-142 in man. *J Hypertens* 3:653, 1985.

70. Blaine EH, Schorn TW, Boger J: Statine-containing renin inhibitor. Dissociation of blood pressure lowering and renin inhibition in sodium-deficient dogs. *Hypertension* 6(Suppl I):I111, 1984.

71. Wood JM, Baum HP, Jobber RA, Neisius D: Sustained reduction in blood pressure during chronic administration of a renin inhibitor in normotensive marmosets. *J Cardiovasc Pharmacol* 10(Suppl 7):S96, 1987.

72. LaCour C, Cazaubon C, Roccon A, et al: Effects of a renin inhibitor SR 43845 and of captopril on blood pressure and plasma active renin in conscious sodium-replete macaca. *J Hypertens* 2(Suppl 7):S33, 1989.

73. Jeunemaitre X, Menard J, Nussberger J, et al: Plasma angiotensinogens, renin and blood pressure during acute renin inhibition by CGP-385560A in hypertensive patients. *Am J Hypertens* 2:819, 1989.

74. Weber MA, Neutel JM, Essinger J, et al: Assessment of renin dependency of hypertension with a dipeptide renin inhibitor. *Circulation* 81:1768, 1990.

75. Kleinert HD, Martin D, Chekal MA, et al: Effects of the renin inhibitor A-64662 in monkeys and rats with varying baseline plasma renin activity. *Hypertension* 11:613, 1988.

76. Gupta SK, Granneman GR, Packer M, Boger RS: Simultaneous modeling of the pharmacokinetic and pharmacodynamic properties of

enalkiren (Abbott-64662, a renin inhibitor). II: A dose-ranging study in patients with congestive heart failure. *J Cardiovasc Pharmacol* 21:834, 1993.

77. Cordero P, Fisher ND, Moore TJ, et al: Renal and endorcrine responses to a renin inhibitor, enalkiren, in normal humans. *Hypertension* 17:510, 1991.

78. Jackson B, Liu G, Perich RB, et al: Haemodynamic, renal and hormonal responses to enalkiren in four patients with post-surgical oliguria. Proceedings of the HBPRCA. *Clin Exp Pharm Physiol* 21:163, 1994.

79. Gupta SK, Granneman GR, Gober RS, et al: Simultaneous modeling of the pharmacokinetic and pharmacodynamic properties of enalkiren (Abbott 64662, a new renin inhibitor): I: Single dose study. *Drug Metab Dispos* 20:821, 1992.

80. Kleinert HD, Baker WR, Stein HH: Renin inhibitors. *Adv Pharmacol* 22:207, 1991.

81. Delabays A, Nussberger J, Porchet M, et al: Hemodynamic and humoral effects of the new renin inhibitor enalkiren in normal humans. *Hypertension* 13:941, 1989.

82. Glassman HN, Kleinert HD, Bogers RS, et al: Clinical pharmacology of enalkiren, a novel dipeptide renin inhibitor. *J Cardiovasc Pharmacol* 16(suppl 4): S76, 1990.

83. Anderson PW, Do YS, Schambelan M, et al: Effects of renin inhibition in systemic hypertension. *Am J Cardiol* 66:1342, 1990.

84. Neutel JM, Luther RR, Boger RS, Weber MA: Immediate blood pressure effects of the renin inhibitor enalkiren and the angiotensin converting enzyme inhibitor enalaprilat. *Am Heart J* 122:1094, 1991.

85. Bursztyn M, Gavras I, Tifft CP, et al: Renin inhibition with A-64662: Effect in blood pressure and hormonal response in man. *J Hypertens* 7(Suppl):S306, 1989.

86. Boger RS, Glassman HN, Cavanaugh JH, et al: Prolonged duration of blood pressure response to enalkiren, the novel dipeptide renin inhibitor, in essential hypertension. *Hypertension* 15(6 Part 2):835, 1990.

87. Fisher N, Allan D, Gaboury C et al: Intrarenal angiotensin II formation in humans. *Hypertension* 25:935, 1995.

88. Admiraal P, Danser A, Jong M et al: Regional angiotensin II production in essential hypertension and renal artery stenosis. *Hypertension* 21:173, 1993.

89. Haber E: Why renin inhibitors? *J Hypertens* 7(Suppl 2):S81, 1989.

90. Kleinert HD, Rosenberg SH, Baker WR, et al: Discovery of a peptide based renin inhibitor with oral bioavailability and efficacy. *Science* 257:1940, 1992.

91. Rosenberg SH, Spina KP, Woods KW, et al: Studies directed toward the design of orally active renin inhibitors. 1. Some factors influencing the absorption of small peptides. *J Med Chem* 36:449, 1993.

92. Wessale JL, Kleinert HD, Calzadilla SV, et al: Effects of renin inhibitor A72517 on hemodynamics and cardiac function in sodium-depleted dogs. *Am J Hypertens* 6:514, 1993.

93. Menard J, Boger RS, Moyse DM, et al: Dose-dependent effects of the renin inhibitor zankiren HCl after a single oral dose in mildly sodium-depleted normotensive subjects. *Circulation* 91:330, 1995.

94. Fisher ND, Hollenberg N: Renal vascular responses to renin inhibition with zankiren in men. *Clin Pharmacol Ther* 57:342, 1995.

95. Kleinert HD, Stein HH, Boyd S, et al: Discovery of well absorbed, efficacious renin inhibitor, A-74273. *Hypertension* 30:768, 1992.

96. Verburg KM, Polakowski JS, Kovar PJ, et al: Effects of high doses of A-74273, a novel nonpeptidic and orally bioavailable renin inhibitor. *J Cardiovasc Pharmacol* 21(1):149, 1993.

97. van Paassen P, deZeeuw D, deJong PE: Renal and systemic effects of the renin inhibitor remikiren in patients with essential hypertension. *J Cardiovasc Pharmacol* 26:39, 1995.

98. Kleinbloesem CH, Weber C, Fahrner E, et al: Hemodynamics, biochemical effects, and pharmacokinetics of the renin inhibitor remikiren in healthy human subjects. *Clin Pharmacol Ther* 53:585, 1993.

99. Greenlee WJ, Weber AE: Renin inhibitors. *Drug News Perspect* 4:332, 1991.

100. Richter WF, Whitby BR, Chou RC: Distribution of remikiren, a potent orally active inhibitor of human renin, in laboratory animals. *Xenobiotica* 26:243, 1996.

101. van Paassen P, de Zeeuw D, Navis G, deJong PE: Renal and systemic effects of continued treatment with renin inhibitor remikiren in hypertensive patients with normal and impaired renal function. *Nephrol Dialysis Transplant* 15:637, 2000.

102. Comenzind E, Nussberger J, Juillert L, et al: Effects of the renin response during renin inhibition: Oral RO42-5892 in normal humans. *J Cardiovasc Pharmacol* 18:299, 1991.

103. Himmelmann A, Bergbrant A, Svensson A, et al: Remikiren (RO 42-5892)—an orally active renin inhibitor in essential hypertension. Effects on blood pressure and the renin-angiotensin-aldosterone system. *Am J Hypertens* 9:517, 1996.

104. Clozel JP, Fischli W: Comparative effects of three different potent renin inhibitors in primates. *Hypertension* 22:9, 1993.

105. Kobrin I, Viskoper RJ, Laszt A, et al: Effects of an orally active renin inhibitor RO 42-5892, in patients with essential hypertension. *Am J Hypertens* 6:349, 1993.

106. Van den Meiracker AH, Admiraal PJ, Man in't Veld AJ, et al: Prolonged blood pressure reduction by orally active renin inhibitor RO 42-5892 in essential hypertension. *Br Med J* 301:205, 1990.

107. Doig JK, MacFadyen RJ, Meredith PA, et al: Neurohormonal and blood pressure responses to low-dose infusion of an orally active renin inhibitor, RO 42-5892 in salt replete men. *J Cardiovasc Pharmacol* 20:875, 1992.

108. Fischli W, Clozel JP, Breu V, et al: Ciprokiren (RO 44-9375): A renin inhibitor with increasing effects on chronic treatment. *Hypertension* 24:163, 1994.

109. Clozel JP, Veniant M, Sprecher U, et al: Acute hemodynamic effects of ciprokiren, a novel renin inhibitor, in sodium-depleted dogs. *J Cardiovasc Pharmacol* 26:674, 1995.

110. Etoh Y, Miyazaki M, Saitoh H, Toda N: KRI-1314: An orally effective inhibitor of human renin. *Jpn J Pharmacol* 63:109, 1993.

111. Shibasaki M, Asano M, Fukunaga Y, et al: Pharmacological properties of YM-21095, a potent and highly specific renin inhibitor. *Am J Hypertens* 4:932, 1991.

112. Shibasaki M, Usui T, Inagaki O, et al: Pharmacokinetics and cardiovascular effects of YM-21095, a novel renin inhibitor, in dogs and monkeys. *J Pharm Pharmacol* 46:68, 1994.

113. Shibasaki M, Shibasaki K, Ichihara M, et al: Pharmacological properties of YM-26365, a low molecular weight, orally active renin inhibitor. *Eur J Pharmacol* 271:341, 1994.

114. Ii Y, Murakami E, Hiwada K: Effect of renin inhibitor, ES-8891, on renal renin secretion and storage in the marmoset: Comparison with captopril. *J Hypertens* 9:1119, 1991.

115. Shannon RP, Friedrich S, Mathier M, et al: Effects of renin inhibition compared to angiotensin converting enzyme inhibition in conscious dogs with pacing-induced heart failure. *Cardiovasc Res* 34(3):464, 1997.

116. Kleinert HD: Hemodynamic effects of rennin inhibitors. *Am J Nephrol* 16:252, 1996.

117. Ryan MJ, Hicks GW, Batley BL, et al: Effect of an orally active renin inhibitor CI-992 on blood pressure in normotensive and hypertensive monkeys. *J Pharmacol Exp Ther* 268:372, 1994.

118. Cook JA, Burger PJ, Michniewicz BM, et al: Pharmacokinetics and pharmacodynamics of CI-992 following intravenous and oral administration to cynomolgus monkeys. *Biopharm Drug Disp* 19:185, 1998.

119. Zimmerman BG: Greater blood pressure-lowering effect of the renin inhibitor EMD 58265 than an angiotensin-converting enzyme inhibitor in two-kidney one-clip Goldblatt rabbit. *Clin Exp Pharm Phys* 27:370, 2000.

120. Sueiras-Diaz J, Jones DM, Szelke M, et al: Potent in vivo inhibitors of rat renin: Analogues of human and rat angiotensinogen sequences containing different classes of pseudodipeptides at the scissile site. *J Peptide Res* 50:239, 1997.

121. Paruszewski R, Jaworski P, Winiecka I, et al: New renin inhibitors with hydrophilic C-terminus. *Pharmazie* 54:102, 1999.

122. Yamada Y, Ando K, Ikemoto Y, et al: Novel renin inhibitors containing (2S,3S,5S)-2-amino-1-cyclohexyl-6-methyl-3,5-heptanediol fragment as a transition-state mimic at the P1-P1' cleavage site. *Chem Pharm Bull* 45:1631, 1997.

123. Lefevre G, Gauron S: Automated quantitative determination of the new renin inhibitor CGP 60536 by high-performance liquid chromatography. *J Chromatog B Biomed Sci Appl* 738:129, 2000.

123a. Nussberger J, Wuerzner G, Jensen C, Brunner HR: Angiotensin II suppression in humans by the orally active renin inhibitor aliskirin (SPP100). *Hypertens* 39:e1, 2002.

124. Simoneau B, Lavallee P, Anderson PC, et al: Discovery of non-peptidic P_2-P_3 butanediamide renin inhibitor with high oral efficacy. *Bioorg Med Chem* 7(3):489, 1999.

125. Bolger G, Vigeant JC, Liard F, et al: The human renin infused rat: use as an in vivo model for the biological evaluation of human renin inhibitors. *Can J Physiol Pharmacol* 77:886, 1999.

126. Jung GL, Anderson PC, Bailey M, et al: Novel small renin inhibitors containing 4,5 or 3,5-dihydroxy-2-substituted-6-phenylhexanamide replacements at the P_2-P_3 sites. *Bioorg Med Chem* 6(12):2317, 1998.

127. Rahuel J, Rasetti V, Maibaum J, et al: Structure-based drug design: The discovery of novel nonpeptide orally active inhibitors of human renin. *Chem Biol* 7(7):493, 2000.

128. Oefner C, Binggeli A, Breu V, et al: Renin inhibition by substituted piperidines: A novel paradigm for the inhibition of monomeric aspartic proteinases? *Chem Biol* 6:127, 1999.

129. Vieira E, Binggeli A, Breu V, et al: Substituted piperidines-highly potent renin inhibitors due to induced fit adaptation of the active site. *Bioorg Med Chem Lett* 9:1397, 1999.

130. Guller R, Binggeli A, Volker B, et al: Piperidine-renin inhibitor compounds with improved physicochemical properties. *Bioorg Med Chem Lett* 9:1403, 1999.

131. Krantz A, Song Y, DeNagel D, et al: Drug pharmacophores covalently linked to the red cell surface are active without prior release. Drug targeting of renin with a synthetic ligand conjugated to red blood cells. *J Drug Target* 7:113, 1999.

132. Krantz A: Red cell-mediated therapy: Opportunities and challenges. *Blood Cells Mol Dis* 23a:58, 1997.

133. Dzau VJ: Tissue renin angiotensin system: Physiologic and pharmacologic implications. *Circulation* 77(6: Suppl I):I1, 1988.

134. Price DA, Porter LE, Gordon M, et al: The paradox of the low-renin state in diabetic nephropathy. *J Am Soc Nephrol* 10(11): 2382, 1999.

135. Schaffer LW, Schorn TW, Winquist RJ, et al: Acute hypotensive responses to peptide inhibitors of renin in conscious monkeys: An effect on blood pressure independent of plasma renin inhibition. *J Hypertens* 8:251, 1990.

136. DeClaviere M, Fourment P, Richaud JP, et al: Haemodynamic effects of the renin inhibitor SR 42128 in conscious baboon. *J Hypertens* 3(Suppl 3):S271, 1985.

137. Kleinert HD, Martin D, Chekal M, et al: Cardiovascular actions of the primate selective renin inhibitor A-62198. *J Pharmacol Exp Ther* 246:975, 1988.

138. Hofbauer KG, Wood JM, Gulati N, et al: Increased plasma renin during renin inhibition: Studies with a novel immunoassay. *Hypertension* 7(Suppl I):I61, 1985.

139. Duan J, Jaramillo J, Jung GL, et al: A novel renal hypertensive guinea pig model for comparing different inhibitors of the renin-angiotensin system. *J Pharmacol Toxicol Methods* 35:83, 1996.

140. Fisher ND, Hollenberg NK. Is there a future for renin inhibitors? *Exp Opin Invest Drugs* 10:417, 2001.

141. Mento PF, Holt WF, Murphy WR, Wilkes BM: Combined renin and converting enzyme inhibition in rats. *Hypertension* 13:741, 1989.

142. Blaine EH, Nelson EJ, Seymour AA, et al: Comparison of renin and converting enzyme inhibition in sodium-deficient dogs. *Hypertension* 7(Suppl I):I66, 1985.

143. Fossa AA, Weinberg LJ, Barber RL, et al: Synergistic effect on reduction in blood pressure with coadministration of the renin inhibitor, CP-80,794, and the angiotensin converting enzyme inhibitor, captopril. *J Cardiovasc Pharmacol* 20:7, 1992.

144. Smith SG, Seymour AA, Mazack EK, et al: Comparison of a new renin inhibitor and enalaprilat in renal hypertensive dogs. *Hypertension* 9:150, 1987.

145. Neisius D, Wood JM: Antihypertensive effect of a renin inhibitor in marmosets with a segmental renal infarction. *J Hypertens* 5:721, 1987.

146. Sweet CS, Ludden CT, Frederick CM, et al: Comparative hemodynamic effects of MK 422, a converting enzyme inhibitor, and a renin inhibitor in dogs with acute left ventricular failure. *J Cardiovasc Pharmacol* 6(6):1067, 1984.

147. Neuberg GW, Kukin ML, Penn J, et al: Hemodynamic effects of renin inhibition by enalkiren in chronic congestive heart failure. *Am J Cardiol* 67:63, 1991.

148. Kleinert HD, Stein HH: Specific renin inhibitors: Concepts and prospects. In: Laragh JH, Brenner BM, eds. *Hypertension: Pathophysiology, Diagnosis and Management*, 2nd ed. New York: Raven Press, 1995:3065–3077.

149. Gavras H, Gavras I, Cannon PJ, et al: Is elevated plasma renin activity of prognostic importance in progressive systemic sclerosis. *Arch Intern Med* 137:1554, 1977.

150. Laragh JH, Baer L, Brunner HR, et al: Renin, angiotensin, and aldosterone system in pathogenesis and management of hypertensive vascular disease. *Am J Med* 52:633, 1972.

151. Laragh JH: The renin system and four lines of hypertension research: Nephron heterogeneity, the calcium connection, and the prorenin vasodilator limb and plasma renin and heart attack. *Hypertension* 20:267, 1992.

152. Giardina WJ, Kleinert HD, Ebert DM, et al: Intraocular pressure lowering effects of the renin inhibitor Abbott-64662 diacetate in animals. *J Ocul Pharmacol* 6:75, 1990.

153. Bursztyn M, Gavras I, Tifft CP, et al: Effects of a novel renin inhibitor in patients with essential hypertension. *J Cardiovasc Pharmacol* 15:493, 1990.

154. Ondetti MA, Cushman DW: Inhibition of the renin angiotensin system. A new approach to the therapy of hypertension. *J Med Chem* 24:355, 1981.

155. Tewksbury DA, Dart RA, Travis J: The amino terminal amino acid sequence of human angiotensinogen. *Biochem Biophy Res Commun* 99:1311, 1981.

CHAPTER 35

Vasopressin and Vasopressin-Receptor Antagonists in the Treatment of Cardiovascular Disease

William H. Frishman

Marc Klapholz

Naveen Acharya

Adam B. Mayerson

In the early 1900s, Cajal first described the nerve connections between the hypothalamus and the neurohypophysis.[1] Subsequently it was discovered that the cell bodies of the hypothalamo-hypophyseal nerve fibers were found in the anterior hypothalamus, while the nerve axons terminated in capillary beds located in the neurohypophysis. Antidiuretic hormone (ADH), which is the same as arginine vasopressin (AVP), and the closely related oxytocin are synthesized in the supraoptic nuclei of the hypothalamus and to a lesser extent in the paraventricular nucleus (Fig. 35-1).[2–5] These hormones are transported from the anterior hypothalamus to the neurohypophysis, where they are stored and later released.[1]

Vasopressin was first isolated by du Vigneaud and Turner in 1951 and was found to be a nonpeptide with a six- member disulfide ring and a three-member tail, with an amidated terminal carboxyl group.[6,7] AVP has been shown to have a wide variety of physiologic activities (Table 35-1),[6–18] the most important of which are its antidiuretic and vasoconstrictive actions, which act to preserve homeostasis volume while maintaining blood pressure. The most important stimuli for vasopressin secretion are an elevated plasma osmolality and reduced circulating blood volume. The plasma AVP levels of normally hydrated humans after an overnight fast are in the range of 2 to 4 pg/mL.[19] A level of approximately 50 pg/mL must be reached before a significant increase in mean arterial pressure is noted in normal conscious human beings.[20] Vasopressin levels are greatly increased in clinical situations associated with reduced circulating blood volume, as seen in patients with dehydration[21,22] and hemorrhage.[23] The highest AVP levels have been found in patients following traumatic surgical procedures and hypotensive hemorrhage.[24]

If AVP secretion or binding are functioning in an abnormal fashion, a marked distortion of fluid balance results, as may be seen with disease states such as the syndrome of inappropriate antidiuretic hormone (SIADH) or diabetes insipidus, though these are usually not associated with systemic hypertension or hypotension. AVP blood levels can be elevated in other pathophysiologic states associated with increased body fluid volumes, such as hepatic cirrhosis and congestive heart failure (CHF).[25,26]

Recently, attention has focused on the role of AVP in the homeostasis of the cardiovascular system and in cardiovascular pathophysiology and therapy. As a therapy, it is now considered an alternative to epinephrine in patients with cardiac arrest. Its contribution to blood pressure, its effect on heart rate and cardiac output, its role as one of the neurohormones activated in CHF, and its recently observed direct effects on vascular smooth muscle– and myocyte-cell hypertrophy are discussed in this chapter. A new class of agents is also discussed, the vasopressin receptor antagonists, which may have potential in treating patients with heart failure who are volume-overloaded and in other disease entities where hyponatremia is a significant problem.

VASOPRESSIN ANALOGUES

Vasopressin analogues were first synthesized in the 1960s for the purpose of creating peptides that were more resistant to degradation while retaining potency. Several analogues were produced, the first of which was desmopressin, a V_2-receptor agonist that mimics vasopressin's antidiuretic effect (Fig. 35-2).[6] Desmopressin is the treatment of choice for neurogenic forms of diabetes insipidus and has also been used as a hemostatic agent because of its pro–platelet aggregation effects and its ability to transiently raise plasma levels of endogenous factor VIII and von Willebrand factor. It has therefore become an attractive alternative to the large numbers of blood transfusions required by patients with hemophilia A, von Willebrand's disease, uremia, cirrhosis, and other diseases with associated platelet dysfunction.

Terlipressin, a V_1-receptor agonist (causing vasoconstriction), is used in the emergency treatment of bleeding from esophageal varices (Fig. 35-2)[6,27,28] and as an alternative to epinephrine in patients with cardiopulmonary arrest.[29,30]

VASOPRESSIN RECEPTORS

All AVP receptors are G protein–coupled receptors with a structure composed of a single polypeptide chain with seven transmembrane domains. Two AVP receptor subtypes, V_1 and V_2, were initially characterized.[31–35] A third "pituitary specific" receptor has been

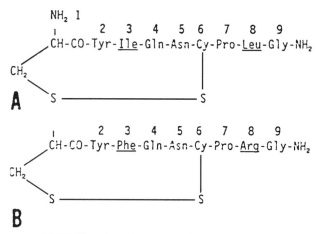

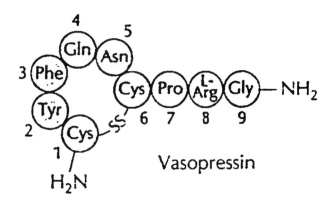

FIGURE 35-1. Oxytocin (A) and arginine vasopressin (B).

designated V_{1b} or V_3[8,36,37]; therefore, the V_1 receptor is now referred to as the V_{1a} receptor.

The V_{1a} receptor has classically been associated with AVP's vasoconstrictor effect; however, the V_{1a} receptor has been found to mediate a multitude of other diverse physiologic actions (Table 35-2).[7,8,33,38,39] The cDNA for the V_{1a} receptor encodes a protein having 394 amino acids with a molecular weight of 44.2 kd.[40] The activation pathway following stimulation of the V_{1a} receptor can be seen in Fig. 35-3.[41] V_{1a}-receptor stimulation shares the same intracellular activation pathway as that of the angiotensin II receptor, consisting of phospholipase C activation, mobilization of intracellular Ca^{2+}, and stimulation of protein kinase C.[42] Most recently, mitogenic and hypertrophic effects of vasopressin, mediated via the V_{1a} receptor, have been observed in both smooth muscle and myocyte cell cultures.[43] Tahara et al. demonstrated that AVP, when added to growth-arrested vascular smooth muscle cells, induced hyperplasia and hypertrophy.[43] The addition of a nonspecific vasopressin antagonist to these cell cultures inhibited AVP-induced increases in intracellular free calcium and the activation of mitogen-activated protein kinase while preventing AVP-induced hyperplasia and hypertrophy.[43] These investigators also observed that vasopressin increased the secretion of vascular endothelial growth factor (VEGF) from human vascular smooth muscle cells. Given VEGF's

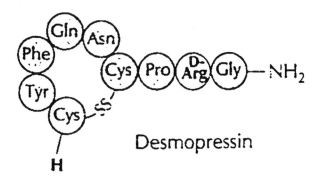

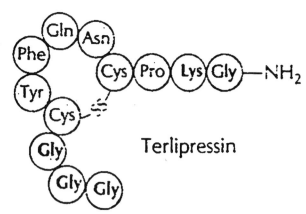

FIGURE 35-2. Changes in the structure of vasopressin can selectively enhance the hormone's antidiuretic or pressor properties. The native hormone (top) is a nonapeptide in which a disulfide bond creates a six-member ring with a three-member tail. Desmopressin differs only in the substitution of a dextroisomer of arginine (D-Arg) for the levoisomer at position 8 and a deamination at position 1, yet its antidiuretic effect is greatly enhanced and prolonged. The change in terlipressin is highlighted (no shading). (*Reproduced with permission from Robertson and Harris.*[6])

known mitogenic capability, it has been suggested that vasopressin might act as a paracrine hormone that could strongly influence the permeability and growth of the overlying vascular endothelium.[44] Additionally, neonatal rat cardiomyocytes have a single population of high-affinity binding sites with the profile of the V_{1a} receptor subtype.[45] When the receptor was blocked, AVP-induced increases

TABLE 35-1. The Actions of Vasopressin

Vasoconstriction
Reabsorption of free water
Intestinal contraction
Hepatic glycogenolysis
Platelet aggregation
Release of factor VIII
Potentiation on pituitary effects of corticotropin-releasing hormone
Aldosterone secretion
Uterine contractility
Neurotransmitter
Role in central thermoregulation in rats
Behavioral response to stress
Autonomic nervous system effects
Central control of thirst
Central control of hypothalamic vasopressin system
Involved in circadian rhythm of melatonin secretion
Osmotically stimulated vasopressin secretion and mediates
Pyrogen-induced febrile response

TABLE 35-2. Location and Effects of Vasopressin Receptor Stimulation

Location	Effect
V_{1a} receptors	
Hepatocytes	Stimulates glycogenolysis
Glomerular mesangial cells	?
Platelets	Promotes aggregation
Vascular smooth muscle cells	Induces vasoconstriction
Adrenals	Stimulates aldosterone secretion
Myometrium	Increases contractility
Endometrium	Mediates release of uterotonic substance
V_2 receptors	
Renal distal tubules	Increases free water reabsorption
Collecting duct	Increases free water reabsorption
Seminal vesicles	?
Vascular smooth muscle	Induces vasodilation
V_3 receptors	
Adenohypophyseal cells	Potentiation of corticotropin-releasing hormone stimulation
Kidney, thymus, heart, lung, spleen, uterus, breast	?

in cytosolic calcium, the activation of MAP kinase, and AVP-induced protein synthesis were inhibited. This has suggested that the antagonism of V_{1a} might be beneficial in preventing the development of cardiomyocyte hypertrophy or mediate its regression.[45] In summary, these recent observations suggest that vasopressin via the V_{1a} receptor might play a role in the regulation of vascular and cardiac function.[44]

The V_2 receptor mediates the antidiuretic effects of AVP in the kidney. The receptor has also been identified in the seminal vesicles of humans, where its role is uncertain.[46] The V_2 receptor has also been implicated in the relaxation of vascular smooth muscle, allowing for the possibility that AVP could have variable effects on the vasculature, which complicates the investigations into AVP's role in the pathophysiology of hypertension and CHF (Table 35-2).[46,47] The V_2 receptor has been cloned and found to encode a protein of 370 amino acids with a weight of 40.5 kd.[48] Signal transduction of the V_2 receptor differs from that of the V_{1a} receptor, working via adenylate cyclase and adenosine 3′, 5′-cyclic phosphate (cAMP).[41]

The V_{1b} receptor or V_3 receptor has been found to have more homology with the oxytocin receptor than with the V_{1a} receptor. Using DNA nucleotide sequences, deKeyzer et al. constructed a phylogenetic tree of AVP receptors, revealing that the V_3 receptor did not diverge from the V_{1a} receptor, as previously thought, but from an earlier ancestor of the human oxytocin receptor.[8]

The molecular cloning of the V_3 receptor was found to yield cDNA encoding a 421–amino acid protein.[49] The mRNA of this receptor is also found in many other tissues, including kidney, thymus, heart, lung, spleen, uterus, and breast, indicating a possible role for the V_3 receptor in the regulation of cellular functions in these organs (Table 35-2).[8,46] The signaling properties of the V_3 receptor have been shown to be identical to those of the V_{1a} receptor,[8] and the activation of the V_3 receptor plays a major role in the regulation of adrenocorticotropin hormone (ACTH) secretion, involved in the physiologic response to stress.[16–18]

Chan et al. reported the unexpected discovery of a potentially novel vasopressin receptor (VP) during an attempt to synthesize new V_2 receptor–selective antagonists.[50] They synthesized four new peptide analogues of vasopressin that caused a significant depressor response when administered in vivo to rats. This effect was resistant to V_{1a}- and V_2-selective antagonists. The peptides did not show any V_{1a}- or V_2-agonist or antagonist activity.

After hormone binding, the AVP receptor-ligand complex is endocytosed and delivered to endosomes. The endosomes are then either joined to lysosomes for degradation or to the plasma membrane for recycling.[41] This endocytosis has been observed for both the V_{1a} and V_2 receptors in vascular smooth muscle, liver, bladder, and kidney cells. Endocytosis is therefore thought to play a role

FIGURE 35-3. Immediate and secondary signals activated by V_1-vascular AVP receptors. PLC = phospholipase C; PLD = phospholipase D; PLA2 = phospholipase A_2; PA = phosphatidic acid; AA = arachidonic acid; PC = phosphatidylcholine; PKC = protein kinase C; ER = endoplasmic reticulum; CO = cyclooxygenase pathway; EPO = epoxygenase pathway; IP3 = 1,4,5-inositol triphosphate; DAG = 1,2-diacylglycerol; Gq = g protein. (*Reproduced with permission from Thibbonier.[41]*)

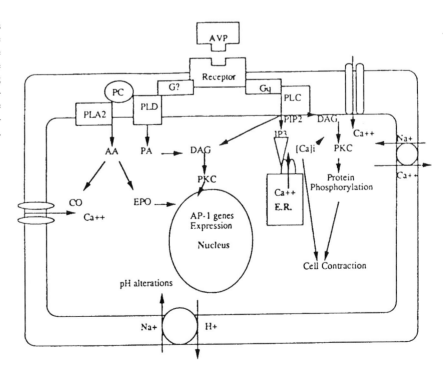

in the desensitization of tissues to vasopressin and to modulate the overall extent of the cellular response to AVP.[51]

OTHER PHYSIOLOGIC EFFECTS OF VASOPRESSIN

Effects on the Autonomic Nervous System

The interaction of AVP with the sympathetic and parasympathetic systems is not well understood, with much species variation in findings. It is generally thought that circulating AVP in the central nervous system lowers sympathetic activity while enhancing efferent vagal tone.[18,52] AVP has been shown to decrease heart rate and renal sympathetic nerve activity via stimulation of the V_{1a} receptor.[53,54] AVP may mediate its effect on the sympathetic nervous system via augmented baroreflex activity,[55] centrally in the central nervous system,[56] or more specifically the area postrema. Lesions produced in the area postrema of rabbits have resulted in reduced effects of AVP in decreasing both renal sympathetic nerve activity and heart rate.[56] These effects are mostly likely mediated via V_{1a}-receptor stimulation.[57]

It has also been postulated that the effects of AVP are due to direct suppression of sympathetic tone in the central nervous system[54,58] or suppression of ganglionic transmission.[53,54] Vasopressin has been implicated as a neurotransmitter in the paraventricular nucleus pathway, affecting cardiovascular function through both pressor actions and sympathetic response.[59]

Effects on the Baroreflex

When arterial pressure falls, there is decreased activity of afferent nerves from the carotid sinus and aortic arch (baroreceptors) that project to the dorsomedial regions of the nucleus tractus solitarius (NTS) via cranial nerves IX and X. Through a series of complex interactions within the brain, the sympathetic nervous system is then activated, leading to increases in peripheral resistance and cardiac output and thereby a rise in blood pressure.[60]

Studies have indicated that baroreceptors may play a permissive role in the sympathoinhibitory effects of AVP.[60] Normal baroreceptor activity would therefore allow AVP to exert its inhibitory influence with chronic elevations in salt intake, allowing for vasodilation and thereby accommodating the increased volume load and permitting natriuresis.

AVP elicits a greater decrease in heart rate for a given increase in arterial pressure than other vasoconstrictors when administered to several species, an action though to be due to baroreflex mechanisms.[61] In rabbits,[61] vasopressin decreased heart rate due to a shift in the baroreflex curve to a lower pressure with no increase in its gain. Furthermore, the actions of AVP on the baroreflex were found to be mediated by V_1 receptors. AVP has also been shown to reduce cardiac output in patients without changing mean arterial pressure.[62] This reduction in cardiac output appears to be partly due to baroreceptor actions and is abolished by sinoaortic denervation in rabbits.[54]

Unger et al. theorized that AVP could sensitize the baroreceptor reflex through V_2 receptors, accessible via the blood, while attenuating the reflex via the central nervous system V_{1a} receptors, which are unreachable via the blood.[63] AVP tonically enhances baroreceptor function through a V_2 receptor in spontaneously hypertensive rats (SHRs).[64] Indeed, systemic administration of the V_2-selective antagonist OPC 31260 attenuates the baroreflex in SHRs,[64] while

V_1 stimulation directly within the blood-brain barrier inhibits the baroreflex in these animals.[63,64] This has suggested a direct interaction between hormonal and neuronal vasopressin in causing AVP's effects.

AVP in the nucleus tractus solitarius (NTS) contributes to the control of peripheral cardiovascular parameters such as blood pressure, heart rate, and sympathetic activity.[65] Sved et al. have demonstrated that AVP contributes to hypertension caused by lesions in the NTS.[66] AVP levels were found to increase more than 10 times after lesions were created in the NTS of rats, and V_{1a} antagonism decreases the arterial pressure in these animals. More recently, Hegarty et al. have shown that the V_{1a} antagonist $d(CH_2)_5Tyr(Me)AVP$ could attenuate the baroreflex control of mean arterial pressure and renal nerve activity in rats.[65] As mentioned previously, microinjection of AVP into the area postrema of rats leads to significant increases in blood pressure.[67] Zhang et al. have shown that AVP receptors in the area postrema modulate the baroreflex control of heart rate and sympathetic efferent discharge.[68] AVP probably also modulates efferent projections from the area postrema to the NTS, thus altering the evoked response from the NTS elicited by aortic and vagal afferent inputs, which ultimately modifies the baroreflex[69] and the exercise pressor reflex.[70] Once again, this mechanism is likely V_{1a} receptor–dependent.

Studies on the effects of AVP on the baroreflex in humans have not been able to validate the results seen in animal models. However, Ebert et al. have reported that AVP helped potentiate the baroreflex in the presence of an angiotensin converting enzyme (ACE) inhibitor, suggesting that an intact renin-angiotensin system masks the effects of AVP on the autonomic nervous system.[62] Attempting to validate this observation, Goldsmith studied the effects of AVP infusion in volunteers subjected to baroreceptor perturbation with head-tilt maneuvers and simultaneous volume infusion in the presence and absence of ACE inhibition.[71] No effects of AVP on the baroreflex were noted, regardless of treatment with an ACE inhibitor. The effects of AVP on the sympathetic nervous system were studied by measuring norepinephrine plasma levels, norepinephrine spillover, and norepinephrine clearance as indirect markers of sympathetic activity, and no changes in adrenergic activity were noted. Evidence for enhanced vagal nerve activity was seen, however, as shown by a fall in heart rate with AVP infusion in the presence of ACE inhibition. It was concluded that long-term ACE inhibition may alter the effects of AVP on the baroreflex.

In summary, there is interaction in the central nervous system between the area postrema, NTS and the baroreflex, and vasopressin appears to play a major role in this interaction. Further research into the interaction between central and peripheral AVP effects may help to elucidate AVP's complex physiologic role in cardiovascular homeostasis.

VASOPRESSIN AS A CARDIOVASCULAR THERAPY

In normotensive patients, a physiologic antidiuretic level of vasopressin does not affect blood pressure. Circulating vasopressin inhibits sympathetic efferents and resets the cardiac baroreflex to a lower pressure via receptors in the medulla oblongata. When blood pressure is compromised, vasopressin-induced vasoconstriction of peripheral vessels helps maintain blood pressure. In patients with baroreflex impairment, the vasoconstrictive effects of vasopressin achieve or exceed those of angiotensin II or norepinephrine and phenylephrine. As vasodilation in shock states is prolonged, smooth muscle becomes poorly responsive to catecholamines, possibly due to down regulation of beta-adrenergic receptors. Exogenous vasopressin helps maintain arterial pressure and prevents cardiovascular collapse.

Vasopressin has been used successfully as a pressor agent in patients with hypovolemia and gastrointestinal hemorrhage. Recently it has also been used as therapy for cardiac arrest and for vasodilatory shock due to sepsis[72,73] or cardiopulmonary bypass.[74,75]

Cardiac Arrest

Epinephrine is the vasopressor of choice in the Advanced Cardiac Life Support (ACLS) guidelines.[76] Vasopressin, however, may also be a viable option in patients who are unresponsive to standard treatment. Vasopressin is recommended as a means to support blood pressure and/or to obtain the return of spontaneous circulation in patients refractory to epinephrine.[29,30] Following ventricular fibrillation arrest, higher serum concentrations of vasopressin have been associated with successful resuscitation, while higher serum concentrations of catecholamines have been associated with a reduced chance of survival.

Epinephrine has some disadvantages in the treatment of cardiac arrest, including increased myocardial oxygen consumption, risk of ventricular arrhythmias, ventilation-perfusion defects, and reduced cerebral blood flow.[29,30,77] These effects may be due to increased myocardial oxygen consumption and lactate production induced by the activation of beta-adrenergic receptors in myocardial and skeletal muscle. Vasopressin increases oxygen delivery to the heart as well as cardiac contractility via the nitric oxide–mediated pathway, thus minimizing these consequences.

Vasopressin has been linked with greater increases in arterial tone and ACTH release, particularly during hypoxia and acidosis.[78] Vasopressin may be beneficial in prolonged or refractory cardiac arrest in which the precipitating acidosis renders catecholamines ineffective in eliciting a pressor response. Vasopressin-mediated vasodilation in cerebral vasculature may help maintain cerebral oxygen delivery and allow survival with fully intact neurologic activity. Vasopressin's duration of action is longer than that of epinephrine, 50 to 100 min versus 5 min.

In a small study of patients with out-of-hospital ventricular fibrillation, a significantly larger number initially treated with intravenous vasopressin 40 U were resuscitated and survived for 24 h versus patients treated with intravenous epinephrine 1 mg.[78a] There was no difference in survival to hospital discharge.

There is preliminary evidence that vasopressin is effective in enhancing the probability of return to spontaneous circulation in patients with ventricular fibrillation. The ACLS guidelines recommend a 40–U bolus of intravenous vasopressin followed by 300 to 360 J of direct current cardioversion to restore spontaneous circulation in patients with ventricular fibrillation arrest refractory to epinephrine.

Vasodilatory Shock

Vasopressin-induced vasoconstriction raises systolic blood pressure by increasing systemic vascular resistance in vasodilatory shock due to sepsis or cardiopulmonary bypass.[72–75,79] Low levels of vasopressin were found in patients during septic shock, possibly due to a defect in the baroreflex-mediated secretion of vasopressin or

a depletion of vasopressin stores during failed attempts to correct hypotension.[80–80b] Supplemental vasopressin may correct this.

Vasopressin may be better than catecholamine pressors in these cases, since vascular smooth muscle is poorly responsive to alpha-adrenergic agonists in septic shock in association with an acidotic state.[72] An increase in urine output often follows vasopressin treatment. Stimulation of vasopressin receptors in efferent arterioles causes constriction. This constriction maintains glomerular filtration rate despite reduced renal blood flow. In contrast, stimulation of catecholamine receptors in afferent arterioles rarely increases urine output even with increased blood pressure.

In a randomized, placebo-controlled trial, Argenziano studied vasopressin in 10 vasodilatory shock patients post left ventricular assist device. Intravenous vasopressin 0.1 U/min led to a significant increase in mean arterial blood pressure from 57 to 84 mm Hg, allowing norepinephrine to be discontinued.[75]

Several preliminary studies have been published using vasopressin to treat vasodilatory septic shock. In patients poorly responsive to catecholamines, low-dose vasopressin infusions at 0.04 U/min for 16 h increased mean arterial pressure, systemic vascular resistance and urine output in patients with vasodilatory shock and limited responsiveness to catecholamines.[72] Vasopressin allows down titration and cessation of catecholamine pressors often times within 24 h. Vasopressin doses can be titrated down to 0.01 U/min over 2 to 11 days before discontinuation. When dose reduction results in decreased blood pressure, arterial pressure can be restored with increasing vasopressin doses.

Therapeutic Monitoring

Since patients receiving vasopressin are inherently hemodynamically unstable, it is important to monitor cardiovascular side effects. Vasopressin causes transient, reversible reductions in cardiac output and heart rate. Coronary vasoconstriction also will decrease coronary blood flow and offsets changes in vagal and sympathetic tone. Patients should be monitored for bradycardia, arrhythmia, myocardial and/or mesenteric ischemia.[81,81a] Vasopressin may exacerbate regional ischemia by reducing collateral-dependent myocardial perfusion. An increased rate of right heart failure in patients using left ventricular assist devices has been observed.

Adverse Events

Data are lacking on adverse events after resuscitation in terms of impaired function of vital organs. Due to the presence of vasopressin receptors in various tissues, there is the potential for reduced regional blood flow in pulmonary, coronary, and splanchnic blood vessels. Vasopressin has not been associated with bowel ischemia or increased liver insufficiency. There is the potential for increased pulmonary arterial pressure and hypertension, although these side effects also have not been observed.

VASOPRESSIN ANTAGONISTS (VAPTANS)

This section provides a brief overview of vasopressin antagonists and specifically focuses on the newer nonpeptide, orally administered AVP antagonists, collectively known as vaptans.

Vincent du Vigneaud, who was the first to isolate and characterize AVP, was also instrumental in creating the first antagonist to the

```
              1              2     3  4  5  6  7  8  9
            CH₂ - CO - Tyr(Me)-Phe-Gln-Asn-Cys-Pro-Arg-Gly-NH₂
       CH₂─CH₂ ╲  │
CH₂            C  A         B         C         D
       CH₂─CH₂ ╱  │
              S ──────────────────────────────── S
```

```
              1     2        3  4  5  6  7  8  9
            CH₂ - CO - Tyr(Alk)- Phe-Val-Asn-Cys-Pro - Z - Gly-NH₂
       CH₂─CH₂ ╲  │
CH₂            C         X         Y
       CH₂─CH₂ ╱  │
              S ──────────────────────────────── S
```

FIGURE 35-4. The chemical structure of a V_1 antagonist—[d(CH₂)₅Tyr(Me)AVP] (top)—and the general structure of V_2 antagonists (bottom).

V_{1a} receptor.[24] This analogue, called OT, is AVP with a methylated hydroxy group on the 2-tyrosine. The most potent V_{1a} antagonists that followed were formulated on the OT model. The most widely used V_{1a} antagonist prior to the development of the nonpeptide antagonists was d(CH₂)₅Tyr(Me)AVP (Fig. 35-4).[24,82] There are now over 70 AVP analogues in development that selectively block the vasopressor activity of AVP.

The general structure of V_2 antagonists is shown in Fig. 35-4.[24] There are over 70 known antagonists of the V_2 receptor, although with much less receptor selectivity than has been achieved with the V_{1a} antagonists. Administration of the V_2 antagonist d(CH₂)₅Tyr(Et) VAVP to dehydrated or normally hydrated rats induced a significant increase in urine volume as well as a reduction in urine osmolality (Fig. 35-5).[83] These changes are dose-dependent.

Initially, all AVP antagonists were peptides having little oral bioavailability. OPC 21268 was one of the first orally effective nonpeptide AVP V_{1a} antagonists to be developed.[84,85] The drug was found to selectively bind to the V_{1a} receptor in a competitive manner, with little if any effect at the renal V_2 receptor.[85] It was shown to block AVP-induced vasoconstriction in rats and in the human forearm vascular bed and to decrease the vasoconstrictor response to intraarterial AVP in normal human subjects.[84,86,87] OPC 21268 was found to mediate V_{1a} antagonism in microvessels in the brain and has also been shown to reduce brain edema and extravasation of protein by reducing the permeability of the blood-brain barrier,[88] suggesting a potential role for this V_{1a} receptor antagonist in the treatment of brain injury caused by the intracerebral release of AVP during trauma.

OPC 31260, an oral nonpeptide, predominant V_2 antagonist,[89] has a renal V_2/hepatic V_{1a} receptor selectivity ratio of 25:1, with some vasodilatory activity.[87] It induces a strong diuretic effect in human beings, increasing urine volume, plasma sodium, and plasma AVP in a dose-dependent manner without altering blood pressure or heart rate.[90] OPC 3120 has demonstrated potential therapeutic usefulness in animal models of SIADH and cirrhosis.[26,91]

Burrell et al. have challenged the receptor selectivity of both OPC 21268 and OPC 31260[92] by demonstrating both variable vasoactive effects of OPC 21268 and significant crossover from V_2 to V_{1a} antagonism with OPC 31260. This was seen in particular in human internal mammary arteries, where OPC 21268 was found to be a partial agonist at the V_{1a} receptor and OPC 31260 (a V_2 antagonist) was found to have V_{1a} antagonist effects.[92] In rat

mesenteric resistance arteries, both nonpeptide antagonists blocked AVP-induced constriction. Previous in vivo studies had shown that OPC 21268 can cause antagonism of the vasoconstrictor responses

FIGURE 35-5. Effects of V_2 antagonist on urine excretion (top) and osmolality (bottom) ($n = 10$). Δ = physiologic NaCl; O = 10-μg/kg antagonist; ● = 30-μg/kg antagonist, □ = Brattleboro homozygous untreated rats; error bars = standard error of the mean. (*Reproduced with permission from Laszlo et al.[83]*)

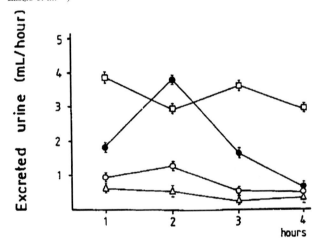

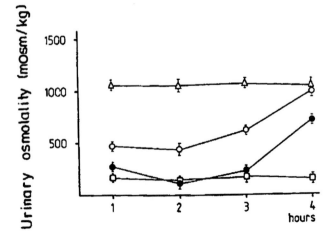

to intraarterial AVP infusion in human subjects.[86,87] These sometimes conflicting results may be related to different experimental methodologies, variable effects of vasopressin on different areas of the vasculature, and/or interspecies variation of vasopressin effects.[93]

Two new orally bioavailable nonpeptide V_2-receptor antagonists have become available. OPC 41061 has recently been developed from the earlier V_2 antagonist OPC 31260 by adding additional moieties to enhance its oral activity.[94] This agent is a specific V_2 receptor antagonist (V_2 versus V_{1a} binding 29:1) whose pharmacologic profile and acute and chronic diuretic effects have been characterized both in vitro and in vivo. In cell cultures expressing cloned AVP receptors, OPC 41061 antagonized AVP binding to the V_2 receptor more potently than OPC 31260 or AVP itself. There was no agonist activity and OPC 41061 did not inhibit AVP binding to human V_{1b} receptors.[94]

The new V_2 antagonist SR 121463A is also more potent than OPC 31260.[95] The compound is more selective for human V_2 receptors and demonstrates virtually no agonist activity. In vivo testing has confirmed its strong aquaretic properties.[95]

In single and multiple dosing studies in rats, OPC 41061 clearly produced a consistent, dose-dependent (1 and 10 mg) aquaretic effect.[94,96] In trials comparing OPC 41061 to the diuretic drug furosemide, OPC 41061 and furosemide produced equivalent dose-dependent increases in urine volume. However, OPC 41061 produced electrolyte-free water clearance, whereas furosemide elevated electrolyte clearance, leading to decreases in serum sodium. Furosemide also significantly activated the renin-angiotensin-aldosterone system (RAAS), as evidence by elevated levels of serum renin and aldosterone activity, whereas OPC 41061 did not activate the RAAS.[96] In addition, in assessing the effects of OPC 41061 on plasma neurohormones in normal conscious dogs, it was observed that in contrast to furosemide, OPC 41061 also does not increase systemic AVP levels, plasma renin levels, or norepinephrine levels.

Another highly potent selective V_{1a} orally active nonpeptide receptor antagonist, SR 49059, has been characterized and found to potently inhibit both second-messenger and physiologic responses of AVP in cultured human aortic vascular smooth muscle cells.[97–99]

In healthy volunteers, SR49059 was assessed in an ascending repeated-dose tolerability trial. Clinical tolerability and biologic safety were excellent for all subjects up to the highest dose of 60 mg. However, SR 49059 appeared to have no effect on AVP plasma levels, hemostasis parameters, blood pressure, heart rate, diuresis, or plasma/urine osmolality.[100] SR 49059 did demonstrate potent antagonistic properties in inhibiting AVP-induced human platelet aggregation and vascular smooth muscle hypertrophy.[101]

An additional new compound, YM087, is a nonpeptide antagonist of both the V_{1a} and V_{1b} receptors and has completed extensive testing in various animal models, where it demonstrated high affinity and antagonistic effect for both the V_{1a} and V_2 receptors.[101a,102] There was no agonist effect and YM087 did not inhibit the binding of AVP to the anterior pituitary (V_{1b} receptors) plasma membranes.[101a,103]

In conscious rats, orally administered YM087 did not affect basal blood pressure, but YM087, in a dose-dependent fashion, inhibited AVP-induced pressor responses. Also, in rats deprived of water for 16 to 18 h, orally administered YM087, in a dose-dependent fashion, increased urine volume and reduced urine osmolality with significantly lower electrolyte excretion versus comparable diuretic doses of furosemide. The diuretic effect of YM087 was still present

at 8 to 10 h postdosing. These studies demonstrated that YM087 is an orally active AVP antagonist with potent and long-lasting effects at both the V_{1a} and V_2 receptors.[104]

In a dog model of congestive heart failure induced by 2 to 3 weeks of rapid right ventricular pacing, intravenous administration of YM087 significantly increased LV contractility (dp/dt) and cardiac output and significantly decreased left ventricular end-diastolic pressure and peripheral vascular resistance. YM087 also increased urine flow and reduced urine osmolality by markedly increasing free water clearance. These results in an animal model of heart failure demonstrated the effectiveness of YM087 by its both improving hemodynamics and promoting a diuresis.[105,106]

Finally, the pharmacokinetic and pharmacodynamic properties of YM087 were characterized in healthy, normotensive subjects. Six subjects were randomly allocated to receive—in an open-label, crossover design—either a single oral (60-mg) or IV (50-mg) dose of YM087. Upon both oral and IV dosing, a marked increase (sevenfold) in urine flow rate and a fall in urine osmolality (from 600 to <100 mosmol/L) with a concomitant increase in plasma osmolality (from 283 to 289 mosmol/L) was observed.[107]

Conivaptan is another dual V_{1A}/V_2 vasopressin antagonist that was administered in intravenous form in a double-blind, placebo-controlled study of 142 patients with symptomatic heart failure compared to placebo. The drug was shown to cause favorable changes in hemodynamics and urine output without affecting blood pressure or heart rate.[107a]

In a Chinese hamster ovarian cell model, the three subtypes of human AVP receptors (human V_{1a}, V_{1b}, and V_2) were cloned, expressed, and characterized by AVP-binding studies. These studies also measured the relative potency of several of the nonpeptide AVP-receptor antagonists in inhibiting AVP binding. At the V_{1a} receptor, the relative order of potency of AVP antagonists was as follows: SR 49059 > YM087 > OPC 31260 > OPC 21268. At the V_2 receptor, the relative potencies were YM087 = OPC 31260 > SR 49059 > OPC 21268.[108] While these observations are pharmacologically important, it is clear, given the foregoing discussion, that binding affinities of the various vasopressin antagonists do not entirely predict their clinical actions.

Studies with AVP antagonists in human beings have thus far been associated with no significant adverse effects.[85,90,109] OPC 21268 was associated with short-lived nonpitting edema in the lower extremities of 1 out of 33 healthy male volunteers.[110] A recent study by Ohnishi et al. found OPC 31260 to cause mild-to-moderate thirst in patients after oral administration of the drug.[90] No serious adverse effects have been reported with these new oral agents. Nicod et al. reported one patient with severe heart failure who was acutely sick and dyspneic on the day of the study and then died of an irreversible episode of ventricular fibrillation 2 h after intravenous administration of the AVP antagonist d(Ch$_2$)$_5$Tyr(Me)AVP.[109] The death was felt to be unrelated to administration of the AVP antagonist; however, caution is advised with the use of an AVP antagonist in acutely unstable patients with CHF.

CLINICAL APPLICATIONS

Systemic Hypertension

Vasopressin's role in the etiology of systemic hypertension has been studied extensively.[111] Animal and human studies have yielded inconsistent results. This section examines vasopressin's participation as an etiologic factor in systemic hypertension and the effects of vaptans as potential antihypertensive agents.

Lowes et al. have shown that microinjections of AVP into the area postrema of rats resulted in statistically significant increases in blood pressure and that such increases in blood pressure were blocked by a V_{1a}-receptor antagonist. These results suggest that circulating AVP may exert its pressor response through V_{1a}-receptor stimulation in the area postrema. In the same study, it was also found that microinjection of a V_2 agonist elicited a depressor response, indicating that a centrally located V_2 receptor may also play a part in cardiovascular homeostasis.[67]

It has also been shown that AVP administered into the cerebral ventricles causes a significant pressor effect in dogs.[112] This study found, in addition, that the V_{1a} receptors are the most likely mediators of this effect in dogs, while stimulation of V_2-like receptors in rats seemed to attenuate this response.

A recent study by Yang et al. supported earlier studies showing that centrally administered relaxin causes an elevation in blood pressure in rats.[113] The study went on to provide evidence that this increase in blood pressure is mediated, at least in part, by centrally-released vasopressin acting on the V_{1a} receptor in the brain. Peripheral plasma levels of vasopressin were also significantly elevated following the central administration of relaxin.[113]

Kremarik et al. have recently implicated the V_{1a} receptor in the fundus striati as a mediator of central blood pressure regulation.[114] Bilateral 100-pmol injections of AVP into the fundi striati of rats induced dose-dependent increases in arterial pressure without affecting heart rate. This increase in blood pressure was successfully blocked by V_{1a} antagonism, again implicating the importance of central V_{1a}-receptor activity.

Spontaneously hypertensive rats (SHRs) have been shown to have higher blood concentrations of AVP than normotensive rats.[115] Increased pressor sensitivity to vasopressin has also been demonstrated in these hypertensive animals.[116–118] However, decreased or unchanged AVP pressor responsiveness has also been demonstrated in other hypertensive animals[111,119] and in humans.[120] A study by Stepniakowski et al.[121] showed that SHRs reacted to AVP bolus injections of 2.5, 5.0, and 10 ng with markedly lower pressor and bradycardic responsiveness. However, in a follow-up study using the same strain of SHRs with a constant AVP infusion of 1.2 ng/kg/min, a significantly increased pressor responsiveness was observed.[122] Stepniakowski et al. hypothesize that this difference may be due to the inability of small boluses of AVP to reach certain target areas in the body that are responsible for increased pressor responsiveness. These target areas include certain areas of the brain involved in the baroreflex response.[123]

Recent evidence suggests that AVP may be involved in the development of systemic hypertension. Naitoh et al.[124] found that OPC 21268 administered to young SHRs between 6 and 10 weeks of age attenuated the development of hypertension in adulthood. Interestingly, V_2 receptor blockade using OPC 31260 during the same developmental period actually augmented hypertension in the adult SHR. These findings implicate AVP in the pathogenesis of hypertension via V_1 receptor stimulation. Naitoh has theorized that V_2 receptor blockade during development may increase hypertension by (1) causing increased endogenous AVP secretion, which augments V_{1a} receptor–mediated vasoconstriction; (2) preventing baroreflex sensitization to AVP by denying intravenous access to centrally located V_2 receptors; and (3) altering tubuloglomerular feedback mechanisms.[124]

dEt_2AVP, a selective V_{1a} antagonist, has been shown to cause a significant decrease in blood pressure and heart rate in the SHR.[125]

However, in normotensive rats, blood pressure and heart rate appear to be maintained after V_{1a} blockade.[122,126] It has been postulated that the cardiovascular effects of V_{1a} blockade may result from unopposed V_2-receptor stimulation, leading to vasodilation and tachycardia.[127]

The orally active vasopressin V_{1a} receptor antagonist OPC 21268 has been shown to lower blood pressure in rats with experimental mineralocorticoid hypertension.[128] This was also observed by Burrell et al.[129] However, a study by Hashimoto et al. found that although OPC 21268 and OPC 31260 (given separately) blocked the vasopressor and antidiuretic actions of exogenously administered vasopressin, respectively, neither treatment decreased blood pressure in Dahl salt-sensitive rats receiving high-salt diets.[130] Hashimoto postulates that this may be due to (1) increased compensatory water intake; (2) increase in plasma Na^+ induced by excretion of free water acting on the central nervous system; (3) blockage of a proposed V_2-mediated vasodilatory effect; and (4) further suppression of an impaired baroreflex function.[130] Others have also suggested a reflex increase in renal sympathetic nerve activity.[53] It is possible that the vasodilating effect of the V_{1a} antagonists were compensated by the enhancement of the baroreflex by AVP, or increased renal sympathetic nerve activity.[53,57,62,128]

As in the case of the animal studies, OPC 21268 was shown not to lower blood pressure in hypertensive patients on different dietary sodium intakes.[131] SR 49059, another V_{1a} antagonist, was studied in 24 untreated patients with stage I and II essential hypertension (12 whites and 12 blacks).[115] In this double-blind, placebo-controlled, crossover-design study, patients received a single 30-mg oral dose of SR 49059 before being stimulated for AVP secretion with a 5% hypertonic saline infusion. This single dose of SR 49059 did not decrease blood pressure before the saline infusion; however, the blood pressure peak at the end of the hypertonic infusion was slightly lower in the presence of SR 49059. Whether vaptans will be effective agents for the treatment of hypertension or heart failure remains to be determined.

Recently, it has been shown that there is a sex-specific difference in response to AVP administration in rats.[132] The decreased antidiuretic activity in female rats is due to the inhibitory effects of estrogens, which mediate the release of prostaglandin E_2 (PGE_2). PGE_2 is a potent inhibitor of the production of cAMP, which ultimately mediates the antidiuretic response of AVP.[133] The increased vasopressor effect in male rats is thought to be due to a sensitizing effect of testosterone via an increase in AVP-binding sites in the walls of most vascular beds through a mechanism that is likely prostaglandin-independent.[133] In rat thoracic aorta, however, contractile responses to AVP in females have been found to be nearly twice as high as those in males.[134] In female rats, contractile tensions develop much more rapidly in response to AVP because of a quicker release of calcium from intracellular stores through a mechanism dependent on IP3 (inositol triphosphate), possibly enhanced by female sex steroids. The slower rise in contractile force in the thoracic aorta of male rats is due to a reliance on mainly extracellular calcium brought into the cytosol via voltage-operated channels, a pathway that may be dependent on androgens.[134]

Selective V_2 agonists have been shown to cause a significant increase in cardiac output and vascular conductance in dogs.[47] This response is inhibited by V_2 but not V_{1a} antagonists.[47] In a 1994 experiment, Liard demonstrated the effects of selective V_2 agonists and their subsequent blunting by the nitric oxide synthase antagonist $N^{(G)}$-nitro-L-arginine methyl ester (L-NAME).[135] Interestingly, V_2-receptor antagonists have also been implicated in vasoconstriction in vitro in certain canine and simian vascular beds,[136,137] while

V_{1a} receptors have been shown to mediate vasodilation in vivo in the carotid arteries of rats.[138]

It appears that, in nonhypertensive individuals, endogenous AVP does not contribute to blood pressure maintenance.[139] Plasma AVP has been shown to be significantly higher in patients with malignant hypertension than in those without hypertension.[140,141] However, AVP levels in essential hypertension have been found to be variable.[19,120,139,140] In an attempt to study this further, Kawano et al. measured AVP levels in normotensive patients and patients with mild essential hypertension under different dietary sodium intakes.[142] They found AVP levels to be similar in both types of patients and concluded that AVP did not play an important role in essential hypertension.

Exogenous AVP, given to create plasma concentrations comparable to those seen in patients with CHF or malignant hypertension, produced only minor changes in blood pressure when given to patients with mild-moderate essential hypertension.[122] When administered to normal subjects at levels up to five times that recorded in patients with malignant hypertension, no effect on blood pressure was seen.[140]

A study by Bursztyn et al. has revealed a significant difference in AVP levels between black and white patients with hypertension.[143] Black hypertensive subjects were found to have significantly higher AVP levels than their white counterparts or control groups. Perhaps vasopressin plays a more important role in blood pressure maintenance in black patients, which might partly explain the decreased effectiveness of antihypertensive treatment with ACE inhibitors and beta blockers observed in black patients.

DePaula et al. compared responsiveness to AVP antagonists in hypertensive patients of different races and ages. The results showed significantly larger decreases in the blood pressure among elderly patients compared to the young as well as in black patients compared to white patients. It is hypothesized that these differences in responsiveness are caused by a greater role of AVP in elderly and black patients due to a greater prevalence of autonomic dysfunction and decreased renin-angiotensin system (RAS) activity, respectively.[144] Bakris et al. compared AVP and PRA (plasma renin activity) levels in white and black hypertensive patients and measured the effectiveness of AVP-receptor antagonism in each population.[145] Black patients had lower levels of plasma renin activity\but higher levels of AVP than whites. Only black patients demonstrated a significant drop in arterial pressure in response to a vasopressin antagonist. These results are consistent with other studies that show a greater role for AVP in patients with low-renin hypertension, such as blacks and the elderly.[50]

The importance of AVP in blood pressure regulation does become more pronounced in situations where the RAS or the sympathetic nervous system is blocked.[146] Blockade of the RAS with captopril and the sympathetic nervous system with clonidine in patients with accelerated hypertension led to an additional average blood pressure drop of 15 mm Hg with AVP antagonism.[147] In these patients, the baseline AVP levels were not correlated with the effect of the AVP antagonist on blood pressure. These observations suggest that the final effects of AVP antagonism on blood pressure are related to the compensatory actions of the RAS and sympathetic nervous system and not to the absolute levels of AVP.[146] An intact sympathetic nervous system has been found to attenuate the pressor response to AVP, mediated mainly by alpha$_1$-adrenergic constriction.[148]

SHRs were treated with the ACE inhibitor cilazapril for a period of 25 days and found to have significantly lower blood pressure and a urine volume that was three to five times that of the control group.[149]

The study group had significantly higher levels of AVP, while plasma concentrations of angiotensin II and aldosterone as well as plasma renin activity did not change significantly. A marked increase in the affinity of the renal V_2 receptor for vasopressin was also noted.[149] These results support the idea that compensatory changes occur among the sympathetic nervous system, the RAS, and AVP.

Further evidence comes from studies showing that an AVP infusion in patients with autonomic dysfunction can lead to a significant increases in blood pressure without much change in heart rate, while an increase in plasma AVP without autonomic dysfunction results in a decrease in heart rate with no change in blood pressure.[20,150] Similarly, in rats with iatrogenic catecholamine depletion, vasopressin levels were found to be significantly elevated.[151] Dogs having ganglionic blockade showed greater blood pressure responsiveness to a vasopressin antagonist than to captopril, implicating AVP as an important backup mechanism for blood pressure maintenance with a blocked sympathetic nervous system.[152]

Congestive Heart Failure

Much work has focused on the neuroendocrine changes that occur in CHF.[153-156] Activation of the sympathetic nervous system, the RAS, and AVP release lead to the vasoconstriction and fluid retention phenomenon that characterizes CHF. Norepinephrine,[157,158] endothelin, atrial natriuretic peptide, and plasma renin activity are also elevated and associated with increased mortality rates in CHF patients.[159-161]

The pathophysiologic role of vasopressin in heart failure appears to be quite variable in human[109,162] and animal models.[163-165] Elevated AVP levels have been recorded in both animals and humans having CHF.[163,166,167] Many studies have found that approximately 33% of patients with CHF have elevated AVP levels.[162,168-170] Patients with hyponatremia and CHF are more likely to have elevated AVP levels than those without hyponatremia.[171,172] Szatalowics et al. found that 30 of 37 patients with both hyponatremia and CHF had significantly increased AVP levels compared to controls.[172] Johnston et al. found elevated AVP levels of 7.8 ± 0.9 pg/mL in patients with severe heart failure compared to normal levels of 2.6 ± 0.2 pg/mL.[171] One study found AVP levels to parallel increased plasma renin activity.[166] It can be generally said that AVP levels tend to be higher in patients with more severe cardiac failure, which probably accounts for the hypoosmolality and hyponatremia that is observed.[171,172]

Secretion of AVP, normally controlled via hypothalamic osmoreceptors and atrial volume receptors, is overridden in CHF by nonosmolar stimuli, allowing for the dilutional hypoosmolality that is seen in CHF.[173] Angiotensin II has been variably found to increase or have no effect on AVP levels.[174-177] Norepinephrine has been shown to decrease AVP levels.[175,176] An impaired baroreflex could lead to maintenance of high AVP levels in CHF in the face of constantly declining osmolality.

It has been shown that in patients without CHF, increased baroreflex activity suppresses AVP levels that have been increased by osmotic stimulation.[178] Recent studies have provided proof of an abnormal baroreflex in CHF patients.[179] Vasopressin release is not impaired in patients with severe CHF, suggesting a defective sympathetic baroreflex control mechanism and implicating AVP as a protective mechanism to maintain blood pressure in patients with severe CHF.[180]

It is generally accepted that the AVP levels present in CHF are adequate to enhance the tubular reabsorption of water.[162] Studies of cardiomyopathic hamsters have revealed increased concentrations of AVP as well as a hypersensitivity of inner medullary collecting duct cells to AVP, as evidenced by the greater formation of cAMP for a given level of AVP.[181]

Even when levels are not elevated, sensitivity to AVP is increased in experimental heart failure, and vasopressin blockade results in vasodilation.[182] Endogenously secreted vasopressin contributes to an increase in systemic vascular resistance in CHF patients having elevated AVP levels,[162] the blockade of which leads to a decrease in systemic vascular resistance.[162,166,169,172]

AVP has been reported to have direct effects on the heart, sinoatrial node, and coronary arteries.[183,184] AVP infusion was found to cause a decrease in heart rate and cardiac output and a dose-dependent increase in total peripheral resistance in healthy young males who had been pretreated with ACE inhibition (to prevent fluctuations in angiotensin II).[62] AVP has also been shown to lead to coronary vasoconstriction with subsequent myocardial ischemia and decrease in cardiac output.[185] These effects were found to be reversible with the V_{1a} receptor antagonist $d(CH_2)_5Tyr(Me)AVP$.[185]

Elevated AVP levels may also contribute to the myocardial hypertrophy associated with heart failure. In vitro studies indicate that AVP increases the rate of protein synthesis in neonatal rat cardiomyocytes.[186] AVP administered to isolated perfused rat adult hearts also accelerated protein synthesis via a mechanism that was sensitive to inhibition of the V_{1a} receptor with OPC 21268.[187] Vasopressin has also been shown to increase production of vascular endothelial growth factor, which can affect the permeability and growth of the overlying vascular endothelium.[44]

Additionally, in vitro studies have shown that AVP can decrease myocardial contractile force in isolated atrial and ventricular preparations from a dog heart.[188] Animal studies in chicks also showed what was probably a direct negative inotropic effect of AVP on the heart.[189] This negative inotropic effect of AVP was suppressed by pretreatment with OPC 21268, a selective V_{1a} receptor. However, in other models, as in the isolated perfused rat heart and in neonatal myocytes, AVP has been shown to have a positive inotropic effect, depending on the test dose used.[190,191] Adult rat ventricular cardiomyocytes, expressing the V_2 receptor three times more than the V_{1a} receptor as a result of infection with a V_2 receptor carrying adenovirus, demonstrated a threefold greater contractile amplitude in response to AVP compared to uninfected cells.[192,193] This implicates the V_2 receptor in the aforementioned positive inotropic effect.

In a study by Arnolda et al., the AVP V_{1a} antagonist $d(CH_2)_5Tyr(Me)AVP$ and ACE inhibition were administered either alone or in combination in rabbits with acute left ventricular failure.[194] No significant change in hemodynamic parameters was noted when the AVP antagonist was given alone. As expected, when the study group was treated with ACE inhibitor alone, a fall in left ventricular end-diastolic pressure was seen. When both of these antagonists were given together (Fig. 35-6),[194] significant increases in cardiac output and total vascular conductance as well as a fall in blood pressure were noted. While the increase in cardiac output can be explained as a summation of two statistically insignificant increases by either antagonist alone, the changes in blood pressure and vascular conductance cannot. Arnolda et al. proposed that these results might be due to the compensatory activation of one system when the other is inhibited, therefore showing no effect unless both systems are blocked from responding. Other studies have shown that the combined effects of ACE inhibitors and AVP antagonists are additive.[171,194,195] For example, the combination of AVP antago-

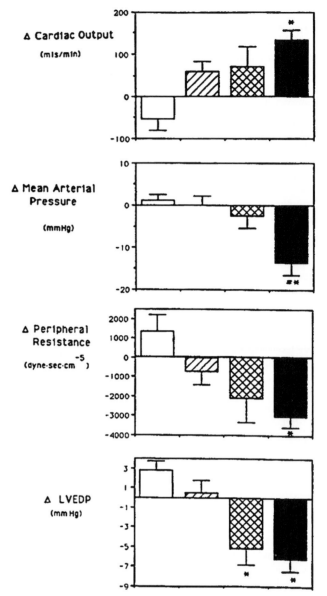

FIGURE 35-6. Changes in cardiac output, blood pressure, peripheral resistance, and left ventricular end-diastolic pressure (posttreatment minus pretreatment values) in rabbits with acute heart failure treated with vehicle (open bars), vasopressin vascular (V_{1a}) antagonist (AVPA, hatched bars), angiotensin converting enzyme inhibitor (ACEi, crosshatched bars) or both (AVPA + ACEi, solid bars). *P <.05 compared with vehicle-treated animals; #P <.05 compared with AVPA or ACEi alone. (*Reproduced with permission from Arnolda et al.[194]*)

nism and ACE inhibition restored intestinal and renal blood flow to near normal levels in animal models of heart failure despite the fall in arterial blood pressure from pretreatment levels, implicating AVP and angiotensin II as important factors in the renal and mesenteric ischemia that accompanies heart failure.

In chronic heart failure, AVP antagonism alone can induce significant vasodilation.[182] The differences found between studies examining acute and chronic heart failure may be due to the abnormal baroreceptor function that is present in chronic heart failure.[179]

In a recent study by Naitoh et al., dogs with CHF from rapid ventricular pacing were present to have elevated plasma AVP levels.[196]

They were then administered the nonpeptide AVP antagonists OPC 21268 (V_{1a} antagonist) and OPC 31260 (V_2 antagonist). As expected, OPC 31260 caused a marked water diuresis in both normal dogs and dogs with CHF, with subsequent increases in serum sodium concentration, plasma renin activity, and plasma concentration of AVP. However, no hemodynamic improvement was noted. Oral administration of OPC 21268 led to a significantly increased cardiac output and improved renal function only in dogs with CHF. No significant changes in serum electrolytes or hormones were noted with the V_{1a} antagonist. Combined V_{1a} and V_2 blockade with both OPC 21268 and OPC 31260 led to additive increases in urine flow rate, glomerular filtration rate, and stimulation of plasma renin activity, AVP, and norepinephrine, and a supraadditive increase in cardiac output.[196] These results implicate AVP in causing elevation of vascular tone and decreased renal function in CHF, while showing its role in retaining free water in both CHF and the normal state. It is possible that with V_2 blockade alone, the effects of preload reduction were counterbalanced by the increases in AVP, plasma renin activity, and norepinephrine.

Naitoh et al. also compared the hemodynamic effects of the V_2-receptor blocker OPC 31260 with the ACE inhibitor ramipril in sheep with pacing-induced CHF.[197] Sheep treated with OPC 31260 demonstrated, within 2 h, an increase in cardiac output and a decrease in right atrial pressure without changes in systemic vascular resistance. The sheep treated with ramipril responded, 2 days after the initiation of treatment, with a significant increase in cardiac output and a decrease in systemic vascular resistance.[197]

In a similar study, the long-term effects of V_{1a} and V_2 blockade were investigated in rats with heart failure induced through the creation of an aortocaval fistula.[198] In untreated rats with heart failure, plasma AVP levels were only slightly higher relative to controls. Rats treated for 4 weeks with OPC 21268 or OPC 31260 did not show any changes in hemodynamic measurements. OPC 31260, however, reduced plasma atrial natriuretic peptide and raised plasma renin activity and AVP levels. Also, left ventricular end-diastolic pressure and right ventricular systolic pressure were markedly reduced in these rats, probably as a result of a diuresis with subsequent reduction of plasma volume. The authors concluded that in this animal model, the interaction of AVP with the V_2 receptor might be the cause of volume overload and subsequent heart failure. Recently it was observed that the selective V_2-receptor blocker VPA-985 decreased urinary aquaporin-2 excretion in patients with heart failure.[199]

Burrell et al. further studied the effects of 6 months of treatment with OPC 31260 on a rat postinfarction model of CHF.[200] They demonstrated no increases in levels of plasma AVP or plasma renin activity, although levels of atrial natriuretic peptide were elevated. Systemic hemodynamics were unaltered and survival was not affected compared to rats with CHF not receiving OPC 31260. Thus, in this model of heart failure, OPC 31260–induced V_2-receptor blockade was not associated with any beneficial effects but also did not worsen mortality or morbidity.

Clinical Studies

In an experimental model of heart failure in pigs, it was shown that although V_{1a} reduced left ventricular loading conditions, only dual receptor blockade resulted in improved left ventricular and myocyte shortening.[201] The V_{1a} antagonist $d(CH_2)_5Tyr(Me)AVP$ was administered to 10 patients who had clinical CHF for at least 3 months. Hemodynamic improvement was seen in only 1 patient,

who was the most acutely ill and symptomatic at the time of administration.[109] He was also the only patient in the study having markedly elevated plasma catecholamine, renin, and AVP levels.

The results of phase II trials with vaptans have generally demonstrated that they reverse the impaired urinary diluting capacity seen in the setting of chronic heart failure, increase free water excretion, correct dilutional hyponatremia, decrease urinary aquaporin-2 excretion, promote peripheral vasodilation, and improve cardiac output.

Three vaptans are being tested in human trials—two are selective V_2 receptor antagonists, WAY-VPA-985 and OPC 41061 (tolvaptan), and the third is a combined V_{1a}/V_2 receptor antagonist, YM087.

WAY-VPA-985 has been tested using a single oral dose in patients with symptomatic heart failure. Twenty-eight patients with chronic left ventricular systolic dysfunction were evaluated in a randomized, double-blind, placebo-controlled trial. All had class III or IV CHF and were either modestly hyponatremic or normonatremic. When they were admitted for the study, the patients' heart failure medications were discontinued and the patients were placed on a fixed intake of sodium and potassium. Average levels of urinary osmolality ranged from 400 to 600 mOsm/kg at baseline. Doses administered were 30, 75, 150, and 250 mg. There was a marked, highly significant, and dose-related decrease in minimal urinary osmolality. At highest doses, minimal urinary osmolality was reduced to <100 mOsm/kg. In addition, there was a marked and highly significant dose-related improvement in urine volume in patients receiving WAY-VPA-985 and a marked reduction in urinary aquaporin-2.

Studies have recently been completed with tolvaptan (OPC 41061), evaluating the effect of this specific V_2-receptor antagonist on changes in body weight in patients with NYHA class I, II, or III CHF who were volume overloaded. The secondary objectives of this study were edema measurements, quality of life, urinary sodium excretion, and urinary volume and osmolality. Patients were randomized in a double-blind placebo-controlled manner with three dosing regimens (30, 45, or 60 mg) of oral tolvaptan once daily versus placebo. All three doses of tolvaptan significantly decreased body weight and maintained the effect for the duration of the study (25 days). Additionally, all three doses of tolvaptan demonstrated significant improvement in the edema score. There was no change in the serum potassium throughout the course of the study, and all doses of tolvaptan significantly increased mean 24-h urinary sodium excretion in the first day of therapy. Additionally, tolvaptan exerted no effect on heart rate or blood pressure. Adverse events tended to be lower with the use of tolvaptan, including a decrease in hospitalizations for heart failure.[202] Trials with YM087 also included class III and IV heart failure patients. Early open-label evaluation required patients to be hyponatremic, with a serum sodium ranging from 120 to 132 mmol/L, and with maximal background medical therapy including continuous intravenous inotropic infusion. In this dose-escalation study, 20, 40, 80, and 120 mg of YM087 were given in two divided doses.

Results demonstrated that compared to the observation period, in which average urinary osmolality was about 450 mOsm/kg, there was a prompt fall in urinary osmolality during the administration of YM087, which was sustained throughout the evaluation and maintenance phases of the study. This fall in urinary osmolality and increase in free water clearance resulted in a correction of the hyponatremia. There was no substantial increase in thirst during the period.[203]

CONCLUSION

Additional investigations are needed before vasopressin's role in the etiology of cardiovascular disease can be entirely delineated. Vasopressin does have important therapeutic effects in hemorrhagic shock, vasodilatory shock, and cardiac arrest. However, with an ever-increasing number of more selective vasopressin antagonists, the outlook for future research in this area also seems promising. The availability of the new nonpeptide orally active antagonists will also provide an opportunity for conducting many future clinical trials.

It seems possible that there will be certain groups of hypertensive patients who may respond best to vasopressin antagonism. Studies showing variability in AVP levels between ages and races may provide some clues as to who these patients might be.[144-146] AVP antagonism may play an important role as an adjunct to standard therapies for hypertension and heart failure, such as ACE inhibitors and beta-blockers. Studies have shown that when the sympathetic nervous system and RAS are blocked, AVP assumes a much more important role in blood pressure maintenance.[20,147-153] Elderly and black patients who are refractory to standard blood pressure treatment may find AVP antagonism to be a reasonable pharmacologic alternative. The development of a screening test for patients with increased AVP levels or increased sensitivity to AVP will be an important step to delineate which patients could benefit most from the vasopressin-receptor antagonists.

The treatment of CHF is also increasingly concentrated on blocking the compensatory changes in the RAS and sympathetic nervous system that take place to support the failing myocardium. Vasopressin antagonists seem ideally suited to help alleviate much of the symptomatology that accompanies the later stages of CHF. V_2 antagonists have been shown to increase free water excretion in normal rats as well as in both normal dogs and those with CHF.[83,183] V_{1a} antagonists have been shown to reduce vascular resistance in both animals and humans with CHF.[163,167,170,173] AVP antagonism may prove most useful in situations where the patients are already on ACE inhibitors and beta-blockers. Studies have shown that concomitant use of ACE inhibitors and AVP antagonists can lead to either additive[172,190] or supraadditive effects on cardiac output.[195] Combined V_{1a} and V_2 blockade may be most useful in combating AVP's effects in CHF on both the vasculature and the kidney. Long-term studies using the new orally active antagonists are now being performed in patients with advanced CHF, where the role of AVP is currently more defined.

AVP's role in the central nervous system has been receiving increasing attention in recent years. Many studies have shown activity in the area postrema, NTS, and baroreflex response. The interaction between peripheral and central vasopressin appears to play an important role in vasopressin's overall effect on the cardiovascular system. Further studies are needed to further explore these interactions.

TABLE 35-3. Potential Uses of Vasopressin Antagonists

Selective V_1-receptor blockade
1. As a vasodilator to treat congestive heart failure, especially in conjunction with angiotensin converting enzyme (ACE) inhibitors and beta-blockers
2. For treatment of systemic hypertension, especially in conjunction with ACE inhibitors and beta-blockers

Selective V_2-receptor blockade
1. Increasing clearance of free water in treatment of congestive heart failure, cirrhosis of the liver, other edematous states

Selective central nervous system AVP antagonists may, in the future, provide another means for understanding this complex interaction.

Vasopressin is involved in a wide variety of cellular processes. As its true importance in different organ systems is better defined, the possible therapeutic uses of AVP agonism and antagonism (Table 35-3) will expand accordingly.

REFERENCES

1. Sachs H: Biosynthesis and release of vasopressin. *Am J Med* 42:687, 1967.
2. Cowley JF, Ausello DA: *Vasopressin Cellular and Integrative Functions.* New York: Raven Press, 1988.
3. Schrier RW: *Vasopressin.* New York: Raven Press, 1985.
4. Schrier RW, Cadnapaphornchai MA, Umenishi F: Water-losing and water-retaining states: Role of water channels and vasopressin receptor antagonists. *Heart Dis* 3:210, 2001.
5. Manning M, Sawyer W: Discovery, development, and some uses of vasopressin and oxytocin antagonists. *J Lab Clin Med* 114:617, 1989.
6. Robertson GL, Harris A: Clinical use of vasopressin analogues. *Hosp Pract* 24:114, 1989.
7. Maggi M, Fantoni G, Peri A, et al: Steroid modulation of oxytocin/vasopressin receptors in the uterus. *J Steroid Biochem Mol Biol* 40:481, 1991.
8. deKeyzer Y, Auzan C, Lenne F, et al: Cloning and characterization of the human V3 pituitary vasopressin receptors. *FEBS Lett* 345:215, 1994.
9. Fahrenholz F, Jurzak M, Gerstberger R, Haase W: Renal and central vasopressin receptors: Immunocytochemical localization. *Ann NY Acad Sci* 689:194, 1993.
10. Phillips M: Functions of angiotensin in the central nervous system. *Annu Rev Physiol* 549:413, 1987.
11. McKinley MJ, Congiu M, Denton DA, et al: The anterior wall of the third cerebral ventricle and homeostatic responses to dehydration. *J Physiol Paris* 79:421, 1984.
12. Zeisberger E: The role of septal peptides in thermoregulation and fever. In: Bligh J, Voigt K, eds. *Thermoreception and Temperature Regulation.* Berlin: Springer-Verlag, 1990:273.
13. Stehle J, Reuss S, Riemann R, et al: The role of arginine vasopressin for pineal melatonin synthesis in the rat: Involvement of vasopressinergic receptors. *Neurosci Lett* 123:131, 1991.
14. Kasting NW: Criteria for establishment of a physiological role for brain peptides. A case in point: The role of vasopressin in thermoregulation during fever and antipyresis. *Brain Res Rev* 14:143, 1989.
15. Meisenberg G, Simmons WH: Hypothermia induced by centrally administered vasopressin in rats. A structure-activity study. *Neuropharmacology* 23:1195, 1984.
16. Whitnall MH: Stress selectively activates the vasopressin-containing subset of corticotropin-releasing hormone neurons. *Neuroendocrinology* 50:702, 1989.
17. Gibbs DM: Vasopressin and oxytocin: Hypothalamic modulators of the stress response. A review. *Psychoneuroendocrinology* 11:131, 1986.
18. Diamant M, DeWied D: Differential effects of centrally injected AVP on heart rate, core temperature and behavior in rats. *Am J Physiol* 264: R51, 1993.
19. Cowley AW, Cushman WC, Quillen EW, et al: Vasopressin elevation in essential hypertension and increased responsiveness to sodium intake. *Hypertension* 3(3 Pt 2):I93, 1981.
20. Mohring J, Glanzer K, Maciel JA Jr, et al: Greatly enhanced pressor response to antidiuretic hormone in patients with impaired cardiovascular reflexes due to idiopathic orthostatic hypotension. *J Cardiovasc Pharmacol* 2:367, 1980.
21. Andrews CE, Brenner BM: Relative contributions of arginine vasopressin and angiotensin II to maintenance of systemic arterial pressure in the anaesthetized water deprived rat. *Circ Res* 48:254, 1981.
22. Woods RL, Johnston CI: Contribution of vasopressin to the maintenance of blood pressure during dehydration. *Am J Physiol* 245(5 Pt 1): F615, 1983.

23. McNeill JR, Stark RD, Greenway CV: Intestinal vasoconstriction after hemorrhage: Roles of vasopressin and angiotensin. *Am J Physiol* 219:1342, 1970.

24. Laszlo FA, Laszlo F Jr, deWied D: Pharmacology and clinical perspectives of vasopressin antagonists. *Pharmacol Rev* 43:73, 1991.

25. Bichet D, Szatalowicz V, Chaimovitz C, Schrier RW: Role of vasopressin in abnormal water excretion in cirrhotic patients. *Ann Intern Med* 96:413, 1982.

26. Tsuboi Y, Ishikawa S, Fujisawa G, et al: Therapeutic efficacy of the non-peptide AVP antagonist OPC 31260 in cirrhotic rats. *Kidney Int* 46:237, 1994.

27. Freeman JG, Cobden I, Lishman AH, Record CO: Controlled trial of terlipressin (glypressin) versus vasopressin in the early treatment of oesophageal varices. *Lancet* 2:66, 1982.

28. Kelsch T, Kikuchi K, Vahdat S, Frishman WH: Innovative pharmacologic approaches to cardiopulmonary resuscitation. *Heart Dis* 3:46, 2001.

29. Wenzel V, Lindner KH, Krismer AC, et al: Repeated administration of vasopressin but not epinephrine maintains coronary perfusion pressure after early and later administration during prolonged cardiopulmonary resuscitation in pigs. *Circulation* 99:1379, 1999.

30. Scharte M, Meyer J, VanAken H. et al: Hemodynamic effects of terlipressin (a synthetic analog of vasopressin) in healthy and endotoxemic sheep. *Crit Care Med* 29:1756, 2001.

31. Chase LR, Aurbach GD: Renal adenyl cyclase: Anatomically separate sites for parathyroid hormone and vasopressin. *Science* 159:545, 1968.

32. Butlen D, Guillon G, Rajerison RM, et al: Structural requirements for activation of vasopressin-sensitive adenylate cyclase, hormone binding, and anti-diuretic actions: Effects of highly potent analogues and competitive inhibitors. *Mol Pharmacol* 14:1006, 1978.

33. Aiyar N, Nambi P, Stassen FL, Crooke ST: Vascular vasopressin receptors mediate phosphatidylinositol turnover and calcium efflux in an established smooth muscle cell line. *Life Sci* 39:37, 1986.

34. Kelly JM, Abrahams JM, Phillips PA, et al: $[^{125}I]$-$[d(CH_2)_3, Sar^7]$ AVP: Selective radioligand for V_1 vasopressin receptors. *J Recept Res* 9:27, 1989.

35. Marchingo AJ, Abrahams JM, Woodcock EA, et al: Properties of $[^3H]$ 1–desamino-8–D-arginine vasopressin as a radioligand for vasopressin V_2 receptors in rat kidney. *Endocrinology* 122:1328, 1988.

36. Antoni FA: Receptors mediating the CRH effects of vasopressin and oxytocin. *Ann NY Acad Sci* 512:195, 1987.

37. Baertschi AJ, Friedli M: A novel type of vasopressin receptor on anterior pituitary corticotrophs. *Endocrinology* 116:499, 1985.

38. Nambi P, Whitman M, Gessner G, et al: Vasopressin-mediated inhibition of atrial natriuretic factor-stimulated cGMP accumulation in an established smooth muscle cell line. *Proc Natl Acad Sci U S A* 83:8492, 1986.

39. Jard S, Lombard C, Marie J, Devilliers G: Vasopressin receptors from cultured mesangial cells resemble V_{1a} type. *Am J Physiol* 253: F41, 1987.

40. Morel A, O'Carroll AM, Brownstein MJ, Lolait SJ: Molecular cloning and expression of a rat V_{1a} arginine vasopressin receptor. *Nature* 356:523, 1992.

41. Thibonnier M: Signal transduction of V_1-vascular vasopressin receptors. *Reg Pept* 38:1, 1992.

42. Nabika T, Velletri PA, Lovenberg W, Beaven MA: Increase in cytosolic calcium and phosphoinositide metabolism induced by angiotensin II and [arg]vasopressin in vascular smooth muscle cell. *J Biol Chem* 260:4661, 1985.

43. Tahara A, Tomura Y, Wada K, et al: Effect of YM087, a potent nonpeptide vasopressin antagonist, on vasopressin-induced hyperplasia and hypertrophy of cultured vascular smooth-muscle cells. *J Cardiovasc Pharmacol* 30(6):759, 1997.

44. Tahara A, Saito M, Tsukada J, et al: Vasopressin increases vascular endothelial growth factor secretion from human vascular smooth muscle cells. *Eur J Pharmacol* 26:89, 1999.

45. Tahara A, Tomura Y, Wada K, et al: Effect of YM087, a potent nonpeptide vasopressin antagonist, on vasopressin-induced protein synthesis in neonatal rat cardiomyocyte. *Cardiovasc Res* 38(1):198, 1998.

46. Maggi M, Baldi E, Genazzani AD, et al: Vasopressin receptors in human seminal vesicles: Identification, pharmacologic characterization, and comparison with the vasopressin receptors present in the human kidney. *J Androl* 10:393, 1989.

47. Liard JF: Peripheral vasodilatation induced by a vasopressin analogue with selective V_2–agonism in dogs. *Am J Physiol* 256:H1621, 1989.

48. Lolait SJ, O'Carroll AM, McBride OW, et al: Cloning and characterization of a vasopressin V_2 receptor and possible link to nephrogenic diabetes insipidus. *Nature* 357:336, 1992.

49. Lolait SJ, O'Carroll AM, Mahan LC, et al: Extrapituitary expression of the rat V_{1b} vasopressin receptor gene. *Proc Natl Acad Sci U S A* 92:6783, 1995.

50. Chang WY, Wo NC, Stoev S, et al: Discovery of novel selective hypotensive vasopressin peptides. A new vasodilating vasopressin receptor? *Adv Exp Med Biol* 449:451, 1998.

51. Kumar R: Endocytosis of the vasopressin receptor. *Semin Nephrol* 14:357, 1994.

52. Cowley AW, Liard JF: Cardiovascular actions of vasopressin. In: Gash DM, Boer GJ, eds. *Vasopressin: Principles and Properties*. New York: Plenum Press, 1987:389.

53. Imaizumi T, Thames MD: Influence of intravenous and intracerebroventricular vasopressin on baroreflex control of renal nerve traffic. *Circ Res* 58:17, 1986.

54. Masaki H, Imaizumi T, Harada S, et al: Effects of a novel orally effective V_1-receptor antagonist OPC 21268, on AVP-induced sympathoinhibition. *Am J Physiol* 264:R1089, 1993.

55. Abboud FM, Aylward PE, Floras JS, Gupta BN: Sensitization of aortic and cardiac baroreceptors by arginine vasopressin in mammals. *J Physiol* 377:251, 1986.

56. Undesser KP, Hasser EM, Haywood JR, et al: Interactions of vasopressin with the area postrema in arterial baroreflex function in conscious rabbits. *Circ Res* 56:410, 1985.

57. Hasser EM, Bishop VS: Reflex effect of vasopressin after blockade of V_1 receptors in the area postrema. *Circ Res* 67:265, 1990.

58. Suzuki S, Takeshita A, Imaizumi T, et al: Central nervous system mechanisms involved in inhibition of renal sympathetic nerve activity induced by arginine vasopressin. *Circ Res* 65:1390, 1989.

59. Malpas SC, Coote JH: Role of vasopressin in sympathetic response to paraventricular nucleus stimulation in anesthetized rats. *Am J Physiol* 266:R228, 1994.

60. Brooks VL, Osborn JW: Hormonal-sympathetic interactions in long-term regulation of arterial pressure: A hypothesis. *Am J Physiol* 268:R1343, 1995.

61. Luk A, Ajaelo I, Wong V, et al: Role of V_1 receptors in the action of vasopressin in the baroreflex control of heart rate. *Am J Physiol* 1993; 265:R524.

62. Ebert TJ, Cowley AW, Skelton M: Vasopressin reduces cardiac function and augments cardiopulmonary baroreflex resistance increases in man. *J Clin Invest* 77:1136, 1986.

63. Unger T, Rohmeiss P, Demmert G, et al: Differential modulation of the baroreceptor reflex by brain and plasma vasopressin. *Hypertension* 8(Suppl II):II-157, 1986.

64. Sampey DB, Burrell LM, Widdop RE: Vasopressin V_2 receptor enhances gain of baroreflex in conscious spontaneously hypertensive rats. *Am J Physiol* 276(3 Pt 2):R872, 1999.

65. Hegarty AA, Felder RB: Antagonism of vasopressin V_1 receptors in NTS attenuates baroreflex control of renal nerve activity. *Am J Physiol* 269:H1080, 1995.

66. Sved AF, Imaizumi T, Talman WT, Reis DJ: Vasopressin contributes to hypertension caused by nucleus tractus solitarius lesions. *Hypertension* 7:262, 1985.

67. Lowes VL, McLean LE, Kasting NW, Ferguson AV: Cardiovascular consequences of microinjection of vasopressin and angiotensin II in the area postrema. *Am J Physiol* 265:R615, 1993.

68. Zhang X, Abdel-Rahman AR, Wooles WR: Vasopressin receptors in the area postrema differentially modulate baroreceptor responses in rats. *Eur J Pharmacol* 222:81, 1992.

69. Qu L, Hay M, Bishop VS: Administration of AVP to the area postrema alters response of NTS neurons to afferent inputs. *Am J Physiol* 272:R519, 1997.

70. Stebbins CL, Bonigut S, Liviakis LR, Munch PA: Vasopressin acts in the area postrema to attenuate the exercise pressor reflex in anesthetized cats. *Am J Physiol* 274:H2116, 1998.

71. Goldsmith SR: Arginine vasopressin and baroreflex function after converting enzyme inhibition in normal humans. *Am J Physiol* 272:E429, 1997.

72. Tsuneyoshi I, Yamada H, Kakihana Y, et al: Hemodynamic and metabolic effects of low-dose vasopressin infusions in vasodilatory septic shock. *Crit Care Med* 29:487, 2001.

73. Gazmuri RJ, Shakeri SA: Low-dose vasopressin for reversing vasodilation during septic shock. *Crit Care Med* 29:673, 2001.

74. Argenziano M, Chen JM, Choudhri AF, et al: Management of vasodilatory shock after cardiac surgery: Identification of predisposing factors and use of a novel pressor agent. *J Thorac Cardiovasc Surg* 116:973, 1998.

75. Argenziano M, Chen JM, Choudhri AF, et al: A prospective randomized trial of arginine vasopressin in the treatment of vasodilatory shock after left ventricular assist device placement. *Circulation* 96(Suppl II):II-286, 1997.

76. Guidelines 2000 for Cardiopulmonary Resuscitation and Emergency Cardiovascular Care. Part 3: Adult basic life support. The American Heart Association in collaboration with the International Liaison Committee on Resuscitation. *Circulation* 102(Suppl). I22, 2000.

77. Wenzel V, Lindner KH, Prengel AW, et al: Vasopressin improves vital organ blood flow after prolonged cardiac arrest with postcountershock pulseless electrical activity in pigs. *Crit Care Med* 27:486, 1999.

78. Kornberger E, Prengel AW, Krismer A, et al: Vasopressin-mediated adrenocorticotropin release increases plasma cortisol concentrations during cardiopulmonary resuscitation. *Crit Care Med* 28:3517, 2000.

78a. Lindner KH, Dirks B, Strohmenger H-U, et al: Randomised comparison of epinephrine and vasopressin in patients with out-of-hospital ventricular fibrillation. *Lancet* 349:535, 1997.

79. Rosenzweig EB, Starc TJ, Chen JM, et al: Intravenous argininevasopressin in children with vasodilatory shock after cardiac surgery. *Circulation* 100(Suppl II):II-182, 1999.

80. Landry DW, Levin HR, Gallant EM, et al: Vasopressin deficiency contributes to the vasodilatation of septic shock. *Circulation* 95:1122, 1997.

80a. Sharshar T, Carlier R, Blanchard A, et al: Depletion of neurohypophyseal content of vasopressin in septic shock. *Crit Care Med* 30:497, 2002.

80b. Hollenberg SM, Tangora JJ, Piotrowski MJ, et al: Impaired microvascular vasoconstrictive responses to vasopressin in septic rats. *Crit Care Med* 25:869, 1997.

81. Lankhuizen IM, van Veghel R, Saxena PR, Schoemaker RG: [Arg^8]-vasopressin-induced responses on coronary and mesenteric arteries of rats with myocardial infarction: the effects of V$_{1a}$ and V$_2$ receptor antagonists. *J Cardiovasc Pharmacol* 36:38, 2000.

81a. Kraft W, Greenberg HE, Waldman SA: Paradoxical hypotension and bradycardia after intravenous arginine vasopressin. *J Clin Pharmacol* 38:283, 1998.

82. Kruszynski M, Lammeck B, Manning M, et al: [1(beta-mercapto-beta-cyclopentamethyl-eneproprionic acid)2-(O-methyl)tyrosine] argine vasopressin and [1-(beta-mercapto-beta, beta-cyclopenta-methyleneproprionic acid)] argine vasopressin, two highly potent antagonists of the vasopressor response to arginine-vasopressin. *J Med Chem* 23:364, 1980.

83. Laszlo FA, Csati S, Balaspiri L: Effect of the vasopressin antagonist d/CH2/5 Tyr/Et/VAVP on the antidiuretic action of exogenous and endogenous vasopressin. *Acta Endocrinol* 106:52, 1984.

84. Yamamura Y, Ogawa H, Chihara T, et al: OPC 21268, an orally effective, nonpeptide vasopressin V$_1$ receptor antagonist. *Science* 252:572, 1991.

85. Burrell LM, Phillips PA, Stephenson J, et al: Characterization of an orally active vasopressin V$_1$ receptor antagonist. *Clin Exp Pharmacol Physiol* 20:388, 1993.

86. Imaizumi T, Harada S, Hirooka Y, et al: Effects of OPC 21268, an orally effective vasopressin V$_1$ receptor antagonist in humans. *Hypertension* 20:54, 1992.

87. Burrell LM, Phillips PA, Stephenson J, et al: Vasopressin and a nonpeptide antidiuretic hormone receptor antagonist (OPC 31260). *Blood Pressure* 3:137, 1994.

88. Bemana I, Nagao S: Treatment of brain edema with a nonpeptide arginine vasopressin V$_1$ receptor antagonist OPC-21268 in rats. *Neurosurgery* 44:148, 1999.

89. Yamamura Y, Ogawa H, Yamashita H, et al: Characterization of a novel aquaretic agent, OPC 31260, as an orally effective nonpeptide vasopressin V$_2$ receptor antagonist. *Br J Pharmacol* 105:787, 1992.

90. Ohnishi A, Orita Y, Takagi N, et al: Aquaretic effect of a potent, orally active, nonpeptide V$_2$ antagonist in men. *J Pharmacol Exp Ther* 272:546, 1995.

91. Fujisawa G, Ishikawa S, Tsuboi Y, et al: Therapeutic efficacy of nonpeptide ADH antagonist OPC 31260 in SIADH rats. *Kidney Int* 44:19, 1993.

92. Burrell LM, Phillips PA, Rolls KA, et al: Vascular responses to vasopressin antagonists in man and rat. *Clin Sci* 87:389, 1994.

93. Liard J-F: Effects of arginine vasopressin on regional circulations. In: Schrier RW, ed. *Vasopressin*. New York: Raven Press, 1985:59.

94. Yamamura Y, Nakamura S, Itoh S, et al: OPC-41061, a highly potent human vasopressin V$_2$–receptor antagonist; pharmacological profile and aquaretic effect by single and multiple oral dosing rats. *J Pharmacol Exp Ther* 287(3): 860, 1998.

95. Serradeil-Le Gal C, Lacour C, et al: Characterization of SR 121463A, a highly potent and selective orally active vasopressin V$_2$ receptor antagonist. *J Clin Invest* 98:2729, 1996.

96. Hirano T, Yamamura Y, Nakamura S, et al: Effects of the V$_{(2)}$-receptor antagonist OPC-41061 and the loop diuretic furosemide alone and in combination in rats. *J Pharmacol Exp Ther* 292(1):288, 2000.

97. Serradeil-Le Gal C, Wagnon J, Garcia C, et al: Biochemical and pharmacological properties of SR 49059, a new, potent, nonpeptide antagonist of rat and human vasopressin V$_{1a}$ receptors. *J Clin Invest* 92:224, 1993.

98. Mechaly I, Laurent F, Poertet K, et al: Vasopressin V$_2$ (SR121463A) and V$_{1a}$ (SR49059) receptor antagonists both inhibit desmopressin vasorelaxing activity. *Eur J Pharmacol* 383(3):287, 1999.

99. Okamura T, Ayajiki K, Fujoka H, Toda N: Mechanisms underlying arginine vasopressin-induced relation in monkey isolated coronary arteries. *J Hypertens* 17(5): 673, 1999.

100. Brouard R, Laporte V, Serradeil Le Gal C, et al: Safety, tolerability, and pharmacokinetics of SR49059, a V$_{1a}$ vasopressin receptor antagonist, after repeated oral administration in healthy volunteers. *Adv Exp Med Biol* 449:455, 1998.

101. Serradeil-Le Gal C, Herbert JM, Delisee C: Effect of SR 49059, a vasopressin V$_{1a}$ antagonist, on human vascular smooth muscle cells. *Am J Physiol* 268:H404, 1995.

101a. Tahara A, Tomura Y, Wada KI, et al: Pharmacological profile of YM087, a novel potent nonpeptide vasopressin V$_{1a}$ and V$_2$ receptor antagonist, in vitro and in vivo. *J Pharmacol Exp Ther* 282:301, 1997.

102. Risvanis J, Naitoh M, Johnston CI, et al: In vivo and in vitro characterization of a nonpeptide vasopressin V$_{1a}$ and V$_2$ receptor antagonist in the rat. *Eur J Pharmacol* 381:23, 1999.

103. Tahara A, Tomura Y, Wada K, et al: Binding characteristics of YM087, an AVP receptor antagonist, in rhesus monkey liver and kidney membranes. *Peptides* 19:691, 1998.

104. Tomura Y, Tahara A, Tsukada J, et al: Pharmacological profile of orally administered YM087, a vasopressin antagonist, in conscious rats. *Clin Exp Pharmacol Physiol* 26:399, 1999.

105. Yatsu T, Tomura Y, Tahara A, et al: Cardiovascular and renal effects of conivaptan hydrochloride (YM087), a vasopressin V$_{1a}$ and V$_2$ receptor antagonist, in dogs with pacing-induced congestive heart failure. *Eur J Pharmacol* 376:239, 1999.

106. Yatsu T, Tomura Y, Tahara A, et al: Pharmacological profile of YM087, a novel nonpeptide dual vasopressin V$_{1a}$ and V$_2$ receptor antagonist in dogs. *Eur J Pharmacol* 321:225, 1997.

107. Burnier M, Fricker AF, Hayoz D, et al: Pharmacokinetic and pharmacodynamic effects of YM087, a combined V$_1$/V$_2$ vasopressin receptor antagonist in normal subjects. *Eur J Clin Pharmacol* 55(9):633, 1999.

107a. Udelson JE, Smith WB, Hendrix GH, et al: Acute hemodynamic effects of conivaptan, a dual V$_{1A}$/V$_2$ vasopressin receptor antagonist, in patients with advanced heart failure. *Circulation* 104:2417, 2001.

108. Tahara A, Saito M, Sugimoto T, et al: Pharmacological characterization of the human vasopressin receptor subtypes stably expressed in Chinese hamster ovary cells. *Br J Pharmacol* 125:1463, 1988.

109. Nicod P, Waeber B, Bussien JP, et al: Acute hemodynamic effect of a vascular antagonist of vasopressin in patients with congestive heart failure. *Am J Cardiol* 55:1043, 1985.

110. Ohnishi A, Ko Y, Fujihara H, et al: Pharmacokinetics, safety, and pharmacologic effects of OPC 21268, a nonpeptide orally active vasopressin V$_1$ receptor antagonist, in humans. *J Clin Pharmacol* 33:230, 1993.

111. Gavras I, Gavras H: Role of vasopressin in hypertensive disorders. In: Laragh JH, Brenner BM, eds. *Hypertension: Pathophysiology, Diagnosis and Management,* 2nd ed. New York: Raven Press, 1995:798.

112. Szczepanska-Sadowsky E, Noszczyk B, Lon S, et al: Central AVP and blood pressure regulation: Relevance to interspecies differences and hypertension. *Ann NY Acad Sci* 689:677, 1993.

113. Yang RH, Bunting S, Wyss JM, et al: Pressor and bradycardic effects of centrally administered relaxin in conscious rats. *Am J Hypertens* 8:375, 1995.

114. Kremarik P, Freund-Mercier MJ, Pittman QJ: Fundus striati vasopressin receptors in blood pressure control. *Am J Physiol* 269:R497, 1995.

115. Thibonnier M, Kilani A, Rahman M, et al: Effects of the nonpeptide V(1) vasopressin receptor antagonist SR49059 in hypertensive patients. *Hypertension* 34:1293, 1999.

116. Mohring J, Kintz J, Schoun J: Studies on the role of vasopressin in blood pressure control of spontaneously hypertensive rats with established hypertension (SHR, stroke-prone strain). *J Cardiovasc Pharmacol* 1:593, 1979.

117. Berecek K, Murray RD, Gross F, Brody MJ: Vasopressin and vascular reactivity in the development of DOCA hypertension in rats with hereditary diabetes insipidus. *Hypertension* 4:3, 1982.

118. Croften T, Share L, Baer PG, et al: Vasopressin secretion in the New Zealand genetically hypertensive rat. *Clin Exp Hypertens* 3:975, 1981.

119. Filep J, Frohlich JC, Fejes-Toth G: Evidence against a vasopressor role of ADH in malignant DOC-salt hypertension. *Clin Exp Hypertens* 7:1457, 1985.

120. Padfield PL, Brown JHJ, Lever AF, et al: Does vasopressin play a role in pathogenesis of hypertension. *Clin Sci* 61(Suppl 7):141s, 1981.

121. Stepniakowski K, Lapinski M, Januszewicz A, et al: Pressor responsiveness to vasopressin in spontaneously hypertensive rats. *Acta Physiol Polonica* 40:2, 1989.

122. Stepniakowski K, Lapinski M, Noszcyk B, et al: Effects of vasopressin and V$_1$ receptors blockade on blood pressure and heart rate in spontaneously hypertensive rats. *Polish J Pharmacol Pharm* 43:487, 1991.

123. Berecek KH, Swords BH: Central role for vasopressin in cardiovascular regulation and the pathogenesis of hypertension. *Hypertension* 16:213, 1990.

124. Naitoh M, Burrell LM, Risvanis J, et al: Modulation of genetic hypertension by short-term V$_{1a}$ or V$_2$ receptor antagonism in young SHR. *Am J Physiol* 272(2 Pt 2):F229, 1997.

125. Manning M, Lammek B, Kruszynski M, et al: Design of potent and selective antagonists of the vasopressor responses to arginine vasopressin. *J Med Chem* 25:408, 1982.

126. Rockhold RW, Share L, Crofton JT, Brooks DP: Cardiovascular responses to vasopressor antagonist administration during water deprivation in the rat. *Neuroendocrinology* 38:139, 1984.

127. Schwartz J, Liard JF, Ott C, Cowley AW Jr: Hemodynamic effects of neurohypophyseal peptides with antidiuretic activity in dogs. *Am J Physiol* 249:H1001, 1985.

128. Burrell LM, Phillips PA, Stephenson JM, et al: Blood pressure lowering effect of an orally active vasopressin V$_1$ receptor antagonist in mineralocorticoid hypertension in the rat. *Hypertension* 23:737, 1994.

129. Burrell LM, Phillips PA, Risvanis J, et al: Attenuation of genetic hypertension after short-term vasopressin V$_{1a}$ receptor antagonism. *Hypertension* 26:828, 1995.

130. Hashimoto J, Imai Y, Minami N, et al: Effects of vasopressin V$_1$ and V$_2$ receptor antagonists on the development of salt-induced hypertension in Dahl rats. *J Cardiovasc Pharmacol* 26:548, 1995.

131. Kawano Y, Matsuoka H, Nishikimi T, et al: The role of vasopressin in essential hypertension. Plasma levels and effects of the V$_1$ receptor antagonist OPC-21268 during different dietary sodium intakes. *Am J Hypertens* 10:1240, 1997.

132. Laszlo FA, Varga CS, Papp A, et al: Difference between male and female rats in vasopressor response to arginine vasopressin. *Acta Physiol Hung* 81:137, 1993.

133. Wang YX, Crofton JT, Share L: Sex differences in the cardiovascular and renal actions of vasopressin in conscious rats. *Am J Physiol* 272(1 Pt 2):R370, 1997.

134. Eatman D, Stallone JN, Rutecki GW, Whittier FC: Sex differences in extracellular and intracellular calcium-mediated vascular reactivity to vasopressin in rat aorta. *Eur J Pharmacol* 20:207, 1998.

135. Liard JF: L-NAME antagonizes vasopressin V$_2$-induced vasodilation in dogs. *Am J Physiol* 26:H99, 1994.

136. Chiba S, Tsukada M: Potent antagonistic action of OPC 31260, a vasopressin V$_2$ receptor antagonist on [Arg^8] vasopressin-induced vasoconstriction in isolated simian femoral arteries. *Eur J Pharmacol* 221;393, 1992.

137. Chiba S, Tsukada M: Blocking effects of OPC 21268 and OPC 31260 (vasopressin V$_1$ and V$_2$-receptor antagonists) on vasopressin-induced constrictions in isolated, perfused dog femoral arteries. *Jpn J Pharmacol* 59:133, 1992.

138. Rutschmann B, Evequoz D, Aubert JF, et al: Vasopressin dilates the rat carotid artery by stimulating V$_1$ receptors. *J Cardiovasc Pharmacol* 32:637, 1998.

139. Bussien JP, Waeber B, Nussberger J, et al: Does vasopressin sustain blood pressure of normally hydrated healthy volunteers? *Am J Physiol* 246: H143, 1984.

140. Padfield PL, Lever AF, Brown JJ, et al: Changes of vasopressin in hypertension: Cause or effect? *Lancet* 1:1255, 1976.

141. Padfield PL, Brown JJ, Lever AF, et al: Blood pressure in acute and chronic vasopressin excess: studies of malignant hypertension and the syndrome of inappropriate antidiuretic hormone secretion. *N Engl J Med* 304:1067, 1981.

142. Kawano Y, Matuoka H, Nishikimi T, et al: The role of vasopressin in essential hypertension. Plasma levels and effects of the V$_1$ receptor antagonist OPC 21268 during different dietary sodium intakes. *Am J Hypertens* 10:1240, 1997.

143. Bursztyn M, Bresnahan M, Gavras I, Gavras H: Pressor hormones in elderly hypertensive persons: Racial differences. *Hypertension* 15(Suppl I):I-88, 1990.

144. DePaula RB, Plavnik FL, Rodrigues CIS, et al: Age and race determine vasopressin participation in upright blood pressure control in essential hypertension. *Ann NY Acad Sci* 689:534, 1993.

145. Bakris G, Bursztyn M, Gavras I, et al: Role of vasopressin in essential hypertension: Racial differences. *J Hypertens* 15:545, 1997.

146. Gavras H: Role of vasopressin in clinical hypertension and congestive cardiac failure: Interaction with the sympathetic nervous system. *Clin Chem* 37:1828, 1991.

147. Ribeiro A, Mulinari R, Gavras I, et al: Sequential elimination of pressor mechanisms in severe hypertension in humans. *Hypertension* 8(Suppl I): I, 1986.

148. Gavras I, Hatinoglou S, Gavras H: The adrenergic system and the release and pressor action of vasopressin. *Hypertension* 8(Suppl II):163, 1986.

149. Nishida N, Ogura Y, Yamauchi T, et al: Treatment with cilazapril, angiotensin converting enzyme inhibitor, changes the affinity of arginine vasopressin receptor in the kidney of the spontaneously hypertensive rat. *Res Commun Chem Pathol Pharm* 84:143, 1994.

150. Khokhar AM, Slater JDH, Ma J, Ramage CM: The cardiovascular effect of vasopressin in relation to its plasma concentration in man and its relevance to high blood pressure. *Clin Endocrinol* 13:259, 1980.

151. Gavras H, Hatzinikolaou P, North WG, et al: Interaction of the sympathetic nervous system with vasopressin and renin in the maintenance of blood pressure. *Hypertension* 4:400, 1982.

152. Houck PC, Fiksen-Olsen MJ, Briton SL, Romero JC: Role of angiotensin and vasopressin on blood pressure of ganglionic blocked dogs. *Am J Physiol* 244:H115, 1983.

153. Parmley WW: Pathophysiology of congestive heart failure. *Am J Cardiol* 55: 9A, 1985.

154. Mancia G: Neurohumoral activation in congestive heart failure. *Am Heart J* 120:1532, 1990.

155. Francis GS: Neurohumoral activation and progression of heart failure: Hypothetical and clinical considerations. *J Cardiovasc Pharmacol* 32(Suppl 1):S16, 1998.

156. Rieffer AJG: Hormones in heart failure-regulation and counterregulation. *Eur Heart J* 12(Suppl D):190, 1991.

157. Thomas JA, Marks BH: Plasma norepinephrine in congestive heart failure. *Am J Cardiol* 41:233, 1978.

158. Levine TB, Francis GS, Goldsmith SR, et al: Activity of the sympathetic nervous system and renin-angiotensin system assessed by plasma hormone levels and their relationship to hemodynamic abnormalities. *Am J Cardiol* 49:1659, 1982.

159. Lee WH, Packer M: Prognostic importance of serum sodium concentration and its modification by converting enzyme inhibition in patients with severe chronic heart failure. *Circulation* 73:257, 1986.

160. Cohn JN, Levine TB, Olivari MT, et al: Plasma norepinephrine as a guide to prognosis in patients with chronic congestive heart failure. *N Engl J Med* 311:819, 1984.

161. Gottlieb SS, Kukin ML, Ahern D, Packer M: Prognostic importance of atrial natriuretic peptide in patients with chronic heart failure. *J Am Coll Cardiol* 13:1534, 1989.

162. Creager MA, Faxon DP, Cutler SS, et al: Contribution of vasopressin in patients with congestive heart failure: Comparison with renin-angiotensin system and the sympathetic nervous system. *J Am Coll Cardiol* 7:758, 1986.

163. Sved AF, Otteweller JE, Tapp WN, et al: Elevated plasma vasopressin in cardiomyopathic hamsters. *Life Sci* 37:2313, 1985.

164. Vari RC, Freeman RH, Davis JO, Sweet WD: Systemic and renal haemodynamic responses to vascular blockade of vasopressin in conscious dogs with ascites. *Proc Soc Exp Biol Med* 179:192, 1985.

165. Cohn JN, Levine TB, Francis GS, Goldsmith S: Neurohumoral control mechanisms in congestive heart failure. *Am Heart J* 102:509, 1981.

166. Goldsmith SR, Francis GS, Cowley AW, et al: Increased plasma arginine vasopressin levels in patients with congestive heart failure. *J Am Coll Cardiol* 1:1385, 1983.

167. Uretsky BF, Verbalis JG, Generalovich T, et al: Plasma vasopressin response to osmotic and hemodynamic stimuli in heart failure. *Am J Physiol* 248:H396, 1985.

168. Gavras H: Pressor systems in hypertension and congestive heart failure: Role of vasopressin. *Hypertension* 16:587, 1990.

169. Riegger GA, Liebau G, Kochsiek K: Antidiuretic hormone in congestive heart failure. *Am J Med* 72:49, 1982.

170. Yamane Y: Plasma ADH levels in patients with chronic congestive heart failure. *Jpn Circ J* 32:745, 1968.

171. Johnston CI, McGrath BP, Phillip P, et al: Vasopressin: Cellular and integrative functions. In: Cowley JA, Liard JF, Ausiello D, eds. *Vasopressin in Congestive Heart Failure: Clinical and Experimental Studies.* New York: Raven Press, 1988:481.

172. Szatalowics VL, Arnold PE, Chaimovitz C, et al: Radioimmunoassay of plasma arginine vasopressin in hyponatremic patients with congestive heart failure. *N Engl J Med* 305:263, 1981.

173. Travill CM, Williams TDM, Pate P, et al: Haemodynamic and neurohumoral response in heart failure produced by rapid ventricular pacing. *Cardiovasc Res* 26:783, 1992.

174. Bojour JP, Malkin RL: Stimulation of AVP release by the renin-angiotensin system. *Am J Physiol* 218:1555, 1970.

175. Cowley AW Jr, Switzer SJ, Skelton MM: Vasopressin, fluid, and electrolyte response to chronic angiotensin II infusion. *Am J Physiol* 240:R130, 1981.

176. Schrier RW, Berl T, Anderson RJ: Osmotic and nonosmotic control of vasopressin release. *Am J Physiol* 236:F321, 1979.

177. Uhlich E, Weber P, Eigler J, Groschel-Stewart U: Angiotensin stimulated AVP-release in humans. *Klin Wochenschr* 53:177, 1975.

178. Goldsmith SR: Baroreceptor mediated suppression of osmotically stimulated vasopressin in normal humans. *J Appl Physiol* 65:1226, 1988.

179. Goldsmith SR: Baroreflex loading maneuvers do not suppress increased plasma arginine vasopressin in patients with congestive heart failure. *J Am Coll Cardiol* 19:1180, 1992.

180. Manthey J, Dietz R, Opherk D, et al: Baroreceptor-mediated release of vasopressin in patients with chronic congestive heart failure and defective sympathetic responsiveness. *Am J Cardiol* 70:224, 1992.

181. Luk JKH, Wong EFC, Wong NLM: Hypersensitivity of inner medullary collecting duct cells to arginine vasopressin and forskolin in cardiomyopathic hamsters. *Cardiology* 83:49, 1993.

182. Arnolda L, McGrath BP, Cocks M, Johnston CI: Vasoconstrictor role for vasopressin in experimental heart failure in the rabbit. *J Clin Invest* 78:674, 1986.

183. Heyndrickx GR, Boettcher DH, Vatner SF: Effects of angiotensin, vasopressin, and methoxamine on cardiac function and blood flow distribution in conscious dogs. *Am J Physiol* 231:1579, 1976.

184. Varma S, Jaju BP, Bhargava KP: Mechanism of vasopressin-induced bradycardia in dogs. *Circ Res* 24:787, 1969.

185. Boyle WA III, Segel LD: Direct cardiac effects of vasopressin and their reversal by a vascular antagonist. *Am J Physiol* 251:H734, 1986.

186. Xu Y, Hopfner RL, McNeill JR, Gopalakrishnan V: Vasopressin accelerates protein synthesis in neonatal rat cardiomyocytes. *Mol Cell Biochem* 195(1–2):183, 1999.

187. Fukuzawa J, Haneda T, Kikuchi K: Arginine vasopressin increases the rate of protein synthesis in isolated perfused adult rat heart via the V_1 receptor. *Mol Cell Biochem* 195(1–2):93, 1999.

188. Furukawa Y, Takayama S, Ren L, et al: Blocking effects of V_1 (OPC 21268) and V_2 (OPC 31260) antagonists on the negative inotropic response to vasopressin in isolated dog heart preparations. *J Pharmacol Exp Ther* 263:627, 1992.

189. Matsui H, Kohomoto O, Hirata Y, Serizawa T: Effects of a nonpeptide vasopressin antagonist (OPC 21268) on cytosolic Ca^{2+} concentration in vascular and cardiac myocytes. *Hypertension* 19:730, 1992.

190. Xu YJ, Gopalakrishnan V: Vasopressin increased cytosolic free $[Ca^{2+}]$ in the neonatal rat cardiomyocyte: evidence for V_1 subtype receptors. *Circ Res* 69:239, 1991.

191. Walker BR, Childs ME, Adams EM: Direct cardiac effects of vasopressin: role of V_1 and V_2 vasopressinergic receptors. *Am J Physiol* 255:H261, 1988.

192. Laugwitz KL, Ungerer M, Schoneberg T, et al: Adenoviral gene transfer of the human V_2 vasopressin receptor improves contractile force of rat cardiomyocytes. *Circulation* 99:925, 1999.

193. Weig H-J, Laugwitz K-L, Moretti A, et al: Enhanced cardiac contractility after gene transfer of V_2 vasopressin receptors in vivo by ultrasound-guided injection or transcoronary delivery. *Circulation* 101:1578, 2000.

194. Arnolda L, McGrath BP, Johnston CI: Systemic and regional effect of vasopressin and angiotensin in acute left ventricular failure. *Am J Physiol* 260:H499, 1991.

195. Arnolda L, McGrath BP, Johnston CI: Vasopressin and angiotensin II contribute equally to the increased afterload in rabbits with heart failure. *Cardiovasc Res* 25:68, 1991.

196. Naitoh M, Suzuki H, Murakami M, et al: Effects of oral AVP receptor antagonists OPC 21268 and OPC 31260 on congestive heart failure in conscious dogs. *Am J Physiol* 267:H2245, 1994.

197. Naitoh M, Power J, Phillips PA, et al: Effects of chronic AVP V_2 blockade in congestive heart failure in sheep. Comparison with chronic ACE inhibition. *Adv Exp Med Biol* 449:445, 1998.

198. Nishikimi T, Kawano Y, Saito Y, Matsuoka H: Effect of long-term treatment with selective vasopressin V_1 and V_2 receptor antagonist on the development of heart failure in rats. *J Cardiovasc Pharmacol* 27:275, 1996.

199. Martin P-Y, Abraham WT, Lieming X, et al: Selective V_2-receptor vasopressin antagonism decreases urinary aquaporin-2 excretion in patients with chronic heart failure. *J Am Soc Nephrol* 10:2165, 1999.

200. Burrell LM, Phillips PA, Risvanis J, et al: Long-term effects of nonpeptide vasopressin V_2 antagonist OPC 31260 in heart failure in the rat. *Am J Physiol* 275:H176, 1998.

201. Clair MJ, King MK, Goldberg AT, et al: Selective vasopressin, angiotensin II, or dual receptor blockade with developing congestive heart failure. *J Pharmacol Exp Ther* 293:852, 2000.

202. Gheorghiade M, Niazi I, Ouyang J, et al: Chronic effects of vasopressin receptor blockade with tolvaptan in congestive heart failure: A randomized, double-blind trial (abstr). *Circulation* 102:II-592, 2000.

203. Abraham WT, Suresh DP, Wagoner LE, et al: Pharmacotherapy for hyponatremia in heart failure: effects of a new dual V_{1a}/V_2 vasopressin antagonist YM087 (abstr). *Circulation* 100:I-299, 1999.

CHAPTER 36

Hormones as Cardiovascular Drugs: Estrogens, Progestins, Thyroxine, Growth Hormone, Corticosteroids, and Testosterone

William H. Frishman

Mardi Gomberg-Maitland

Ruth Freeman

Denise Park

Atif Qureshi

Hormones such as thyroxine, estrogen, and corticosteroids have been used traditionally as replacement therapies for treating hormonal deficiency syndromes such as hypothyroidism, menopause, and Addison's disease. Recently, these hormones were investigated for possible use as drugs to treat and prevent various cardiovascular and cerebrovascular disorders. In this chapter, the pharmacologic profiles of estrogens, progestins, thyroxine, growth hormone, corticosteroids, and testosterone relevant to the cardiovascular system are reviewed, as well as their potential therapeutic use for the prevention and treatment of cardiovascular disease.

ESTROGENS

Women are living more than one-third of their lives after the onset of menopause at increased risk of developing cardiovascular disease. In western society, the death rate from coronary artery disease (CAD) is five to eight times greater in males than in females 25 to 55 years of age.[1] The difference in mortality rate narrows after menopause, suggesting that premenopausal women have a vascular "protective factor" that is lost at menopause (natural or surgically rendered).[2] Estrogen has been implicated as this "factor."[3]

Epidemiologic Evidence for Benefit

The relationship between menopause, estrogen use, and coronary heart disease (CHD) was first discussed in the Framingham Study, which found an increased incidence of CAD in women after menopause.[4] In the same study,[5] an increased risk of cardiovascular disease was observed in postmenopausal women receiving estrogen. After adjustment for several confounding variables, the relative risk of cardiovascular disease in women receiving estrogen was 1.8 times that seen in nonusers. However, on reanalysis of the data,[6] a possible protective effect from estrogen use was described in women 50 to 59 years of age. Most epidemiologic studies, albeit retrospective in

scope, have shown a survival advantage in postmenopausal women who are being treated with estrogen replacement therapy (ERT).[7,8] Colditz et al[8] performed a prospective analysis of the Nurse's Health Study cohort to determine the relationship of menopause and the risk of developing CHD. They found a decrease in the rate of CHD in oophorectomized women receiving estrogen compared to those not receiving treatment.

Low levels of high-density lipoprotein (HDL) are associated with severe coronary artery lesions on angiography.[9] Gruchow and colleagues[10] compared the degree of coronary artery occlusion between users and nonusers of estrogen among 933 women (between the ages of 50 and 75 years) with a diagnosis of chest pain, who were referred for coronary angiography. The investigators found that estrogen users had less-severe coronary artery occlusions than did nonusers. The effect was independent of HDL cholesterol level. The investigators suggested that higher HDL levels among estrogen users may provide a protective effect against CAD.[10] Hong et al[11] examined the effects of estrogen replacement on plasma lipids and on angiographically defined CAD in 90 consecutive postmenopausal women (age greater than 55 years or history of bilateral oophorectomy) undergoing coronary angiography (18 estrogen users and 72 nonusers). The investigators found that estrogen use was associated with an 87% reduction in angiographic prevalence of CAD. Patients given estrogen had a significantly higher mean HDL cholesterol level and lower mean total/HDL cholesterol ratio than did those not given estrogen. In addition, estrogen use, followed by total/HDL cholesterol ratio, was the most powerful predictor of the presence of CAD in these women.

Two additional reports also described a benefit of ERT in postmenopausal women. Henderson and colleagues[12] conducted a prospective evaluation of 8881 postmenopausal women residents of a retirement community using a detailed questionnaire requesting information about estrogen use and cardiac disease. Mean duration of use was 10 years, and patients were followed for 7.5 years. Age-adjusted, all-cause mortality in women with a history of estrogen use was 20% lower than in women who never used estrogen. The mortality rate among current users was 40% lower than among those who had never used estrogen. Those who used estrogen for more than 15 years had a 40% reduction in their overall mortality. The majority of the mortality benefit was attributable to fewer deaths from cardiovascular disease. Estrogen users also had a 20% reduction in mortality from cancer, including breast; however, users had excess of mortality from endometrial cancer. The all-cause mortality risk was 0.79 for estrogen users versus nonusers.

Sullivan and coworkers[13] retrospectively analyzed the relationship between postmenopausal estrogen use and survival in 2268 women undergoing coronary angiography. Patients were grouped based on coronary anatomy: severe (>70% stenosis) in 1178 patients; mild (<70% stenosis) in 644; absent (0% stenosis) in 446 control patients. In the control group, 10-year survival was similar in estrogen users and nonusers. In contrast, estrogen use improved survival in women with CAD. Among patients with severe CAD, 10-year survival was 97% in estrogen users and 60% in nonusers. In the group with mild CAD, the 10-year survival was 95% and 85%, respectively. In addition, the incidence of hyperlipidemia in estrogen users was lower than that in nonusers. Estrogen use in postmenopausal females with CAD was an independent predictor of survival in women.[13]

Other prospective observational and case control studies have demonstrated the decreased risk of ischemic heart disease with the use of estrogen.[14–16] However, the effect of combined therapy with progestins is less-well examined. Stampfer and colleagues looked at data from the Nurses' Health Study and found the relative risk for cardiac disease in the women taking unopposed ERT was 0.56.[14] Although users of ERT were noted to take better care of their health, the beneficial effects of ERT remain even after adjustment for cardiac risk factors such as weight and smoking.

In two reviews,[17,18] estrogen therapy in postmenopausal women reduced the risk of myocardial infarction in users, as compared with nonusers, by 44%. Furthermore, a large case-control study proposed that the longer period over which estrogen is taken, the lower the risk of first myocardial infarction.[19] However, with long-term unopposed estrogen use, there is an increased risk of uterine cancer and possibly breast cancer. Because progestins lessen the benefit of estrogen on HDL, it was considered possible that combined estrogen-progestin therapy would be less cardioprotective than unopposed estrogen. However, it was shown that the addition of progestin does not attenuate the cardioprotective effects of postmenopausal estrogen therapy.[16]

Possible Mechanisms of Cardiovascular Benefit

Estrogens affect many organ systems of the body both directly and indirectly (Table 36-1). Among their actions, estrogens appear to have direct receptor-mediated effects on blood vessels[20] and the myocardium, and indirectly affect lipid and lipoprotein metabolism, systemic blood pressure, coagulation, and carbohydrate metabolism.[20a]

Cardiovascular Estrogen Receptors

Estrogen stimulation of vascular estrogen receptors increases production of prostacyclin and nitric oxide (NO), while it inhibits platelet activation.[21,22] Estrogen also directly affects the receptors in the heart. Estrogen stimulates the myocardium causing a positive inotropic effect.[23] Estrogens have a structural similarity to digoxin and can induce the same nonspecific ST- and T-wave electrocardiogram

TABLE 36-1. Proposed Cardiovascular Protective Effects of Estrogen

Favorable effect on LDL and HDL cholesterol (indirect effects on endothelial function) and antiatherosclerotic effect.

Antioxidant effect (indirect effects on endothelial function)

Indirect effects on peripheral vasomotor tone

Enhancement of nitric oxide activity

Interference with effect of endothelin-1

Calcium-channel blocking effect

Inhibition of α-adrenergic receptor activity on blood vessels

Potentiating production of prostacyclin

Reducing activity of renin-angiotensin system

Enhanced plasma fibrinolytic activity

Reduced smooth-muscle-cell proliferation

Improved fibrinolytic parameters (decreased serum fibrinogen and PAI-1)

Potential for angiogenic effects of fibroblast growth factor, thereby aiding in collateral formation

Direct myocardial benefits (increased stroke volume and contractility)

Body fat redistribution (decreased waist:hip ratio)

Favorable effects on sympathetic innervation (lowered blood pressure)

(ECG) finding[24] seen with the digitalis glycosides.[23] Estrogens may also help in the upregulation of both muscarinic and β-adrenergic receptors in the myocardium.[25]

Estrogen has direct effects on myosin adenosine triphosphatase (ATPase) activity. In ovariectomized animals, a decrease in myosin ATPase activity is observed and estrogen administration corrects this deficit.[26] ERT increases cardiac index and heart rate and decreases systemic blood pressure and systemic vascular resistance.[27] Possible mechanisms for this observation are an increased production of vasodilating prostaglandins and a decreased ability of vessels to react to angiotensin-II, norepinephrine, or vasopressin. This condition is similar to that seen in pregnancy.[28,29]

Effects on Lipids and Lipoproteins

Estrogen causes a modest decrease in both total and LDL-cholesterol levels, while increasing HDL cholesterol and triglycerides in both nondiabetic and diabetic women (Table 36-2, Fig. 36-1).[30,31] Although estrogen has beneficial effects on the lipoprotein profile, only one-third of the observed antiatherogenic benefits of estrogen can be accounted for by the hormone's effects on serum lipid concentrations.[10,12,13,16,22] The proposed mechanism for the lipid effect of estrogen is a hormone-induced reduction in hepatic endothelial lipase, the enzyme responsible for degrading HDL.[32] This effect is seen most prominently with oral estrogens metabolized by first-pass hepatic metabolism. Estrogens may also increase catabolism of LDL. Estrogens appear to increase levels of HDL_2 more than HDL_3.[31] The HDL_2 subfraction contains predominantly

TABLE 36-2. Effects of Estrogen and Progestins on Lipids and Lipoproteins

	Estrogen	Progestin
Total cholesterol	Decrease	Increase
LDL-cholesterol	Decrease	Increase
HDL cholesterol*	Increase	Decrease
Triglycerides	Increase	Decrease

*Major effect is on HDL_2 cholesterol. HDL = high-density lipoprotein; LDL = low-density lipoprotein

Source: From Schwartz J, Freeman R, Frishman W. Clinical pharmacology of estrogens: cardiovascular actions and cardioprotective benefits of replacement therapy in postmenopausal women. *J Clin Pharmacol* 35:314, 1995.

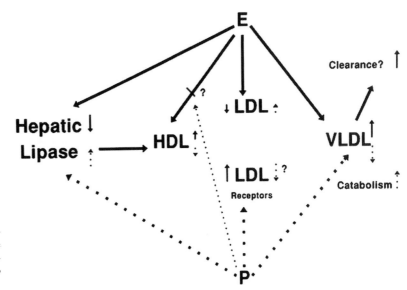

FIGURE 36-1. Effect of hormones on lipoprotein metabolism. E = estrogen; HDL = high density lipoprotein; LDL = low-density lipoprotein; P = progestin; VLDL = very-low-density lipoprotein. (*Adapted with permission from Lobo RA.*[32])

apoprotein I, while the HDL_1 subfraction has both apoproteins I and II.[31] The HDL_2 subfraction can stimulate cholesterol efflux from cultured adipocytes loaded with LDL,[33] and is inversely correlated with the presence of coronary atherosclerosis.[34]

Transdermal estrogens do not appear to be as potent in affecting lipid and lipoprotein parameters as orally active estrogens. The lack of benefit with transdermal estrogen presumably reflects a decreased exposure of estrogen to the liver (compared to oral therapy) due to avoidance of the first-pass effect on the liver. However, when delivering high estrogen concentrations with transdermal formulations over time, there is an effect on serum lipids.[31] In another study in which women were treated for longer periods of time with varying doses of transdermal estradiol, it was found that the total serum cholesterol and LDL concentrations decreased in a dose-dependent fashion after 2 years of therapy.[35] Orally active substituted estrogens, such as ethinyl estradiol, can cause a dramatic rise in blood triglycerides, whereas other oral estrogens cause only a slight increase. Transdermal estrogens usually have no effect at all.[20,31,36] Estrogen-induced plasma triglyceride increases may produce small LDL particles that would be more susceptible to oxidation and, therefore, to atherogenesis.[37]

A recent randomized, crossover trial examined hypercholesterolemic postmenopausal women and compared estrogen and progestin with simvastatin.[38] With high-dose oral-conjugated estrogens combined with continuous medroxyprogesterone acetate (MPA), beneficial changes were seen in the lipoprotein profile: a decrease in both the serum total and LDL-cholesterol, as well as the Lp(a) lipoprotein levels, and an increase in HDL cholesterol levels. Another study directly compared estrogen therapy with treatment with pravastatin, another 3-hydroxy-3-methylglutaryl coenzyme A (HMG-CoA) reductase inhibitor; the study yielded similar results.[39]

In light of the substantial beneficial effects of estrogen on circulating lipids, the National Cholesterol Education Program (NCEP) Expert Panel had, in the past, recommended hormonal therapy as a first-step approach to postmenopausal women requiring pharmacologic treatment of lipid abnormalities.[40] However, in the most recent NCEP guidelines, hormones are no longer recommended as a lipid-modifying treatment.[41]

Effects on Lipoprotein (a)

Epidemiologic and pathophysiologic studies indicate that Lp(a) lipoprotein may also be a powerful, independent predictor of an increased risk of cardiovascular disease.[42] Elevated plasma levels in humans are associated with increased risk of developing CAD, estimated to be two to five times greater than that seen in normal controls. Aging increases Lp(a) in women but not in men.[43] The mode of inheritance of hyperlipoproteinemia (a) is thought to be autosomal codominance. Lp(a) seems to be insensitive to dietary interventions and lipid-lowering treatments, with the exception of omega-3 fatty acids, neomycin, and nicotinic acid.

Estrogen replacement in postmenopausal women has been found to be associated with lower levels of Lp(a).[44,45] A report from the PEPI trial found that estrogen replacement, with or without concomitant progestin regimens, produced consistent reductions in plasma Lp(a) levels by 17 to 23%, which were sustained over a 3-year period.[46] Information involving other therapeutic formulations of estrogens regarding their effects on Lp(a) is not available at this time.

Effects on Blood Pressure

The effect of replacement estrogen on blood pressure remains controversial. In many studies, the presence of hypertension has been a relative contraindication to using ERT because pharmacologic doses of estrogens sufficient to suppress ovulation, as in oral contraceptives, raise blood pressure. Oral estrogen is metabolized in the liver and stimulates the production of renin substrate,[47] angiotensinogen, and a variety of binding globulins (Table 36-3). The induction of high-molecular-weight renin (HMWR) substrate is very dependent on the estrogen formulation.[48]

Shionori and others,[47] found that estrogens induce the synthesis of an electrophoretically immunologically distinct form of renin substrate, HMWR. HMWR is present in normotensive and hypertensive women, but is significantly elevated in normotensive pregnant women at term and in women who have estrogen-induced hypertension. In these women, with the discontinuation of estrogen, blood pressure normalized in all cases, and HMWR decreased to less than 2%. HMWR is not a general marker for hypertension because the protein is not elevated in essential hypertension. Shionori's study

TABLE 36-3. Comparative Effects of Various Estrogen Formulations on Blood Parameters (2 Weeks of Treatment)*

Formulation	Dose (mg)	E1/E2	SHBG-BC	FSH	CBG-BC	Angiotensinogen
Pip E1 sulfate	1.25	30/20	1	1.1	1.0	1
CEE	0.625	>1	3.2	1.4	2.5	3.5
Micronized E2	1.0	>1	1	1.3	1.9	1
DES	0.1	28.4	3.8	70	13	
Ethinyl E2	0.01	614	80–200	1000	232	

*CBG-BC = corticosteroid-binding globulin-binding capacity; CEE = conjugated equine estrogens; DES = diethylstilbestrol; E1/E2 = estrone to estradiol ratio; Ethinyl E2 = ethinyl estradiol; FSH = follicle-stimulating hormone; Micronized E2 = micronized estradiol; Pip E1 sulfate = piperazine estrone sulfate; SHBG-BC = sex hormone-binding globulin-binding capacity

Source: From Mashchak et al,[144] with permission.

had a very small number of patients, and estrogen-induced hypertension was secondary to various oral contraceptive preparations or ethinyl estradiol (50 μg).[47] Occasionally, patients can experience an idiosyncratic estrogen-induced hypertensive response.[49] Other studies involving estrogen and blood pressure show equivocal results: increased blood pressure,[50] decreased blood pressure,[50,51] and no change in blood pressure.[52] In normotensive postmenopausal women, chronic transdermal ERT decreased sympathetic nerve discharge and caused a slight fall in ambulatory blood pressure.[53] Estrogen can also attenuate the development of pressure overload hypertrophy.[54]

Equine estrogens, 60% estrone sulfate and 40% equine estrogens (ring B unsaturated), are derived from the urine of pregnant mares. The ring B unsaturated estrogens are not normally metabolized by enzymes in women, and therefore remain relatively more potent than natural estrogens, which are readily metabolized to other compounds. This may explain the difference in blood pressure response in women.

Blood pressure decreases significantly in the mid-trimester phase of pregnancy; this decrease may be attributed to a massive increase in total estrogen and progesterone production. This fall in blood pressure occurs despite a rise in angiotensin concentration throughout pregnancy, implying that pregnancy makes the peripheral vessels less responsive to the effects of angiotensin.

Thrombosis

Estrogen is associated with an increase in blood coagulability. Blood clots form with changes in blood flow, with enhancement of the coagulation cascade superimposed by intimal damage, and with absence of normal anticoagulant and fibrinolytic activity.

Mechanism   ERT is associated with an increased risk of venous thromboembolism. Estrogens can increase platelet adhesiveness while decreasing those factors that naturally inhibit thrombosis, such as antithrombin III.[49] However, a decrease in antithrombin III activity with estrogens is not associated with increased coagulability.[55] Estrogens can increase fibrinogen, factors VII, IX, X, and XII, and prothrombin. Synthetic estrogens are more potent than natural preparations, and oral estrogen formulations may influence coagulation more than transdermal preparations.[56] However, investigators do not detect an increased coagulability secondary to estrogen as measured by the partial thromboplastin time.[55] Elevations in coagulation factor concentrations with estrogen may not indicate a functional hypercoagulable state because clotting factors circulate as proenzymes or cofactors to other enzymes and are themselves inactive until a suitable clot-promoting surface is available.[57] The

tests that measure the various factors do not differentiate between proenzyme and the activated forms.

Thrombosis is not seen in women given ERT after surgical menopause. After 3 months of treatment, there was no difference in platelet counts, fibrinogen antigen, or fibrin degradation products.[58] In summary, estrogens are probably not direct procoagulant substances in normal women. Thrombosis is likely secondary to an idiosyncratic link to an abnormal clotting protein.[59,60] The PEPI trial supported these findings.[61,62]

Blood Vessel Integrity

Estrogen therapy improves blood vessel integrity,[63,64] and appears to prevent atherosclerosis development.[65,65a] In ovariectomized female monkeys, Williams and others[66] demonstrated endothelial dysfunction in these animals with impaired endothelium-mediated vasodilation. ERT reversed the endothelial dysfunction, and normal vasodilatory activity was restored. Estrogen facilitates the release of NO and inhibits the release of vasoconstrictor substances such as endothelin.[67,68] Estrogens have vascular protective actions that are unrelated to NO.[69,69a] Estrogens appear to decrease lipoprotein-induced smooth-muscle proliferation[70] in blood vessels, and appear to inhibit intimal proliferation associated with mechanical injury to the endothelium.[71] The effects of different estrogen formulations on the vasculature are currently being investigated. A recent clinical study concluded that oral but not transdermal estradiol induces antiatherogenic changes in in vivo endothelium-dependent vasodilation.[72] In addition, when medroxyprogesterone is added to estradiol treatment, the improvement in endothelium-dependent dilation seen with estrogen therapy is diminished.[73]

Blood Flow

In addition to the favorable changes in lipids and lipoproteins, estrogens can increase blood flow in various vascular beds, and can improve exercise capacity.[74] Using Doppler ultrasound techniques, investigators have demonstrated that the impedance to blood flow increases after menopause.[75] Within 6 weeks of transdermal ERT, however, vascular impedance was reduced by 50%.[76]

Effects on the ECG

Approximately 20% of postmenopausal women with a normal baseline stress echocardiogram will have a false-positive exercise ECG response to oral exogenous estrogen therapy.[77] Women also have a longer rate-corrected QT interval and a higher incidence of drug-induced torsades de pointes which may be related to estrogen.[77a]

Other Metabolic Effects

Estrogen may improve insulin sensitivity. This is particularly important considering that many reports suggest that insulin resistance and the resultant hyperinsulinemia predispose to lipid abnormalities and an increased risk of atherosclerosis. In a case-controlled study[78] using conjugated estrogens and progestins in women for more than 20 days, an improvement in glucose tolerance with increased insulin activity was observed. Lobo et al reported that fasting glucose and insulin levels and the insulin response to glucose all decreased in postmenopausal women after 1 year of ERT.[79] In a placebo-controlled study, ERT decreased fasting glucose and C-peptide levels in postmenopausal women with insulin-dependent diabetes mellitus (IDDM).[80]

However, the beneficial effect of estrogen on insulin sensitivity is not confirmed by all studies.[81,82] In the PEPI trial, mean changes in 2 h postchallenge insulin did not differ significantly in any treatment group. An unexplained downward drift in postchallenge insulin levels did occur, but the decrease in insulin was not paralleled by a decrease in postchallenge glucose levels.[62] Moreover, progestins may decrease insulin sensitivity.[83]

Estrogens also have antioxidant effects[84] with chronic use that may protect against ischemic-induced vascular injury.[85] The antioxidant activity of estrogen may diminish lipid peroxidation.[86] In postmenopausal women, both long-term and short-term administration of 17β-estradiol can decrease the oxidation of LDL.[87] Shwaery et al[88] found that the inhibition of LDL oxidation may be mediated by the association of plasma LDL with a derivative of estradiol, probably an ester.

Effect on C-Reactive Protein and the Inflammatory Response

The Women's Health study reported that serum C-reactive protein (CRP), a marker of inflammation, was a strong independent risk factor for cardiovascular disease that added to the predictive value of other factors, such as serum total cholesterol.[88a] Recently, studies have shown that ERT elevates CRP. Ridker et al. observed that among 493 postmenopausal women, median CRP levels were twofold higher among women taking hormone replacement therapy (HRT) as compared to those not using HRT; this difference was noted in all subgroups analyzed and had no association with the type of HRT preparation used (i.e., estrogen alone or estrogen plus progesterone).[89]

In the PEPI trial, CRP levels were measured at baseline and at 12 and 36 months in 365 women.[90] HRT users were found to have an increase in CRP levels as compared to women who received placebo. This increase occurred primarily during the first year of treatment. Final measurements of CRP were 85% higher than baseline. The combination of statins with estrogen can attenuate this hormonal effect on CRP levels.[90a]

More studies are necessary to evaluate the clinical significance of this elevation in CRP with HRT. A proinflammatory effect of estrogen on the vasculature has been proposed to explain part of the prothrombotic actions of the hormone and the apparent lack of benefit of hormone treatment in prospective survival studies, despite the lipid-lowering effect.

Clinical Use of Estrogens in Heart Disease

Prospective Clinical Studies

Currently, ERT is used in postmenopausal women. Although there is much evidence to support estrogen's favorable cardiovascular multiorgan system effects, recommendations regarding its use are still being debated.[91] Estrogen therapy may be associated with breast cancer, but heart disease is the leading cause of death among women in the United States today.[92] Therefore, ERT may still be needed in the female postmenopausal population as a cardiovascular protective agent.

The National Institutes of Health are carrying out the Women's Health Initiative (WHI) Study to examine the clinical outcomes of long-term hormonal replacement in postmenopausal women ages 50 to 80 years: conjugated equine estrogen (CEE) plus MPA given continuously (based on the PEPI study) in women with an intact uterus (CEE alone in women after hysterectomy), and with and without dietary alteration (<22% fat). This 11-year controlled study focuses on diseases of the cardiovascular system, bone (osteoporotic fractures), central nervous system disorders (dementia), and neoplasia (breast, endometrium, and colon). There are 40 study centers nationwide and thousands of subjects are participating. The ultimate goal is to resolve many of the unanswered questions regarding the benefits and risks of hormonal replacement therapy in otherwise healthy postmenopausal women.[93]

A preliminary report from the WHI shows no benefit of HRT on the risk of CAD after 2 years and a slightly greater rate of venoembolic disease as compared to placebo.[94] Recently the estrogen + progestin component of the WHI was terminated because of an increased risk (26% higher) of breast cancer compared to placebo. There was also increased risk of stroke, pulmonary embolism, and coronary heart disease (non-fatal MI and coronary death).[94a] The estrogen only component of the WHI is still ongoing, as is a similar study in Europe.[94b]

Evidence of estrogen's beneficial effects in the secondary prevention of heart disease in women and men has now been called into question because of the negative results of the Heart and Estrogen/Progestin Replacement Study (HERS).[95,95a] In this first large, randomized, placebo-controlled intervention clinical trial examining the use of postmenopausal HRT and risk for cardiovascular disease, 2763 women with established coronary disease were randomly assigned to receive daily CEE plus MPA or placebo. After a mean of 4.1 years of therapy with estrogen plus progestin, no overall effect was seen on the risk of nonfatal myocardial infarction and death from coronary heart disease. Increased venous thromboembolic complications were also observed,[96] and there was no effect of treatment on peripheral arterial events, including stroke.[97,98] There was also an increase in coronary events in the first year in the treated patients and a decrease in coronary events in years 4 and 5. There have been many hypotheses offered to explain the results. There were questions about whether the progestin had offset the effects of estrogen. A proinflammatory vascular effect has also been proposed. Others argued that these findings from a relatively short clinical trial may not reliably predict a long-term benefit, in light of the abundant literature suggesting the benefit of estrogen. In short, the results of HERS are still being interpreted and additional studies are required.

Recently, Herrington and colleagues reported findings on the Estrogen Replacement and Atherosclerosis (ERA) Study.[99] These investigators carried out a randomized, double-blind, placebo-controlled clinical trial assessing the effects of HRT on the progression of coronary atherosclerosis in women. The authors randomly assigned 309 women with angiographically verified coronary heart disease at baseline to receive unopposed estrogen, estrogen plus MPA, or placebo. Of the initial group, 248 women underwent angiography a mean of 3.2 years later. Although both estrogen regimens significantly reduced LDL-cholesterol and significantly increased HDL cholesterol, the researchers discovered that neither treatment had any impact on the progression of coronary atherosclerosis, regardless of disease severity, age, or various clinical characteristics. Moreover, the treatment groups had similar rates of clinical cardiovascular events.

It was recently shown that postmenopausal women who initiate HRT after a recent MI had an increased risk of cardiac events.[100] In women who survived a first MI, there was an increased risk of a recurrent coronary event in the first 60 days and a reduced risk with hormone use for longer than 1 year.[101–103] A recent placebo-controlled study also showed that estradiol in postmenopausal women who had recently had a stroke or transient ischemic attack did not reduce mortality or the recurrence of stroke.[104] Based on the findings to date, HRT should not be prescribed for the express purpose of preventing CAD.[105,105a]

Currently, studies are being done with the selective estrogen-receptor modifying drugs (SERMS), such as raloxifene, in women with known CAD, to determine whether these agents, which have little effect on the breast and uterus, can reduce the risk of cardiovascular mortality.[106–108] SERMS have also been suggested as a treatment in men to reduce the risk of CAD.[107]

Use in Symptomatic Ischemic Heart Disease

Gilligan et al.[109] performed a study in which the acute intra-arterial infusion of 17β-estradiol was shown to potentiate endothelium-dependent vasodilation in the forearm of postmenopausal women with symptomatic ischemic heart disease. However, this effect was not maintained with a 3-week cycle of systemic estradiol administration. The therapy resulted in a lower level of blood estrogen. Acute estrogen administration may have potential use in clinical diseases such as angina pectoris.[110,111]

Acute and chronic estrogen therapy may be useful therapy for syndrome X or microvascular angina with normal coronary angiograms.[112] In premenopausal women with variant angina, the condition appears to be less severe in the follicular phase of the menstrual cycle when the mean level of estradiol is highest.[112a] Estradiol supplementation also suppresses hyperventilation-induced attacks in postmenopausal women with variant angina.[113]

Conclusion

Thus far, there is little evidence in the literature to support the routine use of estrogen in both chronic and acute ischemic heart disease (Table 36-4).[105,113a–113c] Estrogen's vasomotor effects may make it useful in helping to control angina pain or perhaps migraine headache, but this needs to be documented further. Because of its favorable effects on lipids, estrogen may be useful in the primary prevention of CAD, but more definitive data are needed. In July

TABLE 36-4. Potential Uses of Estrogens in Ischemic Heart Disease

Acute use
Angina pectoris
Acute myocardial infarction
Syndrome X
Chronic use
Prevention of atherosclerotic heart disease and its acute complications
Prevention of restenosis following angioplasty and atherectomy

2001, the American Heart Association presented formal guidelines recommending that physicians should not prescribe HRT to prevent heart disease.[114]

Choice of Estrogen

During menopause, cessation of ovarian follicular development causes a decreased production of estradiol and other hormones, leading to a loss of negative feedback to the hypothalamic-pituitary center, causing follicle-stimulating hormone (FSH) and luteinizing hormone (LH) to increase. The major source of estrogen in postmenopausal women is androstenedione, produced in the adrenal cortex, and metabolized to estrone in the liver, fatty tissue, skeletal muscle, kidney, brain, and hair follicles. Although some of the estrone gets converted to estradiol, there still remains a markedly reduced ratio of estradiol to estrone, typically 0.2 to 0.3, as opposed to >1 premenopausally (Table 36-5).[115]

The effect of reduced estradiol production leads to symptoms of vasomotor instability; mood and sleep disturbances; difficulties with memory and concentration; and atrophy of urogenital epithelium resulting in vaginal discomfort, dyspareunia, and urinary frequency. Symptoms appear when plasma estradiol concentration falls below 35 pg/mL. Forty percent of women develop menopausal symptoms serious enough to seek medical assistance.[116] In addition, gradual loss of bone mineral content leads to osteoporosis, alterations in lipid metabolism, decreasing ratio of HDL to LDL, and increase in blood pressure and increased risk of CAD, especially in women with premature menopause, bilateral oophorectomy, or ovarian failure.[117] Estrogen metabolism involves interconversion of estrone sulfate, estrone, and estradiol within various intracellular and extracellular compartments. Estradiol and estrone are largely converted to estrone sulfate, which constitutes the largest pool of estrogen in the body serving as a reservoir primarily for estrone (Fig. 36-2). Ninety percent of estrone sulfate circulates bound to albumin and is inactive. Estrone is cleared by conversion in the liver to estriol, epiestriol, and estrogen conjugates, which are reabsorbed from the enterohepatic circulation, reentering the circulation as estrone. Although the conversion of estrone to estradiol is low in the circulation, a much larger

TABLE 36-5. Typical Production Rates and Plasma Concentrations of Endogenous Estrogen in Premenopausal and Menopausal Women

Stage	Approximate Daily Estradiol Production (μg)	Plasma Concentration ng/L	
		Estradiol	**Estrone**
Premenopausal			
Early follicular	100	40–60	40–60
Mid follicular	96–100	60–100	
Late follicular	320–640	200–400	170–200
Luteal	300	190	100–150
Menopausal	18	5–20	30–70

Source: Reproduced from Good WR, Power MS, Campbell P, Schenkel L. A new transdermal delivery system for estradiol. *J Control Release* 2:89, 1985, with permission.

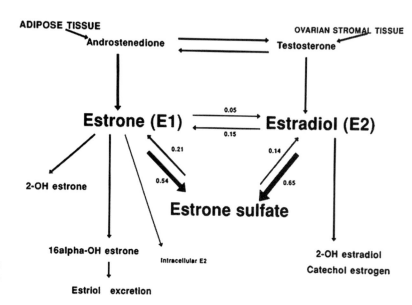

FIGURE 36-2. Estrogen metabolism. Conversion ratios between estradiol, estrone, and estrone sulfate. —OH = hydroxy. (*Adapted with permission from Lobo RA.*[118])

conversion occurs in tissues. The predominant intracellular estrogen is estradiol, which is the most biologically active estrogen.[118]

Estrogen Replacement

Three separate classes of estrogens are used for ERT (Table 36-6, Fig. 36-3): natural estrogens, which include estradiol, estrone, and estriol (used mostly in Europe); CEE; and synthetic substituted estrogens, primarily ethinyl estradiol, quinestrol, and the nonsteroidal estrogen diethylstilbestrol.

Any estradiol administered orally is converted in the liver to estrone via the first-pass effect. During passage through the liver and portal circulation, there is a 30% reduction in bioavailable estrogens. This reduction can be accentuated by certain types of medications, a reaction not seen with systemic administration of estrogen.[119]

TABLE 36-6. Estrogen Formulations

	Components	Doses, mg
Oral formulations		
Natural (similar to normally circulating hormone)		
Micronized estradiol	100% estradiol	1, 2
Estradiol valerate		1, 2
Piperazine estrone sulfate	100% estrone sulfate	0.625, 1.25, 2.5
Natural equine estrogen		
Conjugated estrogens	50%–60% estrone sulfates	0.3, 0.625, 0.9
	20%–35% sodium equilin sulfate	1.25, 2.5
	7.5%–20% unspecified conjugated estrogens	
Substituted estrogens		
Ethinyl estradiol	100% ethinyl estradiol	0.02, 0.05, 0.5
Mestranol		
Quinesterol	Ester of ethinyl estradiol	0.1
Nonsteroidal estrogen (diethylstilbesterol)	100% diethylstilbestrol	0.1, 0.5
Nonoral formulations		
Transdermal system		
17β-Estradiol	Drug layer	
	17β-Estradiol (active component)	
	Alcohol USP gelled with hydroxypropyl cellulose	0.05, 0.1 release mg/d
17β-Estradiol gel		1.5 mg/dose
Vaginal creams		
17β-Estradiol		0.1%
Piperazine estrone sulfate		1.5 mg/g
Conjugated equine estrogen		0.625 mg/g
Diethylstilbestrol		0.01%

Source: Reproduced from Schwartz J, Freeman R, Frishman W. Clinical pharmacology of estrogens: cardiovascular actions and cardioprotective benefits of replacement therapy in postmenopausal women. *J Clin Pharmacol* 35:314, 1995.

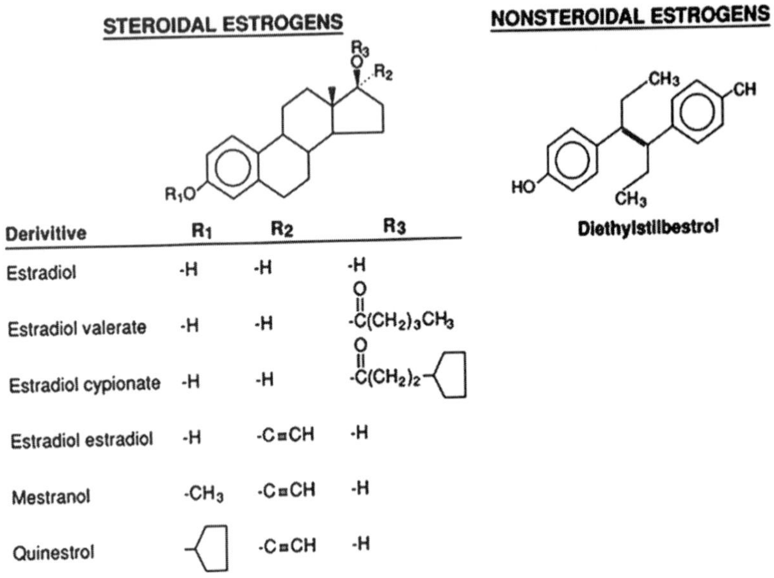

STEROIDAL ESTROGENS

NONSTEROIDAL ESTROGENS

Diethylstilbestrol

Derivitive	R_1	R_2	R_3
Estradiol	-H	-H	-H
Estradiol valerate	-H	-H	$-\overset{O}{\overset{\|}{C}}(CH_2)_3CH_3$
Estradiol cypionate	-H	-H	$-\overset{O}{\overset{\|}{C}}(CH_2)_2$
Estradiol estradiol	-H	-C≡CH	-H
Mestranol	-CH₃	-C≡CH	-H
Quinestrol		-C≡CH	-H

FIGURE 36-3. Structural formulas of selected estrogens.

Adverse Effects of ERT

Endometrial, Ovarian and Colorectal Carcinoma

As per Voigt and others,[120] users of unopposed estrogen incur a risk of endometrial cancer three times greater than that of nonusers. Those who use unopposed estrogen for more than 3 years have a greater than fivefold increase in the risk of endometrial cancer. Hunt and Vessey[121] demonstrated that the predominant type of endometrial cancers seen with unopposed estrogen use are early stage cancers having a good prognosis; ERT users have a better 5-year survival than do nonusers. So, although some reports propose that endometrial carcinoma in these women is less aggressive than usual,[122] other studies show a higher risk of metastases.[123] The risk of endometrial cancer with unopposed estrogen is both duration and dose-dependent. In one study, the relative risk of endometrial cancer increased 17% per year of estrogen therapy, to an odds ratio of greater than 8 after 10 years.[124] The excess risk persisted 5 or more years after cessation of therapy.

The excess risk of endometrial hyperplasia and carcinoma can be reduced or possibly eliminated by the concomitant administration of progestin.[125] In the PEPI trial, unopposed estrogen was associated with a significantly increased risk of adenomatous or atypical hyperplasia (34% vs 1%) and of hysterectomy (6% vs 1%) in comparison with other regimens.[62] In one study,[126] the incidence of endometrial hyperplasia was considerably lower in the group given transdermal estradiol plus cyclic progestin than in the group of women given unopposed transdermal estradiol. When a progestin was used continuously or cyclically for 3 months in women who developed endometrial hyperplasia, in all cases endometrial histology reverted to normal.

It has also been demonstrated that postmenopausal use of estrogen for 10 or more years is associated with an increased risk of ovarian cancer that persisted up to 29 years after cessation of use.[127] In contrast, observational studies suggest a reduced risk of colorectal cancer among women taking postmenopausal hormones.[128]

Breast Cancer

Some investigators have found a slightly increased risk of breast cancer with long-term use of estrogen.[129] Others, however, are unwilling to draw that conclusion because most of the evidence is based on meta-analyses and not on controlled interventional studies.[130] Furthermore, a reanalysis of original data from 51 epidemiologic studies comprising 52,705 women with and 108,411 women without breast cancer found that for each year a woman uses postmenopausal hormones, her risk of breast cancer increases by 2.3%.[131]

The Nurses' Health Study found an increase in breast cancer risk only in women currently taking ERT; past users had a risk that was similar to that in women who had never taken ERT.[132] In the combined analysis of epidemiologic studies, women who had stopped ERT more than 5 years previously were not at increased risk as compared with never users, regardless of the duration of previous ERT.[131] However, there have not been enough data on long-term past users; there may still be a risk associated with past use if the duration was long enough.

Of concern is the recent report from the Breast Cancer Detection Demonstration Project showing a greater risk of breast cancer with combination estrogen and progestin therapy.[133] Similar observations were made in the WHI.[94a]

That progesterone does not downregulate estrogen and progesterone receptors in the breast may contribute to its adverse effects.[134] Moreover, the isoenzyme of 17-hydroxysteroid dehydrogenase induced by progesterone in the breast predominantly catalyzes the conversion of the less potent estrone to the more potent estradiol.[135]

Other Side Effects and Drug Interactions

Common short-term side effects of ERT include mastodynia (breast tenderness), slight salt and water retention, leg edema, increased vaginal secretions, vaginal bleeding, headache, or, in some predisposed individuals, an increase in migraine headaches or abdominal bloating (more likely when coadministered with progestational agents).

Postmenopausal estrogen use can substantially increase a woman's risk of cholecystectomy.[135a] By raising the level of cholesterol in the bile and decreasing bile acid concentration, estrogen can promote the growth of gallstones. Women who currently use estrogen, as well as those who used it in the past, were 50% more likely to develop asthma than those who never used estrogen. An exogenous estrogen has also been shown to inhibit CYP1A2-mediated caffeine metabolism.[136]

Contraindications

Contraindications to ERT include a history of breast or recent uterine cancer, acute liver disease, and active thromboembolic disorders. A family history of premenopausal breast cancer incurs a higher risk, and ERT should not be prescribed unless the patient has demonstrated a normal mammogram. Preexisting leiomyomas could increase in size and careful exams should be performed at regular intervals. Hypertensive patients should be carefully observed if given oral therapy, which is known to affect renin substrate and to possibly cause an idiosyncratic reaction.[137] However, in these patients, nonoral therapies should be considered, such as transdermal estradiol, because the hepatic effects are avoided.[118]

Coadministration with Progesterone

Progestogens have been used to oppose the effects of estrogen on the endometrium. Progestogen effects are antiestrogenic (decrease in receptor number and mitotic activity) and decrease the potency of estrogens by enzymes that aid intracellular effects (dehydrogenase). Although progestogens have been studied far less than estrogens, much is known about the pharmacology and clinical effects of various progestogens. The classes of progestogens include native progestins (progesterone and 17-hydroxyprogesterone) and synthetic progestins [19 nortestosterones (used in oral contraceptives) and C-21 compounds with 17-acetoxy group (MPA, megestrol acetate)].[118]

Clinical Effects

Besides the desired effects of progestins on endometrium, lipid metabolism is the major parameter affected by MPA and norethindrone. No significant effect on binding globulins and negligible effects on clotting parameters have been found.[138] A recent study has demonstrated that progestins can potentiate the vascular procoagulant effects of thrombin by increasing the availability of membrane thrombin receptors.[138a] Several studies show decreased glucose tolerance with progestogen. For example, levonorgestrel causes the greatest perturbation of glucose tolerance followed by norethindrone and MPA. However, most of these studies used oral contraceptives and associated the effect to the androgenic potency of the progestogen.[118]

All progestogens affect lipid metabolism adversely by increasing LDL and/or decreasing HDL, particularly HDL$_2$ (Tables 36-7 and 36-8). However, the type of progestogen and route of administration are important because androgenic potency is the principal factor related to adverse progestational effects. Although MPA has the least androgenic potency of the synthetic progestins, it also decreases

TABLE 36-8. Effects of Progestins

Decrease endometrial hyperplasia
Decrease risk endometrial cancer fivefold
Attenuate estrogen lipid effect on HDL
Increase LDL
Decrease HDL
Antiestrogenic
Antimitotic on endometrium
Common side effects: breast tenderness, bloating, mood changes, chronic vaginal bleeding
Effect on breast unclear

Source: Reproduced with permission from Schwartz J, Freeman R, Frishman W. Clinical pharmacology of estrogens: cardiovascular actions and cardioprotective benefits of replacement therapy in postmenopausal women. *J Clin Pharmacol* 35:314, 1995.

HDL and HDL$_2$ at 10 mg. Both MPA and levonorgestrel decrease HDL levels by 8 to 18%, but MPA lowers HDL-cholesterol much less than levonorgestrel.[139] On the other hand, micronized progesterone seems to have little or no adverse effect on lipid levels.[62,139] Natural progesterone is the only progestin totally devoid of these effects.[139] Progestogens such as MPA may cause minor changes in lipoproteins, but they clearly attenuate the beneficial lipid effects of ERT.[140]

In the PEPI trial,[62] 875 women were randomly assigned to receive placebo, oral estrogen alone, or one of three estrogen-progestin regimens. HDL cholesterol levels were increased and LDL-cholesterol levels were decreased in all the treatment groups. The decreases in LDL-cholesterol levels were similar for all regimens, but the HDL cholesterol levels were significantly less elevated in the women who took estrogen with MPA than in those who took estrogen alone. However, the net effect of oral ERT plus MPA on HDL-cholesterol is, overall, still beneficial, while the addition of a progestin has little effect on the estrogen-induced reduction in LDL-cholesterol.[62,141] A recent study shows that natural progesterone can counteract the vasodilator actions of estrogen.[142]

The most common side effects of progesterone treatment are breast tenderness, bloating, mood changes, and chronic vaginal bleeding.[143]

Recommendations for Using Estrogen and Progesterone as Postmenopausal and Cardioprotective Therapy

Substituted estrogen preparations (i.e., ethinyl estradiol) have demonstrated a potential for increased hepatic and endometrial toxicity and are therefore not recommended.

TABLE 36-7. Percent Change in Lipoproteins with Various Progestins*

	Micronized P 200 mg	MPA 5 mg	MPA 10 mg	NET 1 ng	DL-NG 0.15	DL-NG 0.25
HDL	−1	−6	−6	−10	−14	−18
HDL$_2$	0	−11	−19	−27	−23	−25
HDL$_3$	0	0	−2	−1	0	−8
LDL	0	+3	+7	−1	0	−8
Apo-A1	+1	−5	−11	+10	+6	+1
Apo-B	0	0	+3	+10	−15	+10

*Micronized P = micronized progesterone; MPA = medroxyprogesterone acetate; NET = norethindrone; DL-NG = norgestrel; HDL = high-density lipoprotein, HDL$_2$ = high-density lipoprotein subfraction 2; HDL$_3$ = high-density lipoprotein subfraction 3; LDL = low-density lipoprotein; Apo-A1 = apoprotein A1; Apo-B = aproprotein B. Values given are the percent change during sequential administration compared to the effects of unopposed estrogen.

Source: Lobo RA,[32] with permission.

Natural estrogens, used in equivalent doses, such as piperazine estrone sulfate, and estradiol valerate or micronized estradiol, are not as biologically potent as CEEs.[144] CEEs also appear to have the most favorable actions on plasma lipids and lipoproteins without significant effects on coagulation factors or blood pressure except for rare idiosyncratic responses with a thromboembolic or hypertensive episode. Among the various estrogen-delivery approaches (oral, vaginal, percutaneous, transdermal), oral preparations have the best antilipid effect. Although other estrogen formulations might induce favorable lipid and lipoprotein profiles, after long-term use, nothing surpasses oral treatment.

Transdermal estrogen therapy has potential advantages as compared with oral therapy. The patches are not associated with changes in hepatic proteins[145] and provide more physiologic estradiol and estrone levels. Use of patches avoids first-pass hepatic metabolism of estrogens and avoids gastrointestinal estrogen incompatibility. Finally, the patches appear to reduce adverse effects of estrogens by enhancing the blood concentration-time profile and can increase patient compliance by eliminating multidose treatment schedules. Interpatient differences in absorption of estradiol may also be smaller with the patch.

However, because higher estradiol concentrations are seen with the patch as compared with oral delivery, there may be greater potential for inducing breast changes. This may not be a real problem because estrone is converted to estradiol in body tissues and the intracellular concentrations of estradiol with both oral and transdermal delivery may be similar.

Despite some of the potential advantages of the transcutaneous delivery of estrogens, all of the studies that show a cardiovascular benefit used oral conjugated estrogen. Because there are no definitive data showing the effects of transdermal delivery on cardiovascular outcomes, bone disease, and breast cancer, the authors recommend oral conjugated estrogen as the replacement formulation of choice.

There is no additional benefit from the use of 1.25 mg of conjugated estrogen, and the minimum dose has not been determined. Doses of 0.3 mg/d with supplemental calcium are as effective in maintaining bone mass as 0.625 mg without elemental calcium.[146] Doses of 0.3 mg induce favorable changes in lipids, lipoproteins, and hemostatic factors with no bleeding.[147]

In postmenopausal women with a uterus, it is probably best to use progesterone to reduce the risk of endometrial hyperplasia and neoplasia. The progestin of choice is micronized progesterone in oil at a dose of 200 mg/d. Natural progesterone does not attenuate the effects of estrogens on lipids as do the synthetic progestins. If micronized progesterone is not available, MPA in a low dose of 2.5 mg is recommended because it has low androgenic potency, which may minimize the adverse reactions of treatment while still providing a protective effect on the endometrium.[148]

The exact combination estrogen-progesterone daily regimen or cyclic administration has not been established. Some investigators suggest using daily estrogen with progestin for 12 days of each month. Others use estrogen and progestin continuously to create an atrophic endometrium and decrease the incidence of bleeding. On a continuous regimen, women may have intermittent vaginal bleeding for up to 6 months or longer until the endometrium becomes atrophic,[149] whereas with the cyclical regimen, a monthly menstrual period is more likely at the end of the progesterone course. Even with this regimen, most women will stop bleeding after several years. A specific regimen should ensure patient compliance and needs to be individualized.

PHYTOESTROGENS

Phytoestrogens, a diverse group of compounds found in various plant-derived foods and beverages, can have both estrogenic and antiestrogenic effects.[150] There are three main categories of phytoestrogens: isoflavones, coumestans, and lignans. The isoflavones occur in high concentrations in soybeans, chick peas, and other legumes, as well as bluegrass and clovers. Coumestans are found widely in sprouts of alfalfa and various beans. Cereals and oilseeds such as flaxseed provide a significant source of lignans.[151] These compounds are similar in structure and function to estradiol. Dietary consumption of lignans and isoflavones has been postulated to play a role in the protection of humans against the development of CAD.[152] The estrogenic activity of phytoestrogens was first observed in the 1940s with the outbreak of reproductive disturbances in sheep. The animals were feeding on clover containing formononetin, which is converted by ruminal bacteria to isoflavones.[153]

Isoflavones make up the most common form of phytoestrogens; and they are the best studied. Two of the major isoflavones are genistein and daidzein, which are parent compounds. They are inactive when present in the bound form of glycosides (genistin, daidzin), but as aglycones (genistein, daidzein) they become activated. These compounds undergo fermentation by intestinal microflora, with both metabolites and aglycones being liable to absorption. In the body, the parent compounds are reconjugated to glucuronides and excreted unchanged in the urine.[154]

Evidence suggests the existence of a causal, inverse relationship between phytoestrogens and cardiovascular disease. The lower incidence of cardiovascular diseases and high intakes of dietary phytoestrogens in Asian populations, support the hypothesis that phytoestrogen consumption has a cardioprotective effect.[155]

The major dietary source of phytoestrogens in most populations is soy. Soybeans and their products are consumed by humans in many forms, including whole soybeans, tofu, tempeh, and soy milk. The concentration of genistein in most soy food materials ranges from 1 to 2 mg per g of protein. Many Asian populations that have low rates of breast and prostate cancer consume 20 to 80 mg of genistein per day, almost entirely derived from soy, whereas the dietary intake of genistein in the United States has been estimated at 1 to 3 mg per day.[156] However, as there is significant variation of isoflavone content between varieties of soy beans, the particular crop, and the processing methods, dietary studies can be inconsistent.

Phytoestrogens may have favorable effects on lipid profiles, vascular reactivity, thrombosis and cellular proliferation. The lower incidence of CAD in populations ingesting diets high in phytoestrogen has been attributed to an improved lipid profile. The serum cholesterol and LDL-cholesterol-lowering effects of soy protein-containing food have been investigated in a large number of studies, which have been subjected to a meta-analysis.[157] In summary, a mean intake of 47 g of soy protein daily was associated with a reduction in total cholesterol by 9% and of LDL by 13%, as well as a decrease in triglyceride levels of 10%. However the decrease was directly related to the initial serum cholesterol level, with insignificant changes in individuals with low initial cholesterol (−3.3% in the lowest quartile) and marked reductions in those with the highest levels (−19.6% in the highest quartile).

The mechanism for the hypocholesterolemic effects of phytoestrogens is uncertain. It has been proposed that there is altered hepatic metabolism with augmented LDL and VLDL removal by hepatocytes. Phytoestrogens in soy protein may stimulate the clearance of cholesterol, probably by upregulating LDL receptors, and thereby increasing LDL receptor activity.[158] Lignans may also affect cholesterol homeostasis, as they have been shown to inhibit the activity of cholesterol-7α-hydroxylase, the rate-limiting enzyme, in the formation of primary bile acids from cholesterol.[159]

Isoflavone phytoestrogens may also play a role as antioxidants. Tikkanen et al.[160] observed that consumption of soy-derived isoflavones (total 35 mg genistein and 21 mg daidzein per day) by healthy volunteers for 2 weeks resulted in increased oxidation resistance of LDL isolated at the end of the 2-week period. Purification of LDL from water-soluble contaminants ascertained that the altered oxidation susceptibility was due to alteration in the LDL particles themselves. The LDL fractions contained considerable amounts of the isoflavones and a marked prolongation of the lag time to LDL oxidation was seen, implying antioxidant effect.

The process of atherosclerotic plaque formation is a combination of numerous cellular events. An initial endothelial injury leads to cellular infiltration and proliferation, eventually contributing to the formation of the advanced atherosclerotic lesion. Studies in vitro show that soy-derived isoflavones may favorably alter cellular processes associated with lesion development.[161] Genistein, in particular, exerts antiproliferative effects in human cell lines.[162] Takahashi and colleagues[163] also discovered that genistein is capable of inhibiting the expression of intercellular adhesion molecule (ICAM)-1 and vascular cell adhesion molecule (VCAM)-1 on human endothelial cells cocultured with monocytes. Akiyama and others[164] also reported that genistein is a specific inhibitor of tyrosine kinases.

Phytoestrogens may also have beneficial effects on vascular reactivity. Studies carried out in nonhuman primates with preexisting diet-induced atherosclerosis showed a favorable response in endothelium mediated vasodilation with phytoestrogen treatment.[165] Postmenopausal monkeys on the soy+ diet had normal coronary artery vasodilation following acetylcholine injection whereas the soy− group had a vasoconstrictive response. Vascular reactivity was not markedly different in the soy+ and soy− diet groups among the male monkeys.

The mechanism of action of phytoestrogens on coronary artery vascular tone has been examined.[166] Figtree et al.[167] reported that genistein and its precursor, biochanin A, relax precontracted rabbit coronary artery rings. Other investigators observed that genistein and daidzein relax mesenteric arterial rings of rats in a dose dependent manner.[168] The highly efficacious vasodilator effects of genistein are not dependent on nitric oxide and are independent of endothelium.

Accumulating data from recent studies indicate that phytoestrogen consumption has a favorable effect on the risk of acute coronary events. A recent case-control study took note of the association between the serum enterolactone concentration (a marker for phytoestrogen dietary consumption) with risk for acute coronary events in men.[169] Over a period of 7.7 years, men in the highest enterolactone quartile had a 65% lower risk than did men in the lowest quartile for acute coronary events.

To conclude, the growing body of literature and data surrounding phytoestrogens has suggested that they may confer substantial health benefits. However an exercise in caution is required with the abundant evidence coming primarily from epidemiologic, preclinical, animal, and in vitro studies. Further studies are warranted to better understand the role of phytoestrogens as therapeutic agents and their hormonal actions on the cardiovascular system.

THYROID HORMONE

For many years, a relationship has been recognized between thyroid hormone, the heart, and the peripheral vascular system. In 1786, Parry first described the clinical features of thyrotoxicosis in a patient which included: palpitations, irregular pulse, and dyspnea.[170] Forty-nine years later, Graves provided descriptions of diffuse toxic goiter.[171] The profound cardiac manifestations of thyrotoxicosis led early observers to wrongly conclude that the disease originated within the heart. Eventually, researchers acknowledged that an overactive thyroid gland was the direct cause of the disease.[172] In 1918, Zondek first described a patient with the features of the "myxedema" heart: dilated cardiac silhouette, low electrocardiographic voltage, and slow heart action.[173] This patient's symptoms can be explained by a pericardial effusion, a common entity in hypothyroid patients. Despite the early associations between thyroid disease and the cardiovascular system, it is only recently that thyroid hormone has been considered a potential therapeutic agent in cardiovascular disease. To understand thyroid hormone's potential uses, this chapter first reviews its physiology in normal and disease states, and then examines therapeutic uses of thyroid hormone in cardiovascular disease.

Thyroid Physiology

Synthesis of thyroxine (T_4) and triiodothyronine (T_3) occurs within the thyroid gland. T_4, the primary secretory product, is relatively inactive. Eighty-five percent of T_3, the biologically active compound, is derived from peripheral conversion of T_4 by the 5'-monodeiodinase enzyme.[174] The actions of thyroid hormone occur mostly through T_3 binding with nuclear receptors that regulate expression of thyroid hormone responsive genes.[175] Because T_3 is bound to this receptor with a higher affinity than T_4, this analogue has a higher biologic activity.[174] There are two T_3 receptor genes, α and β, with at least two mRNA splice products for each gene: α_1 and α_2, and β_1 and β_2;[174] α_2 does not bind T_3.[174] T_3 also has some extranuclear actions that occur independent of nuclear T_3-receptor binding or of increases in protein synthesis.[174] Extranuclear effects result in rapid stimulation of amino acid, sugar, and calcium transport.[174]

Changes in cardiac function are mediated by T_3 regulation of cardiac-specific genes.[176] T_3 administration in animals enhances myocardial contractility by stimulating synthesis of the fast α myosin heavy chain and inhibiting the expression of the slow β isoform.[176,177] T_3 in animals also increases sarcoplasmic reticulum (SR) Ca^{2+} ATPase and decreased expression of the Ca^{2+} ATPase regulatory protein phospholamban.[178] T_3 also modulates the expression of heart sodium-potassium ATPase,[179] malic enzyme,[180] atrial natriuretic factor,[181] calcium channels,[182] and the β-adrenergic receptors.[183] Walker et al demonstrated that T_3 enhanced contractility by potentiating β-adrenergic receptor stimulation.[184] Intracellular cyclic AMP levels increased, leading to increased myocyte Ca^{2+} levels, and increased L-type Ca^{2+}-channel density.[184]

Human heart ventricles contain predominantly myosin heavy-chain β,[175] and therefore do not have a myosin shift after T_3 administration.[185] The enhanced contractility in humans is predominantly the result of an elevated expression of SR Ca^{2+} ATPase.[176] Despite the predominance of the β isoform in humans, some investigators have demonstrated an increase in α isoform after T_3 administration.[186] Overall, thyroid hormone increases ATP

TABLE 36-9. Effects of Thyroid Hormone on the Cardiovascular System

Direct	Indirect
Regulation of myocyte-specific genes	Enhanced adrenergic activity
Regulation of thyroid hormone receptor expression	Increased cardiac work
Enhanced cardiac contractility	Cardiac hypertrophy
Lower systemic vascular resistance	Expanded blood volume

Source: Reproduced from Klein I, Ojamaa K: Thyroid hormone and the cardiovascular system: From theory to practice (editorial). *J Clin Endocrin Metab* 78:1026–1027, 1994, with permission.

utilization, with more heat and less contractile energy production.[187] This inefficiency may explain heart failure after prolonged hyperthyroidism.

Contractile performance is also mediated by hemodynamic factors. Left ventricular (LV) function changes with alterations in afterload, preload, and heart rate.[188] A change in myosin heavy chain from β to α is observed in euthyroid rats under cardiac loading conditions.[189] Therefore, a combination of T3 regulation on both cardiac-specific genes and on hemodynamic variables may produce increased cardiac contractility.

Thyroid Hormone and the Cardiovascular System (Table 36-9)

Peripheral Hemodynamic Changes

One of the earliest responses to thyroid hormone administration is a decrease in peripheral vascular resistance.[190] Some investigators propose that thyroid hormone administration increases metabolic activity and oxygen consumption, thereby releasing local vasodilators.[191] These factors, in turn, produce the lowered systemic vascular resistance. A low systemic vascular resistance then decreases diastolic blood pressure, which, in turn, increases cardiac output (Fig. 36-4).[192] This increased cardiac output supports an increased basal metabolic rate[190] and increased oxygen consumption by enhancing the oxygen delivery to the periphery.[193] T_3 administration also increases total blood volume. This produces a rise in right atrial pressure, an increased preload, and thus an elevated cardiac output.[192]

The low peripheral vascular resistance may also be secondary to direct action of thyroid hormone on arteriolar smooth-muscle tone.[193a] T_3 may alter the sodium and potassium flux in smooth-muscle cells, leading to a decrease in smooth-muscle contractility and vascular tone.[194] After T_3 administration, normal animals demonstrate an increase in cardiac output and stroke volume with decreased peripheral vascular resistance.[195] Treatment of postischemic, reperfused animal hearts with T_3 enhanced LV performance in both normothermic[196] and hypothermic[197] models. However, T_3 had no effect on the intrinsic contractility of noninjured animal hearts.[196,197]

Hypothyroid patients hemodynamically manifest low cardiac output, decreased stroke volume, decreased intravascular volume, increased vascular resistance, increased circulation time, and a prolonged diastolic relaxation time.[191,198] Hyperthyroid patients exhibit the opposite hemodynamic picture.[191,198] In fact, T_3 administration to hypothyroid patients reduces the elevated peripheral vascular resistance.[191] The effects of T_3 on the coronary vasculature are presently undetermined, although a study in postischemic dogs found a decrease in coronary vascular resistance after T_3 administration.[196]

Interaction with the Sympathoadrenal System

Hyperthyroid patients have clinical symptomatology similar to that of patients in a hyperadrenergic state. Many investigators speculate that thyroid hormone interacts with catecholamines, such that hyperthyroid patients have an increased sensitivity to catecholamine action.[199] Thyroid hormone administration can increase β-adrenergic receptor expression, and, consequently, β-adrenergic sensitivity. Hormone administration also enhances expression of the stimulatory subunit of the guanosine triphosphate (GTP)-binding protein (Gs).[199] However, in humans, an enhanced sympathetic response with thyroid hormone has been difficult to prove. One study found no change in β-receptor sensitivity with hormone administration.[200] In experimental models, thyroid administration in both isolated myocytes[201] and whole-heart preparations[202] demonstrated effects independent of β-adrenergic receptor stimulation. For instance, it was recently found that thyroid hormone can directly affect the arrhythmogenic activity of pulmonary vein cardiomyocytes.[202a] In contrast, other investigators found increased LV shortening in hyperthyroid patients with β-adrenergic stimulation.[203]

Ventricular Function

Hyperthyroid patients have hypertrophic hearts. Experimental models of hyperthyroidism in animals have reproduced this finding. Within 1 week of T_4 administration, animal hearts exhibit a 135% increase in LV size versus controls.[204] Because thyroid hormone

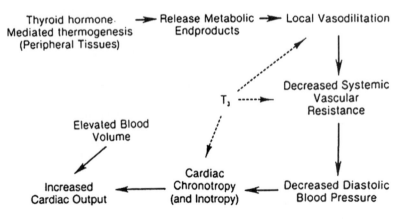

FIGURE 36-4. A model by which thyroid hormone-mediated changes in tissue oxygen consumption and thermogenesis can lead to alterations in cardiovascular hemodynamics. (*Reproduced with permissin from Klein I.*[192])

TABLE 36-10. Proposed Uses of Thyroid Hormone Replacement in Cardiovascular Disease

Congestive heart failure
Cardiopulmonary bypass surgery
Cardiac transplantation
Hyperlipidemia

increases cardiac protein synthesis,[205] this had been the postulated cause of cardiac hypertrophy in hyperthyroid patients. To test this hypothesis, Klein administered propranolol with T_4 to animals.[206] The addition of propranolol prevented both the increased heart rate and hypertrophic response. Klein and Hong demonstrated that cardiac hypertrophy was not observed in a heterotopically-transplanted rat heart without a hemodynamic load.[204] Thyroid hormone had no direct effect on amino acid incorporation, and therefore no measurable effect on myocardial contractile protein synthesis. They concluded that cardiac work mediated cardiac hypertrophy.

Therapeutic Applications (Table 36-10)

Euthyroid Sick Syndrome

The changes in thyroid function that occur in virtually all illnesses and after surgical procedures are referred to as the euthyroid sick syndrome. Patients have normal or decreased free and total T_4, decreased free and total T_3, and, usually, normal thyroid-stimulating hormone.[207] Four proposed mechanisms may explain the pathogenesis of this syndrome.[208] First, the decreased extrathyroidal conversion of T_4 to T_3 secondary to decreased delivery of T_4 to the intracellular deiodinases or a decrease in the deiodinase activity. Second, is a decrease in thyrotropin secretion leading to a fall in thyroidal secretion of T_4 and T_3. The process is potentiated by a fall in T_4 serum concentration, thus producing less substrate for T_3 conversion. Third, the production of thyroxine-binding globulin, transthyretin, and albumin, or their affinity for thyroid hormones may decline. Impaired deiodination results in a decline of total T_4 and T_3 levels and a rise in rT_3. Fourth, tissue uptake of T_4 and T_3 may be decreased, as well as nuclear and postreceptor hormone actions. The medical community assumes that the decrease in T_3 and T_4 with elevated rT_3 has no pathophysiologic consequences. Many believe that the syndrome is an adaptive metabolic response to conserve energy in disease states. However, recent experimental data with T_3 administration questions this assumption.

Congestive Heart Failure

Thyroid hormone metabolism is frequently abnormal in patients with congestive heart failure (CHF). Some CHF patients have been described with the euthyroid sick syndrome.[209] Hypothyroxinemia is a predictor of high mortality in severely ill ICU patients.[210] Given the poor prognosis associated with low thyroid hormone levels, various researchers wondered if supplementation with T_3 could improve clinical outcomes.[211] CHF patients have low cardiac outputs and high systemic vascular resistance. Thyroid hormone administration in depleted patients reverses these abnormalities. Thus, the question was asked, could thyroid hormone ameliorate CHF?

Animal studies preceded studies in humans. Rats with CHF given L-thyroxine demonstrated improved LV performance without alterations in heart rate.[212] Short-term administration with both low and high doses of L-thyroxine produced similar results. In addition, both doses did not alter the cardiac myosin isoenzyme distribution. Rabbits with postmyocardial infarction CHF who were treated

with 3,5-diiodothyropropionic acid (DITPA), a thyroid hormone analogue, demonstrated improved LV performance with reduced end-diastolic pressure.[213] Rabbits also had no significant change in heart rate or in myosin isoenzyme distribution. Mahaffey et al. believed that DITPA could reverse abnormal calcium handling, but that the most likely explanation for the improved performance was the upregulation of thyroid hormone responsive genes such as the SR Ca^{+2}ATPase.[213]

Hamilton et al studied 84 medical intensive care unit patients with advanced heart failure [average ejection fraction (EF) $18 \pm 5\%$].[209] Patients had low T_3 levels, or increased rT_3, with normal fT_4, and investigators determined that a low fT_3/rT_3 index was a negative prognostic factor. The index was associated with lower EFs, higher filling pressures, lower serum sodium, and poor nutritional status. The index was also the strongest predictor of mortality.[209] The authors postulated that the altered thyroid hormone metabolism predicted clinical outcome by indicating disease severity. The low conversion to T_3 may be an adaptive mechanism to decreased catabolism.[209]

Intravenous T_3 therapy may be an effective "bridge" therapy in patients with advanced stages of CHF in cardiogenic shock. T_3 therapy appears to be well tolerated by patients with a New York Heart Association (NYHA) class III or class IV CHF. Hamilton et al. studied 24 patients with class III or class IV CHF who were given 6 h of intravenous T_3 treatment.[214] Patients had no change in heart rate and basal metabolic rate, and no patients experienced angina or ventricular ectopy. Cardiac output increased by >1.0 L/ min in 50% of patients with no significant change in LVEF or filling pressures.[214] They concluded that the CHF patients tolerated the T_3 therapy well, and that the long-term hemodynamic effects produced require further study. Malik et al gave T_3 therapy to 10 patients with class IV CHF who were in cardiogenic shock unresponsive to conventional pharmacologic therapy and mechanical assistance with an intra-aortic balloon pump.[215] The patients had improved hemodynamics at 24 and 36 h, and 9 of 10 lived to receive either a left ventricular assist device and/or heart transplantation. The 6-month and 1-year cohort survival rates were 90% and 80%, respectively, a remarkable result. T_3 therapy in terminal cardiogenic shock appears to be an effective "bridge" to a definitive surgical intervention in endstage heart failure, and deserves further investigation.

L-Thyroxine also appears to be a useful therapy in idiopathic dilated cardiomyopathy (IDC). Exercise tolerance was studied in a randomized, placebo-controlled trial of 20 patients with IDC who were treated with 100 μg/d of L-thyroxine for 1 week.[216] Patients had class II or class III CHF with EF <40%. Patients given L-thyroxine had an improved cardiac output and a drop in systemic vascular resistance, independent of adrenergic influences. The improved exercise performance on the cardiopulmonary exercise stress test was explained by a higher oxygen consumption at peak exercise due to improved oxygen uptake by skeletal muscles, increased musculature perfusion, or improved muscle metabolism by local action of L-thyroxine.

Patients with hyperthyroidism can also develop IDC with both high-output and low-output cardiac failure. Reduction of excess hormone levels may reverse this failure. Umpierrez et al. studied seven patients with hyperthyroidism and low-output cardiac failure and treated them with propylthiouracil or methimazole.[217] Five of the seven patients had echocardiographic resolution of IDC and normalization of LV function. Thus, treatment of hyperthyroidism can reverse related cardiac disease. Although present interest is in treatment of CHF patients with euthyroid sick syndrome and cardiomyopathy, clinicians should not forget about the importance of treatment in the thyrotoxic patient with heart failure.

Investigations using noninvasive imaging continue to advance our knowledge of thyroid heart disease. Positron emission tomography and magnetic resonance imaging suggest a reduced efficiency of cardiac work in patients with hypothyroidism.[218] Hypothyroid patients had an increased LV mass, reduced cardiac oxygen consumption, and contractility with increased peripheral vascular resistance.[218] However, estimates of cardiac work were more severely suppressed than those of oxidative metabolism, which may explain why patients with hypothyroid disease develop CHF. Patients with clinical hyperthyroidism may demonstrate segmental wall abnormalities on echocardiography. Two patients treated with antithyroid medications, beta-blockers, and angiotensin-converting enzyme inhibitors had rapid recovery of function.[219] Myocardial stunning is important to recognize, as it may be reversible with treatment.

Cardiopulmonary Bypass Surgery

Thyroid hormone supplementation has been used to improve hemodynamics after cardiopulmonary bypass surgery (CPBS). Postoperative patients often have a low cardiac output and an elevated systemic vascular resistance, similar to that observed in hypothyroid patients. Additionally, approximately 50 to 75% of patients have a euthyroid sick state for 1 to 4 days postoperatively.[220] If T_3 is a potent vasodilator and inotrope, these patients could benefit from T_3 treatment. Some believe that surgically associated hypothermia, hemodilution, caloric deprivation, and activation of inflammatory mediators[221] decrease T_3 levels.[222] Pigs given 6 μg of T_3 during CPBS showed a beneficial inotropic effect and had improved overall survival.[223] Novitzky et al. performed two randomized, placebo-controlled trials of T_3 therapy in patients undergoing cardiac revascularization surgery.[224] Study 1 evaluated patients with EF <30% and study 2 evaluated patients with EF >40%. Patients with intra- and postoperative T_3 therapy in Study 1 required less adjunctive inotropic agents and diuretics. Study 2 patients with intra- and postoperative T_3 therapy had improved stroke volume and cardiac output, with reduced systemic and pulmonary vascular resistances. The authors concluded that T_3 administration appeared to be beneficial to all patients undergoing open heart surgery, but that patients with a better preoperative cardiovascular status derived greater benefit.

However, present research indicates that although T_3 does exert beneficial inotropic and hemodynamic effects in bypass patients, administration is not recommended. Teiger et al. studied 20 CBPS patients given intravenous T_3 or placebo in a prospective, double-blind, placebo-controlled trial.[225] The doses of T_3 (expressed in μg/kg of body weight) were 0.20, 0.15, 0.10, 0.05, and 0.05. Hormone was administered at the time of aortic cross clamp removal and 4, 8, 12, and 24 h thereafter. Total thyroid levels declined; however, after correction for hemodilution, they failed to demonstrate a decline in the active thyroid hormones. No significant difference was found in postoperative hemodynamics between the two groups. Also, T_3 therapy did not increase the degree of myocardial β-adrenergic responsiveness. Both Teiger and Novitsky's studies were small-scale, nonrandomized studies, and thus provoked further investigation.

A recently published study supports Teiger et al.'s results. Klemperer et al, in a large-scale prospective, placebo-controlled, double-blind trial of high-risk CPBS patients, administered large doses of T_3 (intravenous 0.8 μg/kg followed by 0.113 μg/kg/h for 6 h) at the time of cross-clamp removal and continuously

thereafter.[222] Thirty minutes after the start of CPBS, before T_3 administration, mean serum T_3 levels decreased by approximately 40%. After T_3 infusion, T_3 levels increased twofold in treated patients, with a consequent increase in cardiac output and decline in systemic vascular resistance. Despite supranormal levels of T_3 at surgery, levels normalized by the first postoperative day. The study demonstrated improved cardiovascular performance in the early postoperative period but found no change in inotropic requirements. Klemperer et al concluded that T_3 should not be used as a substitute for recommended drug therapy during and after CPBS. Utiger, in an accompanying editorial, agreed with the authors' recommendation, stating that physicians must realize that patients may have many abnormalities that can affect T_3 and or T_4 levels.[208] However, because replacement doses of hormone in seriously ill patients with low serum thyroxine levels does not hasten recovery or improve survival, replacement is not practical. Low levels of thyroid hormones are probably part of a host's defense mechanism.[208]

Use of T_3, despite minor improvements in myocardial performance, was not recommended for routine use in CPBS patients. Neither study measured thyroid-stimulating hormone, which may have proven important.[226] Therefore, replacement therapy with large doses of T_3 in CPBS patients is currently not advised. But it is conceivable that dopamine plus T_3 may have beneficial effects together or that patients with less severe risk may respond more favorably to therapy.

Cardiac Transplantation

The administration of T_3 to brain-dead organ donors has proved successful in maintaining organ viability (low free and total T_3 occurs after brain death in experimental animals[227] and humans[228]). Hemodynamic stability, reduced inotropic agent requirement, and metabolic derangement normalization have been documented in potential organ donors after T_3 therapy.[229] Jeevanandam studied three groups of donors after T_3 intravenous therapy.[229] Groups 1 and 2 were studied in randomized, placebo-controlled trials and group 3 was studied in a matched case control trial. Group 1 donors had a reduced EF, high filling pressures, and needed inotropic support, and group 2 had normal left ventricular function. Group 3 was matched for hemodynamics, age, donor/recipient weight ratio, ischemic time, and thyroid hormone levels. T_3 effectively resuscitated hearts with diminished function and improved recipient myocardial aerobic metabolism. These beneficial clinical results in organ harvesting for cardiac transplant have produced a relative increase in available donors.

Hyperlipidemia

The hormone thyroxine has been used as a hypercholesterolemic agent in euthyroid patients. The stereoisomer dextrothyroxine (D-thyroxine) initially was chosen for clinical use because it was said to have more selective effects on metabolism than levoxythyroxine. D-Thyroxine lowers the concentration of LDL-cholesterol by 10 to 20%, but has little effect on plasma triglycerides or on the concentration of HDL cholesterol.[230] However, in usual therapeutic doses of 4 to 6 mg/dL, D-thyroxine can cause cardiac arrhythmias and hypermetabolic effects in euthyroid patients.[231] In the Coronary Drug Project, D-thyroxine, when compared to placebo, caused a higher incidence of adverse cardiovascular effects;[232] consequently, D-thyroxine treatment was discontinued in the study.

Cardiovascular events may be related to levels of serum free and total T_3 levels. In a recent German study, all patients presenting to the emergency room underwent thyroid function tests.[233] The investigators found a significant correlation (odds ratio, 2.6; CI 95% 1.3 to 5.2) between angina pectoris and myocardial infarction with elevated free and total T_3 levels. These patients also had a threefold higher risk of developing a subsequent coronary event over the next 3 years. More studies need to be completed, but it is still recommended that patients with overt or subclinical hypothyroidism be treated aggressively to lessen their cardiovascular risk.

It can be concluded from the above that thyroxine replacement can favorably alter the lipid and lipoprotein levels of overt and borderline hypothyroid patients. Therefore, screening for these conditions is mandatory when assessing patients with a lipid abnormality. However, the routine use of thyroxine treatment to lower LDL-cholesterol and to raise HDL-cholesterol cannot be recommended in euthyroid patients. The potential for cardiac toxicity, outweighs the beneficial effect. Thyroxine analogues that do not adversely affect the heart are being developed to reduce plasma lipids and to treat CHF without causing cardiotoxicity (see Chap. 46).

Conclusion

Thyroid hormone may have use as a cardiovascular disease therapy. Replacement therapy in patients with cardiovascular disease having both a euthyroid sick state and hemodynamic abnormalities seems promising. However, it is unknown whether the euthyroid sick state is a beneficial adaptation in these patients. Further investigation is needed before routine replacement therapy can be recommended for treatment of CHF, in patients having open-heart surgery, or for cardiac transplant donors to sustain or augment cardiac function. As elevated levels of T_3 appears to correlate with cardiovascular events, aggressive treatment to reduce elevated levels in patients with angina or myocardial infarction is recommended.

RECOMBINANT GROWTH HORMONE

In recent years, there has been a great deal of interest in growth hormone (GH) as an etiologic factor in many cardiovascular disease states, and as a possible therapeutic agent for these conditions.

Physiology

Hypophyseal-Pituitary Axis

GH secretion is regulated by two hypothalamic peptides: GH-releasing factor (GHRF) and somatostatin. Hypothalamic control of GH has been demonstrated in rats[234] and in human beings.[235] Guillemin et al first isolated GHRF, a 44-amino-acid peptide, from a pancreatic tumor that caused acromegaly in a patient.[236] Bohlen et al. later identified this factor in the hypothalamus.[237] In 1975, Brazeau et al. first detected somatostatin, a polypeptide inhibitor of GH, in the ovine hypothalamus.[238] Somatostatin and GHRF neurons reciprocally control each other through direct synaptic connections at the hypothalamus[239] (Fig. 36-5). GHRF and somatostatin travel from the median eminence of the hypothalamus to the anterior pituitary through the portal circulation.[239] These factors reciprocally regulate GH synthesis and secretion by somatotroph cells in the anterior pituitary. A decrease in somatostatinergic tone results in an increase in GHRF and therefore an elevated secretion of GH.[240,240a] Somatostatin inhibits all physiologic and pharmacologic responses to GH secretion.[240a] GH can inhibit its own secretion via three feedback loops: indirectly by inducing the somatotroph to produce

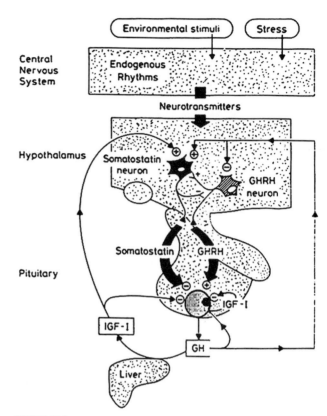

FIGURE 36-5. Representation of GH neuroregulation in man. The central nervous system will exert its regulation over the hypothalamus via specific neurotransmitter pathways. Somatostatin and growth hormone-releasing hormone (GHRH) hypothalamic neurons control each other by direct synaptic connections. The released GHRH and somatostatin will arrive from the hypothalamic median eminence to the somatotrophic cell via portal vessels, stimulating or inhibiting, respectively, GH secretion. GH will inhibit its own secretion by three mechanisms: (a) acting upon the somatotroph cell generating insulin-like growth factor (IGF)-1 locally, which, in turn, inhibits that cell; (b) inhibiting GHRH mRNA synthesis and GHRH release at hypothalamic level; and (c) stimulating both mRNA levels and release of somatostatin. In the long loop, GH will impinge on the liver, generating most of the circulating IGF-l that will inhibit GH secretion by a dual mechanism: (a) direct inhibition of the somatotroph cells and (b) stimulation of somatostatin release. (*Reproduced with permission from Casanueva FF.*[239])

insulin-like growth factor (IGF)-1, by inhibition of GHRF mRNA synthesis and secretion, and by stimulating somatostatin mRNA synthesis and secretion (Fig. 36-6).

Growth Hormone Receptors, Releasing Peptides, and Binding Proteins

The GH receptor (GHR) is a single-chain transmembrane protein consisting of three domains: extracellular, transmembrane, and cytoplasmic.[241] GHRs are most abundant in the liver, but are found in most tissues, including the heart.[242] Purification and sequencing of a serum peptide have identified the GH-binding protein (GHBP).[243] It appears to be a proteolytic cleavage product of the membrane-bound GHR.[243] GHBP resembles the extracellular domain of the GHR and has similar affinity for GH.[243] Thus, GHBPs may serve as intermediary proteins that enhance GH secretion by sequestering GH and thereby slowing the feedback loop. GH-releasing peptides (GHRP) act at the hypothalamus on nonopiate receptors and at the pituitary via non-GHRF receptors.[244] GHRPs act synergistically with GHRF. Clinical disease alters GH secretion by causing destruction of GHRs.

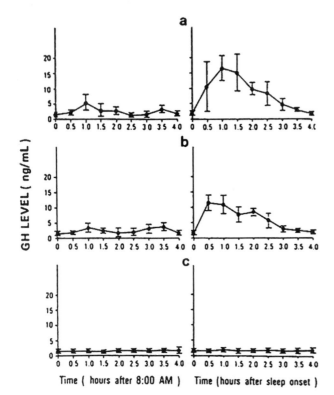

FIGURE 36-6. (*A*) Average serum GH concentration curves for 6 subjects aged 20 to 29 years in both the waking (*left*) and sleeping (*right*) states. (*B*) Average serum GH concentration curves for 6 subjects aged 60 to 79 years with SmC ≤0.64 U/mL in both the waking (diurnal) and sleeping (nocturnal) states. (*C*) Average serum GH concentration curves for 6 subjects aged 60 to 79 years with SmC >0.64 U/mL in both the waking (diurnal) and sleeping (nocturnal) states. Bars represent ± SD. (*Reproduced with permission from Rudman D, et al.*[254])

GHRs are decreased in chronic renal failure, chemically induced diabetes, malnutrition, and fasting. The status of a patient's functional GHRs may be indirectly determined by the concentration of GHBP in serum. The determination of GH responsiveness via GHBP could be useful for determining GH dosing regimens because GH administration in rats results in parallel changes in GHR and GHBP levels.[245] Interestingly, continuous administration yields a greater increase in GHBP than intermittent administration.[245] Measurement of GHBP and GHR in humans may have important implications for the future management of GH treatment.

Secretion

GH is secreted in a pulsatile fashion.[246] Eight pulses are secreted daily. The lowest circulating level of GH is observed in the early morning.[247] Secretion is enhanced by α_2-agonists and inhibited by α_1- and β-agonists.[248] Glucocorticoids also enhance secretion.[248] GH secretion is regulated by daily living activities. A secretory pulse typically occurs within 90 to 120 min of the onset of sleep.[241,240a] Rapid eye movement (REM) sleep suppresses secretion,[249] while slow-wave sleep is associated with the most secretion.[249,240a] GH also increases with daily stress.[240a]

Exercise and GH secretion is a new area of clinical research. In a study of normal males, investigators found that a minimum of 10 min of high-intensity exercise produced peak GH levels, while low-intensity activity produced only minor changes in GH levels.[250] The study found significant subject-to-subject variability in peak

GH levels, and exercise intensity alone could not predict the amplitude and duration of the GH response. Raynaud et al. also concluded that the GH response to exercise showed significant variability among patients. Surprisingly, investigators have observed a larger release of GH with intermittent versus continuous exercise.[251] GH does not improve muscle function, strength, or athletic performance when combined with exercise.[252] However, trained individuals do show an elevated GH response with exercise when compared to untrained subjects.[247] The physiologic significance of this remains undetermined.

GH secretion declines with aging. Aging decreases the number of secretory bursts, the amplitude of bursts, the response to GHRF (secondary to increased somatostatinergic tone), and the response of anterior pituitary cells to secretogogues.[249] Finkelstein et al. demonstrated a decline in spontaneous secretion of GH with age.[253] However, eating and activity levels were confounding variables. After the age of 50 years, patients show a decrease in the number and magnitude of nocturnal peaks, a decrease in GH secretion after exercise, and a decrease in GH secretion in response to direct and indirect stimuli.[253] Studies have also found a negative correlation between subject age and total GH secretion and pulsatile secretion.[254,255] The normal daily serum GH level is >10 ng/mL. Normal values vary among individuals but are defined as a level that produces a physiologic response. Rudman et al. studied 94 male patients of varying ages and concluded that 55% of patients over age 69 had little day or night release of GH (<4 ng/mL).[254] This level produces no physiologic response. They also found a decrease in endogenous GH and plasma somatomedin C (IGF-1) from the third to ninth decades of life (Fig. 36-6). They attributed 67% of somatomedin variability to age and obesity. Rudman's 1985 cross-sectional study of elderly males between the ages of 55 and 85 years in different environmental living situations illustrated the effects of confounding factors such as decreased activity and deconditioning on GH levels.[255] Institutionalized patients were more likely to have GH levels <5 ng/mL (33%) than either free-living patients with chronic disease (20%) or healthy free-living patients (5%).[255] Regardless of the living situation, elderly patients with relative GH deficiency may benefit from GH supplementation. Alarmingly, many elderly citizens appear to be GH deficient.

Role of Insulin-Like Growth Factors

GH exerts its effects either directly or indirectly via IGFs. The presence of this intermediary was first described by Salmon and Daughaday in 1957.[256] They observed sulfate uptake in cartilage by hypophysectomized rats pretreated with bovine GH and no sulfate uptake by cells treated with bovine GH in vitro.[256] They concluded that these actions were mediated by a "sulfation factor." Marquart et al. later redefined this factor as "multiplication stimulating activity."[257] In 1972, Daughaday et al. introduced the term *somatomedin*.[258] However, the terminology quickly changed from somatomedins SM-C and MSA to IGF-1 and IGF-2.[259] Somatomedin was defined as a substance under GH regulation, with insulin-like activity, and with the ability to stimulate growth in one or more tissues.[260] Studies on the molecular biology of IGFs led to the localization of the IGF-1 genes on chromosome 11 and the IGF-2 genes on chromosome 12.[261]

IGF-Receptors, Binding Proteins, and Secretion

IGF-1 and IGF-2 are homologous to proinsulin[262] and have 65% homology to each other.[263] IGFs are synthesized by many tissues and are hypothesized to act in an autocrine and paracrine fashion.[239,262] The IGF-1 receptor is structurally related to the insulin receptor, each having two α and two β subunits.[262] The IGF-2 receptor is homologous to the mannose-6-phosphate receptor, being composed of a single polypeptide chain.[262] Three distinct binding proteins (IGFBP-1 to -3) have been cloned and sequenced. IGF secretion is largely dependent on GH secretion; however, IGF has a longer serum half-life.[241]

Similar to GH, IGF declines with age. Women between the ages of 25 and 34 years have been found to have higher IGF levels than men of the same age. However, between the ages of 55 and 64 years, women have lower levels.[263] In contrast to this study, others have found no gender-dependent difference in IGF levels between the third and seventh decades.[264] Some investigators believe that the age-related decline of IGF may be secondary to the aging process itself and/or a decline in exercise activity with aging.[265] In a recent Swedish study, IGF levels were assessed in both men and women in relation to age, gender, smoking history, coffee consumption, physical activity levels, blood pressure, plasma lipids, fibrinogen, parathyroid-like hormone, and osteoclastin levels.[263] IGF correlated inversely with age, body mass index, systolic blood pressure, and total cholesterol in both sexes. In men, IGF levels positively correlated with fibrinogen and negatively correlated with smoking; in women, IGF levels negatively correlated with coffee consumption. The analysis from this Swedish study of variables that affect IGF levels will allow researchers to improve diagnostic reliability using IGF in the future. Considering the effects of these variables can diminish false positives and negatives. IGF levels can be used with GH levels to examine for deficiency and excess conditions.

Growth Hormone Effects on Organ Systems and Metabolism (Table 36-11)

Normal GH secretion alters the body's homeostasis. GH activates the renin-angiotensin system and has direct actions on the kidneys.[266] Acutely, GH causes the kidneys to conserve water and sodium, but with chronic GH stimulation the body responds with renin-angiotensin axis activation, normalizing fluid homeostasis.[266] Studies on acromegalic patients have demonstrated increased sodium and water retention leading to systemic hypertension, independent of the angiotensin system. Therefore, the expansion of plasma volume may be a direct effect of long-standing GH hypersecretion.[266] GH administration decreases atrial natriuretic peptide, while increasing aldosterone and insulin levels.[267] Some investigators suggest that the expansion of extracellular volume with GH may be secondary to elevated insulin levels.[267] The effects of GH on carbohydrates are both dosage and duration dependent. Acutely, GH causes glucose oxidation to decline secondary to an increase in lipid oxidation, while muscular glucose uptake is suppressed.[268] GH therefore elevates serum glucose levels.

GH administration has beneficial effects on serum lipids. Following GH administration, lipoprotein lipase activity declines resulting in an elevated plasma level of nonesterified fatty acids.[269]

TABLE 36-11. Effects of Growth Hormone on Metabolic Parameters

Increase blood sugar secondary to insulin resistance
Decrease cholesterol and LDL-cholesterol
Decrease adiposity
Increase lean body mass

Three hours after GH administration, there is an elevation of serum glucose and insulin and increased hydrolysis of triglycerides releasing free-fatty acids and glycerol.[239] Small amounts of GH decrease cholesterol to a level comparable to that seen with simvastatin treatment of 3 weeks duration.[270] GH treatment in normal adults prior to elective surgery has been shown to increase the number of LDL receptors, increase VLDL levels, and decrease LDL levels.[270] Body fat deposits decline, and individuals have elevations in lean body mass.[254,264] GH induces positive nitrogen, phosphorus, magnesium, calcium, sodium, and chloride balance.[271] Amino acid uptake is stimulated leading to enhanced protein synthesis.[271]

Effects of GH on the Heart in Human Studies

Theusen et al. studied 11 healthy males to evaluate the effects of rGH on the heart.[272] Two subcutaneous doses of GH were administered: 3.2 IU in the A.M. and 6.4 IU in the P.M., for a total of 7 days. The investigators assessed echocardiographic and hemodynamic measurements before, during, and 1 week after GH treatment. Cardiac output, contractility, heart rate, and fractional shortening were shown to increase, while end-systolic diameter declined. No changes in diastolic parameters were noted after this short course of therapy. The effect of long-term GH treatment in a normal population needs further investigation.

Effects of IGF on the Heart in Animal Studies

IGF produces hypertrophy of myocardial cells in vitro[273] and appears to inhibit cardiac apoptosis.[274] This is not surprising because IGF-1 has a direct hypertrophic effect on cultured cardiomyocytes and can cause increased gene transcription of myosin light-chain 2 (MLC-2) and troponin I.[275] IGF-1 may act with IGFBP-3 to regulate cardiac hypertrophy.[275] Vetter et al. studied the effects of IGF and insulin on rat neonatal myocytes[276] and found that supranormal levels of insulin elevate myocardial contractility. They proposed that IGF acts to stimulate calcium release from the terminal or subsarcolemmal cisternae. The amount of calcium available for contraction is increased, causing an enhanced myocardial contractile response.[276] Lastly, loading conditions such as systemic hypertension, lead to elevated expression of cardiac IGF-1 mRNA, independent of the renin-angiotensin system.[277] Increases in right ventricular volume cause increases in both GHR mRNA and IGF-1 mRNA.[278] IGF-1 may be important in the initiation of GH-induced cardiac hypertrophy. Further studies need to be done to determine whether this same relationship exists in humans.

Pathophysiology

Excess Growth Hormone

Acromegalic patients often develop cardiovascular disease.[279] Intraventricular conduction defects, hypertension, congestive heart failure, atherosclerosis, diabetes, and coronary artery disease frequently occur in acromegalic patients and contribute to patient mortality.[280,281] Only 30% of acromegalic patients are found to be free of concomitant disease.[280] The heart reacts to excess GH by concentric hypertrophy. At first, the peripheral vasculature dilates with GH to diminish resistance, but as the disease progresses, the heart hypertrophies.[280] Hypertension in acromegalics applies more stress on the heart. In normotensive acromegalics, ventricular hypertrophy correlates with disease duration.[282] Acromegalic patients also have alterations in both left and right ventricular diastolic function.[283] This diastolic dysfunction usually progresses to clinical heart failure.

Animal Studies The contractile properties of the heart significantly change with excess GH secretion. Molecular studies in rats with GH-secreting tumors demonstrate a change in protein expression of myosin genes.[284] Hearts that have been exposed to GH treatment have an increased concentration of V3 isomyosin relative to V1 isomyosin.[284] The V1 isotype is more common and has a higher ATPase activity relative to V3. Researchers have observed a normal or supranormal contraction with increased force and normal shortening speed in V3-enriched hearts.[284] On the molecular level, the number of crossbridges between actin and myosin increase, the contractile proteins increase their sensitivity to calcium, and more calcium becomes available for myofilament contraction.[284] These compensatory changes in the heart produce a more economical and efficient contractile state. Mayoux et al. verified these findings in his study of chronic GH secretion on isolated rat cardiac muscle fibers.[285] V1 to V3 conversion correlated with an increase in the number of crossbridges, an increased attachment time, and, simultaneously, an increase in active tension and force. Other investigators corroborated these findings by demonstrating a longer action potential duration with elevated calcium influx after GH treatment.[286] Intrinsic changes in the molecular properties of the heart may help it to preserve its function in excess GH states.

Reversal with Octreotide Octreotide, a somatostatin analogue, has been used to demonstrate the reversibility of body changes related to chronic GH secretion. The peptide inhibits GH release and abolishes residual GH pulsatile secretion.[287] In an echocardiographic study of acromegalic patients with and without left ventricular hypertrophy, octreotide decreased left ventricular mass in patients with hypertrophy within 1 week,[288] but it had no effect on ventricular mass in patients without hypertrophy. Left ventricular mass continued to decline at 2 months, but never reached normal levels.[288] In patients with hypertrophy, blood pressure, left ventricular dimension, and fractional shortening did not change with octreotide treatment.[288] The authors concluded that some components of cardiac response to GH hypersecretion are reversible and advocated aggressive treatment in early acromegalic disease to prevent irreversible cardiac changes. Merola et al. studied octreotide treatment in normotensive acromegalic patients and observed similar hemodynamic changes with improved left and right ventricular filling and decreased isovolumic relaxation time.[289] Octreotide appears to be an effective treatment for early and intermediate myocardial changes seen in acromegalic hearts.

It is not known if chronic treatment is necessary to improve myocardial function. Medical therapy with octreotide, surgical therapy, or surgical treatment with continued octreotide therapy are the treatment options available. In a recent open matched (healthy patients) prospective trial, acromegalics treated for 5 years with either surgery or surgery and octreotide had improved left ventricular function in response to exercise compared to controls.[290] Sixty percent of the acromegalics not controlled with either therapy showed no improvement myocardial performance.[290] Long-term suppression, with either therapy appears to be necessary to reverse cardiac abnormalities.

DEFICIENCY OF GROWTH HORMONE

For many years it has been recognized that hypophysectomized patients and pituitary dwarfs can have an increased risk for cardiovascular disorders. In a retrospective study of 333 patients in Sweden between the years 1956 and 1987, GH-deficient patients had both an increased mortality rate and an increased incidence of cardiovascular problems.[291] Patients demonstrated levels of elevated serum triglyceride and total cholesterol and lower HDL cholesterol levels as compared with controls,[292] a profile increasing the risk for development of cardiovascular disease. The hearts of GH-deficient patients responded to inadequate hormone activity with decreased myocardial work and contractility.[293] The degree of this cardiac impairment correlates directly with the severity and duration of the GH deficiency.[294] A complete understanding of the GH deficiency state is necessary in order to safely treat patients with HRT.

Heart and Exercise GH treatment for GH-deficient patients can cause favorable effects on both the heart and peripheral vasculature. Most studies have used a low-dose daily regimen to prevent the consequences of GH excess described earlier. In a 6-month double-blind, crossover study evaluating both pulmonary and cardiovascular function after GH replacement with 0.5 U/kg/wk (.07 daily), treated patients had improved cardiovascular parameters. Patients demonstrated an increase in cardiac output, stroke volume, and left ventricular mass.[295] No impairment in left ventricular relaxation, blood pressure, ventricular wall thickness, or pulmonary hemodynamic states were observed.[295] GH also had favorable effects on the vasculature, producing a decrease in peripheral vascular resistance. With an increase in peripheral blood flow and improved cardiac function, patients experienced an improvement in their exercise capacity.[295] GH replacement therapy for 6 months with 10 μg/kg/d, 3 days per week, was shown to increase myocardial contractility, to decrease peripheral vascular resistance, and to increase left ventricular end-diastolic pressure.[293] Patients reported an increase in exercise tolerance, a decrease in weakness and fatigue, and an improved quality of life.[293]

GH-deficient patients often suffer from muscle weakness, and consequently they may need to limit their activities. Some investigators suggest that the cardiac manifestations of GH deficiency can, in part, be accounted for by the increased muscle weakness in patients.[296] Therefore, GH replacement could help cardiovascular function by increasing muscle strength and exercise capacity. In a 1991 double-blind, placebo-controlled study by Cuneo et al. of 24 patients receiving .07 μg/kg/d of GH for 6 months or placebo, exercise tolerance, oxygen consumption, and musculature changes were evaluated.[297] GH resulted in an increase in hip flexor and limb girdle muscle strength, an increase in lean tissue and skeletal muscle mass, and an increase in the cross-sectional area of the thigh and quadriceps muscles.[297] Oxygen consumption and power improved, with no change in heart rate.[298] Cardiac output rose in direct correlation with left ventricular and skeletal muscle mass.[298] However, the study findings disagree as to the functional consequences of replacement therapy. In a double-blind, placebo-controlled study of 36 patients using .02 to .05 IU daily of GH for 6 months, exercise tolerance increased with GH but no change was observed in isometric strength in any muscle group, in left ventricular mass, in blood pressure, in cardiac output, or in stroke volume.[299] Whitehead et al. corroborated the findings of Cuneo et al. by showing that GH increased lean tissue, oxygen consumption, thigh muscle volume, and exercise capacity, with no measurable increase in quadriceps strength.[300] GH replacement in GH-deficient patients has favorable effects on the cardiovascular system, illustrating the importance of GH in normal cardiac performance.

GH replacement improves diastolic function after improving exercise tolerance. Initially after treating hypopituitary patients with 6 months of .04±.01 IU/kg/d of GH replacement, researchers observed some improved muscle strength, but no change in diastolic function.[301] However, after 1 year, the impaired diastolic function improved. Untreated diastolic dysfunction can progress to systolic dysfunction, and eventually to congestive heart failure. Low-dose GH replacement can improve diastolic function, thereby halting this progression.

The long-term effects of GH replacement therapy are presently unknown.[302] Replacement at physiologic doses has shown no adverse effects on cardiac muscle in the short-term.[302] However, no set physiologic dose has been determined because individual and age-dependent factors affect dosage. Although, at present, no individuals receiving GH replacement become acromegalic, the cardiac complications of this state must be prevented. Careful monitoring of both GH and IGF levels, and an awareness of the clinical signs of acromegalic heart disease, should prevent undesired effects with GH replacement.

GH appears to regulate the quantity and responsiveness of β receptors.[303] GH increases contractility and can decrease the reliance on sympathetic control to increase blood pressure. Therefore, GH appears to be required for the development of normal contractile capabilities of cardiac and vascular tissues and has a regulatory effect on both β and α-adrenoceptor-mediated responses. Human studies have not yet assessed these phenomena.

Vascular Disease   GH-deficient patients have elevated levels of both fibrinogen and plasminogen activator inhibitor (PAI) (Table 36-12), and demonstrate abnormal vascular reactivity.[304] Patients also have higher waist-to-hip ratios and serum triglycerides.[305] These factors correlate with an increased risk of atheromatous disease. Ultrasonography of the vasculature often demonstrates premature atherosclerosis in GH-deficient patients.[306] Patients have an increase in cholesterol, LDL, and triglycerides. Treatment of GH-deficient patients can reduce levels of fibrinogen, PAI, cholesterol, LDL, and triglycerides,[306] and raise HDL.[307]

Cardiomyopathy   GH deficiency may also play a role in the pathogenesis of cardiomyopathy.[308] Patients with long-term IGF-1 deficiency have reduced cardiac dimensions and output, but normal LVEF at rest and LV contractile reserve following stress.[309]

Renin-Angiotensin   Replacement therapy in GH-deficient patients produces sodium and water retention.[310] Renin levels elevate with no change in aldosterone after a GH replacement dose of

.07 μg/kg/d.[310] With a dose of .5 μg/kg/d, extracellular volume increases, but by decreasing the dose to .25 μg/kg/d, fluid balance reverts to normal levels.[311] Sodium retention usually is seen early, and declines with continued treatment.[310,311] A sodium transport inhibitor is thought to be triggered by volume expansion, thus decreasing total body water.[311] This effect is a normal homeostatic adjustment to an increase in serum GH.

Replacement Doses

Most studies have used what is considered to be low-dose therapy; however, one appropriate dose for the population has not been determined. Low-dose GH therapy decreases energy expenditure and lipid oxidation, while increasing nitrogen excretion and insulin sensitivity in both deficient and normal patients.[312] IGF levels measured after 2 weeks of GH regimens of either 2, 4, or 6 IU/kg/d suggested that optimal IGF levels are achieved after 4 IU/kg/d.[313] The 2 IU/kg/d treatment produced IGF levels that were too low, while the 4 IU/kg/d treatment produced constant physiologic IGF levels.[313] The increment to 6 IU/kg/d only demonstrated a marginal elevation in IGF levels versus the 4 IU/kg/d treatment. Moller et al studied GH doses of 1, 2, and 4 IU/kg/d during three consecutive 4-week periods. Normal levels were achieved with both 1 and 2 IU regimens.[314] Blood glucose levels were not affected by these doses. However, the 4 IU/kg/d dose produced supranormal levels of IGF and patients experienced fluid retention.[314] Low-dose therapy can reverse the adverse consequences of GH deficiency. However, because patients respond to all drugs differently, regardless of dose used, downward titration may be required. Presently, GH sensitivity cannot be determined. Repeated measurements of IGF-1 and IGFBP-3 levels may help to determine adequate dosing in the future.[302]

Adverse Effects

Fluid and sodium retention are the most frequent adverse effects seen in deficient patients receiving GH supplementation (Table 36-13).[302] Patients may experience arthralgias, carpal tunnel syndrome, and muscle stiffness.[302] Non-insulin-dependent diabetes is associated with GH use in children.[315] Rarely, hypertension, atrial fibrillation, headache, and tinnitus may occur.[302] GH elevation has been implicated as a risk factor for colon cancer,[315a] malignant melanoma, but no melanoma cases have yet been reported in patients receive GH supplementation.[316] Leukemia is also thought to be associated with GH treatment; however, GH-treated patients have

---

TABLE 36-12. Metabolic Data, Fibrinogen, Plasminogen Activator Inhibitor-1 Activity, Blood Pressure, and Waist-to-Hip Circumference Ratio in Adult Patients with Growth Hormone Deficiency and Healthy Control Subjects

Variable	Patients (n = 20)	Control Subjects (n = 20)	*p*
Fasting blood glucose, mmol/L	4.0±0.5	4.4±0.7	.042
Fasting plasma insulin, mU/L	7±2	8±2	.839
Cholesterol, mmol/L	6.3±1.2	5.8±1.2	.266
Triglycerides, mmol/L	1.5±0.5	1.1±0.5	.019
Fibrinogen, g/L	3.2±0.7	2.4±0.6	.0001
PAI-1 activity, U/mL	13.2±10.6	6.8±4.3	.013
Systolic blood pressure, mm Hg	136±22	130±13	.319
Diastolic blood pressure, mm Hg	79±7	81±7	.360
Waist/hip circumference ratio	0.97±0.03	0.87±0.09	.0001

PAI-1 = plasminogen activator inhibitor-1. Values are mean ± standard deviation.

Source: Reproduced with permission from Johansson et al.[305]

TABLE 36-13. Types of Side Effects Observed during Growth Hormone Replacement Therapy in 105 Adult Growth Hormone-Deficient Patients

Side Effects	# of Patients
Fluid retention	22
Carpal tunnel syndrome	13
Arthralgia	9
Muscle stiffness	3
Miscellaneous	
Hypertension	1
Atrial fibrillation	1
Encephalocele	1
Headache	1
Tinnitus	1

Source: Reproduced with permission from De Boer et al.[302]

been observed to have an incidence of leukemia lower than the general population.[316]

Therapeutic Implications for Cardiac Disease and Prevention

GH has been suggested as a treatment for various cardiovascular conditions (Table 36-14). It is currently approved by the FDA for treatment of cachexia in patients with AIDS. The use of GH has been studied in small numbers of patients with congestive cardiomyopathy and renal failure.[317,318]

Congestive Heart Failure

GH has many physiologic and biochemical properties that could be useful in the treatment of chronic CHF.[319,320] The typical patient with advanced heart failure would have a dysfunctional left ventricle, decreased cardiac output, increased peripheral vascular resistance, and an abnormal vasoconstrictor response to acetylcholine. Patients are weak and fatigued, having poor exercise tolerance and skeletal muscle function. GH replacement in both normal[272] and deficient patients[321,322] has been shown to augment myocardial contractility, cardiac output, and stroke volume, to correct endothelial dysfunction, and to reduce peripheral vascular resistance (Table 36-15). GH can also increase lean body mass and muscle strength, and improve psychological well being. Many patients with CHF are thought to be GH deficient and could respond favorably to GH replacement therapy.

The hearts of CHF patients exhibit decreased myocardial force and contractility. The cycling rate of individual myocardial crossbridges and the number of crossbridges decline.[323] GH replacement in rats increases the force of contraction by increasing the number of crossbridges and the amount of available calcium.[284] GH increases oxygen-carrying capacity by improving peripheral blood flow. Replacement can improve skeletal muscle metabolic efficiency and therefore exercise tolerance.[324] CHF patients have a 10% lower lean body mass than do their healthy counterparts.[325] Some investigators believe that physical deconditioning in CHF is caused by an intrinsic muscle abnormality and not by diminished blood flow.[325]

TABLE 36-14. Proposed Uses of Growth Hormone Replacement in Cardiovascular Disease

Congestive heart failure
Prevention of ventricular aneurysms
Prevention of coronary artery disease in the high-risk geriatric population

TABLE 36-15. Hemodynamic Effects in Congestive Heart Failure after Growth Hormone Treatment

↑ Cardiac output, cardiac index, ejection fraction, stroke volume
↓ Peripheral vascular resistance, left ventricular end-diastolic pressure
↔ Mean arterial pressure, heart rate

↑ = increase; ↓ = decrease; ↔ = no change.

GH treatment can address both concerns by increasing percent lean body mass and peripheral blood flow.

Acquired GH resistance has been implicated as a possible mechanism for symptoms in patients with CHF.[326] Low levels of IGF-1 with high GH levels suggest resistance.[327] Investigators tested the role of IGF-1 on cardiac myocytes. Adult cardiac myocytes from normal and CHF conditions were tested to determine whether IGF-1 had direct inotropic effects.[328] IGF-1 improved contractility in both failing and nonfailing myocytes by increasing the availability of Ca^{2+} to the myofilaments.[328] This may explain GH's beneficial effects in CHF. CHF patients with low IGF-1 levels have lower lean body mass and altered cytokine (TNFα) and neuroendocrine activation, demonstrating the importance of both components.[329] The possible benefit to both the cardiovascular system and the whole-body composition warrants a clinical study of GH and or IGF-1 as treatments for CHF.[330]

A few small-scale studies investigated GH as a treatment in patients with dilated cardiomyopathy (DCM). The first study, an open trial, evaluated seven patients with DCM and moderate-to-severe CHF studied at baseline, after 3 months of therapy with human GH, and 3 months after the discontinuation of GH.[331] Standard therapy for heart failure was continued throughout the study. When administered at a dose of 14 IU per week, GH doubled the serum concentrations of IGF. GH increased myocardial mass, and reduced the size of the left ventricular chamber, resulting in improvement in hemodynamics, myocardial energy metabolism, and clinical status (Fig. 36-7, Tables 36-16 and 36-17).[331] This led to a 22-patient randomized placebo-controlled trial in class II and class III patients.[332] Surprisingly, patients had no change in left ventricular function or left ventricular structure, but GH appeared safe. Osterziel et al.'s randomized placebo-controlled study of 50 patients with dilated cardiomyopathy also demonstrated no change in ventricular

FIGURE 36-7. Effect of growth hormone on ventricular mechanical efficiency at rest and during bicycle exercise in patients with idiopathic dilated cardiomyopathy. (*Reproduced with permission from Fazio S et al.[331]*)

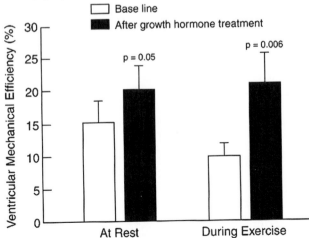

TABLE 36-16. Doppler Echocardiographic Data Before, Immediately After, and 3 Months After Growth Hormone Treatment

Variable	At Baseline	Immediately After Therapy	p Value	3 Months After Therapy	p Value
Cardiac size and shape					
LVED dimension, mm	65±1	61±1	<0.001	63±1	0.05
LVES dimension, mm	52±1	46±1	<0.001	49±1	0.004
Posterior wall thickness, mm	10.0±0.6	12.9±0.8	<0.001	11.4±0.8	0.02
Relative wall thickness	0.31±0.01	0.41±0.02	<0.001	0.35±0.01	0.006
LV mass, g	275±11	326±12	0.007	304±12	0.03
Systolic function					
EF, %	34±1.5	47±1.9	<0.001	40±2.4	0.02
Shortening velocity, circ/s	0.68±0.03	0.90±0.06	<0.001	0.79±0.06	0.002
Mean aortic acceleration, m/s^2	7.8±0.6	10.9±1	0.009	8.2±0.6	NS
ES wall stress, dyne/cm^2	144±11	85±8	<0.001	107±10	<0.001
Diastolic function					
Isovolumic relaxation time, ms	121±9	99±5	0.02	113±6	NS
Ratio of early to late filling velocity	1.17±0.25	1.27±0.21	NS	1.07±0.14	NS

± values are means standard deviation. P values are for comparisons with baseline values. EF = ejection fraction; Circ/s = circumferences per second; LVED = left ventricular end-diastolic; LVES = left ventricular end-systolic; NS = $P > .05$.

Source: Reproduced with permission from Fazio S et al.[331]

function, but patients given GH had an increase in LV mass and IGF-1 levels.[333] A recent dog study showed no benefit of GH treatment during the development of heart failure using a dose that increased body weight and plasma IGF-1 levels.[334] These variable results indicate that further research is needed before GH therapy can become standard of care in these patients.[335,335a]

Prevention of Ventricular Aneurysms After Myocardial Infarction

GH appears to be an effective treatment for prevention of ventricular aneurysms after myocardial infarction. GH given to rats after induced myocardial infarction preserved the collagen framework of myocytes.[336] Untreated rats had gross destruction of intracellular discs, nuclei, contraction bands, mitochondria, tubules, and collagen within 48 h after infarction.[336] Thirty-two percent of untreated rats developed aneurysms, while only 10% of treated rats developed aneurysms.[337] Electron microscopy of untreated rat hearts illustrated complete disarray of myofibers within 72 h, while treated rat hearts displayed less significant disarray.[336] The investigators concluded that perimyocytic and intermyocytic collagen are necessary to avoid ventricular aneurysm formation. The authors suggested that GH prevents aneurysm development by preserving this collagen framework. Prior to this study, a similar study tested GH treatment versus GH and beta-blocker treatment in rats after myocardial infarction.[337]

TABLE 36-17. Effects of Growth Hormone on Hemodynamic Variables in Patients with Congestive Heart Failure Measured Invasively with the Patient at Rest and During Submaximal Exercise

Variable	At Baseline	Immediately After Therapy	p Value
Pulmonary arterial pressure, mm Hg			
At rest	21±3	15±1.5	0.03
During exercise	39±7	31±6	0.02
Pulmonary capillary wedge pressure, mm Hg			
At rest	14±3	8±1	0.05
During exercise	24±5	18±4	0.003
Pulmonary vascular resistance, dyne-sec-cm^{-5}			
At rest	118±16	107±26	NS
During exercise	170±45	132±34	NS
Cardiac output, L/min			
At rest	4.9±0.4	5.7±0.6	0.04
During exercise	7.4±0.7	9.7±0.9	0.003
Systemic vascular resistance, dyne-sec-cm^{-5}			
At rest	1666±136	1466±152	NS
During exercise	1270±125	988±98	0.05
Ventricular mechanical work, kg·m/min			
At rest	5.4±0.6	6.7±0.8	0.03
During exercise	9.2±1.2	13.7±1.8	0.008
Coronary blood flow, mL/min			
At rest	153±18	140±14	NS
During exercise	421±42	297±36	0.01

± values are mean standard deviation. NS = $P > .05$.

Source: Reproduced with permission from Fazio S et al.[331]

Ventricular aneurysm formation decreased with GH versus controls, but increased in rats treated with both GH and beta-blockers. Investigation in human subjects is still in the early stage.

Myocardial Infarction

GH may have clinical use in the treatment of myocardial infarction.[338] Early studies with rats demonstrated improved ejection fraction and cardiac index, with lessening of the pathologic increases in left ventricular end-systolic and -diastolic diameters.[339] GH has been shown to enhance contractile reserve and intracellular calcium transients in myocytes from rats with postinfarction heart failure.[340] GH also decreased noradrenaline and normalized plasma brain natriuretic protein.[339] Rabbits pretreated with either placebo, GH, or GHRP-2 for 2 weeks before myocardial infarction had preserved diastolic function only in those treated with GHRP-2.[341] Surprisingly, only the GH secretagogue appeared protective.

GH has not been given to humans during the clinical presentation of myocardial infarction, but a recent study evaluated 6 months of GH therapy in 10 patients with postischemic CHF as compared to 10 matched controls.[342] This small study demonstrated improved exercise tolerance without significant change in LV thickness, but may have indicated some risk (death or worsening CHF) in patients with severely enlarged left ventricles (signifying severe disease). The study is too small to make justified conclusions. GH levels were measured in 52 patients presenting with acute myocardial infarction to determine its prognostic significance.[343] Patients with persistently elevated levels had higher cardiac enzymes and left ventricular dysfunction. Patients who died within 2 years appeared to be GH resistant (higher GH levels with lower IGF-1 levels).[342] GH therapy appears to have potential use and may prognosticate risk, but again, further investigation is necessary.

Vascular Disease

GH-deficient patients have elevated levels of fibrinogen and PAI, and thus an increased risk for myocardial infarction and stroke. GH at physiologic doses decreases the levels of these peptides and reduces intimal thickening and plaque formation.[306] Also, by decreasing LDL, total cholesterol, adipose tissue, and waist-to-hip ratios in deficient patients, cardiovascular morbidity and mortality risk may also be reduced. Patients on GH have improved physical well-being, decreased atherosclerosis, as well as reduction in other coronary artery disease risk factors. The prevalence of cardiovascular disease in elderly populations may be attributed, in part, to a relative deficiency of GH. Treatment of deficient patients with low-dose GH has beneficial effects on the peripheral vasculature and helps to retard progression of the disease. The extrapolation of these data to large-scale use in elderly populations has exciting implications.

Elderly

GH supplementation in the geriatric population appears to be an effective measure to prevent cardiovascular morbidity and mortality. Rudman et al., as previously discussed, demonstrated declines in GH secretion with age.[254,255] In a 1990 study of 26 normal patients between the ages of 61 and 81 years, GH replacement of .03 mg/kg given three times weekly significantly reduced adipose tissue.[344] Lean body mass and vertebral bone density increased, and IGF-1 levels rose to "youthful" parameters. A few patients showed a slight increase in both glucose and systolic blood pressure.[344] Serum levels of GH were not evaluated prior to treatment, which might have prevented these adverse effects. Elderly patients have diminished GH and IGF-1 levels, but they are still able to respond to rGH supplementation.[345] One week of daily GH achieved a steady state of IGF-1, with a decrease in total cholesterol.[345] Patients with elevated waist-to-hip ratio measurements are at increased risk for myocardial infarction, angina, cerebrovascular accidents, and death.[346] However, others argue that this measurement cannot be used as an independent predictor of cardiovascular disease and death because of confounding factors such as blood pressure and cholesterol.[346] Papadakis et al. found body composition improvement in healthy elderly men after 6 months of thrice weekly rhGH (0.03 mg/kg) administration.[347] Nevertheless, GH supplementation in the elderly decreases waist-to-hip ratios and overall adipose mass, as well as the proposed confounding factors. Thus, GH might be expected to prevent cardiovascular disease states in older subjects.

Although the geriatric population may derive the greatest benefit from replacement therapy, it is also the population at greatest risk for development of mildly elevated systolic blood pressure and blood glucose.[345] More studies need to assess the adverse effects of long-term GH administration. Not all elderly patients are "deficient" and each individual's sensitivity to administration will make it impossible to administer one standard dose to every geriatric patient. The surrogate clinical end-points to follow in dosing GH (e.g., adiposity, muscle mass, strength, endurance) need to be determined.

Dose and Duration

Most clinical studies have simulated physiologic levels with low-dose GH supplementation. The safety, however, of these doses needs to be evaluated for longer periods of time.[348] Interestingly, the anabolic effects of GH and IGF-1 are enhanced when used together[349] (Fig. 36-8). Compared with GH alone, insulin resistance is delayed by combination GH-IGF-1 therapy.[349]

Clinical investigators have evaluated different therapeutic approaches to declining GH and IGF-1 in the elderly. Iovino et al. demonstrated that repetitive intravenous dosing of older subjects with GHRH could restore the suppressed GH response to GHRH often noted in older subjects.[350] Corpas et al. similarly noted that twice daily subcutaneous doses of GHRH increased GH and IGF-1 levels in older men.[351] GHRH is a small molecule making oral, nasal, or transdermal administration likely in the future. Use of GHRH facilitates control of counterregulatory hormones, thus decreasing adverse effects.[351] GHRH can also simulate the pulsatile night-time release of GH, which is diminished in the elderly.[351] The effects of GHRH can be enhanced by concurrent use of low-dose oral arginine.[352] The advantage of this approach is that there appears to be no effect on blood pressure, pulse, temperature, or blood glucose.[352] Oral GHRP may also be an alternative therapy. The onset of oral GHRP action is delayed slightly relative to GH, but patient compliance may be improved because it is a small molecule that can be administered in oral or transdermal forms.[353]

Conclusion

GH deficiency results in a decrease in LV mass, a decreased EF, a dilated cardiomyopathy, and a decrease in exercise tolerance, whereas GH excess produces an increase in cardiac mass, an increase in blood pressure, coronary artery disease, arrhythmias, and heart failure. Thus, it is apparent that GH, in physiologic amounts, is essential for normal cardiac performance.

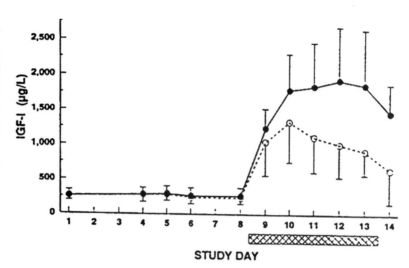

FIGURE 36-8. Changes in serum IGF-1 concentration in response to GH/IGH-1 (●—●) or IGF-1 (O − O) treatments. IGF-1 and GH were administered in the following manner: IGF-1 was given by continuous infusion (12 μg/kg IBW/h) for 16 h, on days 8 to 12 between the hours of 1600 and 0800 and on day 13 between the hours of 0800 and 2400; for the combination therapy, IGF-1 was administered as per the above protocol and GH was given by subcutaneous injection (0.05 mg/kg IBW) at 1600 h on days 8 to 12, and at 0800 h on day 13. Blood samples for measurement of IGF-1 by radioimmunoassay were collected at 0700 h, 1 h before the end of each IGF-1 infusion on days 9 to 13, and 7 h after the end of the infusion on day 14. The results are expressed as the mean ± standard deviation for 7 subjects. The differences in IGF-1 concentrations between treatment groups were significant ($P < .01$) on days 11 to 14. Treatment interval = XXXX. (*Reproduced with permission from Kupfer SR et al.*[349])

Clinical trials are ongoing using GH as a cardiovascular therapy. It has hemodynamic and metabolic effects that could be useful in the prevention and treatment of cardiovascular disease. The patient with CHF may have the most to gain in the short-term from this treatment. Use of GH for prevention of ventricular aneurysms and during and after myocardial infarction also seems promising. The beneficial effects of GH replacement on body composition and the vasculature have prompted multiple investigations on its use as a body maintenance therapy in the geriatric population. Cardiovascular deaths continue to increase in this population and GH may be a means to halt preexisting disease and to improve cardiovascular risk, and thus lower morbidity and mortality. The exact GH dose and duration of treatment still require further study.

GLUCOCORTICOIDS

In the last 30 years, the clinical scope of glucocorticoid use has multiplied. Few therapeutic agents are as effective in such a large number of clinical situations.[354] Glucocorticosteroids comprise all natural steroid hormones produced by the adrenal cortex, and are capable of stimulating hepatic glycogen deposition and gluconeogenesis.[354] Glucocorticoids prevent or suppress many immunologic processes, including inflammation.[355] Over the last 25 years, glucocorticoids have also been evaluated as a first-line therapy in specific cardiovascular disease processes. This section describes glucocorticoid actions, and the experiences with glucocorticoids as a cardiovascular therapy.

Physiology

Mechanisms of Action

Molecular

Glucocorticoids circulate in the blood either freely or bound to cortisol-binding globulin. The free form diffuses through cell plasma membranes and binds to cytoplasmic glucocorticoid receptors.[355] These receptors have three domains: immunogenic, DNA-binding, and ligand-binding. Once the ligand binds the receptor, the complex is activated, and translocates to the nucleus to bind "acceptor sites."[355] The bound complex modulates transcription of genes that encode proteins necessary for glucocorticoid actions.

Cellular

Glucocorticoids affect many immune system modulators. Glucocorticoids inhibit migration of leukocytes to sites of inflammation. Two-thirds of normal lymphocytes recirculate between lymphoid tissue and the vascular compartment.[356] Glucocorticoids redistribute lymphocytes to lymphoid compartments, creating an apparent lymphopenia.[354] The mechanism of this redistribution is unknown.[354] Glucocorticoids also cause a redistribution of monocytes leading to an apparent monocytopenia, and cause an eosinopenia by an uncertain mechanism.[354] Glucocorticoids inhibit IL-2 production and action, thus impairing lymphocyte function.[354] Neutrophil functioning is relatively resistant to glucocorticoid actions. Lysosomal enzymes are marginally affected, but nonlysosomal enzymes, such as collagenase, elastase, and plasminogen activator, are inhibited.[354] Macrophages have diminished response to macrophage activation and migration inhibitor factors, but glucocorticoids do not inhibit the production of these factors. B cells are relatively resistant to glucocorticoids.[354,355] Glucocorticoids minimally affect B cell activation and differentiation into immunoglobulin-secreting plasma cells.[357] However, 2 to 4 weeks of high-dose prednisone treatment will decrease immunoglobulin production.[358] Glucocorticoids suppress fibroblast proliferation and growth factor-induced DNA and protein synthesis.[354] Glucocorticoids inhibit IL-1 and TNFα. Lastly, by stimulating the protein lipomodulin, a phospholipase A inhibitor, production of prostaglandins and leukotrienes is inhibited.[354]

Vascular

Glucocorticoids are necessary for maintenance of basal vascular tone. Steroid-responsive hypotension in septic shock and Addisonian crisis demonstrates glucocorticoids' vasoconstrictive properties.[354] In the 1960s, Sambhi et al. studied the effects of glucocorticoids on hemodynamic measurements in normal patients and patients with shock.[359] Glucocorticoids increased cardiac output and decreased peripheral vascular resistance in both groups.

Septic shock is also implicated in causing ventricular dysfunction, but at the same time protects against ischemia-reperfusion injury. The proposed mechanism of action is by production of inducible nitrous oxide synthase generated in response to cytokines released during sepsis.[360] In a study conducted by Spanier and McDonough, dexamethasone prevented both sepsis-induced cardiac dysfunction and sepsis-induced protection of the heart from ischemia-reperfusion injury.[360]

Effects on the Heart

Glucocorticoids enhance myocardial contractility after acute administration in vivo and in vitro and can increase cardiac mass when administered in doses between .03 and 100 mg/kg for 5 to 14 days.[361] Glucocorticoids also influence cardiac myosin isoenzyme distribution. Sheer and Morkin demonstrated the dependence of myosin V1 and V3 levels on corticosteroids.[362] Adrenalectomy diminished rat V1 levels 33%, while hydrocortisone administration reversed the decline. Czerwinski et al. studied the permanence of cardiac hypertrophy and the correlation between hypertrophy and cardiac myosin heavy-chain synthesis rates.[363] Rats were given placebo or hydrocortisone 21-acetate for 1, 3, 7, 11, or 15 days. It was found that myosin heavy-chain synthesis decreased at day 7 when peak ventricular mass size occurred. After 11 days of treatment, a 10% shift from V1 to V3 occurred with a decline in myosin heavy-chain synthesis (40 to 50%) occurred.[361,362] The authors concluded that cardiac hypertrophy after glucocorticoid administration is not permanent. The downregulation of myosin heavy-chain synthesis and total protein synthesis are early steps that accompany the change from an anabolic to a catabolic state.[363] These changes precede muscle loss by more than 1 week. The results suggested that the heart cannot sustain an anabolic state during prolonged exposure to high steroid levels.

Therapeutic Uses

To Prevent Extension of Myocardial Infarction

In the early 1970s, researchers began to assess the reduction of myocardial infarct size by utilizing pharmacologic interventions that altered the metabolic environment of the ischemic myocardium. Glucocorticoids were thought to be a therapeutic candidate because of their ability to stabilize lysosomal and cellular membranes, limiting the spread of lysosomal acid hydrolases. Early experiments in dogs demonstrated a decline in infarct size after glucocorticoid administration 30 min and 6 h after coronary artery occlusion.[364] Other canine experiments also demonstrated a decrease in coronary vascular resistance after an acute myocardial infarction with increased coronary arterial blood flow after glucocorticoid treatment.[365] Studies in patients treated with steroids after acute myocardial infarction demonstrated a reduction in mortality,[366] but others have not verified these findings.[367] Time-to-administration postinfarction, dose, and initial infarct size differed in all studies. Morrison et al. studied infarct size postmyocardial infarction after 2-g intravenous methylprednisolone treatment given within 7 to 14 h after the initial rise in serum creatine phosphokinase (CPK).[368] The study consisted of 20 control and 19 treated patients. The authors demonstrated a decline in predicted infarct size after early treatment with glucocorticoids, suggesting their use as a possible myocardial salvage therapy.

Others reported, however, that glucocorticoids could impair healing in patients after myocardial infarction.[369] In an animal model, glucocorticoid treatment increased the myocardial infarct size in rats with ischemia reperfusion injury.[370] Roberts et al. demonstrated deleterious effects of corticosteroids in patients given methylprednisolone after myocardial infarction.[371] Treated patients were given either single or multiple doses of steroid and compared to controls (30 mg/kg intravenously once or every 6 h). Patients receiving multiple doses had an increased incidence of ventricular dysrhythmias, with increased couplets and runs of ventricular tachycardia and premature ventricular contractions (increased by 57%). Multiple doses also increased infarct size 84% greater than predicted. The study suggested that multiple doses impaired healing and potentiated injury. Prior to these studies, glucocorticoids had been recommended for immediate postmyocardial infarction control of arrhythmias, heart block, and infarct extension.[372] The findings of increased ventricular dysrhythmias, increased infarct size, and increased risk of aneurysm formation halted further study of glucocorticoids in human patients after myocardial infarction.

Acute Inflammatory Myocarditis

The efficacy and necessity of glucocorticoid treatment for patients with acute inflammatory myocarditis is unclear.[372a] Early lab investigations suggested many potential adverse effects of glucocorticoid therapy.[373] It was suggested that immunosuppressive agents inhibit interferon synthesis, which may exacerbate viral pathogenesis.[373] Because the diagnosis of myocarditis is predominantly a clinical diagnosis of uncertain validity,[374] and because its pathogenesis is equally uncertain, investigators have questioned the negative effects of treatment. Mason et al. were the first to demonstrate a response to prednisone alone or in combination with azathioprine.[375] The study consisted of 10 patients with unexplained congestive heart failure and endomyocardial biopsies positive for inflammatory myocarditis. There was no control group. Evidence demonstrated that treatment may eliminate infiltrates and thereby improve myocardial performance.[375] However, due to its small scale and lack of controls, the study was viewed as inconclusive.

Dec et al. studied 27 patients with acute dilated cardiomyopathy of less than 6 months duration to assess the relationship between histologic and clinical features of myocarditis.[376] Two-thirds of patients had some sign of active inflammation on endomyocardial biopsy. Biopsies were more likely to be positive during early disease. Forty percent of patients had a rise in left ventricular ejection fraction and some improvement in heart failure. Nine patients received immunosuppressive drugs, two received prednisone, and seven received a combination of prednisone and azathioprine; four patients improved.[376] Improvement showed no relation to clinical course or biopsy results. Parillo et al. studied patients with dilated cardiomyopathy, with a mean of 8 months of high-dose prednisone versus placebo.[377] After 3 months of prednisone, ejection fraction increased by 5.5%, but by 9 months, levels had returned to baseline. They concluded that early treatment is necessary in dilated cardiomyopathy patients.

The Dallas criteria, established in 1984 by eight pathologists, histologically classifies myocarditis.[378] Myocarditis is defined as myocardial inflammatory infiltrates with necrosis or degeneration of adjacent myocytes not typical of ischemic damage associated with coronary artery disease.[379] Borderline myocarditis is defined as myocardial inflammatory infiltrates without evidence of concomitant myocyte damage.[378] Borderline myocarditis may be a form of subacute myocardial autoimmunity.[379] If this is true, the borderline patients should benefit most from immunosuppressive therapy. Twenty patients with decreased left ventricular function, 9 with endomyocardial biopsy-proven myocarditis, and 11 with borderline myocarditis received 6 to 8 weeks of treatment with prednisone 1.0 mg/kg/d and azathioprine 1.5 mg/kg/d.[380] At the conclusion of the treatment, a repeat biopsy and reevaluation of left ventricular function were performed. Left ventricular function improved and ventricular dilation decreased more in borderline patients than in myocarditis patients.[380]

The Myocarditis Treatment Trial, the first prospective, large-scale, multicenter, placebo-controlled trial to assess the benefit of immunosuppression therapy in myocarditis and to identify immunologic markers of disease severity, was recently completed.[381] The study randomized 111 patients with a histopathologic diagnosis of myocarditis and left ventricular ejection fraction of less than 45% into control or treatment groups. Treatment consisted of azathioprine 1 mg/kg twice daily for 24 weeks, or cyclosporin 5 mg/kg twice daily and titrated to varying levels over 24 weeks. Prednisone was started at a dose of 1.25 mg/kg/d in divided doses and was maintained at that level for 1 week. The dose was then decreased by approximately 0.08 mg/kg/wk until the dose was 0.33 mg/kg/d at the end of week 12. This reduced dose was maintained through the end of week 20, after which it was reduced by 0.08 mg/kg/wk until the week 24, when the drug was discontinued. Immunosuppressive therapy did not improve survival and did not improve left ventricular ejection fraction at 28 weeks.[381] Researchers demonstrated elevated levels of IgG antibody, indicative of an inflammatory response. A higher level of IgG antibodies was associated with a higher left ventricular ejection fraction, a smaller left ventricular size, and a lower pulmonary capillary wedge pressure.[381] This finding suggested that an immune response may be beneficial in patients with myocarditis, and not the cause of the disease. Higher levels of helper T cells were associated with more severe initial disease, as indicated by a greater use of heart failure therapy. Also, higher levels of CD^{2+} T cells were associated with a greater risk of death.[381] The authors concluded that in some patients, a heightened T-cell activity may be deleterious. A retrospective study was done by researchers in Japan to devise a scoring system to predict the outcome of patients with acute myocarditis, employing six parameters: patients were given scores from −2 to +2 for each parameter. It was found that in patients with total scores from 0 to +6, steroid therapy succeeded.[382] A case study on idiopathic giant-cell myocarditis has also been reported in the literature, with resolution of the disease process as a result of combined immunosuppressive therapy.[383]

Thus, some myocarditis patients may benefit from timed immunosuppressive therapy.[384] Glucocorticoid treatment also suppressed the life-threatening ventricular tachyarrhythmias in chronic myocarditis by decreasing the lymphocytic infiltration, and probably decreases HLA expression on endothelial and interstitial cells.[385]

Studies of myocarditis in pediatric patients have also shown a benefit with steroid therapy in combination with azathioprine.[386] In another study, dual therapy with cyclosporine and steroids was found to improve the outcome in a pediatric population with dilated cardiomyopathy secondary to myocarditis.[387] In a study done in 70 children over the period of 12 years, rheumatic carditis was found to respond to treatment with glucocorticoids.[388] Recently, steroids were found to cause hypertrophic cardiomyopathy in preterm infants, which resolved with discontinuation of treatment.[389]

Recurrent Pericarditis

Glucocorticoids are recommended in the treatment of recurrent pericarditis in extremely ill patients who are unresponsive to nonsteroidal anti-inflammatory agents. Patients are treated with high-dose prednisone for a few days, followed by a medication taper. Fowler et al., in a study of 31 patients with recurrent pericarditis, observed that symptoms recurred if the prednisone dose was below 10 to 15 mg/d.[390] Of the 31 patients, 26 required prednisone to relieve symptoms. Intrapericardial instillation of steroids in autoreactive pericarditis prevented recurrence in 13 of 14 cases after 3 months and in 12 of 14 cases after 1 year.[391] Other studies also prove steroid

therapy beneficial in myopericarditis.[392] Others, however, believe that steroids prolong the disease process.[393] Thus, glucocorticoid therapy is recommended in nonsteroidal anti-inflammatory drug-resistant pericardial disease, but therapy should be quickly tapered after a response is observed.

Coronary Artery Bypass Surgery (CABG)

The complications of major surgery include persistent inflammation which can lead to multisystem organ failure. Polymorphonuclear leukocyte resistance to apoptosis may contribute to this process. Glucocorticoid therapy has been proposed to attenuate the postoperative inflammatory response associated with CABG, with no apparent benefit being seen.[394]

Intravenous methylprednisolone has been used prophylactically to reduce the risk of postpericardiotomy syndrome with limited benefit.[395]

Conclusion

Glucocorticoids are used to treat a wide spectrum of diseases. However, the use of glucocorticoids in cardiovascular disease is limited. Glucocorticoids fail to limit the size of myocardial infarction, but appear to have a limited role in the treatment of both myocarditis and recurrent pericarditis.

TESTOSTERONE AND OTHER ANDROGENS (ANABOLIC STEROIDS)

Androgens are important steroids in men in all stages of life. From a quantitative standpoint, the most important androgen is testosterone, which is produced in testicular Leydig cells and in small amounts by the adrenal glands. Testosterone and other anabolic steroids have been used to increase muscle size and strength, and it has been suggested that they could be used therapeutically to increase vitality and muscle strength in aging men and in patients with cachectic diseases such as chronic CHF.[396] Testosterone has also been associated with an increased risk of coronary artery disease by adversely affecting the plasma lipid and lipoprotein profile.[397] One study showed decreased risk of coronary artery disease related to endogenous testosterone levels.[398]

In this section, testosterone and other anabolic steroids are examined as therapeutic agents in cardiovascular disease, taking into consideration the possible cardiovascular risks of such treatment.

Physiologic Function

The function of androgens in humans includes appropriate differentiation of internal and external male genital system during fetal development. In puberty, androgens mediate sexual maturation of external genitalia, stimulate skeletal muscle growth, growth of the larynx and epiphysis cartilaginous plates, cause growth of pubic, axillary, and sexual (beard, mustache, chest, abdomen, and back) hair, and increase sebaceous gland activity. Androgens also stimulate erythropoiesis and maintain adult bone mass.[399,400]

Males between the ages of 40 and 70 years of age lose about 10% of total testosterone concentration in the plasma.[401] Although this is only a modest fall in total testosterone levels, there is a change in balance between sex-hormone-binding globulin (SHBG) and albumin as the carrier of testosterone in plasma with age. There is an increase in SHBG-bound testosterone and a fall in albumin-bound testosterone.[401] The net effect could be a loss of net free testosterone in plasma because SHBG binds testosterone with a greater affinity than albumin; and free testosterone is the biologically active component of plasma testosterone.[402]

Cardiovascular and Metabolic Actions

Because of this age-related reduction in plasma testosterone, it has been proposed that the hormone be replaced in men to maintain vitality. However, it has been reported that testosterone can cause acute myocardial infarction in young body builders taking anabolic steroids.[403] Androgens affect plasma lipids and lipoproteins, thrombosis and vascular reactivity, and cardiac hypertrophy.

Effects on Lipids and Lipoproteins

On average, men have lower plasma levels of HDL cholesterol and higher levels of triglyceride, LDL-cholesterol, and VLDL than do premenopausal women.[404]

Patients enrolled in Multiple Risk Factor Intervention Trial (MRFIT) were followed over 13 years. The decrease in testosterone in aging was associated with an increase in triglycerides and decrease in HDL cholesterol, but little relationship was found with blood pressure and LDL-cholesterol.[405]

A study was done on Black and white school boys between the ages of 10 and 15 years to assess whether there were racial differences regarding the effects of testosterone and estradiol on plasma lipids.[406] Estradiol levels were higher in Black boys, but free testosterone levels were not different. Black boys had lower triglycerides and apolipoprotein B and higher HDL cholesterol as compared with white boys. Testosterone was found to be positively related to HDL cholesterol, and apolipoprotein (apo)-B and estradiol were inversely related to total cholesterol, triglycerides, LDL-cholesterol, apo-B, and LDL-cholesterol/HDL-cholesterol ratio, which could contribute to the racial differences in the atherogenic lipid profile.[406]

In young, healthy males who were given gonadotropin-releasing hormone (GnRH) antagonists, HDL cholesterol levels, apo-A-I and apo-A-II increased.[407,408] In another group who received GnRH antagonists plus physiologic doses of testosterone, these changes in the lipid profile were prevented.[407] In hypogonadal men, substitution of exogenous androgens increased total cholesterol and LDL-cholesterol and decreased HDL cholesterol.[409]

In elderly patients with CAD who were administered intramuscular testosterone undecenoate, total cholesterol levels and triglycerides decreased, while HDL cholesterol increased.[410] Similarly, in a study of men older than 56 years of age, it was shown that intramuscular testosterone enanthate given in doses to raise plasma testosterone levels to middle-normal adult male range, reduced both total cholesterol and LDL-cholesterol by 11%. There was a tendency for HDL cholesterol to fall, but the change from baseline was not significant.[411]

The majority of studies that have evaluated the effects of exogenous androgens on plasma lipids have shown reductions of HDL cholesterol.[412] The mechanism for this reduction may relate to increases in hepatic triglyceride lipase that can catabolize HDL.[413] Despite this unfavorable effect on HDL cholesterol, a direct association between exogenous androgen use and an increased risk of coronary artery disease has yet to be shown in men. Furthermore, it was demonstrated that bodybuilders who used anabolic androgenic steroids had a favorable reduction in Lp(a) levels.[414]

Effects on Clotting

Androgens may have direct effects on the coagulation (fibrinolytic) system.[415] Some androgens increase plasminogen activator activity and serum plasminogen, protein C, and antithrombin III, which could protect against myocardial infarction. However, thromboxane A_2 (TXA2) receptor activity and increased platelet aggregability have been described with testosterone replacement.[416] Fibrinogen levels may be augmented by unbound free testosterone in the blood.[417]

Despite these varied effects on coagulation factors, a direct cause-and-effect relationship between androgenic steroids and coronary thrombosis has not been proven, and the exact role that replacement or supplementary androgens play in the thrombotic process itself remains undefined.[415]

Effects on Cardiac Hypertrophy

Animals can develop ventricular hypertrophy with anabolic steroids,[418] which is reversible upon discontinuation of therapy.[419] The administration of methandrostenolone to female rats is associated with the appearance and increase of intermediate-size filaments and ultrastructural changes similar to those found in the early stages of congestive heart failure.[420] In a study conducted on male rats treated chronically with 17α-methytestosterone, the heart showed decreased static compliance which limited stroke volume. This may be related to enhanced activity of lysyl oxidase, which resulted in an increased crosslink formation between collagen strands in the extracellular matrix.[421]

Effects on Vascular Tone and Blood Pressure

It has been proposed that androgens may increase vascular reactivity.[422] Androgens may affect the release of nitric oxide.[423] In an experimental model, testosterone was shown to increase the tendency of the coronary arteries to develop vasoconstriction and vasospasm.[424] Testosterone impairs exercise-induced augmented capillarization, which leads to an imbalance between myocardial oxygen supply and demand.[425] Androgen exposure is also associated with increased monocyte adhesion to endothelial cells, a proatherogenic effect that is partly mediated by an increased endothelial cell-surface expression of vascular cell adhesion molecule-1 (VCAM-1).[426] However, there are reports demonstrating antianginal and antiatherosclerotic effects of testosterone in humans,[427,428] and evidence from other experimental models that testosterone may increase vascular relaxation.[422] In one study, a lower level of endogenous androgens was associated with the presence of atherosclerosis when compared with patients with no evidence of CAD on angiograms.[429] Other studies were not able to give conclusive evidence of the role of endogenous testosterone level in patients with CAD.[430]

Endogenous levels of testosterone in males have an inverse relation to systolic blood pressure and diastolic blood pressure levels.[431] In obese men receiving testosterone undecenoate, a reduction in blood pressure was noted.[432] An acute pressure natriuresis was shown to be blunted in spontaneously hypertensive male rats and gonadectomized female rats receiving testosterone, as compared with females and castrated males, which suggests its role in mediating high blood pressure in this group.[433]

Development of atherosclerosis in males and females is the result of complex hormonal interbalance.[434] Further studies are needed to completely define the role of these hormones in both genders. The therapeutic role of testosterone in the treatment of peripheral vessel atherosclerosis is also not of proven benefit.[435]

Other Metabolic Effects

There is an inverse relationship between endogenous testosterone levels and plasma insulin levels.[436] In a study of middle-aged obese men receiving low levels of testosterone undecenoate, increased insulin sensitivity was noted with a euglycemic (hyperinsulinemic) glucose clamp technique.[432] One study reported a diminished glucose tolerance and insulin resistance in weight lifters who used testosterone.[437] In another study, young, healthy men receiving replacement or supplementary doses of testosterone enanthate or 14-nortestosterone were found to show no change in fasting blood-sugar-plasma insulin levels.[438]

Middle-aged men were followed for a period of 7 to 10 years and the levels of testosterone and SHBG levels were measured at the time of enrollment and after 7 to 10 years. The study showed that the decreasing level of testosterone and SHBG was inversely related to the development of insulin resistance and the subsequent development of type 2 diabetes.[439] However, in another study done on patients with idiopathic hypogonadotrophic hypogonadism, exogenous testosterone did not affect the insulin resistance.[440]

Investigators in one study examined the effects of testosterone, administered at different doses and time periods, and using different formulations, on plasma insulin and glucose tolerance.[441] A single intramuscular injection of 500 mg of testosterone enanthate significantly impaired glucose tolerance. When only 250 mg of testosterone enanthate was given, insulin concentration decreased. When testosterone undecenoate was given at 40 mg four times daily, there was a borderline decrease in plasma insulin. Testosterone gel applied to the skin at a dose of 250 mg caused a decrease in insulin and an improved glucose tolerance.[441]

Effects on Skeletal Muscle and Strength

Testosterone and other anabolic steroids do prompt transient nitrogen retention, and supraphysiologic doses of testosterone, when combined with strength training in normal men, can increase fat-free mass and muscle size.[442] Androgens can increase whole-body protein synthesis and may inhibit the catabolic effects of glucocorticoids.[442] They act through the androgen receptor to cause hypertrophy of skeletal muscle cells without increasing their number.[442] Androgens do not, by themselves, increase aerobic capacity. It is this action that has suggested the possible use of supplementary androgens in patients having congestive heart failure with muscle weakness and cachexia. Their use in heart failure may be limited by salt- and water-retaining effects; however, the edema produced is responsive to diuretic agents.

At this juncture, various androgen formulations, including those used in veterinary medicine, are being employed by both men and women to enhance athletic performance. However, there are little data available regarding the long-term consequences of such an approach.

Aging

Serum testosterone levels are reduced in men with age[439,443] and are associated with decreased muscle strength and mass.[444] Androgen-replacement therapy has been suggested as a treatment for increasing body weight, well-being, and blood volume, and for reducing bone loss.[444,445] Older individuals, however, may develop sleep apnea and secondary polycythemia as a result of this treatment.[446,447]

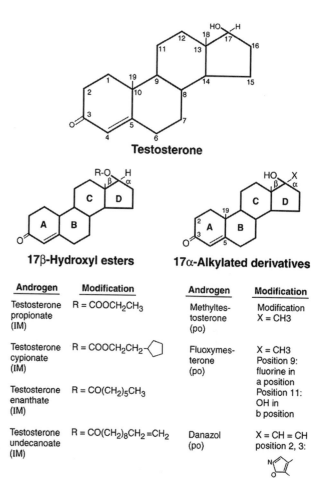

FIGURE 36-9. The structures of testosterone and its modifications in clinical use. IM = intramuscular; po = oral. (*Adapted with permission from Bagatell CJ et al.*[397])

Pharmacologic Replacement

Various androgen formulations are available for treating hypogonadism in adults, delayed puberty, various hematologic disorders, and hereditary angioedema (Fig. 36-9). Androgens have also been proposed as a treatment for aging males and potentially as a treatment for cachexia and muscle weakness in congestive heart failure.

Testosterone is metabolized quickly in the liver, and needs to be reformulated for medicinal use. Testosterone is esterified at the 17α-hydroxy position, which makes the substance hydrophobic, and it is released gradually from injection sites as natural testosterone.[397] Testosterone esters are usually administered in oil by intramuscular injection in weekly injections for up to 24 weeks.[397] In the study by Bhasin et al.,[396] weekly injections of testosterone enanthate were given for 10 weeks, a dose six times that recommended for replacement therapy. Testosterone can also be alkylated at the 17α-hydroxy position, which interferes with hepatic metabolism, allowing for oral testosterone use.

Transdermal patches that are worn on the scrotum and replaced daily are available and a new patch that can be worn on nonscrotal skin is approved for clinical use.[448]

Other available formulations include crystalline testosterone, which can be used in implantable pellets for very long-term use.[449] Experimental formulations include testosterone biciliate, with a duration of up to 16 weeks,[450] and injectable long-acting microcapsules of testosterone.[451]

Testosterone is metabolized to form both dihydrotestosterone, the intracellular form that acts on a defined androgen receptor, and by aromatization to form estradiol, which acts on estrogen receptors. Testosterone formulations that are metabolized to form more estrogen appear to have lesser effects on HDL cholesterol.

Clinical Recommendations

It appears from the available data that normal physiologic levels of testosterone (12.1 to 34.7 nmol/L) may protect against cardiovascular disease[411] and replacement therapy in men may be safe to administer.[452] However, exogenous testosterone administered in supraphysiologic doses may be associated with changes in lipids and lipoproteins, insulin resistance, and myocardial infarction. It is recommended that replacement therapy in older men return testosterone levels to the midrange of normal physiologic levels. Therefore, testosterone replacement therapy should only be administered to men whose plasma levels fall in the low range of normal because they would be most responsive to treatment.[441,453]

Replacement therapy does have its risks. There may be an increased risk of prostatic cancer, benign prostatism, erythrocytosis, and edema.[453] There are no long-term data on the cardiovascular safety of replacement and supraphysiologic doses of testosterone; however, short-term courses of treatment appear to be safe and could be considered as a treatment for patients with congestive heart failure and diminished muscle strength, cachexia, and a poor sense of well being. Drug-induced edema can be treated with diuretics. The dose, duration, and formulation used needs to be established in clinical trials of patients with congestive heart failure.

Androgens have also been used to increase lean body mass in patients receiving chronic dialysis.[454]

Androgens in Women

Androgen therapy is also used as a performance enhancer in women and could be considered as a treatment in congestive heart failure. However, the long-term cardiovascular effects of androgen replacement in women have not been established. Testosterone's role in the development of CAD in women is still not completely understood.[455,456] One study demonstrated the positive relationship of free testosterone level with hypertension[457] and another showed a positive correlation with HDL cholesterol and CAD.[458] One study demonstrated improvement in endothelium-dependent and endothelium-independent (glyceryl trinitrate) brachial artery vasodilatation in postmenopausal women receiving HRT and testosterone.[459] In one study, testosterone administration by implants was given for 2 years to patients complaining of severe premenstrual symptoms (PMS) as compared with age-matched patients.[460] In treated group, apo-AI and HDL cholesterol were significantly decreased; also noted was an increase in VLDL-cholesterol. No significant change was found in the levels of total cholesterol, LDL-cholesterol, apo B, Lp(a), lecithin:cholesterol acyl transferase, and cholesteryl transfer protein activity. There was no difference in the clotting factors of both groups, which included prothrombin time, fibrinogen activator inhibitor, β-thromboglobulin, and prothrombin fragments 1.2. There was also no change in the architecture of the ovaries.[460]

Conclusion

Although testosterone has been studied as a replacement and supplementary therapy for other medical conditions, its long-term effects on CAD risk factors require further study. Testosterone may potentially improve skeletal muscle strength and functional capacity in advanced heart failure.

REFERENCES

1. Ryan KJ: Estrogens and atherosclerosis. *Clin Obstet Gynecol* 19:805, 1976.
2. Schillaci G, Verdecchia P, Borgioni C, et al: Early cardiac changes after menopause. *Hypertension* 32:764, 1998.
3. Mendelsohn ME, Karas RH: The protective effects of estrogen on the cardiovascular system. *N Engl J Med* 340:1801, 1999.
4. Gordon T, Kannel WB, Hjortland MC, et al: Menopause and the coronary artery disease. *Ann Intern Med* 89:157, 1978.
5. Wilson PWF, Garrison RJ, Castelli WP: Post-menopausal estrogen use, cigarette smoking, and cardiovascular morbidity in women over 50. The Framingham Study. *N Engl J Med* 313:1038, 1985.
6. Eaker ED, Catelli WP: Differential risk for coronary heart disease among women in the Framingham Study. In: Eaker E, Pakard B, Wenger N, Clarkson T, Tyroler HA, eds. *Coronary Heart Disease in Women.* New York: Haymarket Doyma, 1987:122.
7. Stampfer MJ, Colditz GA: Estrogen replacement therapy and coronary heart disease: a quantitative assessment of the epidemiologic evidence. *Prev Med* 20:47, 1991.
8. Colditz GA, Willett WC, Stampfer MJ, et al: Menopause and the risk of coronary heart disease in women. *N Engl J Med* 316:1105, 1987.
9. Pearson TA, Bulkley BH, Achuff SC, et al: The association of low levels of HDL-cholesterol and arteriographically defined CA. *Am J Epidemiol* 109:285, 1979.
10. Gruchow HW, Anderson AJ, Barboriak JJ, Sobocinski KA: Post-menopausal use of estrogen and occlusion of coronary arteries. *Am Heart J* 115:954, 1988.
11. Hong MK, Romm PA, Reagan K, et al: Effects of estrogen replacement therapy on serum lipid values and angiographically defined coronary artery disease in postmenopausal women. *Am J Cardiol* 69:176, 1992.
12. Henderson BE, Paganini-Hill A, Ross RK: Decreased mortality in users of estrogen replacement therapy. *Arch Intern Med* 151:75, 1991.
13. Sullivan JM, Vander Zwaag R, Hughes JP, et al: Estrogen replacement and coronary artery disease. *Arch Intern Med* 150:2557, 1990.
14. Stampfer MJ, Colditz GA, Willett WC, et al: Postmenopausal estrogen therapy and cardiovascular disease: Ten-year follow-up from the Nurses' Health Study. *N Engl J Med* 325:756, 1991.
15. Varas-Lorenzo C, Garcia-Rodriguez LA, Perez-Gutthann S, Duque-Oliart A: Hormone replacement therapy and incidence of acute myocardial infarction. A population-based nested case-control study. *Circulation* 101:2572, 2000.
16. Grodstein F, Manson JE, Colditz GA, et al: A prospective, observational study of postmenopausal hormone therapy and primary prevention of cardiovascular disease. *Ann Intern Med* 133:933, 2000.
17. Manson JE, Tosteson H, Ridker PM, et al: Review article: The primary prevention of myocardial infarction. *N Engl J Med* 326:1406, 1992.
18. Grady D, Rubin S, Petitti DB, et al: Hormone therapy to prevent disease and prolong life in postmenopausal women. *Ann Intern Med* 117:1016, 1992.
19. Heckbert SR, Weiss NS, Koepsell TD et al: Duration of estrogen replacement in relation to the risk of incident myocardial infarction in postmenopausal women. *Arch Intern Med* 157:1330, 1997.
20. Losardo DW, Hearney M, Kim EA: Variable expression of the estrogen receptor in normal and atherosclerotic coronary arteries of premenopausal women. *Circulation* 89:1501, 1994.
20a. Mendelsohn ME: Protective effects of estrogen on the cardiovascular system. *Am J Cardiol* 89:12E, 2002.
21. Stefano GB, Prevot V, Beauvillain J-C, et al: Cell-surface estrogen receptors mediate calcium-dependent nitric oxide release in human endothelia. *Circulation* 101:1594, 2000.
22. Thompson LP, Pinkas G, Weiner CP: Chronic 17β-estradiol replacement increases nitric oxide-mediated vasodilation of guinea pig coronary microcirculation. *Circulation* 102:445, 2000.
23. Barrett-Connor E, Wilcosky T, Wallace RB, Heiss G: Resting and exercise electrocardiographic abnormalities associated with hormone use in women. *Am J Epidemiol* 123:81, 1986.

24. Pines A, Fisman EZ, Levo Y, et al: The effects of hormone replacement therapy in normal postmenopausal women: measurements of Doppler-derived parameters of aortic flow. *Am J Obstet Gynecol* 164:806, 1991.

25. Klangkalya B, Chan A: The effects of ovarian hormones on beta-adrenergic and muscarinic receptors in rat heart. *Life Sci* 42:2307, 1988.

26. Scheuer J, Malhotra A, Schaible TF, Capasso A: Effects of gonadectomy and hormonal replacement on rat hearts. *Circ Res* 61:12, 1987.

27. La Sala GB, Gaddi O, Bruno G, et al: Noninvasive evaluation of cardiovascular hemodynamics during multiple follicular stimulation, late luteal phase, and early pregnancy. *Fertil Steril* 51:796, 1989.

28. Chang WC, Nakao J, Orimo H, et al: Stimulation of prostaglandin cyclooxygenase and prostaglandin synthetase activities by estradiol in rat aortic smooth muscle cells. *Biochem Biophys Acta* 620:472, 1980.

29. Paller MS: Mechanism of decreased pressor responsiveness to angiotensin II, norepinephrine, and vasopressin in pregnant rats. *Am J Physiol* 247:H100, 1984.

30. Binder EF, Williams DB, Schechtman KB, et al: Effects of hormone replacement therapy on serum lipids in elderly women. A randomized, placebo-controlled trial. *Ann Intern Med* 134:754, 2001.

31. Walsh BW, Schiff I, Rosner B, et al: Effects of postmenopausal estrogen replacement on the concentrations and metabolism of plasma lipoproteins. *N Engl J Med* 325:1196, 1991.

32. Lobo RA: Clinical review 27: Effects of hormonal replacement on lipids and lipoproteins in postmenopausal women. *J Clin Endocrin Metab* 73:925, 1991.

33. Barbaras R, Puchois P, Fruchart JC, Ailhaud G: Cholesterol efflux from cultured adipose cells is mediated by Lp AI particles but not by LpAI:AII particles. *Biochem Biophys Res Commun* 142:63, 1987.

34. Puchois P, Kandoussi A, Fievet P, et al: Apolipoprotein A-I containing lipoproteins in coronary artery disease. *Atherosclerosis* 68:35, 1987.

35. Ory, SJ, Field, CS, Herrmann, RR, et al: Effects of long-term transdermal administration of estradiol on serum lipids. *Mayo Clin Proc* 73:735, 1998.

36. Crook D, Cust MP, Gangar KF, et al: Comparison of transdermal and oral estrogen-progestin replacement therapy: Effects on serum lipids and lipoproteins. *Am J Obstet Gynecol* 166:950, 1992.

37. Wakatsuki A, Ikenoue N, Okatani Y, Fukaya T: Estrogen-induced small low density lipoprotein particles may be atherogenic in postmenopausal women. *J Am Coll Cardiol* 37:425, 2001.

38. Darling GM, Johns JA, McCloud PI, Davis SR: Estrogen and progestin compared with simvastatin for hypercholesterolemia in postmenopausal women. *N Engl J Med* 337:595, 1997.

39. Davidson MH, Testolin Lisa, Maki KC, et al: A comparison of estrogen replacement, pravastatin, and combined treatment for the management of hypercholesterolemia in postmenopausal women. *Arch Intern Med* 157:1186, 1997.

40. Summary of the Second Report of the National Cholesterol Education Program (NCEP) Expert Panel on Detection, Evaluation, and Treatment of High Blood Cholesterol in Adults (Adult Treatment Panel II). *JAMA* 269:3015, 1993.

41. Executive Summary of the Third Report of the National Cholesterol Education Program (NCEP) Expert Panel on Detection, Evaluation and Treatment of High Blood Cholesterol in Adults (Adult Treatment Panel III). *JAMA* 285:2486, 2001.

42. Cremer P, Nagel D, Labrot B, et al: Lipoprotein Lp(a) as predictor of myocardial infarction in comparison to fibrinogen, LDL cholesterol and other risk factors: Results from the prospective Gottingen Risk Incidence and Prevalence Study (GRIPS). *Eur J Clin Invest* 24:444, 1994.

43. Sandkamp M, Assman G: Lipoprotein (a) in PROCAM participants and young myocardial infarction survivors. In: Scanv AM, ed. *Lipoprotein(a): 25 Years of Progress.* New York: Academic Press, 1990:205.

44. Lobo R, Notelovitz M, Bernstein L, et al: Lp(a) lipoprotein: Relationship to cardiovascular disease risk factors, exercise, and estrogen. *Am J Obstet Gynecol* 166:1182, 1992.

45. Shlipak MG, Simon JA, Vittinghoff E, et al: Estrogen and progestin, lipoprotein(a) and the risk of recurrent coronary heart disease events after menopause. *JAMA* 283:1845, 2000.

46. Espeland MA, Marcovina SM, Miller V, et al: for the PEPI investigators: Effect of postmenopausal hormone therapy on lipoprotein(a) concentration. *Circulation* 97:979, 1998.

47. Shionori H, Eggena P, Barrett JD, et al: An increase in high-molecular weight renin substrate associated with estrogenic hypertension. *Biochem Med* 29:14, 1983.

48. Cacciabaudo JM, August P: Female sex hormones and cardiovascular disease: Implications for therapy. In: Laragh JH, Brenner BM, eds. *Hypertension: Pathophysiology, Diagnosis and Management, 2nd ed.* New York: Raven Press, 1995:2391.

49. Hazzard WR: Estrogen replacement and cardiovascular disease: Serum lipids and blood pressure effects. *Am J Obstet Gynecol* 161:1847, 1989.

50. Wren BG, Routledge AD: The effect of type and dose of oestrogen on the blood pressure of post-menopausal women. *Maturitas* 5:135, 1983.

51. Scuteri A, Bos AJG, Brant LJ, et al: Hormone replacement therapy and longitudinal changes in blood pressure in postmenopausal women. *Ann Intern Med* 135:229, 2001.

52. Utian WH: Effect of postmenopausal estrogen therapy on diastolic blood pressure and body weight. *Maturitas* 1:3, 1978.

53. Vongpatanasin W, Tuncel M, Mansour Y, et al: Transdermal estrogen replacement therapy decreases sympathetic activity in postmenopausal women. *Circulation* 103:2903, 2001.

54. van Eickels M, Grohé C, Cleutjens JPM, et al: 17β-Estradiol attenuates the development of pressure-overload hypertrophy. *Circulation* 104:1419, 2001.

55. Notelovitz M: Coagulation, oestrogen and the menopause. *Clin Obstet Gynecol* 4:107, 1977.

56. Chetkowski RJ, Meldrum DR, Steingold KA, et al: Biologic effects of transdermal estradiol. *N Engl J Med* 314:1615, 1986.

57. Notelovitz M: Exercise, nutrition, and the coagulation effects of estrogen replacement on cardiovascular health. *Obstet Gynecol Clin North Am* 14:121, 1987.

58. Notelovitz M, Kitchens CS, Ware MD: Coagulation and fibrinolysis in estrogen-treated surgically menopausal women. *Obstet Gynecol* 63:621, 1984.

59. Bloemenkamp KWM, Rosendaal FR, Helmerhorst FM, Vandenbrouke JP: Higher risk of venous thrombosis during early use of oral contraceptives in women with inherited clotting defects. *Arch Intern Med* 160:49, 2000.

60. Psaty BM, Smith NL, Lemaitre RN, et al: Hormone replacement therapy, prothrombotic mutations, and the risk of incident nonfatal myocardial infarction in postmenopausal women. *JAMA* 285:906, 2001.

61. Devor M, Barrett-Connor E, Renvall M, et al: Estrogen replacement therapy and the risk of venous thrombosis. *Am J Med* 92:275, 1992.

62. PEPI Trial Writing Group: Effects of estrogen or estrogen/ progestin regimens on heart disease risk factors in post menopausal women [The Postmenopausal Estrogen/Progestin Intervention (PEPI) Trial]. *JAMA* 273:199, 1995.

63. Scuteri A, Vaitkevicius PV, Bos AJ, Fleg JL: Estrogens but not progestins reduce age-associated increase in arterial stiffness and blood pressure in post-menopausal women. *Circulation* 100:I, 1999.

64. Brouchet L, Krust A, Dupont S, et al: Estradiol accelerates reendothelialization in mouse carotid artery through estrogen receptor-α but not estrogen receptor-β. *Circulation* 103:423, 2001.

65. McCrohon JA, Nakhla S, Jessup W, et al: Estrogen and progesterone reduce lipid accumulation in human monocyte-derived macrophages. A sex-specific effect. *Circulation* 100:2319, 1999.

65a. Hodis HN, Mack WJ, Lobo RA, et al: Estrogen in the prevention of atherosclerosis: A randomized, double-blind, placebo-controlled trial. *Ann Intern Med* 135:939, 2001.

66. Williams JK, Adams MR, Klopfenstein HS: Estrogen modulates responses of atherosclerotic coronary arteries. *Circulation* 81:1680, 1990.

67. Webb CM, Ghatei MA, McNeill JG, Collins P: 17β-Estradiol decreases endothelin-1 levels in the coronary circulation of postmenopausal women with coronary artery disease. *Circulation* 102:1617, 2000.

68. Huang A, Sun D, Koller A, Kaley G: 17β-Estradiol restores endothelial nitric oxide release to shear stress in arterioles of male hypertensive rats. *Circulation* 101:94, 2000.

69. Tolbert T, Thompson JA, Bouchard P, Oparil S: Estrogen-induced vasoprotection is independent of inducible nitric oxide synthase

expression. Evidence from the mouse carotid artery ligation model. *Circulation* 104:2740, 2001.

69a. Campisi R, Nathan L, Hernandez Pampaloni M, et al: Noninvasive assessment of coronary microcirculatory function in postmenopausal women and effects of short-term and long-term estrogen administration. *Circulation* 105:425, 2002.

70. Fischer-Dzoga K, Wissler RW, Vesselinovitch D: The effect of estradiol on the proliferation of rabbit aortic medial tissue culture cells induced by hyperlipemic serum. *Exp Mol Pathol* 39:355, 1983.

71. Sudoh N, Toba K, Akishita M, et al: Estrogen prevents oxidative stress-induced endothelial cell apoptosis in rats. *Circulation* 103:724, 2001.

72. Vehkavaara S, Hakala-Ala-Pietilä T, Virkamäki A, et al: Differential effects of oral and transdermal estrogen replacement therapy on endothelial function in postmenopausal women. *Circulation* 102:2687, 2000.

73. Kawano H, Motoyama T, Hirai N, et al: Effect of medroxyprogesterone acetate plus estradiol on endothelium-dependent vasodilation in postmenopausal women. *Am J Cardiol* 87:238, 2001.

74. Redberg RF, Nishino M, McElhinney DB, et al: Long-term estrogen replacement therapy is associated with improved exercise capacity in postmenopausal women without known coronary artery disease. *Am Heart J* 139:739, 2000.

75. Gangar KF, Vyas S, Whitehead M, et al: Pulsatility index in internal carotid artery in relation to transdermal oestradiol and time since menopause. *Lancet* 338:839, 1991.

76. Bourne T, Hillard TC, Whitehead MI, et al: Oestrogens, arterial status and postmenopausal women. *Lancet* 335:1470, 1990.

77. Rovang KS, Arouni AJ, Mohiuddin SM, et al: Effect of estrogen on exercise electrocardiograms in healthy postmenopausal women. *Am J Cardiol* 86:477, 2000.

77a. Pham TV, Sosunov EA, Gainullin RZ, et al: Impact of sex and gonadal steroids on prolongation of ventricular repolarization and arrhythmias induced by I_k-blocking drugs. *Circulation* 103:2207, 2001.

78. Barrett-Connor E, Laakso M: Ischemic heart disease risk in postmenopausal women: Effects of estrogen use on glucose and insulin levels. *Arteriosclerosis* 10:531, 1990.

79. Lobo RA, Pickar JH, Wild RA, et al: Metabolic impact of adding medroxy-progesterone acetate to conjugated estrogen therapy in postmenopausal women. *Obstet Gynecol* 84:987, 1994.

80. Cucinelli F, Paparella P, Soranna L, et al: Differential effect of transdermal estrogen plus progestogen replacement therapy on insulin metabolism in postmenopausal women: Relation to their insulinemic secretion. *Eur J Endocrinol* 140:215, 1999.

81. Elkind-Hirsch KE, Sherman LD, Malinak R: Hormone replacement therapy alters insulin sensitivity in young women with premature ovarian failure. *J Clin Endocrinol Metab* 76:472, 1993.

82. Duncan AC, Lyall H, Roberts RN, et al: The effect of estradiol and a combined estradiol/progestogen preparation on insulin sensitivity in healthy postmenopausal women. *J Clin Endocrinol Metab* 84:2402, 1999.

83. Godsland IF, Crook D, Simpson R, et al: The effects of different formulations of oral contraceptive agents on lipid and carbohydrate metabolism. *N Engl J Med* 323:1375, 1990.

84. Wassmann S, Bäumer AT, Strehlow K, et al: Endothelial dysfunction and oxidative stress during estrogen deficiency in spontaneously hypertensive rats. *Circulation* 103:435, 2001.

85. Gey KF: On the antioxidant hypothesis with regard to arteriosclerosis. *Bibl Nutr Dieta* 37:53, 1986.

86. Massafra, Buonocore G, Gioia D, et al: Effects of estradiol and medroxy-progesterone-acetate treatment on erythrocyte antioxidant enzyme activities and malondialdehyde plasma levels in amenorrheic women. *J Clin Endocrinol Metab* 82:173, 1997.

87. Sack MN, Rader DJ, Cannon RO: Oestrogen and inhibition of oxidation of low-density lipoproteins in postmenopausal women. *Lancet* 343:269, 1994.

88. Shwaery GT, Vita JA, Keaney JF Jr, et al: Antioxidant protection of LDL by physiological concentration of 17β-estradiol: Requirement for estradiol modification. *Circulation* 95:1378, 1997.

88a. Ridker PM, Buring JE, Shih J, et al: Prospective study of C-reactive protein and the risk of future cardiovascular events among apparently healthy women. *Circulation* 98:731, 1998.

89. Ridker PM, Hennekens CH, Buring JE, Rifai N: C-reactive protein and other markers of inflammation in the prediction of cardiovascular disease in women. *N Engl J Med* 342:836, 2000.

90. Cushman M, Legault C, Barrett-Connor E, et al: Effect of postmenopausal hormones on inflammation-sensitive proteins: The Postmenopausal Estrogen/Progestin Interventions (PEPI) Study. *Circulation* 100:717, 1999.

90a. Koh KK, Schenke WH, Waclawiw MA, et al: Statin attenuates increase in C-reactive protein during estrogen replacement therapy in postmenopausal women. *Circulation* 105:1531, 2002.

91. Roussouw JE: Estrogens for the prevention of CHD. *Circulation* 94:2982, 1996.

92. Lieberman EH, Gerhard MD, Akimi E, et al: Estrogen improves endothelium-dependent flow-mediated vasodilation in postmenopausal women. *Ann Intern Med* 121:936, 1994.

93. The Women's Health Initiative Study Group. Design of the Women's Health Initiative Clinical Trial and Observational Study. *Control Clin Trials* 19:61, 1998.

94. Frishman WH: HRT for CAD prevention: Panacea or problem? *Cardiol Rev* 18:39, 2001.

94a. Womens Health Initiative Investigators: Risks and benefits of estrogen plus progestin in healthy postmenopausal women. Principal results from the Womens Health Initiative Randomized Controlled Trial. *JAMA* 288:321, 2002.

94b. Enserink M: Despite safety concerns, U.K. hormone study to proceed. *Science* 297:492, 2002.

95. Hulley S, Grady D, Bush T, et al: Randomized trial of estrogen plus progestin for secondary prevention of coronary heart disease in postmenopausal women. *JAMA* 280:605, 1998.

95a. Grady D, Herrington D, Bittner V, et al: Cardiovascular disease outcomes during 6.8 years of hormone therapy. Heart and Estrogen/Progestin Replacement Study follow-up (HERS II). *JAMA* 288:49, 2002.

96. Grady D, Wenger NK, Herrington D, et al for the Heart and Estrogen/progestin Replacement Study Research Group: Postmenopausal hormone therapy increases risk for venous thromboembolic disease. The Heart and Estrogen/progestin Replacement Study. *Ann Intern Med* 132:689, 2000.

97. Hsia J, Simon JA, Lin F, et al for the HERS Investigators: Peripheral arterial disease in randomized trial of estrogen with progestin in women with coronary heart disease. The Heart and Estrogen/Progestin Replacement Study. *Circulation* 102:2228, 2000.

98. Simon JA, Hsia J, Cauley JA, et al for the HERS Research Group: Postmenopausal hormone therapy and risk of stroke. The Heart and Estrogen-progestin Replacement Study (HERS). *Circulation* 103:638, 2001.

99. Herrington DM, Reboussin DM, Brosnihan KB, et al: Effects of estrogen replacement on the progression of coronary-artery atherosclerosis. *N Engl J Med* 343:522, 2000.

100. Alexander KP, Newby K, Hellkamp AS, et al: Initiation of hormone replacement therapy after acute myocardial infarction is associated with more cardiac events during follow up. *J Am Coll Cardiol* 38:1, 2001.

101. Heckbert SR, Kaplan RC, Weiss NS, et al: Risk of recurrent coronary events in relation to use and recent initiation of postmenopausal hormone therapy. *Arch Intern Med* 161:1709, 2001.

102. Rossouw JE: Early risk of cardiovascular events after commencing hormone replacement therapy. *Curr Opin Lipidol* 12:371, 2001.

103. Grodstein F, Manson JE, Stampfer MJ: Postmenopausal hormone use and secondary prevention of coronary events in the Nurses' Health Study. *Ann Intern Med* 135:1, 2001.

104. Viscoli CM, Brass LM, Kernan WN, et al: A clinical trial of estrogen-replacement therapy after ischemic stroke. *N Engl J Med* 345:1243, 2001.

105. Manson JE, Martin KA: Postmenopausal hormone-replacement therapy. *N Engl J Med* 345:34, 2001.

105a. Laine C: Postmenopausal hormone replacement thrrerapy: How could we have been so wrong? *Ann Intern Med* 137:290, 2002.

106. Goldfrank D, Haytoglu T, Frishman WH, Zalt M: Raloxifene, a new selective estrogen receptor modulator. *J Clin Pharmacol* 39:767, 1999.

107. Clarke SC, Schofield PM, Grace AA, et al: Tamoxifen effects on endothelial function and cardiovascular risk factors in men with advanced atherosclerosis. *Circulation* 103:1497, 2001.

108. Mosca L, Barrett-Connor E, Wenger NK, et al: Design and methods of the Raloxifene Use for the Heart (RUTH) study. *Am J Cardiol* 88:392, 2001.

109. Gilligan DM, Badar DM, Panza JA, et al: Effects of estrogen replacement therapy on peripheral vasomotor function in postmenopausal women. *Am J Cardiol* 75:264, 1995.

110. Sanderson JE, Haines CJ, Yeung L, et al: Anti-ischemic action of estrogen-progestogen continuous combined hormone replacement therapy in postmenopausal women with established angina pectoris: a randomized, placebo-controlled, double-blind, parallel-group trial. *J Cardiovasc Pharmacol* 38:372, 2001.

111. Rosano GMC, Webb CM, Chierchia S, et al: Natural progesterone but not medroxy-progesterone acetate enhances the beneficial effect of estrogen on exercise-induced myocardial ischemia in postmenopausal women. *J Am Coll Cardiol* 36:2154, 2000.

112. Sarrel PM, Lindsay D, Rosano GMC, Poole-Wilson PA: Angina and normal coronary arteries in women: Gynecological findings. *Am J Obstet Gynecol* 167:467, 1992.

112a. Kawano H, Motoyama T, Ohgushi M, et al: Menstrual cycle variation of myocardial ischemia in premenopausal women with variant angina. *Ann Intern Med* 135:977, 2001.

113. Kawano H, Motoyama T, Hirai N, et al: Estradiol supplementation suppresses hyperventilation-induced attacks in postmenopausal women with variant angina. *J Am Coll Cardiol* 37:735, 2001.

113a. Langer RD: Hormone replacement and the prevention of cardiovascular disease. *Am J Cardiol* 89:36E, 2002.

113b. Petitti DB: Hormone replacement therapy for prevention. More evidence, more pessimism (editorial). *JAMA* 288:99, 2002.

113c. Nelson HD, Humphrey LL, Nygren P, et al: Postmenopausal hormone replacement therapy. Scientific Review. *JAMA* 288:872, 2002.

114. Mosca L, Collins P, Herrington DM, et al: Hormone replacement therapy and cardiovascular disease. A statement for healthcare professionals from the American Heart Association. *Circulation* 104:499, 2001.

115. Balfour JA, Heel RC: Transdermal estradiol: A review of its pharmacodynamic and pharmacokinetic properties, and therapeutic efficacy in the treatment of menopausal complaints. *Drugs* 40(4):561, 1990.

116. Carr BR, Bradshaw KD. Disorders of the ovary and female reproductive tract. In: Braunwald E, Fauci AS, Kasper DL, et al, eds. *Harrison's Principles of Internal Medicine*. 15th ed. New York: McGraw-Hill 2001:2154–2167.

117. Lobo RA: Cardiovascular implications of estrogen replacement therapy. *Obstet Gynecol* 75(Suppl):18S, 1990.

118. Lobo RA: Absorption and metabolic effects of different types of estrogen and progestogens. *Obstet Gynecol Clin North Am* 14:143, 1987.

119. Campbell S, Whitehead MI: Potency and hepatocellular effects of oestrogens after oral percutaneous and subcutaneous administration. In: Van Keep PS, Utian WH, Vermeulen A, eds. *The Controversial Climacteric*. Lancaster, UK: MTP Press, 1982.

120. Voigt LF, Weiss NS, Chu J, et al: Progestogen supplementation of exogenous oestrogens and risk of endometrial cancer. *Lancet* 338:274, 1991.

121. Hunt K, Vessey M: Mortality from cancer and cardiovascular disease and hormonal substitution therapy. In: L'Hermite M, ed. *Update on Hormonal Substitution Treatment in the Menopause. Progress in Reproductive Biology and Medicine*. Basel: Karger, 1989:13:63.

122. Chu J, Schweid AI, Weiss NS: Survival among women with endometrial cancer: A comparison of estrogen users and nonusers. *Am J Obstet Gynecol* 143:569, 1982.

123. Shapiro S, Kelly JP, Rosenberg L, et al: Risk of localized and widespread endometrial cancer in relation to recent and discontinued use of conjugated estrogens. *N Engl J Med* 313:969, 1985.

124. Weiderpass E, Adami HO, Baron JA, et al: Risk of endometrial cancer following estrogen replacement with and without progestins. *J Natl Cancer Inst* 91:1131, 1999.

125. Pike MC, Peters RK, Cozen W, et al: Estrogen-progestin replacement therapy and endometrial cancer. *J Natl Cancer Inst* 89:1110, 1997.

126. Clisham PR, Cedars MI, Greendale G, et al: Long-term transdermal estradiol therapy: Effects on endometrial histology and bleeding patterns. *Obstet Gynecol* 79:196, 1992.

127. Rodriguez C, Patel AV, Calle EE, et al: Estrogen replacement therapy and ovarian cancer mortality in a large prospective study of US women. *JAMA* 285:1460, 2001.

128. Grodstein F, Newcomb PA, Stampfer MJ: Postmenopausal hormone therapy and the risk of colorectal cancer: A review and meta-analysis. *Am J Med* 106:574, 1999.

129. Clemons M, Goss P: Estrogen and the risk of breast cancer. *N Engl J Med* 344:276, 2001.

130. Lando JF, Heck KE, Brett KM: Hormone replacement therapy and breast cancer risk in a nationally representative cohort. *Am J Prev Med* 17:176, 1999.

131. Collaborative Group on Hormonal Factors in Breast Cancer. Breast cancer and hormonal replacement therapy: Collaborative reanalysis of data from 51 epidemiological studies of 52,705 women with breast cancer and 108,411 women without breast cancer. *Lancet* 350:1047, 1997.

132. Colditz GA, Hankinson SE, Hunter DJ, et al: The use of estrogens and progestins and the risk of breast cancer in postmenopausal women. *N Engl J Med* 332:1589, 1995.

133. Schairer C, Lubin J, Troisi R, et al: Menopausal estrogen and estrogen-progestin replacement therapy and breast cancer risk. *JAMA* 283:485, 2000.

134. Hargreaves DF, Knox F, Swindell R, et al: Epithelial proliferation and hormone receptor status in the normal post-menopausal breast and the effects of hormone replacement therapy. *Br J Cancer* 78:945, 1998.

135. Poutanen M, Isomaa V, Peltoketo H, Vihko R: Role of 17-hydroxysteroid dehydrogenase type 1 in endocrine and intracrine estradiol biosynthesis. *J Steroid Biochem Mol Biol* 55:525, 1995.

135a. Hulley S, Furberg C, Barrett-Connor E, et al: Noncardiovascular disease outcomes during 6.8 years of hormone therapy. Heart and Estrogen/Progestin Replacement Study follow-up (HERS II). *JAMA* 288:58, 2002.

136. Pollack BG, Wylie M, Stack JA, et al: Inhibition of caffeine metabolism by estrogen replacement therapy in postmenopausal women. *J Clin Pharmacol* 39:936, 1999.

137. Sitruk-Ware R: Estrogen therapy during menopause: practical treatment recommendations. *Drugs* 39:203, 1990.

138. Conard J, Cazenave B, Samama M, et al: Antithrombin III content and antithrombin activity in oestrogen-progestogen and progestogen-only treated women. *Thromb Res* 18:675, 1980.

138a. Herkert O, Kuhl H, Sandow J, et al: Sex steroids used in hormonal treatment increase vascular procoagulant activity by inducing thrombin receptor (PAR-1) expression. Role of the glucocorticoid receptor. *Circulation* 104:2826, 2001.

139. Ottosson UB, Johansson BG, von Schoultz B: Subfractions of high-density lipoprotein cholesterol during estrogen replacement therapy: A comparison between progestogens and natural progesterone. *Am J Obstet Gynecol* 151:746, 1985.

140. Martin KA, Freeman MW: Postmenopausal hormone replacement therapy (editorial). *N Engl J Med* 328:1115, 1993.

141. Medical Research Council's General Practice Framework. Randomised comparison of oestrogen versus oestrogen plus progestogen replace therapy in women with hysterectomy. *BMJ* 312:473, 1996.

142. Mercuro G, Pitzalis L, Podda A, et al: Effects of acute administration of natural progesterone on peripheral vascular responsiveness in healthy postmenopausal women. *Am J Cardiol* 84:214, 1999.

143. Hillard TC, Siddle NC, Whitehead MI, et al: Continuous combined conjugated equine estrogen-progestogen therapy: Effects of medroxyprogesterone acetate and norethindrone acetate on bleeding patterns and endometrial histologic diagnosis. *Am J Obstet Gynecol* 167:1, 1992.

144. Mashchak CA, Lobo RA, Dozono-Takano R, et al: Comparison of pharmacodynamic properties of various estrogen formulations. *Am J Obstet Gynecol* 144:511, 1982.

145. Judd H: Efficacy of transdermal estradiol. *Am J Obstet Gynecol* 156:1326, 1987.

146. Archer DF, Dorin M, Lewis V, et al: Effects of lower doses of conjugated equine estrogens and medroxyprogesterone acetate on endometrial bleeding. *Fertil Steril* 75:1080, 2001.

147. Lobo RA, Bush T, Carr BR, Pickar JH: Effects of lower doses of conjugated equine estrogens and medroxyprogesterone acetate on plasma lipids and lipoproteins, coagulation factors, and carbohydrate metabolism. *Fertil Steril* 76:1324, 2001.

148. Gibbons WE, Moyer DL, Lobo RA, et al: Biochemical and histologic effects of sequential estrogen/progestin therapy on the endometrium of postmenopausal women. *Am J Obstet Gynecol* 154:456, 1986.

149. Hargrove JT, Maxson WS, Wentz AC, Burnett LS: Menopausal hormone replacement therapy with continuous daily oral micronized estradiol and progesterone. *Obstet Gynecol* 73:606, 1989.

150. Glazier MG, Bowman MA: A review of the evidence for the use of phytoestrogens as a replacement for traditional estrogen replacement therapy. *Arch Intern Med* 161:1161, 2001.

151. Thompson LU, Robb P, Serraino M, Cheung F: Mammalian lignan production from various foods. *Nutr Cancer* 16:43, 1991.

152. Hertog MG, Kronhout D, Aravonis C, et al: Flavanoid intake and long-tern risk of coronary heart disease and cancer in the seven countries study. *Arch Intern Med* 155:381, 1995.

153. Bennetts HW, Underwood EJ, Shier FL: A specific breeding problem of sheep on subterranean clover pastures in Western Australia. *Aust Vet J* 22:2, 1975.

154. Adlercruetz H, Hockerstedt K, Bannwart C, et al: Effect of dietary components, including lignans and phytoestrogens, on enterohepatic circulation and liver metabolism of estrogens and on sex hormone binding globulin. *J Steroid Biochem* 27:1135, 1987.

155. Keys A, Menotti A, Aravanis C, et al: The seven countries study: 2,289 deaths in 15 years. *Prev Med* 13:141, 1984.

156. Barnes S, Peterson TG, Coward L: Rationale for the use of genistein-containing soy matrices in chemoprevention trials for breast and prostate cancer. *J Cell Biochem* 22:181, 1995.

157. Anderson JW, Johnstone BM, Cook-Newell ME: Meta-analysis of the effects of soy protein intake on serum lipids. *N Engl J Med* 333:276, 1995.

158. Sirtori CR, Lovati MR, Manzoni C, et al: Soy and cholesterol reduction: Clinical experience. *J Nutr* 125:598S, 1995.

159. Hirose N, Inoue T, Nishihara K, et al: Inhibition of cholesterol absorption and synthesis in rats by sesamin. *J Lipid Res* 32:629, 1991.

160. Tikkanen MJ, Wähälä K, Ojala S, et al: Effect of soybean phytoestrogen intake on low density lipoprotein oxidation resistance. *Proc Natl Acad Sci U S A* 95:3106, 1998.

161. Raines EW, Ross R: Biology of atherosclerotic plaque formation: Possible role of growth factors in lesion development and the potential impact of soy. *J Nutr* 125:624S, 1995.

162. Fotsis T, Pepper M, Adlercreutz H, et al: Genistein, a dietary ingested isoflavonoid, inhibits cell proliferation and in vitro angiogenesis. *J Nutr* 125:790, 1995.

163. Takahashi M, Ikeda U, Masuyama JI, et al: Monocyte-endothelial cell interaction induces expression of adhesion molecules on human umbilical cord endothelial cells. *Cardiovasc Res* 32:422, 1996.

164. Akiyama T, Ishida J, Nakagawa S, et al: Genistein, a specific inhibitor of tyrosine-specific protein kinases. *J Biol Chem* 262:5592, 1987.

165. Honoré EK, Williams JK, Anthony MS, Clarkson TB: Soy isoflavones enhance coronary vascular reactivity in atherosclerotic female macaques. *Fertil Steril* 67:148, 1997.

166. March JD: Phytoestrogens and vascular therapy (editorial, comment). *J Am Coll Cardiol* 35:1986, 2000.

167. Figtree GA, Griffiths H, Lu Y-A, et al: Plant-derived estrogens relax coronary arteries in vivo by a calcium antagonistic mechanism. *J Am Coll Cardiol* 35:1977, 2000.

168. Nevala R, Korpela R, Vapaatalo H: Plant-derived estrogens relax rat mesenteric artery in vivo. *Life Sci* 63:95, 1998.

169. Vanharanta M, Voutilainen S, Lakka TA, et al: Risk of acute coronary events according to concentration of enterolactone: A prospective population-based case-control study. *Lancet* 354:2112, 1999.

170. Parry CH: *Collections from the Unpublished Works of the late Caleb Hillier Parry.* Vol 1. London: Underwood, 1786:478.

171. Graves RF: Newly observed affection of the thyroid gland in females. *Lond Med Surg J* 7:516, 1835.

172. Sandler G, Wilson GM: The nature and prognosis of heart disease in thyrotoxicosis. *Quart J Med* 28:247, 1959.

173. Zondek H: Das myxodemherz. *Muench Med Wochenschr* 65:1180, 1918.

174. Levey GS, Klein I: Disorders of the thyroid. In: Stein J, ed. *Stein's Textbook of Medicine.* 2d ed. Boston: Little Brown, 1994:1383.

175. Brent GA: The molecular basis of thyroid hormone action. *N Engl J Med* 331:847, 1994.

176. Dillman WH: Biochemical basis of thyroid hormone action in the heart. *Am J Med* 88:626, 1990.

177. Morkin E: Regulation of myosin heavy chain genes in the heart. *Circulation* 87:68, 1993.

178. Kiss E, Jakab G, Kranias EG, Edes I: Thyroid hormone-induced alterations in phospholamban protein expression. Regulatory effects on sarcoplasmic reticulum Ca^{2+} transport and myocardial relaxation. *Circ Res* 75:245, 1994.

179. Kamitani T, Ikeda U, Muto et al: Regulation of Na-K-ATPase gene expression by thyroid hormone in rat cardiocytes. *Circ Res* 71:1457, 1992.

180. Dozin B, Manguson MA, Nikodm VM: Thyroid hormone regulation of malic enzyme synthesis. *J Biol Chem* 261:10290, 1986.

181. Landenson PW, Block KD, Seidman JG: Modulation of atrial natriuretic factor by thyroid hormone: messenger ribonucleic acid and peptide levels in hypothyroid, euthyroid, and hyperthyroid rat atria and ventricles. *Endocrinol* 123:652, 1988.

182. Kim D, Smith TW, Marsh JD: Effect of thyroid hormone on slow calcium channel function in cultured chick cells. *J Clin Invest* 80:88, 1987.

183. Stiles GL, Lefkowitz RJ: Thyroid hormone modulation of agonist-beta-adrenergic receptor interactions in the rat heart. *Life Sci* 28:2529, 1981.

184. Walker JD, Crawford RA Jr, Mukherjee R, Spinale FG: The direct effects of 3,5,3'-triiodo-L-thyronine (T_3) on myocyte contractile processes. Insights into mechanisms of action. *J Thoracic Cardovasc Surg* 110(5):1369, 1995.

185. Manger JA, Clark W, Allenby P: Congestive heart failure and sudden death in a young women with thyrotoxicosis. *West J Med* 8:55, 1990.

186. Landenson PW, Sherman SI, Baughman KL, et al: Reversible alterations in myocardial gene expression in a young man with dilated cardiomyopathy and hypothyroidism. *Proc Natl Acad Sci U S A* 89:5251, 1993.

187. Alpert NR, Nulieri LA: Thermomechanical energy of hypertrophied hearts. In: Alpert NR, ed. *Perspectives in Cardiovascular Research: Myocardial Hypertrophy and Failure.* New York: Raven Press, 1983:619.

188. Guyton AC: The relationship of cardiac output and arterial pressure control. *Circulation* 64:1079, 1981.

189. Ojamaa K, Klein I: In vivo regulation of recombinant cardiac myosin heavy chain gene expression by thyroid hormone. *Endocrinol* 132:1002, 1993.

190. Klein I: Thyroid hormone and the cardiovascular system. *Am J Med* 88:631, 1990.

191. Klein I: Thyroid hormone and high blood pressure. In: Laragh JH, Brenner BM, Kaplan NM, eds. *Endocrine Mechanisms in Hypertension.* Vol 2. New York: Raven Press, 1989:61.

192. Klein I: Thyroid hormone and blood pressure regulation. In: Laragh JH, Brenner BM, Kaplan NM, eds. *Endocrine Mechanisms in Hypertension.* Vol 2. New York: Raven Press, 1989:1661.

193. Dillman WH: Cardiac function in thyroid disease: Clinical features and management considerations. *Ann Thorac Surg* 56:S9, 1993.

193a. Napoli R, Biondi B, Guardasole V, et al: Impact of hyperthyroidism and its correction on vascular reactivity in humans. *Circulation* 104: 3076, 2001.

194. Ismail-Beigi F, Haber RS, Loeb JN: Stimulation of active Na and K transport by thyroid hormone in a rat liver cell line: Role of enhanced Na entry. *Endocrinol* 119:2527, 1986.

195. Kapitola J, Vilimovska D: Inhibition of the early circulatory effects of triiodothyronine in rats by propranolol. *Physiol Bohemoslov* 30:347, 1981.

196. Dyke CM, Yek T Jr, Lehman JD, et al: Thiodinone-enhanced left ventricular function after ischemic injury. *Ann Thorac Surg* 52:14, 1991.

197. Klemperer JD, Zelano J, Helm R, et al: Triiodothyronine improves left ventricular function without oxygen wasting effects following global hypothermic ischemia. *J Thorac Cardiovasc Surg* 109:457, 1995.

198. Amidi H, Leon DF, Degroot WJ, et al: Effect of the thyroid state on myocardial contractility and ventricular ejection rate in man. *Circulation* 38:229, 1968.

199. Levey GS, Klein I: Catecholamine-thyroid hormone interactions and the cardiovascular manifestations of hyperthyroidism. *Am J Med* 88:642, 1990.

200. Liggett SB, Shah SD, Cryer PE: Increased fat and skeletal muscle β-adrenergic receptors but unaltered metabolic and hemodynamic sensitivity to epinephrine in vivo in experimental human thyrotoxicosis. *J Clin Invest* 83:803, 1989.

201. Walker JD, Crawford FA, Mukherjee R, et al: Direct effects of acute administration of 3,5,3'-triiodo-L-thyronine on myocyte function. *Ann Thoracic Surg* 58:851, 1994.

202. Ririe DG, Butterworth JF 4th, Royster RL, et al: Triiodothyronine increases contractility independent of β-adrenergic receptors of stimulation of cyclic-3',5'-adenosine monophosphate. *Anesthesiology* 82:1004, 1995.

in Lp(a) and HDL concentrations. *Arterioscler Thromb* 13:296, 1993.

308. Wannenburg T, Khan AS, Sane DC, et al: Growth hormone reverses age-related cardiac myofilament dysfunction in rats. *Am J Physiol* 281:H915, 2001.

309. Feinberg MS, Scheinowitz M, Laron Z: Echocardiographic dimensions and function in adults with primary growth hormone resistance (Laron syndrome). *Am J Cardiol* 85:209, 2000.

310. Cuneo RC, Salomon F, Wilmshurst P, et al: Cardiovascular effects of growth hormone treatment in growth-hormone-deficient adults: Stimulation of the renin-aldosterone system. *Clin Sci (Colch)* 81:587, 1991.

311. Bengtsson B-A, Eden S, Lonn L, et al: Treatment of adults with growth hormone (GH) deficiency with recombinant human GH. *J Clin Endocrinol Metab* 76(2):309, 1993.

312. Jorgensen JOL, Moller J, Alberti KGMM, et al: Marked effects of sustained low growth hormone (GH) levels on day-to-day fuel metabolism: studies in GH-deficient patients and healthy untreated subjects. *J Clin Endocrinol Metab* 77(6):1589, 1993.

313. Jorgensen JOL, Flyvbjerg A, Lauritzen T, et al: Dose-reponse studies with biosynthetic human growth hormone (GH) in GH-deficient patients. *J Clin Endocrinol Metab* 67:36, 1988.

314. Moller J, Jorgensen JOL, Lauersen T, et al: Growth hormone dose regimens in adult GH deficiency: Effects on biochemical growth markers and metabolic parameters. *Clin Endocrinol (Oxf)* 39:403, 1993.

315. Jeffcoate W: Can growth hormone therapy cause diabetes (commentary)? *Lancet* 355:589, 2000.

315a. Swerdlow AJ, Higgins CD, Adlard P, Preece MA: Risk of cancer in patients treated with human pituitary growth hormone in the UK, 1959–85: A cohort study. *Lancet* 360:273, 2002.

316. Ritzen EM: Does growth hormone increase the risk of malignancies? *Horm Res* 39:99, 1993.

317. Vance ML, Mauras N: Growth hormone therapy in adults and children. *N Engl J Med* 341:1206, 1999.

318. Jensen PB, Ekelund B, Nielsen FT, et al: Changes in cardiac muscle mass and function in hemodialysis patients during growth hormone treatment. *Clin Nephrol* 53:25, 2000.

319. Volterrani M, Manelli F, Cicoira M, et al: Role of growth hormone in chronic heart failure. Therapeutic implications. *Drugs* 60:711, 2000.

320. King MK, Gay DM, Pan LC, et al: Treatment with a growth hormone secretagogue in a model of developing heart failure. Effects on ventricular and myocyte function. *Circulation* 103:308, 2001.

321. Genth-Zotz S, Zotz R, Geil S: Recombinant growth hormone therapy in patients with ischemic cardiomyopathy: Effects on hemodynamics, left ventricular function, and cardiopulmonary exercise capacity. *Circulation* 99:18, 1999.

322. Beer N: Beneficial effects of growth hormone in patients with Chagas cardiomyopathy and dilated cardiomyopathy of unknown etiology. Clinical trial and review of the literature. *Cardiovasc Rev Rep* Sept:57, 1998.

323. Hasenfuss G, Mulieri LA, Leavitt BJ, et al: Contractile protein function in failing and nonfailing human myocardium. *Basic Res Cardiol* 87:107, 1992.

324. Arnolda L, Brosnan J, Rajagopalan B, Radda GK: Skeletal muscle metabolism in heart failure in rats. *Am J Physiol* 261:H434, 1992.

325. Massie B, Conway M, Yonge R, et al: Skeletal muscle metabolism in patients with congestive heart failure: Relation to clinical severity and blood flow. *Circulation* 76:1009, 1987.

326. Anker SD, Volterrani M, Pflaum C-D, et al: Acquired growth hormone resistance in patients with chronic heart failure: Implications for therapy with growth hormone. *J Am Coll Cardiol* 38:443, 2001.

327. Giustina A, Volterrani M, Manelli F, et al: Endocrine predictors of acute hemodynamic effects of growth hormone in congestive heart failure. *Am Heart J* 137:1035, 1999.

328. Kinugawa S, Tsutsui H, Ide T, et al: Positive inotropic effect of insulin-like growth factor-1 on normal and failing cardiac myocytes. *Cardiovasc Res* 43(1):157, 1999.

329. Niebauer J, Pflaum CD, Clark AL, et al: Deficient insulin-like growth factor I in chronic heart failure predicts altered body composition, anabolic deficiency, cytokine and neurohormonal activation. *J Am Coll Cardiol* 32(2):393, 1998.

330. Osterziel KJ, Ranke MB, Strohm O, Dietz R: The somatotrophic system in patients with dilated cardiomyopathy: Relation of insulin-like growth factor-1 and its alterations during growth hormone therapy to cardiac function. *Clin Endocrinol (Oxf)* 53:61, 2000.

331. Fazio S, Sabatini D, Capaldo B, et al: A preliminary study of growth hormone in the treatment of dilated cardiomyopathy. *N Engl J Med* 334:809, 1996.

332. Isgaard J, Bergh CH, Caidahl K, et al: A placebo-controlled study of growth hormone in patients with congestive heart failure. *Eur Heart J* 19(11):1704, 1998.

333. Osterziel KJ, Strohm O, Schuler J, et al: Randomised, double-blind, placebo-controlled trial of human recombinant growth hormone in patients with chronic heart failure due to dilated cardiomyopathy. *Lancet* 351(9111):1233, 1998.

334. Shen Y-T, Woltmann RF, Appleby S, et al: Lack of beneficial effects of growth hormone treatment in conscious dogs during development of heart failure. *Am J Physiol* 274:H456, 1998.

335. Ross J Jr: Growth hormone, cardiomyocyte contractile reserve, and heart failure. *Circulation* 99:15, 1999.

335a. Isley WL: Growth hormone therapy for adults: Not ready for prime time? *Ann Intern Med* 137:190, 2002.

336. Castagnino HE, Toranzos FA, Milei J, et al: Preservation of the myocardial collagen framework by human growth hormone in experimental infarctions and reduction in the incidence of ventricular aneurysms. *Int J Cardiol* 35:101, 1992.

337. Castagnino HE, Milei J, Toranzos FA, et al: Bivalent effects of human growth hormone in experimental myocardial infarcts. *Jpn Heart J* 31:45, 1990.

338. Conti E, Andreotti F, Schihbasi A, et al: Markedly reduced insulin-like growth factor-1 in the acute phase of myocardial infarction. *J Am Coll Cardiol* 38:26, 2001.

339. Omerovic E, Bollano E, Mobini R, et al: Growth hormone improves bioenergetics and decreases catecholamines in postinfarct rat hearts. *Endocrinology* 141:4592, 2000.

340. Tajima M, Weinberg EO, Bartunek J, et al: Treatment with growth hormone enhances contractile reserve and intracellular calcium transients in myocytes from rats with postinfarction heart failure. *Circulation* 99:127, 1999.

341. Weekers F, Van Herck E, Isgaard J, Van den Berghe G: Pretreatment with growth hormone-releasing peptide-2 directly protects against the diastolic dysfunction of myocardial stunning in an isolated, blood-perfused rabbit heart model. *Endocrinology* 141:3993, 2000.

342. Spallarossa P, Rossettin P, Minuto F, et al: Evaluation of growth hormone administration in patients with chronic heart failure secondary to coronary artery disease. *Am J Cardiol* 84(4):430, 1999.

343. Friberg L, Werner S, Eggertsen G, Ahnve S: Growth hormone and insulin-like growth factor-1 in acute myocardial infarction. *Eur Heart J* 21(18):1547, 2000.

344. Rudman D, Feller AG, Nagraj HS, et al: Effects of human growth hormone in men over 60 years old. *N Engl J Med* 323:1, 1990.

345. Marcus R, Butterfield G, Holloway L, et al: Effects of short term administration of recombinant human growth hormone to elderly people. *J Clin Endocrinol Metab* 70(2):519, 1990.

346. Larsson B, Svardsudd K, Welin L, et al: Abdominal adipose tissue distribution, obesity and risk of cardiovascular disease and death: 13-year follow up of participants in the study of men born in 1913. *Br Med J* 288:1401, 1984.

347. Papadakis MA, Grady D, Black D, et al: Growth hormone replacement in healthy older men improves body composition but not functional ability. *Ann Intern Med* 124:708, 1996.

348. Takala J, Ruokonen E, Webster NR, et al: Increased mortality associated with growth hormone treatment in critically ill adults. *N Engl J Med* 341:785, 1999.

349. Kupfer SR, Underwood LE, Baxter RC, Clemmons DR: Enhancement of the anabolic effects of growth hormone and insulin-like growth factor I by use of both agents simultaneously. *J Clin Invest* 91:391, 1993.

350. Iovino M, Monteleone P, Steardo L: Repetitive growth hormone-releasing hormone administration restores the attenuated growth hormone (GH) response to GH-releasing hormone testing in normal aging. *J Clin Endocrinol Metab* 69:910, 1989.

351. Corpas E, Hartman SM, Pincyro MA, et al: Growth hormone (GH)-releasing hormone (1-29) twice daily reverses the decreased GH and insulin like growth factor-1 levels in old men. *J Clin Endocrinol Metab* 75:530, 1992.

352. Ghigo E, Ceda GP, Valcavi R, et al: Effect of 15-day treatment with growth hormone-releasing hormone alone or combined with different doses of arginine on the reduced somatotrope responsiveness to the neurohormone in normal aging. *Eur J Endocrinol* 132:32, 1995.

353. Hartman ML, Farello G, Pezzoli SS, Thorner MO: Oral administration of growth hormone (GH)-releasing peptide stimulates GH secretion in normal men. *J Clin Endocrinol Metab* 74:1378, 1992.

354. Mueleman J, Katz P: The immunologic effects, kinetics, and use of glucocorticoids. *Med Clin North Am* 69:805, 1985.

355. Bompras DT, Chousos GP, Wilder RL, et al: Glucocorticoid therapy for immune-mediated diseases: Basis and clinical correlates. *Ann Intern Med* 119:1198, 1993.

356. Fauci AS, Dale DC, Balow JE: Glucocorticosteroid therapy: mechanisms of action and clinical considerations. *Ann Intern Med* 84:304, 1976.

357. Cupps TR, Gerrard TL, Falkoff RJ, et al: Effects of an in vitro corticosteroid on B cell activation, proliferation, and differentiation. *J Clin Invest* 75:754, 1985.

358. Butler WT, Rossen RD: Effects of corticosteroids on immunity in man: Decreased serum IgG concentration caused by 3 or 5 days of high doses of methylprednisolone. *J Clin Invest* 52:2629, 1973.

359. Sambhi MP, Weil MH, Udohoji VN: Acute pharmacodynamic effects of glucocorticoids. Cardiac output and related hemodynamic changes in normal subjects and patients in shock. *Circulation* 31:523, 1965.

360. Spanier AJ, McDonough KH: Dexamethasone blocks sepsis-induced protection of the heart from ischemia-reperfusion injury. *Proc Soc Exp Biol Med* 223(1):82, 2000.

361. Kurowski TT, Czerwinski SM: Glucocorticoid modulation of cardiac mass and protein. *Med Sci Sports Exerc* 22:312, 1990.

362. Sheer D, Morkin E: Myosin isoenzyme expression in rat ventricle: effects of thyroid hormone analogs, catecholamines, glucocorticoids, and high carbohydrate diet. *J Pharmacol Exp Ther* 229:872, 1984.

363. Czerwinski SM, Kuowski TT, McKee EE, et al: Myosin heavy chain turnover during cardiac mass changes by glucocorticoids. *J Appl Physiol* 70:300, 1991.

364. Libby P, Maroko PR, Bloor CM, et al: Reduction of experimental myocardial infarct size by corticosteroid administration. *J Clin Invest* 52:599, 1973.

365. Hinshaw LB: Effects of methylprednisolone on myocardial performance, hemodynamics, and metabolism in normal and failing hearts (abstr.). *Clin Res* 21:196, 1973.

366. Barzilai D, Plavnick J, Hazani A, et al: Use of hydrocortisone in the treatment of myocardial infarction. *Chest* 61:488, 1972.

367. Scientific Subcommittee of the Scottish Society of Physicians. Hydrocortisone in severe myocardial infarction. *Lancet* 2:785, 1964.

368. Morrison J, Maley T, Reduto L, et al: Effect of methyl-prednisolone on predicted myocardial infarction size in man. *Crit Care Med* 3:94, 1975.

369. Kloner RA, Fishbein MC, Lew H, et al: Mummification of the infarcted myocardium by high dose corticosteroids. *Circulation* 57(1):56, 1978.

370. Scheuer DA, Mufflin SW: Chronic corticosterone treatment increases myocardial infarct size in rats with ischemia-reperfusion injury. *Am J Physiol* 272(6 pt 2):R2017, 1997.

371. Roberts R, DeMello V, Sobel BE: Deleterious effects of methylprednisolone in patients with myocardial infarction. *Circulation* 53:I, 1976.

372. Dall JLC, Buchanan J: Steroid therapy in heart block following myocardial infarction. *Lancet* 2:8, 1962.

372a. Myocarditis article.

373. Kilbourne ED, Smart KM, Pokorny BA: Inhibition by cortisone of the synthesis and action of interferon. *Nature* 190:650, 1961.

374. Parillo JE, Aretz HT, Palacios I, et al: The results of transvenous endomyocardial biopsy can frequently be used to diagnose myocardial disease in patients with idiopathic heart failure: Endomyocardial biopsies in 100 consecutive patients revealed a substantial incidence of myocarditis. *Circulation* 69:93, 1984.

375. Mason JW, Billingham ME, Ricci DR: Treatment of acute inflammatory myocarditis assisted by endomyocardial biopsy. *Am J Cardiol* 45:1037, 1980.

376. Dec Jr GW, Palacios IF, Fallon JT, et al: Active myocarditis in the spectrum of acute dilated cardiomyopathies. Clinical features, histologic correlates, and clinical outcome. *N Engl J Med* 312:885, 1985.

377. Parillo JE, Cunnion RE, Epstein SE, et al: A prospective, randomized, controlled study of prednisone for dilated cardiomyopathy. *N Engl J Med* 321:1061, 1989.

378. Aretz HT, Billingham ME, Edwards WD, et al: Myocarditis, a histopathologic definition and classification. *Am J Cardiovasc Pathol* 1:3, 1986.

379. Jones SR, Herskowitz A, Hutchins GM, Baughman KL: Effects of immunosuppressive therapy in biopsy-proved myocarditis and borderline myocarditis on left ventricular function. *Am J Cardiol* 68:370, 1991.

380. Zee-Cheng C, Tsai CC, Palmer DC, et al: High incidence of myocarditis by endomyocardial biopsy in patients with idiopathic congestive cardiomyopathy. *J Am Coll Cardiol* 3:63, 1984.

381. Mason JW, O'Connell JB, Herskowitz A, et al: A clinical trial of immunosuppressive therapy for myocarditis. *N Engl J Med* 333:269, 1995.

382. Kodama M, Okura Y, Hirono S, et al: A new scoring system to predict the efficacy of steroid therapy for patients with active myocarditis—a retrospective study. *Jpn Circ J* 62(10):715, 1998.

383. Menghini VV, Savcenko V, Olson LJ, et al: Combined immunosuppression for the treatment of idiopathic giant cell myocarditis. *Mayo Clin Proc* 74(12):1221, 1999.

384. Ensley RD, Ives M, Zhao L, et al: Effects of alloimmune injury on contraction and relaxation in cultured myocytes and intact cardiac allografts. *J Am Coll Cardiol* 24:1769, 1994.

385. Vester EG, Klein RM, Kuhl U, et al: Immunosuppressive therapy for effective suppression of life-threatening ventricular tachyarrhythmias in chronic myocarditis (German). *Zeitschrift fur Kardiologie* 86(4):298, 1997.

386. Schmaltz AA, Demel KP, Kallenberg R, et al: Immunosuppressive therapy of chronic myocarditis in children: Three cases and the design of a randomized prospective trial of therapy. *Pediatr Cardiol* 19:235, 1998.

387. Kleinert S, Weintraub RG, Wilkinson JL, et al: Myocarditis in children with dilated cardiomyopathy: incidence and outcome after dual therapy immunosuppression. *J Heart Lung Transplant* 16:1248, 1997.

388. Herdy GV, Pinto CA, Olivaes MC, et al: Rheumatic carditis treated with high dose of pulse therapy methylprednisolone. Results in 70 children over 12 years. *Arq Bras Cardiol* 72(5):601, 1999.

389. Miranda-Mallea J, Perez-Verdu J, Gasco-Lacalle B: Hypertrophic cardiomyopathy in preterm infants treated with dexamethasone. *Eur J Pediatr* 156:394, 1997.

390. Fowler NO, Harbin D: Recurrent acute pericarditis: Follow up study of 31 patients. *J Am Coll Cardiol* 7:300, 1986.

391. Maisch B, Pankuweit S, Brilla C, et al: Intrapericardial treatment of inflammatory and neoplastic pericarditis guided by pericardioscopy and epicardial biopsy-results from a pilot study. *Clin Cardiol (Oxf)* 22(Suppl 1):117, 1999.

392. Gurevich MA, Mravian SR, Grigor'eva NM: Myopericarditis: Clinical picture, diagnosis and treatment [Russian]. *Klin Med (Mosk)* 77(7):33, 1999.

393. Clementy J, Jambert H, Dallacchio M: Les pericardites aigues recidivantes: 20 observations. *Arch Mal Coeur Vaiss* 72:857, 1979.

394. Rumalla V, Calvano SE, Spotnitz AJ, et al: The effects of glucocorticoid therapy on inflammatory responses to coronary artery bypass graft surgery. *Arch Surg* 136:1039, 2001.

395. Mott AR, Fraser CD Jr., Kusnoor AV, et al: The effect of short-term prophylactic methylprednisolone on the incidence and severity of postpericardiotomy syndrome in children undergoing cardiac surgery with cardiopulmonary bypass. *J Am Coll Cardiol* 37:1700, 2001.

396. Bhasin S, Storer TW, Berman N, et al: The effects of supra-physiologic doses of testosterone on muscle size and strength in normal men. *N Engl J Med* 335:1, 1996.

397. Bagatell CJ, Bremner WJ: Androgens in men—uses and abuses (review article). *N Engl J Med* 334:707, 1996.

398. Phillips GB, Pinkernell BH, Jing T-Y: The association of hypotestosternemia with coronary artery disease in men. *Arterioscler Thromb Vasc Biol* 14:701, 1994.

399. Degroot LJ, ed. *Endocrinology*. 3rd ed. Philadelphia: WB Saunders, 1995.

400. Snyder PJ, Peachey H, Berlin JA, et al: Effects of testosterone replacement in hypogonadal men. *J Clin Endocrinol Metab* 85(8):2670, 2000.

401. Harman SM, Metter EJ, Tobin JD, et al: Longitudinal effects of aging on serum total and free testosterone levels in healthy men. *J Clin Endocrinol Metab* 86:724, 2001.

402. Mendel CN: The free hormone hypothesis: A physiologically based mathematical model. *Endocr Rev* 10:232, 1989.

403. Bowman S, Tanna S, Fernando S, et al: Anabolic steroids and infarction. *BMJ* 299:632, 1989.

404. Heiss G, Tamir I, Davis CE, et al: Lipoprotein-cholesterol distributions in selected North American populations: The Lipid Research Clinics Program Prevalence Study. *Circulation* 61:302, 1980.

405. Zmuda JM, Cauley JA, Kriska A, et al: Longitudinal relation between endogenous testosterone and cardiovascular disease risk factors in middle-aged men. A 13-year follow-up of former Multiple Risk Factor Intervention Trial participants. *Am J Epidemiol* 146(8):609, 1997.

406. Morrison JA, Sprecher DL, Biro FM, et al: Estradiol and testosterone effects on lipids in black and white boys aged 10 to 15 years. *Metabolism* 49(9):1124, 2000.

407. Bagatell C, Knopp RH, Vale W, Rivier JE, Bremner W: Physiologic testosterone levels in normal men suppress high-density lipoprotein cholesterol level. *Ann Intern Med* 116(12 pt 1):967, 1992.

408. Bucher D, Behre HM, Kleisch S, et al: Effects of testosterone suppression in young men by the gonadotropin releasing hormone antagonist cetrorelix on plasma lipids, lipolytic enzymes, lipid transfer proteins, insulin and leptin. *Exp Clin Endocrinol Diabetes* 107(8):522, 1999.

409. Jockenhovel F, Bullmann C, Schubert M, et al: Influence of various modes of androgen substitution on serum lipids and lipoproteins in hypogonadal men. *Metabolism* 48(5):590, 1999.

410. Wu S, Weng X: Therapeutic effects of andriol on serum lipids and apolipoproteins in elderly male coronary heart disease patients. *Chin Med Sci J* 7:137, 1992.

411. Tenover JS: Effects of testosterone supplementation in the aging male. *J Clin Endocrinol Metab* 75:1092, 1992.

412. Broeder CE, Quindry J, Brittingham K, et al: Physiological and hormonal influences of androstenedione supplementation in men 35 to 65 years old participating in a high-intensity resistance training program. *Arch Intern Med* 160:3093, 2000.

413. Bagatell CJ, Heiman JJR, Matsumoto AM, et al: Metabolic and behavioral effects of high dose, exogenous testosterone in healthy men. *J Clin Endocrinol Metab* 79:561, 1994.

414. Cohen LI, Hartford CG, Rogers GG: Lipoprotein (a) and cholesterol in body builders using anabolic androgenic steroids. *Med Sci Sports Exerc* 28:176, 1996.

415. Ferenchick GS: Anabolic/androgenic steroid abuse and thrombosis: Is there a connection? *Med Hypotheses* 35:27, 1991.

416. Ajayi AAL, Mahur R, Halushka PV: Testosterone increases human platelet thromboxane A2 receptor density and aggregation responses. *Circulation* 91:2742, 1995.

417. Yang X, Jing TJ, Resnick LM, Philips GB: Relation of hemostatic risk factors to other risk factors for coronary heart disease and to sex hormone in men. *Arterioscler Thromb Vasc Biol* 13:467, 1993.

418. Ramo P: Anabolic steroids alter the haemodynamic responses of the canine left ventricle. *Acta Physiol Scand* 130:209, 1987.

419. Pesola MK: Reversibility of the haemodynamic effects of anabolic steroids in rats. *Eur J Appl Physiol* 58:125, 1988.

420. Behrendt H: Effect of anabolic steroids on rat heart muscle cell. *Cell Tissue Res* 180:303, 1977.

421. LeGros T, McConnell D, Murry T, et al: The effects of 17-alpha-methyl-testosterone on myocardial function in vitro. *Med Sci Sports Exerc* 32(5):897, 2000.

422. Ong RJ, Patrizi G, Chong WC, et al: Testosterone enhances flow-mediated brachial artery reactivity in men with coronary artery disease. *Am J Cardiol* 85(2):269, 2000.

423. Green D, Cable NT, Rankin JM, Fox C, Taylor RR: Anabolic steroids and vascular responses. *Lancet* 342:863, 1993.

424. Quan A, Teoh H, Man RY: Acute exposure to a low level of testosterone impairs relaxation in porcine coronary arteries. *Clin Exp Pharmacol Physiol* 26(10):830, 1999.

425. Tagarakis CV, Bloch W, Hartmann G, et al: Testosterone-propionate impairs the response of the cardiac capillary bed to exercise. *Med Sci Sports Exerc* 32(5):946, 2000.

426. McCrohon JA, Jessup W, Handelsman DJ, Celermajer DS: Androgen exposure increases human monocyte adhesion to vascular endothelium and endothelial cell expression of vascular cell adhesion molecule-1. *Circulation* 99:2317, 1999.

427. English KM, Steeds RP, Jones TH, et al: Low-dose transdermal testosterone therapy improves angina threshold in men with chronic stable angina: A randomized, double-blind, placebo controlled study. *Circulation* 102(16):1906, 2000.

428. Hanke H, Lenz C, Hess B, et al: Effect of testosterone on plaque development and androgen receptor expression in the arterial vessel wall. *Circulation* 103:1382, 2001.

429. English KM, Mandour O, Steeds RP et al: Men with coronary artery disease have lower level of androgens than men with normal coronary angiograms. *Eur Heart J* 21(11):890, 2000.

430. Kabakci G, Yildirir A, Can I, et al: Relationship between endogenous sex hormone levels, lipoproteins and coronary atherosclerosis in men undergoing coronary angiography. *Cardiology* 92(4):221, 1999.

431. Barrett-Connor E, Khaw K: Endogenous sex hormones and cardiovascular disease in men: A prospective population-based study. *Circulation* 78:539, 1988.

432. Marin P, Holmang S, Jonsson L, et al: The effect of testosterone treatment on body composition and metabolism in middle-aged obese men. *Int J Obes Relat Metab Disord* 16:991, 1992.

433. Reckelhoff JF, Granger JP: Role of androgens in mediating hypertension and renal injury. *Clin Exp Pharmacol Physiol* 26(2):127, 1999.

434. Bruck B, Brehme U, Gugel N, et al: Gender-specific differences in the effects of testosterone and estrogen on the development of atherosclerosis in rabbits. *Arterioscler Thromb Vasc Biol* 17(10):2192, 1997.

435. Price JF, Leng GC: Steroid sex hormones for lower limb atherosclerosis. *Cochrane Database Syst Rev* (2):CD000188, 2000.

436. Haffner SM, Valdez RA, Mykkanen L, et al: Decreased testosterone and dehydroepiandrosterone sulfate concentrations are associated with increased insulin and glucose concentrations in nondiabetic men. *Metabolism* 43:599, 1994.

437. Cohen JC, Hickman R: Insulin resistance and diminished glucose tolerance in powerlifters ingesting anabolic steroids. *J Clin Endocrinol Metab* 64:960, 1987.

438. Friedl KE, Jones RE, Hannan CJ, Plymate SR: The administration of pharmacological dose of testosterone or 19-nortestosterone to normal men is not associated with increased insulin secretion or impaired glucose tolerance. *J Clin Endocrinol Metab* 68:971, 1989.

439. Stellato RK, Feldman HA, Hamdy O, et al: Testosterone, sex hormone binding globulin, and the development of type 2 diabetes in middle-aged men: prospective results from the Massachusetts male aging study. *Diabetes Care* 23(4):490, 2000.

440. Tripathy D, Shah P, Lakshmy R, et al: Effect of testosterone replacement on whole body glucose utilization and other cardiovascular risk factors in males with idiopathic hypogonadotrophic hypogonadism. *Horm Metab Res* 30(10):642, 1998.

441. Marin P, Krotkiewski M, Bjorntorp P: Androgen treatment of middle-aged, obese men: Effect on metabolism, muscle and adipose tissues. *Eur J Med* 1:329, 1992.

442. Griggs RC, Kingston W, Jozefowicz RF, et al: Effect of testosterone on muscle mass and muscle protein synthesis. *J Appl Physiol* 66:498, 1989.

443. Testosterone: the male HRT for andropause. *Drug Ther Perspect* 16(10): 9, 2000.

444. Tenover JS: Effects of testosterone supplementation in the aging male. *J Clin Endocrinol Metab* 75:1092, 1992.

445. Morley JE: Andropause, testosterone therapy, and quality of life in aging men. *CleveClin J Med* 67:880, 2000.

446. Cistulli PA, Grunstein RR, Sullivan CE: Effect of testosterone administration on upper airway collapsability during sleep. *Am J Respir Crit Care Med* 149:530, 1994.

447. Drinka PJ, Jochen AL, Cuisinier M, et al: Polycythemia as a complication of testosterone replacement therapy in nursing home men with low testosterone levels. *J Am Geriatr Soc* 43:899, 1995.

448. McClellan KJ, Goa KL: Transdermal testosterone. *Drugs* 55:253, 1998.

449. Handelsman DJ, Conway AJ, Boylan LM: Pharmacokinetics and pharmacodynamics of testosterone pellets in man. *J Clin Endocrinol Metab* 71:216, 1990.

450. Joss EE, Mullis PE: Delayed puberty in boys. In: Bardin CW, ed. *Current Therapy in Endocrinology and Metabolism.* 5th ed. St. Louis: Mosby Year Book, 1994:299.

451. Bhasin S, Swerdloff RS, Steiner BS, et al: A biodegradable testosterone microcapsule formulation provides uniform eugonadal levels of testosterone for 10-11 weeks in hypogonadal men. *J Clin Endocrinol Metab* 74:75, 1992.

452. Basaria S, Dobs AS: Hypogonadism and androgen replacement therapy in elderly men. *Am J Med* 110:563, 2001.

453. Shapiro J, Christiana J, Frishman WH: Testosterone and other anabolic steroids as cardiovascular drugs. *Am J Ther* 6(3):167, 1999.

454. Johansen KL, Mulligan K, Schambelan M: Anabolic effects of nandrolone decanoate in patients receiving dialysis. A randomized controlled trial. *JAMA* 281:1275, 1999.

455. Worboys S, Kotsopoulos D, Teede H, et al: Evidence that parenteral testosterone therapy may improve endothelium-dependent-and-independent vasodilation in postmenopausal women already receiving estrogen. *J Clin Endocrinol Metab* 86:158, 2001.

456. Miller KK: Androgen deficiency in women. *J Clin Endocrinol Metab* 86:2395, 2001.

457. Phillips GB, Jing TY, Laragh JH: Serum sex hormone levels in postmenopausal women with hypertension. *J Hum Hypertens* 11(8):523, 1997.

458. Phillips GB, Pinkernall BH, Jing TY: Relationship between serum sex hormones and coronary artery disease in postmenopausal women. *Arterioscler Thromb Vasc Biol* 17(4):695, 1997.

459. Worboys S, Kotsopoulos D, Teede H, et al: Evidence that parenteral testosterone therapy may improve endothelium-dependent and endothelium-independent vasodilation in postmenopausal women already receiving estrogen. *J Clin Endocrinol Metab* 86(1):158, 2001.

460. Buckler HM, McElhone K, Durrington PN: The effects of low-dose testosterone treatment on lipid metabolism, clotting factors and ultrasonographic ovarian morphology in women. *Clin Endocrinol (Oxf)* 49(2):173, 1998.

CHAPTER 37

Innovative Pharmacologic Approaches to the Treatment of Myocardial Ischemia

William H. Frishman

Avi Retter

John Misailidis

Amanda Ganem

Jessica Sekhon

Rajesh Mohandas

David Khaski

Farooq Sheikh

Donald Orlic

Piero Anversa

A variety of innovative pharmacologic approaches for managing myocardial ischemia are currently under investigation (Table 37-1). These approaches, which are discussed in this chapter, include the sinus node inhibitors, potassium-channel openers, agents to improve myocardial metabolism and energetics, cytoprotective anti-ischemic drugs, chelating agents, complement inhibitors, and growth factors to stimulate myocardial regeneration.

SINUS NODE INHIBITORS

In 1973, investigators began a drug research program to develop a new class of agents (sinus node inhibitors) that could selectively reduce the heart rate without affecting myocardial contractility, conduction velocity and refractoriness, or arterial blood pressure. A structural modification of the calcium-channel blocker verapamil led to the development of the benzolactame-derivative falipamil (AQ-A39), a prototype drug that selectively lowered the heart rates of dogs (Fig. 37-1).[1]

Concurrently, investigations with clonidine derivatives began. One agent, alinidine (ST-567), had a selective heart rate-lowering action with minimal central nervous system (CNS) side effects.[2–4] It was investigated in patients with angina pectoris, but its use was limited by ocular toxicity. Two new alinidine analogues, TH91:21 and TH91:22, were investigated in a rat model of ischemia and found to demonstrate a cardioprotective effect by decreasing the incidence of ischemic and reperfusion-induced ventricular arrhythmias. TH91:21 also showed anti-ischemic and antiarrhythmic effects. However, clinical trials have yet to demonstrate the clinical efficacy of these new analogues in ischemic heart disease.[5]

Additional studies with falipamil confirmed its heart rate-lowering effect to be independent of calcium-channel and β-adrenergic blockade.[1] However, the agent did appear to have some class III antiarrhythmic properties.[1] It was demonstrated to prolong repolarization and electrocardiogram (ECG) QT interval prolongation.[1] Consequently, falipamil was modified further by manipulation of its phthalimidine structure, resulting in a second generation bradycardic agent, zatebradine (ULFS 49), a benzazepinone derivative.[6,7] In animal studies, zatebradine (Fig. 37-1) was shown to be more potent than falipamil in reducing heart rate, and to be more specific as a bradycardic agent.[7] Because of its pharmacologic profile, the drug was developed as a specific bradycardic agent (sinus node inhibitor) for the treatment of patients with angina pectoris.

Zatebradine acts as a bradycardic agent because of its ability to directly decrease the rate of spontaneous depolarization in the sinoatrial node.[8] It is believed to block the I_f or ion membrane channel, which is a cyclic AMP-dependent Na^+/K^+ channel that can be influenced by vagal and sympathetic inputs.[9–11] It is postulated that zatebradine changes this ionophose, which governs the autonomic control of heart rate.[12–14] The subsequent slowing of spontaneous depolarization with zatebradine is heart rate-dependent; that is, there is a greater rate reducing effect the higher the heart rate.[13] Investigators have shown that the selective blockade of the I_f channel by zatebradine is reversible, and the drug seems to bind to the inside of the sinoatrial cell.[14]

In addition, there is evidence that zatebradine can interact with the L-type calcium ion channel, but this is only seen with drug

TABLE 37-1. Innovative Approaches for Treating Myocardial Ischemia

Sinus node inhibitors
Potassium channel openers (see Chap. 28)
Coenzyme Q_{10}
L-Carnitine
Cytoprotective agents (ranolazine, trimetazadine)
Rho-Kinase inhibition (fasudil)
Aldose reductase inhibitors
Drugs to enhance angiogenesis and coronary collateralization
   (see Chap. 38)
Growth factors for myocardial regeneration
Chelators
Complement inhibition
Protein kinase C activators (JTV 519)
Nitric oxide and nitric oxide donors (see Chap. 33)
Adenosine receptor activators (see Chap. 32)

concentrations well out of the therapeutic range.[15] Overall, zate-bradine's mechanism of action produces a unique pharmacologic effect: slowing of spontaneous depolarization without altering the magnitude of the subsequent triggered depolarization.

In vitro comparative studies demonstrated that zatebradine was able to decrease the spontaneous depolarization rate of the sinus node at concentrations significantly lower than those required to affect contractility or maximal driving frequency, a measure of the effective refractory period.[16] This type of bradycardic selectivity with zatebradine could not be demonstrated with calcium-channel blockers or even with the other sinus node inhibitors (alinidine and falipamil). Zatebradine, in intravenous and orally active bradycardic doses, was found to have little or no effect on left ventricular developed pressure, myocardial contractility, myocardial relaxation, and coronary vascular tone.[8,17,18] It also has no effect on left ventricular ejection times.[18]

In vivo animal studies showed that the drug reduced heart rate without any changes in cardiac output and without peripheral vascular resistance occurring.[19] There were no changes in the surface ECG other than a bradycardic effect (PR and QRS intervals were unchanged).[20] Any changes in hemodynamics that occurred with the drug related to bradycardia could be reversed by pacing.[21]

FIGURE 37-1. Chemical structures of zatebradine (ULFS 49 CL) and fali-pamil.

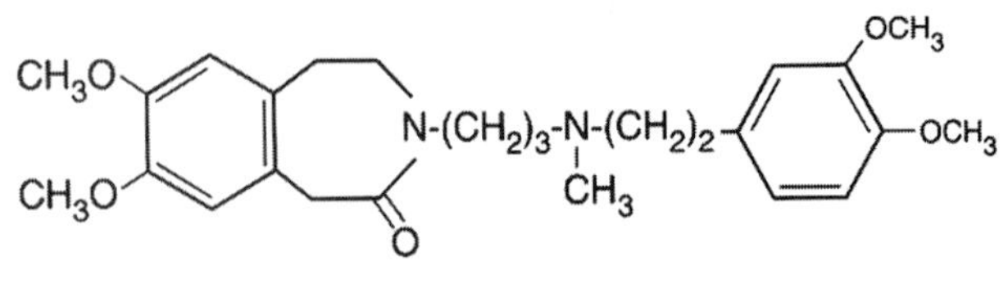

ZATEBRADINE

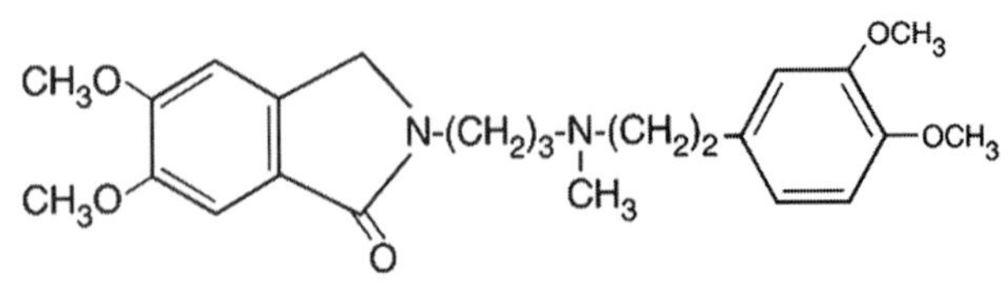

FALIPAMIL

In interaction studies, the drug was also found to antagonize isoproterenol-induced increases in sinus node depolarization rate in a noncompetitive fashion, without having any effect on contractility, unlike the observations with β-adrenergic blockers.[22] The combination of propranolol with zatebradine provided no further heart rate reduction than with zatebradine alone, suggesting a common effect on the I_f channel. When zatebradine was combined with either nifedipine or diltiazem, a blood pressure-lowering effect was seen with both calcium-channel blockers, an effect not seen with zatebradine alone. In addition, nifedipine could raise the heart rate in zatebradine-treated patients. Zatebradine does not appear to interfere with the effects of digoxin.

From animal experiments, functionally, zatebradine is a sinus node inhibitor working as an entity separate from beta-blockers, cholinergics, and calcium-channel blockers, having no negative inotropic effects, blood pressure-lowering effect, or other major electrophysiologic activity. From animal studies, the hemodynamic effects of zatebradine as compared to propranolol are shown in Fig. 37-2.

Having an agent that could selectively reduce HR during rest and exercise made it a possible alternative to beta-blockers and rate-lowering calcium-channel blockers for the treatment of angina pectoris.

FIGURE 37-2. Effects of ULFS 49 CL (0.5 mg/kg intravenous) and propranolol (1 mg/kg intravenous) on hemodynamic and functional parameters during treadmill exercise in dogs. Exercise at maximal workload: mean values of percentage changes after drug administration in comparison to the corresponding moment of control exercise (= 100%). Open columns = propranolol; hatched columns = ULFS 49 CL; CO = cardiac output; HR = heart rate; LV dp/dt max = maximal rate of increase in left ventricular pressure; SV = left ventricular stroke volume; WT_{LAD} = left ventricular systolic wall thickening. (*Reproduced with permission from Krumpl G, Winkler M, Schneider W, Raberger G: Comparison of the haemodynamic effects of the selective bradycardic agent ULFS 49 CL, with those of propranolol during treadmill exercise in dogs. Br J Pharmacol 94:55–64, 1988.*)

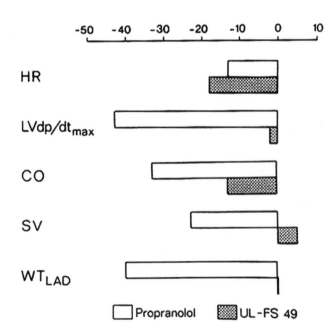

Changes during maximal exercise (%)

HR
LVdp/dt$_{max}$
CO
SV
WT$_{LAD}$

□ Propranolol ▓ UL-FS 49

Preliminary studies in animals and humans suggested that zatebradine had antianginal and anti-ischemic effects that were related to its bradycardic activity.[22-27] These studies suggested that the bradycardic effects of zatebradine not only reduced myocardial oxygen demands, but could affect perfusion of ischemic areas in a favorable manner. A series of placebo-controlled trials were then begun in the United States, Canada, and overseas in patients with effort angina pectoris to compare very low doses of zatebradine in twice-daily dosing to placebo, diltiazem, and as an add-on medication to nifedipine. The results from these trials show that zatebradine, despite heart rate-lowering effects at rest and exercise, was no different than placebo as an antianginal and anti-ischemic drug.[28-30] It produced no additional benefit on exercise tolerance in patients receiving nifedipine,[28] despite a reduction in heart rate at rest and exercise similar to that seen with combinations of dihydropyridines and beta-blockers, which have added efficacy in angina.[31,32] In addition, there is an increased incidence of ocular toxicity with zatebradine as compared with placebo and diltiazem.[28,29] Based on these studies, the sponsor has discontinued the development of zatebradine as an antianginal drug although the compound has been investigated as a rate-lowering drug in patients with congestive heart failure.[33,34] Specifically, Japanese investigators demonstrated a beneficial effect of zatebradine-induced bradycardia in 14 heart-failure patients. The altered cardiac energetics and mechanics created by the lowered heart rate helped via an oxygen-saving effect, contributing to the benefit. More clinical trials are necessary to further support these findings.[35]

Investigations are ongoing with two new bradycardic agents: tedisamil, which has type III antiarrhythmic actions,[36-40] and Zeneca D7288, a calcium blocker derivative.[41,42] Specifically, tedisamil was studied in a prospective, double-blind, placebo-controlled study of 203 patients with stable angina and showed clinically significant dose-dependent anti-ischemic and antiarrhythmic effects compared to placebo.[43] These beneficial effects are not due entirely to the drug's bradycardic effect. The results of a recent study of tedisamil in an ischemic rat model suggest that tedisamil may produce its anti-ischemic and antiarrhythmic effects by a concentration-dependent stimulation of $Na^+ K^+$-ATPase enzymatic activity and an additional protective mechanism that maintains enzyme activity in the presence of ischemia.[44] Other studies are in progress to further elucidate the exact mechanisms of benefit of this agent.

A New Theory for Explaining Antianginal Drug Actions

Although heart rate is a known determinant of myocardial oxygen consumption, drug-induced HR reduction alone with sinus node inhibitors both at rest and exercise in patients with chronic angina pectoris does not contribute to any important anti-anginal or anti-ischemic benefit. The benefit of β-adrenergic blockers and the rate-lowering calcium blockers may therefore not come from heart rate reduction alone but from their effects on contractility and/or regional myocardial metabolism, physiologic functions that are not easily measured. To test this hypothesis, an antianginal drug would need to be tested that only has the negative inotropic effects of beta-blockers or calcium-entry blockers without effects on heart rate, blood pressure, and coronary resistance. It now appears from the clinical experiences of our group and others that an effective antianginal drug must have negative inotropic effects (beta-blockers), or be a coronary vasodilator (nitrates, dihydropyridine calcium blockers), or demonstrate both properties (rate-lowering calcium blockers, diltiazem, and verapamil) (Table 37-2). Drug-induced heart rate and blood pressure reductions alone do not appear to confer important benefits in patients with chronic stable angina.

Conclusion

Heart rate reduction during rest and exercise has been considered an important mechanism for the antianginal and anti-ischemic effects of β-adrenergic blocking drugs and the rate-lowering calcium entry blockers (diltiazem, verapamil). A new class of drugs, the sinus node inhibitors, has provided the opportunity to examine the antianginal and anti-ischemic effects of heart rate reduction alone, because these new agents have bradycardic actions without effects on myocardial contractility, blood pressure, ejection times, or peripheral and coronary vascular resistances. In spite of some early success with a prototype agent [zatebradine (ULFS 49 CL)] in animal studies demonstrating possible anti-ischemic activity, a series of placebo and active-control treatment studies in patients has revealed no demonstrable antianginal or anti-ischemic activities of the drug in spite of reductions in both rest and exercise heart rate. The implication of these findings is that heart-rate reduction alone may play a small role, if any, in the antianginal actions of drugs such as beta-

TABLE 37-2. Effects of Various Cardiovascular Drugs as Antianginal Drugs: Effects on Determinants of Myocardial Oxygen Demand and Supply

CLASS	HR	BP (wall tension)	LVC	CBF	AAE
α-Adrenergic blockers	↔	↓	↔	↔	−
ACE inhibitors	↔	↓	↔	↔	−
β-Adrenergic blockers	↓↓	↓↔	↓	↔	+
β-Adrenergic blockers + pacer	↓	↓	↓	↔	+
Calcium blockers (rate lowering)	↓	↓	↓	↑	+
Calcium blockers (dihydropyridines)	↔	↓	↔	↑	+
Calcium blockers (bepridil, lidoflazine)	↓↔	↔	↓	↑	+
Diuretics	↔	↓	↔	↔	−
Nitrates	↔	↓	↔	↑	+
Serotonin blockers	↔	↓	↔	↔	−
Sinus node inhibitors	↓	↔	↔	↔	−

AAE = antianginal effect; BP = blood pressure; CBF = coronary blood flow; HR = heart rate; LVC = left ventricular contractility;

↑ = increase; ↓ = decrease; ↔ = no change; + = favorable effect; − = no effect.

Source: Reproduced with permission from Frishman WH et al.[45]

blockers and rate-lowering calcium blockers, and that the negative inotropic actions of these agents may be more important in their antianginal and anti-ischemic mechanism than previously thought.[45]

POTASSIUM CHANNEL OPENERS

A group of compounds that selectively activate and open the ATP-dependent potassium channel have been developed as drugs[46] to treat systemic hypertension (e.g., pinacidil, diazoxide, minoxidil) and myocardial ischemia (e.g., nicorandil, BMS-180448, BMS-182264, EMD 56431). Other agents in this class include cromakalim, aprikalim, and bimakalim (see Chap. 28). Nicorandil was the first agent in this drug class to be evaluated for treatment of myocardial ischemia on a large scale.[47,47a]

Nicorandil

Nicorandil [*N*-(2-hydroxyethyl)-nicotinamide nitrate] is the first potassium-channel-opening drug (see Chap. 28) to become clinically available in Europe and Asia for the treatment of ischemic heart disease (Fig. 37-3). The different antianginal pharmacologic therapies currently in common use, while efficacious in many cases, present several problems, establishing the need for a new class of drugs to treat this disease entity. The effectiveness of nitrates is often severely compromised by the development of tolerance.

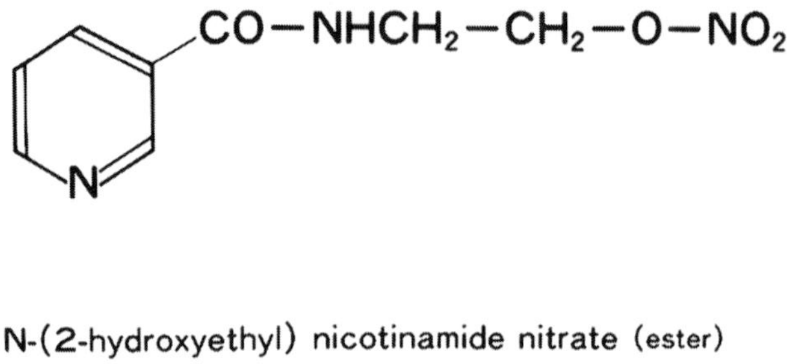

$$CO-NHCH_2-CH_2-O-NO_2$$

N-(2-hydroxyethyl) nicotinamide nitrate (ester)

FIGURE 37-3. Chemical structure of nicorandil.

Calcium antagonists frequently lead to reflex tachycardia, hypotension and edema. Beta-blockers, while remarkably effective, are associated with several contraindications and unpleasant side effects. Nicorandil's efficacy in reducing angina likely results from a combination of increased coronary blood flow via dilatation of large coronary arteries and collateral vessels and a reduction in myocardial oxygen demand via decreased preload and afterload.[48–50] This vasodilator appears to relax vascular smooth-muscle cells through a dual mechanism. Nicorandil increases potassium conductance by opening ATP-regulated potassium ion channels on the sarcolemma and mitochondria, leading to membrane hyperpolarization and closure of calcium ion channels.[51] In addition, in a manner very similar to nitrates, it increases intracellular levels of cyclic guanosine monophosphate (GMP) (Fig. 37-4).[52] Unlike nitrates,

FIGURE 37-4. Proposed mechanisms of action of nicorandil (MLCKase = myosin light-chain kinase).

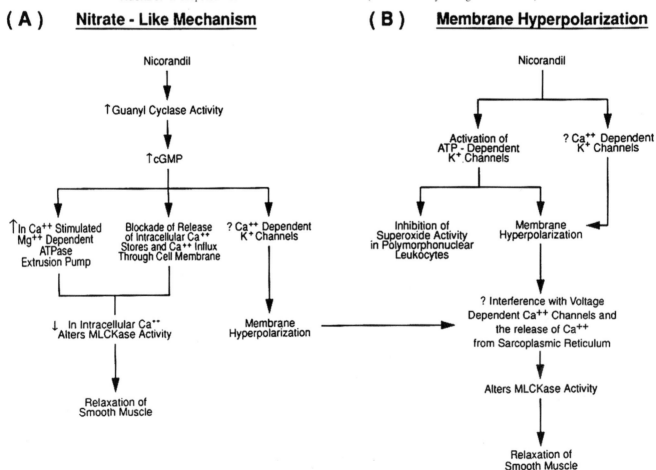

there is less tolerance to nicorandil and no cross-tolerance to nitrates has been observed.[53,54] Some researchers also suggest that the drug exhibits cardioprotective effects apart from its vasodilatory properties.[55–58,58a]

The bulk of the clinical experience with nicorandil has been reported on from studies in Europe and Japan where it has been used primarily for the treatment of patients with angina pectoris of effort. However, nicorandil's strong antispasmodic properties also suggest a possible benefit in Prinzmetal's angina.[59]

Pharmacodynamics

Although nicorandil is classified in the group of potassium-channel-opening agents, it is clear that many of nicorandil's vasodilatory properties do not arise solely from potassium-channel-mediated hyperpolarization of vascular smooth muscle. Unlike other potassium-channel activators, such as cromakalim, nicorandil is able to augment the vasodilatory effects of nitroprusside in the presence of specific potassium-channel antagonists.[60] Several investigators have shown that nicorandil, in a nitrate-like manner, causes an increase in intracellular cyclic GMP. The chemical structure of nicorandil combines nicotinamide with a nitrate ($O\text{-}NO_2$ group), which is thought to react with a sulfhydryl group in smooth-muscle cells to either activate guanylate cyclase or to facilitate the release of nitric oxide, leading to increased cyclic GMP.[50] Through changes in calcium channels, this "second messenger," in turn, leads to decreased intracellular calcium, which is thought to alter myosin light-chain kinase activity, thereby causing dephosphorylation of the myosin light chain and relaxation of vascular smooth muscle.[60–62]

Nicorandil's ability to decrease intracellular calcium via increased cyclic GMP stems from at least two mechanisms. The increased cyclic GMP appears to block release of intracellular calcium stores and calcium influx through the cell membrane. In addition, work by Morimoto et al demonstrated that nicorandil, like nitroglycerin, can dose-dependently block the increase of intracellular calcium caused by such powerful vasoconstrictors as angiotensin-II and prostaglandin $F_{2\alpha}$ through the activation of a calcium-stimulated, magnesium-dependent ATPase calcium extrusion pump.[63]

Nicorandil exhibits a dual pharmacodynamic mechanism. Several studies suggest that in addition to increasing cyclic GMP, nicorandil increases potassium conductance and produces pharmacodynamically relevant membrane hyperpolarization of vascular smooth muscle (see Fig. 37-4). Kreye et al directly demonstrated, by using ^{86}Rb as a marker for potassium, that nicorandil's hyperpolarizing effects stem from specific activation of glibenclamide-sensitive ATP-dependent potassium channels.[64] The hyperpolarization induces vasorelaxation by interfering with voltage-dependent calcium channels and the release of calcium from the sarcoplasmic reticulum.[64] Reduced intracellular calcium, as explained above, results in dephosphorylation of myosin light chains and relaxation of smooth muscle.

ATP-dependent potassium channels may, in fact, be physiologically important in the natural coronary vasodilatory response to cardiac ischemia. Daut et al, in studies of isolated perfused guinea pig hearts, showed that glibenclamide, a specific blocker of ATP-dependent potassium channels, blocks the coronary vasodilation resulting from hypoxic perfusion of the myocardium.[65] Nicorandil, therefore, by activating these channels, may be reinforcing an innate reactive mechanism to coronary ischemia.

It has also been suggested that nicorandil may cause some hyperpolarization by affecting calcium-dependent potassium channels through its nitrate-like increase in cyclic GMP. Robertson and coworkers demonstrated that calcium-activated potassium channels

in arterial smooth muscle are activated by cyclic GMP-dependent protein kinase.[66]

Nicorandil's increase in potassium efflux is perhaps not a novel mechanism, but rather mimics physiologic processes. Acetylcholine accomplishes hyperpolarization and suppression of the sinus node's action potential through the opening of specific muscarinic channels, and perhaps via the release of endothelium-derived hyperpolarizing factor, which relaxes smooth muscle through increased potassium conduction.[67,68] From microelectrode experiments, Furukawa et al showed that nicorandil produces membrane hyperpolarization in a variety of mammalian smooth muscle tissues.[69] In canine atrial and Purkinje fibers, nicorandil, in a manner similar to acetylcholine, produces a shortening of the action potential, and at high concentrations, produces a negative inotropic effect.[70–73] When tetraethylammonium, a nonspecific potassium channel blocker, is added, this hyperpolarization is abolished in the mesenteric artery of dogs and in the trachea of dogs and guinea pigs.[74,75]

Kukovetz et al elucidated the relative contributions of hyperpolarization and nitrate-like effects of nicorandil's vasodilatation by studying bovine coronary smooth muscles in the presence and absence of potassium-channel blockers and inhibitors of guanyl cyclase.[60] This study found that concentrations of nicorandil less than 50 μmol/L produce relaxation primarily through hyperpolarization, while higher concentrations produce relaxation through cyclic GMP. Such results suggest that at therapeutic doses, nicorandil causes vasodilatation principally through its nitrate-like effect.

Apart from its vasodilatory effects, nicorandil may be beneficial in myocardial ischemia by protecting tissues from free radical injury and apoptosis.[75a] In concentrations that produce vasodilatation, Gross et al demonstrated that nicorandil caused a marked inhibition of superoxide activity in both canine and human polymorphonuclear leukocytes.[58a] This inhibition was not demonstrated with nitroglycerin, but was shown with the selective potassium channel enhancer EMD 52692, thus implicating a role for nicorandil's activation of ATP-dependent potassium channels in providing cardioprotection from free radicals.

Animal Hemodynamic Studies

Previous studies in dogs showed that nicorandil reduces ventricular preload and afterload while increasing large coronary artery diameter and redistributing coronary blood flow to the subendocardium.[76–78] After a 20-minute intravenous infusion of 3 to 30 μg/kg/min in dogs, Huckstorf and Bassenge showed a dose-dependent increase in heart rate and coronary artery diameter accompanied by a small decrease in mean arterial pressure.[79] A dose of 100 μg/kg produced substantial hypotension, reflex tachycardia, and a decrease of coronary artery response to dilation. After 5 days of constant intravenous infusion at 10 μg/kg/min, no tolerance was demonstrated as the changes witnessed acutely were maintained during the entire 5-day period. This is in marked contrast to the findings with a long-term nitroglycerin infusion, which causes a slow, continuous decrease in coronary artery vasodilatation.[80,81] Nicorandil's markedly short half-life may also contribute to the relative absence of observed tolerance with the drug. Lastly, no cross-tolerance to nitroglycerin was noted with nicorandil, which may relate to nicorandil's effect on potassium ion permeability.[79,82,83]

Because of nicorandil's favorable hemodynamic actions, several investigators suggested that nicorandil could be effective in limiting or preventing myocardial ischemia or infarction. Lamping and coworkers showed cardioprotection against ischemic injury in infarcted and stunned myocardium.[84,85] Gross et al directly demonstrated in canine models that both nicorandil and EMD 52692 (another potassium-channel-opening agent) reduce myocardial infarct size and improve percent myocardial segment shortening, while nifedipine and nitroprusside had no effect on those same parameters.[58a] Moreover, in an isolated, globally ischemic rat heart, nicorandil produced a greater recovery of isovolumic left ventricular minute work when compared with control values in untreated hearts. However, some of these same studies also suggest that nicorandil's benefits may actually be independent of hemodynamic or coronary vasodilatory effects because the limitation of infarct size did not occur with the known afterload reducer nifedipine and the improvement in stunned myocardium occurred independently of nitroprusside. In animals treated with nicorandil or nifedipine, arterial blood pressure and coronary flow were similarly affected; however, only nicorandil reduced infarct size and improved myocardial shortening.[85] Consequently, Gross et al has postulated that nicorandil's beneficial cardiac effects in ischemia stem from modulation of the potassium channel and/or its antifree radical activity rather than from specific hemodynamic changes.[58a]

Human Hemodynamic Studies

Several studies examined nicorandil's effects on systolic blood pressure, peripheral vascular resistance, left ventricular end-diastolic pressure, and left ventricular end-systolic pressure in humans.[86–91] Table 37-3 summarizes the acute hemodynamic parameters of nicorandil treatment as compared to nifedipine and nitrates.[92]

Suryapranata and MacLeod further examined the acute hemodynamic effects of nicorandil in 10 patients with coronary artery disease after administering 20 mg of the drug sublingually.[93] As seen in previous studies, a reduction in left ventricular end-diastolic pressure and peripheral resistance of 43% and 29%, respectively, was observed with an improved ejection fraction and without spontaneous changes in heart rate (Table 37-4). Because nicorandil has no direct inotropic or β-adrenergic activity, the increased ejection fractions were thought to stem primarily from a reduction in ventricular afterload.[93,94] Regarding coronary hemodynamics, no change in coronary sinus blood flow was demonstrated despite a decrease in aortic pressure, which suggested that coronary vasodilation had occurred although no statistical decrease in calculated coronary vascular resistance was found.[93] The anti-ischemic properties of nicorandil in patients were demonstrated by a significant decrease in myocardial oxygen consumption and in the calculated pressure-rate product of 14% and 19%, respectively. A reduction in pulmonary artery wedge pressure was seen in patients with effort angina, but not in those with a previous myocardial infarction.[95] Suryapranata

TABLE 37-4. Cardiovascular Profile of Nicorandil (20 mg) in Patients with Cardiovascular Disease

Clinical Parameter	Before	After	% Change
Heart rate (bpm)	73±5	78±5	+7
LV pressure (mm Hg)	138±9	121±5	−12*
LV end-diastolic pressure (mm Hg)	12.2±1.4	7±1.5	−43*
Mean arterial pressure (mm Hg)	104±4	90±4	−13*
Coronary sinus blood flow (mL/min)	115±12	109±12	−5
Coronary vascular resistance (mm Hg/mL/min)	1.0±0.1	0.9±0.1	−10
Pressure-rate product (mm Hg/bpm/100)	10.0±0.7	8.1±0.6	−19*
Myocardial oxygen consumption	10.2±0.9	8.8±0.9	−14*

*$P < .05$

Source: Adapted with permission from Bossaller C, et al. Relaxation of human coronary artery and arteria mammaria by K(+)-channel openers. *J Cardiovasc Pharmacol* 20(Suppl 3):S13, 1992.

and MacLeod[93] have theorized that the reduction in left ventricular filling pressure in patients with angina may not necessarily be related to hemodynamic changes with the drug, but may be due to an improvement in ischemic regional wall functioning, as reported by Thormann et al[94] and Kambara[96] in their studies of pacing-induced myocardial ischemia in patients with coronary artery disease.

In patients treated with nitrates, the additional administration of nicorandil was more useful in increasing coronary blood flow than was the additional administration of nitrates.[48]

Clinical Experiences: Angina Pectoris

Because comparisons with placebo are considered unethical in many countries, and, as yet, few clinical trials have been conducted in the United States, the efficacy and safety of oral nicorandil has been principally evaluated overseas against known, well-documented antianginal medications. Several small trials, which compared nicorandil to either a placebo baseline or known antianginal medication, reported varying results with regard to improvement in subjective symptoms and exercise tolerance tests. Kinoshita and coworkers assessed the efficacy of nicorandil by conducting a single-blind trial comparing a single 30-mg dose of nicorandil to 60 and 120 mg of diltiazem, 40 mg of propranolol, and placebo in 12 patients with chronic stable angina.[97] Exercise stress tests were performed 30 min after nicorandil treatment, 120 min after propranolol, and 180 min after both diltiazem and placebo. When compared to placebo, the time to onset of angina and total exercise duration were significantly increased for all of the active medications, with no significant differences between them. Furthermore, nicorandil appeared more effective in patients with one vessel coronary artery disease, while propranolol appeared more effective in those with multivessel disease. Similar results were obtained in a double-blind, double-crossover study reported by Wagner in which 22 patients with stable coronary artery disease were given 10 to 20 mg of nicorandil twice daily for 4 weeks.[98] Exercise time to onset of 0.1 mV ST-segment depression increased from baseline values, and total ST-segment depression at identical workloads decreased significantly 2 and 12 h after dosage. The time to onset of chest pain increased significantly from the 10 and 20 mg doses at 2 h, but not for the 20 mg dose at 12 h. Another study by Falcone et al randomized 41 patients to nicorandil (10 mg twice daily for 3 weeks, followed by 20 mg twice daily for 3 weeks) or isosorbide dinitrate slow release (40 mg twice daily for 6 weeks), and found no

TABLE 37-3. Comparison of Nicorandil to Nifedipine and Nitrates

Hemodynamic Parameters	Nicorandil	Nifedipine	Nitrates*
Wall tension	↓	↓	↓
Ventricular volume	↓	↓	↓
Heart rate	↑↔	↑	↑
Contractility	↔	↔	↔
Coronary blood flow	↑↔	↑	↑
Coronary vascular resistance	↓	↓	↓
Diastolic perfusion time	↓↔	↓	↓
Collateral blood flow	?	↑	↑
Mean arterial pressure	↓	↓	↓

*Nitrates are associated with tolerance; ? = unknown; ↑ = increase; ↓ = decrease; ↔ = no change.

Source: Reproduced with permission from Goldschmidt M et al.[92]

difference in prolongation of time to ischemic threshold on exercise stress testing between the two groups.[99]

A larger study by Meeter and coworkers compared the efficacy and safety of nicorandil to propranolol in a randomized, double-blind, parallel trial involving 77 patients with stable angina pectoris.[100] Initial doses were 10 mg twice daily and 40 mg thrice daily for nicorandil and propranolol, respectively, and were doubled after 3 weeks if the original doses were well tolerated. Nicorandil at both doses was as effective as propranolol in reducing spontaneous anginal attacks (3.5 to 1.0 and 2.9 to 0.7, respectively). No tolerance was observed with nicorandil. Furthermore, the termination of an exercise stress test from angina pectoris 2 h after administration of nicorandil decreased in numbers of patients by approximately 50%, while the percentage reporting fatigue as the limiting factor increased despite no change in exercise capacity as measured by maximal workload. A similar shift from chest pain to fatigue in exercise stress test stoppage was also observed with propranolol treatment. Objective signs of myocardial ischemia were less frequent in both groups, as indicated by a decrease in maximal ST-segment depression and the prolongation of time to ST-segment, although the prolongation was only significant for nicorandil 2 h after its administration in contrast to 2 and 12 h for propranolol. Thus, part of nicorandil's anti-ischemic efficacy in this study was relatively short-lived as compared to propranolol. The exact mechanism for nicorandil's antianginal effect was unclear, because no change in either heart rate or blood pressure occurred with prolonged administration. Meeter et al attributes its effect to epicardial vasodilation and perhaps a reduction of preload.[100]

Two large double-blind studies by Doring were undertaken to establish the antianginal efficacy of nicorandil as compared either to isosorbide dinitrate or to isosorbide-5-mononitrate.[51] Previous studies that compared nitrates to nicorandil had demonstrated that nicorandil caused a greater decrease in ventricular afterload while producing a smaller decrease in preload.[89] However, in contrast to nitroglycerin, nicorandil was found to increase resting coronary sinus flow and cardiac index, but did not increase heart rate or promote myocardial sympathetic activity, as measured by myocardial norepinephrine release.[101] A total of 129 patients with stable New York Heart Association functional class II or class III coronary heart disease were enrolled in the two studies: a crossover trial in which 20 mg of nicorandil and isosorbide-5-mononitrate were administered twice daily for 4 weeks, and a parallel study in which nicorandil and isosorbide dinitrate were given, with regular 8-h dosing intervals, at 10 mg thrice daily for 2 weeks and then 20 mg thrice daily for 4 weeks.[51] Total exercise duration, time to onset of angina, and time to onset of ST-segment depression of 0.1 mV were prolonged significantly from baseline with all medications in both studies, with the prolongation of time to ST-segment depression averaging approximately 1.5 to 2 min. A significant decrease in weekly anginal attack rates with greater efficacy at higher doses was noted for all medications. However, no significant differences were recorded when comparing the drugs in either study, and no tolerance was observed for nicorandil despite the higher-than-recommended dose of 10 to 20 mg twice daily used in previously described studies.

Studies have compared nicorandil twice daily to amlodipine once daily[102] and nifedipine twice daily,[103] and comparable antianginal efficacy was demonstrated.

A placebo-controlled, double-blind trial evaluated monotherapy with nicorandil at 10 to 20 mg twice daily in 83 participants with reproducible exercise-induced angina on the treadmill.[104] After 1 week of single-blind placebo therapy, patients were randomly assigned in a double-blind manner to receive either twice daily nicorandil at 10 mg or placebo. After 1 week, the dose of medication was doubled, and after another week, symptom-limited exercise tests were repeated before and 1, 4, and 8 h after the morning dose of the medication. The anginal attack rate during daily activities was similar with placebo and nicorandil therapies. When compared to placebo, nicorandil neither improved exercise performance nor increased time to ischemia in patients with stable angina pectoris. Consequently, the investigators in this study concluded that despite previous claims, twice-daily nicorandil therapy at this dose was ineffective monotherapy for treating patients with effort-induced angina. However, perhaps more frequent dosing at higher dose levels or the use of a sustained-release formulation might have provided benefit for these same patients.

The effect of nicorandil on clinical outcome was assessed in 5126 patients with stable angina and previous myocardial infarction or coronary artery bypass graft.[105,105a] Patients were randomized to nicorandil 10 mg increasing to 20 mg twice daily, or placebo. Patients randomized to nicorandil had a significant reduction in the primary end point of a combination of coronary heart disease death, nonfatal myocardial infarction, and unplanned hospitalizations for cardiac chest pain compared with patients randomized to placebo. Nicorandil was also associated with a 21% reduction in secondary end point of coronary heart disease and myocardial infarction, but this difference did not achieve significance.

Coronary Artery Vasospasm

The possible role of nicorandil for prevention of coronary artery vasospasm was assessed by LaBlanche and coworkers in a randomized, placebo-controlled, double-blind, double-crossover study of 16 patients with angiographically documented coronary artery spasm.[59] Using ergometrine-induced coronary vasospasm that had previously been shown to be of good sensitivity and specificity in reproducing spontaneous spasm and in predicting clinical outcome, 30 mg of nicorandil and 10 mg of nifedipine were compared against one another and against placebo.[106-109] Nicorandil was found to be as effective as nifedipine in preventing ergometrine-induced coronary artery spasm, thus offering a unique method for prevention of vasospasm other than calcium-channel blockers or nitrates.[59] Aizawa et al obtained a similar result in which 5 mg of nicorandil in patients provided relief of spontaneous and ergometrine-induced vasospasm within 30 to 140 seconds.[110] The efficacy and safety of nicorandil in patients with unstable angina are currently being evaluated in a large European multicenter trial.

Unstable Angina

Oral or intravenous nicorandil improves the control of unstable angina in patients already receiving alternative treatments. A large multicenter, placebo-controlled trial compared the acute effects of oral nicorandil to placebo for this condition.[111] Nicorandil was shown to cause fewer episodes of silent or painful ischemia and fewer arrhythmias.

Myocardial Infarction

Several clinical trials have investigated the short-term effects of intravenous or intracoronary nicorandil on myocardial recovery from ischemic damage caused by acute myocardial infarction.[112-116] In many of the trials, the drug was given as an adjunct to percutaneous transluminal coronary angioplasty (PTCA) and its effects were compared with control groups not receiving the drug.

Nicorandil was associated with significantly improved echocardiographic assessments of myocardial function.

Coronary Bypass Grafting

Recently Hayashi et al showed that the administration of nicorandil during coronary artery bypass grafting (CABG) enhanced the myocardial protective effects against ischemia-reperfusion.[116a] However, other investigators have reported severe peripheral vasodilation and hypotension with nicorandil, requiring vasopressors during open heart surgery.[116b,116c]

Side Effects

In pharmacologic doses, nicorandil has relatively few side effects. The most frequently reported symptom is headache, which is usually of mild to moderate severity, has an incidence comparable to that of nitrates and nifedipine, and is experienced during the first 2 weeks of treatment with rapid dissipation thereafter.[48,53,100,103,117] In the large Doring trial, only 3 of 95 patients withdrew because of headache,[53] while Meeter et al reported only 2 of 38 patients terminating their study for the same reason.[100] When compared to nifedipine, fewer side effects from peripheral vasodilatation, such as edema, flushing, and palpitations, have been noted.[103] Other adverse events occur rarely and include gastrointestinal disturbances, consisting of abdominal pain or vomiting, dizziness, asthenia, mouth and anal ulcers, and musculoskeletal pain.[53,118,118a]

Conclusion

Nicorandil appears to be a potent peripheral and coronary vasodilating drug with a unique dual pharmacodynamic mechanism.[101,119] Many of its vasodilatory properties are similar to nitrates, with the notable exception of tolerance, which appears to be absent in the vast majority of studies. Its use would be indicated in the treatment of angina when reduction of both ventricular preload and afterload, in addition to direct, flow-independent dilatation of large epicardial arteries, are desirable. Its potential clinical role incorporates the prevention of both effort-induced and vasospastic angina. Nicorandil may also have a cardioprotective capacity by inhibiting free radical activity and by enhancement of ischemic preconditioning. Animal studies have shown clear evidence of its hemodynamic action; clinical results, however, are not homogeneous as to the drug's effectiveness relative to other pharmacologic therapies. Differing clinical results may be attributable to dosing issues, the presence of single- versus multivessel disease, or experimental error. More and larger-scale studies are probably needed before nicorandil can be considered as a wide-scale alternative therapy for coronary artery disease. Its relatively mild side-effect profile and absence of known drug-drug interactions give it a distinct advantage over other antianginal drugs. Its use as an antianginal agent, however, may be limited by its short duration of action, which will require more frequent dosing regimens and/or the development of an extended-release formulation.

COENZYME Q$_{10}$ (CoQ)

CoQ$_{10}$ (2,3-dimethoxy-5-methyl-6-decaprenyl benzoquinone), also known as ubiquinone, is an endogenous cellular membrane constituent that has antioxidant properties that may be useful in preventing cellular damage due to myocardial ischemia and reperfusion injury.[120–122] A clinical experience has already been developed with this naturally occurring substance in various cardiovascular and noncardiovascular disorders.

CoQ is a mitochondrial component that is known to have antioxidant and membrane stabilizing properties.[123] Its central physiologic role is in mediating electron transport between nicotinamide adenine dinucleotide (NADH) and succinate dehydrogenases and the cytochrome system. CoQ scavenges free radicals produced by lipid peroxidation.[121,122,124–126] It also may protect against protein and DNA oxidation.[127] Ultrastructurally, CoQ prevents mitochondrial deformity caused by ischemia. CoQ reduces the depletion of nucleosides and lessens Ca^{2+} overload, which is observed in states of hypoxia. These and possibly other protective functions aimed against free radical-induced damage may account for the reported beneficial effects of ubiquinone in both experimental and clinical situations.[128]

CoQ was first identified in 1940, and in 1957, it was demonstrated that CoQ played an important role as a redox carrier in the mammalian respiratory transport chain.[129] Its structure was determined by Folkers and his colleagues.[130] CoQ was found to be identical to that of a quinone earlier described[131] and was called ubiquinone due to its ubiquitous occurrence in various tissues and in microorganisms, plants, and animals. Yamamura et al first used oral CoQ in the therapy of cardiovascular disease in the 1960s.[132] Folkers et al subsequently demonstrated a deficiency of this substance in the myocardium of patients with various cardiac disorders.[130]

Chemistry and Biologic Actions

CoQ (Fig. 37-5) is classified as a fat-soluble quinone with characteristics common to vitamins. Its chemical structure is similar to that of Vitamin K. It is found naturally in the organs of various animal species.[133,134] CoQ has an isoprenoid side chain. The number of isoprene units in the side chain varies with each species of animal. CoQ in humans has 10 isoprene units, hence the designation coenzyme Q$_{10}$. In humans, CoQ is found in relatively high concentrations in the heart, liver, kidney, and pancreas.[135] Total body content of CoQ is estimated to be 0.5 to 1.5 g. Serum levels are approximately 1.0 mg/L.[136] The kinetics of exogenously administered CoQ are poorly understood. Data from recent animal studies revealed that the liver is the target organ for CoQ regardless of intravenous or oral route or delivery vehicle used. Cardiac tissue levels were impacted with intravenous and high oral-dosing regimens in this same model.[137] The intracellular distribution of CoQ is as follows: nucleus 25 to 30%; mitochondria 40 to 50% (inner mitochondrial membrane); microsomal 15 to 20% (Golgi apparatus); and cytosolic 5 to 10%.[138] CoQ in its active form appears to be protein bound. There are at least three classes of CoQ-binding proteins that have not been fully characterized:[139,140] QPs, a Q-binding protein that converts succinate to succinyl-CoQ reductase; QPc, which participates in electron transfer in the cytochrome b-cl complex; and, QPn, which is involved in NADH-Q (reduced form). In mammalian cells, ubiquinone is synthesized via the convergence of the tyrosine

FIGURE 37-5. Chemical structure of coenzyme Q$_{10}$.

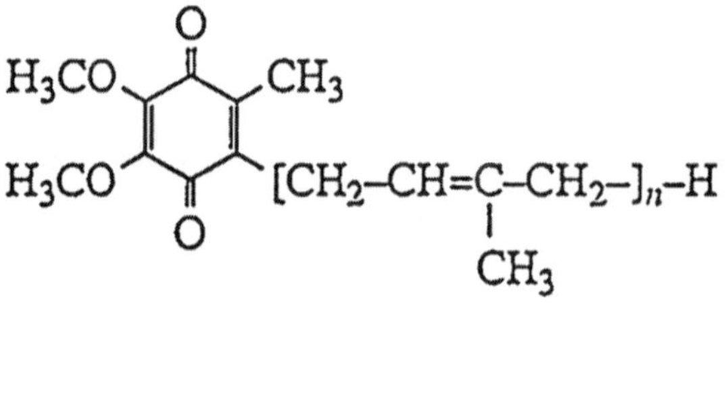

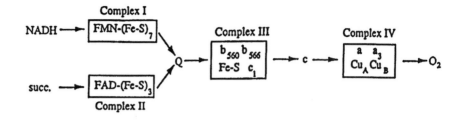

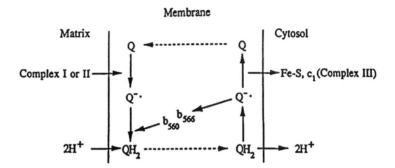

FIGURE 37-6. Role of coenzyme Q_{10} in the respiratory chain.

and acetyl-CoA pathways (mevalonate). According to current evidence, ubiquinone synthesis begins in the endoplasmic reticulum and is completed in the Golgi membranes. In both animals and humans, there appears to be an age-related decline in tissue levels of ubiquinone.[141,142]

From a biochemical standpoint, CoQ appears to serve several functions. Endogenous CoQ plays a pivotal role in oxidative respiration (Fig. 37-6). It has a direct regulatory role on succinyl and NADH dehydrogenases. It serves as a catalyst and has an integral role in regulating the cytochrome *b-cl* complex. Furthermore, CoQ may have direct membrane-stabilizing properties separate from its role in oxidative phosphorylation. CoQ may have mitogenic properties.[143] It may function in membrane secretion,[144] which would explain the occurrence of high concentrations of CoQ in the Golgi apparatus. Relatively little is known about the biodegradation of ubiquinone. The turnover rate of CoQ in various tissues ranges from 50 to 125 h.[145,146]

Pharmacokinetics

There have been few pharmacokinetic studies of CoQ. Following ingestion of 100 mg of CoQ, peak plasma levels occur between 5 and 10 h.[147] The mean time to maximal concentration (T_{max}) of 6.5 h (range, 5 to 10 h) with CoQ indicates slow absorption from the gastrointestinal tract, possibly due to its high molecular weight and low water solubility. The mean plasma levels after a single 100-mg oral dose of CoQ in human subjects is 1.004 ± 0.37 mg/mL. The mean steady state level of CoQ after thrice-daily administration of 100 mg is estimated to be 5.4 mg/mL, approximately four to seven times the level of endogenous CoQ. A new, solubilized form of CoQ, Q-Gel, appears to be more readily bioavailable than standard forms.[148] Approximately 90% of the steady-state concentration can be achieved after 4 days of dosing. Because oral CoQ appears to have a low clearance rate from the plasma, it has a relatively long plasma half-life of 33.9 ± 5.32 h. Exogenously administered CoQ does not appear to

alter endogenous levels.[149] The metabolic fate of CoQ has not been fully characterized. Following absorption from the gastrointestinal tract, CoQ is taken up by chylomicrons. The major portion of an exogenous dose of CoQ is deposited in the liver and packaged into very-low-density lipoprotein (VLDL).[150] It has also been shown that 2-months supplementation of Q_{10} (90 mg daily) more than doubles plasma and VLDL plus low-density lipoprotein (LDL) concentrations of CoQ.[151] Following this step, CoQ appears to be concentrated in certain specific sites that include adrenal, spleen, lung, kidney, and myocardial tissues. The excretion of CoQ is predominantly via the biliary tract.[152] Approximately 62.5% of orally administered CoQ can be recovered in the feces during chronic dosing.

Mechanisms of Action in Myocardial Ischemia

Studies examining CoQ as a therapeutic agent indicate that one major mechanism of action is protection of ischemic tissue from reperfusion damage. CoQ is an established antioxidant and free radical scavenger in vitro. CoQ prevents the initiation and propagation of lipid peroxy radicals (LOO·) either via direct elimination of this species or through the regeneration of vitamin E from the α-tocopheroxyl radical.[153]

Ubiquinol is an effective lipid soluble antioxidant in liposomes.[154] CoQ appears to be capable of stabilizing cellular membranes and preventing depletion of metabolites necessary for the resynthesis of adenosine 5′-triphosphate (ATP). CoQ may also induce DT diaphorase, a potent inhibitor of free-radical formation.[155]

Niibori et al[156] studied the effects of a liposomal suspension of CoQ in the treatment of ischemia/reperfusion injuries in rats. The goal of the study was to determine (a) whether the liposomal suspension acutely raised serum and myocardial levels of CoQ and (b) whether CoQ assists in the recovery of function, myocardial efficiency, and oxidant injury after cardiac ischemia and reperfusion. Sprague-Dawley rats were either given placebo or pretreated with CoQ 15, 30, and 60 min before serum and myocardial measurements of CoQ were made. The rats were also subject to ischemia/reperfusion injury after these time periods. It was found that serum and myocardial levels of CoQ were acutely raised by the liposomal suspension, and that acute intravenous CoQ improves function and efficiency after ischemia/reperfusion, as measured by the percent recovery of developed pressure. Myocardial efficiency improved the most in those rats receiving the intravenous suspension 30 min prior to the ischemic insult.

Nayler used a Langendorff preparation to demonstrate that CoQ protects the ischemic myocardium.[157] When compared to controls, it was shown that animal hearts pretreated with CoQ had significantly less depletion of ATP and reduced mitochondrial O_2 utilization. Ultrastructural studies revealed that animal hearts pretreated with CoQ maintained mitochondrial architecture when compared with the ultrastructural findings of control animals. Controls showed edema, cell membrane disruption, mitochondrial lysis, and disorganization of myofibrils. Ohara also demonstrated the protective effects of CoQ on isolated perfused rat heart muscle.[158] In this study, male Wistar rats were pretreated with CoQ and examined following ischemia and reperfusion. CoQ pretreated hearts demonstrated improved mechanical performance as measured by percent recovery of developed tension. Total ATP concentration following ischemia was significantly higher in the CoQ-treated group when compared with controls. Similar results were reported by Sugiyama et al[159] when coronary artery ligation studies were performed in dogs.

In one study, cultured adult rat cardiomyocytes showed improved survival of cells pretreated with CoQ and subsequently rendered anoxic.[160] Kishi et al demonstrated a cardiostimulatory effect of exogenously administered CoQ on cardiac cells, postulating stimulation of ATP formation.[161] Other experimental data indicate that CoQ may influence prostaglandin metabolism, specifically prostacyclin.[162,163] Furthermore, CoQ appears to possess direct membrane-stabilizing properties separate from its ability to neutralize free-radical species. Numerous in vitro models demonstrate CoQ's membrane-stabilizing properties, which appear to be due to phospholipid-protein interactions.[164,165] Several lines of evidence support a role for CoQ as an antioxidative agent for human LDL, which are discussed later.[166,167]

CoQ's role as a free-radical scavenger and membrane stabilizer could explain why its major activity is demonstrated under conditions of ischemic reperfusion. These basic actions provide the rationale for the experimental and clinical use of CoQ in cardiovascular disorders (Table 37-5).

Although much research has been done investigating CoQ's role in mitigating reperfusion injury, other theories to explain its

TABLE 37-5. Possible Therapeutic Mechanisms of Coenzyme Q_{10} in Cardiovascular Disease

- Correction of Q_{10} deficiency state
- Direct free radical scavenger via semiquinone species
- Direct membrane stabilizing activity due to phospholipid protein interactions
- Correction of mitochondrial "leak" of electrons during oxidative respiration
- Possible effects on prostaglandin metabolism
- Inhibition of intracellular phospholipases
- Preservation of myocardial Na^+/K^+-ATPase activity
- Stabilization of integrity of Ca^{2+}-dependent slow channels
- Mitogenic properties
- Possible role in membrane secretory activity
- Possible inhibition of platelet aggregation

TABLE 37-6. Potential Therapeutic Uses of Coenzyme Q_{10}

Stable angina pectoris
Unstable anginal syndromes
Myocardial preserving agent during mechanical or pharmacologic thrombolysis
Myocardial-preserving agent for cardiac surgery
Congestive heart failure
Toxin-induced cardiotoxicity
Diastolic dysfunction
Essential hypertension
Ventricular arrhythmia
Mitral valve prolapse
Potential imaging agent
Peripheral vascular disease
Cerebral ischemia

mechanism of action exist. Serebrauny et al[168] examined whether CoQ had an inhibitory effect on platelets. In this study, participants took oral CoQ in addition to their usual diet for 20 days. Platelet receptor expression was measured by flow cytometry. Vitronectin receptor expression was significantly inhibited, and a reduction of platelet size was noted. These findings are not fully explained by the antioxidative and bioenergetic properties of CoQ, and more studies must be conducted to completely elucidate its effect on platelets.

Clinical Applications

CoQ has been studied in a variety of clinical settings, including congestive heart failure, hyperlipidemia, hypertension, atherosclerosis, and angina pectoris. Table 37-6 lists the clinical uses for CoQ.

Congestive Heart Failure

The results of clinical trials testing the efficacy of CoQ in the treatment of congestive heart failure (CHF) have been inconsistent. It has been proposed that free-radical injury may promote myocardial decompensation, and that antioxidants may be useful in preventing free-radical damage.[169] Furthermore, CoQ may help to replenish myocardial ATP stores, and thus improve the heart's energy production.[170] Some studies confirm these beneficial effects. In 1997, Sacher et al[171] studied the clinical and hemodynamic effects of CoQ in congestive cardiomyopathy. In this open-label study consisting of 17 patients with New York Heart Association (NYHA) class III and IV heart failure, patients were given 4 months of CoQ therapy (30 mg thrice daily). Significant improvement occurred in a number of areas, including NYHA functional class, left ventricular ejection fraction, and cardiac output. In a recent meta-analysis that evaluated eight randomized controlled trials, Soja et al[170] demonstrated significant improvement in a number of hemodynamic heart parameters, including stroke volume, cardiac output, and ejection fraction. Furthermore, numerous published case studies have touted the benefits of incorporating CoQ as part of the treatment regimen of heart-failure patients.[172,173] The agent is approved for clinical use in heart failure patients in many countries.

However, some recent studies have cast doubts regarding CoQ's efficacy in treating CHF. In 1999, Watson et al[173] conducted a randomized, double-blind study comparing oral CoQ to placebo for patients with ischemic or idiopathic dilated cardiomyopathy and chronic left ventricular dysfunction. In this study, 30 patients randomly received 33 mg CoQ three times daily or placebo for 3 months. Cardiac output, echocardiographic left ventricular volumes, and quality of life indices were measured at baseline and after treatment. There were no improvements in any of the cardiac parameters with CoQ at the study's conclusion. More recently, Khatta et al[174] conducted a randomized, double-blind controlled trial to determine the effect of CoQ on peak O_2 consumption, exercise duration, and ejection fraction in 55 patients with NYHA class III and IV symptoms. Patients were given 200 mg/d of CoQ or placebo for 6 months. Left ventricular ejection fraction (measured by left ventricular radionuclide ventriculography), peak oxygen consumption, and exercise duration were measured at baseline and at the end of the 6-month trial. All three of these parameters remained unchanged at the end of the study period. The authors concluded that there is no clinical benefit in adding CoQ to standard heart-failure regimens.

Proponents of CoQ have argued that the two aforementioned studies included patients with late stage CHF, in whom little benefit would be expected from CoQ; the sample sizes were too small; the studies were too short; and the dosage of CoQ was too low.[175,176] Researchers who found little benefit with CoQ therapy argue that although studies should be done on patients with early stage CHF, it would be difficult to recruit patients when there is already effective standard therapy, and that previous studies that have demonstrated a benefit of CoQ were small, anecdotal, and inconsistent.[177,178] It is hoped that more randomized, double-blind, controlled trials will be performed to fully determine whether CoQ_{10} is efficacious in treating CHF.

Lipids and Atherosclerosis

The effect of CoQ in the prevention of the oxidative modification of lipids has strongly interested CoQ researchers. Free-radical modification of low-density lipoprotein (LDL)-cholesterol is thought to be an important step in the pathogenesis of atherosclerosis, and CoQ is a lipophilic antioxidant for the protection of lipid oxidizability.[179,180] The role of CoQ in the prevention of free-radical damage has already been discussed. Aejmelaeus et al[179] found that LDL antioxidant defenses decrease with age. When humans were given CoQ supplements, the LDL-ubiquinol concentration increased significantly. It is theorized that an increase in LDL ubiquinol may help to prevent the oxidation of LDL, and thus help to prevent coronary artery disease. Kontush et al[180] attempted to determine whether the level of ubiquinol-10 in plasma can discriminate between healthy subjects, and patients who are expected to be subject to an increased oxidative stress in vivo. The plasma ubiquinol was measured in hyperlipidemic patients and healthy subjects. The oxidizability of the plasma samples from hyperlipidemic patients were increased compared to control subjects, suggesting that the hyperlipidemic individuals are subject to a higher oxidative stress in vivo. It was found that the hyperlipidemic patients had significantly less ubiquinol-10, expressed as a percentage of total ubiquinol-10 plus ubiquinone-10 normalized to plasma lipids, as compared with healthy subjects. The researchers concluded that plasma ubiquinol-10 levels may represent an early indicator of oxidative damage.

However, other researchers have garnered contradictory results regarding CoQ's role in modifying lipids. Kaikkonen et al[181] examined the effects of CoQ supplementation or placebo in 60 male smokers. Although CoQ significantly increased in plasma, the 2-month Q_{10} supplementation did not increase the oxidative resistance of the VLDL+LDL fraction. Cleary et al[182] tested whether the levels of major lipophilic antioxidants in the blood of patients with advanced atherosclerosis are different than those in age-matched controls. All patients had severe coronary artery disease, as evidenced by coronary angiography, as compared with the controls.

Plasma ubiquinol-10 (the reduced form of ubiquinone), total CoQ, and CoQ redox status were slightly lower in the atherosclerotic patients, but the differences between patients and controls were not statistically significant. The researchers concluded that plasma and LDL levels of lipophilic antioxidants were not depleted in patients suffering from severe atherosclerosis, and that CoQ does not serve as a diagnostic indicator of disease. It is also noted, however, that the oxidative stress may have occurred during an earlier stage of disease, and may have been compensated for by some adaptive response.

One study examined the role of CoQ in directly lowering lipids. In a recent randomized, double-blind placebo-controlled trial, Singh et al[183] examined the effects of CoQ on lipoprotein (a). Recent studies have indicated that lipoprotein (a) is a genetically determined risk factor for premature coronary artery disease (CAD), and that CoQ is present predominantly in LDL-cholesterol and possibly in the apo lipoprotein (a) fraction. Patients with a clinical diagnosis of acute myocardial infarction, unstable angina or angina pectoris with a moderately raised lipoprotein (a) were randomized to CoQ or placebo. At the end of the 28-day study, the CoQ group showed a significant reduction in lipoprotein (a), as well as a significant increase in HDL cholesterol.

Oxidative modification of LDL has been suggested to be a step in the development of atherosclerosis.[184] Therefore, CoQ may help prevent atheromas from forming by preventing the LDL from becoming oxidized. Singh et al[185] studied the effects of CoQ on experimental atherosclerosis in rabbits. In this randomized, single-blind, controlled trial, rabbits were either given CoQ or placebo over 24 weeks. At the end of the study, aortic and coronary plaque sizes, coronary atherosclerosis index, and aortic and coronary atherosclerosis scores were significantly lower in the CoQ group. Furthermore, a better quality of atheroma was identified in the CoQ group as compared with the placebo group. However, van de Vijver et al[184] sought to determine whether plasma CoQ levels corresponded with the risk of coronary atherosclerosis. A case-control study was performed to examine the relation between unsupplemented concentrations of plasma CoQ and coronary atherosclerosis. The plasma CoQ was measured in 71 males with angiographically documented severe coronary atherosclerosis and in 69 healthy male controls free from symptomatic cardiovascular disease. Differences in CoQ levels between the two groups did not reach significance, and it was concluded that an unsupplemented CoQ level is not related to a risk of coronary atherosclerosis.

Although vitamin E has been studied extensively as a means of preventing CAD, it has been proposed that α-tocopherol can also act as a pro-oxidant.[186] CoQ supplementation may help to reduce the oxidized form of vitamin E, thus promoting the antioxidant function of this vitamin. Again, this may be important in preventing lipids from becoming oxidized. Finally, the effects of lipid-lowering drugs upon the serum CoQ concentration has been studied. The biosynthesis of cholesterol and CoQ are completed through the mevalonate pathway (Fig. 37-7). Hydroxymethylglutaryl coenzyme A (HMG-CoA) inhibitors appear to inhibit the formation of CoQ. Mortensen et al[187] examined the effects of HMG-CoA inhibitors on serum CoQ levels. In a randomized, double-blind study, 45 hypercholesterolemic patients were either given lovastatin or pravastatin over 18 weeks. A dose-related decline of serum CoQ was noted in both groups, although the decline was more pronounced in the lovastatin group. The group cautions that a decline in CoQ may reduce myocardial function, and that the long-term use of statins must be investigated more thoroughly. In addition, decreased serum Q production with statins may also contribute to the skeletal muscle myalgia and myopathy

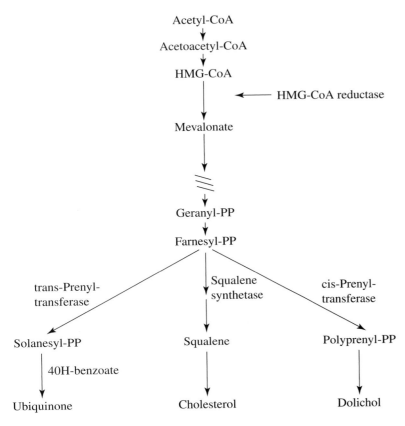

FIGURE 37-7. The mevalonate pathway. Illustration shows the branching point and the synthesis of the end-products: cholesterol, dolichol and coenzyme Q_{10}. (*Reproduced with permission from Mortensen et al.*[187])

seen with these drugs. Whether CoQ supplementation could alleviate these problems needs to be determined.

de Lorgeril et al[151] examined the effects of simvastatin and fenofibrate on serum ubiquinone. Simvastatin, while lowering LDL more than fenofibrate, lowered the serum ubiquinone level. Fenofibrate, which lowered triglycerides and fibrinogen more than simvastatin, actually increased the amount of ubiquinone per LDL molecule. It is suggested that the two drugs may complement each other.

Hypertension

The role of CoQ in the treatment of hypertension has been studied since the 1970s. Many studies have shown a decrease in both systolic and diastolic blood pressure associated with CoQ use. Researchers hypothesize different theories as to CoQ's mode of action, including that CoQ acts directly on the vasculature to decrease peripheral resistance; it acts as a superoxide antagonist; and it may decrease the cytoplasmic redox potential.[188] Recently, Lonnrot et al[189] demonstrated the control of arterial tone after long-term CoQ supplementation in senescent rats. In this study of 16-month-old rats, a control group was kept on a standard diet while the other group was supplemented with Q. The rats supplemented with Q demonstrated improved endothelium-dependent vasodilation and enhanced β-adrenoceptor-mediated relaxation. The group believes that CoQ may have augmented endothelial production of prostacyclin (PGI_2), increased sensitivity of smooth muscle to PGI_2, or both.

In a recent human study, Singh et al[190] examined the effect of CoQ supplementation in 59 patients with hypertension, who were receiving conventional antihypertensive drugs and presenting with coronary artery disease. In this randomized, double-blind study, patients randomly received either CoQ or a B-vitamin complex for

8 weeks. After 8 weeks of follow-up, systolic and diastolic blood pressure was significantly reduced. The group concluded that CoQ reduces blood pressure by decreasing oxidative stress, a possible pathophysiologic mechanism in the development of hypertension.

Angina Pectoris

Animal studies demonstrate that CoQ pretreatment may provide protection for the ischemic myocardium,[157,158,191–194] suggesting a rationale for its use in chronic ischemic cardiovascular syndromes. The results from a limited number of clinical trials using CoQ in chronic stable angina have been reported. In 1984, Hiasa et al[195] evaluated exercise tolerance in a placebo-controlled trial using intravenous CoQ 1.5 mg/kg once daily for 7 days versus placebo in 18 patients with chronic stable angina. The mean exercise time in the CoQ group at day 7 was significantly increased as compared to placebo treatment. The heart rate, blood pressure, and double product showed little change in either treatment group.

In 1985, Kamikawa et al[196] reported the results of a double-blind, randomized, crossover study that compared oral CoQ to placebo in 12 patients with chronic stable angina. In this study, patients randomly received oral CoQ (150 mg/d) or placebo for 4 weeks. This was followed by a crossover to the opposing treatment regimen for another 4 weeks. Patients underwent baseline exercise testing, which was repeated at the end of each 4-week treatment phase. Overall, exercise time significantly increased from 340 $\pm$ 126 seconds at baseline to 406 $\pm$ 114 seconds in the CoQ-treated group. During exercise testing in the CoQ treatment group, heart rate and rate-pressure product did not differ from baseline values.

Schardt et al[197] studied the effects of CoQ on ischemic ECG ST-segment depression in 15 patients with chronic stable angina. Patients entered a double-blind crossover study designed to compare the effects of 600 mg oral CoQ daily to placebo, and the combination of pindolol (7.5 mg) and isosorbide dinitrate (30 mg) daily. Treatment with CoQ caused a significant reduction in cumulative exercise-induced ST-segment depression when compared to placebo. However, there was no difference observed in this parameter when comparing CoQ treatment and combined pindolol and isosorbide dinitrate therapy in patients. In this study, CoQ caused a reduction in exercise systolic blood pressure from placebo values without an observable change in diastolic blood pressure or heart rate.

Finally, in a multicenter placebo-controlled double-blind trial, Wilson et al[198] reported a significant prolongation of treadmill exercise duration to the onset of angina in patients with chronic stable angina who were treated with 300 mg/d of CoQ. These results occurred in the absence of a significant change in the peak rate-pressure product.

The mechanism for improved exercise capacity in patients with angina pectoris treated with CoQ is poorly understood. Experimental studies showing protection of the ischemic myocardium favor a role for CoQ in maintaining oxidative phosphorylation.[157] It has been proposed that CoQ's antianginal action results from either enhanced resynthesis of ATP, a direct membrane protection mechanism,[199] or through reduction of free-radical species.[200] It is clear that CoQ has actions that differ from conventional antianginal agents such as nitrates, β-adrenergic blockers, and calcium antagonists. CoQ does not appear to have appreciable hemodynamic effects. Treatment with CoQ may allow ischemic tissue to reach higher levels of energy expenditure prior to the onset of clinically manifest symptoms or exercise-induced ST changes.

Myocardial Infarction

Singh et al[201] recently conducted a randomized, double-blind, placebo-controlled trial to examine the effects of CoQ in 144 patients with an acute myocardial infarction (MI). CoQ or placebo was given for 28 days to patients with acute MI. After treatment, the rates of angina pectoris, total arrhythmias and poor left ventricular function were significantly reduced in the CoQ group. Furthermore, cardiac deaths and nonfatal infarctions were also significantly reduced in the CoQ group. The authors suggest that CoQ may provide a rapid protective effect in patients with acute MI if administered near the onset of symptoms.

Myocardial Protection (Cardioplegia and Open-Heart Surgery)

The bulk of published data on CoQ as a modifier of cardiac ischemia points to a predominant role of CoQ during the myocardial reperfusion phase. Whether its mechanism of action is as a direct membrane-stabilizing agent or as free-radical scavenger is unclear. Given its ability to protect myocardial tissue during ischemic reperfusion, it is not surprising that CoQ has been evaluated in patients undergoing cardiac surgery. It has been proposed that free radicals and their metabolites derived from molecular oxygen may contribute to myocardial dysfunction during ischemia and reperfusion.[202] A recent study examined CoQ's effect on free radicals formed during cardiac surgery. Zhou et al[202] tested the use of CoQ as myocardial protection in 24 patients undergoing cardiac valve replacement surgery. Twelve patients received intravenous and intracoronary CoQ before, during, and after their operations, while the other 12 patients did not receive CoQ. Plasma malondialdehyde (MDA), erythrocyte superoxide dismutase and myocardial muscle creatine-kinase isoenzyme (CK-MB), hypothesized as indicators of free-radical damage, were measured pre- and postoperatively in both patients and controls. Findings included lower plasma MDA concentrations, serum creatine-kinase (CK)-levels in the CoQ group, as

well as hydroxyl scavenging activity. Furthermore, the erythrocyte superoxide dismutase (SOD) activity was significantly higher in the CoQ group, indicating an upregulation of this enzyme. The researchers concluded that intravenous and intracoronary CoQ may play a protective role during cardiac valve replacement surgery by modifying free-radical formation. In a similar study, Chello et al[203] examined the role of CoQ in protecting tissues from free-radical-mediated reperfusion injury during abdominal aortic cross-clamping. In this study, patients either received oral CoQ or placebo for 7 days prior to the operation. The hemodynamic profile of each patient was measured during clamping and declamping of the abdominal aorta. Indicators of free-radical activity were measured; again, free-radical activity was significantly lower in the CoQ group, suggesting a protective role of CoQ during routine vascular procedures.

One randomized study compared the effectiveness of preoperative CoQ to a control group in preventing low cardiac output states following cardiac surgery.[204] The CoQ-treated group had a significantly lower incidence of low cardiac output states postoperatively when compared to controls. Sunamori et al[205] evaluated CoQ in patients just prior to coronary artery bypass surgery, and compared the effectiveness of this regimen to controls. They found the CoQ-treated group had significantly higher left ventricular stroke work indices, lower requirements for inotropic support, and significantly lower levels of serum CPK-MB in the postoperative state.

Judy et al[206] studied 20 high-risk cardiac surgical patients, half of whom were treated with 100 mg/d CoQ for 14 days preoperatively and 30 days postoperatively. Cardiac index and ejection fraction were improved in the CoQ-treated group when compared to controls. Overall, postoperative recovery time was also lessened with CoQ treatment. Chello et al,[207] using an oral CoQ regimen of 150 mg/d for 7 days preoperatively in patients undergoing elective coronary artery bypass surgery, showed similar results, as well as a reduction in reperfusion arrhythmias.

The effects of CoQ have been studied in the rejection of transplanted hearts in humans. Kucharska et al[208] assessed the CoQ levels in 28 endomyocardial biopsies from 22 patients and 61 blood samples from 31 patients after heart transplantation with histologically confirmed signs of rejection. The values were compared to 14 patients with cardiomyopathies who were candidates for heart transplantation. Blood analyses were compared with 50 healthy patients. Myocardial and blood coenzyme CoQ concentrations were significantly decreased in the incipient phase of rejection; the levels of CoQ decreased in correspondence with the severity of rejection. The authors conclude that supplementary CoQ may be beneficial in patients after heart transplantation by enhancing cellular bioenergetics and preventing cardiac damage.

The effects of CoQ have also been evaluated in animal heart transplant models. Matsumoto et al[209] demonstrated that left ventricular function was better preserved in whole animals treated with CoQ as compared to cold cardioplegia. Furthermore, the combination of CoQ and cold cardioplegia was even better than either regimen alone. Similar results were found by Okamuto et al[210] when using intravenous and intracoronary CoQ to enhance cardioplegia.

The prevailing opinion suggests that CoQ may have a potential role for protecting myocardium that is rendered ischemic and subsequently reperfused. The exact mechanism of action is not well understood. CoQ may prevent lipid peroxidation, making sarcolemmal membranes less sensitive to conformational changes induced by ischemia/reperfusion. From a clinical standpoint, it appears that CoQ might have a role as an ischemia modifier in several ischemic cardiac syndromes, including unstable angina, acute myocardial infarction, following clot lysis by mechanical or fibrinolytic means, and during surgical procedures such as cardiac valve replacement, coronary artery bypass grafting, and, possibly, heart transplantation.

Other Clinical Uses

Recently, ^{11}C-labeled CoQ_{10} was synthesized for use in positron emission tomographic (PET) studies,[211] and was demonstrated to be a desirable agent for myocardial imaging. Because CoQ plays an important role in oxidative phosphorylation, it has the potential to aid in the evaluation of metabolic processes that cannot be directly examined by conventional tracers, such as [18]FDG (fluorodeoxyglucose). Initial studies have demonstrated the feasibility of using [11]C CoQ_{10} and indicate its potential role in imaging the myocardium in states of abnormal metabolic activity.

Adverse Effects

In pharmacologic doses, CoQ is relatively devoid of major side effects. The adverse reactions that have been reported in patients include epigastric discomfort in 0.39%, loss of appetite in 0.23%, nausea in 0.16%, and diarrhea in 0.12%.[212–214] Asymptomatic elevations of lactate dehydrogenase have been seen in patients taking 300 mg of CoQ, as has mild subclinical elevations in serum glutamic oxaloacetic transaminase (SGOT). There are few documented drug interactions with CoQ. However, certain oral hypoglycemic agents are known to inhibit some CoQ enzymes and, thus, theoretically, might be inhibitory to exogenously administered CoQ.[215] As discussed, HMG-CoA inhibitors such as lovastatin lower CoQ levels.[216] Further study is required to clarify whether or not other drug-drug interactions exist for CoQ.

Conclusion

CoQ appears to have potential use as a treatment for myocardial ischemic syndromes and congestive heart failure, and its clinical use for these indications is increasing outside the United States. Additional work must be done in determining reliable Q_{10} levels for clinical purposes. Kaikkonen et al[217] studied a variety of factors that had possible effects upon CoQ levels. In addition to cholesterol and triglycerides, several other factors, including gender, alcohol consumption, age, and intensity of exercise, can affect CoQ levels. Additional work with CoQ needs to be done regarding dose (300 mg/d is the dose used in most studies) and establishing clinical efficacy before a recommendation can be made regarding its use in treating various cardiovascular disorders as a primary or adjunctive treatment.

L-CARNITINE

L-Carnitine (the physiologically required form of carnitine) is a nitrogenous constituent of muscle that plays a primary role in the oxidation of fatty acids in mammals (Fig. 37-8). Because the mammalian heart uses fatty acids as its primary source of energy,

FIGURE 37-8. Chemical formula of L-carnitine.

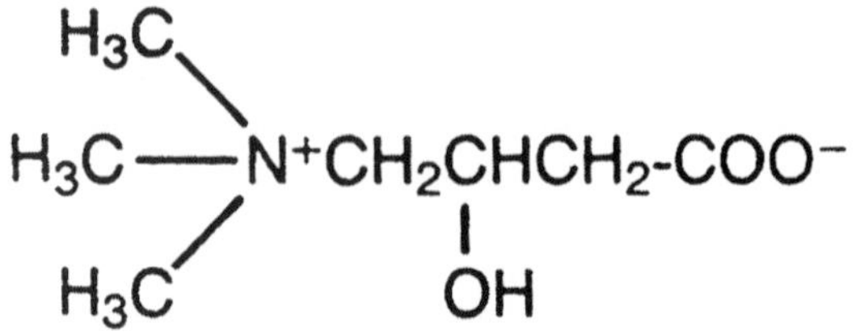

TABLE 37-7. Potential Therapeutic Benefits from Exogenous Treatment with L-Carnitine in Cardiovascular Disease

- Correction of carnitine-deficiency state
- Facilitation of fatty acid and glucose oxidation in situations of limited oxygen availability
- Removal from mitochondria of harmful fatty acyl groups that accumulate as a result of normal and pathological metabolism
- Free-radical scavenger following reperfusion of ischemic myocardium

it is understandable that a deficiency in the supply of carnitine can result in various cardiac abnormalities.

In addition, clinical and experimental studies have shown the therapeutic usefulness of L-carnitine and its derivative, propionyl-L-carnitine (PLC), in the treatment of various cardiovascular diseases, including ischemic heart disease, congestive heart failure, arrhythmia, and peripheral vascular disease (Table 37-7).

History of Carnitine

Carnitine was first identified as a nitrogenous constituent of muscle in 1905. The role it plays in the oxidation of long-chain fatty acids in mammals was established in the laboratories of Fritz and Bremer in the late 1950s.[218]

Carnitine (*levocarnitine;* CARNITOR) was approved by the Food and Drug Administration in 1986, in both its intravenous and oral forms, as an orphan drug for the treatment of primary carnitine deficiency. It is also used in the treatment of patients with conditions known to produce secondary carnitine deficiency (e.g., renal failure and various cardiovascular diseases). One to two g/d orally in divided doses is adequate for most therapeutic purposes. Intravenous doses range from 40 to 100 mg/kg. For children, oral L-carnitine is given at 100 mg/kg/d.

Physiologic Actions

Carnitine has many physiologically important roles. It is most important for the oxidation of long-chain fatty acids. It also allows for the removal of short- and medium-chain fatty acids from the cell. Carnitine also facilitates the aerobic metabolism of carbohydrates,[219,220] and enhances the rate of oxidative phosphorylation.

Carnitine's role in fatty acid oxidation is the following (Fig. 37-9): fatty acids are activated in the outer mitochondrial membrane upon conjugation to a molecule of CoA. They must then enter the mitochondrial matrix to be oxidized. Long-chain fatty acyl-CoA molecules, however, are unable to traverse the inner mitochondrial membrane. Therefore, a special transport system is needed. An activated long-chain fatty acid is able to cross the inner mitochondrial membrane by conjugating itself to a carnitine molecule producing an acylcarnitine. The enzyme for this reaction is carnitine acyltransferase I, which is found on the outer mitochondrial membrane. The acylcarnitine is then shuttled across the inner mitochondrial membrane by a translocase. At this point, the long-chain fatty acid reconjugates with a CoA molecule found in the matrix and it is now ready to undergo oxidation. This reconjugation is catalyzed by carnitine acyltransferase II. The free carnitine molecule is shuttled back to the mitochondrial cytosol by a translocase in exchange for a new incoming acylcarnitine. This specialized transport system is commonly known as the *carnitine shuttle.*

Carnitine also facilitates removal from the mitochondria of short- and medium-chain fatty acids that accumulate there as a result

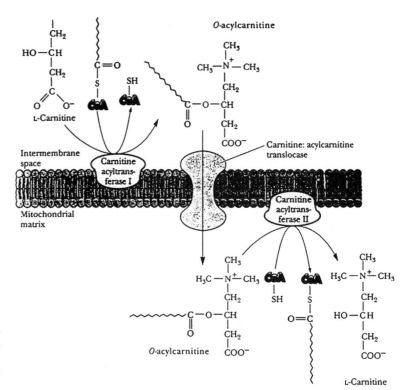

FIGURE 37-9. The formation of acylcarnitines and their transport across the inner mitochondrial membrane — the carnitine "shuttle." (*Reproduced with permission from Garrett RH, Grisham CM: Biochemistry. Fort Worth, TX: Saunders College Publications, 1995:739.*)

of normal and pathologic metabolism. These acyl-CoA groups possess detergent-like properties and are therefore harmful to cellular and intracellular membranes. The short- and medium-chain fatty acyl-CoAs are transesterified to carnitine and are then transported out of the mitochondria by the carnitine-acylcarnitine translocase. This allows the "freeing up" of CoA molecules in the mitochondria under conditions where short- and medium-chain fatty acids are being produced at a rate that is faster than they can be used.

In addition, as carnitine conjugates with these acyl groups, it lowers the mitochondrial acetyl-CoA/CoA ratio, and glucose oxidation is stimulated. This happens because a decrease in the ratio of acetyl-CoA/CoA stimulates the pyruvate dehydrogenase complex, which catalyzes the rate limiting step of glucose oxidation.[219]

Carnitine is a physiologic modulator of the mitochondrial acetyl-CoA/CoA ratio, thus it can influence many biologic processes.

Carnitine Requirements and Biosynthesis

Carnitine is widely distributed, but is particularly abundant in muscle. It is synthesized from the amino acids lysine and methionine in the liver and kidney. Four micronutrients are needed for the various enzymatic steps: iron, niacin, ascorbic acid, and pyridoxine. Adult carnitine requirements are satisfied by dietary sources and biosynthesis. The primary dietary sources of carnitine are meat and dairy products.[221]

Primary carnitine deficiency is usually seen in a group of uncommon genetic disorders (e.g., Barth's disease, which is an X-linked recessive disorder). Lipid metabolism is severely affected resulting in storage of fat in muscle and serious functional abnormalities of cardiac and skeletal muscle. There are two types of disorders caused by primary carnitine deficiency: systematic and myopathic. Systematic disorders are manifested by low levels of carnitine in liver, plasma, and muscle. There are variable symptoms. Myopathic disorders are characterized primarily by muscle weakness. Storage

of nonmetabolized fat and low carnitine levels are seen upon biopsy of muscle. Plasma carnitine levels, however, are normal.

There are secondary forms of carnitine deficiency as well. These include renal tubular disorders,[222] in which carnitine excretion may be excessive, and chronic renal failure,[223] in which hemodialysis may cause excessive losses of carnitine as well. Patients with metabolic disorders in which circulating concentrations of organic acids are increased can also develop carnitine deficiency. Diseases in which there is a leakage of carnitine into the plasma, such as ischemic heart disease, can also be the cause of a secondary carnitine deficiency.

Absorption, Fate, and Excretion

Almost all of dietary L-carnitine is absorbed from the intestine. This is mainly accomplished via a saturable transport mechanism. Therefore, as oral dosage of L-carnitine is increased, absolute absorption decreases. Oral bioavailability is considerably less than following a comparable intravenous dosage.[224] Transport of L-carnitine into cells occurs mainly through an active mechanism.[225]

D-Carnitine is absorbed in a similar way and can therefore inhibit the uptake of L-carnitine. Administration of exogenous D-carnitine can produce a syndrome similar to myasthenia gravis. Carnitine is, for the most part, not metabolized, and most of it is excreted in the urine as acylcarnitine. Renal tubules can reabsorb more than 90% of free unesterified carnitine.[226]

A Comparison of L-Carnitine and Propionyl-L-Carnitine

There are studies that have concluded that the administration of PLC, a naturally occurring analogue of L-carnitine, is considerably more effective in the treatment of carnitine deficiency and cardiomyo- pathies than is the administration of exogenous L-carnitine.[227–229] The reason for this is not completely understood.

It is thought to be, in part, because of the anaplerotic utilization of its propionate group as a source of tricarboxylic acid (TCA) cycle intermediates[227,229] in the presence of an optimal amount of ATP and free L-carnitine, leading to suppression of toxic hydroxyl radicals and increased energy production. The propionate group alone, however, is not the reason, as it has been shown that PLC is significantly more effective in myocardial protection than propionate alone.[227-229]

Ischemic Heart Disease

Myocardial ischemia[230] causes an accumulation of fatty acid esters, primarily because of the inhibition of β-oxidation, but also because of an increased formation of endogenous fatty acids from phospholipid hydrolysis. Because of their detergent properties, these compounds are damaging to cellular and intracellular membranes. Additionally, the high levels of fatty acids inhibit glucose metabolism, further depleting energy reserves. Carnitine protects against these negative effects by decreasing these fatty acyl-CoA esters through formation of corresponding acylcarnitine compounds, which are considerably less harmful to the cell.[231] Also, short- and medium-chain acylcarnitines are able to diffuse across the cell membrane and can be eliminated into the blood and urine.

In ischemic heart disease, however, carnitine levels are very low either due to leakage from damaged tissue or secondary to the high rate of esterification. Several experimental and clinical studies suggest that the administration of exogenous carnitine following ischemic events has a beneficial effect on cardiac function.

Several animal trials show the effects of carnitine treatment on ischemic subjects. Liedtke et al[232] tested the influence of PLC on adolescent swine subjected to 45 min of regional ischemia. Test results indicate that those hearts treated with PLC show significantly smaller decreases of muscle shortening in the ischemic zone, suppression of ventricular fibrillation, and improved metabolic and mechanical work.

Broderick et al[233] showed that L-carnitine reverses the inhibition of glucose oxidation that occurs with the build-up of fatty acyl-CoA molecules during ischemia in normal and diabetic rat hearts.

Paulson et al[234] studied the protective effects of PLC in the ischemic diabetic rat heart. After inducing diabetes in male Sprague-Dawley rats, the study showed that PLC significantly improved the ability of control and diabetic hearts to recover cardiac contractile performance with chronic treatment; however, this recovery was more effective in the diabetic hearts.

Clinical studies show that carnitine plays a protective role in humans with ischemic heart disease. Bohles et al[235] showed that 40 patients treated with oral and intravenous carnitine before coronary bypass surgery had increased myocardial ATP levels and reduced lactate concentrations when compared with those patients not given carnitine treatment.

Corbucci et al[236] compared carnitine and bicarbonate administration in 230 patients undergoing extracorporeal circulation. Ischemic changes were noted in the bicarbonate group and absent in the carnitine group.

Bartels et al[237] studied the effects of PLC on ischemia-induced myocardial dysfunction in men with angina pectoris. The placebo-controlled study consisted of 31 fasting, untreated male patients with ischemic heart disease. The patients were given either 15mg/kg of PLC or placebo. Hemodynamic, metabolic, and nuclear angiographic studies were done before, during, and after pacing stress test. The results of the study showed that PLC prevents ischemia-induced ventricular dysfunction not by improving myocardial oxygen supply (no vasodilatory effects were seen), but as a result of its intrinsic metabolic actions (i.e., esterifying acyl groups) stimulating the pyruvate dehydrogenase complex and increasing tricarboxylic acid cycle intermediate flux.

Iliceto et al[238] conducted a randomized, double-blind, placebo-controlled study on the effect of L-carnitine administration on long-term left ventricular dilation in patients with acute anterior myocardial infarction. The study included 472 patients with a first acute myocardial infarction. The patients were treated with either L-carnitine or placebo within 24 h after onset of chest pains. The dosage was 9 g/d intravenously for the first 5 days and 6 g/d orally for 12 months. The result of the trial showed that those patients treated with L-carnitine had a significant decrease in left ventricular dilation over those in the placebo group. It was also noted that death from congestive heart failure after discharge was approximately 30% less in those treated with L-carnitine.

Similar findings were observed by Singh et al[239] in a randomized, double-blind, placebo-controlled trial of L-carnitine in patients with suspected acute myocardial infarction. These investigators found a reduction in total cardiac events, including cardiac death and nonfatal infarction, during the first 28 days in patients receiving L-carnitine.

Another study[240] evaluated the effects of PLC on the exercise tolerance of 12 patients with stable exertional angina in a double-blind, randomized, placebo-controlled, crossover protocol using serial exercise tests to measure exercise capacity. Patients treated with PLC had significantly improved total work, exercise time, and time-to-ischemia threshold, as compared with patients receiving placebo. Also, the amount of ST segment depression was significantly reduced.

Cacciatore et al[241] conducted a randomized trial of 200 adult males with stable angina. One group (n = 100) was given a daily dose of 2 g oral carnitine for 6 months; the other group was given placebo. The carnitine group showed increased exercise capacity and better NYHA functional classes than did the placebo group.

Rizzon et al[242] administered L-carnitine or placebo to patients suffering from acute myocardial infarction. They then measured urine levels of free carnitine, long-chain acylcarnitine esters, and short-chain acylcarnitine esters. The results of the urine analyses indicated that those patients treated with L-carnitine showed higher levels of acylcarnitine esters in their urine than did those patients treated with placebo. This may be explained as a result of the transesterification between the administered exogenous carnitine and the acyl-CoA groups within the cells. This allows the "washout" of harmful excess acyl groups which are accumulating in the cell due to the postischemic decrease of fatty acid oxidation. These acyl groups conjugate to carnitine and are eventually excreted in the urine.

Although there have been a number of trials showing carnitine administration to be of little or no benefit in the treatment of ischemic disease,[227,243,244] the majority of the studies have shown potential benefit, which warrants further investigation.

Congestive Heart Failure

Several studies show that in situations of cardiac hypertrophy and congestive heart failure, myocardial carnitine levels are significantly decreased, and plasma and urinary free and acyl-carnitine levels are significantly increased.[245-248] It is therefore logical that the restoration of normal carnitine levels through the administration of exogenous carnitine would be of therapeutic value when treating these cardiomyopathies.[249] Interestingly, it has also been shown that the therapeutic value of carnitine treatment extends beyond the restoration of normal carnitine levels, also affecting improvement in cardiac function through other metabolic pathways.[250,251]

Several experimental and clinical studies have shown that carnitine can improve cardiac function in subjects with hypertrophied hearts and those with heart failure.

Schonekess et al[219,252] studied the effects of PLC on hypertrophied rat hearts. The results of the study showed that those rats treated with PLC had a significant increase in contractile function and cardiac work. The study noted that while those hearts treated with PLC showed a sharp rise in their glucose oxidation rate, the increases in fatty acid oxidation rates were not significant. This allows for the possibility that the primary effect of carnitine administration in hypertrophied hearts is an increase in carbohydrate oxidation. The mechanism for this increase is (as mentioned before in great detail) the conjugation of carnitine with acetyl groups, thereby lowering the acetyl-CoA/CoA ratio. This, in turn, stimulates the enzyme PDH, the rate-limiting step of glucose oxidation. Additionally, the anaplerotic effect of the propionyl group in PLC feeds intermediates into the TCA cycle. Another proposed explanation of the improvement of cardiac function is that somehow PLC increases the efficiency of translating ATP production into cardiac work.[246] Either way, data from these experiments seem to indicate that the beneficial effect of PLC on the mechanical functioning of hypertrophied hearts does not result merely from normalization of fatty acid oxidation.[253]

Kobayashi et al[254] studied the myocardial carnitine levels and therapeutic efficacy of L-carnitine in BIO 14.6 hamsters with cardiomyopathies, and in patients with chronic congestive heart failure. The results of the study showed that both cardiomyopathic hamsters and patients with heart failure had reduced free carnitine levels and increased levels of acylcarnitine esters. It was also shown that significant myocardial damage in the cardiomyopathic hamsters was prevented by the intraperitoneal administration of L-carnitine in the early stages of the cardiomyopathy. Similarly, 55% of the patients with congestive heart failure moved to a lower NYHA class and 66% showed an overall improvement in their condition.

A large-scale clinical trial was carried out[255] in which 574 patients with heart failure (NYHA class II and III) and left ventricular ejection fraction <40% were randomized to carnitine versus placebo. Exercise tolerance was significantly improved in the patients with left ventricular ejection fraction of 30 to 40% in the carnitine group. However, the overall mortality rate was slightly higher (3.0% vs 1.9%), as well as the subsequent follow-up admission rate (6.3% vs 5.3%), in the carnitine group.

Additional clinical investigations included a double-blind, phase II study of PLC versus placebo in a group of 60 patients with mild to moderate (NYHA class II and III) congestive heart failure.[256] The group was made up of men and women between the ages of 48 and 73 years who were chronically treated with digitalis and diuretics for at least 3 months, and who still displayed symptoms. Thirty randomly chosen patients were given an oral dosage of 500 mg of PLC, three times daily for 180 days. After 30, 90, and 180 days, the maximum exercise time was evaluated, as was left ventricular ejection fraction. Throughout the period of testing, the patients treated with PLC showed significant increases in the values of both tests. On the basis of these results, the authors concluded that PLC is a drug of undoubted therapeutic interest in patients with congestive heart failure.[256]

Pucciarelli et al[257] also conducted a randomized, double-blind study of PLC versus placebo. The study included 50 patients of both

sexes between the ages of 48 and 69 suffering from mild to moderate congestive heart failure. Results of the study demonstrated that those patients in the PLC group had a greater maximum exercise time and an increased left ventricular ejection fraction.

Peripheral Vascular Disease and Atherosclerosis

The normal nonischemic diabetic heart shows abnormal fat metabolism with excesses of long-chained acyl-CoA and acylcarnitine. There are also reductions in free and total carnitine concentrations.[258] These resultant hyperlipidemic states lead to atherosclerosis and peripheral vascular disease.

Multiple experimental and clinical studies have assessed the therapeutic benefits of L-carnitine administration to patients with peripheral vascular disease. Spagnoli et al[259] studied the beneficial effects of PLC on the progression of atherosclerotic lesions in aged hyperlipidemic rabbits. For 9 months, two groups of rabbits received a hypercholesterolemic diet—one group with PLC administration and one without. The observed results showed that the group treated with PLC in addition to the hypercholesterolemic diet exhibited a marked decrease in plasma triglycerides, VLDL and intermediate-density lipoproteins (IDL), while plasma cholesterol was slightly reduced in comparison to the control group. In addition, the PLC-treated rabbits showed a reduction in both plaque thickness and extent. A decline in macrophage and smooth-muscle-derived foam cells was also noted. These results indicate a decrease in plaque cell formation and in the severity of atherosclerotic lesions with carnitine treatment.

Corsico et al[260] studied the therapeutic effect of PLC on rats with long-lasting chemically induced peripheral arteriopathy. They injected sodium laurate in both femoral arteries of rats, causing arteriopathy by thickening the intima, thereby narrowing the lumen. They then evaluated the walking capacity of the rats at different times up to 5 weeks after sodium laurate injection. The experimental results showed that those rats given long-term treatment (4 weeks) of PLC at a dosage of 250 mg/kg had a significant increase in walking capacity throughout the entire period.

Several clinical studies also assessed the efficacy of carnitine treatment in patients with peripheral vascular disease and/or atherosclerosis. Ghidini et al[261] showed that daily oral doses of carnitine in patients with heart failure significantly decreased their serum triglyceride levels. An additional study showed decreases in serum cholesterol and HDL levels.[262]

Patients with peripheral vascular disease have a reduced exercise capacity due to reduced oxidation and buildup of lactic acid in the ischemic muscle. Through the action of carnitine acetyltransferase, carnitine boosts mitochondrial oxidation by depleting acetyl-CoA and releasing free CoA and acylcarnitine. This acyl-scavenging process becomes crucial in conditions of limited oxygen availability. Therefore, the more severe the ischemic disease or the higher the level of exercise, the greater the accumulation of CoA esters in the damaged tissue, and, consequently, the greater the amount of carnitine needed for their removal.[263]

Brevetti et al[264] studied the effects of carnitine treatment in patients with intermittent claudication and diminished exercise capacity. In a double-blind, placebo-controlled, multicenter study, 245 patients suffering from peripheral vascular disease were randomly assigned to receive PLC or placebo. Brevetti had already determined PLC was more effective than L-carnitine.[265] The initial dosage was 1 g/d and was increased at 2 month intervals to

2 g/d and then 3 g/d. Analysis of results showed that those patients treated with PLC had a significant improvement in maximal walking distance and a marked increase in distance walked at onset of claudication.[265] It was also noted that this improvement took place without affecting regional hemodynamics, suggesting that the role that carnitine plays in metabolism is credited with the benefit.

The efficacy of carnitine in peripheral vascular disease and hyperlipidemia has been strongly demonstrated in both animal studies and clinical trials.[266,267]

Arrhythmia

Both animal studies and clinical trials demonstrate carnitine's antiarrhythmic properties. Experimental studies done in both rat and rabbit hearts show that PLC acts as an antiradical agent protecting myocardial cells from free radicals produced during ischemia and reperfusion.[268,269] This is important because these free radicals are implicated in the development of reperfusion-induced arrhythmias.[270]

Rizzon et al[242] measured the occurrence of left ventricular arrhythmia in patients suffering from acute myocardial infarction treated with L-carnitine or placebo. They noted a significant reduction of left ventricular arrhythmia in those patients receiving L-carnitine. In a study by Palazzuoli et al[271] of 30 patients with ischemic heart disease and extrasystolic ventricular multifocal arrhythmia on dynamic electrocardiograms, L-carnitine was shown to significantly reduce the arrhythmic activity of the ischemic myocardium, with an even better response seen when carnitine was added to propafenone treatment.

Conclusion

Carnitine is an endogenous, naturally occurring, substance with several very important physiologic roles. Exogenous carnitine administration is beneficial to those patients who, for a variety of reasons, are deficient in carnitine.

Specifically, animal studies and clinical trials, performed both abroad and in the United States, indicate that carnitine is effective in treating patients with various cardiovascular diseases such as ischemic heart disease, congestive heart failure, peripheral vascular disease, arrhythmia, and hyperlipemia. Carnitine appears to "boost" fatty acid and carbohydrate oxidation in the cell, while helping to remove harmful substances (i.e., excess acyl groups, free radicals) from the cell. However, the exact mechanisms responsible for carnitine's therapeutic actions are not completely agreed upon. Further studies are warranted.

CYTOPROTECTIVE AGENTS (PARTIAL FATTY ACID OXIDATION INHIBITORS)

Distinct classes of agents known as metabolic modulators and myocardial cytoprotective agents have been available since the 1970s for the treatment of angina pectoris. In contrast to other current pharmacologic approaches to angina, including calcium-channel blockers, nitrates, and beta-blockers, these metabolic modulators do not alter hemodynamics. Furthermore, these drugs do not appear either to reduce myocardial oxygen requirements or to enhance myocardial perfusion, and do not dilate coronary or peripheral arteries. Prototype agents include ranolazine and trimetazidine, and drugs of this class are also known as partial fatty acid oxidation (pFOX) inhibitors.

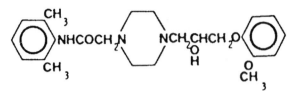

FIGURE 37-10. Chemical structure of ranolazine.

Ranolazine

Biochemistry of Myocardial Ischemia

When there is an adequate supply of oxygen to the heart, both the Krebs cycle and oxidative phosphorylation provide a myocardial cell with high levels of ATP and citrate, thereby blocking glycolysis (Fig. 37-10).[272] During mild ischemia, falling ATP and citrate levels stimulate glycolysis principally through the increased activity of phosphofructokinase, an enzyme allosterically activated by fructose 2,6-biphosphate and AMP, but inhibited by ATP and citrate.[273] This feedback mechanism is known as the *Pasteur effect* (Fig. 37-11). However, during severe ischemia, protons and lactate accumulate due to poor washout which inhibits both phosphofructokinase and glyceraldehyde 3-phosphate dehydrogenase, another enzyme that regulates the glycolytic rate. The inhibition of these enzymes decreases myocardial glucose uptake and shifts substrate myocardial utilization to lactate and free fatty acids, which accumulate from both the impairment of mitochondrial β-oxidation secondary to hypoxia and from the high levels of catecholamines released during ischemia.

A decrease in the glycolytic rate severely impairs a tissue's capacity to survive ischemia because fatty acid oxidation requires approximately 12% more oxygen to produce the same amount of ATP as glucose.[272] Moreover, as Weiss and Lamp suggest, loss of ATP from key glycolytic enzymes located in the sarcolemma or cytoskeleton may predispose the heart to arrhythmias through the

FIGURE 37-11. (*A*) In the normally oxygenated heart, tissue citrate and ATP are high and inhibit glycolysis. (*B*) When coronary flow is mildly decreased (mild ischemia), the Pasteur effect results. (*C*) In severe ischemia (severe deprivation of both oxygen and coronary flow), the accumulation of lactate and protons inhibits glycolysis despite any tendency to accumulate by a low cardiac content of ATP. (*Reproduced with permission from Opie.*[272])

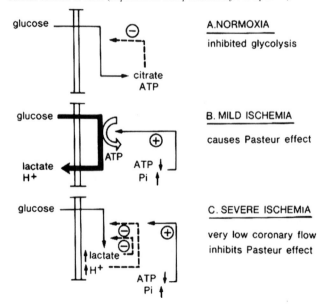

opening of ATP-sensitive potassium channels.[274] The accumulation of lipid metabolites also appears to predispose the heart to arrhythmias, possibly through blockade of membrane functions such as the sodium pump and phospholipid cycles, and to futile cycles that waste ATP with no apparent benefit for the ischemic myocardium.[272] Thus, despite its inadequacy in supplying the total energy needs of a myocardial cell, anaerobic glycolysis may be vital in sustaining critical ion gradients and membrane functions.

Ranolazine, ($\pm$)N-2(2,6-dimethylphenyl)-4-[2-hydroxy-3-(2-methoxyphenoxy) prophyl]-1-piperazineacetamide, is a novel agent that has unique pharmacologic properties that might be useful for the medical management of patients with myocardial ischemia and in patients undergoing renal transplantation.[275–279] Although its mechanism of action is unknown, ranolazine is surmised to alter cellular metabolism, principally because of its negligible effects on cardiovascular hemodynamics and known cellular receptors.[280] Such an antianginal agent could be useful for patients unable to tolerate other medications that cause deleterious effects on myocardial conduction and contractility.

Pharmacologic Actions

The discovery of ranolazine's anti-ischemic properties was based on initial screening tests that showed beneficial effects in several animal disease models. However, few studies have documented the pharmacologic profile of ranolazine. It was shown that ranolazine has negligible to low affinity for α- and β-adrenoreceptors, as well as for D1, D2, M1, M2, A1, A2, and serotonin receptors.[280] Weak calcium antagonist effects with selectivity for heart muscle were seen with ranolazine, but no effects on potassium channels or on resting membrane potentials were noted. Ferrandon and coworkers demonstrated that ranolazine's cardioprotective effects following reperfusion injury were not augmented by coadministration of free-radical scavengers, suggesting a mechanism of action other than neutralization of free radicals.[281]

Because ranolazine has little effect on known cellular drug pharmacoreceptors but does have favorable effects on biochemical indices of ischemia, a modulation of myocardial metabolism has been proposed as the basis for ranolazine's antianginal actions (Table 37-8). Insight into this potential mechanism was provided by Allely and coworkers who studied ranolazine's effect on α_1 receptors.[282] These receptors, which are increased in number during hypoxia and possibly after cardiac hypertrophy, may cause positive inotropic effects via increased intracellular calcium and sensitivity of contractile proteins to calcium.[283,284] An increase in the concentration of sarcolemmal, long-chain acylcarnitines during ischemia may also induce an increase in externalized α_1 receptors, as suggested by data showing sodium 2-[5-(4-chlorophenyl)-pentylene]-oxiran-2-carboxylate (POCA), a carnitine palmityl transferase I inhibitor (CPT 1) blocking such an increase.[284] Allely et al found that palmityl carnitine increased α_1 adrenoreceptor density, while pretreatment with POCA prevented this effect.[282] Ranolazine at 500 μg/kg administered intravenously 15 min before a left anterior descending occlusion or 500 μg/kg twice daily for 3 days and 15 min before occlusion, similarly blocked upregulation of α_1 adrenoreceptors due to

TABLE 37-8. Proposed Mechanisms of Action of Ranolazine During Myocardial Ischemia

- Blocks upregulation of myocardial α_1-adrenergic receptors
- Inhibits uptake of free fatty acids and fatty acid oxidation
- Reverses inhibition of NADH dehydrogenase, thereby improving metabolic efficiency and reducing oxygen waste

ischemia. However, ranolazine does not inhibit CPT 1 directly, thus suggesting that ranolazine modulates the metabolism of ischemic myocardial cells by decreasing the uptake of free fatty acids.

Further evidence of ranolazine's ability to favorably alter myocardial metabolism was shown in a placebo-controlled study of 45 patients with chronic stable angina randomized to receive 50 to 250 μg/kg of ranolazine intravenously.[276a] Hemodynamic data and blood samples were obtained on these patients in a basal state and during pacing at 130 bpm (beats per minute). No effects on coronary resistance, coronary sinus blood flow, arterial pressure, cardiac function or metabolism were seen in the basal state with ranolazine. However, during pacing with plasma levels of ranolazine >150 ng/mL, glucose uptake significantly increased by a median of 70 μmol/min, while fatty acid uptake significantly decreased by a median of 20 μmol/min. Lactate uptake and production remained unchanged. Myocardial oxygen uptake also increased during pacing with no significant differences observed between both groups. Thus, ranolazine appears, whether directly or indirectly, to shift myocardial metabolism toward anaerobic glycolysis during increased oxygen demand.

Finally, Stanley and coworkers noted that the treatment of myocardial ischemia with ranolazine required the presence of sufficient residual oxygen delivery to the myocardium such that it would support some level of oxidative metabolism.[277] Without sufficient Kreb's cycle activity, lactate production cannot be reduced. Thus, it was postulated that ranolazine's effect is maximized with demand-induced ischemia, such as that seen with exercise, or during postischemic reperfusion. In instances of myocardial infarction where the tissue has become completely anoxic, ranolazine may be minimally effective, or not effective at all.

Pharmacokinetics

Very little published information exists to describe ranolazine's pharmacokinetic properties. However, what is known is that ranolazine has a plasma half-life of 2 h.[275] In addition, it is inferred that ranolazine is metabolized hepatically because coadministration with diltiazem resulted in elevated ranolazine plasma concentrations.[275] From early clinical studies with immediate-release ranolazine, an apparent plasma concentration threshold was observed for antianginal efficacy.[275,285,286] Trough ranolazine levels (approximately 8 h postdose) were associated with decreased antianginal activity as compared with peak levels (1 h postdose).[285] Consequently, it was suggested that a sustained-release formulation of ranolazine be developed. Recently completed and ongoing clinical studies have used the sustained-release formulation, which is given every 12 h.[287,288]

Clinical Studies

In a preliminary clinical study by Jain et al,[289] ranolazine significantly prolonged exercise time for patients with chronic stable angina. This was a single-blind, placebo-controlled study that involved 14 patients with reproducible effort-induced angina of at least 3 months' duration, with associated treadmill-induced chest pain and at least 1 mm or more ST segment depression. Antianginal medication was discontinued 14 days before the initial screening visit. This was followed by a 2-week placebo phase, which was followed with consecutive treatments of 30 mg and 60 mg of ranolazine three times daily for 2 weeks each. Exercise treadmill tests were performed at the end of the washout, placebo, and the two active phases 1.5 h (peak), and 7 hours (trough) after the dose. The time to onset of angina symptoms or time to 1 mm of ST segment depression was recorded. The results showed an increase in exercise tolerance from 6.9 min (placebo) to 7.8 min following a single dose of 30 mg ranolazine ($P < .05$). A subsequent increase in exercise time to 8.2 min was noted following continuous administration of ranolazine for 2 weeks ($P < .002$). However, increasing the dose from 30 to 60 mg did not increase exercise time any further. The time to onset of angina showed similar increases in the treatment groups at peak and trough time points compared to placebo ($P \leq .005$). Time to ST segment depression did not change significantly, except for the trough period in the 30-mg group when compared to placebo ($P < .01$). There were also no significant changes observed in either resting or exercise peak heart rates and blood pressure. The results of this initial pilot study helped to establish the potential benefits of ranolazine for the treatment of chronic stable angina.

In a larger safety trial, Cocco et al[275] studied the effects of a single oral dose of ranolazine on exercise duration in 104 patients with chronic stable angina who were on stable therapy with beta-blockers or calcium-channel blockers. The study was a double-blind crossover design, comparing placebo with single doses of ranolazine at 10 mg, 60 mg, 120 mg, or 240 mg. On study days, subjects received placebo or one of the four possible doses of ranolazine in addition to their regular antianginal medications. Subjects underwent bicycle exercise testing to determine the time until the onset of 0.1 mV ST-segment depression or onset of angina. The results showed that ranolazine at doses of 10 mg, 60 mg, and 120 mg had no significant effect on exercise duration as compared with placebo. However, there was a significant improvement in exercise duration (+36.6 seconds) found with ranolazine 240 mg ($P < .004$). The benefits were greater for patients receiving beta-blockers (+39.4 seconds; $P = .02$) than for those receiving diltiazem (+33.8 seconds; $P = .08$). There were also significant improvements in time to angina (+41 seconds; $P = .01$) and in time to 0.1 mm ST-segment depression (+36.5 seconds; $P = .04$), with the 240-mg dose as compared with placebo. Ranolazine peak plasma levels over 500 ng/mL showed improved time to angina compared with plasma levels below 500 ng/mL. There was no effect of the ranolazine 240 mg dose on resting, submaximal, or maximal exercise blood pressure or heart rate. The results of this study suggest that higher doses of ranolazine may be needed to produce significant antianginal and anti-ischemic effects in patients with angina who are already receiving concomitant therapy with beta-blockers or calcium-channel blockers.

A randomized, double-blind, placebo-controlled crossover study of 158 patients with angina was conducted comparing the effects on exercise duration of either ranolazine base 342 mg (equivalent to 400 mg of ranolazine dihydrochloride) three times daily, atenolol 100 mg every day, or placebo for a period of 1 week.[290] Both ranolazine and atenolol significantly increased exercise time, time to angina, and time to 1 mm ST-segment depression as compared with placebo ($P < .001$). In addition, ranolazine was associated with a significantly longer exercise duration than with atenolol (453 ± 5 seconds vs 432 ± 6 seconds; $P = .006$). Atenolol was associated with a decrease in the maximal pressure rate product (PRP), which is common index of cardiac work, when compared to both placebo and ranolazine ($P < .001$). Ranolazine was associated with an increase in the maximal PRP when compared to both placebo and atenolol ($P < .05$ and $P < .001$, respectively). Therefore, by increasing both cardiac work and prolonging exercise duration and time until angina, ranolazine is likely improving myocardial energy efficiency.

Thadani at al[286] compared the safety and antianginal effects of monotherapy with ranolazine 30, 60, and 120 mg every 8 h and placebo in a randomized, multicenter, double-blind study of 4 weeks' duration. The investigators enrolled 318 patients with both a 3-month history of stable angina and 1 mm ST-segment depression on exercise treadmill testing. Treadmill tests were performed at peak (1 h postdose) and trough (8 h postdose) on the last day of the 4-week treatment period. There was no difference between any ranolazine dose and placebo in exercise duration, time to ST-segment depression, or time to onset of angina at both peak and trough time points. Peak ranolazine plasma concentrations ranged from 110 to 597 ng/mL for 30- to 120-mg doses. The lack of benefit with ranolazine treatment in this study has been attributed to the relatively low doses and consequent low plasma concentrations.[285]

A more recent trial by Pepine et al[285] studied the efficacy of ranolazine at higher doses in a group of patients who were responsive to conventional antianginal drugs. This was a multicenter, single-blind, placebo-controlled study that randomized 312 patients with chronic angina to either placebo or ranolazine given as either 267 mg three times daily, 400 mg twice daily, or 400 mg three times daily, in addition to their usual antianginal medications. Patients first underwent a qualifying phase in which one antianginal medication was removed and single-blind placebo initiated if the time to onset of angina on treadmill testing was between 3 and 13 min. After 1 to 2 weeks, the patient returned for another exercise treadmill test and an additional antianginal medication was discontinued if a decrease in time to onset of angina was not greater than 1 minute. If there was a decrease in exercise time of ≥ 1 minute, the patient was initiated on study treatment. Long-acting nitrates were removed first, then beta-blockers, and last calcium-channel blockers. End-points measured in the treatment groups were onset of angina, maximum exercise time, and time to 1 mm ST-segment depression. At peak concentrations, the results favored ranolazine versus placebo. The increase in the time to onset of angina ranged from 0.32 to 0.39 min ($P < .02$), and the increase in time to onset of 1 mm ST-segment depression ranged from 0.28 to 0.41 min ($P < .05$) for each of the ranolazine regimens as compared with placebo. For all ranolazine regimens combined, total exercise duration was increased compared to placebo ($P = .013$). During trough concentrations, only the time to 1 mm ST-segment depression was improved for all ranolazine regimens combined versus placebo ($P = .047$). Improvements in exercise parameters were seen for patients receiving ranolazine both in combination with beta-blockers and calcium-channel blockers, as well as in monotherapy, when compared to placebo. The investigators noted that the magnitude of benefit was greater with ranolazine monotherapy; however, specific information was not provided. No comparisons were made between ranolazine dosage groups. There were no significant differences in heart rate or blood pressure between placebo and each of the ranolazine doses at peak plasma concentrations. This study demonstrates that antianginal effects are associated with higher concentrations (peak levels) of ranolazine and that these higher concentrations must be maintained throughout the dosing interval to provide adequate antianginal and anti-ischemic activity.

The MARISA (Monotherapy Assessment of Ranolazine in Stable Angina) study examined the benefit of ranolazine for patients with chronic stable angina not receiving any other antianginal drugs.[287] This study was a phase III randomized, double-blind, placebo-controlled crossover trial that enrolled 191 patients to receive placebo or sustained-release ranolazine twice daily at doses of 500 mg, 1000 mg, and 1500 mg. When compared to placebo, ranolazine taken twice daily at all three doses demonstrated significant increases in exercise duration, time to onset of angina, and time to 1 mm ST-segment depression at both peak (4 h postdose) and trough (12 h postdose) plasma concentrations ($P \leq .005$). Similar to previous studies, this study demonstrated improvements in exercise performance with no meaningful effect on heart rate and blood pressure. As compared with previous studies, this trial demonstrated clinical benefit with ranolazine as monotherapy throughout the dosing interval using the higher dosage, sustained-release formulation.

Two separate subanalyses of the MARISA study compared patients with diabetes and patients with CHF to patients without the respective condition.[288,291] At both peak and trough ranolazine concentrations, the benefits in exercise duration, time to onset of angina, and time to 1 mm ST-segment depression were similar between diabetic and nondiabetic patients.[288] In addition, ranolazine had no effect on blood glucose or triglyceride levels in patients with diabetes. At trough ranolazine concentrations, the magnitude of benefit was similar between CHF patients and non-CHF patients.[291] However, at peak ranolazine concentrations, both the exercise duration and the time to 1 mm ST-segment depression were increased to a greater extent versus placebo in CHF patients than in non-CHF patients ($P < .01$).

The results of the MARISA study and the majority of the previous studies[275,287,289,290] suggest a clinical benefit of ranolazine without significantly affecting heart rate and blood pressure. A larger, double-blind, multicenter trial called CARISA (Combination Assessment of Ranolazine in Stable Angina) was recently completed. This trial examined the safety and efficacy of ranolazine in combination with other antianginal drugs in more than 823 patients with exercise-induced angina.[292] Patients received either 750 mg or 1000 mg of ranolazine or placebo twice daily in combination with one of three other antianginal agents over a period of 12 weeks. Exercise treadmill time was the primary end point of this study.[293] The study results showed a greater benefit of ranolazine at both doses compared to placebo regarding exercise tolerance, exercise time to angina, exercise time to ST-segment depression, and the number of angina episodes per week. Serious side effects occurred in 6% of patients in the placebo group and 7% in the ranolazine group.[293]

A phase II study of ranolazine in the treatment of CHF is also under way. Although the details for this study have not been published, the rationale for this study is based on preclinical data showing increases in left ventricular ejection fraction and stroke volume with ranolazine in an animal model.[294–296]

Tolerability

Ranolazine appears to be well tolerated even at doses of 1500 mg twice daily. In the MARISA study, side effects that occurred more often with ranolazine than with placebo included dizziness, nausea, asthenia, and constipation. The adverse event rate for the 500-mg dose was identical to placebo, and was 6% higher than placebo for the 1000-mg dose. At the 1500-mg dose, the adverse event rate was 18% higher than with placebo.[297] The results of earlier clinical studies showed similar adverse effects between ranolazine and placebo. However, gastrointestinal complaints, headache, dizziness, and fatigue were reported more frequently with ranolazine than with placebo, and their incidence was dose related.[275,285,286,289] In addition, there were no clinically significant abnormalities in lipids, glucose, and renal or liver function. Overall, ranolazine seems to be well tolerated at lower and higher doses up to 1500 mg twice daily, although the long-term safety of ranolazine has not been established.

Conclusion

Ranolazine is a new antianginal drug with a unique mechanism of action . It is believed to inhibit fatty acid oxidation, thereby converting myocardial energy production from fatty acid oxidation to the more energy-efficient glucose oxidation, which requires less oxygen than the oxidation of fatty acids. Clinical data thus far support a role for ranolazine in the treatment of chronic stable angina as either monotherapy or as adjunct therapy to existing antianginal regimens, because the drug increases exercise tolerance and decreases angina in these settings. The use of ranolazine for other cardiac conditions, long-term safety, and the effect of ranolazine on morbidity and mortality remain to be determined.

Trimetazidine

Similar to ranolazine, trimetazidine demonstrates a number of potentially useful cytoprotective actions, including a limitation of mitochondrial and membrane damage caused by oxygen-free radicals,[298–300] a reduction of intracellular acidosis,[301] and an inhibitory effect on neutrophil infiltration in the perfused myocardium.[302] Kantor et al also demonstrated that trimetazidine exerts its antianginal effects by inhibiting long-chain 3-ketoacyl-CoA thiolase, which increases pyruvate dehydrogenase activity, and subsequently increases glucose oxidation rates.[303]

In multiple clinical studies, trimetazidine has been demonstrated to have significant anti-ischemic actions.[303a–303d] In patients with chronic stable angina, trimetazidine reduces angina attack frequency and nitroglycerin consumption, while increasing treadmill exercise time and the time to the development of 1 mm ST segment depression on the exercise ECG.[304] The drug is as effective as propranolol[305] and nifedipine[302] on both angina and exercise parameters, and can provide additional benefit when added to diltiazem,[306] nifedipine,[307] or beta-blockers.[308] Trimetazidine also reduces the numbers of ischemic episodes in patients with angina pectoris who undergo ambulatory ECG monitoring.[309] These studies also indicate that trimetazidine has no effect on renal function, blood glucose, or plasma lipids, and does not produce any hemodynamic side effects such as hypotension, bradycardia, or fatigue.[310]

Clinical studies have also examined the effects of trimetazidine administration prior to and during interventional cardiac procedures. A double-blind, placebo-controlled study conducted by Kober et al evaluated the role of trimetazidine in myocardial cytoprotection in patients undergoing PTCA.[311] All 20 patients that were enrolled in the trial underwent PTCA of the left anterior descending coronary artery. During the PTCA, the patients underwent three balloon inflations, receiving either placebo or 6 mg trimetazidine following the second balloon inflation. Intracoronary electrocardiograms were subsequently done. The administration of trimetazidine was shown to cause a significant decrease in the amplitude of maximum ST segment shift, a decrease in peak T-wave amplitude, as well as a decrease in the total area-under-the-curve of the ST segment. In comparison, the placebo did not affect any of these parameters. In the presence of trimetazidine, it was also noted that there were no changes in heart rate, systemic blood pressure, or mean poststenotic intracoronary occlusion pressures. These results suggested that trimetazidine has a direct cytoprotective effect on the myocardium, without any alterations in hemodynamics.

Fabiani et al[312] conducted a trial in patients undergoing cardiac surgery. Three weeks prior to surgery the patients were treated with trimetazidine 20 mg three times daily, and then during the procedure, trimetazidine was added to the cardioplegic solution. The accumulation of malondialdehyde, a marker of lipid peroxidation induced by oxygen free radicals, was measured in the coronary sinus 20 min following reperfusion. It was thus concluded that trimetazidine played a beneficial role in coronary artery bypass surgery by decreasing ischemic reperfusion damage.

In experimental studies, trimetazidine has been shown to reduce predicted myocardial infarction size in rabbits when compared to control.[313] The drug also has a myocardial preserving effect in the isolated arrested rat heart.[314] In a large, controlled clinical trial [EMIP-FR (European Myocardial Infarction Project—Free Radicals)], intravenous trimetazidine did not reduce mortality in patients with MI undergoing thrombolytic therapy; however, it may have some beneficial effect in nonthrombolysed patients.[314a]

Conclusion

Similar to ranolazine, trimetazidine appears to have cytoprotective properties that make it a potentially useful drug for treating myocardial ischemia. In addition, like ranolazine, trimetazidine produces these anti-ischemic effects without affecting cardiovascular hemodynamics, making it an appealing addition to patients refractory to treatment with conventional antianginal therapy. Evidence from several clinical trials support the role for trimetazidine both as a monotherapy and in combination therapy for the treatment of ischemic heart disease.

RHO-KINASE INHIBITION

It has recently been demonstrated that the enzyme rho-kinase plays an important role in calcium sensitization for vascular smooth muscle contraction. Inappropriate coronary artery vasoconstriction due to increased rho-kinase in the vascular system may be involved in the pathogenesis of exercise-induced myocardial ischemia and spontaneous coronary artery spasm.[314b,314c]

An orally active selective rho-kinase inhibitor, fasudil, has been shown to be effective in patients with stable effort angina. In a dose-related fashion, the drug was shown to prolong the maximum exercise time and the time to the onset of 1 mm ST-segment depression on the treadmill exercise test. Blood pressure and heart rate during exercise were comparable before and after the fasudil treatment. The beneficial action of the drug has been attributed to coronary vasodilation.

Fasudil was also shown to prevent acetylcholine-induced coronary spasm, chest pain, and ischemic ECG changes.[314c] Fasudil did not affect vasoconstrictor responses at the nonspastic segments.

Rho-kinase inhibition appears to provide a unique pharmaceutical approach to the treatment of ischemic heart disease and further clinical development is indicated.

ALDOSE REDUCTASE INHIBITION (ZOPOLRESTAT)

Alterations in myocardial metabolism and ion transport at the cellular level have been implicated as the cause for the ischemic complications of diabetes.[315,316] These abnormalities have been associated with an impairment of Na^+K^+-ATPase activity and an elevation of intracellular sodium and calcium. The decrease in sodium pump activity in many tissues in diabetics has been attributed to increases in ion flux via the aldose reductase pathway or by depletion of intracellular myoinositol.[317,318] In peripheral nerves it has been shown that Na^+K^+-ATPase activity is normalized in diabetic animals treated with aldose reductase inhibitors or by reducing blood glucose.[317–319]

The consequence of impaired Na^+K^+-ATPase activity and the rise in intracellular sodium during myocardial ischemia is an increase in intracellular calcium with increased ischemic injury. It has been hypothesized that aldose reductase inhibition could normalize Na^+K^+-ATPase activity in the heart, and. as a consequence, protect the ischemic myocardium by reducing the rise in intracellular sodium and calcium.[320]

Furthermore, aldose reductase inhibition preserves the tissue redox ratio of nicotinamide-adenine dinucleotide to the reduced form of NAD (NAD/NADH),[321] which can be protective in myocardial ischemia. In experimental isolated heart studies using diabetic rats, the aldose reductase inhibitor zopolrestat preserved ATP during global ischemia, reduced ischemic injury as indicated by CPK release, and improved functional recovery of the myocardium after reperfusion.[321] In addition, aldose reductase inhibition with zopolrestat in the isolated diabetic rat heart model increased Na^+K^+-ATPase activity with limitation in the rise of intracellular sodium, and, hence, the intracellular calcium rise during ischemia and reperfusion.[322]

Additional animal studies were conducted in rabbit hearts having undergone regional ischemia. Although zopolrestat reduced infarct size by 61%,[323] this reduction in infarct size was less than that achieved by ischemic preconditioning. The studies concluded that zopolrestat produced a concentration-dependent reduction in infarct size, both in vitro and in vivo, and that cardioprotection was implemented without changes in hemodynamic parameters.

Conclusion

Table 37-9 summarize the theoretical benefits of using oral zopolrestat as an antianginal remedy. The current data suggest employing aldose reductase inhibition in both diabetic and nondiabetic patients with chronic stable angina to see whether exercise tolerance could be prolonged and ischemic ECG changes postponed or eliminated. An initial clinical trial was done to investigate oral zopolrestat in comparison to placebo on exercise and ischemia parameters in patients with chronic stable angina, which demonstrated no significant difference between placebo and zopolrestat. Because zopolrestat is effective in preventing diabetic complications in animals, even though the results from clinical studies have been disappointing, it has been proposed that the drug has poor potency in humans. Additional studies are examining the enzyme-inhibitor interactions and focusing on creating more potent and specific inhibitors.[324,325]

CHELATION THERAPY

In general terms, chelation therapy is a process of using specific molecules (chelating agents) to form complexes that inactivate heavy metals (metal ions), which can then be safely excreted in

TABLE 37-9. Theoretical Benefits of Using Zoprolestat as an Antianginal Remedy

- Preservation of ATP during global myocardial ischemia
- Preservation of normal Na^+K^+-ATPase activity during myocardial ischemia, protecting against increased intracellular calcium influx
- Preservation of a normal redox ratio of NAD/NADH
- Improved functional recovery of the ischemic myocardium during reperfusion

the urine. The most popular application of this therapy has been in heavy-metal toxicity where the binding of chelating agents to these metals forms soluble, inactive complexes that are eliminated via the urine.[326–328] The aforementioned use of chelation therapy is a well-established and accepted treatment approach.

However, a more intriguing and controversial aspect of chelation therapy lies in its use in the treatment of human diseases,[329–332] particularly atherosclerotic diseases. The management of cardiovascular disease with this therapy involves the multiple administrations of intravenous ethylenediaminetetraacetic acid (EDTA) supplemented with some "nutrients" (vitamins C, B complex, B$_6$, heparin, and magnesium sulfate)[333–335] and was initiated in the early to mid 1950s when a group from Michigan first reported on its use in the treatment of atherosclerotic cardiovascular diseases.[329,333] This initial report generated tremendous controversy regarding the benefits of chelation therapy that have continued to this day. The focus of the arguments for and against chelation therapy have related to efficacy, safety, and mechanisms of benefit of this treatment.[329,333,334,336–340] Despite the ongoing controversies, it is estimated that chelation therapy accounts for more than 800,000 patient visits in the United States each year.[341]

Chelation can be defined as a situation in which a metal ion is bound by a complex organic molecule with affinity for that metal ion and that serves as the chelating agent or ligand. Usually the chelating agent has a heterocyclic ring structure where the metal ion is bound by two or more ions within the complex molecule.[326,342]

This section briefly summarizes some of the arguments for and against the use of chelation therapy with EDTA and deferoxamine (iron chelation) in the treatment of cardiovascular diseases and presents clinical experiences where its use has been applied or advocated.

EDTA

EDTA is a known chelating agent that has the capability of binding divalent ions such as calcium. It is not specific for this metal as it can also bind other divalent and trivalent cations, as well as trace elements such as zinc, copper, lead and iron, transporting them in a bound form out of the body via the urine.[326,343,344] However, it is the ability of EDTA to displace and immobilize calcium ions by chelation that has prompted its use in atherosclerotic vascular diseases, as is discussed below. Proponents of chelation therapy for the treatment of cardiovascular diseases (especially atherosclerosis mediated) agree that vascular injury and smooth-muscle cell proliferation initiate the atherosclerotic cascade, with proteins, carbohydrates, and lipids (cholesterol esters) as major components of atherosclerotic plaques. However, they also believe there are other critical factors in this pathogenesis, including mineral metabolism—specifically calcium deposition. Calcium is very highly integrated with cholesterol in atheromatous lesions.[329,333,343,345]

Evidence supporting the importance of calcium deposition in atherosclerotic disease served as the theoretical background for using chelation therapy (EDTA) to decalcify complex atherosclerotic plaque in blood vessels. This same evidence would allow EDTA to serve as a therapeutic approach in patients with angina pectoris, intermittent claudication, and other atherosclerosis-mediated cardiovascular diseases.[329,333,344]

Another rationale for EDTA chelation therapy in cardiovascular diseases is that it can decrease platelet aggregability by either irreversibly altering the platelet calcium ratio or by altering a critical pathway in platelet aggregation that requires increased calcium (e.g., the platelet glycoprotein GP IIb/IIIa), and this inhibition of aggregation is obviously important in reducing complications from atherosclerotic disease.[346–348]

Free-radical reduction with EDTA is another proposed mechanism that is believed to be important for the treatment of cardiovascular diseases. EDTA reduces iron and copper levels from cell membranes. These metals are important catalysts in the lipid peroxidation of long-chain unsaturated fatty acids and oxidation of LDL, which generate free radicals that disrupt membrane architecture and consequently promote cellular injury and atherosclerosis.[349,350] Furthermore, some investigators have reported that chelation therapy, by removing calcium, results in a demonstrable increase in vascular dilation, a decrease in peripheral resistance, and an increase in blood flow.[351] EDTA also stimulates parathormone release, which, in turn, might mobilize calcium from the plaques and retard progressive calcification.[352] EDTA may also has an indirect effect by lowering serum iron levels and serum cholesterol.[353,354]

Arguments made against these proposed beneficial actions of EDTA and its use in the management of heart diseases include the contention by critics[338–340] that although calcium is seen in atherosclerotic plaques, its role in stabilizing the plaque may not be significant enough to warrant it being the target of therapy for heart disease. For instance, it is contended that because most stabilized atherosclerotic lesions contain cholesterol and its esters, collagen, lipoproteins, proteoglycans, and elastic fibers as primary components, with calcification occurring only as the final step in chronic atherosclerosis, agents that mobilize serum calcium (like EDTA) may not be effective in altering the initiation or progression of atherosclerotic disease.

Clinical Experiences with EDTA

Peripheral Vascular Disease

Several studies have utilized intravenous EDTA infusions to treat patients with peripheral vascular disease (PVD) and intermittent claudication. Most of the reports have been either retrospective experiences or individual case studies describing how EDTA infusions were able to relieve or improve the symptoms of PVD.[343,355–357] In one of these studies, Casdorph and Farr[357] described how four patients with severe PVD and facing possible amputation of their lower extremities were successfully treated with intravenous and topical antibiotics, debridement, hyperbaric oxygen, and multiple EDTA infusions. Only one patient ended up with amputation of three toes. The investigators believe that EDTA was the main therapeutic ingredient of the treatment regimen.

In a large retrospective study, Olszewer and Carter[332] evaluated 2870 patients with symptomatic vascular disease who received EDTA, and found that these subjects had significant improvement of their clinical symptoms. The drawback of the study was the lack of controls and its retrospective design. However, this same group then set out to conduct a controlled, double-blind study of sodium/magnesium EDTA in PVD. They started with 10 male patients with known PVD from diabetes or atherosclerosis. All patients had intermittent claudication but no rest pain or gangrene. The parameters they used to follow the effects of EDTA included peripheral vascular signs (skin disturbances, temperature, hair changes, etc), kidney function, blood pressure, and blood pressure index comparing the ankle systolic blood pressure to the arm systolic blood pressure, and time exercising on walking and bicycle stress tests. The 10 patients were randomly and equally divided into 2 groups, receiving ampules of 10 mL of EDTA or distilled water. Both treatment groups also received the usual administered nutritional additives to the intravenous solution, which included vitamin C, B complex, B_6, heparin, and magnesium sulfate. Disodium EDTA was used in a dose of 1.5 g for each infusion. After 10 treatments (chelation and placebo), the results indicated that some patients were improving significantly, while others were not. The investigators then broke the study code and realized that the experimental group (those receiving EDTA infusions) showed significant improvement while the placebo group did not. The study was then switched to a single-blind and all patients received EDTA treatment. After this switch, the placebo group improvement was comparable to the EDTA-treated group, as measured by the distance walked and the arm-ankle BP index. This study was significant in supporting earlier descriptive and less-objective studies that showed basically the same results.

In contrast, in a large, double-blind multicenter study of 153 patients with PVD, half of whom received placebo or EDTA, it was concluded from the results that there were no differences in symptomatic relief between control and treatment groups.[358] The same investigators also studied 30 patients on EDTA and followed their treatment with angiograms and transcutaneous oxygen-tension measurements, and reported no positive benefits with chelation therapy.[359] In addition, the results of a single-center, double-blind, randomized, controlled trial[337] failed to show any benefit from chelation therapy in a group of patients with intermittent claudication. In this study, 32 patients were randomized into treatment and control groups. The investigators used subjective measurements of patient improvement combined with the objective measurements of walking distance and ankle/brachial pulse indices.

Coronary Artery Disease

The first clinical use of chelation therapy for cardiovascular disease was for treatment of angina pectoris secondary to coronary artery disease.[333] The rationale for the study was based on the observation that coronary artery atheromas (the pathologic basis for angina) are formed by calcium-cholesterol integration in a matrix that includes proteoglycans and lipoproteins.

EDTA was used because of its known ability to bind and remove calcium.[329,333,343] In this first study,[333] a total of 20 patients with established angina pectoris were treated with a solution of 5 g disodium EDTA in 500 mL of 5% glucose or normal saline given intravenously. Each treatment solution was infused for 2.5 to 4 h, using a regimen of 5 g/d times 5 days a week. Each patient received 35 infusions. It was demonstrated that 19 of the 20 patients treated with these infusions were relieved of their symptoms. Furthermore, the ECG abnormalities associated with old myocardial infarcts that were present in some patients before EDTA were normalized after treatment.

Kitchell et al[360] treated 38 patients with severe angina for 1 to 2 months with repeated infusions of EDTA. Patient progress was based on individual perception of improvement and measured exercise tolerance. The investigators reported significant symptomatic relief in approximately 75% of the patients, and 40% showed evidence of ECG improvement between 6 and 12 of beginning EDTA therapy. However, by 18 months, 32% of the patients had died from their disease and only approximately 40% still maintained their achieved benefit from EDTA treatment. These same investigators then attempted a placebo-controlled study of EDTA in nine relatively sick angina patients and found that only two of these patients showed consistent improvement from the chelation treatment. The investigators concluded that EDTA had no significant benefit in the treatment of coronary artery disease.[360]

In another group of 18 patients with angina pectoris associated with coronary artery disease, EDTA infusions improved clinical symptoms.[360] The patient response to treatment was assessed by documenting clinical symptoms and measuring left ventricular (LV) ejection fraction via cardiac nuclear scintigraphy with technetium-99m before and after EDTA treatment. Twenty infusions of EDTA in 3-g doses led to complete clinical improvement and complete cessation of the anginal pain in all but two patients. There was also a significant (6%) improvement in LV ejection fraction.

In 1993, Hancke and Flytlie,[361] in a retrospective study of 470 patients, reported on the dramatic benefit obtained with EDTA treatment on patients previously scheduled to undergo coronary artery bypass for their coronary artery disease. Of 92 patients referred for surgical management of their diseases, only 10 required surgical intervention after EDTA chelation therapy. This report also described a series of coronary artery disease patients whose abnormal exercise ECG ST segments normalized after EDTA treatment. Furthermore, the authors went on to imply that EDTA chelation therapy was safe because after 6 years of follow-up, no serious side effects were observed. The findings of Van der Schaar[362] showed that patients with various atherosclerotic vascular diseases receiving EDTA had better exercise tolerance than control patients, suggesting a benefit from chelation therapy.

In a case report, a patient with angina secondary to atherosclerosis of the right coronary artery was described in whom EDTA therapy provided both symptomatic relief and a normalized treadmill ECG stress test after 5 months of therapy. However, the patient's symptoms later became worse, requiring angioplasty. These investigators believed that EDTA was not effective in dissolving the "blockade," as angiography of the arteries pre- and postangioplasty showed significant occlusion. They concluded that EDTA chelation therapy is not beneficial.[339]

Other Cardiovascular Diseases

In 1961, Soffer and colleagues performed an uncontrolled study that looked at the effects of EDTA or chelation therapy in patients with arrhythmia.[363] In that study, the investigators administered EDTA infusions to 58 patients with different dysrhythmias for approximately 28 months. They found that chelation therapy abolished ventricular premature contractions in 12 of 18 patients, increased the ventricular rate in all patients with complete heart block, and improved arteriovenous (AV) conduction in 6 of 12 patients. Furthermore, they found that EDTA treatment slowed the ectopic atrial rate in patients with atrial tachycardia. In 9 of 11 patients with atrial fibrillation who were receiving digitalis, the addition of EDTA further slowed the ventricular rate. The therapeutic principle behind the effect of EDTA on digitalis toxicity was based on the effective binding of calcium in serum, because calcium is known to affect cell membrane permeability, especially in the presence of digitalis. The conclusion at that time was that EDTA could abolish ectopic ventricular beats, terminate ventricular tachycardia and improve AV nodal conduction in patients with heart block.[363] However, additional studies and the advent of better and more effective medications for dysrhythmias and digitalis toxicity ultimately countered these findings.[339] Twenty-three years after his initial report, Soffer, one of the early chelation proponents, wrote an editorial condemning the use of this treatment for cardiovascular disease for lack of scientific proof of its efficacy.[364]

Clinical Recommendations

The major questions concerning EDTA chelation revolve around its efficacy and safety. The perception is that there is no generally accepted scientific evidence from well-conducted studies to justify its universal use, even though some studies show that it may be efficacious. In a meta-analysis, it was found that there was evidence to support the use of EDTA in the treatment of cardiovascular diseases.[365] However, most of the studies included in the analysis were not controlled, and in 2001, not a single reputable cardiovascular society has endorsed chelation therapy for the treatment of cardiovascular disease, including the recent ACC/AHA guidelines for the management of patients with stable angina pectoris.[366] At the same time, how safe is chelation therapy? The concerns regarding the safety of EDTA treatment have been addressed by the proponents of this therapy with the publication of guidelines for its safe use.[335] However, it is well known that EDTA is not a benign drug when high doses are administered over a short period of time. Some of the adverse effects that have been reported with high doses of EDTA include nephrotoxicity, bone marrow depression, and hypocalcemic tetany; allergic reactions, insulin shock, hypotension, thromboemboli, ECG changes including cardiac arrhythmias; and prolongation of the prothrombin time.[339,342,367,368]

It seems that the general acceptance of EDTA chelation therapy in the treatment of cardiovascular diseases certainly needs more mainstream basic science studies and better-designed clinical research studies to establish its efficacy and safety. Recently, the results of the Canadian Program to Assess Alternative Treatment Strategies to Achieve Cardiac Health (PATCH) trial showed no benefit with chelation therapy in patients with CAD regarding exercise-tolerance and quality of life measurements.[368a] In addition, a large definitive, placebo-controlled, multicenter RCT trial in 2300 patients has been initiated by the NIH to assess EDTA with regard to clinical symptoms, clinical outcomes, health care utilization, and plasma markers of oxidative stress and endothelial activation.[368b] The use of ultrafast CT scan to evaluate the efficacy of EDTA on coronary artery calcification with clinical correlations has been suggested as a means to evaluate treatment efficacy in future chelation trials. At the present time, chelation therapy with EDTA should remain a last resort choice for cardiovascular disease treatment, and certainly not as a replacement for accepted medical and surgical therapies.[368c,d]

Deferoxamine and Deferiprone

There has been much interest regarding the role of iron in the pathogenesis of atherosclerosis, particularly coronary artery disease. Several epidemiologic studies have found an association between markers of increased iron stores and increased risk of coronary artery disease and acute coronary events.[369,370] Salonen et al followed 1931 randomly selected men with no clinical evidence of coronary artery disease at the time of inclusion in a 5-year observational study.[369] They found that men with serum ferritin 200 μg/L had a 2.2-fold (95% CI, 1.2 to 4.0; $P < .01$) risk factor-adjusted risk for acute myocardial infarction when compared with men with a lower serum ferritin. The dietary intake of iron also showed a significant and direct correlation with the incidence of acute coronary events. The adverse effects of iron seem to be independent of or potentiated by other risk factors such as hypercholesterolemia. Morrison et al[370] also found an increased risk of fatal myocardial infarction in male as well as female patients with increased serum iron levels.

Studies have also shown an increased risk of acute myocardial infarction in carriers of the hemochromatosis gene Cys 282 Tyr mutation.[371] These epidemiologic observations are not surprising, considering that iron is an important element in cellular metabolism and growth. Iron is found in many enzymes and proteins, which are involved in electron shuttling and oxygen binding and transport. Besides its normal physiologic activity, iron has an important role in the generation of oxygen free radicals, specifically the highly reactive hydroxyl radical generated by the superoxide driven Haber-Weiss reaction.[372] Iron can also directly activate platelets.[373] Its activation is mediated by hydroxyl radical formation and involves pyruvate kinase activity.

However, a theoretical link associating iron and atherosclerosis is still not clear. A Canadian study failed to show any relation between serum ferritin levels and angiographically confirmed coronary artery disease.[374] Another study from Iceland followed men and women for up to 8.5 years, and found no association between risk of myocardial infarction and elevated serum ferritin levels.[375]

Deferoxamine is the most widely used iron chelator and has been used experimentally in non-iron overload conditions to interfere with free-radical production during myocardial reperfusion after an ischemic injury and in other cardiovascular conditions.[376] Besides its role as an iron chelator and antioxidant, some authors suggest that deferoxamine might have an effect on vascular smooth-muscle proliferation.[377]

Clinical Use

In animal studies and in small patient trials, deferoxamine preserved myocardial function and energy metabolism after postischemic reperfusion. From these studies, there is evidence of reduced oxygen free-radical generation as a possible mechanism of benefit.[378–380] However, not all studies have shown benefit in protecting against myocardial ischemia-reperfusion injury.[381]

There is a reported case of a patient with severe iron overload cardiomyopathy who was treated successfully with chelation therapy.[382] In addition, chelation therapy with oral deferiprone can be used to improve heart function (LV ejection fraction) in patients with thalassemia major who are transfusion dependent.[383]

Deferoxamine has also been tried as a treatment to prevent or limit cardiotoxicity associated with anthracycline chemotherapy. One mechanism proposed for anthracycline cardiomyopathy is the generation of oxygen free radicals by anthracycline-iron-complexes. Deferoxamine and other iron chelators appear to prevent anthracycline cardiotoxicity while preserving the tumoricidal effects of chemotherapy.[378]

Clinical Recommendation

As with EDTA, the experience with deferoxamine in prevention and treatment of cardiovascular disease needs to be established with more substantial clinical trials before it can be recommended. Deferoxamine is also associated with substantial toxicity involving multiple organ systems.[376]

Conclusion

Although there is a theoretical basis for the use of various chelation therapies for the prevention and treatment of cardiovascular disease, its therapeutic use still remains investigational until more definitive clinical studies show whether the treatment is efficacious and safe.

COMPLEMENT INHIBITION

Reperfusion therapy is beneficial in reducing mortality following acute myocardial infarction. Earlier and more complete reperfusion is related to improved survival. There is, however, evidence that reperfusion itself may result in deleterious adverse effects, including myocyte necrosis, microvascular injury, myocardial stunning, and arrhythmias.[384–386] There is some debate about the clinical relevance of these phenomena. The actual mechanism of reperfusion injury has not been fully characterized but is believed to be caused by several different mechanisms: the formation of oxygen free radicals, changes in intracellular calcium homeostasis, recruitment of neutrophils, complement activation, distributed endothelial function, impaired cellular energetics, and damage to the extracellular collagen matrix.

The pathogenesis of myocardial ischemia/reperfusion (MIR) injury was investigated in a rat model of MIR injury during which it was noted that anti-C5 therapy significantly inhibited cell apoptosis, necrosis, and polymorphonuclear leukocyte infiltration, despite C3 deposition. The authors concluded that the terminal components C5a and C5b-9 were key mediators of tissue injury in MIR injury.[387,388] The results from these experiments demonstrate the potential efficacy of anti-C5 monoclonal antibody (MAb) therapy in reducing the initial tissue damage, as well as the reperfusion inflammatory reaction, in patients with acute myocardial infarction.

Complement can be activated through either the classical or alternative pathways. These merge to a final common pathway in which C5 plays a critical role and is cleaved to form C5a and C5b. C5a is the most potent anaphylatoxin known, and has potent proinflammatory properties. It induces changes in smooth muscle and vascular tone, as well as increasing vascular permeability. It also activates both neutrophils and endothelial cells. C5 cleavage also leads to the formation of C5b-9 or the membrane attack complex, which cause vesiculation of platelets and endothelial cells, formation of prothrombotic microparticles, and activation of leukocytes and endothelial cells.

Complement Inhibitors

h5G1.1-scFv is an anti-C5 monoclonal antibody that is designed to prevent the cleavage of C5 into its pro-inflammatory byproducts.[389] At the same time, blockade of the complement system at C5 preserves the patient's ability to generate C3b, which is critical for opsonization of pathogenic microorganisms and immune complex clearance.[390]

Cardiopulmonary bypass induces a systemic inflammatory response that can cause substantial morbidity. Activation of complement during cardiopulmonary bypass contributes significantly to this inflammatory response. In a recent clinical trial, it was reported that the single-chain antibody for human C5(h5G1.1-scFv) was a safe and effective inhibitor of pathologic complement activation in patients undergoing cardiopulmonary bypass. In addition to reducing sC5b-9 formation and leukocyte CD11b formation, C5 inhibition significantly attenuated postoperative myocardial injury, cognitive defects, and blood loss.[390] Side effects include fever, atrial fibrillation, and nausea. Patients with myocardial infarction have elevated levels of C5b-9 upon arrival at the emergency room. Levels remain elevated for 24 h and then begin to decrease by 48 h. It is proposed that complete complement suppression with C5(h5G1.1-scFv) be achieved for approximately 24 h to achieve possible clinical benefit on infarct size and morbidity and mortality.

Currently there are two ongoing study evaluating the efficacy and safety of intravenous bolus and bolus and infusion treatment with h5G1.1-scFv in the setting of either thrombolysis or angioplasty reperfusion therapy within 6 h of an acute myocardial infarction. It has been shown that h5G1.1scFv treatment does not interfere with those components of the proximal complement cascade that are necessary to prevent infection.

Soluble human complement receptor I (scR1), a recombinant form, is a potent inhibitor of both the classic and alternative pathways of complement activation.[391] It reduces infarct size in rats and limits reperfusion edema after lung transplantation.[392,393] In combination with heparin-bonded cardiopulmonary bypass circuits in pigs, it also optimizes recovery during the revascularization of ischemic myocardium.[393a] Complement inhibition with the Cl 1-1 esterase inhibitor has also been shown to protect ischemic tissue from reperfusion damage. However, high doses are associated with significant toxicity related to a procoagulatory action.[393a]

PROTEIN KINASE C ACTIVATORS

A new 1,4-benzothiazepine derivative, JTV519, has a strong protective effect against calcium overload-induced myocardial injury. It has been shown that JTV519 protects against ischemia/reperfusion injury by activating protein kinase C through a receptor-independent mechanism.[394] This agent provides a novel pharmacologic approach for the treatment of patients with acute coronary diseases via a subcellular mechanism that mimics ischemic preconditioning.[394]

CELLULAR THERAPY FOR CARDIAC REGENERATION: EFFECTS OF GROWTH FACTORS ON STEM CELLS

Despite major advances in diagnosis and treatment, coronary heart disease continues to be the leading cause of morbidity and mortality among both men and women. Current clinical interventions achieve varying degrees of success but none has been capable of regenerating infarcted myocardium. A new class of therapy, stem cell transplantation, has emerged as a potentially novel tool in the clinician's armamentarium against myocardial infarction.

Stem cells have long been regarded as undifferentiated cells capable of self-renewal, production of a large number of differentiated progeny, and the regeneration of tissues.[395] Stem cells have been traditionally divided into two groups: (a) embryonic stem cells, the cells capable of differentiating into the three germ layers, and (b) adult stem cells, the organ/tissue-specific stem cells that are responsible for the production of certain cell types. It is these adult stem cells that are needed to maintain a tissue's homeostasis in response to cellular senescence and injury. Adult stem cells have long been observed in tissues such as the skin, intestines, and the bone marrow (hematopoietic system). Recent discoveries in stem cell biology suggest that the behavior of stem cells may be more complex than had ever been envisioned. In a series of remarkable studies, bone marrow-derived stem cells (BMSCs) have been shown to be capable of differentiating into skeletal and cardiac myocytes,[396–400] neurons,[401,402] hepatocytes,[403,404] epithelial cells,[405] and vascular endothelium.[406] This stem cell "plasticity" has tremendous implications as a new therapeutic pathway to regenerate tissues damaged by disease and injury.[407,408] The heart, an organ less-well equipped to deal with injury, appears to be the perfect candidate for this new therapeutic strategy.

Bone Marrow Cells Can Regenerate Infarcted Myocardium

The possibility that BMSCs could regenerate infarcted myocardium was first demonstrated by Orlic and colleagues,[398] in a murine model of left ventricular infarction. BMSCs were injected 3 to 5 h after left coronary artery ligation in adult mice. The stem cell injections were made in the peri-infarcted areas of the left ventricle. The infarcted tissue was replaced by newly formed cardiac myocytes within 9 days postinfarction. The regenerated myocardium occupied 68% + 11% of the infarcted region (from epicardial to endocardial surface) and it extended across the entire region of the infarct to the spared myocardium. The BMSCs were capable not only of regenerating new myocytes but also capillaries and coronary arterioles. The developing cardiac myocytes resembled fetal and neonatal myocytes in size and gene expression. Early acting cardiac-specific transcription factors (GATA-4, MEF2, and Csx/Nkx2.5) were expressed in cells that were also positive for myocyte-specific markers such as sarcomeric α-actin. In addition, the regenerated myocytes expressed connexin 43, a molecular component of gap junctions, suggesting that the regenerating heart tissue was beginning to become electrically coupled. The regenerated myocytes had an impact on function as well. Hemodynamic parameters such as left ventricular end-diastolic pressure (LVEDP) improved by 36% in those subjects who were treated with BMSCs.

After they demonstrated that BMSCs were capable of regenerating myocardium, Orlic and colleagues[409] designed a protocol to explore this BMSC potential in a more clinically relevant manner. In an effort to identify a noninvasive approach to cardiac regeneration, they tested the hypothesis that a large number of circulating BMSCs would home to the infarcted heart and repair the damaged tissue. Normally, BMSCs are rare in the circulation. However, with the use of cytokines, they can be mobilized from the bone marrow to circulate in the peripheral blood in large numbers. Based on their previous work,[410] Orlic and colleagues decided to use a cytokine cocktail of granulocyte-colony stimulating factor (G-CSF) and stem cell factor (SCF) to mobilize the maximum possible number of BMSCs. The ability of hematopoietic growth factors to mobilize BMSCs into the blood has substantially impacted on clinical bone marrow transplantation and high-dose chemotherapy procedures.[411] In the clinical setting, the preferred modality of mobilization of BMSCs is the use of G-CSF.[412] G-CSF (filgrastim/lenograstim) is a naturally occurring glycoprotein that has proved to be extremely efficacious in mobilizing BMSCs from normal donors. These circulating BMSCs can be collected by apheresis and used as an alternative to bone marrow for patients undergoing allogeneic transplants.[413,414] The short-term effects of G-CSF are well-known and manageable. They include fever, headache, and bone pain. The long-term effects are still not well understood. SCF is an essential hematopoietic growth factor with proliferative and antiapoptotic functions.[415] In clinical studies, SCF has been associated with cases of anaphylaxis.[415] However, because the combination of G-CSF and SCF mobilizes the greatest number of BMSCs in animals[410,416] and humans,[417] Orlic and colleagues[409] decided to use both cytokines in their study of acute myocardial infarct regeneration. The cytokine-mobilized BMSCs were capable of a tremendous degree of cardiac tissue regeneration as seen 27 days later. The cytokine-induced myocardial repair reduced infarct size by 40% (as compared to nontreated controls). All left-ventricular hemodynamic functions tested were improved including EF, which was 114% higher in the cytokine-treated mice. The most gratifying result was that the cytokine-treated animals demonstrated a 68% decrease in mortality when compared to the nontreated controls. The most exciting possibility raised by this finding is that the use of cytokines may one day offer the clinician a noninvasive method to direct BMSCs to the site of myocardial injury with the rapidity and ease necessary to treat an acutely ill myocardial infarction survivor and thereby improve the patient's morbidity and mortality.

Future Directions

Before cellular therapy for myocardial infarction (and other cardiovascular pathology) can become a clinical reality, many important concerns must be addressed. One concern is whether or not the BMSC plasticity demonstrated in the murine model can be translated to larger animals in further preclinical trials.[417a] A second concern is whether or not the newly formed cardiac myocytes seen in these reports are capable of surviving and maturing into cardiac tissue that is properly integrated into the existing myocardial wall.[418] The regenerated cardiac tissue must work in conjunction with the existing myocardium in order to improve the overall function of the infarcted heart. In addition, the molecular mechanisms that are involved in stem cell plasticity must be elaborated. To accelerate the use of stem cells as a therapeutic tool, scientists must identify the mechanisms by which BMSCs respond to alternative environmental cues. In addition, the cytokine cocktail that will achieve optimum delivery of the proper population of stem cells into the peripheral circulation at the right time (i.e., immediately after an infarct) must also be elucidated.

Although adult BMSCs offer the clinician a promising tool for cardiac regeneration, are there alternative cells that may be considered the cells of choice for cardiac repair?[419] Recent evidence by Anversa and colleagues demonstrates significant proof of an intrinsic capability of cardiac myocytes to regenerate themselves in the face of end-stage heart failure,[420] myocardial infarction,[421] and cardiac transplantation.[422] New data suggest that a population of cardiac stem cells (CSCs) exist and that they can be a source of tissue renewal.[419] If their existence can be confirmed, the possibility of mobilizing CSCs to treat patients with ischemic heart disease must also be addressed.

The current reports of cardiac regeneration with BMSCs are important proofs of principle.[423,424] A new approach to therapeutic strategies can now be examined and studied scientifically. These new findings may one day lead to a new method of managing myocardial infarction and other cardiovascular disorders.

CONCLUSION

Ischemic heart disease remains the number one cause of major morbidity and mortality in the United States. Innovative strategies, such as those described in this chapter, are being developed to address this problem. At the same time, these pharmacologic approaches serve as biologic probes that will provide a better understanding of pathophysiology and future therapeutic directions.

REFERENCES

1. Kobinger W, Lillie C: AQ-A 39 (5,6-dimethoxy-2-3[[alpha-(3,4-dimethoxy)-phenylethyl] methylamino] propyl] phthalimidine) a specific bradycardic agent with direct action on the heart. *Eur J Pharmacol* 72:153, 1981.
2. Kobinger W: Central alpha-adrenergic systems as targets for hypotensive drugs. *Rev Physiol Biochem Pharmacol* 81:39, 1987.

3. Kobinger W, Lille C, Pichler L: Cardiovascular actions of *N*-allyl clonidine (ST 567), a substance with specific bradycardic action. *Eur J Pharmacol* 58:141, 1979.

4. Simoons ML, Tummers J, Meurs-van Woezik H, Van Domburg R: Alinidine, a new agent which lowers heart rate in patients with angina pectoris. *Eur Heart J* 13:542, 1982.

5. Challinor-Rogers JL, Rosenfeldt FL, et al: Anti-ischemic and antiarrhythmic activities of some novel alinidine analogs in the rat heart. *J Cardiovasc Pharmacol* 29:499, 1997.

6. Reiffen M, Eberlein W, Muller P, et al: Specific bradycardic agents. Chemistry, pharmacology and structure-activity relationships of substituted benzazepinones, a new class of compounds exerting anti-ischemic properties. *J Med Chem* 33:1496, 1990.

7. Lillie C: ULFS 49 CL, a prototype of a novel pharmacological concept. In: Hjalmarson A, Remme WJ, eds. *Sinus Node Inhibitors*. New York: Springer-Verlag, 1991:9–19.

8. Kobinger W, Lille C: Cardiovascular characterization of ULFS 49, 1,3,4,5-tetrahydro 7,8-dimethoxy-3-[3-[[2-(3,4-dimethoxyphenyl) ethyl] methylimino] propyl] 2H-3-benzazepin-2-on hydrochloride, a new "specific bradycardic agent." *Eur J Pharmacol* 104:9, 1984.

9. DiFrancesco D: Properties of the hyperpolarizing activated current (I_f) in cells isolated from the rabbit sinoatrial node. *J Physiol* 377:61, 1986.

10. DiFrancesco D: Muscarinic modulation of cardiac rate at low acetylcholine concentrations. *Science* 243:669, 1989.

11. Noma A, Kotake H, Irisawa H: Slow inward current and its role mediating the chronotropic effect of epinephrine in the rabbit sinoatrial node. *Pflugers Arch* 388:1, 1980.

12. van Bogaert PP, Goethals M: Pharmacological influence of specific bradycardic agents on the pacemaker current of sheep cardiac Purkinje fibers. A comparison between three different molecules. *Eur Heart J* 8(Suppl L):35, 1987.

13. Goethals M, Raes A, Bogaert PP: Use-dependent block of the pacemaker current I_f in rabbit sinoatrial node cells by zatebradine (UL FS 49) (abstr.). *Circulation* 88(pt 1):2389, 1993.

14. van Bogaert PP, Goethals M: Blockade of the pacemaker current by intracellular application of UL FS49 CL and UL AH99 in sheep cardiac Purkinje fibers. *Eur J Pharmacol* 229:55, 1992.

15. Doerr T, Trautwein W: On the mechanism of the "specific bradycardic action" of the verapamil derivative UL FS 49 CL. *Naunyn Schmiedebergs Arch Pharmacol* 341:331, 1990.

16. Kobinger W, Lillie C: Specific bradycardic agents — a novel pharmacological class? *Eur Heart J* 8(Suppl L):7, 1987.

17. van Woerkens LJ, van der Giessens WJ, Verdouw PD: The selective bradycardic effects of zatebradine (UL FS 49) do not adversely affect left ventricular function in conscious pigs with chronic coronary artery occlusion. *Cardiovasc Drug Ther* 6:59, 1992.

18. Johnston WE, Vinten-Johansen J, Tommasi E, Little WC: UL FS 49 causes bradycardia without decreasing right ventricular systolic and diastolic performance. *J Cardiovasc Pharmacol* 18:528, 1991.

19. Breall JA, Watanabe J, Grossman W: Effect of zatebradine on contractility, relaxation and coronary blood flow. *J Am Coll Cardiol* 21:471, 1993.

20. Riley D, Gross G, Kampine J, Warltier D: Specific bradycardic agents. A new therapeutic modality for anesthesiology: Hemodynamic effects of UL FS 49 and propranolol in conscious and isoflurane-anesthetized dogs. *Anesthesiology* 67:707, 1987.

21. Miura M, Miyazaki S, Guth BD, et al: Influence of the force-frequency relation on left ventricular function during exercise in conscious dogs. *Circulation* 86:563, 1992.

22. Indolfi C, Guth BD, Miura T, et al: Mechanisms of improved ischemic regional dysfunction by bradycardia. Studies on UL FS 49 CL in swine. *Circulation* 80:983, 1989.

23. Daemmgen JW, Lamping KA, Gross GJ: Actions of two new bradycardic agents, AQ AH 208 and UL FS 49 on ischemic myocardial perfusion and function. *J Cardiovasc Pharmacol* 7:71, 1985.

24. Canty JM, Giglia J, Kandath D: Effect of tachycardia on regional function and transmural myocardial perfusion during graded coronary pressure reduction in conscious dogs. *Circulation* 82:1815, 1990.

25. Indolfi C, Guth BD, Miyazaki S, et al: Heart rate reduction improves myocardial ischemia in swine: Role of interventricular blood flow redistribution. *Am J Physiol* 261:H910, 1991.

26. O'Brien P, Drage D, Saeian K, et al: Regional redistribution of myocardial perfusion by UL FS 459, a selective bradycardic agent. *Am Heart J* 123:566, 1992.

27. Schulz R, Rose J, Skyschally A, Heusch G: Bradycardic agent UL FS 49 attenuates ischemic regional myocardial dysfunction and reduces infarct size in swine: Comparison with the β blocker atenolol. *J Cardiovasc Pharmacol* 25:216, 1995.

28. Frishman WH, Pepine CJ, Weiss R, Baiker WM for the Zatebradine Study Group: The addition of a direct sinus node inhibitor (zatebradine) provides no greater exercise tolerance benefit to patients with angina pectoris treated with extended-release nifedipine: Results of a multicenter, randomized, double-blind, placebo-controlled, parallel group study. *J Am Coll Cardiol* 26:305, 1995.

29. Waters D, Baird M, Maranda C, et al: A randomized, double-blind, placebo-controlled trial of zatebradine and diltiazem SR in chronic stable angina: Efficacy and safety (abstr.). *J Am Coll Cardiol* 25(2):208A, 1995.

30. Glasser SP, Michie DD, Thadani U, et al: Effects of zatebradine (ULFS49CL), a sinus node inhibitor, on heart rate and exercise duration in chronic stable angina pectoris. *Am J Cardiol* 79:1401, 1997.

31. Findlay IN, MacLeod K, Ford M, et al: Treatment of angina pectoris with nifedipine and atenolol: Efficacy and effect on cardiac function. *Br Heart J* 55:240, 1986.

32. Davies RF, Habibi H, Klinke WP, et al: Effect of amlodipine, atenolol, and their combination on myocardial ischemia during treadmill exercise and ambulatory monitoring. *J Am Coll Cardiol* 25:619, 1995.

33. Williams R, Nichols WW, Chen L, et al: Myocardial and coronary vascular protection after coronary occlusion and reperfusion by selective sinoatrial node inhibition (abstr.). *J Am Coll Cardiol* 25(2):356A, 1995.

34. Murphy JD, Pepine CJ: Sinus node inhibitors: zatebradine and other agents. In: Messerli FH, ed. *Cardiovascular Drug Therapy*. 2d ed. Philadelphia: WB Saunders, 1996:1386.

35. Shinke T, Takeuchi M, Takaoka H, Yokoyama M: Beneficial effects of heart rate reduction on cardiac mechanics and energetics in patients with left ventricular dysfunction. *Jpn Circ J* 63:957, 1999.

36. Mitrovic V, Oehm E, Liebrich A, et al: Hemodynamic and anti-ischemic effects of tedisamil in humans. *Cardiovasc Drug Ther* 6:353, 1992.

37. Thormann J, Mitrovic V, Riedel H, et al: Tedisamil (KC 8857) is a new specific bradycardic drug: Does it also influence myocardial contractility? Analysis by the conductance (volume) technique in coronary artery disease. *Am Heart J* 125:1233, 1993.

38. Bargheer K, Bode F, Klein HU, et al: Prolongation of monophasic action potential duration and the refractory period in the human heart by tedisamil, a new potassium-blocking agent. *Eur Heart J* 15:1409, 1994.

39. Wallace AA, Stupienski III RF, Baskin EP, et al: Cardiac electrophysiologic and antiarrhythmic actions of tedisamil. *J Pharmacol Exp Ther* 273:168, 1995.

40. Adaikan G, Beatch GN, Lee TL, et al: Anti-arrhythmic actions of tedisamil: Studies in rats and primates. *Cardiovasc Drug Therap* 6:345, 1992.

41. BoSmith RE, Briggs I, Sturgess NC: Inhibition of the hyperpolarisation activated cationic current (I_F) by ICI D7288 in guinea-pig isolated sinoatrial node cells. *Br J Pharmacol* 108:126P, 1993.

42. Marshall PW, Bramley J, Briggs I: The effects of ICI D7288, a novel sinoatrial node modulating agent, on guinea pig isolated atria. *Br J Pharmacol* 107:134P, 1992.

43. Fox KM, Henderson JR, Kaski JC, et al: Antianginal and anti-ischaemic efficacy of tedisamil, a potassium channel blocker. *Heart* 83:167, 2000.

44. Dzurba A, Ziegelhöffer Z, Okruhlicová L, et al: Salutary effect of tedisamil on post-ischemic recovery rat heart: involvement of sarcolemmal (NaK)-ATPase. *Mol Cell Biochem* 215:129, 2000.

45. Frishman WH, Gabor R, Pepine C, Cavusoglu E: Heart rate reduction in the treatment of chronic stable angina pectoris: Experience with a sinus node inhibitor. *Am Heart J* 131:204, 1996.

46. Atwal KS: Pharmacology and structure activity relationships for KATP modulators-tissue selective KATP openers. *J Cardiovasc Pharmacol* 24(Suppl 4):S12, 1994.

47. Frampton J, Buckley MM, Fitton A: Nicorandil: A review of its pharmacology and therapeutic efficacy in angina pectoris. *Drugs* 44:625, 1992.

47a. Gomma AH, Purcell HJ, Fox KM: Potassium-channel openers in myocardial ischaemia. Therapeutic potential of nicorandil. *Drugs* 61:1705, 2001.

48. Markham A, Plosker GL, Goa KL: Nicorandil. An updated review of its use in ischaemic heart disease with emphasis on its cardioprotective effects. *Drugs* 60:955, 2000.

49. Nakae I, Matsumoto T, Horie H, et al: Effects of intravenous nicorandil on coronary circulation in humans: Plasma concentration and action mechanism. *J Cardiovasc Pharmacol* 35:919, 2000.

50. Okamura A, Rakugi H, Ohishi M, et al: Additive effects of nicorandil on coronary blood flow during continuous administration of nitroglycerin. *J Am Coll Cardiol* 37:719, 2001.

51. Sato T, Sasaki N O'Rourke B, Marbán E: Nicorandil, a potent cardioprotective agent, acts by opening mitochondrial ATP-dependent potassium channels. *J Am Coll Cardiol* 35:514, 2000.

52. Taira N: Nicorandil as a hybrid between nitrates and potassium channel activators. *Am J Cardiol* 63:18J, 1989.

53. Doring G: Antianginal and anti-ischemic efficacy of nicorandil in comparison with isosorbide-5-mononitrate and isosorbide dinitrate: Results from two multicenter, double-blind, randomized studies with stable coronary heart disease patients. *J Cardiovasc Pharmacol* 20(Suppl 3): S74, 1992.

54. Rajaratnam R, Brieger DB, Hawkins R, Freedman SB: Attenuation of anti-ischemic efficacy during chronic therapy with nicorandil in patients with stable angina pectoris. *Am J Cardiol* 83:1120, 1999.

55. Horinaka S, Kobayashi N, Higashi T, et al: Nicorandil enhances cardiac endothelial nitric oxide synthase expression via activation of adenosine triphosphate-sensitive K channel in rat. *J Cardiovasc Pharmacol* 38:200, 2001.

56. Hayashi Y, Sawa Y, Ohtake S, et al: Controlled nicorandil administration for myocardial protection during coronary artery bypass grafting under cardiopulmonary bypass. *J Cardiovasc Pharmacol* 38:21, 2001.

57. Kato T, Kamiyama T, Maruyama Y, et al: Nicorandil, a potent cardioprotective agent, reduces QT dispersion during coronary angioplasty. *Am Heart J* 141:940, 2001.

58. Ito H, Taniyama Y, Iwakura K, et al: Intravenous nicorandil can preserve microvascular integrity and myocardial viability in patients with reperfused anterior wall myocardial infarction. *J Am Coll Cardiol* 33:654, 1999.

58a. Gross GJ, Auchampach JA, Maruyama M, et al: Cardioprotective effects of nicorandil. *J Cardiovasc Pharmacol* 20(Suppl 3):S22, 1992.

59. Lablanche J-M, Bauters C, Leroy F, Bertrand ME: Prevention of coronary spasm by nicorandil: Comparison with nifedipine. *J Cardiovasc Pharmacol* 20(Suppl 3):S82, 1992.

60. Kukovetz WR, Holzmann S, Poch G: Molecular mechanism of action of nicorandil. *J Cardiovasc Pharmacol* 20(Suppl 3):S1, 1992.

61. Holzmann S: Cyclic GMP as possible mediator of coronary arterial relaxation by nicorandil (SG-75). *J Cardiovasc Pharmacol* 5:364, 1983.

62. Schmidt K, Reich R, Kukovetz WR: Stimulation of coronary guanylate cyclase by nicorandil (SG-75) as a mechanism of its vasodilating action. *J Cycl Nucl Prot Phosph Res* 10:43, 1985.

63. Morimoto S, Koh E, Fukuo K, et al: Effect of nicorandil on the cytosolic free calcium concentration and microsomal (Ca + Mg)-ATPase activity of vascular smooth muscle cells. *J Cardiovasc Pharmacol* 10(Suppl 8): S31, 1987.

64. Kreye VAW, Lenz T, Pfrunder D, Theiss U: Pharmacological characterization of nicorandil by ^{86}Rb efflux and isometric vasorelaxation studies in vascular smooth muscle. *J Cardiovasc Pharmacol* 20(Suppl 3): S8, 1992.

65. Daut J, Maier-Rudolph W, von Beckerath N, et al: Hypoxic dilation of coronary arteries is mediated by ATP-sensitive potassium channels. *Science* 247:1341, 1990.

66. Robertson BE, Schubert R, Hescheler J, Nelson MT: cyclic GMP-dependent protein kinase activates Ca-activated K channels in cerebral artery smooth muscle cells. *Am J Physiol* 265:C299, 1993.

67. Opie LH: *The Heart: Physiology and Metabolism.* 2d ed. New York: Raven Press, 1991:109, 277.

68. Taylor SG, Weston AG: Endothelium-derived hyperpolarizing factor: A new endogenous inhibitor from the vascular endothelium. *Trends Pharmacol* 9:272, 1988.

69. Furukawa K, Itoh T, Kajiwara M, et al: Vasodilating actions of 2-nicotinamide ethyl nitrate on porcine and guinea pig coronary arteries. *J Pharmacol Exp Ther* 218:248, 1981.

70. Hamilton TC, Buckingham RE, Clapham JC, et al: BRL 3495, a novel antihypertensive agent with potassium channel activity properties. *Cardiovasc Drugs Ther* 1:244, 1987.

71. Imanishi S, Arita M, Kiyosue T, Aomine M: Effects of SG-75 (nicorandil) on electrical activity of canine cardiac Purkinje fibers: Possible increase in potassium conductance. *J Pharmacol Exp Ther* 225:198, 1983.

72. Waters DD, Szlachcic J, Theroux P, Dauwe F, Mizgala HF: Ergonovine testing to detect spontaneous remission of variant angina during long-term treatment with calcium antagonist drugs. *Am J Cardiol* 47:179, 1981.

73. Yanagisawa T, Taira N: Effect of 2-nicotinamidothyl nitrate (SG-75) on the membrane potential of left atrial muscle fibres of the dog. *Naunyn Schmiedebergs Arch Pharmacol* 312:69, 1980.

74. Allen SL, Boyle JP, Cortijo J, et al: Electrical and mechanical effects of BRL 3495 in guinea pig isolated trachealis. *Br J Pharmacol* 89:395, 1986.

75. Inoue R, Ito Y, Takeda T: The effects of 2-nicotinamidoethyl nitrate on smooth muscle cells of the dog mesenteric artery and trachea. *Br J Pharmacol* 80:459, 1983.

75a. Akao M, Teshima Y, Marbán E: Antiapoptotic effects of nicorandil mediated by mitochondrial ATP-sensitive potassium channels in cultured cardiac myocytes. *J Am Coll Cardiol* 40:803, 2002.

76. Hashimoto K, Kinoshita M, Ohbayashi Y: Coronary effects of nicorandil in comparison with nitroglycerin in chronic conscious dogs. *Cardiovasc Drugs Ther* 5:131, 1991.

77. Kinoshita M, Sakai K: Pharmacology and therapeutic effects of nicorandil. *Cardiovasc Drugs Ther* 4:1075, 1990.

78. Lamping KA, Gross GJ: Comparative effects of a new nicotinamide nitrate derivative, nicorandil (SG-75), with nifedipine and nitroglycerin on true collateral blood flow following an acute coronary occlusion in dogs. *J Cardiovasc Pharmacol* 6:601, 1984.

79. Huckstorf C, Bassenge E: Effects of long-term nicorandil application on coronary arteries in conscious dogs. *J Cardiovasc Pharmacol* 20(Suppl 3): S29, 1992.

80. Munzel T, Huckstorf C, Bassenge E: Effects of long-term sydnonimine infusion on endothelium-dependent and independent vasodilation of large coronary arteries (abstr.). *FASEB J* 5:A1729, 1991.

81. Stewart DJ, Holtz J, Bassenge E: Long-term nitroglycerin treatment: Effect on direct and endothelium-mediated large coronary artery dilation in conscious dogs. *Circulation* 75:847, 1987.

82. Tsutamoto T, Kinoshita M, Hisanaga T, et al: Comparison of hemodynamic effects and plasma cyclic guanosine monophosphate of nicorandil and nitroglycerin in patients with congestive heart failure. *Am J Cardiol* 75:1162, 1995.

83. Tabone X, Funck-Brentano C, Billon N, et al: Comparison of tolerance to intravenous nitroglycerin during nicorandil and intermittent nitroglycerin patch in healthy volunteers. *Clin Pharmacol Ther* 56(6 pt 1):672, 1994.

84. Lamping KA, Gross GJ: Improved recovery of myocardial segment function following a short coronary occlusion in dogs by nicorandil, a potent new antianginal agent, and nifedipine. *J Cardiovasc Pharmacol* 7:158, 1985.

85. Lamping KA, Christensen CW, Pelc LR, et al: Effects of nicorandil and nifedipine on protection of ischemic myocardium. *J Cardiovasc Pharmacol* 6:536, 1984.

86. Belz GG, Matthews JH, Heinrich J, Wagner G: Controlled comparison of the pharmacodynamic effects of nicorandil (SG-75) and isosorbide dinitrate in man. *Eur J Clin Pharmacol* 26:681, 1984.

87. Belz GG, Beermann C: Venodilatory effects of nicorandil in healthy volunteers. *J Cardiovasc Pharmacol* 20(Suppl 3):S57, 1992.

88. Coltart DJ, Signy M: Acute hemodynamic effects of single-dose nicorandil in coronary heart disease. *Am J Cardiol* 63:34J, 1989.

89. Murakami M, Takeyama Y, Matsubara H, et al: Effects of intravenous injection of nicorandil on systemic and coronary hemodynamics in patients with old myocardial infarction. A comparison with nifedipine and isosorbide dinitrate (abstr.). *Eur Heart J* 10(Suppl 1):426, 1989.

90. Cohen-Solal A, Jaeger P, Bouthier J, et al: Hemodynamic action of nicorandil in chronic congestive heart failure. *Am J Cardiol* 63:44J, 1989.

91. Tice FD, Binkley PF, Cody RJ, et al: Hemodynamic effects of oral nicorandil in congestive heart failure. *Am J Cardiol* 65:1361, 1990.

92. Goldschmidt M, Landzberg BR, Frishman WH: Nicorandil. *J Clin Pharmacol* 35:559, 1996.

93. Suryapranata H, MacLeod D: Nicorandil and cardiovascular performance in patients with coronary artery disease. *J Cardiovasc Pharmacol* 20(Suppl 3):S45, 1992.

94. Thormann J, Schlepper M, Kramer W, et al: Effectiveness of nicorandil (SG-75), a new long-acting drug with nitroglycerin effects, in patients with coronary artery disease: Improved left ventricular function and regional wall motion and abolition of pacing-induced angina. *J Cardiovasc Pharmacol* 5:371, 1983.

95. Ohnishi M, Maeda K, Fukuzaki W, et al: Antianginal mechanism of nicorandil: Study on exercise invasive hemodynamics and thallium-201 myocardial perfusion images. *J Jpn Coll Angiol* 27:191, 1987.

96. Kambara H, Nakamura Y, Tamaki S, Kawai C: Beneficial effects of nicorandil on cardiovascular hemodynamics and left ventricular function. *Am J Cardiol* 53:56J, 1989.

97. Kinoshita M, Hashimoto K, Ohbayashi Y, et al: Comparison of antianginal activity of nicorandil, propranolol and diltiazem with reference to the antianginal mechanism. *Am J Cardiol* 63:71J, 1989.

98. Wagner G: Selected issues from an overview on nicorandil: Tolerance, duration of action, and long-term efficacy. *J Cardiovasc Pharmacol* 20(Suppl 3):S86, 1992.

99. Falcone C, Auguadro C, Chioffi M, et al: A double-blind comparison of nicorandil and isosorbide dinitrate slow release in patients with stable angina pectoris (abstr.). *Eur Heart J* 14(Suppl I):376, 1993.

100. Meeter K, Kelder JC, Tijssen JGP, et al: Efficacy of nicorandil versus propranolol in mild stable angina pectoris of effort: A long-term, double-blind, randomized study. *J Cardiovasc Pharmacol* 20(Suppl 3): S59, 1992.

101. Kobayashi K, Hakuta T: Effects of nicorandil on coronary hemodynamics in ischaemic heart disease: Comparison with nitroglycerin, nifedipine, and propranolol. *J Cardiovasc Pharmacol* 10(Suppl 8):S109, 1987.

102. Swan Study Group: Comparison of the anti-ischaemic and antianginal effects of nicorandil and amlodipine in patients with symptomatic stable angina pectoris: The SWAN study. *J Clin Basic Cardiol* 2:213, 1999.

103. Ulvenstam F, Diderholm E, Frithz G, et al: Antianginal and anti-ischemic efficacy of nicorandil compared with nifedipine in patients with angina pectoris and coronary heart disease: A double-blind, randomized, multicenter study. *J Cardiovasc Pharmacol* 20(Suppl 3):S67, 1992.

104. Thadani U, Strauss W, Glasser SP, et al: Evaluation of antianginal and anti-ischemic efficacy of nicorandil: Results of a multicenter study (abstr.). *J Am Coll Cardiol* 23(Suppl A):276A, 1994.

105. For first time, an antianginal agent shown to improve clinical outcomes. *Formulary* 37:47, 2002.

105a. IONA Study Group: Effect of nicorandil on coronary events in patients with stable angina: The Impact of Nicorandil in Angina (IONA) randomised trial. *Lancet* 359:1269, 2002.

106. Bertrand ME, LaBlanche JM, Tilmant PY, et al: Frequency of provoked coronary arterial spasm in 1089 consecutive patients undergoing coronary arteriography. *Circulation* 65:1299, 1982.

107. Previtali M, Panciroli C, DePonti R, et al: Time-related decrease in sensitivity to ergonovine in patients with variant angina. *Am Heart J* 117:92, 1989.

108. Theroux P, Waters DD, Affaki GS, et al: Provocative testing with ergonovine to evaluate the efficacy of treatment with calcium antagonists in variant angina. *Circulation* 60:504, 1979.

109. Curry RC, Pepine CJ, Sabom MB, Conti CR: Similarities of ergonovine-induced and spontaneous attacks of variant angina. *Circulation* 52:307, 1979.

110. Aizawa T, Ogasawara K, Nakamura F, et al: Effect of nicorandil on coronary spasm. *Am J Cardiol* 63:75J, 1989.

111. Patel DJ, Purcell HJ, Fox KM: Cardioprotection by opening of the KATP channel in unstable angina. Is this a clinical manifestation of myocardial preconditioning? Results of a randomized study with nicorandil. CESAR 2 Investigation. Clinical European Studies in Angina and Revascularization. *Eur Heart J* 20:51, 1999.

112. Sen S, Neuss H, Berg G, et al: Beneficial effects of nicorandil in acute myocardial infarction: A placebo-controlled, double-blind pilot safety study. *Br J Cardiol* 5:208, 1998.

113. Ito H, Taniyama Y, Iawakura K, et al: Intravenous nicorandil can preserve microvascular integrity and myocardial viability in patients with reperfused anterior wall myocardial infarction. *J Am Coll Cardiol* 33:654, 1999.

114. Kobayashi Y, Goto Y, Daikoku S, et al: Cardioprotective effect of intravenous nicorandil in patients with successful reperfusion for acute myocardial infarction. *Jpn Circ J* 62:183, 1998.

115. Sakata Y, Kodama K, Komamura K, et al: Salutary effect of adjunctive intracoronary nicorandil administration on restoration of myocardial blood flow and functional improvement in patients with acute myocardial infarction. *Am Heart J* 133:616, 1997.

116. Nameki M, Ishibashi I, Miyazaki Y, et al: Cardioprotective effect of nicorandil (ATP-sensitive potassium channel opener) as an adjunct to primary PTCA for acute myocardial infarction compared with magnesium: a prospective randomized trial. *Circulation* 100(Suppl): 284, 1999.

116a. Hayashi Y, Sawa Y, Ohtake S, et al: Controlled nicorandil administration for myocardial protection during coronary artery bypass grafting under cardiopulmonary bypass. *J Cardiovasc Pharmacol* 38:21, 2001.

116b. Falase BA, Bajaj BS, Wall TJ, et al: Nicorandil-induced peripheral vasodilation during cardio-pulmonary bypass. *Ann Thorac Surg* 36:1158, 1999.

116c. Montgomery H, Suneray M, Carr C, et al: Sinus arrest and severe peripheral vasodilation following cardiopulmonary bypass in a patient taking nicorandil. *Cardiovasc Drugs Ther* 11:81, 1997.

117. Dunn N, Freemantle S, Pearce G, et al: Safety profile of nicorandil. Prescription-event monitoring (PEM) study. *Pharmacoepidemiol Drug Saf* 8:197, 1999.

118. Reichert S, Antunes A, Trechot P, et al: Major aphthous stomatitis induced by nicorandil. *Eur J Dermatol* 7:132, 1997.

118a. Watson A, Ozairi OA, Fraser A, et al: Nicorandil associated anal ulcers. *Lancet* 360:546, 2002.

119. Purcell H, Patel DJ, Mulcahy D, Fox K: Nicorandil. In: Messerli FH, ed. *Cardiovascular Drug Therapy*. 2d ed. Philadelphia: WB Saunders, 1996:1638.

120. Takeshige K, Takayanagi K, Minakami S: Reduced coenzyme Q_{10} as an antioxidant of lipid peroxidation in bovine heart mitochondria. In: Yamamura Y, Folkers K, Ito Y, eds. *Biomedical and Clinical Aspects of Coenzyme Q*. Vol 2. Amsterdam: Elsevier/North Holland Biomedical Press, 1980:15.

121. Tran MT: Role of coenzyme Q_{10} in chronic heart failure, angina, and hypertension. *Pharmacotherapy* 21:797, 2001.

122. Mortensen SA: Perspectives on therapy of cardiovascular diseases with coenzyme Q_{10} (ubiquinone). *J Clin Invest* 71:S116, 1993.

123. Beyer, RE, Nordenbrand K, Ernster L: The role of coenzyme Q as a mitochondrial antioxidant. A short review. In: Folkers K, Yamamura Y, eds. *Biomedical and Clinical Aspects of Coenzyme Q*. Vol 5. Amsterdam: Elsevier, 1986:17.

124. Chance B, Erecinska M, Radder G: 12-19-anthracyl-stearic acid, a fluorescent probe for the ubiquinone region of the mitochondrial membrane. *Eur J Biochem* 54:521, 1975.

125. Spinsi A, Masotti L, Lenaz G, et al: Interactions between ubiquinones and phospholipid bilayers. A spin-label study. *Arch Biochem Biophys* 190:454, 1978.

126. Kobayashi M, Shimomura Y, Suzuki H, et al: Structural effects of ubiquinones on the mitochondrial inner membrane. *J Appl Biochem* 2:270, 1980.

127. Hofman-Bangc C, Rehnquist N, Swedberg K for the Q_{10} Study Group: Coenzyme Q_{10} as an adjunctive treatment of congestive heart failure (abstr.). *J Am Coll Cardiol* 19:216A, 1992.

128. O'Mathúna DP: Coenzyme Q_{10} to enhance aerobic exercise. *Alt Med Alert* 5:5, 2002.

129. Crane FL, Hatefi Y, Lester RL, Widmer G: Isolation of a quinone from beef heart mitochondria. *Biochem Biophys Acta* 25:220, 1957.

130. Folkers K, Littani G, Ho L, et al: Evidence for a deficiency of coenzyme Q_{10} in human heart disease. *Int J Vitam Nutr Res* 38:380, 1970.

131. Festenstein GN, Heaton FW, Lowe JS, Morton RA: A constituent of the unsaponifiable portion of animal tissue lipids. *Biochem J* 59:558, 1955.

132. Yamamura Y, Ishiyama T, Yamogami T, et al: Clinical use of coenzyme Q for treatment of cardiovascular disease. *Jpn Circ J* 31:168, 1967.

133. Lowe JS, Morton RA, Vernon J: Unsaponifiable constituents of kidney in various species. *Biochem J* 67:228, 1957.

134. Cunningham NF, Morton FA: Unsaponifiable constituents of liver: Ubiquinone and substance SC in various species. *Biochem J* 72:92, 1959.

135. Linn BO, Page AC, Wong EL, et al: Isolation and distribution of coenzyme Q_{10} in animal tissues. *J Am Chem Soc* 81:4007, 1959.

136. Triolo L, Lippa S, Oradei A, DeSole P, Mori R: Serum coenzyme Q_{10} in uremic patients on chronic hemodialysis. *Nephron* 66:153, 1994.

137. Scalori V, Allesandri MG, Giovannini L, Bertelli A: Plasma and tissue concentrations of coenzyme Q_{10} in the rat after intravenous, oral and topical administrations. *Int J Tissue React* XII(3):149, 1990.

138. Sustry PS, Jayaraman J, Ramasarma T: Distribution of coenzyme Q in rat liver cell fractions. *Nature* 189:577, 1961.

139. King TE: Ubiquinone proteins and cardiac mitochondria. In: Trumpower BL, ed. *Function of Quinones in Energy Conserving Systems*. New York: Academic Press, 1982:3–15.

140. King TE: Ubiquinone proteins. In: Lenaz G, ed. *Coenzyme Q*. New York: John Wiley & Sons, 1985:391–408.

141. Beyer RE, Burnett BA, Cartwright KJ, et al: Tissue coenzyme Q (ubiquinone) and protein concentrations over the life span of the laboratory rat. *Mech Aging Dev* 32:267, 1985.

142. Kalen A, Appelkvist EL, Dallner G: Age-related changes in the lipid compositions of rat and human tissues. *Lipids* 24:579, 1989.

143. Crane FL, Sun IL, Sun EE, et al: Cell growth stimulation by plasma membrane electron transport. *FASEB J* 5:A1624, 1991.

144. Rodriguez M, Moreau P, Paulik M, et al: NADH activated cell-free transfer between Golgi apparatus and plasma membranes of rat liver. *Biochim Biophys Acta* 1107:131, 1992.

145. Thelin A, Schedin S, Dallner G: Half-life of ubiquinone-9 in rat tissues. *FEBS Lett* 313:118, 1992.

146. Rengo F, Abete P, Landino P, et al: Role of metabolic therapy in cardiovascular disease. *J Clin Invest* 71:S124, 1993.

147. Tomono Y, Hasegawa J, Seki T, Morishita N: Pharmacokinetic study of deuterium-labelled coenzyme Q_{10} in man. *Int J Clin Pharmacol Ther Toxicol* 24(10):536, 1986.

148. Chopra, R: Relative bioavailability of coenzyme Q10 formulations in human subjects. *Int J Vitam Nutr Res* 68(2):109, 1998.

149. Kishi H, Kanamori N, Nishii S, et al: Metabolism of exogenous coenzyme Q_{10} in vivo and the bioavailability of coenzyme Q_{10} preparation in Japan. In: Folkers K, Yamamura Y, eds. *Biomedical and Clinical Aspects of Coenzyme Q*. Vol 4. , Amsterdam: Elsevier Science, 1984:131.

150. Yuzuriha T, Takada M, Katayama K: Transport of C^{14} coenzyme Q_{10} from the liver to other tissues after intravenous administration to guinea pigs. *Biochem Biophys Acta* 759:286, 1983.

151. De-Lorgeril, M, Salen P, Bontemps L, et al: Effects of lipid-powering drugs on left ventricular function and exercise tolerance in dyslipidemic coronary patients. *J Cardiovasc Pharmacol* 33:473, 1999.

152. Lucker PF, Wetzelsberger N, Hennings G, Rehn D: Pharmacokinetics of coenzyme ubidecarenone in healthy volunteers. In: Folkers K, Yamamura Y, eds. *Biomedical and Clinical Aspects of Coenzyme Q*. Vol 4. Amsterdam: Elsevier Science, 1984:143.

153. Scalori V, Allesandri MG, Giovannini L, Bertelli A: Plasma and tissue concentrations of coenzyme Q_{10} in the rat after intravenous, oral and topical administrations. *Int J Tissue React* XII(3):149, 1990.

154. Lea CH, Kwietny A: Antioxidant action of ubiquinones and related compounds. *Chem Ind* 24:1245, 1962.

155. Ernster L, Nelson BD: Functions of coenzyme Q. In: Folkers K, Yamamura Y, eds. *Biomedical and Clinical Aspects of Coenzyme Q*. Vol. 3. Amsterdam: Elsevier/North Holland Biomedical Press, 1981:159.

156. Niibori K, Yokoyama H, Crestanello JA, Whitman GJ: Acute administration of liposomal coenzyme Q10 increases myocardial tissue levels and improves tolerance to ischemia reperfusion injury. *J Surg Res* 79:141, 1998.

157. Nayler WG: The use of coenzyme Q_{10} to protect ischaemic heart muscle. In Yamamura Y, Folkers K, Ito Y, eds. *Biomedical and Clinical Aspects of Coenzyme Q*. Vol. 2. Amsterdam: Elsevier/North Holland Biomedical Press, 1980:409.

158. Ohhara H, Kanaide H, Yoshimura R, et al: A protective effect of coenzyme Q_{10} on ischemia and reperfusion of the isolated perfused rat heart. *J Mol Cell Cardiol* 13:65, 1981.

159. Sugiyama S, Ozawa T, Kato T, Suzuki S: Recovery time course of ventricular vulnerability after coronary reperfusion in relation to mitochondrial function in ischemic myocardium. *Am Heart J* 100:829, 1980.

160. Yamamura K, Nohara M, Kinoshita T, Tanimura A: Effects of coenzyme Q_{10} on anoxia-induced changes in cultured adult rat cardiomyocytes. *Kurume Med J* 32:163, 1985.

161. Kishi T, Okamoto T, Takahashi T, et al: Cardiostimulatory action of coenzyme Q homologues on cultured myocardial cells and their biochemical mechanisms. *J Clin Invest* 71:71, 1993.

162. Yasumoto K, Inada Y: Effect of coenzyme Q_{10} on endotoxin shock in dogs. *Crit Care Med* 14:570, 1986.

163. Ham EA, Eagan R, Soderman D: Peroxidase-dependent deactivation of prostacyclin synthetase. *J Biol Chem* 254:2191, 1979.

164. Gwak S, Yu L, Yu S: Studies of protein-phospholipid interaction in isolated mitochondrial ubiquinone-cytochromic reductase. *Biochim Biophys Acta* 809:187, 1985.

165. Ondarroa M, Quinn P: Proton magnetic resonance spectroscopic studies of the interaction of ubiquinone-10 with phospholipid membranes. *Int J Biochem* 155:353, 1986.

166. Kontush A, Hubner C, Finckh B, et al: Antioxidative activity of ubiquinol-10 at physiologic concentrations in human low density lipoprotein. *Biochim Biophys Acta* 1258:177, 1995.

167. Stocker R, Bowry VW, Frei B: Ubiquinol 10 protects human low density lipoprotein more efficiently against lipid peroxidation than does alpha-tocopherol. *Proc Natl Acad Sci U S A* 88:1645, 1991.

168. Serebrauny V, Ordonez J, Herzog W, et al: Dietary coenzyme Q10 supplementation alters platelet size and inhibits human vitronectin (CD51/CD61) receptor expression. *J Cardiovasc Pharmacol* 29:16, 1997.

169. Keith M, Geranmayegan A, Sole MJ, et al: Increased oxidative stress in patients with congestive heart failure. *J Am Coll Cardiol* 31:1352, 1998.

170. Soja AM, Mortensen SA: Treatment of congestive heart failure with coenzyme Q10 illuminated by meta-analyses of clinical trials. *Mol Aspects Med* 18(Suppl):S159, 1997.

171. Sacher HL, Sacher ML, Landau SW, et al: The clinical and hemodynamic effects of coenzyme Q10 in congestive cardiomyopathy. *Am J Ther* 4 2-3):66, 1997.

172. Sinatra ST: Coenzyme Q10: A vital therapeutic nutrient for the heart with special application in congestive heart failure. *Conn Med* 61:707, 1997.

173. Watson PS, Scalia GM, Galbraith A, et al: Lack of effect of coenzyme Q on left ventricular function in patients with congestive heart failure. *J Am Coll Cardiol* 33:1549, 1999.

174. Khatta M, Alexander BS, Krichten CM, et al: The effect of coenzyme Q_{10} in patients with congestive heart failure. *Ann Intern Med* 132:636, 2000.

175. Sinatra S: Coenzyme Q_{10} and congestive heart failure (letter). *Ann Intern Med* 133:745, 2000.

176. Mortensen SA: Coenzyme Q_{10} as an adjunctive therapy in patients with congestive heart failure (letter). *J Am Coll Cardiol* 36:304, 2000.

177. Gottlieb S, Khatta M, Fisher M: Response to S. Sinatra: Coenzyme Q_{10} and Congestive Heart Failure. *Ann Intern Med* 133:745, 2000.

178. Watson P, Scalia G, Galbraith A, et al: Response to S. Mortensen: coenzyme Q_{10} as an adjunctive therapy in patients with congestive heart failure. *J Am Coll Cardiol* 36(1):304, 2000.

179. Aejmelaeus R, Metsa-Ketela T, Laippala P, et al: Ubiquinol-10 and total peroxyl radical trapping capacity of LDL lipoproteins during aging: The effects of Q-10 supplementation. *Mol Aspects Med* 18(Suppl):S113, 1997.

180. Kontush A, Reich A, Baum K, et al: Plasma ubiquinol-10 is decreased in patients with hyperlipidemia. *Atherosclerosis* 129:119, 1997.

181. Kaikkonen J, Nyyssonen K, Porkkala-Sarataho E, et al: Effect of oral coenzyme Q10 supplementation on the oxidation resistance of human VLDL+LDL fraction: Absorption and antioxidative properties of oil and granule-based preparations. *Free Radic Biol Med* 22:1195, 1997.

182. Cleary J, Mohr D, Adams MR, et al: Plasma and LDL levels of major lipophilic antioxidants are similar in patients with advanced atherosclerosis and age-matched controls. *Free Radic Res* 26(2):175, 1997.

183. Singh RB, Niaz MA: Serum concentration of lipoprotein (a) decreases on treatment with hydrosoluble coenzyme Q_{10} in patients with coronary artery disease: Discovery of a new role. *Intl J Cardiol* 68:23, 1999.

184. Van de Vijver L, Weber C, Kardinaal A, et al: Plasma coenzyme Q_{10} concentration are not decreased in male patients with atherosclerosis. *Free Radic Res* 30:165, 1999.

185. Singh RB, Shinde SN, Chopra RK, et al: Effect of coenzyme Q_{10} on experimental atherosclerosis and chemical composition and quality of atheroma in rabbits. *Atherosclerosis* 148:275, 1999.

186. Thomas SR, Neuzil J, Stocker R: Inhibition of LDL oxidation by ubiquinol-10. A protective mechanism for coenzyme Q in atherogenesis? *Mol Aspects Med* 18(Suppl):S85, 1997.

187. Mortensen SA, Leth A, Agner E, Rohde M: Dose-related decrease of serum coenzyme Q_{10} during treatment with HMG-CoA reductase inhibitors. *Mol Aspects Med* 18(Suppl):S137, 1997.

188. McCarty MF: Coenzyme Q_{10} versus hypertension: Does CoQ decrease endothelial superoxide generation? *Med Hypotheses* 53(4): 300, 1999.

189. Lonnrot K, Porsti I, Alho H, et al: Control of arterial tone after long-term coenzyme Q_{10} supplementation in senescent rats. *Br J Pharmacol* 124:1500, 1998.

190. Singh RB, Niaz MA, Rastogi SS, et al: Effect of hydrosoluble coenzyme Q_{10} on blood pressures and insulin resistance in hypertensive patients with coronary artery disease. *J Hum Hypertens* 13:203, 1999.

191. Arita M, Kiyousue T, Imanishi S, Aomine M: Electrophysiological and inotropic effect of coenzyme Q_{10} on guinea pig ventricular muscle depolarized by potassium and hypoxia. *Jpn Heart J* 23:961, 1982.

192. Konishi T, Nakamura Y, Kanishi T, Kawai C: Improvement in recovery of left ventricular function during reperfusion with coenzyme Q_{10} in isolated working rat heart. *Cardiovasc Res* 19:38, 1984.

193. Atar D, Mortensen SA, Flachs H, Herzog WR: Coenzyme Q_{10} protects ischemic myocardium in an open-chest swine model. *J Clin Invest* 71:S103, 1993.

194. Hano O, Thompson-Gorman SL, Zweier JL, Lakatta EG: Coenzyme Q_{10} enhances cardiac functional and metabolic recovery and reduces Ca^{2+} overload during postischemic reperfusion. *Am J Physiol* 266:H2174, 1994.

195. Hiasa Y, Ishida T, Maeda T, et al: Effects of coenzyme Q_{10} on exercise tolerance in patients with stable angina pectoris. In: Folkers K, Yamamura Y, eds. *Biomedical and Clinical Aspects of Coenzyme Q.* Vol 4. Amsterdam: Elsevier Science, 1984:291.

196. Kamikawa T, Kobayashi A, Yamashita T, et al: Effects of coenzyme Q_{10} on exercise tolerance in chronic stable angina pectoris. *Am J Cardiol* 56:247, 1985.

197. Schardt F, Welzel D, Schiess W, Toda K: Effect of coenzyme Q_{10} on ischaemia-induced ST-segment depression: A double-blind, placebo-controlled, crossover study. In: Folkers K, Yamamura Y, eds. *Biomedical and Clinical Aspects of Coenzyme Q.* Vol 5. Amsterdam: Elsevier Science, 1985:385.

198. Wilson M, Frishman WH, Giles T, et al: Coenzyme Q_{10} therapy and exercise duration in stable angina. In: Folkers K, Littaru GP, Yamagami T, eds. *Biomedical and Clinical Aspects of Coenzyme Q.* Vol 6. Amsterdam: Elsevier Science, 1991:339.

199. Kobayashi M, Schimomura Y, Suzuki H, et al: Structural effects of ubiquinones on the mitochondrial inner membrane. *J Appl Biochem* 2:270, 1980.

200. Sugiyama S, Kitazawa M, Ozawa T, et al: Antioxidative effect of coenzyme Q_{10}. *Experientia* 36:1002, 1980.

201. Singh RB, Wander GS, Rastogi A, et al: Randomized, double-blind placebo-controlled trial of coenzyme Q_{10} in patients with acute myocardial infarction. *Cardiovasc Drugs Ther* 12:347, 1998.

202. Zhou M, Zhi Q, Tang Y, et al: Effects of coenzyme Q_{10} on myocardial protection during cardiac valve replacement and scavenging free radical activity in vitro. *J Cardiovasc Surg (Torino)* 40:355, 1999.

203. Chello M, Mastroroberto P, Romano R, et al: Protection by coenzyme Q_{10} of tissue reperfusion injury during abdominal aortic cross-clamping. *J Cardiovasc Surg (Torino)* 37:229, 1996.

204. Tanaka J, Tominaga R, Yoshitoshi MD, et al: Coenzyme Q_{10}: The prophylactic effect on low cardiac output following cardiac valve replacement. *Ann Thorac Surg* 33(2):145, 1982.

205. Sunamori M, Okamura T, Amano J, Suzuki A: Clinical application of coenzyme Q to coronary artery bypass graft surgery. In: Folkers K, Yamamura Y, eds. *Biomedical and Clinical Aspects of Coenzyme Q.* Vol 4. Amsterdam: Elsevier Science, 1984:333.

206. Judy WV, Stogsdill WW, Folkers K: Myocardial preservation by therapy with coenzyme Q_{10} during heart surgery. *J Clin Invest* 71:S155, 1993.

207. Chello M, Mastroroberto P, Romano R, et al: Protection by coenzyme Q_{10} from myocardial reperfusion injury during coronary artery bypass grafting. *Ann Thorac Surg* 58:1427, 1994.

208. Kucharska J, Gvodjakova A, Mizera S, et al: Participation of coenzyme Q_{10} in the rejection development of the transplanted heart: A clinical study. *Physiol Res* 47:399, 1998.

209. Matsumoto H, Matsunaga H, Kawauchi M, et al: The effect of coenzyme Q_{10} pretreatment on myocardial preservation. *Heart Transp*III(2): 160, 1984.

210. Okamuto F, Allen B, Buckberg G, et al: Studies of controlled reperfusion after ischemia. Reperfusate composition: supplemental role of intravenous and intracoronary CoQ_{10} in avoiding reperfusion damage. *J Thorac Cardiovasc Surg* 92:572, 1986.

211. Ishiwata K, Miura Y, Takahashi T, et al: C-coenzyme Q_{10}: A new myocardial imaging tracer for positron emission tomography. *Eur J Nucl Med* 11:162, 1985.

212. Hiasa Y, Ishida T, Maeda T, et al: Effects of coenzyme Q_{10} on exercise tolerance in patients with stable angina pectoris. In: Folkers K, Yamamura Y, eds. *Biomedical and Clinical Aspects of Coenzyme Q.* Vol 4. Amsterdam: Elsevier Science, 1984:291.

213. Kamikawa T, Kobayashi A, Yamashita T, et al: Effects of coenzyme Q_{10} on exercise tolerance in chronic stable angina pectoris. *Am J Cardiol* 56:247, 1985.

214. Baggio E, Gandini R, Plancher AC, et al: Italian multicenter study on the safety and efficacy of coenzyme Q_{10} as adjunctive therapy in heart failure. *Mol Aspects Med* 15(Suppl):S287, 1994.

215. Kishi T, Kishi H, Watanabe T, Folkers K: Bioenergetics in clinical medicine. XI. Studies on coenzyme Q and diabetes mellitus. *J Med* 7:307, 1976.

216. Folkers K, Langsjoen Per, Willis R, et al: Lovastatin decreases coenzyme Q levels in humans. *Proc Natl Acad Sci U S A* 87:8931, 1990.

217. Kaikkonen J, Nyyssonen K, Tuomainen T, et al: Determinants of plasma coenzyme Q_{10} in humans. *FEBS Lett* 443:163, 1999.

218. Rebouche CJ: Carnitine function and requirements during the life cycle. *FASEB J* 6(15):3379, 1992.

219. Schonekess BO, Allard MF, Lopaschuk GD: Propionyl L-Carnitine improvement of hypertrophied heart function is accompanied by an increase in carbohydrate oxidation. *Circ Res* 77(4):726, 1995.

220. Reggiani C, Canepari M, Micheletti R, et al: Effect of propionyl-L-carnitine on the kinetic properties of the myofibrillar system in pressure overload cardiac hypertrophy. *Ann N Y Acad Sci* 752:204, 1995.

221. Murray MK: *Harper's Biochemistry.* Norwalk, CT: Appleton and Lange, 1993:221.

222. Zales VR, Benson DW Jr Reversible cardiomyopathy due to carnitine deficiency from renal tubular wasting. *Pediatr Cardiol* 16:76, 1995.

223. van Es A, Henny FC, Kooistra MP, et al: Amelioration of cardiac function by L-carnitine administration in patients on haemodialysis. *Contrib Nephrol* 98:28, 1992.

224. Harper P, Elwin CE, Cederblad S: Pharmacokinetics of intravenous and oral bolus doses of L-carnitine in healthy subjects. *Eur J Clin Pharmacol* 35:555, 1987.

225. Marcus R, Coulston AM: The vitamins. In: Hardman JG, Limbird LE, eds. *Goodman & Gilman's The Pharmacological Basis of Therapeutics,* 10th ed. New York: McGraw-Hill, 2001:1745.

226. Goa KL, Brogden RN: L-Carnitine. A preliminary review of its pharmacokinetics, and its therapeutic use in ischaemic cardiac disease and primary and secondary carnitine deficiencies in relationship to its role in fatty acid metabolism. *Drugs* 34(1):1, 1987.

227. Sundqvist KE, Vuorinen KH, Peuhkurinen KJ, Hassinen IE: Metabolic effects of propionate, hexanoate and propionyl carnitine in normoxia, ischaemia and reperfusion. Does an anaplerotic substrate protect the ischaemic myocardium? *Eur Heart J* 15:561, 1994.

228. Ferrari R, Ceconi C, Curello S, et al: Protective effect of propionyl-L-carnitine against ischemia and reperfusion damage. *Mol Cell Biochem* 88:161, 1989.

229. Di Lisa F, Menabo R, Barbato R, Siliprandi N: Contrasting effects of propionate and propionyl-L-carnitine on energy linked processes in ischemic hearts. *Am J Physiol* 267(2 pt 2):H455, 1994.

230. Jacoba KGC, Abarquez Jr RF, Topacio GO: Effect of L-carnitine on the limitation of infarct size in one month postmyocardial infarction cases. *Clin Drug Invest* 11(2):90, 1996.

231. Siliprandi D, Biban C, Testa S, et al: Effects of palmityl CoA and palmityl carnitine on the membrane potential and Mg^{2+} content of rat heart mitochondria. *Mol Cell Biochem* 116:117, 1992.

232. Liedtke AJ, DeMaison L, Nellis SH: Effects of L-propionyl carnitine on mechanical recovery during reflow in intact hearts. *Am J Physiol* 255:H169, 1988.

233. Broderick TL, Quinney HA, Barker CC, Lopaschuk GD: Beneficial effects of carnitine on mechanical recovery of rat hearts reperfused

after a transient period of global ischemia is accompanied by a stimulation of glucose oxidation. *Circulation* 87:972, 1993.

234. Paulson DJ, Shug AL, Zhao J: Protection of the diabetic ischemic heart by L-propionyl-carnitine therapy. *Mol Cell Biochem* 116:131, 1992.

235. Bohles H, Noppeney T, Akcetin Z, et al: The effect of preoperative L-carnitine supplementation on myocardial metabolism during aorto-coronary bypass surgery. *Curr Ther Res* 30:429, 1986.

236. Corbucci GG, Menichetti A, Cogliatti A, Ruvolo C: Metabolic aspects of acute tissue hypoxia during extracorporeal circulation and their modification induced by L-carnitine treatment. *Int J Clin Pharmacol Res* 12:149, 1992.

237. Bartels GL, Remme WJ, Pillay M, et al: Effects of L-propionyl carnitine on ischaemia induced myocardial dysfunction in men with angina pectoris. *Am J Cardiol* 74:125, 1994.

238. Iliceto S, Scrutinio D, Bruzzi P, et al: Effects of L-carnitine administration on left ventricular remodeling after acute myocardial infarction: The L-carnitine (CEDIM) trial. *J Am Coll Cardiol* 26:380, 1995.

239. Singh RB, Niaz MA, Agarwal P, et al: A randomised, double-blind, placebo-controlled trial of L-carnitine in suspected acute myocardial infarction. *Postgrad Med J* 72:45, 1996.

240. Lagioia R, Scrutinio D, Mangini SG, et al: Propionyl-L-carnitine: A new compound in the metabolic approach to the treatment of effort angina. *Int J Cardiol* 34:167, 1992.

241. Cacciatore L, Cerio R, Ciarimboli M, et al: The therapeutic effect of L-carnitine in patients with exercise-induced stable angina: A controlled study. *Drugs Exp Clin Res* 17:225, 1991.

242. Rizzon P, Biasco G, Di Biase M, et al: High doses of L-carnitine in acute myocardial infarction: Metabolic and antiarrhythmic effects. *Eur Heart J* 10:502, 1989.

243. Yamada KA, Dobmeyer DJ, Kanter EM, et al: Delineation of the influence of propionyl carnitine on the accumulation of long-chain acylcarnitines and electrophysiologic derangements evoked by hypoxia in canine myocardium. *Cardiovasc Drugs Ther* 5(Suppl 1):67, 1991.

244. Duncker DJ, Sassen LM, Bartels GL, et al: L-Propionyl carnitine does not affect myocardial metabolic or functional response to chronotropic and inotropic stimulation after repetitive ischemia in anesthetized pigs. *J Cardiovasc Pharmacol* 22:488, 1993.

245. Regitz V, Shug AL, Fleck E: Defective myocardial carnitine metabolism in congestive heart failure secondary to dilated cardiomyopathy and to coronary, hypertensive and valvular heart diseases. *Am J Cardiol* 65:755, 1990.

246. Pierpont ME, Judd M, Goldenberg IF, et al: Myocardial carnitine in end-stage congestive heart failure. *Am J Cardiol* 64:56, 1989.

247. Masmura M, Kobayashi A, Yamazaki N: Myocardial free carnitine and fatty acylcarnitine levels in patients in patients with chronic heart failure. *Jpn Circ J* 54:1471, 1990.

248. Matsui S, Sugita T, Matoba M: Urinary carnitine excretion in patients with heart failure. *Clin Cardiol* 17:301, 1994.

249. Yang XP, Samaja M, English E, et al: Hemodynamic and metabolic activities of propionyl-L-carnitine in rats with pressure-overload cardiac hypertrophy. *J Cardiovasc Pharm* 20:88, 1992.

250. Micheletti R, Giacalone G, Canepari M, et al: Propionyl-L-carnitine prevents myocardial mechanical alterations due to pressure overload in rats. *Am J Physiol* 266:H2190, 1994.

251. Ferrari R, Di Lisa F, de Jong, JW, et al: Prolonged propionyl-L-carnitine pre-treatment of rabbit: biochemical, hemodynamic and electrophysiological effect on myocardium. *J Mol Cell Cardiol* 24:219, 1992.

252. Schonekess BO, Allard MF, Lopaschuk GD: Propionyl L-carnitine improvement of hypertrophied rat heart function is associated with an increase in cardiac efficiency. *Eur J Pharm* 286:155, 1995.

253. el Alaoui-Talibi Z, Bouhaddioni N, Moravec J: Assessment of the cardiostimulant action of propionyl-L-carnitine on chronically volume-overloaded rat hearts. *Cardiovasc Drugs Ther* 7:357, 1993.

254. Kobayashi A, Masmura Y, Yamazaki N: L-Carnitine treatment for congestive heart failure. *Jpn Circ J* 56:86, 1992.

255. De Giuli F, Pasini E, Opasich C, et al: Effects of propionyl-L-carnitine in patients with heart failure (abstr.). *J Mol Cell Cardiol* 27:V44, 1995.

256. Mancini M, Rengo F, Lingetti M, et al: Controlled study on the efficacy of propionyl-L-carnitine in patients with congestive heart failure. *Arzneimittelforschung* 42(9):1101, 1992.

257. Pucciarelli G, Mastursi M, Latte S, et al: The clinical and hemodynamic effects of propionyl-L-carnitine in the treatment of congestive heart failure. *Clin Ter* 141(11):379, 1992.

258. Broderick TL, St. Laurent R, Rousseau-Migneron S, et al: Beneficial effects of exercise training on cardiac long-chain acylcarnitine levels in diabetic rats. *Diabetes Res* 14:33, 1990.

259. Spagnoli LG, Orlandi A, Marino B, et al: Propionyl-L-carnitine prevents the progression of atherosclerotic lesions in aged hyperlipemic rabbits. *Atherosclerosis* 114:29, 1995.

260. Corsico N, Nardone A, Lucreziotti MR, et al: Effect of propionyl-L-carnitine in a rat model of peripheral arteriopathy. *Cardiovasc Drugs Ther* 7(2):241, 1993.

261. Ghidini O, Azzurro M, Vita G, Sartori G: Evaluation of the therapeutic efficacy of L-carnitine in congestive heart failure. *Int J Clin Pharmacol Ther Toxicol* 26:217, 1988.

262. Pola P, Savi L, Grilli M, et al: Carnitine in the therapy of dyslipidemic patients. *Curr Ther Res* 27:208, 1980.

263. Hiatt WR, Nawaz D, Brass EP: Carnitine metabolism during exercise in patients with peripheral vascular disease. *J Appl Physiol* 62(6):2383, 1987.

264. Brevetti G, Perna S, Sabba C, et al: Propionyl-L-carnitine in intermittent claudication. *J Am Coll Cardiol* 26:1411, 1995.

265. Brevetti G, Perna S, Sabba A, et al: Superiority of L-propionyl carnitine vs L-carnitine in improving walking capacity in patients with peripheral vascular disease: An acute, intravenous, double-blind, crossover study. *Eur Heart J* 13:251, 1992.

266. Arsenian MA: Carnitine and its derivatives in cardiovascular disease. *Prog Cardiovasc Dis* 40(3):265, 1997.

267. Brevetti G, Di Lisa F, Perna S, et al: Carnitine-related alterations in patients with intermittent claudication. *Circulation* 93:1685, 1996.

268. Reznick AZ, Kagan VE, Ramsey R, et al: Antiradical effects in propionyl-L-carnitine protection of the heart against ischemia-reperfusion injury: the possible role of iron chelation. *Arch Biochem Biophys* 296(2):394, 1992.

269. Packer L, Valenza M, Serbinova E, et al: Free radical scavenging is involved in the protective effect of L-propionyl carnitine against ischemia-reperfusion injury of the heart. *Arch Biochem Biophys* 288:533, 1991.

270. Hearse DJ, Tosaki A: Free radicals and reperfusion-induced arrhythmias: Protection by spin trap agent PBN in the rat heart. *Circ Res* 60(3):375, 1987.

271. Palazzuoli V, Mondillo S, Faglia S, et al: The evaluation of the antiarrhythmic activity of L-carnitine and propafenone in ischemic cardiopathy. *Clin Ther* 142(2):155, 1993.

272. Opie LH: *The Heart: Physiology and Metabolism.* 2d ed. New York: Raven Press, 1991:208, 425.

273. Taegtmeyer H: Energy metabolism of the heart: from basic concepts to clinical applications. *Curr Prob Cardiol* 19(2):57, 1994.

274. Weiss JN, Lamp ST: Glycolysis preferentially inhibits ATP-sensitive potassium channels in isolated guinea pig cardiac myocytes. *Science* 238:67, 1987.

275. Cocco G, Rousseau MF, Bouvy T, et al: Effects of a new metabolic modulator, ranolazine, on exercise tolerance in angina pectoris patients treated with beta blocker or diltiazem. *J Cardiovasc Pharmacol* 20:131, 1992.

276. Jain D, Dasgupta P, Hughes LO, et al: Ranolazine (RS-43285): A preliminary study of a new anti-anginal agent with selective effect on ischaemic myocardium. *Eur J Clin Pharmacol* 38:111, 1990.

276a. Pouleur H, Hue L, Harlow BJ, Rousseau MF: Metabolic pathway modulation: A new approach to treat myocardial ischemia (abstr.)? *Circulation* 80(Suppl II):II52, 1989.

277. Stanley WC, Lopaschuk GD, Hall JL, McCormack JG: Regulation of myocardial carbohydrate metabolism under normal and ischaemic conditions: Potential for pharmacological interventions. *Cardiovasc Res* 33:243, 1997.

278. Anderson JR, Khou S, Nawarskas JJ: Ranolazine: A potential new treatment for chronic stable angina. *Heart Dis* 3:263, 2001.

279. Goldschmidt M, Frishman WH: Ranolazine: A new anti-ischemic drug which affects myocardial energetics. *Am J Ther* 2:269, 1995.

280. McCormack JG, Barr RL, Wolff AA, Lopaschuk GD: Ranolazine stimulates glucose oxidation in normoxic, ischemic, and reperfused ischemic rat hearts. *Circulation* 93:135, 1996.

281. Ferrandon P, Chaylat C, Armstrong JM: Free radical scavengers fail to increase the protective effects of ranolazine in isolated working rat

hearts after ischemia and reperfusion. *Br J Pharmacol* 93(Suppl):247, 1988.

282. Allely MC, Brown CM, Kenny BA, et al: Modulation of alpha$_1$-adrenoceptors in rat left ventricle by ischaemia and acyl carnitines: Protection by ranolazine. *J Cardiovasc Pharmacol* 21:869, 1993.

283. Benfey BG: Function of myocardial alpha adrenoceptors. *Life Sci* 46:743, 1990.

284. Heathers GP, Yamada KA, Kanter EM, Corr PB: Long-chain acylcarnitines mediate the hypoxia induced increases in alpha-1 adrenergic receptors on adult canine myocytes. *Circ Res* 61:735, 1987.

285. Pepine CJ, Wolff AA: A controlled trial with a novel anti-ischemic agent, ranolazine, in chronic stable angina pectoris that is responsive to conventional antianginal agents. *Am J Cardiol* 84:46, 1999.

286. Thadani U, Ezekowitz M, Fenney L, et al: Double-blind efficacy and safety study of a novel anti-ischemic agent, ranolazine, versus placebo in patients with chronic stable angina pectoris. *Circulation* 90:726, 1994.

287. Wolff AA for the MARISA investigators. MARISA. Monotherapy Assessment of Ranolazine in Stable Angina (abstr.). *J Am Coll Cardiol* 35:408A, 2000.

288. DeQuattro V, Skettino S, Chaitman BR, et al: Comparative antianginal efficacy and tolerability of ranolazine in diabetic and nondiabetic patients: Results of the MARISA trial (abstr.). *J Am Coll Cardiol* 37:338A, 2001.

289. Jain D, Dasgupta P, Hughes LO, et al: Ranolazine (RS-43285): A preliminary study of a new anti-anginal agent with selective effect of ischaemic myocardium. *Eur J Clin Pharmacol* 38:111, 1990.

290. Rousseau MF, Visser FG, Bax JJ, et al: Ranolazine: Antianginal therapy with a novel mechanism: Placebo controlled comparison versus atenolol. *Eur Heart J* 15:95, 1994.

291. Chaitman BR, Skettino S, DeQuattro V: Improved exercise performance on ranolazine in patients with chronic angina and a history of heart failure: The MARISA trial (abstr.). *J Am Coll Cardiol* 37:149A, 2001.

292. CV Therapeutics, Inc. CV Therapeutics completes CARISA patient enrollment. Accessed April 10, 2001. Available at http://prnewswire.com/gh/cnoc/comp/166425.html.

293. Ranolazine enhances exercise performance when added to standard medications. *Formulary* 37:48, 2002.

294. Sabbah HN, Mishima T, Biesiadecki BJ, et al: Ranolazine improves left ventricular performance in dogs with chronic heart failure (abstr.). *J Am Coll Cardiol* 34:218A, 2000.

295. CV Therapeutics, Inc. CV Therapeutics announces preclinical data evaluating ranolazine and dobutamine in a model of CHF. Accessed March 19, 2000. Available at http://prnewswire.com/gh/cnoc/comp/166425.html.

296. CV Therapeutics Inc. CV Therapeutics initiates ranolazine Phase II congestive heart failure trial. Accessed December 18, 2000. Available at http://prnewswire.com/gh/cnoc/comp/166424.html.

297. CV Therapeutics presents Phase III results for new drug candidate to treat chronic angina at the 49th annual meeting of the American College of Cardiology. Available at http://prnewswire.com/gh/cnoc/comp/166425.html. Accessed March 15, 2000.

298. Maridonneau-Parini I, Harpey C: Effect of trimetazidine of membrane damage induced by oxygen free radicals in human red cells. *Br J Clin Pharmacol* 20:148, 1985.

299. Veitch K, Maisin L, Hue L: Trimetazidine effects on the damage to mitochondrial functions caused by ischemia and reperfusion. *Am J Cardiol* 76:25B, 1995.

300. Demaison L, Fantini E, Sentex E, et al: Trimetazidine: In vitro influence on heart mitochondrial function. *Am J Cardiol* 76:31B, 1995.

301. Renaud JF: Internal pH, Na$^+$ and Ca^{2+} regulation by trimetazidine during cardiac cell acidosis. *Cardiovasc Drug Ther* 1:677, 1988.

302. Dalla Volta S, Maraglino G, Della-Valentina P, et al: Comparison of trimetazidine with nifedipine in effort angina: A double-blind crossover study. *Cardiovasc Drug Ther* 4:853, 1990.

303. Kantor PF, Lucien A, Kozak R, Lopaschuk GD: The antianginal drug trimetazidine shifts cardiac energy metabolism from fatty acid oxidation to glucose oxidation by inhibiting mitochondrial long-chain 3-ketoacyl coenzyme A thiolase. *Circ Res* 86:580, 2000.

303a. Desideri A, Celegon L: Metabolic management of ischemic heart disease: Clinical data with trimetazidine. *Am J Cardiol* 82:50K, 1998.

303b. Lopaschuk GD: Treating ischemic heart disease by pharmacologically improving cardiac energy metabolism. *Am J Cardiol* 82:14K, 1998.

303c. Sentex E, Sergiel JP, Lucien A, Grynberg A: Is the cytoprotective effect of trimetazidine associated with lipid metabolism? *Am J Cardiol* 82:18K, 1998.

303d. Lu C, Dabrowski P, Fragasso G, Chierchia SL: Effects of trimetazidine on ischemic left ventricular dysfunction in patients with coronary artery disease. *Am J Cardiol* 82:898, 1998.

304. Sellier P: Chronic effects of trimetazidine on ergometric parameters of effort angina. *Cardiovasc Drug Ther* 4:822, 1990.

305. Detry JM, Sellier P, Pennaforte S, et al: Trimetazidine: A new concept in the treatment of angina. Comparison with propranolol in patients with stable angina. *Br J Clin Pharmacol* 37:279, 1994.

306. Levy S, and the Group of South France Investigators. Combination therapy of trimetazidine with diltiazem in patients with coronary artery disease. *Am J Cardiol* 76:12B, 1995.

307. Montpere C, Brochier M, Demange J, et al: Combination of trimetazidine with nifedipine in effort angina. *Cardiovasc Drug Ther* 4:824, 1990.

308. Michaelides AP, Vyssoulis GP, Bonoris PE, et al: Beneficial effects of trimetazidine in men with stable angina under beta blocker treatment. *Curr Ther Res* 46:565, 1989.

309. Detry J-MR, Leclercq PJ on behalf of the TEMS Steering Committee. Trimetazidine European Multicenter Study versus propranolol in stable angina pectoris: Contribution of Holter electrocardiographic ambulatory monitoring. *Am J Cardiol* 76:8B, 1995.

310. Manchanda SC, Krishnaswami S: Combination treatment of trimetazidine and diltiazem in stable angina pectoris. *Heart* 78:353, 1997.

311. Kober G, Buck T, Sievert H, Vallbracht C: Myocardial cytoprotection during percutaneous transluminal coronary angioplasty: Effects of trimetazidine. *Eur Heart J* 13:1109, 1992.

312. Fabiani JN, Ponzio O, Emerit I, et al: Cardioprotective effect of trimetazidine during coronary artery graft surgery. *J Cardiovasc Surg* 38:486, 1992.

313. Noble MIM, Belcher PR, Drake-Holland AJ: Limitation of infarct size by trimetazidine in the rabbit. *Am J Cardiol* 76:41B, 1995.

314. Kay L, Finelli C, Aussedat J, et al: Improvement of long-term preservation by the isolated arrested rat heart by trimetazidine: Effects on the energy state and mitochondrial function. *Am J Cardiol* 76:45B, 1995.

314a. The EMIP-FR Group: Effect of 48-h intravenous trimetazidine on short- and long-term outcomes of patients with acute myocardial infarction, with and without thrombolytic therapy. A double-blind, placebo-controlled, randomized trial. *Eur Heart J* 21:1537, 2000.

314b. Shimokawa H, Iinuma H, Kishida H: Antianginal effect of fasudil-a rho-kinase inhibitor, in patients with stable effort angina: A multicenter study (abst). *Circulation* 104(Suppl): II-601, 2001.

314c. Masumoto A, Mohri M, Shimokawa H, et al: Suppression of coronary artery spasm by the rho-kinase inhibitor fasudil in patients with vasospastic angina. *Circulation* 105:1545, 2002.

315. Schaffer SW: Cardiomyopathy associated with non-insulin-dependent diabetes. *Mol Cell Biochem* 107:1, 1991.

316. Williamson JR, Chang K, Frangos M, et al: Perspectives in diabetes. *Diabetes* 42:801, 1993.

317. Greene DA, Lattimer SA, Sima AAF: Sorbitol, phosphoinositides and sodium-potassium ATPase in the pathogenesis of diabetic complications. *N Engl J Med* 316:599, 1987.

318. Beyer-Mears A: The polyol pathway, sorbinil, and renal dysfunction. *Metabolism* 35(Suppl 1):46, 1986.

319. Pfeifer MA: Clinical trials of sorbinil on nerve function. *Metabolism* 35(Suppl 1):78, 1986.

320. Karmazyn M, Ray M, Haist JV: Comparative effects of Na$^+$/H$^+$ exchange inhibitors against cardiac injury produced by ischemia/reperfusion, hypoxia/reoxygenation, and the calcium paradox. *J Cardiovasc Pharmacol* 21:172, 1993.

321. Ramasamy R, Schaefer S, Oates P: Improved ischemic tolerance in diabetic hearts treated with an aldose reductase inhibitor. Presented at 55th Annual Meeting of American Diabetes Assn. Atlanta, GA, June 10–13, 1995.

322. Ramasamy R, Liu H, Schaefer S: Aldose reductase inhibition limits the rise in intracellular sodium and calcium and protects diabetic hearts from ischemic injury. Presented at the 56th Annual Meeting of the American Diabetes Assn. San Francisco, CA, June 8, 1996.

323. Tracey WR, Magee WP, Ellery CA, et al: Aldose reductase inhibition alone or combined with an adenosine A(3) agonist reduces ischemic myocardial injury. *Am J Physiol* 279:H1447, 2000.

324. Hohman TC, El-Kabbani O, Malamas MS, et al: Probing the inhibitor-binding site of aldose reductase with site-directed mutagenesis. *Eur J Biochem* 256:310, 1998.

325. Hotta N, Toyota T, Matsuoka K, et al: Clinical efficacy of fidarestat, a novel aldose reductase inhibitor, for diabetic peripheral neuropathy. *Diabetes Care* 24:1776, 2001.

326. Cranton EM, ed: A textbook on EDTA chelation therapy. *J Adv Med* 2:1, 1989.

327. Diagnostic and therapeutic technology assessment: chelation therapy. *JAMA* 250:672, 1983.

328. Elihu N, Anandasabapathy S, Frishman WH: Chelation therapy in cardiovascular disease: Ethylenediaminetetraacetic acid and deferoxamine. *J Clin Pharmacol* 38:101, 1998.

329. Clarke NE, Clarke CN, Mosher RF: The "in vivo" dissolution of metastatic calcium: an approach to atherosclerosis. *Am J Med Sci* 229:142, 1955.

330. Blumer W, Cranton EM: Ninety percent reduction in cancer mortality after chelation therapy with EDTA. *J Adv Med* 2:183, 1989.

331. Olszewer E, Carter JC: EDTA chelation therapy in chronic degenerative disease. *Med Hypotheses* 27:41, 1988.

332. Olszewer E, Carter JP: EDTA chelation therapy a retrospective study of 2870 patients. *J Adv Med* 2:197, 1989.

333. Clarke NE, Clarke C, Mosher R: Treatment of angina pectoris with disodium ethylene tetraacetic acid. *Am J Med Sci* 232:654, 1956.

334. Morgan K: Myocardial ischemia treated with nutrients and intravenous EDTA chelation. Report of two cases. *J Adv Med* 4:47, 1991.

335. Cranton EM: *Protocol of the American College of Advancement in Medicine for the Safe and Effective Administration of EDTA Chelation Therapy.* Laguna Hills, CA: American College of Advancement in Medicine, 1989.

336. Godfrey ME: EDTA chelation as a treatment of arteriosclerosis. *N Z Med J* 103:162, 1990.

337. van-Rij AM, Solomon C, Parker SG, Hopkins WG: Chelation therapy for intermittent claudication: A double-blind, randomized, controlled trial. *Circulation* 90:1194, 1994.

338. Soffer A: Chelation therapy for atherosclerosis. *JAMA* 233:1206, 1975.

339. Wirebaugh SR, Geraets DR: Apparent failure of edetic acid chelation therapy for treatment of coronary atherosclerosis. *DICP* 24:22, 1990.

340. Rathmann KL, Golithly LK: Chelation therapy of atherosclerosis. *Drug Intell Clin Pharm* 8:1000, 1984.

341. Eisenberg et al: Trends in alternative medicine use in the United States, 1990–1997: Results of a follow-up national survey. *JAMA* 280:1569, 1998.

342. Magee P: Chelation treatment for atherosclerosis. *Med J Aust* 142:514, 1985.

343. Boyle AJ, Clarke NE, Mosher RE, McCann DS: Chelation therapy in circulatory and sclerosing diseases. *Fed Proc* 29:243, 1961.

344. Olszewer E, Sabbag FC, Carter JA: A pilot double-blind study of sodium-magnesium EDTA in peripheral vascular disease. *J Natl Med Assoc* 82:173, 1990.

345. Ross R: The pathogenesis of atherosclerosis — an update. *N Engl J Med* 314:488, 1986.

346. Peerscke EL, Grant RA, Zucker MB: Decreased association of 45 calcium with platelets unable to aggregate due to thrombasthenia or prolonged calcium deprivation. *Br J Haematol* 46:247, 1980.

347. Kindness G, Frackelton JP: Effect of ethylene diamine tetraacetic acid (EDTA) on platelet aggregation in human blood. *J Adv Med* 2:519, 1989.

348. Fitzgerald LA, Phillips DR: Calcium regulation of the platelet membrane glycoprotein IIb/IIIa complex. *J Biol Chem* 260:11366, 1985.

349. Cranton EM, Frackelton JP: Free radical pathology in age-associated diseases: Treatment with EDTA chelation, nutrition and antioxidants. *J Hol Med* 6:6, 1984.

350. Deucher DP: EDTA chelation: An antioxidant strategy. *J Adv Med* 1:182, 1988.

351. Walker M, Gordon G: *The Chelation Answer. How to Prevent Hardening of the Arteries and Rejuvenate Your Cardiovascular System.* New York: M Evans, 1982.

352. Mallette LE, Hollis BW, Dunn K, et al: Ten weeks of intermittent hypocalcemic stimulation does not produce functional parathyroid hyperplasia. *Am J Med Sci* 302(3):138, 1991.

353. Perry HM, Schroeder HA: Depression of cholesterol levels in human plasma following ethylenediamine tetraacetate and hydralazine. *J Chron Dis* 2:520, 1995.

354. Rudolph CJ, McDonagh EW, Barber RK: Effect of EDTA chelation on serum iron. *J Adv Med* 4:39, 1991.

355. Lamar CP: Chelation therapy of occlusive arteriosclerosis in diabetic patients. *Angiology* 15:379, 1964.

356. Lamar CP: Chelation endarterectomy for occlusive atherosclerosis. *J Am Geriatr Soc* 14:272, 1966.

357. Casdorph HR, Farr CH: EDTA chelation therapy: III. treatment of peripheral arterial occlusion, an alternative to amputation. *J Hol Med* 5:3, 1983.

358. Guldager B, Jelnes R, Jorgensen SJ, et al: EDTA treatment of intermittent claudication: A double-blind, placebo-controlled study. *J Intern Med* 231:261, 1992.

359. Sloth-Nielsen J, Guldager B, Mouitzen C, et al: Arteriographic findings in EDTA chelation therapy on peripheral arteriosclerosis. *Am J Surg* 162:122, 1991.

360. Kitchell JR, Palmon F Jr, Aytan N, Meltzer LE: The treatment of coronary artery disease with disodium EDTA: a reappraisal. *Am J Cardiol* 11:501, 1963.

361. Hancke C, Flytlie K: Benefits of chelation therapy in atherosclerosis: A retrospective study of 470 patients. *J Adv Med* 6:161, 1993.

362. Van der Schaar P: Exercise tolerance in chelation therapy. *J Adv Med* 2:563, 1989.

363. Soffer A, Toribara T, Sayman A: Myocardial responses to chelation. *Br Heart J* 23:690, 1961.

364. Soffer A: Chelation clinics. *Arch Intern Med* 144:1741, 1984.

365. Chappell LT, Stahl JP: The correlation between EDTA chelation therapy and improvement in cardiovascular function: A meta-analysis. *J Adv Med* 6:139, 1993.

366. ACC/AHA/ACP-ASIM guidelines for the management of patients with chronic stable angina. A report from the American College of Cardiology/American Heart Association Task Force on Practice Guidelines (Committee on Management of Patients with Chronic Stable Angina). *J Am Coll Cardiol* 33:2092, 1999.

367. Riordan HD, Cheraskin E, Dirks M, Schultz M, Brizendine P: Electrocardiographic changes associated with EDTA chelation therapy. *J Adv Med* 1:191, 1988.

368. Riordan HD, Cheraskin E, Dirks M, et al: EDTA chelation/hypertension study: Clinical patterns as judged by the Cornell Medical Index questionnaire. *J Ortho Med* 4:91, 1989.

368a. Knudtson ML, Wyse DG, Galbraith PD, et al: Chelation therapy for ischemic heart disease. A randomized, controlled trial. *JAMA* 287:481, 2002.

368b. Holden C: NIH trial to test chelation therapy. *Science* 297:1109, 2002.

368c. Quan H, Ghali WA, Verhoef MJ, et al: Use of chelation therapy after coronary angiography. *Am J Med* 111:686, 2001.

368d. Frishman WH: Chelation therapy for coronary artery disease: panacea or quackery (editorial)? *Am J Med* 111:729, 2001.

369. Salonen JT, Nyyssonen K, Korpela H, et al: High stored iron levels are associated with excess risk of myocardial infarction in eastern Finnish men. *Circulation* 86:803, 1992.

370. Morrison HI, Semenciw RM, Mao Y, Wigle DT: Serum iron and risk of fatal acute myocardial infarction. *Epidemiology* 5:243, 1994.

371. Tuomainen TP, Kontula K, Nyyssonen K, et al: Increased risk of acute myocardial infarction in carriers of the hemochromatosis gene Cys282Tyr mutation: A prospective cohort study in men in eastern Finland. *Circulation* 100(12):1274, 1999.

372. Maza SR, Frishman WH: Therapeutic options to minimize free radical damage and thrombogenicity in ischemic/reperfused myocardium. *Med Clin North Am* 72:227, 1988.

373. Pratico D, Pasin M, Barry OP, et al: Iron-dependent human platelet activation and hydroxyl radical formation: involvement of protein kinase C. *Circulation* 99(24):3118, 1999.

374. Solymoss BC, Marcil M, Gilfix BM, et al: The place of ferritin among risk factors associated with coronary artery disease. *Coron Artery Dis* 5(3):231, 1994.

375. Magnusson MK, Sigfusson N, Sigvaldason H, et al: Low iron-binding capacity as a risk factor for myocardial infarction. *Circulation* 89(1):102, 1994.

376. Voest EE, Vreugdenhil G, Marx JJM: Iron-chelating agents in non-iron overload conditions. *Ann Intern Med* 120:490, 1994.

377. Porreca E, Ucchino S, Di Febbo C, et al: Antiproliferative effect of desferrioxamine on vascular smooth muscle cells in vitro and in vivo. *Arterioscler Thromb* 14(2):299, 1994.

378. DeBoer D, Clark R: Iron chelation in myocardial preservation after ischemia-reperfusion injury: The importance of pretreatment and toxicity. *Ann Thorac Surg* 53:412, 1992.

379. Ambrosio G, Zweier J, Jacobus W, et al: Improvement of postischemic myocardial function and metabolism induced by administration of deferoxamine at the time of reflow: The role of iron in the pathogenesis of reperfusion injury. *Circulation* 76:906, 1987.

380. Menasche P, Antebi H, Alcindor LG, et al: Iron chelation by deferoxamine inhibits lipid peroxidation during cardiopulmonary bypass in humans. *Circulation* 82(Suppl IV):IV390, 1990.

381. Reddy BR, Wynne J, Kloner RA, Przyklenk K: Pretreatment with the iron chelator deferoxamine on transferrin receptors: The cell cycle and growth rates of human leukaemic cells. *Cardiovasc Res* 25:711, 1991.

382. Rudolph CJ, McDonagh EW, Barber RK: Effect of EDTA chelation on serum iron. *J Adv Med* 4:39, 1991.

383. Anderson LJ, Wonke B, Prescott E, et al: Comparison of effects of oral deferiprone and subcutaneous desferrioxamine on myocardial iron concentrations and ventricular function in beta-thalassaemia. *Lancet* 360:516, 2002.

384. Hall RI, Smith MS, Rocker G: The systemic inflammatory response to CPB. *Anesth Analg* 85:766, 1997.

385. Califf RM, Abdelmeguid AE, Kuntz RE, et al: Myonecrosis after revascularization procedures. *J Am Coll Cardiol* 31:241, 1998.

386. Salama A, Hugo F, Heinrich D: Disposition of terminal C5b-9 complement complexes on erythrocytes and leukocytes during cardiopulmonary bypass. *N Engl J Med* 318:408, 1988.

387. Rinder CS, Rinder HM, Smith Br, et al: Blockade of C5a and C5b-9 generation inhibits leukocyte and platelet activation during extracorporeal circulation. *J Clin Invest* 96:1564, 1995.

388. Vakeva AP, Agah A, Rollins SA, et al: Myocardial infarction and apoptosis after myocardial ischemia and reperfusion. *Circulation* 97:2259, 1998.

389. Thomas TC, Rollins SA, Rother RP et al: Inhibition of complement activity by humanized anti-C5 antibody and single-chain Fv. *Mol Immunol* 33:1389, 1996.

390. Fitch JCK, Rollins S, Matis L, et al: Pharmacology and biological efficacy of a recombinant, humanized, single-chain antibody C5 complement inhibitor in patients undergoing coronary artery bypass graft surgery with cardiopulmonary bypass. *Circulation* 100:2499, 1999.

391. Weisman HF, Bartow T, Leppo MK, et al: Soluble human complement receptor type I. in vivo inhibitor of complement suppressing postischemic myocardial inflammation and necrosis. *Science* 249:146, 1990.

392. Lazar HL, Bao Y, Gaudiani J, et al: Total complement inhibition. An effective strategy to limit ischemic injury during coronary revascularization on cardiopulmonary bypass. *Circulation* 100:1438, 1999.

393. Schmid RA, Zollinger A, Singer T, et al: Effect of soluble complement receptor type I on reperfusion edema and neutrophil migration after lung allotransplantation in swine. *J Thorac Cardiovasc Surg* 116:90, 1998.

393a. Horstick G, Berg O, Heimann A, et al: Application of C1-esterase inhibitor during reperfusion of ischemic myocardium. Dose-related beneficial versus detrimental effects. *Circulation* 104:3125, 2001.

394. Inagaki K, Kihara Y, Hayashida W, et al: Anti-ischemic effect of a novel cardioprotective agent, JTV 519, is mediated through specific activation of δ- isoform of protein kinase C in rat ventricular myocardium. *Circulation* 101:797, 2000.

395. Blau, HM et al: The evolving concept of a stem cell: Entity or function. *Cell* 105(7):829, 2001.

396. Ferrari G, Cusella-De Angelis G, Coletta M, et al: Muscle regeneration by bone marrow-derived myogenic progenitors. *Science* 279(5356):1528, 1998.

397. Gussoni E, Soneoka Y, Strickland CD, et al: Dystrophin expression in the mdx mouse restored by stem cell transplantation. *Nature* 401(6751):390, 1999.

398. Orlic D, Kajstura J, Chimenti S, et al: Bone marrow cells regenerate infarcted myocardium. *Nature* 410(6829):701, 2001.

399. Jackson KA, Majka SM, Wang H, et al: Regeneration of ischemic cardiac muscle and vascular endothelium by adult stem cells. *J Clin Invest* 107(11):1395, 2001.

400. Hakuno D, Fukuda K, Makino S, et al: Bone marrow-derived regenerated cardiomyocytes (CMG Cells) express functional adrenergic and muscarinic receptors. *Circulation* 105:380, 2002.

401. Brazelton TR, Rossi FM, Keshet GI, Blau HM: From marrow to brain: expression of neuronal phenotypes in adult mice. *Science* 290(5497):1775, 2000.

402. Mezey E, Chandross KJ, Harta G, et al: Turning blood into brain: Cells bearing neuronal antigens generated in vivo from bone marrow. *Science* 290(5497):1779, 2001.

403. Lagasse E, Connors H, Al-Dhalimy M, et al: Purified hematopoietic stem cells can differentiate into hepatocytes in vivo. *Nat Med* 6(11):1229, 2000.

404. Theise ND, Badve S, Saxena R, et al: Derivation of hepatocytes from bone marrow cells in mice after radiation-induced myeloablation. *Hepatology* 31(1):235, 2000.

405. Krause DS, Theise ND, Collector MI, et al: Multi-organ, multilineage engraftment by a single bone marrow-derived stem cell. *Cell* 105(3):369, 2001.

406. Kocher AA, Schuster MD, Szabolcs MJ, et al: Itescu neovascularization of ischemic myocardium by human bone-marrow-derived angioblasts prevents cardiomyocyte apoptosis, reduces remodeling and improves cardiac function. *Nat Med* 7(4):430, 2001.

407. Anderson DJ, Gage FH, Weissman IL: Can stem cells cross lineage boundaries? *Nat Med* 7(4):393, 2001.

408. Weissman IL: Translating stem and progenitor cell biology to the clinic: Barriers and opportunities. *Science* 287(5457):1442, 2000.

409. Orlic D, Kajstura J, Chimenti S, et al: Mobilized bone marrow cells repair the infarcted heart, improving function and survival. *Proc Natl Acad Sci U S A* 98(18):10344, 2001.

410. Bodine DM, Seidel NE, Gale MS, et al: Efficient retrovirus transduction of mouse pluripotent hematopoietic stem cells mobilized into the peripheral blood by treatment with granulocyte colony-stimulating factor and stem cell factor. *Blood* 84(5):1482, 1994.

411. Kronenwett R, Martin S, Haas R: The role of cytokines and adhesion molecules for mobilization of peripheral blood stem cells. *Stem Cells* 18(5):320, 2000.

412. Begley CG, Basser R, Mansfield R, et al: Enhanced levels and enhanced clonogenic capacity of blood progenitor cells following administration of stem cell factor plus granulocyte colony-stimulating factor to humans. *Blood* 90(9):3378, 1997.

413. Gutierrez-Delgado F, Bensinger W: Safety of granulocyte colony-stimulating factor in normal donors. *Curr Opin Hematol* 8(3):155, 2001.

414. Demetri GD, Griffin JD: Granulocyte colony-stimulating factor and its receptor. *Blood* 78(11):2791, 1991.

415. Smith MA, Court EL, Smith JG: Stem cell factor: Laboratory and clinical aspects. *Blood Rev* 15(4):191, 2001.

416. Andrews RG, Briddell RA, Knitter GH, et al: In vivo synergy between recombinant human stem cell factor and recombinant human granulocyte colony-stimulating factor in baboons enhanced circulation of progenitor cells. *Blood* 84(3):800, 1994.

417. Horsfall MJ, Hui CH, To LB, et al: Combination of stem cell factor and granulocyte colony-stimulating factor mobilizes the highest number of primitive haemopoietic progenitors as shown by pre-colony-forming unit (pre-CFU) assay. *Br J Haematol* 109(4):751, 2000.

417a. Toma C, Pittenger MF, Cahill KS, et al: Human mesenchymal stem cells differentiate to a cardiomyocyte phenotype in the adult murine heart. *Circulation* 105:93, 2002.

418. Rosenthal N: High hopes for the heart. *N Engl J Med* 344(23):1785, 2001.

419. Anversa P, Nadal-Ginard B: Myocyte renewal and ventricular remodelling. *Nature* 415(6868):240, 2002.

420. Kajstura J, Leri A, Finato N, et al: Myocyte proliferation in end-stage cardiac failure in humans. *Proc Natl Acad Sci U S A* 95(15):8801, 1998.

421. Beltrami AP, Urbanek K, Kajstura J, et al: Evidence that human cardiac myocytes divide after myocardial infarction. *N Engl J Med* 344(23):1750, 2001.

422. Quaini F, Urbanek K, Beltrami AP, et al: Chimerism of the transplanted heart. *N Engl J Med* 346(1):5, 2002.

423. Frishman WH, Anversa P: Stem cell therapy for myocardial regeneration: The future is now. *Heart Disease* 4:205, 2002.

424. Penn MS, Francis GS, Ellis SG, et al: Autologous cell transplantation for the treatment of damaged myocardium. *Prog Cardiovasc Dis* 45:21, 2002.

CHAPTER 38

Therapeutic Angiogenesis: A New Treatment Modality for Ischemic Heart Disease

William H. Frishman

Amanda Ganem

Michael A. Nelson

Jonathan Passeri

Coronary artery disease is the leading cause of death in industrialized nations. Atherosclerotic plaque build up, both with and without accompanying thrombosis, often causes occlusion and is the leading cause of ischemia, which is, in turn, the most common cause of myocardial hypoxia.[1] Angiogenesis, the formation of new blood vessels by sprouting from preexisting vessels, offers the potential to increase collateral blood flow to tissue at risk of hypoxic injury because of limited perfusion. While therapeutic attempts in humans are still in their infancy, angiogenesis has shown promising results in animal models of ischemia. In addition, while much remains uncertain, there has recently been a vast improvement in our understanding of the mechanisms underlying angiogenesis and the various factors that determine whether, and under what conditions, it will best occur.

In recognition of the limits of modern therapy, both pharmacologic and invasive, a considerable amount of research has been focused on using angiogenesis in conjunction with or in place of current therapeutic measures to treat ischemic events. The angiogenic process offers the potential for improved blood flow to nearly all ischemic areas. However, in light of the overwhelming prevalence and incidence of myocardial events in our society, the clinical aspects of this review focus on the angiogenic process as it applies to the heart.

REGULATION OF ANGIOGENESIS

Angiogenesis is a highly controlled process, and the rate at which it occurs is dependent on the intricate balance of factors that, on the one hand, promote angiogenesis, and on the other, inhibit it. In human adults and in most animals, angiogenesis is usually quiescent. However, while angiogenesis occurs at very low or even undetectable levels in the normal human adult, it can be markedly increased under certain physiologic and pathologic conditions. The clearest physiologic example of increased angiogenesis is the female menstrual cycle. In this process, the development of new blood vessels is critical to the maintenance and survival of new tissue. The pathologic settings in which angiogenesis is markedly increased include solid tumor growth, metastatic tumor spread, wound healing, inflammation, and ischemic hypoxia.[2]

Ischemia, both acute and chronic, has been clearly shown to stimulate angiogenesis in many experimental models. The decrease in blood flow to tissue, which defines ischemia, results in a diminished supply of necessary substrates, such as oxygen and glucose, and an excess accumulation of metabolic waste products. Hypoxia and hypoglycemia have both been shown to lead to increased expression of several angiogenic growth factors including transforming growth factor (TGFβ)-1, platelet-derived growth factor (PDGF), fibroblast growth factor (FGF)-1 and -2, placental growth factor (PlGF), and vascular endothelial growth factor (VEGF) and its receptors KDR/flk-1 and flt-1.[3–6] These alterations in gene expression appear to be mediated by activation of the transcription factor hypoxia-inducible factor (HIF)-1. One very recent study demonstrated increased levels of HIF-1 mRNA preceding increased levels of VEGF mRNA in the human heart during acute ischemia.[7]

Angiogenic growth factors are also upregulated after acute myocardial infarction. One study of rats by Li et al demonstrated that VEGF expression is increased in remaining viable myocardial tissue following myocardial infarct.[8] Postinfarct myocardial stretching, a means to compensate for the lost myocardium, was proposed as the mechanism by which VEGF expression was elevated. This stretch-induced increase in VEGF expression was found to be mediated, at least in part, by TGF-β. Furthermore, in a rat model of chronic bradycardia, using alinidine, Zheng et al showed that the angiogenic response of the myocardium is dependent on VEGF not bFGF. This stretch model demonstrates that mechanical factors selectively stimulate VEGF, suggesting that bFGF expression occurs only in a hypoxic model.[9] A more recent model of myocardial stretch used carvedilol in a series of 16 patients with congestive heart failure (CHF), and also found an increase in plasma VEGF. This suggests that the clinical benefits of such medications in CHF may be due to increased VEGF production with bradycardia and subsequent collateral formation.[10] Thus, mechanical mechanisms and hypoxia serve as vital stimuli for the production of VEGF. With respect to hypoxia-induced VEGF production, one study reported that myocardial oxygen deprivation induces VEGF mRNA upregulation[11] and another found that systemic hypoxia induces increased heart VEGF expression.[12] A recent study examined VEGF levels in acute myocardial infarction (MI) and its relationship to infarct size as compared to patients with stable angina and placebo.[13] The data show a significant increase in VEGF levels in acute MI as compared with stable angina and placebo, with a bimodal pattern of elevation: VEGF was elevated immediately post MI and 1 to 2 weeks post MI. These investigators suggest that the second rise in VEGF reflects collateral formation with higher levels associated with larger infarct areas and a need for more collateral formation.[13] Kranz et al also determined VEGF levels, specifically VEGF-A, in patients with acute MI and unstable angina pectoris.[14] They discovered that VEGF was also elevated in the setting of acute MI, but not in unstable angina pectoris. Additionally, they noted that the level of circulating VEGF-A is related to the number of platelets. Thus, the source of VEGF-A in acute myocardial ischemia may not be myocardial in origin, despite its role as an endogenous activator of coronary collateral formation.[14]

VEGF expression has also been shown to be increased both in vitro and in vivo by the presence of reactive oxygen intermediates, which are often found in the myocardium secondary to postischemic attempts at reperfusion.[15,16] One study involving pig hearts exposed to a cardioplegic solution followed by reperfusion found an increase in myocardial VEGF mRNA expression.[17] Furthermore, a study of isolated rat hearts has demonstrated that the addition of VEGF attenuates myocardial ischemia-reperfusion injury.[18] These various studies reveal an elevated level of myocardial VEGF expression under conditions of ischemia and hypoxia as a manifestation of the body's attempt to restore blood and oxygen flow. Additionally, the cardioprotective effects of ischemic preconditioning appear to be related to the enhanced expression of VEGF. More specifically, a recent study showed that expression of VEGF mRNA in infarcted cardiomyocytes is enhanced by protein kinase C (PKC)-e nuclear translocation.[19]

Exercise may also contribute to the stimulation of angiogenesis. One interesting clinical study demonstrated that in the period immediately following a single bout of dynamic exercise, skeletal muscle expression of VEGF mRNA increased by an average of 178%, while FGF-2 levels were unchanged as determined by muscle biopsy.[20] These results, in conjunction with those of a study which reported that exercise training in swine promotes capillary angiogenesis in the heart,[21] may warrant future clinical trials analyzing the potential of exercise to induce myocardial angiogenesis.

Whereas enhancement of angiogenesis might prevent ischemia, inhibition of angiogenesis may arrest tumor growth and metastasis. Without access to an effective blood supply, it is thought that tumors cannot receive the nutrients they need to maintain growth. Likewise, if a tumor does not have access to the blood stream, then metastatic growth cannot occur via the hematogenous route. This would transform previously prolific tumors into much weaker local growths. This inhibition of angiogenesis would appear most effective against sarcomas which typically spread through the blood stream, and less effective against carcinomas which have a tendency to spread through the lymphatic system.[2]

MECHANISMS OF ANGIOGENESIS

The process of angiogenesis involves a number of steps each of which involves the interplay of intricate factors that are just now coming to light. Endothelial cells line all blood vessels and, as such, play a central role in angiogenesis. As illustrated in Fig. 38-1, angiogenesis involves each of the following steps: endothelial cells degrade their basement membrane; the cells detach from their neigh-

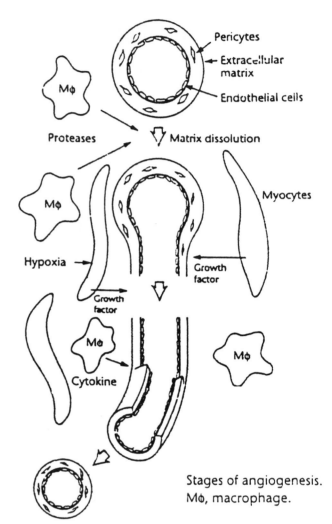

FIGURE 38-1. Stages of angiogenesis. (*Reproduced with permission from Ware JA et al.*[159])

boring cells and the underlying matrix and invade the extravascular space; these cells then migrate and proliferate toward a stimulus, further invading and dissolving the extravascular matrix; and then the endothelial cells restructure themselves, forming a lumen, and secreting new basement membrane.

Remodeling and degradation of the extracellular matrix are important early aspects of angiogenesis because they allow capillary formation to occur. Microvascular endothelial cells synthesize matrix metalloproteinases (MMPs), which enzymatically digest the individual parts of the body matrix in a selective fashion. The presence of MMPs is necessary to enable the migration of endothelial cells through the matrix to the site of new vessel formation during angiogenesis. At the same time, endothelial cells also produce tissue inhibitors of metalloproteinases (TIMPs), which combat the effects of MMPs. The intricate balance between these antagonistic products thus determines whether the scale tips in favor of or against angiogenesis. If MMPs are produced in excess of TIMPs, then matrix degradation will be favored, promoting angiogenesis; if TIMPs are produced in excess of MMPs, then angiogenesis is inhibited.[22] However, numerous factors can enhance, attenuate or even reverse the trends one would predict from considering this simple equation in isolation from other events simultaneously occurring. For instance, mechanical flow, hyperlipidemia, and inflammatory cells can each alter the angiogenic response.[23] Hyperlipidemia presents an interesting challenge to investigators because in vivo studies have shown differing results. One study showed that hyperlipidemia may augment the angiogenic response to VEGF by increasing capillary tube formation.[24] Another study demonstrated that hypercholesterolemia and oxidized low-density lipoprotein (LDL) increased the number of progenitor endothelial cells, but functionally they were unable to fully participate in the angiogenic process.[25] Interestingly, oral folic acid supplementation in the hypercholesterolemic state helps to restore impaired angiogenesis in the ischemic state by increasing the bioactivity of nitric oxide.[26] Similarly, hyperhomocystinemia impairs collateral vessel formation and ischemia-induced angiogenesis by decreasing the bioavailability of nitric oxide.[27] Although one might imagine that the logical course clinically would be to treat with standard hydroxymethylglutaryl coenzyme A (HMG-CoA) reductase inhibitors to reduce the cholesterol burden, one study showed that these inhibitors interfere with VEGF signaling by blocking integrin cross-talk.[28] Another study by Celletti et al examined the effects of rhVEGF 165 on atherosclerotic plaque in rabbits. The data show that rhVEGF can induce plaque neovascularization, and thus, plaque progression, making the plaque exquisitely vulnerable to intraplaque hemorrhage and rupture, leading to unstable angina pectoris.[29] The therapeutic implications of these findings have yet to be determined.

Role of Endothelial Cells

Endothelial cells are the central players in angiogenesis. Embryologically, endothelial cells arise during the third week of development from a specific group of mesenchymal cells known as angioblasts.[30] These angioblasts aggregate to form angiogenic cell clusters at the periphery of what have been termed isolated blood islands with hematopoietic stem cells at the island centers.[31] The angioblasts flatten, at which point they are termed endothelial cells, which form the primitive endothelium.

Similarly, the primitive cardiovascular system, including the heart and great vessels, forms from mesenchymal cells. Endothelial heart tubes develop and begin to fuse into a single primitive heart tube before the end of the third week. The tubular heart begins to beat and has blood circulating through it by day 22 of development. Considering the vital role it plays throughout life, it seems appropriate that the cardiovascular system is the first organ system to reach a functional state in the developing fetus.[30]

In adults, endothelial cells are normally quiescent and nonproliferative under physiologic conditions. However, there are a number of circumstances in which the cells convert to a proliferative state. In fact, normal endothelial cells have three critical functions requiring their proliferation which, if compromised, would lead to pathologic conditions. First, the cells must be able to regenerate following a denuding injury thereby assuring that the endothelial monolayer remains intact at all times. Second, if appropriately signaled, the endothelium must be able to create a new branch while maintaining the monolayer. Finally, during angiogenesis, the endothelial cells must maintain both lumen patency and the intact monolayer, while simultaneously forming a new pathway for the flow of blood.[32] Recently, Wang et al demonstrated that endothelial cell migration, adhesion, and eventual vessel formation is dependent on PKC-α, making this isoenzyme pivotal in angiogenesis.[33]

Considering the central role that endothelial cells play, an analysis of the factors that control their activation is necessary in order to understand the mechanisms underlying angiogenesis. While not

mutually exclusive, there are two major theories as to how endothelial cells are converted from their normal, quiescent state to their proliferative state. One theory suggests that cell-cell and cell-matrix interactions are critical determinants of this transition state, while the second theory proposes that soluble growth factors ultimately control this process.[32]

Role of Cell-Cell and Cell-Matrix Interactions

That cell-cell and cell-matrix interactions determine the state of endothelial activity seems appropriate considering that one of the critical functions of endothelial cells is to maintain the integrity of the monolayer. Under normal conditions contact inhibition of the intact monolayer prevents endothelial cell proliferation and the basement membrane forms a physical barrier separating the endothelium from the extravascular space. When the normal cell-cell interaction is removed, for example by denuding injury or non-denuding desquamation, there is a sudden potential for endothelial cell replication. After the monolayer is again intact, the baseline quiescent state is restored.[32] A recent study using cardiac fibroblasts confirmed the contact-dependent inhibition of angiogenesis.[34]

Certain classes of molecules act to strengthen and stabilize intercellular contact, thereby maintaining the endogenous inhibition that prevents angiogenesis. Cell adhesion molecules (CAMs) promote the binding of one cell to another, while substrate adhesion molecules (SAMs) are the membrane components responsible for adherence of cells to the extracellular matrix. Perhaps the most well characterized SAMs are transmembrane glycoproteins, called integrins, which contain extracellular domains that bind to matrix components and intracellular domains that interact with cytoskeleton components and signal cell attachment, locomotion, or differentiation. Still other molecules located in the cellular cytoplasm, called cytoplasmic junctional molecules (CJMs), act to link the CAMs and the SAMs with the cytoskeleton. These molecules contribute to stabilization of the cell junction and inhibit angiogenesis in quiescent endothelium, while in proliferating endothelium the junctional complexes are lost. Quiescent endothelial cells also contain a peripheral "dense band" of actin filaments associated with adherens complexes. This peripheral dense band is absent in regenerating endothelial cells but returns when the cells revert to the quiescent state. Vascular cadherin (V-CAD) was the first CAM to be identified in endothelial cells and is responsible for calcium-dependent adherence of endothelial cells. Angiogenic growth factors have been shown to inhibit V-CAD activity, cause loss of the peripheral dense band, and prevent, at least in vitro, the establishment of quiescence in endothelial cells.[32]

Components of the extracellular matrix itself may also play an important role in determining the state of endothelial cells. Fibronectin is a multifunctional glycoprotein that binds to a number of other extracellular matrix components and to cells via integrin receptors. Fibronectin contributes to the attachment, spreading, and migration of endothelial cells and its expression correlates directly with angiogenesis. Additionally, fibronectin enhances endothelial cell sensitivity to growth factors.[35] However, laminin and type IV collagen are expressed in the basement membranes of mature vessels and contribute to stability of the quiescent endothelium.[32]

While regenerating the monolayer might seem to require endothelial replication, this is not necessarily the case as there are times when regeneration occurs by cellular movement without accompanying cell replication. Thus, angiogenic factors, which promote maintenance of the endothelial structure need not be mitogenic in nature. It follows that any endothelial mitogenesis that might occur would be a secondary consequence of the primary goal of maintaining an intact monolayer.[32]

Role of Angiogenic Growth Factors

There has been a vast amount of research concerning growth factors and their role in angiogenesis. Analyzing growth factors in the process of angiogenesis is a formidable task considering the number that exist and their overlapping functions. To further complicate matters, it is often difficult to ascertain which cell releases a particular growth factor, as various inflammatory cells and resident cells are located in the area of interest.

Growth factors enhance angiogenesis via several mechanisms. Induction of angiogenesis by growth factors results in an inflammatory-like reaction, including vasodilation, increased permeability, and accumulation of monocytes and macrophages. These cells, along with endothelial cells, when stimulated by growth factors, release proteolytic enzymes that disrupt cell-cell junctional complexes, degrade the extracellular matrix and basement membrane allowing for migration of endothelial cells. Moreover, angiogenic growth factors are endothelial cell mitogens that trigger the proliferation of endothelial cells, a necessary early step in the extension of new blood vessels.

It was believed that the various growth factors and cytokines promoting angiogenesis were released in a paracrine fashion by infiltrating inflammatory cells such as macrophages.[36] However, more recent evidence strongly suggests that endothelial cells themselves play a critical role in promoting the angiogenic process via an autocrine mechanism of action.[36] The autocrine nature of angiogenic stimulation makes one ponder how endothelial cells can ever be in a state of quiescence when they are bathed in a sea of angiogenic factors of their own making. One explanation suggests that the presence of growth factors is critical for the maintenance of the microvasculature as it is found in the physiologic state. Thus, what has been termed "quiescence" is actually baseline activity that is generated by the presence of growth factors. It follows that, in the absence of growth factors, normal microvasculature would simply fail to exist. Some studies of vascular endothelial growth factor (VEGF) have lent support to this theory. A more widely accepted theory states that some form of endogenous inhibition is normally present, which effectively prevents angiogenesis from occurring. Although the precise nature of this inhibition has yet to be determined several endogenous inhibitors have been identified. These inhibitors, which circulate in the blood and may also exist in the matrix surrounding endothelial cells, include thrombospondin-1 and -2, platelet factor-4, interferon-α, and the previously mentioned tissue inhibitors of metalloproteinase. As discussed above, mechanical factors also inhibit angiogenesis and this inhibition can be overcome by disrupting cell-cell contact.

Experimental evidence suggests that endothelial growth is controlled by a two-step mechanism. The administration of an exogenous growth factor (i.e., exogenous FGF-2) apparently disrupts cell-cell interactions or may overcome the activity of circulating inhibitors, thereby removing the endogenous inhibition and allowing endothelial cells to become more responsive to the mitogenic effects of endogenous growth factors (i.e., endogenous FGF-2).[31] The seemingly dual role of FGF-2 as an exogenous and endogenous growth factor becomes clear once a distinction is made between a growth-requiring and a growth-enhancing substance. This difference is best appreciated by removing both substances and observing the effect on growth. When a growth-requiring substance is removed, no further growth is possible, whereas in the absence of a

growth-stimulating agent, growth can still occur but at a diminished rate compared to levels attained with the stimulant present.[32] Additionally, even an infinite amount of a growth-stimulating substance cannot cause growth in the absence of a growth-requiring substance.

It appears that endogenous FGF-2 is a growth-requiring substance, whereas exogenous FGF-2 is growth-stimulating.[32] Thus, under normal adult physiologic conditions, the endogenous inhibitors effectively block the action of endogenous FGF-2 and prevent angiogenesis. Even an infinite amount of exogenous FGF-2 will not stimulate angiogenesis due to the inhibition of endogenous FGF-2 under these conditions. However, if endogenous inhibition is somehow removed then endogenous FGF-2 is effective. Angiogenesis will now occur even in the absence of exogenous FGF-2, but will occur at an enhanced rate in its presence.

In addition to the great interest in the mechanisms by which specific growth factors enhance angiogenesis, there have also been exhaustive efforts to discover the numerous individual growth factors that play a role in the angiogenic process. These efforts have culminated in a continuously growing labyrinth of interacting factors. Table 38-1 presents most of the currently known angiogenic inhibitors and promoters. The numerous angiogenesis-promoting

TABLE 38-1. Factors Regulating Angiogenesis

Angiogenic Inhibitors
Angiopoietin-2 (Ang 2)
Angiostatin
Angiotensin II via AT_2 receptor
Antineoplastic agents
Interferon-alpha (IFNα)
Interferon-beta (IFNβ)
Interferon-inducible protein 10 (IP-10)
Interleukin-12 (IL-12)
Platelet factor-4
Thrombospondin-1 (TSP-1)
Thrombospondin-2 (TSP-2)
Tissue inhibitor of metalloproteinases (TIMP)
TNP-470

Angiogenic Promoters
Acidic fibroblast growth factor
Angiopoietin-1 (Ang 1)
Angiotensin II via AT_1 receptor
Basic fibroblast growth factor
CD44
Diiodothyroproprionic acid (DITPA)
Endothelin
Fibrin
Granulocyte-macrophage colony-stimulating factor (GM-CSF)
Hepatocyte growth factor (HGF) or scatter factor
Human heme oxygenase (HO-1)
Interleukin-1 beta (IL-1-B)
Interleukin-8 (IL-8)
Matrix metalloproteinase (MMP)
Nitric oxide (NO)
Platelet-derived growth factor (PDGF)
Thyroxine
Transforming growth factor-alpha (TGFα)
Transforming growth factor-beta (TGFβ)
Tryptase
Tumor necrosis factor-alpha (TNFα)
Vascular endothelial growth factor (VEGF) or vascular permeability factor
Insulin-like growth factor I (IGF-I)

Source: Reproduced with permission from Nelson MA, Passeri J, Frishman WH. Therapeutic angiogenesis: a new treatment modality for ischemic heart disease. *Heart Dis* 2:314, 2000.

factors produced by the endothelial cells themselves include FGF, VEGF, TGFα, TGFβ, TNFα, and IGF-1. FGF and VEGF act by directly stimulating endothelial cell migration and proliferation, while TGFβ and TNFα act by stimulating endothelial cell differentiation. Additionally, TGFβ, TNFα, and angiogenin each stimulate angiogenesis indirectly by activating secondary cells to produce their own angiogenic factors.[23]

Vascular Endothelial Growth Factor

VEGF, also called vascular permeability factor (VPF), is a potent selective endothelial cell mitogen and monocyte/macrophage chemotactic factor. Five isoforms of human VEGF have been identified: VEGF-121, VEGF-145, VEGF-165, VEGF-189, and VEGF-206.[37–39] The VEGF gene, located on chromosome 6p21.3, spans approximately 14 kilobases (kb) and contains 8 exons separated by 7 introns.[40] The different isoforms are the result of alternative splicing of VEGF mRNA.[38] Related but distinct peptides include PlGF-1 and -2, VEGF-B, VEGF-C/VEGF-related peptide (VRP), and VEGF-D.

The ability to bind heparin and the extracellular matrix distinguish the different isoforms of VEGF.[41] VEGF-121 lacks both exons 6 and 7, is the only weakly acidic isoform, and does not bind heparin or extracellular matrix. VEGF-165, the major isoform, is a basic glycoprotein and unlike VEGF-121, it contains a 44-amino-acid peptide encoded by exon 7, which confers on it the ability to bind heparin. VEGF-145 alternatively contains a 21-amino-acid peptide encoded by exon 6. This peptide consists of a second independent heparin-binding domain, as well as elements that enable VEGF-145 to bind to the extracellular matrix. VEGF-189 and VEGF-206 contain peptides encoded by both exons 6 and 7 and bind heparin with greater affinity than VEGF-165. These isoforms are largely sequestered by heparin-sulfate proteoglycans on cell surfaces and/or the extracellular matrix leading to decreased bioavailability and probably accounts for the fact that VEGF-189 has been shown to be less active in vivo than either VEGF-121 or VEGF-165.[42] Proteases such as plasmin can cleave the larger isoforms and produce a bioactive 110-amino-acid fragment (VEGF-110).[43,44] However, loss of heparin binding, whether it is due to alternative splicing or to proteolytic cleavage, results in a substantial loss of mitogenic activity. VEGF-110 and VEGF-121 are fiftyfold less active than VEGF-165.[45]

VEGF functions through interaction with two high-affinity protein kinase receptors, the *fms*-like tyrosine kinase (flt-1) and the kinase domain region (KDR), which is the human homologue of the murine fetal-liver kinase (flk-1) receptor.[46–49] These receptors comprise a subfamily of protein tyrosine kinases that are distinguished by the presence of seven immunoglobulin-like loops extracellularly and a split tyrosine kinase intracellularly.[50,51] Both receptors are necessary for proper development of embryonic vasculature. Previously the KDR/flk-1 receptor and not the flt-1 receptor was thought to mediate the mitogenic and chemotactic effects of VEGF, suggesting that these receptors have different signal transduction properties.[52] However, recent in vivo data obtained by Marchand et al in mice now demonstrate the integral roles of both Flk-1 and Flt-1 receptors in VEGF-mediated angiogenesis.[53]

Reports indicate that VEGF binding to the KDR/flk-1 receptor activates MAP kinase, which stimulates the phospholipase C-γ (PLC-γ) pathway leading to the generation of inositol 1,4,5-trisphosphate, mobilization of Ca^{2+} from intracellular stores, and activation of protein kinase C. In contrast, MAP kinase is not activated by binding to the flt-1 receptor. It is possible, therefore, that MAP kinase activation is responsible for the mitogen-signaling pathway.[54,55] There is evidence to suggest that the chemotactic response to VEGF binding of KDR may occur through stimulation of

the focal adhesion kinase (FAK) phosphorylation pathway, affecting actin cytoskeleton reorganization and cell migration.[56] A recent study examined VEGF and KDR levels in canine peripheral muscle versus myocardial ischemia and revealed a marked difference in the skeletal and myocardial response to acute ischemia. In the peripheral muscle bed, VEGF and KDR initially increased and subsequently decreased in response to ischemia, whereas in the myocardial bed, KDR consistently decreased while VEGF remained elevated. This suggests that each vascular tissue has a unique cellular response to ischemia, and, thus, clinical application of VEGF might differ considerably between the two locations of ischemia.[57]

VEGF also plays a role in maintaining normal vascular function and has been reported to act as a survival factor. There is evidence implying that VEGF mediates its activity as a survival factor through the phosphatidylinositol 3′(PI3)-kinase/serine-threonine kinase Akt signaling pathway.[58,59] It has also been shown that this pathway is needed for angiopoietin-1-induced in vitro angiogenesis, which ultimately results in the activation of e-nitric oxide synthase (eNOS).[60] In a recent study, Akt expression, as well as Bcl-2 expression, were markedly increased in a mouse model of chronic alcohol consumption. Because these factors are putative inhibitors of apoptosis, these results suggest that cardiac preconditioning with ethanol may be related to these as well as other pathways.[61] Likewise, Gu et al also showed that the cardioprotective effect of moderate ethanol consumption is partly mediated through the induction of VEGF production and subsequent angiogenesis.[62] VEGF augments nitric oxide (NO) production from normal quiescent adult vascular endothelium, probably through mobilization of Ca^{2+} stores,[62a] suggesting that VEGF has a role in maintaining normal density of the microvasculature independently of its effects on endothelial cell proliferation. Recent findings, however, suggest that the nitric oxide pathway may also be a mediator of the angiogenic inducing capability of VEGF, but not FGF-2.[63,64] In fact, one study of myocardial ischemia demonstrated that VEGF induction of coronary collateral formation is contingent on the production of nitric oxide, suggesting that nitric oxide is a part of the signal pathway that regulates VEGF expression.[65]

In addition to its mitogenic effect on endothelial cells, VEGF has several other proangiogenic effects. As mentioned earlier, VEGF is chemotactic for monocytes and macrophages. Recently, Heil et al suggested that VEGF promotes monocyte interaction with the endothelium because monocytes express the VEGF receptor Flt-1.[66] Additionally, the data show that this monocyte recruitment and subsequent collateral development are secondary to the upregulation of MAC-1 and LFA-1, two B2 integrins on monocytes.[66] These inflammatory cells release cytokines and other growth factors that promote angiogenesis. VEGF upregulates the expression of urokinase-type plasminogen activator and matrix metalloproteinases in endothelial cells. As discussed previously, these enzymes dissolve extracellular matrix, an important step in the process of angiogenesis. VEGF also increases vascular permeability, hence its alternate name VPF. In fact, on a molar basis, VEGF is 50,000 times more potent than histamine in increasing vessel permeability.[67] VEGF may account for baseline permeability of the microvasculature through induction of nitric oxide release. Evidence supporting this role of VEGF in physiologic states comes from studies of renal glomeruli, which possess exceptionally permeable vascular beds and have correspondingly elevated VEGF expression.[67] It has also been proposed that increased microvascular permeability is crucial for angiogenesis.[68] Increased permeability allows the leakage of plasma proteins leading to an extravascular fibrin-rich substrate that, in turn, promotes proliferation of macrophages, fibroblasts, and endothelial cells, that, in turn, enhances angiogenesis.

VEGF produces transient tachycardia, hypotension, and decreased cardiac output when injected intravenously into rats.[69] These effects appear to be due largely to NO-mediated vasodilation. This hemodynamic response to VEGF may complicate its use clinically. However, Sato et al examined the intracoronary administration of VEGF 165 in a porcine model of chronic myocardial ischemia and found that the hypotensive effect was blunted by the concomitant use of NG-nitro-L-arginine methyl ester (L-NAME).[70] Additionally, the study showed that the intracoronary group, unlike the intravenous group, demonstrated via coronary angiography a significant increase in blood flow to ischemic myocardium and an improvement in the collateral index 3 weeks after infusion.[70]

Fibroblast Growth Factor

The FGF family is known to contain at least nine subtypes. Of particular importance are FGF-1 (acidic FGF) and FGF-2 (basic FGF). FGF-1 and FGF-2 have a number of similarities. Both FGF-1 and FGF-2 are single-chain polypeptides containing three exons separated by two introns. Exocytosis is one of a number of proposed mechanisms by which they are released from cells. FGF-1 and FGF-2 both bind heparin and have been shown in numerous cell cultures to be potent stimulators of DNA synthesis and cellular division. Finally, FGF-1 and FGF-2 are chemotactic for endothelial cells, thus influencing their migration into areas of compromised endothelium.

As we have seen, endothelial cell migration is a key component in angiogenesis, which is dependent on remodeling of the extracellular matrix and on the expression of cell-surface receptors. Cell-culture studies have shown that FGF-2 induces expression of integrins which function in the adherence of endothelial cells to the extracellular matrix thereby increasing migration of endothelial cells and enhancing angiogenesis.[71]

The FGF family has both high-affinity and low-affinity FGF receptors. At least four distinct high-affinity receptors exist, all of which encode membrane-bound glycoproteins with tyrosine kinase activity and contain three immunoglobulin-like domains within the extracellular region. These various isoforms have the unusual property of arising from the same gene by the processes of internal polyadenylation, which results in truncated products, and alternative mRNA splicing.[71] The low-affinity receptor has been identified as a syndecan. Syndecans are a family of transmembrane proteoglycans that possess membrane-spanning core proteins. The intracellular domain of the syndecans interact with actin while the extracellular domain binds FGF and serves as a coreceptor[72] necessary for FGF to bind to the high-affinity receptor.[71]

Additionally, a recent study showed that the bFGF activated signaling pathway that results in nitric oxide production is a syndecan-4-dependent pathway via PKC-a activation.[73]

A number of comparisons between VEGF and FGF can be made. Both VEGF and FGF are heparin-binding endothelial cell mitogens that potently induce angiogenesis in a direct fashion. Unlike VEGF, however, which is highly specific for endothelial cells, FGF also stimulates smooth-muscle cells and fibroblasts. It is therefore more difficult to limit the effects of FGF to the endothelium and to predict the precise nature of adverse reactions that might occur. Nonetheless, while it is less specific, FGF-2 is a more potent promoter of endothelial cell replication than is VEGF.[67] To date, it is not clear whether FGF-2 or VEGF is the more effective growth factor and this lack of clear preference is reflected in animal studies and clinical trials, which have employed VEGF and FGF equally as often.

THERAPEUTIC APPROACHES FOR STIMULATING ANGIOGENESIS

Gene Therapy

An improved understanding of angiogenic mechanisms has led to various in vitro, preclinical, and clinical applications of angiogenesis. These studies have attempted to introduce either exogenous growth factors known to promote angiogenesis or the genes that encode them by different methods of delivery. For example, in some studies, pure growth factor-encoding DNA was injected into the area being analyzed, while other studies have delivered similar DNA through vectors such as adenoviruses. Still other researchers have introduced the growth factors themselves into the tissue of interest by either direct injection or implantation of a slow-release capsule into the target tissue.

A review of gene therapy is provided in Chap. 41.

Treatment of Ischemia

Animal Studies

A number of investigators have tested the possibility of using growth factors such as VEGF and FGF as therapeutic agents in a variety of animal models of acute and chronic ischemia. Studies using FGF-1 (acidic FGF) in these models have produced somewhat conflicting results. Unger et al showed there was no efficacy of FGF-1 in a canine ameroid-occluder model of chronic ischemia.[74] In this study, the internal mammary artery (IMA) was implanted into the area of ischemic myocardium and continuous infusion of either FGF-1 plus heparin or heparin alone was given. As compared with heparin infusion alone, FGF-1 plus heparin did not improve collateral flow from the IMA to the myocardium. Another study by Unger demonstrated that continuous infusion of FGF-1 into the left main coronary artery did not improve blood flow into ischemic myocardium produced by gradual occlusion of the left circumflex artery (LCX).[75]

Other investigators have had contrary results with FGF-1. Schlaudraff et al demonstrated angiographic evidence of aorta-to-myocardium collateral formation in rats implanted with FGF-1-coated sponges between the aorta and myocardium. No collateral formation was evident in rats implanted with uncoated sponges.[76] It is important to note that a different preparation of recombinant FGF-1 was used in this study. Using a rabbit hind limb ischemia model, other investigators found improved collateral flow in those animals treated with FGF-1 as compared with control.[77] Lopez et al used FGF-1 with a serine residue substituted for one of its cysteines (S^{117}-FGF-1) in a porcine ameroid ischemia model.[78] This substitution increases the active half-life of FGF approximately tenfold. In this study, S^{117}-FGF-1 delivered via a sustained-release polymer resulted in improved regional perfusion and wall motion in the ischemic area, as well as improved global wall motion.[78] Nabel et al determined that FGF-1 encoding DNA injected directly into porcine arteries resulted in intimal hyperplasia and promoted angiogenesis.[79] The use of FGF-1 in animal models of ischemia has produced varying results, however, this variation may be due to the differences in animal models and preparations of FGF used.

Experiences with FGF-2 (basic FGF) have been more consistent than those with FGF-1. In 1992, a landmark study by Yanagisawa-Miwa et al demonstrated the effectiveness of FGF-2 as a therapeutic agent in acute ischemia.[80] Dogs received intracoronary infusions of recombinant FGF-2 at 30 min and 6 h after occlusion of the left anterior descending artery (LAD). Treated animals had reduced infarct size, increased collateral formation, and improved left ventricular systolic function at 1 week as compared to controls. Angiogenesis is a relatively slow process, occurring over days to weeks, whereas myocardial cell death from coronary occlusion is a rapid process, taking only hours. Thus, the reduction of infarct size must result, in part, from some nonangiogenic effect of FGF-2. In a canine model of acute coronary occlusion followed by intracoronary injection of either placebo or FGF-2, Horrigan et al showed that myocardial necrosis was significantly limited by FGF-2, even in a time period too brief for angiogenesis to have occurred.[81] Possible mechanisms for this effect include increased flow from dilation of preexisting collateral vessels or a direct protective effect on ischemic myocardial cells independent of blood flow.[82,83]

There also exists much evidence indicating the efficacy of FGF-2 in models of chronic ischemia. Shou et al showed that injecting FGF-2 into canine models of chronic single-vessel occlusion effectively enhances angiogenesis as compared to controls.[84] While these results were noted at the 5-week point, long-term 6-month analysis of collateral blood flow revealed no significant difference between control and experimental groups. In a canine ameroid ischemia model, FGF-2 given by intracoronary bolus injection or continuous left atrial infusion produced increased angiogenesis and improved regional perfusion.[85,86] Likewise, FGF-2 administered via heparin alginate pellets in a porcine ameroid ischemia model resulted in increased collateral formation and improved perfusion and left ventricular function.[87,88] Additionally, more studies in porcine models have focused on the safety and efficacy of the delivery mechanisms for the introduction of bFGF. Naimark et al demonstrated that direct endocardial delivery resulted in good deposition, with little or no systemic retention.[89] Similarly, Rezaee et al showed that selective retrograde catheter-based infusion of bFGF via the anterior interventricular vein was a safe and efficient delivery route, noting a significant improvement in the regional myocardial blood flow.[90] In a similar study, Rezaee et al showed that percutaneous intramyocardial delivery is safe and efficient for protein delivery.[91] A third study proved the efficacy of both transepicardial and transendocardial delivery of bFGF as compared with intravenous and intracoronary infusions; there was a lower systemic recirculation and greater deposition in the myocardium.[92] The current data reveal the role for bFGF as an important therapeutic growth factor required for angiogenesis and resultant protection of ischemic myocardium. In addition to proangiogenesis and resultant protection of ischemic myocardium, a recent study in pigs showed that bFGF infusion via the anterior interventricular vein decreased the inducibility of monomorphic ventricular tachycardia in chronic ischemia. These data suggest that bFGF could be an important future treatment modality to decrease the arrhythmogenicity of ischemic cardiac myocytes.[93]

The results of FGF-2 in the rabbit hind limb ischemia model is consistent with the myocardial ischemia models. Baffour et al demonstrated that intramuscular injections of FGF-2 increased collateral formation and decreased tissue necrosis in the ischemic limb.[93a] There is a great deal of evidence demonstrating the usefulness of FGF-2 as a therapeutic agent in acute and chronic ischemia via its effects as a proangiogenic growth factor and its apparent direct protective effects on ischemic tissue.

Thus far, there is limited experience with the use of FGF-5 as a therapeutic agent. In one study, Giordano et al investigated adenovirus-mediated transfer of the human FGF-5 gene in a porcine ameroid ischemia model. The adenovirus was delivered via intracoronary injection. Two weeks later, increased collateral formation

and improved perfusion and left ventricular function was evident in the treatment group and persisted for 12 weeks.[94]

Several studies using a rabbit hind limb ischemia model have demonstrated the efficacy of VEGF-165. Takeshita et al showed that intramuscular, intra-arterial, and intravenous administration of VEGF-165 all resulted in improved perfusion, angiographically visible collateral vessel formation, and histologically increased capillary density in the area of ischemia.[95–97] Later studies by the same investigators demonstrated that site-specific introduction of the VEGF gene without adjunctive vector, so-called "naked" DNA, resulted in similar benefits.[98] This response was equivalent with DNA encoding for the 121-, 165-, and 189-isoforms but not for the 206-isoform of VEGF.[99] Successful gene transfer in these studies was accomplished with direct intramuscular injection of the DNA, as well as delivery with the DNA applied to a hydrogel-coated angioplasty balloon.

Although VEGF is clearly useful as a therapeutic agent in animal models of peripheral ischemia, the effectiveness of VEGF in models of myocardial ischemia is less convincing. Schwarz et al, using a rat model of myocardial ischemia, evaluated the direct intramyocardial injection of the plasmid encoding VEGF 165.[100] Their results showed no improvement in relative regional myocardial blood flow and it induced vascular malformations. In contrast, one study, using a canine ameroid myocardial ischemia model, indicated that 28 days of daily intracoronary VEGF injections resulted in improved regional perfusion and increased density of small vessels.[101] Likewise, another study demonstrated that 28 days of continuous infusion of VEGF and heparin via a minipump in a porcine ameroid ischemia model improved regional perfusion and contractile function and increased capillary density.[102] A recent study by Tio et al in a porcine model of chronic ischemia showed improvement in myocardial perfusion and an increase in collateral formation after direct intramyocardial injection of naked DNA VEGF 165.[103] Another study used adenoviral vector for the direct injection of VEGF 121.[104] These investigators found that epicardial and transendocardial injections were equally effective and safe, but highly operator dependent. In a comparative study of VEGF and FGF-2, however, Lazarous et al found improved maximal collateral flow with 7 days of left atrial injections of FGF-2, but no significant improvement with VEGF.[105] Thus, VEGF appears to be effective in peripheral skeletal muscle ischemia and although VEGF may have a potential role in myocardial ischemia, the evidence at this time is not conclusive.

The above studies used minithoracotomies as the delivery mechanism for VEGF. Recent data showed that catheter-based direct intramyocardial injection in a porcine model of ischemia was a safe and effective way of administering a VEGF-121 adenoviral vector.[106]

Other proangiogenic substances are under investigation. Hypoxia-inducible factor (HIF)-1 has shown promise in a rabbit hind limb ischemia model.[106a] In both a rabbit hind limb ischemia model and a hamster cardiomyopathic model, delivery of the gene encoding for hepatocyte growth factor (HGF) has yielded good results.[107,108]

A recent study examined the safety of HGF DNA plasmid administration in the ischemic canine heart.[109] The role of HGF in acute ischemia and its mechanisms of action are currently being investigated in humans. Yasuda et al examined HGF in 40 patients in the setting of acute MI. They suggest that cardiac HGF may have a beneficial role in the process of ventricular remodeling post-MI by attenuating ventricular enlargement and thus increasing cardiac function. Interestingly, they proposed that HGF might directly counteract the actions of BNP, a marker of remodeling and left ventricular dysfunction in acute MI.[110,111] Likewise, recent data suggest that HGF functions as a survival factor in acute MI by preventing endothelial cells death.[112] These investigators also found that elevations in HGF seen a few days post-MI may represent the induction of angiogenesis and subsequent remodeling to preserve cardiac function.[112]

Soeki et al compared the role of VEGF and HGF in 20 acute MI, stable angina pectoris, and patients with old MIs, and found both levels to be elevated in the serum of the acute MI patients.[113] However, they also showed that VEGF, not HGF, was elevated in the stable angina pectoris group, suggesting that VEGF may be more reflective of change in myocardial ischemia than HGF. Another investigator proposed that the benefits of angiotensin-converting enzyme (ACE) inhibitors post-MI, with respect to ventricular remodeling, may be due to decreased VEGF expression in myofibroblasts in the healing infarct tissue.[114]

Local transplantation of autologous bone marrow cells increased collateral vessel formation in a rabbit hind limb ischemia model.[115] When transplanted into a cardiac scar, these bone marrow cells induced both cardiomyogenesis and angiogenesis and improved cardiac function.[116] Similar results with autologous bone marrow transplants were seen in porcine models of myocardial ischemia; that is, it induced angiogenesis, increased collateral circulation, and improved global cardiac function.[117,118] Likewise, bone marrow-derived mononuclear cell transplants were recently described as resulting in increased blood flow in chronically ischemic pig hearts, and improved peak stress score for regional left ventricular wall motion.[119] Aside from bone marrow cell transplants, some investigators are examining the utility of skeletal muscle transplant in the ischemic heart. Susuki et al showed that the use of a single-fiber skeletal myocyte transplant was sufficient to improve ischemia-induced heart failure.[120] A more recent study, using a mouse model of hind limb ischemia, delivered rVEGF via genetically modified skeletal myoblasts.[121] This bioartificial muscle tissue (BAM), when injected subcutaneously adjacent to ischemic tissue, was found to increase capillary density in both the BAM and adjacent ischemic tissue. There was no serum elevation of mVEGF, and no hemangioma formation at 6 weeks. The subcutaneous injection of the BAM tissue might prove to be an effective and efficient vehicle for the long-term delivery of growth factors.[121]

Local gene transfer into the vascular wall offers a promising alternative for the treatment of restenosis after percutaneous transcoronary angioplasty and coronary stenting.[122] Restenosis after angioplasty occurs by 6 months in many patients, leading to obstruction in 20 to 35% of them.[123] The pathogenesis of restenosis depends on endothelial damage, which also predisposes arteries to other pathologic conditions, such as spasm or thrombosis. Inhibition of restenosis could be based on strategies that reinforce endothelial cell protection or stimulate endothelial repair. Studies support the use of endothelial growth factors or vascular gene transfer for this purpose.[124] Reendothelialization in balloon-injured rat carotid artery was accelerated by a single dose of recombinant VEGF injected into the bloodstream or locally.[125,126] Likewise, in balloon-injured rabbit femoral arteries, site-specific VEGF-165 gene transfer accelerated reendothelialization and reduced neointimal thickening.[127] Vessel status was also improved by injection of VEGF plasmid into adventitial surface of rabbit carotid arteries.[128] Additionally, a recent study found that catheter-based prostacyclin synthase gene transfer in rabbits prevented stent restenosis by accelerating endothelial recovery. It is thought that prostacyclin synthase functions via an adenosine $3',5'$-cyclic phosphate (cyclic AMP)-

mediated activation of VEGF.[129] Although evidence indicates intravascular gene transfer in the arterial wall is not very efficient,[130] administration of genes encoding for secreted proteins such as VEGF could still be useful in therapeutic gene transfer trials using infusion-perfusion catheters[131] or histamine-induced increase of endothelial permeability.[132] One study demonstrated that delivery of recombinant VEGF via channel-gated balloon catheter after stent implantation in rabbit iliac arteries accelerated stent endothelialization and reduced in-stent thrombosis.[133] Because VEGF and VEGF-C share one receptor (KDR/flk-1) but differ in the other receptor, VEGF-C and VEGF-165 might have overlapping but distinct effects in the vessel wall. VEGF-C gene transfer inhibits intimal thickening early, and the protective effect is at least equal to that seen with VEGF-165 gene transfer.[134]

Although VEGF and FGF have impressive potential in therapeutic angiogenesis, it remains to be determined whether the injection of the growth factor or its encoding DNA is more therapeutically effective. Advocates of gene transfer allude to the potential for an optimal level of growth factor production that remains consistent over time and limited to the specific cells targeted. Maintaining local production avoids the potential problems associated with systemically elevated growth factor levels, namely, acute-onset severe hypotension and edema, as well as stimulation of growth in undetected latent tumors. Although it has been shown that VEGF is sufficient to promote growth but not malignant proliferation or metastasis,[135] thus confirming that angiogenesis is necessary but not sufficient for malignant growth to occur,[136] these studies do not debunk the notion that growth factors can exacerbate preexisting latent local tumor growth and metastasis. The cell specificity of gene transfer avoids these potential problems. An additional, yet unproven, benefit is that gene transfer might be more effective than a single, larger dose of VEGF from both a safety and bioactivity standpoint.[137]

Proponents of growth factor administration counter that gene transfer risks protooncogene to oncogene transformation. Additionally, with questions concerning DNA transfer efficiency and no proven therapeutic advantage of gene transfer, then why bother with DNA? This issue is now being vigorously debated within the scientific community.

Clinical Trials

The greater understanding of angiogenic mechanisms and the promising results with angiogenesis in animal models have led to human studies using different methods of growth factor delivery (Tables 38-2 and 38-3). Most clinical trials have involved introduction of either a growth factor or its encoding DNA into human hosts. Recognizing that there are many patients with vascular insufficiency for whom medications and surgical bypass are ineffective, Isner et al described a clinical protocol to be used in patients with peripheral artery disease.[138] The authors attempt to safely achieve therapeutic angiogenesis via percutaneous catheter-based delivery of the gene encoding VEGF in patients with peripheral artery disease by using a protocol similar to that employed in their rabbit study. Results in one patient with an ischemic limb who underwent this procedure indicate that angiogenesis was promoted. However, edema and other side effects were noted by the patient. Nonetheless, while adjustments to minimize side effects are needed, these encouraging results have prompted other clinical trials.[139]

VEGF-165 and VEGF-121 are being studied in clinical trials of patients with severe angina pectoris, with the substance being injected directly into the coronary circulation and peripherally.[140,141] In one placebo-controlled study with intracoronary and intravenous

TABLE 38-2. Outcomes Measures for Therapeutic Myocardial Angiogenesis/Neoarteriogenesis

Histology/Histochemistry/Molecular Techniques
 Number of vessels/HPF, area of vessels/HPF, total perimeter of
  vessels/HPF, myocyte-to-capillary ratio, average number
  of vessels adjacent to a muscle fiber
 Infarct size
 Quantitative analysis of endothelial cell markers by Western analysis
 Assessment of vascular cell (in particular endothelial cell) proliferation
  (BrdU uptake)
Angiography
 Quantification of collateral vessels
 Assessment of flow
Perfusion
 Microsphere flow analysis
 Nuclear perfusion techniques (thallium or technetium single-photon
  emission tomography, at rest and with exercise or pharmacologic
  stress)
 Magnetic resonance perfusion techniques
Microvascular Function
 Response of coronary resistance and flow to acute exposure to
  endothelium-dependent receptor-mediated agonists (ADP,
  serotonin, nitric oxide donor, growth factors)
Left Ventricular Function
 Echocardiography
 Nuclear techniques
 Magnetic resonance imaging
 Left ventriculogram with contrast angiography
Clinical End Points
 Degree of angina, exercise tolerance, freedom of myocardial
  (re)infarction, length of survival

Source: Reproduced with permission from Helisch A, Ware JA. Therapeutic angiogenesis in ischemic heart disease. *J Thromb Hemostat* 82:772, 1999.

infusion of VEGF, the procedure was found to be safe and well tolerated, but the results were inconclusive.[140,142,143] In other studies, naked DNA containing the VEGF gene was injected directly into sites in the myocardium identified by angiography.[144] Access was obtained via minithoracotomy. This approach was associated with benefit in a small pilot study.[145,146] These same investigators injected the VEGF gene into cardiac muscle aboard a disarmed adenovirus vector during coronary artery bypass surgery or during

a minithoracotomy.[147,148] Patients in this study reported reduced symptoms and tolerated the procedure well. Moreover, dobutamine single-photon emission computed tomography sestamibi imaging revealed reduced ischemia in 11 of 12 patients studied. Some short-term preliminary studies have revealed clinical benefit in patients with severe angina pectoris, with evidence of increased blood flow to the heart. Some investigators have suggested that intramyocardial, but not intravenous VEGF can improve regional myocardial perfusion.[149] In a randomized, double-bind, placebo-controlled study, Laitinen et al demonstrated that intracoronary administration of VEGF plasmid/liposome during percutaneous transluminal coronary angioplasty (PTCA) via a perfusion-infusion catheter is safe and well tolerated.[150] Patients did not develop acute MI, cerebrovascular accident, angina pectoris, or hypotension up to 48 h after discharge. Although there was no change in the degree of stenosis at 6 months, this form of genetic transmission may be applicable in future clinical trials.[150]

FGF-2 has been administered to humans with angina pectoris and severe coronary artery disease by direct intracoronary injection.[151] Patients had improved exercise tolerance, reduced angina, and improved regional perfusion and wall motion. Two of 10 patients in the high-dose treatment group developed severe hypotension. Intramyocardial delivery of naked DNA containing the FGF gene and delivery of the FGF gene by adenovirus have also been used. Laham et al recently completed a double-blind placebo-controlled study using FGF-2 in patients undergoing coronary artery bypass grafting (CABG). Patients were randomized to receive heparin alginate microbeads coated with either high-dose FGF-2, low-dose FGF-2, or no growth factor. Improved perfusion to the target area was noted in all of the high-dose FGF patients, but in less than half of the patients who received low-dose FGF or placebo. Likewise, regional wall motion was improved only in patients who received the high-dose FGF. Global wall motion was improved in all patients and no patients had side-effects related to FGF administration.[152] Early results with FGF have been promising, and larger studies are in progress.

To assess whether growth factor treatment could enhance coronary collateral growth and relieve myocardial ischemia, a multicenter, randomized, double-blind placebo-controlled trial of Ad5-FGF-4 gene transfer therapy was carried out in patients with stable angina pectoris.[153] Patients received placebo or ascending doses

TABLE 38-3. Clinical Trials of Therapeutic Myocardial Angiogenesis

Growth Factor	Delivery	Phase	Patients Treated with Active Agent/Placebo
FGF-1	Intramyocardial	I	20/20
FGF-2	Intracoronary	I	
FGF-2	Local (polymer)	I	16/8
FGF-2	Intracoronary	I	52/0
FGF-2	Intravenous	I	14/0
FGF-2	Intracoronary	II	251/86
FGF-4	Intracoronary (adenovirus)	I	
VEGF$_{165}$	Intracoronary	I	15/0
VEGF$_{165}$	Intravenous	I	27/0
VEGF$_{165}$	Intracoronary/intravenous	II	
VEGF$_{165}$	Intramyocardial (plasmid)	I	13/0*
VEGF$_{121}$	Intramyocardial (adenovirus)	I	7/0*
HIP-1α	Intramyocardial (adenovirus)	I	

* Enrollment not complete at this time.

Source: Reproduced with permission from Frishman WH. Recent advances in cardiovascular pharmacology. *Heart Dis* 1:81, 1999.

of FGF-4 that were administered by one-time intracoronary injections. Five ascending dose groups in one-half log steps were tested (3.2×10^8 up to 3.2×10^{10} viral particles). Subjects were followed for at least 3 min after treatment. There was evidence of a beneficial anti-ischemic effect in Ad5-FGF-4-treated patients compared to placebo, with greater improvement in exercise duration. The greatest anti-ischemic effects were seen in patients with more baseline impairment of exercise and lower baseline-neutralizing adenovirus antibody titers. The occurrence of fever (highest dose group) and the occasional rise in liver function tests suggest a dosing limit and raises some concerns for safety. Several other limitations of the AGENT trial should also be noted, including study size and the lack of radionuclide demonstration of an anti-ischemic benefit.[153]

rFGF-2 has been evaluated as a treatment for intermittent claudication in the TRAFFIC study (Therapeutic Angiogenesis with Recombinant Fibroblast Growth Factor-2 for Intermittent Claudication).[154] In this placebo-controlled study, patients with claudication received injections of placebo of FBF-2 into both legs at days 1 and 30. At day 90, patients receiving FGF-2 had an increased walking time and an increase in their ankle-brachial index when compared with the placebo group. At day 180, there was no difference between either treatment group. The rFGF-2 therapy was well tolerated and no significant safety concerns were raised.

A single bolus intracoronary infusion of rFGF-2 seemed to be safe and potentially efficacious in an open-label, Phase I clinical trial. In the placebo-controlled FGF Initiating Revascularization Trial (FIRST) in patients with angina pectoris and CAD, rFGF-2 did not improve exercise tolerance or myocardial perfusion, but did cause a trend toward symptomatic improvement at 90 but not 180 days.[154a]

Angiogenic growth factors may also have other benefits in patients with CHF. It has been demonstrated that skeletal-muscle VEGF levels are reduced in patients with CHF.[155] In a recent study, VEGF delivery to ischemic skeletal muscle was shown to cause myoblast-mediated angiogenesis and improved exercise tolerance.[156]

THE FUTURE OF ANGIOGENESIS

Despite the incredible progress that has been made, much remains to be learned about angiogenesis. For instance, there are still considerable gaps in our understanding of the mechanisms by which angiogenesis occurs and of the numerous factors that regulate this process. Questions also remain concerning the long-term efficacy of therapeutic angiogenesis. Additionally, it is not known whether angiogenic therapy has deleterious late sequelae, which might appear years after treatment. These and other questions need to be addressed in order to maximize benefit and minimize risk in patient care.[157]

However, while much remains unknown, ongoing research continues to forge closer to the answers. As more is learned about the underlying mechanisms, a more complete picture of angiogenesis will emerge to shed light on currently hazy issues. New angiogenic growth factors will likely be discovered and greater details about existing growth factors will surface. Preclinical and clinical trials will incorporate the newly discovered growth factors and determine which ones are most therapeutically effective and at what doses. Long-term safety and efficacy, the optimal mode of delivery, and whether to employ growth factors or DNA will likely be determined. Other potential therapeutic roles for VEGF might become apparent.

For example, Torry et al suggest that mRNA VEGF expression may play an important role in creating capillary endothelial cell changes that promote allograft survival after cardiac transplant.[158] Another potential approach is the use of autologous transplantation of bone-marrow cells.[158a]

One significant hurdle must be overcome for progress to continue in a timely fashion. There is a current lack of agreement within the scientific community as to which criteria should serve as the ultimate end points by which to measure the efficacy of therapy.[159] Magnetic resonance imaging, arteriograms, invasive procedures, blood flow measurements, and histologic evidence are a mere sampling of end points measured in various labs. A recent study by Fuchs et al used a porcine model of myocardial ischemia to assess the correlation between tissue perfusion, myocardial function and angiographic assessment of collaterals.[160] This study showed no correlation between angiographic assessment of collaterals and myocardial function and perfusion, suggesting that primary end points should not be based solely on angiography. Additionally, Bradley et al looked at stress echocardiography and nuclear perfusion imaging as a means to evaluate clinical angiogenesis end points in the patients enrolled in the VIVA trial.[161] Despite improvements in angina score and treadmill time, these two imaging modalities did not demonstrate any difference between the VEGF and placebo groups. SPECT imaging on 30 patients who received naked DNA for VEGF-2 via thoracotomy and direct intramyocardial injection showed an improvement in perfusion in some patients, with maximal difference seen in the rest, as opposed to stress scans.[162] They also noted that patients who received higher doses of VEGF-2 demonstrated a greater difference in perfusion as compared to placebo on the resting scans. These data suggest that the scientific and medical communities have yet to discover a sensitive and specific modality of objectively evaluating therapeutic angiogenesis.

Should a single end point or a combination of measurements serve as the "gold standard" through which to measure therapeutic effectiveness? Which end points are the appropriate ones to choose? Whichever ones are chosen, it is critical that there be widespread acceptance within the scientific community so that a true "gold standard" is created. The lack of an accepted standard hinders current progress, as results from various studies are difficult to correlate with one another due to the different end points measured. Cohesiveness within the scientific community in this regard will allow for maximization of the therapeutic potential of angiogenesis.

REFERENCES

1. Cotran RS, Kumar V, Robbins SL, eds: Cellular injury and cellular death. In: *Pathologic Basis of Disease.* 5th ed. Philadelphia: WB Saunders, 1994:3.
2. Cotran RS, Kumar V, Robbins SL, eds: Neoplasia. In: *Pathologic Basis of Disease.* 5th ed. Philadelphia: WB Saunders, 1994: 250.
3. Shweiki D, Itin A, Soffer D, Keshet E: Vascular endothelial growth factor induced by hypoxia may mediate hypoxia-initiated angiogenesis. *Nature* 359:843, 1992.
4. Maltepe E, Schmidt JV, Baunoch D, et al: Abnormal angiogenesis and responses to glucose and oxygen deprivation in mice lacking the ARNT. *Nature* 386:403, 1997.
5. Levy AP, Levy NS, Wegner S, Goldberg M: Transcriptional regulation of the rat vascular endothelial growth factor gene by hypoxia. *J Biol Chem* 270:13333, 1995.
6. Li J, Brown LF, Hibberd MG, et al: VEGF, flk-1, and flt-1 expression in a rat myocardial infarction model of angiogenesis. *Am J Physiol* 270:H1803, 1996.

7. Lee SH, Wolf PL, Escudero R, et al: Early expression of angiogenesis factors in acute myocardial ischemia and infarction. *N Engl J Med* 342:626, 2000.

8. Li J, Hampton T, Morgan JP, Simons M: Stretch-induced VEGF expression in the heart. *J Clin Invest* 100 (1):18, 1997.

9. Zheng W, Brown MD, Brock TA, et al: Bradycardia-induced coronary angiogenesis is dependent on vascular endothelial growth factor. *Circ Res* 85:192, 1999.

10. DeBoer R, Siebelink HJ, Tio RA, et al: Carvedilol increases plasma vascular endothelial growth factor (VEGF) in patients with chronic heart failure. *Eur J Heart Fail* 3:331, 2001.

11. Hashimoto E, Ogita T, Nakaoka T, et al: Rapid induction of vascular endothelial growth factor expression by transient ischemia in rat heart. *Am J Physiol* 267:H1948, 1994.

12. Marti HH, Risau W: Systemic hypoxia changes the organ-specific distribution of vascular endothelial growth factor and its receptors. *Proc Natl Acad Sci U S A* 95(26):15809, 1998.

13. Ogawa H, Suefuji H, Soejima H: Increased blood vascular endothelial growth factor levels in patients with acute myocardial infarction. *Cardiology* 93:93, 2000.

14. Kranz A, Rau C, Kochs M, Waltenberger J: Elevation of vascular endothelial growth factor-A serum levels following acute myocardial infarction. Evidence for its origin and functional significance. *J Mol Cell Cardiol* 32:65, 2000.

15. Kuroki M, Voest EE, Amano S, et al: Reactive oxygen intermediates increase vascular endothelial growth factor expression in vitro and in vivo. *J Clin Invest* 98 (7):1667, 1996.

16. Detmar M, Brown LF, Berse B, et al: Hypoxia regulates the expression of vascular permeability factor/vascular endothelial growth factor (VPF/VEGF) and its receptors in human skin. *J Invest Dermatol* 108(3):263, 1997.

17. Tofukuji M, Metais C, Li J, et al: Myocardial VEGF expression after cardio-pulmonary bypass and cardioplegia. *Circulation* 98 (Suppl 19):II242, discussion II247, 1998.

18. Luo Z, Diaco M, Murohara T, et al: Vascular endothelial growth factor attenuates myocardial ischemia-reperfusion injury. *Ann Thorac Surg* 64:993, 1997.

19. Kawata H, Yoshida K-i, Kawamoto A, et al: Ischemic preconditioning upregulates vascular endothelial growth factor mRNA expression and neovascularization via nuclear translocation of protein kinase C-e in the rat ischemic myocardium. *Circ Res* 88:696, 2001.

20. Gustafsson T, Puntschart A, Kaijser L, et al: Exercise-induced expression of angiogenesis-related transcription and growth factors in human skeletal muscle. *Am J Physiol* 276 (2 pt 2):H679, 1999.

21. White FC, Bloor CM, McKirnan MD, Carroll SM: Exercise training in swine promotes growth of arteriolar bed and capillary angiogenesis in heart. *J Appl Physiol* 85(3):1160, 1998.

22. Ziegelhoeffer T, Hoefer IE, van Royen N, Buschmann IR: Effective reduction in collateral formation through matrix metalloproteinase-inhibitors (abstr). *Circulation* 100(Suppl I):I-705, 1999.

23. Griendling KK, Alexander RW: Endothelial control of the cardiovascular system: recent advances. *FASEB J* 10(2):283, 1996.

24. Han Z, Duquaine D, Addison C, et al: Hyperlipidemia potentiates in vitro angiogenesis with vascular endothelial growth factor (abstr.). *J Am Coll Cardiol* 27(Suppl A):228A, 2001.

25. Kalka C, Masuda H, Wolf N, et al: Hypercholesterolemia stimulates endothelial progenitor cell kinetics but impairs their functional properties (abstr.). *Circulation* 102 (Suppl II):II-64, 2000.

26. Duan J, Shintani S, Sasaki K-I, et al: Rescue of hypercholesterolemia-related impairment of angiogenesis by oral folic acid supplementation (abstr.). *Circulation* 102(Suppl II):II-741, 2000.

27. Duan J, Sasaki K-I, Shintani S, et al: Hyperhomocystinemia impairs angiogenesis and collateral vessel formation in response to hind limb ischemia (abstr.). *Circulation* 102(Suppl II):II-309, 2000.

28. Kong D, Park H-J, Tang D, Galper JB: HMG-CoA reductase inhibitors interfere with VEGF signaling in human endothelial cells (abstr.). *Circulation* 102(Suppl II):II-64, 2000.

29. Celletti F, Hilfiker PR, Ghafouri P, Dake MD: Effect of human recombinant vascular endothelial growth factor 165 on progression of atherosclerotic plaque. *J Am Coll Cardiol* 37:2126, 2001.

30. Moore KL, Persaud TVN, eds: *The Developing Human: Clinically Oriented Embryology.* 6th ed. Philadelphia: WB Saunders, 1998.

31. Asahara T, Murohara T, Sullivan A, et al: Isolation of putative progenitor endothelial cells for angiogenesis. *Science* 275:964, 1997.

32. Schwartz SM, Liaw L: Growth control and morphogenesis in the development and pathology of arteries. *J Cardiovasc Pharmacol* 21(Suppl 1):S31, 1993.

33. Wang A, Ware A: PKC-α is required for endothelial cell adhesion migration, MAP kinase activation and vessel formation. *Circulation* 102(Suppl II):II-64, 2000.

34. Nehls V, Herrmann R, Huhnken M, Palmetshofer A: Contact-dependent inhibition of angiogenesis by cardiac fibroblasts in three-dimensional fibrin gels in vitro: implications for microvascular network remodeling and coronary collateral formation. *Cell Tissue Res* 293(3):479, 1998.

35. Cotran RS, Kumar V, Robbins SL, eds: Cellular growth and differentiation: normal regulation and adaptations. In: *Pathologic Basis of Disease.* 5th ed. Philadelphia: WB Saunders, 1994:42.

36. Kozian DH, Ziche M, Augustin HG: The activin-binding protein follistatin regulates autocrine endothelial cell activity and induces angiogenesis. *Lab Invest* 76(2):267, 1997.

37. Leung D, Cachianes G, Kuang W, et al: Vascular endothelial growth factor is a secreted angiogenic mitogen. *Science* 246:1306, 1989.

38. Houck K, Ferrara N, Winer J, et al: The vascular endothelial growth factor family-identification of a fourth molecular species and characterizations of alternative splicing of RNA. *Mol Endocrinol* 5:1806, 1991.

39. Poltorak Z, Cohen T, Sivan R, et al: VEGF$_{145}$: A secreted VEGF form that binds to extracellular matrix. *J Biol Chem* 272:7151, 1997.

40. Vincenti V, Cassano C, Rocchi M, Persico G: Assignment of the vascular endothelial growth factor gene to the human chromosome 6p21.3. *Circulation* 93:1493, 1996.

41. Park J, Keller G, Ferrara N: Vascular endothelial growth factor (VEGF) isoforms — differential deposition into the subepithelial extracellular matrix and bioactivity of extracellular matrix-bound VEGF. *Mol Biol Cell* 4:1317, 1993.

42. Cheung SY, Nagane M, Huang HJS, Cavenee WK: Intracerebral tumor-associated hemorrhage caused by overexpression of the vascular endothelial growth factor isoforms VEGF(121) and VEGF(165) but not VEGF(189). *Proc Natl Acad Sci U S A* 94:12081, 1997.

43. Plouet J, Moro F, Bertagnolli S, et al: Extracellular cleavage of the vascular endothelial growth factor 189 amino acid form by urokinase is required for its mitogenic effect. *J Biol Chem* 272:13390, 1997.

44. Houck K, Leung D, Rowland A, et al: Dual regulation of vascular endothelial growth factor bioavailability by genetic and proteolytic mechanisms. *J Biol Chem* 267:26031, 1992.

45. Keyt B, Berleau L, Nguyen H, et al: The carboxyl-terminal domain (111–165) of VEGF is critical for mitogenic potency. *J Biol Chem* 271:7788, 1996.

46. deVries C, Escobedo J, Ueno H, et al: The fms-like tyrosine kinase, a receptor for vascular endothelial growth factor. *Science* 255:989, 1992.

47. Terman B, Dougher-Vermazen M, Carrion M, et al: Identification of the KDR tyrosine kinase as a receptor for vascular endothelial growth factor. *Biochem Biophys Res Commun* 187:1579, 1992.

48. Matthews W, Jordan CT, Gavin ME, et al: A receptor tyrosine kinase cDNA isolated from a population of enriched primitive hematopoietic cells and exhibiting close genetic linkage to c-kit. *Proc Natl Acad Sci U S A* 88:9026, 1991.

49. Millauer B, Wizigmann-Voos S, Schurch H, et al: High affinity binding and developmental expression suggest Flk-1 as a major regulator of vasculogenesis and angiogenesis. *Cell* 72:835, 1993.

50. Fournier E, Birnbaum D, Borg JP: Receptors for factors of the VEGF family. *Bull Cancer* 84:397, 1997.

51. Barleon B, Totzke F, Herzog C, et al: Mapping of the sites for ligand binding and receptor dimerization at the extracellular domain of the vascular endothelial growth factor receptor FLT-1. *J Biol Chem* 272(16):10382, 1997.

52. Waltenberger J, Claesson-Welsh L, Siegbahn A, et al: Different signal transduction properties of KDR and Flt1, two receptors for vascular endothelial growth factor. *J Biol Chem* 269:26988, 1994.

53. Marchand GS, Noiseux N, Tanguay JF, Sirois MG: Blockade of in vivo VEGF-mediated angiogenesis by antisense gene therapy: Role of Flk-1 and Flt receptors. *Am J Physiol* 282:H194, 2002.

54. Brock TA, Dvorak HF, Senger DR: Tumour-secreted vascular permeability factor increases cytosolic Ca^{2+} and von Willebrand factor release in human endothelial cells. *Am J Pathol* 138:213, 1991.

55. Kroll J, Waltenberger J: The vascular endothelial growth factor receptor KDR activates multiple signal transduction pathways in porcine aortic endothelial cells. *J Biol Chem* 272:32521, 1991.

56. Abedi H, Zachary I: Vascular endothelial growth factor stimulates tyrosine phosphorylation and recruitment to new focal adhesions of focal adhesion kinase and paxillin in endothelial cells. *J Biol Chem* 272:15442, 1997.

57. Miraliakbari R, Francalancia NA, Lust RM, et al: Differences in myocardial and peripheral VEGF and KDR levels after acute ischemia. *Ann Thorac Surg* 69:1750, 2000.

58. Gerbert H-P, McMurtrey A, Kowalski J, et al: Vascular endothelial growth factor regulates cell survival through the phosphatidylinasitol 3′-kinase/Akt signal transduction pathway. *J Biol Chem* 273:30336, 1998.

59. Luo Z, Kureishi Y, Fijio Y, Walsh K: Akt1/PKB signaling in endothelial cells is sufficient for blood vessel growth in ischemic hind limb (abstr.). *Circulation* 102(Suppl II):II-44, 2000.

60. Teichert-Kuliszewska K, Jones N, Dumont DJ, et al: Angiopoietin-1 induces angiogenesis by activation of the phosphatidylinositol 3-kinase/AKT pathway and increase in nitric oxide production (abstr.). *Circulation* 102(Suppl II):II-44, 2000.

61. Zhou HZ, Karliner JS, Gray MO: Moderate alcohol consumption induces sustained cardiac protection by activating PKC-epsilon and Akt. *Am J Physiol* 283:H165, 2002.

62. Gu J-W, Elam J, Sartin A, et al: Moderate levels of ethanol induce expression of vascular endothelial growth factor and stimulate angiogenesis. *Am J Physiol* 281:R365, 2001.

62a. van der Zee R, Murohara T, Luo Z, et al: Vascular endothelial growth factor/vascular permeability factor augments nitric oxide release from quiescent rabbit and human vascular endothelium. *Circulation* 95(4):1030, 1997.

63. Ziche M, Morbidelli L, Choudhuri R, et al: Nitric oxide synthase lies downstream from vascular endothelial growth factor-induced but not basic fibroblast growth factor-induced angiogenesis. *J Clin Invest* 99(11):2625, 1997.

64. Post MJ, Sato K, Bao J, et al: In vivo role of PAF and NO in angiogenesis induced by FGF-2 and VEGF165 (abstr.). *Circulation* 102(Suppl II):II-248, 2000.

65. Matsunaga T, Warltier DC, Weihrauch DW, et al: Ischemia-induced coronary collateral growth is dependent on vascular endothelial growth factor and nitric oxide. *Circulation* 102:3098, 2000.

66. Heil M, Clauss M, Suzuki K, et al: Vascular endothelial growth factor (VEGF) stimulates monocyte migration through endothelial monolayers via increased integrin expression. *Eur J Cell Biol* 79:850, 2000.

67. Senger DR, Van de Water L, Brown LF, et al: Vascular permeability factor (VPF, VEGF) in tumor biology. *Cancer Metastasis Rev* 12(3–4):303, 1993.

68. Dvorak HF, Harvey VS, Estrella P, et al: Fibrin containing gels induce angiogenesis: Implications for tumor stroma generation and wound healing. *Lab Invest* 57:673, 1987.

69. Yang R, Thomas GR, Bunting S, et al: Effects of VEGF on hemodynamics and cardiac performance. *J Cardiovasc Pharmacol* 27:838, 1996.

70. Sato K, Wu T, Laham RJ, et al: Efficacy of intracoronary or intravenous VEGF165 in a pig model of chronic myocardial ischemia. *J Am Coll Cardiol* 37:616, 2001.

71. Slavin, J. Fibroblast growth factors: At the heart of angiogenesis. *Cell Biol Int* 19(5):431, 1995.

72. Alberts B, Bray D, Lewis J, et al (eds): Cell junctions, cell adhesion, and the extracellular matrix. In: *Molecular Biology of the Cell.* 3rd ed. New York: Garland Publishing, 1994:977.

73. Partovian C, Horowitz A, Murakami M, et al: Basic fibroblast growth factor (FGF-2) activates eNOS through a syndecan-4 dependent pathway (abstr.). *Circulation* 102(Suppl II):II-64, 2000.

74. Unger EF, Shou M Sheffield CD, et al: Extracardiac to coronary anastomoses support left ventricular function in dogs. *Am J Physiol* 264:H1567, 1993.

75. Unger EF, Banai S, Shou M, et al: A model to assess interventions to improve collateral blood flow: Continuous administration of agents into the left coronary artery in dogs. *Cardiovasc Res* 27:785, 1993.

76. Schlaudraff K, Schumacher B, von Specht BU, et al: Growth of "new" coronary vascular structures by angiogenic growth factors. *Eur J Cardiothorc Surg* 7:637, 1993.

77. Pu LQ, Sniderman AD, Brassard R, et al: Enhanced revascularization of the ischemic limb by means of angiogenic therapy. *Circulation* 88:208, 1993.

78. Lopez JJ, Edelman ER, Stamler A, et al: Angiogenic potential of perivascularly delivered aFGF in a porcine model of chronic myocardial ischemia. *Am J Physiol* 274 (3 pt 2):H930, 1998.

79. Nabel E, Yang ZY, Plautz G, et al: Recombinant fibroblast growth factor-1 promotes intimal hyperplasia and angiogenesis in arteries in vivo. *Nature* 362(6423):844, 1993.

80. Yanagisawa-Miwa A, Uchida Y, Nakamura F, et al: Salvage of infarcted myocardium by angiogenic action of basic fibroblast growth factor. *Science* 257(5075):1401, 1992.

81. Horrigan MC, Malycky JL, Ellis SG, et al: Reduction in myocardial infarct size by basic fibroblast growth factor following coronary occlusion in a canine model. *Int J Cardiol* 68(Suppl 1):S85, 1999.

82. Pauda RR, Sethi R, Dhalla NS, Kardami E: Basic fibroblast growth factor is cardioprotective in ischemia-reperfusion injury. *Mol Cell Biochem* 143:129,1995.

83. Huang Z, Chen K, Huang PL, et al: BFGF ameliorates focal ischemic injury by blood flow-independent mechanisms in eNOS mutant mice. *Am J Physiol* 272:H1401, 1997.

84. Shou M, Thirumurti V, Rajanayagam S, et al: Effect of basic fibroblast growth factor on myocardial angiogenesis in dogs with mature collateral vessels. *J Am Coll Cardiol* 29:1102, 1997.

85. Unger EF, Banai S, Shou M, et al: Basic fibroblast growth factor enhances myocardial collateral flow in a canine model. *Am J Physiol* 266:H1588, 1994.

86. Lazarous DF, Scheinowitz M, Shou M, et al: Effects of chronic systemic administration of basic fibroblast growth factor on collateral development in the canine heart. *Circulation* 91:145, 1995.

87. Harada K, Grossman W, Friedman M, et al: Basic fibroblast growth factor improves myocardial function in chronically ischemic porcine hearts. *J Clin Invest* 94:623, 1994.

88. Lopez JJ, Edelman ER, Stamler A, et al: Basic fibroblast growth factor in a porcine model of chronic myocardial ischemia: A comparison of angiographic, echocardiographic and coronary flow parameters. *J Pharmacol Exp Ther* 282:385, 1997.

89. Naimark W, Kavanaugh WM, Palasis M, et al: Characterization of ^{125}-I recombinant fibroblast growth factor 2 retention and distribution following direct intramyocardial injection (abstr.). *J Am Coll Cardiol* 37(Suppl A):7A, 2001.

90. Rezaee M, Herity NA, Lo S, et al: Therapeutic angiogenesis by selective delivery of basic fibroblast growth factor in the anterior interventricular vein (abstr.). *J Am Coll Cardiol* 37(Suppl A):47A, 2001.

91. Rezaee M, Yeung AC, Altman P, et al: Evaluation of the percutaneous intramyocardial injection for local myocardial treatment. *Catheter Cardiovasc Intero* 53:271, 2001.

92. Laham R, Post MJ, Selke FW, Simons M: Tissue and myocardial distribution of endocardial vs epicardial intramyocardial delivery of 125-I labeled basic fibroblast growth factor (bFGF): Is epicardial delivery obsolete (abstr.)? *J Am Coll Cardiol* 37(Suppl A):227A, 2001.

93. Day JD, Rezaee M, Chun SH, et al: Basic fibroblast growth factor may attenuate susceptibility to ventricular tachyarrhythmias in chronically ischemic porcine myocardium (abstr.). *J Am Coll Cardiol* 37(Suppl A):135A, 2001.

93a. Baffour R, Berman J, Garb JL, et al: Enhanced angiogenesis and growth of collaterals by in vivo administration of recombinant basic fibroblast growth factor in a rabbit model of acute lower limb ischemia: Dose-response effect of basic fibroblast growth factor. *J Vasc Surg* 16:181, 1992.

94. Giordano FJ, Ping P, McKirnan MD, et al: Intracoronary gene transfer of fibroblast growth factor-5 increases blood flow and contractile function in an ischemic region of the heart. *Nat Med* 2(5):534, 1996.

95. Takeshita S, Pu LQ, Stein LA, et al: Intramuscular administration of vascular endothelial growth factor induces dose-dependent collateral artery augmentation in a rabbit model of chronic limb ischemia. *Circulation* 90:II228, 1994.

96. Takeshita S, Zheng LP, Brogi E, et al: Therapeutic angiogenesis. A single intraarterial bolus of vascular endothelial growth factor augments revascularization in a rabbit ischemic hind limb model. *J Clin Invest* 93:622, 1994.

97. Bauters C, Asahara T, Zheng LP, et al: Site-specific therapeutic angiogenesis after systemic administration of vascular endothelial growth factor. *J Vasc Surg* 21:314, 1995.

98. Takeshita S, Weir L, Chen D, et al: Therapeutic angiogenesis following arterial gene transfer of vascular endothelial growth factor on a rabbit model of hind limb ischemia. *Biochem Biophys Res Commun* 227:628, 1996.

99. Takeshita S, Tsurumi Y, Couffinahl T, et al: Gene transfer of naked DNA encoding for three isoforms of vascular endothelial growth factor stimulates collateral development in vivo. *Lab Invest* 75(4):487, 1996.

100. Schwarz ER, Speakman MT, Patterson M, et al: Evaluation of the effects of intramyocardial injection of DNA expressing vascular endothelial growth factor (VEGF) in a myocardial infarction model in the rat-angiogenesis and angioma formation. *J Am Coll Cardiol* 35:1323, 2000.

101. Banai S, Jaklitsch MT, Shou M, et al: Angiogenic-induced enhancement of collateral blood flow to ischemic myocardium by vascular endothelial growth factor in dogs. *Circulation* 89:2183, 1994.

102. Harada K, Friedmann M, Lopez JJ, et al: Vascular endothelial growth factor administration in chronic myocardial ischemia. *Am J Physiol* 270:H1791, 1996.

103. Tio RA, Tkebuchava T, Scheuermann TH, et al: Intramyocardial gene therapy with naked DNA encoding vascular endothelial growth factor improves collateral flow to ischemic myocardium. *Hum Gene Ther* 10:2953, 1999.

104. Post MJ, Laham RJ, Sato K, et al: Adenovirus mediated gene therapy through intramyocardial injection: Percutaneous intramyocardial versus surgical epicardial delivery (abstr.). *Circulation* 102(Suppl II): II-206, 2000.

105. Lazarous DF, Shou M, Scheinowitz M, et al: Comparative effects of basic fibroblast growth factor and vascular endothelial growth factor on coronary collateral development and the arterial response to injury. *Circulation* 94:1074, 1996.

106. Kornowski R, Leon MB, Fuchs S, et al: Electromagnetic guidance for catheter-based transendocardial injection: A platform for intramyocardial angiogenesis therapy. *J Am Coll Cardiol* 35:1031, 2000.

106a. Shyu K-G, Vincent KA, Luo Y, et al: Naked DNA encoding an hypoxia-inducible factor 1α (HIF-1α)/VP16 hybrid transcription factor enhances angiogenesis in rabbit hind limb ischemia: An alternate method for therapeutic angiogenesis utilizing a transcriptional regulatory system. *Circulation* 98(Suppl I):I-68, 1998.

107. Taniyama Y, Morishita R, Nakagami H, et al: Potential contribution of a novel antifibrotic factor, hepatocyte growth factor, for prevention of myocardial fibrosis by angiotensin II blockade in cardiomyopathic hamsters. *Circulation* 102:246, 2000.

108. Morishita R, Nakamura S, Hayashi S, et al: Therapeutic angiogenesis induced by human recombinant hepatocyte growth factor in rabbit hind limb ischemia model as cytokine supplement therapy. *Hypertension* 33:1379, 1999.

109. Funatsu T, Sawa Y, Ootake S, et al: Hepatocyte growth factor DNA plasmid injection induces optimal angiogenesis in ischemic canine heart: safe and effective strategy for a clinical trial. *Circulation* 102(Suppl II):II-206, 2000.

110. Yasuda S, Goto Y, Baba T, et al: Enhanced secretion of cardiac hepatocyte growth factor from an infarct region is associated with less severe ventricular enlargement and improved cardiac function. *J Am Coll Cardiol* 36:115, 2000.

111. DeLemos JA, Morrow DA, Bentley JH, et al: The prognostic value of B-type natriuretic peptide in patients with acute coronary syndromes. *N Engl J Med* 345:1014, 2001.

112. Kapetanios KI, Pitsavos CE, Economou EV, et al: Hepatocyte growth factor: Potential role of a novel vascular modulator in acute myocardial infarction patients (abstr.). *J Am Coll Cardiol* 37(Suppl A):312A, 2001.

113. Soeki T, Tamura Y, Shinohara H, et al: Role of circulating vascular endothelial growth factor and hepatocyte growth factor in patients with coronary artery disease. *Heart Vessels* 15:105, 2000.

114. Wickline S, Zhu Q, Lewis H, et al: Angiotensin converting enzyme inhibitor reduces VEGF expression by cardiac myofibroblasts in healing infarct scar tissue and attenuates ventricular remodeling (abstr.). *J Am Coll Cardiol* 37(Suppl A):337A, 2001.

115. Shintani S, Murohara T, Ueno T, et al: Local transplantation of autologous bone marrow-derived mononuclear cells augments collateral vessel formation in ischemic hind limb in rabbits (abstr). *Circulation* 100(Suppl I):I-406, 1999.

116. Tomita S, Li RK, Weisel RD, et al: Autologous transplantation of bone marrow cells improves damaged heart function. *Circulation* 100 (1 Suppl):II247, 1999.

117. Tomita S, Li R-K, Weisel RD, et al: Bone marrow cells transplanted into a porcine infarct region induced angiogenesis and improved heart failure. *Circulation* 102(Suppl II):II-650, 2000.

118. Nishiue T, Kamihata H, Matsubara H, et al: Bone marrow-derived mononuclear cell secretes angiogenic factors and its intramyocardial autologous transplantation enhances collateral perfusion in pigs with myocardial ischemia. *Circulation* 102(Suppl II):II-21, 2000.

119. Ueno T, Coussement PK, Murohara T, et al: Therapeutic angiogenesis by bone marrow-derived cell transplantation in pigs with coronary constrictor-induced chronic myocardial ischemia. *J Am Coll Cardiol* 37(Suppl A):48A, 2001.

120. Suzuki K, Murtuza B, Jayakumar J, Suzuki N: Feasibility of single fiber of skeletal muscle as a novel graft for cell transplantation to the heart. *Circulation* 102(Suppl II):II-650, 2000.

121. Lu Y, Shansky J, Del Tatto M, et al: Recombinant vascular endothelial growth factor secreted from tissue-engineered bioartificial muscles promotes localized angiogenesis. *Circulation* 104:594, 2001.

122. Ferrara N, Alitao K: Clinical applications of angiogenic growth factors and their inhibitors. *Nat Med* 5:1359, 1999.

123. Bittle JA: Advances in coronary angioplasty. *N Engl J Med* 335:1290, 1996.

124. Yla-Herttuala S: Vascular gene transfer. *Curr Opin Lipidol* 8:72, 1997.

125. Asahara T, Bauters C, Pastore C, et al: Local delivery of vascular endothelial growth factor accelerates reendothelialization and attenuates intimal hyperplasia in balloon-injured rat carotid artery. *Circulation* 91:2793, 1995.

126. Burke PA, Lehmann-Bruinsma K, Powell JS: Vascular endothelial growth factor causes endothelial proliferation after vascular injury. *Biochem Biophys Res Commun* 297:348, 1995.

127. Asahara T, Chen D, Tsurumi S, et al: Accelerated restitution of endothelial integrity and endothelium-dependent function following phVEGF-165 gene transfer. *Circulation* 94:3291, 1996.

128. Laitinen M, Zachary I, Breier G, et al: VEGF gene transfer reduces intimal thickening via increased production of nitric oxide in carotid arteries. *Hum Gene Ther* 8:1737, 1997.

129. Harada M, Numaguchi Y, Toki Y, et al: Catheter-based prostacyclin synthase gene transfer prevents in-stent restenosis in atheromatous rabbits: A potential strategy for therapeutic angiogenesis via vascular endothelial growth factor (abstr). *J Am Coll Cardiol* 37(Suppl A):49A, 2001.

130. Laitinen M, Makinen K, Manninen H, et al: Adenovirus-mediated gene transfer to lower limb artery of patients with chronic critical leg ischemia. *Hum Gene Ther* 9:1481, 1998.

131. Camenzind E, Kint PP, DiMario C, et al: Intracoronary heparin delivery in humans. Acute feasibility and long-term results. *Circulation* 92:2463, 1995.

132. Greenlish JP, Su LT, Lankford EB, et al: Stable restoration of the sarcoglycan complex in dystrophic muscle perfused with histamine and a recombinant adeno-associated viral vector. *Nat Med* 5:439, 1999.

133. Van Belle E, Tio FO, Couffinhal T, et al: Stent endothelialization: Time course, impact of local catheter delivery, feasibility of recombinant protein administration, and response to cytokine expedition. *Circulation* 95:438, 1997.

134. Hiltunen MO, Laitinen M, Turunen M-P, et al: Intravascular adenovirus-mediated VEGF-C gene transfer inhibits neo-intima formation in balloon-denuded rabbit aorta. *Circulation* 102:2262, 2000.

135. Ferrara N, Winer J, Burton T, et al: Expression of vascular endothelial growth factor does not promote transformation but confers a growth advantage in vivo to Chinese hamster ovary cells. *J Clin Invest* 91(1): 160, 1992.

136. Folkman J, Shing Y: Angiogenesis. *J Biol Chem* 267:10931, 1992.

137. Isner JM, Walsh K, Symes J, et al: Arterial gene therapy for therapeutic angiogenesis in patients with peripheral artery disease. *Circulation* 91(11):2687, 1995.

138. Isner JM, Pieczek A, Schainfeld R, et al: Clinical evidence of angiogenesis after arterial gene transfer of phVEGF165 in patient with ischaemic limb. *Lancet* 348(9024):370, 1996.

139. Makinen K, Laitinen M, Manninen H, et al: Catheter-mediated VEGF gene transfer to human lower limb arteries after PTA (abstr). *Circulation* 100(Suppl I):I-770, 1999.

140. Henry TD, Annex BH, Azrin MA, et al: Final results of the VIVA Trial of rhVEGF for human therapeutic angiogenesis (abstr). *Circulation* 100(Suppl I):I-476, 1999.

141. Freedman B, Vale PR, Kalka C, et al: Plasma VEGF levels after intramyocardial and intramuscular VEGF gene transfer in patients with coronary artery and peripheral artery disease. *Circulation* 102(Suppl II):II-10, 2000.

142. Henry TD, Annex BH, Azrin MA, et al: Double blind, placebo-controlled trial of recombinant human vascular endothelial growth factor—the VIVA trial (abstr). *J Am Coll Cardiol* 33(Suppl A):384A, 1999.

143. Henry TD, McKendall GR, Azrin MA, et al: VIVA trial: One year follow up. *Circulation* 102(Suppl II):II-309, 2000.

144. Rosengart TK, Lee LY, Patel SR, et al: Angiogenesis gene therapy. Phase I assessment of direct intramyocardial administration of an adenovirus vector expressing VEGF121 cDNA to individuals with clinically significant severe coronary artery disease. *Circulation* 100:468, 1999.

145. Losordo DW, Vale PR, Hendel RC, et al: Phase 1/2 placebo-controlled, double-blind, dose-escalating trial of myocardial vascular endothelial growth factor 2 gene transfer in patients with chronic myocardial ischemia. *Circulation* 105:2012, 2002.

146. Vale PR, Symes JF, Esakof DD, et al: Direct myocardial gene transfer of VEGF-165 in patients with endstage coronary artery disease: 12 month results of a phase I/II clinical trial. *J Am Coll Cardiol* 37(Suppl A):285A, 2001.

147. Vale PR, Losordo DW, Dunnington CH, et al: Direct intramyocardial injection of VEGF results in effective gene transfer for patients with chronic myocardial ischemia (abstr). *J Am Coll Cardiol* 33(Suppl A):384A, 1999.

148. Fortuin FD Jr, Vale P, Losordo DW, et al: Direct myocardial gene transfer of vascular endothelial growth factor-2 (VEGF-2) naked DNA via thoracotomy relieves angina pectoris and increases exercise time: One year follow up of a completed dose-escalated phase I study (abstr.). *J Am Coll Cardiol* 37(Suppl A):285A, 2001.

149. Hughes CG, Biswas SS, Yin B, et al: Intramyocardial but not intravenous vascular endothelial growth factor improves regional perfusion in hibernating porcine myocardium (abstr). *Circulation* 100(Suppl I): I-476, 1999.

150. Laitenen M, Hartikainen J, Hiltunen MO, et al: Catheter-mediated vascular endothelial growth factor gene transfer to human coronary arteries after angioplasty. *Hum Gene Ther* 11:263, 2000.

151. Laham RJ, Chronos NA, Pike M, et al: Intracoronary basic fibroblast growth factor (FGF-2) in patients with severe ischemic heart disease: Results of a phase I open-label dose escalation study. *J Am Coll Cardiol* 36:2132, 2000.

152. Laham RJ, Sellke FW, Ware JA, et al: Results of a randomized, double-blind, placebo-controlled study of local perivascular basic fibroblast growth factor (bFGF) treatment in patients undergoing coronary artery bypass surgery (abstr). *J Am Coll Cardiol* 33(Suppl A):383A, 1999.

153. Grines CL, Watkins MW, Helmer G, et al: Angiogenic gene therapy (AGENT) trial in patients with stable angina pectoris. *J Am Coll Cardiol* 38:600, 2001.

154. Lederman RJ, Mendelsohn FO, Anderson RD, et al: Therapeutic angiogenesis with recombinant fibroblast growth factor-2 for intermittent claudication: Results of the TRAFFIC study. *J Am Coll Cardiol* 38:601, 2001.

154a. Simons M, Annex BH, Laham RJ, et al: Pharmacological treatment of coronary artery disease with recombinant fibroblast growth factor-2. Double-blind, randomized, controlled clinical trial. *Circulation* 105:788, 2002.

155. Kraus WE, Duscha BD, Thompson MA, et al: Vascular endothelial growth factor levels in skeletal muscle are reduced in patients with congestive heart failure (abstr.). *Circulation* 100(Suppl I):I-246, 1999.

156. Cherwek DH, Hopkins MB, Hutcheson KA, et al: Relieving exercise intolerance secondary to heart failure: Myoblast-mediated angiogenesis via VEGF delivery to ischemic skeletal muscle (abstr.). *Circulation* 100(Suppl I):I-657, 1999.

157. Ware JA, Simons M: *Angiogenesis and Cardiovascular Disease*. New York: Oxford University Press, 1999.

158. Torry R, Bai L, Miller SJ, et al: Increased vascular endothelial growth factor expression in human hearts with microvascular fibrin. *J Mol Cell Cardiol* 33:175, 2001.

158a. Tateishi-Yuyama E, Matsubara H, Murohara T, et al: Therapeutic angiogenesis for patients with limb ischaemia by autologous transplantation of bone-marrow cells: A pilot study and a randomised controlled trial. *Lancet* 360:427, 2002.

159. Ware JA, Simons M: Angiogenesis in ischemic heart disease. *Nat Med* 3:158, 1997.

160. Fuchs S, Shou M, Baffour R, et al: Lack of correlation between angiographic grading of collateral and myocardial perfusion and function: Implications for the assessment of angiogenic response. *Coron Artery Dis* 12:173, 2001.

161. Bart BA, Herzog CA, Boisjolie CR, et al: Stress echocardiography and nuclear perfusion imaging to assess response to angiogenesis therapy. A double-blind, placebo-controlled clinical trial (abstr.). *J Am Coll Cardiol* 37(Suppl A):7A, 2001.

162. Hendel RC, Vale PR, Losordo DW, et al: The effects of VEGF-2 gene therapy on rest and stress myocardial perfusion: Results of serial SPECT imaging. *Circulation* 102(Suppl II):II-769, 2000.

CHAPTER 39

Innovative Drug Targets for Treating Cardiovascular Disease: Adhesion Molecules, Cytokines, Neuropeptide Y, Calcineurin, Bradykinin, Urotensin, and Heat Shock Protein

William H. Frishman

Avi Retter

Daniel Mobati

Mariana Fernandez

Sameet A. Palkhiwala

Fay Rim

Andre Scott Jung

Shadi Qasqas

Christos Vavasis

Recent advances in vascular and molecular biology have helped to identify groups of molecular entities that can influence normal vascular tone, cardiac function, and the thrombotic process. These substances can also influence various pathophysiologic conditions such as systemic hypertension, left ventricular hypertrophy, congestive heart failure (CHF); vasospasm; unstable angina; acute myocardial infarction, restenosis following angioplasty, reperfusion injury, transplant arteriosclerosis, atherosclerosis, and inflammation. These biologic targets include nitric oxide, thromboxane, prostacyclin, calcineurin, caspases, natriuretic peptides; adenosine, endothelin, vascular active neuropeptides, tissue growth factors, adhesion molecules; osteopontin; tyrosine kinase, protein kinase C, complement, heat shock proteins, and various cytokines. Many of these substances and their biologic receptors are being targeted as possible drug therapies for cardiovascular disease.

Nitric oxide and drugs to potentiate or sustain its action are being investigated for various cardiovascular conditions including myocardial ischemia, erectile dysfunction, and pulmonary hypertension. Endothelin receptor antagonists are being evaluated in patients with systemic hypertension and CHF, and an agent in this class is approved for use in pulmonary hypertension (see Chap. 31). Prostacyclin is now available for the treatment of pulmonary hypertension (see Chap. 25). Thromboxane receptor antagonists are being evaluated as anticoagulant therapies (see Chap. 18). Tissue growth factor inhibitors are being evaluated for prevention of atherosclerosis and myocardial infarction (see Chap. 18). Adenosine is available for the treatment of arrhythmias and is being evaluated for the treatment of ischemic heart disease (see Chap. 32).

In this chapter, adhesion molecules, cytokines, neuropeptide Y, calcineurin, bradykinin, heat shock proteins and their receptors are discussed as examples of possible biologic targets for future drug development. In addition, other innovative targets for future drug development are proposed (Table 39-1).

ADHESION MOLECULES

Adhesion molecules and adhesion receptors are a contributing factor in many cardiovascular disease processes, including thrombosis, restenosis following percutaneous transluminal coronary angioplasty (PTCA), atherosclerosis, and reperfusion injury (Table 39-2). In this section, we review the clinically relevant families of adhesion molecules and elucidate their possible role in cardiovascular therapeutics.

Integrins

Integrins are cell-surface proteins that participate in cell-to-cell and cell-to-matrix communication (Table 39-3).[1] These proteins "integrate" the activities of the extracellular matrix and the cytoskeleton. Each member of this family is composed of a noncovalently linked heterodimer consisting of an α and a β chain (Fig. 39-1).[1-3] Both the α and β subunits are transmembrane proteins with short cytoplasmic tails. Different types of cells assemble and express different α-β complexes. The combination of α and β subunits

TABLE 39-1. Some Potential Biologic Targets for Possible Future Drug Development

Autocrine, Paracrine, and Endocrine Substances	Type of Drug	Disease
Bradykinin	Receptor agonists or metabolism inhibitors	HTN, CHF
Renin (see Chap. 34)	Inhibitors	HTN, CHF
Endothelin (see Chap. 31)	Receptor inhibitors	HTN, CHF, pulmonary HTN
Nitric oxide (see Chap. 33)	NO synthase activators, stabilizers, releasers	IHD, pulmonary HTN, CHF
Natriuretic peptides (see Chap. 27)	Metabolism inhibitors, releasers	HTN, CHF
Adenosine (see Chap. 32)	Adenosine receptor agonists, releasers	IHD, HTN
Vasodilating neuropeptides (see Chap. 27)	Releasers, metabolic inhibitors	HF, HTN
Neuropeptide Y	Receptor inhibitors	HTN, CHF
Serotonin (see Chap. 29)	Receptor, selective	CAD, HTN
Cell adhesion molecules (integrins, selectins, immunoglobulin superfamily)	Inhibitors of receptor activity and binding	IHD, myocarditis
Cytokines (anti-inflammatory substances)	Inhibitors of activity	CHF, MI
Osteopontin	Inhibitors of activity	CHF
Complement	C1-esterase inhibitors	IHD
Intracellular Signal Transduction and Muscle Contraction		
Phospholipase	Inhibitors	HTN
Myosin light-chain kinase	Inhibitors	IHD, CHF
Calmodulin	Inhibitors	IHD, CHF
Protein kinase C	Stimulators	IHD, CHF
Protein phosphatase 2	Inhibitors	IHD
Cyclic AMP and cyclic GMP	Inhibitors of metabolism	IHD, CHF
Tyrosine kinase	Inhibitors	IHD
Cell Growth		
Tissue growth factor (see Chap. 18)	Inhibitors	Restenosis
Tissue growth inhibitors	Stimulation	Atherosclerosis
Calcineurin	Inhibitors	HTN, cardiac hypertrophy
Urotensin	Inhibitors	HTN, CHF

CHF = congestive heart failure; HTN = hypertension; IHD = ischemic heart disease; MI = myocardial infarction.

determines the ligand and specificity. By generating specific subsets of α and β components, the cell can select specific ligands for recognition.

Integrins are components of both "outside-in" and "inside-out" signaling systems.[2] In the "outside-in" signaling pathway, binding of extracellular matrix proteins to the integrins will change gene expression and affect cellular proliferation and differentiation. "Inside-out" signal transduction occurs when leukocytes are recruited during inflammatory responses. Locally derived endothelial chemoattractants generate signals in the leukocyte, which result in an increase in leukocyte integrin affinity for endothelial ligands. This is caused by a conformational change in the extracellular domains of integrins on the cell membrane, resulting in greater affinity for immunoglobulin family member ligands. This process dramatically increases the adhesiveness of leukocytes for endothelium. For example, a discrete site within the I domain of integrin alpha M beta 2 is found and it modulates the adhesion capacity of this receptor.[4] Targeting such sites for the activation of integrins may represent a way to inhibit adhesion of leukocytes to the endothelium.

TABLE 39-2. Role of Adhesion Molecules in Cardiovascular Pathology

Adhesion Molecule	Alteration	Pathology
ICAM, VCAM, selectins, β_2-integrins	Elevation	Atherosclerosis
ICAM, P, and E selectins, integrins	Elevation	Ischemia-reperfusion injury
ICAM, VCAM, E selectins	Elevation	Uncomplicated hypertension
ICAM, VCAM, E selectin	Elevation	Dyslipidemia
PECAM, P selectin, E selectin	Elevation	Congestive heart failure

ICAM = intercellular adhesion molecule; PECAM = platelet endothelial cell adhesion molecule; VCAM = vascular cell adhesion molecule.

Immunoglobulin Superfamily

Members of the immunoglobulin superfamily bind to integrins expressed on leukocytes and play an important role in adhesion strengthening (Table 39-4).[2] Intercellular adhesion molecular-1 (ICAM-1) was found to bind to the leukocyte integrin $\alpha_1\beta_2$ (LFA-1).[2] This interaction serves as a paradigm for other similar

TABLE 39-3. Major Subfamilies of Integrin Molecules and Ligands

Integrin Subfamilies	Ligands	RGD
LA Integrins (β_1 Subfamily, VLAβ, GPIIa, CD29)		
$\alpha_1\beta_1$ (VLA-1, CD49a)	Laminin, collagen	−
$\alpha_2\beta_1$ (VLA-2, GPIa, CD49b)	Collagen, laminin	+
$\alpha_3\beta_1$ (VLA-3, CD49c)	Fibronectin, laminin, collagen	+
$\alpha_4\beta_1$ (VLA-4, CD49d)	Fibronectin, VCAM-1, PP HEV	−
$\alpha_5\beta_1$ (VLA-5, GPIc, CD49e)	Fibronectin	+
$\alpha_6\beta_1$ (VLA-6, GPIc, CD49f)	Laminin	−
Leukocyte Integrins (VLA-5, GPIc, CD49e)		
$\alpha_L\beta_2$ (LFA-1, CD11a)	ICAM-1, ICAM-2	−
$\alpha_M\beta_2$ (Mac-1, CD11b)	ICAM-1, iC3b, fibrinogen	−
	Factor X	
$\alpha_x\beta_2$ (p150, CD11c)	Fibrinogen, iC3b?	−
Cytoadhesions (β_3 Subfamily, Cytoadhesins, GPIIIa, CD61)		
$\alpha_{IIb}\beta_3$ (GPIIb, CD41)	Fibrinogen, fibronectin, vitronectin, von Willebrand factor	+
$\alpha_v\beta_3$ (vitronectin receptor, CD51)	Vitronectin, fibrinogen, von Willebrand factor, thrombospondin, osteopontin	+

CD = cluster determinant; GP = glycoprotein; ICAM = intercellular adhesion molecule; iC3b = breakdown product of third component of complement; LFA = lymphocyte function-associated antigen; VCAM = vascular cell adhesion molecule; VLA = very late after activation.

Source: Modified from Shimizu Y, Shaw L. Lymphocyte adhesion mediated by VLA (beta 1) integrins. In: Hogg N, ed. *Integrins and ICAM-1 in Immune Responses. Chemical Immunology.* Vol 50. Basel: Karger, 1991:34.

interactions between members of the immunoglobulin family and integrins. Intercellular adhesion molecule-2 (ICAM-2) binds to the same integrin.[2] Vascular cell adhesion molecule-1 (VCAM-1) is another member of this family that serves as an endothelial adhesion molecule.[2] VCAM-1 binds to the integrin $\alpha_4\beta_1$ (VLA-4) and $\alpha_4\beta_7$ (LPAM-1). In contrast to ICAM-1 and ICAM-2, VCAM-1 is dramatically induced by inflammatory cytokines in endothelial cells and selectively binds lymphocytes and monocytes. Platelet endothelial cell adhesion molecule-1 (PECAM-1) is involved in the process of leukocyte transmigration[5] and thrombosis.[6]

Selectins

Selectins are a family of adhesion molecules that mediate leukocyte rolling, a prerequisite for later adhesion and migration to the site of inflammation. This leukocyte rolling is mediated by the interaction between selectins on the surface of leukocytes and glycosylated proteins such as GlyCAM on the surface of endothelial cells.[7] Three major types of selectins have been identified: L, P, and E. The N-terminal lectin domain of selectins is important for calcium-dependent binding to their oligosaccharide ligands.[8]

FIGURE 39-1. Four major classes of adhesion receptors, shown embedded in a putative plasma membrane. (*Reproduced with permission from Frenette PS, et al.[2]*)

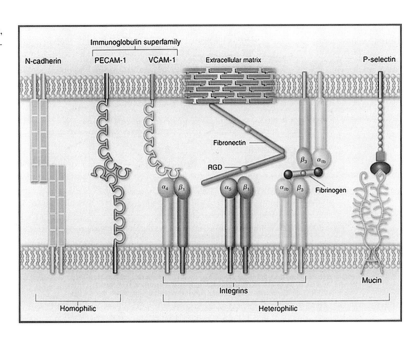

TABLE 39-4. Immunoglobulin Superfamily

Major Glycoprotein	Primary Distribution	Counter-Receptor	Time of Maximal Expression
ICAM-1	Endothelial cells, fibroblasts, epithelial cells, hematopoietic cells	LFA-1, Mac-1	12–24 h
ICAM-2	Same as above	LFA-1	Constitutive
VCAM-1	Endothelial cells, smooth-muscle cells	VLA-4	4–10 h
PECAM-1 (CD31)	Intercellular junction of endothelial cells, platelets		

ICAM = intercellular adhesion molecular; LFA = lymphocyte function-associated antigen; PECAM = platelet endothelial cell adhesion molecule; VCAM = vascular cell adhesion molecule.

Source: Reproduced with permission from Faruqi RM, Dicorleto PE. Mechanisms of monocyte recruitment and accumulation. *Br Heart J* 69(Suppl):S19, 1993.

A selectin is named according to the cell type on which it was originally identified (Table 39-5).[9] L-selectin is found on lymphocytes, neutrophils, and monocytes and mediates lymphocyte homing to lymph nodes.[2,10] E-selectin, found on endothelial cells (expressed on activated vascular endothelium), supports rolling and participates in the adhesion of neutrophils, monocytes, and a subpopulation of memory T lymphocytes to endothelial cells that have been activated by inflammatory cytokines [interleukin-1 (IL-1) and tumor necrosis factor (TNF)] and bacterial endotoxin.[11] P-selectin is stored in α-granules of platelets[12] and Weibel-Palade bodies[13] of endothelial cells, but is rapidly redistributed to the plasma membrane on activation by thrombin or other mediators.[2] P-selectin mediates the adhesion of leukocytes to activated platelets and endothelial cells.[14] Eriksson et al demonstrated that leukocyte rolling can be almost abolished by antibodies blocking the function of P-selectins.[15] P-selectin glycoprotein ligand-1 (PSGL-1) is expressed on the surface of most leukocytes and it is a high affinity ligand for P-selectin. The P-selectin/PSGL-1-mediated interaction between leukocytes and activated platelets or endothelial cells plays an important role in thrombosis and inflammation. Recombinant P-selectin glycoprotein ligand-Ig (rPSGL-Ig) may be useful in preventing reperfusion injury following myocardial ischemia/reperfusion.[16] rPSGL-Ig acts as a P-selectin antagonist by binding to cell-associated P-selectin and inhibiting the P-selectin-mediated cell interaction. In a porcine model, it has been demonstrated that administration of rPSGL-Ig in combination with thrombolytic therapy provides a safe therapeutic method in accelerating thrombolysis, improving reperfusion

and reducing acute reocclusion.[17] A placebo-controlled clinical trial is now in place evaluating the safety and efficacy of recombinant P-selectin glycoprotein ligand-Ig in combination with thrombolytic therapy in patients with acute myocardial infarction. Also a small peptide based on the lectin domain of the three classes of selectins can be used effectively to inhibit leukocyte rolling in vivo.[8] An in vivo model of the leukocyte-endothelium interaction has demonstrated cytokine-induced leukocyte rolling that is critically dependent on P-selectins and modulated by E-selectins and integrins.[15] Alterations in the levels of selectins may regulate PMN-endothelial interaction in vivo.

Cadherins

The cadherin superfamily molecules are known to be involved in many biologic processes, such as cell recognition, cell signaling, cell communication, morphogenesis, angiogenesis, and possibly even neurotransmission.[18] The cadherins are major mediators of calcium-dependent cell-cell adhesion[18a] and are also involved in cell-signaling pathways during development (Table 39-6).

The cadherins form a superfamily with at least six subfamilies, which can be distinguished on the basis of protein domain composition, genomic structure, and phylogenetic analysis of the protein sequences. These subfamilies include classical or type I cadherins, atypical or type II cadherins, desmocollins, desmogleins, protocadherins, and Flamingo cadherins. In addition, several cadherins clearly occupy isolated positions in the cadherin superfamily

TABLE 39-5. Selectins: Nomenclature and Expression

	Cell Distribution	Regulation	Binds to
L-selectin activated cells	All leukocytes	Constitutive surface expression; modulation of activity; shed after cellular activation	LNHEV, endothelial
E-selectin	Activated endothelial cells	IL-1, TNF, LPS; inducible expression(h); RNA; protein synthesis	Neutrophils, monocytes, some T cells
P-selectin	Platelets, Weibel-Palade bodies of endothelial cells	Thrombin, histamine; others from storage granules (min); cytokine inducible (?)	Neutrophils, monocytes, some T cells

IL-1-interleukin-1; LNHEV = lymph node high endothelial venules; LPS = lipopolysaccharide; RNA = ribonucleic acid; TNF = tumor necrosis factor.

Source: Modified from Bevilacqua MP. Endothelial leukocyte adhesion molecules. *Ann Rev Immunol* 11:767, 1993.

TABLE 39-6. Cadherins Relevant to Cardiovascular System: Nomenclature and Expression

Cadherin	Cell Expression
T-cadherin	Smooth-muscle cell
E/VE-cadherin	Endothelial cells
N-cadherin	Endothelial cells

(cadherin-13, -15, -16, -17, Dachsous, RET, FAT, MEGF1).[19] The classic cadherins family is comprised of the N, P, R, B, and E cadherins.

The role of cadherins in cardiovascular physiology and pathophysiology is currently being studied. Smooth-muscle cells (SMCs) have been shown to express T-cadherin (T-cad), an unusual GPI-anchored member of the cadherin family of adhesion molecules. It has been suggested that a phenotype-associated expression of T-cad may be relevant to control of the normal vascular architecture and its remodeling during atherogenesis.[20] Endothelial cells express two major cadherins, VE and N, but only the former consistently participates in adherens junction organization. Down-expression of vascular endothelial (VE) cadherin expression in areas of neovascularization may be related to the accumulation of immunocompetent anti-inflammatory cells within atherosclerotic plaque.[21] Bobryshev et al studied whether the cell adhesion molecule E-cadherin is involved in atherogenesis.[22] The E-cadherin expression in carotid artery and aorta was examined by comparative analysis of consecutive sections and by a double immunostaining procedure. It was found that no E-cadherin + cells were found in normal nonatherosclerotic intima, but E-cadherin + cells were present in 96% of the atherosclerotic lesions. In atherosclerotic intima, E-cadherin was expressed by intimal cells showing varying degrees of transformation into foam cells. Further investigation into the role of cadherins will help to develop a better understanding of their function in cardiovascular disease, and examining them as possible pharmacologic targets.

Role in Thrombosis

Thrombus plays an important role in atherosclerosis, in restenosis after PTCA, as well as in acute myocardial infarction and unsta-

ble angina. Cell adhesion molecules are involved in thrombus formation through the coagulation pathway with leukocyte integrins[23] and through platelet adhesion and aggregation with β_1 and β_3 integrin.[24,25]

Platelets function in normal hemostasis by adhering to subendothelial surfaces after blood vessels have been damaged and then aggregating to form a thrombus.[26] Platelets have a number of cell adhesion molecules (Table 39-7).[27] The GPIb/2a receptor mediates the initial binding of platelets at rest to von Willebrand factor.[24] This interaction induces the transition of the GPIIb/IIIa receptor from an inactive state to an active state, which leads to platelet aggregation. Platelet aggregation is mediated by ligand binding to GPIIb/IIIa. On platelet stimulation with numerous agonists, GPIIb/IIIa becomes activated such that it can bind fibrinogen and several other ligands, including fibronectin, vitronectin, von Willebrand factor, and thrombospondin. The activation and occupancy of GPIIb/IIIa is the final common pathway leading to platelet aggregation. A number of triggers, such as thrombin, subendothelial collagen, or stainless steel from intracoronary stents, can cause exposure of GPIIb/IIIa and platelet aggregation, even if the arachidonic acid pathway is completely blocked by aspirin (via reduction of thromboxane A_2, a potent trigger of platelet activation) or other inhibitors.[28]

Adhesion between platelets and polymorphonuclear leukocytes is an important event in thrombosis. Activated polymorphonuclear leukocyte β_2 integrin binds to the counter-receptor on platelets. Adhesion of platelets to polymorphonuclear leukocytes results in binding of monoclonal antibody (MoAb 24) known as β_2 integrin "activation receptor." It has been shown that anti-CD18 and anti-CD11b inhibitory antibody blocks platelet-polymorphonuclear leukocyte adhesion.[25]

Recently, investigators identified an important role for antiplatelet therapy using a monoclonal antibody directed against GPIIb/IIIa.[29,30] More than 33,000 patients have been evaluated in large-scale, placebo-controlled trials of GPIIb/IIIa receptor antagonist (see Chap. 18). There has been an ongoing effort to develop new and specific antagonists for adhesion molecules. The GPIIb/IIIa receptor antagonists include abciximab (a chimeric monoclonal antibody), eptifibatide (a synthetic peptide), and tirofiban, lamifiban, xemilofiban, sibrafiban, and lefradafiban. Currently, parenteral agents in this class are being used in the treatment of unstable

TABLE 39-7. Platelet Membrane Glycoproteins and Their Receptor Function

Glycoprotein Receptor	Ligand	Platelet Function
GPIIb/IIIa ($\alpha_{IIb}\beta_3$)	Fibrinogen, von Willebrand factor, fibronectin, thrombospondin, vitronectin	Aggregation, adhesion
Vitronectin receptor ($\alpha_v\beta_3$)	Vitronectin, von Willebrand factor, fibronectin, fibrinogen, thrombospondin	Adhesion
GPIa/IIa ($\alpha_2\beta_1$)	Collagen	Adhesion
GPIc/IIa ($\alpha_5\beta_1$)	Fibronectin	Adhesion
GPIc/IIa ($\alpha_6\beta_1$)	Laminin	Adhesion
GPIb/IX	von Willebrand factor, thrombin	Adhesion
GPV	Thrombin substrate	?
GPIV (GPIIIb)	Thrombospondin, collagen	Adhesion
P-selectin leukocyte	Sialyated Lewis X	Platelet-interaction
PECAM (CD31) platelet	PECAM	Platelet-binding

PECAM = platelet endothelial adhesion molecule.

angina and myocardial infarction (MI), and as an adjunct treatment for high-risk angioplasty.

Role in Vascular Inflammation

During reperfusion of ischemic myocardium, there is a well-orchestrated interplay between the coronary vascular endothelium and the circulating neutrophils.[31] This interplay involves the initial slowing or "rolling" of neutrophils along the endothelium during the early moments of reperfusion, followed by firm attachment and amplification of the neutrophil response, and culminating with the diapedesis of neutrophils into the myocardial parenchyma where neutrophil-myocyte interaction contributes to the process of inflammation and necrosis. Adhesion molecules play a significant role in the inflammatory process. Monoclonal antibody blockade studies have demonstrated the functional importance of intercellular adhesion molecules, selectins, and integrins with inflammation.[32] Also, it has been demonstrated that there is an alteration of the expression of various adhesion molecules during inflammation and in a variety of cardiovascular disease processes.[33] Altering the adhesion molecule expression on neutrophils, monocytes, and endothelium may serve as a target for pharmacologic therapy. Furthermore, monitoring the levels of selected adhesion molecules may be of value as a predictor of endothelial injury such as restenosis.

There is strong evidence that chronic inflammation may be playing a role in patients with ischemic heart disease. Patients with coronary artery disease have been shown to have increased levels of ICAM-1 and decreased L-selectin levels, which are indicative of chronic inflammation.[34] From pathologic studies in atherosclerotic plaques, the expression of the leukocyte adhesion molecules (ICAM-1, VCAM-1) on neovasculature and nonendothelial cells was associated with increased intimal leukocyte accumulation.[35] In ApoE-deficient mice, Patel et al demonstrated that α_4 integrin and ICAM-1 play an important role in recruitment of macrophages to atherosclerotic plaques. E-selectin, however, did not appear to be a major contributor to macrophage recruitment.[36] These findings suggest that leukocyte recruitment into the arterial wall may have an important role in the pathogenesis of atherosclerosis.[35] Patients with dyslipidemia have been shown to have significantly higher levels of VCAM-1, ICAM-1, and E-selectin (of soluble cell adhesion molecules) when compared to controls,[37] suggesting that these adhesion molecules may be useful as a marker for atherosclerosis. Aggressive lipid-lowering therapy had limited effects on these levels.

Adhesion molecules may play a role in the pathogenesis of hypertension. In a clinical study, circulating levels of ICAM-1, VCAM-1, and E-selectins are elevated in men with uncomplicated essential hypertension.[38]

P-selectin is elevated in patients with unstable angina and coronary spasm.[39,40] P-selectin mediates platelet-leukocyte and endothelial cell-leukocyte adhesive interactions. Similarly, neutrophil and monocyte CDIIb/CD18 adhesion molecules show a higher expression in the coronary sinus blood of patients having unstable angina.[25,41] There is also an increase in plasma soluble ICAM-1 levels.[42,43]

Leukocyte activation with platelet adhesion occurs following angioplasty.[44] Also coronary angioplasty stimulates cellular activation with an inflammatory response that could contribute to vascular injury, leading to restenosis.[45] An increased expression of CDIIb on monocytes and neutrophils occurs in patients following angioplasty.[45] There is an increase in the expression of neutrophil

CD18 and CD11, monocyte CD14, and platelet GP IIb/IIIa expression, and a decrease in neutrophil L-selectin expression, 15 min after coronary angioplasty.[45] CDIIb promotes the adhesion of monocytes and neutrophils to endothelial cells, extracellular matrix, and smooth-muscle cells. This increased adhesion occurs despite aspirin and heparin therapy, and can predict which patients will have clinical events following angioplasty. ICAM-1 plays an important role in postangioplasty restenosis. It is shown that cytokine TNFα regulates the expression of ICAM-1 in human coronary endothelial cells, which contributes to the inflammatory and immune response after angioplasty.[46] There is also an upregulation of neutrophil adhesion molecule MAC-1 at 48 h after PTCA,[47] as well as significant increase from baseline E-selectin levels in patients who restenose following PTCA, when compared with those who patients who do not restenose.[48] These adhesion molecules may represent markers for endothelial damage and a predictor of subsequent restenosis. In ischemia-reperfusion injury, the functional importance of I-CAM and integrins such as β_2 integrin has been demonstrated by monoclonal antibody blockade studies.[32]

There is evidence to suggest that CHF is a state of immune activation and inflammation involving adhesion molecules on both neutrophils, the vascular endothelium, and the activation of cytokines and nitric oxide. Patients with CHF have increased levels of stimulated ICAM-1, which may relate to increased production of cytokines. In a majority of patients with severe CHF, levels of PECAM-1, P-selectin, and E-selectin are elevated, which might suggest enhanced platelet-endothelial interaction modulated by PECAM-1.[49] In another clinical study, treatment of CHF patients with angiotensin type 1 receptor agonist (candesartan cilexetil) decreased the elevated plasma levels of immune markers such as ICAM-1, VCAM-1, TNFα and IL-6.[50] Serum-soluble ICAM-1 is elevated in patients with transplant coronary artery disease (CAD), posttransplant ischemic events, and cardiac graft failure.[51] Osteopontin activity is also elevated in patients with heart failure. Osteopontin is an extracellular matrix protein that can act as an adhesion molecule, affecting cellular function by interacting with integrins and modulating the expression of inducible nitric oxide synthetase. Angiotensin-II stimulates osteopontin and angiotensin-converting enzyme (ACE) inhibitors may inhibit its production.[52]

Inflammation may play an important role in the pathophysiology of acute MI by causing plaque instability. The soluble adhesion molecule ICAM-1 is expressed on activated endothelial cells, and the plasma level of this molecule is increased in patients with acute MI.[53]

Monoclonal antibodies directed toward selectins and their associated ligands substantiate their role in the dynamic process of neutrophil-mediated reperfusion injury and provide therapeutic targets for interfering with inflammation in myocardial ischemia.[3]

Silver and colleagues[54] demonstrated that selectin blockade with CY1503, given as an adjunct to thrombolytic therapy, interfered with the inflammatory response after ischemia-reperfusion, and significantly reduced infarct size and myocardial neutrophil infiltration well beyond that of thrombolysis alone in the electrolytic canine model. In other rabbit models following angioplasty, blockage of selectins with an analogue of Sialyl-Lewis(x), resulted in larger lumen area, smaller intima area, and a smaller percent area stenosis.[55] These data suggest that selectin blockade could be extremely effective at reducing ischemia-reperfusion injury, MI size, and postangioplasty restenosis.[56]

A study carried out by Ma and colleagues[57] in a cat reperfusion model showed that administration of a monoclonal antibody against

ICAM-1 10 min before reperfusion led to significantly less myocardial necrosis than that occurring in control animals. Recent studies support the finding that ICAM-1 is a critical adhesion molecule in the pathogenesis of ischemia-reperfusion injury, and that the use of monoclonal antibodies raised against ICAM-1 can represent a useful tool for the prevention of ischemia-reperfusion damage.[58]

In a dog infarction model, antibodies against neutrophil adhesion protein CD18 were administered before reperfusion and were found to limit myocardial infarct size by nearly 50%, and preserved global and regional left ventricular function after 48 h of reperfusion.[59]

In studies in rabbits, it was found that leukocyte accumulation in the ischemic zone following left anterior descending coronary artery occlusion aggravated arrhythmogenesis. By inhibiting leukocyte adhesion, arrhythmogenesis was reduced.[60]

Activation of the complement cascade has been observed in many different diseases, including MI and reperfusion injury. C1-esterase inhibitor belongs to the serine protease inhibitor family. It is a major inhibitor of the classical complement pathway. It is also found to have anti-inflammatory properties. C1-esterase inhibitor is consumed in severe inflammation and is beneficial in preventing postoperative myocardial dysfunction due to reperfusion injury.[61,62] The mechanism for this benefit appeared to be inhibition of leukocyte adhesion to the endothelium.[63] Also, recombinant variants of the complement receptor 1, SCRI-SLex, are found to inhibit selectin-mediated interactions of neutrophils and lymphocytes with the endothelium.[61] In an immunohistochemical analysis of ischemic-reperfused myocardial tissue in rat models, it was shown that the classical complement pathway was activated. This led to deposition of C1 on cardiac myocytes and cardiac vessels. Following reperfusion of the ischemic myocardium, there was expression of P-selectin and ICAM-1 on the cardiac vasculature. The C1-esterase inhibitor administration abolished the expression of P-selectins and ICAM-1, in addition to blocking complement activation.[64] Clinical trials using C1-esterase inhibitors in patients undergoing coronary bypass surgery are now in progress.

Conclusion

Cell adhesion molecules play important roles in many cardiovascular processes, including coronary thrombosis, postangioplasty restenosis, MI, and reperfusion injury. Much of the recent attention has been given to the inhibitors of GPIIb/IIIa as an antithrombotic therapy for coronary artery disease. These inhibitors will continue to be tested in randomized trials in patients with MI and unstable angina, as well as in those patients undergoing coronary angioplasty.

Therapies that are targeted at different points in the leukocyte trafficking and adhesion processes may reduce the inflammatory response involved in vascular lesion progression or the initiation of acute ischemia events (Table 39-8). Such strategies include

TABLE 39-8. Clinical Situations in Which Adhesion Molecule Inhibition Could be Beneficial

Unstable angina
Acute myocardial infarction (reducing extent of myocardial injury)
Reperfusion injury
Prevention of restenosis following angioplasty and/or stent placement
Prevention of atherosclerosis
Preventing transplantation rejection

antagonists of leukocyte adhesion molecules such as selectins and ICAM-1.[65,66]

Although a number of important issues with anticell adhesion molecular therapy, such as safety and side effects, have not been adequately addressed in patients, selected monoclonal antibodies or peptide inhibitors against cell adhesion molecules have been evaluated in clinical trials in combination with angioplasty or thrombolysis.

Another strategy (discussed in the next section) is to block certain cytokines that potentiate the inflammatory process, such as TNFα and specific interleukin molecules.[92,93]

CYTOKINES

Cytokines are a group of small pleiotropic endogenous peptides produced by a variety of cell types in response to a variety of different stimuli. (TNFα), interleukin-1-alpha (IL-1α), interleukin-1-beta (IL-1β), and interleukin- (IL-6) are classified as "proinflammatory" cytokines. These substances are responsible for initiating the primary host response to bacterial infections, as well as initiating the repair of injured tissue.[67]

Cytokines are involved in augmenting the expression of adhesion molecules described in the previous section and for enhanced cell-to-cell interactions involved in inflammation. In addition, the proinflammatory cytokines are able to affect cardiovascular functioning by promoting left ventricular remodeling, by causing ventricular dysfunction, and by uncoupling myocardial β receptors.[67] They are elevated in the serum in various cardiovascular disorders and are often a marker of disease severity.[68]

A potential pharmacologic strategy is to inhibit these cytokines and with it the inflammatory response, which could be useful in mitigating reperfusion injury, transplant rejection, CHF, and acute coronary ischemic syndromes. Chronic inhibition of cytokines might impact on the atherosclerotic process and prevent atherosclerotic plaque rupture.

Tumor Necrosis Factor-α

Biologic Role of TNFα

TNFα is a proinflammatory cytokine that was originally discovered, in 1975, as a protein with necrotizing effects in certain transplantable mouse tumors.[69] This cytokine exerts a spectrum of pleiotropic effects in many different cell types.[70] The major biologic role for TNFα is thought to be a host response to systemic infections, most notably gram-negative sepsis.[71] In fact, TNFα levels are considerably elevated in patients with septic shock, and TNFα is implicated as an important mediator in the lethal effect of endotoxin, possibly causing the symptoms characteristic of the "shock state" (Table 39-9).[72] Currently, this cytokine has also been implicated in a variety of cardiac disease states that are not considered to be attributable to bacterial infections, including acute viral myocarditis, cardiac allograft rejection, CHF, and MI (Table 39-10).[73,74]

Three theories are offered as to the source of elevated serum TNF levels in cardiac disease. The first suggests that immune system activation is responsible and that the stimulus is some form of tissue injury resulting in systemic cytokine production.[74] The second theory is that proinflammatory cytokines such as TNF are manufactured by the myocardium itself under conditions of insult and stress, and that elevated serum TNF levels represent a spillover of

TABLE 39-9. Abridged List of the Pathogenic Effects of TNFα Implicated in Septic Shock

System	Effects
Cardiovascular	Hypotension
	Myocardial suppression
	Decreased peripheral vascular resistance
	Decreased pulmonary capillary wedge pressure
	Capillary leakage syndrome
Pulmonary	Adult respiratory distress syndrome
	Capillary leakage with edema
	Leukocyte margination
	Endothelial activation
	Respiratory arrest

Source: Modified from Tracey KJ. The acute and chronic pathophysiological effects of TNF: mediation of septic shock and wasting. In: Beutler B, ed. *Tumor Necrosis Factors: The Molecules and Their Emerging Role in Medicine.* New York: Raven Press, 1992:257.

cytokines produced in the cardiac tissue.[75] The final theory suggests that elevated serum TNF levels occur as a result of the underperfusion of systemic tissues.[76] It is likely that a combination of these theoretical mechanisms is responsible for the elevation of TNF in the peripheral bloodstream.

Many experimental and clinical studies have shown an association between depressed myocardial function and elevated levels of TNFα. However, the nature of this association is not yet clear or agreed upon. There are studies that suggest that the elevated levels of TNFα play a major role in causing myocardial depression, while other studies conclude that TNFα is likely to play a part in the alleviation of this condition.[77] A third school of thought suggests that the elevated levels of TNFα are merely a marker that may indicate the stage of progression of the disease.

TNFα Receptors and Signal Transduction Pathways

The actions of TNFα are initiated by the binding of TNFα to two receptors: a 55-kd, lower affinity receptor (TNFR-1) and a 75-kd, higher affinity receptor (TNFR-2).[71] Both types of receptors have been identified in the human heart and have been immuno-localized in the adult human cardiac myocyte, providing a possible signaling pathway for the negative inotropic effects associated with TNFα.[78]

The nature of the TNFα signaling pathway has not been elucidated in its entirety. However, the involvement of G-proteins has been suggested based on the induction of guanosine triphosphate (GTP) binding activity and the inhibiting effects of pertussis toxin on TNF.α[79] This is followed by the elevation of adenosine 3,5-cyclic

TABLE 39-10. Possible Pathogenic Effects of TNFα in Cardiovascular Disease

Heart failure
   Left ventricular dysfunction
   Left ventricular remodeling
   Cardiomyopathy
   Cachexia
   Abnormalities in myocardial metabolism
   Exercise intolerance
Myocardial Infarction
Pulmonary edema
Atherosclerosis
Allograft rejection
Acute viral myocarditis

monophosphate (cyclic AMP), as evidenced by the fact that pharmacologic agents, which increase intracellular cyclic AMP concentrations, have rendered cells more sensitive to TNF toxicity. TNF also activated a serine kinase.[80] The involvement of tyrosine kinases is unclear, with conflicting evidence being reported.[81,82] Figure 39-2 illustrates the systems activated by TNF which are involved in signal transduction.

An interesting aspect of the TNF receptor is that mammalian cells seem to "shed" their TNF receptors following exposure to certain stimuli, including high levels of TNFα and lipopolysaccharide, seen in patients with heart failure.[83] These soluble truncated versions of the TNF receptors are found in human serum and urine. Several hypotheses have been proposed to explain the function of and reason for the existence and role of these soluble receptors.[84] One suggestion is that the shedding of TNF receptors with high circulating levels of the cytokine functions as an adaptive response that effectively neutralizes the biologic actions of TNFα in heart failure.[85] This is true because the circulating receptors can bind the TNFα, blocking its effects on target cells.[86–88] Along this line of thought, it is logical to devise a therapeutic strategy to infuse these soluble receptors to treat the heart disease associated with elevated levels of TNFα. However, some suggest that these soluble receptors act to enhance, rather than to block, the actions of TNF in pathologic states. Effectively, they claim, the release of these receptors into the bloodstream acts to establish a circulating "pool" of stabilized, biologically active TNF molecules that can be slowly released into the circulation. Along these lines it is possible that these shed receptors may provide a short-term benefit by buffering the deleterious effects of TNF. However, in the long-term, these receptors may be quite harmful. Finally, some investigators claim the soluble receptors neither neutralize nor enhance the actions of TNF. They act, rather, as "markers" for the interaction of the cytokine with its target cell.[87]

Pathophysiology

The exact mechanism(s) responsible for TNF-induced cardiac damage is controversial. There is, however, increasing evidence that TNFα's role in the production of nitric oxide (NO), a potent vasodilator, is responsible for the delayed negative inotropism.[89] It is believed that TNFα stimulates the expression of the inducible form of nitric oxide synthase (iNOS), which controls the conversion of L-arginine to NO. The role that NO plays in the negative inotropism is not clear. Some mechanisms proposed are that (a) NO acts to increase levels of cyclic GMP leading to altered calcium homeostasis;[90] (b) NO leads to a defect in β-adrenergic-stimulated generation of cyclic AMP involved in a G-protein-mediated signal transduction pathway;[91] (c) TNFα stimulation of NO in neonatal myocytes leads to a decrease in the second messenger molecule inositol triphosphate (IP3).[92]

There are several other suggested theories as to the mechanism of TNF-induced myocardial damage. One possibility is that TNF serves to disrupt the handling of calcium in the myocardium independent of its relationship with nitric oxide. This may lead to dysfunctional excitation-contraction coupling, thereby causing systolic/diastolic dysfunction.[70]

Another interesting theory is that TNF induces myocardial, apoptosis, or programmed cell death. Cardiac myocyte apoptosis is characterized by cell death with the maintenance of cell-membrane integrity. Thus, these myocytes do not release creatine kinase and are able to exclude dyes such as Tryptan blue.[93] This may result in the underestimation of cell death during myocardial infarction.

FIGURE 39-2. Tumor necrosis factor (TNF) signal transduction pathways. A cycl. = adenylate cyclase; AP-1 = nuclear transcription factor; cap = cap-binding protein; DAG = diacylglycerol; EGF-R = epidermal growth factor receptor; hsp = heat shock protein; I_kB = inhibitor of NF = $_kB$; NF-$_kB$ = nuclear factor kappa B; P = phosphate; PC = phosphatidylcholine; PC-PL-C/D = PC-specific phospholipase C or D; PL = phospholipids; PLA$_2$ = phospholipase A$_2$; PKA = protein kinase A; PKC = protein kinase C; Ser/Thr PK = serine-threonine protein kinase; TRE = phorbol ester-responsive element; TR60 = TNF receptor type I, 55 to 60 kd; TR80 = TNF receptor type II, 75 to 80 kd. (*Reproduced with permission from Pfizenmaier K, Himmler, Schutze S, et al. TNF receptors and TNF signal transduction. In: Beutler B, ed. Tumor Necrosis Factors: The Molecules and Their Emerging Role in Medicine. New York; Raven Press, 1992:457.*)

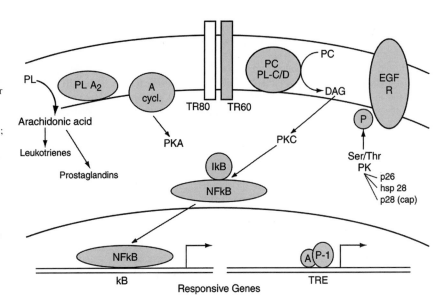

TNF causes apoptosis in various cell types, including cardiac myocytes,[93] through several different mechanisms.

Other possible mechanisms are direct cytotoxicity and oxidant stress.

It seems that TNF induces cardiac dysfunction in a biphasic manner (Fig. 39-3). The early phase occurs minutes after the insult, and the delayed phase seems to occur hours after exposure to TNF. Because it is unlikely that a sufficient quantity of NO is made within minutes of TNF exposure to account for a substantial degree of cardiac insult,[94] it is likely that at least this early phase occurs via a nitrous oxide-independent mechanism.

Role of TNFα in Heart Failure and Atherosclerotic Heart Disease

The expression of TNFα is highly tissue specific. It is expressed under normal conditions in tissue such as the spleen, liver, thymus, and kidney. However, following various types of stimulation (e.g., bacterial sepsis), TNF can be expressed at extremely high levels. In addition, under conditions of myocardial stress, as well as pressure and volume overload, TNF is produced in large quantities in the heart.[88,95] Myocardial TNF is manufactured by macrophages, as well as by cardiac myocytes.[75]

Were it simply for the association of elevated levels of TNFα in patients with advanced heart failure, the scientific rationale for studying TNFα in heart failure would be logical but not intuitively satisfying. However, because there is increasing evidence that suggests that TNFα may play a broad pathophysiologic role in heart failure and that many of the clinical hallmarks of heart failure, including left ventricular dysfunction and remodeling, cardiomyopathy, and pulmonary edema, can be explained by the known biologic effects of TNFα, the rationale for studying TNFα in heart failure is more compelling.[96] TNFα production is increased by the failing heart, which has dynamically regulated receptors,[97] and in myocardial ischemia and reperfusion.[98]

Numerous experimental and clinical studies show the presence of elevated levels of TNF in advanced heart disease.[98a] Historically, a prominent feature in end-stage heart failure is a state called *cachexia,* which is a marked state of constitutional disorder and generalized "wasting away." Cachexia is characterized by a profound reduction of body weight and anorexia, leading to severe muscle wasting and consequent immobility. TNFα is thought to be responsible for many of the cachexic symptoms (Table 39-11). Levine et al[74] assessed the potential role of TNF in the pathogenesis of cardiac cachexia and the severity of heart failure. They measured the serum TNF in 33 patients with heart failure and in 33 age-matched controls. The results of these tests showed that serum levels of TNF were considerably higher in patients with heart failure than in the healthy controls. In addition, the patients with significantly elevated levels of TNFα were more cachexic than those patients with lower levels, and had more advanced heart failure (as evidenced by their higher value for plasma-renin activity). It has been suggested that as heart failure worsens and renal blood flow declines, and the kidney releases prostaglandins into circulation to regulate glomerular filtration and systemic vascular resistance, and that it is these prostaglandins (specifically prostaglandin E$_2$) that stimulate the production of TNF.[99] As production of TNF is increased far in excess of its receptors, there is a spillover of TNFα into the bloodstream. This spillover seems to be responsible for the observed cachexia, increased coagulability, and hypotension often seen in end-stage heart disease.[67] Other studies have also linked TNF to cardiac cachexia.[100] A substudy from the Studies on Left Ventricular Dysfunction (SOLVD) showed that patients with symptomatic heart failure had progressively higher circulating TNF.[101]

Suffredini et al[102] showed that injection of endotoxin into humans results in elevations of TNFα, which leads to depressed left ventricular ejection performance. Current studies also indicate that TNFα produces both immediate and delayed negative inotropic effects on myocardial contractility.[103]

It has also been shown that infusion of high levels of TNFα into dogs produces significant left-ventricular dilatation.[102] This is characterized by an increase in left ventricular unstressed dimension (diastolic creep), a right shift in the left ventricular end-diastolic pressure-volume relationship, and a left shift in the left ventricular end-diastolic pressure-strain relationship. These observations suggest that TNFα alters the diastolic viscoelastic properties of the ventricle, resulting in an increase in left ventricular chamber dimension and a resultant decrease in chamber compliance. The biochemical mechanism for these findings has not been clarified. It is notable that TNFα stimulates the expression of extracellular matrix proteins

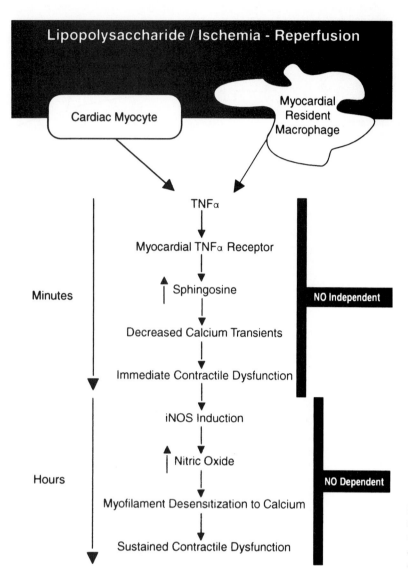

FIGURE 39-3. Myocardial TNF production by both cardiac myocytes and resident macrophages contribute to two phases of contractile dysfunction. (*Reproduced with permission from Meldrum DR. Tumor necrosis factor in the heart. Am J Physiol 274:R577, 1998.*)

such as collagen and regulates the expression of enzymes such as collagenase, which degrade the extracellular matrix.[104] Thus TNFα may play an important role in the remodeling and dilatation of the left ventricle.

Vaddi et al[105] studied the possible role played by TNFα in the triggering and perpetuation of atherosclerosis. The study concluded that TNFα might have a bearing on increased free-radical generation, endothelial injury, recruitment of neutrophils in ischemic-reperfused tissues, and, possibly, the progression of coronary atherosclerosis. Barath et al[106] localized TNFα in a majority of human atherosclerotic tissues.

In addition, TNFα may cause endothelial dysfunction by decreasing levels of the constitutive form of nitric oxide synthase (cNOs), thereby inhibiting endothelial vasodilation. Interestingly, we previously mentioned that TNF may exert a negative inotropic effect on the myocardium by increasing the production of the inducible form of nitric oxide synthase (iNOs). For this reason, it has been suggested that TNFα may contribute importantly to the severe limitation of exercise tolerance characteristic of patients with advanced heart failure via several mechanisms involving the nitric oxide production pathway.[107]

Elevated levels of TNFα have also been observed in patients with pulmonary edema,[108] cardiac allograft rejection,[109] and acute viral myocarditis.[110] Additionally, Pilz et al used TNF and TNF receptor levels together with APACHE (Acute Physiology and Chronic Health Evaluation) scores to prognosticate the hospital course of postcardiac surgical patients.[111]

TNFα's Potential as a Therapeutic Target

Because a strong association and possibly causative relationship exists between TNFα levels and myocardial damage, various drug trials have looked at TNFα and its possible metabolic pathways as therapeutic targets in the treatment of heart disease.[112] Table 39-12 summarizes the possible strategies for preventing toxicity from TNFα.

Fakade et al[113] developed anti-TNFα antibodies and conducted a double-blinded, placebo-controlled study that included 29 control patients and 26 patients suffering from septic shock-like symptoms (hypotension, declining peripheral resistance, etc) that were accompanied by increased levels of TNFα. After injection with the anti-TNFα antibodies and placebo, the study results revealed that those patients treated with antibodies had a significantly reduced

TABLE 39-11. Pathogenic Effects of TNFα Implicated in Cachexia

System	Effects
Cardiovascular	Capillary leakage syndrome
	Dehydration
Gastrointestinal	Decreased motility and absorption
	Increased liver size
	Increased hepatic lipogenesis
	Acute phase protein biosynthesis
	Stimulation of glucagon-mediated amino
	acid uptake by hepatocytes
Central nervous	Anorexia
Metabolic	Suppression of lipoprotein lipase
	Hypertriglyceridemia
	Increased whole-body lipolysis
	Net insulin resistance
	Release of catabolic stress hormones
	Increased whole-body protein turnover
	Net losses of whole-body nitrogen
	and protein
	Hyperaminoacidemia
	Increased amino acid release from
	skeletal muscle
	Net losses of muscle glycogen
	Development of "euthyroid sick" syndrome

Source: Reproduced with permission from Tracey KJ. The acute and chronic pathophysiological effects of TNF: Mediation of septic shock and wasting. In: Beutler B, ed. *Tumor Necrosis Factors: The Molecules and Their Emerging Role in Medicine.* New York: Raven Press, 1992:257.

incidence and severity of shock-like symptoms and undetectable levels of TNFα. It is therefore plausible that these antibodies would be effective in treating those cases of heart disease that are possibly induced by elevated levels of TNFα. Abraham et al showed that mice infected with encephalomyocarditis virus had improved survival and myocardial lesions when monoclonal anti-TNF antibodies were given 1 day prior to virus inoculation.[114] It is, therefore, possible that pretreatment of certain patients (cardiac surgery, etc) with anti-TNF antibodies may prevent the untoward effects of the cytokine. The monoclonal anti-TNF antibody infliximab (Remicade)

TABLE 39-12. Strategies for Preventing Tumor Necrosis Factor (TNF) Toxicity in Critical Care Illnesses

Strategy	Agents
Neutralize bioactive TNF	Chimeric inhibitors, anti-TNF antibodies, soluble TNF receptor, soluble TNF-receptor fusion proteins
Suppress TNF biosynthesis	Glucocorticoids, pentoxifylline, amrinone, cyclosporine A, G-CSF, IL-10, prostaglandin E$_2$, LIF, adenosine, β-agonists
Reduce responsiveness to TNF	Low-dose TNF, low-dose lipopolysaccharide, hydralazine
Inhibit secondary mediators	IL-1, IL-6, interferon-γ, platelet-activating factor, eicosanoid, nitric oxide

G-CSF = granulocyte-colony stimulating factor; IL = interleukin; LIF = leukemia inhibitory factor.

Source: From Frishman WH, Weisen S, Lerro KA, et al. Innovative drug targets for treating cardiovascular disease: Adhesion molecules, cytokines, neuropeptide Y and bradykinin. In: Frishman WH, Sonnenblick EH, eds. *Cardiovascular Pharmacotherapeutics.* New York: McGraw-Hill 1997:892.

has been studied as a treatment in a large randomized clinical trial of patients with heart failure. Upon review of preliminary results, a higher incidence of mortality and hospitalization for worsening heart failure were seen in patients treated with infliximab. Seven of 10 patients treated with infliximab died, as compared to no deaths among the 49 patients on placebo. This drug currently has indications in the treatment of rheumatoid arthritis as well as Crohn's disease, and the drug is contraindicated for use in patients with CHF.

TNFα synthesis can be inhibited by agents that increase intracellular cyclic AMP, which may explain the mechanism by which vesnarinone and amrinone reduce TNFα production.[115] Amrinone inhibition of TNF production is associated with decreased TNF mRNA accumulation. Corticosteroids and pentoxifylline may act by the same mechanism to reduce TNF synthesis, but appear less potent.[116] Simultaneous treatment with both amrinone and corticosteroids can cause additive inhibition of TNF synthesis, suggesting that they also may work by different mechanisms.[117]

Feldman et al[118] conducted a trial treating patients suffering from heart failure with vesnarinone, a quinolinone derivative that inhibits the lipopolysaccharide-stimulated production of TNFα, which is seen in heart failure.[119] The drug improves hemodynamic indexes and exercise capacity. It is possible that part of the efficacy of this pharmacologic intervention on hemodynamics is the inhibition of TNF production with its damaging myocardial effects. In a recent study, however, vesnarinone was shown to increase mortality; consequently, it is no longer being evaluated as a treatment for heart failure.

Other pharmacologic approaches include hydralazine sulfate, which can inhibit some of the biologic effects of TNF,[120] dietary fish oil, which decreases TNF and IL-1 production,[121] nonsteroidal anti-inflammatory drugs, which prevent production of eicosanoids, resulting in the blunting of TNF effects,[117] β-agonists,[122] adenosine,[123] and agents that inhibit platelet-activating factor, a powerful chemoattractant.[117]

It was suggested earlier that TNFα effects its negative inotropism through its role in increasing the production of NO. Therefore, Pinsky et al[124] studied the possibility of blocking the lethal effects of cytokine-induced NO on cardiac myocytes in rats using nitric oxide synthase antagonists (NO synthase is the enzyme whose increased production is induced by TNFα). Results of the study showed that there was significantly less cardiac myocyte death in those rats given the NO synthase antagonist.

As noted earlier, the soluble receptors "shed" by cells may play a role in neutralizing the effects of TNFα. Therefore, it has been suggested that infusions of these soluble receptors might be therapeutically beneficial in the treatment of heart disease aggravated by TNFα.[124a]

Deswal et al used a soluble p75 TNF receptor fusion protein (etanercept) that binds to TNF and neutralized the effect of the cytokine in 12 patients with advanced heart failure. The results of the study showed that there was an improvement in the functional status and quality of life of those patients treated.[125] Recently, a randomized, double-blind, placebo-controlled study assessed the long-term effects and efficacy of etanercept in the treatment of 47 patients with advanced heart failure. The results of this study showed that treatment with etanercept for 3 months was safe and well tolerated, and it resulted in a significant dose-dependent improvement in left ventricular structure and ejection fraction as well as functional status.[126] Multicenter trials have been carried out to assess whether the beneficial effects of etanercept can be sustained over longer periods of time and in larger patient populations. These trials are the

Randomized Etanercept North American Strategy to Study Antagonism of Cytokines (RENAISSANCE), Research into Etanercept Cytokine Antagonism in Ventricular Dysfunction (RECOVER), and Randomized Etanercept Worldwide Evaluation (RENEWAL). Although these studies initially generated some excitement, the trial results have been disappointing.

Finally, the enzyme that processes precursor TNFα has been identified as a microsomal metalloproteinase called TNFα-converting enzyme (TACE). TACE presents a novel target for therapeutic intervention in that inhibitors of the enzyme block TNFα production.

Conclusion

TNFα, a proinflammatory cytokine, has a definite associative and possible causative relationship with heart failure and other states of cardiovascular dysfunction. At this point, we are left with at least two important questions. First, does the increased release of TNFα act to prolong and exacerbate heart failure or does it act to attenuate the symptoms of heart failure after they are already established? Second, what are the "trigger" mechanisms that lead to the sustained release of TNFα in heart failure and other cardiovascular diseases? A deeper understanding of the exact role played by TNFα in these disease states will allow us to better use it as a source or target of therapy.

As of now, pharmacologic approaches to inhibit TNFα activity have not shown clinical benefit in patients with heart failure.

Interleukins

Interleukins represent a broad family of cytokines that are made by hematopoietic cells and act primarily on leukocytes. IL-1 is a cytokine that helps mediate the systemic immune response via the production of prostaglandins.[127] Although almost every cell type in the body can produce the substance under the appropriate conditions, monocytes are considered the main source.[127] IL-1 is produced and released in response to different stimuli, including lipopolysaccharide, microbial toxins, components of the clotting system, and IL-1 itself.[127]

IL-1 is composed of two polypeptides, IL-1α and IL-1β, which are produced by two polypeptide precursors each 270 amino acids long. In turn, the precursors are cleaved to yield the active circulating peptides.[127]

Both IL-1α and IL-1β bind to common receptors and thus have similar biologic effects.[127] Recent studies suggest the presence of two distinct receptors (high and low affinity) for IL-1, each coded for by a single gene. The low-affinity receptor is a surface glycoprotein and a member of the immunoglobulin superfamily.[127]

The effects of IL-1 are mediated through a G-protein-coupled mechanism.[127] An endogenous IL-1 receptor inhibitor exists (IL-1ra); it can block the effects of IL-1.[128]

IL-2 and IL-4 are cytokines associated with the regulation of lymphocyte function. They may regulate lymphocyte activation, growth, and differentiation.[129] IL-2 is also used as an antineoplastic agent that has significant cardiovascular toxicity. Prominent features of this cardiotoxicity that are seen are diffuse capillary leak syndrome, hypotension, tachycardia, and left ventricular dysfunction.[130]

IL-6 is another multipurpose cytokine that mediates both immune and inflammatory responses.[127] It is produced by a variety of different cell types, including mononuclear phagocytes, vascular endothelial cells, and fibroblasts. It is released in response to both TNFα and IL-1, which are thought to induce IL-6 gene expression by the release of nuclear binding protein NF-KB. Increased activity of NF-KB can also induce a coordinated upregulation in the expression of adhesion molecules such as VCAM-1 and various chemokines.[65] IL-6 is also thought to be a major inducer of acute phase reactants. In vitro studies show that IL-6 induces C-reactive protein, serum amyloid A, α-macroglobulin, and fibrinogen by human hepatocytes.[131]

The IL-6 receptor is also a member of the immunoglobulin gene superfamily and appears to interact with another membrane glycoprotein to transmit the intracellular signal.[127]

IL-8 may also be involved in "proinflammatory" responses affecting the cardiovascular system by its effects on chemotaxis and surface receptor expression on leukocytes.[132] Some investigators describe an inhibitory effect of this cytokine on inflammation, but studies using IL-8 antibodies demonstrate that IL-8 inhibition can reduce the extent of vascular injury in experimental models.[132]

IL-10 is a cytokine that is a negative regulator of immune responses as well as an activator of macrophages during cell-mediated immune responses.[133]

IL-18 is a potent proinflammatory cytokine that may play a role in atherosclerotic plaque instability.[133a]

Interleukins in Heart Disease

Recent studies suggest that IL-1 plays a significant role in the pathogenesis of several forms of myocardial dysfunction.[134] It has also been observed to be produced by myocardial cells themselves, in response to injury.[134,134a] Of particular note is IL-1β, which is associated with ischemic heart disease as a trigger for restenosis[135] and as a prothrombotic cytokine, suggested by its elevation in unstable angina.[136]

In patients with mild to moderate heart failure secondary to ischemic or idiopathic dilated cardiomyopathy, an elevation in IL-6 levels were also observed, with no increase in IL-1α levels.[137] Neurohumoral activation could not explain the elaboration of proinflammatory cytokines in heart failure.

In patients with acute MI who were reperfused, there was evidence for cardiac release of the cytokines IL-6 and IL-8.[132] In another study in humans, monocyte-related cytokines were found to increase during acute MI.[138]

Finally, there is also evidence for an endogenous cytokine antagonism system that is amplified during myocardial ischemia.[127,128] In patients with acute MI and unstable angina, elevations in the plasma levels of the anticytokine molecules, α-melanocyte-stimulating hormone and IL-1 receptor antagonist (IL-ra), are found. It is presumed that during myocardial ischemia, anticytokine molecules are released from the myocardium and reduce the amount of inflammation induced by cytokines and other mediators of inflammation.[128]

The explanation for interleukin release in MI and unstable angina is probably related to the inflammatory process triggered by myocardial cell injury.[132] The explanation for why cytokines are elevated in chronic CHF is less clear, but a chronic inflammatory process has been proposed.[87]

In addition to their proinflammatory effects, there is evidence that IL-1 and IL-6 can also have their own unfavorable effects on myocardial function.[139] IL-1 has been shown to upregulate nitric oxide synthetase in cardiac myocytes.[139] Nitric oxide elevations could, in turn, depress the myocardium.[140]

IL-6 elevation in CHF is associated with a poor prognosis. Plasma IL-6 concentrations are related to decreasing functional status of the patient and inversely related to left ventricular ejection fraction.[141] It is also a strong predictor of risk of serious coronary events in patients with unstable angina pectoris.[136,142] Elevated serum IL-6 levels also suggest ongoing infective endocarditis and might be used to aid in diagnosis and monitoring of treatment of the disease.[143] Data relating previous exposure to cytomegalovirus (CMV) with the IL-6 response was a better predictor of cardiac mortality.[144] Increasing titers of CMV correlated with increasing levels of IL-6. Patients with elevated IL-6 levels and CMV had an increased risk of future cardiac death as compared to those patients without IL-6 elevations but CMV seropositivity.

IL-2 and IL-2 receptors are significant in heart disease in terms of cardiotoxicity, as well as have a role in transplant rejection, as IL-2 is an inducer of T lymphocytes in immune response. T lymphocytes have been found in significant numbers in atherosclerotic plaques, indicating immune and inflammatory mechanisms in the pathogenesis of atherosclerosis.[145] A recent study also determined a relationship between T lymphocytes and ischemic heart disease.[146] These data also showed an increase in circulating IL-2 plasma levels in patients with ischemic heart disease. Another study showed that mean levels of IL-2 and soluble IL-2 receptor were significantly higher in patients with stable angina than in those patients with unstable angina.[147] Obviously, the contribution of IL-2 in the development of ischemic heart disease requires further investigation.

IL-4 is a less-studied cytokine with lymphocyte functions associated with cardiac inflammation. Afansyeva et al found that experimental autoimmune myocarditis induced in A/J mice exhibit a Th2-like phenotype.[148] They also found that blocking IL-4 with anti IL-4 monoclonal antibody reduced the severity of myocarditis. The reduction in severity is thought to be associated with a shift from a Th2-like phenotype to a Th1-like one. IL-4-deficient mice develop an enhanced Th1-like phenotype response to *Borrelia burgdorferi* infection.[149] This is thought to control the extent of the cardiac inflammation. The IL-4-deficient mice displayed significantly higher levels of interferon-γ, TNFα, and IL-10.

Not all cytokines may be unfavorable on the myocardium. IL-10 is a potent anti-inflammatory cytokine. Recently, it was proposed that IL-10 inhibits inducible nitric oxide synthase (iNOS) activity after myocardial ischemia-reperfusion and consequently exerts cardioprotective effects.[150] It has been found that deficiency of IL-10 in a knock-out animal model results in significantly larger infarct size than in wild-type hearts. This study also showed that deficiency of both IL-10 and iNOS yielded significantly larger infarct sizes when compared to the wild-type. This suggests that the cardioprotective effects of IL-10 are not dependent on the presence or absence of iNOS. Deficiency if IL-10 also enhances the infiltration of neutrophils into the myocardium after ischemia-reperfusion. IL-10 may also be cardioprotective in the pathogenesis of bacterial endocarditis. Data shows that IL-10 is an important factor in downregulation of monocyte tissue factor activity.[151,151a] Monocyte tissue factor activity is thought to activate the coagulation system and maintain established vegetations.

Proinflammatory Interleukins as Therapeutic Targets

The cardiac inflammatory process may play an important role in reperfusion injury following myocardial infarction and may also increase the short-term risk of recurrent myocardial ischemia. By blocking cytokine production, inhibiting the activity or proinflammatory cytokines with antibodies or soluble receptors, or directly blocking the interleukin receptors, the extent of reperfusion injury could potentially be modified by attenuating cell-to-cell interactions that are amplified by these cytokines. Natural anticytokine substances could also be used to accomplish the same outcome. Interleukins may also be used as treatments for infectious illness, such as myocarditis.[152]

We have already discussed how anti-IL-4 antibody may be beneficial in myocarditis.[148] Cyclosporin, a drug used posttransplant, inhibits IL-2 expression by blocking calcium-dependent signal transduction and inhibits IL-2 receptor expression on T-helper cells and cytotoxic T lymphocytes. There is also a IL-2 receptor monoclonal antibody with antagonist properties. These two drugs are primarily used for reducing rejection in postcardiac transplantation.[153] However, given more research and data on the role of IL-2 in atherosclerosis, they may also be modified for the treatment of ischemic heart disease.

Tranilast, an antiallergic drug that suppresses the release of cytokines, such as platelet-derived growth factor, transforming growth factor-β1, and IL-1β, and prevents keloid formation after skin injury, is in clinical trials. In a preliminary study, treatment with this drug showed a reduced restenosis rate after PTCA; however, a long-term trial showed no apparent benefit.[154]

Commonly used drug therapies may already favorably affect these immunologic or inflammatory parameters. One study examined the effect of high versus low-dose angiotensin-converting enzyme inhibitor on cytokine levels in chronic heart failure.[155] This study showed a significant decrease in IL-6 in patients with severe CHF receiving high-dose enalapril therapy. However, despite treatment, a persistent immune activation existed in these patients, emphasizing the importance of cytokines in the pathogenesis of CHF and a need for better drug therapies for the control of CHF.

Conclusion

The proinflammatory interleukins and TNFα appear to play an important role in amplifying the inflammatory reaction to acute cardiac cellular injury. In addition, these cytokines have their own direct and indirect detrimental effects on both acute and chronic myocardial function. An exciting and potential approach for the future management of cardiovascular injury is to attenuate the effects of proinflammatory cytokines or upregulating cardioprotective cytokines. What is not understood, however, is what effects cytokine inhibition might have on the normal inflammatory response, and, more importantly, whether cytokine release may have some protective effect in patients with cardiac dysfunction. Another area of contention is whether the cytokines are simply markers or are active in causing cardiac injury.

NEUROPEPTIDE Y

Neuropeptide Y is a neurotransmitter that may have significance in the pathophysiology of various cardiovascular diseases, and may serve as an innovative pharmacologic target.[156]

Biochemistry and Physiology

Neuropeptide Y (NPY) functions as a neurotransmitter and modulator of other neurotransmitters, playing a role in cardiovascular control, anxiety, consummatory behavior such as eating, and other processes.[156a] It belongs to a multigene family, together with peptide YY and pancreate polypeptide.[157] Neuropeptide Y is 36 amino

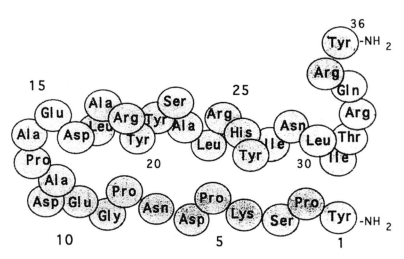

FIGURE 39-4. Structure of neuropeptide Y.

acids long, with a tyrosine residue at the N-terminus and a tyrosine amide at the C-terminus, and folds into a hairpin-like structure with an N-terminal polyproline helix closely apposed to a C-terminal α helix (Fig. 39-4). Neuropeptide Y is very abundant in mammals, and is found centrally in the amygdala, hippocampus, hypothalamus, and locus ceruleus, where it is co-stored with a number of different neurotransmitters.[157] It is also found in the sympathetic nervous system where it is co-stored with norepinephrine in large secretory vesicles and released in response to high-frequency stimulation of postganglionic neurons. In contrast, norepinephrine alone is released from small vesicles in response to low-frequency stimulation. Six mammalian NPY receptor types have been identified, five of which have been cloned to date (Y1, Y2, Y4, Y5, and Y6).[157]

The receptor subtypes are located in target tissues that include a variety of anatomic brain regions, many sympathetic and parasympathetic axons, and postsynaptic smooth-muscle cells of the sympathetically innervated arterial and venous beds.[157] Of the different NPY receptors, it is mainly NPY Y1 and NPY Y2 receptors that have been suggested to be involved in sympathetic vascular control (Table 39-13).

TABLE 39-13. Hemodynamic Effects of Neuropeptide Y

Effect	Target
Peripheral Nervous System	
Y1 Receptor	
Vasoconstriction	Blood vessels
Potentiation of vasoconstriction by other pressors	Blood vessels
Inotropy? (positive, negative)	Myocardium
Y2 Receptor	
Vasoconstriction	Certain blood vessels
Suppression of transmitter release	Sympathetic nerve fibers, parasympathetic nerve fibers, sensory C fibers
Central Nervous System	
Y2 Receptor	
Decrease in heart rate, blood pressure	Nucleus tractus solitarius
Increase in mean arterial pressure and renal vascular resistance	Posterior hypothalamic nucleus and area postrema

The Y1 receptor is a member of the 7-transmembrane α-helix family of membrane proteins, and the substance K receptor is its closest homologue, with 30% sequence identity.[158] The Y1 is the main receptor mediating vasoconstrictive responses in the peripheral nervous system.[158] It is found on postsynaptic smooth-muscle cells of many arteries and veins, where it mediates vasoconstriction and potentiates the vasoconstricting effects of norepinephrine, histamine, angiotensin, and serotonin.[159] Binding of neuropeptide Y is associated with inhibition of adenylate cyclase and/or an increase in intracellular calcium concentration.[157] The Y2 receptor also mediates vasoconstriction in the periphery, where it is presynaptic in location, but notably it is the predominant receptor for neuropeptide Y in the brain where it appears to be coupled to inhibition of adenylate cyclase and suppression of glutamate and norepinephrine release in the locus ceruleus, and suppression of norepinephrine release in the hippocampus.[157] Y3 receptors have been less-well characterized, but may be involved in vasoconstriction in the periphery and function through inhibition of adenylate cyclase and elevation of intracellular calcium levels.[157] The NPY Y4 subtype is present in the periphery, including the heart, skeletal muscle, lung, and intestine, and centrally in the hypothalamus, thalamus, and amygdala; its function is unknown. The NPY Y5 subtype is found centrally in the hypothalamus, where it is related to the regulation of feeding behavior. The characteristics of the Y6 receptor are yet to be identified.

Neuropeptide Y causes vasoconstriction in situ in the human arm, and is released from sympathetic postganglionic axons to mediate vasoconstriction in the coronary, cerebral, renal, and mesenteric vascular beds.[160,161] It is also released from the adrenal medulla, but this site of production and release is not thought to appreciably affect plasma levels, which are determined mainly by sympathetic tone.[156] Neuropeptide Y raises mean arterial pressure and renal vascular resistance and decreases renal blood flow when administered to animals intravenously, in physiologic doses. In general, arteries are more responsive than veins, smaller arteries are more responsive than larger arteries, and larger veins are more responsive than smaller veins.[160] Neuropeptide Y also binds to postsynaptic Y1 receptors to modulate the vasoconstrictive activities of norepinephrine and angiotensin, even in tissues that are insensitive to neuropeptide Y alone.[160] Furthermore, neuropeptide Y binds to presynaptic Y2 receptors to inhibit release of itself and norepinephrine, in a negative feedback control mechanism to dampen down sympathetic tone. Similarly, norepinephrine acts at presynaptic α₂ receptors to inhibit release of itself and neuropeptide Y. Neuropeptide Y can also inhibit release of transmitters from parasympathetic and sensory nerve terminals. Indirect cardiac effects of neuropeptide Y include an increase in preload via venoconstriction and an increase in afterload via arterioconstriction, effects that take place in the peripheral circulation. It also might have direct effects on cardiac myocytes, and studies of cardiac preparations from different species have reported either no inotropic response, a positive inotropic response, or a negative inotropic response.[160] The positive inotropic effect on myocytes is proposed to be produced by inhibition of a vagally mediated negative inotropic response.[156]

The control of cardiovascular physiology by neuropeptide Y is not limited to the periphery; neuropeptide Y is abundant in central nervous system sites known to be important in blood pressure maintenance.[161] Microinjection of neuropeptide Y in the nucleus tractus solitarius results in a fall in blood pressure and heart rate, and application to the posterior hypothalamic nucleus or the area postrema increases mean arterial pressure and resistance in the renal vascular bed.[160]

Role in Heart Disease

The role of neuropeptide Y in the pathophysiology of systemic hypertension is under active investigation in different areas. Stress raises the plasma levels of neuropeptide Y and norepinephrine in humans.[157] In hypertensive patients, sympathetic nervous activity is often increased relative to normotensive controls, which is reflected by increased plasma levels of norepinephrine and neuropeptide Y in a subset of patients. Although the elevated plasma neuropeptide Y levels are at least partially due to increased production and release, the role of altered clearance has not yet been examined.[160] Perhaps more importantly than developing increased plasma levels of neuropeptide Y and norepinephrine, hypertensives demonstrate enhanced vascular reactivity to both neuropeptide Y and catecholamines, which parallels the elevation in blood pressure. However, some studies comparing hypertensive and normotensive patients showed no significant differences in the degree of vasoconstriction with a neuropeptide Y infusion.[162]

It appears that neuropeptide Y is acting to amplify noradrenergic vascular reactivity and to prevent desensitization to norepinephrine in hypertension. There is also evidence for central nervous system downregulation of neuropeptide Y in the cardiovascular control centers of spontaneously hypertensive rats and in rats after myocardial infarction,[163] with decreased sensitivity to neuropeptide Y in their brain centers.[157] Thus, it seems plausible that central and/or peripheral neuropeptide Y plays some role in the pathophysiology of hypertension, although the relative importance in the overall disease process is unclear.

Elevated plasma levels of neuropeptide Y have been found in patients with CHF. However, these elevated levels are not a sensitive marker for early CHF[164] because the neuropeptide Y response decreases with age.[165] In studies of patients with CHF, vascular reactivity to neuropeptide Y seems to vary. Compared to controls, one trial showed a significant increase in venoconstriction as a response to exogenous neuropeptide Y in patients with diminished left ventricular ejection fractions,[166] whereas another trial showed a decreased venoconstrictive response as compared with controls.[167] The expression of Y1 receptors decreases in patients with heart failure, similar to the alterations in adrenergic receptor activity.[168]

Neuropeptide Y may play a role in myocardial ischemia and MI.[163] After the occlusion of the left anterior descending artery in

TABLE 39-14. Possible Roles of NPY in Disease

Cardiovascular	Hypertension
	Hypovolemic and endotoxic shock
	Congestive heart failure
	Pheochromocytoma
	Coronary artery disease
Noncardiovascular	Anticonvulsant
	Anxiety
	Depressive disorders
	Analgesia
	Memory enhancing (Alzheimer's dementia)
	Obesity
	Anorexia nervosa

pigs, a slight but significant increase in neuropeptide Y was seen.[169] In patients with coronary artery disease, the plasma levels of neuropeptide Y directly correlated with the degree and duration of ST segment depression after an exercise test.[170]

Neuropeptide Y may be important in angiogenesis during tissue development and repair. Neuropeptide Y appears to have growth factor properties on cardiac myocytes via G(1) protein coupled to Y5 receptors. In vitro, neuropeptide Y has been shown to promote vessel sprouting, adhesion, migration, proliferation, and capillary tube formation by human endothelial cells mediated by the Y1 and Y2 receptors. Besides being the site of action for neuropeptide Y, the endothelium contains the peptide, its mRNA, and the enzymes related to its activity.[171] Neuropeptide Y could also participate in the development of cardiac hypertrophy during chronic sympathetic stimulation by potentiating α adrenergic signals.[172]

Neuropeptide Y as a Pharmacologic Target

Neuropeptide Y is being actively pursued as a pharmacologic target for the control of hypertension and other cardiovascular and noncardiovascular illnesses (Table 39-14). In the future, centrally acting neuropeptide Y agonists and antagonists, selective for receptor subtypes, could be used emergently to modulate hemodynamic parameters during general anesthesia for management of shock states, or perhaps for long-term control of blood pressure in hypertension. In the periphery, neuropeptide Y antagonists, which do not cross the blood-brain barrier, might be used to control blood pressure in hypertension by dampening sympathetic tone through blockade of the direct and indirect vasoconstrictive effects of neuropeptide Y. Furthermore, neuropeptide Y antagonists might be useful in the management of pheochromocytoma, other hypertensive crises, and vasospastic and atherosclerotic coronary artery disease.

Several peptidic and nonpeptidic antagonists of neuropeptide Y were recently developed (Table 39-15). Compound 1229U91 is

TABLE 39-15. NPY Antagonists Under Investigation

BIBP3226	Selective anti-Y1
BIBO3304	Selective anti-Y1
SR-120819A	Selective anti-Y1
H 409/22	Selective anti-Y1
GW1229(1129U91 or GR23118)	Nonselective (anti-Y1 + agonist-Y4)
BIIE246	Selective anti-Y2
T4-[NPY33-36]4	Selective anti-Y2
CGP71683A	Selective anti-Y2
SYNAPTIC 28	anti-Y5
SYNAPTIC 34	anti-Y5

a nonapeptide dimer that is a potent, highly specific antagonist that binds to Y1 and Y2 receptors.[173] The drug was able to antagonize the neuropeptide Y-mediated elevation in intracellular calcium concentration in HEL cells, and the increase in blood pressure with administration of neuropeptide Y to rats, both Y1-mediated events.[174] However, this compound had no effect on resting blood pressure of kidney perfusion in rats or dogs. A heptapeptide mimic of neuropeptide Y corresponding to residues 22 to 27 was recently shown to antagonize the neuropeptide Y pressor responses and to decrease the resting arterial blood pressure in anesthetized and spontaneously hypertensive rats. Three nonpeptide Y1 selective antagonists (BIBP3226, BRL-672, SR120819A) have also been developed.[175,176] The latter drug, when administered as an oral preparation, is capable of blocking the hypertensive effect of neuropeptide Y in anesthetized guinea pigs 4 h after administration.[176]

Future Directions

Additional clinical research is needed to evaluate the safety and efficacy of the drugs targeting neuropeptide Y receptors and related proteins in the treatment of cardiovascular and noncardiovascular illness.

CALCINEURIN

Cardiac hypertrophy is an important compensatory response by the heart. The heart often responds to a wide array of intrinsic and extrinsic stimuli by increasing the size and mass of individual cardiomyocytes without an increase in cell number. Although initially thought to be beneficial, prolonged pathologic hypertrophy is a major risk factor for dilated cardiomyopathy, heart failure, arrhythmias, and sudden death.[177,178] Thus, it would be of benefit to elucidate the mechanisms for the development of cardiac hypertrophy and possible sites of intervention.[178,179]

A variety of intrinsic and extrinsic pathologic stimuli are responsible for the development of the hypertrophic response in the heart. Extrinsic stimuli consist of pressure overload, volume overload, extracellular factors (Table 39-16) that are either of neuroendocrine origin (e.g., the catecholamines) or those synthesized and

released locally by the myocytes and nonmyocytes in the heart (e.g., endothelin-1 and angiotensin-II).[180] Intrinsic stimuli include contractile abnormalities resulting from altered expression or mutations of sarcomeric proteins. Mutations in myosin heavy chain (MHC), two myosin light chains, α-tropomyosin, troponin-T and -I, myosin-binding protein C, and cardiac α-actin have been identified in patients with hypertrophic cardiomyopathies.[178,179,181] Similarly, overexpression, misexpression, or deletion of several sarcomeric and cytoskeletal proteins in the hearts of transgenic mice result in forms of hypertrophy that mimic human heart disease.

It is well established that cardiomyocytes carrying mutant sarcomeric proteins show alterations in calcium handling and contractility.[182] Because of its well-known role in excitation-contraction coupling, increased calcium concentration has been suggested to be an intrinsic factor that plays an essential role in gene expression and growth in cardiomyocytes.[183] Molkentin et al[184] have provided evidence that the calcium/calmodulin (CaM)-dependent phosphoprotein phosphatase calcineurin plays a significant role in cardiomyocyte hypertrophy. An overexpressed calcineurin leads to cardiac hypertrophy in transgenic mice.[179] This suggests an intimate connection between calcium and calcineurin in the process of cardiac hypertrophy.[185] Since then, many research studies have been conducted to elucidate the importance of calcineurin and the potential effects of calcineurin inhibition by the drugs cyclosporin A and FK506 to prevent pathologic cardiac hypertrophy and subsequent heart failure.

Calcineurin and Its Signaling Pathway

Calcineurin is a universally expressed serine- and threonine-protein phosphatase dependent on calcium and CaM for activation. It is a heterodimer of a 60-kd CaM-binding catalytic A subunit and a 19-kd calcium-binding regulatory B subunit. The enzyme resides primarily in the cytoplasm.[186] All calcineurin A isoforms include N-terminal and C-terminal variable domains, a catalytic domain, and a regulatory domain. The regulatory domain contains a calcineurin B-binding helix, a CaM-binding domain, and an autoinhibitory region that binds to the active site preventing enzymatic activity at low calcium concentrations. There are two catalytic subunit genes and one regulatory subunit gene in mice and humans. Only one of the

TABLE 39-16. Extracellular Stimuli of Ventricular Myocyte Hypertrophy

Agonist Type	Examples	Point of Action
Vasoactive peptides → nPKCs	ET-1, Ang II	$G\alpha 9/G\alpha 11 \rightarrow$ PtdlnsP$_2$ hydrolysis
α1-adrenergic agonist → nPKCs?	NE/E, phenylephrine	$G\alpha 9/G\alpha 11 \rightarrow$ PtdlnsP$_2$ hydrolysis
Direct activators of PKC	Tumor promoting phorbol esters	nPKCs/cPKCs
Peptide growth factors	FbGF, IGF-1	Receptor protein tyrosine kinases
Cytokines	Cardiotrophin-1	GP130/IL-6 receptor
Arachidonate metabolites	PGF$_{2a}$	JNKs
Mechanical stretch	Autocrine/paracrine factors (ET-1, Ang II or PGF$_{2a}$)	PtdlnsP$_2$ hydrolysis/PKCs/JNKs?
Cell contact	Not known	Not known

Ang = angiotensin; NE = norepinephrine; cPKC = classical isoform of protein kinase C; E = epinephrine; ET = endothelin; FbGF = fibroblast growth factor; GP = glycoprotein; IGF = insulin-like growth factor; IL = interleukin; nPKC = novel isoform of protein kinase C; PGF$_{2a}$ = prostaglandin F$_{2a}$.

Source: Reproduced with permission from Sugden PH. Signaling in myocardial hypertrophy: Life after calcineurin? *Circ Res* 84:633–646, 1999.

catalytic subunit genes has been knocked-out in mice.[187] These mutant mice are viable and do not show any cardiac defects.

Many studies support the premise that calcium is a primary signal for cardiac hypertrophy. Hypertrophic agonists, such as angiotensin-II, phenylephrine, and endothelin-1, activate calcium-dependent signaling systems.[188] In addition, myocyte stretch, increased loads on working heart preparations, use of calcium-channel agonists, treatment with calcium ionophores, and electrical pacing can also elevate calcium and induce cardiomyocyte hypertrophy.[189] It is the prolonged increases in basal concentrations of calcium, but not transient calcium spikes during each phase of contraction/relaxation that are responsible for the activation of calcineurin. It is likely that calcium pools are compartmentalized in cardiomyocytes such that calcium pools that signal the hypertrophic response are distinct from those involved in excitation/contraction coupling in the sarcoplasmic reticulum. This notion is supported by the ability of calcium-channel blockers, which act at the cell membrane, to attenuate the hypertrophic response. There must be a specific role for calcium in the area of the cell membrane for hypertrophic signaling, because changes in calcium concentration at the cell membrane are dramatically less than in the region of the sarcoplasmic reticulum during contraction/relaxation.

Calcineurin is involved in NFAT (nuclear factor of activated T cells)-mediated T-lymphocyte activation. NFATs are a family of Rel homology transcription factors, a group that also includes nuclear factor kappa B. There are four known NFAT proteins: NFAT1, NFAT2, and NFAT4 are expressed at the highest levels in immune cells and skeletal muscle, whereas NFAT3 is expressed in a wide range of tissues, including the adult heart. In the inactive state, NFATs are phosphorylated and are located in the cytoplasm. NFATs are tightly associated with calcineurin (independent of their phosphorylation state). When T lymphocytes bind to antigen-presenting cells through T-lymphocyte receptors, cytoplasmic calcium concentrations increase and calcineurin is activated, causing NFAT dephosphorylation[186,190] (Fig. 39-5). Then NFAT complexed to calcineurin[191] migrates into the nucleus and upregulates the transcription of a number of genes, such as those for interleukin-2 (an autocrine growth factor in T-lymphocytes) and other lymphocyte growth factors. The transcription factor GATA4 is present in adult heart and a limited number of other tissues.[192] Molkentin et al[184] reported that GATA4 synergized with calcineurin and NFAT3 activates the brain natriuretic peptide (BNP) promoter in neonatal rat cardiomyocytes and that a high-affinity NFAT binding site within the BNP promoter was required for synergistic activation by GATA4 and NFAT3. Other than BNP, GATA4 causes a positive regulation of hypertrophic marker genes, including atrial natriuretic factor (ANF), and β-MHC.[188,193] Overexpression of calcineurin or constitute nuclear NFAT3 mutant produces substantial hypertrophy that rapidly progresses to heart failure.[194]

There is clear evidence that the calcineurin/NFAT pathway interacts with other signaling pathways. NFATs interact with the activator protein-1 (AP-1) transcription factor complex to bind to the 5'-regulatory region of the interleukin-2 gene in the nucleus, and the MAPK cascades and Ras superfamily control AP-1 transactivating activity.[195] In addition, there are examples of an interaction of calcium with the ERK and JNK cascades in myocytes.[196] Another study suggests that the PKC → Ras → Raf → MKK1/-2 → ERK pathway may cause changes in calcium transients similar to those seen in cardiac hypertrophy and heart failure[197] (Fig. 39-6).

Effects of Anticalcineurin Therapy

Studies suggest that calcineurin is involved in pathologic cardiac hypertrophy. Indubitably, agents that target calcineurin have been explored. Immunosuppressant drugs cyclosporin A (CsA) and tacrolimus (FK506) inhibit enzymatic activity, thereby decreasing T-cell receptor signaling.[198,198a] These drugs interact specifically with the cytoplasmic immunophilin proteins, cyclophilins, and FK506 binding protein-12 (FKBP12), respectively, to form inhibitory complexes that bind the calcineurin A subunit.[199] CsA and FK506 do not affect early biochemical events associated with signaling at the cell membrane, for example, phosphatidylinositol turnover, calcium mobilization, and protein kinase C (PKC) activation.[200] Therefore, they can be used to discriminate the roles of such signals from calcineurin activation in cellular responses, like hypertrophy. Another immunosuppressant, rapamycin also binds

FIGURE 39-5. Calcineurin signaling in T cells. Activation of the T-cell receptor leads to elevation of [Ca^{2+}] and activation of calcineurin, which dephosphorylates NFAT proteins. On removal of phosphate (indicated by circled P), NFAT proteins translocate to the nucleus and activate gene expression together with AP-1. CsA and FK506 interact with the cytoplasmic binding proteins cyclophilin (CyP) and PKBP12, respectively, to form complexes that inhibit calcineurin activity. (*Reproduced with permission from Olson EN, Molkentin JD. Prevention of cardiac hypertrophy by calcineurin inhibition: hope or hype? Circ Res 84:625, 1999.*)

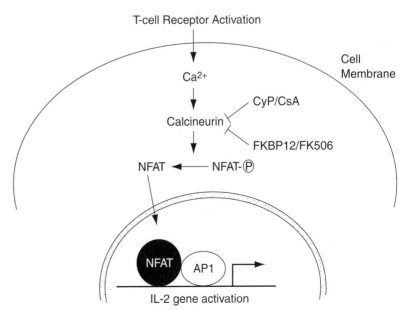

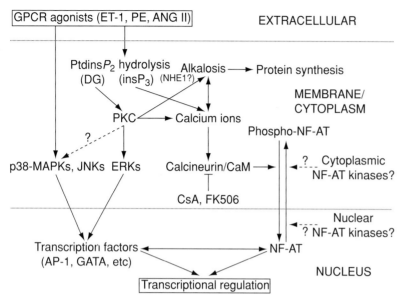

FIGURE 39-6. Putative interactions between the MAPK and calcineurin signaling pathways. GPCR agonists activate MAPs, with at least the ERKs being activated by a mechanism involving hydrolysis of membrane $PtdInsP_2$ and PKC. MAPKs then mediate the phosphorylation of nuclear transcription factors. In addition, activation of PKC leads to changes in calcium handling (through phosphorylation of channels and pumps), and increases in pH_1 [possibly mediated by the Na^+/H^+ exchanger 1 (NHE1)]. The significance of $InsP_3$ (from $PtdInsP_2$ hydrolysis) in cardiac calcium handling is unclear. Increases in calcium concentrations of pH_1 lead to increased binding of calcium to effector proteins such as calcineurin and CaM. Activation of calcineurin dephosphorylates NFAT, which translocates into the nuclear to interact with other transcription factors to regulate transcription. Poorly characterized NFAT kinases phosphorylate NFAT, causing its return to or retention in the cytoplasm. Furthermore, small increases in pH_1 stimulate protein synthesis at the level of translation by a poorly understood mechanism. (*Reproduced with permission from Sugden PH. Signaling in myocardial hypertrophy: Life after calcineurin? Circ Res 84:633–646, 1999.*)

FKBP12 but does not inhibit calcineurin activity,[192] which shows that formation of immunophilin-ligand complex is not sufficient to inhibit calcineurin.

Molkentin et al[184] demonstrated that calcineurin plays a vital role in the development of cardiac hypertrophy and that the calcineurin inhibitors CsA and FK506 could prevent cardiac hypertrophy in activated calcineurin transgenic mice and in humoral factor induced hypertrophy of cultured cardiomyocytes of neonatal rats. Sussman et al[179] also reported that several transgenic mice models that show hypertrophic cardiomyopathy could be treated with CsA. It should be noted that CsA did not prevent the cardiac hypertrophy induced by cardiospecific expression of an activated retinoic acid receptor. This implies that some forms of myocardial hypertrophy may be mediated by calcineurin-independent signaling pathways[179] or that there may be multiple mediators in cardiac hypertrophy, one of which is calcineurin. Sussman et al[179] reported decrease in cardiac hypertrophy on mice models with intrinsic and extrinsic stimuli upon treatment with CsA and FK506. Lim et al[280] also showed prevention of cardiac hypertrophy in pressure-overloaded mice models with CsA. Haines et al[201] reported possible synergistic effects in improving postischemic cardiac function with the calcineurin inhibitor FK506 and the free radical scavenger Egb 761.

Zhang et al[202] tested the ability of calcineurin inhibitors to prevent pressure-overload left ventricular hypertrophy using two widely accepted rat models: the spontaneously hypertensive rat and suprarenal aortic banding. Notably, these investigators studied multiple time points in the hypertrophy process and different times for initiation of drug administration. Despite elevated calcineurin phosphatase activity in the hearts of the two rodent hypertrophy models and nearly complete inhibition (90%) of phosphatase activity by CsA in the hypertrophied myocardium of the treated groups, neither the amount of cardiac hypertrophy nor cardiac function was appreciably changed. Ding et al[203] also reported on the effects of CsA administration regarding the degree of pressure-overload hypertrophy induced by 4 weeks of ascending aortic banding in mice and similarly, they failed to observe any increase in the amount of cardiac hypertrophy between CsA-treated and control banded mice, despite comparable elevations of left ventricular systolic pressure. In contrast to all prior studies, they measured a decrease in cal-

cineurin phosphatase activity in hypertrophied hearts, as compared with normal hearts, that was further reduced by CsA administration. Later on, Megura et al[204] demonstrated the effects of calcineurin inhibition by CsA on the degree of hypertrophy produced by transverse aortic banding in mice. Calcineurin phosphatase activity in the myocardium did not differ between hypertrophied and control hearts but was decreased by CsA administration. These differences may be attributable to variations in experimental technique or to the time course of hypertrophy in pressure-overload models. More importantly, it is not clear whether administration of CsA during the decompensated phase of hypertrophy/heart failure (rather than prophylactic use) is beneficial.

CsA and FK506 are currently used to prevent allograft tissue rejection after organ transplantation. They have been anticipated to have positive or negative effects on cardiac hypertrophy. However, the clinical data correlating CsA treatment with cardiac function are inconclusive.[205] A number of studies in transplant patients have examined the association of cardiac hypertrophy with the use of CsA. Although some studies failed to detect a convincing association,[206] other studies show that CsA may actually induce cardiac hypertrophy through its hypertensive side effects.[207] Additionally, CsA is a relatively toxic drug that can cause problems of immunosuppression (increased opportunistic infections and skin malignancies) and nephrotoxicity that may be caused by its interference with the calcineurin-dependent regulation of convoluted tubule Na^+/K^+-ATPase.[208] Its use is also associated with hypertension, possibly because of the nephrotoxic side effects involving renal vasoconstriction,[209] neural effects (tremor and fits), hepatotoxicity, and gingival hypertrophy/hyperplasia. Also, Hojo et al[210] demonstrated that CsA may directly induce cancer progression (a known complication of this form of immunosuppressive therapy after orthotopic transplantation) by stimulating the production of transforming growth factor-beta (TGFβ). The mechanism for enhanced TGFβ production is unknown, but the cardiotrophic effects of this growth factor may offset the results of CsA inhibition of calcium calcineurin-NFAT3-GATA4 in vivo. Although FK506 may cause fewer side effects, it is more expensive than CsA[209].

Other innovative strategies to inhibit calcineurin and therefore the hypertrophic process include the use of a myocyte-enriched calcineurin-interacting protein[211] and gene therapy to express calcineurin inhibitory protein domains.[212]

The evolving information regarding the potential role of the calcineurin pathway in the production of cardiac hypertrophy and failure shows the importance of multidisciplinary studies in this area. Shimoyama et al[213] suggested that calcineurin plays an important role in the development of load-induced cardiac hypertrophy, which is most often observed clinically. Additionally, Lim et al[214] demonstrated that calcineurin is activated in the heart in human heart failure. It may not be realistic to use calcineurin inhibitors (CsA and FK506) in their present formulations because of their potential harmful side effects. However, because the possibility exists that inhibition of calcineurin may prevent not only the development of cardiac hypertrophy but also that of heart failure, it should be worthwhile to develop novel calcineurin inhibitors, and to develop drug systems of delivery that are specific to the cardiac tissues. It is unlikely that a single signaling pathway is responsible for the overall hypertrophic response. That is why, interaction of the calcineurin pathway with other signaling pathways, like the MAPK pathways, should be examined in detail. An extensive study in the signaling pathways may also reveal other possible sites for drug intervention.

BRADYKININ AND THE KININ-KALLIKREIN SYSTEM

Bradykinin is a vasoactive kinin that is liberated from its substrate kininogen by the action of kallikrein, and is known to be involved in a wide range of biologic processes.[215] It may play an important role in blood pressure regulation and the maintenance of normal blood flow. Moreover, in various pathologic states of the cardiovascular system, it appears to provide protective actions against ischemic injury, ventricular hypertrophy, congestive heart failure, and thrombosis (Fig. 39-7).[215]

Bradykinin is a potent vasodilator that acts through endothelial B2 kinin receptors to stimulate the release of nitric oxide and endothelium-derived hyperpolarizing factor.[216] Bradykinin deficiency states may play a role in some forms of hypertension,[215] and a relative deficiency in bradykinin may be a contributing factor to worsening heart failure. Experimental studies revealed that mice

lacking the B2-receptor gene were more likely to develop hypertension, cardiac hypertrophy, and myocardial damage.[217] It seems quite clear that bradykinin has the potential to be an important pharmacologic target for treatment of cardiovascular disease.[218]

Kinin Physiology

Kinins exert several biologic actions. They are involved in nociception, inflammation, capillary permeability, reactive hyperemia, and stimulation of cellular glucose uptake.[219] Bradykinin is a polypeptide that circulates in the plasma in very low concentrations in comparison with the amount of bradykinin found in various body tissues.[215] Kininogens (α_2 globulins) are synthesized in the liver and circulate at high concentrations in the plasma. There are two kininogenases that convert kininogens into bradykinin: plasma kallikrein, also known as Fletcher factor, and glandular kallikrein, also known as tissue kallikrein.[215] The two kallikreins are distinct enzymes with different molecular weights.[215] Plasma kallikrein forms bradykinin from high-molecular-weight kininogen and glandular kallikrein forms lys-bradykinin from both high- and low-molecular-weight kininogen.[215] The kinins have very short half-lives in the plasma and are rapidly degraded[215] by various kinases. Kinase-1 is a plasma carboxypeptidase which is synthesized in the liver. Kinase-2 is an angiotensin-converting enzyme that converts angiotensin-I to angiotensin-II and also inactivates other peptides.[215] Other kinases, such as neutral endopeptidase, also destroy the natriuretic peptides and endothelin. Plasma kinin levels have been shown to not change much even when all the known kinases are inhibited, suggesting that undiscovered substances may also be contributing to bradykinin degradation.[215,220]

Bradykinin Receptors

Bradykinin receptors have been characterized by use of various bradykinin analogues.[215] These receptors, known as B1 and B2, cause the various physiologic actions of bradykinin through different second messengers and mediators (nitric oxide, prostaglandins).[221] Both receptors are predominantly coupled to the same Gα subunit, leading to the release of inositol phosphates and, thereby, to an increase in intracellular calcium upon ligand stimulation.[222]

FIGURE 39-7. Mechanism of kinin generation and effects of kinins, either directly or via various intermediates (EDRF, EDHF, eicosanoids, and t-PA). [*Reproduced with permission from Carretero OA. Kinins: Local hormones in regulation of blood pressure and renal function. Choices Cardiol 7 (Suppl 1):10, 1993.*]

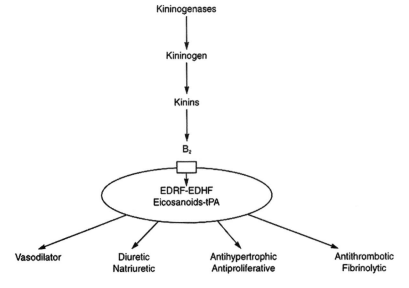

The B1 receptors are expressed de novo mainly under pathologic conditions such as inflammation and sepsis.[222] B1 agonists are available that include des-Arg[9]-bradykinin.

The B2 receptors are ubiquitously expressed in many tissues and cell lines.[222] These receptors mediate most of the effects of bradykinin and lys-bradykinin. They are transmembrane G-protein-linked serpentine receptors, and are also divided into B2A and B2B subtypes.[223] The synthetic nonspecific B2-antagonist HOE 140, a long-acting potent agent, has been extremely helpful in delineating the body's physiologic activities mediated through B2-receptor activity.[224] Other antagonists and agonists are available.[225]

The binding of kinins to B2 receptors on plasma membranes leads to G-protein-coupled stimulation of phospholipase-C, which catalyzes the hydrolysis of phosphatidal inositol 4-5 diphosphate (PIP2) to inositol triphosphate (IP3) and diacylglycerol (DAG). IP3 diffuses to the endoplasmic reticulum and causes the release of calcium ions to cause various physiologic effects, such as stimulation of phospholipase A2, leading to the release of arachidonic acid from membrane phospholipids. In vascular tissue, most of the arachidonic acid is converted into vasodilator prostaglandins (PGI_2, PGE_2), which, in turn, are responsible for some of the vasodilating actions of kinins. Nitric oxide production is also enhanced, which contributes to the vasodilatory actions of bradykinin.[226]

The B2 receptor was recently cloned,[227] and much work is being done with various B2-receptor antagonists and agonists to further elucidate bradykinin's physiologic activity, as well as providing the test compounds for possible future drugs.

Potential Clinical Applications of Bradykinin Augmentation and Blockade

Enhancement of the kallikrein system may have important clinical value in the treatment of hypertension, ischemic heart disease, and congestive heart failure. There is experimental evidence that bradykinin levels are elevated in cardiac ischemia, myocardial in-

farction, and congestive heart failure.[228] It is believed that these elevated levels of bradykinin play a protective role. Approaches to enhancing the activity of bradykinin can come from inhibition of its degradation by using drugs such as ACE inhibitors, neutral endopeptidase (NEP) inhibitors, and their combination, or by using agents that act directly to stimulate the B2 receptor. Bradykinin infusion would be too short-lived because of its rapid degradation in the body.

Possible strategies for targeting the kallikrein-kinin system to treat cardiovascular disease are (a) to develop more sensitive assays for measurement of kinins to identify patients with a deficiency state; (b) to develop long-acting kinin analogues to stimulate B2 receptors; (c) to indirectly potentiate bradykinin activity by the combined use of ACE inhibitors and NEP inhibitors; (d) to develop even more inclusive kinase inhibitors to potentiate bradykinin's actions; (e) to bypass the kallikrein-kinin system by potentiating the actions of nitric oxide and/or prostacyclin; and (f) to use gene therapy for treating patients with either kallikrein-kinin defective or deficient genes.

Systemic Hypertension

The kallikrein-kinin system plays an important role both in the kidneys and vascular tissues in helping to regulate blood pressure.[215] Kinins are involved in the blood pressure-lowering effects of ACE inhibitors in all forms of hypertension associated with stimulation of the renin-angiotensin system.[229] Through its effects on PGE_2, prostacyclin, and endothelium-derived relaxing factor (EDRF), bradykinin exerts natriuretic and diuretic effects in the kidney and a vasodilator action on peripheral blood vessels.[215,230] Exogenous bradykinin injected intravenously or intra-arterially can induce an immediate and dose-related dilatation of the vessels, resulting in decreases in total peripheral resistance and systemic blood pressure (Fig. 39-8), as well as an increase in venous pooling and a reduced cardiac preload.[229] Exogenous kinin administration may also lower blood pressure by increasing renal blood flow and natriuresis.[231] One can see how an impaired kallikrein-kinin system in the tissue (Fig. 39-9) could be an important etiologic factor in hypertension

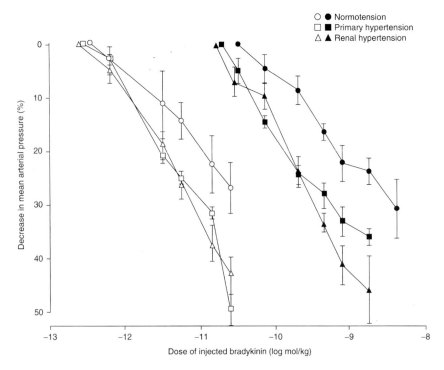

FIGURE 39-8. Bradykinin-induced reduction in mean arterial pressure in six healthy volunteers, five patients with primary hypertension, and five patients with renal hypertension. Pretreatment with captopril 50 mg (open symbols) clearly shifted the dose response curve of the control experiment (closed symbols) to the left. Mean values ± SEM are shown. [*Reproduced with permission from Bonner G, Schunk U, Preis S, et al. Effect of bradykinin on systemic and pulmonary circulation in healthy and hypertensive humans. J Cardiovasc Pharmacol 15(Suppl 6):S46–S56, 1990.*]

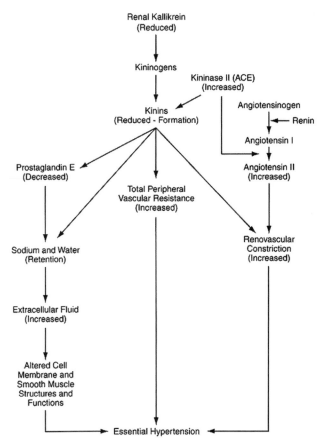

FIGURE 39-9. A hypothetical potentiation of the involvement of the renal kallikrein-kinin, prostaglandin and renin-angiotensin systems in the pathophysiology of essential hypertension. (*Reproduced with permission from Su JB, et al.[237]*)

and why an ACE inhibitor might be an important drug to use for blood pressure control in these patients. The importance of the kallikrein-kinin system on blood pressure control has been elucidated using ACE inhibitors and B2-receptor blockers in various experiments.[232,233] ACE inhibitors potentiate actions of both endogenous and exogenous bradykinin by about fiftyfold.[229] ACE inhibitors inhibit the degradation of endogenous bradykinin and the blood pressure-lowering activity of the drugs can be inhibited by use of the B2-receptor blocker HOE 140.[232] In one study, rats with renovascular hypertension were pretreated with ACE inhibitors. The rats were then infused with bradykinin receptor antagonists, resulting in a 25 to 30% decrease in the antihypertensive effect of the ACE inhibitor.[229]

Differences exist regarding the role of bradykinin in the acute versus chronic hypotensive effects of ACE inhibitors. Bradykinin appears to contribute only to the acute (1 week) hypotensive effect of ACE inhibitors, and not to the chronic (4 weeks) hypotensive effect.[233]

Hypotension

It is of interest that a deficiency of kinase-1 activity and an increase in kinin activity has been identified in patients with orthostatic hypotension.[234] An increased production of kallikrein may be the cause of vasodilation and hypotension in gram-negative sepsis. Thus, there may be a role for the B2 antagonists as a therapeutic agent for these conditions.

Myocardial Ischemia

Endogenous bradykinin has an important role in mediating normal vasomotor responses in both resistance and epicardial coronary arteries under basal and flow-stimulated conditions in the normal human coronary circulation.[216] The use of HOE 140, a specific B2-receptor blocker, was shown to cause an increase in coronary vascular resistance and a decrease in coronary blood flow, actions that were inhibited by acetylcholine.[216] The bradykinin-induced coronary vasodilatation appears to be mediated via nitric oxide.[235] In addition, bradykinin can stimulate plasminogen activation release through B2-receptor-dependent, nitric oxide synthase-independent, and cyclooxygenase-independent pathways.[236] B1-receptor stimulation may also produce vasodilatation, which is mediated by nitric oxide and not modulated by ACE.[237]

Based on these observations, one might consider the use of bradykinin potentiation through ACE inhibition as a means for treating angina pectoris. However, ACE inhibitors are not very effective as antianginal agents, because bradykinin's effects on coronary flow may not be as appreciable in the face of atherosclerotic disease where local nitric oxide and prostacyclin release may be inhibited.[216] Because bradykinin works through these substances to cause vascular dilation, its use as a coronary dilator in atherosclerotic vessels may be limited.

However, in the face of ischemia, kinins have a protective effect. They decrease creatine kinase and lactate release, increase neovascularization (β_1 receptor), and prevent the rapid consumption of energy-rich phosphates via improved cellular metabolism.[220,237a] The mechanisms for this favorable effect of kinins have yet to be elucidated.[229]

ACE inhibitors can protect survivors of an acute myocardial infarction from recurrent events and some are being evaluated for this indication, suggesting that the antithrombotic and prothrombolytic effects of bradykinin may be important in this regard. Bradykinin is a potent stimulus to tissue-type plasminogen activation (t-PA) secretion in animal models; some studies suggest the same is true in hypertensive humans.[236] This stimulatory effect of bradykinin on t-PA release is augmented by an ACE inhibitor.[238]

Bradykinin has an important role in reducing the extent of myocardial reperfusion injury after the reversal of ischemia.[239] Myocardial B2 receptors are upregulated during myocardial ischemia in both the infarcted and noninfarcted areas of the heart.[240] In experimental models, perfusion with bradykinin or the use of ACE inhibition to potentiate the action of bradykinin can reduce both the incidence and duration of ventricular fibrillation, improve ventricular functioning, and reduce infarct size following coronary artery occlusion and reperfusion[218,241] (Fig. 39-10). In myocardial infarct, the potentiation of kinins via ACE inhibitors is involved in the reduction of infarct size and the improvement in cardiac function.[218] These protective effects of bradykinin can be reversed by B2 receptor blockade or by inhibition of nitric oxide synthase.[237] These favorable effects on reperfusion injury can be potentiated by ACE inhibition therapy and not by angiotensin-II-receptor blockers, again demonstrating the importance of bradykinin in protecting against reperfusion injury and the importance of bradykinin in providing the protective effects of ACE inhibition.

It was recently demonstrated, in an experimental model, that kallikrein gene delivery could protect against myocardial infarction and apoptosis during ischemia/reperfusion injury via a kinin-cyclic GMP signal pathway.[242]

ACE is not the only kinin-degrading enzyme. Aminopeptidase P has been shown to participate in myocardial kinin metabolism to the

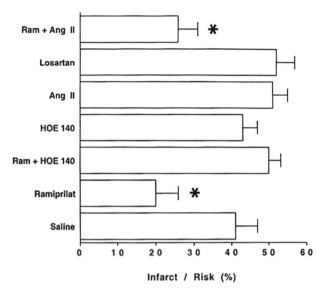

FIGURE 39-10. Study comparing effects of ACE inhibitor ramipril (ram) + angiotensin-II (Ang II), losartan, Ang II, HOE 140 (B2 antagonist), ram + HOE 140, ramiprilat, and saline on infarct size in experimental myocardial infarction. (*Reproduced with permission from Hartman JC. The role of bradykinin and nitric oxide in the cardioprotective action of ACE inhibitors. Ann Thorac Surg 60:789, 1995.*)

same extent as ACE. Apstatin, a specific inhibitor of aminopeptidase P, reduced infarct size in an in vivo model of acute myocardial ischemia and reperfusion.[243]

Bradykinin and B2-receptor stimulation have an important role in the phenomenon of "ischemic preconditioning,"[241,244–246] with effects similar to those seen with adenosine. Using both inhibitors of protein kinase C and B2 receptors (HOE 140) in experimental models, it was demonstrated that bradykinin participates in the trigger phase of ischemic preconditioning, but not in the mediation phase. In addition, it was shown that protein kinase C, and not nitric oxide or prostaglandin, plays an important role in the signal-transduction cascade of bradykinin. A threshold level of protein kinase C must be reached before protection can be triggered. It is proposed by investigators that both adenosine and bradykinin work through redundant pathways to activate protein kinase C to insure that exposure to ischemia will induce the protective adaptive phenomenon.[244]

Left Ventricular Hypertrophy and Vascular Remodeling

Left ventricular hypertrophy is an independent predictor for increased morbidity and mortality from cardiac disease. In experimental models, ACE inhibitors can prevent or cause regression of ventricular hypertrophy[231,247] induced by aortic banding, an effect that can be inhibited by HOE 140.[231] Bradykinin's antimitogenic effects may be mediated by both nitric oxide and prostacyclin. Angiotensin-II-receptor blockade with losartan did not have as impressive an effect on left ventricular regression as did the ACE inhibitors.[247]

Endothelial cell injury can lead to smooth muscle proliferation in the media and neointima formation (vascular remodeling). In experimental models, ACE inhibition can inhibit neointimal proliferation more effectively than either losartan or control. As with left ventricular hypertrophy, the effect of ACE inhibition on vascular remodeling can be inhibited by HOE 140, suggesting a bradykinin mediated effect.[231,247] In experimental models of vascular remodeling postmyocardial infarction, both AT1 blockers and ACE

inhibitors had similar beneficial effects.[248] Surprisingly, the therapeutic actions of both classes of drugs are mediated by bradykinin.[248] The mechanism of bradykinin's antimitogenic actions may come from local release of nitric oxide and prostacyclin, both of which have their own effects to inhibit proliferation of vascular smooth muscles.[249] It was recently demonstrated that the B1 receptor may mediate a reduction of neointimal formation via the promotion of reendothelialization and inhibition of vascular smooth-muscle cell proliferation.[250]

Congestive Heart Failure

In congestive heart failure, various vasoconstrictive and fluid conserving neurohumoral systems come into play including the renin-angiotensin-aldosterone system, the adrenergic nervous system, endothelin, and vasopressin, which are counteracted by vasodilatory prostaglandins, natriuretic peptides, and bradykinin. It has been demonstrated that plasma levels of bradykinin are elevated in animal models of congestive heart failure.[228] The actions of endogenous bradykinin, mediated via the B2 kinin receptor, include coronary and systemic vasodilatation, and improvement of left ventricular relaxation, filling, and contractile performance.[228] This suggests that endogenous bradykinin may blunt the detrimental effects of other neurohormonal systems in congestive heart failure.[228,251] Thus bradykinin may play an important role in preserving cardiovascular function in congestive heart failure.[228]

Regarding the therapy of congestive heart failure, ACE inhibition has important action in reducing both morbidity and mortality in patients with left ventricular dysfunction.[252] What remains unresolved is the role that bradykinin plays with ACE inhibition in this benefit. Bradykinin as a vasodilating substance with diuretic and natriuretic actions, mediated by prostacyclin and nitric oxide, should have an important role to play in the beneficial actions of ACE inhibition.[247,253] In experimental studies, ACE inhibition appears to have advantages over angiotensin-II-receptor blockade alone in preventing hypertrophy and ventricular remodeling, and in reducing infarct size.[226,247] This differential benefit is lost in the presence of a B2-receptor antagonist.

Part of the benefit of ACE inhibitors in treatment of congestive heart failure may be the result of upregulation of β-adrenergic receptors. A recent study concluded that this upregulation of β-adrenergic receptors is mediated in part by bradykinin B2-receptor stimulation.[254]

Cereport, a bradykinin agonist, was recently studied in conscious dogs with pacing-induced heart failure. This study found cereport to be a potent systemic and coronary vasodilator, with hemodynamic effects mediated via nitric oxide.[255]

The combined use of ACE inhibitors and NEP inhibitors can cause additive potentiation of the kinin system and is another useful approach being applied for patients with both hypertension and congestive heart failure.[255a] The combination of ACE/NEP inhibitors leads to an increase of nitric oxide production in heart-failure models. This increase in nitric oxide is completely abolished by HOE-140, suggesting a bradykinin-mediated event.[256]

Adverse Effects

Increased bradykinin activity and its potentiating effects on prostaglandins and nitric oxide can cause various side effects. Adverse effects of ACE inhibitors, namely cough and angioneurotic edema, may be the result of increased kinin levels in tissues and plasma.[257] However, there are few reliable published data to support such a relationship.[229] Increased levels of bradykinin have been shown to increase microvascular leakage in mouse airways via the release of tachykinins from terminals of primary sensory neurons.[257] Bradykinin can induce orthostatic hypotension. Because bradykinin is so ubiquitous, it can affect multiple organ systems, including the vascular smooth muscle of GI and bronchial muscles. Kinins are among the local mediators in the inflammatory process that cause increased vascular permeability and edema, causing induction of pain both in the visceral organs and the skin. The actions could be potentiated with bradykinin enhancement at B receptors.

Bradykinin increases exocytotic release of endogenous norepinephrine from cardiac sympathetic neurons via activation of presynaptic B2 receptors.[258] The norepinephrine-releasing action of bradykinin is likely to be enhanced in myocardial ischemia, when protons accumulate, C-fibers become activated, and the production of bradykinin and prostaglandins increases.[259] Because norepinephrine is a major arrhythmogenic agent, the activation of this interneuronal signaling system between sensory and adrenergic neurons may have the potential to contribute to ischemic dysrhythmias and sudden cardiac death.[259]

Conclusion

Kinins as autocoids have been found in nearly every organ of the body. Kinins act via receptors, and stimulation of the B2 receptors appears to mediate formation of prostaglandins, nitric oxide, t-PA and endothelial-derived hyperpolarized factor (ENHF). These substances have various cardioprotective functions in improving the metabolic milieu of the heart, reducing left ventricular hypertrophy, causing peripheral and coronary artery vasodilation, augmenting natriuresis and diuresis, and reducing postischemic reperfusion injury and myocardial infarct size. Bradykinin is a central substance in cardiac ischemia preconditioning, and in addition, decreases the risk of ischemia-induced arrhythmias. Inhibition of B2 receptors can reverse all of these potentially beneficial actions.

Augmentation of the kallikrein-kinin system does appear to be a useful pharmacologic target if it can be done safely. Kinins themselves circulate in very low concentrations in the plasma, and have relatively short half-lives. Measurement of plasma kinin is also difficult.[260] These issues make it difficult to establish a deficiency state of the kallikrein-kinin system in the body or to assess the effects of an intervention on bradykinin production.

Table 39-17 lists the potential and proven approaches for augmenting the kallikrein-kinin system. Blockade of the system may be useful in patients with orthostatic hypotension.

Pharmacologic manipulation of the kallikrein-kinin system may not only provide innovative new treatments for hypertension, hypotension, heart failure, and ischemic heart disease, but it will

TABLE 39-17. Pharmacologic Approaches for Enhancing Kinin Activity

- Enhancement of bradykinin by inhibiting its metabolism (selective kinase inhibition with ACE inhibition, NEP inhibition).
- Use of more inclusive kinase inhibition with combined ACE-NEP inhibition.
- USE of long-acting kinin analogues (B2-receptor agonists).
- Bypassing kallikrein-kinin system by augmenting kinin mediators, nitric oxide, prostaglandins.
- Use of gene therapy for defective and deficient kallikrein-kinin system.

provide greater insights into the normal physiologic functioning of the cardiovascular system and pathophysiology of various disease processes.

UROTENSIN

Urotensin II has been recognized as an important hormone of the caudal neurosecretory system of teleost fish for more than 30 years.[261] The recent detection of this potent vasoconstrictor in human tissue and the identification of its receptor, however, have made it a major focus of current clinical research and a potential target for future pharmacotherapy.

Structure

The urophysis is a terminal organ of the teleost fish caudal neurosecretory system, a neurohemal endocrine organ morphologically and functionally similar to the mammalian hypothalamoneurohypophysial complex.[261] The two major regulatory peptides isolated from this organ are urotensin I, a 41-amino-acid residue peptide homologous to mammalian corticotropin-releasing factor, and urotensin II (U-II), a 12-amino-acid residue peptide that exhibits some sequence similarity with somastatin-14.[262] Several structural forms of U-II have been identified in different species of mollusks, fish, amphibians, and mammals.[263]

Like many vasoactive peptides, mature U-II is derived from a larger precursor prepropeptide. In humans, two prepropeptides of U-II have been identified, 124 (alpha) and 139 (gamma) residue alternate splice variants.[264,265] Both precursors give rise to an identical mature 11-amino-acid U-II following the cleavage of a conserved polybasic proteolytic processing site (Lys/Arg-Lys-Arg) by prohormone-converting enzymes.[264] The C-terminal region of the precursor, which includes the U-II peptide, exhibits significant sequence identity among species. This region includes the cyclic hexapeptide, which is essential for the biologic activity of U-II, which has been conserved across all species (Fig. 39-11). The N-terminal flanking region of the precursor, however, has no significant similarity between species and is highly variable. The conserved sequence has some structural similarities to the active central region of somatostatin-14 (-Phe-Trp-Lys-Thr-).[266] However, cloning and sequence analysis of both peptides' precursors has shown that the sequence identity with preprosomatostatin-II outside the conserved region is poor as compared to preprourotensin-II, suggesting that these two peptides are unlikely to be derived from a common ancestral precursor.[267]

Human Urotensin II Receptor

Initially, the existence of the sequence similarities within the cyclic region of U-II and somatostatin has led to the hypothesis that these two compounds share a common binding site.[268] However, functional and radioligand binding studies demonstrate that U-II mediates its action through a unique "U-II-specific" receptor.[269] This receptor was identified by Ames and colleagues in 1999 as an orphan human G-protein-coupled receptor homologous to rat GPR14, which is identical to the rat SENR (sensory epithelial neuropeptide-like receptor).[265] This intronless, 389-residue novel receptor is encoded on chromosome 17q25.3[270] and has 75% homology with the rat 386-residue GPR14. The rat GPR14 shares the most sequence

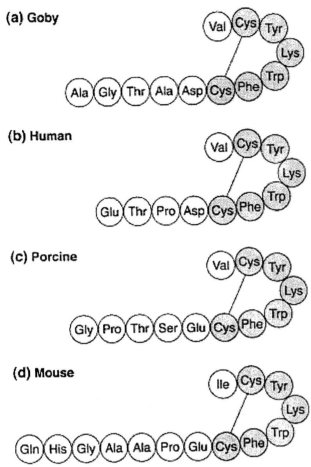

FIGURE 39-11. Amino-acid sequences for (a) goby, (b) human, (c) porcine, and (d) the predicted sequence for mouse, urotensin II (U-II). A second isoform of porcine U-II, differing only by a proline for threonine substitution at the third residue, has also been identified. The deduced sequence of rat U-II differs from the mouse by a threonine for alanine substitution in the fourth residue. Shading indicates the C-terminal cyclic hexapeptide sequence, which is conserved across species. (*Adapted with permission from Davenport AP, Maguire JJ. Urotensin II: Fish neuropeptide catches orphan receptor. TIPS 21:80, 2000.*)

identity with the somatostatin receptor, SSTR4 (<27%), and with the opioid receptors (<25%).[271] The first and second extracellular loops of the seven-transmembrane motifs contain cystine residues that are thought to be crucial in achieving the correct tertiary configuration (Fig. 39-12).[265] There are two potential glycosylation sites in the N-terminal domain of the receptor, Asn29 and Asn33, and two cysteine residues in the C-terminal that are potential site for post-translational palmitate addition.[272] Binding of U-II to the human GPR14 was selective. Somatostatin-1 to -14, urotensin I, neuropeptide Y, and angiotensin-II did not compete for binding.

Physiologic Role

Evolutionary pressures to conserve the active moiety of U-II isoforms across all species imply that this peptide plays a crucial role in their physiology. In addition, the wide distribution of its production and its site of action also suggest that U-II affects multiple

organ systems and it may have alternative physiologic roles besides its cardiovascular actions.

Vasoconstrictor Activity

Human U-II (hU-II) is the most potent mammalian vasoconstrictor identified to date, six- to twenty-eightfold more potent than endothelin-1 in nonhuman primates[273] (Table 39-18). Although reactivity is seen in a diverse range of species, the activity of hU-II is dependent upon the anatomic origin of the vessel studied and the species from which it was isolated (Table 39-19). In rats, hU-II vasoconstrictor activity was limited to the thoracic aorta, carotid artery,[273] and coronary arteries,[274] sparing the abdominal aorta, femoral arteries, and renal arteries from contraction.[269] In nonhuman primates, however, hU-II caused constriction in all arterial vessels studied, both elastic and muscular types.[265] Vasoconstriction has been observed mainly in the arterial vasculature, which is consistent with the expression of GPR14 in cardiac and arterial tissue but not in venous blood vessels.[265] However, Maguire and colleagues recently reported that U-II contracted human coronary, mammary and radial arteries, in addition to saphenous and umbilical veins.[275] The endothelium in these vessels, however, was mechanically removed prior to study. Urotensin-II was 50 times more potent in arteries and less than 10 times more potent in veins than enothelin-1 (ET-1) but the maximal response to U-II (20% of control KCl) was significantly less than the maximal response to ET-1 (80% of control KCl). In contrast, Hillier et al studied the effects of hU-II on intact human blood vessels that include small subcutaneous resistance arteries, internal mammary arteries, saphenous veins, and small subcutaneous veins and found it to have no vasoconstrictor action on these vessels, bringing into question its role in human cardiovascular regulation.[276] Paysant and colleagues, however, showed that hU-II constricted three of eight human mammary arteries in vitro, and two of three human radial arteries, with no response detected in human saphenous veins.[277] More studies are needed to assess hU-II's role as a vasoconstrictor in vivo.

The vasoconstrictor effect of hU-II appears to be mediated through a phospholipase C-dependent increase in inositol phosphates, suggesting that the peptide acts through a G_q protein-coupled receptor.[278] Activation of phospholipase C leads to elevation of intracellular calcium, which causes contraction in vascular smooth muscle. Although it has been reported that U-II-induced release of arachidonic acid might be a potential mechanism of vasoconstriction,[279] the cyclooxygenase inhibitor indomethacin did not affect hU-II induced vasoconstriction in rabbit aorta.[278] In addition, because U-II can cause contraction in endothelium-denuded vessels, it appears that the GPR14 receptor is located on vascular smooth-muscle cells and not on the endothelium.

It has been postulated that the intracellular signaling pathway of hU-II involves the small GTPase RhoA, which is recognized as a major regulator of smooth muscle contraction involved in maintaining arterial tone.[280] Sauzeau et al demonstrated that hU-II activates small GTPase RhoA and its target, Rho-kinase, in arterial smooth muscle.[281] The contracting takes place through the phosphorylation and the consequent inhibition of the myosin light-chain phosphatase, leading to an increased myosin light-chain phosphorylation, and tension, at constant Ca^{2+} concentration.[280] This same signaling pathway is likely to be responsible for hU-II-induced actin stress fiber formation and cytoskeletal organization. In addition, hU-II activation of RhoA/Rho-kinase pathway has also been shown

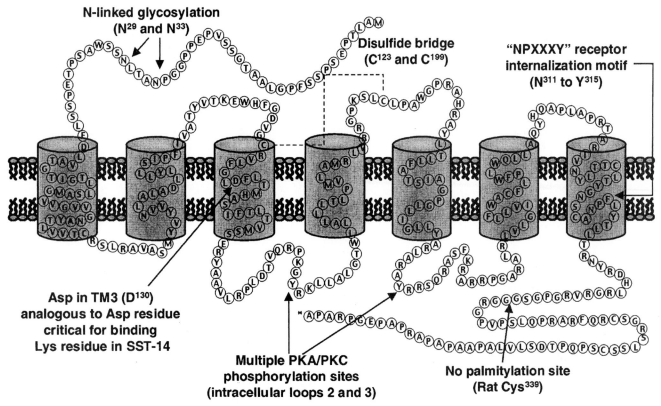

FIGURE 39-12. Representation of the G-protein-coupled receptor (GPR14) that selectively binds human urotensin II. In addition to the lipophilic seven-transmembrane spanning motifs of the GPCR superfamily, human GPR14 also possesses several structural motifs characteristic of a GPCR, including potential N-linked glycosylation sites, intraloop disulfide bridge, and putative intracellular PKA/PKC phosphorylation sites. Although an "NPXXY" consensus motif is retained in TM7 of both rat and human GPR14 (required for receptor internalization), the putative palmitiylation site (Cys339) present in rat GPR14 is absent in the human receptor. (*Reproduced with permission from Douglas SA, Ohlstein EH. Human urotensin-II, the most potent mammalian vasoconstrictor identified to date, as a therapeutic target for the management of cardiovascular disease. Trends Cardiovasc Med 10:229–237, 2000.*)

TABLE 39-18. Relative Contractile Potency of Human U-II in Nonhuman Primates

Vessel	hU-II -log[EC$_{50}$]	Endothelin-1 -log[EC$_{50}$]	Relative Potency
Arterial tissue			
Left anterior descending coronary	9.39±0.40	8.20±0.32*	15
Left circumflex coronary	9.56±0.05	n.d.	
Mesenteric	9.35±0.26	8.24±0.28*	13
Pulmonary	9.29±0.16	7.84±0.06†	28
Renal	9.59±0.36	8.83±0.24	6
Proximal descending thoracic aorta	8.96±0.24	n.d.	
Distal descending thoracic aorta	9.06±0.22	n.d.	
Distal abdominal aorta	9.37±0.13	n.d.	
Basilar	10.00±0.16	n.d.	
Common carotid	9.16±0.08	n.d.	
Internal mammary	9.30±0.08	n.d.	
Venous tissue			
Portal vein	<7.00	7.00±0.77	
Jugular vein	<7.00	8.88±0.21	

All values are mean ± sem (n = 3-4). Statistical comparisons made by analysis of variance (post hoc Fisher's least squares difference) * = $P < .05$; † = $P < .001$; n.d. = not determined.

Source: Reproduced with permission from Ames RS.[265]

TABLE 39-19. Synopsis of the Regional and Species Differences in Vascular Reactivity to Human U-II

Vessels	Rat	Mouse	Dog	Pig	Marmoset	C. Monkey	Human
Arterial							
Thoracic aorta	+++	0	0	++	+	+++	
Abdominal aorta	+	0	0	+	+	+++	
LCX coronary			+++	0		+++	
LAD coronary	++		+++			+++	+
Pulmonary	++		0	++		+++	++
Renal			0	0		+++	
Internal mammary			0	0		+++	+
Femoral			0	+	0	+++	
Basilar	0		0			+++	
Common carotid	++		0	0	+	+++	
Mesenteric	+		0	++	+	+++	
Venous							
Pulmonary			+			++	
Saphenous			0	0		0	++
Jugular	0		0			0	
Umbilical	0		0			0	+

Reactivity is classified as follows: +++ = $IR_{max} \geq$ 75% KCl response; ++ = $R_{max} \geq$ 20% KCl and $\leq$ 75% KCl response; + = $R_{max} \leq$ 20% KCl response; 0 = unresponsive. Where no symbol is provided, reactivity has not been assessed.

Source: Reproduced with permission from Douglas SA, Ohlstein EH, Human urotensin-II, the most potent mammalian vasoconstrictor identified to date, as a therapeutic target for the management of cardiovascular disease. *Trends Cardiovasc Med* 10:229–237, 2000.

to promote arterial SMC proliferation, giving hU-II a possible role in the development of atherosclerosis.

Vasodilator Activity

Gibson et al described how at low concentrations (0.1 to 0.5 nM) U-II caused endothelium-dependent relaxation of rat aortic strips[282] and at higher concentrations (1 to 10 nM) caused endothelium-independent contraction. Because the vasoconstrictor effects are modulated by endothelium-dependent vasodilators, U-II may play a bigger role in states of endothelium dysfunction. As with U-II vasoconstrictive action, there are clear anatomic differences in the response of different vascular beds to hU-II-induced vasodilatation. Recent studies show that although hU-II is a potent vasoconstrictor of the rat main pulmonary artery, it is unable to contract smaller pulmonary arteries of the rat or human.[283] The vasoconstrictor effect of hU-II in the small pulmonary arteries may be masked by the potent vasodilator effect of human U-II. Stirrat and colleagues were the first to demonstrate a vasodilatory response to ET-1 precontracted vessels of the small pulmonary arteries and abdominal-resistant arteries.[284] Although the study conducted by Ames et al illustrates hU-II capability to constrict all nonhuman primate arteries, the arteries investigated in this study were all large conduit arteries.[265] Stirrat et al showed that a vasodilatory response may predominate in certain human-resistant arteries,[284] suggesting the possibility of a second receptor subtype for hU-II, similar to the two receptor subtypes that carry out the vasoconstrictor and vasodilator action of ET-1. In fact, hU-II was found to be just as potent a vasodilator of the above mentioned arteries as adrenomedullin, which was believed to be the most potent vasodilator of small pulmonary arteries, and a more potent vasodilator than sodium nitroprusside and acetylcholine.

Urotensin II also elicits sustained vasodilatation in the coronary arteries of isolated perfused rat heart.[285] There is an initial short lasting (less than 1 minute) vasoconstricting effect of U-II followed by a rapid recovery with sustained (up to 20 min) vasodilatation of the coronary arteries. Diclofenac, a cyclooxygenase inhibitor, NG-nitro-L-arginine (L-NNA), a nitric oxide inhibitor, and 25 mM KCl (which inhibits endothelium-derived hyperpolarizing factors, EDHF),[274] significantly decreased vasodilatation as compared to controls, suggesting that U-II vasodilatory effect may be mediated by nitric oxide, eicosanoids, as well as EDHF.

Cardiohemodynamic Effects

In the anesthetized rat, U-II induces systemic vasodepression.[286] This may be due to the restricted contractile action, which is limited only to the rat's thoracic aorta and is attenuated in vessels distal to the aortic arch. Such selective contraction may be insufficient to elevate total peripheral resistance in vivo. On the other hand, hU-II (300 pmol/kg) causes as much as a threefold increase in total peripheral resistance in anesthetized primates.[265] Unlike the rat, primates exhibit a spasmogenic response to hU-II in all large conduit arteries. Ames et al have shown that hU-II elicited a complex dose-dependent hemodynamic response that culminated in severe myocardial depression and fatal circulatory collapse. At doses <30 pmol per kg (intravenous), hU-II slightly increased cardiac output and reduced regional vascular resistance, with little or no change in arterial pressure. At doses >30 pmol per kg, hU-II decreased myocardial function and increased vascular resistance. There is a dose-dependent decrease in cardiac output as a result of the combination of a mild drop in heart rate and a more significant drop in stroke volume. In addition, myocardial contractility was severely depressed, but mean arterial pressure was only moderately reduced, despite the marked decrease in cardiac output. This is most likely due to the threefold increase in total peripheral resistance. Furthermore, left ventricular end-diastolic pressure increased in a dose-dependent manner, indicating systemic vasoconstriction. Echocardiography showed grossly attenuated septal and free-wall motion and electrocardiogram readings showed ST segment changes. It is uncertain whether these ECG changes are secondary to myocardial ischemia or due to a direct electrophysiologic effect by hU-II.[286] Although this response to hU-II might appear maladaptive,

TABLE 39-20. [³H] Thymidine Incorporation into Vascular Smooth-Muscle Cell DNA

Control	$100 \pm 5\%$
UII (10 nmol/L)	$100 \pm 3\%$
Endothelin-1 (10 nmol/L)	$139 \pm 21\%$
Angiotensin II (10 nmol/L	$136 \pm 16\%$
MoxLDL (100 ng/mL)	$114 \pm 7\%$
UII (10 nmol/L) + moxLDL (100 ng/mL)	$345 \pm 37\%*$
Endothelin-1 (10 nmol/L) + moxLDL (100 ng/mL)	$287 \pm 12\%*$
Angiotensin II (10 nmol/L) + moxLDL (100 ng/mL)	$277 \pm 21\%*$

Values are mean $\pm$ SEM. $100 \pm 5\% = 222 \pm 10$ counts per minute. $*P < .0001$ vs moxLDL.

Source: Reproduced with permission from Wantanabe T, et al.[287]

it should be remembered that this response is a pharmacologic one caused by bolus intravenous administration of the peptide. The true (patho)physiogic role might be better studied with the development of hU-II or GPR14 antagonists.[286]

Atherosclerosis Formation

Vasoconstrictors such as endothelin-1 and angiotensin-II, and oxidized LDL (oxLDL) accelerate atherosclerosis by inducing vascular SMC proliferation.[287] This fact, coupled to the identification of U-II immunostaining of coronary atherosclerotic plaques (most intense in lipid-laden smooth-muscle cells and macrophage-rich regions), suggests a possible role of U-II in atheroma formation.[265] Under physiologic conditions, LDL is less likely to be fully oxidized into oxLDL because of antioxidants circulating in the plasma. Under these conditions, LDL is more likely to undergo only partial oxidation, forming mildly oxidized LDL (moxLDL). This form of LDL is the most potent type in atherosclerosis formation when compared to oxLDL and to nonoxidized LDL.[288] The study done by Watanabe and colleagues looked at the combination of U-II (10 nmol/L) and moxLDL (100 nmol/L) for inducing vascular SMC proliferation and compared it to other LDL/vasoconstrictor combinations.[287] They found the pairing of U-II/moxLDL to be the most potent combination capable of inducing vascular SMC proliferation as compared to cells incubated with U-II/LDL, U-II/oxLDL, ET-1/moxLDL, and angiotensin-II/moxLDL (Table 39-20). Furthermore, this synergistic interaction was abolished when inhibitors of PKC, c-Src tyrosine kinase, or MAPK were added to the incubated cells, suggesting the PKC/c-Src tyrosine kinase/MAPK pathway to be the most likely intercellular signaling mechanism by which U-II and moxLDL induce vascular SMC proliferation.

Cardiac and Vascular Remodeling

The results of recent studies suggest that hU-II may have a function in the remodeling of the vasculature. Using cultured rat neonatal fibroblasts, which express both prepro-U-II mRNA and GPR14 mRNA, Tzanidis and colleagues showed that hU-II elevates α (I)-procollagen mRNA expression.[289] This raises the possibility that hU-II may regulate cardiac and peripheral vascular fibrosis under (patho)physiologic settings, as is the case with other vasoconstrictors (ET-1, angiotensin-II, and norepinephrine).

Conclusion

Urotensin II is a recently discovered neuropeptide whose expression in humans has been found in nearly every organ of the body, with most of the experimental attention being focused on its expression in the cardiovascular system, CNS, endocrine organs, and the kidney. The urotensin-II receptor expression, on the other hand, is mostly limited to the CNS, arterial vasculature, and the heart. Its cardiovascular action exhibits both species-specific and anatomy-specific variations. Urotensin-II has been described as the most potent vasoconstrictor known to date, mediating its action through the G-coupled protein receptor, GPR14, which mobilizes Ca^{2+} through the activation of the inositol phosphates. Interestingly, U-II also acts as a vasodilator in small pulmonary and resistant mesenteric arteries by a nitric oxide, eicosanoids, and/or an EDHF-mediated mechanism. The dual vasoactive action of U-II raises the possibility of a second type of receptor, which explained the dual action of ET-1. Furthermore, in nonhuman primates, hU-II provides regional vasoconstriction accompanied by profound cardiac depressor actions. Urotensin-II potentiates atherosclerosis in the presence of moxLDL and is believed to play a role in cardiovascular remodeling. In addition to its roles in cardiovascular (patho)physiology, U-II appears to be an important player in endocrine and metabolic function, CNS-mediated behavioral and motor activity, osmoregulation, renal disease, and portal hypertension.

Augmentation of the U-II/GPR14 interaction appears to be a useful pharmacologic target. This will also help define the pathophysiologic position of U-II/GPR14 in humans. Urotensin could also provide an effective vasoconstrictor drug. Given the wide distribution and all the possible physiologic roles of the urotensin-II system and the evolutionary pressures to conserve the active peptide among all species it has been identified in, blocking U-II's action safely is a major challenge to overcome. The two possible targets appear to be blocking the preprourotensin-II-"converting enzymes" and direct blockage of GPR14. One may need to develop multiple pharmacologic blockers because the existence of multiple U-II receptor subtypes is still a distinct possibility. In the meantime, measuring U-II levels in different disease states, such as hypertension, coronary artery disease, and congestive heart failure, will give us more insight to the possible role of U-II in these conditions. Identifying the factors that trigger U-II release and GPR14 expression will also aid in this task.

Pharmacologic manipulation of U-II and its receptor(s) could not only provide innovative new treatment for hypertension, hypotension, heart failure, and ischemic heart disease, but it will also provide greater insight into the normal physiologic function of the cardiovascular, endocrine, and central nervous systems, in addition to the pathophysiology of various disease processes.

ADVANCED GLYCATION END-PRODUCT CROSSLINK BREAKERS (ALT-711)

Arterial stiffening with increased pulse pressure is a leading risk factor for cardiovascular disease in the elderly. ALT-711, a thiazolium derivative, is the first of a new pharmaceutical class that catalytically breaks advanced glycosylation end-product (AGE) crosslinks.[290] ALT-711 improves arterial distensibility in aged and diabetic animals.[291,292]

Artery compliance is determined by ambient mean pressure, endothelial function, vessel tone, and artery structure and composition. Current antihypertensive therapies focus on the first three factors,[293] yet this can run the risk of reducing diastolic pressure while inadequately lowering pulse pressure.[293,294] Treatments targeting structural factors remain largely unexplored. Among the latter

TABLE 39-21. Major Eukaryotic Heat Shock Proteins

Family	Members	Prokaryotic Homologue	Functional Role	Comments
Hsp90	Hsp100, Hsp90, Grp94	C62.5 (*E.coli*)	Maintenence of proteins such as steroid receptor. Src in an inactive form until appropriate.	*Drosophila* and yeast homologues of hsp90 are known as hsp83
Hsp70	Grp78 (=Bip) Hsp72, Hsp 73 Hsx70	dna K (*E. coli*)	Protein folding and unfolding; assembly of multimeric complexes	Hsx70 only in primates
Hsp60	Hsp60	gro EL (*E. coli*) mycobacterial 65 kd antigen	Protein folding and unfolding; organelle translocation.	Major antigen of many bacteria and parasites which infect man.
Hsp56	Hsp56	—	Protein folding, component of steroid receptor complex.	Binds FK506 (tacrolimus) and is also known as FK BP56
Hsp32	Hsp32	—	Cleaves heme to yield carbon monoxide and the protective antioxidant molecule, biliverdin.	Also known as heme oxygenase-1
Hsp27	Hsp27, Hsp26, etc	Mycobacterial 18kd antigen	Unclear	Very variable in size and number in different organisms
Ubiquitin	Ubiquitin	none	Protein degradation	Also conjugated to histone H2A in the nucleus leading to potential role in gene regulation

Source: Reproduced with permission from Snoeckx LHEH et al.[298]

are alterations in matrix proteins within the vessel wall from nonenzymatic crosslinks between glucose (or other reducing sugars) and amino groups that generate AGE.[295] AGE accumulate slowly on the long-lived proteins such as collagen and elastin to stiffen both arteries and the heart, and decreasing these crosslinks can enhance vessel and cardiac compliance in experimental animals.[291,292,296]

The effects of oral ALT-711 210 mg/d on arterial compliance and blood pressure were evaluated in patients with both systolic hypertension and a wide blood pressure.[297] In this placebo-controlled trial, pulse pressure declined significantly with 8 weeks of active treatment as compared with placebo (-5.6 vs -0.5 mm Hg, $P = .024$). Mean arterial pressure trended downward slightly in both groups (2 to 5 mm Hg), but neither systemic vascular resistance nor cardiac output was altered. ALT-711 improved arterial compliance and distensibility 11 to 18% ($P < .02$ vs placebo for both) and the effect was significant after accounting for concomitant changes in mean artery pressure. In conclusion, ALT-711 improves arterial distensibility in older patients with vascular stiffening. This may represent a novel therapeutic approach for patients with arterial stiffening associated with aging, diabetes, and isolated systolic hypertension.

HEAT SHOCK PROTEINS

Human cells have the capability of defending themselves from various stressors by activating a genetic program with the production of substances known as heat shock proteins and their regulatory partners, the heat shock transcription factors.[298] The heat shock proteins protect against cell damage by maintaining proper protein assembly, folding, and transport. They also protect against cell apoptosis. Heat shock proteins are increased in the presence of cardiovascular stress stimuli, such as ischemia, hypoxia, oxidative injury, and endotoxemia.[298] It has been proposed that heat shock proteins and factors would be attractive pharmacologic targets for stimulating endogenous protective mechanisms in various cardiovascular diseases.

Heat shock proteins were so named because heat shock was the trigger for turning on the genetic machinery to produce these

substances.[298] The various proteins are classified by their function and size. Those heat shock proteins most associated with cardiovascular disease are hsp27, hsp60, hsp65, hsp70, and hsp90 (Table 39-21). Heat shock factors control the stress-inducible expression of heat shock protein genes. The most important heat shock factor in acute cell injury appears to be hsf1.[298]

Pathophysiology

Members of the families of heat shock proteins are usually found in a specific locality in the unstressed cell. However, with stress, they can be translocated to other cellular compartments.[298] Heat shock proteins are rapidly synthesized after the onset of stress.[298]

Multiple investigations have demonstrated an elevation in heat shock proteins in patients with systemic hypertension, coronary artery disease, and carotid atherosclerosis.[298–300] There are also elevations in heat shock proteins during acute myocardial ischemia and infarction and a decreased heat shock protein response with aging.[298] Elevations in heat shock proteins with hypertension and atherosclerosis suggest a possible etiologic role in these conditions because of their proinflammatory actions.[301–303]

It has been shown that inducible hsp70 protects against ischemic cardiac damage. After global ischemia, the hearts of transgenic mice overexpressing heat shock proteins were shown to have a decrease in myocardial infarction size and improved contractile recovery compared to wild-type litter mates.[304] In addition, Hunter et al demonstrated a similar correlation between the amounts of hsp70 and the ability to limit the size of the infarct following exposure of the heart to ischemia and subsequent reperfusion.[305] Heat shock proteins have been suggested as the means by which drugs such as adenosine provide their ischemic preconditioning actions.[298]

Currie demonstrated that the exposure of isolated rat hearts to ischemia or elevated perfusion temperature on a Langendorff perfusion apparatus resulted in the induction of heat shock protein.[306] Currie and colleagues later determined that heat shock protein induction could protect the heart against subsequent exposure to a more severe stress. They exposed rats to elevated temperatures and then removed their hearts and exposed them to ischemia using a Langendorff perfusion apparatus.[307] The hearts exposed to an elevated temperature showed improved recovery of contractile function following ischemia and reperfusion as compared with control hearts. These were the first findings demonstrating heat shock protein induction in the intact heart was able to produce a protective effect against subsequent exposure to ischemia and reperfusion.[308] By using antisense technology, it was also determined that the inhibition of heat shock proteins decreased the tolerance to stress compared to control cells.[298]

Therapeutic Implications

The potential for the therapeutic targeting of heat shock proteins with drugs remains a promising yet elusive goal. Much work still needs to be done regarding heat shock protein-gene transcription and heat shock protein translation mechanisms in human blood vessels and in the myocardium.[308a] With known heat shock protein synthesis initiators, it has been shown that cytoprotection appears at the earliest 6 to 12 h later, which would make acute myocardial infarction a less-likely target for this type of therapy.

There are drugs that can influence heat shock protein expression and/or heat shock factor regulation, including geranylgeranyl acetone and bimoclomol, which can induce hsp70 expression and provide cytoprotective effects in experimental settings.[309,310] Gene therapy approaches are also being used that target heat shock factor and hsp70 production.[311,312]

OTHER POTENTIAL TARGETS

In an experimental model, cardiac allograft arteriosclerosis was prevented by use of a protein tyrosine kinase inhibitor selective for the platelet-derived growth factor receptor.[313]

Fostriecin, an inhibitor of protein phosphatase 2A, limits MI size even when administered after the onset of ischemia.[314]

REFERENCES

1. Hynes RO: Integrins: Versatility, modulation, and signaling in cell adhesion. *Cell* 69:11, 1992.
2. Frenette PS, Wagner DD: Adhesion molecules: Part I. *N Engl J Med* 334:1526, 1996.
3. Krieglstein CF, Granger DN: Adhesion molecules and their role in vascular disease. *Am J Hypertens* 14:44S, 2001.
4. Zhang L, Plow EF: A discrete site modulates activation of I domains. Application to integrin alpha-beta2. *J Biol Chem* 271:47, 1996.
5. Muller WA, Weigl SA, Deng X, Phillips DM: PECAM-1 is required for transendothelial migration of leukocytes. *J Exp Med* 178:449, 1993.
6. Newman P, Hillery CA, Albrecht R, et al: Activation-dependent changes in human platelet PECAM-1: Phosphorylation, cytoskeletal association, and surface membrane redistribution. *J Cell Biol* 119:239, 1992.
7. Johnson-Leger C, Aurrand Lions M, Imhif BA: The parting of the endothelium: miracle, or simply a junctional affair? *J Cell Sci* 113:921, 2000.
8. Norman KE, Scheding C, Kunkel EJ: Peptides derived from the lectin domain of selectin adhesion molecules inhibit leukocyte rolling in vivo. *Microcirculation* 3:29, 1996.
9. Bevilacqua MP, Nelson RM: Selectins. *J Clin Invest* 91:379, 1993.
10. Picker LJ: Mechanisms of lymphocyte homing. *Curr Opin Immunol* 4:277, 1992.
11. Yoshida M, Szente BE, Kiely JM, et al: Phosphorylation of the cytoplasmic domain of E-selectin is regulated during leukocyte-endothelial adhesion. *J Immunol* 161:933, 1998.
12. Israels SJ, Gerrard JM, Jacques YV, et al: Platelet dense granule membranes contain both granulophisin and P-selectin (GMP-140). *Blood* 80:143, 1992.
13. Johnston GI, Cook RG, McEver RP: Cloning of GMP-140, a granule membrane protein of platelets and endothelium: sequence similarity to proteins involved in cell adhesion and inflammation. *Cell* 56:1033, 1989.
14. Hirose M, Kawashima H, Miyasaka M: A functional epitope on P-selectin that supports binding of P-selectin to P-selectin glycoprotein ligand-1 but not to sialyl Lewis X oligosaccharides. *Int Immunol* 10:639, 1998.
15. Eriksson EE, Werr J, Guo Y, et al: Direct observation in vivo on the role of endothelial selectins and alpha(4) integrin in cytokine-induced leukocyte-endothelium interactions in mouse aorta. *Circ Res* 86:526, 2000.
16. Théorêt J-F, Bienvenu J-G, Kumar A, Merhi Y: P-selectin antagonism with recombinant P-selectin glycoprotein ligand-1 (rPSGL-Ig) inhibits circulating activated platelet binding to neutrophils induced by damaged arterial surfaces. *J Pharmacol Exp Ther* 298:658, 2001.
17. Kumar A, Villani MP et al: Recombinant soluble form of PSGL-1 accelerates thrombolysis and prevents reocclusion in a porcine model. *Circulation* 99:1363, 1999.
18. Angst BD, Marcozzi C, Magee AI: The cadherin superfamily: Diversity in form and function. *J Cell Sci* 114:629, 2001.
18a. Boggon TJ, Murray J, Chappuis-Flament S, et al: C-Cadherin ectodomain structure and implications for cell adhesion molecules. *Science* 296:1308, 2002.
19. Nollet F, Kools P, van Roy F: Phylogenetic analysis of the cadherin superfamily allows identification of six major subfamilies besides several solitary members. *J Mol Biol* 299:551, 2000.
20. Ivanov D, Philippova M, Antropova J et al: Expression of cell adhesion molecule T-cadherin in the human vasculature. *Histochem Cell Biol* 115:231, 2001.
21. Bobryshev YV, Cherian SM, Inder SJ, Lord RS: Neovascular expression of VE-cadherin in human atherosclerotic arteries and its relation to intimal inflammation. *Cardiovasc Res* 43:1003, 1999.
22. Bobryshev YV, Lord RS, Watanabe T, Ikezawa T: The cell adhesion molecule E-cadherin is widely expressed in human atherosclerotic lesions. *Cardiovasc Res* 40:191, 1998.
23. Ott I, Neumann F-J, Gawaz M: Increased neutrophil-platelet adhesion in patients with unstable angina. *Circulation* 94:1239, 1996.
24. Jang Y, Lincoff M, Plow EF, Topol EJ: Cell adhesion molecules in coronary artery disease. *J Am Coll Cardiol* 24:1591, 1994.
25. Evangelista V, Manarini S, Rotondo S, et al: Platelet/polymorphonuclear leukocyte interaction in dynamic conditions: Evidence of adhesion cascade and cross talk between P-selectin and Beta 2 integrin CD11b/CD18. *Blood* 88:4183, 1996.
26. Coller BS: Platelets and thrombolytic therapy. *N Engl J Med* 322:33, 1990.
27. Kieffer N, Phillips DR: Platelet membrane glycoproteins: Functions in cellular interaction. *Ann Rev Cell Biol* 6:329, 1990.
28. Frishman WH, Burns B, Atac B, et al: Novel antiplatelet therapies for treatment of patients with ischemic heart disease. Inhibitors of platelet glycoprotein IIb/IIIa integrin receptor. *Am Heart J* 130:877, 1995.
29. EPIC Investigators. Use of monoclonal antibody directed against the platelet glycoprotein IIb/IIIa receptor in high-risk coronary angioplasty. The EPIC Investigators. *N Engl J Med* 330:956, 1994.
30. Lincoff AM, Califf RM, Topol EJ: Platelet glycoprotein IIb/IIIa receptor blockade in coronary artery disease. *J Am Coll Cardiol* 35:1103, 2000.
31. Sheridan FM, Cole PG, Ramage D: Leukocyte adhesion to the coronary microvasculature during ischemia and reperfusion in an in vivo canine model. *Circulation* 93:1784, 1996.
32. Dragun D, Haller H: Diapedesis of leukocytes: Antisense oligonucleotides for rescue. *Exp Nephrol* 7:185, 1999.
33. Blankenberg S, Rupprecht HJ, Bickel C, et al for the AtheroGene Investigators. Circulating cell adhesion molecules and death in patients with coronary artery disease. *Circulation* 104:1336, 2001.
34. Haught WH, Mansour M, Rothlein R, et al: Alterations in circulating intercellular adhesion molecule-1 and L-selectin: Further evidence for

chronic inflammation in ischemic heart disease. *Am Heart J* 132:1, 1996.

35. O'Brien KD, McDonald TO, Chait A, et al: Neovascular expression of E-selectin, intercellular adhesion molecule-1, and vascular cell adhesion molecule-1 in human atherosclerosis and their relation to intimal leukocyte content. *Circulation* 93:672, 1996.

36. Patel SS, Thiagarajan R, Willerson JT, Yeh ETH: Inhibition of alpha 4 integrin and ICAM-1 markedly attenuate macrophage homing to atherosclerotic plaques in ApoE-deficient mice. *Circulation* 97:75, 1998.

37. Hackman A, Abe Y, Insult W Jr, et al: Levels of soluble cell adhesion molecules in patients with dyslipidemia. *Circulation* 93:1334, 1996.

38. DeSouza CA, Dengel DR, Macko RF, et al: Elevated levels of circulating cell adhesion molecules in uncomplicated essential hypertension. *Am J Hypertens* 10:1335, 1997.

39. Ikeda H, Takajo Y, Ichiki K, et al: Increased soluble form of P-selectin in patients with unstable angina. *Circulation* 92:1693, 1995.

40. Kaikita K, Ogawa H, Yasue H, et al: Soluble P-selectin is released into the coronary circulation after coronary spasm. *Circulation* 92:1726, 1995.

41. DeServi S, Mazzone A, Ricevuti G, et al: Clinical and angiographic correlates of leukocyte activation in unstable angina. *J Am Coll Cardiol* 26:1146, 1995.

42. Ogawa H, Yasue H, Miyao Y et al: Plasma soluble intercellular adhesion molecule-1 levels in coronary circulation in patients with unstable angina. *Am J Cardiol* 83:39, 1999.

43. O'Malley T, Ludlam CA, Riemermsa RA, Fox KAA: Early increase in levels of soluble intercellular adhesion molecule-1 (sICAM-1). Potential risk factor for the acute coronary syndromes. *Eur Heart J* 22:1226, 2001.

44. Mickelson K, Lakkis NM, Villarreal-Levy G, et al: Leukocyte activation with platelet adhesion after coronary angioplasty: A mechanism for recurrent disease? *J Am Coll Cardiol* 28:345, 1996.

45. Serrano CV Jr, Ramires JA, Venturinelli M, et al: Coronary angioplasty results in leukocyte and platelet activation with adhesion molecule expression. Evidence of inflammatory responses in coronary angioplasty. *J Am Coll Cardiol* 29:1276, 1997.

46. Voisard R, Osswald M, Baur R, et al: Expression of intercellular adhesion molecule-1 in human coronary endothelium and smooth muscle cells after stimulation with tumor necrosis factor-alpha. *Coron Artery Dis* 9:737, 1998.

47. Inoue T, Sakai Y, Morooka S, et al: Expression of polymorphonuclear leukocyte adhesion molecules and its clinical significance in patients with percutaneous transluminal coronary angioplasty. *J Am Coll Cardiol* 28:1127, 1996.

48. Belch JJ, Shaw JW, Kirk G, et al: The white blood cell adhesion molecule E-selectin predicts restenosis in patients with intermittent claudication undergoing percutaneous transluminal angioplasty. *Circulation* 95:2027, 1997.

49. Serebruany VL, Murugesan SR, Pothula A, et al: Increased soluble platelet/endothelial cellular adhesion molecule-1 and osteonectin levels in patients with severe congestive heart failure. Independent of disease etiology and antecedent aspirin therapy. *Eur J Heart Fail* 1:243, 1999.

50. Tsutamoto T, Wada A, Mabuchi N, et al: Angiotensin II type 1 receptor antagonist decreases plasma levels of tumor necrosis factor alpha, interleukin-6 and soluble adhesion molecules in patients with chronic heart failure. *J Am Coll Cardiol* 35:714, 2000.

51. Labarrere CA, Nelson DR, Miller SJ, et al: Value of serum-soluble intercellular adhesion molecule-1 for the noninvasive risk assessment of transplant coronary artery disease, posttransplant ischemic events, and cardiac graft failure. *Circulation* 102:1549, 2000.

52. Singh K, Sirokman G, Communal C, et al: Myocardial osteopontin expression coincides with the development of heart failure. *Hypertension* 33:663, 1999.

53. Siminiak T, Dye JF, Egdell RM, et al: The release of soluble adhesion molecules ICAM-1 and E-selectin after acute myocardial infarction and following coronary angioplasty. *Int J Cardiol* 61:113, 1997.

54. Silver MJ, Sutton JM, Hook S, et al: Adjunctive selectin blockade successfully reduces infarct size beyond thrombolysis in the electrolytic canine coronary artery model. *Circulation* 92:492, 1995.

55. Barron MK, Lake RS, Buda AJ, Tenaglia AN: Intimal hyperplasia after balloon injury is attenuated by blocking selectins. *Circulation* 96:3587, 1997.

56. Smyth SS, Reis ED, Zhang W, et al: β_3-Integrin-deficient mice but not P-selectin-deficient mice develop intimal hyperplasia after vascular injury. Correlation with leukocyte recruitment to adherent platelets 1 h after injury. *Circulation* 103:2501, 2001.

57. Ma XL, Lefer DJ, Lefer AM, Rothlein R: Coronary endothelial and cardiac protective effects of a monoclonal antibody to intercellular adhesion molecule-1 in myocardial ischemia and reperfusion. *Circulation* 86:937, 1992.

58. Hartman JC, Anderson DC, Wiltse AL, et al: Protection of ischemic/reperfused canine myocardium by CL18/6, a monoclonal anti-body to adhesion molecule ICAM-1. *Cardiovasc Res* 30:47, 1995.

59. Arai M, Lefer DJ, So T, et al: An anti-CD18 antibody limits infarct size and preserves left ventricular function in dogs with ischemia and 48-h reperfusion. *J Am Coll Cardiol* 27:1278, 1996.

60. Dhein S, Schott M, Gottwald E, et al: The contribution of neutrophils to reperfusion arrhythmias and a possible role of anti-adhesive pharmacological substances. *Cardiovasc Res* 30:881, 1995.

61. Asghar SS, Pasch MC: Therapeutic inhibition of the complement system. Y2K update. *Front Biosci* 5:63, 2000.

62. Bauernschmitt R, Böhrer H, Hagl S: Rescue therapy with C1-esterase inhibitor concentrate after emergency coronary surgery for failed PTCA. *Intensive Care Med* 24:635, 1998.

63. Muerke M, Murohara T, Lefer AM: Cardioprotective effects of a C1 esterase inhibitor in myocardial ischemia and reperfusion. *Circulation* 91:393, 1995.

64. Buerke M, Prufer D, Dahm M, et al: Blocking of classical complement pathway inhibits endothelial adhesion molecule expression and preserves ischemic myocardium from reperfusion injury. *J Pharmacol Exp Ther* 286:429, 1998.

65. Gibbons GH, Dzau VJ: Molecular therapies for vascular diseases. *Science* 272:689, 1996.

66. Frenette PS, Wagner DD: Adhesion molecules—Part II: blood vessels and blood cells. *Mol Med* 335:43, 1996.

67. Mann DL, Young JB: Basic mechanisms in congestive heart failure: Recognizing the role of proinflammatory cytokines. *Chest* 105:897–904, 1994.

68. Biasucci LM, Vitelli A, Liuzzo G: Elevated levels of interleukin-6 in unstable angina. *Circulation* 94:874, 1996.

69. Carswell EA, Old LJ, Kassel RL, et al: An endotoxin-induced serum factor that causes necrosis of tumors. *Proc Natl Acad Sci U S A* 72:3666, 1975.

70. Yokoyama T, Vaca L, Rossen RD, et al: Cellular basis for the negative inotropic effects of tumor necrosis factor-alpha in the adult mammalian heart. *J Clin Invest* 92:2303, 1993.

71. Bazzoni F, Beutler B: The tumor necrosis factor ligand and receptor families. *N Engl J Med* 334:1717, 1996.

72. Tracey KJ, Beutler B, Lowry SF, et al: Shock and tissue injury induced by recombinant human cachectin. *Science* 234:470, 1986.

73. Latini R, Bianchi M, Correale E, et al: Cytokines in acute myocardial infarction: Selective increase in circulating tumor necrosis factor, its soluble receptor and interleukin-1 receptor antagonist. *J Cardiovasc Pharmacol* 23:1, 1994.

74. Levine B, Kalman J, Mayer L, et al: Elevated circulating levels of tumor necrosis factor in severe chronic heart failure. *N Engl J Med* 323:236, 1990.

75. Kapadia S, Oral H, Lee J, et al: Tumor necrosis factor-alpha gene and protein expression in adult feline myocardium after endotoxin administration. *J Clin Invest* 96:1042, 1995.

76. Sindhwani R, Yuen J, Hirsch H, et al: Reversal of low flow states attenuates immune activation in sever decompensated congestive heart failure. *Circulation* 88:255, 1993.

77. Katz SD, Rao R, Berman JW, et al: Pathophysiological correlates of increased serum tumor necrosis factor in patients with congestive heart failure: Relation to nitric oxide dependent vasodilation in the forearm circulation. *Circulation* 90:12, 1994.

78. Torre-Amione G, Kapadia S, Lee J, et al: Expression and functional significance of tumor necrosis factor receptors in human myocardium. *Circulation* 92:1487, 1995.

79. Imamura K, Sherman Ml, Spriggs D, et al: Effect of tumor necrosis factor on GTP binding and GTPase activity in HL-60 and L929 cells. *J Biol Chem* 263:10247, 1988.

80. Zhang YH, Lin JX, Yip YK, et al: Enhancement of cyclic AMP levels and of protein kinase activity by TNF and IL-1 in human fibroblasts:

Role in the induction of IL-6. *Proc Natl Acad Sci U S A* 85:6802, 1988.

81. Foxwell B, Barrett K: Introduction to cytokine receptors: Structure and signal transduction. *Int Rev Exp Pathol* 34B:105, 1993.

82. Foxwell B, Barrett K, Feldmann M: Cytokine receptors: Structure and signal transduction. *Clin Exp Immunol* 90:161, 1992.

83. Ferari R, Bachetti T, Confortini R, et al: Tumor necrosis factor soluble receptors in patients with various degrees of congestive heart failure. *Circulation* 92:1479, 1995.

84. Packer M: Is tumor necrosis factor an important neurohormonal mechanism in chronic heart failure. *Circulation* 92:1379, 1995.

85. Engemann GL, Novick D, Wallach D: Two tumor necrosis factor-binding proteins purified from human urine. *J Biochem* 265:1531, 1990.

86. Mohler KM, Torrance DS, Smith CA, et al: Soluble TNF receptors are effective therapeutic agents in lethal endotoxemia and function simultaneously as both TNF carriers and TNF antagonists. *J Immunol* 151:1548, 1993.

87. Diez-Ruiz A, Tilz GP, Zangerle R, et al: Soluble receptors for TNF in clinical laboratory diagnosis. *Eur J Haematol* 54:1, 1995.

88. Kapadia S, Lee JS, Torre-Amione G, Mann DL: Soluble TNF binding proteins modulate the negative inotropic properties of TNF-α in vitro. *Am J Physiol* 268:H517, 1995.

89. Habib FM, Springall DR, Davies GJ, et al: Tumor necrosis factor and inducible nitric oxide synthase in dilated cardiomyopathy. *Lancet* 347:1151, 1996.

90. Mery P-F, Pavoine C, Belhassen L, et al: Nitric oxide regulates Ca^{2+} current. *J Biol Chem* 268:26286, 1993.

91. Balligand J-L, Ungereanu D, Kelly RA, et al: Abnormal contractile function due to induction of nitric oxide synthesis in rat cardiac myocytes follows exposure to activated macrophage-conditioned medium. *J Clin Invest* 91:2314, 1993.

92. Reithmann C, Werdan K: TNF-α decreases inositol phosphate formation and phosphatidylinositol-biphosphate synthesis in rat cardiomyocytes. *Naunyn Schmiedebergs Arch Pharmacol* 349:175, 1994.

93. Krown KA, Page MT, Nguyen D, et al: Tumor necrosis factor alpha-induced apoptosis in cardiac myocytes: Involvement of the sphingolipid signal cascade in cardiac cell death *J Clin Invest* 98:2854, 1996.

94. Oral H, Dorn WG, Mann DL: Sphingosine mediates the immediate negative inotropic effects of tumor necrosis factor-alpha in the adult mammalian myocardium. *J Biol Chem* 272:4836, 1997.

95. Kapadia S, Oral H, Lee J, et al: Hemodynamic regulation of tumor necrosis factor-alpha gene and protein expression in adult feline myocardium. *Circ Res* 81:187, 1997.

96. Kadokami T, McTiernan CF, Kubota T, et al: Sex-related survival differences in murine cardiomyopathy are associated with differences in TNF-receptor expression. *J Clin Invest* 106:589, 2000.

97. Torre-Amione G, Kapadia S, Lee J, et al: Tumor necrosis factor-α and tumor necrosis factor receptors in the failing human heart. *Circulation* 93:704, 1996.

98. Gurevitch J, Frolkis I, Yuhas Y, et al: Tumor necrosis factor-alpha is released from the isolated heart undergoing ischemia and reperfusion. *J Am Coll Cardiol* 28:247, 1996.

98a. Grossman GB, Rohde LE, Clausell N: Evidence for increased peripheral production of tumor necrosis-factor-α in advanced congestive heart failure. *Am J Cardiol* 88:578, 2001.

99. Renz H, Gong J-H, Schmidt A, et al: Release of TNFα from macrophages: Enhancement and suppression are dose-dependently regulated by prostaglandin E$_2$ and cyclic nucleotides. *J Immunol* 141:2388, 1988.

100. McMurray J, Abdullah I, Dargie HJ, Shapiro D: Increased concentration of TNF in "cachetic" patients with severe chronic heart failure. *Br Heart J* 66:356, 1991.

101. Torre-Amione G, Kapadia S, Benedict C, Oral H, Young JB, Mann DL: Proinflammatory cytokine levels in patients with depressed left ventricular ejection fraction: A report from the Studies of Left Ventricular Dysfunction (SOLVD). *J Am Coll Cardiol* 27:1201, 1996.

102. Suffredini AF, Fromm RE, Parker MM, et al: The cardiovascular response of normal humans to the administration of endotoxin. *N Engl J Med* 321; 280, 1989.

103. Pagani FD, Baker LS, Hsi C, et al: Left ventricular systolic and diastolic dysfunction after infusion of TNF-α in conscious dogs. *J Clin Invest* 90:389, 1992.

104. Dayer J-M, Beutler B, Cerami A: Cachectin/TNF stimulates collagenase and prostaglandin E$_2$ production by human synovial cells and dermal fibroblasts. *J Exp Med* 162:2163, 1985.

105. Vaddi K, Nicolini FA, Mehta P, Mehta JL: Increased secretion of TNF-α and interferon-gamma by mononuclear leukocytes in patients with ischemic heart disease. *Circulation* 90:694, 1994.

106. Barath P, Fishbein MC, Cao J, et al: Detection and localization of TNF in human atheroma. *Am J Cardiol* 65:297, 1990.

107. Yoshizumi M, Perrella MA, Burnett JCJ, et al: Tumor necrosis factor downregulates an endothelial nitric oxide synthase mRNA by shortening its half-life. *Circ Res* 73:205, 1993.

108. Millar AB, Foley NM, Singer M, et al: Tumor necrosis factor in bronchopulmonary secretions of patients with adult respiratory distress syndrome. *Lancet* 2:712, 1989.

109. Arbustini E, Grasso M, Diegoli M, et al: Expression of TNF in human acute cardiac rejection. *Am J Pathol* 139:709, 1991.

110. Satoh M, Nakamura M, Satoh H, et al: Expression of tumor necrosis factor-alpha converting enzyme and tumor necrosis factor-alpha in human myocarditis. *J Am Coll Cardiol* 36:1288, 2000.

111. Pilz G, Fraunberger P, Appel R, et al: Early prediction of outcome in score-identified, postcardiac surgical patients at high risk for sepsis, using soluble tumor necrosis factor receptor-p55 concentrations. *Crit Care Med* 24:595, 1996.

112. Kadokami T, Frye C, Lemster B, et al: Anti-tumor necrosis factor-α antibody limits heart failure in a transgenic model. *Circulation* 104:1094, 2001.

113. Fakade D, Knox K, Hussein K, et al: Prevention of Jarisch-Herxheimer reactions by treatment with antibodies against TNF-α. *N Engl J Med* 335:311, 1996.

114. Abraham E, Wunderlink R, Silverman H: Efficacy and safety of monoclonal antibody to human tumor necrosis antibody to human tumor necrosis factor alpha in patients with sepsis syndrome. *JAMA* 273:934, 1995.

115. Giroir BP, Beutler B: Effect of amrinone on tumor necrosis factor pro-duction in endotoxic shock. *Circ Shock* 36:200, 1992.

116. Strieter RM: Cellular and molecular regulation of tumor necrosis-alpha production by pentoxifylline. *Biochem Biophys Res Commun* 155:1230, 1988.

117. Han J: Dexamethasone and pentoxifylline inhibit endotoxin-induced cachectin/TNF synthesis at separate points in the signaling pathway. *J Exp Med* 172:391, 1990.

118. Feldman AM, Bristow MR, Parmley WW, et al: Effects of vesnarinone on morbidity and mortality in patients with heart failure. *N Engl J Med* 326:149, 1993.

119. Matsumori A, Shioi T, Yamada T, et al: Vesnarinone, a new inotropic agent, inhibits cytokine production by stimulated human blood from patients with heart failure. *Circulation* 89:955, 1994.

120. Hughes TK, Cadet P, Larned CS, et al: Modulation of tumor necrosis factor activities by a potential anti-cachexia compound, hydralazine sulfate. *Int J Immunopharmacol* 11:501, 1989.

121. Endres S, Ghorbani R, Kelley VE, et al: The effect of dietary supplementation with n-3 polyunsaturated fatty acids on the synthesis of interleukin-1 and tumor necrosis factor by mononuclear cells. *N Engl J Med* 320:265, 1989.

122. Yoshimura T, Kurita C, Nagoa T, et al: Inhibition of tumor necrosis factor and interleukin-1 beta production by beta adrenoreceptor agonists from lipopolysaccharide-stimulated human peripheral blood mononuclear cells. *Pharmacology* 54:144, 1997.

123. Wagner DR, Combes A, McTiernan CF, et al: Adenosine inhibits lipopolysaccharide-induced cardiac expression of tumor necrosis factor-alpha. *Circ Res* 82:47, 1998.

124. Pinsky DJ, Cai B, Yang X, et al: The lethal effects of cytokine-induced nitric oxide on cardiac myocytes are blocked by nitric oxide synthase antagonism or transforming growth factor- beta. *J Clin Invest* 95:677, 1995.

124a. Fichtlscherer S, Rössig L, Breuer S, et al: Tumor necrosis factor antagonism with etanercept improves systemic endothelial vasoreactivity in patients with advanced heart failure *Circulation* 104:3023, 2001.

125. Deswal A, Bozkurt B, Seta Y, et al: Safety and efficacy of a soluble P75 tumor necrosis factor (Etanercept) in patients with advanced heart failure. *Circulation* 99:3224, 1999.

126. Bozkurt B, Torre-Amione G, Warren MS, et al: Results of targeted anti-tumor necrosis factor therapy with etanercept in patients with advanced heart failure. *Circulation* 103:1044, 2001.

127. Mann DL, Young JB: Basic mechanisms in congestive heart failure: Recognizing the role of proinflammatory cytokines. *Chest* 105:897, 1994.

128. Airaghi L, Lettino M, Manfredi MG, et al: Endogenous cytokine antagonists during myocardial ischemia and thrombolytic therapy. *Am Heart J* 130:204, 1995.

129. Cotran RS, Kumar V, Collins T (eds): *Robbins Pathologic Basis of Disease*. 6th ed. Philadelphia: WB Saunders, 1999.

130. Feenstra J, Grobbee DE, Remme WJ: Drug-induced heart failure. *J Am Coll Cardiol* 33:1152, 1999.

131. Borden EC, Chin P: Interleukin-6: A cytokine with potential diagnostic and therapeutic role. *J Lab Clin Med* 123:824, 1994.

132. Neumann F-J, Ott I, Gawaz M, et al: Cardiac release of cytokines and inflammatory responses in acute myocardial infarction. *Circulation* 92:748, 1995.

133. Smith DA, Irving SD, Sheldon J, et al: Serum levels of the antiinflammatory cytokine interleukin-10 are decreased in patients with unstable angina. *Circulation* 104:746, 2001.

133a. Mallat Z, Corbaz A, Scoazec A, et al: Expression of interleukin-18 in human atherosclerotic plaques and relation to plaque instability *Circulation* 104:1598, 2001.

134. Long CS: Role of interleukin-1 in the failing heart. *Heart Fail Rev* 6(2):81, 2001.

134a. Hwang M.W, Matsumori A, Furukawa Y, et al: Neutralization of interleukin-1β in the acute phase of myocardial infarction promotes the progression of left ventricular remodeling. *J Am Coll Cardiol* 38:546, 2001.

135. Oemar BS: Is interleukin-1β a triggering factor for restenosis? *Cardiovasc Res* 44(1):17, 1999.

136. Simon AB, Yazdani S, Wang W, et al: Circulating levels if IL-1β, a prothrombotic cytokine, are elevated in unstable versus stable angina. *J Thromb Thrombolysis* 9(3):217, 2000.

137. Munger MA, Johnson B, Amber IJ, et al: Circulating concentrations of proinflammatory cytokines in mild or moderate heart failure secondary to ischemic or idiopathic dilated cardiomyopathy. *Am J Cardiol* 77:723, 1996.

138. Tashiro H, Shimokawa H, Yamamoto K, et al: Monocyte-related cytokines in acute myocardial infarction. *Am Heart J* 130:446, 1995.

139. Okusawa G, Gelfand JA, Ikejma T, et al: Interleukin-1 induces a shock-like state in rabbits: Synergism with tumor necrosis factor and the effect of cyclooxygenase inhibition. *J Clin Invest* 81:1162, 1988.

140. LaPointe MC, Sitkins JR: Mechanisms of interleukin-1β-regulation of nitric oxide synthase in cardiac myocytes. *Hypertension* 27(pt 2):709, 1996.

141. Raymond RJ, Dehmer GJ, Theoharides TC, Deluargynis EN: Elevated IL-6 levels in patients with asymptomatic left ventricular systolic dysfunction. *Am Heart J* 141(3):435, 2001.

142. Koukkunen H, Penttila K, Keuppaina A, et al: C-reactive protein, fibrinogen, IL-6, and tumor necrosis factor-alpha in prognostic classification of unstable angina pectoris. *Ann Med* 33:37, 2001.

143. Rawczynska-Englert I: Evaluation of serum cytokine concentration in patients with infective endocarditis. *J Heart Valve Dis* 9(5):705, 2000.

144. Blankenberg S, Ruprecht HJ, Bickel C, et al: Cytomegalovirus infection with IL-6 response predicts cardiac mortality in patients with coronary artery disease. *Circulation* 103:2915, 2001.

145. Ross R: Atherosclerosis is an inflammatory disease. *Am Heart J* 138(5):S419, 1999.

146. Mazzone A: Plasma levels of IL-2, 6, 10 and phenotypic characterization of circulating T-lymphocytes in ischemic heart disease. *Atherosclerosis* 145(2):369, 1999.

147. Simon AD, Yazdani S, Wang W, et al: Elevated plasma levels of IL-2 and soluble IL-2 receptor in ischemic heart disease. *Clin Cardiol* 24:253, 2001.

148. Afansyeva M, Wang Y, Kaya Z, et al: Experimental autoimmune myocarditis in A/J mice is a IL-4 dependent disease with a Th2-phenotype. *Am J Pathol* 159(1):193, 2001.

149. Satoskar AR: IL-4 deficient BALB/C mice develop an enhanced Th-1-like response but control cardiac inflammation following *Borrelia burgdorferi* infection. *FEMS Microbiol Lett* 183:319, 2000.

150. Jones SP, Trocha SD, Lefer DJ: Cardioprotective actions of endogenous IL-10 are independent of iNOS. *Am J Physiol* 281:H48, 2001.

151. Veltrop MH, Langermans JA, Thompson J, Bancsi MJ: IL-10 regulates the tissue factor activity of monocytes in an in vitro model of bacterial endocarditis. *Infect Immun* 69(5):3197, 2001.

151a. Bolger AP, Sharma R, von Haehling S, et al: Effect of interleukin-10 on the production of tumor necrosis factor-alpha by peripheral blood mononuclear cells from patients with chronic heart failure. *Am J Cardiol* 90:384, 2002.

152. Kanda T, Wilson McManus JE, Nagai R, et al: Modification of viral myocarditis in mice by interleukin-6. *Circ Res* 78:848, 1996.

153. Beniaminovitz A, Hesin S, Lietz K: Prevention of rejection in cardiac transplantation by blockade of the IL-2 receptor with a monoclonal antibody. *N Engl J Med* 342:613, 2000.

154. Tamai H, Katoh O, Suzuki S, et al: Impact of tranilast on restenosis after coronary angioplasty: Tranilast Restenosis Following Angioplasty Trial (TREAT). *Am Heart J* 138(5):968, 1999.

155. Gullestad L, Aukrust P, Ueland T, et al: Effect of high- verus low-dose angiotensin converting enzyme inhibitor on cytokine levels in chronic heart failure. *J Am Coll Cardiol* 34:2068, 1999.

156. Munglani R, Hudspith MJ, Hunt SPL: The therapeutic potential of neuropeptide Y. Analgesic, anxiolytic and antihypertensive. *Drugs* 52:371, 1996.

156a. Correia MLG, Morgan DA, Sivitz WI, et al: Hemodynamic consequences of neuropeptide-y-induced obesity. *Am J Hypertens* 15:137, 2002.

157. Grundemar L, Hakanson R: Neuropeptide Y effector systems: Perspectives for drug development. *Trends Pharmacol Sci* 15:153, 1994.

158. Serone AP, Wright CE, Angus JA: Role of NPY Y1 receptors in cardiovascular control in the conscious rabbit. *J Cardiovasc Pharmacol* 35:315, 2000.

159. Abrahamsson C: Neuropeptide Y1- and Y2- receptor-mediated cardiovascular effects in the anesthetized guinea pig, rat, and rabbit. *J Cardiovasc Pharmacol* 36:451, 2000.

160. Michel MC, Rascher W: Neuropeptide Y: A possible role in hypertension? *J Hypertens* 13:385, 1995.

161. Matsumura K, Tsuchihashi T, Abe I: Central cardiovascular action of neuropeptide Y in conscious rabbits. *Hypertension* 36:1040, 2000.

162. Nilsson T, Hrafnkelsdottir T, Edvinsson L, et al: Forearm blood flow responses to neuropeptide Y, noradrenaline and adenosine $5'$-triphosphate in hypertensive and normotensive subjects. *Blood Press* 9:126, 2000.

163. Basu S, Sinha SK, Shao Q, et al: Neuropeptide Y modulation of sympathetic activity in myocardial infarction. *J Am Coll Cardiol* 27:1796, 1996.

164. Daggubati S, Parks JR, Overton RM, et al: Adrenomedullin, endothelin, neuropeptide Y, atrial, brain, and C-natriuretic prohormone peptides compared as early heart failure indicators. *Cardiovasc Res* 36(2):246, 1997.

165. Lambert ML, Callow ID, Feng QP, et al: The effects of age on human venous responsiveness to neuropeptide Y. *Br J Clin Pharmacol* 47:83, 1999.

166. Feng Q, Lambert ML, Callow ID, Arnold JM: Venous neuropeptide Y receptor responsiveness in patients with chronic heart failure. *Clin Pharmacol Ther* 67:292, 2000.

167. Feng Q, Sun X, Lu X, et al: Decreased responsiveness of vascular postjunctional alpha1-alpha2-adrenoceptors and neuropeptide Y1 receptors in the rats with heart failure. *Acta Physiol Scand* 166(4):285, 1999.

168. Gullestad L, Aass H, Ross H, et al: Neuropeptide Y receptor 1 (NPY-Y1) expression in human heart failure and heart transplantation. *J Auton Nerv Syst* 70(1-2):84, 1998.

169. Mertes PM, el-Abbassi K, Jaboin Y, et al: Consequences of coronary occlusion on changes in regional interstitial myocardial neuropeptide Y and norepinephrine concentrations. *J Mol Cell Cardiol* 28(9):1995, 1996.

170. Gullestad L, Jorgensen B, Bjuro T, et al: Postexercise ischemia is associated with increased neuropeptide Y in patients with coronary artery disease. *Circulation* 102(9):987, 2000.

171. Zukowska-Grojec Z, Karwatowska-Prokopczuk E, Rose W, et al: Neuropeptide Y: A novel angiogenic factor from the sympathetic nerves and endothelium. *Cir Res* 83(2):187, 1998.

172. Pellieux C, Sauthier T, Domenighetti A, et al: Neuropeptide Y (NPY) potentiates phenylephrine-induced mitogen-activated protein kinase activation in primary cardiomyocytes via NPY Y5 receptors. *Proc Natl Acad Sci U S A* 97:1595, 2000.

173. Tadepalli AS, Harrington WW, Hashim MA, et al: Hemodynamic characterization of a novel neuropeptide Y receptor antagonist. *J Cardiovasc Pharmacol* 27:712, 1996.

174. Daniels AJ, Matthews JE, Slepetis RJ, et al: High-affinity neuropeptide Y receptor antagonists. *Proc Natl Acad Sci U S A* 92:9067, 1995.

175. Doods HN, Wienen W, Entzeroth M, et al: Pharmacological characterization of the selective nonpeptide neuropeptide Y Y1 receptor antagonist BIBP3226. *J Pharmacol Exp Ther* 275:136, 1995.

176. Serradeil-Le Gal C, Valette G, Rouby P-E, et al: SR120819A, an orally active and selective neuropeptide Y Y1 receptor antagonist. *FEBS Lett* 362:192, 1995.

177. Levy D, Garrison RJ, Savage DD, et al: Prognostic implications of echocardiographically determined left ventricular mass in the Framingham heart study. *N Engl J Med* 322:1561, 1990.

178. Olson E, Molkentin J: Prevention of cardiac hypertrophy by calcineurin inhibition: hope or hype? *Circ Res* 84:623, 1999.

179. Sussman M, Lim H, Gude N, et al: Prevention of cardiac hypertrophy in mice by calcineurin inhibition. *Science* 281:1690, 1998.

180. Hachamovitch R, Sonnenblick EH, Strom JA, Frishman WH: Left ventricular hypertrophy in hypertension and the effects of antihypertensive drug therapy. *Curr Probl Cardiol* 13:375, 1988.

181. Watkins H, Seidman JG, Seidman CE: Familial hypertrophic cardiomyopathy: A genetic model of cardiac hypertrophy. *Hum Mol Genet* 1721, 1995.

182. Bottinelli R, Coviello DA, Redwood CS, et al: Mutant tropomyosin that causes hypertrophic cardiomyopathy is expressed in vivo and associated with an increased Ca^{2+} sensitivity. *Circ Res* 82:106, 1997.

183. Berridge MJ: Ca^{2+} signaling and cell proliferation. *Bioassay* 17:491, 1995.

184. Molkentin JD, Lu J-R, Antos C, et al: A calcineurin-dependent transcriptional pathway for cardiac hypertrophy. *Cell* 93:215, 1998.

185. Eto Y, Yonekura K, Sonoda M, et al: Calcineurin is activated in rat hearts with physiological left ventricular hypertrophy induced by voluntary exercise training. *Circulation* 101:2134, 2000.

186. Klee CB, Ren H, Wang X: Regulation of the calmodulin-stimulated protein phosphatase, calcineurin. *J Biol Chem* 273:13367, 1998.

187. Zhang BW, Zimmer G, Chen J, et al: T-cell responses in calcineurin A alpha-deficient mice. *J Exp Med* 183:413, 1996.

188. Grepin C, Dagnino LL, Robitaille L, et al: A hormone-encoding gene identifies a pathway for cardiac but not skeletal muscle gene transcription. *Mol Cell Biol* 14:3115, 1994.

189. Hongo K, White E, Gannier F, et al: Effect of stretch on contraction and the Ca^{2+} transient in ferret ventricular muscles during hypoxia and acidosis. *Am J Physiol* 269:C690, 1995.

190. Rao A, Luo C, Hogan PC: Transcription factors of the NFAT family: regulation and function. *Annu Rev Immunol* 15:707, 1997.

191. Shibasaki F, Price ER, Milan D, McKeon F: Role of kinases and the phosphatase calcineurin in the nuclear shuttling of transcription factor NF-AT4. *Nature* 382:370, 1996.

192. Molkentin JD, Olson EN: GATA4: A novel transcriptional regulator of cardiac hypertrophy? *Circulation* 96:3833, 1997.

193. Hasegawa K, Lee SJ, Jobe SM, et al: Cis-acting sequences that mediate induction of beta-myosin heavy chain expression during left ventricular hypertrophy due to aortic constriction. *Circulation* 96:3943, 1997.

194. Lim H, De Windt L, Steinberg L, et al: Calcineurin expression, activation, and function in cardiac pressure-overload hypertrophy. *Circulation* 101:2431, 2000.

195. Chen L, Glover JNM, Hogan PG, et al: Structure of the DNA-binding domains from NFAT, Fos and Jun bound specifically to DNA. *Nature* 392:42, 1998.

196. McDonough PM, Hanford DS, Sprenkle AB, et al: Collaborative roles for c-Jun N-terminal kinase, c-Jun, serum response factor and Sp1 in calcium-regulated myocardial gene expression. *J Biol Chem* 272:24046, 1997.

197. Ho PD, Zechner DK, He H, et al: The Raf-MEK-ERK cascade represents a common pathway for the alteration of intracellular calcium by Ras and protein kinase C in cardiac myocytes. *J Biol Chem* 273:21730, 1998.

198. Henning SW, Cantrell DA: GTPases in antigen receptor signaling. *Curr Opin Immunol* 10:322, 1998.

198a. Parasrampuria DA, Lantz MV, Birnbaum JL, et al: Effect of calcineurin inhibitor therapy on P-gp expression and function in lymphocytes of renal transplant patients: A preliminary evaluation. *J Clin Pharmacol* 42:304, 2002.

199. Schreiber SL: Chemistry and biology of the immunophilins and their immunosuppressive ligands. *Science* 251:283, 1991.

200. Emmel EA, Verweij CL, Durand DB, et al: Cyclosporin A specifically inhibits function of nuclear proteins involved in T cell activation. *Science* 246:1617, 1989.

201. Haines DD, Bak I, Ferdinandy P, et al: Cardioprotective effects of calcineurin inhibitor FK 506 and the PAF receptor antagonist and free radical scavenger, Egb 761, in isolated ischemic/reperfused rat hearts. *J Cardiovasc Pharmacol* 35:37, 2000.

202. Zhang W, Kowal RC, Rusnak F, et al: Failure of calcineurin inhibitors to prevent pressure-overload left ventricular hypertrophy in rats. *Circ Res* 84:722, 1999.

203. Ding B, Price RL, Borg TK, et al: Pressure overload induces severe hypertrophy in mice treated with cyclosporine, an inhibitor of calcineurin. *Circ Res* 84:729, 1999.

204. Meguro T, Hong C, Asai K, et al: Cyclosporine attenuates pressure-overload hypertrophy in mice while enhancing susceptibility to decompensation and heart failure. *Circ Res* 84:735, 1999.

205. O'Connor CM, Gattis WA, Swedberg K: Current and novel pharmacologic approaches in advanced heart failure. *Am Heart J* 135(6 pt 2 Suppl):S249, 1998.

206. Rowan RA, Billingham ME: Pathologic changes in the long-term transplanted heart: A morphometric study of myocardial hypertrophy, vascularity and fibrosis. *Hum Pathol* 21:767, 1990.

207. Ventura HO, Lavie CJ, Messerli FH, et al: Cardiovascular adaptation to cyclosporine-induced hypertension. *J Hum Hypertens* 8:233, 1994.

208. Aperia A, Ibarra F, Svensson LB, Klee C, Greengard P: Calcineurin mediates alpha-adrenergic stimulation of Na$^+$/K$^+$-ATPase activity in renal tubule cells. *Proc Natl Acad Sci U S A* 89:7394, 1992.

209. Radermacher J, Meiners M, Bramlage C, et al: Pronounced renal vasoconstriction and systemic hypertension in renal transplant patients treated with cyclosporin versus FK506. *Transpl Int* 11:3, 1998.

210. Hojo M, Morimoto T, Maluccio M, et al: Cyclosporine induces cancer progression by a cell-autonomous mechanism. *Nature* 397:530, 1999.

211. Rothermel BA, McKinsey TA, Vega RB, et al: Myocyte-enriched calcineurin-interacting protein, MCIP1, inhibits cardiac hypertrophy in vivo. *Proc Natl Acad Sci U S A* 98:3328, 2001.

212. De Windt LJ, Lim HW, Bueno OF, et al: Targeted inhibition of calcineurin attenuates cardiac hypertrophy in vivo. *Proc Natl Acad Sci U S A* 98:3322, 2001.

213. Shimoyama M, Hayashi D, Takimoto E, et al: Calcineurin plays a critical role in pressure overload-induced cardiac hypertrophy. *Circulation* 100:2449, 1999.

214. Lim HW, Molkentin JD. Calcineurin and human heart failure. *Nat Med* 5:246, 1999.

215. Carretero OA, Scicli AG: The kallikrein-kinin system as a regulator of cardiovascular and renal function. In: Laragh JH, Brenner BM, eds. *Hypertension: Pathophysiology, Diagnosis and Management.* New York: Raven Press, 1995:983.

216. Groves P, Kurz S, Just H, Drexler H: Role of endogenous bradykinin in human coronary vasomotor control. *Circulation* 92:3424, 1995.

217. Madeddu P, Emanueli C, Maestri R, et al: Angiotensin II type 1 receptor blockade prevents cardiac remodeling in bradykinin B2 receptor knockout mice. *Hypertension* 2000(1 pt 2):391.

218. Dell'Italia LJ, Oparil S: Bradykinin in the heart. Friend or foe? *Circulation* 100:2305, 1999.

219. Ito K, Zhu YZ, Zhu YC, et al: Contribution of bradykinin to the cardioprotective action of angiotensin converting enzyme inhibition in hypertension and after myocardial infarction. *Jpn J Pharmacol* 75(4):311, 1997.

220. Kokkonen JO, Kuoppala A, Saarinen J, et al: Kallidin- and bradykinin-degrading pathways in human heart. Degradation of kallidin by aminopeptidase M-like activity and bradykinin by neutral endopeptidase. *Circulation* 99:1984, 1999.

221. Regoli D, Rhaleb NE, Drapeau G, et al: Basic pharmacology of kinins: pharmacologic receptors and other mechanisms. *Adv Exp Med Biol* 247A:399, 1989.

222. Faussner A, Bathon JM, Proud D: Comparison of the responses of B and B2 kinin receptors to agonist stimulation. *Immunopharmacology* 45:13, 1999.

223. Regoli D, Gobeil F, Nguyen QT, et al: Bradykinin receptor types and B2 subtypes. *Life Sci* 55:735, 1994.

224. McEachern AE, Shelton ER, Bhakta S, et al: Expression cloning of a rat B2 bradykinin receptor. *Proc Natl Acad Sci U S A* 88(17):7724, 1991.

225. Burch RM, Farmer SG, Steranka LR: Bradykinin receptor antagonists. *Med Res Rev* 10:237, 1990.

226. Schror K: Role of prostaglandins in the cardiovascular effects of bradykinin and angiotensin-converting enzyme inhibitors. *J Cardiovasc Pharmacol* 20(Suppl 9):S68, 1992.

227. Regoli D, Rhaleb NE, Dion S, Drapeau G: New selective bradykinin receptor antagonists and bradykinin B2 receptor characterization. *Trends Pharmacol Sci* 11:156, 1990.

228. Cheng CP, Onishi K, Ohte N, et al: Functional effects of endogenous bradykinin in congestive heart failure. *J Am Coll Cardiol* 31:1679, 1998.

229. Bonner G: The role of kinins in the antihypertensive and cardioprotective effects of ACE inhibitors. *Drugs* 54(Suppl 5):23, 1997.

230. Yamasaki S, Sawada H, Komatsu S, et al: Effects of bradykinin on prostaglandin I_2 synthesis in human vascular endothelial cells. *Hypertension* 36:201, 2000.

231. Sharma JN: Interrelationship between the kallikrein-kinin system and hypertension: A review. *Gen Pharmacol* 19:177, 1988.

232. Bouaziz H, Joulin Y, Safar M, Benetos A: Effects of bradykinin B2 receptor antagonism on the hypotensive effects of ACE inhibition. *Br J Pharmacol* 113:717, 1994.

233. Gainer JV, Morrow JD, Loveland A, et al: Effect of bradykinin-receptor blockade on the response to angiotensin-converting-enzyme inhibitor in normotensive and hypertensive subjects. *N Engl J Med* 339:1285, 1998.

234. Streeten DH, Kerr CB, Kerr LP, Prior JC, Dalakos TG: Hyperbradykininism: A new orthostatic syndrome. *Lancet* 2(7786):1048, 1972.

235. Miura H, Liu Y, Gutterman DD: Human coronary arteriolar dilation to bradykinin depends on membrane hyperpolarization. Contribution of nitric oxide and Ca^{2+}-activated K^+ channels. *Circulation* 99:3132, 1999.

236. Brown NJ, Gainer JV, Murphey LJ, Vaughan DE: Bradykinin stimulates tissue plasminogen activator release from human forearm vasculature through B2 receptor-dependent, NO synthase-independent, and cyclooxygenase-independent pathway. *Circulation* 102:2190, 2000.

237. Su JB, Houël R, Héloire F, et al: Stimulation of bradykinin B1 receptors induces vasodilation in conductance and resistance coronary vessels in conscious dogs. Comparison with B2 receptor stimulation. *Circulation* 101:1848, 2000.

237a. Emanueli C, Salis MB, Stacca T, et al: Targeting kinin β_1 receptor for therapeutic neovascularization. *Circulation* 105:360, 2002.

238. Minai K, Matsumoto T, Horie H, et al: ACE inhibitor augments the release of tissue plasminogen activator induced by bradykinin in the human coronary circulation (abstr.). *J Am Coll Cardiol* 37(Suppl A):293A, 2001.

239. Brew EC, Mitchell MB, Rehring TF, et al: Role of bradykinin in cardiac functional protection after global ischemia-reperfusion in rat heart. *Am J Physiol* 269(4 pt 2):H1370, 1995.

240. Tschöpe C, Heringer-Walther S, Koch M, et al: Myocardial bradykinin B2-receptor expression at different time points after induction of myocardial infarction. *J Hypertens* 18:223, 2000.

241. Linz W, Wiemer G, Scholkens BA: Beneficial effects of bradykinin on myocardial energy metabolism and infarct size. *Am J Cardiol* 80(3A):118A, 1997.

242. Yoshida H, Zhang JJ, Chao L, Chao J: Kallikrein gene delivery attenuates myocardial infarction and apoptosis after myocardial ischemia and reperfusion. *Hypertension* 35:25, 2000.

243. Wolfrum S, Dendorfer A, Tempel K, et al: Apstatin, a new inhibition of aminopeptidase P, reduces myocardial infarction size by a kinin-dependent pathway (abstr.). *J Am Coll Cardiol* 37(Suppl A):330A, 2001.

244. Goto M, Liu Y, Yang XM, et al: Role of bradykinin in protection of ischemic preconditioning in rabbit hearts. *Circ Res* 77:611, 1995.

245. Schulz R, Post H, Vahlhaus C, Heusch G: Ischemic preconditioning in pigs: A graded phenomenon: its relation to adenosine and bradykinin. *Circulation* 98:1022, 1998.

246. Leesar MA, Stoddard MF, Manchikalapudi S, Bolli R: Bradykinin-induced preconditioning in patients undergoing coronary angioplasty. *J Am Coll Cardiol* 34:639, 1999.

247. Stauss HM, Zhu YC, Redlich T, et al: Angiotensin-converting enzyme inhibition in infarct-induced heart failure in rats: Bradykinin versus angiotensin II. *J Cardiovasc Risk* 1:255, 1994.

248. Holtz J: Role of ACE inhibition or AT1 blockade in the remodeling following myocardial infarction. *Basic Res Cardiol* 93(Suppl 2):92, 1998.

249. Ishigai Y, Mori T, Ikeda T, et al: Role of bradykinin-NO pathway in prevention of cardiac hypertrophy by ACE inhibitor in rat cardiomyocytes. *Am J Physiol* 273(6 pt 2):H2659, 1997.

250. Agata J, Miao RQ, Yayama K, et al: Bradykinin B1 receptor mediates inhibition of neointima formation in rat artery after balloon angioplasty. *Hypertension* 36:364, 2000.

251. Su JB, Barbe F, Houel R, et al: Preserved vasodilator effect of bradykinin in dogs with heart failure. *Circulation* 98:2911, 1998.

252. The SOLVD Investigators: Effect of enalapril on survival in patients with reduced left ventricular ejection fractions and congestive heart failure. *N Engl J Med* 325:293, 1991.

253. Liu Y-H, Yang X-P, Mehta D, et al: Role of kinins in chronic heart failure and in the therapeutic effect of ACE inhibitors in kininogen-deficient rats. *Am J Physiol* 278:H507, 2000.

254. Yonemochi H, Yasunaga S, Teshima Y, et al: Mechanism of beta-adrenergic receptor upregulation induced by ACE inhibition in cultured neonatal rat cardiac myocytes: Roles of bradykinin and protein kinase C. *Circulation* 97:2268, 1998.

255. Mathier MA, Bartus RT, Shannon RP: Bradykinin agonist, Cereport, is a potent systemic and coronary vasodilator in conscious dogs with pacing induced heart failure (abstr.). *Circulation* 100:I-299, 1999.

255a. Witherow FN, Dawson P, Ludlam CA, et al: Marked bradykinin-induced tissue plasminogen activator release in patients with heart failure maintained on long term angiotensin-converting enzyme inhibitor therapy. *J Am Coll Cardiol* 40:961, 2002.

256. Zhang X, Recchia FA, Bernstein R, et al: Kinin-mediated coronary nitric oxide production contributes to the therapeutic action of angiotensin-converting enzyme and neutral endopeptidase inhibitors and amlodipine in the treatment in heart failure. *J Pharmacol Exp Ther* 288:742, 1999.

257. Emanueli C, Grady EF, Madeddu P, et al: Acute ACE inhibition causes plasma extravasation in mice that is mediated by bradykinin and substance P. *Hypertension* 31:1299, 1998.

258. Kurz T, Tolg R, Richardt G: Bradykinin B2-receptor-mediated stimulation of exocytotic noradrenaline release from cardiac sympathetic neurons. *J Mol Cell Cardiol* 29:2561, 1997.

259. Seyedi N, Maruyama R, Levi R: Bradykinin activates a cross-signaling pathway between sensory and adrenergic nerve endings in the heart: A novel mechanism of ischemic norepinephrine release? *J Pharmacol Exp Ther* 290:656, 1999.

260. Pellacani A, Brunner HR, Nussberger J: Antagonizing and measurement: approaches to understanding of hemodynamic effects of kinins. *J Cardiovasc Pharmacol* 20(Suppl 9):S28, 1992.

261. Bern HA, Pearson D, Larson BA, et al: Neurohormones from fish tails: The caudal neurosecretory system. I: "Urophysiology" and the caudal neurosecretory system in fishes. *Recent Prog Horm Res* 41:533, 1985.

262. Pearson D, Shively JE, Clark BR, et al: Urotensin II: A somatostatin-like peptide in the caudal neurosecretory system of fishes. *Proc Natl Acad Sci U S A* 77:5021, 1980.

263. Conlon JM, O'Harte F, Smith DD, et al: Isolation and primary structure of urotensin II from the brain of a tetrapod, the frog *Rana ridibunda*. *Biochem Biophys Res Commun* 188:578, 1992.

264. Coulouarn Y, Lihrmann I, Jegou S, et al: Cloning of the cDNA encoding the urotensin II precursor in frog and human reveals intense expression of the urotensin II gene in motoneurons of the spinal cord. *Proc Natl Acad Sci U S A* 95:15803, 1998.

265. Ames RS, Sarau HM, Chambers JK, et al: Human urotensin-II is a potent vasoconstrictor and agonist for the orphan receptor GPR14. *Nature* 401:282, 1999.

266. Conlon JM, Tostivint H, Vaudry H: Somatostatin- and urotensin II-related peptides: Molecular diversity and evolutionary perspectives. *Regul Pept* 69:95, 1997.

267. Ohsako S, Ishida I, Ichikawa T, et al: Cloning and sequence analysis of cDNAs encoding precursors of urotensin II-alpha and -gamma. *J Neurosci* 6:2730, 1986.

268. Conlon JM, Yano K, Waugh D, et al: Distribution and molecular forms of urotensin II and its role in cardiovascular regulation in vertebrates. *J Exp Zool* 275:226, 1996.

269. Itoh H, McMaster D, Lederis K: Functional receptors for fish neuropeptide urotensin II in major rat arteries. *Eur J Pharmacol* 149:61, 1988.

270. Protopopov A, Kashuba V, Podowski R, et al: Assignment of GPR14 gene coding for the G-protein-coupled receptor 14 to human chromosome 17q25.3 by fluorescent in situ hybridization. *Cytogenet Cell Genet* 88:312, 2000.

271. Marchese A, Heiber M, Nguyen T, et al: Cloning and chromosomal mapping of three novel genes, GPR9, GPR10, and GPR14, encoding receptors related to interleukin 8 neuropeptide Y, and somatostatin receptors. *Genomics* 29:335, 1995.

272. Davenport AP and Maguire JJ: Urotensin II: fish neuropeptide catches orphan receptor. *Trends Pharmacol Sci* 21:80, 2000.

273. Douglas SA, Sulpizio AC, Piercy V, et al: Differential vasoconstrictor activity of human urotensin-II in vascular tissue isolated from the rat, mouse, dog, pig, marmoset and cynomolgus monkey. *Br J Pharmacol* 131:1262, 2000.

274. Bottrill FE, Douglas SA, Hiley CR, et al: Human urotensin-II is an endothelium-dependent vasodilator in rat small arteries. *Br J Pharmacol* 130:1865, 2000.

275. Maguire JJ, Kuc RE, Davenport AP: Orphan-receptor ligand human urotensin II: receptor localization in human tissues and comparison of vasoconstrictor responses with endothelin-1. *Br J Pharmacol* 131:441, 2000.

276. Hillier C, Berry C, Petrie MC, et al: Effects of urotensin II in human arteries and veins of varying caliber. *Circulation* 13:1378, 2001.

277. Paysant J, Rupin A, Simonet S, et al: Comparison of the contractile responses of human coronary bypass grafts and monkey arteries to human urotensin-II. *Fundam Clin Pharmacol* 15(4):227, 2001.

278. Opgaard OS, Nothacker HP, Ehlert FJ, et al: Human urotensin II mediates vasoconstriction via an increase in inositol phosphates. *Eur J Pharmacol* 406:265, 2000.

279. Mori M, Sugo T, Abe M, et al: Urotensin II is the endogenous ligand of a G-protein-coupled orphan receptor, SENR (GPR14). *Biochem Biophys Res Commun* 265:123, 1999.

280. Somlyo AP, Somlyo AV: Signal transduction by G-proteins, rho-kinase and protein phosphatase to smooth muscle and non-muscle myosin II. *J Physiol* 522:177, 2000.

281. Sauzeau V, Le Mellionnec E, Bertoglio J, et al: Human urotensin II-induced contraction and arterial smooth muscle cell proliferation are mediated by rhoA and rho-kinase. *Cir Res* 88:1102, 2001.

282. Gibson A: Complex effects of Gillichthys urotensin II on rat aortic strips. *Br J Pharmacol* 91:205, 1987.

283. Maclean MR, Alexander D, Stirrat A, et al: Contractile response to human urotensin-II in rat and human pulmonary arteries: Effect of chronic hypoxia in the rat. *Br J Pharmacol* 123:201, 2000.

284. Stirrat A, Gallagher M, Douglas SA, et al: Potent vasodilator responses to human urotensin-II in human pulmonary and abdominal resistance arteries. *Am J Physiol Heart Circ Physiol* 280:H925, 2001.

285. Katano Y, Ishihata A, Tomomi A, et al: Vasodilator effect of urotensin I, one of the most potent vasoconstricting factors, on rat coronary arteries. *Euro J Pharmacol* 402:209, 2000.

286. Douglas SA, Ohlstein EH: Human urotensin-II, the most potent mammalian vasoconstrictor identified to date, as a therapeutic target for the management of cardiovascular disease. *Trends Cardiovasc Med* 10:229, 2000.

287. Watanabe T, Pakal R, Katagiri T, et al: Synergistic effect of urotensin II with mildly oxidized LDL on DNA synthesis in vascular smooth muscle cells. *Circulation* 104:16, 2001.

288. Watanabe T, Pakala R, Benedict CR, et al: Lysophosphatidylcholine and reactive oxygen species mediate the synergistic effect of mildly oxidized LDL with serotonin on vascular smooth muscle cell proliferation. *Circulation* 103:1440, 2001.

289. Tzanidis A, Hannan RD, Krum H: Urotensin-II stimulates collagen synthesis by cardiac fibroblasts in vitro: Implications for myocardial remodeling. *Eur Heart J* 21:72, 2000.

290. Vasan S, Zhang X, Kapurniotu A, et al: An agent cleaving glucose-derived protein crosslinks in vitro and in vivo. *Nature* 382:275, 1996.

291. Wolffenbuttel BH, Boulanger CM, Crijns FR, et al: Breakers of advanced glycation end products restore large artery properties in experimental diabetes. *Proc Natl Acad Sci U S A* 95:4630, 1998.

292. Vaitkevicius PV, Lane M, Spurgeon H, et al: A cross-link breaker has sustained effects on arterial and ventricular properties in older rhesus monkeys. *Proc Natl Acad Sci U S A* 98:1171, 2001.

293. Safar ME: Epidemiological findings imply that goals for drug treatment of hypertension need to be revised. *Circulation* 103:1088, 2001.

294. Safar ME, Rudnichi A, Asmar R: Drug treatment of hypertension: The reduction of pulse pressure does not necessarily parallel that of systolic and diastolic blood pressure. *J Hypertens* 18:1159, 2000.

295. Lee AT, Cerami A: Role of glycation in aging. *Ann N Y Acad Sci* 663:63, 1992.

296. Corman B, Duriez M, Poitevin P, et al: Aminoguanidine prevents age-related stiffening and cardiac hypertrophy. *Proc Natl Acad Sci U S A* 95:1301, 1998.

297. Kass DA for the Study Investigators: A placebo-controlled safety and pharmacology study of ALT-711 in older patients with stiffened cardiovasculature (abst.). *J Am Coll Cardiol* 38:602:2001.

298. Snoeckx LHEH, Cornelussen RN, Van Nieuwenhoven FA, et al: Heat shock proteins and cardiovascular pathophysiology. *Physiol Rev* 81:1461, 2001.

299. Frostegard J, Lemne C, Andersson B, et al: Association of serum antibodies to heat shock protein 65 with borderline hypertension. *Hypertension* 29:40, 1997.

300. Pockley AG, Wu R, Lemne C, et al: Circulating heat shock protein 60 is associated with early cardiovascular disease. *Hypertension* 36:303, 2000.

301. Zhu J, Quyyumi AA, Rott D, et al: Antibodies to human heat shock protein 60 are associated with the presence and severity of coronary artery disease: Evidence for an autoimmune components of atherogenesis. *Circulation* 103:1071, 2001.

302. Xu Q, Schett G, Perschinka H, et al: Serum soluble heat shock protein 60 is elevated in subjects with atherosclerosis in a general population. *Circulation* 102:14, 2000.

303. Prohaszka Z, Duba J, Horvath L, et al: Comparative study on antibodies to human and bacterial 60 kDa heat shock proteins in a large cohort of patients with coronary heart disease and healthy subjects. *Eur J Clin Invest* 31:285, 2001.

304. Martin JL, Mestril R, Hilal-Dandan R, et al: Small heat shock proteins and protection against ischemic injury in cardiac myocytes. *Circulation* 96:4343, 1997.

305. Hunter MM, Sievers RE, Barbosa V, Wolfe C: Heat shock protein induction in rat hearts. A direct correlation between the amount of heat shock protein induced and the degree of myocardial protection. *Circulation* 89:353, 1994.

306. Currie RW: Effects of ischemia and perfusion temperature on the synthesis of stress-induced (heat shock) proteins in isolated and perfused rat hearts. *J Mol Cell Cardiol* 19:795, 1987.

307. Currie RW, Karmazyn M, Kloc M: Heat shock response is associated with enhanced postischemic ventricular recovery. *Circ Res* 63:543, 1988.

308. Latchman DS: Heat shock proteins and cardiac protection. *Cardiovasc Res* 51:637, 2001.

308a. Pockley AG: Heat shock proteins, inflammation, and cardiovascular disease. *Circulation* 105:1012, 2002.

309. Yamagami K, Yamamoto Y, Ishikawa Y, et al: Effects of geranyl-geranyl-acetone administration before heat shock preconditioning for conferring tolerance against ischemia-reperfusion injury in rat livers. *J Lab Clin Med* 135:465, 2000.

310. Jednakovits A, Ferdinandy P, Jaszlits L, et al: In vivo and in vitro acute cardiovascular effects of bimoclomol. *Gen Pharmacol* 34:363, 2000.

311. Emiliusen L, Gough M, Bateman A, et al: A transcriptional feedback loop for tissue-specific expression of highly cytotoxic genes which incorporates an immunostimulatory components. *Gene Ther* 8:987, 2001.

312. Christians ES, Yan L-J, Benjamin IJ: Heat shock factor 1 and heat shock proteins: Critical partners in protection against acute cell injury. *Crit Care Med* 30(Suppl):S43, 2002.

313. Sihvola R, Koskinen P, Myllärniemi M, et al: Prevention of cardiac allograft arteriosclerosis by protein tyrosine kinase inhibitor selective for platelet-derived growth factor receptor. *Circulation* 99:2295, 1999.

314. Weinbrenner C, Baines CP, Liu G-S, et al: Fostriecin, an inhibitor of protein phosphatase 2A, limits myocardial infarct size even when administered after onset of ischemia. *Circulation* 98:899, 1998.

Pharmacologic Therapies for the Prevention of Restenosis Following Percutaneous Coronary Artery Interventions

William H. Frishman

Brian R. Landzberg

Melvin Weiss

The introduction of percutaneous transluminal coronary angioplasty (PTCA) by Andreas Gruntzig, in 1979, has had a tremendous impact on the management of patients with coronary artery disease (CAD).[1] Interventional cardiologists are now able to rapidly and directly alleviate coronary obstruction with a remarkably low morbidity and mortality.[2] The applications of this procedure have extended from its original use in stable angina for single-vessel disease to include higher risk patients with multivessel disease, total occlusion, complex lesions, unstable angina, and acute myocardial infarction, while the overall in-hospital success rate has been increasing over the last decade, from 67 to 88% per lesion, with 91% realizing improvement in at least one dilated segment.[3] Abrupt closure in the first 24 h after the procedure, occurring in less than 6% of cases, can be effectively reversed in over half of those cases. Comparisons of sequential National Heart Lung and Blood Institute (NHLBI) Angioplasty Registries demonstrate that acute complications, including hospital deaths, myocardial infarctions, and emergency bypass surgery, have greatly declined, with estimated current rates of 1%, 4.3%, and 1.8%, respectively. Much of this improvement is attributed to the aggressive use of antispasmodic agents, anticoagulants, thrombolysis, and new mechanical devices, including perfusion balloons and intravascular stents. Such favorable results have led to the current performance level of over 300,000 such procedures annually in the United States.

Although the occurrence of acute complications has been greatly reduced,[4] it has become increasingly apparent that the rate of chronic recurrence of occlusions after angioplasty and stenting, or restenosis, has been relatively unaffected, and are currently estimated at 30 to 50%.[8] Rates range widely, depending on which clinical or angiographic criteria are used,[9] and are substantially higher in patients undergoing second and third courses of PTCA.[10] The marked prevalence of restenosis clearly compromises the long-term benefits associated with percutaneous procedures and has far-reaching consequences. In a recent 10-year follow-up study of coronary angioplasty, patients with restenosis 6 months after PTCA had a lower rate of survival and higher rates of coronary artery bypass grafting (CABG), repeat PTCA, and infarction as compared to patients without restenosis.[11] From the patient's perspective, it is certainly distressing to experience similar anginal symptomatology before and after an invasive procedure. Finally, the advantage of purportedly lower costs of PTCA relative to CABG has been

greatly diminished by the expense of repeat diagnostic and therapeutic catheterizations caused by restenosis.[12]

Myriad investigations, therefore, have been conducted to evaluate various forms of adjuvant medical therapy directed at preventing restenosis after PTCA and the placement of a coronary stent (Table 40-1). After discussing the current theories regarding the pathogenesis of restenosis, this article reviews both animal and clinical studies of various preventive pharmacotherapies used against restenosis. The litany of pharmacologic approaches considered for reducing restenosis has come to include antiplatelet agents, antithrombotics, anticoagulants, thrombolytics, antiproliferatives, anti-inflammatory drugs, vasodilators, antioxidants, lipid-lowering regimens, chimeric toxins, and gene therapies. Although few agents have met with undisputed success in preventing restenosis, this chapter highlights those that currently show the most promise.

Several mechanical devices, including atherectomy systems, which use rapidly rotating cutting devices to reduce plaques,[13] intravascular stents,[14,15] and laser technology,[16] have come into clinical testing and use for the types of lesions for which they are particularly suited. While showing some benefit with regard to acute complications, some of these procedures may offer distinct advantages in avoiding restenosis. Disappointing results were reported from the Coronary Atherectomy Versus Angioplasty (CAVA) and Coronary Angioplasty Versus Excisional Atherectomy (CAVEAT) trials, the latter of which suggested that directional atherectomy yields a mild reduction in early angiographic restenosis over PTCA, but with higher rates of early complications, increased cost, and no apparent clinical benefit after 6 months of follow up.[17–19] Somewhat more positive results in mildly reducing restenosis rates were suggested by the large Belgium Netherlands Stent Trial (BENESTENT) and Stent Restenosis Study (STRESS) trials of Palmaz-Schatz Stents (Johnson & Johnson, Warren, NJ) versus balloon angioplasty, but again, thrombotic and hemorrhagic complications were of concern.[20,21] In addition, there is significant evidence to show that the late loss of luminal diameter was actually greater in stented vessels, and that the reduced restenosis observed in the STRESS trial stemmed from superior initial procedural gain rather than reduction in late intimal hyperplasia.[22] A recent study showed that stent replacement, when compared with balloon angioplasty, did yield superior results in procedural outcome, larger luminal gain, and reduction in major cardiac events, but, more importantly, did

TABLE 40-1. Outline of Pharmacologic Approaches to the Prevention of Restenosis

Antiplatelet Agents and Antithrombotics
  Aspirin
  Dipyridamole
  TXA_2 receptor antagonists (vapiprost, sulotroban, S-1452)
  TXA_2 synthetase inhibitors
  TXB_2 synthetase inhibitors (ridogrel)
  Prostacyclin and prostacyclin analogs (ciprostene, beraprost)
  Fish oils (omega-3 fatty acids, eicosapentaenoic acid, Maxepa)
  Ticlopidine
  Dextran
  Heparin (unfractionated)
  Low-molecular-weight heparin (enoxaparin, ardeparin, reviparin, dalteparin, nadroparin)
  Exogenous antithrombin III
  Direct thrombin antagonists (hirudin, Hirulog, antistasin)
  Factor Xa inhibitors (antistasin, tick anticoagulant peptide)
  Tissue factor pathway inhibitor (rTFPI)
  Vitamin K antagonists (warfarin)
  Early coagulation cascade inhibitors (rTFPI, DEGR-VIIa)
  Thrombolytic agents (tissue plasminogen activator, urokinase)
  IIb/IIIa receptor antagonists (c7E3 fab, abciximab, integrelin, tirofiban, xemilofiban, RGD and KCD peptides)
  Ib receptor antagonists (VCL)
  Defibrinogenating agents (ancrod)
  Cyclic AMP phosphodiesterase inhibitors (cilostazol)

Anti-Inflammatory Drugs
  Steroids
  NSAIDs (ebselen, sulfinpyrazone)
  Antiallergic agents (tranilast)
  Interleukin-10
  P-selectin inhibition
  α_v/β_3 integrin receptor blockade
  Inhibition of 12-lipoxygenase
  Ubiquitin-proteosome inhibition (MG132)

Growth Factor Antagonists
  PDGF antagonists (trapidil, PDGF receptor tyrosine kinase inhibitor, polyclonal α-PDGF antibodies)
  Pituitary growth hormone antagonists (angiopeptin, octreotide, lanreotide)
  Serotonin antagonists (ketanserin)
  ACE inhibitors (cilazapril, captopril, fosinopril, enalapril, quinapril)
  Angiotensin II receptor blocker (irbesartan, valsartan)
  Estrogen
  α-Adrenergic receptor antagonists (prazosin, urapidil)
  β_1-Adrenergic receptor antagonists (carvedilol)
  Nitric oxide donors (L-arginine, nitrosated albumin, linsidomine, molsidomine)
  Leukocyte and endothelial adhesion molecule antagonists (α-CD11) CD18 adhesion complex antibodies)
  Insulin sensitizing agents (troglitazone)
  Folic acid

Endothelial Growth Factors
  VEGF
  (Human) HGF

Vasodilators
  Calcium-channel antagonists (diltiazem, nifedipine, nisoldipine, amlodipine, verapamil)
  Minoxidil
  Bradykinin-1-receptor stimulation

Antiproliferatives and Antineoplastics
  Microtubule stabilizers (colchicine, paclitaxel)
  Other antineoplastics (etoposide, vincristine, dactinomycin, cyclosporine, azathioprine, methotrexate)
  Sirolimus [cyclin-dependent kinase (Cdk) inhibitor]

  Flavopiridol (oral cdk inhibitor)
  8-chloro-cyclic AMP
  Vascular remodeling agents
  Matrix metalloproteinase inhibitor
  Cytochalasin B

Lipid-Lowering Agents
  HMG-CoA reductase inhibitors (lovastatin, pravastatin, fluvastatin)
  Probucol

Antioxidants
  Vitamins E, C
  Probucol
  AGI-1067

Molecular Strategies
  Recombinant chimeric toxins
  ASODNs (c-myc, c-myb, PCNA, nonmuscle myosin)
  Nucleic acid based drugs (ribozymes, DZs)
  Gene therapy (thymidine kinase, retinoblastoma gene product, inhibition of central inflammatory mediator nuclear factor κB)

Note: Drugs have been classified according to what is thought to be their principal pharmacodynamic mechanism in reducing restenosis, although there is certainly overlap among the categories, with several antithrombotic agents, for example, having also been found to have direct antiproliferative effects on smooth muscle cells.

PCNA = proliferating cell nuclear antigen.

Source: Adapted from Landzberg BR, Frishman WH, Lerrick K. Pathophysiology and pharmacological approaches for prevention of coronary artery restenosis following coronary artery balloon angioplasty and related procedures. *Prog Cardiovasc Dis* 39(4):361–398, 1997.

not show a significant benefit in the rate of angiographic restenosis at 6 months follow-up.[23]

There has been a veritable explosion of research in new technologies, which also include thermal balloons,[24] intravascular ultrasound guidance,[25,26] radiotherapeutic implants,[27–31] and drug-eluting stents.[32] However, this chapter focuses its discussion mainly on pharmacologic interventions related to PTCA and stenting, which is, in itself, a vast subject. The impact of stent type on the restenosis has been well reviewed by Kastrati et al.[33]

DEFINITIONS OF POSTANGIOPLASTY RESTENOSIS

Exact definitions of restenosis have been widely debated. The literature speaks of angiographic restenosis and clinical restenosis, with the former being considered the gold standard to be used for evaluating the merit of pharmacologic interventions after PTCA. The NHLBI's extensive registry precisely defines criteria for angiographic restenosis including an increase of at least 30% in occlusive diameter from the immediate post-PTCA stenosis on follow-up angiography or a loss of at least 50% of the gain from PTCA[5] (Table 40-2). The latter angiographic definition is probably the most commonly used; however, careful angiographic follow-up studies by Serruys et al[6] showed the NHLBI percentage criteria to be somewhat arbitrary with a significant lack of overlap among them, and suggested that only changes in absolute quantitative measurements of minimal luminal diameter be used. Other investigators simply use the definition of greater than 50% stenosis on follow-up angiography. One might also argue, however, that clinical restenosis, that is, recurrent ischemic symptoms within 6 months after PTCA, is the more important variable, as more frequently this is the end-point followed in clinical practice. Repeat angiograms and PTCA are usually not considered in the asymptomatic patient. A problem arises, however, when using the presence or absence of recurrent chest pain

TABLE 40-2. Definitions of Restenosis and End-Points Used in Clinical Trials

Angiographic

    NHLBI I: Increase of $\geq 30\%$ from immediate post-PTCA stenosis to follow-up

    NHLBI II: Immediate post-PTCA stenosis diameter of $<50\%$ increasing to $\geq 70\%$ at follow-up

    NHLBI III: Increase in stenosis severity at follow up to 10% below the predilated diameter stenosis or higher at follow-up

    NHLBI IV: Loss of $\geq 50\%$ of the gain in luminal diameter after PTCA

    Presence of $>50\%$ diameter stenosis in dilated vessel at follow-up

    Late loss index equals late loss/acute gain

    Relative losses in MLD

    Decrease in MLD of >0.72 mm when compared with post-PTCA angiogram

Clinical

    Symptomatology (return of angina symptoms)

    Exercise stress testing (evidence of pain and ischemic ECG changes)

    Need for repeat revascularizations

    MI and death

ECG = electrocardiogram; MI = myocardial infarction; MLD = minimal lumen diameter; PTCA = percutaneous transluminal coronary angioplasty.

Source: Reproduced with permission from Landzberg BR, Frishman WH, Lerrick K. Pathophysiology and pharmacological approaches for prevention of coronary artery restenosis following coronary artery balloon angioplasty and related procedures. *Prog Cardiovasc Dis* 39(4):361–398, 1997.

as a marker of restenosis in that the correlation is far from absolute. Recurrent pain, usually reported in 20% of patients, may reflect disease in other coronary vessels, vasospasm, or even noncardiac pain. Conversely, absence of pain may reflect silent ischemia. The NHLBI group found that 44% of patients with probable or definite recurrent angina did not have angiographic restenosis of the revascularized coronary artery and that 14% of the patients without chest pain did have restenosis.[5]

An excellent angiographic study of 1353 patients by Rensing et al.[34] suggests that restenosis is not simply an undesirable side effect that occurs in a minority of cases, but rather a process that occurs to some extent in virtually all patients, following a gaussian distribution. Therefore, precise definitional criteria of restenosis are very important in understanding the magnitude of the problem.

When does restenosis occur? Objective serial angiographic studies have confirmed the common clinical finding that the vast majority of restenosis occurs in the first 6 months after PTCA. Nobuyoshi et al.[35] found restenosis rates in 229 patients to be 12.7% at 1 month, 43% at 3 months, 49.4% at 6 months, and 52.5% at 1 year. Similar results were found in the serial angiographic study of 342 patients by Serruys et al.[6] This knowledge that restenosis peaks between 1 and 3 months after the procedure gives clues into possible pathogenetic processes and highlights the period in which pharmacologic intervention would be most essential. Recently an observation was made that as part of the history of restenosis, a small number of subjects can spontaneously regress without treatment.[36]

PATHOPHYSIOLOGIC CHARACTERISTICS OF RESTENOSIS

The elusiveness of a definitive prophylactic treatment for restenosis after PTCA is most likely due to the incredible difficulty of elucidating the pathogenesis of the problem. Clearly, there is a role for vascular injury and platelet aggregation, procedural factors, anatomic

variation, clinical variables, hemodynamic effects and inflammation, but the relative contributions of these are unclear. The process bears many similarities and distinctions from the more gradual process of primary atherosclerosis. It appears to differ grossly from the process of early closure, which most frequently incorporates vasoconstriction, intimal flap formation, mural thrombus formation, and subintimal hemorrhage.[37]

Before discussing the proposed theories of the pathogenesis of restenosis, it is probably appropriate to comment on what is thought to be the mode of action of PTCA. How does it achieve improved coronary diameter? Based on clinical and experimental evidence, Ip et al.[38] suggest four possible mechanisms. The balloon may create a "controlled injury," leading to rents and cracks in the atherosclerotic plaque that enlarge the channel through which blood can flow. Alternatively, the balloon may tear the plaque at the point of least resistance, that is, through the intima and into the media, enlarging luminal caliber; with continued inflation, the media and adventitia may distend along the contour of the balloon. Third, the balloon may redistribute and compress the plaque. Fourth, in the presence of an eccentric plaque, the balloon may distend only the disease-free arc of the vessel. Ultrasound studies show that rotational atherectomy increases lumen size by selective ablation of hard, calcific, atherosclerotic plaques, with tissue destruction and arterial expansion occurring much less frequently than with PTCA.[39] However, the procedure very frequently requires adjunct balloon angioplasty.

The most widely held theory in the literature on the pathophysiology of restenosis begins with vascular and plaque injury and bears many similarities to the process of wound healing[40] (Fig. 40-1). After balloon inflation, platelets very rapidly adhere to the traumatized surface, probably to an extent proportional to the amount of injury.[41] The platelets then release thromboxane A_2 (TXA2), a powerful stimulus for platelet aggregation and vasoconstriction,[42] leading to further platelet disposition. In a recent study of markers of the coagulation-fibrinolysis system, patients with restenosis were shown to exhibit higher levels of P-selectin and β-thromboglobulin, implying a role for activated platelets.[43] Furthermore, the patients also had higher levels of plasminogen activator inhibitor type-1 and lower levels of plasmin-plasmin inhibitor complex, suggesting a role for impaired fibrinolysis in the pathogenesis of restenosis.

Platelets, coronary endothelium, inflammatory cells, and vascular smooth muscle operationally contribute a large host of mitogens, including, but not limited to, platelet-derived growth factor (PDGF), adenosine diphosphate (ADP), thrombin, epinephrine, endothelial and fibroblast growth factors, angiotensin-II, serotonin, thrombospondin, free oxygen radicals, tumor necrosis factor-alpha, transforming growth factor-beta, insulin-like growth factor, and several interleukins[37] (Fig. 40-2). These mitogens, most notably PDGF, stimulate migration and proliferation of smooth-muscle cells from the media into the intima, followed by the formation of fibrocellular tissue with an abundant proteoglycan matrix.[44] A recent study found that deposition of PG-M/versican, an important extracellular matrix proteoglycan of the vessel wall, was greatest, as measured by immunohistochemistry, when restenosis detected by angiography progresses most rapidly.[45] The net result is an enlarging mass of neointimal hyperplasia that compromises the coronary lumen and induces ischemic symptoms. Some investigators relate the process to an exaggerated healing response analogous to the formation of a hypertrophied scar after skin injury. In addition to the presence of mitogens after injury, there also probably exists a failure of secretion of inhibitory substances on smooth-muscle cell proliferation, such as

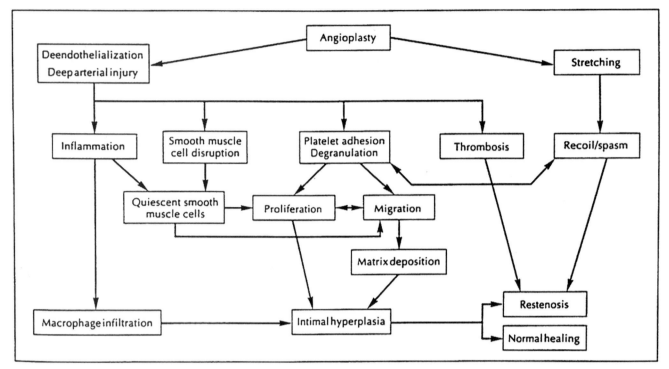

FIGURE 40-1. This figure depicts the postulated phases in the widely held "wound-healing" theory of the pathogenesis of restenosis. Various elements are identified, including platelet aggregation, thrombus formation, smooth-muscle cell disruption, and inflammation, which are triggered by balloon vascular injury and stretch. By the secretion of various mitogens, these elements probably induce smooth muscle cell migration from the media, proliferation and matrix formation. The net result is intimal hyperplasia, the key element of restenosis. Recoil and arterial remodeling also play a like role in determining ultimate luminal diameter. (*Reprinted with permission from Franklin SM, Faxon DP: Pharmacologic prevention of restenosis after coronary angioplasty: Review of the randomized clinical trials. Coron Artery Dis 4:232–242, 1993.*)

nitric oxide, heparin sulfate, and prostacyclin, which are normally released by intact endothelium[37] (Fig. 40-3).

This overall theory has been supported by postmortem evidence such as the study by Nobuyoshi et al,[46] who examined 28 coronary lesions in 20 patients autopsied who had experienced restenosis after PTCA. In agreement with other similar studies, intimal proliferation of smooth-muscle cells was histopathologically determined to be the principal cause of restenosis in 84 to 100% of specimens. Ohara et al,[47] in an electron microscopic study of coronary artery specimens, was able to demonstrate the migration of smooth-muscle cells from the media into the intima by visualizing the cells stretching through fenestrae in the internal elastic lamella in patients who died 1 to 6 days after PTCA. In specimens obtained 1 to 3 months postangioplasty, smooth-muscle cell proliferation had developed with abundant collagen and elastic fibers. Tissue taken in clinical atherectomy specimens from patients with restenosis after either PTCA or primary directional atherectomy exhibit essentially the identical histology of neointimal proliferation, suggesting a similar pathogenesis for restenosis after both types of procedures.[48] From the histologic evidence, it would appear that all theories as to pathogenesis of restenosis should share the final common pathway of smooth-muscle cell migration and proliferation.

There is also almost certainly a role for inflammatory cells, particularly macrophages, in the natural response to injury and the pathogenesis of restenosis. Their histologic presence has been documented in areas of vascular injury within several days after PTCA, and they have been noted to exist in much larger quantity in clin-

ical atherectomy specimens taken from restenotic versus primary coronary artery lesions.[49] Mononuclear cells, including monocytes, macrophages, and foam cells, can secrete potent substances that induce platelet aggregation and proliferation of vascular smooth muscle, in addition to a host of other effects. Their importance is supported by the experimental evidence that immunologically blocking monocyte chemotactic proteins significantly inhibits neointimal formation after balloon-catheter vascular injury.[50] The relevance of these leukocyte activities in restenosis suggests a potential role for anti-inflammatory drugs such as steroids. Some investigators have gone so far as to suggest that the process of restenosis may involve an autoimmune mechanism based on the finding that patients with restenosis tend to have increased levels of immunoglobulin M (IgM)-anticardiolipin antibodies.[51] One group of investigators from Japan, citing the possibility of a genetically determined immune response in restenotic patients, looked at the relationship between human leukocyte antigens (HLA) and restenosis.[52] In a cross-sectional study of 65 patients with coronary artery stenosis, they discovered that the HLA-C Cw1 locus was negatively related to restenosis, with an odds ratio of 0.19, and concluded that the Cw1 locus may be a useful marker for prediction of restenosis after PTCA. Another recent study of 54 patients found that the patients who subsequently developed restenosis showed an increased level of baseline E-selectin, a cell adhesion molecule that is only expressed on activated endothelial cells. These data support a possible role for white blood cell/endothelial interaction in restenosis.[53]

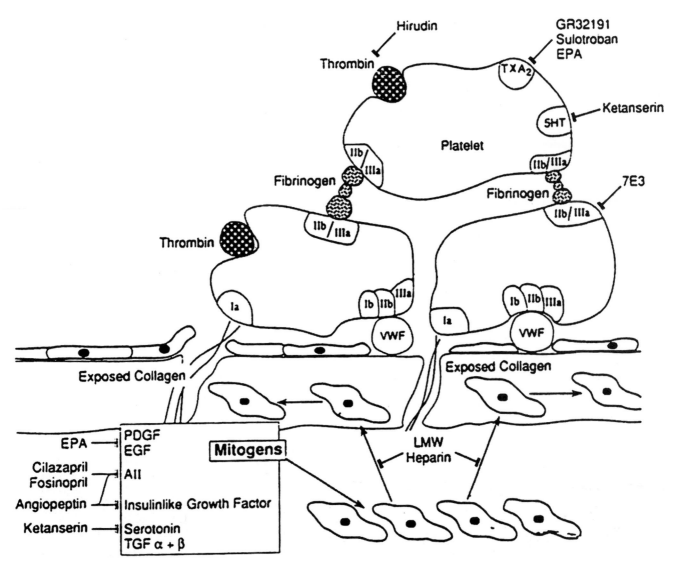

FIGURE 40-2. This figure depicts many of the biologic processes underlying restenosis. It underscores the important elements in platelet-endothelial and platelet-platelet interactions, and identifies many of the salient proplatelet and prothrombotic elements and smooth-muscle cell growth factors involved in restenosis. The sites of action of prototypic drugs in several of the pharmacologic approaches for prevention of restenosis are indicated. 5HT = serotonin; AII = angiotensin-II; EGF = epidermal growth factor; EPA = eicosapentaenoic acid; 7E3 = murine monoclonal antibody to glycoprotein IIb/IIIa receptor; LMW = low molecular weight; PDGF = platelet-derived growth factor; TGF = transforming growth factor; TXA$_2$ = thromboxane A$_2$; VWF = von Willebrand's factor. (*Reprinted with permission from Popma JJ, Califf RM, Topol EJ: Clinical trials of restenosis after coronary angioplasty (editorial). Circulation 84:1426–1436, 1991.*)

Although widely accepted, the theory that restenosis is an exaggerated healing response to injury is not entirely undisputed. If stimulated myointimal hyperplasia were the major factor, one would expect to find larger and softer plaque masses with restenotic as compared with de novo lesions. In fact, ultrasound comparisons have frequently demonstrated the precise opposite, with restenotic lesions being statistically smaller and with increased noncompliant (calcium and dense fibrous) tissue composition.[54] Furthermore, Waller et al., in necropsy studies of restenotic lesions,[55,56] found that while most of the specimens had evidence of intimal hyperplasia, 40% of the specimens showed densely fibrotic calcified plaques with no intimal proliferation or any morphologic evidence of PTCA injury. This finding can be explained by two alternative theories of restenosis (Figs. 40-4 and 40-5).

First, elastic recoil may make a significant contribution to restenosis. Although recoil has been commonly used to explain acute closure after PTCA, its role in more chronic reocclusion may be attributed to death or "stunning" of smooth-muscle cells which, after weeks or months, recover or are replaced and recoil the vessel diameter. This process is probably favored in restenosis cases in which the original dilatation resulted from the disproportionate distention of disease-free vessel wall adjacent to eccentric plaques.[55,56] In fact, some work has demonstrated an increased incidence of restenosis in dilated vessels with eccentric lesions.[57] Any role recoil might play in restenosis would favor the use of vasodilatory pharmacologic interventions and nondistending percutaneous revascularization procedures such as atherectomy or thermal dilation.

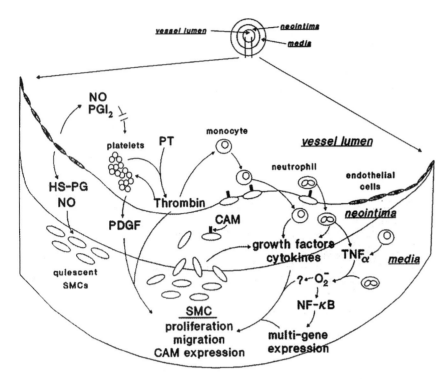

FIGURE 40-3. This schematic drawing identifies some of the interactive biologic processes between platelets, inflammatory cells, endothelial cells, cytokines and growth factors in the response to vascular injury and the development of coronary restenosis. In addition to including several of the myriad mitogens involved, this diagram includes some of the naturally occurring inhibitors to platelet aggregation and smooth-muscle cell (SMC) proliferation, including nitric oxide (NO), prostacyclin (PGI_2), and heparin sulfate proteoglycans (HS-PG). CAM = cellular adhesion molecule; NF-κB = nuclear factor κB; O_2 = superoxide ion; PDGF = platelet-derived growth factor; PT = prothrombin; TNFα = tumor necrosis factor α. (*Reprinted with permission from Epstein SE, Speir E, Unger EF, et al: The basis of molecular strategies for treating coronary restenosis after angioplasty. J Am Coll Cardiol 23:1278–1288, 1994.*)

The absent intimal hyperplasia in the 40% of restenotic lesions described by Waller et al. can also be explained by a third theory of restenosis involving "accelerated atherosclerosis." However, Waller's group believe that this etiology is highly unlikely given the histopathologic maturity of the plaques, as evidenced by dense and calcified fibrosis and a lack of dichotomy between old and new plaque in outer versus inner layers.[55,56]

If vascular injury were the root cause of restenosis, one would expect minimization of trauma to the vessel to yield lower restenosis rates. Shawl has coined the term "minimally invasive angioplasty" to describe the use of lowest possible inflation pressures during PTCA.[58] In fact, both Nobuyoshi et al.[46] and Waller et al.,[55] in examining necropsy specimens, did find that intimal proliferation was greater when there was evidence of injury extending from the intima into the media and adventitia. However, the importance of the severity of vascular insult is not undisputed, as a few large study groups have shown no increase in restenosis in dilated lesions that had angiographically visible dissection.[59] Similarly, a large randomized trial at Duke University was unable to generate any significant differences in restenosis or adverse clinical events at follow up in patients who received angioplasty with gradual and prolonged rather than standard balloon inflation, although initial angiographic appearance was somewhat better.[60] The issue of reducing procedural trauma relates to the vast spectrum of new mechanical technologies, which are not further reviewed here; however, the lack of unanimity among the trials on this issue casts a doubt on whether extent of vascular injury correlates with restenosis.

The theory of injury, platelet aggregation, and subsequent vascular smooth-muscle proliferation also does not explain the frequent clinical finding that, in so many cases of restenosis after PTCA, there is an 80 to 90% occlusive lesion, that is, one that does not completely obstruct the artery. Myocardial infarction from restenosis is generally rare, seen in less than 2% of cases. A simple process of platelet-stimulated accumulation of smooth muscle would logi-

cally lead to frequent total occlusion. Rather, this implies a dynamic molding and/or recoil of coronary lumina in response to flow and probably shear forces, which is clearly not perceivable in autopsy specimens. Kakuta et al.,[61] based on pathologic specimens taken from animal restenosis models, lends support to the importance of remodeling. In rabbits with experimental restenosis killed 4 months after balloon angioplasty, investigators observed that although the intimal cross-section area had increased, so had the area circumscribed by the internal elastic lamina.[61] Furthermore, animals with and without luminal restenosis by criteria had virtually identical intimal areas (2.41 vs 2.49 mm^2, respectively), with the difference in luminal diameter resulting from the fact that the latter group had developed a significantly larger internal elastic lamina area (2.56 vs 3.22 mm^2, respectively). In restenotic animals, the ratio of internal elastic lamina area increase to intimal area increase was <1, while the ratio in the nonrestenotic specimens was >1. This animal study suggests that intimal hyperplasia occurs almost invariably after vascular injury, but that the presence or absence of restenosis reflects differences in capacity for compensatory vessel enlargement rather than differences in actual intimal formation. Some recent intravascular ultrasound studies after balloon angioplasty, rotational and directional atherectomy, and laser angioplasty in humans have, in fact, confirmed this exact finding in the clinical setting.[62–64]

Glagov,[65] based on sound evidence from human cadaver and animal experiments, postulated that restenosis is a remodeling process in which the critical factors are wall shear stress and wall tensile stress. Wall shear stress is proportionate to blood flow velocity and viscosity, and inversely proportional to the cube of the vessel radius in the state of laminar flow. The theory holds that a decrease in wall shear stress will induce a decrease in luminal radius, such as is accomplished by neointimal formation, and an increase in flow velocity until wall shear stress is normalized, whereas the opposite holds for cases of increased shear stress. Angioplasty of stenotic lesions abruptly introduces a new relation between diameter and

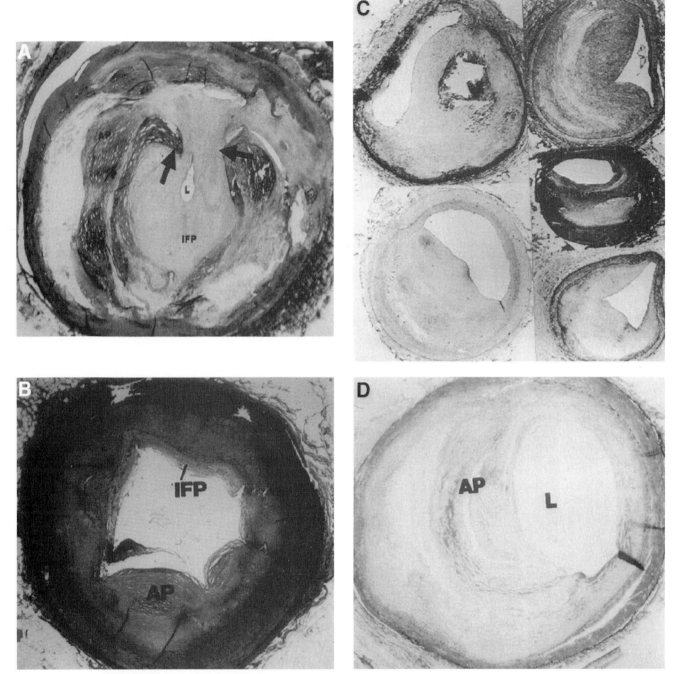

FIGURE 40-4. In keeping with the theory of restenosis as an exaggerated healing response to injury, (*A*) depicts exuberant intimal-fibrous proliferation (IFP) in a specimen of proximal left anterior descending coronary artery examined 4.3 months post-PTCA. Arrows identify cracks resulting from balloon vascular injury (L = lumen); and (*B*) depicts a left anterior descending coronary artery 6.8 months post-PTCA, with minimal balloon dilatation, and with evidence of only superficial intimal injury and proportionally minimal IFP. To the contrary, restenotic coronary vessels in (*C*) and (*D*), essentially all left anterior descending arteries (except *bottom right* photo, which depicts a right coronary artery) ranging from 3.4 to 14.5 months after PTCA, show no evidence of prior dilatation, vascular injury (such as cracks, breaks, or tears), healed lesion, or IFP. These vessels all contain eccentric atherosclerotic plaques with arcs of essentially disease-free wall. It can be inferred from this photo evidence that overdistention of disease-free wall was the likely mechanism for improved diameter at PTCA in these patients, and that elastic recoil of these same segments was the probable etiology of restenosis. Arrows identify a normal medial thickness in the eccentric wall. (*A*) Magnification 10×, reduced by 46%; elastic trichrome stain. (*B*) Magnification 10×, reduced by 14%, elastic trichrome stain. (*C*) Magnification 10×, reduced by 30%; elastic trichrome stain. (*D*) Magnification 10×, reduced by 14%; movat stain. [*Adapted from Waller BF, et al: Status of the major epicardial coronary arteries 80 to 150 days after percutaneous transluminal coronary angioplasty: analysis of 3 necropsy patients. Am J Cardiol 51:81–84, 1983; Waller BF, et al: Morphologic evidence of accelerated left main coronary disease: A late complication of percutaneous transluminal coronary angioplasty of the proximal left anterior descending coronary artery. J Am Coll Cardiol 9:1019–1023, 1987; and Waller BF, et al: Morphologic observations late (>30 days) after clinically successful coronary balloon angioplasty: An analysis of 20 necropsy patients and review of 41 necropsy patients with coronary angioplasty restenosis. Circulation 83(Suppl I):I28–I41, 1991.*]

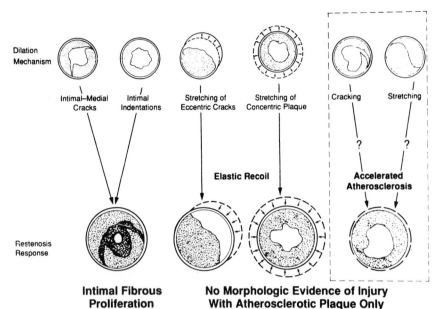

Intimal Fibrous Proliferation   **No Morphologic Evidence of Injury With Atherosclerotic Plaque Only**

FIGURE 40-5. This figure depicts two histopathologic types of coronary restenosis specimens seen at autopsy: (*A*) those with evidence of vascular injury and intimal hyperplasia, and (*B*) those with only atherosclerotic plaques, frequently eccentric, and with no evidence of vascular injury or smooth muscle cell proliferation. The figure identifies two explanations for the latter finding, which explanations deviate from the widely held "wound-healing" theory of restenosis. These are elastic recoil of disease-free (eccentric plaques) or diseased wall (concentric plaques) and accelerated atherosclerosis. Accelerated atherosclerosis has been put in a dashed line box as the investigators feel this etiology is very unlikely, given the histopathologic maturity of the plaques as evidenced by dense and calcified fibrosis, and a lack of dichotomy between "old" and "new" plaque. [*Reprinted with permission from Waller BF, et al: Morphologic observations late (>30 days) after clinically successful coronary balloon angioplasty: An analysis of 20 necropsy patients and review of 41 necropsy patients with coronary angioplasty restenosis. Circulation 83(Suppl I): 128–141, 1991.*]

flow, which, depending on the nature of the vessel geometry, can cause compensatory increases or decreases in lumen size. By this theory the benefit realized in nonrestenotic cases reflects an increase in flow resulting from the procedure sufficient to raise wall shear stress above baseline values, leading to further increases in vessel radius. Conversely, if flow is insufficiently increased to raise wall shear stress above baseline, vessel radius will decrease and restenosis will result. However, the bulk of the evidence in the literature refutes geometric remodeling as the primary mechanism behind restenosis. Evidence from a correlative angiographic-histomorphometric study of atherosclerotic arteries in rabbits showed a significant increase in luminal cross-sectional area narrowing by plaque after angioplasty, with no difference in overall arterial cross-sectional area restenotic sites.[66]

Nevertheless, recent studies have gathered more support for the role of remodeling in the restenotic process. A recent review highlighted evidence of gene transcription factors that can regulate gene expression in response to physical forces such as shear stress.[67] Another group of investigators, testing the possible effects of long-term constriction remodeling in restenosis, used serial intravascular ultrasonography and quantitative angiographic examination to characterize remodeling changes after coronary angioplasty or atherectomy.[68] Post et al., using the atherosclerotic pig model, showed that late lumen loss postangioplasty correlated strongly with geometric remodeling and weakly with intimal hyperplasia area.[69] Several studies suggest a fundamental difference in the pathophysiology of post-PTCA and in-stent restenosis, with geometric remodeling dominating in the former, and intimal hyperplasia and smooth-muscle cell proliferation dominating in the latter.[69,70] Faxon et al. postulate that at least 60% of restenosis may be explained by unfavorable remodeling with vessel constriction stemming mostly from alterations in cellular matrix metabolism.[71] Furthermore, a multicenter study by Kern et al.,[72] using Doppler-tipped angioplasty guidewires in 121 patients, found evidence to the contrary of Glagov's theory, demonstrating that lower postprocedural distal coronary flow did not appear to correlate with the development of restenosis.

Considering the many proposed theories, the subtotal occlusion clinically observed with restenosis probably reflects a complex equilibrium of natural stimulatory and inhibitory factors for smooth muscle cell growth into which hemodynamic factors give substantial input.

Finally, some investigators have pointed to the possible role of infectious agents in the restenotic process. Speier et al.,[73] at the National Institutes of Health, reported a possible contribution of human cytomegalovirus (CMV) infection. In examining restenotic coronary lesions, they found that many of the proliferating smooth-muscle cells were infected with the virus and elaborated CMV protein IE84. This viral protein both inactivated and led to increased levels of p53, a human tumor-suppressor protein. Subsequently, the human CMV immediate-early protein IE2 was postulated to interact with p53 through its C-terminal domain, possibly functioning as a transcriptional repressor of p53 in reducing its transactivation activity.[74] Speir et al. postulated that CMV infection of smooth muscle cells generated reactive oxygen intermediates, which facilitates CMV immediate-early gene expression and viral replication. However, three recent studies failed to show any association between prior CMV infection and the risk of clinical restenosis after PTCA.[75–77] On a different front, a recent study of 112 patients from Italy found that *Helicobacter pylori* seropositivity was independently predictive of restenosis, perhaps due to a systemic low-grade inflammatory response to common infective agents.[78] The precise role, if any, of infective agents in the restenotic process remains to be seen.

PHARMACOLOGIC APPROACHES TO PREVENT RESTENOSIS

Antiplatelet and Antithrombotic Agents

Given the extensive role probably played by platelets and thrombus in inducing smooth-muscle migration and proliferation, antiplatelet agents would certainly seem a fertile area for pharmacologic intervention. Indeed, antiplatelet drugs are at the forefront in the research for an effective prophylactic agent against restenosis. The known interaction between TXA_2 and platelets, leading to formation of

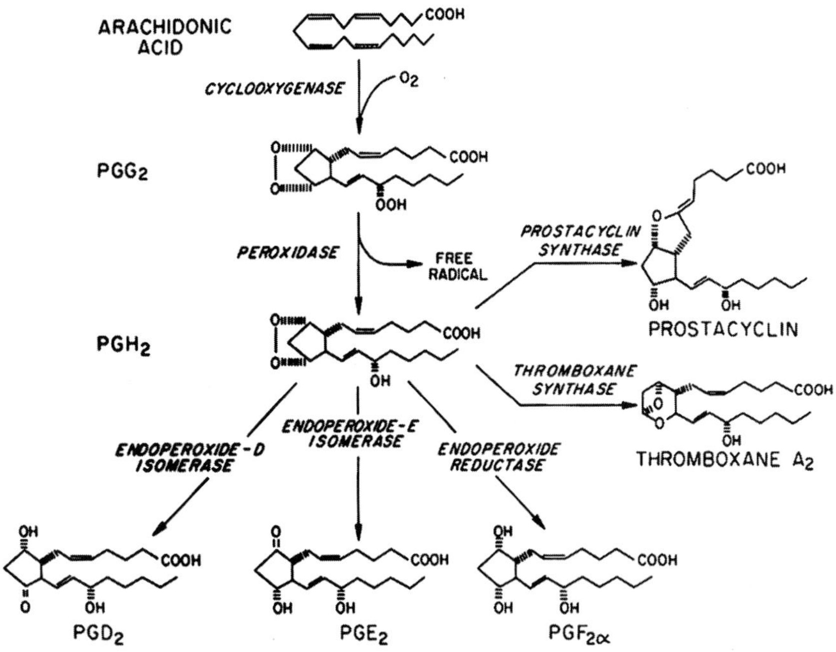

FIGURE 40-6. This figure depicts the pathway of arachidonic acid metabolism, which leads to the production of eicosanoids particularly relevant to platelet aggregation and restenosis. It is included to demonstrate the multiple potential sites of pharmacotherapeutic intervention. It becomes apparent that by blocking cyclooxygenase, aspirin reduces the production of the proplatelet agent A2, but also reduces the formation of the antiplatelet agent prostacyclin. Approaches that antagonize thromboxane A_2 receptors naturally spare prostacyclin production. Pharmacologic attempts to block thromboxane synthetase would reduce thromboxane A_2 levels, while increasing prostacyclin levels by the channeling of precursors into prostacyclin formation. Arachidonic acid is also metabolized by lipoxygenase to form leukotrienes and other related substances, however, this is not shown. (*Reprinted with permission from Oates JA, et al: Clinical implications of prostaglandin and thromboxane A_2 formation. N Engl J Med 319:689–698, 1988.*)

thrombus, vasospasm, and, ultimately, smooth-muscle cell proliferation, has directed many of the antiplatelet approaches toward various points in the arachidonic acid pathway. TXA_2 appears to be a key element in restenosis, as it has been shown to be released during angioplasty[79] and to induce smooth-muscle cell proliferation both indirectly through proplatelet effects, thus activating leukocytes,[80,81] and through direct mitogenic effects on cultured smooth-muscle cells.[82]

Aspirin, one of the oldest pharmacologic agents in this class, has been the subject of several restenosis trials. By irreversibly blocking cyclooxygenase, it has been shown to clinically reduce the upregulated synthesis of TXA_2 that regularly occurs after vascular injury and stimulates platelet activation[83] (Fig. 40-6). Aspirin, frequently combined with dipyridamole, is already routinely used both periprocedurally for PTCA and for long-term therapy. However, although it has reduced the incidence of acute complications of PTCA in clinical trials,[84] it has not generally been shown to reduce restenosis. This is despite very positive results in animal restenosis models.[85] In fact, a well-designed clinical trial in Canada involving 376 patients demonstrated virtually identical restenosis rates in placebo and aspirin-treated groups (38.6% vs 37.7%, NS).[86] However, this important study did corroborate the reduction of periprocedural MI with this antiplatelet regimen. In a study by Taylor et al.[87] in 216 subjects, aspirin was suggested to offer only minor benefit over placebo in reducing restenosis (35% vs 43%, NS) with statistical significance achieved only when comparing per lesion restenosis rates (25% vs 38%). Several other smaller studies of aspirin, with or without dipyridamole, have been performed, the net results of which, upon meta-analysis, offer a relative risk of restenosis of 0.932 with aspirin as compared with placebo treatment.[88] The Antiplatelet Trialists' Collaboration, in an analysis of several clinical trials involving about 800 patients, found that allocation to 6 months of antiplatelet therapy, usually consisting of aspirin and dipyridamole, reduced the occurrence of restenosis by only 4% in patients.[89] Despite these rather disappointing results in reduction of frequency of restenosis, there is some sound clinical evidence, based on reexamination of data from the Canadian study by Schwartz et al.,[90] that

aspirin and dipyridamole may significantly lower the severity of the reocclusions when they do occur.

Some investigators believe that the ineffectiveness of aspirin in these trials was due to inadequate dosing. A study by Darius et al.[91] in 256 patients has shown superior results in reducing restenosis with 500 mg once daily of aspirin as compared with 100 mg or 40 mg once daily. To the contrary, Mufson et al.[92] found no significant differences in restenosis rates in 495 patients randomized to 80 or 1500 mg daily of aspirin after PTCA, however, this study was limited by a very low frequency of angiographic follow up (166 patients). A meta-analysis of several studies of aspirin dosing and restenosis, including the ones mentioned, showed no significant difference in restenosis rates in patients administered higher doses of aspirin, and even suggested that higher doses of aspirin might exert a detrimental effect, with a relative risk of restenosis of 1.2.[88]

Aspirin is probably a relatively weak inhibitor of platelet aggregation because thromboxane is only one of many potential platelet activators, including ADP, epinephrine, thrombin, and collagen. In addition, by blocking cyclooxygenase, aspirin also blocks the potentially beneficial antiplatelet effects of prostacyclin production in platelets as well as in intimal tissue; this might also explain the declining benefit of high-dose aspirin in the meta-analysis mentioned above. Some research suggests that aspirin given at lower doses and higher dosing intervals confers more selective suppression of thromboxane over prostacyclin.

Dipyridamole, whose mechanism of action has been well reviewed by FitzGerald,[93] is believed to affect vasodilation and platelet antagonism by three mechanisms, namely, potentiation of prostacyclin's inhibition of platelets by blocking platelet phosphodiesterase and increasing cyclic adenosine monophosphate (AMP), the direct stimulation of prostacyclin release from the vascular endothelium, and the effects on adenosine metabolism. It is a natural complement to aspirin therapy as its ability to increase cyclic AMP may compensate for aspirin's undesired suppression of prostacyclin production. However, there is no suggestion in the literature that the addition of dipyridamole to aspirin achieves any benefit in preventing restenosis. One group of investigators, in fact, showed that dipyridamole conferred no added benefit to aspirin therapy, even in pretreatment for acute complications of PTCA, where it is already frequently used.[94]

Given the relative failure of the aspirin/dipyridamole combination, which blocks the production of both thromboxane and the beneficial prostacyclin, attention has turned to the use of more specific thromboxane antagonism. For example, selectively blocking TXA_2 receptor probably not only blunts the effects of TXA_2 with sparing of prostacyclin function, but also blocks some of the other eicosanoid intermediaries, including prostaglandins G_2 and H_2, which are also felt to activate the TXA_2 receptor. Despite excellent results observed in patients post-CABG,[95] clinical restenosis trials using this line of therapy after percutaneous interventions have yielded mostly negative results. The Coronary Artery Restenosis Prevention on Repeated Thromboxane-Antagonism (CARPORT) trial, having randomized 697 post-PTCA patients to receive either vapiprost (thromboxane-receptor antagonist) or placebo, both in combination with aspirin, was an extremely well-designed trial with a large sample size and precise quantitative angiographic follow-up examinations.[96] However, it failed to reveal any difference in restenosis or clinical outcome between the treatment groups. A study of long-term vapiprost therapy in 1192 patients post-PTCA, showed a 21% reduction in ischemic clinical events at 65 months, especially MI, and the need for repeat PTCA ($P = .02$), but did not provide information regarding angiographic restenosis.[97] In a small clinical trial of 78 patients, a novel TXA_2 receptor antagonist named S-1452 has been suggested as offering some benefit in reducing restenosis relative to aspirin at 6-month follow-up, especially in a subset of patients with post-MI angina; however, it is unclear from the abstract if statistical significance was achieved.[98] The large, Multi-Hospital Eastern Atlantic Restenosis Trial (M-HEART II) sought to determine the effectiveness of 6 months of therapy with sulotroban, another thromboxane inhibitor, relative to aspirin and to placebo.[99] The results in the patients who were followed up to the 6-month angiographic examination revealed no difference in angiographic restenosis rates across the three arms of the study.[100]

Another approach toward specific thromboxane antagonism has come in the form of inhibitors of thromboxane synthetase, which block the production of thromboxanes and favor the channeling of precursors into the formation of prostacyclin. After a TXA_2 synthase inhibitor was found to reduce platelet aggregation better than aspirin or heparin in an animal vascular injury model,[101] two small clinical restenosis trials were performed. The first, a nonrandomized study by Yabe et al.,[102] suggested a TXA_2 synthetase inhibitor to offer some benefit, with restenosis rates of 22.2% in 18 actively treated patients, as compared with 53.3% in a historical placebo group. Because of the nature and small size of the study, no satisfying statistical significance was achieved. Another group in Japan randomized 80 patients to thromboxane synthetase inhibitor therapy or placebo and showed no benefit from active treatment.[103] Ridogrel, a TXB_2 synthetase inhibitor, has also been considered for restenosis, although the importance of TXB_2 in restenosis is not yet clear. This drug has been clinically tested in combination with heparin for short-term therapy with PTCA, found to be safe and well tolerated, and generated favorable restenosis rates.[104] However, there are no randomized clinical restenosis trials for ridogrel in the current literature. As a class, thromboxane synthetase inhibitors have not generated the large clinical trials that have been performed with the receptor antagonists; however, such trials are certainly needed to fully determine the merits of pharmacologic approaches in preventing restenosis.

Prostacyclin is a naturally occurring eicosanoid that has very much the opposite effects of TXA_2. It is a vasodilator produced by endothelial cells as a natural defense against platelet aggregation on normal vascular endothelium.[42] Some research suggests that endothelial prostacyclin production may be deficient in cases of restenosis.[105] Consequently, pharmacologic supplementation of prostacyclin has been considered for restenosis prevention. One group evaluating the short-term use of prostacyclin in a randomized clinical trial of 286 patients failed to demonstrate any statistically significant benefit from the drug over placebo, when taken in combination with aspirin and dipyridamole, in preventing angiographic restenosis.[106] Similarly, negative results were observed by Gershlick et al.[107] in a randomized clinical trial of 135 patients in which prostacyclin was unable to significantly reduce angiographic restenosis at 6-month follow-up or alter platelet aggregation (as determined by aortic and coronary sinus blood sampling) after PTCA. However, related work with ciprostene, a stable analogue of prostacyclin, showed some mildly positive but significant results in early clinical testing relative to placebo, mostly in PTCA patients with unstable angina.[108] A larger trial with ciprostene, involving 311 patients, found the eicosanoid analogue to reduce clinical markers of restenosis (repeat PTCA, coronary bypass surgery, MI, or death) that occurred in 23% of actively-treated patients versus 39% of the placebo group.[109] These clinical results were corroborated by favorable retrospective angiographic findings.[110] However, larger trials with more formal prospective angiographic follow-up are required to accurately evaluate the efficacy of ciprostene. If positive results were confirmed from the use of exogenous prostacyclin or its analogues,[111] these drugs could serve as a potentially complementary therapy to aspirin, whose action reduces the endogenous levels of this natural antiplatelet substance.

Omega-3 ($n - 3$) fatty acids from salt-water-fish oils, by competitively interfering with arachidonic acid metabolism, appear to lower platelet thromboxane production and leukotriene formation (see Chap. 23). They are also believed to have a beneficial effect on serum lipid profiles, reducing low-density lipoprotein cholesterol (LDL-C) and very-LDL-C and triglycerides, and raising high-density lipoprotein cholesterol (HDL-C).[112] Fish oils also are reported to increase bleeding times owing to alterations in the platelet membrane. These cardiovascular and hematologic effects have been suggested to contribute to the low incidence of ischemic heart disease seen in Eskimos. Several clinical restenosis trials have been performed with fish oils, with far from unanimous results. Bairati et al[113] randomized 205 patients undergoing first-time PTCA to receive either 15 g of fish oil or olive oil daily, starting 3 weeks before the procedure. At 6-month angiographic follow-up examination, restenosis occurred in 22 to 35.6% (depending on the definition of restenosis) of the fish oil group, and 40 to 53.3% in the olive oil group. By most definitions the fish oil group had less-frequent restenosis. Dehmer et al.[114] ran a small unblinded clinical trial with 82 high-risk male patients, in which patients treated with fish oil in addition to aspirin and dipyridamole enjoyed a significant reduction in restenosis. Another small clinical study of 110 patients showed eicosapentaenoic acid, the active element in fish oil, to reduce restenosis relative to placebo, but not better than aspirin and dipyridamole.[115] In a study by Milner et al.[116] of 194 patients randomized to receive fish oil, dietary supplements generated significant benefit in patients who completed the entire regimen, with restenosis rates (by clinical criteria) of 19% in the active-treated group and 35% in the placebo group. Angiographic follow-up examination was lacking in this study, and compliance was a major problem, with 12% of the patients refusing to continue the supplements after the first week secondary to unpleasant side effects. In contrast to these trials, a German study in which 204 patients, after successful angioplasty, were randomized in a double-blind trial to receive daily fish oil or olive oil for 4 months, demonstrated no significant differences in restenosis rates between the groups.[117] Several other trials with patient enrollments between 100 and 200 also found no benefit with fish oil over olive oil in reducing restenosis.[118–121]

However, the final word on dietary fish oil supplementation is probably provided by the large-scale Enoxaparin and Maxepa for the Prevention of Angioplasty Restenosis (EMPAR) study,[122] Fish Oil Restenosis Trial (FORT),[123] and the Coronary Angioplasty Restenosis Trial (CART).[124] EMPAR randomized 814 patients in 4 centers to receive 5.4 g of omega-3 polyunsaturated fatty acids or placebo daily, starting an average of 6 days before PTCA and continuing for 18 weeks; there was no reduction in restenosis with active treatment.[122] The FORT investigators, hypothesizing that higher doses and earlier pretreatment might be necessary to achieve efficacy, randomized 551 patients to high-dose omega-3 fatty acids (8 g daily) or corn oil, starting a minimum of 12 days before PTCA and continuing for 6 months.[123] The occurrence of restenosis, whether defined as loss of half of the gain or >30% increase in post-PTCA stenosis, was no different between the groups. Similarly, supplementation with 5.1 g of n-3 fatty acids prior to angioplasty in CART showed no benefit on restenosis.[124] The almost identical restenosis rates and narrow confidence limits of these three very large and well-designed trials make it highly unlikely that fish oil has any benefit in reducing restenosis.

Ticlopidine is an antithrombotic agent whose pharmacologic mechanism remains largely unknown. After conversion of the prodrug to its active form, the inhibition of platelet von Willebrand's factor and the fibrinogen receptor probably plays a central role in its action. The occasional incidence of reversible neutropenia and thrombotic thrombocytopenia purpura makes ticlopidine somewhat less desirable than other antiplatelet agents. Although ticlopidine is used as a stroke prophylaxis in aspirin-intolerant patients, it has been considered for various cardiac ailments including unstable angina, MI prophylaxis, and restenosis. A randomized multicenter trial by White et al.[125] involving 236 patients did not find ticlopidine to reduce angiographic or clinical restenosis relative to aspirin or placebo. A Spanish clinical trial of 179 patients[126] and the French Ticlopidine Angioplasty Coronary Trial (TACT) study of 266 patients[127] agreed with the previous negative findings regarding restenosis reduction relative to placebo, but the latter trial did find ticlopidine therapy to be useful in reducing acute events relative to placebo, with acute closure in actively treated patients occurring in 5.1%, versus 16.2% of the placebo group.

Dextran is another antiplatelet agent whose mechanism of action is unclear. It appears to antagonize the interaction of factor VII with von Willebrand's factor. It is used with PTCA to prevent acute complications of the procedure. A study in dogs showed the drug to decrease platelet adhesion and deposition in balloon-dilated coronary arterial segments;[128] however, there is little evidence of benefit with dextran in reducing either acute complications of the procedure or restenosis. In fact, a clinical trial involving 152 patients by Swanson et al.[129] suggested that dextran during PTCA conferred no added benefit to aspirin and dipyridamole therapy in clinical outcome. However, the results of this placebo-controlled, randomized study are somewhat suspect, as the drug was probably not administered early enough prior to PTCA to exert maximal benefit. Second, the coadministration of aspirin and dipyridamole may

likely have masked the potentially beneficial antiplatelet effects of dextran. Proper clinical trials for restenosis and acute complication prevention are certainly in order for this drug, which is already being used clinically.

Heparin is routinely used with PTCA to reduce the acute complications of the procedure, especially coronary thrombosis and abrupt vessel closure, which can be frequently triggered by an intimal dissection. Its antithrombotic effects stem from its binding with antithrombin III, a natural inhibitor of coagulation. Once bound, the heparin induces a conformational change in antithrombin III, dramatically increasing its affinity to bind and inactivate thrombin (factor IIa) and factor Xa. Heparin, however, has also been known for some time to have direct inhibitory effects on vascular smooth-muscle cell proliferation independent from its anticoagulant and antithrombotic properties.[130] It antiproliferative mechanism is largely unknown, but it is felt to be selective for smooth-muscle cells, and to involve rapid membrane uptake and incorporation into cell nuclei, inhibition of DNA and RNA synthesis, and prevention of the cell from entering S phase.[131] In fact, some work has shown that there may exist endogenous heparin-like molecules, which serve to regulate smooth-muscle cell growth.[132] However, the largest of the randomized trials ($n = 416$) to query whether heparinization extended to 18 to 24 h could reduce restenosis at 6 months following PTCA was unable to demonstrate any such benefit.[133] It also noted more bleeding complications in the patients with extended heparin therapy. Similar findings regarding the rate of restenosis were observed in a study using subcutaneous heparin over 4 months.[134] Recent studies that might explain the lack of efficacy for heparin in preventing restenosis found that heparin may displace or activate basic fibroblast growth factor (bFGF), a potent mitogen for arterial smooth-muscle cells. bFGF becomes deposited on injured vessel walls, thereby contributing to the pathogenesis of restenosis.[135] Heparin, in light of it's stimulatory effects on bFGF, may exert its antiproliferative effects through multiple effects, including blocking the cell cycle at early and late checkpoints.

Heparin is actually composed of an assortment of glycosaminoglycans, ranging in weight between 2 and 50 kd, with an average of 15 kd. The low-molecular-weight fractions of heparin, ranging from 2 to 5 kd, were recently considered for restenosis prophylaxis due to their similar, if not stronger, effect on smooth-muscle cell proliferation, with less anticoagulant effect and, therefore, fewer bleeding complications relative to unfractionated heparin.[136] While still exhibiting anti-Xa activity, their anti-IIa activity is much reduced. They also have the benefit of a much longer elimination half-life than heparin (3 to 5 h vs 0.6 h).[137] After promising results with low-molecular-weight heparin in vitro in animal restenosis studies,[137,138] and in humans for deep-vein thrombosis prophylaxis,[139] early clinical studies showed a low incidence of restenosis in patients who received reviparin.[140,141] However, hope for this line of therapy was largely dispelled by the multicenter, double-blind Enoxaparin Restenosis (ERA) trial in which 458 patients, after successful angioplasty, were randomized to receive daily subcutaneous injections of 40 mg of enoxaparin or placebo for 1 month.[142] No significant improvement in restenosis was realized with active treatment. The EMPAR study, an even larger multicenter trial, randomized 653 patients to receive 30 mg of enoxaparin twice daily for 6 weeks or placebo, and similarly demonstrated no difference in restenosis.[122] Subsequently, a study using the low-molecular-weight heparin reviparin for 28 days failed to show any difference from placebo in the incidence of restenosis post-PTCA; however, fewer acute ischemic events occurred with active treatment.[143] The REDUCE Trial, an international double-blind trial enrolling 625 patients, showed that reviparin used during and after coronary angioplasty did not reduce the occurrence of angiographic restenosis at median follow-up of 184 days after PTCA.[144] Furthermore, although reviparin treatment resulted in a 52% reduction in the acute-phase adverse outcome, it did not reduce the occurrence of major clinical events over 30 weeks, the primary clinical end-point of the study. Similar effects on restenosis were seen with subcutaneous ardeparin used for 3 months after PTCA.[144a] Recently, a study of 118 patients using certoparin, a different low-molecular-weight heparin, did show a tendency to prevent restenosis,[145] as did the local delivery of enoxaparin just prior to angioplasty and stenting.[146] However, most recently it was shown that the intramural delivery of nadroparin with a microporous catheter after stent deployment had no effect in reducing restenosis.[147]

It is possible that the studies' failure to generate positive results may reflect a problem of low-molecular-weight heparin dosage. Trialists used the highest doses found to be safe and effective in orthopedic trials for deep-vein thrombosis prophylaxis,[142] however, these may fall below the therapeutic window for restenosis prophylaxis. Several animal studies have revealed that heparin's antiproliferative effects are dose-related. It is also possible that more benefit could be realized by starting the drug earlier prior to PTCA. Alternatively, one study that compared smooth-muscle cells cultured from primary bypass surgery and revision surgery for restenosis showed that the restenotic smooth-muscle cells did not grow faster than the primary lesion cells, but were remarkably more resistant to the inhibitory effects of heparin.[148] The same heparin resistance was found in smooth-muscle cells taken from apparently normal veins in the restenotic patients, suggesting that heparin resistance is a property of the patient rather than the lesion. This finding might explain why only some patients appear to benefit from heparin therapy as well as the marked differences between the results of animal restenosis studies and clinical trials.

Due to heparin's unwanted anticoagulant effects, β-cyclodextrin tetradecasulfate (CDT), a nonanticoagulant synthetic heparin mimic, was recently investigated as a possible treatment of restenosis. CDT caused a dose-dependent inhibition of human smooth-muscle cell proliferation and migration in vitro and reduced experimental restenosis in the double injury atherosclerotic rabbit model in vivo.[149] A periadventitially applied sulfated cyclodextrin inhibited intimal thickening in the rat carotid model, possibly by binding to heparin-binding growth factors.[150] Studies are currently underway to evaluate the effects of oral and local administration of cyclodextrins in the porcine coronary model.

One group has tested the use of exogenous human antithrombin III in swine coronary models of vascular injury.[151] Surprisingly, administration of this naturally occurring inhibitor of thrombin's effects on platelet aggregation and smooth-muscle cell proliferation has not received much research attention. An early animal study with exogenous human antithrombin III did demonstrate a marked reduction in restenosis after both balloon and stent injury. However, in a prospective, double-blind, randomized trial of 615 patients, adjunctive intracoronary antithrombin III did not have any effect on restenosis outcome or on acute complications during PTCA after conducting a subgroup analysis of patients with a high risk for thrombotic complications.[152] On the other hand, a more recent study of the effects of antithrombin III in atherosclerotic swine showed that supraphysiologic antithrombin III levels in combination with heparin inhibited the reduction in minimal lumen diameter and reduced the percentage area stenosis in coronary arteries subjected

to oversized balloon injury.[153] Most recently, a controlled, randomized, double-blind pilot study of 50 patients undergoing PTCA for unstable angina pectoris showed that antithrombin III supplementation resulted in less coagulation activation, measured as elevations of fibrin d-dimer, as well as a tendency toward less restenosis, although not statistically significant.[154] Furthermore, measurements of prothrombin fragment $1 + 2$, thrombin-antithrombin complexes, and soluble fibrin were similar in patients who developed restenosis and those who did not, suggesting a need to further clarify the mechanism by which antithrombin III might reduce restenosis.[155]

Inhibition of tissue factor with recombinant tissue-factor pathway inhibitor (rTFPI) prevents thrombosis and intimal hyperplasia after vascular injury in experimental animals.[156]

Hirudin, a specific thrombin inhibitor, is a 65-amino-acid polypeptide. Originally identified in the salivary glands of the leech, *Hirudo medicinalis,* it is currently produced in microbes. Its pharmacodynamic mechanism is more direct than that of heparin, as it appears to bind directly to and inactivate thrombin without the use of an antithrombin III intermediary, leading to more reliable dose responses. It also offers the distinct advantages of being able to inhibit thrombin that is already bound to clots or extracellular matrices, which is usually resistant to heparin, and it is not inhibited by activated platelets, which release platelet factor IV and other substances that largely inactivate heparin.[157] Its antithrombotic effects are empirically more potent than heparin's in vitro, and hirudin has been shown to more effectively prevent coronary thrombus formation during PTCA.[158] In two separate studies conducted by Sarembock and colleagues to probe the mechanism by which hirudin acts, it was first shown that, while angioplasty resulted in a marked increase in cellular proliferation peaking at 72 h, a 2-h infusion of hirudin failed to reduce early ^{3}H-thymidine labeling, suggesting that hirudin does not exert its effect by inhibition of cellular proliferation.[159] Subsequently, it was shown that the same 2-h infusion of hirudin resulted in prolonged 24-h suppression of arterial wall thrombin activity, which may account for the reduction in restenosis.[160] Hirudin and the smaller (20-amino-acid) related substance, hirulog, have therefore come into consideration as anticoagulant substitute for heparin during the PTCA procedure.

Promising results with hirudin and hirulog were attained from earlier studies using vascular injury restenosis animal models.[161] More recently, though, a study comparing the effects of acute versus chronic administration of recombinant desulfatohirudin (r-hirudin) in cholesterol-fed rabbits showed that prolonged treatment with r-hirudin neither inhibited vascular smooth-muscle cell proliferation after angioplasty nor reduced the size of neointimal lesions, and that prolonged treatment might even impair endothelial cell function.[162] Another study on the effects of r-hirudin in different animal models showed interspecies variation in susceptibility to reduction of neointimal growth by inhibition of thrombin after arterial injury.[163] Nevertheless, most animal studies still point to a potential/promising role for hirudin/hirulog in reducing restenosis. In a porcine coronary stent-angioplasty model, a novel long-lasting polyethleneglycol-conjugated hirudin reduced maximal neointimal thickness as well as neointimal area, with prolonged treatment showing the same effect.[164] Abendschein et al. demonstrated a marked reduction of lumen stenosis in r-hirudin-treated minipigs subsequent to arterial injury, and suggest that a brief interval of profound, direct inhibition of thrombin may be effective in attenuating clinical restenosis after balloon angioplasty.[165] In another study, a 2-h infusion of hirulog at the time of angioplasty effectively reduced restenosis in atherosclerotic rabbits as compared with heparin controls.[166]

Both studies confirm a specific role for thrombin in restenosis after angioplasty.

Two clinical trials exist in the literature regarding the use of hirudin in relation to the acute complications of PTCA.[167,168] Although a number of clinical trials with positive results have been reported with the thrombin inhibitors used in patients with deep-vein thrombosis,[169] acute MI,[170] unstable angina,[171] and acute complications of PTCA,[167,168] there were no reports in the literature of clinical restenosis trials until the Hirudin in a European Trial versus Heparin in the Prevention of Restenosis after PTCA (HELVETICA), which randomized 1141 patients with unstable angina undergoing PTCA to 24-h hirudin infusion (subcutaneous injections of hirudin or placebo for 3 days), or heparin infusion for 24 h with subcutaneous placebo.[172] This very large trial found virtually identical results in event-free survival and minimal lumen diameter across all groups at 7-month follow-up examination, although the addition of subcutaneous hirudin for 3 days did somewhat reduce acute complications. Similarly, hirulog was shown to be no more effective than heparin in patients postangioplasty.[173] At 4 months, the restenosis rate in heparin-treated patients was 61% versus 68% with hirulog.

Taken together, these results with hirudin and hirulog are disappointing, especially considering the size of the HELVETICA trial. However, even though the HELVETICA trial showed that short-term hirudin was not superior to heparin in preventing restenosis in the particular subset of patients, the use of antithrombin regimens may as yet still be a meaningful avenue to explore. As the authors note, thrombin inhibition was incomplete at the doses of hirudin used in the study deemed to be safe. There can very well be another antithrombin agent which can more completely inhibit thrombin at doses which are safe clinically. Moreover, very beneficial insights can still be gained into the vascular growth response from analyzing the effects of thrombin inhibition after arterial injury.[174] Future studies can be aimed at elucidating the mechanism by which thrombin stimulates intimal growth and antithrombin agents such as hirudin inhibit that growth; at analyzing inhibition at different levels of the coagulation cascade; at determining the role of plaque composition and how tissue factor increases with higher levels of cholesterol; and at answering the question of why studies show that brief infusions of hirudin for 2 h can cause prolonged reduction in growth response of much longer duration.[174] The last suggests that profound responses at the time of vessel injury may reduce delayed growth responses.[174] The distinct possibility of multiple mechanisms of thrombin-induced intimal growth suggests that the lack of usefulness of an antithrombin agent as demonstrated by a large trial may not translate into a lack of usefulness of the agent for an individual. Furthermore, the potential importance of the extrinsic coagulation pathway suggests that thrombin may not be the only relevant coagulation protein in the restenotic process.[175]

Recombinant antistasin, also originally found in leeches, and tick anticoagulant peptide (TAP), are substances related to hirudin that are also being considered for restenosis. These are believed to be factor Xa inhibitors; they significantly reduced restenosis in early animal studies.[176] Recombinant TAP successfully prevented thrombus formation and reduced platelet deposition in balloon-injured vessel segments in atherosclerotic rabbits.[177] These compounds will likely be the subject of much future research.

Warfarin, a frequently used anticoagulant, is an antagonist of vitamin K and therefore reduces the formation of clotting factors II, VII, IX, and X, whose production depends on the cofactor. In a randomized study of 248 patients, warfarin, administered so as to raise prothrombin time to 2 to 2.5 times control, was not found to yield any benefit on restenosis relative to 325 mg daily aspirin, and was found to lead to worse outcomes than aspirin in patients with a longer history of angina and in whom compliance was a problem.[178] A smaller trial of 110 patients suggested some benefit of warfarin on restenosis, but the result did not reach statistical significance.[179] A problem with both these studies is that warfarin was only started on the day of PTCA; therefore, therapeutic prothrombin times were probably not achieved until 2 to 3 days after the procedure, a time period essential to platelet adherence and thrombus formation. A large trial with therapy starting 2 to 3 days before PTCA is needed to accurately determine the potential value of warfarin in restenosis; however, the small clinical studies in the literature do not show much promise for this line of therapy, especially when considering the issue of compliance.

A study by Jang et al. evaluated the effect of blockade of specific levels of coagulation cascade on neointimal hyperplasia in the atherosclerotic rabbit arterial injury model.[175] Active-site inactivated factor VIIa (DEGR-VIIa) blocks the binding of factor VIIa to tissue factor. rTFPI binds factor Xa and inhibits the tissue-factor VIIa complex and factor Xa. Both agents were shown to reduce angiographic restenosis and decrease neointimal hyperplasia as compared to controls. This study highlights the potential importance of the early initiators of the extrinsic coagulation pathway on restenosis. A more recent study hypothesized that the efficacy of antithrombin agents in previous studies may have been limited by persistent activation of factors IX and X by the complex of tissue factor and VIIa.[180] This study showed that rTFPI inhibition of tissue factor-mediated coagulation for 24 h after balloon-induced injury in minipigs markedly attenuated subsequent neointimal formation and stenosis.

The thrombolytic agent tissue plasminogen activator has also been tested in animal models of restenosis with positive results in reducing neointimal hyperplasia achieved with both low- and high-dose therapy.[181–183] Further study into the potential role of fibrinolytic components in the process of restenosis revealed that there was induction of plasminogen activator inhibitor-1 (PAI-1) and urokinase-type plasminogen activator receptor (u-PAR) in cells exposed to transforming growth factor beta (TGF-β) and thrombin,[184] and that neointimal progression is increased in PAI-1-deficient vessels and decreased in u-PA-deficient vessels.[185] Subsequently, free PAI-1 levels after PTCA in patients with restenosis were found to be significantly higher than those in patients without restenosis,[186] and several components of the plasminogen activator system were shown to modulate smooth-muscle cell migration and invasion in vitro.[187] However, to date, clinical studies on the effects of tissue-PA as well as urokinase-PA have been negative. In a double-blind, randomized trial of 199 patients to evaluate the benefits of urokinase on the initial success of angioplasty, urokinase treatment was found to be safe and did not increase complications, but it also demonstrated no significant benefits over placebo, as well as demonstrating similar overall incidence of restenosis.[188] A study to determine the efficacy of three dosing regimens of intracoronary urokinase for facilitated angioplasty of chronic total native coronary artery occlusions showed that lower doses of urokinase are equally effective and safe and result in fewer bleeding complications, but again had no effect on restenosis rate.[189] Finally, a prospective randomized trial of 280 patients showed no beneficial effect of intracoronary urokinase infusion on procedural outcome, even in subgroups of patients with a high risk of thrombotic complications.[190] Nevertheless, recent studies suggest that impaired fibrinolysis may yet play a role in the pathogenesis of restenosis.[43] One group studying 138 patients in Japan measured the pre- and post-PTCA levels of lipoprotein (a) [Lp(a)], which structurally resembles plasminogen in the fibrinolytic system, binds to fibrin and fibrinogen competitively with plasminogen in vitro, and inhibits thrombolysis.[191] Lp(a) levels were found to be significantly higher before PTCA in patients who subsequently developed restenosis, but significantly reduced in the same restenotic patients 1 day after PTCA. The authors hypothesize that plasma concentration of Lp(a) may decrease due to its role in thrombus formation in the coronary artery wall after PTCA. These recent results indicate that the thrombolytic line of therapy needs further animal and clinical studies.

With the failure of essentially all of the approaches involving arachidonic acid metabolites, thrombin, and vitamin K antagonism, researchers turned to other antiplatelet strategies. Some of the most positive results in restenosis prophylaxis have come with the use of a monoclonal antibody Fab fragment (c7E3 Fab), also known as abciximab, directed against the platelet IIb/IIIa integrin receptor, essentially the final common pathway in platelet aggregation (see Chap. 18).[192,193] This platelet receptor has the capacity to bind von Willebrand's factor, fibrinogen, fibronectin, and collagen; these circulating proteins, in turn, at different sites, simultaneously bind other platelet IIb/IIIa receptors, causing platelet aggregation (Fig. 40-2). Many of the stimulants for platelet aggregation, such as thromboxane, ADP, and epinephrine, increase the affinity of these receptors. If this receptor is blocked, or is congenitally absent, as in the bleeding diathesis Glanzmann's disease, platelet aggregation is essentially made impossible, while platelet adhesion is, fortunately, spared. This marks a clear pharmacodynamic improvement over previous agents, which only block one potential avenue of platelet activation, permitting other molecules, including thrombin, collagen, thromboxane, and ADP, to work as platelet agonists.[194] A study by Reverter et al. concluded that thrombin generation initiated by tissue factor in the presence of platelets is significantly inhibited by c7E3 Fab, and that this effect may contribute to its antithrombotic properties.[195]

Remarkable reductions in platelet aggregation by c7E3 Fab in animal models led to the Evaluation of 7E3 for the Prevention of Ischemic Complications (EPIC) study, in which 2099 patients at 56 centers, undergoing angioplasty or directional atherectomy, were randomized to receive c7E3 Fab or placebo in addition to aspirin and heparin.[192,193] Enrollees were confined to those requiring "high risk" revascularization procedures because of unstable angina, evolving MI, or difficult angiographic morphology. Both abrupt closure and clinical restenosis (as determined by need for repeat revascularization or major ischemic event at 6-month follow-up) were significantly reduced in the antibody-treated group, demonstrating a clear benefit of the drug in high-risk angioplasty. At 6 months, patients who had an initially successful angioplasty enjoyed a 26% reduction in target vessel revascularizations and a 23% reduction in all ischemic events with bolus and infusion c7E3 Fab therapy as compared with placebo.

An economic analysis of the EPIC trial results demonstrated that this 26% reduction in the 6-month rate of restenosis achieved with c7E3 treatment translates into a saving per patient of more than $1000 in medical costs, reflecting reduced incidence in rehospitalization and declines in need for repeat angioplasty and bypass surgery.[196] In addition, subsequent analysis of patients in the EPIC trial who underwent direct PTCA for acute myocardial infarction and rescue PTCA after failed thrombolysis also revealed benefit for glycoprotein IIb/IIIa receptor blockade during PTCA in decreasing acute ischemic events and clinical restenosis.[197]

The EPIC trial stands out as one of the exceedingly rare large-scale clinical trials to show a promising reduction in restenosis.[193] However, its conclusions and implications for the use of c7E3 Fab in the general angioplasty population are limited by several factors. The inclusion criteria of "high risk" patients as described above, probably select a group of patients with acute coronary syndromes in which intravascular thrombosis and platelet aggregation play an inordinately large role and who would therefore receive exceptional benefit from antiplatelet therapy. Restenosis in the more stable angina patients in the study was also apparently reduced, but more formal testing is necessary. In addition, unlike essentially all of the restenosis trials discussed here, this study did not include formal 6 month angiographic follow-up examination for determination of restenosis. The investigators favored clinical criteria for restenosis as they felt that mandated repeat angiograms lead some asymptomatic patients with recurrent target vessel stenosis to undergo elective repeat revascularizations that would not otherwise undergo this procedure in clinical practice. Given the rare incidence of death and MI in post-PTCA patients, the investigators felt that the recurrence of angina and need for repeat revascularizations were the best clinical end-points to follow. Although this format is probably a better simulation of clinical practice, one can only infer that the improved clinical results stem from reduction in restenosis of dilated vessels. Therefore another study is necessary to provide angiographic confirmation of the apparent clinical benefit. One final factor limiting the application of the study is the mild increase in bleeding events with treatment.[198] In high-risk patients benefit clearly outweighs risk; however, in the general angioplasty population, this may not hold true. Additionally, bleeding complications, which were greater in lower body weight patients, may have been reduced by more careful heparin dosing, which was not weight adjusted in the EPIC study. Similar studies have been carried out with other agents in this class.[199]

Another method of IIb/IIIa antagonism may lie in peptides extracted from certain snake venoms. Peptides, including the sequences Arg-Gly-Asp (RGD) and Lys-Gly-Asp (KGD), antagonize the IIb/IIIa receptor and have yielded positive results in reducing neointimal hyperplasia when locally delivered to injured rat carotid arteries.[200] The Integrelin to Minimize Platelet Aggregation and Prevent Coronary Thrombosis (IMPACT) investigators produced a clinical trial of IIb/IIIa-receptor antagonism using integrelin, a cyclic heptapeptide derived from the pit viper, with a short half-life, which is believed to inhibit the essential platelet glycoprotein more specifically than does c7E3 Fab.[201] By randomizing 150 patients at several centers to periprocedural active treatment or placebo, in combination with aspirin and heparin, investigators found the former group to enjoy a reduction in serious acute complications at 1-month follow-up, with only a mild increase in minor bleeding. However, in a larger study of 4010 patients (IMPACT-II), there was no improvement in minimal luminal diameter or rate of restenosis when compared with placebo 6 months postangioplasty, despite a trend toward improvement at 30 days in some ischemic heart disease patients.[202,203] In a review of the EPIC, EPILOG, IMPACT II, and RESTORE trials, the three agents—abciximab, integrelin, and tirofiban—all appeared to improve clinical outcomes following percutaneous intervention, with clinical benefit extending to all patient categories, and bleeding risks minimized by minor changes in standard patient care algorithms.[204] However, in the RESTORE trial, there was no apparent benefit of tirofiban therapy on the rate of restenosis at 6 months postangioplasty.[205]

It was recently demonstrated that the combined inhibition of integrins, α_{IIb}/β_3 and α_v/β_3 with G3580 significantly reduced neointimal development after experimental angioplasty.[206] In the Evaluation of Reo-Pro and Stenting to Prevent Restenosis (ERASER) study, there was no benefit of the drug abciximab on the rate of in-stent restenosis.[207] A similar observation was made in the Intracoronary Stenting and Antithrombotic Regimen-2 (ISAR-2) trial in patients who underwent stent implantation within 48 h of an acute MI.[208]

Ancrod, a peptide also obtained from the pit viper, is a potent defibrinogenating agent that, in combination with aspirin and heparin, reduces neointimal formation in a porcine coronary injury model.[209] Clearly, more animal studies are in order, particularly regarding the safety and bleeding complications associated with this agent.

Cilostazol is a new synthetic platelet-aggregation inhibitor that inhibits cyclic AMP phosphodiesterase; it was recently approved for clinical use for intermittent claudication. In a recent study from Japan, 213 lesions dilated by balloon angioplasty were randomized to cilostazol or aspirin.[210] Three-month follow- up showed significantly lower restenosis and revascularization rates in the cilostazol group. Additional studies with longer follow-ups have continued to show a benefit to using cilostazol alone or in combination with probucol.[211–213] A study evaluating cilostazol in patients undergoing stent placement showed no benefit on the restenosis rate.[214]

Anti-Inflammatory Drugs

With the apparent correlations between restenosis and exaggerated wound healing in response to injury,[215] and the potential role played by inflammatory cells and the mitogens and chemoattractants they secrete, some investigators have considered the use of anti-inflammatory drugs, in particular corticosteroids, for preventing restenosis. After some success with steroids in reducing skeletal muscle cell proliferation in animal vascular-injury models,[216] a small clinical placebo-controlled study was undertaken by Stone et al in a subset of patients undergoing repeat PTCA after restenosis, to determine whether periprocedural high-dose methylprednisolone used intramuscularly and orally administered prednisone for 1 week could effectively reduce the incidence of restenosis over placebo.[217] This study showed almost no reduction in the per-lesion incidence of angiographic restenosis in the treated group. There were somewhat more positive results in the treated group with regard to clinical correlates of restenosis, namely incidence and severity of angina, positive treadmill stress tests, nonfatal infarctions and deaths; however, these failed to reach statistical significance. Similarly, negative results were achieved in a trial of methylprednisolone versus placebo for 1 week in 66 patients undergoing PTCA with restenosis rates of 33%.[218]

Inspired by the mildly positive clinical results of the study of Stone et al.,[217] which was clearly limited by small sample size, an extremely large multicenter study was undertaken by Pepine et al.[219] to query whether prophylactic corticosteroids could elicit a significant reduction in restenosis. To that end, 915 patients were randomized to receive either 1 g of methylprednisolone intravenously or placebo on the day prior to PTCA. No statistical difference was noted between groups, with angiographic restenosis occurring in 40% (117/291 lesions) after steroid treatment and 39% (120/307 lesions) after placebo. Similarly, the use of intravenous methylprednisolone before coronary stenting had no effect on the restenosis rate at 6 months.[220] The results of these large, well-designed clinical trials indicate that there is no likely role for short-term steroids in restenosis prevention,[221] although the use of more chronic, orally administered corticosteroids has not been evaluated. A study is now in

progress evaluating the antirestenosis efficacy of a dexamethasone-eluting stent.[32]

Some investigators have also looked into the use of nonsteroidal anti-inflammatory drug (NSAIDs), which, unlike aspirin, competitively inhibit platelet cyclooxygenase. Ebselen, a selenium-containing heterocyclic NSAID, is believed to have an additional antioxidant capacity, and has been found to reduce activation of leukocytes and peroxidation of lipids. It was tested in a small clinical trial of 80 patients undergoing PTCA with positive results. Angiographic restenosis at 3-month follow-up was found to occur in 18.6% of actively treated patients, and in 38.2% of placebo-treated patients ($P < .05$).[222] Clearly, trials with more patients and longer follow-up are in order, but early clinical results are promising. Sulfinpyrazone, an older NSAID, shows positive results in reducing neointimal formation in animal models;[223] however, there are no clinical trials in the literature that demonstrate a reduction in restenosis in angioplasty patients using this agent.

The drug tranilast represents another anti-inflammatory approach that has come into consideration. It is a drug, originally used in allergic disorders, which has also been known to reduce keloid formation by suppression of monocyte/macrophages and fibroblasts.[224–226] Tranilast exhibited prominent inhibitory effects on the migration and proliferation of cultured vascular smooth-muscle cells and on vascular smooth-muscle cell collagen synthesis in the thoracic aorta of rats.[227] Tranilast also inhibited PDGF- and TGF-β_1-induced collagen synthesis, migration, and proliferation in vascular smooth-muscle cells from spontaneously hypertensive rats.[228] A subsequent study suggested that tranilast inhibited the proliferation, migration, c-myc gene expression, and collagen synthesis of human vascular smooth-muscle cells.[229] Tranilast was further shown to suppress intimal hyperplasia after vascular injury in the rat[230] and pig,[231] and to suppress vascular intimal hyperplasia after balloon injury in rabbits fed on a high-cholesterol diet, suggesting the usefulness of tranilast in the prevention of restenosis after PTCA of patients, including those with clinical risk of hypercholesterolemia.[232] Other animal studies show that tranilast antagonizes angiotensin-II, which is thought to possibly potentiate neointimal formation.[233] Finally, tranilast restores cytokine-induced nitric oxide production and its antiproliferative effect in the presence of PDGF.[234]

In the placebo-controlled, randomized Tranilast Restenosis Following Angioplasty Trial (TREAT), investigators demonstrated a significant reduction in restenosis rates at 3-month follow-up in patients receiving tranilast, with restenosis rates of 14.7% in patients treated with tranilast 600 mg once daily versus 46.5% in the placebo group ($P < .001$).[235] However, the results of the recent Prevention of Restenosis with Tranilast and Its Outcomes (PRESTO) study showed no benefit of the drug on the restenosis and clinical event rates in a placebo-controlled trial of 11,484 patients who underwent angioplasty (85% stenting).[236]

Other anti-inflammatory approaches to prevent restenosis that are under investigation include the use of the anti-inflammatory cytokine interleukin-10, selective inhibition of the α_v/β_3-integrin receptor by XT199, inhibition of P-selectin 12-lipoxygenase, an arachidonic metabolite with proliferative effects on vascular smooth muscle and macrophage depletion by clodronate-containing liposomes.[237–240a] The ubiquitin-proteasome system is the major intracellular protein degradation pathway in eukaryotic cells, regulating central mediators of proliferation, inflammation and apoptosis, which are fundamental mechanisms in the development of vascular restenosis. The proteasome inhibitor M6132 inhibited neointimal formation in a balloon-injury model in the rat carotid artery.[241]

Specific Growth Factor Antagonists

In light of the clear importance of growth factors in restenosis, some groups have investigated the impact of specific antagonism of such substances on restenosis. PDGF is secreted by platelets, endothelium, smooth muscle, and monocyte/macrophages, and is a strong chemoattractant and mitogen for vascular smooth muscle. It is the smooth-muscle cell growth factor currently believed to play the most important role in restenosis. Trapidil, a PDGF antagonist, significantly reduces smooth-muscle cell proliferation in vitro and in animal restenosis models.[242] Trapidil-treated rabbits showed a significant reduction in luminal renarrowing after vascular injury as compared with those treated with placebo. A small clinical study of trapidil showed significant reductions in angiographic restenosis relative to aspirin and dipyridamole therapy (19.4% vs 41.7% of patients, respectively).[243] This effect was more pronounced in patients with high post-PTCA residual stenosis. These findings were corroborated by the larger Italian Studio Trapidil versus Aspirin nella Restenosi Coronarica (STARC) trial.[244] Among the 254 patients who completed this study, angiographic restenosis at 6 months occurred in 24.2% of those actively treated, and in 39.7% of the placebo group. Similar results were obtained from a study of 160 patients randomized to receive trapidil or dipyridamole, both in combination with aspirin for 6 months, with restenosis rates of 20% and 38%, respectively.[245] These results invite confirmation by a large multicenter trial.

RPR101511A is an orally active inhibitor of the PDGF-receptor tyrosine kinase and that inhibits postangioplasty restenosis in the swine coronary artery.[246]

Immunology provides another potential approach to PDGF antagonism. Polyclonal PDGF antibodies have already been shown to dramatically reduce neointimal formation after vascular injury in an animal model.[247] Further animal and early clinical testing are currently in order to determine the potential usefulness of this line of therapy.

It has also been suspected that pituitary hormones exert an influence on smooth-muscle cell proliferation in restenosis. Fingerle et al.[248] demonstrated that hypophysectomy reduced neointimal hyperplasia after balloon injury in animal models. Although it is not clear which pituitary hormones are responsible for these effects, growth hormone and somatomedin intermediaries are believed to be involved. In an attempt to manipulate the pituitary endocrine axis, synthetic analogues of somatostatin, including angiopeptin, octreotide, and lanreotide, have been developed. Similar to the endogenous substance, these agents act on the pituitary to reduce growth hormone secretion and can prevent an increase in insulin-like growth factor (IGF-1), an important serum and tissue component responsible for cell proliferation in various tissues, including the vascular wall. Angiopeptin inhibited myointimal thickening in animal restenosis models, but only when angiopeptin was given prior to or during angioplasty, with no benefit achieved with treatment commencing more than 8 h postangioplasty.[249] This approach has also been subjected to a number of clinical trials in PTCA patients. Angiopeptin yielded very promising results in the Scandinavian Angiopeptin Study of 112 PTCA patients, in which restenosis rates at 6-month angiographic follow-up were significantly lower in the actively treated group versus placebo (7.5% vs 37.8%, respectively), with late losses in luminal diameter of 0.10 versus 0.52 mm, respectively.[250] However, a larger trial by Emanuelsson et al[251] involving 554 patients was unable to demonstrate a reduction in angiographic restenosis with angiopeptin, as compared with placebo,

but was able to generate a clear reduction in major clinical events at 6-month follow-up. The incidence of repeat percutaneous revascularizations was reduced by almost half in the actively treated group (9% vs 16%). In the largest angiopeptin trial to date ($n = 1246$), patients were randomized to receive twice daily subcutaneous injections of placebo or 1 of 3 varying doses of angiopeptin for 10 days after PTCA.[252] All groups in this trial exhibited virtually identical angiographic restenosis rates, making it very unlikely that angiopeptin has much efficacy in this regard.

Nevertheless, questions remain regarding adequate dosage of angiopeptin due to its short half-life; therefore, further studies are ongoing. A recent study of the porcine coronary in-stent restenosis model did indicate that systemic, continuous subcutaneous treatment with angiopeptin after stent implantation did significantly reduce intimal hyperplasia and restenosis as compared to the control group.[252] However, a major limitation of this study is that the systemic treatment group did not have a sham local delivery catheter insertion, thereby making it difficult to compare results with other groups, which most likely experienced additional injury through local delivery catheter.

Similar to the results with angiopeptin, a clinical trial showed octreotide having no benefit on the postangioplasty restenosis rate.[253]

Despite its name, serotonin is a vasoregulatory substance found mostly in association with platelets rather than free in the serum. Serotonin released from platelet granules after vascular injury is believed to contribute to the process of restenosis, both by direct mitogenic effects on smooth-muscle cells and by stimulating platelet activation and vasoconstriction.[254] In vitro it increases proliferation, migration, and contraction of vascular smooth-muscle cells. Although a relatively weak direct platelet activator and proproliferative, it probably potentiates the effect of other factors, including ADP, TXA2, and PDGF. Ketanserin is a serotonin S2-receptor antagonist that is known to block many of the above effects in animal models. Therefore, the 658-patient Dutch Multicenter Post-Angioplasty Restenosis Ketanserin (PARK) trial was undertaken to evaluate ketanserin relative to placebo (in combination with aspirin) for prevention of restenosis.[255] The results of this study showed active treatment to have no effect on angiographic restenosis or clinical outcome. The results of smaller clinical trials in Austria and Germany agreed with this outcome regarding restenosis; however, the former also suggested that the drug may have some benefit on acute PTCA complications.[256,257]

Angiotensin-converting enzyme (ACE) inhibitors have been considered for restenosis prophylaxis since local neointimal ACE and angiotensin-II activity were shown to be increased in injured arteries.[258] Although this drug class is most widely known for its vasodilatory efficacy, it is included in the section of growth factor antagonists because locally produced angiotensin-II stimulates DNA synthesis in and promotes migration and growth of arterial smooth muscle.[259] Further study suggests that angiotensin-II induces the gene for thrombospondin I, which is required for matrix interactions in neointimal formation, as well as other protooncogenes and growth factors in vascular smooth-muscle cells.[260] In addition to blocking the effects of angiotensin-II mentioned above, ACE inhibitors are thought to reduce neointimal proliferation by increasing bradykinin levels, leading to increased vascular nitric oxide production, which, in turn, generates cyclic guanosine monophosphate (GMP), a potent smooth-muscle cell-growth inhibitor.[258–265] Such effects on proliferation of vascular smooth muscle and, perhaps, myocardium, have already been documented in response to hypertension and diabetes, and are postulated in the pathogenesis of restenosis. Interestingly, certain genotypes of ACE, which lead to greater angiotensin-II levels, are disproportionately prevalent in patients with restenosis.[260,262–264]

In several animal models, cilazapril and captopril strongly reduced smooth-muscle cell proliferation and neointimal formation after vascular balloon injury in a way that other vasodilators, including hydralazine and calcium antagonists, have not, although several animal studies have shown no benefit.[260,262–264]

In humans, a retrospective analysis of PTCA patients showed that those patients discharged on ACE inhibitors had a significantly reduced incidence of restenosis when compared to those patients not on drug (3% vs 30%).[266] These positive results led to the initiation of the large, prospective, Multicenter European Research Trial with Cilazapril after Angioplasty to Prevent Transluminal Coronary Obstruction and Restenosis (MERCATOR) trial.[267] In the 595 patients who completed this study to long-term angiographic follow-up examination, cilazapril 5 mg twice daily for 6 months neither reduced angiographic restenosis nor improved clinical outcome to any statistically significant degree. Similarly negative results were obtained in a Belgian study of 509 patients using fosinopril,[268] in an Indian study of 95 patients using enalapril,[269] and in a French study of 345 patients undergoing coronary stenting using quinapril.[270]

It is very possible that the failure of these clinical studies relative to the animal results reflects a problem of dose. This concept is corroborated by Rakugi et al.,[259] who treated rats with varying doses of quinapril. They found that the drug's suppression of serum and tissue ACE activity, and, indeed, neointimal formation, is clearly dose dependent and occurs at a therapeutic window well above levels needed for antihypertensive purposes. They also found that suppression of tissue ACE activity correlated much more closely with prevention of restenosis than did serum ACE activity or blood pressure. To address this need, the Multicenter American Research Trial with Cilazapril after Angioplasty to Prevent Transluminal Coronary Obstruction and Restenosis (MARCATOR) group[271] tested doses of 2.5, 5, and 10 mg twice daily of cilazapril for a 6-month course against placebo (in addition to aspirin) after successful PTCA in an otherwise very similar study to the MERCATOR study. Among the 1436 patients enrolled, no real benefit in reducing restenosis was observed with active therapy at any of the doses. Perhaps doses in excess of 20 mg twice daily would prove to reduce restenosis; however, systemic hypotension clearly becomes a limiting factor. These results invite further research to clinically test higher doses of ACE inhibitors and to develop systems for local delivery of ACE inhibitors to suppress tissue ACE activity and minimize systemic hypotension.

Recently, the question was raised whether angiotensin contributes in a major way to the process of postangioplasty restenosis.[272] Investigators could not demonstrate any benefit in using subtype selective and balanced angiotensin-II-receptor antagonists in a porcine coronary artery model of vascular restenosis.[273]

There is evidence that 17-estradiol can inhibit neointima formation after coronary angioplasty in swine,[274] and retrospective evidence in humans suggests that chronic estrogen replacement can reduce late loss after PTCA and atherectomy.[275] Estrogens appear to have actions to reduce the risk of atherosclerotic disease,[276] and two recent studies used the hormone as an antiproliferative agent following balloon injury to the carotid arteries of ovariectomized rats. In one study, estrogen inhibited the adventitial contribution to the vascular injury response.[277] In the other study, rats were randomized to

estrogen, irbesartan, estrogen/irbesartan, and placebo.[278] Irbesartan is a selective type 1 angiotensin-II (AT1) antagonist, while the type 2 angiotensin-II (AT2) receptor is estrogen responsive and mediates antiproliferative effects. Interestingly, both estrogen and irbesartan significantly inhibited neointimal formation but did not show an additive effect, suggesting a common mechanism shared by the two agents. These studies merit further investigation of estrogen and angiotensin-II-receptor blockers as potential therapeutic agents for preventing restenosis.[278a]

Catecholamines apparently have trophic influences on vascular smooth-muscle cells. An earlier study of the rat carotid artery showed that α-adrenergic receptor antagonists such as urapidil and prazosin reduced neointimal formation.[279,280] Subsequently, a study of the novel multiple-action antihypertensive agent carvedilol showed that it inhibited human vascular smooth-muscle cell proliferation at a level similar to that of the calcium antagonist verapamil, and that it had an apparent relative selectivity for restenosis-derived cells.[281] However, in a study with carvedilol, using 50 mg daily of the drug, when compared to placebo, in patients undergoing angioplasty, there was no effect of active treatment in preventing restenosis.[282] The work on the class of growth factor inhibitors is early in its development, though, and further studies are warranted.

Another approach, which is in its early stages of research development, involves accentuating certain naturally occurring inhibitors to smooth-muscle cell proliferation. Nitric oxide (NO), secreted by intact endothelial cells, in addition to locally regulating vasomotor tone, probably exerts a natural defense to intimal overgrowth by direct smooth-muscle cell cytostasis and by reducing platelet and inflammatory cell adhesion.[283] Studies demonstrate that nitric oxide synthase, which joins L-arginine and oxygen to form nitric oxide, has an important presence after vascular injury and may be deficient in cases of restenosis.[284] The potential role of nitric oxide and nitric oxide synthase in the restenotic process has been reviewed.[285] Although nitric oxide suppresses smooth-muscle cell proliferation in vivo, its remarkably short half-life makes it impractical for use in restenosis prevention. To circumvent this problem, a number of nitric oxide donors, including DETA/NO,[286] nitrosated albumin (which can contribute nitric oxide),[287] and L-arginine,[288] have been tested in animal vascular-injury models with remarkable success in reducing neointimal formation. More recently, one study found that chronic inhalation of NO inhibits neointimal formation after balloon-induced arterial injury in the rat carotid model.[289] Another study found that a novel, single, local intramural administration of L-arginine enhances vascular nitric oxide generation and inhibits lesion formation.[290]

The positive results of these animal studies led to the first major clinical restenosis trial of nitric oxide donors.[291] This trial randomized 700 patients undergoing generally lower-risk PTCA to nitric oxide donor therapy (consisting of periprocedural intravenous linsidomine followed by molsidomine therapy for 6 months), or diltiazem treatment, both in combination with aspirin. Nitric oxide donor-treated patients were found at 6-month follow-up to have superior minimal luminal diameters (1.54 vs 1.38 mm), lower late-loss indices (late loss/acute gain: 0.35 vs 0.46), and lower restenosis rates by 50% stenosis criterion (38% vs 36.5%) than diltiazem-treated patients. This study is one of the very few large-scale clinical trials to show a significant reduction in restenosis; however, the significance is largely statistical, due to the high power of the study, rather than clinical, as the actual reduction in restenosis is minute. These results should be corroborated by other large studies; however, they demonstrate nitric oxide donors to have a very promising role in restenosis prevention.

One of the most modern approaches lies in the antagonism of leukocyte and endothelium adhesion molecules necessary for cell accumulation and function. PTCA has been shown to induce a rise in concentration of certain cell adhesion molecules in serum,[292] and the importance of cell adhesion molecules in restenosis has been reviewed.[293] Investigators also found that interleukin-1β (IL-1β), a pleiotropic cytokine involved in the development of restenosis, was a potent inducer for ICAM-1 and VCAM-1 expression in human vascular smooth-muscle cells.[294] The identification of more adhesion molecules, as well as cytokines involved in cell-cell interaction, presents an ever-greater opportunity for immunologic and other molecular methods of combating restenosis. One group has shown an in vivo reduction in neointimal proliferation in a rabbit carotid injury model by immunologically blocking the leukocyte CD11/CD18 adhesion complex with specific monoclonal antibodies.[295] However, a larger animal investigation by Guzman et al.,[296] using a rabbit femoral artery balloon-injury model, found no reduction in neointimal proliferation. The presence of mixed results on this issue certainly invites further animal testing, although the latter group's findings are probably more indicative. Other groups have demonstrated in vivo reductions in neointimal hyperplasia after immunologically blocking intercellular adhesion molecule and leukocyte function-associated antigen-1, molecules essential to leukocyte adhesion.[297] Investigation of the importance of endothelial adhesion molecules, including the family of selectins, is just beginning.[239,298] A recent study found that baseline E-selectin levels were higher in patients who restenosed when compared with those patients who did not.[53] This approach is still in its early stages, and given the diversity of adhesion molecules in endothelial, inflammatory, and smooth-muscle cells, it is likely to be the subject of a large body of investigative work in the future.

Diabetic patients have a higher frequency of in-stent restenosis than do nondiabetic patients. It has been reported that the insulin-sensitizing agent troglitazone reduces neointimal tissue proliferation after coronary stent implantation in patients with type II diabetes.[299]

Endothelial Growth Factors

A related, albeit different, focus of investigators is the interaction between endothelial cells and smooth-muscle cells in the modulation of the healing process and the role of endothelial dysfunction as one of the major regulatory elements in the restenotic process.[300] Instead of focusing on inhibiting vascular smooth-muscle cell proliferation through the use of growth factor antagonists, alternatively, smooth-muscle cell proliferation might be indirectly inhibited by facilitating reendothelialization of sites exposed to balloon-induced arterial injury. Vascular permeability factor, a natural growth factor responsible for vessel permeability and microvascular angiogenesis, stimulated rabbit endothelial cell proliferation in vitro and accelerated regeneration of endothelium in vivo.[301] Another group of investigators discovered that application of vascular endothelial growth factor, an EC-specific growth regulatory molecule, to the left carotid artery of rats after balloon injury effectively increased the extent of reendothelialization and attenuated neointimal thickening to a statistically significant degree.[302] On the other hand, seeding with autologous venous endothelial cells restored the endothelial monolayer, but failed to attenuate intimal hyperplasia in balloon-injured rabbit arteries.[303] Reendothelialization using transfection of human HGF, a novel potent member of endothelium-specific growth factors, significantly inhibited neointimal formation in the rat restenosis model, accompanied by a rise in nitric oxide levels.[304] Gene therapy approaches using VEGF-C and PhVEGF165, in both animals and humans, are currently being evaluated.[32] More studies are necessary to assess this potentially useful approach for preventing restenosis.

Vasodilators

The finding that restenosis occurs more frequently in patients with vasospastic angina along with the potential contributions of recoil, deficiencies in compensatory vessel enlargement, and flow/stress considerations, suggest a role for vasodilators in the prevention of restenosis.[305] Calcium antagonists are already used routinely during PTCA to avert acute complications such as vasospasm and to reduce myocardial oxygen demand. There is also some evidence, however, to suggest that this class of drugs, in addition to affecting acute and chronic vasodilation, reduces growth factor-dependent proliferation and migration of smooth-muscle cells.[306] The long-acting calcium antagonist benidipine arrests growth on vascular smooth-muscle cells in vivo, as well as in vitro, in the porcine model.[307]

There have been several good randomized trials on the subject of calcium antagonists and restenosis in patients without variant angina that have arrived at divergent results. Placebo-controlled studies involving 201 patients and 92 patients with high-dose diltiazem (in combination with aspirin and dipyridamole), and a study of 241 patients with nifedipine, all showed no benefit in long-term angiographic findings or clinical events over placebo-treated patients.[308–310] In contrast, the Verapamil Angioplasty Study (VAS), having randomized 196 patients, found calcium antagonism (in combination with aspirin and dipyridamole) to yield a lower angiographic restenosis rate than the placebo group in compliant patients (47.4% vs 63.9%, respectively).[311] Further analysis of the data revealed that benefit was preferentially derived by patients with stable angina (37.8% vs 63.2%), whereas patients who had unstable angina or who had suffered an infarction realized no reduction in restenosis from verapamil therapy (55.8% vs 62.2%). A trial of 170 patients by Unverdorben et al.[312] found diltiazem to reduce angiographic restenosis better than placebo, with highest benefit in patients with diabetes mellitus and hypercholesterolemia. A meta-analysis performed by Hillegass et al.[313] of several trials as an aggregate suggests a 30% reduction in the odds of angiographic restenosis by calcium antagonism. These promising results, notably with verapamil, certainly invite a large multicenter trial on this subject for more conclusive results. A long-term trial with nisoldipine CC after coronary angioplasty showed no benefit on postangioplasty restenosis.[314] Similarly, amlodipine had no effect on restenosis, but it did reduce clinical events, including repeat PTCA.[315] Clearly, in studies with some of the calcium antagonists, angiographic restenosis must be the primary end-point, as the negative inotropic and chronotropic effects of verapamil and diltiazem could reduce ischemic symptoms resulting from restenosis through reduction in myocardial oxygen demand. In addition, the extent to which calcium antagonists fail in this regard probably lowers the probability of a major contribution by recoil or vasospasm in restenosis.

Other vasodilator approaches used to prevent postangioplasty restenosis in experimental models include bradykinin receptor stimulation and the use of minoxidil.[316,316a]

Antiproliferatives, Antineoplastics, and Antibiotics

Rather than focus on platelet or growth factor antagonism, some researchers have turned toward nonspecific antiproliferatives and antineoplastic agents, attempting to block cell division in smooth-muscle cells, essentially the final common pathway of restenosis. In fact, the proliferation of smooth-muscle cell in restenosis and the growth factors involved bear many similarities to benign neoplasias.[317] Rapamycin (Sirolimus), a macrolide antibiotic, inhibits porcine aortic smooth-muscle cell migration in vivo and neointimal formation, and inhibits both human and rat aortic smooth-muscle cell proliferation in vitro.[318,319] Rapamycin causes cyclin-CdK complex inhibition and cell-cycle arrest,[320] and in clinical trials where it was used in a drug-eluting stent, it inhibited neointimal formation.[320–322b]

Although severe toxicity probably prohibits the use of most antimitogenic and antineoplastic therapies, colchicine has been considered as a potential inhibitor of leukocyte and smooth-muscle cell migration and proliferation. This plant alkaloid interrupts mitotic spindle formation by interfering with microtubule formation. It arrests cell division in metaphase, in addition to blocking a host of microtubule-dependent functions, including the release of inflammatory and chemoattractant factors stored in secretory vesicles, and pseudopodial activity needed for smooth-muscle cell migration. Its potency in reducing inflammation and fibrosis has extended its role from its traditional use in gout to include consideration for treatment of cirrhosis and acute leukemia. Colchicine has yielded positive results in animal restenosis models,[323] but the dose-dependent reduction in postinjury neointimal formation occurred at arterial wall drug concentrations probably unachievable and systemically intolerable by conventional routes of administration in human beings. When clinically tested, 1.2 mg of colchicine daily for 6 months yielded no benefit over placebo in an angiographically determined restenosis trial of 197 patients.[324] In addition, approximately 7% of the actively treated patients withdrew because of gastrointestinal side effects. Similarly, negative results were obtained in a randomized study of 253 patients receiving colchicine 1 mg daily for 1 month, which used clinical variables and exercise thallium tests as restenosis end-points.[325] In consideration of the possibility that the lack of clinical efficacy reflected limitations on adequate dosing of the drug, animal studies have been performed using colchicine with or without steroids, locally delivered via coated microparticles intramurally injected; however, these have also generally failed to demonstrate positive results.[326]

Paclitaxel (Taxol), a more potent microtubule-stabilizing agent, inhibits smooth-muscle cell proliferation in vitro and in vivo postvascular injury in rat carotid artery models after intraperitoneal delivery of the drug.[327] Local delivery of paclitaxel, using a microcapsule system, reduces intimal thickening in the same model relative to control microcapsules. While promising in suggesting a workable route of delivery that minimizes the drug's very toxic side effects, this study is limited by the absence of a control group of animals who did not receive locally delivered microcapsules at all. It is not uncommon in local delivery studies to find that the vascular injury resulting from the trauma of introducing drug-impregnated microspheres is greater than the potential benefit of the therapy. Recently, paclitaxel was shown to inhibit human smooth-muscle cell proliferation and migration even in the presence of mitogens.[328] Local delivery through microporous balloons significantly reduced intimal area and degree of restenosis in rabbits after balloon angioplasty,

making paclitaxel a promising candidate for local therapy of restenosis.

More favorable results on neointimal proliferation have been observed in various animal models using drug-eluting stents containing paclitaxel.[329–332a] The European Evaluation of Paclitaxel Eluting Stent Trial (ELUTES) demonstrated a significant reduction in restenosis that was dose related.[332b] Similarly, benefit was observed with a drug-delivery stent containing 7-hexanolytaxol (QP2, a taxane analogue).[333]

Other potent antimitotic agents used for cancer chemotherapy are being considered for restenosis prophylaxis; their tremendous toxicity, however, is a limiting factor. Such agents have been tested in animal trials but have not yet reached the point of clinical testing. In vitro, etoposide reduces proliferation of smooth-muscle cells cultured from restenotic lesions.[334] Barath et al.[335] administered low-dose vincristine and dactinomycin to rabbits, some of which underwent balloon dilatation of the aorta and some of which did not. By examining electron microscopic findings at 3 days postprocedure, they were able to show a selective in vivo suppression of smooth-muscle cell proliferation without injury to normal smooth-muscle cells. However, studies using standard animal restenosis models and angiographic end-points with cyclosporin, azathioprine, and both locally and systemically administered methotrexate, have failed to generate significant reductions in restenosis, when compared with controls.[336–338] The effects of actinomycin D on restenosis are currently being evaluated in a drug-eluting stent [Actinomycin Eluting Stent Improves Outcomes by Reducing Neointimal Hyperplasia (ACTION)].[32] Other antimitotic agents being evaluated for prevention of restenosis in experimental studies include 8-chloro-cyclic AMP and the oral CdK inhibitor flavopiridol.[339,340]

Lipid-Lowering Agents and Antioxidants

In addition to these novel pharmacotherapeutic approaches, researchers have not forgotten traditional secondary prevention for coronary disease, which includes diet, exercise, and pharmacologic modification of serum cholesterol, particularly reducing LDL-C and raising HDL-C. A study by Shah et al.[341] of the relation of restenosis to serum lipid fractions found that a low HDL fraction was independently and strongly related to the risk of restenosis and the brevity of the time interval to restenosis. Restenosis occurred in 64% of patients with HDL $\leq$40 mg/dL as opposed to 17% of patients with HDL >40 mg/dL.

A number of clinical studies suggest that high serum Lp(a), in particular, confers an increased risk for restenosis, as it probably does for coronary artery disease in general.[342,343] The LDL-Apheresis Angioplasty Restenosis Trial (L-ART) group in Japan achieved positive results in reducing restenosis by LDL apheresis, a method that uses a dextran sulfate cellulose column to reduce plasma Lp(a) and LDL-C levels.[344] In the L-ART trial, those patients whose plasma Lp(a) levels were reduced by more than 50% with apheresis had restenosis rates of 21.2%, in contrast to a rate of 52.4% in a control group. Effects were naturally greatest in patients starting out with high Lp(a) levels.

A number of trials have attempted to reduce the incidence of restenosis with 3-hydroxy-3-methylglutaryl-coenzyme A (HMG-CoA) reductase inhibitors.[344a] Studies of hypercholesterolemic rabbits showed clear reduction in neointimal hyperplasia after balloon vascular injury with lovastatin therapy.[345] However, it has become apparent that the drug's efficacy in this regard may not stem from lipid-lowering effects; application of lovastatin to cultured smooth-muscle cells that have been stimulated by PDGF shows a clear and dose-dependent direct suppression of smooth-muscle cell proliferation.[346] It has been postulated that HMG-CoA reductase inhibitors exert this effect by reducing the biosynthesis of mevalonate, a precursor of nonsterol compounds essential in cell proliferation. A clinical trial by Sahni et al.,[347] randomizing 157 PTCA patients to lovastatin treatment or placebo, found the former group to have significantly less frequent restenosis (12% vs 44%, respectively). However, compliance and loss to follow-up were major problems in this study, with only 50% of patients undergoing repeat angiography. The multicenter Lovastatin Restenosis Trial Study Group, with an enrollment of 404 patients, found that treatment with lovastatin starting 7 to 10 days before PTCA and extending for 6 months conferred no reduction in restenosis over placebo, using percent stenosis of the index lesion at 6-month angiographic follow-up as the primary endpoint.[348] Restenosis rates were essentially identical despite a 42% reduction in serum LDL-C in the active-treated group. A small study in Japan found pravastatin to similarly yield no reduction in restenosis despite profound reductions in total serum cholesterol.[349] A small study from Brazil showed similar results with lovastatin.[350] Results of the Fluvastatin Angioplasty Restenosis (FLARE) trial, a placebo-controlled, randomized, multicenter trial of 1054 patients that tested the efficacy of fluvastatin,[351] showed that the drug exerted more neointimal suppression than other drugs in this class in an earlier study. In the FLARE trial, fluvastatin therapy appeared to decrease the incidence of death and nonfatal MI, as well as total cholesterol, LDL, and triglyceride levels. Unfortunately, examination of the minimal lumen diameter, the primary end-point of the study, showed no significant differences in initial gain, late loss, or late gain, as compared to placebo. A more recent study using pravastatin demonstrated that after 2 years the postangioplasty restenosis rate was considerably reduced.[352] The investigators in this study concluded that 6 months was too short a time to demonstrate a benefit from lipid-lowering therapy in patients undergoing balloon angioplasty.

A study by Walter et al. also demonstrated the benefit of statin therapy in reducing restenosis development following coronary stenting.[353]

Probucol, another lipid-lowering agent, has the capacity to reduce total and LDL-C, and also possesses antioxidant action.[354] The latter mechanism may be important because free radicals, generated by vascular injury and frequently associated with macrophages and foam cells, are reported as playing a role in activating the cascade of growth factors and mitogens responsible for restenosis. This is in addition to the reported importance of oxidative modification of LDL-C contributing to deposition in vessel walls.[355] Studies with probucol and porcine coronary injury models show positive results and suggest that it is probably its antioxidant rather than hypercholesterolemic efficacy that is responsible for its reduction of neointimal proliferation.[356,357]

An early randomized clinical trial by Setsuda et al.[358] involving 67 patients, suggested a reduction in restenosis with probucol relative to dipyridamole therapy. In a larger study of 118 patients, probucol was administered from more than 7 days before PTCA until 3 months after PTCA, at which time coronary angiography was conducted.[359] The restenosis rate of the probucol treated group was statistically lower (19.7%) when compared with the control group (39.7%). Serum total cholesterol and LDL-C were comparable in the two groups, suggesting the antirestenotic effect was not due to the lowering of cholesterol levels. On the other hand, the Angioplasty plus Probucol/Lovastatin Evaluation Trial reduced total and LDL-cholesterol, but did not prevent restenosis or clinical restenosis at 6 months follow-up.[360]

The seemingly contradictory results would be cleared up in the double-blind, placebo-controlled, randomized trial of 317 patients by the Multivitamin and Probucol Study Group.[361] In this trial to test the effectiveness of antioxidants in reducing restenosis, the patients were randomly assigned to receive one of four treatments (placebo, probucol, multivitamins, or multivitamins plus probucol), starting at 4 weeks before PTCA until the angiographic follow-up at 6 months. As compared to placebo, probucol treatment resulted in decreases of 68% in the late reductions in luminal diameter, 47% in the proportion of dilated coronary artery segments with restenosis, and 58% percent in the need for repeated angioplasty. The investigators postulate that the initiation of treatment 1 month before angioplasty is crucial, citing data suggesting that probucol accumulates slowly in tissue.[362] This might also explain why the Probucol/Lovastatin study failed to show any effect on restenosis prevention. These results with probucol represent one of the first pharmacologic approaches shown to conclusively reduce restenosis. Recently, a subgroup analysis of this trial showed that probucol was effective in reducing lumen loss and restenosis rate in small coronary arteries, which have higher restenosis rates than do larger arteries after PTCA.[363] In addition, the investigators undertook an intravascular ultrasound substudy during the trial to assess the mechanism of probucol's action. Probucol appears to exert its antirestenotic effects by improving vascular remodeling after angioplasty, while lumen loss after PTCA appears to be due to inadequate remodeling in response to tissue hyperplasia.[364] It should be noted that probucol appears to adversely reduce the HDL-C concentration and will probably exert adverse effects if prolonged administration is required.[365] Therefore, further follow-up study is necessary to demonstrate whether cessation of probucol treatment after 6 months causes subsequent lumen narrowing.

Recently, it was shown in the Canadian Antioxidant Restenosis Trial (CART-1) that AG-1067, with oxidant properties similar to probucol, reduced restenosis at a rate similar to probucol.[366] In contrast to probucol, AG-1067 does not prolong the QT interval.

Other antioxidants have been considered, including vitamin E and α-tocopherol, which are thought to also have a direct antiproliferative efficacy. An in vivo animal study by Lafont, using balloon-injured vessels in rabbits, found vitamin E to significantly improve minimal lumen diameter at 28-day angiographic follow-up relative to controls, 1.7 versus 1.07 mm.[367] The reduction of intimal hyperplasia was then confirmed by histologic examination. In a porcine model, vitamin E in combination with vitamin C was found to increase postinjury lumina not by decreasing neointimal area but by increasing total vessel area, suggesting a beneficial effect on vascular remodeling.[368] A clinical trial with vitamin E at Emory University suggested some benefit in reducing angiographic and clinical restenosis, but was unable to generate statistically significant differences due to a small sample size.[369] A parenteral bolus of β-carotene, a lipid-soluble antioxidant, failed to reduce either intimal hyperplasia or late lumen loss after angioplasty in cholesterol-fed rabbits.[370] Finally, in the aforementioned Multivitamin and Probucol Study Group, which showed beneficial effects of probucol on angiographic restenosis, multivitamin treatment, using a regimen including β-carotene, vitamin C, and vitamin E, showed no significant effect on either restenosis or major clinical end-points.[361] Because probucol and multivitamins are both antioxidants, the disparate results call for the elucidation of the agents' mechanism of action. Two possibilities that the authors suggest are that probucol may be a stronger antioxidant or that the vitamins may act as a prooxidant. The likely role of active oxygen species in the restenotic process and the potential therapeutic potential of antioxidants is corroborated by a study showing hydrogen peroxide to be a potent mitogen for smooth-muscle cells and probucol to be an inhibitor of this process.[371] Nevertheless, future studies may yield new mechanisms unrelated to antioxidants effects, which may account for the differential effects of antioxidant treatment on restenosis.

LOCAL DRUG DELIVERY

As hypothesized, the relative failure of many of these pharmacologic interventions in human studies, when compared with animal studies, may not stem from pharmacodynamic mechanism but from inadequate concentration of drug in the human coronary vasculature due to limitation by systemic intolerance.[372] Attention, therefore, has been focused on the concept of local delivery of drugs to injured coronary epithelium. With such an approach, extremely high concentrations of drug can be achieved at the target site with minimal systemic side effects. Such a route of delivery also averts or minimizes the potential problems of poor oral bioavailability, rapid clearance, and protease degradation. Some forms of local delivery offer the additional advantage of prolonged administration of drug. As local drug delivery already has noncardiac clinical usage in the form of progesterone-coated intrauterine devices and conjunctival pilocarpine reservoirs for glaucoma, for example, it is only natural to consider its role in the prevention of restenosis. Its use in other cardiac diseases is currently under investigation; there already

exist pacemaker leads with dexamethasone reservoirs to reduce the fibrosis, which frequently leads to long-term increases in pacing thresholds.[373] Also being studied are drug-impregnated controlled-release polymeric matrices for ventricular arrhythmias and bioprosthetic valve calcification.[374]

Early animal studies demonstrated the effectiveness of local drug delivery for restenosis by surgically implanting reservoirs of various agents adjacent to the external surface of an injured vessel with the drug diffusing from the adventitia to the intima.

A pioneer animal study by Edelman et al.[375] showed similarly reduced neointimal proliferation in the injured carotid vessels of rats treated both systemically and locally with local heparin. However, rats treated with an adventitial matrix exhibited no change in laboratory coagulation profiles, establishing desired efficacy without undesirable systemic effects. Of course, surgical implantation of epicardial reservoirs is impractical as a treatment for restenosis, therefore attention has turned to systems which can be placed percutaneously. Devices under investigation currently include porous and infusion balloon catheters, polymeric or coated stents, techniques for "facilitated diffusion," and coated microspheres, but clearly a discussion of this technology is beyond the scope of this chapter. These devices are well reviewed by Lincoff et al.[372] An explosion of studies has been generated using stent-based local-drug-delivery percutaneous devices and include matrix metalloproteinase inhibitors, actinomycin-D, rapamycin, paclitaxel, QP2, and steroids (Table 40-3).[32,321,322b,332,333,376–379]

TABLE 40-3. Stent-Based Drug Delivery for In-Stent Restenosis

Drug Type/Drug	Animal Studies		
	Animal Model	Polymer	Effect
Anti-inflammatory			
Methylpredisone	Pig	PFM	23% AS reduction
Dexamethasone	Pig	PLLA	nil
Colchicine	Pig	PLLA	nil
Antiproliferative			
Sirolimus	Pig	NK	39%–45% reduction*
Paclitaxel	Rabbit	pLA/pCL	42% NI reduction
	Pig	NA	39.5% NI reduction
Other			
Prostacyclin analog	Pig	PLLA	22.9% RA reduction
PTK inhibitor	Pig	PLLA	47% AS reduction
Angiopeptin	Pig	POPZ	29% MLD reduction
	Human Studies		
Drug	Mechanism	Pt. #	Restenosis Rate/Trial
Sirolimus	Cdk inhibitor	30	10.4–11.0 ± 3.0 NI%
Sirolimus	Cdk inhibitor	238	(RAVEL) 0% restenosis rate >50%
Paclitaxel/QP2	Microtubule stabilizer	14	14% ± 15% CSN%
Paclitaxel/QP2	Microtubule stabilizer	32	13% CSA stenosis in13/13
Paclitaxel/QP2	Microtubule stabilizer	400	SCORE†
Batimastat	MMP-1 inhibitor	350	†
Actinomycin D	Multiple	350	ACTION†
Methylprednisolone	Multiple	70	STRIDE†

*Injury scores varied between treatment and control; †ongoing studies.

ACTION = actinomycin-eluting stent improves outcomes by reducing neointimal hyperplasia trial; AS = area stenosis; CSN = cross-sectional narrowing (neointimal area/stent area); MLD = minimal lumen diameter; MMP = matrix metalloproteinase inhibitor; NI = neointima; NK = not known; PC = phosphorylcholine; PFM = fluororinated polymethacrylate; PLA/PCL = poly(lactide-10-∑-caprolactone); PLLA = poly-L-lactic acid; POPZ = polyorganophosphazene; RA = restenosis area; RAVEL = rapamycin-eluting versus plain polymer stents trial; SCORE = Study to Compare Restenosis Rates with Paclitaxel Following Stenting; STRIDE = Study of Antirestenosis with the BiodiviYsio Dexamethasone Eluting Stent.

Source: Adapted with permission from Lowe HC, et al.[32]

However, the process of local delivery is not without its problems.[380] It has been observed that stent-based drug delivery results in marked spatial variation in delivered drug dose,[381] and there are reports of late stent thrombosis with paclitaxel stents.[382] A study by Hodgson et al.[382a] showed that the local infusion of ethanol, suramin (an antiproliferative) or even saline after PTCA caused more smooth-muscle cell proliferation than that found in animal vessels thta had angioplasty alone. Another study using doxorubicin locally delivered suggested a reduction in restenosis when compared with locally delivered saline, but not when compared with rabbits that received angioplasty alone, implying that any potential benefit of the drug was outweighed by endothelial injury and inflammation caused by the local delivery system.[382b] Some work suggests that the addition of steroids to the local delivery vehicle might reduce the inflammatory response, but this remains in early testing.

The promise of the field of local drug delivery with stents has spurred many recent studies on numerous therapeutic agents as well as delivery systems. Local drug delivery is currently limited by low delivery efficiency, short intramural retention, and potential safety issues.[383] To overcome the variability of local drug delivery, Topol's group successfully tested a single, local intraluminal infusion of a novel sustained-release, biodegradable nanoparticle.[384] Administration of nanoparticles with incorporated dexamethasone significantly reduced neointimal formation in the rat carotid model. The same group recently used a novel polymer-coated eluting stent to achieve sustained, site-specific delivery of dexamethasone to the porcine coronary artery wall.[385] Most recently, site-specific intracoronary drug delivery in humans was demonstrated, using a special coil balloon to deliver radiolabeled heparin, which allows on-line visualization and off-line quantification through radioisotopic assessment.[386] This technology has tremendous potential in facilitating the site-specific delivery of optimized doses of therapeutic agents.[32] In light of recent positive results with local delivery of therapeutic agents.[290] promising novel drug-eluting delivery stents, as well as the potential of photodynamic therapy and brachytherapy, the site-specific approach of administering therapeutic agents may represent the most significant pharmacologic developments for preventing restenosis.

MOLECULAR STRATEGIES

The exciting future of restenosis prophylaxis probably lies in molecular biology. A large body of research and literature has been devoted to use of chimeric toxins using recombinant DNA, antisense approaches, and the ultimate application of molecular biology, gene therapy, to suppress smooth-muscle cell proliferation.[32,386a] However, most of this work is still in the animal testing stage, although preliminary clinical trials have begun. Before reviewing these approaches, it is appropriate to first highlight some of the molecular processes believed to be pathogenetically at work in restenosis.

Growth factors and chemoattractants contributed by platelets, smooth-muscle cells, and monocytes induce quiescent vascular smooth-muscle cells to proliferate after injury by the activation of several stimulatory pathways and the curtailment of inhibitory pathways. These ligands bind to cell-surface receptors and activate several signal transduction pathways, which ultimately move the smooth-muscle cells from the quiescent G_0 stage into the cell cycle. The goals of molecular therapies, therefore, are to intervene at any of the mentioned steps in order to stop the migration and proliferation of smooth-muscle cells.

One molecular approach to reducing smooth-muscle cell proliferation, the use of recombinant chimeric toxins, has actually been borrowed from cancer research where it is already in phase I/II clinical trials.[387] In this approach, a gene encoding a potent cellular toxin that is lethal to essentially all cells, such as a bacterial exotoxin, is mutated and fused to a gene encoding a ligand, frequently a growth factor. The ultimate protein produced by this compound gene, composed of both a toxin and a ligand moiety, is selectively bound and internalized by cells with receptors for the encoded ligand. Epstein et al.[387a] likened the concept to a Trojan horse. Once the chimeric protein is taken in, the toxin moiety poisons the cell; in the case of pseudomonas exotoxin, for example, this is accomplished by stopping protein synthesis through inactivation of elongation factor.[388]

The success of this approach in cancer probably reflects the large upregulation of certain growth factor receptors in neoplasia. A similar effect has also been seen in proliferating smooth-muscle cells in which receptors for PDGF, epidermal growth factor, fibroblast growth factor, and insulin-like growth factor-1 have all been noted to be upregulated.[387a] After selective killing of proliferating smooth-muscle cells in vitro was achieved,[389,390] an in vivo animal study was performed with a chimeric toxin composed of fibroblast growth factor and saporin (a ribosome inactivator from plants), which specifically inhibited neointimal proliferation after balloon injury without affecting uninjured arteries.[391] Since then, large-scale purification and characterization of the recombinant fibroblast growth factor-saporin mitotoxin has been undertaken for preclinical evaluation of restenosis models.[392] Other groups have achieved similarly positive in vivo results postexperimental vascular injury with an interleukin-2-receptor-specific toxic agent linked to epidermal growth factor and interleukin-2.[393] Isner's group showed that DAB389EGF, a recombinant fusion protein in which the receptor-biding domain of diphtheria toxin is replaced by human epidermal growth factor, inhibited neointimal hyperplasia in the balloon-injured rat carotid artery.[394] Moreover, local administration of DAB389EGF caused an even more pronounced reduction in intimal area and also avoided systemic toxicity. The results are certainly promising, but this work is still in early testing with more data needed regarding safety and efficacy before clinical testing can be undertaken.

The use of antisense oligodeoxynucleotides (ASODN) has also received great attention.[32] This is a means of blocking the expression of genes integral to cell migration and proliferation, frequently oncogenes.[395] All of the gene products needed for cell division, DNA replication, and transcription and growth factors, and their receptors, are potential targets for ASODN therapy. In this strategy, one introduces synthetic short DNA segments or oligodeoxynucleotides into the cell. These are generated to complement target mRNA molecules ("sense") and will hybridize with them.

Hybridization is thought to block translation of the mRNA in ribosomes, and hence to prevent gene expression. This novel strategy in combating restenosis received a big boost when initial in vitro experiments showed successful suppression of smooth-muscle cell migration and proliferation using ASODN therapy directed against proliferating cell nuclear antigen, c-myc, and c-myb, which are necessary for nuclear transcription, and nonmuscle myosin, which is necessary for cell division.[396–399] These results led to in vivo studies with ASODN against c-myc, c-myb, and proliferating cell nuclear antigen with very positive outcomes in reducing postinjury neointimal formation.[376,400–402] One group showed that c-myc ASODN delivered locally via single-transcatheter administration reduced neointimal formation in denuded porcine coronary arteries.[403]

In spite of these early impressive studies, Stein and Cheng[404] cautioned that for antisense to be useful clinically, it must possess absolute specificity as well as consistent uptake and stability in target cells. To address the former concern, a study was conducted to confirm that ASODN directed against c-myb results in a specific antiproliferative effect.[405] In vitro experiments using rat, dog, and human aortic smooth-muscle cells, as well as in vivo experiments with the rat carotid model, showed a lack of specificity and consistency in growth inhibitory effects, suggesting that an antisense mechanism against c-myb was not responsible for the suppression.[405] Rather, the study found that growth was invariably inhibited by oligomers containing a contiguous four-guanosine residue motif. At about the same time, another study using ASODN directed against c-myc as well as c-myb, also showed that inhibition of skeletal muscle cell proliferation was not caused by a hybridization-dependent antisense mechanism, but rather by phosphorothioate oligonucleotides containing at least two sets of three or four consecutive guanosine residues.[406] While these results call into question many of the previous studies using antisense sequences, they also represent the identification of a potential new class of antirestenotic compounds.

To improve uptake in cells, investigators encapsulated antisense molecules in viral-coated liposomes.[407] Viral liposome-mediated delivery of a combination of CDC2 kinase and cyclin B1 oligonucleotides produced sustained inhibition of neointimal hyperplasia in the rat carotid model. Another group examined the uptake and distribution of phosphorothioate oligonucleotides into vascular smooth-muscle cells in rabbit arteries after intraluminal administration and found that oligonucleotides easily penetrated the arterial wall of balloon-injured arteries and accumulated in medial smooth-muscle cells, suggesting the usefulness of local delivery without liposome facilitation.[408] More recently, in a study of oligonucleotide processing by human vascular smooth-muscle cells,[409] cationic liposomes increased oligonucleotide uptake but not intracellular bioavailability.

Clearly, many questions remain regarding the mechanism as well as the clinical practicality of ASODN therapy.[410] First, nonspecific effects of oligonucleotides need to be considered when using antisense agents to define specific biologic roles of genes. Second, before clinical use, the agents need to have clearly defined pharmacokinetics, systemic effects, and toxicity of breakdown products. Finally, the best targets for antisense therapy are still largely unidentified. This is shown by the aforementioned experiments showing that inhibition of smooth-muscle cell proliferation by antisense nucleotides to c-myc and c-myb involved the guanosine repeats encoded in the oligonucleotides, not by a specific hybridization-dependent antisense mechanism.[405,406] Antisense strategies have also been directed against the rat PDGF α-receptor mRNA,[411] as well as against the p65 subunit of NF-B, a pleiotropic transactivator of genes implicated in the cellular response to inflammation.[412] In both studies, the respective antisense agents suppressed vascular smooth-muscle cell proliferation. These and other agents represent potential targets of ASODN, and more experiments are needed to verify their specificity before clinical trials. The single center, randomized ITALICS trial, which assessed the effectiveness of local delivery of antisense oligonucleotide LR-3280 against c-myc for the prevention of in-stent restenosis[413] showed no benefit.

Other nucleic acid-based therapies include the use of ribozyme oligonucleotides. Ribozymes are RNA-based molecules that cleave their target messenger RNA in an enzymatic fashion. A ribozyme targeting transforming growth factor B was shown to inhibit neointimal formation in a rat model.[414] An additional strategy has been the development of DNAzymes, which are single-stranded DNA molecules with catalytic domains capable of RNA cleavage. DNAzymes are useful in inhibiting the restenosis process.[415]

In addition to blocking the expression of genes with antisense strategies, blocking of factors necessary to cellular migration and proliferation can also occur at the protein level. A group of researchers from Finland found that a synthetic D-amino-acid peptide structurally resembling the D-domain of insulin-like growth factor-1 (IGF-1) blocked the growth factors interaction with IGF-1 receptor and reduced intimal smooth-muscle cell replication by 60 to 70%,[416] suggesting that the IGF-1/IGF-1R interaction is a rate-limiting step for skeletal muscle cell replication.

The ultimate application of molecular biology is gene therapy (see Chap. 41), which is defined as the in vivo delivery, by means of a vector, of a functional gene for expression in somatic cells in order to cure disease.[417] It has already been clinically tested in noncardiac cases in a few pediatric patients suffering from immunodeficiency from adenosine deaminase deficiency, with positive results.[418] The list of genes potentially introducible into vascular smooth muscle for restenosis prevention extends from those coding for growth factors and their receptors and components of signal transduction pathways to vasodilators, antiplatelet agents, antithrombotics, and antiproliferatives such as nitric oxide synthase, tissue-type plasminogen activator, hirudin, prostaglandin H synthase, and tumor suppression gene (Table 40-4).[387a] Early success with gene transfer into the arterial wall stimulated a surge of research in this area.[419] Some investigators garnered positive results from animal injury models; that is, reduced neointimal formation by gene transfer of human calponin gene into injured rabbit carotid arteries and aortas.[420,421] This gene encodes a smooth-muscle actin-binding protein, possibly deficient in restenosis,[422] that is felt to inhibit smooth-muscle cell migration and proliferation. One group of investigators in Italy studied the effects of ras as a possible key player in the transduction of mitogenic signals from the membrane to the nucleus in proliferating smooth-muscle cells in the arterial wall in response to local injury.[423] Local gene delivery of ras transdominant-negative mutants in balloon-injured rat carotid artery reduced neointimal formation. However, progress in gene therapy for restenosis was held up due to extremely low transfection efficacy. Transfection rates with retroviral vectors and liposomes (lipid envelopes surrounding DNA fragments) ranged from 1 in 10,000 to 1 in 1000 cells.[424] Some investigators have tried, with some success, to improve transfection rates by seeding the artery with endothelial or smooth-muscle cells that had been infected in vivo.[425] The technical difficulty of delivering the genes to the target cells has been largely overcome by the advent of adenoviral vectors that yield a much higher rate of transfection.[32,426] A pharmacokinetic study of adenoviral vector-mediated gene delivery using a β-galactosidase reporter system, found that the addition of poloxamer 407, a biocompatible polyol, further improved transfection rates, perhaps by maintaining a high pericellular concentration of the vector.[427]

Ohno et al.,[428] using adenoviral vectors, were among the first to achieve promising results in an animal restenosis model, albeit with a very different approach. They infected porcine artery smooth-muscle cells after balloon injury with adenoviral vectors containing the herpes virus thymidine kinase gene. The cells, subsequently susceptible to the drug ganciclovir, exhibited reduced intimal hyperplasia after treatment with the nucleoside analogue without apparent local or systemic toxicity. More recently, similar results were obtained with adenoviral transfer of the same gene into balloon-injured rat carotids,[429] as well as in a rabbit model of angioplasty of

TABLE 40-4. Gene Transfer Therapies for Restenosis

Predominant Mechanism	Animal Studies			
	Gene Target	Animal Model	Vector	%NI Inhibition
Cell proliferation	P53	Rat	HVJ	>80
	Fas ligand	Rat	AV	60
	Cecropin	Pig	L	>90
	PDGF β R	Rat	AV	>50
Cell migration	TIMP-1	Rat	RV	40
	MMP-2	Rat	AV	53
Thrombosis	Hirudin	Rat	AV	35
	Plasmin	Rat	AV	53*
Endothelium	eNOS	Rat	HVJ/L	70
	VEGF-C	Rabbit	AV	33*†
	PhVEGF$_{165}$	Rabbit	Naked	60%
	PGI$_2$	Rat	P/L	>80

Human Studies				
Gene Target	Setting	Pt. #	Delivery Method	Vector	Effect
---	---	---	---	---	---
Lac Z	Peripheral artery	18	Dispatch catheter	AV	Uptake in <5% cells
VEGF	Coronary stenting	10	Dispatch catheter	P/L	Nil
	Peripheral artery PTA	19	Hydrogel balloon	Naked DNA	14/19 minimal NI hyperplasia

* These studies showed diminished effects at later timepoints; † neointima:media ratio inhibition.

AV = adenovirus; HVJ-L = hemagglutinating virus of Japan/liposome; MMP = matrix metalloproteinase; NI = neointima; PDGF-β R = platelet-derived growth factor-β receptor; P/L = plasmid/lipid; PG = prostaglandin; RV = retrovirus; TIMP = tissue inhibitor of metalloproteinase; VEGF = vascular endothelial growth factor.

Source: Reproduced with permission from Lowe HC, et al.[32]

atheromatous iliac arteries.[430] Another group has achieved in vitro and in vivo success in reducing postinjury neointimal formation in rat carotids with adenoviral transfer of a constitutive retinoblastoma gene, an important negative regulator of cell-cycle progression.[431] More recently, adenoviral transfer of the Gax (growth arrest homeobox) gene, which is normally downregulated in vascular tissue following balloon injury, inhibited both mitogen-induced proliferation of vascular smooth-muscle cells in vitro and neointimal formation in denuded rat carotid arteries in vivo.[432] Isner's group found that simultaneous balloon injury and gene transfer of phVEGF165 (encoding an isoform of vascular endothelial growth factor) in rabbits accelerated reendothelialization within 1 week, leading to inhibition of neointimal thickening, as well as restoration of other important endothelial functions.[433] Because cloning and identification of recombinant adenoviruses remain difficult and time-consuming, one group of researchers from Germany demonstrated that a complex consisting of the reporter plasmid encoding firefly luciferase, polycationic liposomes, and replication-deficient adenovirus yielded high in vitro transfection of human smooth-muscle cells, up to 1000-fold, when compared with lipofection.[434] Subsequently, human smooth-muscle cells cotransfected with a RSV-CD (cytosine deaminase) expression plasmid and the luciferase reporter plasmid in the presence of 5-FC [which is deaminated by CD to the toxic 5-fluorouracil (5-FU)], showed twofold less luciferase activity as compared to cells transfected with a non-CD-coding plasmid. Transient expression of CD was shown to sufficiently reduce protein synthesis in human smooth-muscle cells. The authors postulate that this method of adenovirus-assisted lipofection for transfer of a target gene with a luciferase reporter gene can be used in vivo to target genes to the vascular wall to inhibit smooth-muscle cell proliferation.

Recently it was shown that inhibition of the central inflammatory mediator NF-κB could favorably influence postangioplasty restenosis by the use of adenovirus carrying human IκBα.[435]

The in vivo success of adenoviral vectors has opened up a wide and exciting range of potential applications for gene therapy (see Chap. 41). Nevertheless, certain technical issues need to be resolved before this method of gene therapy can be used effectively in a clinical setting.[436,437] First, recombinant adenoviruses elicit host immune responses that may lead to toxicity. Second, the low efficiency of gene transfer to atherosclerotic arteries needs to be considered. To this end, some investigators are studying nonviral gene-delivery systems using more efficient liposome-delivery systems as well as receptor-mediated gene transfer.[438] Finally, the multifactorial nature of restenosis most likely necessitates a broad-based therapeutic strategy involving many genetic players, and hence the search continues to identify the most essential genes involved in restenosis.

CONCLUSION

Although the vast majority of pharmacologic approaches aimed at preventing postangioplasty restenosis have shown no benefit in clinical trials, there are a number of avenues that do show promise and include probucol and statins. Innovative strategies also under investigation include drug-eluting stents that use paclitaxel and sirolimus, nucleic acid-based drugs, and gene therapy.

Perhaps the relative lack of success of various pharmacotherapies in preventing restenosis relates to a mistaken understanding of its pathogenesis. If, as Glagov has suggested,[65] restenosis reflects a restoration of hemodynamic equilibria between flow, shear stress, and tensile stress, then attempts to simply block smooth-muscle cell proliferation are likely to remain fruitless. Alternatively, as the heterogeneous autopsy specimens examined by Waller et al.[55,56] have demonstrated, there may be different pathogenetic mechanisms leading to restenosis in different individuals. Therefore, one pharmacologic agent is unlikely to prevent the problem across the board. The EPIC trial, one of the few major clinical trials to generate successful results, besides using an extremely potent antiplatelet agent, was targeted to a population for which thrombosis probably played an exceptionally important role.[193] Therefore, future successes in restenosis prevention may lie in tailoring specific pharmacodynamic approaches to specific subsets of patients, that is, those in whom thrombosis, elastic recoil, vasospasm or hyperlipidemia may be the chief factors. Alternatively, if risk factors could be clearly elucidated in the future, they could identify patients who do not require therapy at all or who might be in most need of preventive therapy against restenosis. They might also entirely exclude subsets of patients from percutaneous procedures, relegating them to medical therapy or surgery. However, risk factors are poorly defined, widely debated, and certainly depend on which of the many definitions of angiographic restenosis are used.

Another drug approach that might warrant consideration in the future is combination therapy. Using more than one agent would seem indicated because there may be more than one pathogenetic mechanism at hand, and it would also allow the possibility of synergy, for example, two drugs working at different points in the same pathway. Additive effects might also permit the use of lower dosages of drugs, achieving adequate efficacy without systemic intolerance. In the nonrandomized, nonplacebo-controlled Mevacor, ACE inhibitor, colchicine (BIG-MAC) study by Freed et al.,[439] which administered a daily cocktail of enalapril 2.5 mg, lovastatin 20 to 40 mg, and colchicine 0.6 mg after PTCA, restenosis occurred in 33% to 47% of the 50 study patients. However, another nonrandomized, nonblinded trial by Kitazume et al. in 297 patients, observed a significant reduction in the incidence of angiographic restenosis in patients administered a combination of aspirin, ticlopidine, and nicorandil versus aspirin and ticlopidine or aspirin alone after PTCA (16.3% vs 26.5% vs 37.8%, respectively).[440] Such combinations certainly warrant testing in large placebo-controlled, double-blind trials.

The occurrence of restenosis has certainly reduced the benefit of percutaneous coronary revascularization procedures. The overall merits of the approach in reducing angina and improving exercise tolerance have been well documented.[441] Therefore, it is crucial to overcome the obstacle of restenosis after percutaneous revascularization procedures if these interventions are to remain as long-term viable alternatives for the management of ischemic heart disease.[442]

REFERENCES

1. Gruntzig AR, Senning AS, Siegenthaler WE: Nonoperative dilatation of coronary artery stenosis-percutaneous transluminal coronary angioplasty. *N Engl J Med* 301:61 1979.
2. Bredlau Ce, Roubin GS, Leimgruber PP, et al: In hospital morbidity and mortality in patients undergoing elective coronary angioplasty. *Circulation* 72:1044, 1985.
3. Detre K, Holubkov R, Kelsey S, et al: Percutaneous transluminal coronary angioplasty in 1985–1986, 1977–1981. The National Heart, Lung and Blood Institute Registry. *N Engl J Med* 318:265, 1988.
4. Holmes DR Jr, Simpson JB, Berdan LG, et al: Abrupt closure: The CAVEAT I Experience. *J Am Coll Cardiol* 26:1494, 1995.
5. Holmes DR, Vlietstra RE, Smith HC, et al: Restenosis after percutaneous transluminal coronary angioplasty (PTCA): A report from the PTCA Registry of the National Heart, Lung and Blood Institute. *Am J Cardiol* 53:77C, 1984.
6. Serruys PW, Luijten HE, Beatt KJ, et al: Incidence of restenosis after successful coronary angioplasty: a time related phenomenon. *Circulation* 77:361, 1988.
7. Roubin GS, King SB III, Douglas JS Jr: Restenosis after percutaneous transluminal coronary angioplasty: The Emory University Hospital experience. *Am J Cardiol* 60:39B, 1987.
8. Gruntzig AR, King SB III, Schlumpf M, et al: Long-term follow up after percutaneous transluminal coronary angioplasty. The early Zurich experience. *N Engl J Med* 316:1227, 1987.
9. Kastrati A, Schömig A, Elezi S, et al: Prognostic value of the modified American College of Cardiology/American Heart Association stenosis morphology classification for long-term angiographic and clinical outcome after coronary stent placement. *Circulation* 100:1285, 1999.
10. Glazier JJ, Varricchione TR, Ryan TJ, et al: Outcome in patients with recurrent restenosis after percutaneous transluminal balloon angioplasty. *Br Heart J* 61:485, 1989.
11. Espindola-Klein C, Rupprecht HJ, Erbel R, et al: Impact of restenosis ten-years after coronary angioplasty. *Eur Heart J* 19:1047, 1998.
12. Reeder GS, Krishan I, Nobrega FT, et al: Is percutaneous coronary angioplasty less expensive than bypass surgery? *N Engl J Med* 311:1157, 1984.
13. Warth DC, Leon MB, O'Neill W, et al: Rotational atherectomy multicenter registry: Acute results, complications and 6 month angiographic follow up in 709 patients. *J Am Coll Cardiol* 24:641, 1994.
14. Faxon DP, Williams DO, Yeh W, et al: Improved in-hospital outcome with expanded use of coronary stents: Results from the NHLBI dynamic registry (abstr.). *J Am Coll Cardiol* 33(Suppl A):91A, 1999.
15. Al Suwaidi J, Berger P, Holmes DR: Coronary artery stents. *JAMA* 284:1828, 2000.
16. Köster R, Hamm CW, Seabra-Gomes R, et al for the Laser Angioplasty of Restenosed Stents (LARS) Investigators. Laser angioplasty of restenosed coronary stents: Results of a multicenter surveillance trial. *J Am Coll Cardiol* 34:25, 1999.
17. Topol EJ, Leya F, Pinkerton CA, et al: A comparison of directional atherectomy with coronary angioplasty in patients with coronary artery disease. The CAVEAT Study Group. *N Engl J Med* 329:221, 1993.
18. Feld H, Schulhoff N, Lichstein E, et al: Coronary atherectomy versus angioplasty: The CAVA Study. *Am Heart J* 126:31, 1993.
19. Holmes DR, Topol EJ, Califf RM, et al: A multicenter, randomized trial of coronary angioplasty versus directional atherectomy for patients with saphenous vein bypass graft lesions. *Circulation* 91:1966, 1995.
20. Serruys PW, deJaegere P, Kiemeneji F, et al: A comparison of balloon expandable stent implantation with balloon angioplasty in patients with coronary artery disease. Benestent Study Group. *N Engl J Med* 331:489, 1994.
21. Fischman DL, Leon MB, Baim DS, et al: A randomized comparison of coronary stent placement and balloon angioplasty in the treatment of coronary artery disease. Stent Restenosis Study Investigators. *N Engl J Med* 331:496, 1994.
22. Fischman D, Savage M, Leon M, et al: Acute and late angiographic results of the Stent Restenosis Study (STRESS) (abstr.). *J Am Coll Cardiol* 23(Suppl I):60A, 1994.
23. Savage MP, Douglas JS Jr, Fischman DL, et al: Stent placement compared with balloon angioplasty for obstructed coronary bypass grafts. *N Engl J Med* 337:740, 1997.
24. Deutsch E, Martin JL, Makowski S, et al: Acute and chronic outcomes after physiologic low stress angioplasty (PLOSA) of de novo coronary stenoses: Results of the Phase I trial (abstr.). *Circulation* 88(Suppl I):646, 1992.
25. Hoffman R, Mintz GS, Dussaillant RG, et al: Patterns and mechanisms of in-stent restenosis: a serial intravascular ultrasound study. *Circulation* 94:1247, 1996.
26. Nakamura M, Yock PG, Bonneau HN, et al: Impact of peri-stent remodeling on restenosis. A volumetric intravascular ultrasound study. *Circulation* 103:2130, 2001.
27. Teirstein PS, Massullo V, Jani S, et al: Catheter-based radiotherapy to inhibit restenosis after coronary stenting. *N Engl J Med* 336:1697, 1997.
28. Raizner AE, Oesterle SN, Waksman R, et al: Inhibition of restenosis with beta-emitting radiotherapy: Report of the Proliferation Reduction with Vascular Energy Trial (PREVENT). *Circulation* 102:951, 2000.
29. Teirstein PS, Massullo V, Jani S, et al: Three-year clinical and angiographic follow up after intracoronary radiation: Results of a randomised clinical trial. *Circulation* 101:360, 2000.

30. Verin V, Popowski Y, de Bruyne B, et al: Endoluminal beta-radiation therapy for the prevention of coronary restenosis after balloon angioplasty. *N Engl J Med* 344:243, 2001.

31. Cannon RO III: Restenosis after angioplasty. *N Eng J Med* 346:1182, 2002.

32. Lowe HC, Oesterle SN, Khachigian LM: Coronary in-stent restenosis: current status and future strategies. *J Am Coll Cardiol* 39:183, 2002.

33. Kastrati A, Mehilli J, Dirschinger J, et al: Restenosis after coronary placement of various stent types. *Am J Cardiol* 87:34, 2001.

34. Rensing BJ, Hermans WR, Decker JW, et al: Luminal renarrowing after percutaneous transluminal coronary angioplasty following gaussian distribution. A quantitative angiographic study in 1,445 successfully dilated lesions. *J Am Coll Cardiol* 19:939, 1992.

35. Nobuyoshi M, Kimura T, Osaka H, et al: Restenosis after successful percutaneous transluminal coronary angioplasty: Serial angiographic follow up of 229 patients. *J Am Coll Cardiol* 12:616, 1988.

36. Mehta VY, Jorgensen MB, Raizner AE, et al: Spontaneous regression of restenosis: An angiographic study. *J Am Coll Cardiol* 26:696, 1995.

37. Frishman WH, Chiu R, Landzberg BR, Weiss M: Medical therapies for the prevention of restenosis after percutaneous coronary interventions. *Curr Probl Cardiol* 23:533, 1998.

38. Ip JP, Fuster V, Israel D, et al: The role of platelets, thrombin and hyperplasia in restenosis after coronary angioplasty. *J Am Coll Cardiol* 17:77B, 1991.

39. Kovach JA, Mintz GS, Pichard AD, et al: Sequential intravascular ultrasound characterization of the mechanisms of rotational atherectomy and adjunct balloon angioplasty. *J Am Coll Cardiol* 22:1024, 1993.

40. Forrester JS, Fishbein M, Helfant R, et al: A paradigm for restenosis based on cell biology: clues for the development of new preventive therapies. *J Am Coll Cardiol* 17:758, 1991.

41. Wilentz JR, Sanborn TA, Haudenschild CC, et al: Platelet accumulation in experimental angioplasty: Time course and relation to vascular injury. *Circulation* 75:636, 1987.

42. Oates JA, FitzGerald GA, Branch RA, et al: Clinical implications of prostaglandin and thromboxane A2 formation. *N Engl J Med* 319:689, 1988.

43. Ishiwata S, Tukada T, Nakanishi S, et al: Postangioplasty restenosis: Platelet activation and the coagulation-fibrinolysis system as possible factors in the pathogenesis of restenosis. *Am Heart J* 133:387, 1997.

44. Liu MW, Roubin GS, King SB III: Restenosis after coronary angioplasty: Potential biologic determinants and role of intimal hyperplasia. *Circulation* 79:1374, 1989.

45. Matsuura R, Isaka N, Imanaka-Yoshida K, et al: Deposition of Pg/M/versican is a major cause of human coronary restenosis after percutaneous transluminal coronary angioplasty. *J Pathol* 180:311, 1996.

46. Nobuyoshi M, Kimura T, Ohishi H, et al: Restenosis after percutaneous transluminal coronary angioplasty: Pathologic observations in 20 patients. *J Am Coll Cardiol* 17:433, 1991.

47. Ohara T, Kodama K, Mishima M, et al: Ultrastructural findings of proliferating and migrating smooth muscle cells at the site of percutaneous transluminal coronary angioplasty (abstr.). *J Am Coll Cardiol* 11(2):131A, 1988.

48. Garratt KN, Holmes DR, Bell MR, et al: Restenosis after directional coronary atherectomy: differences between primary atheromatous and restenosis lesions and influence of subintimal tissue resection. *J Am Coll Cardiol* 16:1665, 1990.

49. Moreno PR, Falk E, Fuster V, et al: Increased macrophage content of restenotic coronary plaque tissue (abstr.). *Circulation* 90(Suppl I):378, 1994.

50. Guzman LA, Whitlow PL, Beall CJ, et al: Monocyte chemotactic protein antibody inhibits restenosis in the rabbit atherosclerotic model (abstr.). *Circulation* 88(Suppl I):371, 1993.

51. Eber B, Schumacher M, Auer-Grumbach P, et al: Increased IgM-anticardiolipin antibodies in patients with restenosis after percutaneous transluminal coronary angioplasty. *Am J Cardiol* 69:1255, 1992.

52. Watanabe Y, Yamada N, Yokoi H, et al: Relationship between HLA-C locus and restenosis after coronary artery balloon angioplasty. *JAMA* 277:983, 1997.

53. Belch JJ, Shaw JW, Kirk G, et al: The white blood cell adhesion molecule E-selectin predicts restenosis in patients with intermittent claudication undergoing percutaneous transluminal angioplasty. *Circulation* 95:2027, 1997.

54. Mintz GS, Douek PC, Bonner RF, et al: Intravascular ultrasound comparison of de novo and restenotic coronary artery lesions (abstr.). *J Am Coll Cardiol* 22:118A, 1993.

55. Waller BF, Pinkerton CS, Orr CM, et al: Restenosis 1 to 24 months after clinically successful coronary balloon angioplasty: A necropsy study of 20 patients. *J Am Coll Cardiol* 17:58B, 1991.

56. Waller BF, Pinkerton CA, Orr CM, et al: Morphologic observations late (>30 days) after clinically successful coronary balloon angioplasty: An analysis of 20 necropsy patients and review of 41 necropsy patients with coronary angioplasty restenosis. *Circulation* 83(Suppl I):I28, 1991.

57. Deutsch E, Gerber RS, Martin JL, et al: Initial lesion eccentricity predicts restenosis after successful coronary angioplasty (abstr.). *J Am Coll Cardiol* 21(Suppl A):34A, 1993.

58. Shawl FA. Minimally invasive angioplasty: An editorial. *J Invasive Cardiol* 5:119, 1993.

59. Hermans WR, Rensing BJ, Foley DP, et al: Therapeutic dissection after successful coronary balloon angioplasty: No influence on restenosis or on clinical outcome in 693 patients. The MERCATOR Study Group (Multicenter European Research Trial with Cilazapril after Angioplasty to Prevent Transluminal Coronary Obstruction and Restenosis). *J Am Coll Cardiol* 20:767, 1992.

60. Ohman EM, Marquis JF, Ricci DR, et al: A randomized comparison of the effects of gradual prolonged versus standard primary balloon inflation on early and late outcome. Results of a multicenter clinical trial (Perfusion Balloon Catheter Study Group). *Circulation* 89:1118, 1994.

61. Kakuta T, Currier JW, Haudenschild CC, et al: Differences in compensatory vessel enlargement, not intimal formation, account for restenosis after angioplasty in the hypercholesterolemic rabbit model. *Circulation* 89:2809, 1994.

62. Mintz GS, Kovach JA, Pichard AD, et al: Geometric remodeling is the predominant mechanism of clinical restenosis after coronary angioplasty (abstr.). *J Am Coll Cardiol* 23(Suppl I):138A, 1994.

63. Bier JD, Kakuta T, Currier JW, et al: Arterial remodeling: importance in primary versus restenotic lesions (abstr.). *J Am Coll Cardiol* 23(Suppl I):139A, 1994.

64. Mintz GS, Matar FA, Kent KM, et al: Chronic compensatory arterial dilatation following coronary angioplasty: An intravascular ultrasound study (abstr.). *J Am Coll Cardiol* 23(Suppl I):139A, 1994.

65. Glagov S: Intimal hyperplasia, vascular modeling and the restenosis problem. *Circulation* 89:2888, 1994.

66. Gertz SD, Gimple LW, Banai S, et al: Geometric remodeling is not the principal pathogenetic process in restenosis after balloon angioplasty. Evidence from correlative angiographic-histo-morphometric studies of atherosclerotic arteries in rabbits. *Circulation* 90:3001, 1994.

67. Cowan DB, Langille BL: Cellular and molecular biology of vascular remodeling. *Curr Opin Lipidol* 7:94, 1996.

68. Kimura T, Kaburagi S, Tamura T, et al: Remodeling of human coronary arteries undergoing coronary angioplasty or atherectomy. *Circulation* 96:475, 1997.

69. Post MJ, deSmet B, van der Helm Y, et al: Arterial remodeling after balloon angioplasty or stenting in an atherosclerotic experimental model. *Circulation* 96:996, 1997.

70. Virmani R, Farb A: Pathology of in-stent restenosis. *Curr Opin Lipidol* 10:499, 1999.

71. Faxon DP, Coats W, Currier J: Remodeling of the coronary artery after vascular injury. *Prog Cardiovasc Dis* 40(2):129, 1997.

72. Kern MJ, Anderson HV, Talley JD, et al: Relationship of post-procedural distal coronary flow dynamics with restenosis after coronary angioplasty: Results of a multicenter pilot study (abstr.). *J Am Coll Cardiol* 23(Suppl I):137A, 1994.

73. Speier M, Modali R, Huang ES, et al: Potential role of human cytomegalovirus and p53 interaction in coronary restenosis (abstr.). *Science* 265:391, 1994.

74. Tsai HL, Kou GH, Chen SC, et al: Human cytomegalovirus immediate-early protein IE2 tethers a transcriptional repression domain to p53. *J Biol Chem* 271:3534, 1996.

75. Manegold C, Alwazzeh M, Jablonowski H, et al: Prior cytomegalovirus infection and the risk of restenosis after percutaneous transluminal coronary balloon angioplasty. *Circulation* 99:1290, 1999.

76. Bertrand ME, Bauters C: Cytomegalovirus infection and coronary restenosis (editorial). *Circulation* 99:1278, 1999.

77. Carlsson J, Karl-Heinz M, Miketic S, et al: Prior cytomegalovirus infection and the risk of restenosis after PTCA: Results from the VERAS study (abstr.). *Circulation* 96(Suppl I):650, 1997.

78. Buffon A, Liuzzo GM Caligiuri G, et al: Association between prior *Helicobacter pylori* infection and the risk of restenosis after coronary angioplasty (abstr.). *Circulation* 96(Suppl I):650, 1997.

79. Peterson MB, Machaj V, Block PC, et al: Thromboxane release during percutaneous transluminal coronary angioplasty. *Am Heart J* 111:1, 1986.

80. Nichols WW, Mehta J, Wargovich TJ, et al: Reduced myocardial neutrophil accumulation and infarct size following thromboxane synthetase inhibitor or receptor antagonist. *Angiology* 40:209, 1989.

81. Wargovich TJ, Mehta J, Nichols WW, et al: Reduction in myocardial neutrophil accumulation and infarct size following administration of thromboxane inhibitor U-63,557A. *Am Heart J* 114:1078, 1987.

82. Hanasaki K, Nakano T, Arita H: Receptor mediated mitogenic effect of thromboxane A2 in vascular smooth muscle cells. *Biochem Pharmacol* 40:2535, 1990.

83. Ciabattoni G, Ujang S, Sritara P, et al: Aspirin, but not heparin, suppresses the transient increase in thromboxane biosynthesis associated with cardiac catheterization or coronary angioplasty. *J Am Coll Cardiol* 21:1377, 1993.

84. Bourassa MG, Schwartz L, Lesperance J, et al: Prevention of acute complications after percutaneous transluminal coronary angioplasty. *Thromb Res* 12(Suppl:)51, 1990.

85. Faxon DP, Sanborn TA, Haudenschild CC, et al: Effect of antiplatelet therapy on restenosis after experimental angioplasty. *Am J Cardiol* 53:72C, 1984.

86. Schwartz L, Bourassa MG, Lesperance J, et al: Aspirin and dipyridamole in the prevention of restenosis after percutaneous transluminal coronary angioplasty. *N Engl J Med* 318:1714, 1988.

87. Taylor RR, Gibbons FA, Cope GD, et al: Effects of low-dose aspirin on restenosis after coronary angioplasty. *Am J Cardiol* 68:874, 1991.

88. Herrman JPR, Hermans WRM, Vos J, et al: Pharmacologic approaches to the prevention of restenosis following angioplasty (part 1). *Drugs* 46:18, 1993.

89. Antiplatelet Trialists' Collaboration: Collaborative overview of randomized trials of antiplatelet therapy. II. Maintenance of vascular graft or arterial patency by antiplatelet therapy. *BMJ* 308:159, 1994.

90. Schwartz L, Lesperance J, Bourassa MG, et al: The role of antiplatelet agents in modifying the extent of restenosis following percutaneous transluminal coronary angioplasty. 119(2 pt 1):232, 1990.

91. Darius H, Sellig S, Belz GG, et al: Aspirin 500 mg daily is superior to 100 and 40 mg daily for prevention of restenosis following PTCA (abstr.). *Circulation* 90(Suppl I):651, 1994.

92. Mufson L, Black A, Roubin G, et al: A randomized trial of aspirin in PTCA: effect of high-vs low-dose aspirin on major complications and restenosis (abstr.). *J Am Coll Cardiol* 11(Suppl I):236A, 1988.

93. FitzGerald GA: Dipyridamole. *N Engl J Med* 316:1247, 1987.

94. Lembo NJ, Black AJ, Roubin GS, et al: Effect of pretreatment with aspirin versus aspirin plus dipyridamole on frequency and type of acute complications of percutaneous transluminal coronary angioplasty. *Am J Cardiol* 65:422, 1990.

95. Torka MC, Hacker RW, Yukseltan I, et al: Reduction of the vein graft occlusion rate after coronary artery bypass surgery by treatment with a thromboxane receptor antagonist (abstr.). *Eur Heart J* 9(Suppl I):325, 1988.

96. Serruys PW, Rutsch W, Heyndrickx GR, et al: Prevention of restenosis after percutaneous transluminal coronary angioplasty with thromboxane A2 receptor blockade. A randomized, double-blind, placebo-controlled trial. Coronary Artery Restenosis Prevention on Repeated Thromboxane Antagonism Study (CARPORT). *Circulation* 84:1568, 1991.

97. Feldman RL, Bengtson JR, Pryor DP, et al: The GRASP study: Use of a thromboxane A2 receptor blocker to reduce adverse clinical events after coronary angioplasty (abstr.). *J Am Coll Cardiol* 19:259A, 1992.

98. Yabe Y, Nakano H, Muramatsu T, et al: Could a novel TXA2 receptor antagonist (S-1452) reduce restenosis after PTCA in patients with post infarction angina (abstr.). *Circulation* 90(Suppl I):651, 1994.

99. Savage MP, Goldberg S, MacDonald RG, et al: Multi-Hospital Eastern Atlantic Restenosis Trial II: A placebo-controlled trial of thromboxane blockade in the prevention of restenosis following coronary angioplasty. *Am Heart J* 122:1239, 1991.

100. Savage MP, Goldberg S, Bove A, et al: Effects of thromboxane A2 blockade on clinical outcome and restenosis after successful coronary angioplasty: Multi-Hospital Eastern Atlantic Restenosis Trial. *Circulation* 92:3194, 1995.

101. Sanborn TA, Ballelli LM, Faxon DP, et al: Inhibition of ^{51}Cr-labelled platelet accumulation after balloon angioplasty in rabbits: Comparison of heparin, aspirin and CGS 13080, a selective thromboxane synthetase inhibitor (abstr.). *J Am Coll Cardiol* 7:213A, 1986.

102. Yabe Y, Okamoto K, Oosawa H, et al: Does a thromboxane A2 synthetase inhibitor prevent restenosis after PTCA? (abstr.) *Circulation* 80(Suppl II):260, 1989.

103. Hattori R, Kodama K, Takatsu F, et al: Randomized trial of a selective inhibitor of thromboxane A2 synthetase (E) 7-phenyl-7-(3-pyridyl)-6-heptenoic acid (CV-4151) for prevention of restenosis after coronary angioplasty [in English]. *Jpn Circ J* 55:324, 1991.

104. Timmermans C, Vrolix M, Vanhaecke J, et al: Ridogrel in the setting of percutaneous transluminal coronary angioplasty. *Am J Cardiol* 68:463, 1991.

105. Kanaka S, Takenouchi S, Tajima T, et al: Increased platelet-derived growth factor and reduced prostacyclin production in patients with restenosis after percutaneous transluminal coronary angioplasty (abstr.). *Circulation* 78(Suppl II):290, 1988.

106. Knudtson ML, Flintoft VF, Roth DL, et al: Effect of short-term prostacyclin administration on restenosis after percutaneous transluminal coronary angioplasty. *J Am Coll Cardiol* 15:691, 1990.

107. Gershlick AH, Spriggins D, Davies SW, et al: Failure of epoprostenol (prostacyclin PGI$_2$) to inhibit platelet aggregation and to prevent restenosis after coronary angioplasty: Results of a randomised placebo-controlled trial. *Br Heart J* 71:7, 1994.

108. Darius H, Nixdorff U, Zander J, et al: Effects of ciprostene on restenosis rate during therapeutic transluminal coronary angioplasty. *Agts Actions* 37(Suppl):305, 1992.

109. Raizner A, Hollman J, Demke D, et al: Beneficial effects of ciprostene in PTCA: A multicenter, randomized, controlled trial (abstr.). *Circulation* 78(Suppl II):290, 1988.

110. Raizner AE, Hollman J, Abukhalil J, et al: Ciprostene for restenosis revisited: Quantitative analysis of angiograms (abstr.). *J Am Coll Cardiol* 21:321A, 1993.

111. Isogaya M, Yamada N, Koike H, et al: Inhibition of restenosis by beraprost sodium (a prostaglandin I$_2$ analogue) in the atherosclerotic rabbit artery after angioplasty. *J Cardiovasc Pharmacol* 25:947, 1995.

112. Leaf A: Cardiovascular effects of fish oils. Beyond the platelet. *Circulation* 82:624, 1990.

113. Bairati I, Roy L, Meyer F: Double-blind, randomized, controlled trial of fish oil supplements in prevention of recurrence of stenosis after coronary angioplasty. *Circulation* 85:950, 1991.

114. Dehmer GJ, Popma JJ, van den Berg EK, et al: Reduction in the rate of early restenosis after coronary angioplasty by a diet supplemented with omega-3 fatty acids. *N Engl J Med* 319:733, 1988.

115. Nye ER, Ablett MB, Robertson MC, et al: Effect of eicosapentaenoic acid on restenosis rate, clinical course and blood lipids in patients after percutaneous transluminal coronary angioplasty. *Aust N Z J Med* 20:549, 1990.

116. Milner MR, Gallino RA, Leffingwell A, et al: Usefulness of fish oil supplements in preventing clinical evidence of restenosis after percutaneous transluminal coronary angioplasty. *Am J Cardiol* 64:294, 1989.

117. Franzen D, Schannwell M, Oette K, et al: A prospective, randomized and double-blind trial on the effect of fish oil on the incidence of restenosis following PTCA. *Catheter Cardiovasc Diagn* 28:301, 1993.

118. Bellamy CM, Schofield PM, Faragher EB, et al: Can supplementation of diet with omega-3 polyunsaturated fatty acids reduce coronary angioplasty restenosis rate? *Eur Heart J* 13:1626, 1992.

119. Kaul U, Sanghvi S, Bahl VK, et al: Fish oil supplements for prevention of restenosis after coronary angioplasty. *Int J Cardiol* 35:87, 1992.

120. Reis GJ, Boucher TM, Sipperly ME, et al: Randomised trial of fish oil for prevention of restenosis after coronary angioplasty. *Lancet* 2:177, 1989.

121. Grigg LE, Kay TW, Valentine PA, et al: Determinants of restenosis and lack of effect of dietary supplementation with eicosapentaenoic

acid on the incidence of coronary artery restenosis after angioplasty. *J Am Coll Cardiol* 13:665, 1989.

122. Cairns JA, Gill JB, Morton B, et al: Fish oils and low-molecular-weight heparin for the reduction of restenosis after percutaneous transluminal coronary angioplasty. The EMPAR Study. *Circulation* 94:1553, 1996.

123. Leaf A, Jorgensen MB, Jacobs AK, et al: Do fish oils prevent restenosis after coronary angioplasty? *Circulation* 90:2248, 1994.

124. Johansen O, Brekke M, Seljeflot I, et al: n-3 Fatty acids do not prevent restenosis after coronary angioplasty: Results from the CART study. *J Am Coll Cardiol* 33:1619, 1999.

125. White CW, Knudson M, Schmidt D, et al: Neither ticlopidine nor aspirin-dipyridamole prevents restenosis post PTCA: Results from a randomized, placebo-controlled, multicenter trial (abstr.). *Circulation* 76(Suppl 4):213, 1987.

126. Iniguez RA, Macaya MC, Hernandez AR, et al: The effects of ticlopidine administration at low doses on the incidence of restenosis following percutaneous transluminal coronary angioplasty. *Rev Esp Cardiol* 44:366, 1991.

127. Bertrand ME, Allain H, Lablanche JM, et al: Results of a randomized trial of ticlopidine versus placebo for prevention of acute closure and restenosis after coronary angioplasty (abstr.). *Circulation* 82(Suppl 3):190, 1990.

128. Pasternak RC, Baughman KL, Fallon JT, et al: Scanning electron microscopy after coronary transluminal angioplasty of normal canine coronary arteries. *Am J Cardiol* 5:91, 1980.

129. Swanson KT, Vlietstra RE, Holmes DR, et al: Efficacy of adjunctive dextran during percutaneous transluminal coronary angioplasty. *Am J Cardiol* 54:447, 1984.

130. Clowes AW, Karnovsky MJ: Suppression of heparin of smooth muscle cell proliferation in injured arteries. *Nature* 265:625, 1977.

131. Castellot JJ Jr, Wong K, Herman B, et al: Binding and internalization of heparin by vascular smooth muscle cells. *J Cell Physiol* 124:13, 1985.

132. Castellot JJ Jr, Addonizio ML, Rosenberg R, et al: Cultured endothelial cells produce a heparinlike inhibitor of smooth muscle cell growth. *J Cell Biol* 90:372, 1981.

133. Ellis SG, Roubin GS, Wilentz J, et al: Effect of 18–24 h heparin administration for prevention of restenosis after uncomplicated coronary angioplasty. *Am Heart J* 117:777, 1989.

134. Brack MJ, Ray S, Chauhan A, et al: The Subcutaneous Heparin and Angioplasty Restenosis Prevention (SHARP) Trials: Results of a multicenter randomized trial investigating the effects of high dose unfractionated heparin on angiographic restenosis and clinical outcome. *J Am Coll Cardiol* 26:947, 1995.

135. Medalion B, Merin G, Aingorn H, et al: Endogenous basic fibroblast growth factor displaced by heparin from the luminal surface of human blood vessels is preferentially sequestered by injured regions of the vessel wall. *Circulation* 95:1853, 1997.

136. Guyton JR, Rosenberg RD, Clowes AW, et al: Inhibition of rat arterial smooth muscle cell proliferation by heparin. In vivo studies with anticoagulant and nonanticoagulant heparin. *Circ Res* 46:625, 1980.

137. Currier JW, Pow TK, Haudenschild CC, et al: Low-molecular-weight heparin (enoxaparin) reduces restenosis in the hypercholesterolemic rabbit. *J Am Coll Cardiol* 17:118B, 1991.

138. Buchwald AB, Unterberg C, Nebendahl K, et al: Low-molecular-weight heparin reduces neointimal proliferation after coronary stent implantation in hypercholesterolemic minipigs. *Circulation* 86:531, 1992.

139. Turpie AG, Levine MN, Hirsh J, et al: A randomized controlled trial of a low molecular weight heparin to prevent deep vein thrombosis in patients undergoing elective hip surgery. *N Engl J Med* 315:925, 1986.

140. Schmid KM, Preisack M, Voelker W, et al: First clinical experience with low molecular weight heparin LU 47311 (reviparin) for prevention of restenosis after percutaneous transluminal coronary angioplasty. *Semin Thromb Hemostasis* 19(Suppl 1):155, 1993.

141. Preisack MB, Karsch KR: Experimental and early clinical experience with reviparin-sodium for prevention of restenosis after percutaneous transluminal coronary angioplasty. *Blood Coagul Fibrinolysis* 4(Suppl 1): S55, 1993.

142. Faxon DP, Spiro TE, Minor S, et al: Low-molecular-weight heparin in prevention of restenosis after angioplasty: Results of enoxaparin restenosis (ERA) trial. *Circulation* 90:908, 1994.

143. Karsch KR, Preisack MB, Bonan R, et al: Low-molecular-weight heparin, reviparin, in prevention of restenosis after PTCA (abstr.). *J Am Coll Cardiol* 27:113A, 1996.

144. Karsch KR, Preisack MB, Baildon R, et al: Low-molecular-weight heparin (reviparin) in percutaneous transluminal coronary angioplasty. *J Am Coll Cardiol* 28:1437, 1996.

144a. Gimple LW, Herrmann HC, Winnifrod M, et al: Usefulness of subcutaneous low molecular weight heparin (ardeparin) for reduction of restenosis after percutaneous transluminal coronary angioplasty. *Am J Cardiol* 83:1524, 1999.

145. Grassman ED, Leya FS, Fareed J, et al: A randomized trial of the low-molecular-weight heparin certoparin to prevent restenosis following coronary angioplasty. *J Invasive Cardiol* 13:723, 2001.

146. Kiesz RS, Buszman P, Martin JL, et al: Local delivery of enoxaparin to decrease restenosis after stenting: Results of initial multicenter trial. Polish-American Local Lovenox NIR Assessment Study (The POLONIA Study). *Circulation* 103:26, 2001.

147. Meneveau N, Schiele F, Grollier G, et al: Local delivery of nadroparin for the prevention of neointimal hyperplasia following stent implantation: Results of the IMPRESS Trial. A multicentre, randomized, clinical, angiographic and intravascular ultrasound study. *Eur Heart J* 21:1767, 2000.

148. Chan P, Patel M, Munro E, et al: Human restenosis: An in vitro correlation to vascular smooth muscle proliferation (abstr.). *Eur Heart J* 14(Suppl):276, 1993.

149. Okada SS, Kuo A, Muttreja MR, et al: Inhibition of human vascular smooth muscle cell migration and proliferation by beta-cyclodextrin tetradecasulfate. *J Pharmacol Exp Ther* 273:948, 1995.

150. Bachinsky WB, Barnathan ES, Liu H, et al: Sustained inhibition of intimal thickening. In vitro and in vivo effects of polymeric beta-cyclodextrin sulfate. *J Clin Invest* 96:2583, 1995.

151. Ali NM, Mazur W, Kleiman NS, et al: Inhibition of restenosis by antithrombin III in atherosclerotic swine (abstr.). *Circulation* 90(Suppl I):239, 1994.

152. Schachinger V, Allert M, Kasper W, et al: Adjunctive intracoronary infusion of antithrombin III during percutaneous transluminal coronary angioplasty. Results of a prospective, randomized trial. *Circulation* 90:2258, 1994.

153. Ali MN, Mazur W, Kleiman NS, et al: Inhibition of coronary restenosis by antithrombin III in atherosclerotic swine. *Coron Artery Dis* 7:851, 1996.

154. Grip L, Blomback M, Egberg N, et al: Antithrombin III supplementation for patients undergoing PTCA for unstable angina pectoris. A controlled randomized double-blind pilot study. *Eur Heart J* 18:443, 1997.

155. Huber K, Maurer G. Adjunctive infusion of antithrombin III during percutaneous transluminal coronary angioplasty. *Eur Heart J* 18:362, 1997.

156. Roqué M, Reis ED, Fuster V, et al: Inhibition of tissue factor reduces thrombus formation and intimal hyperplasia after porcine coronary angioplasty. *J Am Coll Cardiol* 36:2303, 2000.

157. Johnson PH. Hirudin: clinical potential of a thrombin inhibitor. *Ann Rev Med* 45:165, 1994.

158. Heras M, Chesebro JH, Penny WJ, et al: Effects of thrombin inhibition on the development of acute platelet-thrombus deposition during angioplasty in pigs. Heparin versus recombinant hirudin, a specific thrombin inhibitor. *Circulation* 79:657, 1989.

159. Ragosta M, Barry WL, Gimple LW, et al: Effect of thrombin inhibition with desulfatohirudin on early kinetics of cellular proliferation after balloon angioplasty in atherosclerotic rabbits. *Circulation* 93:1194, 1996.

160. Barry WL, Gimple LW, Humphries JE, et al: Arterial thrombin activity after angioplasty in an atherosclerotic rabbit model: Time course and effect of hirudin. *Circulation* 94:88, 1996.

161. Sarembock IJ, Gertz SD, Gimple LW, et al: Effectiveness of recombinant desulphatohirudin in reducing restenosis after balloon angioplasty of atherosclerotic femoral arteries in rabbits. *Circulation* 84:232, 1991.

162. Hadoke PW, Wadsworth RM, Wainwright CL, et al: Subcutaneous infusion of r-hirudin does not inhibit neointimal proliferation after angioplasty of the subclavian artery in cholesterol-fed rabbits. *Coron Artery Dis* 7:599, 1996.

163. Gerdes C, Faber-Steinfeld V, Yalkinoglu O, et al: Comparison of the effects of the thrombin inhibitor r-hirudin in four animal models of

neointima formation after arterial injury. *Arterioscler Thromb Vasc Biol* 16:1306, 1996.

164. Buchwald AB, Hammerschmidt S, Stevens J, et al: Inhibition of neointimal proliferation after coronary angioplasty by low-molecular-weight heparin (clivarine) and polyethyleneglycol hirudin. *J Cardiovasc Pharmacol* 28:481, 1996.

165. Abendschein DR, Recchia D, Meng YY, et al: Inhibition of thrombin attenuates stenosis after arterial injury in minipigs. *J Am Coll Cardiol* 28:1849, 1996.

166. Sarembock IJ, Gertz SD, Thome LM, et al: Effectiveness of hirulog in reducing restenosis after balloon angioplasty of atherosclerotic femoral arteries in rabbits. *J Vasc Res* 33:308, 1996.

167. Topol EJ, Bonana R, Jewitt D, et al: Use of a direct anti-thrombin, Hirulog, in place of heparin during coronary angioplasty. *Circulation* 87:1622, 1993.

168. Van den Bos AA, Deckers JW, Heyndrickx GR, et al: Safety and efficacy of recombinant hirudin (CGP 39 393) versus heparin in patients with stable angina undergoing coronary angioplasty. *Circulation* 88:2058, 1993.

169. Schiele F, Vuillemenot A, Kramarz P, et al: A pilot study of subcutaneous recombinant hirudin (HBW 023) in the treatment of deep vein thrombosis. *Thromb Haemost* 71:558, 1994.

170. Cannon CP, McCabe CH, Henry TD, et al: A pilot trial of recombinant desulfatohirudin compared with heparin in conjunction with tissue-type plasminogen activator and aspirin for acute myocardial infarction: results of the Thrombolysis in Myocardial Infarction (TIMI) 5 trial. *J Am Coll Cardiol* 23:993, 1994.

171. Lidon RM, Theroux P, Juneau M, et al: Initial experience with a direct antithrombin, Hirulog, in unstable angina. Anticoagulant, antithrombotic and clinical effects. *Circulation* 88:1495, 1993.

172. Serruys PW, Herrmann J-PR, Simon R, et al: A comparison of hirudin with heparin in the prevention of restenosis after coronary angioplasty. *N Engl J Med* 333:757, 1995.

173. Burchenal JEB, Marks DS, Tift Mann J, et al: Effect of direct thrombin inhibition with bivalirudin (hirulog) on restenosis after coronary angioplasty. *Am J Cardiol* 82:511, 1998.

174. Stouffer GA, Runge MS. Thrombin and restenosis: Has the question been answered? *J Am Coll Cardiol* 28:1856, 1996.

175. Jang Y, Guzman LA, Lincoff AM, et al: Influence of blockade at specific levels of the coagulation cascade on restenosis in a rabbit atherosclerotic femoral artery injury model. *Circulation* 92:3041, 1995.

176. Ragosta M, Gimple LW, Gertz SD, et al: Specific factor Xa inhibition reduces restenosis after balloon angioplasty of atherosclerotic femoral arteries of rabbits. *Circulation* 89:1262, 1994.

177. Lyle EM, Fujita T, Conner MW, et al: Effect of inhibitors of factor Xa or platelet adhesion, heparin, and aspirin on platelet deposition in an atherosclerotic rabbit model of angioplasty injury. *J Pharmacol Toxicol Methods* 33:53, 1995.

178. Thornton MA, Gruentzig AR, Hollman J, et al: Coumadin and aspirin in the prevention of restenosis after transluminal coronary angioplasty: A randomized study. *Circulation* 69:721, 1984.

179. Urban P, Buller N, Fox K, et al: Lack of effect of warfarin on the restenosis rate on clinical outcome after balloon coronary angioplasty. *Br Heart J* 60:485, 1988.

180. Oltrona L, Speidel CM, Recchia D, et al: Inhibition of tissue factor-mediated coagulation markedly attenuates stenosis after balloon-induced arterial injury in minipigs. *Circulation* 96:646, 1997.

181. Kanamasa K, Ishida N, Kato H, et al: Recombinant tissue plasminogen activator prevents intimal hyperplasia after balloon angioplasty in hypercholesterolemic rabbits. *Jpn Circ J* 60:889, 1996.

182. Kanamasa K, Ishida N, Kato H, et al: TPA infusion for seven days prevents restenosis following balloon angioplasty in atherosclerotic rabbit (abstr.). *Circulation* 86(Suppl I):I-188, 1992.

183. Kanamasa K, Ishida N, Kato H, et al: Seven-day t-PA or heparin administration prevents intimal hyperplasia following balloon angioplasty in atherosclerotic rabbits (abstr.). *Circulation* 90(Suppl I):I-157, 1994.

184. Lundgren CH, Sawa H, Sobel BE, Fujii S: Modulation of expression of monocyte/macrophage plasminogen activator activity and its implications for attenuation of vasculopathy. *Circulation* 90:1927, 1994.

185. Carmeliet P, Collen D: Gene targeting and gene transfer studies of the plasminogen/plasmin system: Implications in thrombosis, hemostasis, neointima formation, and atherosclerosis. *FASEB J* 9:934, 1995.

186. Sakata K, Miura F, Sugino H, et al: Impaired fibrinolysis early after percutaneous transluminal coronary angioplasty is associated with restenosis. *Am Heart J* 131:1, 1996.

187. Okada SS, Grobmyer SR, Barnathan ES: Contrasting effects of plasminogen activators, urokinase receptor, and LDL receptor-related protein on smooth muscle cell migration and invasion. *Arterioscler Thromb Vasc Biol* 16:1269, 1996.

188. Mehan VK, Meier B, Urban P: Influence on early outcome and restenosis of urokinase before elective coronary angioplasty. *Am J Cardiol* 72:106, 1993.

189. Zidar FJ, Kaplan BM, O'Neill WW, et al: Prospective, randomized trial of prolonged intracoronary urokinase infusion for chronic total occlusions in native coronary arteries. *J Am Coll Cardiol* 27:1406, 1996.

190. Schachinger V, Kasper W, Zeiher AM: Adjunctive intracoronary urokinase therapy during percutaneous transluminal coronary angioplasty. *Am J Cardiol* 77:1174, 1996.

191. Horie H, Takahashi M, Izumi M, et al: Association of an acute reduction in lipoprotein(a) with coronary artery restenosis after percutaneous transluminal coronary angioplasty. *Circulation* 96:166, 1997.

192. Topol EJ, Califf RM, Weisman HF, et al: Randomised trial of coronary intervention with antibody directed against platelet IIb/IIIa integrin for reduction of clinical restenosis: Results at six months. *Lancet* 343:881, 1994.

193. EPIC Investigators: Use of a monoclonal antibody directed against the platelet glycoprotein IIb/IIIa receptor in high risk coronary angioplasty. *N Engl J Med* 330:956, 1994.

194. Frishman WH, Burns B, Atac B, et al: Novel antiplatelet therapies for treatment of patients with ischemic heart disease. *Am Heart J* 130:877, 1995.

195. Reverter JC, Beguin S, Kessels H, et al: Inhibition of platelet-mediated, tissue factor-induced thrombin generation by the mouse-human chimeric 7E3 antibody. Potential implications for the effect of c7E3 Fab treatment on acute thrombosis and "clinical restenosis." *J Clin Invest* 98:863, 1996.

196. Califf RM. Restenosis: the cost to society. *Am Heart J* 130:680, 1995.

197. Lefkovits J, Ivanhoe RJ, Califf RM, et al: Effects of platelet glycoprotein IIb/IIIa receptor blockade by a chimeric monoclonal antibody (abciximab) on acute and six-month outcomes after percutaneous transluminal coronary angioplasty for acute myocardial infarction. EPIC investigators. *Am J Cardiol* 77:1045, 1996.

198. Aguirre FJ, Topol EJ, Ferguson JJ, et al: Bleeding complications with the chimeric antibody to platelet glycoprotein IIb/IIIa integrin in patients undergoing percutaneous coronary intervention. EPIC Investigators. *Circulation* 91:2882, 1995.

199. Kereiakes DJ, Kleiman NS, Ambrose J, et al: Randomized, double-blind, placebo-controlled dose-ranging study of tirofiban (MK-383) platelet IIb/IIIa blockade in high risk patients undergoing coronary angioplasty. *J Am Coll Cardiol* 27:536, 1996.

200. Slepian MJ, Massia SP: Local delivery of a cyclic RGD peptide inhibits neointimal hyperplasia following balloon injury (abstr.). *Circulation* 88(Suppl I):372, 1994.

201. Tcheng JE, Harrington RA, Kottke-Marchant K, et al: Multicenter, randomized, double-blind, placebo-controlled trial of the platelet integrin glycoprotein IIb/IIIa blocker integrelin in elective coronary intervention. *Circulation* 91:2151, 1995.

202. Lincoff AM, Tcheng JE, Ellis SG, et al: Randomized trial of platelet glycoprotein IIb/IIIa inhibition with integrelin for prevention of restenosis following coronary intervention. The IMPACT-Angiographic Substudy (abstr.). *Circulation* 92:I, 1995.

203. Ferguson JJ: Integrelin for PTCA (abstr.). *Circulation* 92:I-2362, 1995.

204. Tcheng JE: Glycoprotein IIb/IIIa receptor inhibitors: Putting the EPIC, IMPACT II, RESTORE, and EPILOG trials into perspective. *Am J Cardiol* 78:35, 1996.

205. Gibson CM, Goel M, Cohen DJ, et al for the RESTORE Investigators: Six-month angiographic and clinical follow up of patients prospectively randomized to receive either tirofiban or placebo during angioplasty in the RESTORE Trial. *J Am Coll Cardiol* 32:28, 1998.

206. Chico TJA, Chamberlain J, Gunn J, et al: Effect of selective or combined inhibition of integrins α_{IIb}/β_3 and α_v/β_3 on thrombosis and neointima after oversized porcine coronary angioplasty. *Circulation* 103:1135, 2001.

207. The ERASER Investigators: Acute platelet inhibition with abciximab does not reduce in-stent restenosis (ERASER Study). *Circulation* 100:799, 1999.

208. Neumann F-J, Kastrati A, Schmitt C, et al: Effect of glycoprotein IIb/IIIa receptor blockade with abciximab on clinical and angiographic restenosis rate after the placement of coronary stents following acute myocardial infarction. *J Am Coll Cardiol* 35:915, 2000.

209. Simari RD, Camrud AR, Jorgenson MA, et al: Ancrod and heparin reduce reactive neointimal hyperplasia in a porcine coronary injury model (abstr.). *Circulation* 88(Suppl I):657, 1993.

210. Tsuchikane E, Fukuhara A, Sumitsuji S, et al: Cilostazol reduces restenosis following coronary balloon angioplasty (abstr.). *Circulation* 96(Suppl I):324, 1997.

211. Take S, Matsutani M, Ueda H, et al: Effect of cilostazol in preventing restenosis after percutaneous transluminal coronary angioplasty. *Am J Cardiol* 79:1097, 1997.

212. Sekiya M, Funada J, Watanabe K, et al: Effects of probucol and cilostazol alone and in combination on frequency of poststenting restenosis. *Am J Cardiol* 82:144, 1998.

213. Tsuchikane E, Fukuhara A, Kobayashi T, et al: Impact of cilostazol on restenosis after percutaneous coronary balloon angioplasty. *Circulation* 100:21, 1999.

214. Park S-W, Lee CW, Kim H-S, et al: Effects of cilostazol on angiographic restenosis after coronary stent placement. *Am J Cardiol* 86:499, 2000.

215. MacDonald RG, Panush RS, Pepine CJ: Rationale for the use of glucocorticoids in modification of restenosis after percutaneous transluminal coronary angioplasty. *Am J Cardiol* 60:56B, 1987.

216. Berk BC, Gordon JB, Alexander RW, et al: Pharmacologic roles of heparin and glucocorticoids to prevent restenosis after coronary angioplasty. *J Am Coll Cardiol* 17(Suppl B):111B, 1991.

217. Stone GW, Rutherford BD, McConahay DR, et al: A randomized trial of corticosteroids for the prevention of restenosis in 102 patients undergoing repeat coronary angioplasty. *Catheter Cardiovasc Diagn* 18:227, 1989.

218. Rose TE, Beauchamp BG: Short-term high-dose steroid treatment to prevent restenosis in PTCA (abstr.). *Circulation* 76(Suppl IV):371, 1987.

219. Pepine CJ, Hirshfeld JW, MacDonald RG, et al: A controlled trial of corticosteroids to prevent restenosis after coronary angioplasty. *Circulation* 81:1753, 1990.

220. Lee CW, Chae J-K, Lim H-Y, et al: Prospective randomized trial of corticosteroids for the prevention of restenosis after intracoronary stent implantation. *Am Heart J* 138:60, 1999.

221. Kong DF: Steroids for restenosis: strike three! (editorial). *Am Heart J* 138:3, 1999.

222. Hirayama A, Nanto S, Ohara T, et al: Preventive effect on restenosis after PTCA by ebselen: a newly synthesized anti-inflammatory agent (abstr.). *J Am Coll Cardiol* 19:259A, 1992.

223. Faxon DP, Sanborn TA, Haudenschild CC, et al: Effect of anti-platelet therapy on restenosis after experimental angioplasty. *Am J Cardiol* 53:72C, 1984.

224. Suzawa H, Kikuchi S, Arai N, et al: The mechanism involved in the inhibitory action of tranilast on collagen biosynthesis of keloid fibroblasts. *Jpn J Pharmacol* 60:91, 1992.

225. Suzawa H, Kikuchi S, Ichikawa K, et al: Inhibitory action of tranilast, an anti-allergic drug, on the release of cytokines and PGE2 from human monocytes-macrophages. *Jpn J Pharmacol* 60:85, 1992.

226. Kawano Y, Noma T: Cell action mechanism of tranilast-effect on the expression of HLA-class II antigen. *Int J Pharmacol* 15:487, 1993.

227. Tanaka K, Honda M, Kuramochi T, Morioka S: Prominent inhibitor effects of tranilast on migration and proliferation of and collagen synthesis by vascular smooth muscle cells. *Atherosclerosis* 107:179, 1994.

228. Miyazawa K, Kikuchi S, Fukuyama J, et al: Inhibition of PDGF- and TGF-beta 1-induced collagen synthesis, migration and proliferation by tranilast in vascular smooth muscle cells from spontaneously hypertensive rats. *Atherosclerosis* 118:213, 1995.

229. Fukuyama J, Miyazawa K, Hamano S, Ujiie A: Inhibitory effect of tranilast on proliferation, migration, and collagen synthesis on human vascular smooth muscle cells. *Can J Physiol Pharmacol* 74:80, 1996.

230. Kikuchi S, Umemura K, Kondo K, Nakashima M: Tranilast suppresses intimal hyperplasia after photochemically induced endothelial injury in the rat. *Eur J Pharm* 295:221, 1996.

231. Ishiwata S, Verheye S, Robinson KA, et al: Inhibition of neointima formation by tranilast in pig coronary arteries after balloon angioplasty and stent implantation. *J Am Coll Cardiol* 35:1331, 2000.

232. Fukuyama J, Ichikawa K, Hamano S, Shibata N: Tranilast suppresses the vascular intimal hyperplasia after balloon injury in rabbits fed on a high-cholesterol diet. *Eur J Pharmacol* 318:327, 1996.

233. Miyazawa, K, Fukuyama J, Misawa K, et al: Tranilast antagonizes angiotensin II and inhibits its biological effects in vascular smooth muscle cells. *Atherosclerosis* 121:167, 1996.

234. Hishikawa K, Nakaki T, Hirahashi J, et al: Tranilast restores cytokine-induced nitric oxide production against platelet-derived growth factor in vascular smooth muscle cells. *J Cardiovasc Pharmacol* 28:200, 1996.

235. Tamai H, Katoh O, Suzuki S, et al: Impact of tranilast on restenosis after coronary angioplasty: Tranilast Restenosis Following Angioplasty Trial (TREAT). *Am Heart J* 138:968, 1999.

236. Holmes DR Jr, Savage M, LaBlanche J-M, et al: Results of Prevention of Restenosis with tranilast and its outcomes (PRESTO) trial. *Circulation* 106:1243, 2002.

237. Feldman LJ, Aguirre L, Ziol M, Bridou J-P, et al: Interleukin-10 inhibits intimal hyperplasia after angioplasty or stent implantation in hypercholesterolemic rabbits. *Circulation* 101:908, 2000.

238. Bishop GG, McPherson JA, Sanders JM, et al: Selective α_v/β_3 receptor-blockade reduces macrophage infiltration and restenosis after balloon angioplasty in the atherosclerotic rabbit. *Circulation* 103:1906, 2001.

239. Hayashi S-i, Watanabe N, Nakazawa K, et al: Role of P-selectin in inflammation, neointimal formation, and vascular remodeling in balloon-injured rat carotid arteries. *Circulation* 102:1710, 2000.

240. Wang K, Zhou Z, Zhou X, et al: Prevention of intimal hyperplasia with recombinant soluble P-selectin glycoprotein ligand-immunoglobulin in the porcine coronary artery balloon injury model. *J Am Coll Cardiol* 38:577, 2001.

240a. Danenberg HD, Fishbein I, Gao J, et al: Macrophage depletion by clodronate-containing liposomes reduces neointimal formation after balloon injury in rats and rabbits. *Circulation* 106:599, 2002.

241. Meiners S, Laule M, Rother W, et al: Ubiquitin-proteasome pathway as a new target for the prevention of restenosis. *Circulation* 105:483, 2002.

242. Liu MW, Roubin GS, Robinson KA, et al: Trapidil in preventing restenosis after balloon angioplasty in the atherosclerotic rabbit. *Circulation* 81:1089, 1990.

243. Okamoto S, Inden M, Setsuda M, et al: Effects of trapidil (triazolopyrimidine), a platelet-derived growth factor antagonist, in preventing restenosis after percutaneous transluminal coronary angioplasty. *Am Heart J* 123:1439, 1992.

244. Maresta A, Balducelli M, Cantini L, et al: Trapidil (triazolopyrimidine), a platelet-derived growth factor antagonist, reduces restenosis after percutaneous transluminal coronary angioplasty: Results of the randomized, double-blind STARC study. *Circulation* 90:2710, 1994.

245. Nishikawa H, Ono N, Motoyasu M, et al: Preventive effects of trapidil on restenosis after PTCA (abstr.). *Circulation* 86(Suppl I):53, 1992.

246. Bilder G, Wentz T, Leadley R, et al: Restenosis following angioplasty in the swine coronary artery is inhibited by an orally active PDGF-receptor tyrosine kinase inhibitor, RPR101511A. *Circulation* 99:3292, 1999.

247. Ferns GA, Raines EW, Sprugel KH, et al: Inhibition of neointimal smooth muscle accumulation after angioplasty by an antibody to PDGF. *Science* 253:1129, 1991.

248. Fingerle J, Faulmuller A, Muller G, et al: Pituitary factors in blood plasma are necessary for smooth muscle cell proliferation in response to injury in vivo. *Arterioscler Thromb* 12:1488, 1992.

249. Hong MK, Kent KM, Mehran R, et al: Continuous subcutaneous angiopeptin treatment significantly reduces neointimal hyperplasia in a porcine coronary in-stent restenosis model. *Circulation* 95:449, 1997.

250. Eriksen UH, Amtorp O, Bagger JP, et al: Continuous angiopeptin infusion reduces coronary restenosis following balloon angioplasty (abstr.). *Circulation* 88(Suppl I):594, 1993.

251. Emanuelsson H, Bagger JP, Balcon R, et al: Long-term effects of angiopeptin treatment in coronary angioplasty: Reduction of clinical events but not of angiographic restenosis. *Circulation* 91:1689, 1995.

252. Kent KM, Williams DO, Cassagneau B, et al: Double-blind, controlled trial of the effect of angiopeptin on coronary restenosis following balloon angioplasty (abstr.). *Circulation* 88(Suppl I):506, 1993.

253. von Essen R, Ostermaier R, Grube E, et al for the VERAS Investigators: Effects of octreotide treatment on restenosis after coronary angioplasty. Results of the VERAS Study. *Circulation* 96:1482, 1997.

254. Willerson JT, Eidt JF, McNatt J, et al: Role of thromboxane and serotonin as mediators in the development of spontaneous alterations in coronary blood flow and neointimal proliferation in canine models with chronic coronary artery stenosis and endothelial injury. *J Am Coll Cardiol* 17:101B, 1991.

255. Serruys PW, Klein W, Tijssen JP, et al: Evaluation of ketanserin in the prevention of restenosis after percutaneous transluminal coronary angioplasty. A multicenter randomized double-blind placebo-controlled trial. *Circulation* 88:1588, 1993.

256. Klein W, Eber B, Dusleag J, et al: Ketanserin prevents early restenosis following percutaneous transluminal coronary angioplasty. *Clin Physiol Biochem* 8(Suppl 3):101, 1990.

257. Heik SCW, Bracht M, Benn HP, et al: No prevention of restenosis after PTCA with ketanserin. A controlled prospective randomized double-blind study (abstr.). *Circulation* 86(Suppl I):53, 1992.

258. Rakugi H, Kim DK, Krieger JE, et al: Induction of angiotensin converting enzyme in the neointima after vascular injury. Possible role in restenosis. *J Clin Invest* 93:339, 1994.

259. Rakugi H, Wang DS, Dzau VJ, et al: Potential importance of tissue angiotensin-converting enzyme inhibition in preventing neointima formation. *Circulation* 90:449, 1994.

260. Lehmann K, Powell JS: Effect of cilazapril on the proliferative response after vascular damage. *J Cardiovasc Pharmacol* 22(Suppl 4):S19, 1993.

261. Beohar N, Prather A, Yu QT, et al: Angiotensin-converting enzyme genotype DD is a potent risk factor for coronary artery disease and restenosis post percutaneous transluminal angioplasty (abstr.). *Circulation* 90(Suppl I):145, 1994.

262. Powell JS, Clozel JP, Muller RK, et al: Inhibitors of angiotensin-converting enzyme prevent myointimal proliferation after vascular injury. *Science* 245:186, 1989.

263. Powell JS, Muller RKM, Baumgartner HR: Suppression of the vascular response to injury: The role of angiotensin-converting enzyme inhibitors. *J Am Coll Cardiol* 17:137B, 1991.

264. Huber KC, Schwartz RS, Edwards WD, et al: Effects of angiotensin converting enzyme inhibition on neointimal proliferation in a porcine coronary injury model. *Am Heart J* 125:695, 1993.

265. Reddy BH, Farrar MA Yip DS, et al: Kinin B2 receptor antagonism reverses angiotensin converting enzyme inhibition in postangioplasty vascular neointimal proliferation (abstr.). *J Am Coll Cardiol* 23(Suppl I): 233A, 1994.

266. Brozovich FV, Morganroth J, Gottlieb NB, et al: Effect of angiotensin converting enzyme inhibition on the incidence of restenosis after percutaneous transluminal coronary angioplasty. *Catheter Cardiovasc Diagn* 23:263, 1991.

267. Multicenter European Research Trial with Cilazapril after Angioplasty to Prevent Transluminal Coronary Obstruction and Restenosis (MERCATOR) Study Group. Does the new angiotensin-converting enzyme inhibitor cilazapril prevent restenosis after percutaneous transluminal coronary angioplasty? Results of the MERCATOR study: A multicenter, randomized, double-blind, placebo-controlled trial. *Circulation* 86:100, 1992.

268. Desmet W, Vrolix M, DeScheerder I, et al: Angiotensin-converting enzyme inhibition with fosinopril sodium in the prevention of restenosis after coronary angioplasty. *Circulation* 89:385, 1994.

269. Kaul U, Chandra S, Bahl VK, et al: Enalapril for prevention of restenosis after coronary angioplasty. *Indian Heart J* 45:469, 1993.

270. Meurice T, Bauters C, Hermant X, et al: Effect of ACE inhibitors on angiographic restenosis after coronary stenting (PARIS): A randomised, double-blind, placebo-controlled trial. *Lancet* 357:1321, 2001.

271. Faxon DP, The Multicenter American Research Trial with Cilazapril after Angioplasty to Prevent Transluminal Coronary Obstruction and Restenosis (MARCATOR) Study Group. Effect of high dose angiotensin-converting enzyme inhibition on restenosis: Final results of the MARCATOR study, a multicenter, double-blind, placebo-controlled trial of cilazapril. *J Am Coll Cardiol* 25:362, 1995.

272. Pratt RE, Dzau VJ: Pharmacologic strategies to prevent restenosis: Lessons learned from blockade of the renin-angiotensin system (editorial). *Circulation* 93:848, 1996.

273. Huckle WR, Drag MD, Acker WR, et al: Effects of subtype selective and balanced angiotensin II receptor antagonists in a porcine coronary artery model of vascular restenosis. *Circulation* 93:1009, 1996.

274. Levine RL, Anderson PG, Lyle K, et al: 17-Estradiol inhibits neointima formation after coronary angioplasty in swine (abstr.). *J Am Coll Cardiol* 27:320A, 1996.

275. O'Brien JE, Peterson ED, Keeler GP, et al: Relation between estrogen replacement therapy and restenosis after percutaneous coronary interventions. *J Am Coll Cardiol* 28:1111, 1996.

276. Schwartz J, Freeman R, Frishman W: Clinical pharmacology of estrogens: Focus on their cardiovascular actions and cardioprotective benefits of replacement therapy in postmenopausal women. *J Clin Pharmacol* 35:314, 1995.

277. Oparil S, Chen SJ, Chen YF, et al: Estrogen reduces cellular proliferation following carotid artery balloon injury in ovariectomized rats (abstr.). *Circulation* 96(Suppl I):607, 1997.

278. Chen SJ, Osbakken MD, Chen YF, et al: Angiotensin II type I (ATI) receptor antagonist irbesartan and estrogen have profound but non-additive effects on neointimal formation in balloon injured carotid arteries of ovariectomized rats (abstr.). *Circulation* 96(Suppl I):608, 1997.

278a. Peters S, Götting B, Trümmel M, et al: Valsartan for prevention of restenosis after stenting of Type B2/c lesions: The Val-Prest Trial. *J Invasive Cardiol* 13:93, 2001.

279. Fingerle J, Sanders KH, Fotev Z: Alpha-1 receptor antagonists urapidil and prazosin inhibit neointima formation in rat carotid artery induced by balloon catheter injury. *Basic Res Cardiol* 86(Suppl 1):75, 1991.

280. Gregorini L, Marco J, Bernies M, et al: The alpha-1-adrenergic blocking agent urapidil counteracts postrotational atherectomy "elastic recoil" where nitrates have failed. *Am J Cardiol* 79:1100, 1997.

281. Patel MK, Chan P, Betteridge LJ, et al: Inhibition of human vascular smooth muscle cell proliferation by the novel multiple-action antihypertensive agent carvedilol. *J Cardiovasc Pharmacol* 25:652, 1995.

282. Desmet WJ, DeScheerder IK, Emanuelsson H, et al: Carvedilol in the prevention of restenosis after coronary angioplasty (abstr.). *Circulation* 92:I-345, 1995.

283. Folts JD, Stamler J, Keaney JF Jr: Coating stenosed intimally damaged dog coronary arteries with nitrosated albumin prevents platelet adhesion-aggregation and thrombus formation (abstr.). *Circulation* 90(Suppl I):345, 1994.

284. Myers PR, Webel R, Thondapu V, et al: Restenosis is associated with decreased coronary artery nitric oxide synthase. *Int J Cardiol* 55:183, 1996.

285. Cooke VP, Dzau VJ: Nitric oxide synthase: role in genesis of vascular disease. *Ann Rev Med* 48:489, 1997.

286. Mooradian DL, Hutsell TC, Keefer LK. Nitric oxide (NO) donor molecules: Effect of NO release rate on vascular smooth muscle cell proliferation in vitro. *J Cardiovasc Pharmacol* 25:674, 1995.

287. Marks DS, Vita JA, Folts JD, et al: Inhibition of neointimal proliferation in rabbits after vascular injury by a single treatment with a protein adduct of nitric oxide. *J Clin Invest* 96:2630, 1995.

288. Tarry WC, Bettinger DA, Makhoul RG: L-Arginine, the nitric oxide precursor, reduces intimal hyperplasia following endothelial injury independent of early smooth muscle cell proliferation (abstr.). *Circulation* 88(Suppl I):367, 1993.

289. Lee JS, Adrie C, Jacob HJ, et al: Chronic inhalation of nitric oxide inhibits neointimal formation after balloon-induced arterial injury. *Circ Res* 78:337, 1996.

290. Schwarzacher SP, Lim TT, Wang B, et al: Local intramural delivery of L-arginine enhances nitric oxide generation and inhibits lesion formation after balloon angioplasty. *Circulation* 95:1863, 1997.

291. Lablanche J-M, Grollier G, Lusson J-R, et al: Effect of the direct nitric oxide donors linsidomine and molsidomine on angiographic restenosis after coronary balloon angioplasty. The ACCORD study. *Circulation* 95:83, 1997.

292. Kurz RW, Graf B, Gremmel F, et al: Increased serum concentrations of adhesion molecules after coronary angioplasty. *Clin Sci* 87:627, 1994.

293. Jang Y, Lincoff AM, Plow EF, Topol EJ: Cell adhesion molecules in coronary artery disease. *J Am Coll Cardiol* 24:1591, 1994.

294. Wang X, Feuerstein GZ, Gu JL, et al: Interleukin-1 beta induces expression of adhesion molecules in human vascular smooth muscle

cells and enhances adhesion of leukocytes to smooth muscle cells. *Atherosclerosis* 115:89, 1995.

295. Golino P, Ambrosio G, Ragni M, et al: Inhibition of neutrophil adhesion proteins reduces neointimal hyperplasia following artery injury in rabbit carotid arteries (abstr.). *Circulation* 90(Suppl I):85, 1994.

296. Guzman LA, Villa AE, Forudi F, et al: Effect of anti-CD18 adhesion glycoprotein monoclonal antibody on restenosis following balloon angioplasty in the rabbit atherosclerotic model (abstr.). *J Am Coll Cardiol* 23(Suppl I):20A, 1994.

297. Ishizaka N, Ohno M, Mochida S, et al: Coadministration of anti-ICAM/anti-LFA-1 suppresses neointimal hyperplasia of balloon injured rat carotid artery (abstr.). *Circulation* 90(Suppl I):84, 1994.

298. Shebuski RJ, Humphrey WR, Simmons CA, et al: Role of P-selectin in animal models of thrombosis and restenosis (abstr.). *Circulation* 90(Suppl I):142, 1994.

299. Takagi T, Akasaka T, Yamamuro A, et al: Troglitazone reduces neointimal tissue proliferation after coronary stent implantation in patients with non-insulin dependent diabetes mellitus. *J Am Coll Cardiol* 36:1529, 2000.

300. Meurice T, Vallet B, Bauters C, et al: Role of endothelial cells in restenosis after coronary angioplasty. *Fundam Clin Pharmacol* 10:234, 1996.

301. Callow AD, Choi ET, Trachtenberg JD, et al: Vascular permeability factor accelerates endothelial regrowth following balloon angioplasty. *Growth Factors* 10:223, 1994.

302. Asahara T, Bauters C, Pastore C, et al: Local delivery of vascular endothelial growth factor accelerates reendothelialization and attenuates intimal hyperplasia in balloon-injured rat carotid artery. *Circulation* 91:2793, 1995.

303. Conte MS, Choudhry RP, Shirakowa M, et al: Endothelial cell seeding fails to attenuate intimal thickening in balloon-injured rabbit arteries. *J Vasc Surg* 21:413, 1995.

304. Nakamura S, Moriguchi A, Morishita R, et al: Re-endothelialization therapeutics for restenosis: In vivo gene transfer of human hepatocyte growth factor (HGF) gene resulted in an inhibition of neointimal formation after balloon injury, accompanied by restore of nitric oxide (NO) (abstr.). *Circulation* 96(Suppl I):608, 1997.

305. Leisch F, Schutzenberger W, Kerschner K, et al: Influence of a variant angina on the results of percutaneous transluminal coronary angioplasty. *Br Heart J* 56:341, 1986.

306. Hoberg E, Kubler W: Calcium antagonist in preventing restenosis following coronary angioplasty *Cardiology* 36(12 Suppl 1):225, 1991.

307. Ide S, Kondoh M, Satoh H, Karasawa A: Anti-proliferative effects of benidipine hydrochloride in porcine cultured vascular smooth muscle cells and in rats subjected to balloon catheter-induced endothelial denudation. *Biol Pharm Bull* 17:627, 1994.

308. O'Keefe JH, Giorgi LV, Hartzler GO, et al: Effects of diltiazem on complications and restenosis after coronary angioplasty. *Am J Cardiol* 67:373, 1991.

309. Corcos T, David PR, Val PG, et al: Failure of diltiazem to prevent restenosis after percutaneous transluminal coronary angioplasty. *Am Heart J* 109:926, 1985.

310. Whitworth HB, Roubin GS, Hollman J, et al: Effect of nifedipine on recurrent restenosis after percutaneous transluminal coronary angioplasty. *J Am Coll Cardiol* 8:1271, 1986.

311. Hoberg E, Dietz R, Frees U, et al: Verapamil treatment after coronary angioplasty in patients at high risk of recurrent stenosis. *Br Heart J* 71:254, 1994.

312. Unverdorben M, Kunkel B, Leucht M, et al: Reduction of restenosis by diltiazem (abstr.)? *Circulation* 86(Suppl I):53, 1992.

313. Hillegass WB, Ohman EM, Leimberger JD, et al: A meta-analysis of randomized trials of calcium antagonists to reduce restenosis after coronary angioplasty. *Am J Cardiol* 73:835, 1994.

314. Dens JA, Desmet WJ, Coussement P, et al: Usefulness of nisoldipine for prevention of restenosis after percutaneous transluminal coronary angioplasty (Results of the NICOLE Study). *Am J Cardiol* 87:28, 2001.

315. Jørgensen B, Simonsen S, Endresen K, et al: Restenosis and clinical outcome in patients treated with amlodipine after angioplasty: Results from the Coronary AngioPlasty Amlodipine REStenosis Study (CAPARES). *J Am Coll Cardiol* 35:592, 2000.

316. Agata J, Miao RQ, Yayama K, et al: Bradykinin B1 receptor mediates inhibition of neointima formation in rat artery after balloon angioplasty. *Hypertension* 36:364, 2000.

316a. Li Z, Nater C, Kinsella J, et al: Minoxidil inhibits proliferation and migration of cultured vascular smooth muscle cells and neointimal formation after balloon catheter injury. *J Cardiovasc Pharmacol* 36:270, 2000.

317. Muller DWM, Ellis SG, Topol EJ: Colchicine and antineoplastic therapy for the prevention of restenosis after percutaneous coronary interventions. *J Am Coll Cardiol* 17:126B, 1991.

318. Poon M, Marx SO, Gallo R, et al: Rapamycin inhibits vascular smooth muscle cell migration. *J Clin Invest* 98:2277, 1996.

319. Suzuki T, Kopia G, Hayashi S-I, et al: Stent-based delivery of sirolimus reduces neointimal formation in a porcine coronary model. *Circulation* 104:1188, 2001.

320. Marx SO, Marks AR: Bench to bedside. The development of rapamycin and its application to stent restenosis. *Circulation* 104:852, 2001.

321. Sousa JE, Costa MA, Abizaid A, et al: Lack of neointimal proliferation after implantation of sirolimus-coated stents in human coronary arteries. A quantitative coronary angiography and three-dimensional intravascular ultrasound study. *Circulation* 103:192, 2001.

322. Morice M-C, Serruys PW, Sousa JE, et al: A randomized comparison of sirolimus-eluting stent with a standard stent for coronary revascularization. *N Engl J Med* 346:1773, 2002.

322a. Nieman K, Ligthart JMR, Serruys PW, de Feyter PJ: Left main rapamycin-coated stent. Invasive versus noninvasive angiographic follow up. (On-line article.) *Circulation* 105:e130, 2002.

322b. Degertekin M, Serruys PW, Foley DP, et al: Persistent inhibition of neointimal hyperplasia after sirolimus-eluting stent implantation. Long-term (up to 2 years) clinical, angiographic, and intravascular ultrasound follow-up. *Circulation* 106:1610, 2002.

323. Gradus-Pizlo I, Wilensky RL, March KL, et al: Local delivery of biodegradable microparticles containing colchicine or a colchicine analogue: Effects on restenosis and implications for catheter-based drug delivery. *J Am Coll Cardiol* 26:1549, 1995.

324. O'Keefe JH, McCallister BD, Bateman TM, et al: Ineffectiveness of colchicine for the prevention of restenosis after coronary angioplasty. *J Am Coll Cardiol* 19:1597, 1992.

325. Grines CL, Rizik D, Levine A, et al: Colchicine angioplasty restenosis trial (CART) (abstr.). *Circulation* 84(Suppl II):365, 1991.

326. Dev V, Eigler N, Fishbein MC, et al: Local arterial wall delivery of dexamethasone and colchicine via biodegradable micro-spheres does not prevent intimal hyperplasia in rabbit (abstr.). *Circulation* 90(Suppl I): 157, 1994.

327. Sollott SJ, Cheng L, Pauly RR, et al: Taxol inhibits neointimal smooth muscle cell accumulation after angioplasty in the rat. *J Clin Invest* 95:1869, 1995.

328. Axel DI, Kunert W, Goggelmann C: Paclitaxel inhibits arterial smooth muscle cell proliferation and migration in vitro and in vivo using local drug delivery. *Circulation* 96:636, 1997.

329. Heldman AW, Cheng L, Jenkins GM, et al: Paclitaxel stent coating inhibits neointimal hyperplasia at 4 weeks in a porcine model of coronary restenosis. *Circulation* 103:2289, 2001.

330. Herdeg C, Oberhoff M, Baumbach A, et al: Local paclitaxel delivery for the prevention of restenosis: biological effects and efficacy in vivo. *J Am Coll Cardiol* 35:1969, 2000.

331. Drachman DE, Edelman ER, Seifert P, et al: Neointimal thickening after stent delivery of paclitaxel: Change in composition and arrest of growth over six months. *J Am Coll Cardiol* 36:2325, 2000.

332. Farb A, Heller PF, Shroff S, et al: Pathological analysis of local delivery of paclitaxel via a polymer-coated stent. *Circulation* 104:473, 2001.

332a. Kolodgie FD, John M, Khurana C, et al: Sustained reduction of in-stent neointimal growth with the use of a novel systemic nanoparticle paclitaxel. *Circulation* 106:1195, 2002.

332b. Progress in Clinical Trials: ELUTES (European Evaluation of Paclitaxel Eluting Stent). *Clin Cardiol* 25:38, 2002.

333. Honda Y, Grube E, de la Fuente LM, et al: Novel drug-delivery stent. Intravascular ultrasound observations from the first human experience with the QP2-eluting polymer stent system. *Circulation* 104:380, 2001.

334. Voisard R, D'Artsch PC, Seitzer U, et al: Human cell culture as pre-screening system for a pharmacological approach to the prevention of restenosing events after angioplasty (abstr.)? *Circulation* 84(Suppl II): 71, 1991.

335. Barath B, Arakawa K, Cao J, et al: Low dose of antitumor agents prevents smooth muscle cell proliferation after endothelial injury (abstr.). *J Am Coll Cardiol* 13(Suppl):252A, 1989.

336. McKenney PA, Currier JW, Haudenschild CC, et al: Cyclosporine A does not inhibit restenosis in experimental angioplasty (abstr.). *Circulation* 85(Suppl II):70, 1991.

337. Muller DWM, Topol EJ, Abrams G, et al: Intramural methotrexate therapy for the prevention of intimal proliferation following porcine carotid balloon angioplasty (abstr.). *Circulation* 82(Suppl III):429, 1990.

338. Murphy JG, Schwartz RS, Edwards WD, et al: Methotrexate and azathioprine fail to inhibit porcine coronary restenosis (abstr.). *Circulation* 82(Suppl III):429, 1990.

339. Ruef J, Meshel AS, Hu Z, et al: Flavopiridol inhibits smooth muscle cell proliferation in vitro and neointimal formation in vivo after carotid injury in the rat. *Circulation* 100:659, 1999.

340. Indolfi C, Di Lorenzo E, Rapacciuolo A, et al: 8-chloro-cyclic AMP inhibits smooth muscle cell proliferation in vitro and neointimal formation induced by balloon injury in vivo. *J Am Coll Cardiol* 36:288, 2000.

341. Shah PK, Amin J: Low high-density lipoprotein level is associated with increased restenosis rate after coronary angioplasty. *Circulation* 85:1279, 1992.

342. Miyata M, Biro S, Arima S, et al: High serum concentration of lipoprotein(a) is a risk factor for restenosis after percutaneous transluminal coronary angioplasty in Japanese patients with single vessel disease. *Am Heart J* 132:269, 1996.

343. Yamamoto H, Imazu M, Yamabe T, et al: Risk factors for restenosis after percutaneous transluminal coronary angioplasty: Role of lipoprotein (a). *Am Heart J* 130:1168, 1995.

344. Daida H, Lee YJ, Yokoi H, et al: Prevention of restenosis after percutaneous transluminal coronary angioplasty by reducing lipoprotein(a) levels with low density lipoprotein apheresis. Low Density Lipoprotein Apheresis Angioplasty Restenosis Trial (L-ART) Group. *Am J Cardiol* 73:1037, 1994.

344a. Bunch TJ, Muhlestein JB, Anderson JL, et al: Effects of statins on six-month survival and clinical restenosis frequency after coronary stent deployment. *Am J Cardiol* 90:299, 2002.

345. Gellman J, Ezekowitz MD, Sarembock IJ, et al: Effect of lovastatin on intimal hyperplasia after balloon angioplasty: A study in an atherosclerotic, hypercholesterolemic rabbit. *J Am Coll Cardiol* 17:251, 1991.

346. Constantinescu DE, Banka VS, Tulenko TN: Lovastatin inhibits proliferation of arterial smooth muscle and endothelial cells. Indication in atherosclerosis and prevention of restenosis (abstr.). *Eur Heart J* 13(Suppl):82, 1992.

347. Sahni R, Maniet AR, Voci G, et al: Prevention of restenosis by lovastatin after successful coronary angioplasty. *Am Heart J* 121:1600, 1991.

348. Weintraub WS, Boccuzzi SJ, Klein JL, et al: Lack of effect of lovastatin on restenosis after coronary angioplasty. *N Engl J Med* 331:1331, 1994.

349. Onaka H, Hirota Y, Kita Y, et al: The effect of pravastatin on prevention of restenosis after successful percutaneous transluminal coronary angioplasty [in English]. *Jpn Circ J* 58:100, 1994.

350. Tanajura L, Cano M, Nunes G, et al: A prospective randomized trial of lovastatin for prevention of coronary restenosis (abstr.). *Circulation* 92(Suppl I):I-345, 1995.

351. Foley DP, Bonnier H, Lackson G, et al: Prevention of restenosis after coronary balloon angioplasty: Rationale and design of the Fluvastatin Angioplasty Restenosis (FLARE) trial. *Am J Cardiol* 73:50D, 1994.

352. Mulder HJGH, Bal ET, Jukema JW, et al: Pravastatin reduces restenosis two years after percutaneous transluminal coronary angioplasty (REGRESS Trial). *Am J Cardiol* 86:742, 2000.

353. Walter DH, Schachinger V, Elsner M, et al: Effect of statin therapy on restenosis after coronary stent implantation. *Am J Cardiol* 85:962, 2000.

354. Zimetbaum P, Eder H, Frishman W: Probucol: Pharmacology and clinical application. *J Clin Pharmacol* 30:3, 1990.

355. Marshall JJ, Wu KX, Peterson TE, et al: Superoxide anions, produced by regenerated endothelium, contribute to impaired endothelium-dependent relaxations following balloon injury (abstr.). *Circulation* 88(Suppl I):467, 1993.

356. Schneider JE, Berk BC, Gravanis MB, et al: Probucol decreases neointimal formation in a swine model of coronary artery balloon injury. A possible role for antioxidants in restenosis. *Circulation* 88:628, 1993.

357. Ferns GA, Forster L, Stewart-Lee A, et al: Probucol inhibits neointimal thickening and macrophage accumulation after balloon injury in the cholesterol-fed rabbit. *Proc Natl Acad Sci U S A* 89:11312, 1992.

358. Setsuda M, Inden M, Hiraoka N, et al: Probucol therapy in the prevention of restenosis after successful percutaneous transluminal coronary angioplasty. *Clin Ther* 15:374, 1993.

359. Watanabe K, Sekiya M, Ikeda S, et al: Preventive effects of probucol on restenosis after percutaneous transluminal coronary angioplasty. *Am Heart J* 132:23, 1996.

360. O'Keefe JH Jr, Stone GW, McCallister BD Jr, et al: Lovastatin plus probucol for prevention of restenosis after percutaneous transluminal coronary angioplasty. *Am J Cardiol* 77:649, 1996.

361. Tardif JC, Cote G, Lesperance J, et al: Probucol and multivitamins in the prevention of restenosis after coronary angioplasty. *N Engl J Med* 337:365, 1997.

362. Reaven PD, Parthasarathy S, Beltz WF, Witztum JL: Effect of probucol dosage on plasma lipid and lipoprotein levels and on protection of low density lipoprotein against in vitro oxidation in humans. *Arterioscler Thromb* 12:318, 1992.

363. Rodés, Côté G, Lespérance J, et al: Prevention of restenosis after angioplasty in small coronary arteries with probucol. *Circulation* 97:429, 1998.

364. Côté G, Tardif J-C, Lespérance J, et al: Effects of probucol on vascular remodeling after coronary angioplasty. *Circulation* 99:30, 1999.

365. Libby P, Ganz P: Restenosis revisited—new targets, new therapies (editorial). *N Engl J Med* 337:418, 1997.

366. Progress in Clinical Trials: CART-1 (Canadian Antioxidant Restenosis Trial). *Clin Cardiol* 25:38, 2002.

367. Lafont AM, Whitlow PL, Cornhill JF, et al: Alpha-tocopherol 5 reduced restenosis after femoral artery angioplasty in a rabbit model of experimental atherosclerosis (abstr.). *Circulation* 86(Suppl I):747, 1992.

368. Nunes GL, Sgoutas DS, Redden RA, et al: Combination of vitamins C and E alters the response to coronary balloon injury in the pig. *Arterioscler Thromb Vasc Biol* 15:156, 1995.

369. DeMaio SJ, King III SB, Lembo NJ, et al: Vitamin E supplementation, plasma lipids and incidence of restenosis after percutaneous transluminal coronary angioplasty. *J Am Coll Nutr* 11:68, 1992.

370. Burchenal JE, Keaney JF Jr, Curran-Celentano J, et al: The lack of effect of beta-carotene on restenosis in cholesterol-fed rabbits. *Atherosclerosis* 123:157, 1996.

371. Herbert JM, Bono F, Savi P: The mitogenic effect of H202 for vascular smooth muscle cells is mediated by an increase of the affinity of basic fibroblast growth factor for its receptor. *FEBS Lett* 395:43, 1996.

372. Lincoff AM, Topol EJ, Ellis SG: Local drug delivery for the prevention of restenosis. *Circulation* 90:2070, 1994.

373. Radovsky AS, Van Vleet JF: Effects of dexamethasone elution on tissue reaction around stimulating electrodes of endocardial pacing leads in dogs. *Am Heart J* 117:1288, 1989.

374. Sintov A, Scott WA, Gallagher KP, et al: Conversion of ouabain induced ventricular tachycardia in dogs with epicardial lidocaine: Pharmacodynamics and functional effects. *Pharm Res* 7:28, 1990.

375. Edelman ER, Adams DH, Karnovsky MJ, et al: Effect of controlled adventitial heparin delivery on smooth muscle cell proliferation following endothelial injury. *Proc Natl Acad Sci U S A* 87:3773, 1990.

376. Simons M, Edelman ER, DeKeyser KL, et al: Antisense c-myb oligonucleotides inhibit intimal arterial smooth muscle cell accumulation in vivo. *Nature* 359:67, 1992.

377. Villa AE, Guzman LA, Chen W, et al: Local delivery of dexamethasone for prevention of neointimal proliferation in a rat model of balloon angioplasty. *J Clin Invest* 93:1243, 1994.

378. Laporte S, Escher E: Neointima formation after vascular injury is angiotensin II mediated. *Biochem Biophy Res Commun* 187:1510, 1992.

379. Sirois MG, Simons M, Edelman ER: Antisense oligonucleotide inhibition of PDGFR-β receptor subunit expression directs suppression of intimal thickening. *Circulation* 95:669, 1997.

380. Hwang C-W, Wu D, Edelman ER: Physiological transport forces govern drug distribution for stent-based delivery. *Circulation* 104:600, 2001.

381. Hwang C-W, Wu D, Edelman ER: Stent-based delivery is associated with marked spatial variations in drug distribution (abstr.). *J Am Coll Cardiol* 37:1A, 2001.

382. Liistro F, Colombo A: Late acute thrombosis after paclitaxel eluting stent implantation. *Heart* 86:262, 2001.

382a. Hodgson J, Cacchione J, Bryant L, et al: Local intramural delivery of suramin or ethanol does not inhibit cellular proliferation in atherosclerotic lesions following angioplasty (abstr.). *Eur Heart J* 14(Suppl):277, 1993.

382b. Currier JW, Kalan JM, Franklin SM, et al: Effects of local infusion of doxorubicin or saline on restenosis following angioplasty in atherosclerotic rabbits (abstr.). The Restenosis Summit IV, Cleveland Clinic Foundation, May 28, 1992, Cleveland, Ohio.

383. Bailey SR: Local drug delivery: Current applications. *Prog Cardiovasc Dis* 40(2):183, 1997.

384. Guzman LA, Labhasetwar V, Song C, et al: Local intraluminal infusion of biodegradable polymeric nanoparticles. A novel approach for prolonged drug delivery after balloon angioplasty. *Circulation* 94:1441, 1996.

385. Lincoff AM, Furst JG, Ellis SG, et al: Sustained local delivery of dexamethasone by a novel intravascular eluting stent to prevent restenosis in the porcine coronary injury model. *J Am Coll Cardiol* 29:808, 1997.

386. Camenzind E, Bakker WH, Reijs A, et al: Site-specific intracoronary heparin delivery in humans after balloon angioplasty. *Circulation* 96:154, 1997.

386a. Rutanen J, Markkanen J, Ylä-Herttuala S: Gene therapy for restenosis. Current Status. *Drugs* 62:1575, 2002.

387. Woodworth TG, Nichols JC: Recombinant fusion toxins—a new class of targeted biologic therapeutics. *Cancer Treat Res* 68:145, 1993.

387a. Epstein SE, Speir E, Unger EF, et al: The basis of molecular strategies for treating coronary restenosis after angioplasty. *J Am Coll Cardiol* 23:1278, 1994.

388. Kreitman RJ, Fitzgerald D, Pastan I: Targeting growth factor receptors with fusion toxins. *Int J Immunopharmacol* 14:465, 1992.

389. Fu YM, Mesri EA, Yu ZX, et al: Cytotoxic effects of vascular smooth muscle cells of the chimeric toxin, heparin binding TGF-alpha-pseudomonas exotoxin. *Cardiovasc Res* 27:1691, 1993.

390. Epstein SE, Siegall CB, Biro S, et al: Cytotoxic effects of a recombinant chimeric toxin on rapidly proliferating vascular smooth muscle cells. *Circulation* 84:778, 1991.

391. Casscells W, Lappi DA, Olwin BB, et al: Elimination of smooth muscle cells in experimental restenosis: Targeting of fibroblast growth factor receptors. *Proc Natl Acad Sci U S A* 89:7159, 1992.

392. McDonald JR, Ong M, Shen C, et al: Large-scale purification and characterization of recombinant fibroblast growth factor-saporin mitotoxin. *Protein Expr Purif* 8:97, 1996.

393. Miller DD, Paige SB, Tio FO, et al: Lymphocyte/monocyte interleukin-2 receptor targeted fusion toxin therapy with DAB 486IL2 prevents proliferative post-angioplasty restenosis (abstr.). *Circulation* 84(Suppl II): II-70, 1991.

394. Pastore CJ, Isner JM, Bacha PA, et al: Epidermal growth factor receptor-targeted cytotoxin inhibits neointimal hyperplasia in vivo. Results of local versus systemic administration. *Circ Res* 77:519, 1995.

395. Prins J, DeVries EG, Mulder NH: Antisense of oligonucleotides and the inhibition of oncogene expression. *Clin Oncol* 5:245, 1993.

396. Biro S, Fu YM, Yu ZX, et al: Inhibitory effects of antisense oligodeoxynucleotides targeting c-myc mRNA on smooth muscle cell proliferation and migration. *Proc Natl Acad Sci U S A* 90:654, 1993.

397. Speir E, Epstein SE: Inhibition of smooth muscle cell proliferation by an antisense oligo-deoxynucleotide targeting the mRNA encoding PCNA. *Circulation* 86:538, 1992.

398. Simons M, Rosenberg RD: Antisense nonmuscle myosin heavy chain and c-myb oligonucleotides suppress smooth muscle cell proliferation in vitro. *Circ Res* 70:835, 1992.

399. Shi Y, Hutchinson HG, Ha DJ II, et al: Downregulation of c-myc expression by antisense oligonucleotides inhibits proliferation of human smooth muscle cells. *Circulation* 88:1190, 1993.

400. Morishita R, Gibbons GH, Ellison KE, et al: Single intraluminal delivery of antisense cdc2 kinase and proliferating cell nuclear antigen oligonucleotides result in chronic inhibition of neointimal hyperplasia. *Proc Natl Acad Sci U S A* 90:8474, 1993.

401. Bennett MR, Anglin S, McEwan JR, et al: Inhibition of vascular smooth muscle proliferation in vitro and in vivo by c-myc antisense oligodeoxynucleotides. *J Clin Invest* 93:822, 1994.

402. Azrin MA, Mitchel JF, Pedersen C, et al: Inhibition of smooth muscle cell proliferation in vivo following local delivery of antisense oligonucleotides to c-myb during angioplasty (abstr.). *J Am Coll Cardiol* 23(Suppl I):396A, 1994.

403. Shi Y, Fard A, Galeo A, et al: Transcatheter delivery of c-myc antisense oligomers reduces neointimal formation in a porcine model of coronary artery balloon injury. *Circulation* 90:944, 1994.

404. Stein CA, Cheng YC: Antisense oligonucleotides as therapeutic agents—is the bullet really magical? *Science* 261:1004, 1993.

405. Villa AE, Guzman LA, Poptic EJ, et al: Effects of antisense c-myb oligonucleotides on vascular smooth muscle cell proliferation and response to vessel wall injury. *Circ Res* 76:505, 1995.

406. Burgess TL, Fisher EF, Ross SL, et al: The antiproliferative activity of c-myb and c-myc antisense oligonucleotides in smooth muscle cells is caused by a nonantisense mechanism. *Proc Nat Acad Sci U S A* 92:4051, 1995.

407. Morishita R, Gibbons GH, Kaneda Y, et al: Pharmacokinetics of antisense oligodeoxy-ribonucleotides (cyclin B1 and CDC2 kinase) in the vessel wall in vivo: Enhanced therapeutic utility for restenosis by HVJ-liposome delivery. *Gene* 149:13, 1994.

408. Farrell CL, Bready JV, Kaufman SA, et al: The uptake and distribution of phosphorothioate oligonucleotides into vascular smooth muscle cells in vitro and in rabbit arteries. *Antisense Res Dev* 5:175, 1995.

409. Pickering JG, Isner JM, Ford CM, et al: Processing of chimeric antisense oligonucleotides by human vascular smooth muscle cells and human atherosclerotic plaque. Implications for antisense therapy of restenosis after angioplasty. *Circulation* 93:772, 1996.

410. Bennett MR, Schwartz SM: Antisense therapy for angio rest. Some critical considerations. *Circulation* 92:1981, 1995.

411. Sugiki H: Suppression of vascular smooth muscle cell proliferation by an antisense oligo-nucleotide against PDGF receptor. *Hokkaido Igaku Zasshi* 70:485, 1995.

412. Autieri MV, Yue TL, Ferstein GZ, Ohlstein E: Antisense oligonucleotides to the p65 subunit of NF-B inhibit human vascular smooth muscle cell adherence and proliferation and prevent neointima formation in rat carotid arteries. *Biochem Biophys Res Commun* 213(3):827, 1995.

413. Serruys PW, Kutryk MJB, Bruining N, et al: Antisense oligonucleotide against c-myc administered with the transport catheter for the prevention of in-stent restenosis: Results of the randomised ITALICS trial (abstr.). *Circulation* 98:I-1909, 1998.

414. Yamamoto K, Morishita R, Tomita N, et al: Ribozyme oligonucleotides against transforming growth factor-β inhibited neointimal formation after vascular injury in rat model. Potential application of ribozyme strategy to treat cardiovascular disease. *Circulation* 102:1308, 2000.

415. Lowe HC, Fahmy RG, Kavurma MM, et al: Catalytic oligodeoxynucleotides define a critical regulatory role for early growth response factor-1 in porcine coronary in-stent restenosis. *Circ Res* 89:670, 2001.

416. Hayry P, Myllarniemi M, Aavik E, et al: Stabile D-peptide analog of insulin-like growth factor-1 inhibits smooth muscle cell proliferation after carotid ballooning injury in the rat. *FASEB J* 9:1336, 1995.

417. Mitani K, Clemens PR, Moseley AB, et al: Gene transfer therapy for heritable disease: Cell and expression targeting. *Philos Trans R Soc Lond B Biol Sci* 339:217, 1993.

418. Blaese RM: Development of gene therapy for immunodeficiency: Adenosine deaminase deficiency. *Pediatr Res* 33 (1 Suppl):S49, 1993.

419. Nabel EG, Plautz G, Nabel GJ: Site-specific gene expression in vivo by direct gene transfer into the arterial wall. *Science* 249:1285, 1990.

420. Takahashi K, Fukui R, Kato O, et al: Percutaneous transluminal transfer of the human calponin gene for expression of intimal hyperplasia following arterial balloon injury: A model for successful gene therapy for restenosis after coronary angioplasty (abstr.). *Circulation* 88(Suppl I): 657, 1993.

421. Hiltunen MO, Laitinen M, Turunen MP, et al: Intravascular adenovirus-mediated VEGF-C gene transfer reduces neointima formation in balloon-denuded rabbit aorta. *Circulation* 102:2262, 2000.

422. Negoro N, Fukui R, Tsutikani E, et al: Down expression of calponin in smooth muscle of coronary artery lesions identifies a group of lesions

at high risk for restenosis after atherectomy: Implications for human gene therapy by direct calponin gene transfer (abstr.). *Circulation* 90(Suppl I): 142, 1994.

423. Indolfi C, Avvedimento EV, Rapacciuolo A, et al: Inhibition of cellular ras prevents smooth muscle cell proliferation after vascular injury in vivo. *Nat Med* 1:541, 1995.

424. Flugelman MY, Jaklitsch MT, Newman KD, et al: Low level in vivo gene transfer into the arterial wall through a perforated balloon catheter. *Circulation* 85:1110, 1992.

425. Plauta G, Nabel EG, Nabel GJ: Introduction of vascular smooth muscle cells expressing recombinant genes in vivo. *Circulation* 83:578, 1991.

426. Guzman RJ, Lemarchand P, Crystal RG, et al: Efficient and selective adenovirus-mediated gene transfer into vascular neointima. *Circulation* 88:2838, 1993.

427. March KL, Madison JE, Trapnell BC: Pharmacokinetics of adenoviral vector-mediated gene delivery to vascular smooth muscle cells: Modulation by poloxamer 407 and implications for cardiovascular gene therapy. *Hum Gene Ther* 6:41, 1995.

428. Ohno T, Gordon D, San H, et al: Gene therapy for vascular smooth muscle cell proliferation after artery injury. *Science* 265:781, 1994.

429. Guzman RJ, Hirschowitz EA, Brody SL, et al: In vivo suppression of injury-induced vascular smooth muscle cell accumulation using adenovirus-mediated transfer of the herpes simplex virus thymidine kinase gene. *Proc Nat Acad Sci U S A* 91:10732, 1994.

430. Steg PG, Tahlil O, Aubailly N, et al: Reduction of restenosis after angioplasty in an atheromatous rabbit model by suicide gene therapy. *Circulation* 96:408, 1997.

431. Chang MW, Barr E, Seltzer J, et al: Cytostatic gene therapy for vascular proliferative disorders with a constitutively active form of the retinoblastoma gene product. *Science* 267:518, 1995.

432. Maillard L, Walsh K: Growth-arrest homeobox gene Gax: A molecular strategy to prevent arterial restenosis. *Schweiz Med Wochenscht Suppl* 126:1721, 1996.

433. Asahara T, Chen D, Tsurumi Y, et al: Accelerated restitution of endothelial integrity and endothelium-dependent function after phVEGF165 gene transfer. *Circulation* 94:3291, 1996.

434. Kreuzer J, Denger S, Reifers F, et al: Adenovirus-assisted lipofection: Efficient in vitro gene transfer of luciferase and cytosine deaminase to human smooth muscle cells. *Atherosclerosis* 124:49, 1996.

435. Breuss JM, Cejna M, Bergmeister H, et al: Activation of nuclear factor κB significantly contributes to lumen loss in a rabbit iliac artery balloon angioplasty model. *Circulation* 105:633, 2002.

436. Feldman LJ, Tahlil O, Steg G: Perspectives of arterial gene therapy for the prevention of restenosis. *Cardiovasc Res* 32:194, 1996.

437. Steg PG, Tahlil O, Aubailly N: Reduction of restenosis after angioplasty in an atheromatous rabbit model by suicide gene therapy. *Circulation* 96:408, 1997.

438. Kaneda Y: Development of non-viral gene delivery system and its applications. *Nippon Rinsho* 54:2829, 1996.

439. Freed MS, Sfian MA, Safian RD, et al: An intensive polypharmaceutical approach to the prevention of restenosis: the Mevacor, ACE Inhibitor, Colchicine (BIG-MAC) Pilot Trial (abstr.). *J Am Coll Cardiol* 21:33A, 1993.

440. Kitazume H, Kubo I, Iwama T, et al: Combined use of aspirin, ticlopidine and nicorandil prevented restenosis after coronary angioplasty (abstr.). *Circulation* 78(Suppl II):II-633, 1988.

441. Parisi A, Foiland ED, Hartigan P, et al: A comparison of angioplasty with medical therapy in the treatment of single-vessel coronary disease. *N Engl J Med* 326:10, 1992.

442. Lefkovits J, Topol EJ: Pharmacological approaches for the prevention of restenosis after percutaneous coronary intervention. *Prog Cardiovasc Dis* 40(2):141, 1997.

CHAPTER 41

Gene Transfer in the Cardiovascular System

Jeffrey A. Medin

Peter M. Buttrick

It has been slightly more than 13 years since the first "proof-of-concept" studies were done in 1989 demonstrating the feasibility of gene transfer into the heart and vasculature of experimental animals. In this interval, enormous strides have been made both in the nature and sophistication of gene-targeting techniques and it is clear that many of the necessary tools are now established and nearly ready for potential clinical applications. The initial unrealistically high expectations for gene therapy have been tempered by investigators (also by the media and by the general public) and are now being replaced by systematic and rigorous experiments to better define targets for therapy and to synthesize reproducible and safe methods to accomplish treatment. Although gene therapy in the cardiovascular arena has lagged behind that in some other organ systems, novel, genetically encoded therapeutic agents are currently being developed, and appropriate cell targets are being investigated as the molecular participants and mechanisms in key cardiovascular pathways are identified by biochemical, cell biologic, and genome studies. Importantly, cardiovascular investigators are also recognizing some of the limitations of gene therapy (largely involving the efficiency of the gene delivery vehicles and the inadequate physical methods for getting the vector to its target site) and are developing novel therapeutic strategies. It is now quite clear, to paraphrase Friedmann,[1] that in the cardiovascular system, the immature genie that is gene therapy is now very much out of the bottle.

As an example of the promise and problems in gene therapy for the cardiovascular system, consider delivery of an angiogenic factor to improve blood flow to ischemic tissue. Studies in animals show that the addition of vascular endothelial growth factor (VEGF), either as a recombinant protein or as a result of gene transfer, can lead to development of collateral vessels in myocardial and hind limb ischemia models in rabbits and pigs (for review see Ferrara[2]). Based on these results, transfer of VEGF was one of the first clinical gene therapy trials for cardiovascular disease[3] and the first patient who received a plasmid vector encoding human VEGF applied to the polymeric coating of an angioplasty balloon demonstrated an increase in collateral vessels in an ischemic limb compartment at 4 and 12 weeks posttreatment and had an increase in resting and maximal blood flow. A companion study demonstrated improved distal flow in 8 of 10 limbs of multiple patients injected intramuscularly with this plasmid vector along with new collateral blood vessels in 7 of 10 limbs.[4] Despite these initial successes, it has become clear that the therapy is compromised by both technical and biologic problems. Expression of VEGF protein must achieve certain minimal levels for an effect and this is difficult to achieve with the current gene delivery systems. Systemic administration can potentially cause both hypotension and unwanted angiogenesis at distant sites (especially in the kidney and eye) and may expedite undiagnosed tumor growth.[5] Thus, peripheral toxicities exist and indiscriminate expression of this highly potent factor might be detrimental. In addition, short-term diffuse expression of VEGF does not have long-term efficacy. These issues all speak to the fact that biologic and therapeutic advances are necessarily linked, one cannot meaningfully precede the other. They also acknowledge the complex technical features of gene delivery, which must recognize the site, duration and extent of expression in a highly contextual fashion.

GENE DELIVERY AND EXPRESSION METHODS

At the outset, it is important to acknowledge a few fundamental issues: (a) Gene therapy, at this point in its evolution, is actually gene augmentation, wherein a correct gene or factor is coexpressed with the incorrect or missing gene in key target cells. Gene augmentation has two semantic subsets: gene addition and gene insertion. Gene addition describes expression of a corrective factor that is nonintegrating and carried as an episome within the host cell. Gene insertion involves insertion of the correct gene sequence into the genome of the target cell, either randomly or specifically. This is not to say that some therapies designed for actual correction of sequence defects at the genomic level (i.e., actual gene replacement) are not being pursued;[6,7] it is just an acknowledgment that those approaches are still being refined, and are not yet ready for clinical application. (b) Effective gene delivery still remains the bottleneck for the general application of this therapeutic approach. Cells in culture, and even in some small-animal models, can be targeted quite efficiently. Yet major limitations exist in the extrapolation of these results to large animals and especially to humans. Problems also remain in targeting expression or ensuring physiologic levels of the corrective factor at an appropriate time and place. Compounding this is the additional complication of the physical restraints of delivering the gene transfer vehicle in the cardiac system without undue trauma to the recipient. Gene therapy is also currently directed only to somatic cells as issues, both ethical and technical in nature, involving germ-line cell gene transfer have not been resolved.

GENE TRANSFER

Rather than detailing the types and uses of gene delivery vehicles (for which other reviews exist, see for example Miller,[8] Mulligan,[9]

TABLE 41-1. Characteristics of Various Vectors Used for Gene Tranfer

Liposome/Lipofectant	HVJ + liposome	RNA Virus (retrovirus)	DNA Virus (adenovirus)	DNA Virus (adeno-associated)
Easy to prepare	Easy to prepare	Complex preparation process; low titer	Complex preparation process; high titer	Complex preparation process; modest titer
No size constraints	No size constraints	Significant size constraints	Large size capacity	Modest size constraint
Targets many cell types	Targets many cells types	Targets dividing cells	Targets nondividing cells	Targets nondividing cell; ? tropism for muscle
Most likely transient transformation	Most likely transient transformation	Stable transformation (integration)	Transient transformation (episomal)	Transient transformation (episomal)
Low transfection efficiency	Adequate transfection efficiency	High transfection efficiency	High transfection efficiency	High transfection efficiency
Nonimmunogenic	Low immunogenicity	Immunogenic	Very immunogenic with brisk inflammation	Can be modified so as to have minimal immune reactivity
No potential vector related toxicity	Little vector-related toxic potential	Potential toxicity: tumor virus recombination; insertional mutagenesis	Little vector-related toxic potential	Little vector-related toxicity

HVJ = hemagglutinating virus of Japan.

Ledley,[10] Crystal[11]), we briefly mention the salient features and persistent problems of each vector system and outline a few current studies that suggest potential improvements in that vehicle as a gene delivery apparatus. Some details are summarized in Table 41-1. One fact that seems to be emerging is that a single delivery vector for all applications is not likely; rather, delivery will be modified for the specific requirements of each inherited and acquired disease.

Delivery methods employ either infectious or noninfectious approaches and are orchestrated towards ex vivo or in vivo applications of therapy. Noninfectious delivery is most often mediated by the addition to target cells of plasmid DNA or antisense oligonucleotides that either encode the sequence for the therapeutic factor or, in the case of antisense oligonucleotides, block translation of undesired protein products (such as viral or neoplastic gene components). For plasmid DNA, after uptake into cells, expression of the corrective factor occurs from an exogenous promoter contained in the plasmid. For delivery, the DNA is packaged by itself (naked DNA) or in complexes with viral coat proteins (such as those from the hemagglutinating virus of Japan) and/or with cationic lipid vesicles (liposomes). Plasmid DNA, along with these associated transfer-facilitating compounds, has the advantage that large genes or complex sequences can be transferred. Also the tropism is broad as a variety of cells including those that are proliferating and nonproliferating can be transfected. Recipient cells do not integrate the DNA into their genome so the risk of insertional mutagenesis, by the activation of oncogenes or the downregulation of expression of tumor-suppressor genes, is minimal. The host immune response to the delivery of naked DNA is also not generally an issue. The central problem for this type of gene delivery is efficiency, as most of the transferred DNA is degraded. Also, as the internalized plasmid DNA does not integrate, expression of the transfected gene is transient (although transient expression is sometimes actually desirable). As cells have developed methods to internalize various macromolecules they also have developed methods to screen or limit uptake of these agents and therefore large amounts of DNA/liposome complexes must be added on a per cell basis to achieve measurable transfection. The use of high levels of DNA/liposome complexes for in vivo delivery has a potential toxicity due to contaminating bacterial DNA carried along in the preparations.[12] Current research is focused on addressing a number of these issues.[13] For example, investigators are adding targeting ligands or endosome-disrupting peptides to

liposome complexes,[14] or generating pH-sensitive liposomes,[15] which can increase transfection efficiencies. Other investigators, examining the effect of serum, which reduces transfer efficiency in vivo and in vitro, have established that larger liposome/DNA complexes can possibly overcome this effect.[16] Lastly, some investigators are pursuing the idea that virosomes can be created that combine beneficial features from the above system along with the opportunity for genomic integration of the transfer agent (see below) and thus provide the possibility of actual long-term expression of the therapeutic factor.[17,18]

Since the late 1960s and early 1970s, when it was first recognized that correction of inherited or acquired diseases might be effected by gene transfer approaches (for a concise history see Friedmann[19]), investigators have focused on the use of viruses for delivery of therapeutic genes. Viruses have evolved very efficient methods to infect cells and even to integrate their carrier genetic sequence into the chromosomes of recipients. Harnessing these desired traits and minimizing those that are deleterious has involved substantial modification of potential candidate viruses. A wide variety of viruses or some of their components or properties have been adapted to gene delivery, including such diverse agents as vaccinia,[20] herpes,[21] influenza,[22] and other RNA viruses.[23] For this review, however, we focus only on a few of the most commonly used viral gene-delivery vectors.

The initial recombinant viral vector used for gene transfer was derived from modified murine retroviruses. These are single-stranded RNA molecules that are reverse transcribed into DNA, most often in the cytoplasm of recipient cells, and then imported into the nucleus and integrated into the host genome through an integrase function provided as part of the recombinant virion. Replication-deficient retroviruses are constructed by supplying the necessary functions for packaging of the vector in trans in packaging cells and not from the coding sequence or backbone of the virus itself. The first types of retroviruses to be adapted for therapy were "simple" retroviruses. Their genomes are small and very well characterized, comprised of the coding sequences for only a few polypeptides. Inherent in this biology are major limitations, including size, the efficiency of infection, and the fact that they do not infect nondividing cells.[24] In the cardiovascular system, cardiomyocytes are terminally differentiated and nondividing, and therefore not approachable using retroviruses, although other key target cells such as the vascular endothelium and smooth muscle are proliferative. Another problem is the reduced transfer capacity of recombinant retroviruses and the fact that retroviruses packaged in murine-based cells are very efficiently inactivated by human complement, thus limiting the possibility of in vivo delivery. Murine onco-retroviruses (which are simple retroviruses) also have an approximately 7-kb constraint on the amount of foreign DNA that they are able to package, which means that large, complex genes cannot be packaged. As a result, recent investigations have centered on the use of lentiviruses (such as recombinant HIV) where infection of nondividing cells (although they must pass through the $G1_b$ phase of mitosis)[25] has been demonstrated.[26] Lentiviruses are now commonly pseudotyped with the vesicular stomatitis virus-G protein,[27] which can increase the range of cells able to be infected and allows concentration of virions by ultracentrifugation, thereby allowing higher multiplicity of infection when incubated with target cells. Beating cardiac myocytes and differentiated multinucleated myofibers have been successfully transduced with these vectors.[28] Investigators are also performing ex vivo viral infections in the presence of protein fragments[29] or on positively charged surfaces,[30] which may help colocalize viral particles and recipient cells. Recently, some "humanized" packaging cells have been developed that are of primate[31] and nonprimate origin,[32] which may allow virions to be produced which will survive in vivo delivery into patients. In spite of these incremental advances, retroviruses remain fairly inefficient gene-delivery vehicles. Moreover, they also have the potential problem of insertional mutagenesis, which could activate oncogenes or shut down expression of tumor-suppressor genes, although this concern remains theoretical and has not manifested in any animal experiment or human protocol.

Current research on retroviruses has mostly centered on developing and refining HIV-based vectors or HFV-based vectors[33] to increase transduction frequencies, although no clinical protocol has yet been approved that employs these complex delivery agents. Investigators are also developing methods to sort transduced cells following infection[34,35] either to increase the fraction of positive cells returned to patients or to select positive cells in vivo by the addition of cytotoxic molecules that transduced cells are protected against.[36] Very recently, some important studies were undertaken to develop methods to actually expand transduced cells. One way this is done is by adding genes for monomeric tyrosine kinase receptors that can be activated by the addition of narrowly acting dimerizing reagents.[37,38] Cells have also developed ways to shutdown expression of inserted retroviral promoters through methylation, so some effort is directed toward abrogating this effect[39,40] or to add chromosomal architectural elements to retroviral vectors that can sustain transcription.[41]

A viral delivery system that has received a great deal of study, especially in the cardiovascular system, is recombinant adenovirus. Adenovirus contains a double-stranded linear DNA genome approximately 36 kb in length and can transfer large single-gene sequences or gene complexes with expression driven from a number of promoters. More than 40 human serotypes of human adenovirus are known, although serotypes 2 and 5 have been used most often for creation of recombinant gene transfer vectors. The major strength of adenovirus is that it infects a wide variety of cells, including quiescent cells, with great efficiency. In fact, adenovirus shows high tropism for smooth-muscle cells, cardiomyocytes, and vascular endothelium. The infecting recombinant adenovirus does not integrate into the host genome but remains episomal and can persist though diluted through multiple cell divisions. This vector can also be produced at very high titers (at levels of $>10^{12}$ plaque-forming units/mL). The major problem

with adenovirus, however, is the brisk immune response that it engenders. This complicates repeat delivery of the gene-transfer vehicle, shortens the duration of therapeutic gene expression, and risks immune-mediated host-cell damage. In fact, some investigators have observed that infection with adenovirus can actually induce arterial inflammation and thickening, which countermands a major therapeutic goal.[42] A high percentage of the human population have preexisting antibody titers to the serotypes commonly used for gene delivery. Tragically, manifestations of this potent immune response to the recombinant adenoviral delivery vector likely contributed to the first death directly attributed to gene therapy.[43,44] Production of recombinant replication-incompetent adenovirus for clinical protocol administration is also likewise not trivial as replication competent virus can appear through recombination.

A number of approaches have been undertaken to reduce the immune response generated to recombinant adenoviral vectors and to improve methods of viral production. The general approach has been to remove as much of the wild-type adenoviral genome as possible while maintaining the infectious function. This is especially important in view of a recent study that has shown that first-generation adenoviral vectors (lacking E1 and E3 sequences) affect the normal cell cycle progression and cyclin expression leading to a G_2/M arrest.[45] Next-generation vectors have been engineered by removing most of the E4 region as well, supplying the necessary ORF6 sequence as an inducible product in the packaging line.[46] Vectors have recently been constructed that have internal inverted repeats that generate recombination and produce small particles that can be packaged and are infectious.[47] Another group has shown that recombinant adenoviral vectors that are lacking viral genes can persist almost 3 months in vivo in muscle tissue as long as an immune response to the therapeutic or marking transfer product is reduced.[48] A helper-dependent adenovirus vector system has been created where the helper virus genome was not packaged due to removal of its packaging signal using the Cre/*lox* recombinase system.[49] Other investigators have designed next-generation helper cells or helper virus along with novel recombinant adenoviral backbones that minimize the chance of recombination leading to replication competent virus.[50,51] One group has even added "insulator" elements from the chicken globin gene locus to recombinant adenoviruses to overcome the interference of gene expression from viral regulatory elements.[52] Important to the context of this review, recent experiments have also shown low inflammatory responses in adenovirus-perfused cardiac isografts in mice,[53] even in the presence of a systemic vector-specific immune response. This is encouraging and indicates that this organ system may be less susceptible than others (such as the liver) to damage caused by this gene transfer vehicle.

Adeno-associated virus (AAV) is another major viral system that has received study as an agent for gene transfer to the heart, skeletal muscle, and vasculature. AAV is a small single-stranded DNA parvovirus with five serotypes that has not, by itself, been associated with any disease, although a high proportion of the human population has circulating antibody to the AAV coat protein. AAV infects through heparin sulfate proteoglycan receptors and integrates into the genome with relatively high frequency. Advantages of this delivery system are the relative simplicity of the genome and a comparative lack of immunogenicity or toxicity. Foreign DNA sequences are cloned between dual 145-bp inverted terminal repeats (ITRs) and are expressed off exogenously added promoters. Expression of viral replication and capsid proteins is driven by cotransfected plasmids. Problems with AAV have been mostly technical in nature, as production of recombinant virus requires associated helper viral functions, which then must be removed prior to administration to patients. These helper functions are usually generated by coinfection of producer cells by adenovirus (or HSV). AAV is also somewhat limited in the size of the insert that can be packaged (up to about 5 kb). Interestingly, wild-type AAV shows preferential integration to specific sites in human chromosome 19, which may decrease the possibility of insertional mutagenesis, although recombinant AAV may not show the same preference. AAV also appears to have a particular tropism for muscle tissue after subcutaneous delivery.[54] Some unresolved issues concerning AAV are whether recombinant vectors are truly nonpathogenic in humans and if these engineered constructs affect the cell cycle of infected cells—as the wild-type virus does.[55] Efficiency of transduction and production of high quantities of the transfer agent are issues, especially since in vivo delivery requires large numbers of recombinant AAV particles ($> 10^{10}$ viral particles/mouse) in some studies.[56,57] Nonetheless, the sustained expression of genes delivered using modified AAV in skeletal muscle of immunologically competent hosts is a very encouraging development.

Recent work on AAV has centered on improving production of viral stocks and enhancing infection efficiency.[58] Helper virus-free packaging of AAV is a major goal,[59] as appreciable amount of helper virus in clinical grade AAV preparations will elicit significant immune responses. Several groups have expressed adenoviral-derived packaging proteins E2A, VAI, and E4 from a cotransfected plasmid and have observed high vector yield and little replication-competent AAV.[60,61] Others have created inducible packaging cell lines (necessary because continual overexpression of the AAV rep protein is toxic to cells) that abrogate the need for cotransfection of a replication-containing plasmid along with the therapeutic gene-containing plasmid.[62] Lastly, an interesting hybrid vector has been created that combines AAV ITRs, flanking a reporter gene, placed within a recombinant adenovirus. Rearranged vector genomes are produced without cytotoxic viral proteins that infect recipient cells at efficiencies similar to those seen using recombinant AAV vectors[63] and may be simpler to produce.

One major area of emphasis for all delivery vectors is the effort to target transfer to certain cell types with the assumption that increasing cell specificity will limit undesirable peripheral effects. Despite this, efforts at targeting in general have been largely unsuccessful. As an example, efforts directed toward altering envelope proteins of recombinant retroviruses to focus targeting to CD34+ cells (which are primitive stem/progenitor cells) in the hematopoietic system have been quite disappointing.[64] It appears that the interaction between the viral *env* protein and the cellular receptor is constrained by both amino acid sequence and restrictive spatial considerations. Furthermore, although more virus can be bound to cells expressing the CD34 cell-surface antigen, viral entry was not facilitated indicating that other interactions are important for productive fusion events. Modest success has been obtained in targeting vascular lesions by remodeling the viral *env* protein to express a collagen-binding domain from von Willebrand clotting factor,[65] and recently, Boerger et al[66] described a receptor-ligand bridge protein that can be preloaded onto recombinant virions and that allows specific infection. Perhaps viral-delivery vehicles other than recombinant retroviruses will be more amenable to targeting. In support of this, targeting of recombinant adenoviruses has been addressed by a couple of methods, including the use of bridge proteins (antibody-receptor) and by altering the viral fiber protein,[67] but these strategies remain to be adapted into general use. Some recent studies

on AAV targeting have shown that nonpermissive cells can be transduced by using a bispecific antibody that facilitates interaction between the AAV vector and specific receptors on target cells.[68] In this case, binding to the alternate receptor did not affect internalization and transduction as it did with the modified retroviruses.

EX VIVO AND IN VIVO DELIVERY IN CARDIOVASCULAR GENE THERAPY

The application of gene therapy approaches to cardiovascular diseases has lagged behind that in some other organ systems. Most work in the cardiovascular area has been "proof-of-principle" in nature, and has involved tagging constructs in order to track expression in cells in culture or in animal models. In retrospect, considering the limited clinical successes observed in other organ systems, this caution seems warranted and even fortuitous. The limited cardiovascular studies to date can basically be split into two conceptual areas. The first is the ex vivo modification of cells followed by subsequent transplant. This is most appropriate for targeting disorders, such as familial hypercholesterolemia, in which a long-term corrective strategy is necessary. The second is the direct in vivo placement of the transfer vector into the desired locale. This is more appropriate for disorders such as restenosis following vascular damage, where the biologic process leading to the disease is transient. Both ex vivo and in vivo approaches have limitations and strengths. Manipulating (culturing and infecting) cells ex vivo can affect phenotype and subsequent function. On the other hand, ex vivo gene transfer increases the efficiency of delivery since selection strategies can be employed and higher amounts of the transfer vehicle can be specifically directed to the recipient cells of interest. Furthermore, the likelihood that the transfer agent will target the desired cell type is clearly increased (if it can be cultured) and the potential recipient immune effects are abrogated. In vivo approaches are, of course, handicapped by delivery, efficiency, and targeting issues. For in vivo correction, optimization of delivery of the gene transfer agent is paramount and often quite difficult to achieve. Some physical methods being explored for this type of delivery are discussed in a following section.

Delivery of Ex Vivo Modified Cells

Ex vivo modification of cells followed by reimplantation in the cardiovascular system was first reported in three studies in 1989. Two employed recombinant retroviruses that engineered expression of a reporter gene, in this case, β-galactosidase (β-gal). In the first study, Nabel et al[69] tagged endothelial cells which were then infused into porcine arteries and persistent reporter gene expression was detected in a limited area lining the blood vessel for up to 4 weeks. In the second study,[70] modified cells were grown on a vascular graft, which was then implanted. Reporter expression was detected at 5 weeks. In the third, cells expressing a potentially therapeutic gene [tissue plasminogen activator (t-PA)] were attached to an implantable device with the goal of making the hardware less thrombogenic,[71] an attractive theoretic approach that thus far has been clinically disappointing.

Other early approaches focused on modifying cells such as myoblasts that, after implantation within skeletal or possibly cardiac muscle, could repopulate infarcted areas or become platforms for systemic drug delivery. Initial studies using this approach were performed in the early 1990s where expression and detection in serum of proteins, such as the human growth hormone[72] and factor IX,[73] were shown. A later study[74] demonstrated that modified myoblasts placed in microcapsules and implanted into mice could secrete factor IX into the circulation. In a modification of this approach, cardiocytes themselves have been injected directly into hearts of adult syngeneic animals where they have integrated into a functional muscle syncytium.[75] This work opened the door for the possibility of genetic modification of these cells prior to implantation. A cautionary note is that incomplete electrical coupling or coordinate mechanical activity may result and could certainly be harmful to the recipient, and this issue will need to be more convincingly addressed as myoblasts or stem cells are considered for therapeutic myoplasty. Hematopoietic cells have been modified with the intent of creating systemic delivery platforms or circulating delivery vehicles as well. As an example, for lysosomal storage disorders that have cardiovascular effects including Fabry disease (see below), relevant enzymes in the deficient metabolic pathways are often secreted by cells engineered for overexpression. This allows metabolic cooperativity or "cross-correction" of bystander cells and has been demonstrated in cell culture and animal models.[76–79] Lastly, hepatocytes have been a major target for ex vivo gene transfer and appear to have provided the first clinical demonstration of efficacy from a gene transfer trial. This involved transfer of the low-density lipoprotein receptor into hepatocytes from a young woman with familial hypercholesterolemia followed by reimplantation.[80] A significant and sustained decrease in serum cholesterol occurred in that trial, although the levels never reached therapeutic clinical goals.

Some problems for ex vivo modification and reimplantation were mentioned above. Another important consideration for the cardiovascular system is the long-term effect of overexpression of certain factors on transplanted cells. In a recent study, a decrease in the expression of a putative therapeutic factor (t-PA) was observed over time as transplanted endothelial cells were exposed to local shear forces due to vascular flow.[81] One plausible explanation for this was that overexpression of the factor in the local context actually weakened cellular attachments and the modified cells became untethered. Nonetheless, ex vivo modification of cells followed by implantation is a strategy that will certainly be pursued for a number of disorders, although direct targets in the realm of cardiovascular gene therapy may actually turn out to be few.

Physical Methods for In Vivo Delivery of the Gene Transfer Agent to the Heart or Associated Vessels

For applications involving in vivo delivery, once a vector has been chosen and assembled, actual methods for the physical delivery of the vehicle to the cardiovascular system need to be formulated. Unlike in the hematopoietic system where cell delivery is pretty straight forward, in vivo delivery issues here add considerable complexity. Cardiologists are generally comfortable with catheter-based systems, so these have been adapted to facilitate delivery of gene-correction agents to arteries.[82] One of the first demonstrations of gene delivery directly to cells in the cardiovascular system was from Nabel et al,[83] who, in 1990, used a double-balloon catheter to deliver a retroviral vector encoding a reporter gene to a region of the porcine iliac artery. Expression persisted for months at the site of delivery and was not detected outside the target region. One problem with this type of delivery is that the mechanism of transfer, passive diffusion, is relatively slow, which increases the chance of tissue ischemia. Furthermore, if a vessel branch point exists between the balloons the chance of leakage into surrounding areas is high. To abrogate the first

problem investigators have modified perfusion catheters to allow distal perfusion and minimal ischemia.[84,85] To abrogate the second, that of delivery of the gene transfer vehicle to undesired locations through leakage and/or an effective diluting of the vehicle, investigators have developed balloon catheters coated with a variety of polymers containing the vector (usually recombinant adenovirus).[86] In fact, this type of delivery was used in the VEGF clinical study mentioned earlier.[3] Despite the theoretic appeal of this approach, loss of the delivery vehicle as a result of interactions with the bloodstream occurs, and limitations exist as to how much vector can be placed in the hydrophilic polymer and how much can be released through contact with the vessel wall. Other types of balloon catheters have also been used for gene delivery, including porous[87] and channeled.[88] One study compared surgical and catheter-based delivery techniques for the delivery of recombinant adenovirus[89] and found that different target cells were infected at a higher rate depending on the delivery technique. For example, the double-balloon catheter was most effective at infecting intimal cells and the polymer-coated catheter was most effective at targeting smooth muscle cells.

Other methods of in vivo delivery have been examined. Periadventitial nonocclusive polyethylene or silicon cuffs have been used to facilitate delivery. The gene-transfer agent then diffuses passively from the outside into the artery. Because the cuff fits around the vessel and blood flow is not interrupted, tissue damage and spurious leakage of the vector to surrounding tissues can be minimized. Antisense oligonucleotides have been delivered using this method to prevent the onset of neointimal hyperplasia in rats.[90]

Hemagglutinating virus of Japan (HVJ)-liposomes harboring β-gal-expressing plasmids have been infused into the myocardium through coronary arteries of rats and evidence of cell infection seen in a high percentage of myocytes.[91] Direct injection and other surgical approaches to the delivery of recombinant adenoviruses into the myocardium have also been explored.[92,93] Direct intramyocardial injection of naked VEGF DNA resulted in modest levels of gene expression, increased myocardial blood flow, and enhanced collateral formation in pigs that had mechanical coronary artery constriction.[94] Surgical isolation techniques, using clamps and ligatures, followed by injection of a plasmid engineering expression of a decoy RNA affecting the fibronectin mRNA-binding protein prevented closure of the ductus arteriosus in fetal lambs.[95] A final, novel and intriguing strategy for percutaneous transluminal gene delivery involves continuous pressure-regulated selective retroinfusion of coronary veins.[96] In this study, antegrade and retrograde delivery (via the great cardiac vein) were compared with and without ischemia in pigs, by using recombinant adenoviruses engineered to express luciferase and β-gal. It was found that retrograde delivery improved myocardial gene transfer during ischemia, perhaps by prolonging viral adhesion time, and vector distribution as measured by PCR, was limited to the targeted left anterior descending artery distribution.

The ideal physical delivery system will allow efficient and localized delivery of the corrective agent to a specific site while still allowing therapeutic manipulations of a different nature to occur if needed. Furthermore no harm should occur from the delivery regimen itself. With this in mind, two recent reports bear mentioning. In the first, investigators exploring delivery of cationic liposomes complexed with a β-gal-expressing plasmid into rabbit hearts, observed myocardial damage possibly due to macroaggregates of the transfer vector composite,[97] and false-positive readings of the β-gal reporter were also seen at the microinfarction site. In the second study, Hughes et al[98] examined gene transfer with a recombinant adenoviral vector into pigs that had received left thoracotomy followed by transmyocardial laser revascularization (TMR). They found that the TMR procedure limited transgene expression, as opposed to direct injection of the vector alone, possibly due to an increased localized immune response.

CURRENT AND FUTURE TARGETS FOR GENE THERAPY IN THE CARDIOVASCULAR SYSTEM

We now briefly review a few key cardiovascular defects for which gene-transfer approaches have been initiated, distinguishing between disorders in which the therapy can alter the disease course itself, and disorders in which the cardiovascular defects are secondary to other clinical manifestations. One issue that emerges, especially for conditions such as restenosis after arterial injury and angiogenesis, is the lack of consensus as to what factor is appropriate for gene transfer, as the processes that govern these disorders are not fully understood or suitably modeled. This will, undoubtedly, be clarified in the future, as the underlying mechanisms become better elucidated.

Restenosis

Angioplasty or other interventions that involve injury of the arterial wall induces a complex series of cellular and biochemical events, the result of which is intimal thickening and narrowing of the lumen of the vessel. Animal models have been extensively employed to study these effects. These generally rely on injury to previously normal vessels and may not be directly reflective of effects to damaged atherosclerotic tissues.[99] Thus identification of clear targets for gene therapy-based intervention for patients is not unambiguous. Another caution is the possibility that treatments that are too aggressive or sustained may lead to formation of aneurysmal dilatation, especially in the context of an intrinsically abnormal vessel. Nonetheless, transfer of a wide variety of therapeutic factors has been examined and many have been shown to have desirable effects (see Chap. 40). As comparative studies are performed in the future, appropriate targets, that have maximal therapeutic outcomes and minimal detrimental side effects, will be elucidated. It may even be possible that combinations of gene transfer approaches, employing both recombinant adenoviruses and antisense oligonucleotides together, targeted toward different moments in the biologic process, may be most effective.[99a]

Acknowledging the above caveats, several studies have examined adenoviral gene transfer of cytotoxic agents such as the HSV-tk (herpes simplex virus thymidine kinase)/ganciclovir system to injured vessels of atherosclerotic rabbits and pigs.[100,101] The idea behind this approach is that actively dividing cells will be specifically killed through the incorporation of phosphates into the ganciclovir molecule by cells that express HSV-tk, which then becomes a nucleoside analogue, leading to DNA chain termination. This strategy results in a decrease in the intimal/media (I/M) ratio after delivery. Cytosine deaminase, delivered by recombinant adenovirus, and the prodrug 5-fluorocytosine have been used as "suicide" gene therapy as well.[102] HSV-tk gene transfer has been used successfully in the clinic for the treatment of graft-versus-host disease after bone marrow transplantation.[103] Furthermore, a bystander effect exists,[104] which is useful in this cardiovascular context, as the effector chain termination molecule can be transferred to nearby uncorrected cells. Thus, if dividing, these cells can also be lysed, which broadens the

scope of the effect and reduces the requirement of high gene-transfer efficiency for effective therapy.

Cell-cycle modulators have also been studied in the context of reducing neointimal thickening. A number of genes regulate the transitions through the various checkpoints in the cell cycle in smooth muscle and endothelial cells. One interesting candidate gene that has received attention is the retinoblastoma (RB) gene product. This polypeptide, when unphosphorylated, affects cells at the transition point from G_1/S phase by binding to the transcription factor E2F. Phosphorylation of RB initiates a disengagement from E2F and allows cells to proceed through mitosis. In 1995, investigators transferred a constitutively active form of RB into the vessel wall and demonstrated a significant reduction of the I/M ratio in both rat and pig arteries.[105] This same group also demonstrated that adenovirus-mediated transfer of the p21 protein, which is a multifunctional cyclin-dependent kinase inhibitor involved in proliferation, also led to a reduction of the I/M ratio in rat arteries.[106] Recently, in additional studies, transfer of the same constitutively active RB product has also been shown to reduce neointimal thickening in vein grafts.[107] Other gene products involved in the cell cycle have been transferred as well. These include the p27 gene, which is another cyclin-dependent kinase inhibitor,[108] and the p53 gene, which interacts with p21.[109] There are also transcription factors such as Gax (growth arrest homeobox) that, when overexpressed, may decrease proliferation by arresting cells at the G_0/G_1 transition point. Overexpression of this factor in vivo also reduces the I/M ratio in rat arteries.[110]

Rather than only overexpressing factors that will stall progression through the cell cycle, studies have been performed to examine the possibility of decreasing cellular proliferation by blocking the upregulation or induction of cell proliferation signals using antisense oligonucleotides. This approach is limited by the efficiency of delivery and the specificity of targeting, but has shown some success in model systems. c-Myc and c-myb have been targeted by this approach,[111,112] as have cdc2 kinase and PCNA (proliferating cell nuclear antigen) in tandem.[113] Gene transfer of all of these has shown reductions in neointimal area in models of local vascular injury. Transcription factors have been targeted similarly, including a subunit of NF-βB (p65),[90] as have growth factors themselves, including basic fibroblast growth factor (bFGF),[114] and even cyclins targeted by using recombinant retroviruses expressing antisense sequences.[115] A significant reduction in medial hyperplasia was observed when a dominant negative form of H-ras was transferred into rat arteries by adenoviral gene transfer following endothelial injury.[116]

Lastly, amidst this plethora of potential therapeutic targets, some additional applications merit mention. VEGF itself, surprisingly, may have a possible use in this domain. The idea here is that overexpression of VEGF can initiate full and rapid recovery of endothelial cells at the injury site and that this will lead to a reduction in injury-related stimuli and decreased neointimal formation. This phenomenon has been demonstrated in the rat artery model.[117] VEGF also can modulate the nitric oxide system, which is a major target itself, as NO has antiproliferative properties and is a strong vasodilator. It also reduces platelet aggregation and the migration of leukocytes. Indeed, a number of investigators have transferred components of the NO synthase system to arteries in vivo by HVJ complexes and liposomes,[118,119] retroviruses,[120] and adenoviruses,[121,122] all with a resultant reduction in neointimal formation. Finally, in a true paradigm shift, Santiago et al[123] recently created an actual DNA-based enzyme targeted to the transcription regulator Egr-1 and demonstrated catalytic inhibition of Egr-1 and neointimal formation in rat carotid arteries.

Therapeutic Angiogenesis

Angiogenesis is the formation of new vessels from existing ones and the use of angiogenesis to facilitate the delivery of oxygen and nutrients to ischemic peripheral tissues and the myocardium is an important goal of therapy in the cardiovascular system (see Chap. 38). The delivery of VEGF is a major focus with which to implement these aims. VEGF has a number of effects.[2] It is a fairly specific mitogen, acting on vascular endothelial cells but not on smooth-muscle cells. It interacts with receptors including KDR, Flt-1, and RTK,[124] which causes dimerization and the activation of various signal transduction pathways. Numerous studies have examined the effect of VEGF, delivered either as a recombinant protein or expressed from gene delivery vehicles (usually adenovirus or plasmid DNA). One such study tested delivery of a single dose of recombinant VEGF protein into rabbit hind limbs.[125] This led to enhanced collateral vessel formation and improved tissue perfusion. Similar effects were observed when other isoforms of VEGF were transferred.[126] Transfer of VEGF plasmids directly into the ischemic myocardium has been suggested to reduce angina,[127] and the transfer of recombinant adenovirus expressing VEGF into rat iliac artery imparts some protection against vascular occlusion.[128] Amelioration of peripheral neuropathy (present in a high percentage of patients with limb ischemia) has also been demonstrated following intramuscular transfer of VEGF in the rabbit ischemic hind limb model.[129] As mentioned earlier, limited clinical trials have been performed with plasmid DNA encoding VEGF,[3,4] and modest improvements in blood flow and vascular function have been observed. Recombinant adenovirus has also been used for the direct intramyocardial delivery of VEGF in patients with coronary artery disease.[130] In that Phase I study, no adverse events were reported and very marginal improvement in clinical parameters were found, including in angina class and treadmill exercise assessments. On a related side note, an interesting conceptual hypothesis was recently presented in a study by Kanno et al.[131] These authors demonstrate that low-intensity electrical stimulation of skeletal muscle can up-regulate VEGF production and enhance local angiogenesis. This approach may actually turn out to be less expensive and less invasive than vector delivery, and it may even allow the possibility of multiple administrations with reduced associated systemic side effects.

Other factors in the angiogenic schema are also targets for gene therapy, either alone or in combination. bFGF is a broader mitogen than VEGF, acting on fibroblasts and smooth-muscle cells, as well as the endothelium. It also is a potent synergistic partner of VEGF.[132] bFGF improves collateral flow to chronically ischemic porcine myocardium and improves myocardial function.[133] Acidic FGF (FGF-1) was recently examined in coronary heart disease patients.[134] Twelve weeks postinjection, neovascularization was suggested by subtraction angiography. Angiopoietin-1 recruits smooth-muscle cells to the walls of new vessels[135] and has been transferred by intramuscular plasmid injection into rabbits; it also has facilitated hind limb revascularization.[136] Lastly, hepatocyte growth factor (HGF), which acts on endothelial cells (among others) but not on smooth-muscle cells, was recently transfected by HVJ-liposome-mediated delivery into the myocardium of rats and results in an increase in PCNA-positive cells and in the number of vessels around the injection site.[137]

Other Direct Targets in Cardiovascular Gene Therapy

Atherosclerosis leading to cardiovascular and cerebrovascular disease is a major cause of death. Reduced high-density lipoprotein (HDL) levels and increased low-density lipoprotein (LDL) levels correlate with a high risk of disease. On the other hand, high levels of HDL seem to have an antiatherogenic effect.[138] Studies employing gene transfer technology have been undertaken to impact the pathophysiologic processes involved in the progression of this disorder. One of the first genes to receive substantial study was apolipoprotein A-I (apoA-I), a component of the HDL complex. In 1994, two studies were published demonstrating that overexpression of apoA-I reduced the formation of atherosclerotic lesions in apoE-deficient mice.[139,140] Another study, in a similar model, indicated that increasing HDL through this mechanism has a direct effect on the vascular wall,[141] and in a very recent study, investigators showed that long-term adenovirus-based expression of apoA-I results in a marked antiatherogenic effect.[142] Other potential antiatherogenic targets include lecithin:cholesterol acyltransferase (LCAT), as overexpression of this enzyme prevents diet-induced atherosclerosis,[143] and the scavenger receptor class B, type I (SR-BI), which enhances reverse cholesterol transport and cholesterol removal from the body.[138] In fact, overexpression of SR-BI, which is a cell-surface LDL receptor in mice, by using recombinant adenovirus, significantly reduces LDL levels in plasma.[144] Combining some of the above candidates may also prove to be fruitful in the long run and to this end, polycistronic recombinant retroviruses were recently created that express both apoA-I and LCAT.[145]

A role for gene therapy can also be envisioned in transplantation[146] and some recent studies have been designed to address the tolerance and rejection issues that limit the long-term success of organ transplantation. In the first study, retroviral gene transfer was used to facilitate transplantation across species. Xenoreactive antibodies bind specific carbohydrate epitopes on donor tissues. Bracy et al[147] found that transfer of the specific porcine galactosyltransferase to murine bone marrow cells induced molecular chimerism and abrogated production of xenoreactive antibodies, thereby opening the door for the direct modulation of B cell tolerance. Another group[148] found that antisense oligonucleotides, which were directed against intracellular adhesion molecule (ICAM)-1 and transferred into hearts ex vivo using a hyperbaric transfection procedure, increased allogeneic recipient survival especially when an antibody to leukocyte function-associated antigen was also included. The "suicide" approach mentioned above has been used to demonstrate tolerance of cardiac allografts in discordant strains of mice when host T cells are specifically killed with ganciclovir.[149]

Gene therapy may also have a role in the treatment of heart failure itself, although the heterogeneity of the clinical disorder suggests that no single biochemical approach would be appropriate for all patients. However, it does appear as if abnormal intracellular calcium sequestration and a reduction in β-adrenergic receptor expression and function seem to be related to the progression to end-stage heart failure in a number of circumstances. Two very recent studies, both using recombinant adenoviruses as the gene-delivery vehicle, have addressed these issues. In the first,[150] investigators demonstrated that transfer of the β_2-adrenergic receptor in vivo, by injection of vector into the left ventricular cavity of normal rabbits while the aorta was cross-clamped, improved cardiac physiology for up to 21 days as measured by in vivo hemodynamics. In vitro studies in failing rabbit ventricular cardiomyocytes, in that same report, demonstrated that transfer of this receptor could rescue some level of cyclic AMP signaling in ventricular cardiocytes. In the second study,[151] the transferred gene was the sacroplasmic reticulum (SR) Ca^{2+} ATPase (SERCA 2a), which is downregulated in animal models and humans with heart failure. Here in vitro gene transfer into cardiomyocytes from patients with failing hearts restored contraction and relaxation parameters of the cells. These effects certainly warrant further study, as does the pursuit of other candidate genes[151a] that effect important regulatory moments in excitation-contraction coupling such as use of a dominant negative phospholamban. Important here, too, are considerations about the duration of expression needed to fully sustain corrective effects and whether repeat administration of the vector will be needed. It will also be critical to modulate gene and protein expression carefully so that unwanted effects of over expression, such as dysregulation of cytosolic calcium, can be avoided.

Gene therapy has been suggested for other cardiovascular aberrations as well.[151b] Antithrombotic factors, including cyclooxygenase[152] and t-PA,[153] have been expressed within the vascular endothelium to enhance clot lysis and/or to prevent platelet aggregation, although to date the biologic impact of these strategies has been modest at best. Antisense strategies using AAV-based vectors to block angiotensinogen expression and to treat secondary hypertension have been initiated with initial success in animal models.[154] In addition, myocardial reperfusion injury has been proposed as a therapeutic objective[155] and a number of potential gene targets have been suggested. Thus far, intracoronary transfer of the fibroblast growth factor-5 gene has been shown to improve contractile function and blood flow in ischemic hearts[156] and others have begun to explore the possibility of using free radical scavengers to prevent secondary tissue damage.

Targets with Secondary Effects on the Cardiovascular System

Other classes of disorders exist in which the defect manifests itself in the cardiovascular system through a secondary mechanism. An example is Fabry disease, a lysosomal storage disorder, which has an atypical variant that can selectively effect the heart.[157] Patients with this disorder accumulate lipid deposits with terminal galactosyl residues (such as globotriaosylceramide; Gb3) and develop left ventricular hypertrophy and heart failure. These patients often go undiagnosed because of the lack of clinical suspicion and any other coincident clinical manifestations. This form of the disorder may be a prototypic target for gene therapy as these patients have some residual lysosomal hydrolase enzyme activity, in contrast to typical Fabry patients, and may need only a small enhancement of enzyme activity to fully ameliorate the cardiac symptoms.[158,159] To effect this, it ought to be possible to target noncardiocytes so as to enhance secretion of the hydrolase activity that can then be taken up by bystander cells either in vivo or in vitro.[160] Indeed, one of us recently demonstrated in a murine model of Fabry disease that genetic correction of bone marrow cells allows metabolic cooperativity effects that largely abrogate the enzyme deficiency and Gb3 storage in the hearts (and other organs) of Fabry animals.[77] Indeed enzyme levels in the plasma at 6 months posttransplant were greater than levels seen in normal animals even with a fairly low percentage of corrected cells. Secondarily transplanted Fabry animals receiving bone marrow from the original corrected animals also showed correction in the heart.

The converse approach is to use cardiac or skeletal muscle not as a target tissue but rather as a platform from which to deliver therapeutic proteins or hormones. Some years ago, Dhawan et al.[72] and Barr et al[161] separately demonstrated that myoblasts could be cultured from skeletal muscle, transformed in culture, and then reimplanted into muscle and successfully maintained. A similar strategy was proposed by Sounda et al,[75] who showed that fetal syngenic myocytes could be directly injected into adult cardiac muscle where they could persist for an extended period of time, and even establish junctional links with adjacent cells so as to participate in the contractile unit. A potential application of this work is that myocytes could be functionally altered ex vivo prior to implantation and then used to deliver a gene product to the circulation and in fact the feasibility of this concept was confirmed by showing that human growth hormone could be secreted from a skeletal muscle "platform," albeit at relatively low levels.

CONCLUSION/FUTURE DIRECTIONS

The past decade of cardiovascular gene therapy has been one of enormous promise and excitement but has also been marked by relatively few and modest clinical successes. Technical issues related to vector design and efficiency of gene transfer remain and there is still an incomplete appreciation of the biology of the complex biologic processes that are being targeted. Given this, what does the future hold? Can this therapy move from infancy to adolescence and ultimately to maturity? The enormous power of the technologies and the explosive advances in our understanding of basic biology makes it almost a foregone conclusion that the field will move forward, that the "genie will escape." The links between academia and the biotech industry, which are more prevalent in this area (and perhaps more problematic) than almost any other,[162] will likely lead to the development of new vectors and delivery systems that successfully overcome issues of efficiency and immunogenicity. The remarkable recent advances in cellular and molecular biology will certainly identify novel and plausible targets for genetic manipulation.[163,164] However each advance will likely engender a critical reappraisal of the morality of the new technology. In the future, we can anticipate scrutiny of the ethics of tissue and organ generation from mesenchymal stem cells,[165] of the use of artificial chromosomes as nonviral gene-delivery agents that can effect persistent gene expression gene,[166] and the delivery of genes in utero[167] to correct congenital anomalies. Indeed, the future of gene therapy is bright, but the path is uncertain.

REFERENCES

1. Friedmann T: Human gene therapy-an immature genie, but certainly out of the bottle. *Nat Med* 2:144, 1996.
2. Ferrara N, Alitalo K: Clinical applications of angiogenic growth factors and their inhibitors. *Nat Med* 5:1359, 1999.
3. Isner JM, Pieczek A, Scainfeld R, et al: Clinical evidence of angiogenesis after arterial gene transfer of phVEGF165 in patient with ischaemic limb. *Lancet* 348:370, 1996.
4. Baumgartner I, Pieczek A, Manor O, et al: Constitutive expression of phVEGF165 after intramuscular gene transfer promotes collateral vessel development in patients with critical limb ischemia. *Circulation* 97:1114, 1998.
5. Springer ML, Chen AS, Kraft PE, et al: VEGF gene delivery to muscle: Potential role for vasculogenesis in adults. *Mol Cell* 2:549, 1998.

6. Cole-Strauss A, Yoon K, Xiang Y, et al: Correction of the mutation responsible for sickle cell anemia by an RNA-DNA oligonucleotide. *Science* 273:1386, 1996.

7. Alexeev V, Yoon K: Stable and inheritable changes in genotype and phenotype of albino melanocytes induced by an RNA-DNA oligonucleotide. *Nat Biotechnol* 16:1343, 1998.

8. Miller AD: Human gene therapy comes of age. *Nature* 357:455, 1992.

9. Mulligan RC: The basic science of gene therapy. *Science* 260:926, 1993.

10. Ledley FD: Non-viral gene therapy. *Curr Opin Biotech* 5:626, 1994.

11. Crystal RG: Transfer of genes to humans: early lessons and obstacles to success. *Science* 270:404, 1995.

12. McLachlan G, Stevenson BJ, Davidson DJ, Porteous DJ: Bacterial DNA is implicated in the inflammatory response to delivery of DNA/DOTAP to mouse lungs. *Gene Ther* 7:384, 2000.

13. Li S, Huang L: Nonviral gene therapy: promises and challenges. *Gene Ther* 7:31, 2000.

14. Simoes S, Slepushkin V, Gaspar R, et al: Gene delivery by negatively charged ternary complexes of DNA, cationic liposomes and transferrin or fusogenic peptides. *Gene Ther* 5:955, 1998.

15. Budker V, Gurevich V, Hagstrom JE, et al: pH-sensitive, cationic liposomes: A new synthetic virus-like vector. *Nat Biotechnol* 14:760, 1996.

16. Ross PC, Hui SW: Lipoplex size is a major determinant of in vitro lipofection efficiency. *Gene Ther* 6:651, 1999.

17. Hodgson CP, Solaiman F: Virosomes: Cationic liposomes enhance retroviral transduction. *Nat Biotechnol* 14:339, 1996.

18. Schoen P, Chonn A, Cullis PR, et al: Gene transfer mediated by fusion protein hemagglutinin reconstituted in cationic lipid vesicles. *Gene Ther* 6:823, 1999.

19. Friedmann T: *The Development of Human Gene Therapy.* Cold Spring Harbor, NY: Cold Spring Harbor Laboratory Press, 1999.

20. Uzendoski K, Kantor JA, Abrams SI, et al: Construction and characterization of a recombinant vaccinia virus expressing murine intercellular adhesion molecule-1: Induction and potentiation of antitumor responses. *Hum Gene Ther* 8:851, 1997.

21. Glorioso JC, DeLuca NA, Fink DJ: Development and application of herpes simplex virus vectors for human gene therapy. *Ann Rev Microbiol* 49:675, 1995.

22. Palese P, Zheng H, Engelhardt OG, et al: Negative-strand RNA viruses: Genetic engineering and applications. *Proc Natl Acad Sci U S A* 93:11354, 1996.

23. Hewson R: RNA viruses: Emerging vectors for vaccination and gene therapy. *Mol Med Today* 6:28, 2000.

24. Miller DG, Adam MA, Miller AD: Gene transfer by retrovirus vectors occurs only in cells that are actively replicating at the time of infection. *Mol Cell Biol* 10:4239, 1990.

25. Korin YD, Zack JA: Progression to the G_1b phase of the cell cycle is required for completion of human immunodeficiency virus type 1 reverse transcription in T cells. *J Virol* 72:3161, 1998.

26. Naldini L, Blomer U, Gallay P, et al: In vivo gene delivery and stable transduction of nondividing cells by a lentiviral vector. *Science* 272:263, 1996.

27. Burns JC, Friedmann T, Driever W, et al: Vesicular stomatitis virus G glycoprotein pseudotyped retroviral vectors: Concentration to very high titer and efficient gene transfer into mammalian and nonmammalian cells. *Proc Natl Acad Sci U S A* 90:8033, 1993.

28. Sakoda T, Kasahara N, Hamamori Y, Kedes L: A high-titer lentiviral production system mediates efficient transduction of differentiated cells including beating cardiac myocytes. *J Mol Cell Cardiol* 31:2037, 1999.

29. Hanenberg H, Xiao XL, Dilloo D, et al: Colocalization of retrovirus and target cells on specific fibronectin fragments increases genetic transduction of mammalian cells. *Nat Med* 2:876, 1996.

30. Hennemann B, Chuo JY, Schley PD, et al: High-efficiency retroviral transduction of mammalian cells on positively charged surfaces. *Hum Gene Ther* 11:43, 2000.

31. Cosset FL, Takeuchi Y, Battini JL, et al: High-titer packaging cells producing recombinant retroviruses resistant to human serum. *J Virol* 69:7430, 1995.

32. Mason JM, Guzowski DE, Goodwin LO, et al: Human serum-resistant retroviral vector particles from galactosyl (α1-3) galactosyl containing nonprimate cell lines. *Gene Ther* 6:1397, 1999.

33. Trobridge GD, Russell DW: Helper-free foamy virus vectors. *Hum Gene Ther* 9:2517, 1998.

34. Medin JA, Karlsson S: Selection of retrovirally transduced cells to enhance the efficiency of gene therapy. *Proc Assoc Am Phys* 109:111, 1997.

35. Pawliuk R, Bachelot T, Wise RJ, et al: Long-term cure of the photosensitivity of murine erythropoietic protoporphyria by preselective gene therapy. *Nat Med* 5:768, 1999.

36. Allay JA, Persons DA, Galipeau J, et al: In vivo selection of retrovirally transduced hematopoietic stem cells. *Nat Med* 4:1136, 1998.

37. Blau CA, Peterson KR, Drachman JG, Spencer DM: A proliferation switch for genetically modified cells. *Proc Natl Acad Sci U S A* 94:3076, 1997.

38. Jin L, Siritanaratkul N, Emery DW, et al: Targeted expansion of genetically modified bone marrow cells. *Proc Natl Acad Sci U S A* 95:8093, 1998.

39. Robbins PB, Skelton DC, Yu XJ, et al: Consistent, persistent expression from modified retroviral vectors in murine hematopoietic stem cells. *Proc Natl Acad Sci U S A* 95:10182, 1998.

40. Wang L, Robbins PB, Carbonaro DA, Kohn DB: High-resolution analysis of cytosine methylation in the 5′ long terminal repeat of retroviral vectors. *Hum Gene Ther* 9:2321, 1998.

41. Dang Q, Auten J, Plavec I: Human beta interferon scaffold attachment region inhibits de novo methylation and confers long-term, copy number-dependent expression to a retroviral vector. *J Virol* 74:2671, 2000.

42. Newman K, Dunn P, Owens J, et al: Adenovirus-mediated gene transfer into normal rabbit arteries results in prolonged vascular cell activation, inflammation, and neointimal hyperplasia. *J Clin Invest* 96:2955, 1996.

43. Lehrman S: Virus treatment questioned after gene therapy death. *Nature* 401:517, 1999.

44. Marshall E: Gene therapy death prompts review of adenovirus vector. *Science* 286:2244, 1999.

45. Wersto RP, Rosenthal ER, Seth PK, et al: Recombinant, replication-defective adenovirus gene transfer vectors induce cell cycle dysregulation and inappropriate expression of cyclin proteins. *J Virol* 72:9491, 1998.

46. Brough DE, Lizonova A, Hsu C, et al: A gene transfer vector-cell line system for complete functional complementation of adenovirus early regions E1 and E4. *J Virol* 70:6497, 1996.

47. Steinwaerder DS, Carlson CA, Lieber A: Generation of adenovirus vectors devoid of all viral genes by recombination between inverted repeats. *J Virol* 73:9303, 1999.

48. Chen HH, Mack LM, Kelly R, et al: Persistence in muscle of an adenoviral vector that lacks all viral genes. *Proc Natl Acad Sci U S A* 94:1645, 1997.

49. Parks RJ, Chen L, Anton M, et al: A helper-dependent adenovirus vector system: Removal of helper virus by Cre-mediated excision of the viral packaging signal. *Proc Natl Acad Sci U S A* 93:13565, 1996.

50. Fallaux FJ, Bout A, van der Velde I, et al: New helper cells and matched early region 1-deleted adenovirus vectors prevent generation of replication-competent adenoviruses. *Hum Gene Ther* 9:1909, 1998.

51. Sandig V, Youil R, Bett AJ, et al: Optimization of the helper-dependent adenovirus system for production and potency *in vivo. Proc Natl Acad Sci U S A* 97:1002, 2000.

52. Steinwaerder DS, Lieber A: Insulation from viral transcriptional regulatory elements improves inducible transgene expression from adenovirus vectors in vitro and in vivo. *Gene Ther* 7:556, 2000.

53. Chan SY, Li K, Piccotti JR, et al: Tissue-specific consequences of the anti-adenoviral immune response: implications for cardiac transplants. *Nat Med* 10:1143, 1999.

54. Donahue BA, McArrthur JG, Spratt SK, et al: Selective uptake and sustained expression of AAV vectors following subcutaneous delivery. *J Gene Med* 1:31, 1999.

55. Winocour E, Callaham MF, Huberman E: Perturbation of the cell cycle by adeno-associated virus. *Virol* 167:393, 1988.

56. Kessler PD, Podsakoff GM, Chen X, et al: Gene delivery to skeletal muscle results in sustained expression and systemic delivery of a therapeutic protein. *Proc Natl Acad Sci U S A* 93:14082, 1996.

57. Herzog RW, Hagstrom JN, Kung S-H, et al: Stable gene transfer and expression of human blood coagulation factor IX after intramuscular

injection of recombinant adeno-associated virus. *Proc Natl Acad Sci U S A* 94:5804, 1997.

58. Rabinowitz JE, Samulski J: Adeno-associated virus expression systems for gene transfer. *Curr Opin Biotech* 9:470, 1998.

59. Monahan PE, Samulski RJ: AAV vectors: Is clinical success on the horizon? *Gene Ther* 7:24, 2000.

60. Xiao X, Li J, Samulski RJ: Production of high-titer recombinant adeno-associated virus vectors in the absence of helper adenovirus. *J Virol* 72:2224, 1998.

61. Collaco RF, Cao X, Trempe JP: A helper virus-free packaging system for recombinant adeno-associated virus vectors. *Gene* 238:397, 1999.

62. Inoue N, Russell DW: Packaging cells based on inducible gene amplification for the production of adeno-associated virus vectors. *J Virol* 72:7024, 1998.

63. Lieber A, Steinwaerder DS, Carlson CA, Kay MA: Integrating adenovirus-adeno-associated virus hybrid vectors devoid of all viral genes. *J Virol* 73:9314, 1999.

64. Benedict CA, Tun RYM, Rubinstein DB, et al: Targeting retroviral vectors to CD34-expressing cells: Binding to CD34 does not catalyze virus-cell fusion. *Hum Gene Ther* 10:545, 1999.

65. Hall FL, Gordon EM, Wu L, et al: Targeting retroviral vectors to vascular lesions by genetic engineering of the MoMLV gp70 envelope protein. *Hum Gene Ther* 8:2183, 1997.

66. Boerger AL, Snitkovsky S, Young JA: Retroviral vectors preloaded with a viral receptor-ligand bridge protein are targeted to specific cell types. *Proc Natl Acad Sci U S A* 96:9867, 1999.

67. Curiel DT: Strategies to adapt adenoviral vectors for targeted delivery. *Ann N Y Acad Sci* 886:158, 1999.

68. Bartlett JS, Kleinschmidt J, Boucher RC, Samulski RJ: Targeted adeno-associated virus vector transduction of nonpermissive cells mediated by a bispecific F(ab'γ)2 antibody. *Nat Biotechnol* 17:181, 1999.

69. Nabel EG, Plautz G, Boyce FM, et al: Recombinant gene expression in vivo within endothelial cells of the arterial wall. *Science* 244:1342, 1989.

70. Wilson JM, Birinyi LK, Salomon RN, et al: Implantation of vascular grafts lined with genetically modified endothelial cells. *Science* 244:1344, 1989.

71. Dichek D, Neville RF, Zwiebel JA, et al: Seeding of intravascular stents with genetically engineered endothelial cells. *Circulation* 80:1347, 1989.

72. Dhawan J, Pabn LC, Pavlath GK, et al: Systemic delivery of human growth hormone by injection of genetically engineered myoblasts. *Science* 254:1509, 1991.

73. Yao SN, Kurachi K: Expression of human factor IX in mice after injection of genetically modified myoblasts. *Proc Natl Acad Sci U S A* 89:3357, 1992.

74. Hortelano G, Al-Hendy A, Ofosu FA, Chang PL: Delivery of human factor IX in mice by encapsulated recombinant myoblasts: A novel approach towards allogeneic gene therapy of hemophilia B. *Blood* 87:5095, 1996.

75. Sounpa MH, Koh GY, Klug MG, Field LJ: Formation of nascent intercalated disks between grafted fetal cardiocytes and host myocardium. *Science* 264:98, 1994.

76. Wolfe JH, Sands MS, Barker JE, et al: Reversal of pathology in murine mucopolysaccharidosis type VII by somatic cell gene transfer. *Nature* 360:749, 1992.

77. Takenaka T, Murray GJ, Qin G, et al: Long-term enzyme correction and lipid reduction in multiple organs of primary and secondary transplanted Fabry mice receiving transduced bone marrow cells. *Proc Natl Acad Sci U S A* 97:7515, 2000.

78. Fairbairn LJ, Lashford LS, Spooncer E, et al: Long-term in vitro correction of α-L-iduronidase deficiency (Hurler syndrome) in human bone marrow. *Proc Natl Acad Sci U S A* 93:2025, 1996.

79. Takenaka T, Hendrickson CS, Tworek DM, et al: Enzymatic and functional correction along with long-term enzyme secretion from transduced bone marrow hematopoietic stem/progenitor and stromal cells derived from patients with Fabry disease. *Exp Hematol* 27:1149, 1999.

80. Grossman M, Raper SE, Kozarsky K, et al: Successful ex vivo gene therapy directed to liver in a patient with familial hypercholesterolemia. *Nat Genet* 6:335, 1994.

81. Dunn PF, Newman KD, Jones M, et al: Seeding of vascular grafts with genetically modified endothelial cells: Secretion of recombinant

t-PA results in decreased seeded cell retention in vitro and in vivo. *Circulation* 93:1439, 1996.

82. Feldman LJ, Steg G: Optimal techniques for arterial gene transfer. *Cardiovasc Res* 35:391, 1997.

83. Nabel EG, Plautz G, Nabel GJ: Site-specific gene expression in vivo by direct gene transfer into the arterial wall. *Science* 249:1285, 1990.

84. Mitchel JF, Fram DB, Palme DF, et al: Molecular and cellular cardiology: Enhanced intracoronary thrombolysis with urokinase using a novel local drug delivery system: in vitro, in vivo, and clinical studies. *Circulation* 91:785, 1995.

85. Tahlil O, Brami M, Feldman LJ, et al: The dispatch catheter as a delivery tool for arterial gene transfer. *Cardiovasc Res* 33:181, 1997.

86. Steg PG, Feldman LJ, Scoazec J-Y, et al: Arterial gene transfer to rabbit endothelial and smooth muscle cells using percutaneous delivery of an adenoviral vector. *Circulation* 90:1648, 1994.

87. Wolinsky H, Thung SN: Use of a perforated balloon catheter to deliver concentrated heparin into the wall of the normal canine artery. *J Am Coll Cardiol* 15:475, 1990.

88. Feldman LJ, Steg PG, Zheng LP, et al: Low efficiency of percutaneous adenovirus-mediated arterial gene transfer in the atherosclerosis rabbit. *J Clin Invest* 95:2662, 1995.

89. Willard JE, Landau C, Glamann B, et al: Genetic modification of the vessel wall: Comparison of surgical and catheter-based techniques for delivery of recombinant adenovirus. *Circulation* 89:2190, 1994.

90. Autieri MV, Yue T, Ferstein GZ, Ohlstein E: Antisense oligonucleotides to the p65 subunit of NF-κB inhibit humans vascular smooth muscle cell adherence and proliferation and prevent neointima formation in rat carotid arteries. *Biochem Biophys Res Commun* 213:827, 1995.

91. Sawa Y, Kaneda Y, Bai HZ, et al: Efficient transfer of oligonucleotides and plasmid DNA into the whole heart through the coronary artery. *Gene Ther* 5:1472, 1998.

92. French BA, Mazur W, Geske RS, Bolli R: Direct in vivo gene transfer into porcine myocardium using replication-deficient adenoviral vectors. *Circ Res* 90:2414, 1994.

93. Magovern CJ, Mack CA, Zhang J, et al: Direct in vivo gene transfer to canine myocardium using a replication-deficient adenovirus vector. *Ann Thorac Surg* 62:425, 1996.

94. Tio RA, Tkebuchava T, Scheuermann TH, et al: Intramyocardial gene therapy with naked DNA encoding vascular endothelial growth factor improves collateral flow to ischemic myocardium. *Hum Gene Ther* 10:2953, 1999.

95. Mason CAE, Bigras J-L, O'Blenes SB, et al: Gene transfer in utero biologically engineers a patent ductus arteriosus in lambs by arresting fibronectin-dependent neointimal formation. *Nat Med* 5:176, 1999.

96. Boekstegers P, von Degenfeld G, Giehrl W, et al: Myocardial gene transfer by selective pressure-regulated retroinfusion of coronary veins. *Gene Ther* 7:232, 2000.

97. Wright MJ, Rosenthal E, Stewart L, et al: β-Galactosidase staining following intracoronary infusion of cationic liposomes in the in vivo rabbit heart is produced by microinfarction rather than effective gene transfer: a cautionary tale. *Gene Ther* 5:301, 1998.

98. Hughes GC, Annex BH, Yin B, et al: Transmyocardial laser revascularization limits in vivo adenoviral-mediated gene transfer in porcine myocardium. *Cardiovasc Res* 44:81, 1999.

99. Libby P: Gene therapy of restenosis: Promises and perils. *Circ Res* 82:404, 1998.

99a. Rutanen J, Markkanen J, Ylä-Herttuala S: Gene therapy for restenosis: Current status. *Drugs* 62:1575, 2002.

100. Simari RD, San H, Rekhter M, et al: Regulation of cellular proliferation and intimal formation following balloon injury in arthrosclerotic rabbit arteries. *J Clin Invest* 98:225, 1996.

101. Steg PG, Tahlil O, Aubailly N, et al: Reduction of restenosis after angioplasty in an atheromatous rabbit model by suicide gene therapy. *Circulation* 96:408, 1997.

102. Harrell RL, Rajanayagam S, Doanes AM, et al: Inhibition of vascular smooth muscle cell proliferation and neointimal accumulation by adenovirus-mediated gene transfer of cytosine deaminase. *Circulation* 96:621, 1997.

103. Bonini C, Ferrari G, Verzeletti S, et al: HSV-tk gene transfer into donor lymphocytes for control of allogeneic graft-versus-leukemia. *Science* 276:1719, 1997.

104. Freeman SM, Abboud CN, Whartenby KA, et al: The "bystander effect": Tumor regression when a fraction of the tumor mass is genetically modified. *Cancer Res* 53:5274, 1993.

105. Chang MW, Barr E, Seltzer J, et al: Cytostatic gene therapy for vascular proliferative disorders with a constitutively active form of the retinoblastoma gene product. *Science* 267:518, 1995.

106. Chang MW, Barr W, Lu MM, et al: Adenovirus-mediated overexpression of the cyclin/cyclin-dependent kinase inhibitor, p21, inhibits vascular smooth muscle cell proliferation and neointima formation in the rat carotid artery model of balloon angioplasty. *J Clin Invest* 96:2260, 1995.

107. Schwartz LB, Moawad J, Svensson EC, et al: Adenoviral-mediated gene transfer of a constitutively active form of the retinoblastoma gene product attenuates neointimal thickening in experimental vein grafts. *J Vasc Surg* 29:874, 1999.

108. Chen D, Krasinski K, Chen D, et al: Downregulation of cyclin-dependent kinase 2 activity and cyclin αA promoter activity in vascular smooth muscle cells by p21^{kip1}, an inhibitor of neointima formation in the rat carotid artery. *J Clin Invest* 99:2334, 1997.

109. Yonemitsu Y, Kaneda Y, Tanaka S, et al: Transfer of wild-type p53 gene effectively inhibits vascular smooth muscle cell proliferation in vitro and in vivo. *Circ Res* 82:147, 1998.

110. Maillard L, van Belle E, Smith RC, et al: Percutaneous delivery of the Gax gene inhibits vessel stenosis in a rabbit model of balloon angioplasty. *Cardiovasc Res* 35:536, 1997.

111. Shi Y, Fard A, Galeo A, et al: Cellular, molecular, biological, and immunological research: Transcatheter delivery of c-myc antisense oligomers reduces neointimal formation in a porcine model of coronary artery balloon injury. *Circulation* 90:944, 1994.

112. Gunn J, Holt CM, Francis SE, et al: The effect of oligonucleotides to c-myb on vascular smooth muscle cell proliferation and neointima formation after porcine coronary angioplasty. *Circ Res* 80:520, 1997.

113. Morishita R, Gibbons GH, Ellison KE, et al: Single intraluminal delivery of antisense cdc2 kinase and proliferating-cell nuclear antigen oligonucleotides results in chronic inhibition of neointimal hyperplasia. *Proc Natl Acad Sci U S A* 90:8474, 1993.

114. Hanna AK, Fox JC, Neschis DG, et al: Antisense basic fibroblast growth factor gene transfer reduces neointimal thickening after arterial injury. *J Vasc Surg* 25:320, 1997.

115. Zhu NL, Wu L, Liu PX, et al: Downregulation of cyclin G1 expression by retrovirus-mediated antisense gene transfer inhibits vascular smooth muscle cell proliferation and neointima formation. *Circulation* 96:628, 1997.

116. Ueno H, Yamamoto H, Ito S, et al: Adenovirus-mediated transfer of a dominant-negative H-ras suppresses neointimal formation in balloon-injured arteries in vivo. *Arterioscler Thromb Vasc Biol* 17:898, 1997.

117. Asahara T, Bauters C, Pastore C, et al: Molecular and cellular cardiology: Local delivery of vascular endothelial growth factor accelerates reendothelialization and attenuates intimal hyperplasia in balloon-injured rat carotid artery. *Circulation* 91:2793, 1995.

118. von der Leyen HE, Gibbons GH, Morishita R, et al: Gene therapy inhibiting neointimal vascular lesion: In vivo transfer of endothelial cell nitric oxide synthase gene. *Proc Natl Acad Sci U S A* 92:1137, 1995.

119. Veit K, Boissel JP, Buerke M, et al: Highly efficient liposome-mediated gene transfer of inducible nitric oxide synthase in vivo and in vitro in vascular smooth muscle cells. *Cardiovasc Res* 43:808, 1999.

120. Chen L, Daum G, Forough R, et al: Overexpression of human endothelial nitric oxide synthase in rat vascular smooth muscle cells in balloon-injured carotid artery. *Circ Res* 82:862, 1998.

121. Shears LL, Kibbe MR, Murdock A, et al: Efficient inhibition of intimal hyperplasia by adenovirus-mediated inducible nitric oxide synthase gene transfer to rats and pigs in vivo. *J Am Coll Surg* 187:295, 1998.

122. Varenne O, Pislaru S, Gillijns H, et al: Local adenovirus-mediated transfer of human endothelial nitric oxide synthase reduces luminal narrowing after coronary angioplasty in pigs. *Circulation* 98:919, 1998.

123. Santiago FS, Lowe HC, Kavurma MM, et al: New DNA enzyme targeting Egr-1 mRNA inhibits vascular smooth muscle proliferation and regrowth after injury. *Nat Med* 5:1264, 1999.

124. Neufeld G, Cohen T, Gengrinovitch S, Poltorak Z: Vascular endothelial growth factor (VEGF) and its receptors. *FASEB J* 13:9, 1999.

125. Takeshita S, Zheng LP, Brogi E, et al: Therapeutic angiogenesis: A single intraarterial bolus of vascular endothelial growth factor augments revascularization in a rabbit ischemic hind limb model. *J Clin Invest* 93:662, 1994.

126. Takeshita S, Tsurumi Y, Couffinahl T, et al: Gene transfer of naked DNA encoding for three isoforms of vascular endothelial growth factor stimulates collateral development in vivo. *Lab Invest* 75:487, 1996.

127. Losordo DW, Vale PR, Symes JF, et al: Gene therapy for myocardial angiogenesis: Initial clinical results with direct myocardial injection of phVEGF165 as sole therapy for myocardial ischemia. *Circulation* 98:2800, 1998.

128. Mack CA, Magovern CJ, Budenbender KT, et al: Salvage angiogenesis induced by adenovirus-mediated gene transfer of vascular endothelial growth factor protects against ischemic vascular occlusion. *J Vasc Surg* 27:699, 1998.

129. Schratzberger P, Schratzberger G, Silver M, et al: Favorable effect of VEGF gene transfer on ischemic peripheral neuropathy. *Nat Med* 6:405, 2000.

130. Rosengart TK, Lee LY, Patel SR, et al: Angiogenesis gene therapy: Phase I assessment of direct intramyocardial administration of an adenovirus vector expressing VEGF121 cDNA to individuals with clinically significant severe coronary artery disease. *Circulation* 100:468, 1999.

131. Kanno S, Oda N, Abe M, et al: Establishment of a simple and practical procedure applicable to therapeutic angiogenesis. *Circulation* 99:2682, 1999.

132. Pepper MS, Ferrara N, Orci L, Montesano R: Potent synergism between vascular endothelial growth factor and basic fibroblast growth factor in the induction of angiogenesis in vitro. *Biochem Biophys Res Commun* 3:211, 1992.

133. Harada K, Grossman W, Friedman M, et al: Basic fibroblast growth factor improves myocardial function in chronically ischemic porcine hearts. *J Clin Invest* 94:623, 1994.

134. Schumacher MD, Pecher MD, von Specht BU, et al: Induction of neoangiogenesis in ischemic myocardium by human growth factors: First clinical results of a new treatment of coronary heart disease. *Circulation* 97:645, 1998.

135. Suri C, Jones PF, Patan S, et al: Requisite role of angiopoietin-1, a ligand for the TIE2 receptor, during embryonic angiogenesis. *Cell* 87:1171, 1996.

136. Shyu K-G, Manor O, Magner M, et al: Direct intramuscular injection of plasmid DNA encoding angiopoietin-1 but not angiopoietin-2 augments revascularization in the rabbit ischemic hind limb. *Circulation* 98:2081, 1998.

137. Aoki M, Morishita R, Taniyama Y, et al: Angiogenesis induced by hepatocyte growth factor in non-infarcted myocardium and infarcted myocardium: Up-regulation of essential transcription factor for angiogenesis, ets. *Gene Ther* 7:417, 2000.

138. Acton SL, Kozarsky KF, Rigotti A: The HDL receptor SR-BI: A new therapeutic target for atherosclerosis? *Mol Med Today* 5:518, 1999.

139. Paszty C, Maeda N, Verstuyft J, Rubin EM: Apolipoprotein AI transgene corrects apolipoprotein E deficiency-induced atherosclerosis in mice. *J Clin Invest* 94:899, 1994.

140. Plump AS, Scott CJ, Breslow JL: Human apolipoprotein A-I gene expression increases high density lipoprotein and suppresses atherosclerosis in the apolipoprotein E-deficient mouse. *Proc Natl Acad Sci U S A* 91:9607, 1994.

141. de Geest B, Zhao Z, Collen D, Holvoet P: Effects of adenovirus-mediated human apo A-I gene transfer on neointima formation after endothelial denudation in apo E-deficient mice. *Circulation* 98:2081, 1998.

142. Benoit P, Emmanuel F, Caillaud JM, et al: Somatic gene transfer of human apo A-I inhibits atherosclerosis progression in mouse models. *Circulation* 99:105, 1999.

143. Hoeg JM, Santamarina-Fojo S, Berard AM, et al: Overexpression of lecithin:cholesterol acyltransferase in transgenic rabbits prevents diet-induced atherosclerosis. *Proc Natl Acad Sci U S A* 93:11448, 1996.

144. Kozarsky KF, Donahee MH, Rigotti A, et al: Overexpression of the HDL receptor SR-BI alters plasma HDL and bile cholesterol levels. *Nature* 387:414, 1997.

145. Fan L, Owen JS, Dickson G: Construction and characterization of polycistronic retrovirus vectors for sustained and high-level

co-expression of apolipoprotein A-I and lecithin-cholesterol acyl-transferase. *Atherosclerosis* 147:139, 1999.

146. Giannoukakis N, Thomson A, Robbins P: Gene therapy in transplantation. *Gene Ther* 6,1499, 1999.

147. Bracy JL, Sach DL, Iacomini J: Inhibition of xenoreactive natural antibody production by retroviral gene therapy. *Science* 281:1845, 1998.

148. Poston AS, Mann MJ, Hoyt EG, et al: Antisense oligonucleotides prevent acute cardiac allograft rejection via a novel, nontoxic, highly efficient transfection method. *Transplant* 68:825, 1999.

149. Braunberger E, Raynal-Raschilas N, Thomas-Vaslin V, et al: Tolerance induced without immunosuppression in a T-lymphocyte suicide-gene therapy cardiac allograft model in mice. *J Thorac Cardiovasc Surg* 119:46, 2000.

150. Maurice JP, Hata JA, Shah AS, et al: Enhancement of cardiac function after adenoviral-mediated in vivo intracoronary β_2-adrenergic receptor gene delivery. *J Clin Invest* 104:21, 1999.

151. del Monte F, Harding SE, Schmidt U, et al: Restoration of contractile function in isolated cardiomyocytes from failing human hearts by gene transfer of SERCA 2a. *Circulation* 100:2308, 1999.

151a. Ikeda Y, Gu Y, Iwanaga Y, et al: Restoration of deficient membrane proteins in the cardiomyopathic hamster by in vivo cardiac gene transfer. *Circulation* 105:502, 2002.

151b. Lim B-K, Choe S-C, Shin J-O, et al: Local expression of interleukin-1 receptor antagonist by plasmid DNA improves mortality and decreases myocardial inflammation in experimental Coxsackieviral myocarditis. *Circulation* 105:1278, 2002.

152. Zoldhelyi P, McNatt J, Xu X-M, et al: Prevention of arterial thrombosis by adenovirus-mediated transfer of the cyclooxygenase gene. *Circulation* 93:10, 1996.

153. Carmeliet P, Moons L, Dewerchin M, et al: Insights in vessel development and vascular disorders using targeted inactivation and transfer of vascular endothelial growth factor, the tissue factor, and the plasminogen system. *Ann N Y Acad Sci* 811:191, 1997.

154. Tang X, Mohuczy D, Zhang YC, et al: Intravenous angiotensinogen antisense in AAV-based vector decreases hypertension. *Am J Phys* 277:H2392, 1999.

155. Das DK, Engelman RM, Maulik N, et al: Molecular targets of gene therapy. *Ann Thorac Surg* 68:1929, 1999.

156. Giordano FJ, Ping P, McKirnan MD: Intracoronary gene transfer of fibroblast growth factor-5 increases blood flow and contractile function in an ischemic region of the heart. *Nat Med* 2:534, 1996.

157. Sakuraba H, Yanagawa Y, Igarashi T, et al: Cardiovascular manifestations in Fabry's disease. *Clin Genet* 29:276, 1986.

158. Eng CM, Guffon N, Wilcox WR, et al for the International Collaborative Fabry Disease Study Group: Safety and efficacy of recombinant human α-galactosidase a replacement therapy in Fabry's disease. *N Engl J Med* 345:9, 2001.

159. Frustaci A, Chimenti C, Ricci R, et al: Improvement in cardiac function in the cardiac variant of Fabry's disease with galactose-infusion therapy. *N Engl J Med* 345:25, 2001.

160. Gahl WA: New therapies for Fabry's disease (editorial). *N Engl J Med* 345:55, 2001.

161. Barr E, Leiden JM: Systemic delivery of recombinant proteins by genetically modified myoblasts. *Science* 254(1278,2002):1507, 1991.

162. Rosenberg LE, Schechter AN: Gene therapist, heal thyself. *Science* 287:1751, 2000.

163. Asahara T, Murohara T, Sullivan A, et al: Isolation of putative progenitor endothelial cells for angiogenesis. *Science* 275:964, 1997.

164. Shi Q, Rafii S, Wu MH, et al: Evidence for circulating bone marrow-derived endothelial cells. *Blood* 92:362, 1998.

165. Pittenger MF, Mackay AM, Beck SC, et al: Multilineage potential of adult human mesenchymal stem cells. *Science* 284:143, 1999.

166. Harrington JJ, Van Bokkelen G, Mays RW, et al: Formation of de novo centromeres and construction of first-generation human artificial microchromosomes. *Nat Genet* 15:345, 1997.

167. Zanjani ED, Anderson WF: Prospects for in utero human gene therapy. *Science* 285:2084, 1999.

CHAPTER 42

Inhibition of Myocardial Apoptosis as a Therapeutic Target: Focus on Caspase Inhibition

William H. Frishman

Nils Guttenplan

Christine Leehealey

Edmund H. Sonnenblick

Piero Anversa

Apoptosis is an essential biologic process that removes excess, unwanted, or damaged cells from an organism or cell population in order to maintain homeostasis. Excessive apoptotic cell death has been implicated in the pathogenesis of a wide range of disease entities, and it has been shown that apoptosis is responsible for a significant proportion of the cell death that occurs in chronic, as well as in acute, cardiovascular disease, including that seen with ischemic heart disease, ischemia-reperfusion injury, atherosclerosis, and congestive heart failure.[1–6] In light of these findings, current research has focused on ways of inhibiting or terminating the apoptotic death process in the hopes of preventing myocyte cell death and its ramifications. In this chapter, the caspases and other pharmacologic approaches are emphasized as potential therapeutic targets for inhibiting apoptosis.[7]

CASPASE

Key elements in the apoptotic cascade include a family of cysteine proteases called caspases. Originally known as interleukin-1β-converting enzyme, they contain a cysteine residue in their catalytic center. These proteases are triggered in response to proapoptotic signals and function to cleave key cellular proteins that ultimately result in the disassembly of a cell. Caspase was initially discovered as the mammalian homologue to CED-3, which was a gene product known to be required for programmed cell death in the nematode *Caenorhabditis elegans*.[8] There have been 14 caspase enzymes characterized to date, and most of these play an integral part in the apoptotic process.

Caspases are located in the cytoplasm of cells as proenzyme or zymogens, which require both localization to the nucleus and proteolytic cleavage into two subunits for activation. Several unique features of caspases include the observations that they must be cleaved after an aspartic acid for appropriate activation, that they must cleave their target proteins after specific aspartic acids, and that recognition of four amino acids at the N-terminus to the cleavage site is also required for proper activation.[9] The caspase molecule consists of three general domains: an amino-terminal domain, a large subunit (20 kd) and a small subunit (10 kd). Activation involves cleavage between the domains and interaction between the two subunits to form a heterodimer, two of which associate to form a tetramer with two separate catalytic sites.[10]

How Do the Caspases Work?

Apoptosis of a cell has several characteristic features: cell shrinkage, DNA fragmentation, chromatin condensation, membrane blebbing into apoptotic bodies or vesicles, the lack of a surrounding inflammatory response, and, finally, the phagocytic engulfment of these vesicles by neighboring myocytes, fibroblasts, and macrophages. This sequence is usually complete within 30 to 60 min. Caspases fit into two different subsets in the overall mechanism of apoptosis: as initiators, which activate cell disassembly in response to proapoptotic signals, and as effectors, which actually carry out the disassembly process (Fig. 42-1).

The initiator caspases (including caspases 2, 8, 9, and 10) generally inactivate those antiapoptotic cellular proteins that function to keep the cell from undergoing apoptosis. One such example is the Bcl-2 proteins, which function to protect the cell from apoptosis when it sustains cytotoxic insults such as suboptimal growth conditions, ultraviolet irradiation, cytokine withdrawal, or chemotherapeutic drugs.[11] Caspases cleave Bcl-2 proteins, which not only inactivates them, but also produces a fragment that is further involved in apoptosis.[12] Another example where caspase initiation is necessary is with Icad/DFF45, the inhibitor of a caspase-activated deoxyribonuclease (Icad), which is responsible for DNA fragmentation (DFF). Caspase inactivates Icad so that the nuclease is no longer inhibited and can begin its job in cell destruction.[13]

The effector caspases (including caspases 3, 6, and 7) directly contribute to the final disassembly of the cell during apoptosis by targeting more than 40 cellular proteins involved in the general maintenance function of the cell. For instance, PAK2 is a serine/threonine kinase that is involved in the regulation of the actin cytoskeleton. It is activated by caspase cleavage and helps to reorganize the

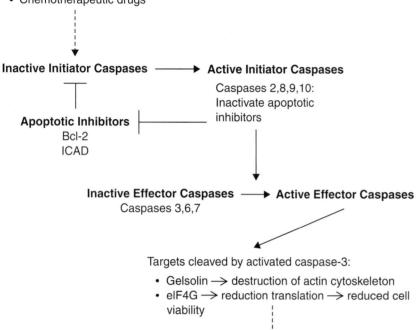

Apoptotic Stimuli

- Suboptimal growth conditons
- UV irradiation
- Cytokine withdrawal
- Chemotherapeutic drugs

Inactive Initiator Caspases ⟶ **Active Initiator Caspases**

Caspases 2,8,9,10:
Inactivate apoptotic
inhibitors

Apoptotic Inhibitors
Bcl-2
ICAD

Inactive Effector Caspases ⟶ **Active Effector Caspases**
Caspases 3,6,7

Targets cleaved by activated caspase-3:

- Gelsolin ⟶ destruction of actin cytoskeleton
- eIF4G ⟶ reduction translation ⟶ reduced cell viability

Apoptosis

FIGURE 42-1. Diagram of selected aspects of the caspase cascade. Initiator caspases generally function to inactivate cellular antiapoptotic proteins. Effector caspases carry out apoptosis by targeting cellular proteins involved in the general maintenance function of the cell. → = activation via cleavage; ⊢ = negative regulation; eIF4G = eukaryotic initiation factor 4G; ICAD = inhibition of caspase-activated deoxyribonuclease. (*Reproduced with permission from Guttenplan N, Lee C, Frishman WH: Inhibition of myocardial apoptosis as a therapeutic target in cardiovascular disease prevention: Focus on caspase inhibition. Heart Dis 3:313, 2001.*)

shrinking cell into apoptotic bodies.[14] Gelsolin is another cytoskeletal protein that is a substrate for caspase; its cleavage by caspase-3 causes deconstruction of the actin cytoskeleton. Gelsolin-deficient smooth-muscle cells grown in vitro showed significant resistance to proapoptotic factors.[15] Caspase-3 is also necessary for the degradation of eukaryotic initiation factor 4G during apoptosis. This factor is part of the cellular machinery necessary for translating messenger RNA into cytosolic proteins, and its breakdown signifies the loss of cell viability.[16] In yet another example occurring during apoptosis, caspases disassemble the structural scaffolding for chromatin by cleaving the nuclear lamina, resulting in its collapse with an end result of chromatin condensation.[17] Effector caspases are also involved in the inactivation of parts of the cell's regulatory machinery, such as mRNA splicing factors, DNA replication proteins, and DNA repair enzymes. Caspase-3 is involved in cleaving DNA-dependent protein kinase, and poly ADP-ribose polymerase during apoptosis.[18]

How Are the Caspases Regulated?

Activation of initiator caspases requires specific cofactors that bind the zymogen form of caspase when triggered by a proapoptotic signal (Fig. 42-2). Procaspase-9 binds with the cofactors APAF-1, mitochondria-released cytochrome C, and dADP.[19,20,20a] Cytochrome C, in addition to its role as a cofactor, may even act to amplify the caspase cascade during apoptosis.[21] The requirement of several cofactors to activate caspases ensures that the apoptotic signal cannot be easily triggered. Initiator caspases go on to activate the effector caspases, which results in cell disassembly.

Caspase regulators also come in the form of inhibitors, which compete with procaspases for the binding of their cofactors, thus preventing caspase activation. Procaspase-8 activation requires the association with cofactor FADD (Fas-associated protein with death domain) through the death-effector domain.[22] FADD-like interleukin-1B-converting enzyme inhibitory proteins were recently discovered;[23] these proteins are similar in sequence to procaspase-8 and compete for binding to cofactor FADD, thus ensuring that procaspase-8 is not activated constitutively. Other inhibitors have been identified: the inhibitors of apoptosis proteins,[24] which function to selectively inhibit effector caspases even when they are overexpressed in vitro,[25] and an apoptosis repressor with a caspase recruitment domain, which selectively targets certain caspases in skeletal and cardiac muscle for inhibition.

Caspase-3

The expression of caspase-3 (CPP32/apopain) is widespread in a variety of mammalian cell types.[26] By using an in vivo immunohistochemical analysis of procaspase-3 expression, it was found to be located in both the cytosol and mitochondria at different levels of intensity depending on the tissue. The highest levels were found in tonsil, spleen, thymus, and colon tissues, while intermediate levels were found in cardiomyocytes, the adrenal gland, and in the pancreas. This difference may reflect the important role that spontaneous apoptosis plays in various tissues, such as lymphoid and intestinal tissues, which generate more cell turnover than the myocardium.[27] These findings may not reflect pre- or postapoptotic levels,

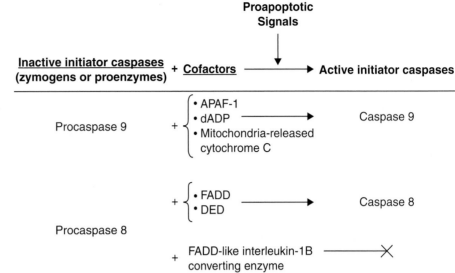

FIGURE 42-2. Regulation of caspases. The requirement of several cofactors to activate caspases ensures that the apoptotic signal cannot be easily triggered. Competitive inhibitors of cofactors also prevents the constitutive activation of caspases. → = activation via cleavage; APAF-1 = apoptotic protease-activating factor-1; dADP = deoxyadenosine diphosphate; DED = death effector domain; FADD = fas-associated protein with death domain; X = competitive inhibition. (*Reproduced with permission from Guttenplan N, Lee C, Frishman WH: Inhibition of myocardial apoptosis as a therapeutic target in cardiovascular disease prevention: Focus on caspase inhibition. Heart Dis 3:313, 2001.*)

however, as procaspase-3 expression is likely upregulated acutely prior to apoptosis, and is rapidly cleared away as the apoptotic bodies are phagocytized.[28] In a knock-out mouse model, caspase-3 null mice were born at a lower frequency rate and with pronounced developmental abnormalities resulting in the death of animals during the neonatal period. Caspase-2 null strains were deficient in female germ-cell death, but were able to survive beyond the neonatal period.[29]

Caspase-3 is a distal protease along the effector pathway, and has a wide range of cellular targets that contribute to disassembly of the cell, among them gelsolin, eukaryotic initiation factor 4G, poly-ADP-ribose polymerase, and DNA-dependent protein kinase, whose mechanisms of action were mentioned above. In vitro studies using rat neonatal cardiac myocytes demonstrated that apoptosis was induced with staurosporine as identified by TUNEL (in situ nick end-labeling) staining and DNA laddering on an agarose gel electrophoresis. Based on substrate analysis, the major component of caspases activated in these myocytes was caspase-3, which suggests that it has a major involvement in cardiomyocyte apoptosis.[30] Current data from brain and cardiovascular research studies also suggest that caspase-3 is a central component of the proteolytic cascade during apoptosis, particularly in studies of cerebral and myocardial ischemia.[31,31a]

Increased caspase-3 expression and evidence of apoptosis by TUNEL studies was shown in explanted human hearts with end-stage ischemic or dilated cardiomyopathy when compared to normal controls. The end-stage hearts also exhibited a fifteen- to twenty-fold higher release of cytochrome C into the cytoplasm of myocytes than normals, further strengthening the evidence that cytochrome C is a cofactor in the activation of caspase-3. Although the presence of caspase-3 confirms that the apoptotic cascade is activated, ultrastructural characteristics of apoptosis in the nuclei were not observed in these end-stage hearts, further suggesting that there may be a preapoptotic stage, with a dissociation of cytoplasmic and nuclear processes of apoptosis.[32]

Induced by a Fas ligand (the death receptor), caspase-3 is also critical for the increased apoptosis found in atherosclerotic lesions, namely endothelial cells of the intimal layer, and smooth-muscle cells that migrated from the medial layer. Traditional models of atherosclerosis have described a necrotic lipid core with

cell debris, fibrosis, and dead cells in the atheroma. Recent work, however, shows that proinflammatory cytokines, such as tumor necrosis factor, interleukin-1, and interferon-γ, released from local macrophages and T cells around the lesion may trigger apoptosis, leading to decreased stability of the atherosclerotic plaque, a highly tenuous condition that could easily lead to myocardial infarction.[33] Many cells in the atheromatous lesion show characteristic apoptotic markers even though necrosis may also occur predominantly in the lipid core.[33,34]

Acute coronary occlusion was induced in rats to produce a regional myocardial ischemia. Caspase-3 immunoreactivity levels were substantially elevated and colocalized with TUNEL-positive staining to this region, indicating that acute ischemia of the myocardium induces caspase-3-mediated apoptosis. Measuring these factors after both occlusion and reperfusion time showed that apoptosis substantially increased in a time-dependent fashion, which suggests that apoptosis may also be induced by reactive oxygen species and tumor necrosis factor released during reperfusion injury.[35]

Chronic forms of cardiomyopathy have also been shown to have a pathologic level of apoptosis, which contributes to the progressive deterioration of the myocardium into heart failure.[36,36a] Chronic ischemic heart failure induced for 6 months in a sheep model has been shown to activate caspase-3 as well as caspase-2.[37] Moderate heart failure, defined as a left ventricular ejection fraction of less than 35%, was induced via intracoronary microembolization. These hearts showed a 2.6-fold increase in expression of caspase-3 when compared to normal samples. The activity of DNAse I, an enzyme that cleaves chromatin at internucleosomal sites during apoptosis, was also measured in this experiment, and showed an increased expression in the failing hearts as compared to normals. This demonstrates a possible role of apoptosis in the chronic ischemia pathologic state.[37]

Therapeutic Potential of Caspase Inhibitors in Cardiovascular Disease

Through modulation of the caspase-associated apoptotic process, apoptosis is attenuated, allowing significantly injured myocardium to survive until the insult is removed and the tissue can undergo repair and remodeling efforts.

Caspase inhibitors interfere with apoptosis after proapoptotic signals have been sent. Benzyloxycarbonyl-valine-alanine-aspartate fluoromethylketone (zVAD-fmk), an irreversible inhibitor of caspases, reduced the amount of induced apoptosis in several models of cardiomyocyte injury, whether it be secondary to chemotherapeutic agents such as staurosporine,[32] ischemia,[35] or reperfusion injury.[35,38] In a rat model, coronary occlusion was induced for 30 min, followed by 24-h of reperfusion. zVAD-fmk was administered intravenously before occlusion and ending after reperfusion. The myocardial infarct size/ischemic areas were characterized by apoptosis and increased caspase levels, as seen with TUNEL methods and DNA laddering. The experimental group receiving the caspase inhibitor not only had decreased left ventricular end diastolic pressure, but also had significantly reduced infarct size/ischemic areas. The number of TUNEL-positive cells were significantly fewer, effectively reflecting reduced reperfusion injury which could be partially attributed to the attenuation of apoptosis in the injured myocytes.[38]

A similar study using coronary occlusion in a rat model also examined the effect of caspase inhibitors on apoptosis.[39] In this study, the coronary arteries were similarly occluded for 30 min, followed by only a 6-h period of reperfusion. A less broad-spectrum caspase inhibitor, Ac-Asp-Glu-Val-Asp-aldehyde (DEVD-CHO) was administered 5 min prior to occlusion of the coronary arteries. Unlike the previous study, the caspase inhibitor was withheld during the reperfusion period. Caspase-3 activity was measured at 4 h into the reperfusion period and found to be reduced significantly in the treatment group. The percentage of TUNEL-positive cells was also significantly reduced. However, there were important differences between these studies. In this study,[39] there was no beneficial effect of the treatment on hemodynamic variables, and infarct size was not reduced. The authors noted that caspase-3 levels were not elevated at 1 h into the reperfusion period; however, there were already ultrastructural changes evident in both the cell membrane and mitochondria. If caspase-3 is activated after cellular damage has taken place, the benefit of caspase inhibitors, specifically on infarct size, may be limited.[39] Given the discrepancy between these two similar studies, it is possible that the specific selection of the caspase inhibitor is crucial. Other caspases may be activated earlier in the apoptosis caspase than caspase-3, and perhaps zVAD-fmk is more effective than DEVD-CHO in preventing these early ultrastructural changes. The mode of administration may also influence outcome. Superior results were seen in the study that administered the caspase inhibitor in both the pre- and postocclusion periods.[38]

The effects of two caspase inhibitors were documented in an investigation of hypoxia-induced apoptosis in a neonatal rat cardiac myocyte model.[40] The purpose of the study was to investigate whether glucose uptake and glycolysis prevents hypoxia-induced apoptosis of neonatal rat cardiac myocytes. This study demonstrated that hypoxia-induced apoptosis occurred within 3 to 8 h in cultures deprived of glucose. Glucose uptake and glycolysis were shown to be protective against hypoxia-induced apoptosis. Furthermore, the study showed that caspase-3 activation was accompanied by cytochrome C translocation to the cytosol. The effects of preincubation with the caspase inhibitors zVAD-fmk and benzyloxycarbondyl-Asp-Glu-Val-Asp-fluoromethylketone (zDEVD-fmk) were also studied. Preincubation with zVAD-fmk in myocytes subjected to long-term hypoxia in the presence of glucose completely prevented the DNA laddering indicative of apoptosis. DNA repair enzymes are another target of caspases. The DNA repair enzyme poly(ADP-ribose) polymerase is a known target of caspase-3. The effects of preincubation of myocytes with the broad-spectrum caspase inhibitor, zVAD-fmk, and the more caspase-3-specific inhibitor, zDEVD-fmk, were studied. Both agents significantly reduced the cleavage of PARP. However, zDEVD-fmk had the greater protective effect. DNA laddering was also completely prevented by both agents. Another interesting difference between these two agents is that zDEVD-fmk was able to block cytochrome C release in the glucose-deprived hypoxic cells, whereas zVAD-fmk did not have this effect.[40]

A similar study of glucose deprivation in cardiac myocytes also demonstrated that zVAD-fmk blocks DNA fragmentation. Similarly, zVAD-fmk was also unable to prevent cytochrome C release in the glucose-deprived myocytes.[41] These studies demonstrate that the currently used caspase inhibitors have different antiapoptotic properties. These differences may play a role in their potential therapeutic applicability and can perhaps be exploited to target unique aspects of various cardiovascular diseases. For instance, chronic congestive heart failure is associated with elevated nitric oxide levels.[42] zVAD-fmk was employed in an in vitro study using neonatal myocytes, and was found to attenuate apoptosis triggered by nitric oxide production.[43]

zVAD-fmk has also been studied as a potential treatment to prevent postangioplasty restenosis in an animal model. Significant inhibition of balloon injury-mediated apoptosis of arterial smooth muscle cells was achieved with local administration of the drug, resulting in a significant decrease in both neointimal formation and media proliferation.[44]

Gene therapy represents another research methodology being considered in the search for antiapoptotic therapies. Apoptosis regulator with caspase recruitment (ARC) is a gene predominantly expressed in cardiac and skeletal muscle tissues that has the capability of binding caspases and reducing apoptosis.[26] A myogenic rat cell line was transfected to overexpress ARC and was then subjected to a hypoxic environment. The transfected cells were able to suppress caspase-3 activation and PARP cleavage. Moreover, these cells were also able to inhibit the release of mitochondrial cytochrome C into the cytosol. Preincubation of control cells with either zVAD-fmk or zDEVD-fmk did not result in a similar inhibition of cytochrome C release.[45] In vivo studies are needed before the clinical potential of apoptosis inhibition via genetic manipulation can begin to be assessed.

One such in vivo study was performed with transgenic mice overexpressing insulin-like growth factor 1 (IGF-1). IGF-1 may also be a possible therapeutic inhibitor of caspase-3. Apoptosis was induced with in vitro cardiomyocytes using serum withdrawal and doxorubicin incubation, and increased caspase-3 levels were found. With IGF-1 treatment, myocytes showed enhanced viability, suppressed DNA fragmentation, and attenuated caspase-3 activation.[46] Transgenic mice overexpressing IGF-1 underwent coronary occlusion and showed decreased cell death as well as less ventricular dilatation and wall stress.[47] Thus, IGF-1 may offer another therapeutic manipulation in the future to prevent cardiomyocyte loss in pathologic disease states of the heart.[48]

Apoptosis has been shown to begin immediately after myocardial infarction and is the predominant method of cell death in the first 24 h. Necrosis, marked by cell disintegration and leakage of intracellular contents, follows apoptosis, with measurable levels evident 6 to 8 h after infarction has commenced. This is currently measured quantitatively by using creatine phosphokinase MB fraction and troponin. Apoptosis by definition preserves the integrity of plasma membranes and does not cause release of intracellular enzymes, and thus probably cannot be measured by a marker within the systemic circulation for detection of myocardial infarction. However, given the immediate onset of apoptosis with impending infarction, a novel diagnostic method might be found in the future that would identify an ongoing infarction by detecting apoptosis, and thus could effectively reduce the time between diagnosis of infarction and treatment.

Future Directions

Although initial experiments in animal models are promising, many questions have yet to be answered before caspase-3 inhibition can be considered as a treatment modality in human cardiovascular disease. The inhibitors of caspase-3 also need to be proven more effective in reducing apoptosis than available drugs, which are described in the next section.

1. Because caspase-3 in vivo expression is widespread, any therapeutic action to inhibit this protease in cardiomyocytes could also have implications for other cell types as well. For instance, given that caspase-3 is constitutively expressed in organs, such as the adult mouse brain,[49] inhibiting apoptosis in nontargeted tissues may cause long-term effects such as cerebral dysfunction. In other organs where an administered caspase inhibitor could reach, malignancy could arise from the inhibition of a cell's "maintenance" apoptosis.[50] A unique regulatory mechanism targeting the cardiovascular organ(s) must be used in order to avoid this risk.
2. Current studies have only described the short-term effects of inhibiting apoptosis in injured myocardial cells. However, apoptosis is also important for the inflammatory and granulation tissue phases which follow myocardial infarction. If these processes are blocked, the findings of abnormal remodeling with fragile granulation tissue in the ventricle may be even more detrimental regarding long-term morbidity and mortality.
3. What is the ultimate fate of those cells in which caspase was inhibited after ischemia/reperfusion injury and then survived? Even if apoptosis is avoided, cells may not maintain their overall viability depending on the extent of injury. Is there a possibility that the inhibition only delays death, and the cell would then undergo a slower nonapoptotic cell death in the long term?
4. What is the fate of cells that were exposed to a caspase inhibitor and were not originally proapoptotic? Would these cells potentially become malignant if they were abnormal?
5. What is the true incidence of apoptosis? Reported values that have been significant have ranged between 0.04% and 35% of total nuclei per section. Better quantitative methods of detection may be needed.
6. The differences in the antiapoptotic mechanisms of caspase-inhibitors need further characterization.[38,51] In the future it may be possible to select specific agents to target unique aspects of cardiovascular disease.[51a] Small molecule inhibitors of caspase proteases or caspase activator proteins may also have a role in the context of acute tissue and organ damage in stroke.[52]
7. There may be a temporal propriety to the mode of administration of the therapy. For example, apoptosis associated with chronic congestive heart failure might respond better to a daily treatment protocol similar to the current use of angiotensin converting

enzyme inhibitors. Ischemia-induced apoptosis may respond best to a peri-infarct treatment.

Perhaps in the future caspase inhibitors will be infused along with t-PA in the treatment of acute myocardial infarction.

OTHER PHARMACOLOGIC APPROACHES

Other pharmacologic approaches that have been found useful in the inhibition of myocardial apoptosis include β-adrenergic blockers, α-adrenergic agonists, angiotensin-converting enzyme inhibitors, angiotensin-I-receptor blockers, calcium-channel blockers, antioxidants, Na^+/H^+ exchangers, mitochondrial K^+-channel openers, insulin growth-factor agonists, and inhibitors of tumor necrosis factor-α.

Experimental studies have shown that exposure to catecholamines can accelerate the rate of apoptosis related to the stimulation of β-adrenergic receptors,[53–56] which could modulate the pathologic transition from myocardial hypertrophy to dilated cardiomyopathy.[57] Antagonism of the β_1-adrenergic receptor is associated with a reduction in myocyte apoptosis,[58–61] which may, in part, be related to effects on the caspase-3 pathway. Beta-blockers may also attenuate the upregulation of both apoptosis-inducing factor and Bak, a proapoptotic member of the Bcl-2 family. Perhaps the benefit of β blockade in heart failure relates to its ability to reduce apoptosis, allowing natural myocardial hyperplastic processes to dominate.

α-Agonists also appear to reduce the rate of myocardial apoptosis by increasing the bclx/bax ratio.[55,62]

Angiotensin-II via the angiotensin-I receptor is known to increase the rate of myocardial apoptosis, and this mechanism may be important in both diabetic and nondiabetic cardiomyopathy.[63–65] Both ACE inhibitors and angiotensin-II-receptor blockers can reduce the rate of apoptosis,[65–68] which may explain the benefit observed with these drugs in the treatment of heart failure.

Increased calcium-ion content in the myocardial cell is associated with increased apoptosis.[69,70] Calcium-channel antagonists have been documented to reduce the risk of apoptosis.[71]

Various antioxidants are useful in reducing the degree of apoptosis in animal models of catecholamine stimulation and adriamycin-induced cardiotoxicity.[72–74]

Intracellular acidosis causes an increased predisposition to cell death and inhibition of the Na^+/H^+ exchanger with various drugs has been shown to reduce myocardial apoptosis.[75] These drugs can prevent the calcium ion accumulation in cells that occurs indirectly by stimulation of the Na^+/H^+ exchanger with enhanced sodium/calcium exchange (see also Chap. 28).

Ischemic preconditioning reduces apoptosis by upregulating the antideath gene Bcl-2.[76] This phenomenon is mediated by opening of the ATP-potassium channel and can be enhanced by drugs such as adenosine and diazoxide.[77,78]

Insulin-like growth factor-1 and insulin have been shown to reduce the rate of myocardial apoptosis.[79,80]

Activation of both MAPK and downstream JNK is associated with an increased rate of apoptosis.[81] Pharmacologic inhibitors of MADK and JNK can reduce the apoptosis rate in experimental models.[82,83]

Other therapies under investigation for reducing apoptosis include inhibitors of tumor necrosis factor-α,[84] antibodies against the C5 complement component,[85] and various gene therapy strategies.[86–88]

TABLE 42-1. Some Potential Approaches to Antiapoptosis Therapy in the Myocardium

Gene Therapy
  Overexpression of dominant inhibitor
  Deficiency of essential mediator
    Antisense
    Ribozyme

Small Molecular Therapy
  Peptide inhibitors of the caspase family
  Inhibition of proximal pathways
    Administration of insulin growth factor-1
    Inhibition of tumor necrosis factor-α pathway
    Angiotensin II receptor blockade
    β-Adrenergic blockade
    Calcium antagonists

CONCLUSION

Apoptosis plays a role in the normal biologic cell death processes and in specific pathophysiologic conditions. Antiapoptotic treatments (Table 42-1) could modify cell loss and preserve organ function, but the safety of this approach needs to be determined.

REFERENCES

1. Hetts SW: To die or not to die. An overview of apoptosis and its role in disease. *JAMA* 279:300, 1998.
2. Olivetti G, Abbi R, Quaini F, et al: Apoptosis in the failing human heart. *N Engl J Med* 336:1131, 1997.
3. Buja LM, Entman ML: Modes of myocardial cell injury and cell death in ischemic heart disease. *Circulation* 98:1355, 1998.
4. Williams RS: Apoptosis and heart failure. *N Engl J Med* 341:759, 1999.
5. Tricot O, Mallat Z, Heymes C, et al: Relation between endothelial cell apoptosis and blood flow direction in human atherosclerotic plaques. *Circulation* 101:2450, 2000.
6. James TN: Apoptosis in cardiac disease. *Am J Med* 107:606, 1999.
7. Schwartz SM: Cell death and the caspase cascade. *Circulation* 97:227, 1998.
8. Yuan J, Shaham S, Ledoux S, et al: The *C. elegans* cell death gene *ced-3* encodes a protein similar to mammalian interleukin-1B-converting enzyme. *Cell* 75:641, 1993.
9. Thornberry N, Rano T, Peterson E, et al: A combinatorial approach defines specificities of members of the caspase family and granzyme B. *J Biol Chem* 272:17907, 1997.
10. Walker N, Talanian R, Brady K, et al: Crystal structure of cysteine protease interleukin-1B-converting enzyme: A (p20/p10)2 homodimer. *Cell* 78:343, 1994.
11. Adams J, Cory S: The Bcl-2 protein family: Arbiters of cell survival. *Science* 281:1322, 1998.
12. Xue D, Horvitz H: *Caenorhabditis elegans* CED-9 protein is a bifunctional cell death inhibitor. *Nature* 390:305, 1997.
13. Enari M, Sakahira H, Yokoyama H, et al: Caspase-activated DNase that degrades DNA during apoptosis, and its inhibitor ICAD. *Nature* 391(6662):43, 1998.
14. Rudel T, Bokoch G: Membrane and morphological changes in apoptotic cells regulated by caspase mediated activation of PAK2. *Science* 276:1571, 1997.
15. Geng Y, Azuma T, Tang J, et al: Caspase-3 induced gelsolin fragmentation contributes to actin cytoskeletal collapse, nucleolysis, and apoptosis of vascular smooth muscle cells exposed to proinflammatory cytokines. *Eur J Cell Biol* 77:294, 1998.
16. Bushell M, McKendrick L, Janicke R, et al: Caspase-3 is necessary and sufficient for cleavage of protein synthesis eukaryotic initiation factor 4G during apoptosis. *FEBS Lett* 451:332, 1999.
17. Takahishi A, Alnemri E, Lazebnik Y, et al: Cleavage of lamin A by Mch2a but not CPP32: Multiple interleukin-1B-converting enzyme-related proteases with distinct substrate recognition properties are active in apoptosis. *Proc Natl Acad Sci U S A* 93:8395, 1996.
18. Cryns V, Yuan J: Proteases to die for. *Genes Dev* 12:1551, 1998.
19. Degli Esposti M, McLennan H: Mitochondria and cells produce reactive oxygen species in virtual anaerobiosis: Relevance to ceramide-induced apoptosis. *FEBS Lett* 430:338, 1998.
20. Wolf C, Eastman A: The temporal relationship between protein phosphatase, mitochondrial cytochrome c release, and caspase activation in apoptosis. *Exp Cell Res* 247:505, 1999.
20a. Kumar S, Vaux DL: A cinderella caspase takes center stage. *Science* 297:1290, 2002.
21. Bossy-Wetzel E, Green D: Caspases induce cytochrome c release from mitochondria by activating cytosolic factors. *J Biol Chem* 274:17484, 1999.
22. Jacobson M, Raff M: Programmed cell death and Bcl-2 protection in very low oxygen. *Nature* 374:814, 1995.
23. Zamzami N, Marchetti P, Castedo M, et al: Inhibitors of permeability transition interfere with the disruption of the mitochondrial transmembrane potential driving apoptosis. *FEBS Lett* 384:53, 1996.
24. Hengartner M, Horvitz H: *C. elegans* cell survival gene *ced-9* encodes a functional homolog of the mammalian proto-oncogene *bcl-2. Cell* 76:665, 1994.
25. Kane D, Sarafian T, Anton R, et al: Bcl-2 inhibition of neural death: Decreased generation of reactive oxygen species. *Science* 262:1274, 1993.
26. Koseki T, Inohara N, Chen S, Nunez G: ARC, an inhibitor of apoptosis expressed in skeletal muscle and heart that interacts selectively with caspases. *Proc Natl Acad Sci U S A* 95(9):5156, 1998.
27. Kumar S: The apoptotic cysteine protease CPP32. *Int J Biochem Cell Biol* 29:393, 1997.
28. Samali A, Zhivotovsky B, Jones D, Orrenius S: Detection of procaspase3 in cytosol and mitochondria of various tissues. *FEBS Lett* 431:167, 1998.
29. Krajewska M, Wang H, Krajewski S, et al: Immunohistochemical analysis of in vivo patterns of expression of CPP32 (caspase-3), a cell death protease. *Cancer Res* 57:1605, 1997.
30. Los M, Wesselborg S, Schulze-Osthoff K: The role of caspases in development, immunity, and apoptotic signal transduction: Lessons from knockout mice. *Immunity* 10:629, 1999.
31. Narula J, Pandey P, Arbustini E, et al: Apoptosis in heart failure: Release of cytochrome C from mitochondria and activation of caspase-3 in human cardiomyopathy. *Proc Natl Acad Sci U S A* 96:8144, 1999.
31a. Condorelli G, Roncarati R, Ross J Jr, et al: Heart-targeted overexpression of caspase 3 in mice increases infarct size and depresses cardiac function. *Proc Natl Acad Sci, U S A* 98:9977, 2001.
32. Yue T, Wang C, Romanic A, et al: Staurosporine induced apoptosis in cardiomyocytes: A potential role of caspase-3. *J Mol Cell Cardiol* 30:495, 1998.
33. Geng Y: Regulation of programmed cell death or apoptosis in atherosclerosis. *Heart Vessels* 12(Suppl):76, 1997.
34. Enari M, Hug H, Nagata S: Involvement of an ICE-like protease in Fas-mediated apoptosis. *Nature* 375:78, 1995.
35. Black S, Huang J, Rezaiefar P, et al: Co-localization of the cysteine protease caspase-3 with apoptotic myocytes after in vivo myocardial ischemia and reperfusion in the rat. *J Mol Cell Cardiol* 30:733, 1998.
36. Leri A, Claudio PP, Li Q, et al: Stretch-mediated release of angiotensin II induces myocyte apoptosis by activating p53 that enhances the local renin-angiotensin system and decreases the Bcl-2-to-Bax protein ratio in the cell. *J Clin Invest* 101:1326, 1998.
36a. Scheubel RJ, Bartling B, Simm A, et al: Apoptotic pathway activation from mitochondria and death receptors without caspase-3 cleavage in failing human myocardium, fragile balance of myocyte survival? *Am J Cardiol* 39:481, 2002.
37. Jiang L, Huang Y, Yuasa T, et al: Elevated DNAase activity and caspase expression in association with apoptosis in failing ischemic sheep left ventricles. *Electrophoresis* 20:2046, 1999.
38. Yaoita H, Ogawa K, Maehara K, Maruyama Y: Attenuation of ischemia/reperfusion injury in rats by a caspase inhibitor. *Circulation* 97:276, 1998.

39. Okamura T, Miura T, Takemura G, et al: Effect of caspase inhibitors on myocardial infarct size and myocyte DNA fragmentation in the ischemia-reperfused rat heart. *Cardiovasc Res* 45:642, 2000.

40. Malhotra R, Brosius FC III: Glucose uptake and glycolysis reduce hypoxia-induced apoptosis in cultured neonatal rat cardiac myocytes. *J Biol Chem* 274:12567, 1999.

41. Bialik S, Cryns VL, Drincic A, et al: The mitochondrial apoptotic pathway is activated by serum and glucose deprivation in cardiac myocytes. *Circ Res* 85:403, 1999.

42. Haywood GA, Tsao PS, von der Leyen HE, et al: Expression of inducible nitric oxide synthase in human heart failure. *Circulation* 93:1087, 1996.

43. Ing DJ, Zang J, Dzau VJ, et al: Modulation of cytokine-induced cardiac myocyte apoptosis by nitric oxide, Bak and Bcl-x. *Circ Res* 84:21, 1999.

44. Beohar N, Flaherty JD, Davidson CJ, et al: Antirestenotic effects of inhibition of balloon injury mediated apoptosis with local delivery of a caspase inhibitor (abstr.). *J Am Coll Cardiol* 39(Suppl A):442A, 2002.

45. Ekhterae D, Lin Z, Lundberg MS, et al: ARC inhibits cytochrome C release from mitochondria and protects against hypoxia-induced apoptosis in heart-derived H9c2 cells. *Circ Res* 85:e70, 1999.

46. Wang L, Ma W, Markovich R: Regulation of cardiomyocyte apoptotic signaling by insulin-like growth factor I. *Circ Res* 83:516, 1998.

47. Li W, Li B, Wang X, et al: Overexpression of insulin-like growth factor I in mice protects from myocyte death after infarction, attenuating ventricular dilation, wall stress, and cardiac hypertrophy. *J Clin Invest* 100:1991, 1997.

48. Leri A, Liu Y, Claudio PP, et al: Insulin-like growth factor-1 induces Mdm2 and downregulates p53, attenuating the myocyte renin-angiotensin system and stretch-mediated apoptosis. *Am J Pathol* 154:567, 1999.

49. Namura S, Zhu J, Fink K, et al: Activation and cleavage of caspase-3 in apoptosis induced by experimental cerebral ischemia. *J Neuroscience* 18:3659, 1998.

50. Bedner E, Smolewski P, Amstad P, Darzynkiewicz Z: Activation of caspases measured *in situ* by binding of fluorochrome-labeled inhibitors of caspases (FLICA): Correlation with DNA fragmentation. *Exp Cell Res* 259:308, 2000.

51. Nevière R, Fauvel H, Chopin C, et al: Caspase inhibition prevents cardiac dysfunction and heart apoptosis in a rat model of sepsis. *Am J Respir Crit Care Med* 163:218, 2001.

51a. Grüenfelder J, Miniati DN, Murata S, et al: Upregulation of Bcl-2 through caspase-3 inhibition ameliorates ischemia/reperfusion injury in rat cardiac allografts. *Circulation* 104(Suppl I):I 202, 2001.

52. Hengartner MO: The biochemistry of apoptosis. *Nature* 407:770, 2000.

53. Communal C, Singh K, Pimentel DR, Colucci WS: Norepinephrine stimulates apoptosis in adult rat ventricular myocytes by activation of the beta-adrenergic pathway. *Circulation* 98:1329, 1998.

54. Shizukuda Y, Buttrick PM, Geenen DL, et al: Beta-adrenergic stimulation causes cardiocyte apoptosis: Influence of tachycardia and hypertrophy. *Am J Physiol* 275(3 pt 2):H961, 1998.

55. Iwai-Kanai E, Hasegawa K, Araki M, et al: α- and β-adrenergic pathways differentially regulate cell type-specific apoptosis in rat cardiac myocytes. *Circulation* 100:305, 1999.

56. Zaugg M, Xu W, Lucchinetti E, et al: β-Adrenergic receptor subtypes differentially affect apoptosis in adult rat ventricular myocytes. *Circulation* 102:344, 2000.

57. Colucci WS, Sawyer DB, Singh K, Communal C: Adrenergic overload and apoptosis in heart failure: Implications for therapy. *J Card Fail* 6(2 Suppl 1):1, 2000.

58. Sabbah HN, Sharov VG, Gupta RC, et al: Chronic therapy with metoprolol attenuates cardiomyocyte apoptosis in dogs with heart failure. *J Am Coll Cardiol* 36:1698, 2000.

59. Romeo F, Li D, Shi M, Mehta JL: Carvedilol prevents epinephrine-induced apoptosis in human coronary artery endothelial cells: Modulation of Fas/Fas ligand and caspase-3 pathway. *Cardiovasc Res* 45:788, 2000.

60. Feuerstein G, Yue TL, Ma X, Ruffolo RR: Novel mechanisms in the treatment of heart failure: Inhibition of oxygen radicals and apoptosis by carvedilol. *Prog Cardiovasc Dis* 41(1 Suppl 1):17, 1998.

61. Todor AV, Sharov VG, Suzuki G, et al: Chronic therapy with metoprolol CR/XL prevents apoptosis inducing factor and downregulates the proapoptotic protein Bak in cardiomyocytes of dogs with heart failure (abstr.). *J Am Coll Cardiol* 39(Suppl A):165A, 2002.

62. Baghelai K, Graham LJ, Wechsler AS, Jakoi ER: Delayed myocardial preconditioning by α_1-adrenoceptors involves inhibition of apoptosis. *J Thorac Cardiovasc Surg* 117:980, 1999.

63. Ravassa S, Fortuno MA, Gonzalez A, et al: Mechanisms of increased susceptibility to angiotensin II-induced apoptosis in ventricular cardiomyocytes of spontaneously hypertensive rats. *Hypertension* 36:1065, 2000.

64. Sato M, Engelman RM, Otani H, et al: Myocardial protection by preconditioning of heart with losartan, an angiotensin II type-1 receptor blocker: Implication of bradykinin-dependent and bradykinin-independent mechanisms. *Circulation* 102(Suppl 3):III346, 2000.

65. Fiordaliso F, Li B, Latini R, et al: Myocyte death in streptozotocin-induced diabetes in rats is angiotensin-II dependent. *Lab Invest* 80:513, 2000.

66. Fortuno MA, Ravassa S, Etayo JC, Diez J: Overexpression of Bax protein and enhanced apoptosis in the left ventricle of spontaneously hypertensive rats: Effects of AT1 blockade with losartan. *Hypertension* 32:280, 1998.

67. White M: Cardioprotective effect of angiotensin II receptor antagonists. *Can J Cardiol* 15(Suppl F):10F, 1999.

68. Goussev A, Sharov VG, Shimoyama H, et al: Effects of ACE inhibition on cardiomyocyte apoptosis in dogs with heart failure. *Am J Physiol* 275:H626, 1998.

69. Muth JN, Bodi I, Lewis W, et al: A Ca^{2+}-dependent transgenic model of cardiac hypertrophy: A role for protein kinase C alpha. *Circulation* 103:140, 2001.

70. Pacher P, Csordas G, Hajnoczky G: Mitochondrial Ca^{2+} signaling and cardiac apoptosis. *Biol Signals Recept* 10:200, 2001.

71. Saito S, Hiroi Y, Zou Y, et al: Beta-adrenergic pathway induces apoptosis through calcineurin activation in cardiac myocytes. *J Biol Chem* 275:34528, 2000.

72. Dhalla NS, Elmoselhi AB, Hata T, Makino N: Status of myocardial antioxidants in ischemia-reperfusion injury. *Cardiovasc Res* 47:446, 2000.

73. Kumar D, Kirshenbaum LA, Li T, et al: Apoptosis in adriamycin cardiomyopathy and its modulation by probucol. *Antioxid Redox Signal* 3:135, 2001.

74. Kotamraju S, Konorev EA, Joseph J, Kalyanavaman B: Doxorubicin-induced apoptosis in endothelial cells and cardiomyocytes is ameliorated by nitrone spin traps and ebselen. Role of reactive oxygen and nitrogen species. *J Biol Chem* 275:33585, 2000.

75. Chakrabarti S, Hoque AN, Karmazyn M: A rapid ischemia-induced apoptosis in isolated rat hearts and its attenuation by the sodium-hydrogen exchange inhibitor HOE 642 (cariporide). *J Mol Cell Cardiol* 29:3169, 1997.

76. Maulik N, Engelman RM, Rousou JA, et al: Ischemic preconditioning reduces apoptosis by upregulating antideath gene Bcl-2. *Circulation* 100(Suppl II):II369, 1999.

77. Vinten-Johansen J, Thourani VH, Ronson RS, et al: Broad spectrum cardioprotection with adenosine. *Ann Thorac Surg* 68:1942, 1999.

78. Xu M, Wang Y, Ayub A, Ashraf M: Mitochondrial K(ATP) channel activation reduces anoxic injury by restoring mitochondrial membrane potential. *Am J Physiol* 281:H1295, 2001.

79. Aikawa R, Nawano M, Gu Y, et al: Insulin prevents cardiomyocytes from oxidative stress-induced apoptosis through activation of PI3 kinase/Akt. *Circulation* 102:2873, 2000.

80. Lee WL, Chen JW, Ting CT, et al: Insulin-like growth factor-1 improves cardiovascular function and suppresses apoptosis of cardiomyocytes in dilated cardiomyopathy. *Endocrinol* 140:4831, 1999.

81. Ma XL, Kumar S, Gao F, et al: Inhibition of p38 mitogen-activated protein kinase decreases cardiomyocyte apoptosis and improves cardiac function after myocardial ischemia and reperfusion. *Circulation* 99:1685, 1999.

82. Mackay K, Mochly-Rosen D: An inhibitor of 38 mitogen-activated protein kinase protects neonatal myocytes from ischemia. *J Biol Chem* 274:6272, 1999.

83. Yue TL, Wang C, Gu JL, et al: Inhibition of extracellular signal-regulated kinase enhances ischemia/reoxygenation-induced apoptosis in cultured cardiac myocytes and exaggerates reperfusion injury in isolated perfused heart. *Circ Res* 86:692, 2000.

84. Agnoletti L, Curello S, Bachetti T, et al: Serum from patients with severe heart failure down-regulates eNOS and is proapoptotic. Role of tumor necrosis factor-α. *Circulation* 100:1983, 1999.

85. Vakeva AP, Agah A, Rollins SA, et al: Myocardial infarction and apoptosis after myocardial ischemia and reperfusion. Role of the terminal complement components and inhibition by anti-C5 therapy. *Circulation* 97:2259, 1998.

86. Hreniuk D, Garay M, Gaarde W, et al: Inhibition of c-Jun N-terminal kinase-1, but not c-J N-terminal kinase-2, suppresses apoptosis induced by ischemia/reoxygenation in rat cardiac myocytes. *Mol Pharmacol* 59:867, 2001.

87. Leri A, Giordaliso F, Setoguchi M, et al: Inhibition of p53 function prevents renin angiotensin system activation and stretch-mediated myocyte apoptosis. *Am J Pathol* 157:843, 2000.

88. Miao W, Luo Z, Kitsis RN, Walsh K: Intracoronary, adenovirus-mediated Akt gene transfer in heart limits infarct size following ischemia-reperfusion injury in vivo. *J Mol Cell Cardiol* 32:2397, 2000.

CHAPTER 43

Matrix Metalloproteinases and Their Inhibitors in Cardiovascular Disease

William H. Frishman

Brian A. Ahangar

Sanjai Sinha

Matrix metalloproteinases (MMP) are a family of enzymes that are important in the resorption of extracellular matrices in both normal physiologic processes and in pathologic states (Table 43-1). Individually, these enzymes digest selective components of the extracellular matrix. Collectively, this family can degrade the entire extracellular matrix.

In the past, MMPs were studied mostly in the context of normal physiologic development, postnatal remodeling, and in the pathologic resorption associated with invasive tumors, periodontal disease, and rheumatoid arthritis. More recently, this area of study expanded to include diseases of the cardiovascular system. Evidence now suggests that MMPs play an important role in maintaining blood vessel integrity.[1–3b] To avoid weakening from the normal mechanical stresses of blood pressure, a vessel must continuously remodel its connective tissue. MMPs contribute to this remodeling by breaking down the extracellular matrix while new matrix is being synthesized.

MMPs may also play an important role in pathologic states involving the coronary arteries. By breaking down the extracellular matrix, MMPs may allow smooth muscle cells to invade and migrate, contributing to pathologic processes such as atherosclerosis and postcoronary angioplasty restenosis. In addition, MMPs may degrade the fibrous cap of an atherosclerotic plaque, thereby contributing to coronary plaque rupture.[3c] Furthermore, MMPs are involved in the pathologic processes that may lead to cardiac rupture or ventricular dilatation following myocardial infarction This chapter discusses the role of MMPs in the pathogenesis of coronary artery disease, abdominal aortic aneurysm, and ventricular dilatation, and introduces potential therapeutic approaches to these disease processes through pharmacologic manipulation of the MMP system.

THE MATRIX METALLOPROTEINASE FAMILY

The MMP family is subdivided into three groups based on substrate preference: the collagenases, gelatinases, and stromelysins (Table 43-2).[4] A fourth group that is gaining recognition is the integral membrane proteins. At present, each MMP can be referred to by either its molecular weight, its order of identification, or its substrate specificity. This chapter uses substrate specificity.

The MMP family of enzymes are calcium-activated zinc endopeptidases that share similarity at the amino acid level. These enzymes have several structural features in common, including a propeptide domain that contains a cysteine switch,[5] a catalytic zinc-binding domain, and a hemopexin-like domain.[6,7]

Production and Regulation

MMPs can be secreted from many cells including immune cells, fibroblasts, tumor cells, endothelial cells, smooth-muscle cells, and foam cells.[8–10] Their synthesis and activity must be closely regulated to prevent any over- or underproduction that may lead to excessive tissue destruction or a fibrotic process. To maintain tight control, MMPs are regulated at three main levels: transcription; activation of latent proenzymes; and inhibition of activity by endogenous inhibitors, which are called tissue inhibitors of MMPs (TIMPs).

The regulation of MMP genes in normal tissue is not thoroughly understood at present. Complicating this area of research are differences between in vitro and in vivo patterns of expression, variation of regulation in different tissues, and evidence of both inducible and constitutive expression of certain MMPs. Individual MMP expression is discussed below.

All members of the MMP family are produced as inactive zymogens that must be cleaved to be active.[11,12] These proteases are thought to be held in the inactive form through coordination of a cysteine in the proregion with the active site zinc ion, thereby blocking access to the active site.[13] Activation of most MMPs involves cleavage of the propeptide, which destabilizes this cysteine-zinc interaction. Plasmin and stromelysin are known physiologic activators.[12,14] Progelatinase A, however, lacks the appropriate protein cleavage site required for enzyme activation.[15] Other mechanisms of activation have been described for gelatinase A, including self-activation[12,16] and receptor-mediated activation.[12,17,18]

Once the zymogen is activated, the major point of control lies with the tissue inhibitors of MMP (TIMP). There are three major members of the tissue inhibitor(s) family: TIMP-1, TIMP-2, and TIMP-3. All three types contain two domains: the N domain, which

TABLE 43-1. Matrix Metalloproteinase Involvement in Tissue Resorption/Degradation

Normal Process	Pathologic Process
Ovulation	Cancer invasion
Endometrial cycling	Tumor metastasis
Blastocyst implantation	Rheumatoid arthritis
Embryogenesis	Osteoarthritic cartilage
Salivary gland morphogenesis	Periodontal disease
Mammary development/involution	Wound/fracture healing
Cervical dilatation	Fibrotic lung disease
Fetal membrane rupture	Liver cirrhosis
Uterine involution	Corneal ulceration
Bone growth plate	Gastric ulcer
Bone remodeling	Dilated cardiomyopathy
Angiogenesis	Aortic aneurysm
Tooth eruption	Atherosclerosis
Hair-follicle cycle	Otosclerosis
Macrophage function	Epidermolysis bullosa
Neutrophil function	Myocardial infarction
	Postangioplasty restenosis

Source: Adapted with permission from Woessner JF Jr. The family of matrix metalloproteinases. *Ann N Y Acad Sci* 732:14, 1994.

reacts with the active site of MMPs, and the C domain, which binds to other components of the MMP.[19] Basically, TIMP-1 and TIMP-2 inhibit the activity of all MMPs, whereas TIMP-3 only inhibits MMP-1, -2, -3, -9, and -13.[20] TIMP-1 is synthesized by macrophages and most connective tissue cells. It acts against all members of the MMP family and is highly inducible by cytokines and hormones. It is ten times more active in inhibiting the activity of MMP-1 than other MMPs.[21] TIMP-2 is the most abundantly expressed TIMP, and has been suggested to provide the basic and constant antimetalloproteinase activity in tissues.[22] TIMP-2 acts more specifically on gelatinase A (MMP-2), and its expression usually follows that of gelatinase A. This inhibitor, along with its substrate, is generally found at a constant level in vascular connective tissue and it is not easily induced. TIMP-3 is anchored in the matrix, and has the additional properties of stimulating cell growth.[23] A recent study[24] demonstrated that TIMP-3 can inhibit endothelial cell migration and angiogenesis in response to the angiogenic factors, basic fibroblast growth factor, and vascular endothelial growth factor. A study done by Butler et al[25] suggested that the effects of TIMP-3 and TIMP-2 might be due to the specific ability of these inhibitors to bind to progelatinase A, as well as to inhibit transmembrane spanning MMP-1 (MT1). They concluded that colocalization of TIMP-3 in the pericellular environment via binding to the extracellular matrix, including heparin sulfate proteoglycans, would place this inhibitor in a key position to inhibit MMPs produced by endothelial cells, thus regulating degradation of the extracellular matrix and release of the angiogenic factors required for migration and angiogenesis. More extensive research is needed to further elucidate the apparently important roles that these inhibitors play. The existence of three additional MMP inhibitor proteins (imp-a, imp-b, and TIMP-4) has been reported; their target substrates, however, have not been elucidated.[26,27] Olson et al[28] isolated genomic DNA containing the human TIMP-4 gene and determined the structure of the exons comprising the gene. Like other members of the TIMP family, the TIMP-4 protein is encoded by five exons. These span 6 kb of genomic DNA, so that TIMP-4 is similar in size to TIMP-1, but considerably smaller than TIMP-2 and TIMP-3. The exon-intron boundaries of TIMP-4 are at locations very similar to those of the other TIMP genes,

demonstrating the high degree of conservation of gene structure in this family. The human and mouse TIMP-4 genes map to comparable locations in the respective genomes, localizing to human chromosome 3p25 and mouse chromosome 6. Dollery et al[29] studied the expression and localization of TIMP-4 in rat carotid arteries that had sustained injuries. These data and the temporal relationship between the upregulation of TIMP-4, its accumulation, and the onset of collagen deposition suggest an important role for TIMP-4 in the proteolytic balance of the vasculature controlling both smooth muscle migration and collagen accumulation in the injured arterial wall.

Recent studies report other actions of TIMP. The increased mitogenic activity of TIMP on human heart endothelial cells in patients who have had angioplasty has provided insight into vessel restenosis.[30] Furthermore, TIMPs also act as growth factors for erythroid precursors.[31]

A fourth regulatory mechanism is being studied involving a negative feedback system (Fig. 43-1). Some research suggests that plasmin can both activate MMPs and may also provide a negative feedback for its degradation response.[32] At low levels, plasmin induces the synthesis and activation of collagenase and stromelysin from smooth-muscle cells.[33] However, plasmin in high concentrations will induce plasminogen activator inhibitor-1 (PAI-1) secretion from smooth-muscle cells. This induction may act as a negative feedback by limiting further plasmin generation, thus reducing further synthesis and activation of MMPs. Proposed mechanisms for plasminogen activator inhibitor-1 induction include mechanical cytoskeletal changes on the smooth-muscle cell from surrounding extracellular matrix breakdown[34] or a receptor-mediated mechanism by extracellular matrix breakdown products. Lijnen et al[35] investigated the potential physiologic role of the plasminogen/plasmin system in activation of the MMP system. They discovered that the addition of plasmin(ogen) to the cell culture medium of fibroblasts did not significantly affect the distribution of active and latent MMP-2, but resulted in an approximately twofold enhancement of the contribution of active MMP-9. In macrophages of plasminogen-deficient mice, active MMP-9 was detected only when the cells were cultured in the presence of plasminogen. These data indicate that activation of proMMP-2 occurs independently of the physiologic plasminogen activators and of plasmin(ogen) in all the cell types evaluated. Activation of proMMP-9 was enhanced in the presence of plasmin(ogen), but active MMP-9 was also detected in fibroblasts of plasminogen-deficient mice, indicating that in vivo activation may occur via plasmin(ogen)-independent mechanisms.

THE METALLOPROTEINASES IN CORONARY ARTERY DISEASE

Atherosclerosis

The classic mechanism for the pathogenesis of atherosclerosis, called the "response to injury hypothesis," states that atherosclerosis is initiated as a response to arterial endothelial injury, mechanical or functional, which allows increased permeability to lipids and monocytes, and permits platelets to adhere to the endothelium.[36] The monocytes then transform into macrophages in the intima and accumulate lipids to become foam cells. These macrophages and platelets at the surface then release multiple factors, including interleukin-1, tumor necrosis factor-α, and platelet-derived growth factor, that may cause migration of medial smooth-muscle cells into the intima

TABLE 43-2. MMPs, Their Substrates, and Native Inhibitors

Enzyme	MMP Classification	Substrate	Native Inhibitor
Collagenases			
Interstitital collagenase	MMP-1	Collagens, I, II, III, VII, X, gelatin, entactin, aggrecan	TIMP-1, -2
Neutrophil collagenase	MMP-8	Collagens I, II, III, aggrecan	TIMP-1, -2
Collagenase 3	MMP-13	Collagens I, III, III, gelatin, fibronectin, laminins, tenascin	
Collagenase 4	MMP-18	Not known	
Gelatinases			
Gelatinase A	MMP-2	Gelatin, collagens I, IV, V, VII, X, fibronectin laminins, aggrecan, tenascin-C, vitronectin	TIMP-2, -1
Gelatinase B	MMP-9	Gelatin, collagens IV, V, XIV, aggrecan, elastin, entactin, vitronectin	TIMP-1, -2
Stromelysins			
Stromelysin 1	MMP-3	Gelatin, fibronectin, laminins, collagens III, IV, IX, X, tenascin-C, nitronectin	TIMP-1, -2
Stromelysin 2	MMP-10	Collagen IV, fibronectin, aggrecan	TIMP-1, -2
Stromelysin 3	MMP-11	Fibronectin, gelatin, laminins, collagen IV, aggrecan	TIMP-1, -2
Membrane Type MMPs			
MT1	MMP-14	Collagens I, II, III, fibronectin, laminins, vitronectin, proteoglycans; activates proMMP-2 and proMMP-13	
MT2	MMP-15	Activates proMMP-2	
MT3	MMP-16	Activates proMMP-2	
MT4	MMP-17	Not known	
MT5	MMP-24	Activates proMMP-2	
MT6	MMP-25		
Others			
Matrilysin	MMP-7	Gelatin, fibronectin, laminins, collagen IV, vitronectin, tenascin-C, elastin, aggrecan	
Metalloelastase	MMP-12	Elastin	
Unnamed	MMP-19	Not known	
Enamelysin	MMP-20	Agrecan	
	MMP-23		
Endometase	MMP-26		

Source: Adapted with permission from Creemers EEJM, et al.[4]

to proliferate and produce the extracellular matrix of the resulting lesion.

It is proposed that the mechanism by which medial smooth-muscle cells migrate to the intima is mediated by MMPs degrading the extracellular matrix surrounding them and the basement membrane separating the media from the intima. This would involve the breakdown of fibronectin and collagen type I found in the extracellular matrix, and collagen type IV, laminin and heparin sulfate proteoglycans found in the basement membrane. It is known that the cytokines secreted by the intimal macrophages can stimulate smooth-muscle cells in vitro to produce MMPs that are capable of degrading these substances.[10] This matrix-degrading activity of MMPs is thought essential for the pathologic arterial remodeling in atherosclerosis and restenosis. Godin et al[37] concluded that MMP-9 induction is associated with the formation of intimal hyperplasia and does not require frank mechanical injury. They also demonstrated that a significant increase in MMP-9 expression preceded the positive geometric remodeling of arteries, suggesting a potentially

beneficial role for this matrix-degrading enzyme. In another study,[38] peripheral blood levels of MMPs were measured in patients with acute coronary syndromes. Serial changes in serum MMP and plasma MMP-9 were documented in these patients. These findings provide further insight into the molecular mechanism of plaque destabilization. Pasterkamp et al[39] aimed to investigate the association between the remodeling mode and the localization of macrophages and MMPs in coronary atherosclerotic segments. More MMP-2 and MMP-9 staining was observed in plaques of expansively remodeled segments as compared with constrictively remodeled segments. In general, MMP-staining was less evident in the adventitial layer as compared with the plaque. They postulated that MMPs within the plaque play a causal role not only in plaque vulnerability (discussed later) but also in de novo atherosclerotic remodeling. Another in vitro study, Fitzgerald et al[40] attempted to determine whether MMP activity is also involved in the induction of smooth-muscle cell phenotypic change by macrophages. They demonstrated that MMPs assist macrophage heparinase-induced smooth-muscle

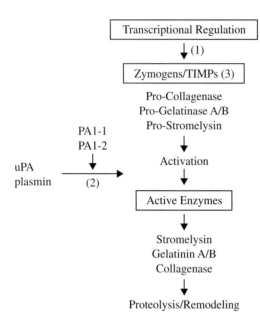

FIGURE 43-1. An illustration of the regulation and activation of MMPs. The three major pathways coordinately regulate the activity that MMPs exert in the extracellular matrix. At the transcriptional level, MMPs contain binding sites in their promoters for both transcriptional activators and repressors, including the stimulatory or inhibitory effects of several cytokines and growth factors. Because MMPs are secreted and stored as latent proenzymes, the evolutionarily conserved plasmin-dependent pathway plays a key role in promoting proteolytic cleavage of zymogens, enabling their activation and subsequent degradation. Lastly, the four TIMPs identified to date bind MMPs with 1:1 stoichiometry and broad specificity to all classes of MMPs. Experimental studies support the general notion that strategic changes in MMP/TIMP interactions could be harnessed beneficially to effect tissue remodeling such as cardiac rupture after myocardial ischemia or maintaining the patency of vein grafts after coronary revascularization. (*Reproduced with permission from Benjamin IJ.*[3a])

cell phenotypic change in vitro. As heparinase and MMPs were present together in the balloon-injured rabbit carotid artery model and in a range of human artery lesions, it is possible that these MMPs act synergistically with heparinase to promote smooth-muscle cell phenotypic change in vivo in a manner distinct from their effects on cell migration, thereby contributing to myointimal thickening and atherosclerosis.

Human smooth-muscle cells in culture respond to interleukin-1 and tumor necrosis factor-α by increasing the secretion and the activity of stromelysin (MMP-3), interstitial collagenase (MMP-1), and gelatinase-B (MMP-9). Stromelysin, among other things, activates procollagenase and progelatinase B. Interstitial collagenase acts by disrupting the native structure of collagen I fibrils found in the media. These degraded fibrils can then be further degraded by either gelatinase A or B (MMP-2 or 9) respectively.

Gelatinase A (MMP-2), TIMP-1, and TIMP-2 were also produced by these smooth-muscle cells before and after stimulation, but their concentration was unaffected by the stimuli. Gelatinase A is the MMP that degrades the collagen found in the basement membranes. In vitro studies show that smooth-muscle cell invasion through basement membrane is dependent on production of gelatinase A and can be inhibited by gelatinase A inhibitors.[41] Although gelatinase A did not increase in concentration following stimulation by interleukin-1 or tumor necrosis factor-α, it was found in a lower molecular weight and a more active form after stimulation.[10] As mentioned previously,

there is usually a constitutive secretion of gelatinase A and its activation is different from the other MMPs. Perhaps this MMP does not increase in concentration in response to stimulation, but becomes more active. Regardless, the ratio of MMP activity to tissue inhibitors of MMP increased following interleukin-1 and tumor necrosis factor-α stimulation to the smooth-muscle cell, favoring the necessary connective tissue and basement membrane breakdown for smooth-muscle cell migration from the media to the intima.

Other in vivo evidence connects MMPs with the atherosclerotic process.[41a] A common polymorphism in the promoter region for stromelysin is associated with a faster progression of coronary atherosclerotic disease in humans.[42] This was again demonstrated by Humphries et al[43] who demonstrated that particular stromelysin-1 promoter polymorphism (5A) was important in the development of coronary artery disease and other polymorphisms (6A) that might place their carriers at a particularly increased risk of rapid progression of coronary artery disease that may need rapid and aggressive treatment with lipid lowering agents. Stromelysin acts on many substrates, including proteoglycans, collagen II, IV, and IX, laminin, fibronectin, and gelatin.[44–47] When 72 patients from the St. Thomas Atherosclerosis Regression Study (STARS) were studied, patients with an altered stromelysin promoter region had a more rapid progression of coronary atherosclerotic disease than did those patients with this altered genotype. It is proposed that MMPs and TIMPs are coordinately regulated in response to cytokines, and thus a change in the transcription of the enzyme and not the inhibitor may disrupt the normal balance. Thus, extracellular matrix degradation would predominate and smooth-muscle cells could migrate faster.

This significant difference, however, was only found in comparing those patients with the least stenosis (<20%) to those with the highest serum low-density lipoprotein cholesterol (plasma LDL >4.2 mmol/L). This finding of significant progression in the least-stenosed vessels is consistent with several other studies that show a more rapid progression in less-stenosed vessels.[48] It is possible that those patients with more severe stenosis were progressing too slowly to detect a significant difference between the rates. The association between low-density lipoprotein cholesterol and cardiovascular disease has been documented in many studies. Interestingly, patients with the altered genotype who were treated with diet and lipid-lowering agents did not exhibit the same rapid progression effects. It is proposed that products of the oxidized low-density lipoprotein produced in the intima may alter cells to produce more cytokines, thus stimulating more MMP production and smooth-muscle cell migration, facilitating atherosclerosis. If oxidized low-density lipoprotein induces this reaction in all patients, possibly patients with this altered genotype have an enhanced response, that is, a genetic predisposition to progress faster.

Another study[49] searched for common functional variations in the MMP-12 gene locus that may be implicated in coronary artery disease. In this study, investigators found a particular allele (A) of the MMP-12 promoter possessing increased transcriptional activity in vitro in monocytes/macrophages that was associated with a smaller coronary artery luminal diameter in vivo in patients with diabetes and manifested in coronary artery disease requiring percutaneous transluminal coronary angioplasty with stent implantation. These findings contradict the studies of aneurysms that showed increased elastolytic activity that led to widened luminal diameter. However, this apparent contradiction can be explained by the linkage that some degradation products of elastin are chemotactic for leukocytes, and thereby, potentially contribute to inflammation and the development of atherosclerosis.[50]

Weitkamp et al[51] researched type VIII collagen, a short-chain collagen that is present in increased amounts in atherosclerotic lesions. Human macrophages synthesize type VIII collagen and MMP-1 (in different ratios) both in vitro and in the atherosclerotic plaque. It is possible that the production of type VIII collagen by macrophages in the plaque counterbalances macrophage production of degradative enzymes. Thus, plaque stability may depend on a balance between these two macrophage functions. If such an interaction exists, it is most likely very complex. Liptay et al[52] demonstrated that collagen production by smooth-muscle cells is not stimulated in the vicinity of macrophage-derived foam cells, whereas nonfoamy macrophages exert a stimulatory effect. Thus, the overall characteristics of a plaque may depend not only on the number of macrophages within the lesion, but also on their degree of activation and localization.[51] Further research is needed to elucidate this mechanism.

Another area for future research is the role of tenascin-C. Wallner et al[53] investigated the pattern of expression of tenascin-C in human coronary atherosclerotic plaques. They demonstrated that the expression of tenascin-C increases with ascending levels of plaque instability, from fibrous through lipid-rich to ruptured plaque. This increased induction was also correlated with the progressive accumulation of macrophages in the plaque. On the basis of this data, the hypothesis was made that macrophages express tenascin-C in advanced human atherosclerotic plaques. The introduction of a small isoform of tenascin into the matrix may generate a dynamic interactive network of matrix proteins that create a microenvironment that affects macrophages and other intimal cells. This microenvironment promotes progression and destabilization of atherosclerotic plaques rather than maintenance and stability.[53]

Postangioplasty Restenosis

Percutaneous transluminal coronary angioplasty is a widely used treatment for angina pectoris and myocardial infarction. It is an attractive procedure because of its limited invasiveness and minimal complication rate when compared with surgery. However, its usefulness is limited by a high restenosis rate. Arterial remodeling after balloon angioplasty has been recognized as a major determinant of restenosis. Perturbation of collagen metabolism might be important. After balloon injury, MMP expression is upregulated.

The pathogenesis of human restenotic lesions after percutaneous transluminal coronary angioplasty is not well defined (see Chap. 40), but there is some consensus regarding the general sequence of events.[54,54a,54b] Degradation of the extracellular matrix may result in clinically silent plaque disruption, causing interplaque thrombosis with a subsequent smooth-muscle cell proliferative response.[49] Within the first 24 h, "recoil" can occur secondary to vessel elasticity[55,56] and thrombi are formed by the exposure of subendothelial structures to blood. Because atherosclerotic lesions vary in composition, their thrombotic potential does as well. Evidence suggest that the highly lipid plaques are the most thrombogenic.[57]

The involvement of smooth-muscle cells in this event is less clear. Evidence suggests medial smooth-muscle cells immediately replicate on day 1,[58] migrate to the intima on day 4, and then may replicate again in the intima and produce an extracellular matrix.[59] As discussed in the development of atherosclerosis, MMPs may play a central role in migration of medial smooth-muscle cells to the intima. This theory is supported by a rise in gelatinase B synthesis and activity in the vessel 1 day after balloon injury, and its continued presence for 6 days post injury.[60]

However, smooth-muscle cells in an artery postpercutaneous transluminal coronary angioplasty are in a strikingly different environment than they were in the development of the de novo atherosclerotic plaque. In injured arteries, there are fewer intact cells, intimal smooth-muscle cells are present from the original atherosclerotic plaque, there are different degrees of thrombus depending on the plaque make up, and there are different cytokines and chemoattractants. Thus, smooth-muscle cells in this postangioplasty environment probably act differently than in the preangioplasty state. Evidence suggests that smooth-muscle cells in an environment similar to a balloon-injured vessel produce less TIMP-1 and 60% more active gelatinase A without any stimulation.[41] In addition, these smooth-muscle cells will migrate and invade a basement membrane when platelet-derived growth factor is added to the medium, whereas smooth-muscle cells in an intact vessel environment will neither migrate nor invade without additional stimulation.

The significance of this smooth-muscle cell migration with platelet-derived growth factor stimulation is unclear. Platelet-derived growth factor is a potent mitogen and chemoattractant for smooth-muscle cells. It is secreted from platelets, endothelium, smooth-muscle cells, and macrophages,[61–63] and it seems to play a role in postangioplasty restenosis. Evidence shows that balloon-catheter arterial injury in rats induces expression of both platelet-derived growth factor and its receptor in the resulting neointimal lesion.[64] In addition, administration of an antiplatelet-derived growth factor antibody before and after balloon artery injury reduces the thickness and cellular content of the neointima lesion by nearly 41%,[65] while infusion of platelet-derived growth factor for 7 days increases the intimal lesion fifteenfold.[66]

Interestingly, when an MMP inhibitor is added to the injury vessel environment in which smooth-muscle cells react to platelet-derived growth factor, invasion of the basement membrane is inhibited but migration is not. Thus, invasion of the basement membrane in the postangioplasty state seems to be MMP-dependent, but the migration of smooth-muscle cells is not, even though both smooth-muscle cell migration and basement membrane invasion are triggered by platelet-derived growth factor in this environment. de Smet et al[67] investigated the effect of batimastat, a nonspecific MMP inhibitor, on late lumen loss, arterial remodeling, and neointima formation after balloon dilation. MMP inhibition by batimastat significantly reduced late lumen loss after balloon angioplasty by inhibiting constrictive arterial remodeling, whereas neointima formation was not inhibited.

In addition, one has to question whether the migration of medial smooth-muscle cells is absolutely necessary to form a restenotic plaque, because intimal smooth muscle cells are already present from the original plaque. In vivo animal studies support this idea by showing that when an MMP inhibitor is given before and after balloon-catheter injury for up to 14 days, the number of intimal smooth-muscle cells is greatly reduced, but not completely obliterated.[68] This reduction correlates to an initial reduction in intimal thickening at 7 to 10 days. However, it does seem that the small number of smooth-muscle cells that did cross the basement membrane were able to increase proliferation to compensate. At day 14, the intimal lesion has the same cell number and size as controls. Thus, it is possible that the small number of intimal smooth-muscle cells present after percutaneous transluminal coronary angioplasty could also compensate by proliferating even if migration of medial cells is completely inhibited.

The role of plasminogen in MMP regulation has already been addressed and is now being studied in the context of restenosis. Both tissue-type plasminogen activator (t-PA) and urokinase-type plasminogen activator (u-PA) are expressed in smooth-muscle cells after arterial injury. u-PA expression in smooth-muscle cells is detectable immediately after arterial balloon injury, and t-PA is detectable at 3 days, around the time of smooth-muscle cell migration.[69] In an attempt to link plasmin with smooth-muscle cell migration, rats infused with a compound that inhibits plasmin production showed a significant reduction in the rate of smooth-muscle cell migration in ballooned arteries.[70,71] This migration could be secondary to either direct matrix degradation by plasmin or by activating MMPs. Smooth-muscle cell migration, in addition to proliferation, contributes to a large extent to the neointima formed in humans after balloon angioplasty or bypass surgery. Plasminogen activator/plasmin-mediated proteolysis is an important mediator of this smooth-muscle cell migration. Quax et al[72] provide evidence that adenoviral transfer of a hybrid protein that binds selectively to the u-PA receptor and inhibits plasmin activity directly on the cell surface is a powerful approach to inhibiting neointima formation and restenosis.

Another study showed that treatment with a heparin fraction (low molecular weight and no anticoagulant function) for 14 days postballoon injury in rats decreased t-PA but not u-PA, and resulted in a 60% reduction in smooth-muscle cell accumulation and intimal thickening.[73] By inhibiting t-PA, heparin may be inhibiting the activation of plasminogen that is required for activation of many latent MMPs, although it is not clear why u-PA would not make up for the lost t-PA function. Alternatively, heparin inhibits collagenase at the level of transcription.[74] This evidence supports the idea that plasmin/plasminogen activators are important in restenosis; however, the molecular mechanism for these effects are unknown and may be unrelated to MMPs. A review done by Christ et al[75] suggested that increases in plasminogen activator inhibitor type-1 (PAI-1) plasma levels after balloon angioplasty or permanently elevated lipoprotein (a) [Lp(a)] plasma levels might be helpful in the prediction of restenosis after coronary angioplasty. In contrast, t-PA plasma levels appear unrelated to restenosis, and data regarding a possible role of u-PA in the circulation are currently unavailable. Furthermore, a new hypothesis was presented on the pathophysiologic role of local PAI-1 overexpression as a beneficial negative feedback mechanism to limit excess cellular proliferation in atherogenesis and restenosis. More research needs to be performed examining this relationship between t-PA and intimal smooth-muscle cell accumulation.

The role of TIMPs in atherosclerosis has not been as well studied as MMPs. However, it has been noted that TIMP-1 synthesis is greatly elevated in the neointima 8 weeks after endothelial removal in a rabbit aorta.[76] This elevation is not well understood. It is probable that TIMPs have functions other than inhibiting MMPs, and may contribute to the development of atherosclerosis. Hayakawa et al[77] demonstrated evidence that TIMPs promote fibroblast and endothelial cell proliferation. More research in this area is needed as well.

Patency of Venografts After Bypass Surgery

Accelerated atherosclerosis of saphenous vein grafts causes premature graft failure in a large number of patients. There is recent evidence that inhibition of MMPs can alter graft patency.[3a] Overexpression of TIMP-3 by adenovirus gene transfer reduces neointimal formation in vein grafts, and increases the rate of apoptosis of vascular smooth-muscle cells.[3a] These observations suggest that selective alterations of MMP/TIMP could be of therapeutic use in decelerating vein graft closure.[3a]

Rupture of Coronary Atherosclerotic Plaques

Rupture of coronary atheromas accounts for most acute myocardial infarctions. These rupture-prone areas (shoulder and core) generally contain accumulations of activated macrophage foam cells and T lymphocytes with few smooth-muscle cells present.[78–80] These areas also contain reduced collagen and glycosaminoglycan concentrations.

It is suggested that MMPs derived from macrophages may digest the extracellular matrix in the fibrous cap, leading to plaque rupture (Fig. 43-2). In vitro studies have certainly shown that macrophages are able to break down fibrous caps and this degradation is correlated to the presence of MMP secretion.[81] In addition, all three subgroups of the MMP family have been identified intracellularly in macrophages accumulated in rupture-prone areas of human

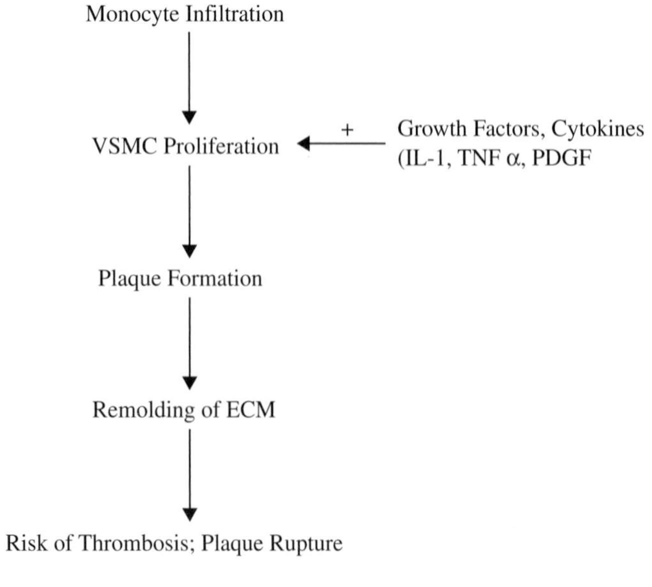

Monocyte Infiltration

↓

VSMC Proliferation ← + ← Growth Factors, Cytokines (IL-1, TNF α, PDGF

↓

Plaque Formation

↓

Remolding of ECM

↓

Risk of Thrombosis; Plaque Rupture

FIGURE 43-2. An early event in the development of atherosclerotic plaque is the infiltration of circulating monocytes, the proliferation of macrophages and vascular smooth-muscle cells (VSMCs), the major constituents in atherosclerotic lesions. Plaque formation leads to obligatory changes and to remodeling of the extracellular matrix (ECM) through the functions of MMPs and TIMPs, the tissue inhibitors of MMPs. MMP-2 may stimulate VSMC migration and penetration in the basement membrane, whereas growth factors and cytokines [e.g., tumor necrosis factor-α (TNFα) interleukin-1 (IL-1), and platelet-derived growth factor (PDGF)] stimulate MMP synthesis and matrix turnover in diseased lesions. Imbalances between matrix formation and distribution may perturb the supporting architecture and circumferential wall stress, alter the distribution of shear stress across the fibrous cap, and contribute to plaque instability or rupture, resulting in coronary thrombosis. Because the major composition of lipid-laden plaques is the ECM, the MMPs and TIMPs are principal targets for future therapeutic interventions, using pharmacologic or gene-based maneuvers, to alter the pathogenesis and clinical course in acute ischemic syndromes. (*Reproduced with permission from Benjamin IJ.*[3a])

atherosclerotic plaques.[82] This intracellular location indicates active synthesis because MMPs are not stored.

Kaartinen et al[83] attempted to define the role of mast cells in plaque destabilization. Unstable coronary syndromes are associated with increased numbers of mast cells in culprit lesions. Activated mast cells were shown to secrete neutral proteases capable of degrading the extracellular matrix and tumor necrosis factor-α, capable of stimulating macrophages to synthesize MMP-9. They suggested that mast cells, in addition to macrophages, contribute to matrix degradation and, hence, to progression of coronary syndromes.

Other studies have only been able to associate gelatinase B with rupture-prone areas in vivo. When atherectomy specimens obtained from patients with unstable angina were compared to specimens from patients with stable angina and normal internal mammary arteries, it was found that gelatinase B was present in 83% of the patients with unstable angina, in 25% of the patients with stable angina, and in 0% of the patients with normal internal mammary arteries.[84] Again, gelatinase B enzyme was found intracellularly in the macrophages. This study shows a strong association between the presence of gelatinase B in human coronary atherosclerosis with the clinical syndrome of unstable angina. It is possible that only 83% of the unstable angina patients were positive because of sampling error inherent in atherectomy procedures, and that 25% of the stable angina patients were positive because they were going to progress to unstable angina.

It is unclear at present which MMPs are involved in coronary plaque rupture and what activates their production. However, because activated macrophage foam cells and T lymphocytes are the dominant cells in vulnerable regions, the interaction between these two cells may be critical to the process of rupture. One study has demonstrated that T lymphocytes that express high levels of CD40 ligand gp39 can stimulate human monocytes to produce gelatinase B.[33] Although macrophages and T lymphocytes are present all over plaques, their accumulation in vulnerable areas and the presence of few smooth-muscle cells make these areas most prone to degradation. Thus, degradation would predominate in these areas. Another study[85] tested the hypothesis that the T-lymphocyte surface molecule CD40 ligand, recently localized in atherosclerotic plaques, regulates the expression of MMPs in human vascular smooth-muscle cells, the most numerous cell type in arteries. This study found that recombinant human CD40 ligand induced de novo synthesis of MMP-1, MMP-3, and MMP-9 on vascular smooth-muscle cells and stimulated the expression of these enzymes to a greater extent than did maximally effective concentrations of tumor necrosis factor-α or interleukin-1β, established agonists of MMP expression. Interferon-γ, another T-lymphocyte-derived cytokine, inhibited the

induction of MMPs by recombinant CD40 ligand. Immunohistochemical analysis of human coronary atheromata colocalized MMP-1 and MMP-3 with CD40-positive smooth-muscle cells. These results demonstrated that CD40 ligand, expressed on T lymphocytes, promoted the expression of matrix-degrading enzymes in vascular smooth-muscle cells, and thus established a new pathway of immune-modulated destabilization in human atheromata.

Other mechanisms of stimulating MMP production in these areas have been proposed as well.[85a] It seems that macrophage foam cells from atherosclerotic lesions secrete stromelysin and collagenase without any stimulation, whereas nonlipid-laden macrophages do not.[86] It is possible that the reactive oxygen radicals and oxidized low-density lipoprotein generated from these foam cells stimulate macrophage secretion of MMPs. Thus, multiple mechanisms of how MMPs could produce rupture in prone areas of atherosclerotic plaques exist. It is probable that different combinations of these mechanisms contribute to each rupture event.

POTENTIAL THERAPEUTIC INTERVENTIONS

The potential for drug therapy to intervene in the actions of MMPs in cardiovascular disease is real. However, target specificity and selectivity will be of primary importance in developing new treatments in this area. As Table 43-1 demonstrates, MMPs are involved in tissue resorption and degradation all over the body. Thus, potential drugs must act in specified local areas and avoid systemic effects.

Novel ideas for the delivery of these potential treatments are being examined. Promising clinical applications include temporary or permanent local delivery devices within the vasculature to enhance bioavailability and target specificity.[54] Some experiments have shown encouraging results with local drug-delivery catheters that use an iontophoretic mechanism to facilitate delivery. This device uses electrical current to enhance the movement of charged molecules through tissue, and results in an even distribution of the drug without significant endothelial damage.[87] To avoid distal ischemia, a reperfusion lumen catheter is also used (Fig. 43-3). Mitchel et al[88] conducted a study to assess the efficacy of intravascular iontophoresis in the local delivery of heparin to balloon angioplasty sites by using a recently designed iontophoretic catheter. They demonstrated that local intramural heparin delivery is feasible with an intravascular iontophoretic catheter. Following intracoronary heparin iontophoresis in the porcine model, intramural drug is detected for at least 24 h. Local delivery of heparin with this technique significantly decreases early platelet deposition following balloon injury in peripheral porcine arteries. Robinson et al[89]

FIGURE 43-3. Representation of the iontophoretic approach to local drug delivery. (*Reproduced with permission from Celentano D and Frishman WH.[127]*)

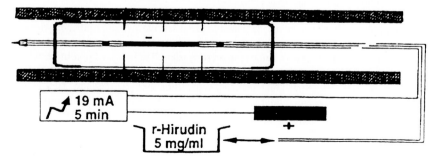

Local iontophoretic delivery device

19 mA
5 min

r-Hirudin
5 mg/ml

Local double balloon delivery device

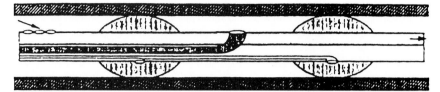

FIGURE 43-4. Representation of the barophoretic approach to local drug delivery. (*Reproduced with permission from Celentano D and Frishman WH.*[127])

also demonstrated the iontophoretic catheter to be a useful device, in their attempt to deliver antisense oligonucleotide to pig coronary arteries after balloon angioplasty. Although further research needs to be done in this field, specifically for use of MMP inhibitors, these studies highlight the tremendous potential regarding this methodology. Interestingly, the efficacy of this method was tested in canine coronary arteries by Hodgkin et al.[90] They demonstrated that an R-wave synchronized iontophoretic field with a response-frequency limiter can be safely used within the canine coronary arterial system at 50% effective refractory period (ERP) with moderate outputs (5 to 10 mA). Increasing the stimulus duration to 75% of ERP increases arrhythmogenesis, but is tolerated at lower output levels (<5 mA).

Another mechanism for achieving high local concentrations in a vessel uses a barophoretic approach.[13] This device uses a double-balloon catheter creating a mini-environment isolated from blood between the balloons where therapeutic agents can be delivered (Fig. 43-4). To avoid distal ischemia, this device also has an internal conduit for the continued flow of blood. Both the iontophoretic and barophoretic systems offer a significant increase in specificity and transfer efficiency over systemic delivery or other local devices being investigated.[54]

In addition to method of delivery, the other primary obstacle to drug therapy intervention is the therapeutic agent to be used. The increased MMP activity during atherosclerotic plaque development and instability must be caused by increased cytokine and growth factor-stimulated gene transcription, elevated zymogen activation, and an imbalance in the MMP:TIMP ratio. It is therefore conceivable that inhibition of MMPs or reestablishing the MMP:TIMP balance may be useful in treating the symptoms of atherosclerosis. Recent studies using synthetic MMP inhibitors and gene therapy have highlighted the potential for such an approach.[91]

A number of agents have been created to inhibit the synthesis, activation, and active sites of MMPs.[92–94] For instance, N-aryl-pyrido-fused isothiazolones are nonpeptidic small molecules that seem to inhibit activation of pro-MMPs by binding to Cys75 in the pro-region of the MMP zymogen. In turn, this binding interferes with the normal activation of these proteases (Fig. 43-5). This inhibition has been documented for MMP-3 and is assumed to inhibit the entire MMP family because they share a common activation mechanism.

Other promising pharmacologic approaches include the use of marimastat. Peterson et al.[95] discovered that marimastat inhibits neointimal thickening in a model of human arterial intimal hyperplasia, and thus has a potential therapeutic role in the prevention of human arterial restenosis. Another interesting study[96] tested the effects of magnesium sulfate on MMP-1 and interleukin-6 levels in patients who were undergoing coronary reperfusion therapy following an acute myocardial infarction. They concluded that increased serum ionized magnesium sulfate may inhibit arrhythmic recurrence and the production of interleukin-6 and MMP-1 after reperfusion and prevent the increase of myocardial lesions caused

by calcium overload on myocytes. They hypothesized that the increased interleukin-6 production may induce MMP-1, leading to tissue organ injury, and that pretreatment with magnesium sulfate may protect the myocardium of acute myocardial infarction patients from reperfusion injuries.

In considering the development of de novo atherosclerotic lesions and their progression, MMPs seem to be most involved in this process by allowing the smooth-muscle cells to migrate to the intima. Because this is a slowly developing process that can continue over the course of a lifetime, an intravascular device seems impractical in this situation. For the same reason, a generalized MMP inhibitor given systemically long-term would probably have far too many toxic side effects to make it useful. In addition, it may prevent plaque reorganization and collateral vessels from forming because evidence strongly suggests that MMPs are necessary in neoangiogenesis and plaque reorganization.[82,97] The use of synthetic MMP inhibitors in balloon-injured arteries has been studied in rats. One study showed that MMP-mediated migration of smooth-muscle cell could be inhibited and cause a temporary decrease in plaque size.[98] However, smooth-muscle cell replication rates were not altered by the inhibitor, known as GM-6001, and neointimal lesion size eventually reached control sizes. Another study demonstrated that dose-dependent inhibition of smooth-muscle cell migration, as well as DNA synthesis of smooth-muscle cells, could be achieved by a synthetic inhibitor (batimastat).[99] As major sources of MMP-9, the blockage of smooth-muscle cell migration could be efficacious in the treatment of coronary artery disease. Although batimastat, in the context of cardiovascular disease, has been studied in abdominal aortic aneurysms (AAA), it appears not only to act as a direct pharmacologic inhibitor of MMPs, but also to interfere with the inflammatory response seen in AAA.[99] Control of the inflammatory response was an unexpected result and may be related to the alterations in feedback mechanisms that are related to extracellular matrix degradation. Because this drug is presently being developed to control the MMP inflammatory response seen with arthritis, this class of drug may soon become available for clinical testing as a pharmacologic treatment of AAA.

A potentially more optimal approach may be one that blocks the specific stimulators in vessels that induce MMP transcription or activation during times of atherosclerosis formation. As discussed in the STARS study, the association of an altered MMP gene with progression of cardiovascular disease only became significant when combined with high levels of serum low-density lipoprotein. Thus, one potential way of preventing MMP induction in vessels is already being used in clinical practice, lowering low-density lipoprotein cholesterol with diet and/or drug therapy. This is an extremely interesting finding in lieu of new research on the beneficial effects of hydroxymethylglutaryl-coenzyme A (HMG-CoA) reductase inhibitors. Aikawa et al[100–102] recently demonstrated that dietary lipid lowering in cholesterol-fed rabbits reduces expression and activity of MMPs and tissue factor

A. Normal Activation

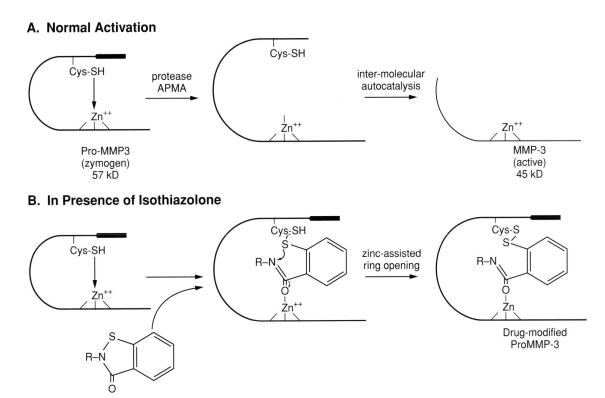

B. In Presence of Isothiazolone

FIGURE 43-5. (*A*) Absence of inhibitor; activation of the propeptide involves the dissociation of the cysteine thiol from the zinc ion, which exposes the active site, allowing bimolecular autolysis to occur. (*B*) Isothiazolones react with the cysteine thiol residue, forming a disulfide bond. This adduct can then act as a ligand for zinc, replacing the cysteine thiol and, in turn, interfering with the normal activation of proMMP-3. APMA = 4-aminophenylmercuric acid. (*Reproduced with permission from Arner EC, et al.*[92])

expression in established atheroma by reducing macrophage number and, in turn, ameliorating smooth-muscle cell activation. Shiomi et al[103] demonstrated that cerivastatin retards progression of atherosclerosis in terms of plaque size and macrophage accumulation in Watanabe heritable hyperlipidemic rabbits. Lipid lowering by HMG-CoA reductase inhibitors may alter the biology of atherosclerotic lesion formation. Among all vascular cell types, macrophages, in particular, are involved in all phases of atherosclerosis from initiation through progression and finally plaque rupture and thrombosis. Aikawa et al,[104] in a recent study, demonstrated that cerivastatin can suppress the growth of macrophages that express proteolytic enzymes and a tissue factor in atheroma of animals with endogenous hypercholesterolemia. Cerivastatin, in a concentration that can be achieved in patients, also suppresses proliferation and activation of macrophages in culture. This study provides new evidence for an effect of HMG-CoA reductase inhibitors on macrophage functions beyond lipid lowering and sheds new light on the mechanisms of plaque stabilization and reduced thrombotic complications in patients treated with HMG-CoA reductase inhibitors. A study by Ganne et al[105] shows that the expression of u-PA and urokinase-receptor induced by oxidized LDL on monocyte surface is suppressed by cerivastatin from as low as 2 nM. This leads to reduced plasmin generation and monocyte adhesion to vitronectin. Furthermore, higher concentrations of cerivastatin (50 to 100 nM) reduce the expression of u-PA and urokinase receptor on unstimulated monocytes. It also inhibits MMP-9 secretion, but has no effect on TIMP-1 secretion, suggesting that the decrease in MMP-9 has a real protective effect

on plaque stabilization. The inhibitory effect of cerivastatin on u-PA expression and MMP-9 secretion can be explained by the inhibition of nuclear factor-kappa B (NF-κB) translocation into the nucleus. Because farnesyl-pyrophosphate reverses the effect of cerivastatin, Ganne et al postulated that these effects could also be due to the inhibition of Ras prenylation. This was confirmed by confocal microscopy, which shows the Ras delocalization from the monocyte membrane. The cerivastatin-induced effects on monocyte functions could explain, at least in part, the protective effect of this drug against atherothrombotic events. Similarly promising data was obtained by Bellosta et al.[106] They studied the effect of fluvastatin on the activity of MMP-9 in mouse and human macrophages in culture. Conditioned media of cells were treated for 24 h with fluvastatin and analyzed by gelatin zymography. In mouse macrophages, fluvastatin (5 to 100 μmol/L) significantly inhibited in a dose-dependent manner MMP-9 activity from 20 to 10% versus control. A concentration as low as 5 μmol/L, inhibited MMP-9 activity (30%) in human monocyte-derived macrophages. Phorbel esters (t-PA, 50 ng/mL) stimulated MMP-9 activity by 50%, and fluvastatin inhibited this enhanced activity by up to 50% as well. These results were confirmed by Western blotting and enzyme-linked immunosorbent assay (ELISA). The inhibitory effect of fluvastatin was overcome by simultaneous addition of exogenous mevalonate (100 μmol/L), precursors of isoprenoids. Fluvastatin's effect was fully reversible and the drug did not cause any cellular toxicity. Similar data were obtained with simvastatin.[106]

The problem of restenosis is theoretically easier to treat due to the acuteness of vessel injury and the isolated location to direct treatment. It is in this situation that an intravascular device may be most beneficial. However, the development of efficacious agents to be used in these devices has failed, mostly due to the paucity of precise information concerning the mechanism of human restenosis. It is probable that development of restenosis occurs by several mechanisms, thus merely blocking one pathway with a drug may initiate compensation by a different pathway.

The experiments discussed have shown that the inhibition of MMPs does not reduce long-term neointimal lesions,[68] although there is some experimental data to suggest that MMP can inhibit late coronary vein bypass neointima formation.[107] Perhaps medial smooth-muscle cell migration is not the correct therapeutic target because human atherosclerotic arteries undergoing percutaneous transluminal coronary angioplasty already possess intimal smooth-muscle cells. It is possible that even with complete suppression of medial smooth-muscle cell migration, intimal smooth-muscle cells can compensate by replicating and producing the extracellular matrix of a new lesion. Thus, a better target may be the prevention of intimal smooth-muscle cell proliferation and the production of extracellular matrix. Potential investigations in the future may involve temporarily implanting a double-balloon barophoretic catheter with a drug or a gene vector to be delivered to the site of injury that would act on these intimal smooth-muscle cells directly after percutaneous transluminal coronary angioplasty.

Therapeutic intervention regarding plaque rupture is complicated by the sudden onset of these events with little warning. Once the plaque has ruptured, intervening with MMPs probably has little effect. Therefore, therapeutic intervention should be aimed at preventing what stimulates macrophage foam cells from synthesizing MMPs that may initiate rupture.[85a] Two areas could address this problem, and prevention of plaque rupture may need to use both of them. The first involves the prevention of T lymphocytes from activating macrophages to secrete MMPs. This has been done in vivo by giving an anti-gp39 antibody to prevent arthritis in mice. However, its long-term effects in humans are unknown. The second involves the other proposed trigger of MMP secretion by macrophages, oxidized low-density lipoprotein. Again, clinicians are already routinely reducing low-density lipoprotein in patients with cholesterol-lowering therapy.

Conclusion

MMP are a family of enzymes that selectively digest individual components of the extracellular matrix. Their function has been studied in both normal physiologic processes and pathologic states. In the blood vessel, MMPs play an important role in maintaining the vessel's integrity by breaking down extracellular matrix while new matrix is being synthesized. This is necessary to avoid weakening of the vessel wall from continuous mechanical stresses. However, in certain environments, these MMPs may contribute to cardiovascular pathologic processes.

Evidence suggests that MMPs contribute to the development of de novo atherosclerotic plaques, atherosclerosis of saphenous vein venografts after bypass surgery, and postangioplasty restenotic plaques by allowing smooth-muscle cells to migrate from the vascular media to the intima. Evidence also suggests that MMPs contribute to the rupture of these plaques by degrading the fibrous cap that surrounds them. With this increased molecular information concerning the pathogenesis of coronary vascular disease, new molecular therapies aimed at altering these processes are being investigated.[108]

THE METALLOPROTEINASES IN ABDOMINAL AORTIC ANEURYSM

Once thought to be purely secondary to atherosclerotic occlusive disease, AAA is no longer seen as merely on a continuum with the former.[108a] The concept of treating AAA as an inflammatory disease has been proposed in the literature. Although the link of AAA with systemic connective tissue disorders is a tenuous one, there is some evidence of similar monogenic mutations in Marfan's syndrome, Ehlers-Danlos' syndrome, and AAA. Given the increasing arsenal of knowledge of the molecular and histopathologic features of AAA, pharmacologic modes of treatment have become a distinct possibility. The impact that early medical management could have on the progression of aneurysm development and growth cannot be overemphasized. Currently, physicians can only monitor the size of small asymptomatic aneurysms but can do nothing about them; this is the so-called "watchful waiting" dilemma. Recent studies have focused on MMP, chemokine, and prostaglandin inhibition as methods to deter aneurysmal degeneration. These studies, as well as proposed mechanisms for drug delivery, are discussed below.

Medical Therapies

Given the literature supporting MMP-9 as a major elastolytic MMP linked with AAA, it is sensible that suppression of this gelatinase could have profound beneficial effects on the disease. Petrinec et al[109] demonstrated that this, indeed, was the case in an elastase-induced rat model of AAA. They found that doxycycline given subcutaneously to the rats resulted in decreased damage to the elastic media and limited aneurysmal dilatation after elastase perfusion of the aorta. Additionally, there was marked suppression of MMP-9 levels in the aortic walls as compared to controls with AAA. The mechanism of metalloproteinase inhibition with doxycycline is distinct from its antimicrobial activity and has proven effective in treatment of other MMP-mediated diseases such as gingivitis and arthritis.[109] Curci et al[110] expanded the use of doxycycline for treatment of AAA to human models. Following their earlier work,[111] and a study done by Boyle et al,[112] they concluded that in addition to its recognized effects as a direct MMP antagonist, doxycycline may influence connective tissue degradation within human aneurysm tissue by reducing monocyte/macrophage expression of MMP-9 mRNA and by suppressing the posttranslational processing (activation) of proMMP-2. Through this complimentary combination of pharmacologic actions, treatment with doxycycline may be a particularly effective strategy for achieving MMP inhibition in patients with an AAA.

Additional investigation is warranted to delineate the mechanism and efficacy of the tetracycline antibiotics as MMP inhibitors. Recently, however, Franklin et al[113] concluded that tetracycline rapidly penetrates AAA walls in vivo and inhibits MMP-9 and monocyte chemotactic proteins (MCP-1) released by AAA explants. However, the concentration achieved may be insufficient to alter collagen turnover through limitation of MMP production or activity. Interestingly, high concentrations of tetracycline inhibited MCP-1 secretion from aneurysm biopsy explants. Other studies show that it also inhibits the expression of inducible nitric oxide synthase and it is active against *Chlamydia pneumoniae* (50% of AAA biopsies are positive with this organism).[111] Thus, its affects and mechanisms are several.[113] The future challenge with use of tetracycline is the development of a formulation that penetrates the aneurysm wall

TABLE 43-3. Matrix Metalloproteinase (MMP) 50% Inhibitory Concentration (IC_{50}) as nmol/L of MMP Inhibitors

	Batimastat	Marimastat	CP-471474	PD-166793	Prinomastat	Tanomastat	Doxycycline
MMP-1	3	5	1170	6100	8.3	>5000	15,000
MMP-2	4	6	0.7	47	0.05	11	—
MMP-3	20	230	16	12	0.03	134	—
MMP-7	6	16	—	8100	54	—	—
MMP-9	10	3	13	9900	0.26	301	<50,000
MMP-13			0.9				

Source: Reproduced with permission from Li YY, Feldman AM. Matrix metalloproteinases in the progression of heart failure: Potential therapeutic implications. *Drugs* 61:1245, 2001.

more effectively to achieve a concentration that both impairs MMP functions and maximizes its anti-inflammatory effects.

Holmes et al used an elastase-induced AAA rat model with indomethacin as the MMP inhibitor.[114] Substrate zymography demonstrated decreased levels of MMP-9 and decreased aortic dilatation in the treated group as compared to the controls, supporting the hypothesis that indomethacin inhibits aneurysmal growth in the rat model.[114] This effect of indomethacin was shown by Miralles et al[115] to be mediated by the inhibition of the COX-2 isoform of cyclooxygenase, which decreases prostaglandin-2 and MMP-9 synthesis. The harmful effects of prostaglandin-2 as a part of the inflammatory response on aortic smooth-muscle cell viability and cytokine secretion were further highlighted by Walton et al,[116] who also demonstrated the benefits of inhibiting COX-2 in patients with asymptomatic AAA.

At present, aneurysms are managed by close observation and vascular reconstruction when the vessels have dilated to a critical size.[116a] It might now be possible by local gene transfer and the use of TIMP-1 overexpression to block aneurysmal expansion and thereby reduce the risk of rupture and the need for surgery.[117] Another possible therapeutic approach may be through the targeted gene disruption of MMP-9 as was proposed by Pyo et al.[118]

A series of low-molecular-weight MMP inhibitors (Table 43-3) with varying efficacy and specificity of MMP inhibition have been developed for the treatment of cancer and AAA with promising results.[119,120]

In a recent study,[121] marimastat was shown to inhibit elastin degradation and MMP-2 activity in a model of aneurysm disease. Marimastat is an agent that acts by competitive inhibition at the zinc active site essential for enzyme activity. Therapeutic concentrations of marimastat appeared to have reduced significantly the experimentally induced elastolysis that occurs in the aortic wall, with the end effect of preservation of medial elastin.

Moore et al[122] tested the effects of RS 132908 on the development of aneurysmal dilation. RS132908 is an oral compound that is designed to antagonize MMP activity in a direct and reversible fashion. It is based on a hydroxamic acid structure capable of interacting with the active site zinc in MMPs. By means of in vitro assays of enzyme activity, RS 132908 blocks the action of several different elastolytic MMPs, including MMP-2, MMP-9, and MMP-12. RS 132908 promoted the preservation of aortic elastin and enhanced a profibrotic response within the aortic wall and was well tolerated by rats. Thus, further investigation into the development of hydroxymate-based MMP antagonists may prove useful and promising.

Another study demonstrated that dose-dependent inhibition of smooth-muscle cell migration, as well as DNA synthesis of smooth-muscle cells, could be achieved by a synthetic inhibitor (batimastat).[123] As major sources of MMP-9, the blockage of smooth-muscle cell migration could be efficacious in aneurysmal tissue. Replication rate of smooth-muscle cells in the intima or inner media may not lead to as much dilatation of the aorta as that seen when smooth muscle cells are in the outer media and adventitia elaborating elastolytic MMPs. In a more recent study, Bigatel et al[99] were able to limit the expansion of AAA in rat models using batimastat. It appears that batimastat acts not only as a direct pharmacologic inhibitor of MMPs, but also interferes with the inflammatory response seen in AAA. Control of the inflammatory response was an unexpected result and may be related to the alterations in feedback mechanisms that are related to extracellular matrix degradation. Because this drug is presently being developed to control the MMP inflammatory response seen with arthritis, this class of drug may soon become available as a pharmacologic treatment of AAA. Hence, there may be utility in drugs similar to batimastat in decreasing aneurysmal degeneration.[68]

Investigators have identified a group of proteins known as monocyte chemoattractant proteins (MCPs), thought to be important in the pathogenesis of atherosclerotic plaques and AAA. Found in <1% of medial cells from normal aortas, mRNA of MCP-1 is expressed in macrophages, lymphocytes, and smooth-muscle cells in inflammatory zones of tissue from degenerative aorta.[123] Greater expression has been found in aneurysmal extracts than in occlusive disease tissue.[124] These proteins may be responsible for trafficking of monocytes through the aortic wall. A recent study by Hernandez-Presa et al[125] examined the effect of ACE inhibition on MCP-1 expression. Angiotensin II activates nuclear factor-kappa B (NF-κB), an agent that controls expression of MCP-1. They found that ACE inhibitors slowed neointimal macrophage infiltration in a rabbit model of accelerated atherosclerosis via control of NF-κB and MCP-1. Whether or not local delivery of ACE inhibitors to early aneurysmal tissue will slow disease progression through similar mechanisms remains to be seen.

Another target in the medical management of AAA aside from MMPs and MCPs involves the prostaglandin (PG) pathways. PGE_2 was localized by immunohistochemical analysis to macrophage-like cells in the inflammatory infiltrate of AAA specimens, but was not expressed significantly in normal specimens. Furthermore, the COX-2 isoform also has been localized to the same area in AAA extracts and is posited to control PGE_2 expression. Hence COX-2 is another potential target for pharmacotherapy.[126]

For potential treatments to be efficacious, they need an efficient delivery system—one that yields high bioavailability and target specificity. Because MMPs are involved in normal physiologic tissue resorption and degradation processes throughout the body (at sites such as bone, endometrium, and hair follicles), systemic toxicity of inhibitor drugs can be quite serious.[127] To alleviate this problem, local drug-delivery systems using intravascular devices have been developed. Placing the device in the infrarenal aorta, where the majority of aneurysmal dilatation occurs, would increase target specificity and theoretically reduce systemic toxicity. Double lumen catheters using iontophoretic and barophoretic mechanisms are examples of devices that use electrical current and pressure differences, respectively, to distribute the drug evenly throughout target areas.[13,127,128] Several important problems may arise, however, with this kind of delivery method. First, it may not be feasible to leave a catheter in a vessel for life-long treatment due to infection, patency, or difficulty in maintenance. Second, normal physiologic MMP function in the aortic wall, such as collateral vessel formation and plaque reorganization, may be suppressed, worsening rather than helping the aortic disease. It may be impossible to ascertain the amount of suppression of MMPs necessary to thwart pathologic processes in the aorta. Furthermore, current data on the efficacy of MMP inhibitors has been based on experimental models. Clinical trials are tantamount to uncovering the true utility of pharmacologic inhibition in AAA. Whether pharmacologic inhibition of the metalloproteinases will ultimately slow or prevent the progression of AAA disease remains to be tested in clinical trials. Nonetheless, the preliminary success with this drug therapy in experimental models is promising.

Conclusion

A plethora of research reports describing the mechanisms of AAA formation, expansion, and rupture currently exists. A variety of investigators have characterized specific enzymes and proteolytic processes that may be responsible for the potentially fatal disease. MMPs are consistently implicated as a major source of the collagen and elastin destruction that occur in AAA. Although most aneurysmal disease of the aorta is associated with preexisting arterial occlusive disease, many studies have found distinguishing features in MMP levels and distribution when comparing the two diseases. These reports suggest that some individuals may be predisposed to aneurysmal disease; however, specific genetic markers have not been clearly identified. In elastase-induced rodent models, MMP inhibition by tetracycline derivatives, as well as by synthetic inhibitors, has proven successful in limiting AAA growth. These findings are welcome, given the lack of treatment for small asymptomatic aneurysms. Methods of delivering the novel therapeutic agents are being refined with the goal of increasing tissue specificity and decreasing adverse effects.

METALLOPROTEINASES IN CONGESTIVE HEART FAILURE AND LEFT VENTRICULAR DILATATION

One new approach to preventing left ventricular (LV) enlargement following myocardial infarction addresses a different side of LV remodeling. Rather than interrupting the neurohormonal cascade, it appears possible to attack the remodeling phenomenon itself within the myocardium. Remodeling of any tissue requires that cells and extracellular matrix change their geometric relations; in the case of LV dilation, this may require that cells slip and slide along the collagenous scaffold of the heart. It has been known for decades that remodeling tissues rely heavily upon MMPs. MMPs are increased in failing hearts of both animal models and patients with heart failure.[129] New data indicate that these enzymes can medi-

ate the LV dilation process. In fact, several orally active MMP inhibitory compounds can inhibit LV dilatation in different animal models,[130–133] and some data suggest that blocking these enzymes may reduce postinfarct rupture of the myocardium.[134] Blockade of MMPs not only prevents postinfarct LV dilatation, but also cardiac enlargement in other heart-failure models, such as rapid pacing tachycardia,[131] suggesting that MMPs are fundamentally involved in the dilation process. These drugs also cause less collagen matrix damage, favorable extracellular matrix remodeling, and improve cardiac function in various heart-failure models.[135]

It is not yet clear at what stage metalloproteinase inhibition should be used, whether LV function improves over the long-term, or whether specific MMPs should be targeted for heart-failure prevention. However, there are literally hundreds of inhibitor compounds already available and it is likely that this approach will reach clinical testing soon.

MMP inhibitory compounds under investigation as possible therapies for heart failure include batimastat, the first synthetic MMP inhibitor; marimastat; prinomastat; tanomastat; PD-166739, a broad-spectrum MMP inhibitor; CP-471474, a selective inhibitor of MMP-2 and MMP-13; RS-113456 and ABT-770; and doxycycline.

Conclusion

Myocardial extracellular matrix remodeling and fibrosis regulated by MMPs are thought to contribute to heart-failure progression. These observations suggest a potential benefit of MMP inhibitors in heart failure as suggested by the favorable results of multiple preclinical studies with these compounds. MMP inhibitors are being considered as possible adjuncts to ACE inhibitors for reducing fibrosis and improving ventricular remodeling after myocardial infarction.

REFERENCES

1. Mignatti P, Tsuboi R, Robbins E, Rifkin DB: In vitro angiogenesis on the human amniotic membrane: Requirement for basic fibroblast growth factor induced proteinases. *J Cell Biol* 108:671, 1989.
2. Schnaper HW, Grant DS, Stetler-Stevenson WG, et al: Type IV collagenases and TIMPs modulate endothelial cell morphogenesis in vitro. *J Cell Physiol* 156:235, 1993.
3. Murphy AN, Unsworth EJ, Stetler-Stevenson WG: Tissue inhibitor of metalloproteinase-2 inhibits FGF-induced human microvasculature endothelial cell proliferation. *J Cell Physiol* 157:351, 1993.
3a. Benjamin IJ: Matrix metalloproteinases: From biology to therapeutic strategies in cardiovascular disease. *J Invest Med* 49:381, 2001.
3b. Jacob M-P, Cazaubon M, Scemama A, et al: Plasma matrix metalloproteinase-9 as a marker of blood stasis in varicose veins. *Circulation* 106:535, 2002.
3c. Schöenhagen P, Tuzcu EM, Ellis SG: Plaque vulnerability, plaque rupture, and acute coronary syndromes. (Multi)-focal manifestation of a systemic disease process. *Circulation* 106:760, 2002.
4. Creemers EEJM, Cleutjens JPM, Smits JFM, Daemen MJAP: Matrix metalloproteinase inhibition after myocardial infarction. *Circ Res* 89:201, 2001.
5. Van Wart HE, Birkedal-Hansen H: The cysteine switch: A principle of regulation of metalloproteinase activity with potential applicability to the entire matrix metalloproteinase gene family. *Proc Natl Acad Sci U S A* 87:5578, 1990.
6. Birkedal-Hansen H, Moore WG, Bodden MK, et al: Matrix metalloproteinase. A review. *Crit Rev Oral Biol Med* 4:197, 1993.
7. Docherty AJP, Murphy G: The tissue metalloproteinase family and the inhibitor TIMP: A study using DNAs and recombinant proteins. *Ann Rheum Dis* 49:469, 1990.

8. Matrisian LM:Matrix metalloproteinases and their inhibitors in connective tissue remodeling. *FASEB J* 6:121, 1991.

9. Unemori EN, Hibbs MS, Amento EP: Constitutive expression of a 92-kd gelatinase by rheumatoid synovial fibroblasts and its induction in normal human fibroblasts by inflammatory cytokines. *J Clin Invest* 88:1656, 1991.

10. Galis ZS, Muszynski M, Sukhova GK, et al: Cytokine-stimulated human vascular smooth muscle cells synthesize a complement of enzymes required for extracellular matrix digestion. *Circ Res* 75:181, 1994.

11. Nagase H, Enghild JJ, Suzuki K, Salvesen G: Stepwise activation mechanisms of the precursor of matrix metalloproteinase-3 by proteinases and mercuric acetate. *Biochem* 29:5783, 1990.

12. Murphy G, Willenbrock F, Crabbe T, et al: Regulation of matrix metalloproteinase activity. *Ann N Y Acad Sci* 732:31, 1994.

13. Meyer BJ, Fernandez Ortiz A, Mailhac A, et al: Local delivery of r-hirudin by a double balloon perfusion catheter prevents mural thrombosis and minimizes platelet deposition after angioplasty. *Circulation* 90:2474, 1994.

14. Dollery CM, McEwan JR, Henney AM: Matrix metalloproteinases and cardiovascular disease. *Circ Res* 77:863, 1995.

15. Okada Y, Morodomi T, Enghild JJ, et al: Matrix metallo-proteinase-2 from human rheumatoid synovial fibroblasts. Purification and activation of the precursor and enzymatic properties. *Eur J Biochem* 194:721, 1990.

16. Crabbe T, Ioannou C, Docherty AJP: Human progelatinase A can be activated by autolysis at a rate that is concentration dependent and enhanced by heparin bound to the C-terminal domain. *Eur J Biochem* 218:431, 1993.

17. Murphy G, Willenbrock F, Ward RV, et al: The C-terminal domain of 72-kDa gelatinase A is not required for catalysis, but is essential for membrane activation and modulates interactions with tissue inhibitors of metalloproteinases. *Biochem J* 283:637, 1992.

18. Overall CM, Sodek J: Concanavalin A produces a matrix-degradative phenotype in human fibroblasts. Induction and endogenous activation of collagenases, 72-kDa gelatinases and PUMP-1 is accomplished by suppression of the tissue inhibitor of matrix metalloproteinases. *J Biol Chem* 265:21141, 1990.

19. Willenbrock FT, Crabbe TM, Slocombe PM, et al: The activity of the tissue inhibitors of metalloproteinases is regulated by C-terminal domain interactions: A kinetic analysis of the inhibition of gelatinase A. *Biochemistry* 32:4330, 1993.

20. Kahari VM, Saarialo-Kere U: Matrix metalloproteinases and their inhibitors in tumor growth and invasion. *Ann Med* 31:34, 1999.

21. Joronen K, Salminen H, Glumoff V, et al: Temporospatial expression of tissue inhibitors of matrix metalloproteinases-1, -2, and -3 during development, growth and aging of the mouse skeleton. *Histochem Cell Biol* 114:157, 2000.

22. Hammani K, Blakis A, Morsette D, et al: Structure and characterization of the human tissue inhibitor of metalloproteinases-2 gene. *J Biol Chem* 271:25498, 1996.

23. Yang TT, Hawkes SP: Role of the 21-kDa protein TIMP-3 in oncogenic transformation of cultured chicken embryo fibroblasts. *Proc Natl Acad Sci U S A* 89:10676, 1992.

24. Anand-Apte B, Pepper MS, Voest E, et al: Inhibition of angiogenesis by tissue inhibitor of matrix metalloproteinase-3. *Invest Opthalmol Visual Sci* 38:817, 1997.

25. Butler GS, Apte SS, Willenbrock F, Murphy G: Human tissue inhibitor of metalloproteinases 3 interacts with both the N- and C-terminal domains of gelatinases A and B. *J Biol Chem* 274:10846, 1999.

26. Werb Z: Matrix metalloproteinases. Proceedings of the IBC's International Conference on Matrix Metalloproteinases in Tissue Remodeling. San Fransisco, CA: May, 1997.

27. Kishnani N, Yang T, Masiarz F, Hawkes S: Identification and characterization of human tissue inhibitor of metalloproteinase-3 and detection of three additional metalloproteinase inhibitor activities in extracellular matrix. *Matrix Biol* 14:479, 1995.

28. Olson TM, Hirohata S, Ye J, et al: Cloning of the human tissue inhibitor of metalloproteinase-4 gene (TIMP4) and localization of the TIMP4 and Timp4 genes to human chromosome 3p25 and mouse chromosome 6, respectively. *Genomics* 51(1):148, 1998.

29. Dollery CM, McEwan JR, Wang M, et al: TIMP-4 is regulated by vascular injury in rats. *Circ Res* 84(5):498, 1999.

30. Tyagi S, Meyer L, Kumar S, et al: Induction of tissue inhibitor of metalloproteinase and its mitogenic response to endothelial cells in human atherosclerotic and restenotic lesions. *Can J Cardiol* 12:353, 1996.

31. Chesler L, Golde DW, Bersch N, Johnson MD: Metalloproteinase inhibition and erythroid potentiation are independent activities of tissue inhibitor of metalloproteinase-1. *Blood* 86:4506, 1995.

32. Lee E, Vaughan DE, Parikh SH, et al: Regulation of matrix metalloproteinases and plasminogen activator inhibitor-1 synthesis by plasminogen in cultured human vascular smooth muscle cell. *Circ Res* 78:44, 1996.

33. Malik N, Greenfield BW, Wahl AF, Kiener PA: Activation of human monocytes through CD40 induces matrix metalloproteinases. *J Immunol* 156:3952, 1996.

34. Lambert CA, Soudant EP, Nusgens BV, Lapiere CM: Pretranslational regulation of extracellular matrix macromolecules and collagenase expression in fibroblasts by mechanical forces. *Lab Invest* 66:444, 1992.

35. Lijnen HR, Silence J, Lemmens G, et al: Regulation of gelatinase activity in mice with targeted inactivation of components of the plasminogen/plasmin system. *Thromb Haemost* 79:1171, 1998.

36. Ross R: The pathogenesis of atherosclerosis. A prospective for the 1990s. *Nature* 362:801, 1993.

37. Godin D, Ivan E, Johnson C, et al: Remodeling of carotid artery is associated with increased expression of matrix metalloproteinases in mouse blood flow cessation model. *Circulation* 102:2861, 2000.

38. Ikeda KH, Yasukawa H, Kai M, et al: Peripheral blood levels of matrix metalloproteases-2 and -9 are elevated in patients with acute coronary syndromes. *J Am Coll Cardiol* 32:368, 1998.

39. Pasterkamp G, Schoneveld AH, Hijnen DJ, et al: Atherosclerotic arterial remodeling and the localization of macrophages and matrix metalloproteases 1, 2 and 9 in the human coronary artery. *Atherosclerosis* 150(2):245, 2000.

40. Fitzgerald M, Hayward IP, Thomas AC, et al: Matrix metalloproteinases can facilitate the heparanase-induced promotion of phenotypic change in vascular smooth muscle cells. *Atherosclerosis* 145(1):97, 1999.

41. Pauly RR, Passaniti A, Bilato C, et al: Migration of cultured vascular smooth muscle cells through a basement membrane barrier requires type IV collagenase activity and is inhibited by cellular differentiation. *Circ Res* 75:41, 1994.

41a. Schoenhagen P, Vince DG, Ziada KM, et al: Relation of MMP-3 found in coronary lesion samples retrieved by directional coronary atherectomy to intravascular ultrasound observations on coronary remodeling. *Am J Cardiol* 89:1354, 2002.

42. Ye S, Watts GF, Mandalia S, et al: Preliminary report: Genetic variation in the human stromelysin promoter is associated with progression of coronary atherosclerosis. *Br Heart J* 73:209, 1995.

43. Humphries SE, Luong L, Talmud PJ, et al: The 5A/6A polymorphism in the promoter of the stromelysin-1(MMP-3 gene predicts progression of angiographically determined coronary artery disease in men in the LOCAT gemfibrozil study. *Atherosclerosis* 139(1):49, 1998.

44. Sandy JD, Boynton RE, Flannery CR: Analysis of the catabolism of aggrecan in cartilage explants by quantitation of peptides from the three globulin domains. *J Biol Chem* 266:8198, 1991.

45. Fosang AJ, Neame PJ, Last K, et al: The interglobulin domain of cartilage aggrecan is cleaved by PUMP, gelatinases and cathepsin B. *J Biol Chem* 267:19470, 1992.

46. Chin JR, Murphy G, Werb Z: Stromelysin, a connective tissue–degrading metalloendopeptidase secreted by stimulated rabbit synovial fibroblasts in parallel with collagenases. *J Biol Chem* 260:12367, 1985.

47. Ogata Y, Enghild JJ, Nagase H: Matrix metalloproteinase-3 (stromelysin) activates the precursor for the human matrix metalloproteinase-9. *J Biol Chem* 267:3581, 1992.

48. Little WC, Constantinescu M, Applegate RJ, et al: Can coronary angiography predict the site of a subsequent myocardial infarction in patients with mild to moderate coronary artery disease? *Circulation* 78:1157, 1988.

49. Jormsjo S, Ye S, Mortiz J, et al: Allele-specific regulation of matrix metalloproteinase-12 gene activity is associated with coronary artery luminal dimensions in diabetic patients with manifest coronary artery disease. *Circ Res* 86:998, 2000.

50. Senior RM, Griffin GL, Mecham RP: Chemotactic activity of elastin-derived peptides. *J Clin Invest* 66:859, 1980.

51. Weitkamp B, Cullen P, Plenz G, et al: Human macrophages synthesize type VIII collagen in vitro and in the atherosclerotic plaque. *FASEB J* 13:1445, 1999.

52. Liptay MJ, Parks WC, Mecham RP, et al: Neointimal macrophages colocalize with extracellular matrix gene expression in human atherosclerotic pulmonary arteries. *J Clin Invest* 91:588, 1993.

53. Wallner K, Li C, Prediman SK, et al: Tenascin–C is expressed in macrophage-rich human coronary atherosclerotic plaque. *Circulation* 99:1284, 1999.

54. Fuster V, Falk E, Fallon JT, et al: The three processes leading to post percutaneous transluminal coronary angiography restenosis: Dependence on the lesion substrate. *Thromb Haemost* 74:552, 1995.

54a. Wentzel JJ, Kloet J, Andhyiswara I, et al: Shear-stress and wall-stress regulation of vascular remodeling after balloon angioplasty. Effect of matrix metalloproteinase inhibition. *Circulation* 104:91, 2001.

54b. Frishman WH, Chiu R, Landzberg BR, Weiss M: Medical therapies for the prevention of restenosis after percutaneous coronary interventions. *Curr Probl Cardiol* 23:533, 1998.

55. Hanet C, Wijns W, Michel X, Schroeder E: Influence of balloon size and stenosis morphology on immediate and delayed elastic recoil after percutaneous transluminal coronary angioplasty. *J Am Coll Cardiol* 18:506, 1991.

56. Hjemdhal-Monsen CE, Ambrose JA, Borrico S, et al: Angiographic patterns of balloon inflation during percutaneous transluminal coronary angioplasty: Role of pressure-diameter curves in studying distensibility and elasticity of the stenotic lesion and the mechanism of dilation. *J Am Coll Cardiol* 16:569, 1990.

57. Fernandez Ortiz A, Badimon JJ, Falk E, et al: Characterization of the relative thrombogenicity of atherosclerotic plaque components: Implications for consequences of plaque rupture. *J Am Coll Cardiol* 23:1562, 1994.

58. Clowes AW, Reidy MA, Clowes MM: Kinetics of cellular proliferation after arterial injury. I: Smooth muscle growth in the absence of endothelium. *Lab Invest* 49:327, 1983.

59. Jackson CL, Raines EW, Ross R, Reidy MA: Role of endogenous platelet-derived growth factor in arterial smooth muscle cell migration after balloon catheter injury. *Arterioscler Thromb* 13:1218, 1993.

60. Bendeck MP, Zempo N, Clowes AW, et al: Smooth muscle cell migration and matrix metalloproteinases expression after arterial injury in the rat. *Circ Res* 75:539, 1994.

61. Ross R, Raines EW, Bowen-Pepe DR: The biology of platelet-derived growth factor (review). *Cell* 46:155, 1986.

62. Heldin CH, Westermark B: Platelet-derived growth factor: Mechanism of action and possible in vivo function. *Cell Res* 1:555, 1990.

63. Reidy MA, Bendeck MP: The development of arterial lesions: A process controlled by multiple factors. In: Goldhaver SZ, ed. *Coronary Restenosis, From Genetics to Therapeutics.* New York: Marcel Dekker, 1997:55–67.

64. Majesky MW, Reidy MA, Bowen-Pope DP et al: PDGF ligand and receptor gene expression during repair of arterial injury. *J Cell Biol* 111:2149, 1990.

65. Ferns GAA, Raines EW, Sprugal KH, et al: Inhibition of neointimal smooth muscle accumulation after angioplasty by an antibody to PDGF. *Science* 253:1129, 1991.

66. Jawien A, Bowen-Pope DF, Lindner V, et al: Platelet-derived growth factor promotes smooth muscle migration and intimal thickening in a rat model of balloon angioplasty. *J Clin Invest* 89:507, 1992.

67. de Smet BJ, de Kleijn D, Hanemaaijer R, et al: Metalloproteinase inhibition reduces constrictive arterial remodeling after balloon angioplasty: A study in the atherosclerotic Yucatan micropig. *Circulation* 101(25):2962, 2000.

68. Bendeck MP, Irvin C, Reidy MA: Inhibition of matrix metalloproteinase activity inhibits smooth muscle cell migration but not neointimal thickening after arterial injury. *Circ Res* 78:38, 1996.

69. Clowes AW, Clowes MM, Au YPT, et al: Smooth muscle cells express urokinase during mitogenesis and tissue-type plasminogen activator during migration in injured rat carotid artery. *Circ Res* 67:61, 1990.

70. Verstraete M: Clinical application of inhibitors of fibrinolysis. *Drugs* 29:236, 1985.

71. Takada A, Takada Y: Inhibition by tranexamic acid of the conversion of single-chain tissue plasminogen activator to its two chain form by plasmin: The presence on tissue plasminogen activator of a site to bind with lysine binding sites of plasmin. *Thromb Res* 55:717, 1989.

72. Quax PH, Lamfers ML, Lardenoye JH, et al: Adenoviral expression of a urokinase receptor-targeted protease inhibitor inhibits neointima formation in murine and human blood vessels. *Circulation* 103:562, 2001.

73. Clowes AW, Clowes MM, Kirkman TR, et al: Heparin inhibits the expression of tissue-type plasminogen activator by smooth muscle cells in injured rat carotid artery. *Circ Res* 70:1128, 1992.

74. Au KP, Kenagy RD, Clowes AW: Heparin selectively inhibits the transcription of tissue-type plasminogen activator in private arterial smooth muscle cells during mitogenesis *J Biol Chem* 267:3438, 1992.

75. Christ G, Kostner K, Zehetgruber M, et al: Plasmin activation system in restenosis: Role in pathogenesis and clinical prediction? *J Thromb Thrombolysis* 7(3):277, 1999.

76. Wang H, Moore S, Alavi MZ: Synthesis of tissue inhibitor of metalloproteinase-1 (TIMP) in rabbit aortic neointima after selective de-endothelialization. *Atherosclerosis* 126:95, 1996.

77. Hayakawa T, Yamashita K, Tunyawa K, et al: Growth promoting activity of tissue inhibitor of metalloproteinases-1 (TIMP-1) for a wide range of cells. A possible new growth factor in serum. *FEBS Lett* 298:29, 1992.

78. Richardson PD, Davies MJ, Born GVR: Influence of plaque configuration and stress distribution on fissuring of coronary atherosclerotic plaques. *Lancet* 2:941, 1989.

79. Cheng GC, Loree HM, Kamm RD, et al: Distribution of circumferential stress in ruptured and stable atherosclerotic lesions: A structural analysis with histopathologic correlation. *Circulation* 87:1179, 1993.

80. Schroeder AP, Falk E: Pathophysiology and inflammatory aspects of plaque rupture. *Cardiol Clin* 14:211, 1996.

81. Shah PK, Falk E, Badimon JJ, et al: Human monocyte-derived macrophages induce collagen breakdown in fibrous caps of atherosclerotic plaques. *Circulation* 95:1565, 1995.

82. Galis ZS, Sukhova GK, Lark MW, Libby P: Increased expression of matrix metalloproteinases and matrix degrading activity in vulnerable regions of human atherosclerotic plaques. *J Clin Invest* 94:2493, 1994.

83. Kaartinen M, van der Wal AC, van der Loos CM, et al: Mast cell infiltration in acute coronary syndromes: Implication for plaque rupture. *J Am Coll Cardiol* 32(3):606, 1998.

84. Brown DL, Hibbs MS, Kearney M, et al: Identification of 92-kd gelatinase in human coronary atherosclerotic lesions, association of active enzyme synthesis with unstable angina. *Circulation* 91:2125, 1995.

85. Schonbeck U, Mach F, Sukhova GK, et al: Regulation of matrix metalloproteinase expression in human vascular smooth muscle cells by T lymphocytes: A role for CD40 signaling in plaque rupture? *Circ Res* 81(3):448, 1997.

85a. Death AK, Nakhla S, Mc Grath KCY, et al: Nitroglycerin upregulates matrix metalloproteinase expression in human macrophages. *J Am Coll Cardiol* 39:1943, 2002.

86. Galis ZS, Sukhova GK, Kranzhofer R, et al: Macrophage foam cells from experimental atheroma constitutively produce matrix-degrading proteinases. *Proc Natl Acad Sci U S A* 92:402, 1995.

87. Fernandez Ortiz A, Meyer BJ, Mailhac A, et al: A new approach for local intravascular drug delivery: Iontophoretic balloon. *Circulation* 89:1518, 1994.

88. Mitchel JF, Azrin MA, Fram DB, et al: Localized delivery of heparin to angioplasty sites with iontophoresis. *Catheter Cardiovasc Diagn* 41(3):315, 1997.

89. Robinson KA, Chronos NA, Schieffer E, et al: Pharmacokinetics and tissue localization of antisense oligonucleotides in balloon-injured pig coronary arteries after local delivery with an iontophoretic balloon catheter. *Cath Cardiovasc Diagn* 41:354, 1997.

90. Hodgkin DD, Pierpont GL, Hildebrand KR, Gornick CC: Electrophysiologic characteristics of a pulsed iontophoretic drug-delivery system in coronary arteries. *J Cardiovasc Pharmacol* 29(1):39, 1997.

91. George SJ: Therapeutic potential of matrix metalloproteinase inhibitors in atherosclerosis. *Expert Opin Investig Drugs* 9:5:993, 2000.

92. Arner EC, Pratta MA, Freimark B, et al: Isothiazolones interfere with normal matrix metalloproteinase activation and inhibit cartilage proteoglycan degradation. *Biochem J* 318:417, 1996.

93. Van Wart HE, Schwartz MA: Synthetic inhibitors of bacterial and mammalian interstitial collagenases. *Prog Med Chem* 29:271, 1992.

94. Chandrasekhar S, Harvey AK, Dell CP, et al: Identification of a novel chemical series that blocks interleukin-1-stimulated metalloproteinase activity in chondrocytes. *J Pharmacol Exp* 273:1519, 1995.

95. Peterson M, Porter KE, Loftus IM, et al: Marimastat inhibits neointimal thickening in a model of human arterial intimal hyperplasia. *Eur J Vasc Endovasc Surg* 19:461, 2000.

96. Shibata M, Ueshima K, Harada M, et al: Effect of magnesium sulfate pretreatment and significance of matrix metalloproteinase-1 and interleukin-6 levels in coronary reperfusion therapy for patients with acute myocardial infarct. *Angiology* 50(7):573, 1999.

97. Zucker S, Conner C, DiMassmo BI, et al: Thrombin induces the activation of progelatinase A in vascular endothelial cells, physiologic regulation of angiogenesis. *J Biol Chem* 40:23730, 1995.

98. Zempo N, Koyama N, Kenagy RD, et al: Regulation of vascular smooth muscle cell migration and proliferation in vitro and in injured rat arteries by a synthetic matrix metalloproteinase inhibitor. *Arterioscler Thromb Vasc Biol* 16:28, 1996.

99. Bigatel DA, Elmore JR, Carey DJ, et al: The matrix metalloproteinase inhibitor BB-94 limits expansion of experimental abdominal aortic aneurysms. *J Vasc Surg* 29:130, 1999.

100. Aikawa M, Rabkin E, Okada Y, et al: Lipid lowering by diet reduces matrix metalloproteinase activity and increases collagen content of rabbit atheroma: A potential mechanism of lesion stabilization. *Circulation* 97:2433, 1998.

101. Aikawa M, Voglic SJ, Sugiyama S, et al: Dietary lipid lowering reduces tissue factor expression in rabbit atheroma. *Circulation* 100:1215, 1999.

102. Aikawa M, Rabkin E, Voglic SJ, et al: Lipid lowering promotes accumulation of mature smooth muscle cells expressing smooth muscle myosin heavy chain isoforms in rabbit atheroma. *Circ Res* 83:1015, 1998.

103. Shiomi M, Ito T: Effect of cerivastatin sodium, a new inhibitor of HMG-CoA reductase, on plasma lipid levels, progression of atherosclerosis, and the lesional composition in the plaques of WHHL rabbits. *Br J Pharmacol* 126:961, 1999.

104. Aikawa M, Rabkin E, Sugiyama S, et al: An HMG-CoA reductase inhibitor, cerivastatin, suppresses growth of macrophages expression matrix metalloproteinases and tissue factor in vivo and in vitro. *Circulation* 103:276, 2001.

105. Ganne F, Vasse M, Beaudeux JL, et al: Cerivastatin, an inhibitor of HMG-CoA reductase, inhibits urokinase/urokinase-receptor expression and MMP-9 secretion by peripheral blood monocytes—a possible protective mechanism against atherothrombosis. *Thromb Haemost* 84:680, 2000.

106. Bellosta S, Via D, Canavesti M, et al: HMG-CoA reductase inhibitors reduce MMP-9 secretion by macrophages *Arterioscler Thromb Vasc Biol* 18:1671, 1998.

107. George SJ, Lloyd CT, Angelini GD, et al: Inhibition of late vein graft neointima formation in human and porcine models by adenovirus-mediated overexpression of tissue inhibitor of metallo-proteinase-3. *Circulation* 101:296, 2000.

108. Sierevogel MJ, Pasterkamp G, Velema E, et al: Oral matrix metalloproteinase inhibition and arterial remodeling after balloon dilation: An intravascular ultrasound study in the pig. *Circulation* 103:302, 2001.

108a. Sinha S, Frishman WH: Matrix metalloproteinase and abdominal aortic aneurysm: A potential therapeutic target. *J Clin Pharmacol* 38:1077, 1998.

109. Petrinec D, Liao S, Holmes DR, et al: Doxycycline inhibition of aneurysmal degeneration in an elastase-induced rat model of abdominal aortic aneurysm: Preservation of aortic elastin associated with suppressed production of 92-kD gelatinase. *J Vasc Surg* 23:336, 1996.

110. Curci JA, Mao D, Bohner DG, et al: Preoperative treatment with doxycycline reduces aortic wall expression and activation of MMP in patients with abdominal aortic aneurysm. *J Vasc Surg* 31:325, 2000.

111. Curci JA, Petrinee D, Liao S, et al:. Pharmacologic suppression of experimental abdominal aortic aneurysms: A comparison of doxycycline and four chemically modified tetracyclines. *J Vasc Surg* 28:1082, 1998.

112. Boyle JR, McDermott E, Crowther M, et al: Doxycycline inhibits elastin degradation and reduces metalloproteinase activity in a model of aneurysmal disease. *J Vasc Surg* 27:354, 1998.

113. Franklin IJ, Harley SL, Greenhalgh RM, Powell JT: Uptake of tetracycline in aortic aneurysms: Influence on inflammation and proteolysis. *Br J Surg* 86:771, 1999.

114. Holmes DR, Petrinec D, Wester W, et al: Indomethacin prevents elastase-induced abdominal aortic aneurysms in the rat. *J Surg Res* 63:305, 1996.

115. Miralles M, Wester W, Sicard GA, et al: Indomethacin inhibits expansion of experimental aortic aneurysms via inhibition of the COX2 isoform of cyclooxygenase. *J Vasc Surg* 29:884, 1999.

116. Walton LJ, Franklin IJ, Bayston T, et al: Inhibition of prostaglandin E$_2$ synthesis in abdominal aortic aneurysms. *Circulation* 100:48, 1999.

116a. The United Kingdom Small Aneurysm Trial Participants: Long-term outcomes of immediate repair compared with surveillance of small abdominal aortic aneurysms. *N Engl J Med* 346:1445, 2002.

117. Allaire E, Forough R, Clowes M, et al: Local overexpression of TIMP-1 prevents aortic aneurysm degeneration and rupture in a rat model. *J Clin Invest* 102:1413, 1998.

118. Pyo R, Lee KL, Shipley M, et al: Targeted gene disruption of matrix metalloproteinase-9 (gelatinase B) suppresses development of experimental abdominal aortic aneurysms. *J Clin Invest* 105:1641, 2000.

119. Skotnicki JS, Zask A, Nelson FC, et al: Design and synthetic considerations of matrix metalloproteinase inhibitors. *Ann N Y Acad Sci* 878:61, 1999.

120. De B, Natchus MG, Cheng M, et al: The next generation of MMP inhibitors. Design and synthesis. *Ann N Y Acad Sci* 878:40, 1999.

121. Treharne GD, Boyle JR, Goodall S, et al:. Marimastat inhibits elastin degradation and matrix metalloproteinase 2 activity in a model of aneurysm disease. *Br J Surg* 86(8):1053, 2000.

122. Moore G, Liao S, Curci JA, Thompson RW, et al: Suppression of experimental abdominal aortic aneurysms by systematic treatment with a hydroxamate-based matrix metalloproteinase inhibitor (RS 132908). *J Vasc Surg* 29:522, 1999.

123. Wilcox JN, Nelken NA, Coughlin SR, et al: Local expression of inflammatory cytokines in human atherosclerotic plaques. *J Atheroscler Thromb* 1(Suppl 1):S10, 1994.

124. Koch AE, Kunkel SL, Pearce WH, et al: Enhanced production of the chemotactic cytokines interleukin-8 and monocyte chemoattractant protein-1 in human AAA. *Am J Pathol* 142(5):1423, 1993.

125. Hernandez-Presa M, Bustos C, Ortego M, et al: ACE-inhibition prevents arterial nuclear factor-kappa B activation, monocyte chemoattractant protein-1 expression, and macrophage infiltration in a rabbit model of early accelerated atherosclerosis. *Circulation* 95:6:1532, 1997.

126. Holmes DR, Wester W, Thompson RW, Reilly JM: Prostaglandin E$_2$ synthesis and cyclooxygenase expression in abdominal aortic aneurysms. *J Vasc Surg* 25:810, 1997.

127. Celentano D, Frishman W: Matrix metalloproteinases and coronary artery disease: A novel therapeutic target. *J Clin Pharmacol* 37:991, 1997.

128. Fernandez OA, Meyer BJ, Mailhac A, et al: A new approach for local intravascular drug delivery: Iontophoretic balloon. *Circulation* 89:1518, 1994.

129. Li YY, Feldman AM, Sun Y, et al: Differential expression of tissue inhibitors of metalloproteinases in the failing human heart. *Circulation* 98:1728, 1998.

130. Rohde LE, Ducharme A, Arroyo LH, et al: Matrix metalloproteinase inhibition attenuates early left ventricular enlargement after experimental myocardial infarction in mice. *Circulation* 99:3063, 1999.

131. Spinale FG, Coker ML, Krombach SR, et al: Matrix metalloproteinase inhibition during the development of congestive heart failure: Effects on left ventricular dimensions and functions. *Circ Res* 85:364, 1999.

132. McMurray J, Pfeffer MA: New therapeutic options in congestive heart failure. Part II. *Circulation* 105:2223, 2002.

133. Chancey AL, Brower GL, Peterson JT, Janicki JS: Effects of matrix metalloproteinase inhibition on ventricular remodeling due to volume overload. *Circulation* 105:1983, 2002.

134. Heymans L, Luttun A, Nuyens D, et al: Inhibition of plasminogen activators or matrix metalloproteinases prevents cardiac rupture but impairs therapeutic angiogenesis and causes cardiac failure. *Nat Med* 5:1135, 1999.

135. Li YY, Feng YQ, Kadokami T, et al: MMP inhibition prevents myocardial fibrosis and improves myocardial function and survival in a transgenic model of heart failure (abstr.). *Circulation* 102:II–132, 2000.

CHAPTER 44

Vasopeptidase Inhibitors: Neutral Endopeptidase Inhibitors and Dual Inhibitors of Angiotensin-Converting Enzyme and Neutral Endopeptidase

William H. Frishman

James Nawarskas

Vikram Rajan

Domenic A. Sica

Atrial natriuretic peptide (ANP) is a 28-residue C-terminal peptide derived from the 126-amino-acid precursor proatrial natriuretic peptide.[1] ANP is produced and stored in atrial myocytes and its release is triggered by volume and pressure changes in the circulation causing atrial distention. It has diuretic, natriuretic, and vasodilatory properties, as well as inhibitory effects on renin, aldosterone, and vasopressin release.[2] Furthermore, ANP improves ventricular relaxation and glomerular filtration rate, while reducing cardiac preload and afterload, as well as urinary potassium excretion.[3–5] ANP produces its effects via a guanylate cyclase-coupled receptor, the NPR-A receptor,[3–5] located in the glomeruli and collecting ducts, as well as extrarenal organs. Activation of such receptors leads to increased intracellular concentrations of the second messenger cyclic guanosine monophosphate (GMP), which subsequently helps to produce the various aforementioned physiologic effects.[6–9] This pathway is similar to that of nitric oxide (NO), where the active catalyst is also cyclic GMP, although in the latter, the receptors are linked to a soluble guanylate cyclase (Fig. 44-1).[6] Elevated plasma ANP levels are found in patients with systemic hypertension, acute myocardial infarction, congestive heart failure (CHF), and chronic renal failure.[10–12] The administration of exogenous ANP for the treatment of these disorders has been attempted with some success.[6,13–16] This mode of therapy, however, is limited by both poor oral absorption of the drug and its rapid clearance from the circulation when administered by intravenous infusion. An intravenous form of recombinant brain natriuretic peptide (rBNP, nesiritide) has been approved for use in heart failure with acute pulmonary edema (see Chap. 27).

ANP is cleared from the circulation via a clearance receptor and, more importantly, inactivated by a Zn-dependent, membrane-bound endopeptidase known as neutral endopeptidase (NEP), classified by the enzyme commission as EC 3.4.24.11.[17,18] NEP bears stereochemical resemblance to angiotensin-converting enzyme (ACE), as both are zinc-containing peptidases with their active sites located at the cell surface.[19] These endopeptidases are located primarily within the brush-border membranes of the kidney, but are also found in the central nervous system, lungs, lymph nodes, and the intestine.[20–25] ANP is cleaved by neutral endopeptidase (NEP) at the CYS-105-Phe-106 and Ser-123-Phe-124 bonds, that is, at the amino terminal of hydrophobic residues, resulting in inactivation of the peptide. It has been demonstrated that the cardiorenal effects of ANP can be potentiated by inhibiting its inactivation,[26–30] which has prompted the development of both orally active NEP inhibitors and dual ACE-NEP inhibitors, which are discussed in this chapter.

NEUTRAL ENDOPEPTIDASE INHIBITORS

Molecular Structure

The inhibitors of ANP endopeptidase have been designed using a simplified model of the active site of metallopeptidases. Stability and selectivity of the inhibitors binding to the enzyme endopeptidase is achieved by a combination of hydrogen bonding, van der Waals forces, and ionic interactions. By introducing various functional groups, four different classes have been identified (Fig. 44-2).

Thiol Inhibitors

This class of inhibitors is represented by thiorphan, the first synthetic inhibitor of endopeptidase to be described.[31–34] It has R and S enantiomers: thiorphan and retrothiorphan. Reduction of the phenyl ring of thiorphan produces a highly selective endopeptidase 24.11 inhibitor, while substituting the glycine for aminoheptanoic acid results in increased selectivity but slightly reduced potency.

Carboxyl Inhibitors

These are represented by SCH 39370 and UK 69578, which contain a hydrophobic moiety in P1, significantly improving the affinity for endopeptidases.[35–40] They are synthesized by introducing an N-terminal carboxyl-bearing group onto the dipeptide Phe-leu.

Phosphoryl and Hydroxamate Inhibitors

These are very potent inhibitors of endopeptidase 24.11 and contain a strong Zn-coordinating bidentate group. One representative of the

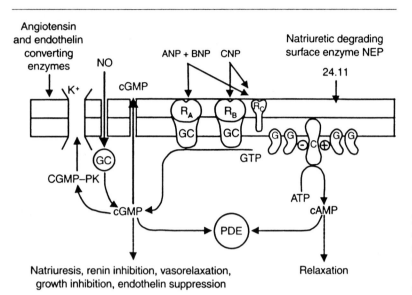

FIGURE 44-1. Illustration of the colocalization of neutral endopeptidase (NEP) and angiotensin-converting enzyme (ACE) on the cell surface and the pathways for signal transduction of the natriuretic peptide and nitric oxide systems. (*Reproduced with permission from Espiner EA. Physiology of natriuretic peptides. J Intern Med 235:527–541, 1994.*)

group, RS kelatorphan, can completely block in vivo enkephalin metabolism. The most potent NEP inhibitor, however, is a tyrosine-containing hydroxamic acid inhibitor, RB 1047.8 ($K_D = 0.05$ nM).

Clinical Pharmacology and Mechanism of Action

NEP inhibitors enhance the effect of ANP[26,27,32,35,37,38] by competitively inhibiting its degradation, prolonging its half-life (2 to 3 min in humans), and hence potentiating its diuretic and natriuretic action. Therefore, they exhibit ANP-like effects in vivo. SCH 39370, SQ 29072, and UK 69578 increased the half-life of exogenous ANP in rats,[32,37–40] prolonging its renal effects, and hence confirming the in vivo metabolism of ANP.

In the conscious, spontaneously hypertensive rat, SQ 29072 and SCH 39370 increased the response to exogenous ANP.[41] None of these inhibitors have any intrinsic antihypertensive effect. In the volume-based model of hypertension (the desoxycorticosterone-acetate-rat),[37] SCH 39370 lowered blood pressure. ANP-immunoreactivity and cyclic GMP in urine were also increased by antihypertensive doses of SCH 39370.[38] UK 69 578[36] raised ANP-like immunoreactivity in the saline-infused rat, and doubled this effect in volunteers. The orally active product, SCH 34826, increased diuresis and cyclic GMP excretion in salt-loaded subjects.[42] NEP inhibitors can also potentiate the activity of ANP by mechanisms independent of altered ANP catabolism (Fig. 44-3).[43] For example, it is thought that NEP inhibitors may potentiate the accumulation of the cardioprotective bradykinin within the kidney.[44] In vitro studies of human cardiac membranes show that the inactivation of bradykinin is mostly mediated by NEP. Thus, inhibition of this enzyme could serve to increase the local concentration of bradykinin in the heart.[45,46] NEP inhibitors also decrease circulating levels of endothelin, a potent endogenous vasoconstrictor.[19,47–50] Furthermore, NEP inhibition may result in an increase in adrenomedullin, a renal vasodilator with natriuretic and diuretic properties.[49]

Use in Systemic Hypertension

Using several NEP inhibitors, animal experiments have demonstrated an acute antihypertensive effect.[37,51,52] Studies on the effects of NEP inhibitors in healthy volunteers using UK 69578[36] and acetorphan[31] showed increased plasma ANP levels and increased natriuresis without any change in blood pressure. This is similar to the response of normal human volunteers to exogenous infusion of ANP.

The response of hypertensive subjects to NEP inhibitors has been mixed. Sybertz reported a blood pressure-lowering effect in patients with low-renin hypertension during 2 weeks of treatment.[53] In another study, however, there was no antihypertensive effect of candoxatril in hypertensive patients on a high-salt diet, despite a documented natriuresis.[54] Richards et al demonstrated with both NEP inhibitors SCH 42495[55] and candoxatril[56] small (7 to 9 mm Hg systolic and 2 to 4 mm Hg diastolic) but statistically significant reductions in blood pressure in mildly hypertensive patients on a normal salt diet. After 8 weeks of treatment with up to 200 mg twice daily of NEP inhibitor SCH 42495, Ogihara et al demonstrated a reduction in systolic blood pressure of 25 mm Hg and a reduction in mean diastolic blood pressure of 16 mm Hg.[57] On the other hand, Bevan et al, in a well-designed study of 40 patients with essential hypertension being treated with 200 mg of candoxatril (UK 79300), demonstrated a reduction in erect systolic pressures only.[58] Further studies show that selective NEP inhibition may only have a limited ability to lower elevated systolic blood pressure, while others demonstrate increases in diastolic blood pressure.[19]

Use in Congestive Heart Failure

Studies in animals demonstrate that the natriuretic and hypotensive effects of ANP infusion are augmented when combined with NEP inhibition.[59] In animal models of heart failure and hypertension, where levels of ANP are increased, NEP inhibition caused a similar increase in sodium excretion.[60,61] In normal subjects and subjects with essential hypertension, in whom ANP is only mildly elevated, a doubling of sodium excretion is seen with NEP inhibition.[62] In hypertensive patients on a high-sodium diet, a state of increased ANP levels with a sixfold increase in sodium excretion was demonstrated.[54] This effect should also be observed in CHF, another state with increased ANP levels.[13] The natriuresis and diuresis achieved with NEP inhibition has the added advantage that it occurs without the associated kaliuresis seen with standard diuretic therapy.

In studies in patients with mild to moderate heart failure, candoxatrilat (UK 69578) and sinorphan reduced pulmonary capillary wedge pressure and right atrial pressure.[63,64] Munzel et al, in a small

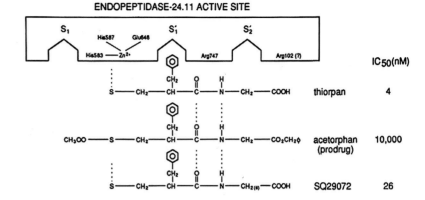

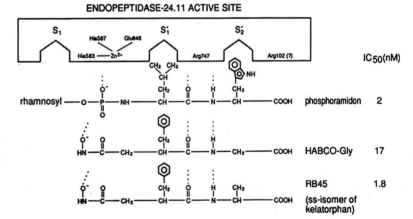

FIGURE 44-2. Endopeptidase 24.11 inhibitors used in ANP studies, shown interacting with a model of the active site of the enzyme. (*Top*) Thiol-containing inhibitors; (*middle*) carboxy-containing inhibitors; (*bottom*) phosphoryl- and hydroxamate-containing inhibitors. (*Adapted with permission from Sybertz EJ, et al.*[41])

open study, showed a reduction in pulmonary capillary wedge pressure and a sixfold increase in sodium excretion in patients with severe chronic heart failure who were treated with repeated doses of candoxatrilat intravenously over a 24-h period.[65] A double-blind,

FIGURE 44-3. Algorithm of the components of the natriuretic peptide system. (*Reproduced with permission from Burnett JC Jr.*[43])

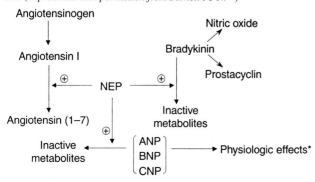

randomized trial by Good et al[66] showed an increase in urinary volume from 263 to 490 mL and increased natriuresis, as compared to placebo, in patients with severe heart failure treated with a single dose of candoxatrilat. Finally, Elsner et al, in a randomized, placebo-controlled, double-blind study of 12 patients with moderately severe CHF treated for 10 days with oral candoxatril, found a decrease in body weight and a decrease in right and left filling pressures.[67] Candoxatril is currently being evaluated as a treatment for congestive heart failure.[68]

Potential Side Effects

The high level of ANP already existent in such disease states as hypertension and heart failure may make pharmacologic tolerance with endopeptidase inhibitors a theoretical possibility, therefore limiting long-term clinical usefulness. Also, behavioral and antidepressant effects similar to D-opioid receptor agonists may result from an increase in enkephalin levels induced by selective inhibition of cerebral endopeptidase 24.11.

DUAL INHIBITORS OF ANGIOTENSIN-CONVERTING ENZYME AND NEUTRAL ENDOPEPTIDASE

Based on the results of recent clinical trials, the clinical utility of NEP inhibitors in the treatment of hypertension has been disappointing and contradictory results have been demonstrated. Although the data regarding the treatment of CHF with NEP inhibitors are somewhat encouraging, a clinical paradox is seen in patients with severe CHF; despite naturally high levels of ANP, fluid retention and edema remain a problem. There is evidence from clinical and experimental studies that decreased responsiveness to exogenous ANP infusion occurs in heart failure.[65,69] It is felt that this attenuation of responsiveness to endogenous and exogenous ANP may be due to activation of the renin-angiotensin-aldosterone system (RAAS) in CHF,[70–73] which has opposing actions on vascular resistance, sodium and water retention, and aldosterone secretion. Angiotensin-II exerts its effects by activating an intracellular phosphodiesterase that subsequently produces a decrease in cyclic GMP.[7–9,74,75] Angiotensin-II may additionally downregulate guanylate cyclase receptors, also leading to a reduction in cyclic GMP. Therefore, it is thought that angiotensin-II, resulting from activation of the RAAS, may directly antagonize the effects of ANP.[76–79] This has prompted the development of agents that both augment the action of ANP, as well as block the RAAS. Support for this idea comes from experimental models of CHF in dogs and rats with high output heart failure and coronary ligation-induced heart failure, and in dogs with pacing-induced heart failure where ACE inhibition restored the natriuretic action of infused ANP.[80,81] A combined NEP-ACE inhibitor may also have application in the treatment of hypertension. In a study of spontaneously hypertensive rats treated with simultaneously administered NEP and ACE inhibitors, it was found that the combination of both agents produced a more pronounced blood pressure effect than either agent alone.[82,83] Similarly, in a study of mild to moderate essential hypertension, sinorphan combined with captopril had a greater effect on blood pressure than did either agent alone.[84] The RAAS has been implicated as an important factor in the proliferation of smooth muscle after vascular injury[85,86] and in arteriosclerosis.[87,88] ACE inhibitors may slow the rate of vascular smooth-muscle proliferation, as well as reducing ventricular remodeling and decreasing LV filling pressures.[7,74,75] In a rabbit model of balloon-injured vasculature, ANP and the potentiation of this peptide via NEP was shown to decrease the degree of intimal proliferation.[89] Therefore, there may be additional vascular benefits to the dual inhibitors beyond the known and suspected effect on volume status, blood pressure, and cardiac remodeling.

The biochemical development of dual NEP-ACE inhibition (also called vasopeptidase inhibition) is based on the fact that the ACE and NEP differ in the relative positions of their Zn-containing catalytic sites. The characteristics of the active sites of these enzymes along with the known structure of the most potent and selective individual inhibitors was used to develop a single effective inhibitor of both enzymes.[90] Fournie-Zaluski et al developed mixanpril (RB105), which was found in oral and intravenous forms to lower blood pressure and to cause a diuresis and natriuresis in spontaneously hypertensive rats.[91] French et al compared their dual-inhibitor MDL 100173 against captopril in renovascular hypertensive high-renin rats, normal renin spontaneously hypertensive rats, and low-renin deoxycortisone acetate-salt hypertensive rats. MDL 100173 effectively lowered blood pressure in all three animal models, with an increase in diuresis and natriuresis, whereas captopril

only lowered blood pressure in the normal and high-renin models of hypertension.[92] Bralet and colleagues demonstrated that alatriopril, a vasopeptidase inhibitor, attenuated myocardial hypertrophy to a greater extent than captopril in rats with experimentally induced myocardial infarction.[93]

OMAPATRILAT

Omapatrilat (Vanlev, BMS 186716) is a mercaptoacyl derivative of a bicyclic thiazepinone dipeptide (Fig. 44-4).[94] Omapatrilat has demonstrated the ability to inhibit NEP and ACE with approximately equal affinity and similar potency. As an antihypertensive agent, omapatrilat appears to decrease blood pressure in animal models irrespective of sodium status or angiotensin II involvement, as determined by the degree of activation of RAAS.[19,88,95,96] In a study using sodium-depleted and sodium-repleted spontaneously hypertensive rats, administration of omapatrilat resulted in a uniform reduction of blood pressure. This suggests that vasopeptidase inhibitors exert their effects regardless of whether the animal model is in a high or low renin state. Further analysis reveals that ACE inhibitors have greater efficacy against high-renin-state animals, while NEP inhibitors are effective against low-renin-state models.[97] NEP and ACE inhibitors function synergistically in reducing blood pressure in intermediate renin activity models.[97] Consequently, omapatrilat appears to be an effect oral antihypertensive agent regardless of sodium and renin levels.[97a] Furthermore, it appears to be more efficacious than either ACE or NEP inhibition alone.[97]

Omapatrilat, in addition to its antihypertensive effects, also increases survival in animal models of heart failure. One study showed a 44% increased survival with omapatrilat, versus a 23% increased survival with an equipotent dose of an ACE inhibitor.[98] In another study of left ventricular failure, administration of omapatrilat improved myocyte contractility and responsiveness to β-adrenergic stimulation as compared to placebo controls. Omapatrilat also reduced the amount of left ventricular dilatation and myocyte length,[99,100] while increasing plasma vasodilator and natriuretic peptide levels.[100a,100b] The results of human trials are equally promising, showing a reduction in both systolic and diastolic blood pressures in a dose-dependent fashion.[101,102]

Clinical Trials

Nawarskas and Anderson have summarized clinical studies assessing the clinical effects of omapatrilat in humans.[103] Briefly, omapatrilat has shown efficacy in treating both hypertension and heart failure. Phase II clinical studies in more than 1800 patients with hypertension demonstrated omapatrilat 80 mg once daily to reduce

FIGURE 44-4. Chemical structure of omapatrilat (BMS 186716), a vasopeptidase inhibitor.

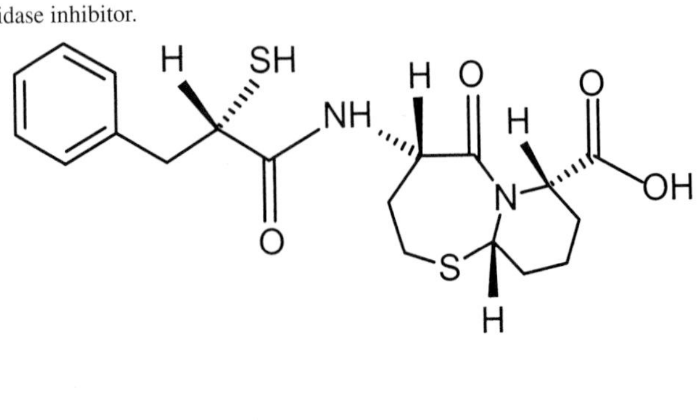

systolic blood pressure (SBP) and diastolic blood pressure (DBP) by 25.8 and 16.9 mm Hg at peak and by 19.5 and 14.2 mm Hg at trough, respectively.[104,105] This same dosage was also shown to result in a greater percentage of patients (71% with a baseline DBP <100 mm Hg and 40% with a DBP between 100 and 110 mm Hg) achieving a BP of <140/<90 mm Hg as compared to lisinopril 20 mg daily (51% and 17%) and amlodipine 10 mg daily (60% and 26%).[105] Omapatrilat, in dosages of 20 mg and 40 mg, has also been shown to be superior to 20 mg lisinopril in reducing SBP in a separate study.[106] Reductions in SBP of 14.3 and 16 mm Hg have been shown with 20 mg and 40 mg omapatrilat, respectively, versus a reduction of 10.5 mm Hg with lisinopril ($P < .05$).[106] Differences between DBP reductions were not statistically significant. Omapatrilat is also beneficial in elderly and African American patients, populations that generally have low-renin hypertension that is somewhat refractory to ACE inhibitors. African American patients receiving omapatrilat 40 mg daily displayed SBP/DBP reductions of 16.8/11.4 mm Hg as compared to reductions of 0.9/5.1 mm Hg with lisinopril. This same dosage also resulted in SBP/DBP reductions of 17.1/10.6 mm Hg as compared to 8.5/10.5 mm Hg with lisinopril in patients older than 65 years of age.

The OCTAVE (Omapatrilat Cardiovascular Treatment Assessment Versus Enalapril) study compared the safety and efficacy of omapatrilat and enalapril in approximately 25,000 patients with hypertension. In this trial, there was significantly greater reduction in BP and higher achieved control rates with omapatrilat than enalapril. In addition, there was more high dose enalapril and adjunctive therapy with enalapril. The overall incidence of angioedema with omapatrilat was 2.17 versus 0.68% for enalapril, and in the case of omapatrilat, occurred in 5.54% of black patients. The angioedema in this series, although potentially life-threatening, required either no treatment or antihistamine therapy alone in 60% of the cases.[107] These data have cast a cloud over the combined ACE-NEP inhibitor class of drugs and as recently as July 2002, the Cardiorenal Advisory Panel of the Food and Drug Administration has voted negatively on the approval of omapatrilat for use in difficult to manage hypertensives. It remains to be determined whether this drug will ever gain regulatory approval.

The Inhibition of Metalloprotease in a Randomized Exercise and Symptoms Study (IMPRESS) compared omapatrilat 40 mg once daily ($n = 289$) to lisinopril 20 mg once daily ($n = 284$) in patients with New York Heart Associations (NYHA) class II to class IV heart failure (mean left ventricular ejection fraction 28%).[108] Following 24 weeks of treatment, exercise tolerance (primary end point) was increased to a similar extent with both drugs. However, the combined end-point of morbidity (hospitalization for worsening heart failure, discontinuation of study medication for worsening heart failure) and mortality was significantly less in the patients receiving omapatrilat (5.5%) versus lisinopril (10.2%); risk ratio 0.52, $P < .04$.

The Omapatrilat Heart Failure Program consisted of two double-blind, lisinopril-controlled trials involving 1242 patients with NYHA class II to class IV heart failure.[109] One trial ($n = 669$) compared omapatrilat 20 mg ($n = 340$) to lisinopril 20 mg ($n = 329$) over 52 weeks; the other study (IMPRESS)[108] is mentioned above. Combined, these trials demonstrated a statistically significant reduction in the combined endpoint of death or hospitalization for worsening heart failure in patients receiving omapatrilat compared to lisinopril (relative risk 0.72, 95% confidence interval 0.53 to 0.97; $P = .03$).

The Omapatrilat Versus Enalapril Randomized Trial of Utility in Reducing Events (OVERTURE) was a double-blind, randomized trial that included 5770 patients with severe heart failure (Class II, III or IV symptoms, LVEF less than 30% and a hospitalization for heart failure within the last 12 months). Patients were all receiving optimal therapies for heart failure—50% were on β-blockers, 40% on spironolactone and 60% on digoxin. Subjects were randomized to enalapril (10 mg bid) or omapatrilat 40 mg once daily. The primary endpoint was all-cause mortality/CHF hospitalizations, which showed a 6% reduction with omapatrilat, but this did not reach statistical significance. Adverse events showed a lower incidence of impaired renal function with omapatrilat and only a slightly increased rate of angioedema compared to enalapril.[110] The promising future for omapatrilat in CHF was not realized per se in this trial and additional studies need to be performed with this compound if its development continues.

Because omapatrilat has not yet been approved for use by regulatory agencies either in the United States or in Europe, the adverse effect profile for this drug has yet to be fully defined. Preliminary studies, however, suggest tolerability similar to placebo.[106,111] The most common side effects experienced in the IMPRESS trial were diarrhea, mild dizziness, and loss of consciousness. Concerns regarding reports of angioedema in patients receiving omapatrilat have delayed the approval of this compound for human use.

OTHER DUAL-INHIBITOR AGENTS

Besides omapatrilat, other vasopeptidase inhibitors currently under investigation for the treatment of hypertension and/or heart failure include sampatrilat, gemopatrilat (BMS 189921), MDL-100240, fasidotril (also known as alatriopril and aladotril [BP 1137]), Z-13752A, and S21402.[112–114]

CONCLUSION

Inhibitors of NEP have limited benefit in the treatment of hypertension and are currently being studied in patients with CHF. In contrast, dual inhibitors of NEP-ACE have potential utility as clinical treatments for systemic hypertension, CHF, and vascular remodeling. Issues regarding the safety of NEP-ACE inhibitors, specifically angioedema, need to be resolved before the widespread utilization of this new class of drugs can be recommended.

REFERENCES

1. Bloch KD, Zisfein JB, Margolies MN, et al: A serum protease cleaves pro ANF into a 14 kilodalton protein and ANF. *Am J Physiol* 252:E147, 1987.
2. Espiner EA, Richards AM: Atrial natriuretic peptide: an important factor in sodium and blood pressure regulation. *Lancet* 1:707, 1989.
3. Chen HH, Burnett JC Jr: C-type natriuretic peptide. The endothelial component of the natriuretic peptide system. *J Cardiovasc Pharmacol* 32(Suppl 3):S22, 1998.
4. Boland DG, Abraham WT: Natriuretic peptides in cardiovascular disease. *CHF* March/April:23, 1998.
5. Stein BC, Levin RI: Natriuretic peptides. Physiology, therapeutic potential, and risk stratification in ischemic heart disease. *Am Heart J* 136:914, 1998.
6. Kelly RA, Smith TW: Drugs used in the treatment of heart failure. In: Braunwald E, ed. *Heart Disease II, A Textbook of Cardiovascular Medicine.* 5th ed. Philadelphia: WB Saunders, 1997:471.

7. Schiffrin E: Vascular protection with new antihypertensive agents. *J Hypertens* 16(Suppl 5):S25, 1998.
8. Susic D, Frohlich ED: Nephroprotective effect of antihypertensive drugs in essential hypertension. *J Hypertens* 16:555, 1998.
9. Cho Y, Somer BG, Amatya A: Natriuretic peptides and their therapeutic potential. *Heart Dis* 1:305, 1999.
10. Sagnella GA, Markandu ND, Shore AC, MacGregor GA: Raised circulating levels of atrial natriuretic peptides in essential hypertension. *Lancet* 1:179, 1986.
11. Burnett JC, Kao PC, Hu DC, et al: Atrial natriuretic peptide elevation in congestive heart failure in the human. *Science* 231:1145, 1986.
12. Rascher W, Tulassay T, Lang RE: Atrial natriuretic peptide in plasma volume-overloaded children with chronic renal failure. *Lancet* 2:303, 1985.
13. Cody R, Atlas SA, Laragh JH, et al: Atrial natriuretic factor in normal subjects and heart failure patients. Plasma levels and renal, hormonal and hemodynamic responses to peptide infusion. *J Clin Invest* 78:1362, 1986.
14. Weidmann P, Gnaidinger MP, Ziswiler HR, et al: Cardiovascular, endocrine and renal effects of atrial natriuretic peptide in essential hypertension. *J Hypertens* 4(S2):S71, 1986.
15. Janssen WM, DeZeeuw D, Van der Hem GK, DeJong PE: Antihypertensive effect of a 5-day infusion of atrial natriuretic factor in humans. *Hypertension* 14:640, 1989.
16. Windus DW, Stokes TJ, Morgan JR, Klahr S: The effects of atrial peptide in humans with chronic renal failure. *Am J Kidney Dis* 13:477, 1989.
17. Kenny AJ, Stephenson SL: Role of endopeptidase 24.11 in the inactivation of atrial natriuretic peptide. *FEBS Lett* 232:1, 1989.
18. Sonnenberg L, Sakane Y, Teng AAY, et al: Identification of protease endopeptidase 24.11 as the major atrial natriuretic factor degrading enzyme in the rat. *Kidney Pept* 9:173, 1987.
19. Robl JA, Trippodo NC, Petrillo EW: Neutral endopeptidase inhibitors and combined inhibitors of neutral endopeptidase and angiotensin-converting enzyme. In: van Zwieten PA, Greenlee WJ, eds. *Antihypertensive Drugs*. Amsterdam: Hardwood Academic Publishers, 1997:113.
20. Granger JP Opgenorth TJ, Salazer J, et al: Long-term hypotensive and renal effects of ANF. *Hypertension* 8(Suppl II):II-112, 1986.
21. Bertrand P, Doble A: Degradation of atrial natriuretic peptides by an enzyme in rat kidney resembling neutral endopeptidase 24.11. *Biochem Pharmacol* 37:3817, 1988.
22. Gee NS, Bowes MA, Buck P, Kenny AJ: An immunoradiometric assay for endopeptidase 24.11 shows it to be a widely distributed enzyme in pig tissues. *Biochem J* 228:119, 1985.
23. Olins GM, Spear KL, Siegel NR, et al: Atrial peptide inactivation by rabbit-kidney brush border membranes. *Eur J Biochem* 170:431, 1987.
24. Shimamori Y, Watanabe T, Fujimoto Y: Specificity of a membrane-bound neutral endopeptidase from rat kidney. *Chem Pharm Bull* 34:275, 1986.
25. Stephenson SL, Kenny AJ: The hydrolysis of α-human atrial natriuretic peptide by pig kidney microvillar membranes is initiated by endopeptidase 24.11. *Biochem J* 243:183, 1987.
26. Margulies KB, Cavero PG, Seymour AA, et al: Neutral endopeptidase inhibition potentiates the renal actions of atrial natriuretic factor. *Kidney Int* 38:67, 1990.
27. Richards M, Espiner E, Frampton C, et al: Inhibition of endopeptidase EC 24-11 in humans: Renal and endocrine effects. *Hypertension* 16(3):269, 1990.
28. Corti R, Burnett JC Jr, Rouleau JL, et al: Vasopeptidase inhibitors. A new therapeutic concept in cardiovascular disease? *Circulation* 104:1856, 2001.
29. Bralet J, Mossiat C, Lecomte J-M, et al: Diuretic and natriuretic responses in rats treated with enkephalinase inhibitors. *Eur J Pharmacol* 179:57, 1990.
30. Cavero PG, Margulies KB, Winaver J, et al: Cardiorenal actions of neutral endopeptidase inhibition in experimental congestive heart failure. *Circulation* 82:196, 1989.
31. Gros C, Souque A, Schwartz J-C, et al: Protection of atrial natriuretic factor against degradation: Diuretic and natriuretic responses after in vivo inhibition of enkephalinase EC 3.4.24.11 by acetorphan. *Proc Natl Acad Sci U S A* 86:7580, 1989.
32. Seymour A, Fennell SA, Swerdel JN: Potentiation of renal effects of atrial natriuretic factor (99–126) by SQ 29,072. *Hypertension* 14:87, 1989.
33. Trapani AJ, Smits GJ, McGraw DE, et al: Thiorphan, an inhibitor of endopeptidase 24-11, potentiates the natriuretic activity of atrial natriuretic peptide. *J Cardiovasc Pharmacol* 14:419, 1989.
34. Fennell SA, Swerdel JN, Delaney NG, Seymour AA: Potentiation of renal and depressor responses to ANP 99-126 by SQ29,072 in conscious dogs (abstr.). *FASEB J* 2:A936, 1988.
35. Samuels GMR, Barclay PL, Peters CJ, Ellis P: Atriopeptidase inhibitors, a novel class of drugs that raises levels of endogenous ANF—the Preclinical Pharmacology of UK 69,578 (abstr.). *J Am Coll Cardiol* 13:75A, 1989.
36. Northridge DB, Alabaster CT, Connell JMC, et al: Effects of UK 69578: a novel atriopeptidase inhibitor. *Lancet* 2:591, 1989.
37. Sybertz EJ, Chiu PJS, Vemulapalli S, et al: SCH 39370, a neutral metalloendopeptidase inhibitor, potentiates biological responses to atrial natriuretic factor and lowers blood pressure in desoxycorticosterone acetate-sodium hypertensive rats. *J Pharmacol Exp Ther* 250:624, 1989.
38. Jardine A, Connell JMC, Dilly SG, et al: Pharmacologic elevation of endogenous ANF in man using the atriopeptidase inhibitor (UK 69,578) (abstr.). *J Am Coll Cardiol* 13:76A, 1989.
39. Barclay PL, Peters CJ, Bennett JA, et al: The diuretic and natriuretic responses to the atriopeptidase inhibitor UK 69,578 in volume expanded rats (abstr.). *J Am Coll Cardiol* 13:824P, 1989.
40. Samuels GMR, Barclay PL, Shepperson NB, Bennett JA: The acute and chronic antihypertensive efficacy of atriopeptidase inhibition in rats (abstr.). *J Am Coll Cardiol* 13:76A, 1989.
41. Sybertz EJ, Chiu PS, Subbairo V, et al: Atrial natriuretic factor—potentiating and antihypertensive activity of SCH 34826: An orally active neutral metalloendopeptidase inhibitor. *Hypertension* 15:152, 1990.
42. Smits GJ, McGraw DE, Trapani AJ: Interaction of ANP and bradykinin during endopeptidase 24-11 inhibition: Renal effects. *Am J Physiol* 258:F1417, 1990.
43. Burnett JC Jr: Vasopeptidase inhibition: A new concept in blood pressure management. *J Hypertens* 17(Suppl 1):S37, 1999.
44. Granger P: Inhibitors of ANF metabolism: Potential therapeutic agents in cardiovascular disease. *Circulation* 82:313, 1990.
45. Kokkonen JO, Kuoppala A, Saarinen J, et al: Kallidin and bradykinin-degrading pathways in human heart: Degradation of kallidin by aminopeptidase M-like activity and bradykinin by neutral endopeptidase. *Circulation* 99:1984, 1999.
46. Dumoulin M-J, Adam A, Rouleau J-L, Lamontagne D: Comparison of a vasopeptidase inhibitor with neutral endopeptidase and angiotensin-converting enzyme inhibitors on bradykinin metabolism in the rat coronary bed. *J Cardiovasc Pharmacol* 37:359, 2001.
47. Margulies KB, Barclay PL, Burnett JC Jr: The role of neutral endopeptidase in dogs with evolving congestive heart failure. *Circulation* 91:2036, 1995.
48. Fink CA: Recent advances in the development of dual angiotensin-converting enzyme and neutral endopeptidase inhibitors. *Exp Opin Ther Patents* 6:1147, 1996.
49. Liay O, Jougasaki M, Schirger JA, et al: Neutral endopeptidase inhibition potentiates the natriuretic actions of adrenomedullin. *Am J Physiol* 275:F410, 1998.
50. Sybertz EJ: Drugs inhibiting the metabolism and inactivation of atrial natriuretic factor. Pharmacologic actions and therapeutic implications. *Cardiovasc Drug Rev* 8:71, 1990.
51. Seymour AA, Swerdel JA, Fennell SA, et al: Potentiation of the depressor responses to atrial natriuretic peptides in conscious SHR by an inhibitor of neutral endopeptidase. *J Cardiovasc Pharmacol* 14:194, 1989.
52. Koepke JP, Tyler LD, Blehm DJ, et al: Chronic atriopeptin regulation of arterial pressure in conscious hypertensive rats. *Hypertension* 16:642, 1990.
53. Sybertz EJ: SCH 34826: An overview of its profile as a neutral endopeptidase inhibitor and ANF potentiator. *Clin Nephrol* 36:187, 1991.
54. Singer DRJ, Markandu ND, Buckley MG, et al: Dietary sodium and inhibition of neutral endopeptidase 24.11 in essential hypertension. *Hypertension* 18:798, 1991.

55. Richards AM, Crozier IG, Kosoglou T, et al: Endopeptidase 24.11 inhibition by SCH 42495 in essential hypertension. *Hypertension* 22:119, 1993.

56. Richards AM, Crozier IG, Espiner EA, et al: Plasma brain natriuretic peptide and endopeptidase 24.11 inhibition in hypertension. *Hypertension* 22:231, 1993.

57. Ogihara T, Rakugi H, Masuo K, et al: Antihypertensive effects of the neutral endopeptidase inhibitor SCH 42495 in essential hypertension. *Am J Hypertens* 7:943, 1994.

58. Bevan EG, Connell JMC, Doyle J, et al: Candoxatril, a neutral endopeptidase inhibitor: efficacy and tolerability in essential hypertension. *J Hypertens* 10:607, 1992.

59. Wilkins MR, Settle SL, Needleman P: Augmentation of the natriuretic activity of exogenous and endogenous atriopeptin in rats by inhibition of 3′,5′-cyclic monophosphate degradation. *J Clin Invest* 85:1274, 1990.

60. Seymour AA, Norman JA, Asaad MM, et al: Antihypertensive and renal activity of SC 28603, an inhibitor of neutral endopeptidase. *J Cardiovasc Pharmacol* 17:296, 1991.

61. Wilkins MR, Settle SL, Stockman PT, Needleman P: Maximizing the natriuretic effect of endogenous atriopeptin in a rat model of heart failure. *Proc Natl Acad Sci U S A* 87:6465, 1990.

62. O'Connel JE, Jardine AG, Davidson G, Connell JMC: Candoxatril, an orally active neutral endopeptidase inhibitor, raises plasma atrial natriuretic factor and is natriuretic in essential hypertension. *J Hypertens* 10:271, 1992.

63. Kahn JC, Patey M, Dubois-Rande JL, et al: Effect of sinorphan on plasma atrial natriuretic factor in congestive heart failure (letter). *Lancet* 335:118, 1990.

64. Northridge DB, Jardine A, Henderson E, et al: Increased circulating atrial natriuretic factor concentrations in patients with chronic heart failure after inhibition of neutral endopeptidase: Effects on diastolic function. *Br Heart J* 68:387, 1992.

65. Munzel T, Kurz S, Holtz J, et al: Neurohormonal inhibition and hemodynamic unloading during prolonged inhibition of ANF degradation in patients with severe chronic heart failure. *Circulation* 86:1089, 1992.

66. Good JM, Peters M, Wilkins M, et al: Renal response to candoxatrilat in patients with heart failure. *J Am Coll Cardiol* 25:1273, 1995.

67. Elsner D, Muntze A, Kromer EP, Riegger GA: Effectiveness of endopeptidase inhibition (candoxatril) in congestive heart failure. *Am J Cardiol* 70:494, 1992.

68. Westheim AS, Bostrøm P, Christensen CC, et al: Hemodynamic and neuroendocrine effects for candoxatril and frusemide in mild stable chronic heart failure. *J Am Coll Cardiol* 34:1794, 1999.

69. Kohzuki M, Hodsman GP, Johnston CL: Attenuated response to atrial natriuretic peptide in rats with myocardial infarction. *Am J Physiol* 256:H533, 1989.

70. Abassi Z, Haramati A, Hoffman A, et al: Effect of converting enzyme inhibition on renal response to ANP in rats with experimental heart failure. *Am J Physiol* 259:R84, 1990.

71. Villarreal D, Freeman RH, Johnson RA: Captopril enhances renal responsiveness to ANF in dogs with compensated high output heart failure. *Am J Physiol* 262:R509, 1992.

72. Raya TE, Lee RW, Westhoff T, Goldman S: Captopril restores hemodynamic responsiveness to atrial natriuretic peptide in rats with heart failure. *Circulation* 80:1886, 1989.

73. Lee RW, Raya TE, Michael U, et al: Captopril and ANP. Changes in renal hemodynamics, glomerular ANP receptors and guanylate cyclase activity in rats with heart failure. *J Pharm Exp Ther* 260:349, 1992.

74. Gibbons GH: Cardioprotective mechanisms of ACE inhibition. The angiotensin II-nitric oxide balance. *Drugs* S4(Suppl 5):1, 1997.

75. Kaplan NM: Treatment of hypertension. Drug therapy. In: Kaplan NM, ed. *Clinical Hypertension.* 8th ed. Philadelphia: Lippincott Williams & Wilkins, 2002:237.

76. Haneda M, Kikkawa R, Maeda S, et al: Dual mechanism of angiotensin II inhibits ANP-induced mesangial cGMP accumulation. *Kidney Int* 40:188, 1991.

77. Smith JB, Lincoln TM: Angiotensin decreases cyclic cGMP accumulation produced by atrial natriuretic factor. *Am J Physiol* 253:C147, 1987.

78. Supaporn T, Wennberg PW, Wei CM, et al: Role for the endogenous natriuretic peptide system in the control of basal coronary vascular tone in dogs. *Clin Sci* 90:357, 1996.

79. Yamamoto K, Burnett JC Jr, Redfield MM: Effect of endogenous natriuretic peptide system on ventricular and coronary function in failing heart. *Am J Physiol* 273:H2406, 1997.

80. Margulies KB, Perrella MA, McKinley LJ, Burnett JC Jr: Angiotensin inhibition potentiates the renal responses to neutral endopeptidase inhibition in dogs with congestive heart failure. *J Clin Invest* 81:1636, 1991.

81. Seymour AA, Asaad MM, Lanoce VM, et al: Systemic hemodynamics, renal function and hormonal levels during inhibition of neutral endopeptidase 3.4.24.11 and angiotensin converting enzyme in conscious dogs with pacing induced heart failure. *J Pharm Exp Ther* 266:872, 1993.

82. Seymour AA, Swerdel JN, Abboa-Offei B: Antihypertensive activity during inhibition of neutral endopeptidase and angiotensin converting enzyme. *J Cardiovasc Pharmacol* 17:456, 1991.

83. Pham I, Gonzalez W, El Amrani A-I, et al: Effects of converting enzyme inhibitor and neutral endopeptidase inhibitor on blood pressure and renal function in experimental hypertension. *J Pharm Exp Ther* 265:1339, 1993.

84. Favrat B, Burnier M, Nussberger J, et al: Neutral endopeptidase versus angiotensin converting enzyme inhibition in essential hypertension. *J Hypertens* 13:797, 1995.

85. Powell JS, Clozel J-P, Muller RK, et al: Inhibitors of angiotensin-converting enzyme prevent myointimal proliferation after vascular injury. *Science* 245:186, 1989.

86. Powell JS, Muller RKM, Baumgartner HR: Suppression of the vascular response to injury: the role of angiotensin converting enzyme inhibitors. *J Am Coll Cardiol* 17(6 Suppl B):137B, 1991.

87. Aberg G, Ferrer P: Effects of captopril on atherosclerosis in cynomolgus monkeys. *J Cardiovasc Pharmacol* 15(Suppl 5):S65, 1990.

88. Chobanian AV, Haudenschild CC, Nickerson C, Drago R: Anti-atherogenic effect of captopril in the Watanabe heritable hyperlipidemic rabbit. *Hypertension* 15:327, 1990.

89. Davis HR Jr, McGregor DG, Hoos L, et al: Atrial natriuretic factor and the neutral endopeptidase inhibitor SCH42495 prevent myointimal proliferation after vascular injury (abstr.). *Circulation* 86:I–220, 1992.

90. Gros C, Noel N, Souque A, et al: Mixed inhibitors of angiotensin converting enzyme (EC 3.4.15.1) and enkephalinase (EC 3.4.24.11): Rational design, properties, and potential cardiovascular applications of glycopril and alatriopril. *Proc Natl Acad Sci U S A* 88:4210, 1991.

91. Fournie-Zaluski M-C, Coric P, Turcaud S, et al: New dual inhibitors of neutral endopeptidase and angiotensin-converting enzyme: Rational design, bioavailability, and pharmacological responses in experimental hypertension. *J Med Chem* 37:1070, 1994.

92. French JF, Anderson BA, Downs TR, Dage RC: Dual inhibition of angiotensin converting enzyme and neutral endopeptidase in rats with hypertension. *J Cardiovasc Pharmacol* 26:107, 1995.

93. Bralet J, Marie C, Mossiat C, et al: Effects of alatriopril, a mixed inhibitor of atriopeptidase and an angiotensin I converting enzyme, on cardiac hypertrophy and hormonal responses in rats with myocardial infarction. Comparison with captopril. *J Pharmacol Exp Ther* 270:8, 1994.

94. Robl JA, Sun CO, Stevenson J, et al: Dual metalloprotease inhibitors. Mercaptoacetyl-based fused heterocyclic neutral endopeptidase. *J Med Chem* 40:1570, 1997.

95. Trippodo NC, Robl JA, Assad MM, et al: Cardiovascular effects of the novel dual inhibitor of neutral endopeptidase and angiotensin-converting enzyme BMS-182657 in experimental hypertension and heart failure. *J Pharmacol Exp Ther* 275:746, 1995.

96. Vera WG, Fournie-Zaluski MC, Pham I, et al: Hypotensive and natriuretic effects of RB 105, a new dual inhibitor of angiotensin converting enzyme and neutral endopeptidase in hypertensive rats. *J Pharmacol Exp Ther* 272:343, 1995.

97. Trippodo NC, Robl JA, Assad MM, et al: Effects of omapatrilat in low, normal, and high renin experimental hypertension. *Am J Hypertens* 11:363, 1998.

97a. Campese VM, Lasseter KC, Ferrario CM, et al: Omapatrilat versus lisinopril. Efficacy and neurohormonal profile in salt-sensitive hypertensive patients. *Hypertension* 38:1342, 2001.

98. Trippodo NC, Fox M, Monticello TM, et al: Simultaneous inhibition of neutral endopeptidase and angiotensin converting enzyme by omapatrilat increased survival in heart failure hamsters greater than ACE inhibition (abstr.). *Circulation* 88:I–761, 1998.

99. Thomas CV, Holzgrefe HH, Mukherjee R, et al: Dual metalloprotease inhibition during the development of left ventricular failure; effects on left ventricular myocyte beta-adrenergic response (abstr.). *Circulation* 98:I–520, 1997.

100. Thomas CV, Holzgrefe HH, Mukherjee R, et al: Dual metalloprotease inhibition during the development of left ventricular failure; effects on left ventricular and myocyte function and geometry (abstr.). *Circulation* 88:I–524, 1997.

100a. McClean DR, Ikram H, Mehta S, et al: Vasopeptidase inhibition with omapatrilat in chronic heart failure. Acute and long-term hemodynamic and neurohumoral effects. *J Am Coll Cardiol* 39:2034, 2002.

100b. Cataliotti A, Boerrigter G, Chen HH, et al: Differential actions of vasopeptidase inhibition versus angiotensin-converting enzyme inhibition on diuretic therapy in experimental congestive heart failure. *Circulation* 105:639, 2002.

101. Vesterqvist O, Liao W, Manning JA, et al: Effects of BMS 1867, a new dual metalloprotease inhibitor, on pharmacodynamic markers of neutral endopeptidase (NEP) and angiotensin converting enzyme (ACE) activity in healthy men (abstr.). *Clin Pharmacol Ther* 61:230, 1997.

102. Liao W, Delaney C, Smith R, et al: Supine mean arterial blood pressure (MAP) lowering and oral tolerance of BMS-186716, a new dual metalloprotease inhibitor of angiotensin converting enzyme (ACE) and neutral endopeptidase (NEP) in healthy male subjects (abstr.). *Clin Pharmacol Ther* 61:229, 1997.

103. Nawarskas J, Anderson JR: Omapatrilat: A unique new agent for the treatment of cardiovascular disease. *Heart Dis* 2:266, 2000.

104. Weber M: Emerging treatments for hypertension: Potential role for vasopeptidase inhibition. *Am J Hypertens* 12:139S, 1999.

105. Waeber B, Zanchetti A, Black HR, et al: Omapatrilat, a vasopeptidase inhibitor, is an effective antihypertensive agent in mild to moderate hypertension (abstr.). *J Hypertens* 17(Suppl 3):S152, 1999.

106. Neutel J, Shepherd A, Pool J, et al: Antihypertensive efficacy of omapatrilat, a vasopeptidase inhibitor, compared with lisinopril (abstr.). *J Hypertens* 17(Suppl 3):S67, 1999.

107. OCTAVE: Omapatrilat in hypertension; 2.17% incidence of angioedema. http://info@theheart.org./index.cfm. Accessed July 14, 2002.

108. Rouleau JL, Pfeffer MA, Stewart DJ, et al: for the IMPRESS Investigators. Comparison of vasopeptidase inhibitor, omapatrilat, and lisinopril on exercise tolerance and morbidity in patients with heart failure: IMPRESS randomized trial. *Lancet* 356:615, 2000.

109. Kostis JB, Rouleau JL, Pfeffer MA, et al: Beneficial effects of vasopeptidase inhibition on mortality and morbidity in heart failure: Evidence from the Omapatrilat Heart Failure Program (abstr.). *J Am Coll Cardiol* 35(Suppl A):240A, 2000.

110. OVERTURE: Omapatrilat no better than enalapril in heart failure. http://info@theheart.org./index.cfm. Accessed July 14, 2002.

111. Klapholz M, Thomas I, Eng C, et al: Omapatrilat, a novel cardiovascular agents, improves hemodynamics in patients with heart failure (abstr.). *Circulation* 98(Suppl):I–105, 1998.

112. Burrell LM, Farina NK, Balding LC, Johnston CI: Beneficial renal and cardiac effects of vasopeptidase inhibition with S21402 in heart failure. *Hypertension* 36:1105, 2000.

113. Weber MA: Vasopeptidase inhibitors. *Lancet* 358:1525, 2001.

114. Chodjania Y, Tharaux P-L, Ragueneau I, et al: Renal and vascular effects of S 21402, a dual inhibitor of angiotensin-converting enzyme and neutral endopeptidase, in healthy subjects with hypovolemia. *Clin Pharmacol Ther* 71:468, 2002.

CHAPTER 45

The Many Faces of Eicosanoids: Prostaglandins, Leukotrienes, and Other Arachidonate Metabolites

Michael Balazy

John C. McGiff

Michal Laniado-Schwartzman

Domenic A. Sica

Eicosanoids[*] exert a pervasive influence on body function as they involve all systems and their effects are heightened by disease states and unphysiologic conditions.[1] Nonetheless, the therapeutic applications of the vast experimental edifice that rests on the multiple arachidonate metabolites arising from three pathways—cyclooxygenases (COX), lipoxygenases (LOX), and cytochrome P450 monooxygenases (CYP)—have been disappointing, with few exceptions. Prominent amongst these exceptions are the uses of aspirin in the prevention of myocardial infarction and acute ischemic stroke.[2] The interval between the discovery in 1971, by Vane,[3] that aspirin inhibits prostaglandin synthesis, and the widespread use of low-dose aspirin as an antiplatelet agent, was more than two decades. This interval should be kept in mind as it is close to the average period of dormancy between discovery and therapy. Indeed, the interval between the discovery of renin[4] and the development of angiotensin-converting enzyme inhibitors to blunt the activity of the renin-angiotensin system was eight decades (1898 to 1977).[5]

The most recent major discoveries in the field of arachidonic acid (AA) metabolism, and elaboration of CYP-derived metabolites of AA, were made two decades ago in the laboratory of Capdevila and Estabrook.[6] Another decade was required to elaborate the unexpected critical functional roles of arachidonate products of CYP in circulatory physiology and in diseases of the cardiovascular system. The critical experimental mass having been achieved in the CYP pathway of AA metabolism, novel therapeutic developments should be realized within the next decade. The availability of selective inhibitors of the ω/ω-1 hydroxylases and epoxygenases[7] allows separating and differentiating the functional effects of epoxyeicosatrienoic acids (EETs) and 19- and 20-hydroxyeicosatetraenoic acids (HETEs), respectively.[8] The studies, based on the use of selective inhibitors developed by Camille Falck, prefigure future developments in therapeutic applications in man. For example, 20-HETE and 11,12 EET act antagonistically on the rat afferent glomerular arteriole.[9] This physiologic antagonism determines afferent arteriolar diameter and thereby glomerular filtration rate in the face of alterations in renal perfusion pressure. A priori, studies directed to novel therapeutic interventions based on natural products such as arachidonate metabolites usually proceed along three lines of experimental exploration: (a) characterization of synthesizing, metabolizing, and catabolizing enzymes involved in the production, transformation, and degradation, respectively, of the eicosanoid/arachidonate product; (b) developing synthetic analogues of arachidonate metabolites; and (c) producing agonists and antagonists of eicosanoid receptors. To these traditional approaches, those based on molecular biologic techniques have and will amplify past findings and facilitate advances into new areas such as carcinogenesis.

PROSTAGLANDIN RECEPTORS

The multiplicity of prostaglandin and thromboxane (TXA_2) receptors and their signaling systems have yielded to a combined molecular biologic, biochemical, and pharmacologic-physiologic approach that has defined their structures, distribution, properties and function. Two groups, led by Shuh Narumiya in Kyoto[10] and Mathew and Richard Breyer in Nashville,[11] have contributed importantly to our understanding of these receptors which are represented by five major types: EP, IP, FP, DP, and TP, corresponding to the five major species of prostanoids arising from COX activity: PGE_2(EP), PGI_2 (IP), $PGF_{2\alpha}$ (FP), PGD_2 (DP), and TXA_2 (TP) (Fig. 45-1).

EP Receptors

PGE_2 acts through four receptors—EP_1, EP_2, EP_3, and EP_4—coupled to G proteins to produce a myriad of biologic effects ranging from production of fever (pyrexia) to regulation of renin secretion and modulation of salt and water excretion.[10,11] The EP_2 and EP_4 receptors coupled to G_s, when activated by PGE_2, stimulate cyclic adenosine monophosphate (AMP) formation, as does activation of DP and IP receptors. Contrariwise, stimulation of the EP_3 receptor inhibits formation of cyclic AMP. Like FP and TP receptors, the EP_1 receptor raises intracellular calcium, perhaps, by regulating Ca^{2+} channel gating, as this effect is dependent on availability of extracellular Ca^{2+}.[10] An alternative mechanism that elevates

---

[*]This review considers eicosanoids (signifying 20 carbon molecules) and arachidonic acid metabolites to be identical.

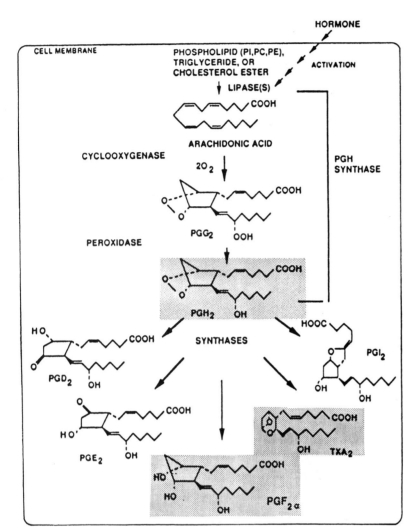

FIGURE 45-1. Hormone-activated prostanoid biosynthesis in a model cell. Although all products of the "cyclooxygenase pathway" are shown, usually only one prostanoid is formed as a major product by a given cell type. PGH = prostaglandin endoperoxide; PI, PC, and PE = phosphatidylinositol, -choline, and -ethanolamine, respectively; PGG_2, PGD_2, PGE_2, and $PGF_{2\alpha}$ = prostaglandins G_2, D_2, E_2, and $F_2\alpha$, respectively; PGI_2 = prostacyclin; TXA_2 = thromboxane A_2. *Stippling* identifies the prohypertensive prostanoids in contrast to PGI_2 and PGE_2, the antihypertensive prostanoids. (*Reproduced with permission from Smith W. Prostanoid biosynthesis and mechanisms of action. Am J Physiol 263:F181, 1992.*)

intracellular Ca^{2+}—phosphatidylinositol hydrolysis—was reported to be negligible in response to stimulation of EP_1 receptors.[12]

The EP receptors, all of which have been cloned, exhibit less sequence homology when compared with each other than when compared with other receptor subtypes. Rather, they are more closely related to other prostanoid receptors that act through "similar signaling mechanisms."[13] For example, the EP_1 receptor resembles TP and FP receptors in its ability to raise cytosolic Ca^{2+} and constrict blood vessels as well as when analyzed in terms of amino acid sequence identity.[11] The renal EP_1 receptor is expressed primarily in the collecting duct; activation of the EP_1 receptor inhibits sodium (Na^+) and water absorption at this site.[14] The vasoconstrictor response to EP_1 stimulation is in keeping with the hypotension observed in EP_1 receptor knock-out mice,[15] and suggests a significant contribution of the EP_1 receptor to blood pressure homeostasis.

Despite an abundance of EP receptor ligands that either block or stimulate EP receptors, none has made it through clinical trials other than misoprostol, a synthetic analogue of PGE_1, which is given to patients at risk to prevent upper gastrointestinal tract ulceration and bleeding.[16] PGE_2, synthesized by the gastric mucosa, on binding to the EP_3 receptor of parietal cells, inhibits acid production and is cytoprotective, two properties that are the basis for its use in prevention and treatment of upper gastrointestinal injury/disease. Of patients treated chronically with aspirin-like drugs, 2 to 4% will

develop a gastric ulcer, bleeding, or perforation, complications that are related to the dose of the nonsteroidal antiinflammatory drugs (NSAIDs).[17,18] These adverse effects are greatly reduced or prevented by misoprostol; its use in pregnancy, however, is contraindicated because of abortifacient properties.[19]

An unmodified prostaglandin, PGE_1, is used in the neonate with some forms of congenital heart disease, in preparation for corrective cardiovascular surgery.[20] PGE_1 is infused intravenously to maintain patency of the ductus arteriosus, which is very sensitive to dilatation by PGE_1. It is intended to "buy time" for infants to improve their preoperative condition and to decelerate their clinical deterioration by promoting pulmonary and/or systemic blood flow.

FP Receptor

Despite the relatively large production of $PGF_{2\alpha}$ by the kidney[21] and the association of altered renal production of $PGF_{2\alpha}$ in response to salt loading,[22] the role of $PGF_{2\alpha}$ in the regulation of salt and water homeostasis is uncertain. The AT_2 receptor has been identified as a component in a mechanism that regulates renal levels of $PGF_{2\alpha}$ by activating a key enzyme, PGE-9-ketoreductase, that increases $PGF_{2\alpha}$ levels by converting PGE_2 to PGF_{2a}.[23] Inhibition of this enzyme increases PGE_2 levels and, thereby, promotes salt and water excretion and decreases renal vascular resistance. Indeed, furosemide inhibits 9-keto reductase,[24] suggesting the potential importance of this enzyme to renal and systemic regulatory mechanisms. The levels of $PGF_{2\alpha}$ in the blood entering the thoracic Great Veins can be substantially increased by input from the renal veins as, for example, after activation of 9-keto reductase ($PGE_2 \to PGF_{2\alpha}$). This consideration, when viewed in terms of the venoconstrictor property of $PGF_{2\alpha}$,[25] underlies linking increased renal PGF_{2a} production to decreased compliance (increased tone) of the great veins and resultant increase in cardiac output.[26] This may be the basis of the mechanism proposed by Hinman in 1967, that $PGF_{2\alpha}$ couples renal function to cardiac performance; that is, $PGF_{2\alpha}$ is released into renal venous effluent in response to depressed renal function in order to increase cardiac output by elevating venous tone.[26] This area of investigation, still unsettled, like so many in the field of eicosanoid research, has been bypassed by the unexpected therapeutic avenues opened on discovery of alternative pathways of AA metabolism and the incredible array of novel eicosanoids they generate.[27] These studies have moved cardiovascular and renal investigation from the phenomenonologic to the mechanistic. For example, circulatory autoregulation, tubuloglomerular feedback (TGF) and ion channel activity have been reexamined in terms of lipid mediators and modulators of CYP origin[28] that invite drug development targeted to selective modification of the activity of key control points in the circulation and transporting epithelia.

A critical nephron segment, the medullary thick ascending limb of the loop of Henle (mTAL) and the site of the primary action of the most potent diuretics, the loop diuretics, such as furosemide, generates eicosanoids via several pathways: CYP and the inducible cyclooxygenase (COX-2).[29,30] The relative contributions of the principal products of these pathways—20-HETE and PGE_2—and their interactions to transport function in the TAL is uncertain. Nonetheless, important connections of TAL arachidonate products have been uncovered relative to Ca^{2+} excretion,[31] cytokine activity, and blood pressure regulation,[32] as well as to the pathophysiology of adrenal insufficiency[33] and renal failure in hepatic cirrhosis (the hepatorenal syndrome).[34] The progression of hepatic cirrhosis is associated with major abnormalities in renal eicosanoid metabolism. The most evident is a sharp increase in excretion of 20-HETE; the intense constriction of the renal vasculature, considered the hallmark of the hepatorenal syndrome, has been proposed to be mediated by 20-HETE.[34] Increased renal TXA_2 production had been considered to contribute to the renal failure in patients with cirrhosis and ascites.[35] The inability to modify the deterioration in renal function in response to cirrhosis by treatment with TXA_2 synthase inhibitors caused abandonment of the proposed role of TXA_2.[36] Furthermore, excretion of 20-HETE was closely correlated with deterioration of renal function in patients with cirrhosis and ascites.[34]

TP Receptors

Although antagonists have been developed for several of the prostaglandin receptors, chiefly the TP receptor, the initial clinical trials have not fulfilled the high expectations in the treatment of cardiovascular disease that were based on the use of TP-receptor antagonists in treating ischemic and thrombotic disease models in experimental animals.[37] Recent studies, however, indicate a reappraisal is in order for TP antagonists in the prevention/treatment of atherogenesis and thrombosis,[37] and of far advanced congestive heart failure.[38] Administration of a TP-receptor antagonist to apolipoprotein (Apo) E-deficient mice inhibited atherogenesis by a "mechanism independent of platelet-derived TXA_2."[39] TP-receptor

antagonism decreased serum levels of an intercellular adhesion molecule-1 (ICAM-1), which was associated with reduced development of atherosclerosis, effects not shared with aspirin, in ApoE-deficient mice. In view of the ability of several arachidonate products, isoprostanes and HETEs, generated during oxidative stress and atherogenesis to activate TP receptors,[37] inhibition of atherogenesis by TP-receptor antagonists may be related to inhibition of formation and/or enlargement of vascular plaques by these arachidonate metabolites, in addition to the principal endogenous agonists of the TP receptor, TXA_2 and the prostaglandin endoperoxide, PGH_2. Increased formation of isoprostanes and 15-HETE and their localization in atherosclerotic plaques would favor adherence and vascular infiltration of monocytes in response to increased expression of adhesion molecules induced by HETEs and isoprostanes.[37,40,41] The study by Cayatte et al[39] has prompted reconsideration of the use of TP-receptor antagonists for both preventing and inducing regression of arteriosclerosis.

Additional impetus for review of the status of TP-receptor antagonists derives from the failure of aspirin and other antiplatelet agents to affect the progression of atherogenesis in contrast to their efficacy in reducing the incidence of the acute ischemic complications of atherosclerosis in the coronary and cerebral circulations.[2,39] Indeed, in the management of vascular disease in which aspirin was considered to be the treatment of choice, for example, prevention of coronary artery restenosis, a TP antagonist may be more efficacious than aspirin because of preservation of endothelial PGI_2 synthesis.[37] The latter should be a therapeutic objective in view of the antiproliferative action of prostacyclin, a property that was reaffirmed in two recent studies: (a) beraprost, an IP-receptor agonist, inhibited restenosis after angioplasty of atherosclerotic rabbit arteries,[42] and (b) a neointimal proliferative response of carotid arteries to balloon injury in rats was prevented by human prostacyclin synthase gene transfer.[43] The relationship of PGI_2 synthesis to inhibition of the initiation and progression of thrombosis has also been addressed in a recent study that indicates the importance of PGI_2 to the prevention of arterial thrombosis: namely, deletion of the gene encoding the IP receptor predisposes mice to arterial thrombus formation.[44]

IP (Prostacyclin) Receptors

In view of the biologic profile of PGI_2—vasodilator, inhibitor of both platelet aggregation and mesenchymal proliferation—as well as its primary localization in the endothelium,[11,37] drug development can also be expected along the lines of prostacyclin analogues that resist rapid degradation, the half-life of PGI_2 being 3 min in aqueous solution. Thus far, the clinical applications in this field rest chiefly on the administration of PGI_2 (epoprostenol) either intravenously or by aerosol to patients having primary pulmonary hypertension (PPH) (see Chap. 25), a uniformly fatal disease.[45] Decreased expression of prostacyclin synthase in the lungs of subjects with PPH provides a rationale for the administration of supplemental PGI_2 to these patients.[46] In contrast to the remarkable improvement produced by intravenous PGI_2 in these patients with PPH who are subject to right ventricular failure,[47] the use of prostacyclin in patients with advanced biventricular failure increased the mortality rate.[48] The different outcomes reflect the underlying disorders; namely, in PPH, an elevation of pulmonary vascular resistance and secondary right-sided heart failure can be reduced by prostacyclin, whereas in biventricular failure, contractile dysfunction and accompanying cardiovascular remodeling predominate[49] and do not benefit from vasodilator therapy.[48] Indeed, a randomized clinical trial endorses the view that vasodilator therapy per se doesn't improve the outcome in patients with chronic heart failure.[48]

ASPIRIN: USES AND LIMITATIONS

The benefit of low-dose aspirin (e.g., 75 mg/d) treatment in the prevention of myocardial infarction and stroke (see Chap. 17) derives from inhibition of platelet generation of TXA_2, which, in addition to activating platelets, elicits vasoconstrictor and proliferative responses of blood vessels.[2] The critical event in the action of aspirin on platelets is the inhibition of PGH_2 production by COX-1 as PGH_2 is the obligatory precursor of TXA_2, the final product of platelet metabolism of AA via COX-1 and thromboxane synthase[50] (Fig. 45-1). Aspirin irreversibly inhibits COX-1 by acetylating the amino acid serine, which occupies position 529 in the peptide chain of COX, in close proximity to the catalytic site of COX.[51] COX-1 inhibition of platelets, the target of low-dose aspirin, persists for 7 to 10 days, the life span of the platelet. As platelets are without nuclei, COX-1, like other platelet proteins, cannot be synthesized. Platelet COX-1 is synthesized by the nucleated precursor of platelets, megakaryocytes, during their maturation in bone marrow.[52]

The beneficial effects of aspirin in the prevention of myocardial infarction, as well as in stroke, as noted, derive from prevention of platelet synthesis of TXA_2 and thereby platelet activation, a contributory factor in the genesis of thrombosis.[2] This is the situation in stable angina. In addition to the already cited failure of aspirin to prevent progression of atherosclerosis, aspirin has been reported to be inefficacious in the treatment of unstable angina.[53] Several factors are operative in unstable angina that limit the effects of low-dose aspirin which is directed at prevention of TXA_2 production by platelets. Namely, extraplatelet sources of TXA_2 are relatively unaffected by low-dose aspirin (when compared to platelets), particularly the vascular lesions of atherogenesis.[54] These sites in arteriosclerotic blood vessels contain both COX enzymes. COX-2, having a relatively short half-life ($\sim$3 h) and, perforce, a rapid turnover,[53] is less vulnerable to once-a-day treatment as aspirin is rapidly hydrolyzed in plasma (half-life 15 to 20 min),[55] thereby limiting the duration of its action on enzymes that are subject to rapid decay and regeneration. That is, COX-2 will be replenished at a time when unbound aspirin is no longer present in extraplatelet sites such as diseased arteries.

In unstable angina, another factor, one that is extraplatelet, is operative; it is responsible for production of TXA_2 by both COX-1 and COX-2 associated with atherosclerotic plaques.[54] In a significant number of patients with unstable angina, thromboxane production is only partially inhibited as reflected in urinary excretion of thromboxane metabolites, this despite virtually complete suppression of TXA_2 production by platelets.[53] Atherosclerotic plaques and contiguous tissue of the diseased arteries are the presumed sources of aspirin-insensitive TXA_2. This proposal was put to the test by treating patients with unstable angina[53] who demonstrated increased excretion of thromboxane metabolites (despite aspirin therapy) with a reversible COX inhibitor, indobufen, having a long half-life (8 h) as compared to that of aspirin (15 to 20 min). It should be noted that indobufen has been reported to be as effective as aspirin plus dipyridamole in preventing occlusion of coronary bypass grafts.[56] Indobufen treatment decreased the rate of TXA_2 synthesis to a greater degree than aspirin, which was interpreted to result from indobufen inhibition of extraplatelet sources of TXA_2 production "unaffected by aspirin because of rapid de novo synthesis" of

COX-2 by diseased arteries during the 24-h interval between administration of aspirin. Finally, it should be noted that any NSAID with a half-life similar to or longer than that of indobufen can be used to achieve the benefits described for indobufen.

To summarize, there are limitations in the use of aspirin in the prevention of heart attacks in patients with unstable angina when compared to NSAIDs having half-lives of several hours or more. These limitations are based on the short half-life of aspirin (of 15 to 20 min) vis-à-vis the rapid turnover of COX-2 in the arterial lesions of atherogenesis.

The second pathway of AA, LOX, makes its greatest mark on the pathophysiology of respiratory diseases. Extensions into the cardiovascular system have received less attention and invite studies that will lead to drug discovery.

LIPOXYGENASES AND LEUKOTRIENES

Biosynthesis of Hydroperoxyacids and Leukotrienes

A second more recently discovered important pathway of AA metabolism involves oxidation catalyzed by LOX enzymes. In contrast to the COX pathway in which prostaglandin products have three oxygen atoms covalently attached to AA from two moles of oxygen, LOX insert one mole of oxygen into the molecular structure of AA.[57,58] The free fatty acid is initially oxidized to a hydroperoxy derivative (hydroperoxyeicosatetraenoic acid, HpETE), which is subsequently reduced by glutathione peroxidase to the corresponding more stable hydroxy acid (HETE). Mammalian and plant (e.g., soybean) LOX have been characterized in detail as iron-containing enzymes that require fatty substrates having a cis, cis-1,4-pentadiene system.[59,60] This structural feature is found in four locations of AA and in other polyunsaturated fatty acids. Consequently, AA can be metabolized to several HpETE and HETE positional isomers by various LOX. Unlike COX, which act comparatively specifically on AA, LOX can efficiently oxidize other fatty acid substrates such as eicosapentaenoic acid. Three different mammalian LOX insert oxygen into either the 5, 12, or 15 position of AA[61] (Fig. 45-2). During the process of oxygen insertion, a proton is removed from a bis allylic methylene group with subsequent formation of a new double bond and hydroperoxy group. LOX stereospecifically control this process because the S configuration is typically observed in the HpETE products. In contrast, spontaneous free radical-mediated autooxidation of AA involves a similar mechanism but leads to racemic mixtures (R and S) of HpETEs. The first LOX product of AA that was described in mammalian system was that occurring in blood platelets, which generate 12(S)-HETE.[62] However, the formation of 5(S)-HpETE is of greater interest, because it is a precursor in the formation of potent biologically active leukotrienes.[57] Although COX is found in almost all mammalian cells, 5-LOX is restricted to a group of cells, mainly neutrophils, eosinophils, monocytes, macrophages, and mast cells.[63] These cells are believed to originate from a common precursor stem cell in the bone marrow. Because all these cells participate in immunologic defense and the inflammatory response, the presence of a common 5-LOX enzyme has been suggested to be of functional significance. LOX enzymes have also been described in blood vessels, brain and other cells.[61] In contrast to COX, which appears to be constantly in an active state, 5-LOX requires a complex multicomponent activation system. For example, the leukocyte 5-LOX is regulated by Ca^{2+},

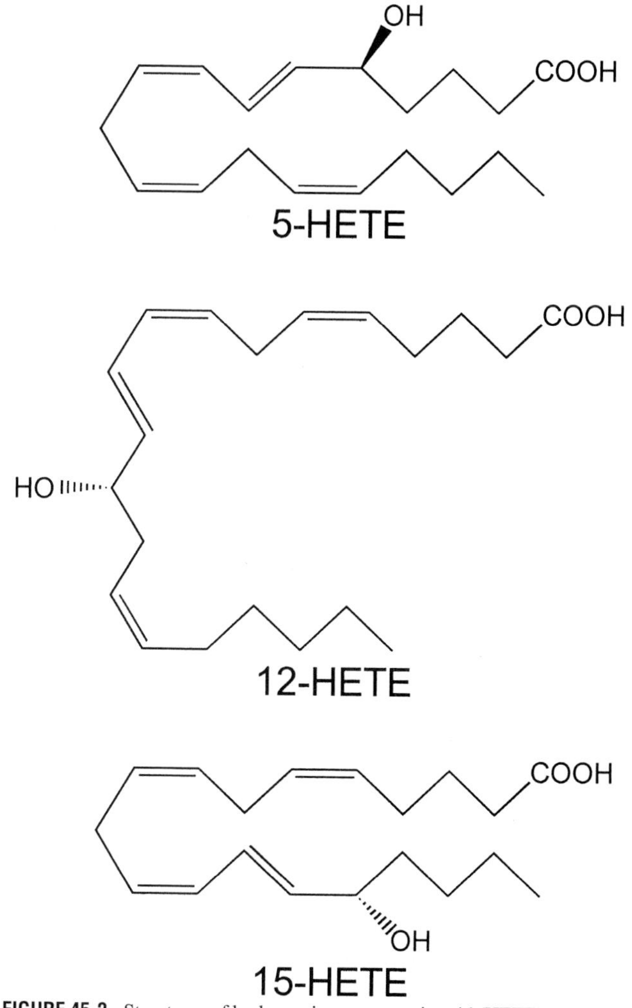

FIGURE 45-2. Structures of hydroxyeicosatetraenoic acid (HETE) products of 5-,12-, and 15-lipoxygenases having the *S* stereoconfiguration of the hydroxyl group.

adenosine 5′-triphosphate (ATP), and at least three nondialyzable factors.[64] Formation of leukotrienes proceeds by the removal of water molecule from 5-HpETE by a specific dehydrase enzyme, leukotriene A_4 (LTA$_4$) synthase, which produces an unstable 5,6-epoxide having three conjugated double bonds (a triene molecule) (Fig. 45-3).[65] This unique structural feature, which produces a characteristic ultraviolet spectrum, combined with the first observation of these triene lipids in the leukocyte, has led Samuelsson to coin the name leukotrienes to describe this type of lipid.[66] As is the case with the endoperoxides in the prostaglandin cascade, the LTA$_4$ plays a similar role of a crucial intermediate in the biosynthesis of two groups of leukotrienes. Enzymatic hydrolysis by a soluble hydrolase leads to leukotriene B_4 (LTB$_4$)[65] (Fig. 45-4). LTA$_4$ can also be hydrolyzed nonenzymatically to a mixture of 5,6- and 5,12-dihydroxy acids, as well as conjugated with glutathione to form leukotriene C_4 (LTC$_4$) (Fig. 45-5)[67] by a distinct form of glutathione S-transferase, which is known as LTC synthase (LTC$_4$S). At least two forms of enzyme have been described, and in humans, LTC$_4$S gene promoter shows significant polymorphism.[68,69] LTC$_4$ can be hydrolyzed by a γ-glutamyl transpeptidase to LTD$_4$, which can be hydrolyzed by cysteinyl glycinase to LTE$_4$. LTC$_4$, D$_4$, and E$_4$ form a group of sulfidopeptide leukotrienes and now

are known as the components of the "slow-reacting substance of anaphylaxis" (SRS-A), an active principal released by pulmonary tissue in response to antigen challenge, first described by Brocklehurst in 1953.[70] The sulfidopeptide leukotrienes account for the biologic activity of SRS-A, which Kellaway and Trethewie described, in the late 1930s, as having a potent "bronchoconstrictor activity" because it contracted smooth muscle of the respiratory tract.[70]

Metabolism of Leukotrienes

Leukotriene metabolism is not understood as well as that of prostaglandins. As previously discussed, specific peptidases rapidly convert LTC$_4$ to LTD$_4$ and then LTD$_4$ to LTE$_4$; all three compounds are biologically active. LTE$_4$ is excreted in urine and its measurement has provided a useful index of systemic leukotriene synthesis. For example, during an anaphylactic attack, urinary LTE$_4$ levels are increased.[71] However, Szczeklik et al have noted that only 10 to 20% of total cysteinyl-leukotriene body production is excreted by the kidney, which may limit the usefulness of urinary LTE$_4$ levels for predicting and defining clinical responses.[72] An active transport system concentrates sulfidopeptide leukotrienes in the hepatocyte, which can further oxidize LTE$_4$ at the C20 terminus.[73,74] Several rounds of β-oxidation further metabolize this ω-carboxy LTE$_4$.[74] Omega-oxidation and subsequent β-oxidation from the methyl terminus appear to be the major metabolites for sulfidopeptide leukotrienes in man.[74] Such metabolites of LTE$_4$ could be useful in assessing in vivo production of sulfidopeptide leukotrienes in humans; yet further quantitative studies are needed to reveal this potential of these metabolites. Sensitive methodologies also have been developed to measure directly sulfidopeptide leukotrienes in the lung lavage.[75] LTB$_4$ is inactivated within those cells in which it is formed[76–78] as well as by hepatocytes.[79,81] A major metabolic process involves ω-hydroxylation by a unique membrane-bound NADH-dependent CYP into 20-hydroxy-LTB$_4$, which can be further oxidized by a distinct dehydrogenase to 20-carboxy-LTB$_4$. These oxidations substantially reduce LTB$_4$ activity, and have been observed in human polymorphonuclear leukocytes and liver. A specific CYP$_{LTB\omega}$ enzyme oxidizes LTB$_4$ in neutrophils,[77] whereas in hepatocytes, CYP from the CYP4F family of enzymes appear to be more specific for LTB$_4$ ω-hydroxylation.[80,81]

Pharmacologic Properties of Leukotrienes

LTC$_4$ and LTD$_4$ cause hypotension in humans by a marked reduction in coronary blood flow.[82] The renal vasculature is resistant to this action of leukotrienes. LTC$_4$ and LTD$_4$ constrict coronary arteries and distal segments of the pulmonary artery at nanomolar concentrations. The sulfidopeptide leukotrienes have prominent effects on the microvasculature. LTC$_4$ and LTD$_4$ appear to act on the endothelium of postcapillary venules to cause plasma exudation. LTC$_4$ and LTD$_4$ are more than 1000-times more potent than histamine in this activity. LTC$_4$ and LTD$_4$ are potent constrictors of bronchial smooth muscles. They activate receptors on smooth muscle in peripheral airways and are much more potent than histamine. Leukotrienes also stimulate bronchial mucus secretion and cause mucosal edema. Immunohistochemical studies of mucosal biopsies from the bronchi of aspirin-intolerant asthmatics show that LTC$_4$S is overrepresented in individuals with this phenotype, and this finding correlates with overproduction of cysteinyl leukotrienes (CysLTs) and lysine-aspirin bronchial hyperreactivity.

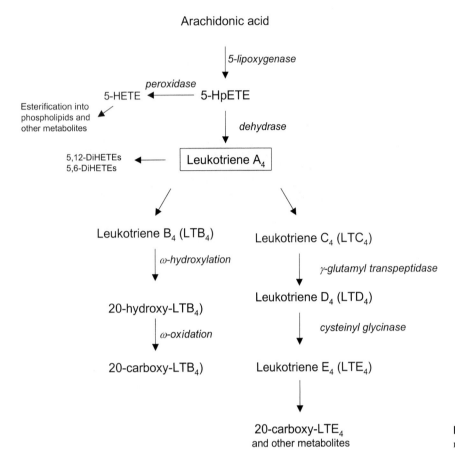

Arachidonic acid

FIGURE 45-3. Schematic steps of arachidonic acid metabolism by 5-lipoxygenase pathway.

LTB$_4$ is a potent chemotactic and chemokinetic lipid for polymorphonuclear (PMN) leukocytes, eosinophils, and monocytes;[83] LTC$_4$ and LTD$_4$ do not show this activity. LTB$_4$ potency is comparable to that of platelet-activating factor and chemotactic peptides. Higher concentrations of LTB$_4$ cause PMN aggregation, degranulation and generation of superoxide, adhesion of neutrophils to vascular endothelium, and *trans*-endothelial migration. LTB$_4$ is biologically important for the clearance of pathogens by activating and recruiting granulocytes to the inflamed lesions. Overproduction of LTB$_4$, however, is also involved in various inflammatory diseases, including bronchial asthma, rheumatoid arthritis, ulcerative colitis, psoriasis, and ischemic reperfusion injury in various tissues.[84]

Leukotriene Receptors

The distinct receptors that bind LTB$_4$, LTC$_4$, and LTD$_4$/LTE$_4$ have been identified in various tissues by radiologic binding techniques and pharmacologically.[85–87] Many leukotriene antagonists of various different structural types have been obtained and studies support the existence of four leukotriene receptors. The biologic actions of CysLTs, including bronchoconstriction, microvascular edema, mucus hypersecretion, and eosinophil chemotaxis, are mediated by CysLT type 1 (CysLT$_1$) and type 2 (CysLT$_2$) receptors distinct from those for LTB$_4$ receptors.[85] The CysLT$_1$ receptor is the molecular target for a recently introduced group of drugs nicknamed "lukasts" (montelukast, zafirlukast, pranlukast, pobilukast) (Fig. 45-6). These drugs do not antagonize the CysLT$_2$ receptor; the actions of CysLTs mediated by this receptor are not yet well characterized. Both receptors, which have been characterized at the molecular level,[88,89] show interesting differences in distribution. Whereas expression of

CysLT$_1$ mRNA has been found mainly in leukocytes, airway smooth muscle, and spleen, large amounts of CysLT$_2$ mRNA have been found in the heart, placenta, spleen, and leukocytes, but not in the lung. CysLTs relax many vessels at very low concentrations (10^{-8} to 10^{-7} M) supposedly via CysLT$_2$ receptor on the vascular endothelium and by the synthesis of nitric oxide and prostanoids. Higher concentrations cause vascular constriction apparently by stimulating the CysLT$_1$ receptor. Activation of CysLT$_1$ receptor appears to mobilize intracellular Ca^{2+}, reduce intracellular ATP, and activate phospholipase C. The possibility that these two receptors may mediate opposing effects of leukotrienes in other tissues is under intense investigation. Further studies that are being directed towards cloning CysLT receptor-deficient animals are likely to yield more clues concerning the pathophysiologic roles of these receptor subtypes.

Two G-protein-coupled receptor types for LTB$_4$ have been cloned and characterized. BLT1 is a high-affinity receptor exclusively expressed in leukocytes,[90] and BLT2 is a low-affinity receptor expressed more widely and found in the spleen, liver, ovary, and leukocytes.[91] Whereas numerous BLT-receptor antagonists have been developed to block LTB$_4$ actions in vitro, no BLT antagonist is available for clinical use. Molecular characterization of these receptors is likely to accelerate research of clinically useful BLT blockers.

Leukotriene Antagonists

5-LOX inhibitors and leukotriene receptor antagonists are newly developed classes of drugs for asthma therapy and related conditions. Early experimental efforts found that inhibition of 5-LOX translocation from the cytosol to the membrane could be an alternative strategy to inhibit leukotriene production.[92,93] The new class of

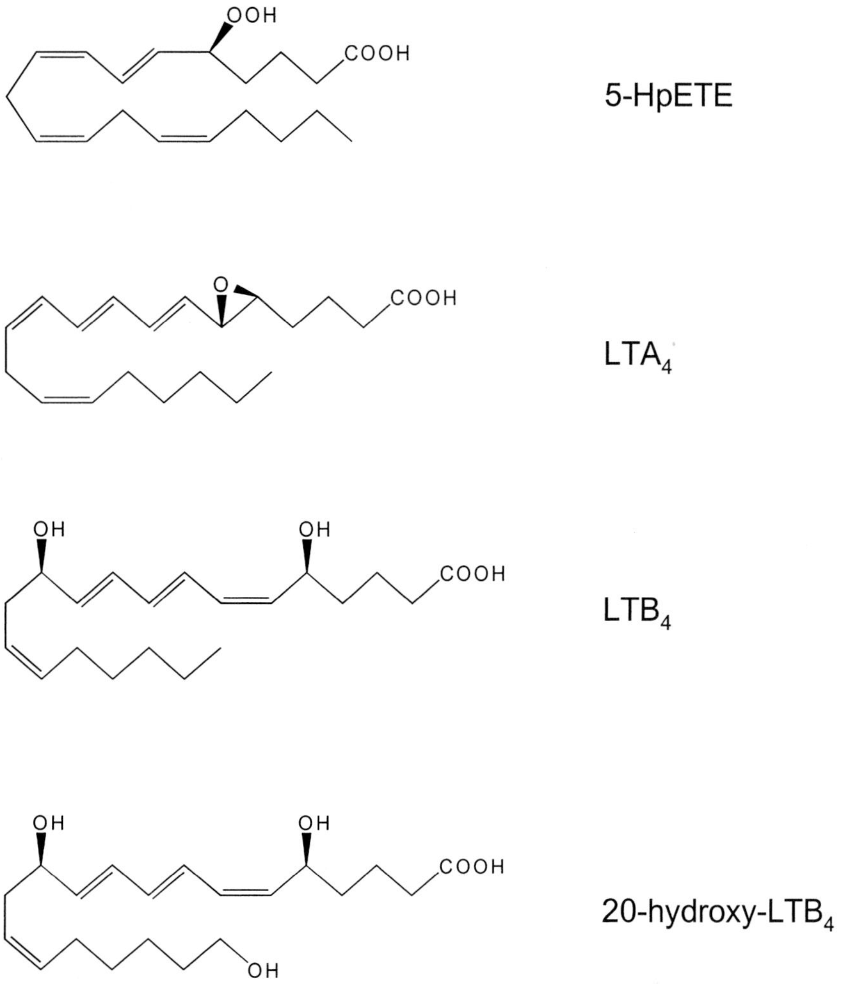

FIGURE 45-4. Structures of 5-HpETE and LTA4, LTB4, and its major metabolite, 20-hydroxy-LTB4.

asthma therapy drugs includes montelukast, zafirlukast, pranlukast, and zileuton[94] (Fig. 45-6). Zileuton is a potent and selective, but short-acting (half-life about 2.5 h), 5-LOX inhibitor, and thus inhibits all 5-LOX-derived lipids. It might seem that a therapy that uses a 5-LOX inhibitor should be more effective because all products that originate from 5-HpETE will be inhibited. However, clinical studies do not support that zileuton is more efficacious than $CysLT_1$-receptor blockers in asthma therapy.[72] Montelukast is a potent, specific leukotriene receptor antagonist. Administered once daily in a tablet form, montelukast reduces the signs and symptoms of chronic asthma in children as young as 2 years of age with a toxicity profile similar to that of the placebo.[95] Additionally, montelukast inhibits exercise-induced bronchoconstriction in asthmatic patients. Interestingly, the effectiveness of montelukast in patients with aspirin-induced asthma is similar to that in aspirin-tolerant asthmatics, suggesting that tachyphylaxis and/or downregulation of LTC receptors may be involved. In some countries, but not in the United States, pranlukast, a $CysLT_1$-receptor antagonist, is used in the treatment of asthma.

Other Lipoxygenases

LOX are abundant enzymes that have been found in numerous tissues and cells, including platelets, leukocytes, and vascular and neural tissue. Typically, several distinct LOX isoforms can synthesize

the same HETE isomer. For example, two types of 12-LOX are known as the "platelet" type and the "leukocyte" type.[96] Recent studies have focused on characterizing the roles of 12-LOX and 12(S)-HETE in cancer growth and angiogenesis.[97,98] Overexpression of 12-LOX in human prostate cells parallels prostate tumor growth and stimulates angiogenesis. In addition, the flavonoid, baicalein, a potent 12-LOX inhibitor, slows metastatic prostate tumor growth and tumor angiogenesis.[99] These studies suggest that 12-LOX and possibly other LOX could be important regulators of tumor angiogenesis via generation of proangiogenic lipids, such as 12(S)-HETE, and that inhibition of 12-LOX could be a novel therapeutic approach for the treatment of prostate cancers.[97]

Binding proteins and receptors for HETEs have been characterized in more detail only recently. For example, a 12(S)-HETE high-affinity binding protein (dissociation constant <1 nM), which has been found in lung carcinoma cells, activates a signaling mechanism involving nuclear receptor coactivator protein, suggesting a role for 12(S)-HETE in gene transcription.[100] Another aspect of the interaction of HETEs with the biologic membrane is that HETEs, unlike prostaglandins, are readily esterified into membrane phospholipids. Thus, HETE molecules may not only influence membrane properties such as permeability, but may also release secondary signaling molecules in a more delayed and hormone-dependent way, for example, following stimulation by phospholipases which releases HETEs from storage in phospholipids. Results indicate that

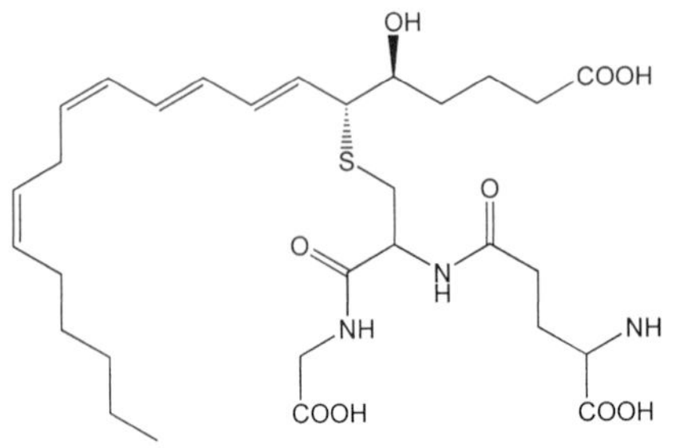

FIGURE 45-5. Structures of cysteinyl leukotrienes.

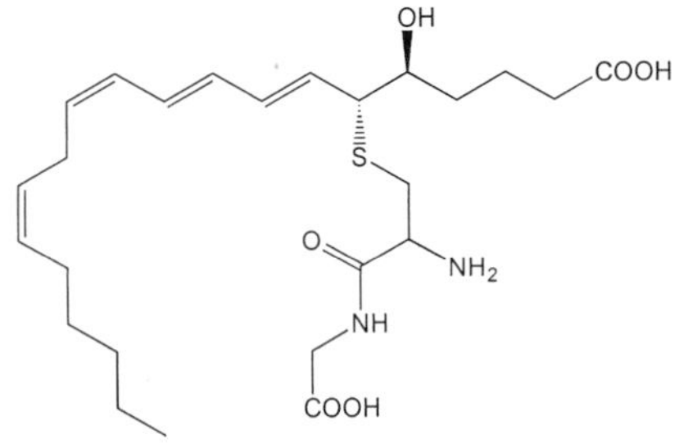

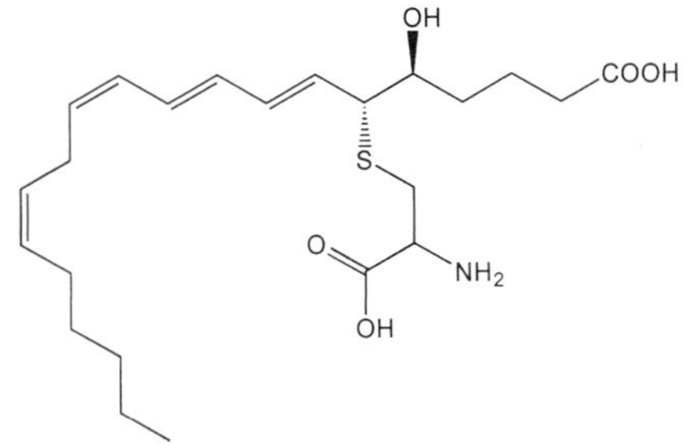

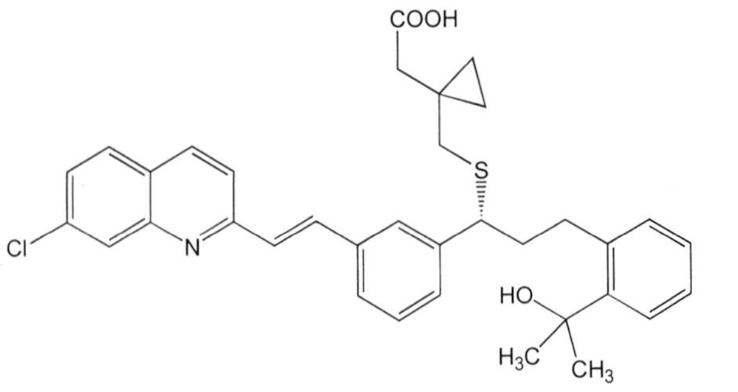

FIGURE 45-6. Inhibitors of leukotrienes.

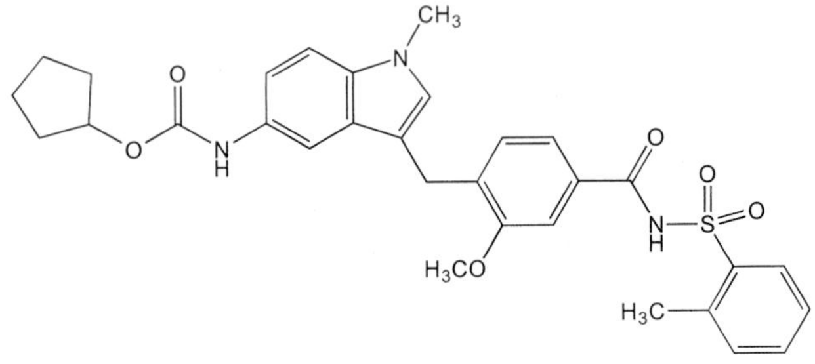

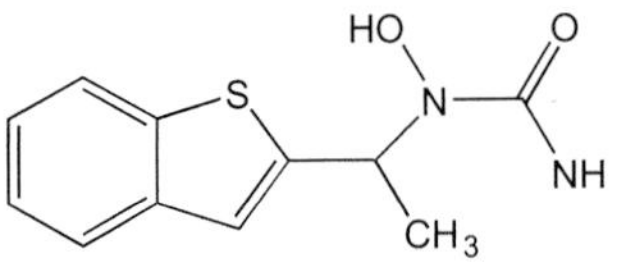

15(S)-HETE is rapidly esterified into phosphatidylinositol of PMNs, from which site the HETE can be mobilized and transformed upon exposure of the cells to a secondary signal.[101] Thus, HETEs, like AA, can be stored by cells, released via signal transduction mechanisms, and further oxygenated to generate alternative profiles of eicosanoids.

Additional studies suggest that 15-LOX may be involved in processes that modify native LDL into an oxidized form that is readily taken up by tissue macrophages. Colocalization of 15-LOX with macrophage-rich arterial lesions and epitopes of modified LDL supports a role of 15-LOX in atherogenesis. Investigations using transgenic animals also suggest that the site of 15-LOX expression may be an important factor in the development of atherosclerotic lesions. Because 15-HpETE has been shown to be a potent inhibitor of PGI_2 biosynthesis, it has been proposed that overproduction of lipid hydroperoxides in the vascular wall by LOX may be an important contributing factor in the development of atherosclerosis.[102] Studies also established that LOX products and enzymes play a role in renin release, aldosterone secretion, vasopressor effects of angiotensin-II (Ang II) and hypertension.[103]

Aspirin, NSAIDs, and Leukotrienes

A side effect of COX inhibition by aspirin and other NSAIDs, is the potentiation of leukotriene production in connection with development of asthmatic, gastrointestinal, and other effects.[104,105] It

appears that COX inhibition results in diversion of AA metabolism to LOX pathways, leading to excess production of vasoconstrictor sulfidopeptide leukotrienes (LTC_4, D_4, and E_4), chemoattractive LTB_4, and various HpETEs and HETEs having numerous biologic effects. Diversion of AA metabolism through LOX could be of additional importance as the effects of leukotrienes are potentiated in conditions of NSAIDs-induced COX inhibition, as removal of prostaglandins, some of which have protective properties, can also promote formation of LOX products. For example, PGE_2 inhibits LOX activity.[106] While there may be beneficial health aspects of aspirin therapy through the inhibition of thromboxane in platelets,[2] it appears that aspirin and other NSAIDs may induce severe disorders, especially in asthmatic patients. Although the mechanism by which NSAIDs induce a syndrome called aspirin-induced asthma (AIA) is not fully understood, it appears that aspirin increases leukotriene levels in these patients.[107] It has been also proposed that platelets may play a critical role in the development of AIA.[108] Although platelets do not synthesize leukotrienes, they are capable of converting LTA_4, originating from leukocytes, into LTC_4 via a *trans*-cellular mechanism.[109] Another aspect of the interactions of NSAIDs with arachidonate metabolism is that aspirin triggers biosynthesis of new lipid mediators related to lipoxins (LX)—LOX interaction products of AA metabolism.[110] While aspirin inhibits the constitutive form of

COX, COX-1, via acetylation of a serine residue in close proximity to the catalytic site, the inducible form of COX, COX-2, is still active following acetylation by aspirin. Although prostaglandin synthesis is blocked, COX-2 can form 15(R)-HETE.[111] While 15(S)-HETE, a product of 15-LOX found in endothelial and lung epithelial cells, can be further metabolized by 5-LOX to lipoxin molecules, recent work by Serhan et al shows that 15(R)-HETE could also be a precursor for a new class of lipids, aspirin-triggered lipoxins (ATL), by a cell-cell interaction and transcellular biosynthesis.[112] ATL-derived drugs may potentially inhibit inflammation and protect in reperfusion injury. Much additional work is needed to understand the potential beneficial aspects of these observations and translate them to therapeutic interventions.

Concluding Remarks

Discovery of the first mammalian LOX in the human platelet triggered intensive research that led to the discovery of leukotrienes, lipoxins, and other LOX-derived mediators. These lipids appear to play an important role in host defense, inflammation, asthma, cancer, and other disorders acting through specific receptor proteins. Much effort has been given to finding new drugs that could function as leukotriene receptor antagonists and 5-LOX inhibitors. Such drugs are now entering clinics and are the first new drugs in almost 20 years developed for the treatment of asthma symptoms and outcomes. Much needs to be learned in the area of LOX AA metabolism, as well as about the function of 5-LOX and other LOX enzymes, and receptors. This area of research has witnessed rapid advances. The recent finding of 5-LOX in the nucleus has raised hypotheses of potentially novel roles for this enzyme.[113] Furthermore, the discovery that LTB$_4$ can act through a nuclear hormone receptor, the peroxisome proliferator-activated receptor,[114] has intensified research into novel aspects of LOX pathways. Recent work also suggests that 12(S)-HETE and 15(S)-HETE can bind and activate BLT2 receptor, suggesting a broader role for these molecules.[91] A recently discovered LOX that can produce HETE molecules of the opposite R configuration,[115] as well as novel forms of LOX,[116] add to the complexity of lipid mediators that can be generated by this pathway. Knowledge of AA metabolism by LOX is extensive at the biochemical level but relatively insufficient in terms of understanding their full role in health and disease.

CYTOCHROME P450 MONOOXYGENASES

The concurrent reports of Brash et al,[6] Oliw et al,[117] and Morrison and Pascoe[118] on the oxidation of AA to metabolites by NADPH-dependent microsomal reactions in rat liver and rabbit kidney introduced CYP as the third enzymatic pathway. The work by the group at New York Medical College brought it to the forefront and invigorated intensive research that has placed these eicosanoids as key regulators of vascular tone and salt and water transport. Their therapeutic potential stems not only from their documented involvement in the regulation of vascular reactivity and ion transport mechanisms but also from the facts that: (a) they are synthesized by a system engaged in metabolism of xenobiotics and drugs; (b) their levels and production may be enhanced following pharmacologic inhibition of COX and LOX, not only because more substrate is available but also because they are readily metabolized by COX and LOX; and (c) their mechanism of action may not be restricted to a conventional receptor interaction. Several review articles have been recently published in this new area of research.[27,28,119,120]

Biosynthesis

CYP represents a superfamily of enzymes which exist in multiple forms differing in substrate specificity, positional specificity and stereospecificity. They are exposed to different regulatory mechanisms resulting in tissue-specific patterns of expression, which yield differences in isoform compositions and activities in various tissues. Across species, more than 500 CYP proteins have been isolated and their cDNAs cloned and sequenced.[121] They are grouped by amino acid sequence homology into gene families, each consisting of several subfamilies differing from each other in their amino acid sequences. A protein in one family is <36% similar to CYP in another gene family, and within a family, a protein in a given subfamily is approximately 40 to 68% similar to a protein in another subfamily.[121] AA, like other fatty acids and their derivatives, is a substrate for CYP-dependent oxidation reactions. While both COX and LOX are dioxygenases and have a minimal cofactor requirement and confined substrate specificity, CYP proteins are monooxygenases with an absolute requirement for nicotinamide adenine dinucleotide phosphate (NADPH)/nicotinamide adenine dinucleotide (NADH) and a flavoprotein, NADPH-CYP (c) reductase and/or cytochrome b$_5$, for substrate activation. This enzyme system catalyzes three types of primary AA oxidation reactions: (a) olefin epoxidation generating four regioisomeric cis-epoxyeicosatrienoic acids (EETs; 5,6-, 8,9-, 11,12-, and 14,15-EETs), each of which can be formed as R, S or S, R stereoisomers; (b) allylic oxidation, resulting in six regioisomeric $cis,trans$-conjugated mono-hydroxy-eicosatetraenoic acids (HETEs; 5-,8-, 9-,11-, 12-, and 15-HETE); and (c) hydroxylations at or near the ω-carbon (C-20) producing 16-,17-, 18-,19-, and 20-hydroxyeicosatetraenoic acids (16-,17-, 18-,19-, and 20-HETEs) (Fig. 45-7). The product specificity depends on tissue-specific isozyme composition, as well as on the pathophysiologic conditions, because CYP isozymes are readily induced by exogenous and endogenous compounds including hydrocarbons, anesthetics, antibiotics, drugs, hormones, and dietary manipulation. CYP-derived eicosanoids have been increasingly recognized as important autocrine and paracrine mediators of cell functions. They have been implicated in the regulation of vascular tone, ion transport mechanisms, inflammation, cell proliferation and differentiation, renal hemodynamics and salt and water excretion. The epoxygenase and ω/ω-1 hydroxylase branches of the CYP-AA pathway are the predominant CYP-catalyzed reactions in most tissues (Fig. 45-7).

Formation of EETs

Epoxidation of AA to EETs is catalyzed by a large number of CYP isoforms from different CYP gene families including 1A1, 1A2, 2B1, 2B4, 2B12, 2C2, 2C9, 2C11, 2C23, 2E1, 2G1, 2J, and 4A.[120,122] These isoforms demonstrate tissue-specific expression and exhibit relative regioselectivity and stereospecificity. For example, the predominant AA epoxygenases in liver and kidney tissues are members of the CYP2C family. CYP2C8, a major epoxygenase in human kidney, is highly regio- and stereospecific as it catalyzes the formation of 11,12-EET and 14,15-EET with 80% of each as the R,S enantiomer.[123] On the other hand, CYP2J isoforms are the predominant arachidonate epoxygenases in the heart; CYP2J2 expressed in human heart lacks regioselectivity and exhibits relatively low

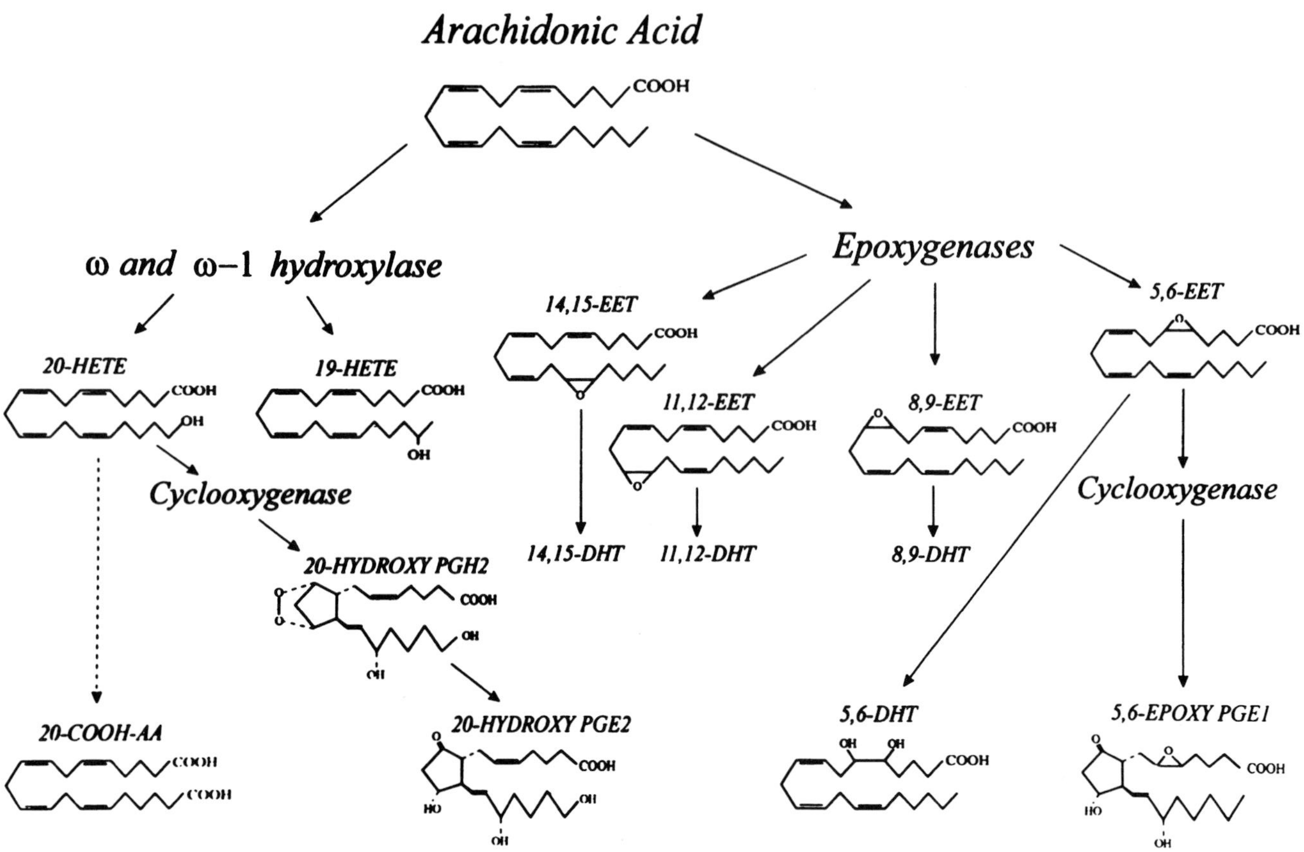

FIGURE 45-7. Arachidonic acid (AA) metabolism by cytochrome P450-dependent monooxygenases to ω and ω-1 hydroxyeicosatetraenoic acids (HETEs), epoxyeicosatrienoic acids (epoxides, EETs) and dihydroxyeicosatrienoic acids (diols, DHTs). 20-HETE and 5,6-EET can be converted by cyclooxygenase to analogs of prostaglandins. (*Reproduced with permission from McGiff JC, Quilley J. 20-HETE and the kidney. Am J Physiol 277:R607, 1999.*)

stereospecificity in producing 14,15-EET.[124] In the vasculature, endothelial cells are believed to be the major source of EETs and both CYP2C and 2J have been shown to contribute to their formation. Other CYP isoforms may become important for EETs formation under conditions where their expression is induced or suppressed. For example, in rats, phenobarbital administration induces CYP2B in the liver leading to increased EET formation,[125] whereas fasting causes a reduction in hepatic CYP2C11 expression and decreased EET formation.[126] In rats on high-salt diet, expression of renal CYP2C23 and urinary EETs are markedly increased,[127] and in rabbits fed high-cholesterol diet, coronary EET production is increased.[128]

Upon formation, EETs are subjected to rapid hydrolysis by epoxide hydrolases to their respective dihydroxyepoxytrienoic acids (DHETs) as well as to esterification primarily to glycerophospholipids. Measurements of EETs in tissues demonstrate that more than 85% is esterified into phospholipids.[129] Several studies implicate phospholipid-containing EETs in the regulation of membrane permeability. The low content of DHET in phospholipids led Weintraub et al[130] to suggest that epoxide hydrolases may play a role in regulating EET incorporation into phospholipids, thereby modulating cellular function. Other metabolic pathways include β- and ω-oxidations as well as conjugation to glutathione. 5,6-EET and 8,9-EET are substrates for COX enzymes,[131,132] and 5,6-EET can be metabolized by 12-LOX in platelets.[133] The vasodilatory effect of 5,6-EET in the rabbit kidney and the vasoconstrictor effect of 8,9-EET in the rat kidney are COX-dependent[131,132] (see Fig. 45-7).

The pathophysiologic significance of EETs and DHETs stem from numerous studies describing potent stereospecific biologic effects on functions such as vascular tone, ion transport, inflammatory response, and cell growth,[120] and from studies indicating that EETs are endogenous constituents of cell membrane phospholipids and biologic fluids.[129] That EET biology is relevant to human pathophysiology is further inferred from studies demonstrating that their urinary excretion is markedly elevated in patients with pregnancy-induced hypertension as well as in patients with unstable coronary disease and following coronary angioplasty.[134,135]

Formation of 20-HETE

20-HETE, the ω-hydroxylation product of AA, is generated primarily by enzymes of the CYP4 gene family. This family encodes multiple structurally and functionally similar CYP proteins that catalyze hydroxylation of the terminal ω-carbon forming 20-HETE and, to a lesser extent, the (ω-1) carbon of AA and other saturated and unsaturated fatty acids, and are controlled by factors such as age, sex hormones and dietary lipids. Hypolipidemic drugs (clofibrate, ciprofibrate, nafenopin), nonsteroidal anti-inflammatory drugs (aspirin, ibuprofen), and dehydroepiandrosterone (DHEA) induce, whereas lipopolysaccharide (LPS) and cytokines reduce, CYP4 proteins.[136,137] The CYP4 gene family comprises about 30 proteins across species in 3 subfamilies: CYP4A, 4B, and 4F; 12 of these proteins catalyze the synthesis of 20-HETE in different organs, including liver, kidney, lung, and brain. Although these isoforms share high sequence similarity and common catalytic properties, they differ with respect to tissue localization and hormonal regulation. For example, in the rat kidney, CYP4A1, CYP4A3, and CYP4A8 are highly expressed in the proximal tubules, whereas CYP4A2 is preferentially expressed in the outer medullary TAL region and is believed to be the major CYP4A isoform expressed in the renal microvasculature.[138,139] Renal CYP4A1 and CYP4A3 can be induced by hypolipidemic drugs such as clofibrate, whereas CYP4A2 is male-specific and is regulated by androgens.[140] In the rat kidney, CYP4A1, 4A2, and 4A3 are the predominant arachidonate ω-hydroxylases, whereas in the human kidney, this activity is mainly driven by CYP4F2.[141] The rabbit lung expresses high levels of CYP4A4, which exhibits high catalytic efficiency for AA ω-hydroxylation and is greatly induced during pregnancy in rabbits.[142]

Upon formation, 20-HETE is also subjected to further metabolism including oxidation by COX, LOX, and CYP to biologically active or inactive metabolites. β-Oxidation is the primary catabolic pathway, whereas esterification into phospholipids creates a reservoir from which 20-HETE can be released upon demand. 20-HETE is readily esterified into phospholipids in liver and kidney tissues but not in the vasculature.[143] This feature, storage of 20-HETE, impedes the efficacy of drugs targeting 20-HETE synthesis because multiple doses are needed to demonstrate reduction in, for example, urinary levels of 20-HETE.

Studies of 20-HETE in humans have been limited to the characterization of its synthesis in human kidney[144,145] and its detection as a glucuronide conjugate in urine of normal individuals.[146] A study by Sacerdoti et al[34] provides some evidence to suggest a role for 20-HETE in human disease. These investigators demonstrated that urinary 20-HETE excretion in patients with hepatic cirrhosis is several-fold higher than that of normal subjects and suggested that excess production of 20-HETE contributes to the renal functional disturbances in cirrhotic patients, particularly the depression of renal hemodynamics that characterizes the hepatorenal syndrome.

Vasculature: Role in the Regulation of Vascular Tone and Homeostasis

The vascular wall expresses numerous CYP proteins, including CYP2C epoxygenases and CYP4A hydroxylases, and has a substantial capacity to produce EETs and 20-HETE. The synthesis of EETs is primarily localized to the endothelium, whereas 20-HETE synthesis is localized to the smooth-muscle cells. EETs and 20-HETE have prominent actions, mostly opposing effects, on the vasculature including vasoreactivity and mitogenicity, further implicating a role for these eicosanoids in the regulation of vascular tone and vascular homeostasis including vascular hypertrophy, inflammation, and angiogenesis.

EETs

EETs dilate and constrict blood vessels and this vasoreactivity is regio- and stereospecific, as well as tissue- and species-specific. In most vascular beds, EETs appear to be direct vasodilators except that 5,6-EET and 8,9-EET can be metabolized by COX to vasodilator or vasoconstrictor prostanoids that modify their actions. Infusion of 5,6-EET or 8,9-EET into the renal artery of the rat increases renal vascular resistance and decreases glomerular filtration rate.[147] The vasoconstrictor effect of both EETs is COX-dependent. In the isolated rabbit kidney preconstricted with phenylephrine, 5,6-EET causes vasodilation due to metabolism by COX

as well as stimulation of PGE_2 and PGI_2 production.[148] 11,12-EET and 14,15-EET dilate preglomerular arterioles, whereas 5,6-EET constricts the preglomerular arterioles, an action that is COX- and endothelium-dependent.[149] COX-dependent vasoactivity of 5,6-EET in the pulmonary circulation, either dilation or constriction, is species-dependent.[150] In the cerebral microcirculation, the vasodilator response to EETs is mainly independent of COX. However, 5,6-EET dilates pial arterioles via COX-dependent generation of free radicals. The vasodilator response to EETs in the cerebral circulation of the newborn pig also has a prostanoid component as it involves PGI_2 receptor activation.[151] 11,12-EET and 14,15-EET, which dilate cerebral microvessels, may contribute to the regulation of cerebral blood flow.[152]

The mechanism of the vasodilator effect of EET in the renal, cerebral, and mesenteric circulations is believed to be related to their ability to open Ca^{2+}-activated K^+ (BK_{Ca}) channels, thus evoking hyperpolarization of vascular smooth-muscle cells. These properties, together with their endothelial origin, are the basis for defining EETs as potential endothelium-derived hyperpolarizing factors (EDHFs).[153] The proposal that one or more EETs are EDHFs is strengthened by studies demonstrating antisense oligonucleotides against CYP2C8/9, major arachidonate epoxygenases in the vasculature, attenuated bradykinin-induced EDHF-mediated hyperpolarization and vasorelaxation in coronary arteries without compromising responses to nitric oxide.[154]

Additional prominent actions of EETs on the vasculature include their ability to promote cell proliferation and to enhance anti-inflammatory responses. In endothelial cells, addition of EETs or overexpression of the human CYP2J2 decreased cytokine-induced adhesion molecules and increased tissue plasminogen activator expression and fibrinolytic activity. EETs, thereby, prevented leukocyte adhesion to the vascular wall that was attributed, at least in part, to the ability of EET to inhibit nuclear factor-kappa B (NF-κB) activation and IκB kinase activity.[155,156] In both endothelial and smooth-muscle cells, addition of 11,12-EET or overexpression of CYP2C8, which catalyzes the conversion of AA to 11,12-EET, activates Erk 1/2 and p38 MAP kinases and stimulates endothelial cell proliferation.[157] Studies by Medhora and Harder demonstrated that EETs produced by astrocytes stimulate an angiogenic response in cerebral microvessel endothelial cells.[158]

20-HETE

The ω-hydroxylation of AA, that is, the formation of 20-HETE, was thought to be a catabolic step in the oxidation and degradation of this fatty acid. Escalante et al were the first to characterize 20-HETE as a potent vasoconstrictor eicosanoid.[159] Subsequently, 20-HETE was established as a potent vasoactive autacoid in several vascular beds. 20-HETE constricts the rat and canine renal and cerebral microvasculatures,[160,161] whereas it relaxes the rabbit renal vasculature and bronchial airways.[162,163] In large arteries, 20-HETE vasoactivity is indomethacin-sensitive and is due to its transformation by COX to the vasoconstrictor 20-hydroxy prostaglandin endoperoxide[159,164,165] (see Fig. 45-7). In pressurized small arterial vessels of the kidney and brain, 20-HETE elicits vascular contraction via a COX-independent mechanism that is triggered by inhibition of large conductance Ca^{2+}-activated K^+ channels leading to vascular smooth-muscle cell depolarization and elevation of cytosolic Ca^{2+}, the latter dependent on activation of L-type Ca^{2+} channels.[160,161,166,167] In small resistance arteries, 20-HETE acts as a functional antagonist of the action of EETs. Endogenous 20-HETE contributes to the mechanisms underlying myogenic constrictor responses in renal and cerebral arterial vessels,[168–170] oxygen-induced constriction of cremaster arterioles,[171,172] phenylephrine-stimulated constriction of small mesenteric arteries,[173] and the renal vasoconstrictor response to endothelin.[174] These effects are potentiated by inhibition of nitric oxide synthesis.[167] Moreover, cyclic guanosine monophosphate (GMP)-independent mechanisms of NO relaxant effects in renal and cerebral arterioles have been attributed to NO-mediated inhibition of 20-HETE synthesis; that is, vascular relaxation is produced by elimination of the vasoconstrictor action of 20-HETE.[167] Muthalif et al demonstrated that 20-HETE can increase mitogen-activated protein kinase (MAPK) and cytosolic PLA$_2$ activities, thus stimulating AA release and causing translocation of Ras in rabbit vascular smooth-muscle cells.[175] They proposed that the signaling mechanism by which norepinephrine, Ang II, and EGF activate the Ras/MAPK pathway are through the generation of a CYP-AA metabolite, that is, 20-HETE. Tyrosine kinase and protein kinase C (PKC) have both been implicated in the vasoconstrictor response to 20-HETE in renal arterioles.[176] A recent study by Alonso-Galicia et al[168] suggested the existence of a binding site or receptor for 20-HETE in the vasculature. Whether this receptor/binding site is a channel, kinase, or other structural protein remains to be defined.

20-HETE formation in the circulatory system is not limited to the blood vessel wall. Human and canine neutrophils produce 20-HETE upon incubation with AA.[177,178] Human myeloid cells in peripheral blood and bone marrow express a variant of CYP4F3, which has a significant capacity to produce 20-HETE.[179] 20-HETE stimulates erythropoiesis[180] and inhibits platelet and neutrophil aggregation via a mechanism that includes blockade of the thromboxane/endoperoxide receptor.[181]

The Cardiovascular System

Kidney

EETs are formed in tubular and vascular structures and contribute to the maintenance of hemodynamic function and fluid and electrolyte homeostasis via their effect on vascular tone and epithelial transport directly or by mediating/modulating the action of Ang II, renin, vasopressin, and endothelin. The relevance of EETs to renal function and blood pressure control has been implicated in numerous studies showing that (a) removal of one kidney resulted in increased production of EETs by the other to maintain renal blood flow and glomerular filtration rate;[182] (b) increasing dietary salt intake in the rat augmented renal epoxygenase activity and urinary EET levels; (c) salt-sensitive hypertension in animal models was associated with an inability to increase EET production;[127,183,184] (d) inhibition of epoxide hydrolase activity to prevent degradation of EETs to DHETs lowered blood pressure in spontaneously hypertensive rats (SHR);[185] and (e) targeted disruption of soluble epoxide hydrolase gene lowered salt-induced increase in blood pressure in mice.[186]

20-HETE was found to constitute a major CYP-AA metabolite.[142,172] 20-HETE formation is localized in the proximal tubules (segments S1, S2, S3),[187,188] mTAL,[189] preglomerular microvessels,[160] and glomeruli.[190] As noted, 20-HETE is excreted in human and rat urine.[34,191] 20-HETE exhibits important renal vascular effects; it constricts isolated renal microvessels,[160,168] mediates vascular responses to constrictor stimuli,[173,174] and modulates the myogenic response of renal arterioles to elevation in transmural pressure.[192] Inhibition of 20-HETE formation blocks the vasoconstrictor response of afferent arterioles to elevation in perfusion pressure, and impairs autoregulation of glomerular capillary

pressure in vitro[192] and autoregulation of renal blood flow in vivo.[193] An important role for 20-HETE in mediating TGF has been suggested from studies demonstrating that perfusion of the loop of Henle with a 20-HETE inhibitor blocked TGF and addition of 20-HETE following blockade of its formation, restored TGF.[194] 20-HETE also affects tubular transport function at several sites; it inhibits proximal tubular Na$^+$/K$^+$-ATPase activity,[195,196] the TAL Na$^+$-K$^+$-2Cl$^-$ cotransporter,[197,198] and K$^+$ efflux via a large conductance (70 ps) K$^+$ channel in the TAL.[199] Inhibitors of 20-HETE formation increase while 20-HETE decreases transepithelial potential and chloride transport in the thick ascending limb of the loop of Henle in vitro[200] and the loop of Henle perfused in vivo.[201] These studies point to a central role for 20-HETE in the regulation of salt and water reabsorption in the kidney.

Several hormones were found to modulate kidney function by controlling the synthesis and release of 20-HETE. In the rabbit, Ang II was found to increase renal efflux of 20-HETE.[143] Endothelin (ET-1) evoked an increase in 20-HETE release from the rat kidney and inhibition of CYP-dependent AA metabolism greatly reduced the renal vascular response to ET-1.[202] These studies suggested that 20-HETE may contribute to the renal vasoconstrictor responses to both ET-1 and Ang II. In addition, parathyroid hormone (PTH) and EGF were found to stimulate the production of 20-HETE,[187] which is thought to serve as a mediator of PTH-induced natriuresis and EGF-stimulated mitogenic activity in the proximal tubules.[195,203] More recently, several reports have shown that the inhibitory action of Ang II and bradykinin on sodium transport in the mTAL can be blocked by inhibitors of CYP, suggesting that 20-HETE acts as a second messenger for these vasoactive peptides.[198,204] For example, the inhibitory effect of a low concentration of Ang II (5 × 10^{-11} M) on the apical K$^+$ channel was found to be mediated via the 20-HETE pathway.[189] In addition, very low Ang II concentrations ($\leq$10^{-12} M) through high-affinity receptor occupancy, maximally inhibit the Na$^+$-K$^+$-2Cl$^-$ cotransporter via diacylglycerol-lipase and CYP-derived products, that is, 20-HETE.[198] The addition of 20-HETE to the bathing medium of the rat microperfused mTAL elicited a significant reduction in Cl$^-$ transport, suggesting that the bradykinin-dependent inhibition of NaCl transport in this region of the nephron is mediated by CYP-dependent AA metabolites.[204] Altogether, these studies suggested that 20-HETE plays an important role in many key elements of renal function (Fig. 45-8).

Inasmuch as renal 20-HETE of vascular and tubular origins has effects that are opposite in their functional outcomes, disturbances of renal vascular and/or tubular CYP4 expression and 20-HETE synthesis may result in abnormalities of fluid volume regulation and blood pressure homeostasis. For example, upregulation of 20-HETE synthesis in renal microvessels may contribute to elevation of blood pressure by promoting increased renal vascular resistance, which, in turn, may bring about sodium retention by causing a rightward shift in the pressure-natriuresis relationship. Likewise, downregulation of CYP4 expression and 20-HETE synthesis in mTAL is expected to promote sodium and chloride reabsorption thereby contributing to the development of hypertension. Thus, inhibition of vascular 20-HETE synthesis decreased blood pressure.[173,205] On the other hand, inhibition of outer medullary 20-HETE synthesis increased blood pressure, presumably by facilitating NaCl absorption by the mTAL,[206] whereas increased outer medullary 20-HETE synthesis lowers blood pressure in female Dahl salt-sensitive rats by reducing NaCl entry at the mTAL.[207] The notion that tubular 20-HETE production is an important determinant of salt sensitivity is further substantiated by studies demonstrating that CYP4A

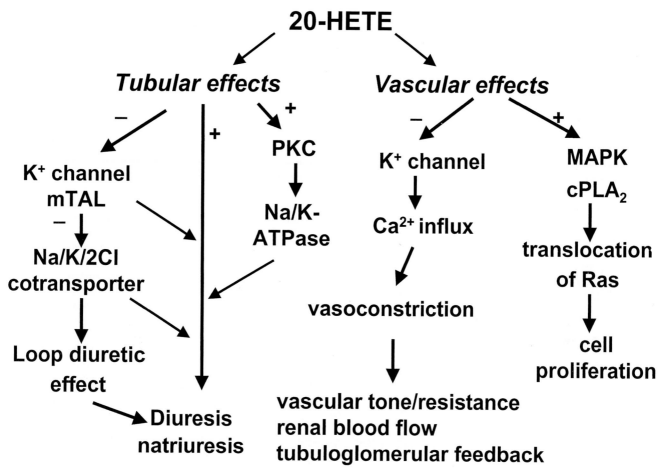

FIGURE 45-8. Biologic activities of 20-HETE in the kidney and their consequences on renal function. Stimulation is denoted as +; inhibition is denoted as −.

genotype cosegregates with the development of salt-induced hypertension in F_2 populations derived from a cross of both SHR and Dahl S rats with normotensive strains.[208,209] Interestingly, disruption of the CYP4A14 in mice causes hypertension that is more severe in the male; male CYP4A14 (−/−) mice show increases in renal CYP4A12 expression (driven by androgen) and 20-HETE synthesis.[210] Collectively, these studies provide substantial evidence that, in the rat, the CYP4A genes and the catalytic activity of their product, ω-thydroxylase, are important factors in the development and/or maintenance of hypertension.

Studies of 20-HETE in humans have been limited to the characterization of its synthesis in the human kidney[144,145] and its detection in urine of normal individuals.[146] As noted earlier, a study by Sacerdoti et al[34] has provided some evidence to suggest a role for 20-HETE in human disease. Urinary 20-HETE excretion in patients with hepatic cirrhosis is several-fold higher than that of normal subjects.

Heart

EETs are produced by atrial and ventricular myocytes, as well as by coronary endothelial and smooth-muscle cells. CYP2J isoforms have been shown to be the primary epoxygenases in the heart.[122] EETs dilate coronary arteries and constitute a major component of bradykinin- and acetylcholine-mediated increase in blood flow. Studies by Miura et al suggested that EETs contribute significantly (more so than NO) to flow-induced dilation in coronary arteries

from healthy subjects.[211] In isolated myocytes, EETs increase cell contractility and intracellular calcium. In canine stenosed coronary arteries and in aorta from rabbit fed a high cholesterol diet, EET production is increased.[128] All together, these studies suggest that EETs function to moderate coronary blood flow as well as to influence cardiac contractility.

The role of 20-HETE in the regulation of cardiac function is unclear although recent studies demonstrated that its levels are increased following ischemic reperfusion injury in dogs and that it relaxes bovine coronary arteries presumably via release of prostacyclin.[128,177,212]

Lung

Many cell types within the lung including ciliated epithelial cells, Clara cells and pneumocytes have the capacity to produce EETs. In rat and human lung, CYP2J isoforms seem to be the primary epoxygenases and 14,15-EET the major metabolite, mainly $14(R),15(S)$-EET. In rabbit lung, CYP2B is the primary epoxygenase and the major epoxide is 14,15-EET. EETs relax airway smooth muscle and alter transepithelial voltage through activation of a chloride conductive pathway in airway epithelial cells, suggesting a role in the control of pulmonary fluid and electrolyte balance.[150]

The lungs of several species produce 20-HETE; CYP4A enzymes are expressed in ciliated and nonciliated airway epithelial cells, in bronchial vascular smooth muscle, and in capillary endothelial cells.[150] In contrast to most vascular beds, 20-HETE dilates human and rabbit pulmonary arteries via endothelium- and COX-dependent mechanisms which include formation and/or release of vasodilatory prostanoids.[150]

Brain

The production of EETs in the brain is localized in the vasculature and astrocytes. In the rat brain, all four EET regioisomers are formed primarily via a CYP2C11, with 14,15-EET being the major EET. As indicated, all EETs dilate the cerebral vasculature primarily via activation of the Ca^{2+}-activated K^+ channels. In cultured astrocytes, EET production is increased in response to the neurotransmitter, glutamate. Harder and coworkers have provided evidence in the rat that EET production in astrocytes is involved in the regulation of cerebral blood flow by affecting vascular tone and promoting formation of new blood vessels.[152,158]

20-HETE synthesis in the brain has been localized primarily to the smooth muscle in the cerebral microcirculation.[213] 20-HETE has been implicated in the autoregulation of cerebral blood flow as it mediates the pressure-induced myogenic constriction of cerebral arteries. 20-HETE, presumably by inhibition of K^+ channel activity, produces membrane depolarization and Ca^{2+} entry through voltage-sensitive Ca^{2+} channels, the basis of the myogenic response. Indeed, inhibitors of 20-HETE synthesis block autoregulation in vivo.[170]

Physiologic and Pharmacologic Inhibitors: Therapeutic Implications

Heme oxygenase is the rate-limiting enzyme in heme degradation. By controlling cellular heme levels, heme oxygenase directs the flow of heme to the CYP hemoproteins. Moreover, heme oxygenase is the sole source of endogenously formed carbon monoxide, which effectively binds to the heme moiety causing enzyme inactivation.[214] Numerous studies documented that among other heme proteins, CYP is particularly susceptible to increased heme oxygenase activity. These features place the heme oxygenase system as a physiologic regulator of CYP. Studies using heme oxygenase induction as the means to reduce CYP activity were the first to suggest a pathophysiologic role for these eicosanoids.[215] Heme oxygenase induction, although effective, is far from being specific. Another enzyme system that controls CYP is the nitric oxide synthase (NOS). Nitric oxide, like carbon monoxide, binds avidly to the heme moiety, thus causing enzymatic inactivation. Increased NOS activity or administration of NO donors inhibit whereas inhibition of NOS activity enhances CYP activity.[216]

The high homology among the CYP isoforms and the ability of many CYP isoforms to use AA as substrate and produce an array of EETs and ω-1,-2,-3 hydroxylated products, pose problems in developing drugs that specifically target the formation of each of these eicosanoids without affecting others. However, recent advances in the knowledge of the chemistry and biochemistry of these eicosanoids have led to the development of a few compounds that demonstrate some kind of specificity and may be suitable therapy for certain diseases, for example, elevation of blood pressure and abnormalities of salt and water excretion. The first of such inhibitors were a series of AA analogues that showed reasonable specificity; for example, the inhibitors of microsomal 20-HETE formation, N-methylsulfonyl-12,12-dibromododec-11-enamide (DDMS) and 12,12-dibromododec-11-enoic acid (DBDD). Also, selective inhibitors of epoxygenases have been developed: 6-(2-propargyloxyphenyl)hexanoic acid (PPOH) and N-methylsulfonyl-6-(2-propargyloxyphenyl)hexanamide (MS-PPOH). However, the in vivo efficacy of these compounds is limited by water insolu-

bility and high binding to albumin and other proteins. A recent study by Miyata et al[217] identified a selective and potent inhibitor of 20-HETE synthesis in vitro and in vivo, namely N-hydroxy-N'-(4-butyl-2-methylphenyl)-formamidine (HET0016). Blockade of 20-HETE formation following in vivo administration with HET0016 attenuates cerebral vasospasm after subarachnoid hemorrhage in the rat,[218] further indicating the therapeutic potential of such inhibitors.

CYCLOOXYGENASE-2, COXIBS AND CARDIOVASCULAR DISEASE

Non-selective NSAIDs, such as ibuprofen, naproxen, and indomethacin inhibit both isoforms of cyclooxygenase (COX-1 and COX-2) over their clinical dose range.[219] In contrast, the coxibs—such as rofecoxib and celecoxib—are selective for only the COX-2 isoform over their clinical dose range.[220–221] In comparing aspirin, non-selective NSAIDs, and COX-2 inhibitors, variation in platelet inhibitory effects may result in different influences on the rate of cardiovascular thrombotic events.[222] This is particularly so for the COX-2 inhibitors in that they lack clinically recognizable effects on platelet-derived thromboxane and platelet aggregation.[223] It has been speculated that selective COX-2 inhibitors might adversely affect hemostatic balance, and even favor thrombosis, by selectively inhibiting COX-2-derived endothelial prostacyclin—a known vasodilation and platelet anti-aggregant—without affecting platelet-derived thromboxane.[224–225] The issue of whether COX-2 inhibitors are prothrombotic remains unresolved.[226] In the Vioxx Gastrointestinal Outcomes Research Study (VIGOR) high-dose rofecoxib (50 mg) was compared to naproxen (1000 mg) in the treatment of rheumatoid arthritis. Thrombotic cardiovascular events were higher in the rofecoxib treatment group.[226] Yet it has now been shown that naproxen—a non-selective NSAID—decreases thrombotic events in relationship to its platelet anti-aggregant effects.[227] This finding with naproxen holds promise in helping to explain at least some of the adverse findings in the VIGOR trial.[227–228] Pending resolution of this issue, patients who are candidates for antiplatelet therapy should receive low-dose aspirin therapy to ensure an antiplatelet effect. Whether the combination of a COX-2 inhibitor and aspirin maintains the advantage of a coxib over a non-selective NSAID with respect to gastrointestinal side-effects remains to be formally tested.[229,230,230a]

Recently it was shown that meloxicam, a preferential COX-2 inhibitor with heparin and aspirin, was superior to heparin and aspirin in reducing adverse outcomes in patients with acute coronary syndromes without ST-segment elevation.[231]

Acknowledgments   This review was supported by NIH grants PPG HL34300 (MB, JCM, MLS); RO1 GM62453 (MB); RO1 HL25394 (JCM); and RO1 EY05613 (MLS).

The authors thank Melody Steinberg for preparation of the manuscript and editorial assistance.

REFERENCES

1. Quilley J, Bell-Quilley CP, McGiff JC: Eicosanoids and hypertension. In: Laragh JH, Brenner BM, eds. *Hypertension: Pathophysiology, Diagnosis, and Management.* 2nd ed. New York: Raven Press, 1995:963.
2. Patrono C, Coller B, Dalen JE, et al: Platelet-active drugs: The relationships among dose, effectiveness, and side effects. *Chest* 114:470S, 1998.

3. Vane JR: Inhibition of prostaglandin synthesis as a mechanism of action for aspirin-like drugs. *Nat New Biol* 231:232, 1971.

4. Tigerstedt R, Bergman PG: Niere und Kreislauf. *Skand Arch Physiol* 8:223, 1898.

5. Cushman DW, Cheung HS, Sabo EF, et al: Design of potent competitive inhibitors of angiotensin-converting enzymes. Carboxyalkanoyl and mercaptoalkanoyl amino acids. *Biochemistry* 16:5484, 1977.

6. Capdevila J, Chacos N, Werringloer J, et al: Liver microsomal cytochrome P-450 and the oxidative metabolism of arachidonic acid. *Proc Natl Acad Sci U S A* 78:5362, 1981.

7. Wang M-H, Brand-Schieber E, Zand BA, et al: Cytochrome P450-derived arachidonic acid metabolism in the rat kidney: Characterization of selective inhibitors. *J Pharmacol Exp Ther* 284:966, 1998.

8. Pomposiello SI, Carroll MA, Falck JR, et al: Epoxyeicostrienoic acid-mediated renal vasodilation to arachidonic acid is enhanced in SHR. *Hypertension* 37:887, 2001.

9. Imig JD, Falck JR, Inscho EW: Contribution of cytochrome P450 epoxygenase and hydroxylase pathways to afferent arteriolar autoregulatory responsiveness. *Br J Pharmacol* 127:1399, 1999.

10. Narumiya S, Sugimoto Y, Ushikubi F: Prostanoid receptors: Structures, properties, and functions. *Physiol Rev* 79:1193, 1999.

11. Breyer MD, Breyer RM: G protein—coupled prostanoid receptors and the kidney. *Annu Rev Physiol* 63:579, 2001.

12. Watabe A, Sugimoto Y, Honda A, et al: Cloning and expression of cDNA for a mouse EP_1 subtype of prostaglandin E receptor. *J Biol Chem* 268:20175, 1993.

13. Toh H, Ichikawa A, Narumiya S: Molecular evolution of receptors for eicosanoids. *FEBS Lett* 361:17, 1995.

14. Guan Y, Zhang Y, Breyer RM, et al: Prostaglandin E_2 inhibits renal collecting duct Na+ absorption by activating the EP1 receptor. *J Clin Invest* 102:194, 1998.

15. Audoly L, Kim H, Patrick J, et al: Mice lacking the prostaglandin E2 EP1 receptor subtype have hypotension, hyperreninemia and altered responses to angiotensin II (abstr.). *FASEB J* 13:A1549, 1999.

16. Monk JP, Clissold SP: Misoprostol: A preliminary review of its pharmacodynamic and pharmacokinetic properties, and therapeutic efficacy in the treatment of peptic ulcer disease. *Drugs* 33:1, 1987.

17. Wolfe MM, Lichenstein DR, Singh G: Medical progress: Gastrointestinal toxicity of nonsteroidal antiinflammatory drugs. *N Engl J Med* 340:1888, 1999.

18. Leonards JR, Levy G, Niemczura R: Gastrointestinal blood loss during prolonged aspirin administration. *N Engl J Med* 289:1020, 1973.

19. Morrow JD, Roberts LJ II: Lipid-derived autocoids: Eicosanoids and platelet-activating factor. In: Hardman JG, Limbird LE, eds. *Goodman & Gilman's: The Pharmacological Basis of Therapeutics.* 10th ed. New York: McGraw-Hill, 2001:679.

20. Braunwald E, Zipes DP, Libby P: *Heart Disease. A Textbook of Cardiovascular Medicine.* 6th ed. Philadelphia: WB Saunders, 2001: 1523.

21. McGiff JC, Miller MJS: Renal functional aspects of eicosanoid-dependent mechanisms. In: Fisher J, ed. *Kidney Hormones.* Vol 3. London: Academic Press, 1986:363.

22. Weber P, Larsson C, Scherer B: Prostaglandin E2-9-ketoreductase as a mediator of salt intake-related prostaglandin-renin interaction. *Nature* 266:65, 1977.

23. Siragy HM, Carey RM: The subtype 2 angiotensin receptor regulates renal prostaglandin F2 alpha formation in conscious rats. *Am J Physiol* 273:R1103, 1997.

24. McGiff JC, Wong P Y-K: Prostaglandins and renal function: Implications for the activity of diuretic agents. In: Cragoe EJ Jr, ed. *Diuretic Agents.* Washington DC: ACS Symposium, 1978:1.

25. Ducharme DW, Weeks JR, Montgomery RG: Studies on the mechanism of the hypertensive effect of prostaglandin $F_{2\alpha}$. *J Pharmacol Exp Ther* 160:1, 1968.

26. Hinman JW: Prostaglandins. *Bioscience* 17:779, 1967.

27. McGiff JC, Quilley J: 20-HETE and the kidney: Resolution of old problems and new beginnings. *Am J Physiol* 277:R607, 1999.

28. Roman RJ: P-450 metabolites of arachidonic acid in the control of cardiovascular function. *Physiol Rev* 82:131, 2001.

29. Escalante B, Erlij D, Falck JR, et al: Effect of cytochrome P450 arachidonate metabolites on ion transport in rabbit kidney loop of Henle. *Science* 251:799, 1991.

30. Ferreri NR, An S-J, McGiff JC: Cyclooxygenase-2 expression and function in the medullary thick ascending limb. *Am J Physiol* 277:F360, 1999.

31. Wang D, McGiff JC, Ferreri NR: Regulation of cyclooxygenase isoforms in the renal thick ascending limb: Effects of extracellular calcium *J Physiol Pharmacol* 51:587, 2000.

32. Ferreri NR, Zhao Y, Takizawa H, et al: Tumor necrosis factor-α-angiotensin interactions and regulation of blood pressure. *J Hypertens* 15:1481, 1997.

33. Vio CP, An S-J, Cespedes C, et al: Induction of cyclooxygenase-2 in thick ascending limb cells by adrenalectomy. *J Am Soc Nephrol* 12:649, 2001.

34. Sacerdoti D, Balazy M, Angeli P, et al: Eicosanoid excretion in hepatic cirrhosis: Predominance of 20-HETE. *J Clin Invest* 100:1264, 1997.

35. Moore K, Ward PS, Taylor GW, et al: Systemic and renal production of thromboxane A2 and prostacyclin in decompensated liver disease and hepatorenal syndrome. *Gastroenterology* 100:1069, 1991.

36. Zipser RD, Kronborg I, Rector W, et al: Therapeutic trial of thromboxane synthesis inhibition in the hepatorenal syndrome. *Gastroenterology* 87:1228, 1984.

37. Pratico D, Cheng Y, FitzGerald GA: TP or not TP. Primary mediators in a close runoff? *Arterioscler Thromb Vasc Biol* 20:1695, 2000.

38. Castellani S, Paladini B, Paniccia R, et al: Increased renal formation of thromboxane A_2 and prostaglandin $F_{2\alpha}$ in heart failure. *Am Heart J* 133:94, 1997.

39. Cayatte AJ, Du Y, Oliver-Krasinski J, et al: The thromboxane receptor antagonist S18886 but not aspirin inhibits atherogenesis in ApoE-deficient mice. *Arterioscler Thromb Vasc Biol* 20:1724, 2000.

40. Van Diest MJ, Herman AG, Verbeuren TJ: Influence of hypercholesterolaemia on the reactivity of isolated rabbit arteries to 15-lipoxygenase metabolites of arachidonic acid: Comparison with platelet-derived agents and vasodilators. *Prostaglandin Leukot Essent Fatty Acids* 54:135, 1996.

41. Pfister SL, Schmitz JM, Willerson JT, et al: Characterization of arachidonic acid metabolism in Watanabe heritable hyperlipidemic (WHHL) and New Zealand White (NZW) rabbit aortas. *Prostaglandins* 36:515, 1988.

42. Isogaya M, Yamada N, Koike H, et al: Inhibition of restenosis by beraprost sodium (a prostaglandin I_2 analogue) in the atherosclerotic rabbit artery after angioplasty. *J Cardiovasc Pharmacol* 25:947, 1995.

43. Todaka T, Yokoyama C, Yanamoto H, et al: Gene transfer of human prostacyclin synthase prevents neointimal formation after carotid balloon injury in rats. *Stroke* 30:419, 1999.

44. Hirata M, Hayashi Y, Ushikubi F, et al: Cloning and expression of cDNA for human thromboxane A2 receptor. *Nature* 349:617, 1991.

45. Hoeper MM, Schwarze M, Ehlerding S, et al: Long-term treatment of primary pulmonary hypertension with aerosolized iloprost, a prostacyclin analogue. *N Engl J Med* 342:1866, 2000.

46. Tuder RM, Cool CD, Geraci MW, et al: Prostacyclin synthase expression is decreased in lungs from patients with severe pulmonary hypertension. *Am J Respir Crit Care Med* 159:1925, 1999.

47. Shapiro SM, Oudiz RJ, Cao T, et al: Primary pulmonary hypertension. Improved long-term effects and survival with continuous intravenous epoprostenol infusion. *J Am Coll Cardiol* 30:343, 1997.

48. Califf RM, Adams KF, McKenna WJ, et al: A randomized controlled trial of epoprostenol therapy for severe congestive heart failure: The Flolan International randomized Survival Trial (FIRST). *Am Heart J* 134:44, 1997.

49. Eichhorn EJ, Bristow MR: Medical therapy can improve the biologic properties of the chronically failing heart: A new era in the treatment of heart failure. *Circulation* 94:2285, 1996.

50. Oyekan A, McGiff JC, Quilley J: Eicosanoids: Do they matter? In: Oparil S, Weber MA, eds. *Hypertension: A companion to Brenner and Rector's The Kidney.* Philadelphia: WB Saunders, 1999:176.

51. Smith WL, DeWitt, DL, Garavito RM: Cyclooxygenases: Structural, cellular, and molecular biology. *Annu Rev Biochem* 69:145, 2000.

52. Kuter DJ: Megakaryopoiesis and thrombopoiesis. In: Beutler E, Coller BS, Lichtman MA, et al, eds. *Williams Hematology,* 6th ed. New York: McGraw-Hill, 2001:1339.

53. Cipollone F, Patrignani P, Greco A, et al: Differential suppression of thromboxane biosynthesis by indobufen and aspirin in patients with unstable angina. *Circulation* 96:1109, 1997.

54. Schonbeck U, Sukhova GK, Graber P, et al: Augmented expression of cyclooxygenase-2 in human atherosclerotic lesions. *Am J Pathol* 155:1281, 1999.

55. Roberts LJ II, Morrow JD: Analgesic-antipyretic and anti-inflammatory agents and drugs employed in the treatment of gout. In: Hardman JG, Limbird LE, eds. *Goodman & Gilman's:*

The Pharmacological Basis of Therapeutics. 10th ed. New York: McGraw-Hill, 2001:700.

56. Rajah SM, Rees M, Walker D, et al: Effects of antiplatelet therapy with indobufen or aspirin-dipyridamole on graft patency one year after coronary artery bypass grafting. *J Thorac Cardiovasc Surg* 107:1146, 1994.

57. Samuelsson B: The discovery of the leukotrienes. *Am J Respir Crit Care Med* 161:S2-S6, 2000.

58. Samuelsson B: From studies of biochemical mechanism to novel biological mediators: Prostaglandin endoperoxides, thromboxanes, and leukotrienes. Nobel Lecture, 8 December 1982. *Biosci Rep* 3:791, 1983.

59. Hamberg M, Samuelsson B: On the specificity of the oxygenation of unsaturated fatty acids catalyzed by soybean lipoxidase. *J Biol Chem* 242:5329, 1967.

60. Percival MD: Human 5-lipoxygenase contains an essential iron. *J Biol Chem* 266:10058, 1991.

61. Spector AA, Gordon JA, Moore SA: Hydroxyeicosatetraenoic acids (HETEs). *Prog Lipid Res* 27:271, 1988.

62. Hamberg M, Samuelsson B: Prostaglandin endoperoxides. Novel transformations of arachidonic acid in human platelets. *Proc Natl Acad Sci U S A* 71:3400, 1974.

63. Samuelsson B: Leukotrienes: Mediators of allergic reactions and inflammation. *Int Arch Allergy Appl Immunol* 66(Suppl 1):98, 1981.

64. Rouzer CA, Samuelsson B: On the nature of the 5-lipoxygenase reaction in human leukocytes: Enzyme purification and requirement for multiple stimulatory factors. *Proc Natl Acad Sci U S A* 82:6040, 1985.

65. Radmark O, Malmsten C, Samuelsson B, et al: Leukotriene A: Stereochemistry and enzymatic conversion to leukotriene B. *Biochem Biophys Res Commun* 92:954, 1980.

66. Samuelsson B: Prostaglandins, thromboxanes, and leukotrienes: Formation and biological roles. *Harvey Lect* 75:1, 1979.

67. Murphy RC, Hammarstrom S, Samuelsson B: Leukotriene C: A slow-reacting substance from murine mastocytoma cells. *Proc Natl Acad Sci U S A* 76:4275, 1979.

68. Penrose JF, Austen KF: The biochemical, molecular, and genomic aspects of leukotriene C_4 synthase. *Proc Assoc Am Physicians* 111:537, 1999.

69. Scoggan KA, Jakobsson PJ, Ford-Hutchinson AW: Production of leukotriene C_4 in different human tissues is attributable to distinct membrane bound biosynthetic enzymes. *J Biol Chem* 272:10182, 1997.

70. Brocklehurst WE: The role of slow-reacting substance in asthma. *Adv Drug Res* 5:109, 1970.

71. Denzlinger C, Haberl C, Wilmanns W: Cysteinyl leukotriene production in anaphylactic reactions. *Int Arch Allergy Immunol* 108:158, 1995.

72. Szczeklik A, Mastalerz L, Nizankowska E, et al: Montelukast for persistent asthma. *Lancet* 358:1456, 2001.

73. Uehara N, Ormstad K, Orrenius S, et al: Active transport of leukotrienes into rat hepatocytes. *Adv Prostaglandin Thromboxane Leukot Res* 11:147, 1983.

74. Sala A, Voelkel N, Maclouf J, et al: Leukotriene E_4 elimination and metabolism in normal human subjects. *J Biol Chem* 265:21771, 1990.

75. Wescott JY, Balazy M, Stenmark KR, et al: Analysis of leukotriene D_4 in human lung lavage by HPLC, RIA and mass spectrometry. *Adv Prostaglandin Thromboxane Leukot Res* 16:353, 1986.

76. Hansson G, Lindgren JA, Dahlen SE, et al: Identification and biological activity of novel ω-oxidized metabolites of leukotriene B_4 from human leukocytes. *FEBS Lett* 130:107, 1981.

77. Sumimoto H, Minakami S: Oxidation of 20-hydroxyleukotriene B_4 to 20-carboxyleukotriene B_4 by human neutrophil microsomes. Role of aldehyde dehydrogenase and requirement for leukotriene B_4 ω-hydroxylase (cytochrome P-450LTB$_\omega$) in leukotriene B_4 ω-oxidation. *J Biol Chem* 265:4348, 1990.

78. Kikuta Y, Kusunose E, Sumimoto H, et al: Purification and characterization of recombinant human neutrophil leukotriene B_4 ω-hydroxylase (cytochrome P450 4F3). *Arch Biochem Biophys* 355:201, 1998.

79. Kikuta Y, Kato M, Yamashita Y, et al: Human leukotriene B_4 ω-hydroxylase (CYP4F3) gene: Molecular cloning and chromosomal localization. *DNA Cell Biol* 17:221, 1998.

80. Kikuta Y, Kusunose E, Kusunose M: Characterization of human liver leukotriene B_4 ω-hydroxylase P450 (CYP4F2). *J Biochem (Tokyo)* 127:1047, 2000.

81. Kikuta Y, Kusunose E, Kondo T, et al: Cloning and expression of a novel form of leukotriene B_4 ω-hydroxylase from human liver. *FEBS Lett* 348:70, 1994.

82. Moncada S, Flower RJ, Vane JR: Prostaglandins, prostacyclin, thromboxane A_2 and leukotrienes. In: Gilman AG, Goodman LS, Rall TW, Murad F, eds. *The Pharmacological Basis of Therapeutics.* 7th ed. New York: Macmillan Publishing, 1985:660.

83. Ford-Hutchinson AW, Bray MA, Doig MV, et al: Leukotriene B, a potent chemokinetic and aggregating substance released from polymorphonuclear leukocytes. *Nature* 286:264, 1980.

84. Samuelsson B, Paoletti R, Folco GC, et al: *Advances in Prostaglandin and Leukotriene Research: Basic Science and New Clinical Applications.* New York: Kluwer Academic Publishers, 2001.

85. James AJ, Sampson AP: A tale of two CysLTs. *Clin Exp Allergy* 31:1660, 2001.

86. Serhan CN, Prescott SM: The scent of a phagocyte: Advances on leukotriene B_4 receptors. *J Exp Med* 192:F5–F8, 2000.

87. Folco GC, Samuelsson B, Murphy RC: *Novel Inhibitors of Leukotrienes.* Boston: Birkhauser, 1999.

88. Martin V, Sawyer N, Stocco R, et al: Molecular cloning and functional characterization of murine cysteinyl-leukotriene 1 (CysLT$_1$) receptors. *Biochem Pharmacol* 62:1193, 2001.

89. Hui Y, Yang G, Galczenski H, et al: The murine cysteinyl leukotriene 2 (CysLT$_2$) receptor: cDNA and genomic cloning, alternative splicing, and in vitro characterization. *J Biol Chem* 276:47489, 2001.

90. Yokomizo T, Izumi T, Chang K, et al: A G-protein-coupled receptor for leukotriene B_4 that mediates chemotaxis. *Nature* 387:620, 1997.

91. Yokomizo T, Kato K, Hagiya H, et al: Hydroxyeicosanoids bind to and activate the low affinity leukotriene B_4 receptor, BLT2. *J Biol Chem* 276:12454, 2001.

92. Ford-Hutchinson AW: FLAP: A novel drug target for inhibiting the synthesis of leukotrienes. *Trends Pharmacol Sci* 12:68, 1991.

93. Jakobsson PJ, Morgenstern R, Mancini J, et al: Membrane-associated proteins in eicosanoid and glutathione metabolism (MAPEG). A widespread protein superfamily. *Am J Respir Crit Care Med* 161:S20–S24, 2000.

94. Undem BJ, Lichtenstein LM: Drugs used in the treatment of asthma. In: Hardman JG, Limbird LE, Goodman LS, Gilman A, eds. *Goodman & Gilman's The Pharmacological basis of Therapeutics.* 10th ed. New York: McGraw-Hill, 2001:740.

95. Knorr B, Franchi LM, Bisgaard H, et al: Montelukast, a leukotriene receptor antagonist, for the treatment of persistent asthma in children aged 2 to 5 years. *Pediatrics* 108:E48, 2001.

96. Funk CD, Funk LB, FitzGerald GA, et al: Characterization of human 12-lipoxygenase genes. *Proc Natl Acad Sci U S A* 89:3962, 1992.

97. Nie D, Tang K, Szekeres K, et al: Eicosanoid regulation of angiogenesis in human prostate carcinoma and its therapeutic implications. *Ann N Y Acad Sci* 905:165, 2000.

98. Tang K, Honn KV: 12(*S*)-HETE in cancer metastasis. *Adv Exp Med Biol* 447:181, 1999.

99. Chen S, Ruan Q, Bedner E, et al: Effects of the flavonoid baicalin and its metabolite baicalein on androgen receptor expression, cell cycle progression and apoptosis of prostate cancer cell lines. *Cell Prolif* 34:293, 2001.

100. Kurahashi Y, Herbertsson H, Soderstrom M, et al: A 12(*S*)-hydroxyeicosatetraenoic acid receptor interacts with steroid receptor coactivator-1. *Proc Natl Acad Sci U S A* 97:5779, 2000.

101. Brezinski ME, Serhan CN: Selective incorporation of 15(*S*)-hydroxyeicosatetraenoic acid in phosphatidylinositol of human neutrophils: Agonist-induced deacylation and transformation of stored hydroxyeicosanoids. *Proc Natl Acad Sci U S A* 87:6248, 1990.

102. Moncada S, Gryglewski RJ, Bunting S, et al: A lipid peroxide inhibits the enzyme in blood vessel microsomes that generates from prostaglandin endoperoxides the substance (prostaglandin X) which prevents platelet aggregation. *Prostaglandins* 12:715, 1976.

103. Lin L, Balazy M, Pagano PJ, et al: Expression of prostaglandin H_2-mediated mechanism of vascular contraction in hypertensive rats. Relation to lipoxygenase and prostacyclin synthase activities. *Circ Res* 74:197, 1994.

104. Szczeklik A, Gryglewski RJ, Vane JR: *Eicosanoids, Aspirin, and Asthma.* New York: Marcel Dekker, 1998.

105. Rainsford KD: *Aspirin and Related Drugs.* New York: Taylor and Francis, 2002.

106. Leitch AG, Corey EJ, Austen KF, et al: Indomethacin potentiates the pulmonary response to aerosol leukotriene C4 in the guinea pig. *Am Rev Respir Dis* 128:639, 1983.

107. Szczeklik A, Stevenson DD: Aspirin-induced asthma: Advances in pathogenesis and management. *J Allergy Clin Immunol* 104:5, 1999.

108. Page CP: Platelets and asthma. *Ann N Y Acad Sci* 629:38, 1991.

109. Maclouf JA, Murphy RC: Transcellular metabolism of neutrophil-derived leukotriene A4 by human platelets. A potential cellular source of leukotriene C4. *J Biol Chem* 263:174, 1988.

110. Serhan CN, Samuelsson B: Lipoxins: A new series of eicosanoids (biosynthesis, stereochemistry, and biological activities). *Adv Exp Med Biol* 229:1, 1988.

111. Lecomte M, Laneuville O, Ji C, et al: Acetylation of human prostaglandin endoperoxide synthase-2 (cyclooxygenase-2) by aspirin. *J Biol Chem* 269:13207, 1994.

112. Claria J, Serhan CN: Aspirin triggers previously undescribed bioactive eicosanoids by human endothelial cell-leukocyte interactions. *Proc Natl Acad Sci U S A* 92:9475, 1995.

113. Peters-Golden M, Brock TG: Intracellular compartmentalization of leukotriene biosynthesis. *Am J Respir Crit Care Med* 161:S36–S40, 2000.

114. Devchand PR, Keller H, Peters JM, et al: The PPARα-leukotriene B4 pathway to inflammation control. *Nature* 384:39, 1996.

115. Boeglin WE, Kim RB, Brash AR: A 12R-lipoxygenase in human skin: mechanistic evidence, molecular cloning, and expression. *Proc Natl Acad Sci U S A* 95:6744, 1998.

116. Brash AR, Jisaka M, Boeglin WE, et al: Investigation of a second 15S-lipoxygenase in humans and its expression in epithelial tissues. *Adv Exp Med Biol* 469:83, 1999.

117. Oliw EH, Lawson JA, Brash AR, et al: Arachidonic acid metabolism in rabbit renal cortex. Formation of two novel dihydroxyeicosatrienoic acids. *J Biol Chem* 256:9924, 1981.

118. Morrison AR, Pascoe N: Metabolism of arachidonate through NADPH-dependent oxygenase of renal cortex. *Proc Natl Acad Sci U S A* 78:7375, 1981.

119. Makita K, Falck JR, Capdevila JH: Cytochrome P450, the arachidonic acid cascade, and hypertension: New vistas for an old enzyme system. *FASEB J.* 10:1456, 1996.

120. Imig JD: Epoxyeicosatrienoic acids. Biosynthesis, regulation, and actions. *Methods Mol Biol* 120:173, 1999.

121. Nelson DR, Koymans L, Kamataki T, et al: P450 superfamily: Update on new sequences, gene mapping, accession numbers and nomenclature. *Pharmacogenetics* 6:1,1996.

122. Zeldin DC: Epoxygenase pathways of arachidonic acid metabolism. *J Biol Chem* 276:36059, 2001.

123. Zeldin DC, DuBois RN, Falck JR, et al: Molecular cloning, expression and characterization of an endogenous human cytochrome P450 arachidonic acid epoxygenase isoform. *Arch Biochem Biophys* 322:76, 1995.

124. Scarborough PE, Ma J, Qu W, et al: P450 subfamily CYP2J and their role in the bioactivation of arachidonic acid in extrahepatic tissues. *Drug Metab Rev* 31:205, 1999.

125. Capdevila JH, Karara A, Waxman DJ, et al: Cytochrome P-450 enzyme-specific control of the regio- and enantiofacial selectivity of the microsomal arachidonic acid epoxygenase. *J Biol Chem* 265:10865,1990.

126. Qu W, Rippe RA, Ma J, et al: Nutritional status modulates rat liver cytochrome P450 arachidonic acid metabolism. *Mol Pharmacol* 54:504, 1998.

127. Makita K, Takahashi K, Karara A, et al: Experimental and/or genetically controlled alterations of the renal microsomal cytochrome P450 epoxygenase induced hypertension in rats fed a high salt diet. *J Clin Invest* 94:2414, 1994.

128. Pfister SL, Falck JR, Campbell WB: Enhanced synthesis of epoxyeicosatrienoic acids by cholesterol-fed rabbit aorta. *Am J Physiol* 261:H843, 1991.

129. Karara A, Dishman E, Falck JR, et al: Endogenous epoxyeicosatrienoyl-phospholipids: A novel class of cellular glycerolipids containing epoxidized arachidonate moieties. *J Biol Chem* 266:7561, 1991.

130. Weintraub NL, Fang X, Kaduce TL, et al: Epoxide hydrolases regulate epoxyeicosatrienoic acid incorporation into coronary endothelial phospholipids. *Am J Physiol* 277:H2098, 1999.

131. Carroll MA, Schwartzman ML, Capdevila J, et al: Vasoactivity of arachidonic acid epoxides. *Eur J Pharmacol* 138:281,1987.

132. Katoh T, Takahashi K, Capdevila J, et al: Glomerular stereospecific synthesis and hemodynamic actions of 8,9-epoxyeicosatrienoic acid in rat kidney. *Am J Physiol* 261:F578, 1991.

133. Balazy M: Metabolism of 5,6-epoxyeicosatrienoic acid by the human platelet. Formation of novel thromboxane analogs. *J Biol Chem* 226:23561, 1991.

134. Catella F, Lawson JA, Fitzgerald DJ, et al: Endogenous biosynthesis of arachidonic acid epoxides in humans: Increased formation in pregnancy-induced hypertension. *Proc Natl Acad Sci U S A* 87:5893, 1990.

135. Catella F, Lawson J, Braden G, et al: Biosynthesis of P450 products of arachidonic acid in humans: Increased formation in cardiovascular disease. *Adv Prostaglandin Thromboxane Leukot Res* 21A:193, 1991.

136. Claire AE, Simpson M: The cytochrome P450 4 (CYP4) family. *Gen Pharmacol* 28:351, 1997.

137. Okita RT, Okita JR: Cytochrome P450 4A fatty acid omega hydroxylases. *Curr Drug Metab* 2:265, 2001.

138. Hardwick JP: CYP 4A subfamily: Functional analysis by immunocytochemistry and in situ hybridization. *Methods Enzymol* 206:273, 1991.

139. Ito O, Alonso-Galicia M, Hopp KA, et al: Localization of cytochrome P-450 4A isoforms along the rat nephron. *Am J Physiol* 274:F395, 1998.

140. Imaoka S, Yamazoe Y, Kato R, et al: Funae Y. Hormonal regulation of rat cytochrome P450s by androgen and pituitary. *Arch Biochem Biophys* 299:179, 1992.

141. Powell PK, Wolf I, Jin R, et al: Metabolism of arachidonic acid to 20-hydroxy-5,8,11,14-eicosatetraenoic acid by P450 enzymes in human liver: Involvement of CYP4F2 and CYP4A11. *J Pharmacol Exp Ther* 285:1327, 1998.

142. Muerhoff AS, Williams DE, Leithauser MT, et al: Regulation of the induction of a cytochrome P450 prostaglandin w-hydroxylase by pregnancy in rabbit lung. *Proc Natl Acad Sci U S A* 84:7911, 1987.

143. Carroll MA, Balazy M, Huang DD, et al: Cytochrome P450-derived renal HETEs: Storage and release. *Kidney Int* 51:1696, 1997.

144. Schwartzman ML, Martasek P, Rios AR, et al: Cytochrome P450-dependent arachidonic acid metabolism in human kidney. *Kidney Int* 37:94, 1990.

145. Lasker JM, Chen WB, Wolf I, et al: Formation of 20-hydroxyeicosatetraenoic acid, a vasoactive and natriuretic eicosanoid in human kidney. Role of Cyp4F2 and Cyp4A11. *J Biol Chem* 275:4118, 2000.

146. Prakash C, Zang JY, Falck JR, et al: 20-hydroxyeicosatetraenoic acid is excreted as a glucuronide conjugate in human urine. *Biochem Biophys Res Commun* 185:728, 1992.

147. Takahashi KJ, Capdevila A, Karara JR, et al: Cytochrome P450 arachidonate metabolites in rat kidney: Characterization and hemodynamic responses. *Am J Physiol* 258:F781, 1990.

148. Carroll MA, Balazy M, Margiotta P, et al: Renal vasodilator activity of 5,6-epoxyeicosatrienoic acid depends upon conversion by cyclooxygenase and release of prostaglandins. *J Biol Chem.* 268:12260, 1993.

149. Imig JD, Navar LG, Roman RJ, et al: Actions of epoxygenase metabolites on the preglomerular vasculature. *J Am Soc Nephrol* 7:2364, 1996.

150. Jacobs ER, Zeldin DC: The lung HETEs (and EETs) up. *Am J Physiol* 280:H1, 2001.

151. Leffler CW, Fedinec AL: Newborn piglet cerebral microvascular responses to epoxyeicosatrienoic acids. *Am J Physiol* 273:H333, 1997.

152. Alkayed NJ, Birks EK, Hudetz AG, et al: Inhibition of brain P-450 arachidonic acid epoxygenase decreases baseline cerebral blood flow. *Am J Physiol* 271:H1541, 1996.

153. Quilley J, McGiff JC: Is EDHF an epoxyeicosatrienoic acid? *Trends Pharmacol Sci* 21:121, 2000.

154. Fisslthaler B, Popp R, Kiss L, et al: Cytochrome P450 2C is an EDHF synthase in coronary arteries. *Nature* 401:493, 1999.

155. Node K, Huo Y, Ruan X, et al: Anti-inflammatory properties of cytochrome P450 epoxygenase-derived eicosanoids. *Science* 285:1276, 1999.

156. Node K, Ruan XL, Dai J, et al: Activation of G alpha s mediates induction of tissue-type plasminogen activator gene transcription by epoxyeicosatrienoic acids. *J Biol Chem* 276:15983, 2001.

157. Fleming I, Fisslthaler B, Michaelis UR, et al: The coronary endothelium-derived hyperpolarizing factor (EDHF) stimulates multiple signalling pathways and proliferation in vascular cells. *Pflugers Arch* 442:511, 2001.

158. Medhora M, Harder D: Functional role of epoxyeicosatrienoic acids and their production in astrocytes: Approaches for gene transfer and therapy (review). *Int J Mol Med* 2:661, 1998.

159. Escalante B, Sessa WC, Falck JR, et al: Vasoactivity of 20-hydroxyeicosatetraenoic acid is dependent on metabolism by cyclooxygenase. *J Pharmacol Exp Ther* 248:229, 1988.

160. Imig JD, Zou A-P, Stec DE, et al: Formation and actions of 20-hydroxyeicosatetraenoic acid in rat renal arterioles. *Am J Physiol* 270:R217, 1996.

161. Harder DR, Gebremedhin D, Narayanan J, et al: Formation and action of a P450 4A metabolite of arachidonic acid in cat cerebral microvessels. *Am J Physiol* 266:H2098, 1994.

162. Carroll MA, Balazy M, Margiotta P, et al: Cytochrome P-450-dependent HETEs: Profile of biological activity and stimulation by vasoactive peptides. *Am J Physiol* 271:R863, 1996.

163. Birks EK, Bousamara M, Presberg K, et al: Human pulmonary arteries dilate to 20-HETE, an endogenous eicosanoid of lung tissue. *Am J Physiol* 272:L823, 1997.

164. Laniado-Schwartzman M, Falck JR, Yadagiri P, et al: Metabolism of 20-hydroxyeicosatetraenoic acid by cyclooxygenase: Formation and identification of novel endothelium-dependent vasoconstrictor metabolites. *J Biol Chem* 264:1165, 1989.

165. Carroll MA, Pilar Garcia M, Falck JR, et al: Cyclooxygenase dependency of the renovascular actions of cytochrome P450-derived arachidonate metabolites. *J Pharmacol Exp Ther* 260:104, 1992.

166. Zou A-P, Fleming JT, Falck JR, et al: 20-HETE is an endogenous inhibitor of the large-conductance Ca^{2+}-activated K^+ channel in renal arterioles. *Am J Physiol* 270:R228, 1996.

167. Sun CW, Alonso-Galicia M, Taheri MR, et al: Nitric oxide-20-hydroxyeicosatetraenoic acid interaction in the regulation of K^+ channel activity and vascular tone in renal arterioles. *Circ Res* 83:1069, 1998.

168. Alonso-Galicia M, Falck JR, Reddy KM, et al: 20-HETE agonists and antagonists in the renal circulation. *Am J Physiol* 277:F790, 1999.

169. Kauser K, Clark JE, Masters BS, et al: Inhibitors of cytochrome P450 attenuate the myogenic response of dog renal arcuate arteries. *Circ Res* 68:1154, 1991.

170. Gebremedhin D, Lange AR, Lowry TF, et al: Production of 20-HETE and its role in autoregulation of cerebral blood flow. *Circ Res* 87:60, 2000.

171. Kerkhof CJ, Bakker EN, Sipkema P: Role of cytochrome P-450 4A in oxygen sensing and NO production in rat cremaster resistance arteries. *Am J Physiol* 277:H1546, 1999.

172. Harder DR, Narayanan J, Birks EK, et al: Identification of a putative microvascular oxygen sensor. *Circ Res* 79:54, 1996.

173. Wang MH, Zhang F, Marji J, et al: CYP4A1 antisense oligonucleotide reduces mesenteric vascular reactivity and blood pressure in SHR. *Am J Physiol* 280:R255, 2001.

174. Oyekan A, Balazy M, McGiff JC: Renal oxygenases: Differential contribution to vasoconstriction induced by ET-1 and ANG II. *Am J Physiol* 273:R293, 1997.

175. Muthalif MM, Benter IF, Karzoun N, et al: 20-Hydroxyeicosatetraenoic acid mediates calcium/calmodulin-dependent protein kinase II-induced mitogen-activated protein kinase activation in vascular smooth muscle cells. *Proc Natl Acad Sci U S A* 95:12701, 1998.

176. Sun CW, Falck JR, Harder DR, et al: Role of tyrosine kinase and PKC in the vasoconstrictor response to 20-HETE in renal arterioles. *Hypertension* 33:414, 1999.

177. Nithipatikom K, DiCamelli RF, Kohler S, et al: Determination of cytochrome P450 metabolites of arachidonic acid in coronary venous plasma during ischemia and reperfusion in dogs. *Anal Biochem* 292:115, 2001.

178. Hill E, Murphy RC: Quantitation of 20-hydroxy-5,8,11,14-eicosatetraenoic acid (20-HETE) produced by human polymorphonuclear leukocytes using electron capture ionization gas chromatography/mass spectrometry. *Biol Mass Spectrum* 21:249, 1992.

179. Christmas P, Jones JP, Patten CJ, et al: Alternative splicing determines the function of CYP4F3 by switching substrate specificity. *J Biol Chem* 276:38166, 2001.

180. Abraham NG, Feldman E, Falck JR, et al: Modulation of erythropoiesis by novel human bone marrow cytochrome P450-dependent metabolites of arachidonic acid. *Blood* 78:1461, 1991.

181. Hill E, Fitzpatrick F, Murphy RC: Biological activity and metabolism of 20-hydroxyeicosatetraenoic acid in the human platelet. *Br J Pharmacol* 106:267, 1992.

182. Takahashi K, Harris RC, Capdevila JH, et al: Induction of renal arachidonate cytochrome P-450 epoxygenase after uninephrectomy: Counterregulation of hyperfiltration. *J Am Soc Nephrol* 3:1496, 1993.

183. Rahman M, Wright JT Jr, Douglas JG: The role of the cytochrome P450-dependent metabolites of arachidonic acid in blood pressure regulation and renal function: A review. *Am J Hypertens* 10:356, 1997.

184. Messer-Letienne I, Bernard N, Benzoni D, et al: Cytochrome P450-dependent arachidonate metabolites and renal functions in the Lyon hypertensive rat. *Clin Exp Pharmacol Physiol* 25:559, 1998.

185. Yu Z, Xu F, Huse LM, et al: Soluble epoxide hydrolase regulates hydrolysis of vasoactive epoxyeicosatrienoic acids. *Circ Res* 87:992, 2000.

186. Sinal CJ, Miyata M, Tohkin M, et al: Targeted disruption of soluble epoxide hydrolase reveals a role in blood pressure regulation. *J Biol Chem* 275:40504, 2000.

187. Omata K, Abraham NG, Laniado-Schwartzman M: Renal cytochrome P450 arachidonic acid metabolism: Localization and hormonal regulation in SHR. *Am J Physiol* 262:F591, 1992.

188. Laniado-Schwartzman M, Abraham NG: The renal cytochrome P450 arachidonic acid system. *Pediat Nephrol* 6:490, 1992.

189. Lu M, Zhu Y, Balazy M, et al: Effect of angiotensin II on the apical K^+ channel in the thick ascending limb of the rat kidney. *J Gen Physiol* 108:537, 1996.

190. Ito O, Roman RJ: Regulation of P450 4A activity in the glomerulus of the rat. *Am J Physiol* 276:R1749, 1999.

191. Laniado-Schwartzman M, Omata K, Lin F, et al: Detection of 20-hydroxyeicosatetraenoic acid in rat urine. *Biochem Biophys Res Commun* 180:445, 1991.

192. Imig JD, Zou A-P, Ortiz-de-Montellano PR, et al: Cytochrome P450 inhibitors alter afferent arteriolar responses to elevations in pressure. *Am J Physiol* 266:H1879, 1994.

193. Zou A-P, Imig JD, Kaldunski M, et al: Inhibition of renal vascular 20-HETE production impairs autoregulation of renal blood flow. *Am J Physiol* 266:F275, 1994.

194. Zou A-P, Imig JD, Ortiz de Montellano PR, et al: Effect of P450 ω-hydroxylase metabolites of arachidonic acid on tubuloglomerular feedback. *Am J Physiol* 266:F934, 1994.

195. Pedrosa CM, Dubay GR, Falck JR, et al: Parathyroid hormone inhibits Na^+-K^+-ATPase through a cytochrome P450 pathway. *Am J Physiol* 266:F497, 1994.

196. Nowicki S, Chen SL, Aizman O, et al: 20-Hydroxyeicosa-tetraenoic acid (20-HETE) activates protein kinase C. Role in regulation of rat renal Na^+,K^+-ATPase. *J Clin Invest* 99:1224, 1997.

197. Escalante B, Erlij D, Falck JR, et al: Cytochrome P450 arachidonate metabolites affect ion fluxes in rabbit medullary thick ascending limb. *Am J Physiol* 266:C1775–C1782, 1994.

198. Amlal H, LeGoff C, Vernimmen C, et al: Ang II controls Na(+)-K+(NH4+)-2Cl-cotransport via 20-HETE and PKC in medullary thick ascending limb. *Am J Physiol* 274:C1047, 1998.

199. Wang W, Lu M: Effect of arachidonic acid on activity of the apical K^+ channel in the thick ascending limb of the rat kidney. *J Gen Physiol* 106:727, 1995.

200. Ito O, Roman RJ: Role of 20-HETE in elevating chloride transport in the thick ascending limb of Dahl SS/Jr rats. *Hypertension* 33:41, 1999.

201. Zou A-P, Drummond HA, Roman RJ: Role of 20-HETE in elevating loop chloride reabsorption in Dahl SS/Jr rats. *Hypertension* 27:631, 1996.

202. Oyekan AO, McGiff JC: Cytochrome P450-derived eicosanoids participate in the renal functional effects of ET-1 in the anesthetized rat. *Am J Physiol* 274:R52, 1998.

203. Lin F, Rios A, Falck JR, et al: 20-hydroxyeicosatetraenoic acid is formed in response to EGF and is a mitogen in rat proximal tubule. *Am J Physiol* 269:F806, 1995.

204. Grider JS, Falcone JC, Kilpatrick EL, et al: P450 arachidonate metabolites mediate bradykinin-dependent inhibition of NaCl transport in the rat thick ascending limb. *Can J Physiol Pharmacol* 75:91, 1997.

205. Wang M-H, Guan H, Nguyen X, et al: Contribution of cytochrome P450 4A1 and 4A2 to vascular 20-hydroxyeicosatetraenoic acid synthesis in the rat kidney. *Am J Physiol* 276:F246, 998.

206. Stec DE, Mattson DL, Roman RJ: Inhibition of renal outer medullary 20-HETE production produces hypertension in Lewis rats. *Hypertension* 29:315, 1997.

207. Roman RJ, Ma Y-H, Frohlich B, et al: Clofibrate prevents the development of hypertension in Dahl salt-sensitive rats. *Hypertension* 21:985, 1993.

208. Stec DE, Deng AY, Rapp JP, et al: Cytochrome P4504A genotype cosegregates with hypertension in Dahl S rats. *Hypertension* 27:564, 1996.

209. Stec DE, Trolleit MR, Krieger JE, et al: Cytochrome P4504A activity and salt sensitivity in spontaneously hypertensive rats. *Hypertension* 27:1329, 1996.

210. Holla VR, Adas F, Imig JD, et al: Alterations in the regulation of androgen-sensitive Cyp 4a monooxygenases cause hypertension. *Proc Natl Acad Sci U S A* 98:5211, 2001.

211. Miura H, Wachtel RE, Liu Y, et al: Flow-induced dilation of human coronary arterioles: important role of Ca(2+)-activated K(+) channels. *Circulation* 103:1992, 2001.

212. Pratt PF, Falck JR, Reddy KM, et al: 20-HETE relaxes bovine coronary arteries through the release of prostacyclin. *Hypertension* 31:237, 1998.

213. Gebremedhin D, Lange AR, Narayanan J, et al: Cat cerebral arterial smooth muscle cells express cytochrome P450 4A2 enzyme and produce the vasoconstrictor 20-HETE which enhances L-type Ca^{2+} current. *J Physiol* 507:771, 1998.

214. Abraham NG, Drummond GS, Lutton JD, et al: Biological significance and physiological role of heme oxygenase. *Cell Physiol Biochem* 61:129, 1996.

215. Sacerdoti D, Escalante B, Abraham NG, et al: Treatment with tin prevents the development of hypertension in spontaneously hypertensive rats. *Science* 243:388, 1989.

216. Morgan ET, Ullrich V, Daiber A, et al: Cytochromes P450 and flavin monooxygenases-targets and sources of nitric oxide. *Drug Metab Dispos* 29:1366, 2001.

217. Miyata N, Taniguchi K, Seki T, et al: HET0016, a potent and selective inhibitor of 20-HETE synthesizing enzyme. *Br J Pharmacol* 133:325, 2001.

218. Kehl F, Cambj-Sapunar L, Maier KG, et al: 20-HETE contributes to the acute fall in cerebral blood flow following subarachnoid hemorrhage in the rat. *Am J Physiol* 282:H1556, 2002.

219. Brooks P, Emery P, Evans JF, et al: Interpreting the clinical significance of the differential inhibition of cyclooxygenase-1 and cyclooxygenase-2. *Rheumatology (Oxford)* 38:779, 1999.

220. Davies NM, McClachlan AJ, Day RO, Williams KM: Clinical pharmacokinetics and pharmacodynamics of celecoxib. A selective cyclooxygenase-2 inhibitor. *Clin Pharmacokinet* 38:225, 2000.

221. Depre M, Ehrich E, Van Hecken A, et al: Pharmacokinetics, COX-2 specificity, and tolerability of supratherapeutic doses of rofecoxib in humans. *Eur J Clin Pharmacol* 56:167, 2000.

222. Catella-Lawson F, Crofford LJ: Cyclooxygenase inhibition and thrombogenicity. *Amer J Med* 110:28S, 2002.

223. FitzGerald GA: Cardiovascular pharmacology of nonselective nonsteroidal anti-inflammatory drugs and coxibs: Clinical considerations. *Am J Cardiol* 89:26D, 2002.

224. Mukherjee D, Nissen SE, Topol EJ: Risk of cardiovascular events associated with selective COX-2 inhibitors. *JAMA* 286:954, 2001.

225. Cheng Y, Austin SC, Rocca B, et al: Role of prostacyclin in the cardiovascular response to thromboxane A2. *Science* 296:539, 2002.

226. Bombardier C, Laine L, Reicin A, et al: Comparison of upper gastrointestinal toxicity of rofecoxib and naproxen in patients with rheumatoid arthritis. VIGOR Study Group. *N Engl J Med* 343:1520, 2000.

227. Watson DJ, Rhodes T, Cai B, Guess HA: Lower risk of thromboembolic cardiovascular events with naproxen among patients with rheumatoid arthritis. *Arch Intern Med* 162:1105, 2002.

228. Konstam MA, Weir MR, Reicin A, et al: Cardiovascular thrombotic events in controlled, clinical trials of rofecoxib. *Circulation* 104:2280, 2001.

229. FitzGerald GA, Patrono C: The coxibs, selective inhibitors of cyclooxygenase-2. *N Engl J Med* 345:433, 2001.

230. Pitt B, Pepine C, Willerson JT: Cyclooxygenase-2 inhibition and cardiovascular events. *Circulation* 106:167, 2002.

230a. Nurmohamed MT, van Halm VP, Dijkmans BAC: Cardiovascular risk profile of antirheumatic agents in patients with osteoarthritis and rheumatoid arthritis. *Drugs* 62:1599, 2002.

231. Altman R, Luciardi HL, Muntaner J, et al: Efficacy assessment of meloxicam, a preferential cyclooxygenase-2 inhibitor, in acute coronary syndromes without ST-segment elevation. The Nonsteroidal Anti-Inflammatory Drugs in Unstable Angina Treatment-2 (NUT-2) Pilot Study. *Circulation* 106:191, 2002.

CHAPTER 46

Innovative Medical Approaches for the Treatment of Hyperlipidemia

William H. Frishman

Andrew Y. Choi

Alice Guh

This chapter discusses innovative drug therapies for hyperlipidemias, including novel approaches toward targeting pathways of dyslipidemias and exciting advances in somatic gene therapy. Also discussed are newer pharmacologic approaches that are still in development, whose goal is to obtain beneficial cholesterol and lipoprotein profiles.

LIFIBROL

Lifibrol is a novel lipid-lowering agent with an unknown mechanism of action. Lifibrol undergoes biotransformation to a glucuronide and exists in the circulation mainly as the glucuronide.[1] Lifibrol can cause dramatic reductions in low-density lipoprotein (LDL)-cholesterol, total cholesterol, apolipoprotein B (apoB), and triglycerides in hypercholesterolemic patients.[2] It does not act as an inhibitor of hydroxymethylglutaryl coenzyme A (HMG-CoA) reductase, but it does inhibit sterol synthesis to the same degree as the HMG-CoA reductase inhibitors without affecting the production of essential compounds in the mevalonate pathway.[3] A study involving hypercholesterolemic patients treated with lifibrol (450 to 900 mg/d) showed decreases in LDL-cholesterol (40%), total cholesterol (35%), and apoB (30%) after 4 weeks.[3] These reductions were similar to the decreases achieved by high doses of HMG-CoA reductase inhibitors. The study also demonstrated a 20% reduction in lipoprotein (a) [Lp(a)] and a 20% decrease in serum triglycerides by 6 weeks. Serum uric acid levels were also decreased by 10 to 15%.

A study done in patients afflicted with severe familial hypercholesterolemia (FH) suggests that lifibrol decreases levels of cholesterol through the enhancement of the LDL-receptor pathway.[1] In addition, this study showed that patients with a severe reduction or complete absence of LDL receptors did not experience reductions in either plasma LDL-apoB or LDL-cholesterol levels after 4 weeks of treatment with lifibrol.[1] This study provides evidence that lifibrol's action is dependent on the expression of LDL receptor. A study of hypercholesterolemic patients measured the net cholesterol balance and the urinary excretion of mevalonic acid to determine whether lifibrol interfered with cholesterol synthesis.[3] There were no significant changes to the net cholesterol balance and the urinary excretion of mevalonic acid in patients treated with lifibrol, in contrast to the decreases in net cholesterol balance and urinary excretion of

mevalonic acid seen with simvastatin. These results led researchers to believe that lifibrol's mechanism of LDL-receptor enhancement is not dependent on the inhibition of HMG-CoA reductase. Another key finding has been the demonstration that lifibrol seems to have a quicker onset of action than the HMG-CoA reductase inhibitors. Separate investigators have shown that lifibrol reaches a maximum effect on LDL-cholesterol reduction at 4 weeks, rather than the 4 to 8 weeks seen with the HMG-CoA reductase inhibitors.[3–6]

Lifibrol also does not seem to act through the inhibition of cholesterol absorption. One study showed that lifibrol increases both the levels and the clearance of apoA-1, a possible factor in the drug's ability to lower LDL-cholesterol.[7] Despite the findings of some earlier studies, it has also been discovered that lifibrol may act as a weak competitive inhibitor of HMG-CoA synthase.[8] In vitro studies were performed comparing the effects of lifibrol on the enzymatic activities of HMG-CoA synthase and HMG-CoA reductase. One study suggests that lifibrol's weak inhibition of HMG-CoA synthase alone is insufficient to explain its LDL-cholesterol-lowering ability.[9] The investigators also demonstrated lifibrol's powerful ability to upregulate LDL receptor expression in an in vitro study. Although lifibrol's definitive mechanism of action is still unknown, recent evidence suggests that the drug's LDL-cholesterol-lowering ability lies in its ability to upregulate LDL expression, with a lesser ability to inhibit HMG-CoA synthase.

No severe adverse side effects were reported during 4 weeks of treatment with this drug. The only statistically significant adverse effects noted were skin reactions observed in 9.8% of patients, as compared to 5.5% of patients taking the placebo.[2] Further studies hope to unlock the key to lifibrol's mechanism of action.

SQUALENE SYNTHASE INHIBITORS

Inhibition of HMG-CoA reductase may prevent formation of essential compounds such as dolichol and ubiquinone (Fig. 46-1), and attempts have been made to pharmacologically inhibit cholesterol synthesis beyond the branch in the final pathway of cholesterol synthesis [inhibition of squalene synthesis from farnesyl pyrophosphate by inhibiting squalene synthase(SQS)].[10,11] HMG-CoA reductase inhibitors occasionally cause adverse effects in patients, including liver damage and myopathy, and researchers are continually

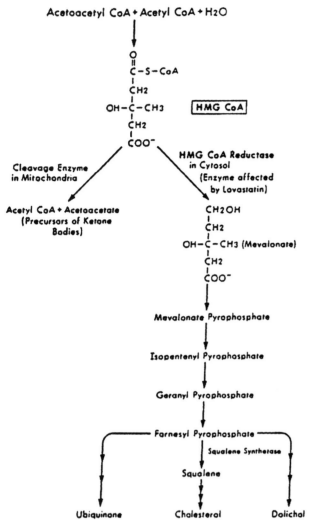

FIGURE 46-1. Branched pathway of cholesterol synthesis. (*Reproduced with permission from Frishman WH: Medical management of lipid disorders: Focus on prevention of coronary artery disease. Mt. Kisco, NY: Futura, 1992.*)

attempting to find newer and safer alternatives to current treatments used in cholesterol management. Investigators have tested several agents that target steps beyond mevalonate formation, such as at squalene epoxidase, oxidosqualene cyclase, and lanosterol demethylase. Researchers found that inhibition of these enzymes resulted in an accumulation of toxic lipophilic substrates in the cell.[12,13] Therefore studies have centered on targeting squalene synthase, an enzyme that catalyzes a key step in sterol biosynthesis. Squalene, a key cholesterol precursor, is formed by the dimerization of two farnesyl pyrophosphate molecules, a reaction catalyzed by squalene synthase.[14] Inhibitors of squalene synthase include the squalestatins and isoprenyl biphosphates, which have been shown to reduce cholesterol synthesis in vivo.[15,16]

ER-27856 is a squalene synthase inhibitor that is reported to have less hepatotoxicity and to result in greater decreases in plasma cholesterol in the rhesus monkey than pravastatin, simvastatin, or atorvastatin.[17] At 4 days of treatment, ER-27856 (30 mg/kg) resulted in a 38% decrease of plasma total cholesterol, as compared to decreases of 5% by pravastatin (30 mg/kg), 19% by simvastatin (30 mg/kg), and 20% by atorvastatin (30 mg/kg) in the rhesus

monkey. As one measure of potential hepatotoxicity, serum alanine aminotransferase (ALT) activity was measured and compared to values before drug treatments. Atorvastatin at 30 and 100 mg/kg, correlated to measured plasma ALT of 232% and 366% of prevalues, while ER-27856 at 30 and 100 mg/kg resulted in ALT values of 136% and 159% of prevalues.

YM-53601 is another squalene synthase inhibitor that is reported to have a greater cholesterol-lowering effect in rhesus monkeys when compared with a HMG-CoA reductase inhibitor.[18] YM-53601 (50 mg/kg) given twice a day for 1 week decreased plasma cholesterol in rhesus monkeys, an effect equal to or greater than pravastatin (25 mg/kg). At the same time, researchers reported there were no indications of hepatotoxicity in the YM-53601-treated monkeys, while observing increased ALT levels in the pravastatin-treated monkeys. YM-53601 also resulted in greater reductions of triglyceride levels in hamsters when compared to a fibric acid derivative (FAD). YM-53601 demonstrated a dose-dependent ability to reduce triglyceride levels at dosages of 10 to 100 mg/kg, with observed triglyceride reductions of 35 to 73%. In comparison, fenofibrate at 10 to 100 mg/kg showed decreases of triglyceride of 15 to 53%. Rare adverse affects, such as rhabdomyolysis, have been documented when an HMG-CoA reductase inhibitor and a FAD are used in tandem to lower both plasma cholesterol and triglyceride levels.[19] YM-53601 may become an agent for use as a powerful combined cholesterol- and triglyceride-lowering agent.

RPR 107393 is a novel squalene synthase inhibitor that is orally effective and extremely potent in both rats and marmosets. It produces a greater reduction in LDL-cholesterol than lovastatin in rats, and a greater reduction in serum cholesterol than either lovastatin or pravastatin in marmosets.[20]

Many squalene synthase inhibitors, however, induce a marked increase in HMG-CoA reductase activity,[21] resulting in an accumulation of a toxic farnesyl-derived dicarboxylic acid.[22] One exception is P3622, an inhibitor that does not increase HMG-CoA reductase activity in cultured human cells.[23] While there is concern of possible toxicity from the use of these compounds, prior studies demonstrate that dicarboxylic acids derived from geraniol are readily excreted in urine.[24] Therefore, many studies conclude that the rapid urinary excretion of toxic dicarboxylic acids would likewise occur with use of squalene synthase inhibitors.[20,25,26]

One study even used the urinary excretion rate of one of the dicarboxylic acids as a measure of the extent of enzyme inhibition by BMS-188494, a squalene synthase inhibitor.[26] The study estimated the clinical pharmacokinetics and pharmacodynamics of BMS-188494 in healthy male volunteers for a total of 4 weeks, with no reported harmful effects.

YM-16638 has a significant ability to inhibit cholesterol biosynthesis in monkey liver and the human hepatoma cell line HepG2.[27] Many recent studies with squalene synthase inhibitors show their enormous potential as potent drugs to aggressively lower cholesterol and triglycerides.

ACYL-COENZYME A TRANSFERASE INHIBITORS

The acyl-coenzyme A transferase (ACAT) enzyme is responsible for the acylation of free cholesterol into cholesteryl esters in the intestine, liver, and adrenal gland, and in macrophages. The intracellular accumulation of cholesteryl esters is an early step in the development of atherosclerosis.[28] Cholesteryl esters accumulate in macrophages and smooth-muscle cells to produce foam cells within the arterial intima. The intracellular cholesteryl ester accumulation and foam cell formation leads to plaque initiation and atherosclerotic progression. It is believed that the inhibition of the enzyme ACAT will lead to antiatherosclerotic effects.[29] ACAT inhibitors may also increase the stability of the atherosclerotic plaque and reduce the risk of plaque rupture. The stability of the atherosclerotic plaque increases as the number of lipid-laden macrophages decreases.[30]

Studies show the existence of several isoforms of ACAT with different expression sites in tissues. ACAT-1 is preferentially expressed in macrophages, the adrenal gland, and in the kidney, while ACAT-2 exists in the liver and intestinal epithelium. Inhibition of ACAT-1 may lead to beneficial reductions in foam cell formation and cholesterol storage within macrophages. Inhibition of ACAT-2 decreases absorption of cholesterol in the intestine and decreases the very-low-density lipoprotein (VLDL) cholesteryl ester content.

The ACAT inhibitor avasimibe (CI-1011) has demonstrated an ability to dramatically reduce plasma lipid concentrations in animals. Avasimibe decreased plasma cholesterol by >56% in cholesterol-fed mice.[31] The mice treated with avasimibe also showed an enrichment of VLDL/LDL with triglycerides. The enrichment and observed decrease in cholesteryl esters in the VLDL/LDL particles results in molecules that are potentially less atherogenic. Mice fed high-cholesterol diets and treated with avasimibe had a 92% reduction of atherosclerotic lesion area measured in cross-sections at the aortic valve area. The avasimibe-treated mice had an average lesion area per section of $7.6 \pm 7 \ \mu^2 \times 1000$ compared to $95.5 \pm 35.2 \ \mu^2 \times 1000$ measured in the control group. The atherosclerotic lesions of the avasimibe-treated mice also contained smaller numbers of foam cells and a reduced lipid pool when compared to the control group. Avasimibe also showed a significant reduction in the number of monocytes adhering to the endothelium. The mechanism by which avasimibe reduces endothelial adhesion is currently unknown.

Currently avasimibe is being evaluated in clinical trials including studies to evaluate the drug's effects on vascular dynamics in patients with myocardial ischemia.

F-1394 is an ACAT inhibitor that is a highly specific and potent inhibitor of both ACAT-1 and ACAT-2. F-1394 decreased intimal lesion areas at the aortic sinus by 39% (low dose) and 45% (high dose) in cholesterol-fed mice.[32] F-1394 also reduced lesion macrophage content and aortic lipid content. The reduction of atherosclerotic lesions may result from macrophages not becoming overloaded with cholesteryl esters and allowing the macrophages to remain relatively small.

CL-283796 is an ACAT inhibitor that may enhance the activity of 7α-hydroxylase, the rate-limiting step in the conversion of cholesterol to bile acid.[33] This could result in the accelerated cholesterol excretion from the liver, in the form of bile. Other ACAT inhibitors have additional properties of lipid peroxidation inhibition and thromboxane A$_2$-binding inhibition.[34]

There are several obstacles to the development of ACAT inhibitors into practical drugs, including poor gastrointestinal tolerability. ACAT inhibitors also have poor bioavailability that may lead to a failure to reach arterial lesions. There is also a concern that inhibiting ACAT will hinder its physiologic role in hormone synthesis with the possibility of inducing adrenal insufficiency. With respect to the mechanisms of this adrenotoxicity, it still remains unclear whether this toxicity is related to ACAT inhibition. It has been suggested that ACAT inhibition increased adrenal cell toxicity due to the build-up of intracellular free cholesterol concentrations.[35,36] However, further investigation is necessary, including data from an adrenal ACAT assay, as well as more detailed molecular biologic aspects of the ACAT enzyme, in order to elucidate the mechanism of adrenotoxicity. Despite reports of adrenotoxicity, there are several ACAT inhibitors that have not been found to be adrenotoxic.

A study of avasimibe administered in high doses to beagles over 2, 13, and 52 weeks addressed this concern. This study concluded that avasimibe had minimal adrenal effects in dogs.[37] Minimal to mild cortical cytoplasmic vacuolization and fibrosis were observed at doses of 300 mg/kg or greater over a 52-week study.

One study contradicting the beneficial effects seen in ACAT inhibition reported no notable reduction in foam cell progression or an actual increase in foam cell progression after specific ACAT-1 inhibition in mice and rabbits.[38] The ACAT-1 inhibitor used in the study, GF1-086, lowered serum cholesterol in rabbits, while concurrently showing an overall increase in xanthoma formation. Current investigations aim to determine whether a safe antithrombotic effect results from partial rather than complete inhibition of ACAT-1 and ACAT-2. Several ACAT inhibitors are in current clinical development, with avasimibe the furthest along. Included in the studies of avasimibe are clinical trials to evaluate the drug's effects on endothelial functioning, hemodynamics and myocardial ischemia, actions that may be unrelated to cholesterol lowering activity.

ILEAL NA+/BILE ACID COTRANSPORTER INHIBITORS

The ileal Na+/bile acid cotransporter (IBAT) contributes to the enterohepatic circulation of bile acids by exchanging bile acids in the ileal brush-border membrane for Na+. IBAT is bile acid specific and Na+ dependent. The bile acid sequestrants interrupt the enterohepatic circulation of bile acids, but are nonspecific anion exchange resins with the bulkiness of the agents being a common patient complaint.

A study using the IBAT inhibitor S-8921, a ligand derivative, showed a dramatic decrease of serum cholesterol concentrations in hamsters.[39] Hamsters treated with S-8921 also showed an increased fecal excretion of bile acids. While S-8921 has a potent cholesterol-lowering activity in vivo, it also has an antioxidative property against LDL oxidation in vitro. S-8921 both inhibits cholesterol absorption and enhances cholesterol elimination, thereby suppressing plasma total and VLDL/LDL-cholesterol levels in rats.[40] A study assessing the effects of the administration of S-8921 in the diet (0.01 to 0.1%) given to hyperlipidemic rabbits showed an increased fecal excretion of measured bile acids of 60 to 180% and a decrease in serum cholesterol of 29 to 37%.[41] The study also found that 0.01% S-8921 suppressed the development of hypercholesterolemia to a greater extent than did 1.5% cholestyramine. This finding suggests that S-8921 may have a greater potency than cholestyramine.

Passive diffusion along the entire intestine or active transport at the terminal ileum accounts for 90% of bile acid absorption. Free bile acids are absorbed to a larger extent via passive diffusion, while conjugated bile acids are mainly absorbed by active transport. S-8921 inhibits the active reuptake of bile acids at the terminal ileum without inhibiting the passive absorption of bile acids.

When the enterohepatic circulation of bile acids is interrupted, the liver increases the biosynthesis of bile acids from cholesterol to compensate for the loss. The liver LDL receptor increases the uptake of plasma LDL-cholesterol. There is also a decrease in the bile acid concentration in bile leading to an overall decreased cholesterol absorption in the intestine. The bile acid sequestrants cholestyramine, colestipol, and colesevelam are the only drugs in clinical use that disrupt the enterohepatic circulation of bile acids. The drugs can effectively lower LDL-cholesterol plasma concentration, but frequently have associated gastrointestinal side effects (cholestyramine and colestipol), and impaired taste is often a common patient complaint. Investigators are seeking drugs that interrupt the enterohepatic circulation of bile acids with higher potency and less gastrointestinal side effects. IBAT inhibitors such as S-8921 show promise as a new class of effective hypocholesterolemic drugs. S-8921 is currently in the preclinical development phase.

BILE ACID SEQUESTRANTS

SK&F 97426 is a bile acid sequestrant that has higher affinity for the trihydroxy bile acids and slower rates of dissociation from this resin when compared to cholestyramine.[42] This property of SK&F 97426 is believed to account for its having threefold greater potency than cholestyramine. In animal models, it increases bile acid secretion and has been shown to reduce total cholesterol by 37 to 58%, LDL-cholesterol by 56 to 75% and VLDL-cholesterol by 25 to 41%.[42a]

GT16-239, a novel bile acid sequestrant, is nonabsorbable, with a unique affinity for binding conjugated primary bile acids. At half the dose of cholestyramine, it was more effective in preventing diet-induced hypercholesterolemia and the development of early aortic atherosclerosis in hamsters.[43]

CHOLESTERYL ESTER TRANSFER PROTEIN INHIBITORS

Cholesteryl ester transfer protein (CETP) was first discovered to be an integral component of lipid transfer in the early 1990s, when data from Japanese families with CETP deficiency showed an increase in high-density lipoprotein (HDL) levels and no evidence of premature atherosclerosis.[44] However, since that time, both proatherogenic and antiatherogenic roles for CETP have been demonstrated. CETP is a hydrophobic glycoprotein that is involved with the exchange of cholesteryl esters, triglycerides and phospholipids between plasma lipoproteins. CETP is mainly found on HDL and is believed to be directly involved in the transfer of cholesterol from HDL to LDL and VLDL. This finding suggests that CETP plays an atherogenic role and that the inhibition of CETP could result in a beneficial increase of HDL while decreasing the levels of cholesterol in other lipoproteins. Additional research in rabbits with chemically inhibited CETP also appeared to decrease both total cholesterol and non-HDL cholesterol levels.[45,46] Researchers postulate that a mechanism exists in the liver for recycling cholesterol through an HDL-mediated route, in addition to the original LDL-mediated route (reverse cholesterol transport pathway). The theory is that if CETP is inhibited, cholesterol will not be transported to LDL and will directly be catabolized in the liver. New research in humans, however, does not support the favorable findings observed in rabbits. Although HDL levels do rise in humans with CETP deficiency, total cholesterol appears to increase. Two possible explanations are that rabbits have a more dominant HDL recycling pathway through the liver or that inhibition of CETP in rabbits creates an upregulation of LDL receptors on the liver for cholesterol recycling.[47]

CETP is an integral component in the reverse cholesterol transport pathway.[48] This process involves the removal of cholesterol from lipid-laden cells by HDL, the transfer of the cholesterol to LDL, and subsequently to the liver where it is converted to bile salts by 7α-hydroxylase. Because this pathway decreases both LDL and total cholesterol, CETP may act as an antiatherogenic substance. If a patient has deficient CETP activity, the reverse cholesterol transfer pathway may be compromised, resulting in an increase in total cholesterol. Another study in patients with CETP deficiency contradicts the theory that genetic CETP deficiency is associated with a decreased risk of coronary heart disease (CHD).[49] Data collected demonstrate that the overall prevalence of CHD in CETP-deficient men is 21%, while only 16% in men without CETP deficiency.[49] CETP-deficient subjects with HDL-cholesterol levels between 41 and 60 mg/dL were at an increased risk of CHD when compared with patients with normal CETP function. However, when the HDL-cholesterol level was greater than 60 mg/dL in both groups of patients, risk of coronary disease was low. Many researchers believe that CETP deficiency may result in an antiatherogenic state only when accompanied by a significant elevation in HDL. Therefore, these studies suggest that CETP inhibitors are only effective in achieving a beneficial reduction in CHD risk if the HDL level is increased sufficiently.

The development of compounds to inhibit CETP is still ongoing. A synthetic isoflavone, CGS-25159, has already been shown to downregulate CETP and to subsequently increase HDL levels.[50] Another study has demonstrated that injection of hog plasma peptides, P28 and P20, into cholesterol-fed rabbits can also suppress activity against CETP.[51]

At this time, conflicting roles exist for CETP in the transfer of cholesterol and theories that support both the inhibition and the enhancement of CETP activity exist as therapeutic targets now. The dominant role of CETP in cholesterol catabolism must be elucidated before definitive CETP-related therapies can be used.

LIPOPROTEIN LIPASE ACTIVATORS

Lipoprotein lipase (LPL) is an important protein involved with regulating the levels of HDL-cholesterol seen in plasma. The enzyme has been cloned, and its regulation is being studied on the molecular level. LPL-mediated lipolysis of chylomicrons and VLDLs contributes to the plasma HDL level. The concentration of HDL-cholesterol also depends on HDL production by the liver and small intestine[52] and CETP metabolism, as mentioned in the previous section. LPL digests chylomicrons and VLDLs into remnants and LDL. Conversion of HDL_3 into a less-dense HDL_2 then ensues.[53] Low levels of HDL_2 have been consistently linked to patients with extensive CHD.[54] LPL is also a strong modulator of triglyceride metabolism. LPL hydrolyses triglycerides within lipoproteins into nonesterified fatty acids and glycerol. The free fatty acids are then absorbed in adjacent tissues by diffusion.[55]

An enhancement of LPL activity could favorably influence the level of triglycerides and other atherogenic lipoproteins in the plasma. A team of researchers recently developed the compound NO-1886, an agent that enhances the activity of LPL.[56] Investigators have demonstrated in the rat, hamster, and rabbit models, that NO-1886 elevates HDL-cholesterol by the selective enhancement of LPL independent of the CETP pathway.[57] NO-1886 given to rabbits for 20 weeks resulted in reductions of aortic atheromatous lesions, with a concomitant increase in HDL and a decrease in triglycerides.[58] NO-1886 also demonstrated a strong ability to decrease triglyceride levels in both normal and streptozotocin induced diabetic rats.[59] Other studies show that NO-1886 results in reduced insulin resistance along with decreased triglyceride levels in rats fed a high-fat diet.[60,61] NO-1886 may be an important drug in the future for diabetics with poor lipid profiles and insulin resistance.

CHOLESTEROL TRANSPORT INHIBITORS

SCH58235 (ezetimibe) is a potent cholesterol transport inhibitor currently progressing through clinical trials. Ezetimibe is a promising drug in the new class of lipid-lowering agents, the cholesterol transport inhibitors. The cholesterol transport inhibitors reduce the intestinal absorption of both dietary and biliary cholesterol. Studies show that ACAT and the pancreatic lipases are not directly inhibited by the cholesterol transport inhibitors. This new drug class does not act by binding bile acids as do bile acid sequestrants. These drugs also do not inhibit HMG-CoA reductase activity.[62] It has been shown that ezetimibe selectively inhibits the transport of radiolabeled cholesterol through the intestinal wall and into the plasma thereafter.[63] The actual mechanism of how these drugs inhibit cholesterol absorption is unknown at present.

One of the first cholesterol transport inhibitors SCH48461 demonstrated the ability to reduce LDL-cholesterol by 15% in humans.[64] SCH48461 undergoes both phase I and phase II metabolism, resulting in polar glucuronide conjugates. Ezetimibe was discovered as the more potent metabolite of its predecessor SCH48461. SCH48461 caused a 70% decrease in cholesterol absorption in the rat model while the bile that contained the metabolites of SCH48461 caused a greater than 95% decrease. Ezetimibe was found to be 400 times as potent as SCH48461 in the rhesus monkey.[65]

In a study with hypercholesterolemic humans, ezetimibe lowered LDL-cholesterol by 18.5% and raised HDL cholesterol by 3.5%.[66] Hamsters with hyperinsulinemia, hyperlipidemia, hypercholesterolemia, and hypertriglyceridemia, similar to the profile observed in obese insulin-resistant and/or type 2 diabetic patients, were treated with ezetimibe. Ezetimibe markedly reduced the combined hyperlipidemia in obese hamsters resulting in an improvement in the HDL/LDL ratio and the complete inhibition of cholesterol absorption.[67] The control groups that were fed high-fat diets showed significant increases in VLDL + IDL, while the ezetimibe treated hamsters fed the same diet, experienced no increases in VLDL + IDL. Another study with rhesus monkeys showed that ezetimibe showed a 41% reduction in apoB100 in LDL, while having little change to the apoB48 concentration in chylomicrons. While the cholesterol content in chylomicrons was reduced, the actual number of chylomicrons was not reduced.[68] The reduction in chylomicron cholesterol content may lead to the reduction in overall cholesterol delivery to the liver and to the periphery. These data suggest that these inhibitors act to indirectly reduce LDL-cholesterol and particle number by reducing cholesterol content in chylomicrons. Therefore, ezetimibe may be a member of a new class of drugs that shows promise for treatment of humans with combined hyperlipidemia, such as in the obese insulin-resistant and/or type 2 diabetic population.

Ezetimibe has been shown to be synergistic with simvastatin or atorvastatin in lowering cholesterol in hypercholesterolemic humans.[68a,68b,68c] Ezetimibe (10 mg/d) and simvastatin (10 mg/d) given for a 2-week period produced a 51.9% reduction in LDL-

cholesterol as compared to a 34.9% reduction with simvastatin (10 mg/d) alone.[69] This combination therapy may be a future option for patients who cannot tolerate or are minimally responsive to current methods of cholesterol lowering.

ENHANCERS OF 7α-HYDROXYLASE

The enzyme 7α-hydroxylase is the regulatory substance in the conversion of cholesterol to bile salts.[70] Bile-acid biosynthesis represents the major route of catabolism and removal of cholesterol in the body. Since reporting the cloning of the regulatory enzyme in 1989,[71] several molecular mechanisms that regulate the enzyme have been described. Bile acids have been shown to bind and activate the farnesoid X receptor (FXR), which represses the transcription of CYP7A1 that encodes 7α-hydroxylase.[72] Downregulation of CYP7A1 transcription can also occur via activation of the JNK/c-Jun pathway,[73] whereas activation of CYP7A1 transcription occurs through the activity of hepatocyte nuclear factor-4.[74] These are significant findings because an understanding of the molecular mechanisms would provide a strategy for developing drugs, such as a FXR antagonist, that could enhance the activation of 7α-hydroxylase. This drug would potentially reduce plasma cholesterol levels while having a preventive influence on gallstone production.

Previous studies showed an increase in the activity of 7α-hydroxylase with the administration of cholestyramine.[75] Recent studies demonstrate that direct augmentation of hepatic 7α-hydroxylase markedly lowers plasma LDL concentrations in animals with diet-induced hypercholesterolemia, as well as in animals that genetically lack LDL receptors.[76] This finding suggests the combination of 7α-hydroxylase gene transfer and a cholesterol synthesis inhibitor might prove useful in familial hypercholesterolemia patients without LDL receptors.

New studies also indicate that polymorphism of the gene encoding hepatic 7α-hydroxylase contribute significantly to the interindividual variation in plasma LDL-cholesterol concentration, and a specific CYP7A1 allele associated with increased plasma LDL-cholesterol concentrations has been identified.[77]

PEROXISOME PROLIFERATOR-ACTIVATED RECEPTOR ACTIVATORS

The peroxisome proliferator-activated receptors (PPARs) are members of the nuclear hormone receptor family that regulate glucose and lipid homeostasis, including receptors for steroid hormones, retinoids, thyroid hormones, vitamin D, and fatty acids.[78,79] The three subtypes identified to date are PPARα, PPARδ (also referred to as PPARβ), and PPARγ.[80] Although the role of PPARδ is unclear, PPARα appears to have a catabolic role in lipid metabolism and PPARγ has an anabolic role.[81] The PPARs form heterodimers with other nuclear receptors (RXRs) and subsequently bind peroxisomal proliferation response elements (PPREs) to their promoters.[80,82] The binding of PPRE agonists leads to the transcription of proteins that are then involved with metabolism of lipid and carbohydrates.

It has been discovered that fibric acid derivatives act at the level of PPARα and that the glitazone drugs target PPARγ.[83] The favorable antiatherogenic properties of fibric acid derivatives are partly a result of PPARα-mediated hepatic gene expression.[84] It has also been recognized that PPARα plays an important role in the downregulation of fibrinogen expression seen with the fibric acid derivatives.[85]

PD 72953, an ether diacid, is a PPAR agonist that is believed to affect PPARα. PD72953 caused the downregulation of apoC-III expression and the consequent reduction of plasma triglyceride levels observed in PD 72953-treated rats.[86] It is known that apoC-III acts to inhibit triglyceride clearance; the reduction of apoC-III seen in the PD 72953 rats was then followed by a reduced level of hypertriglyceridemia.[87] PD72593 also resulted in an elevation of HDL cholesterol in the treated rats.[86] These findings are consistent with the triglyceride reductions and HDL elevations observed with FADs and PPARα activation.

PPARγ activators (glitazones) are used in type 2 diabetics to increase insulin sensitivity and improve glycemic control. Recently, it was learned that while PPARγ is needed in the formation of adipose depots, agonists for PPARγ are used to treat the insulin resistance and hyperglycemia seen in type 2 diabetes.[88] It has also been noted that PPARγ is highly expressed in macrophages and the foam cells of atheromatous lesions.[89,90] PPARγ is involved in the regulation of the influx and efflux of cholesterol esters for macrophages. PPARγ agonists raise HDL cholesterol in humans and their ability to enhance cholesterol efflux from macrophages and endothelial cells may prevent the development of atherosclerosis.[88]

GW501516 was recently developed as a selective PPARδ agonist that may be effective in increasing the reverse cholesterol transport pathway.[91] An 80% increase in HDL cholesterol was seen in GW501516 (3 mg/kg)-treated monkeys. The GW501516 (3 mg/kg)-treated monkeys had significant increases in apoA-I and apoA-II, both components of HDL. GW501516 (3 mg/kg) caused reductions in triglyceride levels and a 50% decrease in VLDL. Interestingly, GW501516 raised serum apoC-III levels while simultaneously experiencing a reduction of serum triglyceride levels. As mentioned above, it is believed that a possible mechanism for the ability of PPARα to reduce levels of triglycerides is by decreasing levels of apoC-III and thereby removing the inhibition of triglyceride clearance. It is believed, therefore, that PPARα and PPARδ operate in different pathways to achieve similar triglyceride reductions.

Researchers are also involved with a new class of drugs that exhibit dual PPARα/γ agonist activity. Propionic acid derivative 8, also known as compound 8, is one of the drugs synthetically designed to stimulate both PPARα and PPARγ.[92] Compound 8 was tested in the diabetic animal model, the EOB mouse. Compound 8 (30 mg/kg), fenofibrate (100 mg/kg), and rosiglitazone (30 mg/kg) were orally dosed in the mouse model for a period of 7 days and then compared to control. These studies showed a 48.4% increase in HDL-cholesterol in the compound 8-treated mice, a greater increase than in the fenofibrate-treated mice. The compound 8-treated mice also showed a greater decrease in plasma glucose level than achieved in the rosiglitazone-treated mice. Serum triglyceride levels were markedly reduced in all the treated mice when compared to control, with the greatest decrease observed in the compound 8-treated mice. Compound 8 shows great promise for a new class of drugs that can result in powerful reductions in hyperglycemia combined with favorable changes in plasma HDL cholesterol and triglyceride levels.

These combined PPARα/γ agonists show potential as important drugs of the future for helping type 2 diabetics achieve manageable serum glucose controls while also addressing their increased risks for coronary heart disease and atherosclerosis. The ability to focus on the PPARs and their subclasses may provide a new class of specific and more powerful drugs in the treatment in both atherosclerosis and diabetes. By targeting the separate PPARs specifically, new drugs with fewer side effects and greater potency can be developed.

HORMONES

Estrogen

Both thyroxine and estrogens have the ability to reduce LDL-cholesterol and are reviewed in Chap. 36. A number of reports have shown possible benefit from estrogen use in preventing CAD in postmenopausal women.[93,94] In contrast, the Heart and Estrogen/Progestin Replacement Study (HERS), a recent randomized clinical trial, demonstrated that estrogen and progestin therapy did not reduce the overall rate of coronary events in postmenopausal women with established coronary disease, despite reductions in total cholesterol and LDL-cholesterol and increases in HDL-cholesterol with estrogen.[95]

Several studies, including HERS, have shown increases in plasma triglyceride concentration by estrogen,[95–97] which can reduce the size of LDL particles.[98] In postmenopausal patients with estrogen-induced hypertriglyceridemia, the resulting reduction in size of LDL particles makes them more susceptible to oxidation, which may counteract the antioxidant effect of estrogen.[99] Future studies are needed to investigate the possible benefit of lowering plasma triglyceride concentrations during hormone replacement therapy on the risk of cardiac events in postmenopausal women with established coronary artery disease.

A current question that has yet to be fully answered is whether estrogen is more effective for primary prevention or for treating atherosclerosis once it is already established. According to results in HERS, estrogen may not be effective for secondary prevention of cardiovascular disease.[95] The Estrogen and Prevention of Atherosclerosis Trial (EPAT) is the first randomized clinical trial of estrogen intervention for atherosclerotic disease in postmenopausal women with elevated LDL-cholesterol levels but no evidence of coronary disease.[100] The newest data from the EPAT study show increased carotid wall thickness in the placebo group, as compared with slight decrease in the estrogen group, suggesting estrogen may be more effective as primary prevention. However, more data from ongoing studies, such as the Women's Health Initiative (WHI) and the Women's International Study of long Duration Oestrogen after Menopause (WISDOM), are needed to clarify the role of HRT in lipid lowering.

Thyroxine Analogues

A thyroxine analogue, CGS 26214, devoid of the cardiovascular effects seen with thyroxine, has been shown in animal models to lower LDL-cholesterol and Lp(a).[101] In hypercholesterolemic rats, it produced a reduction in LDL of 31% at a dose of 1 μg/kg, which was equivalent to that obtained with 25 μg/kg of liothyronine. CGS-26214 also reduced LDL levels and Lp(a) levels by 43% in normal chow-fed monkeys, which was consistent with effects observed in hypothyroid patients receiving thyroid hormones.[102]

Another thyroxine analogue that lacks the undesirable cardiotoxic effects of thyroid hormone is CGS 23425. In hypercholesterolemic rats, it produced a 44% decrease in LDL-cholesterol at a dose of 10 μg/kg. The reduction in plasma cholesterol is mediated by an increase in hepatic LDL receptor activity. In addition, CGS 23425 produces a dose-dependent increase in apoA-I, an activator of LCAT that promotes cholesterol transport from peripheral tissues.[103]

β-SITOSTEROL (PLANT STEROLS)

β-Sitosterol is a plant sterol with a structure similar to that of cholesterol except for the substitution of an ethyl group at C-24 of its side chain. Despite this structural relation to cholesterol, it is poorly absorbed from the intestine. β-Sitosterol is known to compete with cholesterol for incorporation into mixed micelles, thereby reducing intestinal cholesterol absorption.[104,105] β-Sitosterol is also thought to inhibit absorption of endogenous biliary cholesterol.[106–108] The importance of dietary intake of plant sterols on cholesterol absorption and serum cholesterol has been demonstrated in human beings; dietary intake of plant sterols is negatively related to fractional cholesterol absorption and overall cholesterol synthesis.[109–111] Sitosterol may also inhibit 7α-hydroxylase.[112,113]

β-Sitosterol is used for treatment of hypercholesterolemia in Europe. It is quite effective in reducing cholesterol by 5 to 15%.[111] It is a very safe substance, although a high dose is required (6 g), taken before meals and at bedtime. Another plant sterol, β-sitostanol, reduces serum cholesterol more effectively than sitosterol at a lower dose.[114]

Miettinen and colleagues reported on the use of sitostanol ester, a derivative of the plant sterol sitosterol, which reduces the intestinal absorption of cholesterol and serum cholesterol more than sitosterol.[108] In this study, sitostanol ester was dissolved in margarine in a double-blind, randomized trial of men with moderate hypercholesterolemia. The formulation achieved a reduction in serum LDL-cholesterol of 14% with 2.6 g of sitostanol. A more recent study showed significant reduction of serum total cholesterol and LDL-cholesterol even at a dose of 1.6 g of stanol. While the dose of 2.4 g resulted in a slightly greater reduction of serum cholesterol than the dose of 1.6 g, the actual difference was not statistically significant.[115]

Because the inhibition of dietary cholesterol could increase endogenous cholesterol synthesis, several studies investigated the combination of sitostanol with HMG-CoA reductase inhibitors.[115a] Combined administration of a sitostanol ester margarine with a statin increased the net reduction in LDL-cholesterol from 38 to 44% in noninsulin-dependent diabetics[116] and from 35 to 46% in postmenopausal women with coronary heart disease.[106] A larger, more recent study confirmed the effective reduction of total cholesterol and LDL from the administration of a stanol with a stable dose of statin. The study showed a 10% reduction in LDL-cholesterol from the combined therapy of a plant stanol ester spread with either atorvastatin, pravastatin, simvastatin, or lovastatin.[117]

In children with hypercholesterolemia, sitostanol is effective and could be considered a treatment of choice. Replacement of regular daily fat intake by a margarine with a soluble ester form of stanol reduced total cholesterol and LDL-cholesterol levels by 11% and 15%, respectively, and increased HDL-cholesterol by 4% in children with heterozygous familial hypercholesterolemia.[118] The study suggests that familial hypercholesterolemic children with high baseline lathosterol proportions in serum can be expected to be good responders to LDL-cholesterol lowering by dietary sitostanol ester.[118]

Another group of plant compounds, the saponins, also interfere with cholesterol absorption by causing cholesterol precipitation, interference with micelle formation, or bile acid absorption. A synthetic saponin, β-tiogenin cellobioside, was found to reduce plasma cholesterol and LDL-cholesterol in men with hypercholesterolemia.[119] β-Ketotiogenin cellobioside, a derivative, selectively inhibits cholesterol absorption and is being evaluated as a potential replacement for bile acid resins.[119]

POLICOSANOL

Policosanol is an orally active sugar cane mixture of octasanol within other heavy alcohols; it has a confirmed lipid-lowering effect with a platelet antiaggregant action.[120a] It has been demonstrated to inhibit the progression of carotid and coronary atherosclerosis.[121,122] In the cuffed carotid artery of rabbits, policosanol showed better protective effect than did lovastatin against neointima formation through a greater inhibition of smooth-muscle cell proliferation.[123]

In type II hypercholesterolemic patients with two other coronary risk factors, policosanol is effective in lowering LDL-cholesterol and total cholesterol, as well as in increasing HDL-cholesterol.[123] In patients with coronary artery disease, treatment with policosanol results in significant improvements in coronary clinical symptoms and exercise ECG responses with amelioration of myocardial ischemia. With concomitant administration of aspirin, patients show more improvement.[124]

In addition, policosanol does not elevate transaminases, which can occur with other lipid-lowering drugs, and is considered safe and well tolerated in hypercholesterolemic patients.[125]

TOCOTRIENOLS

Tocotrienols exhibit antioxidant and cholesterol biosynthesis inhibitory activities and may be of value as antiatherosclerotic agents. In addition, they may have an antithrombotic effect through suppression of thromboxane B2 and platelet factor 4.[126,127] The tocotrienols are structurally related to the lipid-soluble antioxidant vitamin E (tocopherols); they differ from tocopherols by possessing a farnesyl, rather than phytyl, side chain.[128] The mechanism of their hypolipidemic action involves posttranscriptional suppression of HMG-CoA reductase in a manner mimicking the action of putative nonsterol feedback inhibitors.[128] The mechanisms of their inhibitory action on the generation of foam cells include inhibition of LDL oxidation and inhibition of adhesion molecules surface expression.[102]

Animal model studies suggest tocotrienols exhibit a greater degree of LDL-cholesterol and triglyceride (T_g)-lowering property than do tocopherols in cholesterol-fed rabbits.[129] A small, short-term case-controlled human trial shows that hypercholesterolemic patients on an American Heart Association diet for 8 weeks had a 7% decrease in plasma cholesterol level, but when supplemented for 4 of the 8 weeks with γ-tocotrienol, they demonstrated a significant decrease of 10% in plasma cholesterol level. The major reduction in cholesterol occurred in the LDL fraction, whereas HDL-cholesterol remained essentially unchanged.[126] Another short-term case-controlled study shows that a tocotrienol-rich fraction from specially processed rice bran oil also decreased plasma Lp(a) levels by 17%.[130] Additional long-term intervention studies in humans are required to draw final conclusions about the beneficial effects of tocotrienols on cholesterol levels.

CYCLOPHANES

A chemical cage has been synthesized from two cyclophane molecules that can trap cholesterol molecules in its central cavity while ignoring a similar compound. When cholesterol was added to a cyclophane-water solution, it could accept 190 times more cholesterol than normal. It is proposed that cyclophanes could be incorporated into the membrane of a dialysis machine that could essentially vacuum cholesterol from the blood of patients with hypercholesterolemia.[131]

HDL INFUSION

Several large epidemiologic studies show the inverse relationship between the incidence of coronary heart disease and HDL-cholesterol levels.[132,133] A study was completed in which homologous (rabbit) HDL-VHDL was infused in rabbits to determine the in vivo effects on the development of atherosclerosis.[134] The experimental animals (n = 31) all received a 0.5% cholesterol-rich diet for 8 weeks. During this period, 50 mg/wk of homologous HDL-VHDL protein was intravenously administered to the treatment group; the control group received a matching volume of normal saline. During the study, plasma lipid values were similar in both groups. At the completion of the study, the animals were sacrificed, and atherosclerotic lesions of the intimal aortic surface were less prevalent in the treated group. The values of total and free cholesterol, esterified cholesterol, and phospholipids deposited within the vessel wall were significantly lower in the HDL-treated animals. Cholesterol accumulation in the liver was also significantly less in the treated group.

The investigators concluded that the administration of homologous HDL-VHDL lipoprotein fraction to cholesterol-fed rabbits reduced the extent of aortic fatty streaks and reduced lipid deposition in the arterial wall and liver without modification of the plasma lipid levels. It was suggested that HDL-VHDL infusions could play a role in enhancing reverse cholesterol transport, thus inhibiting the development and/or progression of atherosclerosis.

In response to these findings, another group of investigators studied the effect of homologous (rabbit) HDL and heterologous (human) HDL on development of fatty streaks and plasma lipid levels in cholesterol-fed rabbits under identical conditions as the first study. Different effects of homologous and heterologous HDL injections on the atherosclerotic process in rabbits were found. Human HDL diminished serum cholesterol but had no effect on the degree of intima covered with fatty streaks, whereas rabbit HDL had no influence on plasma lipid levels but significantly reduced the area of intima covered with fatty streaks in cholesterol fed rabbits,[135] as was reported in the first study. These results support a difference in the mode of action between heterologous versus homologous HDL in cholesterol-fed rabbits regarding the development of hyperlipidemia and macroscopically detectable atherosclerosis.

SOMATIC GENE THERAPY

There are several techniques currently being investigated as possible approaches to treat atherosclerosis via gene therapy (see Chap. 41). Gene transfer to somatic cells can be performed by an ex vivo or an in vivo approach. Ex vivo approaches require expensive and complicated procedures that may be unacceptable to the patient. These procedures, for instance, may require a partial hepatectomy, followed by the transfection of target cells in vitro and the reimplantation of the organ. The in vivo approach is conducted in a much-less-invasive manner, involving the direct administration of the gene locally or systemically. The in vivo approach can be performed by using viral or nonviral delivery strategies. An exciting development in gene therapy involves using chimeraplasty as an alternative to viral gene therapy.

Adenoviruses are useful viral vectors for achieving hepatic transgene expression. Human adenovirus is a double-stranded DNA virus, nonenveloped and icosahedral, approximately 36 kb in length. First-generation adenovirus vectors were designed with the E1 region of viral DNA deleted in an effort to inhibit viral gene expression.[136] The results of in vivo experiments demonstrated the occurrence of serious hepatotoxicity and side effects resulting in morbidity and mortality in humans treated with the first-generation adenovirus vectors.[137] This led to the development of second-generation adenovirus vectors that were designed with further deletions of the viral DNA. Recently researchers developed helper-dependent adenoviral vectors designed for the removal of all viral protein genes as an attempt to further decrease toxicity.[138]

Initial experiments demonstrated that adenoviruses could transfer foreign genes to the mouse model for the expression of the human LDL receptor (LDLR) gene.[139] A drawback to adenovirus-mediated gene transfer is the short-lived expression of the transgene. Some studies show after the first week of transduction, gene expression declines greatly.[140] There is evidence that the elicitation of the host's immune responses against the vector and viral proteins expressed by the transduced cells are major factors in the observed drop in gene expression.[141] New studies are in progress to prevent the immune response leading to the loss of adenovirus-mediated gene expression. One study demonstrated long-term cholesterol reduction in LDLR-deficient mice via the transfer of the LDLR gene coupled with a blocking antibody directed against CD154, in order to achieve suppression of the immune response.[142] This study demonstrated that the anti-CD154-treated mice continued to have significant cholesterol reductions 93 days after the adenovirus-mediated transfer of LDLR and anti-CD154.

Further promising studies with adenovirus-mediated gene transfer have observed regression of atherosclerotic lesions in animal models. One group of experimenters observed plaque regression in apoE-deficient mice infected with adenovirus encoding the human apoE gene.[143] ApoE-deficient mice are hypercholesterolemic and develop atherosclerosis spontaneously on a cholesterol-rich diet.[144] Researchers demonstrated dose-dependent reductions in total cholesterol and triglyceride levels, along with atherosclerotic growth regression in the arterial walls of the infected mice. At the time of adenoviral introduction of the human apoE gene, the mice had fatty streak lesions averaging 220 ± 37 mm^2 via histologic analysis. The arterial lesion sizes of mice treated with 5×10^8 and 10^9 pfu of adenovirus measured 147 ± 76 and 28 ± 6 mm^2 at day 199 of the experiment. In comparison, the control mice had an average lesion size of 1172 ± 255 mm^2 at day 199. Histologic analysis demonstrated the complete remodeling and reendothelialization of the arterial wall along with a disappearance of macrophages, foam cells, and cholesterol crystals. This study provides physical evidence of the antiatherogenic potential of adenovirus-mediated gene therapy.

A different strategy to gene therapy involves the inhibition of gene expression of certain genes. Potential use of this technique involves incorporating antisense oligonucleotides to control c-myb and c-myc gene expression and protein synthesis at several points.[145] By this method, it could be possible to inhibit smooth-muscle cell proliferation in the arterial wall to decrease atherosclerosis.

Chimeraplasty, or targeted gene correction, involves the use of synthetic DNA-RNA oligonucleotides (chimeraplasts) for targeted gene repair of mutant genes. Chimeraplasty is a novel approach to gene correction that does not rely on a viral delivery strategy. This method to gene correction uses synthetic DNA-RNA oligonucleotides (chimeraplasts) that target a specific mutated gene sequence.[146] The use of the chimeraplast offers an advantage to traditional gene therapy that normally requires delivery of much larger amounts of genetic material. The chimeraplasts bind to the mutant gene sequence resulting in the activation of the cell's DNA repair machinery.[147] The cell repairs the mutant gene in situ to match the correct version delivered by the chimeraplast. This targeted gene therapy has an advantage over viral vectors because viruses can integrate at random locations in chromosomes, which can make it difficult to regulate gene expression.

Initial studies in chimeraplasty have been successful in gene transfer. Studies provide evidence that targeted gene therapy can restore tyrosinase activity in the melanocytes of albino mice.[148] A recent study also described the correction of the genetic lesion responsible for Crigler-Najjar syndrome in a rat model via chimeraplasty.[149] The scientists observed that in rats previously expressing the faulty gene, there was restoration of normal enzyme expression with consequent improvement in the metabolic abnormality after chimeraplasty.

Chimeraplasty has shown promise in early studies for the correction of the enzymatic defect attributed to be a major cause of type III hyperlipidemia. ApoE has antiatherogenic properties associated with the promotion of cholesterol efflux from cells. Having low levels of apoE is associated with hyperlipidemia and atherosclerosis. ApoE2 is a dysfunctional form of apoE expressed in patients with Type III hyperlipidemia, whereas the wild-type protein, apoE3 is a functional form.[147] Scientists were able to target the apoE gene in the liver of transgenic mice overexpressing human apoE2.[150] The researchers injected 1000 nm of a chimeraplast, the 68-mer oligonucleotide, into the transgenic mice overexpressing human apoE2. The researchers analyzed the DNA taken from the liver of the treated mice 7 days later and determined approximately 25% of the hepatic apoE2 converted to apoE3. This study provides early evidence that chimeraplasty can be used in the future as a possible tool to correct mutant genes in patients with dyslipidemias. One concern of chimeraplasty is the possibility that infusion of the chimeric molecules may lead to the unintentional binding to similar genes with large stretches of DNA identical to the target sequence. Scientists are working on newer ways to deliver the chimeraplasts to the targeted cells, with the hope that the development of these small chimeric molecules will result in a more efficient means of gene transfer.

CHOLESTEROL VACCINES

Cholesterol vaccines have been proposed and tested as a technique for lowering serum cholesterol by enhancing clearance of serum lipoprotein via the reticuloendothelial system.[151–153] Two synthetic antigens containing cholesterol esters covalently coupled as haptens to various carrier proteins (bovine albumin, human β-lipoprotein) were synthesized.[154] Groups of rabbits immunized with these preparations were fed atherogenic diets up to 15 weeks. Reduction in serum cholesterol of 25 to 35% and suppression of atherosclerotic plaque formation up to 90% were observed in immunized animals, as compared with controls.[154] Another study demonstrated inhibition of the neointimal response to balloon injury in hypercholesterolemic rabbits after immunization with homologous oxidized LDL.[155] In the future, cholesterol immunization procedures should be tested for more typical hyperlipidemias occurring in human populations.

CONCLUSION

Researchers are continually discovering innovative lipid-lowering methods that are potentially more efficient and less toxic than current methods. These innovations are coming to light as scientists gain a better understanding of the pathophysiology and metabolic processes that contribute to the atherosclerotic process. Exciting modalities for treatment are also developing together with advances in the field of gene research. Some of the pioneering experimental modalities are aimed at targeting inhibition of cholesterol synthesis; disrupting cholesteryl ester formation and transfer; targeting the LDL receptor; altering macrophage and endothelial lipid content; increasing the plasma HDL-cholesterol levels; enhancing reverse cholesterol transport; inhibiting cholesterol transfer; targeting nuclear receptors; and investigating new vectors and methods of gene transfer. The plethora of novel lipid-lowering agents should ultimately result in further decreases in patient mortality and morbidity from disease processes stemming from atherosclerosis.

REFERENCES

1. Vega G, Von Bergmann K, Grundy S, et al: Effect of lifibrol on the metabolism of low-density lipoproteins and cholesterol. *J Intern Med* 246:1, 1999.
2. Schwandt P, Elsasser, Schmidt C, Gertz B, et al: Safety and efficacy of lifibrol upon four-week administration to patients with primary hypercholesterolaemia. *Eur J Clin Pharmacol* 47:133, 1994.
3. Locker P, Jungbluth G, Francom S, Hughs G Jr, for the Lifibrol Study Group. Lifibrol: A novel lipid-lowering drug for the therapy of hypercholesterolemia. *Clin Pharmacol Ther* 57:73, 1995.
4. Grundy S: HMG-CoA reductase inhibitors for treatment of hypercholesterolemia. *N Engl J Med* 319:24, 1988.
5. Todd P, Goa K: Simvastatin: A review of its pharmacological properties and therapeutic potential in hypercholesterolaemia. *Drugs* 40:583, 1990.
6. McTavish D, Sorkin E: Pravastatin: A review of its pharmacological properties and therapeutic potential in hypercholesterolaemia. *Drugs* 42:65, 1990.
7. Winkler K, Schaefer J, Klima B, et al: HDL steady state levels are not affected, but HDL apo A-I turnover is enhanced by lifibrol in patients with hypercholesterolemia and mixed hyperlipidemia. *Atherosclerosis* 150:113, 2000.
8. Scharnagl H, Marz W, Wieland H: Lifibrol: First member of a new class of lipid-lowering drugs? *Expert Opin Investig Drugs* 6:583, 1997.
9. Scharnagl H, Schliack M, Loser R, et al: The effects of lifibrol (K12.148) on the cholesterol metabolism of cultured cells: Evidence for sterol independent stimulation of the LDL pathway. *Atherosclerosis* 153:69, 2000.
10. Suckling K: Emerging strategies for treatment of atherosclerosis as seen from the patient literature. *Biochem Soc Trans* 21:660, 1993.
11. Biller SA, Forster C, Gordon EM, et al: Isoprenyl phosphyinylformates. New inhibitors of squalene synthetase. *J Med Chem* 34:1912, 1991.
12. Burton P, Swinney D, Heller R, et al: Azalanstat (RS-21607), a lanosterol 14-alpha-demethylase inhibitor with cholesterol-lowering activity. *Biochem Pharmacol* 50:529, 1995.
13. Morand O, Aebi J, Dehmlow H, et al: Ro 48-8.071, a new 2, 3-oxidosqualene:Lanosterol cyclase inhibitor lowering plasma cholesterol in hamsters, squirrel monkeys, and minipigs: comparison to simvastatin. *J Lipid Res* 38:373, 1997.
14. Popjack G, Agnew W: Squalene synthase. *Mol Cell Biochem* 27:97, 1979.
15. Ciosek C Jr, Magnin D, Harrity T, et al: Lipophilic 1, 1-biphosphonates are potent squalene synthase inhibitors and orally active cholesterol lowering agents in vivo. *J Biol Chem* 268:24832, 1993.

16. Baxter A, Fitzgerald B, Hutson J, et al: Squalestatin 1, a potent inhibitor of squalene synthase, which lowers serum cholesterol in vivo. *J Biol Chem* 267:11705, 1992.

17. Hiyoshi H, Yanagimachi M, Ito M, et al: Effect of ER-27856, a novel squalene synthase inhibitor, on plasma cholesterol in rhesus monkeys: Comparison with 3-hydroxy-3-methylglutaryl-coa reductase inhibitors. *J Lipid Res* 41:1136, 2000.

18. Ugawa T, Kakuta H, Moritani H, et al: YM-53601, a novel squalene synthase inhibitor, reduces plasma cholesterol and triglyceride levels in several animal species. *Br J Pharmacol* 131:63, 2000.

19. Abdul-Ghaffar N, el-Sonbaty M: Pancreatitis and rhabdomyolysis associated with lovastatin-gemfibrozil therapy. *J Clin Gastroenterol* 21:340, 1995.

20. Amin D, Rutledge RZ, Needle SN, et al: RPR 107393, a potent squalene synthase inhibitor and orally effective cholesterol-lowering agent: Comparison with inhibitors of HMG-CoA reductase. *J Pharmacol Exp Ther* 281:746, 1997.

21. Peffley DM, Gayen AK: Inhibition of squalene synthase but not squalene cyclase prevents mevalonate-mediated suppression of 3-hydroxy-3-methylglutaryl coenzyme A reductase synthesis at a post-transcriptional level. *Arch Biochem Biophys* 337:251, 1997.

22. Ness GC, Zhao Z, Keller RK: Effect of squalene synthase inhibition on the expression of hepatic cholesterol biosynthetic enzymes, LDL receptor, and cholesterol 7-alpha hydroxylase. *Arch Biochem Biophys* 311:277, 1994.

23. Harwood JH Jr, Barbacci-Tobin EG, Petras SF, et al: 3-(4-Chlorophenyl)-A-pentenonitrile monohydrogen citrate and related analogs. *Biochem Pharmacol* 53:839, 1997.

24. Asano M, Yamakwa T: The fate of branched chain fatty acids in animal body. I. A contribution of the problem of hildebrant acid. *J Biochem* 37:321, 1950.

25. Bergstrom JD, Kurtz MM, Rew DJ, et al: Zaragozic acids: A family of fungal metabolites that are picomolar competitive inhibitors of squalene synthase. *Proc Natl Acad Sci U S A* 90:80, 1993.

26. Sharma A, Slugg PH, Hammett JL, Jusko WJ: Clinical pharmacokinetics and pharmacodynamics of a new squalene synthase inhibitor, BMS-188494, in healthy volunteers. *J Clin Pharmacol* 38:1116, 1998.

27. Goto S, Shimokawa T: Effect of the hypocholesterolemic agent YM-16638 on cholesterol biosynthesis activity and apolipoprotein B secretion in HepG2 and monkey liver. *Jpn J Pharmacol* 79:75, 1999.

28. Ross R: The pathogenesis of atherosclerosis: A perspective for the 1990s. *Nature* 362:801, 1993.

29. Sliskovic D, White A: Therapeutic potential of ACAT inhibitors as lipid lowering and anti-atherosclerotic agents. *Trends Pharmacol Sci* 12:194, 1991.

29a. Rival Y, Junquéro D, Bruniguel F, et al: Anti-atherosclerotic properties of the acyl-coenzyme A: cholesterol acyltransferase inhibitor F 12511 in casein-fed New Zealand rabbits. *J Cardiovasc Tharmocol* 39:181, 2002.

30. Libby P, Geng YJ, Aikawa M, et al: Macrophages and atherosclerotic plaque stability. *Curr Opin Lipidol* 7:330, 1996.

31. Delsing D, Offerman E, van Duyvenvoorde W, et al: Acyl-CoA: cholesterol acyltransferase inhibitor avasimibe reduces atherosclerosis in addition to its cholesterol-lowering effect in ApoE*3-Leiden mice. *Circulation* 103:1778, 2001.

32. Kusunoki J, Hansoty D, Katsumi A, et al: Acyl-CoA: cholesterol acyltransferase inhibition reduces atherosclerosis in apolipoprotein E-deficient mice. *Circulation* 103:2604, 2001.

33. Chong P, Bachenheimer B: Current, new and future treatments in dyslipidaemia and atherosclerosis. *Drugs* 60:55, 2000.

34. Matsuda K: ACAT inhibitors as anti-atherosclerotic agents: Compounds and mechanisms. *Med Res Rev* 14:271, 1994.

35. Tanaka A, Terasawa T, Hagihara H, et al: Inhibitors of acyl-CoA:cholesterol O-acyltransferase. 3. Discovery of a novel series of *N*-alkyl-N-[(fluorophenoxy)benzyl]-N'-arylureas with weak toxicological effects on adrenal glands. *J Med Chem* 41:4408, 1998.

36. Sliskovic DR, Picard JA, O'Brien PM, et al: α-Substituted malonester amides: Tools to define the relationship between ACAT inhibition and adrenal toxicity. *J Med Chem* 41:682, 1998.

37. Roberson D, Breider M: Preclinical safety evaluation of avasimibe in beagle dogs: An ACAT inhibitor with minimal adrenal effects. *Toxicol Sci* 59:324, 2001.

38. Perrey S, Legendre C, Matsuura A, et al: Preferential pharmacological inhibition of macrophage ACAT increases plaque formation in mouse and rabbit models of atherogenesis. *Atherosclerosis* 155:359, 2001.

39. Hara S, Higaki J, Higashino K, et al: S-8921, an ileal Na+/bile acid cotransporter inhibitor decreases serum cholesterol in hamsters. *Life Sci* 60:365, 1997.

40. Ichihashi T, Izawa M, Miyata K, et al: Mechanism of hypocholesterolemic action of S-8921 in rats: S-8921 inhibits ileal bile acid absorption. *J Pharmacol Exp Ther* 284:43, 1998.

41. Higaki J, Hara S, Takasu N, et al: Inhibition of ileal Na+/bile acid cotransporter by S-8921 reduces serum cholesterol and prevents atherosclerosis in rabbits. *Arterioscler Thromb Vasc Biol* 18:1304, 1998.

42. Benson M, Alston DR, Hickey DMB, et al: SK&F 97426-A: A novel bile acid sequestrant with higher affinities and slower dissociation rates for bile acids in vitro than cholestyramine. *J Pharm Sci* 86(1):76, 1997.

42a. Benson GM, Alston DR, Bond BC, et al: SKYF 97426, a more potent bile acid sequestrant and hypercholesterolemic agent than cholestyramine in the hamster. *Atherosclerosis* 101:51, 1993.

43. Wilson TA, Nicolosi RJ, Rogers EJ, et al: Studies of cholesterol and bile acid metabolism, and early atherogenesis in hamsters fed GT16-239, a novel bile acid sequestrant (BAS). *Atherosclerosis* 140:315, 1998.

44. Inazu A, Brown M, Hesler C, et al: Increased high density lipoprotein levels caused by a common cholesteryl-ester transfer protein gene mutation. *N Engl J Med* 323:1234, 1990.

45. Okamoto H, Yonemori F, Wakitani K, et al: A cholesteryl ester transfer protein inhibitor attenuates atherosclerosis in rabbits. *Nature* 406:203, 2000.

46. Sugano M, Makino N, Sawada S, et al: Effect of antisense oligonucleotides against cholesteryl ester transfer protein on the development of atherosclerosis in cholesterol-fed rabbits. *J Biol Chem* 273:5033, 1998.

47. Ken-ichi H, Shizuya Y, Matsuzawa Y: Pros and cons of inhibiting cholesteryl ester transfer protein. *Curr Opin Lipidol* 11:589, 2000.

48. Bruce C, Chouinard RA Jr, Tall AR: Plasma lipid transfer proteins, high-density lipoproteins, and reverse cholesterol transport. *Annu Rev Nutr* 18:297, 1998.

49. Zhong S, Sharp DS, Grove JS, et al: Increased coronary heart disease in Japanese-American men with mutations in the cholesteryl ester transfer protein gene despite increased HDL levels. *J Clin Invest* 97:2917, 1996.

50. Kothari HV, Poirier KJ, Lee WH, et al: Inhibition of cholesterol ester transfer protein CGS 25159 and changes in lipoproteins in hamsters. *Atherosclerosis* 128:59, 1997.

51. Cho KH, Lee JY, Choi MS, et al: A peptide from hog plasma that inhibits human cholesteryl ester transfer protein. *Biochim Biophys Acta* 1391:133, 1998.

52. Eisenberg S: High-density lipoprotein metabolism. *J Lipid Res* 25:1017, 1984.

53. Patsch J, Gotto A Jr, Olivecrona T, Eisenberg S: Formation of high density lipoprotein-like particles lipolysis of very low density lipoproteins in vitro. *Proc Natl Acad Sci U S A* 75:4519, 1978.

54. Lewis B: Relation of high-density lipoproteins to coronary artery disease. *Am J Cardiol* 52:5B, 1983.

55. Eckel R: Lipoprotein lipase: A multifunctional enzyme relevant to common metabolic diseases. *N Engl J Med* 320:1060, 1989.

56. Tsutsumi K, Inoue Y, Shima A, et al: The novel compound NO-1886 increases lipoprotein lipase activity with resulting elevation of high density lipoprotein cholesterol, and long-term administration inhibits atherogenesis in the coronary arteries of rats with experimental atherosclerosis. *J Clin Invest* 92:411, 1993.

57. Tsutsumi K, Inoue Y, Hagi A, Murase T: The novel compound NO-1886 elevates plasma high-density lipoprotein cholesterol levels in hamsters and rabbits by increasing lipoprotein lipase without any effect on cholesteryl ester transfer protein activity. *Metabolism* 46:257, 1997.

58. Chiba T, Miura S, Sawamura F, et al: Antiatherogenic effects of a novel lipoprotein lipase-enhancing agent in cholesterol-fed New Zealand white rabbits. *Arterioscler Thromb Vasc Biol* 17:2601, 1997.

59. Tsutsumi K, Inoue Y, Shima A, Murase T: Correction of hypertriglyceridemia with low high-density lipoprotein cholesterol by the novel

compound NO-1886, a lipoprotein lipase-promoting agent, in STZ-induced diabetic rats. *Diabetes* 44:414, 1995.

60. Hara T, Cameron-Smith D, Cooney GJ, et al: The actions of a novel lipoprotein lipase activator, NO-1886, in hypertriglyceridemic fructose-fed rats. *Metabolism* 47:149, 1998.

61. Kusunoki M, Hara T, Tsutsumi K, et al: The lipoprotein lipase activator, NO-1886, suppresses fat accumulation and insulin resistance in rats fed a high-fat diet. *Diabetologia* 43:875, 2000.

62. Salisbury B, Davis H, Burrier R, et al: Hypocholesterolemic activity of a novel inhibitor of cholesterol absorption, SCH48461. *Atherosclerosis* 115:45, 1995.

63. van Heek M, Farley C, Compton D, et al: Comparison of the activity and disposition of the novel cholesterol absorption inhibitor, SCH58235, and its glucuronide, SCH60663. *Br J Pharmacol* 129:1748, 2000.

64. Dujovne CA, Bays H, Davidson MH, et al: Reduction of LDL cholesterol in patients with primary hypercholesterolemia by SCH 48461: results of a multicenter, dose-ranging study. *J Clin Pharmacol* 41:70, 2001.

65. van Heek M, France C, Compton D, et al: In vivo metabolism-based discovery of a potent cholesterol absorption inhibitor, SCH58235, in the rat and rhesus monkey through the identification of the active metabolites of SCH48461. *J Pharmacol Exp Ther* 283:157, 1997.

66. Bays HE, Moore PB, Drehobl MA, et al: Effectiveness and tolerability of ezetimibe in patients with primary hypercholesterolemia: Pooled analysis of two phase II studies. *Clin Therap* 23:1209, 2001.

67. van Heek M, Austin T, Farley C, et al: Ezetimibe, a potent cholesterol absorption inhibitor, normalizes combined dyslipidemia in obese hyperinsulinemic hamsters. *Diabetes* 50:1330, 2001.

68. van Heek M, Compton D, Davis H: The cholesterol inhibitor, ezetimibe, decreases diet-induced hypercholesterolemia in monkeys. *Eur J Clin Pharmacol* 415:79, 2001.

68a. Gagné C, Gaudet D, Bruckert E for the Ezetimibe Study Group: Efficacy and safety of ezetimibe coadministered with atorvastatin or simvastatin in patients with homozygous familial hypercholesterolemia *Circulation* 105:2469, 2002.

68b. An investigative look: Selective cholesterol absorption inhibitors. Based on a presentation by Evan A, Stein MD, PhD at the Symposium "Reinventing Treatment of Dyslipedemia: Novel Therapeutic Targets," Nov. 10, 2001, Anaheim, Ca. *Cardiol Rev* 19(Suppl):20, 2002.

68c. Preclinical and clinical pharmacology of a new class of lipid management agents. Based on a presentation by Lawrence L, Rundel MD at the Symposium *Cardiol Rev* 19(Suppl):17, 2002.

69. Kosoglou T, Meyer I, Musiol B, et al: Pharmacodynamic interaction between the new selective cholesterol absorption inhibitor SCH 58235 and simvastatin (abstr.). *Atherosclerosis* 151:135, 2000.

70. Edwards PA, Fogelman AM: Cellular enzymes of cholesterol metabolism. *Curr Opin Lipidol* 1:136, 1990.

71. Noshiro N, Nishimoto M, Morohashi K, Okuda K: Molecular cloning of cDNA for cholesterol 7α-hydroxylase from rat liver microsomes. Nucleotide sequence and expression. *FEBS Lett* 257:97, 1989.

72. Chiang JYL, Kimmel R, Weinberger C, Stroup D: Farnesoid X receptor responds to bile acids and represses cholesterol 7α-hydroxylase gene (CYP7A1) transcription. *J Biol Chem* 275(15):10918, 2000.

73. Gupta S, Stravitz RT, Ent P, Hylemon PB: Down-regulation of cholesterol 7α-hydroxylase (CYP7A1) gene expression by bile acids in primary rat hepatocytes is mediated by the c-Jun N-terminal kinase pathway. *J Biol Chem* 276(19):15816, 2001.

74. De Fabiani E, Mitro N, Anzulovich AC, et al: The negative effects of bile acids and tumor necrosis factor-α on the transcription of cholesterol 7α-hydroxylase gene (CYP7A1) converge to hepatic nuclear factor-4. A novel mechanism of feedback regulation of bile acid synthesis mediated by nuclear receptors. *J Biol Chem* 276(33):30708, 2001.

75. Kuroki S, Naito T, Chijiiwa K, Tanaka M: Effects of cholestyramine on hepatic cholesterol 7α-hydroxylase and serum 7α-hydroxycholesterol in the hamster. *Lipids* 34(8):817, 1999.

76. Spady DK, Cuthbert JA, Willard MN, Meidell RS: Overexpression of cholesterol 7α-hydroxylase (CYP7A) in mice lacking the low-density lipoprotein (LDL) receptor gene. LDL transport and plasma LDL concentrations are reduced. *J Biol Chem* 273(1):126, 1998.

77. Wang J, Freeman DJ, Grundy SM, et al: Linkage between cholesterol 7α-hydroxylase and high-plasma low-density lipoprotein cholesterol concentrations. *J Clin Invest* 101(6):1283, 1998.

78. Mangelsdorf D, Evans R: The RXR heterodimers and orphan receptors. *Cell* 83:841, 1995.

79. Xu E, Lambert M, Montana V, et al: Molecular recognition of fatty acids by peroxisome proliferator-activated receptors. *Mol Cell* 3:397, 1999.

80. Schoonjans K, Staels B, Auwerx J: Role of the peroxisome proliferator-activated receptor (PPAR) in mediating the effects of fibrates and fatty acids on gene expression. *J Lipid Res* 37:907, 1996.

81. Willson T, Wahli W: Peroxisome proliferator-activated receptor agonists. *Curr Opin Chem Biol* 1:235, 1997.

82. Schoonjans K, Peinado-Onsurbe J, Lefebvre A, et al: PPARα and PPARγ activators direct a distinct tissue-specific transcriptional response via a PPRE in the lipoprotein lipase gene. *EMBO J* 15:5336, 1996.

83. Willson T, Brown P, Sternbach D, Henke B: The PPARs: From orphan receptors to drug discovery. *J Med Chem* 43:527, 2000.

84. Staels B, Dallongeville J, Auwerx J, et al: Mechanism of action of fibrates on lipid and lipoprotein metabolism. *Circulation* 98:2088, 1998.

85. Kockx M, Gervois P, Poulain P, et al: Fibrates suppress fibrinogen gene expression in rodents via activation of the peroxisome proliferator-activated receptor-α. *Blood* 93:2991, 1999.

86. Bisgaier C, Essenburg A, Barnett B, et al: A novel compound that elevates high-density lipoprotein and activates the peroxisome proliferator-activated receptor. *J Lipid Res* 39:17, 1998.

87. Windler E, Chao Y, Havel R: Regulation of the hepatic uptake of triglyceride-rich lipoproteins in the rat. *J Biol Chem* 255:8303, 1980.

88. Willson T, Lambert M, Kliewer S: Peroxisome proliferator-activated receptor γ and metabolic disease. *Annu Rev Biochem* 70:341, 2001.

89. Tontonoz P, Nagy L, Alvarez J, et al: PPARγ promotes monocyte/macrophage differentiation and uptake of oxidized LDL. *Cell* 93:241, 1998.

90. Ricote M, Huang J, Fajas L, et al: Expression of the peroxisome proliferator-activated receptor gamma (PPARγ) in human atherosclerosis and regulation in macrophages by colony stimulating factors and oxidized low density lipoprotein. *Proc Natl Acad Sci U S A* 95:7614, 1998.

91. Oliver W Jr, Shenk J, Snaith M, et al: A selective peroxisome proliferator-activated receptor δ agonist promotes reverse cholesterol transport. *Proc Natl Acad Sci U S A* 98:5306, 2001.

92. Brooks D, Etgen G, Rito C, et al: Design and synthesis of 2-methyl-{4-[2-(5-methyl-2-aryloxazol-4-yl)ethoxy]phynoxy}propionic acids: A new class of dual PPARα/γ agonists. *J Med Chem* 44:2061, 2001.

93. Schwartz J, Freeman R, Frishman W: Clinical pharmacology of estrogens: focus on their cardiovascular actions and cardioprotective benefits of replacement therapy in postmenopausal women. *J Clin Pharm* 35:314, 1995.

94. Grodstein F, Stampfer MJ, Manson JE, et al: Postmenopausal estrogen and progestin use and the risk of cardiovascular disease. *N Engl J Med* 335:453, 1996.

95. Hulley S, Grady D, Bush T, et al: Randomized trial of estrogen plus progestin for secondary prevention of coronary heart disease in postmenopausal women. *JAMA* 280:7, 1998.

96. Walsh BW, Schiff I, Rosner B, et al: Effects of postmenopausal estrogen replacement on the concentrations and metabolism of plasma lipoproteins. *N Engl J Med* 325:1196, 1991.

97. The Writing Group for the PEPI Trial: Effects of estrogen or estrogen/progestin regimens on heart disease risk factors in postmenopausal women. The postmenopausal estrogen/progestin interventions (PEPI) trial. *JAMA* 273:199, 1995.

98. Wakatsuki A, Ikenoue N, Sagara Y: Effect of estrogen on the size of low-density lipoprotein particles in postmenopausal women. *Obstet Gynecol* 90:22, 1997.

99. Wakatsuki A, Ikenoue N, Okatani Y, Fukaya T: Estrogen-induced small low density lipoprotein particles may be atherogenic in postmenopausal women. *J Am Coll Cardiol* 37(2):425, 2001.

100. Herrington DM, Howard TD, Hawkins GA, et al: Estrogen-receptor polymorphisms and effects of estrogen replacement on high-density

lipoprotein cholesterol in women with coronary disease. *N Engl J Med* 346:967, 2002.

101. Steele RE, Wasvary JM, Dardik BN, et al: CGS 26214, the thyroxine connection revised. In: Woodford FP, Davignon J, Sniderman A, eds. *Atherosclerosis X.* Amsterdam: Elsevier, 1995:321–324.

102. Chong PH, Bachenheimer BS: Current, new and future treatments in dyslipidaemia and atherosclerosis. *Drugs* 60(1):55, 2000.

103. Taylor AH, Stephan ZF, Steele RE, Wong NCW: Beneficial effects of a novel thyromimetic on lipoprotein metabolism. *Mol Pharmacol* 52(3):542, 1997.

104. Ikeda I, Tanaka K, Sugano M, et al: Inhibition of cholesterol absorption in rats by plant sterols. *J Lipid Res* 29:1573, 1988.

105. Ikeda I, Tanaka K, Sugano M, et al: Discrimination between cholesterol and sitosterol for absorption in rats. *J Lipid Res* 29:1583, 1988.

106. Gylling H, Radhakrishnan R, Miettinen TA: Reduction of serum cholesterol in post-menopausal women with previous myocardial infarction and cholesterol malabsorption induced by dietary sitostanol ester margarine. *Circulation* 16:4226, 1997.

107. Hallikainen MA, Uusitupa MIJ: Effects of 2 low-fat stanol ester-containing margarines on serum cholesterol concentrations as part of a low-fat diet in hypercholesterolemic *Am J Clin Nutr* 69:403, 1999.

108. Miettinen TA, Puska P, Gylling H, et al: Reduction of serum cholesterol with sitostanol-ester margarine in a mildly hypercholesterolemic population. *N Engl J Med* 333:1308, 1995.

109. Kesaniemi YA, Miettinen TA: Cholesterol absorption efficiency regulates plasma cholesterol level in the Finnish population. *Eur J Clin Invest* 17:391, 1987.

110. Miettinen TA, Kesaniemi YA: Cholesterol absorption: Regulation of cholesterol synthesis and elimination and within-population variations of serum cholesterol levels. *Am J Clin Nutr* 49:629, 1989.

111. von Bergmann K: Lipid-lowering drugs working in the intestine. *Curr Opin Lipid* 1:48, 1990.

112. Boberg KM, Akerlund J-E, Bjorkhem I: Effects of sitosterol on the rate-limiting enzymes in cholesterol synthesis and degradation. *Lipids* 24:9, 1989.

113. Shefer S, Salen G, Nguyen L, et al: Competitive inhibition of bile acid synthesis by endogenous cholestanol and sitosterol in sitosterolemia with xanthomatosis. Effect of cholesterol 7-alpha hydroxylase. *J Clin Invest* 82:1833, 1988.

114. Heinemann T, Pietruck B, Kullak-Ublick G, von Bergmann K: Comparison of sitosterol and sitostanol on inhibition of intestinal cholesterol absorption. *Agents Actions* 26(Suppl):117, 1988.

115. Hallikainen MA, Sarkkinen ES, Uusitupa MIJ: Plant stanol esters affect serum cholesterol concentrations of hypercholesterolemic men and women in a dose-dependent manner. *J Nutr* 130:767, 2000.

115a. Nguyen TT, Dale LC, von Bergmann K, Croghan IT: Cholesterol-lowering effect of stanol ester in a U.S. population of mildly hypercholesterolemic men and women: Randomized, controlled trial. *Mayo Clin Proc* 74:1198, 1999.

116. Gylling H, Miettinen TA: Effects of inhibiting cholesterol absorption and synthesis on cholesterol and lipoprotein metabolism in hypercholesterolemic non-insulin-dependent diabetic men. *J Lipid Res* 37:1776, 1996.

117. Blair SN, Capuzzi DM, Gottlieb SO, et al: Incremental reduction of serum total cholesterol and low-density lipoprotein cholesterol with the addition of plant stanol ester-containing spread to statin therapy. *Am J Cardiol* 86:46, 2000.

118. Gylling H, Siimes MA, Miettinen TA: Sitostanol ester margarine in dietary treatment of children with familial hypercholesterolemia. *J Lipid Res* 36:1807, 1995.

119. Davignon J: Prospects for drug therapy for hyperlipoproteinemia. *Diabetes Metab* 21:139, 1995.

120. Batista JF, Stusser RJ, Padron R, et al: Functional improvement in coronary artery disease after 20 months of lipid-lowering therapy with policosanol. *Adv Ther* 13:137, 1996.

120a. Gouni-Berthold I, Berthold HK: Policosanol: Clinical pharmacology and therapeutic significance of a new lipid-lowering agent. *Am Heart J* 143:356, 2002.

121. Batista J, Stusser R, Penichet M, Uguet E: Doppler-ultrasound pilot study of the effects of long-term policosanol therapy on carotid-vertebral atherosclerosis. *Curr Ther Res* 56:906, 1995.

122. Batista J, Stusser R, Saez F, Perez B: Effect of policosanol on hyperlipidemia and coronary heart disease in middle-aged patients. A 14-month pilot study. *Int J Pharmacol Ther* 34:134, 1996.

123. Noa M, Mas R, Mesa R: A comparative study of policosanol vs lovastatin on intimal thickening in rabbit cuffed carotid artery. *Pharm Res* 43:31, 2001.

124. Stusser R, Batista J, Padron R, et al: Long-term therapy with policosanol improves treadmill exercise-ECG testing performance of coronary heart disease patients. *Int J Clin Pharmcol Ther* 36(9):469, 1998.

125. Mas R, Castano G, Illnait J, et al: Effects of policosanol in patients with type II hypercholesterolemia and additional coronary risk factors. *Clin Pharmacol Ther* 65(4):439, 1999.

126. Qureshi AA, Bradlow BA, Brace L, et al: Response of hypercholesterolemic subjects to administration of tocotrienols. *Lipids* 30:1171, 1995.

127. Qureshi AA, Qureshi N, Wright JJ, et al: Lowering of serum cholesterol in hypercholesterolemic humans by tocotrienols (Palmvitee). *Am J Clin Nutr* 53(4 Suppl):1021S, 1991.

128. Pearce BS, Parker RA, Deason ME, et al: Inhibitors of cholesterol biosynthesis, hypocholesterolemic, antioxidant activities by analogues of tocotrienols. *J Med Chem* 37:526, 1994.

129. Teoh MK, Chong JM, Monamed J, Phang KS: Protection by tocotrienols against hypercholesterolemia and atheroma. *Med J Malaysia* 49:255, 1994.

130. Qureshi AA, Bradlow BA, Salser WA, Brace LD: Novel tocotrienols of rice bran modulate cardiovascular disease risk parameters of hypercholesterolemic humans. *Nutr Biochem* 8:290, 1997.

131. Bradley D: Crafting a cage for cholesterol. *Science* 266:34, 1994.

132. Miller NE, Forde OM, Thelle DS: for The Tromso Heart Study. High-density lipoproteins and coronary heart disease. A prospective case control study. *Lancet* 1:965, 1977.

133. Gordon T, Castelli WP, Hjortland MC, et al: High density lipoprotein as a protective factor against coronary heart disease: The Framingham Study. *Am J Med* 62:707, 1977.

134. Badimon JJ, Badimon L, Galvez A, et al: High density lipoprotein plasma fractions inhibit aortic fatty streaks in cholesterol-fed rabbits. *Lab Invest* 60:455, 1989.

135. Beitz A, Beitz J: Antiatherosclerotic potency of high density lipoprotein of different origins: A review and some new findings. *Prostaglandins Leukot Essent Fatty Acids* 58(3):221, 1998.

136. Kazuhiro O, Davis A, Chan L: Recent advances in liver-directed gene therapy: implications for the treatment of dyslipidemia. *Curr Opin Lipidol* 11:176, 2000.

137. Lehrman S: Virus treatment questioned after gene therapy death. *Nature* 401:517, 1999.

138. Kockanek S: High-capacity adenoviral vectors for gene transfer and somatic gene therapy. *Hum Gene Ther* 10:2451, 1999.

139. Herz J, Gerard R: Adenovirus-mediated transfer of low density lipoprotein receptor gene acutely accelerates cholesterol clearance in normal mice. *Proc Natl Acad Sci U S A* 90:2812, 1993.

140. Kass-Eisler A, Falck-Pedersen E, Elfenbein D, et al: The impact of developmental stage, route of administration and the immune system on adenovirus-mediated gene transfer. *Gene Ther* 1:395, 1994.

141. Yang Y, Nunes F, Berencsi K, et al: Cellular immunity to viral antigens limits E1-deleted adenoviruses for gene therapy. *Proc Natl Acad Sci U S A* 91:4407, 1994.

142. Stein C, Martins I, Davidson B: Long-term reversal of hypercholesterolemia in low density lipoprotein receptor (LDLR)-deficient mice by adenovirus-mediated LDLR gene transfer combined with CD154 blockade. *J Gene Med* 2:41, 2000.

143. Desurmont C, Caillaud J-M, Emmanuel F, et al: Complete atherosclerosis regression after human apoE gene transfer in apoE-deficient/nude mice. *Arterioscler Thromb Vasc Biol* 20:435, 2000.

144. Plump A, Smith J, Hayek T, et al: Severe hypercholesterolemia and atherosclerosis in apolipoprotein-e-deficient mice created by homologous recombination in ES cells. *Cell* 71:343, 1992.

145. Chong P, Bachenheimer B: Current, new and future treatments in dyslipidaemia and atherosclerosis. *Drugs* 60:55, 2000.

146. Stephenson J: New method to repair faulty genes stirs interest in chimeraplasty technique. *JAMA* 281:119, 1999.
147. Mahley R, Huang Y, Rall S: Pathogenesis of type III hyperlipoproteinemia (dysbetalipoproteinemia). Questions, quandaries, and paradoxes. *J Lipid Res* 40:1933, 1999.
148. Alexeev V, Yoon K: Stable and inheritable changes in genotype and phenotype of albino melanocytes induced by an RNA-DNA oligonucleotide. *Nat Biotechnol* 16:1343, 1998.
149. Kren B, Parashar B, Bandyopadhyay P, et al: Correction of the UDP-glucuronosyltransferase gene defect in the Gunn rat model of Crigler-Najjar syndrome type I with a chimeric oligonucleotide. *Proc Natl Acad Sci U S A* 96:10349, 1999.
150. Tagalakis A, Graham I, Riddell D, et al: Gene correction of the apolipoprotein (apo) E2 phenotype to wild-type apoE3 by in situ chimeraplasty. *J Biol Chem* 276:13226, 2001.
151. Gero S, Gergely J, Jakab L, et al: Inhibition of cholesterol atherosclerosis by immunization with β-lipoprotein (letter). *Lancet* 1:1119, 1961.
152. Bailey JM, Bright R, Tomar R: Immunization with synthetic cholesterol-ester antigen and induced atherosclerosis in rabbits. *Nature* 201:40, 1963.
153. Travis J: Army targets a potential vaccine against cholesterol. *Science* 262:1974, 1975.
154. Bailey JM, Right R, Tomar R, Butler J: Antiatherogenic effects of cholesterol vaccination. *Biochem Soc Trans* 22:433S, 1994.
155. Nilsson A, Calara F, Regnstrom J, et al: Immunization with homologous oxidized low-density lipoprotein reduces neointimal formation after balloon injury in hypercholesterolemia rabbits. *J Am Coll Cardiol* 30:1886, 1997.

PART IV

Special Topics

Use of Alternative/Complementary Medicine in Treating Cardiovascular Disease

Stephen T. Sinatra

William H. Frishman

Stephen J. Peterson

George Lin

For some physicians, complementary therapies as treatment interventions provide a more integrative approach to heart disease. But for others, alternative, unconventional, or "unorthodox" medicine is more often viewed as quackery masquerading as legitimate medicine. Nevertheless, alternative medicine has now become a prominent focus for patients/consumers in the orthodox medical system. For example, Americans spent an estimated $15.7 billion on nutritional supplements alone in the year 2000. In six public opinion surveys, researchers analyzed the responses of 1196 people comprising 235 "regular," 381 "sometimes," and 580 "never" users of dietary supplements. The researchers reported that considerable numbers of patients use dietary supplements without proof of efficacy or safety. The appropriate use and need for regulatory guidelines of these products have now become controversial issues for both patients and physicians.[1] Clearly, modern physicians need to listen to the voice of the public and at least try to become acquainted with alternative methods as part of their continuing medical education.[1a,b] This chapter looks at the scientific revelations as well as the scientific criticisms on the subject, including an evidence-based review of the existing literature on the use of alternative methods in treating cardiovascular disease.

A decade ago, Eisenberg et al.[2] estimated, from national survey data, that in a given year, roughly one-third of English-speaking adults in the United States reported using at least one form of alternative medicine, and one-third of these consulted alternative medicine providers. Those who went to providers of alternative medicine averaged 19 visits a year; paying about $27.60 per visit (not including books, herbs, dietary supplements, medical equipment, or other material), with a majority (55%) paying entirely out of pocket. In 1990, there were more visits to alternative medicine providers than to all primary care physicians (general and family practitioners, pediatricians, and specialties of internal medicine) combined.

Demographically, the use of alternative medicine in the United States is more prevalent among college-educated, non–African American persons between 25 and 49 years of age with annual incomes above $35,000 who live in the western United States. Alternative therapies are most frequently used for back problems, anxiety, headaches, chronic pain, and cancer or tumors.[2a,b] Relaxation techniques, chiropractic, and massage therapy are the most frequently used alternative therapies. Although most (83%) of those who have used alternative medicine for a serious medical condition were also being treated by a medical provider for the same condition, most patients (72%) who used alternative therapies did not inform their medical doctor. In 1997, an estimated 4 of 10 adults incorporated some form of alternative therapy, including herbal medicine, massage, and megavitamins. Startling revelations have also indicated that consumers made more visits to alternative medical practitioners—such as chiropractors, naturopaths, and massage therapists—than they did to primary care physicians: an estimated 629 million versus 386 million visits.[3]

Clearly, the use of alternative medicine is far higher than previously reported. Although most alternative therapies are relatively innocuous, some involve the use of pharmacologically active substances (e.g., herbal medicine, megavitamin therapy, and some folk remedies) that could complicate existing medical therapy or even harm patients. Historically, American medical schools did little to educate their students on complementary therapies; but more recently, 64% of American medical schools offered elective courses in this area.[4] Although an increasing number of physicians are becoming more comfortable with alternative medicine,[5] the widespread use of nutritional supplements with potential pharmacologic activities demands that all physicians not only inquire about their patient's use of alternative medicine but also educate themselves and their patients as to the potential harms and benefits of these remedies. The reluctance of patients to disclose their use of complementary medicines stems from fear of disapproval of these interventions by their physicians and from the belief that natural remedies are harmless.[6] Surveys also indicate that patients fail to discuss the use of dietary supplements with their health care providers because they believe that these practitioners know little or nothing about these products and may even be biased against them.[1]

Rather than dismissing a patient's highly motivated intentions toward health-conscious behaviors or refusing to prescribe for them out of fear of potential drug interactions, it behooves physicians to understand the range of complementary therapies available and when they can be safely integrated into conventional medicine. Thus, they may more effectively counsel their patients in a collaborative and more effective atmosphere of open communication. Physicians' knowledge of nutritional supplement intake is also critical to avoid potentially dangerous interactions with prescribed medication. For example, consider patients taking warfarin who are also ingesting nonprescribed natural blood thinners such as garlic, ginger, fish oil, ginkgo biloba, and even excessive amounts of vitamin E at the same time. Such a combination clearly poses potential risks for both patient and the physician!

This chapter limits its review to some of the pharmacologically active substances most commonly used or that have effects on the cardiovascular system based on the existing scientific literature. Although nonpharmacologic therapies—such as relaxation techniques, biofeedback, and meditation—are known to lower heart rate and blood pressure by decreasing the activity of the sympathetic nervous system, they are not covered here, as they are beyond the scope of this commentary. This chapter also pays particular attention to medicinal plants, which the authors accept to be pharmacologically active substances in a diluted form; however, three other alternative remedies (vitamins/minerals and other micronutrient supplements, homeopathy, and acupuncture) are also examined briefly, in this and in other chapters, since their mechanisms of action are either pharmacologic in nature or beyond the simple central nervous system control of the autonomic nervous system.

MEGAVITAMINS AND OTHER MICRONUTRIENT SUPPLEMENTS

Vitamins and minerals are required in trace amounts for normal bodily functioning. A number of people have subscribed to the notion that "more is better." Ingestion of micronutrient supplements (vitamins and minerals) beyond the "recommended daily allowances" (RDAs) is beneficial in certain deficiency states resulting from inadequate intake, disturbed absorption, or increased tissue requirements[7]; however, routine dietary supplementation of micronutrients in the absence of deficiency states and beyond what one can usually obtain from consumption of a well-balanced diet, has been shown to be of questionable benefit and in some cases may be harmful. Of course, there are exceptions. This section reviews micronutrient supplements with beneficial and harmful effects on the cardiovascular system (see Chap. 24).

THE RATIONALE FOR TARGETED NUTRITIONAL SUPPLEMENTS FOR CARDIOVASCULAR HEALTH

The heart, possessing approximately 5000 mitochondria per cell and functioning in a high-oxygen environment, is one of the most susceptible of all organs to free-radical oxidative stress. Fortunately, it is also highly responsive to the benefits of targeted nutritional agents, such as phytonutrients, antioxidants, and nutriceuticals.

The term *nutriceutical* includes a wide variety of nonprescription nutritional supplements normally found in the body or in natural sources (such as vitamins, amino acids, and herbals).[7a] Strong scientific evidence from large and repeated clinical trials have confirmed their efficacy and safety as well as guidelines for patient selection, dosage, and potential medication interactions.[8]

For example, fat-soluble vitamins (K, E, D, and A) are stored to a variable extent in the body and are more likely to cause adverse reactions than water-soluble vitamins, which are readily excreted in the urine. Excessive vitamin K can cause hemolysis in persons with glucose-6-phosphate dehydrogenase (G6PD) deficiency and anemia (with Heinz bodies), hyperbilirubinemia, and kernicterus

in newborns[9]; moreover, vitamin K can counter the effects of oral anticoagulants by conferring biologic activity on prothrombin and factors VII, IX, and X.[10,11]

Vitamin E

On the other hand, high doses of vitamin E may potentiate the effects of oral anticoagulants by antagonizing vitamin K and prolonging prothrombin time. On the benefit side, vitamin E's antioxidant and anticoagulant properties may offer protection against myocardial infarction and thrombotic strokes. A recent extensive review article assessed the preventive effects of vitamin E on the development of atherosclerosis.[12] Alpha tocopherols are the key lipid-soluble, chain-breaking antioxidants found in tissues and plasma. Oxidation of unsaturated fatty acids in LDL particles, as a pivotal factor in atherogenesis, is widely recognized. Vitamin E, a predominant antioxidant present in the LDL particle, blocks the chain reaction of lipid peroxidation by scavenging intermediate peroxyl radicals.[12,13] Vitamin E supplementation can reduce lipid peroxidation by as much as 40%.[14] Stabilizing plaque, reducing inflammation, decreasing thrombolytic aggregation, reducing the expression of adhesion molecules on the arterial wall, and enhancing vasodilation are key cardioprotective effects of vitamin E.[12,15] However, prospective controlled clinical trials have presented a confusing picture.

The Alpha Tocopherol, Beta Carotene (ATBC) Cancer Prevention Study, a randomized double-blind, placebo-controlled trial involving 29,133 male smokers ages 50 to 69 with a median follow-up of 4.7 years, showed a minor but statistically significant decrease in angina pectoris with vitamin E supplementation of 50 mg per day [relative risk (RR) = 0.91].[16] A nonsignificant (8%) reduction in mortality rate from coronary artery disease was also realized.[12]

In the Cambridge Heart Antioxidant Study (CHAOS), patients with atherosclerosis who received 400 to 800 U of vitamin E daily appreciated a 77% decrease in the relative risk of nonfatal MI[17]; however, there was a nonsignificant increase in death from cardiovascular disease.[12] The Heart Outcomes Prevention Evaluation (HOPE)[18] and the initial GISSI Prevenzioni data[19] failed to establish a clear benefit; however, one researcher's reevaluation of GISSI showed a 20% reduced risk of cardiovascular death.[20]

On the other hand, in one of the investigations of patients with a history of myocardial infarction (MI), mortality was higher when vitamin E was combined with beta carotene.[21] In the most recent review of the major five human trials on vitamin E supplementation—including the ATBC, CHAOS, GISSI, SPACE, and HOPE trials—a statistical reanalysis of the data, including the totality of the evidence, suggests that alpha tocopherol supplementation does not have a place in treating patients with preexisting cardiovascular disease.[20] However it is important to keep in mind that the oxidative modification of low-density lipoprotein (LDL)-cholesterol is only a hypothesis and has yet to be proven,[22] which raises the question of whether or not cardiologists should routinely recommend vitamin E to their patients. In two large prospective Harvard studies (Nurses' Health Study[23] and the Health Professional Study[24]) involving approximately 87,000 women and 40,000 men, investigators attributed reductions in heart disease and stroke to vitamin E rather than other unidentified factors. In another investigation of men with documented coronary heart disease, 100 U or more of vitamin E per day was correlated with decreased progression of coronary artery lesions compared to untreated counterparts.[25] In this study of 156 men 40 to 59 years old with a history of coronary artery bypass surgery, supplemental vitamin E intake was associated with angiographically proven reduction in progression of coronary artery lesions.[25]

Considering the many longitudinal epidemiologic studies and prospective randomized trials in which vitamin E consumption was associated with decreased cardiac risk, it is probably safe to say that some vitamin E supplementation could be considered for those individuals at high risk for coronary artery disease (CAD) or with documented CAD, however, there are no definitive data to support such an approach.[20] In addition, the rationale for vitamin E supplementation in healthy individuals is still open to question. In one investigation into the effects of vitamin E on lipid peroxidation in healthy individuals, vitamin E was supplied as d-alpha-tocopherol capsules. Increased circulating vitamin E levels were not associated with any change in three urinary indices of lipid peroxidation.[26] It would be interesting to note whether administration of a combination of mixed tocopherols and gamma tocopherols would have made any difference in the analysis of lipid peroxidation.

Whenever vitamin E supplements are being considered, gamma tocopherol should be included in the basic formula. Alpha tocopherol in the absence of a gamma tocopherol may be ineffective in inhibiting the oxidative damage caused by the reactive peroxynitrite radicals and, in larger doses, alpha tocopherol can displace gamma tocopherol in plasma.[27,28] Gamma tocopherol can also be obtained in the diet in the form of healthy nuts, such as almonds, sunflower seeds, wheat germ, and wheat germ oil. Vitamin E (alpha tocopherol) and mixed tocopherols, including tocotrienols (other derivatives of vitamin E), may be the best combination of tocopherol biochemistry and may play an even greater role in modifying the oxidation of LDL.[28,29]

Natural forms of vitamin E, but not synthetic, also help to reduce platelet aggregability. In studies looking at healthy volunteers, researchers measured how well platelet cells absorb d-alpha tocopherol, d-alpha tocopherol acetate (both natural forms), and d-l-alpha tocopherol (synthetic form). The research showed that platelets effectively absorbed d-alpha tocopherol acetate and d-alpha tocopherol but not synthetic vitamin E. Both forms of natural vitamin E reduced platelet aggregation by more than 50%, while no significant change was associated with synthetic vitamin E. The researchers determined that vitamin E's anticoagulant effect was unrelated to its antioxidant properties. Vitamin E's anticoagulant effect appears to result from its inhibition of protein kinase C, an enzyme that facilitates blood clotting.[30]

Vitamin E has also been shown to significantly lower levels of C-reactive protein and monocyte interleukin-6, culprits that can also contribute to atherogenesis.[31] Vitamin E is the least toxic of the fat-soluble vitamins, rarely causing adverse reactions even at doses 20 to 80 times the recommended daily requirement taken for extended periods of time. However, malaise, gastrointestinal (GI) complaints, headache, and even hypertension have been reported,[10] and parenteral vitamin E, which has been withdrawn from the market, has been shown to cause pulmonary deterioration, thrombocytopenia, and liver and renal failure in several premature infants.[9]

Previous investigations also suggest that plasma levels of antioxidants like vitamins E and C are a more sensitive predictor of unstable angina than severity of atheroslcerosis.[32] The fact that free-radical activity has been noted to influence the degree of coronary ischemia and spasm[33] suggests that the beneficial effects of antioxidants in patients with CAD may result in part from a favorable influence on vascular reactivity rather than a reduction in atherosclerotic plaque. Results of randomized double-blind, placebo-controlled clinical trials have also indicated that vitamins E and C can prevent nitrate intolerance,[34,35] a major problem for patients who require

long-term treatment with high-dose oral nitrates for relief of anginal symptoms.

Investigational research suggests that nitrate intolerance is associated with increased vascular production of superoxides.[36] When nitric oxide is released during metabolism of nitroglycerin, it reacts with superoxide anions, resulting in lower levels of cyclic guanosine monophosphate, an important intracellular intermediary that promotes vasorelaxation. There are key vitamins that warrant attention for the prevention of nitrate intolerance, including vitamin E, the main lipid-phase antioxidant, and vitamin C, the main aqueous-phase antioxidant. Supplementation with these nutrients boosts the free-radical scavenging ability of the superoxide radical, promoting the prevention of nitrate intolerance. As the primary aqueous antioxidant, vitamin C—the major antioxidant in the aqueous phase—acts as the first line of defense against oxidative stress.

Vitamin C

Vitamin C is not only a scavenger antioxidant but also acts synergistically with vitamin E to reduce the peroxyl radical. In addition to blocking lipid peroxidation by trapping peroxyl radicals in the aqueous phase, vitamin C helps normalize endothelial vasodilative function in patients with heart failure by increasing the availability of nitric oxide.[37] Although the evidence linking vitamin C to human cardiovascular disease is still being evaluated, one study did report that vitamin C slowed the progression of atherosclerosis in men and women older than 55 years.[38] It is also well known that many groups known to be at an increased risk for CAD have lower blood levels of vitamin C, such as men, the elderly, smokers, patients with diabetes, patients with hypertension, and possibly women taking oral estrogen contraceptives.[39] In a recent large, prospective population study, British researchers evaluated the health of almost 20,000 people ages 45 to 79 over 4 years. They found that men and women consuming about 109 to 113 mg of vitamin C daily had about half the risk of death of those consuming only 51 to 57 mg of vitamin C per day. Higher blood levels of vitamin C were directly and inversely related to death from all causes and specifically death from ischemic heart disease in both men and women. The researchers strongly advocated modest consumption of fruits and vegetables, since their results suggested that the equivalent of one extra serving of vitamin C–rich food reduced the risk of death by 20%.[40] However, carotenoids, flavonoids, magnesium, and other health-promoting nutrients affected these data.[40] Because improved endothelial function has been observed with the administration of vitamin C in patients with hypertension, hypercholesterolemia, and diabetes mellitus, some vitamin C supplementation appears warranted.[41] Vitamin C at daily doses of 500 mg has been shown to increase red cell glutathione by 50%.[42] Glutathione is not only the major antioxidant responsible for inhibiting lipid peroxidation but also a key contributing agent in stabilizing immune function.

Megadose vitamin C (>500 mg a day) in patients who are vulnerable to iron overload states should be avoided. Vitamin C supplements may exacerbate iron toxicity by mobilizing iron reserves. Such patients may accumulate harmful excess iron with higher doses of vitamin C, so caution must be employed for those with genetic diseases such as hereditary hemochromatosis, thalassemia major, or other diseases that promote iron overload.[43]

Carotenoids

Serum carotenoids have been extensively studied in the prevention of coronary heart disease. There are approximately 600 carotenoids found in nature, predominantly in fresh fruits and vegetables, with carrots being the primary source of beta carotene and tomatoes being the best source of lycopene. Although lycopene has twice the antioxidant activity of beta carotene, the latter has been the primary focus of study because of its activity as a precursor to vitamin A.

Elevated levels of serum beta carotene have been associated with a lower risk of cancer and overall mortality.[44] However, inconsistent data from randomized clinical trials regarding both beta carotene's antioxidant properties on LDL in vitro[45-47] and its preventive actions on cardiovascular disease cast doubt on the beneficial effects of beta carotene supplementation.

Research has associated a high dietary intake of beta carotene with a reduction in the incidence of cardiovascular disease.[48] One study reported that increased beta carotene stores in subcutaneous fat were correlated with a decreased risk of MI.[49]

However, controlled studies have found that excessive supplemental beta carotene failed to lead to a reduction in rates of lung cancer or cardiovascular disease among heavy smokers.[50] An increased incidence of lung cancer was found in the beta carotene and retinal efficacy trial,[51] halting the study 21 months early when this alarming cancer rate was observed among smokers and workers exposed to asbestos. Similarly, after the Physician's Health Trial[52] demonstrated that alternate-day administration of 50 mg of beta carotene for 12 years showed no positive effects on coronary heart disease events, the enthusiasm for beta carotene as a preventive intervention for cardiovascular disease declined. The male participants in the Physician's Health Study did benefit from a lower risk of prostate cancer if their beta carotene status was low at the beginning of the study. Researchers suggested that beta carotene in moderate concentrations significantly inhibits the growth of three prostate cancer lines in culture medium.[53]

The use of excess synthetic beta carotene, as done in the ATBC and the beta carotene and retinal efficacy trials,[50,51] should be avoided in any high-risk populations because there are yet unidentified elements that may somehow affect cancer growth in vulnerable individuals. It is safer and more efficacious to take is a mixed natural supplement combination of mixed carotenoids including beta carotene, lutein, lycopene, alpha carotene, and beta cryptoxanthin. Beta carotene is responsible for only an estimated 25% of total serum carotenoid activity. Perhaps the lower mortality associated with higher levels of baseline serum beta carotene had more to do with long-term dietary habits of individuals who eat more fruits and vegetables containing multiple carotenoids than with artificial elevation of serum beta carotenes with supplementation. Excessive carotene ingestion is relatively innocuous and results in yellowing of the skin, particularly on the palms and soles but sparing the sclerae. Hypothyroid patients are more susceptible to carotenemia.[10]

The other carotenoids, such as lutein, that enter the LDL and high-density lipoprotein (HDL) particles may retard CAD by their favorable effects on LDL oxidation. In the Toulouse Study,[54] those participants with greater lutein activity in their blood had a lower incidence of CAD. Some researchers consider the lutein found in a diet rich in green and yellow fruits and vegetables to be more responsible for the inhibition of CAD than the red wine benefit referred to as the "French paradox."

Flavonoids

Residents of France—whose diet is steeped in high-fat cheeses, rich sauces, gravies, patés, and other highly-saturated fats—have a lower incidence of coronary heart disease than their American counterparts. This paradoxical situation challenges the belief that a low-fat diet is protective against heart disease. Offsetting the "risk" that we see in the typical French diet is the routine consumption of fresh fruits and vegetables that contain vital phytonutrients, including tocopherols, carotenoids (especially lutein), flavonoids (quercetin), phenols, catechins, and other phytonutrients that may effectively reduce peroxidative tendencies and retard the varied interactions involved in atherogenesis and thrombosis.[55] Red wine consumption could be another factor.

The serum antioxidant activity of red wine was addressed in a small study of volunteers, the results indicating that two glasses of red wind consumed before a meal offered considerable antioxidant protection for at least 4 h.[56] Red wine increased antioxidant activity through a flavonoid-polyphenol effect. In another small investigation performed in the Netherlands, the use of dietary bioflavonoids, phenolic acids, and quercetin showed a reduction in the incidence of heart attack and sudden death.[57] The findings in 64- to 85-year old men showed an inverse relationship between the amount of quercetin ingested and mortality. Quercetin-rich black tea, apples, and onions were the best foods evaluated, as they contain polyphenols in amounts similar to those found in the red grapes used in making wine and grape juice.

A recent study with grape juice in normal volunteers demonstrated favorable effects on platelet aggregation, platelet-derived nitric oxide release, and free oxygen-derived free radical production.[57a] Short- and long-term consumption of black tea was shown to reverse endothelial vasomotor dysfunction in patients with CAD.[58]

Oligomeric proanthocyanidins (OPCs), like carotenoids, are found predominantly in brightly colored fruits and vegetables and represent a safe source of polyphenols and quercetin, which are believed to be the most active protective ingredients in preventing the oxidation of LDL. OPCs are significant free-radical scavengers that inhibit lipid peroxidation and contain anti-inflammatory and antiallergenic properties as well.[59]

Magnesium

Magnesium has a profound influence on coronary vascular tone and reactivity; deficiencies have been shown to produce spasm of the coronary vasculature, pointing to the low-magnesium state as a possible risk factor in nonocclusive MI (see Chap. 12). Hypomagnesemia can result in progressive vasoconstriction, coronary spasm, and even sudden death.[60] In anginal episodes due to coronary artery spasm, treatment with magnesium has been shown to be considerably efficacious.[61]

Magnesium deficiency, which is better detected by mononuclear blood cell magnesium than the standard serum level performed at most hospitals, predisposes to excessive mortality and morbidity in patients with acute MI.[62] Several studies have shown an association between intravenous magnesium supplementation during the first hour of admission for MI and reductions in both morbidity and mortality.[63] Although other trials of magnesium therapy in patients with acute MI have produced inconsistent results, the most efficacious use of magnesium, like thrombolytics, occurs with the earliest administration.[64] Multiple cardioprotective and physiologic activities of magnesium include antiarrhythmic effects, calcium channel–blocking effects, improvement in nitric oxide release from coronary endothelium, and the ability to help prevent serum coagulation, to name a few.[64]

Research into the inhibition of platelet-dependent thrombosis indicates that magnesium may have a positive preventive role for patients with CAD. In one double-blind, placebo-controlled study of 42 patients, median platelet-dependent thrombosis was reduced by 35% in 75% of patients receiving oral administration of magnesium oxide tablets (800–1200 mg daily) for 3 months.[65] This antithrombotic effect occurred despite the use of aspirin therapy in the study population.

Magnesium has also shown considerable efficacy in relieving symptoms of mitral valve prolapse (MVP). In a double-blind study of 181 participants, serum magnesium levels were assessed in 141 patients with symptomatic MVP and compared to those of 40 healthy control subjects; decreased serum magnesium levels were identified in 60% of the patients with MVP, while only 5% of control subjects showed similar decreases.[66] The second leg of the study investigated response to treatment. Subjective results in the magnesium group were dramatic, with significant reductions noted in weakness, chest pain, shortness of breath, palpitations, and even anxiety. Lower levels of epinephrine metabolites were also found in the urine. For patients with MVP, magnesium supplementation offers a reduction in symptomatology and improvement in quality of life. Blood pressure lowering with magnesium, especially when combined with calcium and potassium, has also been reported.[67] Supplemental magnesium and potassium should be avoided in patients with renal insufficiency.

Trace Minerals and the Heart

Cobaltous chloride is sometimes used in the treatment of iron deficiency and chronic renal failure.[9] Excessive cobalt intake may cause cardiomyopathy and congestive heart failure (CHF), with pericardial effusions due to deposition of cobalt-lipoic acid complexes in the heart.[10] High cobalt consumption has also been implicated in thyroid enlargement, polycythemia, neurologic abnormalities, and interference with pyruvate and fatty acid metabolism. Rarely, excessive iron ingestion may cause cardiomyopathy, CHF, and cardiac arrhythmias from hemochromatosis.[68]

Chromium assists in glucose and lipid metabolism. It may bring about regression of cholesterol-induced atherosclerosis.[69] In a double-blind study involving 34 male athletes with elevated cholesterol levels, supplementation with 200 μg of elemental chromium (chromium as niacin-bound chromium complex) significantly lowered serum cholesterol by an average of 14%.[70] In a more recent study of 40 hypercholesterolemic patients (total cholesterol 210–300 mg/dL), a combination of 200 μg of chromium polynicotinate (Cr) and (proanthocyanidin) grape-seed extract (GSE) 100 mg twice daily resulted in profound lowering of LDL and total cholesterol. However, there was no significant change in either HDL or triglyceride level in either the treatment or the placebo group.[71] Since insulin resistance may be the major factor in disturbed lipid metabolism, chromium's favorable action on glucose/insulin metabolism may be the key factor in cholesterol lowering.[72,73] Although no significant adverse reactions from chromium polynicotinate have been observed at the dose of 400 μg per day, massive ingestion of chromium has been associated with renal failure.[9]

Selenium is an antioxidant with immune-enhancing and cancer-fighting properties. In some areas of the world, soil deficiencies in selenium have produced Keshan disease, a disorder of cardiac muscle characterized by multifocal myocardial necrosis that causes cardiomyopathy, CHF, and cardiac arrhythmias.[10] Men with low levels of serum selenium (<1.4 μmol/L) demonstrated increased thickness in the intima and media of the common carotid arteries.[74] Selenium, when combined with coenzyme Q10, may also offer cardioprotective benefits in patients after MI. In one study of 61 patients admitted for an acute MI,[75] 32 subjects in the experimental group received 100 mg of coenzyme Q10 with 500 μg of selenium in the first 24 h of hospitalization followed by daily doses of 100 mg of coenzyme Q10, 100 μg of selenium, 15 mg of zinc, 1 mg of vitamin A, 2 mg of vitamin B$_6$, 90 mg of vitamin C, and 15 mg vitamin E for 1 year. The control group (29 patients) received placebo for the same time period. During their hospital stay, none of the participants in the experimental group showed prolongation of the QT interval, compared to 40% of the control subjects, whose QTC increased 440 milliseconds (about a 10% increase). Although there were no significant differences in early complications between the two groups, 6 (21%) patients in the control group died of recurrent MI, whereas only 1 patient in the study group (3%) died a noncardiac death.[75] Although selenium is quite safe at levels below 200 μg, excessive selenium can result in alopecia, abnormal nails, emotional lability, lassitude, and a garlic odor to the breath.[67] Skin lesions and polyneuritis have been reported in people taking selenium from health food stores.[9]

Copper is a prooxidant that oxidizes LDL and may contribute to the development of atherosclerosis. Men with high serum copper (>17.6 μmol/L) demonstrate increased thickening in the intima and media of the common carotid arteries.[74] Excessive oral intake of copper may cause nausea, vomiting, diarrhea, and hemolytic anemia. Even higher doses can result in renal and hepatic toxicity as well as central nervous system (CNS) disturbances similar to those of Wilson's disease.[10] Any multivitamin with higher than the RDA level of copper (2 mg) should be avoided. Excessive levels of copper in drinking water, especially noted in homes with copper pipes, can also contribute to elevated serum copper levels.

B Vitamins

Clinical cardiologists must be familiar with B vitamin support for their patients. B vitamin depletion commonly occurs as a result of high-dose diuretic therapy used in the treatment of CHF[76] and should be considered in any patient with refractory CHF that is unresponsive to high-dose diuretic therapy. The nocturnal leg cramps associated with diuretic therapy are a hallmark symptom of B vitamin depletion. The involuntary, painful contraction of the calf muscles and other areas of the leg can be alleviated with B vitamin support, resulting in an improved quality of life. A randomized placebo-controlled double-blind study,[77] validated the efficacy of B complex supplementation in the treatment of nocturnal cramps. Of 28 elderly patients, 86% taking vitamin B complex reported remission of prominent symptoms, compared to no benefit in the placebo group.

Most cardiologists are now familiar with the clinical significance of providing B vitamin supplementation to lower hyperhomocysteinemia (see Chap. 23). In 1969, Kilmer McCully[78] first proposed the homocysteine hypothesis, identifying accelerated vascular pathology as a sequela to homocysteinuria, a rare autosomal recessive disease caused by a deficiency in cystathione B-synthetase. Several investigations have confirmed his proposed connection between high plasma homocysteine levels and occlusive arterial disease, including atherosclerosis, peripheral vascular disease, and CAD.[79–85]

Hyperhomocysteinemia may be even more detrimental in women. In one study, women with coronary disease had higher homocysteine levels than matched control subjects.[86] In a study comparing men and women with high homocysteine levels, women demonstrated greater carotid thickening ratios than their male counterparts.[85] In another study involving postmenopausal women, high homocysteine levels in combination with hypertension resulted in an alarming 25 times higher incidence of stroke.[87]

The actual mechanism of action in homocysteine-associated endothelial damage remains unclear. The fact that the injury may be inhibited by the addition of catalase suggests that the process may be the result of free-radical oxidative stress. This theory is strengthened by the fact that free-radical hydrogen peroxide is generated during the oxidation of homocysteine.[88] Homocysteine also enhances thromboxane A_2 and platelet aggregation[89] and increases the binding of lipoprotein Lp(a) and fibrin.[90] Because the association between homocysteine and atherothrombotic vascular events has been shown to be consistent regardless of other factors, high levels of homocysteine are a significant marker for atherothrombotic vascular disease. The relationship between high homocysteine and degree of myocardial injury was studied in 390 consecutive patients who presented with acute coronary syndromes; 205 with MI and 185 with unstable angina. In a multivariate analysis, a homocysteine level in the top quintile (>15.7 μg/L) was an excellent predictor of possible peak cardiac protein troponin T level in patients with acute coronary syndromes and an even stronger predictor in those with unstable angina. The researchers suggest that homocysteine has a causal prothrombotic effect and indicate that further study is needed to assess homocysteine-lowering therapy.[91] Since enzymatic deficiencies occur in as many as 5% of the population[92] and 28% of patients with premature vascular disease have high blood levels of homocysteine,[93] screening for this lethal risk factor should be considered. Should future randomized trials correlate homocysteine lowering with a significant reduction in vascular events, supplementation with B complex therapy must be strongly considered for patients with elevated homocysteine levels.[94]

Certainly, administration of B vitamins at the recommended daily allowance levels (folic acid = 400 μg; B_6 = 2 mg; B_{12} = 6 μg) is safe and can be recommended routinely. Research shows a dose-dependent relationship between higher homocysteine levels and lower serum levels of B vitamins, so much higher doses must be administered to those patients with severe hyperhomocysteinemia and documented CAD.[94,95] It is also encouraging to note that the U.S. Food and Drug Administration (FDA) has required that enriched grains be fortified with folic acid at a concentration that provides the average individual with an extra 100 μg of folic acid per day.

A potential hazard of folic acid therapy is subacute degeneration of the spinal cord with a subclinical vitamin B_{12} deficiency; folic acid may mask the development of hematologic manifestations in these patients.[94] This situation can be avoided by either ruling out B_{12} deficiency before initiating folic acid therapy or by supplementing folic acid with vitamin B_{12}.[94]

High-dose niacin (vitamin B_3) is used in the treatment of hyperlipidemia and hypercholesterolemia (see Chap. 20) and helps curb the development of atherosclerosis.[96] Side effects include cutaneous flushing, pruritus, GI disturbances, exacerbation of asthma, and even acanthosis nigricans. Very high doses can cause liver toxicity.[10] Vasodilation and flushing, the most common side effect of niacin, may help patients who suffer from Raynaud's phenomenon.

In an attempt to find a safer form of niacin with less side effects, investigators have discovered a new, extended-release, once-daily formulation of niacin (Niaspan).[97] This slowly metabolized form of niacin does not reach maximum serum levels for several hours after ingestion, resulting in fewer and less severe side effects.[97,98] Randomized, double-blind, placebo-controlled investigations showed that sustained-released niacin had an impact in decreasing LDL-cholesterol, total cholesterol, and triglycerides while raising HDL-cholesterol at the same time.[97–99]

Niaspan and niacin also play a significant role in reducing lipoprotein Lp(a), a serious risk factor in atherogenesis. In one small study of patients with lipoprotein Lp(a) concentrations greater than 30 mg/dL, the ingestion of 1 g of niacin three times daily demonstrated reduction in lipid levels, with the level of lipoprotein Lp(a) showing the greatest reduction (36.4%).[100]

Coenzyme Q10

Coenzyme Q10 (see Chap. 37), present in most foods, especially organ meats and fish, facilitates electron transport in oxidative metabolism.[101] Its reduced form, ubiquinol, protects membrane phospholipids and serum LDLs from lipid peroxidation as well as mitochondrial membrane proteins and DNA from free radical–induced oxidative damage.[102] Ubiquinol's antioxidant effects on membrane phospholipids and LDL directly antagonizes the atherogenesis process. Vitamin E regeneration is significantly improved by the addition of coenzyme Q10 because of the latter's ability to recycle the oxidized form of vitamin E back to its reduced form. Coenzyme Q10 also prevents the prooxidant effect of alpha tocopherols.[103] Supplemental coenzyme Q may also improve utilization of oxygen at the cellular level, hence benefiting patients with coronary insufficiency.[75,104]

Perhaps coenzyme Q10's most remarkable effects involve tissue protection in the setting of myocardial ischemia and reperfusion.[105–107] The results of a controlled study of patients with acute MI demonstrated reduction in free-radical indices, infarct size, arrhythmia, and cardiac death in those patients receiving coenzyme Q10.[108] Although side effects of coenzyme Q10, such as nausea and abdominal discomfort, are rare,[101] it is not suggested for healthy pregnant or lactating women, as the unborn and the newborn both produce sufficient quantities of the compound.

However, statin drugs cause profound deficiencies in coenzyme Q10, because HMG-CoA reductase inhibitors (statins) block the endogenous production of coenzyme Q10.[109] Coenzyme Q10 treatment has been used successfully to counteract the side effect of myalgia associated with statin therapy.

L-Carnitine

L-carnitine (see Chap. 37) has a synergistic relationship with coenzyme Q10, as it also penetrates the inner mitochondrial membrane. As a trimethylated amino acid, L-carnitine's primary function is in the oxidation of fatty acids. Supplemental L-carnitine has a wide application in cardiovascular disease.

Omega-3 Fatty Acids

Omega-3 fatty acids—such as eicosapentaenoic acid (EPA) and docosahexaenoic acid (DHA)—are found in fish oils (see Chap. 23). They stimulate the production of nitric oxide, which relaxes vascular smooth muscle. Their actions can counteract the impairment of nitric oxide production that is caused by atherosclerotic plaques.[110] In addition, consumption of eicosapentaenoic acid stimulates the production of prostaglandin I_3, an antithrombotic and anti-platelet-aggregating agent similar to prostacyclin. As an anticoagulant, omega-3 fatty acids can increase bleeding time, inhibit platelet adhesiveness, decrease platelet count, and reduce serum thromboxane levels.[111–113] Omega-3 fatty acids can also blunt the vasopressor effects of angiotensin II and norepinephrine and may reduce blood pressure.[111,114,115]

In one recent placebo-controlled trial, an average systolic reduction of 5 mm Hg and a mean diastolic decrease of 3 mm Hg was realized in those participants taking DHA.[116] The triglyceride-lowering effect of these fish oil components may be one of many factors that inhibit the progression of atherosclerosis.[113–115] There are conflicting data from studies regarding the role of omega-3 fatty acids in the reduction of arterial restenosis after coronary angioplasty.[117,118]

In a recent landmark decision, the FDA reported that it would allow products containing omega-3 fatty acids to claim heart health benefits. The FDA based its decision on the wealth of scientific evidence that suggests a correlation between omega-3 fatty acids such as EPA and DHA and a reduced risk of CAD. In the GISSI-Prevenzione trial,[19] Italian investigators reported overwhelming health benefits for participants who were placed on 1 g of omega-3 essential fatty acids a day. After the initial study had been reevaluated, participants on the omega-3 program experienced a 20% reduction in all-cause mortality and a 45% decrease in sudden cardiac death.[119] One case-controlled study showed that those participants eating the equivalent of one fish meal a week had a 50% less chance of sudden cardiac death compared to counterparts whose daily menus did not contain these vital fish oils.[120]

A recent National Institutes of Health (NIH) conference on fatty acids concluded that there is now sufficient evidence of the importance of omega-3 in the diet to recommend 220 mg of DHA per day as an adequate intake (AI) for adults and 300 mg per day for pregnant and lactating females.[121] Attaining this proposed recommendation will require an approximate fourfold increase in omega-3 fatty acid consumption in the United States.[122] Although side effects of fish oils are mostly abdominal upset or burping, excessive intake (greater than 6 g daily of omega-3 fatty acids) may interfere with the effects of oral anticoagulants.

HOMEOPATHY

Homeopathy is a healing system dating back to the 18th Century created by Samuel Christian Hahnemann, a German physician who lost faith in conventional allopathic medicine. He began his investigation around 1785 and by 1810 was 45 years old and practicing homeopathic medicine. Hahnemann based homeopathy on three laws: (1) the law of similars, (2) the law of infinitesimals, and (3) the law of chronic suppressions or law of chronic disease. The law of similars states that a substance that induces complaints in a healthy person resembling the symptoms of the patient can be used to cure the patient. A similar concept is employed in allopathic medicine in the form of vaccination and allergy desensitization. The law of chronic suppressions or chronic disease suggests that in a chronic patient, only his or her disease or syndrome is treated instead of the whole patient. If the treatment of the disease or syndrome is successful, it often happens that a more profound and vital organ may start showing evidence of disease.[123] Diseases that are refractory to therapy are a result of conditions that have been driven

deep into the body by allopathic medicine. This concept is difficult to prove and has generated much controversy, even among homeopaths.

However, the most difficult notion for allopathic physicians to accept is the law of infinitesimals. It states that the more dilute the remedy, the stronger and more potent it becomes when it is combined with a certain shaking technique. Dilutions above 10^{-24} are unlikely to contain even a single molecule of the original substance. Nevertheless, many homeopathic remedies start near 10^{-24} dilution and many solutions go far beyond, even as much as $10^{-20,000}$

Thus, even though homeopathic medicine prepares its medicine by starting initially with a substance, the final product may contain little if any trace of the original substance. Homeopaths concede that many of their medicines may contain no molecules of the original substance but say that their method of succussion (this being the combination of shaking and dilution) leaves some sort of "imprint" on the solvent. Existing physical and chemical laws dictate that a substance diluted beyond 10^{-24} is no more active than placebo. To accept homeopathic theory as the truth would require scientists and physicians to revise long-established laws of physics and chemistry—something most allopathic physicians are unwilling to do.[123a]

Numerous controlled trials have been conducted on homeopathic remedies showing both positive (significant difference between drug and placebo)[124] and negative (no significant difference between drug and placebo)[125] results. One study, however, performed a meta-analysis of 107 controlled trials and weighed them on the basis of scientific methodology.[126] The result showed a positive trend in favor of homeopathy, although the review may have been complicated by the publication bias of certain journals to trials with positive results. In a subsequent analysis combining the data of 89 studies, the authors felt that while there was insufficient evidence that homeopathy is effective for any single clinical situation, the evidence was "not compatible with the hypothesis that the clinical effects are completely due to placebo."[127] In an updated review, two of the same authors looked at 32 trials and continued to conclude that although their methodologic quality was still variable, the case of homeopathy was less convincing. However, overall, homeopathy was statistically significant in relation to placebo.[128] If homeopathic remedies actually do work better than placebos, their pharmacologic mechanisms are unknown.

ACUPUNCTURE

Acupuncture, a drugless therapy that is part of traditional chinese medicine (TCM), consists of stimulation of designated points on the skin by insertion of needles followed by the application of heat, massage, or both. While the main purpose of acupuncture in TCM is to affect body energetics, the primary uses of acupuncture in the West are for relief of chronic pain and management of drug addiction.

However, in 1997, an NIH conference found clear evidence that needle acupuncture is especially effective in postoperative and chemotherapy-induced nausea as well as postoperative dental discomfort.[129] The consensus also stated that although inconclusive, there was promising evidence to support the use of acupuncture for several other medical conditions including back pain, asthma, stroke rehabilitation, fibromyalgia, carpal tunnel syndrome, osteoarthritis, and myofascial pain as well as for the management of addictive disorders.

In one small randomized controlled trial of auricular acupuncture for cocaine dependence, the acupuncture group tested negative for all three urine tests in the final week of the study, suggesting that acupuncture may have a positive effect on this addiction.[130]

Acupuncture's mechanism of action is thought to involve at least two pathways. First, the gate-control theory of pain introduced by Melzack and Wall[131] explains that stimulation of low-threshold myelinated nociceptive afferents (Aa/AB fibers) near the skin can activate inhibitory interneurons, which then suppress projection neurons that relay signals to the brain, thereby reducing the perception of pain. Second, acupuncture may be mediated by the body's endogenous endorphins, based on increasing evidence that acupuncture analgesia can be blocked by naloxone, an opiate-receptor antagonist.[132–134] By these mechanisms, acupuncture may also reduce heart rate and blood pressure by increasing the pain threshold during physical activity and lowering the activity of the sympathetic nervous system.[135] More research is needed to determine whether acupuncture has any long-term potential in affecting the cardiovascular system.[135a,b]

HERBAL MEDICINE

Since the beginning of human civilization, herbs have been an integral part of society, valued for their culinary and medicinal properties. However, with the development of patent medicines in the early part of the twentieth century, herbal medicine lost ground to new synthetic medicines touted by scientists and physicians to be more effective and reliable. Nevertheless, about 3% of English-speaking adults in the United States still report having used herbal remedies in the preceding year.[2] This figure is probably higher among non-English-speaking Americans.

The term *herbal medicine* refers to the use of plant structures, known as phytomedicinals or phytopharmaceuticals. Herbal medicine has become an increasing presence and area of interest to both pharmacists and other health care professionals with the advent of the German commissioned E-monographs, reporting extensive information about the safety and efficacy of herbal preparations.[136]

Herbal medicine has made many contributions to commercial drug preparations manufactured today, including ephedrine from *Ephedra sinica* (ma-huang), digitoxin from *Digitalis purpurea* (foxglove), salicin (the source of aspirin) from *Salix alba* (willow bark), and reserpine from *Rauwolfia serpentina* (snakeroot), to name just a few.[136a] The discovery of the antineoplastic agent paclitaxel (Taxol) from *Taxus brevifolia* (the Pacific yew tree) stresses the role of plants as a continuing resource for modern medicine.

Regulations in the United States

A number of laws exist in the United States affecting the sale and marketing of drugs, including the Food and Drug Act (1906) with its Sherley amendment (1912) and the Federal Food, Drug, and Cosmetic Act (1938) with its many amendments. The amendments passed in 1962, also known as the Kefauver-Harris amendments, required that all drugs marketed in the United States be proved both safe and effective. To evaluate the safety and efficacy of drugs, the FDA turned to the Division of Medical Sciences of the National Academy of Sciences–National Research Council, which then organized a "drug efficacy study" based on reviews of in vitro tests and clinical trials on patients, usually supplied by the companies interested in marketing the drugs. At the time, very few herbs had

their active ingredients isolated and even fewer had undergone clinical trials.[136b] Hence, only a small number of herbs were evaluated, and only for specific indications.[137]

In 1990, the results of the FDA's study on over-the-counter (OTC) medications, which included many herbs and herbal products, were released to the public. A few plant products, such as *Plantago psyllium* (plantago seed), *Cascara sagrada* (cascara bark, *Rhamnus purshiana*), and *Cassia acutifolia* (senna leaf, *Senna alexandrina*), were judged to be "both safe and effective" (category I) for their laxative actions. However, 142 herbs and herbal products were deemed "unsafe or ineffective" (category II), while there was "insufficient evidence to evaluate" (category III) another 116 herbs. Many herbs and herbal products in categories II and III had been grandfathered by the 1938 act and 1962 amendments, since they were already covered in the 1906 act. Thus they were not subject to the requirements of proving both safety and efficacy to be out on the market. However, to deal with these grandfathered OTC products, the FDA declared that any grandfathered drug with claims of efficacy on the package or in the package insert that did not concur with the FDA's OTC study would be considered misbranded and subject to confiscation.[137]

Unfortunately for the herbal industry, complying with the new FDA regulations meant having to remove all but the names of the herbal products from their labels and marketing them as nutritional supplements or food additives. Therefore consumers who wish to obtain factual information regarding the therapeutic use or potential harm of herbal remedies would have to obtain them from books and pamphlets, most of which based their information on traditional reputation rather than existing scientific research. Another major problem is that the marketing of herbal products under their common names, which is usually the case in health food stores, does not allow for proper identification, as there may be many species of herbs with the same common name. Another problem is the lack of dose standardization with herbal medicinals having active pharmacologic ingredients. These problems will remain until herbal medicinals are recognized as the drugs that they are.

One may wonder why the herbal industry never chose simply to prove their products safe and effective with more in vitro tests or clinical trials. The answer is primarily economic. With the cost and time of developing a new drug estimated at $231 million over 12 years (based on a 1990 report from the Center for the Study of Drug Development at Tufts University), most members of the herbal and pharmaceutical industries shy away from such endeavors, especially with the slim chance of obtaining patent protection for the many herbs that have been in use for centuries.[137] Without financial sponsorship from pharmaceutical companies, there is very little financial incentive for doing research to evaluate the merits of herbal remedies, resulting in the paucity of scientific data from the United States. One step in the right direction is the decision by the NIH to allocate $2 million each for 1992 and 1993 and 2.4 million in 2000 for research to validate alternative medical practices; however, if this amount is compared to the estimated cost of developing a single new drug, it is clear this grant allocation is inadequate.

The Effects of Herbal Remedies on the Cardiovascular System

The use of herbal medicine has skyrocketed over the last 5 years. Out-of-pocket therapy is estimated at more than $5 billion in the United States alone.[3] The following review of herbal medicinals

TABLE 47-1. Some Conditions in Which Herbal Medicines Are Used as Cardiovascular Treatments

Conditions	Examples of Herbs Used
Congestive heart failure	*Digitalis purpurea*
	Digitalis lanata
Systolic hypertension	*Rauwolfia serpentina*
	Stephania tetrandra
	Veratrum alkaloids
Angina pectoris	*Crataegus* species
	Panax notoginseng
	Salvia miltiorrhiza
Atherosclerosis	Garlic
Cerebral insufficiency	*Ginkgo biloba*
	Rosmarinus officinalis
Venous insufficiency	*Aesculus hippocastanum*
	Ruscus aculeatus

affecting the cardiovascular system is based on information gleaned from the scientific literature. These herbs are roughly categorized under the primary diseases they are used treat (Table 47-1). Note that most herbal medicinals have multiple cardiovascular effects and that the purpose of this organization is to simplify, not pigeonhole, herbs under specific diseases. In general, the dilution of active components in herbal medicinals results in fewer side effects and toxicities in comparison with the concentration of active components in the allopathic medicines. However, cardiovascular disease is a serious health hazard and no one should attempt to self-medicate with herbal remedies without first consulting a physician.

Congestive Heart Failure

Cardiac Glycosides

A number of herbs contain potent cardioactive glycosides that have positive inotropic effects on the heart. The drugs digitoxin, derived from either *Digitalis purpurea* (foxglove) or *Digitalis lanata,* and digoxin, derived from *D. lanata* alone, have been used in the treatment of CHF for many decades. Cardiac glycosides have a low therapeutic index, and the dose must be adjusted to the needs of each patient. The only way to control dosage is to use standardized powdered digitalis, digitoxin, or digoxin. Treating CHF with nonstandardized herbal agents would be dangerous and foolhardy. Accidental poisonings due to cardiac glycosides in herbal remedies are abundant in the medical literature.[137a] Some common plant sources of cardiac glycosides include: *D. purpurea* (foxglove, already mentioned), *Adonis microcarpa* and *Adonis vernalis* (Adonis), *Apocynum cannabinum* (black Indian hemp), *Asclepias curassavica* (redheaded cotton bush), *Asclepias fruticosa* (balloon cotton), *Calotropis precera* (king's crown), *Carissa acokanthera* (bushman's poison), *Carissa spectabilis* (wintersweet), *Cerbera manghas* (sea mango), *Cheiranthus cheiri* (wallflower), *Convallaria majalis* (lily of the valley, convallaria), *Cryptostegia grandiflora* (rubber vine), *Helleborus niger* (black hellebore), *Helleborus viridus, Nerium oleander* (oleander), *Plumeria rubra* (frangipani), *Selenicereus grandiflorus* (cactus grandiflorus), *Strophanthus hispidus* and *Strophanthus kombé* (strophanthus), *Thevetia peruviana* (yellow oleander), and *Urginea maritime* (squill).[137–146] Even the venom glands of the *Bufo marinus* (cane toad) contain cardiac glycosides.[139] Health providers should be aware of the cross-reactivity of cardiac glycosides from herbal sources with the digoxin radioimmunoassay. Treatment of intoxication with these substances is directed at controlling arrhythmias and hyperkalemia, which are

the usual causes of fatalities. The effects and treatment of digitalis toxicity are reviewed in Chap. 13.

Hypertension

Rauwolfia Serpentina

The root of *Rauwolfia serpentina* (snakeroot), the natural source of the alkaloid reserpine, has been a Hindu Ayurvedic remedy since ancient times. In 1931, Indian literature first described the use of *R. serpentina* root for the treatment of hypertension and psychoses; however, the use of rauwolfia alkaloids in western medicine did not begin until the mid-1940s.[147] Both standardized whole-root preparations of *R. serpentina* and its reserpine alkaloid are officially monographed in the *United States Pharmacopeia*.[148] A 200- to 300-mg dose of powdered whole root taken orally is equivalent to 0.5 mg of reserpine.[149]

Reserpine was one of the first drugs used on a large scale to treat systemic hypertension. It acts by irreversibly blocking the uptake of biogenic amines (norepinephrine, dopamine, and serotonin) in the storage vesicles of central and peripheral adrenergic neurons, thus leaving the catecholamines to be destroyed by the intraneuronal monoamine oxidase in the cytoplasm. The depletion of catecholamines accounts for reserpine's sympatholytic and antihypertensive actions.

Reserpine's effects are long-lasting, since recovery of sympathetic function requires synthesis of new storage vesicles, which takes days to weeks. Reserpine lowers blood pressure by decreasing cardiac output, peripheral vascular resistance, heart rate, and renin secretion. With the introduction of other antihypertensive drugs with fewer CNS side effects, the use of reserpine has diminished. The daily oral dose of reserpine should be 0.25 mg or less, and as little as 0.05 mg if given with a diuretic. Using the whole root, the usual adult dose is 50 to 200 mg per day administered once daily or in two divided doses.[147,149]

Rauwolfia alkaloids are contraindicated for use in patients with previously demonstrated hypersensitivity to these substances, in patients with a history of mental depression (especially with suicidal tendencies), or an active peptic ulcer or ulcerative colitis and in those receiving electroconvulsive therapy (ECT). The most common side effects are sedation and inability to concentrate and perform complex tasks. Reserpine may cause mental depression sometimes resulting in suicide and must be discontinued at the first sign of depression. Reserpine's sympatholytic effect and its enhancement of parasympathetic actions account for its other well-described side effects: Nasal congestion, increased secretion of gastric acid, and mild diarrhea.[147,150]

Stephania Tetrandra

Stephania tetrandra is an herb sometimes used in TCM to treat hypertension. Tetrandrine, an alkaloid extract of *S. tetrandra,* has been shown to be a calcium-channel antagonist, paralleling the effects of verapamil. Tetrandrine inhibits T and L calcium channels, interferes with the binding of diltiazem and methoxyverapamil at calcium-associated sites, and suppresses aldosterone production.[151,152] A parenteral dose (15 mg/kg) of tetrandrine in conscious rats decreased mean, systolic, and diastolic blood pressures for greater than 30 min; however, an intravenous dose of 40 mg/kg killed the rats by myocardial depression. In stroke-prone hypertensive rats, an oral dose of 25 or 50 mg/kg produced a gradual and sustained hypotensive effect after 48 h without affecting plasma renin activity.[153] In addition to its cardiovascular actions, tetrandrine has reported antineoplastic, immunosuppressive, and mutagenic effects.[151]

Tetrandrine is 90% protein-bound with an elimination half-life ($t_{1/2}$) of 88 min according to dog studies; however, rat studies have shown a sustained hypotensive effect for more than 48 h after a 25- or 50-mg oral dose. Tetrandrine causes liver necrosis in dogs orally administered 40 mg/kg of tetrandrine thrice weekly for 2 months, reversible swelling of liver cells at a 20-mg/kg dose, and no observable changes at a 10-mg/kg dose.[151] Given the evidence of hepatotoxicity, many more studies are necessary to establish a safe dosage of tetrandrine in humans.

Lingusticum Wallichii

The root of *Lingusticum wallichii* (chuan-xiong, chuan-hsiung) is used in TCM as a circulatory stimulant, hypotensive agent, and sedative.[154] Tetramethylpyrazine, the active constituent extracted from *L. wallichii*, inhibits platelet aggregation in vitro and lowers blood pressure by vasodilation in dogs. With its actions independent of the endothelium, tetramethylpyrazine's vasodilatory effect is mediated by calcium antagonism and nonselective antagonism of alpha adrenoceptors. Some evidence suggests that tetramethylpyrazine can selectively act on the pulmonary vasculature.[151] Currently, there is insufficient information to evaluate the safety and efficacy of this herbal medicinal.

Uncaria Rhynchophylla

Uncaria rhynchophylla (gou-teng) is sometimes used in TCM to treat hypertension. Its indole alkaloids, rhynchophylline and hirsutine, are thought to be the active principles of *U. rhynchophylla*'s vasodilatory effect. The mechanism of *U. rhynchophylla*'s actions is unclear. Some studies point to an alteration in calcium flux in response to activation, whereas others point to hirsutine's inhibition of nicotine-induced dopamine release.[151] One in vitro study has shown that *U. rhynchophylla* extract relaxes norepinephrine-precontracted rat aorta through endothelium-dependent and -independent mechanisms. For the endothelium-dependent component, *U. rhynchophylla* extract appears to stimulate endothelium-derived relaxing factor/nitric oxide (EDRF/NO) release without involving muscarinic receptors.[155] Also, in vitro and in vivo studies have shown that rhynchophylline can inhibit platelet aggregation and reduce platelet thromboses induced by collagen or ADP plus epinephrine.[151] The safety and efficacy of this agent cannot be evaluated at present owing to a lack of clinical data.

Veratrum

Veratrum (hellebore) is a perennial herb growing in many parts of the world. Varieties include *V. viride* from Canada and the eastern United States, *V. californicum* from the western United States, *V. album* from Alaska and Europe, and *V. japonicum* from Asia. All *Veratrum* plants contain poisonous veratrum alkaloids, which are known to cause vomiting, bradycardia, and hypotension. Most cases of *Veratrum* poisonings are due to misidentification with other plants. Although once a treatment for hypertension, the use of *Veratrum* alkaloids has lost favor owing to a low therapeutic index and unacceptable toxicity as well as the introduction of safer antihypertensive drug alternatives.[156]

Veratrum alkaloids enhance nerve and muscle excitability by increasing sodium conductivity. They act on the posterior wall of the left ventricle and the coronary sinus baroreceptors, causing a reflex hypotension and bradycardia via the vagus nerve (Bezold-Jarisch reflex). Nausea and vomiting are secondary to the alkaloids' actions on the nodose ganglion.[156]

The diagnosis of *Veratrum* toxicity is established by history, identification of the plant, and strong clinical suspicion. Treatment is mainly supportive and directed at controlling bradycardia and hypotension. *Veratrum*-induced bradycardia usually responds to treatment with atropine; however, the blood pressure response to atropine is more variable and may require the addition of pressors. Electrocardiographic (ECG) changes may be reversible with atropine but are sometimes not. Seizures are a rare complication and may be treated with conventional anticonvulsants. For patients with preexisting cardiac disease, the use of beta agonists or pacing may be necessary. Nausea may be controlled with phenothiazine antiemetics. Recovery is usually within 24 to 48 h.[156]

Angina Pectoris

Crataegus

Hawthorn, a name encompassing many *Crataegus* species (such as *C. oxyacantha* and *C. monogina* in the West and *C. pinnatifida* in China), has acquired the reputation on the modern herbal literature as an important tonic for the cardiovascular system, particularly useful for angina. *Crataegus* leaves, flowers, and fruits contain a number of biologically active substances such as oligomeric procyanidins, flavonoids, and catechins. From current studies, *Crataegus* extract appears to have antioxidant properties and can inhibit the formation of thromboxane A_2.[157,158] Also, *Crataegus* extract antagonizes the increases in cholesterol, triglycerides, and phospholipids in LDL and very low density lipoprotein (VLDL) in rats fed a hyperlipidemic diet; thus, it may inhibit the progression of atherosclerosis.[159] According to one study, *Crataegus* extract in high concentrations has a cardioprotective effect on ischemic-reperfused heart without an increase in coronary blood flow.[160] On the other hand, oral and parenteral administration of oligomeric procyanins of *Crataegus* leads to an increase in coronary blood flow in cats and dogs.[161,162] Double-blind clinical trials have demonstrated simultaneous cardiotropic and vasodilatory actions of *Crataegus*.[163] In essence, *Crataegus* increases coronary perfusion, has a mild hypotensive effect, antagonizes atherosclerosis, has positive inotropic and negative chronotropic actions and improves congestive heart failure.[159,164,165] Crataegus lowers blood pressure due to its action in lowering peripheral vascular resistance. Animal studies have also indicated that peripheral and coronary blood flow increases while arterial blood pressure decreases.[166] Hawthorn is relatively devoid of side effects; however, concomitant use of hawthorn and digoxin can markedly enhance the activity of digitalis.[137,167] Therefore hawthorn and digitalis should not be given together.

Panax Notoginseng

Because of its resemblance to *Panax ginseng* (Asian ginseng), *Panax notoginseng* (pseudoginseng; san-qui) has acquired the common name of pseudoginseng, especially since it is often an adulterant of *P. ginseng* preparations. In TCM, the root of *P. notoginseng* is used for analgesia and hemostasis. It is also often used in the treatment of patients with angina and coronary artery disease.[154]

Although clinical trials are lacking, in vitro studies using *P. notoginseng* do suggest possible cardiovascular effects. One study that used purified notoginsenoside R1, extracted from *P. notoginseng*, on human umbilical vein endothelial cells showed a dose- and time-dependent synthesis of tissue-type plasminogen activator (tPA) without affecting the synthesis of plasminogen activating inhibitor (PAI-1), thus enhancing fibrinolytic parameters.[168]

Another study suggests that *P. notoginseng* saponins may inhibit atherogenesis by interfering with the proliferation of smooth muscle cells.[169] In vitro and in vivo studies using rats and rabbits have demonstrated that *P. notoginseng* may be useful as an antianginal agent, since it dilates coronary arteries in all concentrations. The role of *P. notoginseng* in the treatment of hypertension is less certain, since it causes vasodilation or vasoconstriction depending on concentration and the target vessel.[170] The results of these in vitro and in vivo studies are encouraging; however, clinical trials will be necessary to enable more informed decisions regarding the use of *P. notoginseng*. The most common side effects reported with ginseng were insomnia, diarrhea, and skin reactions.[137]

Salvia Miltiorrhiza

Salvia miltiorrhiza (dan-shen), a relative of the Western sage *S. officinalis*, is native to China. In TCM, the root of *S. miltiorrhiza* is used as a circulatory stimulant, sedative, and cooling agent.[154] *S. miltiorrhiza* may be useful as an antianginal agent because, like *P. notoginseng,* it has been shown to dilate coronary arteries in all concentrations. Also, *S. miltiorrhiza* has variable action on other vessels, depending on its concentration, so it may not be as helpful in treating hypertension.[170] In vitro, *S. miltiorrhiza,* in a dose-dependent fashion, inhibits platelet aggregation and serotonin release induced by either ADP or epinephrine, which is thought to be mediated by an increase in platelet cAMP caused by *S. miltiorrhiza's* inhibition of cAMP phosphodiesterase.[171] *S. miltiorrhiza* appears to have a protective effect on ischemic myocardium, enhancing the recovery of contractile force upon reoxygenation.[172] Qualitatively and quantitatively, a decoction of *S. miltiorrhiza* was as efficacious as the more expensive isolated tanshinones.[168] Clinical trials will be necessary to further evaluate the safety and efficacy of *S. miltiorrhiza.*

Atherosclerosis

Allium Sativum

In addition to its use in the culinary arts, *Allium sativum* (garlic) has been valued for centuries in many cultures for its medicinal properties. In recent decades, animal and human data have focused on garlic's use in treating atherosclerosis and hypertension.[173,173a] A number of studies have demonstrated garlic's effects, which include lowering blood pressure, reducing serum cholesterol and triglycerides, enhancing fibrinolytic activity, and inhibiting platelet aggregation.[173b] However, some investigators have been hesitant to endorse the routine use of garlic for cardiovascular disease outright despite positive evidence because many of the published studies had methodologic shortcomings.[174–179] For example, in one of the largest collective reviews of randomized controlled trials of garlic lasting 4 weeks or longer, the researchers concluded that the effects of garlic treatment are tainted by an inadequate definition of active constituents in the study preparations.[179] The pharmacologic properties of garlic are extremely complex, comprising a variety of sulfur-containing compounds that include allicin, alliin, diallyl disulfide, ajoene, s-allylcysteines, and gamma-glutamylpeptides, to mention a few.[180] Many of the previous controlled trials of garlic used different preparations containing all or some of these active pharmacologic factors. This may be the major reason for the variability and confusion found in the research.[179] The definition and delineation of the major active garlic ingredients and their specific mechanisms of action are absolutely necessary before future trials are planned and conducted.

Intact cells of garlic bulbs contain an odorless, sulfur-containing amino acid derivative known as alliin. When garlic is crushed, alliin comes into contact with alliinase, which converts alliin to allicin. Allicin has potent antibacterial properties but is also highly odoriferous and unstable. Ajoenes, self-condensation products of allicin, appear to be responsible for garlic's antithrombotic activity. Most authorities now agree that allicin and its derivatives are the active constituents of garlic's physiologic activity. Fresh garlic releases allicin in the mouth during the chewing process. Dried garlic preparations lack allicin but do contain alliin and alliinase. Since alliinase is inactivated by acids in the stomach, dried garlic preparations should be enteric-coated so that they pass through the stomach into the small intestine, where alliin can be enzymatically converted to allicin. Few commercial garlic preparations are standardized for their allicin yield based on alliin content, hence making their effectiveness less certain.[137,180] However, one double-blind, placebo-controlled study involving 261 patients over 4 months using one 800-mg tablet of garlic powder daily, standardized to 1.3 % alliin content, demonstrated significant reductions in total cholesterol (12%) and triglycerides (17%).[181] In studies that use garlic supplements containing either no allicin or poorly bioavailable allicin, no lipid lowering was realized. Consumption of large quantities of fresh garlic (0.25 to 1 g/kg body weight or about 5 to 20 average-size 4-g cloves in a 175 lb person) does appear to produce beneficial effects.[178] However, in a meta-analysis, it was demonstrated that garlic, in an amount approximating one-half to one clove per day, decreased total serum cholesterol by about 9% in the patients studied.[182] The allicin yield of each 800-mg garlic tablet is equivalent to 2.8 g of fresh garlic—less than one average-size 4-g clove; in other words, therapeutic effectiveness may be seen in doses much lower than five cloves of garlic.[137] In 11 large databases collected from January 1966 through February 2000, various garlic preparations did suggest small reductions in total cholesterol, LDL, and triglyceride, but no statistically significant changes were noted in high-density lipoproteins. Significant reductions in platelet aggregation and insignificant effects on blood pressure outcomes were also observed.[179]

Aside from a garlic odor on the breath and body, moderate garlic consumption causes few adverse effects. Consumption in excess of five cloves daily may result in heartburn, flatulence, and other GI disturbances. Case reports have also described bleeding in patients ingesting large doses of garlic (average of four cloves per day).[183] Because of its antithrombotic activity, garlic should also be used with caution in people taking oral anticoagulants.[137,183] Some individuals have also reported allergic reactions to garlic.

Cerebral and Peripheral Vascular Disease

Ginkgo Biloba

Dating back well over 200 million years, *Ginkgo biloba* (maidenhair tree) was apparently saved from extinction by human intervention, surviving in Far Eastern temple gardens while disappearing for centuries in the West. It was reintroduced to Europe in 1730 and became a favorite ornamental tree.[154,184] Although the root and kernels of *G. biloba* have long been used in TCM, *Ginkgo* gained attention in the West during the twentieth century for its medicinal value after a concentrated extract of *G. biloba* leaves was developed in the 1960s. At least two groups of substances within *G. biloba* extract demonstrated beneficial pharmacologic actions. The flavonoids reduce capillary permeability and fragility and serve as free-radical scavengers. The terpenes (i.e., ginkgolides) inhibit platelet activating factor, decrease vascular resistance, and improve circulatory flow without appreciably affecting blood pressure.[167,185] Continuing research appears to support the primary use of *G. biloba* extract for treating cerebral insufficiency and its secondary effects on vertigo, tinnitus, memory, and mood.[186] In a study evaluating 327 demented patients, 120 mg of *G. biloba* extract produced improvements in dementia, similar to other studies with donepezil and tacrine.[187] However, a more recent study showed no benefit of *G. biloba* on cognitive functioning.[187a] In addition, *G. biloba* extract appears to be useful for treating peripheral vascular disease, including intermittent claudication and diabetic retinopathy.[137,167,185,188–190]

Although approved as a drug in Europe, *Ginkgo* is not approved in the United States and is instead marketed as a food supplement, usually supplied as 40-mg tablets of extract. Since most investigations examining the efficacy of *G. biloba* extracts used preparations such as EGb 761 or LI 1370, the bioequivalence of other *G. biloba* extract products has not been established. The recommended dose in Europe is one 40 mg tablet taken three times daily with meals (120 mg daily).[137,185] Adverse effects of *G. biloba* extract are rare but can include GI disturbances, headache, and skin rash.[137,167] Several case reports of bleeding, including subarachnoid hemorrhage,[191] intracranial hemorrhage,[192] and subdural hematoma[193] have been associated with *G. biloba. G. biloba* should not be used in combination with analgesic agents such as aspirin, ticlopidine, and clopidogrel or anticoagulants such as warfarin, since it undermines the effect of the platelet inhibiting factor.[194]

Rosmarinus Officinalis

Known mostly as a culinary spice and flavoring agent, *Rosmarinus officinalis* (rosemary) is listed in many herbal sources as a tonic and all-around stimulant. Traditionally, rosemary leaves are said to enhance circulation, aid digestion, elevate mood, and boost energy. When applied externally, the volatile oils are supposedly useful for arthritic conditions and baldness.[137]

Although research on rosemary is scanty, some studies have focused on antioxidant effects of diterpenoids, especially carnosic acid and carnosol, isolated from rosemary leaves. In addition to having antineoplastic effects (especially skin), antioxidants in rosemary have been credited with stabilizing erythrocyte membranes and inhibiting superoxide generation and lipid peroxidation.[195,196] Essential oils of rosemary have demonstrated antimicrobial, hyperglycemic, and insulin-inhibiting properties.[197,198] Rosemary leaves contain high amounts of salicylates, and its flavonoid pigment diosmin is reported to decrease capillary permeability and fragility.[167,199,200]

Despite the conclusions derived from in vitro and animal studies, the therapeutic use of rosemary for cardiovascular disorders remains questionable, as few if any clinical trials have been conducted using rosemary. Due to lack of studies, no conclusions can be reached regarding the use of the antioxidants of rosemary in inhibiting atherosclerosis. Although external application may cause cutaneous vasodilatation from the counterirritant properties of rosemary's essential oils, there is no evidence to support any prolonged improvement in peripheral circulation.[137] While rosemary does have some carminative properties, it may also cause GI and kidney disturbances in large doses.[137,200] Until more studies are done, rosemary should probably be limited to its use as a culinary spice and flavoring agent rather than as a medicine.

Venous Insufficiency

Aesculus Hippocastanum

The seeds of *Aesculus hippocastanum* (horse chestnut) have long been used in Europe to treat venous disorders such as varicose veins. The medicinal qualities of horse chestnut reside mostly in its large seeds, which resemble edible chestnuts. The seeds contain a complex mixture of saponins, glycosides, and several other active ingredients. The grouping of most interest is called aesculic acid or aescin. In addition to a high level of flavonoids, horse chestnuts contain several minerals including magnesium, manganese, cobalt, and iodine.[201]

The saponin glycoside aescin from horse chestnut extract (HCE) inhibits the activity of lysosomal enzymes, which are thought to contribute to varicose veins by weakening vessel walls and increasing permeability, resulting in dilated veins and edema.[137] In animal studies, HCE, in a dose-dependent fashion, increases venous tone, venous flow, and lymphatic flow. HCE also antagonizes capillary hyperpermeability induced by histamine, serotonin, or chloroform. HCE decreases edema formation of lymphatic and inflammatory origin. HCE has antiexudative properties, suppressing experimentally induced pleurisy and peritonitis by inhibiting plasma extravasation and leukocyte emigration. HCE's dose-dependent antioxidant properties can inhibit in vitro lipid peroxidation.[202,203] Randomized double-blind, placebo-controlled trials using HCE show a statistically significant reduction in edema, as measured by plethysmography.[204,205] Although still controversial, prophylactic use of HCE does not appear to decrease the incidence of thromboembolic complications of gynecologic surgery.[206]

Standardized HCE is prepared as an aqueous-alcohol extract of 16 to 21% of triterpene glycosides, calculated as aescin. The usual initial dose is 90 to 150 mg of aescin daily, which may be reduced to 35 to 70 mg daily after improvement.[137] Standardized HCE preparations are not available in the United States, but nonstandardized products may be available.

Some manufacturers promote the use of topical preparations of HCE for treatment of varicose veins as well as hemorrhoids; however, at least one study has demonstrated very poor aescin distribution at sites other than the skin and muscle tissues underlying the application site.[207] Moreover, the involvement of arterioles and veins in the pathophysiology of hemorrhoids makes the effectiveness of HCE doubtful, since HCE has no known effects on the arterial circulation. For now, research studies have yet to confirm any clinical effectiveness of topical HCE preparations.

Although side effects are uncommon, HCE may cause GI irritation and facial rash. Parenteral aescin has produced isolated cases of anaphylactic reactions as well as hepatic and renal toxicity.[137,208–210] In the event of toxicity, aescin is completely dialyzable, with elimination dependent on protein binding.[211]

Ruscus Aculeatus

Like *A. hippocastanum, Ruscus aculeatus* (butcher's broom) is known for its use in treating venous insufficiency. *R. aculeatus* is a short evergreen shrub found commonly in the Mediterranean region. Two steroidal saponins, ruscogenin and neurogenin, extracted from the rhizomes of *R. aculeatus* are thought to be its active components.[200] In vivo studies on hamster cheek pouch reveal that topical *Ruscus* extract dose-dependently antagonizes a histamine-induced increase in vascular permeability.[212] Moreover, topical *Ruscus* extract causes dose-dependent constriction on venules without appreciably affecting arterioles.[213] Topical *Ruscus* extract's vascular effects are also temperature-dependent and appear to counter the sympathetic nervous system's temperature-sensitive vascular regulation: Venules dilate at a lower temperature (25°C), constrict at near-physiologic temperature (36.5°C), and further constrict at a higher temperature (40°C); arterioles dilate at 25°C, are unaffected at 36.5°C, and remain unaffected or constricted at 40°C depending on *Ruscus* concentration.[214] Based on the influence of prazosin, diltiazem, and rauwolscine, the peripheral vascular effects of *Ruscus* extract appear to be selectively mediated by effects on calcium channels and alpha-adrenergic receptors.[212,213]

Several small clinical trials using topical *Ruscus* extract support its role in treating venous insufficiency. One randomized double-blind, placebo-controlled trial involving 18 volunteers showed a statistically significant decrease in femoral vein diameter (median decrease of 1.25 mm) using duplex B-scan ultrasonography 2.5 h after applying 4 to 6 g of a cream containing 64 to 96 mg of *Ruscus* extract.[215] Another small trial ($n = 18$) showed that topical *Ruscus* extract may be helpful in reducing venous dilatation during pregnancy.[216] Oral agents may be as useful as topical agents for venous insufficiency, although the evidence is less convincing.[217]

Although capsule, tablet, ointment, and suppository (for hemorrhoids) preparations of *Ruscus* extract are available in Europe, only capsules are available in the United States. These capsules contain 75 mg of *Ruscus* extract and 2 mg of rosemary oil.[200] Aside from occasional nausea and gastritis, side effects from using *R. aculeatus* have rarely been reported, even at high doses.[167] Nevertheless, one should be wary of any drug that has not been thoroughly tested. Although there is ample evidence to support the pharmacologic activity of *R. aculeatus,* there is still a relative deficiency of clinical data to establish its actual safety and efficacy. Until more studies are completed, no recommendations regarding dosage can be offered.

NONCARDIOVASCULAR HERBS WITH NOTEWORTHY CARDIOVASCULAR EFFECTS

For the following noncardiovascular herbs, only cardiovascular actions are emphasized. (Table 47-2).

Tussilago Farfara

Tussilago farfara (coltsfoot, kuan-dong-hua) is a perennial herb that is grown in many parts of northern China, Europe, Africa, Siberia, and North America. Over the years, *T. farfara* has acquired a rep-

TABLE 47-2. Adverse Cardiovascular Reactions Observed with Herbal Medicines Used for Other Indications

Examples	Herbal Medicines
Antithrombotic actions that could potentiate the effects of warfarin	Garlic
Hypertension	*Tussilago farfara*
	Ephedra sinica
Hypotension	*Aconitum* species
Digitalis toxicity	Over 20 herbal substances with activity to digitalis radioimmunoassay
Bradycardia	*Aconitum* species
	Jin-bu-huan

utation as a demulcent antitussive agent due to a throat-soothing mucilage within the herb. Recently, the use of *T. farfara* has lost favor due to several studies that found senkirkine, a pyrrolizidine alkaloid known to cause hepatotoxicity, in all parts of the herb. In addition, rats fed a diet containing *T. farfara* had a high risk of developing hemangioendothelial sarcoma of the liver.[200]

A diterpene isolated from *T. farfara,* named tussilagone, is shown to be a potent respiratory and cardiovascular stimulant. Administered intravenously, tussilagone produces a dose-dependent increase in the peripheral vascular resistance of dogs, cats, and rats without much effect on ventricular inotropy and chronotropy. The LD_{50} in mice with an acute intravenous administration of tussilagone is 28.9 mg/kg.[218]

Ephedra Sinica

Ephedra sinica (joint fir, ma-huang), the natural source of the alkaloid ephedrine, has been used in TCM for over 5000 years as an antiasthmatic and decongestant. *Ephedra* has gained recent notoriety stemming from several fatalities of youths who took an excess of *Ephedra,* which is promoted by some as a "legal high," weight-loss aid, energy booster, and aphrodisiac.[219] In a study involving a review of 140 adverse case reports submitted to the FDA between 1997 and 1999, *Ephedra* alkaloids in dietary supplements caused 10 deaths and 13 permanent disabilities. Most of these tragic events were cardiovascular (e.g., cardiac arrest, arrhythmia) or neurologic (e.g., stroke, seizure).[220]

Ephedrine acts by releasing stored catecholamines from synaptic neurons and nonselectively stimulates alpha- and beta-adrenergic receptors. Ephedrine increases mean, systolic, and diastolic blood pressures by vasoconstriction and cardiac stimulation. Ephedrine's bronchodilating actions may be helpful for the chronic treatment of asthma. Ephedrine enhances the contractility of skeletal muscle. It penetrates the central nervous system and can produce nervousness, excitability, and insomnia. Patients taking monoamine oxidase inhibitors or guanethidine should not be receiving any product containing ephedrine alkaloids. Patients with preexisting CAD, hypertension, and severe glaucoma should also avoid ephedrine alkaloids.[200,221,222]

Commercially synthesized ephedrine in the United States is identical with the alkaloid derived from *Ephedra.* Oral preparations of ephedrine sulfate are supplied as capsules and syrups. The usual adult dose is 25 to 50 mg every 6 h; for children, the dose is 3 mg/kg every 24 h in four divided doses.[222]

Aconitum

The roots of *Aconitum* species, such as *A. kusnezoffii* (cao-wu) and *A. carmichaeli* (chuan-wa), are sometimes used in TCM to treat rheumatism, arthritis, bruises, and fractures. In Europe, *A. napellus* (monkshood, wolfsbane) grows in the wild and is sometime cultivated as an ornamental.[223,224]

Plant parts of *Aconitum* species contain diterpenoid ester alkaloids, including aconitine, which have been linked to several deaths in Hong Kong and Australia. Death usually results from cardiovascular collapse and ventricular tachyarrhythmias induced by aconite alkaloids. These alkaloids activate sodium channels and cause widespread membrane excitation in cardiac, neural, and muscular tissues. Characteristic manifestations of aconite intoxication include nausea, vomiting, diarrhea, hypersalivation, and generalized paresthesias (especially circumoral numbness). Muscarinic activation may cause hypotension and bradyarrhythmias. Transmembrane enhancement of sodium flux during the plateau phase prolongs repolarization and induces afterdepolarizations and triggered automaticity in cardiac myocytes. Aconite-induced cardiac arrhythmias can also lead to cardiac failure in as little as 5 min to as long as 4 days.[223-225]

Management of aconite intoxication consists of symptomatic relief, since no specific antidote exists. Amiodarone and flecainide may be used as antiarrhythmic agents. Intragastric charcoal can decrease alkaloid absorption.[224,225]

A fatal dose can be as little as 5 mL of aconite tincture, 2 mg of pure aconite, or 1 g of plant.[224] Considering their low therapeutic index and unacceptable toxicity, *Aconitum* and its products are not recommended even in therapeutic doses, since an erroneous dose can be fatal.

Jin-Bu-Huan

Often misidentified as a derivative of *Polygala chinensis,* jin-bu-huan is most likely derived from the *Stephania* genus. This herbal remedy contains an active alkaloid known as levotetrahydropalmatine, which is a potent neuroactive substance that produces sedation, naloxone-resistant analgesia, and dopamine-receptor antagonism in animals. Jin-bu-huan is used as an analgesic, sedative, hypnotic, and antispasmodic agent as well as a dietary supplement. It is associated with significant cardiorespiratory toxicity, including respiratory failure and bradycardia requiring endotracheal intubation. There is no specific antidote for the treatment of acute jin-bu-huan overdose. Several cases of hepatitis have also been associated with long-term ingestion of jin-bu-huan. Although it is now banned in the United States, jin-bu-huan is still being imported illegally as jin bu huan anodyne tablets.[6]

CONCLUSION

With the widespread use of alternative medicine in the United States, health practitioners, in taking clinical histories, should remember to ask patients about their alternative health practices and stay informed regarding the beneficial or harmful effects of these treatments. Continuing research is elucidating the pharmacologic activities of many alternative medicines and may stimulate future pharmaceutical development; however, such research is lacking in the United States and may require support from government agencies.[225a,b] Legal surveillance of alternative medicine practices with low safety margins should be instituted for the sake of public health. As more information becomes available regarding the safety and efficacy of alternative medicines, research-supported claims may one day appear on the labels of alternative medicinals.

The integration of proven complementary therapies with conventional treatments in heart disease will allow cardiologists to offer many additional options to their patients. An open mind and a willingness to support conventional methodology while investigating alternatives can improve quality of life and reduce human suffering. Choosing from the best conventional and complementary options is the only logical and ethical thing to do.

REFERENCES

1. Blendon RJ, DesRoches CM, Benson JM, et al: Americans' views on the use and regulation of dietary supplements. *Arch Intern Med* 161:805, 2001.
1a. Sampson W: The need for educational reform in teaching about alternative therapies. *Acad Med* 76:248, 2001.
1b. Frenkel M, Arye EB: The growing need to teach about complementary and alternative medicine: Questions and challenges. *Acad Med* 76:251, 2001.
2. Eisenberg DM, Kessler RC, Foster C, et al: Unconventional medicine in the United States. *N Engl J Med* 238:246, 1993.
2a. Tesch BJ: Herbs commonly used by women: An evidence-based review. *Clin J Womens Health* 1:89, 2001.
2b. Holland JC: Use of alternative medicine—a marker for distress? *N Engl J Med* 340:1758, 1999.
3. Eisenberg DM, Davis RB, Ettner SL, et al: Trends in alternative medicine use in the United States, 1990–1997: Results of a follow-up national survey. *JAMA* 280(18):1569, 1998.
4. Wetzel MS, Eisenberg MD, Kaptchuk TJ: Courses involving complementary and alternative medicines at US medical schools. *JAMA* 280:784, 1998.
5. Fontanarosa PB, Lundberg GD: Alternative medicine meets science. *JAMA* 280:1618, 1998.
6. Horowitz RS, Feldhaus K, Dart RC, et al: The clinical spectrum of *Jin Bu Huan* toxicity. *Arch Intern Med* 156:899, 1996.
7. Omaye ST: Safety of megavitamin therapy. *Adv Exp Med Biol* 177:169, 1984.
7a. Frishman WH: Nutriceuticals as treatments for cardiovascular disease. *Heart Disease* 1:51, 1999.
8. Cooke JP: Nutriceuticals for cardiovascular health. *Am J Cardiol* 82(10A):43S, 1998.
9. McLaren DS: Vitamin deficiency, toxicity, and dependency. In: Berkow R, Fletcher AJ, Bondy PK, et al, eds. *The Merck Manual,* 16th ed. Rahway, NJ: Merck Research Laboratories, 1992.
10. Russell RM: Vitamin and trace mineral deficiency and excess. In: Braunwald E, Fauci A, Kasper D, et al, eds. *Harrison's Principles of Internal Medicine,* 15th ed. New York: McGraw-Hill, 2001:468.
11. O'Reilly RA: Drugs used in disorders of coagulation. In: Katzung BG, ed. *Basic and Clinical Pharmacology,* 6th ed. Norwalk, CT: Appleton & Lange, 1995.
12. Pryor WA: Vitamin E and heart tissue: Basic science to clinical intervention trials. *Free Radic Biol Med* 28:141, 2000.
13. Ingold KU, Webb AC, Witter D, et al: Vitamin E remains the major lipid-soluble chain-breaking antioxidant in human plasma even in individuals suffering from severe vitamin E deficiency. *Arch Biochem Biophys* 258:224, 1987.
14. Reaven PD, Khouw A, Belz WF, et al: Effects of dietary antioxidant combinations in humans. Protection of LDL by vitamin E but not by beta carotene. *Arterioscler Thromb* 13(4):590, 1993.
15. Chan AC: Vitamin E and atherosclerosis. *J Nutr* 128:1593, 1998.
16. Rapola JM, Virtamo J, Haukka JK, et al: Effect of vitamin E and beta carotene on the incidence of angina pectoris. A randomized, double-blind, controlled trial. *JAMA* 275(9):693, 1996.
17. Stephens NG, Parsons A, Schofield PM, et al: Randomized controlled trial of vitamin E in patients with coronary disease: Cambridge Heart Antioxidant Study. *Lancet* 347:781, 1996.
18. Yusuf S, Sleight P, Pogue J, et al: Effects of an angiotensin-converting-enzyme inhibitor, ramipril, on cardiovascular events in high-risk patients. *N Engl J Med* 342:145, 2000.
19. Gruppo Italiano per lo Studio della Sopravvivenza nell'Infarto miocardioco. Dietary supplementation with n-3 polyunsaturated fatty acids and vitamin E after myocardial infarction: Results of the GISSI Prevenzione trial. *Lancet* 354:447, 1999.
20. Jialal I, Traber M, Deveraj S: Is there a vitamin E paradox? *Curr Opin Lipidol* 12:49, 2001.
21. Rapola JM, Virtamo J, Ripatti S, et al: Randomized trial of alpha-tocopherol and beta carotene supplements on incidence of major coronary events in men with previous myocardial infarction. *Lancet* 349:1715, 1997.
22. Ewy GA: Antioxidant therapy for coronary artery disease. *Arch Intern Med* 159:1279, 1999.

23. Stampfer MJ, Hennekens CH, Manson JE, et al: Vitamin E consumption and the risk of coronary disease in women. *N Engl J Med* 328:1444, 1993.

24. Rimm EB, Stempfer MJ, Ascherio A, et al: Vitamin E consumption and the risk of coronary disease in men. *N Engl J Med* 328:1450,1993.

25. Hodis HN, Mack WJ, LaBree L, et al: Serial coronary angiographic evidence that antioxidant vitamin intake reduces progression of coronary atherosclerosis. *JAMA* 273(23):1849, 1995.

26. Meagher EA, Barry OP, Lawson JA, et al: Effects of vitamin E on lipid peroxidation in healthy persons. *JAMA* 285(9):1178, 2001.

27. Cooney R, Franke A, Harwood P, et al: Gamma-tocopherol detoxification of nitrogen dioxide: Superiority to alpha-tocopherol. *Proc Natl Acad Sci U S A* 90:1771, 1993.

28. Wolf G: Gamma-tocopherol: An efficient protector of lipids against nitric oxide-initiated peroxidative damage. *Nutr Rev* 55(10):376, 1997.

29. Moore AS, Papas AM: Biochemistry and health significance of vitamin E. *J Advance Med* 9(1):11, 1996.

30. Freedman JE, Cheney K, Eaney JR: Vitamin E inhibition of platelet aggregation is independent of antioxidant activity. *J Nutr* 131:374S, 2000.

31. Devaraj S, Jialal I: LDL post-secretory modification, monocyte function and circulating adhesion molecules in type 2 diabetic patients with and without macrovascular complications: Effect of alpha tocopherol supplementation. *Circulation* 102:191, 2000.

32. Kostner K, Hornykewycz S, Yang P, et al: Is oxidative stress casually linked to unstable angina pectoris? A study in 100 CAD patients and matched controls.*Cardiovas Res* 36:330, 1997.

33. Gill J: The pathophysiology and epidemiology of myocardial infarction. A review. *Drugs* 42(2):1, 1991.

34. Watanabe H, Kakihana M, Ohtsuka S, et al: Randomized, double-blind, placebo-controlled study of the preventive effect of supplemental oral vitamin C on attenuation of development of nitrate tolerance. *J Am Coll Cardiol* 31(6):1323, 1998.

35. Watanabe H, Kakihana M, Ohtsuka S, et al: Randomized, double-blind, placebo-controlled study of supplemental vitamin E on an attenuation of the development of nitrate tolerance. *Circulation* 96:2545, 1997.

36. Munzel T, Sayegh H, Freeman B, et al: Evidence for enhanced vascular superoxide anion-production in nitrate tolerance. *J Clin Invest* 95:187, 1995.

37. Watanabe H, Kakihana M, Ohtsuka S, et al: Randomized, double-blind, placebo-controlled study of ascorbate on the preventive effect of nitrate tolerance in patients with congestive heart failure. *Circulation* 97:886, 1998.

38. Kritchevsky SB, Shimakawa T, Tell GS, et al: Dietary antioxidants and carotid artery wall thickness: The ARIC Study. *Circulation* 92:2142, 1995.

39. Simon JA: Vitamin C and cardiovascular disease: A review. *J Am Coll Nutr* 11:107, 1992.

40. Kaw KT, Bingham S, Welch A, et al: Relation between plasma ascorbic acid and mortality in men and women in EPIC-Norfolk Prospective Study: A prospective population study. *Lancet* 357:657, 2001.

41. Ting HH, Creager MA, Ganz P, et al: Vitamin C improves endothelium-dependent vasodilation in forearm resistance vessels of humans with hypercholesterolemia. *Circulation* 95:2617, 1997.

42. Johnson C, Meyer C, Srilakshmi J: Vitamin C elevates red blood cell glutathione in healthy adults. *Am J Clin Nutr* 58:103, 1993.

43. Herbert V: Does mega-C do more good than harm, or more harm than good? *J Am Diet Assoc* 92:1502, 1992.

44. Greenberg ER, Baron JA, Karagas MR, et al: Mortality associated with low plasma concentration of beta carotene and the effect of oral supplementation. *JAMA* 275:699, 1996.

45. Jialal I, Norkus EP, Cristol L, et al: B-carotene inhibits the oxidative modification of low-density lipoprotein. *Biochem Biophys Acta* 1086:134, 1991.

46. Reaven PD, Khouw A, Belz WF, et al: Effects of dietary antioxidant combinations in humans. Protection of LDL by vitamin E but not by beta carotene. *Arterioscler Thromb* 13(4):590, 1993.

47. Gaziano JM, Hatta A, Flynn M, et al: Supplementation with beta carotene in vivo and in vitro does not inhibit low density lipoprotein oxidation. *Artherosclerosis* 112:187, 1995.

48. Gey FK, Puska P: Plasma vitamin E and A inversely correlated to mortality from ischemic heart disease in cross-cultural epidemiology. *Ann NY Acad Sci* 570:268, 1989.

49. Kardinaal AF, Kok FJ, Ringstad J, et al: Antioxidants in adipose tissue and risk of myocardial infarction: The EURAMIC Study. *Lancet* 342:1379, 1993.

50. The Alpha-Tocopherol, Beta-Carotene Therapy Cancer Prevention Study Group: The effect of vitamin E and beta carotene on the incidence of lung cancer and other cancers in male smokers. *N Engl J Med* 330:1029, 1994.

51. Omenn GS, Goodman GE, Thornquist MD, et al: Effects of a combination of beta carotene and vitamin A on lung cancer and cardiovascular disease. *N Engl J Med* 334(18):1150, 1996.

52. Hennekens CH, Buring JE, Manson JE, et al: Lack of effect of long-term supplementation with beta carotene on the incidence of malignant neoplasms and cardiovascular disease. *N Engl J Med* 334(18):1145, 1996.

53. Williams AW, Boileau TW, Zhou JR, et al: Beta carotene modulates human prostate cancer cell growth and may undergo intracellular metabolism to retinol. *J Nutr* 130:728, 2000.

54. Howard AN, Williams NR, Palmer CR, et al: Do hydroxy-carotenoids prevent coronary heart disease? A comparison between Belfast and Toulouse. *Int J Vit Nutr Res* 66(2):113, 1996.

55. Renaud S, de Lorgeril M: Wine, alcohol, platelets and the French paradox for coronary heart disease. *Lancet* 339:1523, 1992.

56. Maxwell S, Cruickshank A, Thorpe D: Red wind and antioxidant activity in serum. *Lancet* 344:193, 1994.

57. Hertog MC, Feskens EJ, Hollman PC, et al: Dietary antioxidant flavonoids and risk of coronary heart disease: The Zutphen Elderly Study. *Lancet* 342:1007, 1993.

57a. Freedman JE, Parker C 3rd, Li L, et al: Select flavonoids and whole juice from purple grapes inhibit platelet function and enhance nitric oxide release. *Circulation* 103:2792, 2001.

58. Duffy SJ, Keaney JF, Holbrook M, et al: Short- and long-term black tea consumption reverses endothelial dysfunction in patients with coronary artery disease. *Circulation* 104:151, 2001.

59. Havsteen B: Flavonoids, a class of natural products of high pharmacological potency. *Biochem Pharmacol* 32(7):1141, 1983.

60. Turlapaty PDMV, Altura BM: Magnesium deficiency produces spasms of coronary arteries: Relationship to etiology of sudden death ischemic heart disease. *Science* 208:198, 1980.

61. McLean RM: Magnesium and its therapeutic uses: A review. *Am J Med* 96:63, 1994.

62. Elin RJ: Magnesium metabolism in health and disease. *Dis Mon* 34:161,1988.

63. Shechter M, Kaplinsky E, Rabinowitz B: The rationale of magnesium supplementation in acute myocardial infarction: A review of the literature. *Arch Intern Med* 152:2189, 1992.

64. Shechter M: Oral magnesium in coronary artery disease: Fresh insight on thrombus inhibition. *Magn Rep* 1, 1999.

65. Shechter M, Merz CN, Paul-Labrador M, et al: Oral magnesium supplementation inhibits platelet-dependent thrombosis in patients with coronary artery disease. *Am J Cardiol* 84(2):152, 1999.

66. Lichodziejewska B, Klos J, Rezler J, et al: Clinical symptoms of mitral valve prolapse are related to hypomagnesemia and attenuated by magnesium supplementation. *Am J Cardiol* 79(6):768, 1997.

67. Kendler BS: Recent nutritional approaches to the prevention and therapy of cardiovascular disease. *Prog Cardiovasc Nurs* 12(3):3, 1997.

68. Powell LW, Isselbacher KJ: Hemochromatosis. In: Braunwald E, Fauci A, Kasper D, et al, eds. *Harrisons Principles of Internal Medicine,* 15th ed. New York: McGraw-Hill, 2258, 2001.

69. Abraham AS, Sonnenblick M, Eini M, et al: The effect of chromium on established atherosclerotic plaques in rabbits. *Am J Clin Nutr* 33:2294,1980.

70. Lefavi RG, Wilson D, Keith RE, et al: Lipid lowering effects of a dietary chromium (III)-nicotinic acid complex in male athletes. *Nutr Res* 13:239,1993.

71. Preuss HG, Wallerstedr' D, Talpur N, et al: Effects of niacin-bound chromium and grape seed proanthocyanidins extract on the lipid profile of hypercholesterolemic subjects: A pilot study. *J Med* 31(5&6):227, 2000.

72. Grundy SM: Hypertriglyceridemia, insulin resistance, and the metabolic syndrome. *Am J Cardiol* 83:25F, 1999.

73. Grundy SM: Cholesterol management in the era of managed care. *Am J Cardiol* 85:3A, 2000.

74. Salonen JT, Salonen R, Seppanen K, et al: Interactions of serum copper, selenium, and low density lipoprotein cholesterol in atherogenesis. *BMJ* 302:756, 1991.

75. Kuklinski B, Weissenbacher E, Fahnrich A, et al: Coenzyme Q10 and antioxidants in acute myocardial infarction. *Mol Aspects Med* 15:S143, 1994.

76. Leslie D, Gheorghiade M: Is there a role for thiamine supplementation in the management of heart failure? *Am Heart J* 131:1248, 1996.

77. Chan P, Huang TY, Chen YJ, et al: Randomized, double-blind, placebo-controlled study of the safety and efficacy of vitamin B complex in the treatment of nocturnal leg cramps in elderly patients with hypertension. *J Clin Pharmacol* 38(12):1151, 1998.

78. McCully KS: Vascular pathology of homocysteinemia: Implications for the pathogenesis of arteriosclerosis. *Am J Pathol* 56:111, 1969.

79. Clark R, Daly L, Robinson K, et al: Hyperhomocysteinemia: An independent risk factor for vascular disease. *N Engl J Med* 324(17):1149, 1991.

80. Nygard O, Nordrehaug JE, Refsum H, et al: Plasma homocysteine levels and mortality in patients with coronary artery disease. *N Engl J Med* 337:230, 1997.

81. Selhub J, Jacques PF, Wilson PW, et al: Vitamin status and intake as primary determinants of homocysteinemia in an elderly population. *JAMA* 270:2693, 1993.

82. Kang SS, Wong PWK, Norusis M: Homocysteinemia due to folate deficiency. *Metabolism* 36:458, 1987.

83. Stampfer MJ, Malinow MR, Willett WC, et al: A prospective study of plasma homocyst(e)ine and risk of myocardial infarction in US physicians. *JAMA* 268(7):877, 1992.

84. Wald NJ, Watt HC, Law MR, et al: Homocysteine and ischemic heart disease: results of a prospective study with implications regarding prevention. *Arch Intern Med* 158:862, 1998.

85. Malinow RM, Nieto J, Szklo M, et al: Carotid artery intimal-medial wall thickening and plasma homocyst(e)ine in asymptomatic adults: The Atherosclerosis Risk in Communities Study. *Circulation* 87:1107, 1993.

86. Selhub J, Jacques PF, Bostom AG, et al: Association between plasma homocysteine concentrations and extracranial carotid artery disease. *N Engl J Med* 332:286, 1995.

87. Ridker PM, Manson JE, Buring JE, et al: Homocysteine and risk of cardiovascular disease among post-menopausal women. *JAMA* 281(19):1817, 1999.

88. Starkebaum G, Harlan JM: Endothelial cell injury due to copper-catalyzed hydrogen peroxide generation from homocysteine. *J Clin Invest* 77:1370, 1986.

89. Durand P, Lussier-Cacan S, Blanche D: Acute methionine load-induced hyperhomocysteinemia enhances platelet aggregation, thromboxane biosynthesis, and macrophage-derived tissue factor activity in rats. *FASEB J* 11:1157, 1997.

90. Stamler JS, Osborne JA, Jaraki O, et al: Adverse vascular effects of homocysteine are modulated by endothelium-derived relaxing factor and related oxides of nitrogen. *J Clin Invest* 91:303, 1993.

91. Al-Obaidi MK, Stubbs PJ, Collinson P, et al: Elevated homocysteine levels are associated with ischemic myocardial injury in acute coronary syndrome. *J Am Coll Cardiol* 36:1217, 2000.

92. McCully KS: Homocysteine and vascular disease. *Nat Med* 2:386, 1996.

93. Boushey CJ, Beresford SA, Omenn GS, et al: A quantitative assessment of plasma homocysteine as a risk factor for vascular disease. Probable benefits of increasing folic acid intakes. *JAMA* 274:1049, 1995.

94. Hankey GJ, Eikeboom JW: Homocysteine and vascular disease. *Lancet* 354: 407, 1999.

95. Homocysteine Lowering Trialists' Collaboration. Lowering blood homocysteine with folic acid based supplements: Meta-analysis of randomized trials. *BMJ* 316:894, 1998.

96. Malloy MJ, Kane JP: Agents used in hyperlipidemia. In: Katzung BG, ed. *Basic and Clinical Pharmacology,* 6th ed. Norwalk, CT: Appleton & Lange, 1995.

97. Morgan JM, Capuzzi DM, Guyton JR: A new extended-release niacin (Niaspan): Efficacy, tolerability, and safety in hypercholesterolemic patients. *Am J Cardiol* 82:29U, 1998.

98. Goldberg A, Alagona P Jr, Capuzzi DM, et al: Multiple-dose efficacy and safety of an extended-release form of niacin in the management of hyperlipidemia. *Am J Cardiol* 85:1100, 2000.

99. Goldberg AC: Clinical trial experience with extended-release niacin (Niaspan) dose escalation study. *Am J Cardiol* 82(12A):35U, 1998.

100. Seed M, O'Connor B, Perombelon N, et al: The effect of nicotinic acid and acipimox on lipoprotein(a) concentration and turnover. *Atherosclerosis* 101(1):61, 1993.

101. Greenberg S, Frishman WH: Co-enzyme Q10: A new drug for cardiovascular disease. *J Clin Pharmacol* 30:596, 1990.

102. Ernster L, Dallner G: Biochemical, physiological and medical aspects of ubiquinone function. *Biochem Biophys Acta* 127:195, 1995.

103. Thomas SR, Neuil J, Stocker R: Co-supplementation with coenzyme Q prevents the pro-oxidant effect of alpha-tocopherol and increases the resistance of LDL to mental-dependent oxidation initiation. *Arteriothromb Vasc Biol* 16(5):687, 1996.

104. Wilson MF, Frishman WH, Giles T, et al: Coenzyme Q10 therapy and exercise duration in stable angina. In: Folkers K, Littarru GP, Yamagami T, eds. *Biochemical and Clinical Aspects of Coenzyme Q.* Vol 9. Amsterdam: Elsevier Science Publishing, 1991.

105. Langsjoen PH, Langsjoen AM: Overview of the use of CoQ10 in cardiovascular disease. *Biofactors* 9:273, 1999.

106. Chen YF, Lin YT, Wu SC: Effectiveness of coenzyme Q10 on myocardial preservation during hypothermic cardioplegic arrest. *J Thorac Cardiovasc Surg* 107(1):242, 1994.

107. Chello M, Mastroroberto P, Romano R, et al: Protective effect of coenzyme Q10 from myocardial reperfusion injury during coronary artery bypass grafting. *Ann Thorac Surg* 58(5):1427, 1994.

108. Singh RB, Wander GS, Rastogi A, et al: Randomized, double-blind placebo-controlled trial of coenzyme Q10 in patients with acute myocardial infarction. *Cardiov Drugs Ther* 12:347, 1998.

109. Bliznakov EG, Wilkins DJ: Biochemical and clinical consequences of inhibiting coenzyme Q biosynthesis by lipid-lowering HMG-CoA reductase inhibitors (statins): A critical overview. *Adv Ther* 15:218, 1998.

110. Braunwald E: Cellular and molecular biology of cardiovascular disease. In: Isselbacher KJ, Braunwald E, Wilson JD, et al, eds. *Harrison's Principles of Internal Medicine,* 13th ed. New York: McGraw Hill, 1994.

111. Lorenz R, Spengler U, Fischer S, et al: Platelet function, thromboxane formation and blood pressure control during supplementation of the western diet with cod liver oil. *Circulation* 67:504, 1983.

112. Li XL, Steiner M: Fish oil: A potent inhibitor of platelet adhesiveness. *Blood* 76:938, 1990.

113. Weiner BH, Ockene IS, Levine PH, et al: Inhibition of atherosclerosis by cod liver oil in hyperlipidemic swine model. *N Eng J Med* 315: 841, 1986.

114. Kenny D, Warltier DC, Pleuss JA, et al: Effect of omega-3 fatty acids on the vascular response to angiotensin in normotensive men. *Am J Cardiol* 70:1347, 1992.

115. Kestin M, Clifton P, Belling GB, et al: N-3 fatty acids of marine origin lower systolic blood pressure and triglycerides but raise LDL cholesterol compared with n-3 and n-6 fatty acids from plants. *Am J Clin Nutr* 51:1028, 1990.

116. Mori TA, Bao DQ, Burke V, et al: Docosahexaenoic acid but not eicosapentaenoic acid lowers ambulatory blood pressure and heart rate in humans. *Hypertension* 34(2):253, 1999.

117. Leaf A, Jorgensen MB, Jacobs AK, et al: Do fish oils prevent restenosis after coronary angioplasty? *Circulation* 90:2248, 1994.

118. Dehmer GJ, Popma JJ, van den Berg EK, et al: Reduction in the rate of early restenosis after coronary angioplasty by a diet supplemented with n-3 fatty acids. *N Engl J Med* 319:733, 1988.

119. O'Keefe J, Harris W: Omega-3 fatty acids: Time for clinical implementation? *Am J Cardiol* 85:1239, 2000.

120. Albert CM, Hennekens CH, O'Donnell CJ, et al: Fish consumption and risk of sudden cardiac death. *JAMA* 279:23, 1998.

121. Simopoulos AP, Leaf A, Salem N Jr, et al: Workshop on the essentiality of and recommended dietary intakes for omega-6 and omega-3 fatty acids. *J Am Coll Nutr* 18(5):487, 1999.

122. Kris-Etherton PM, Taylor DS, Yu-Poth S, et al: Polyunsaturated fatty acids in the chain in the United States. *Am J Clin Nutr* 71(1 Suppl):179S, 2000.

123. Hahnemann S: *Organon of Medicine,* 6th ed. Kunzli J, Naude A, Pendle P, trans. Los Angeles: JP Tarcher, 1982.

123a. Vandenbroucke JP, de Craen AJM: Alternative medicine: A "mirror image" for scientific reasoning in conventional medicine. *Ann Intern Med* 135:507, 2001.

124. Reilly DT, Taylor MA, McSharry C, et al: Is homeopathy a placebo response? Controlled trial of homeopathic potency, with pollen in hay fever as model. *Lancet* 2:881, 1986.

125. Shipley M, Berry H, Broster G, et al: Controlled trial of homeopathic treatment of osteoarthritis. *Lancet* 1:97, 1983.

126. Kleijnen J, Knipschild P, ter Riet G: Clinical trials of homeopathy. *BMJ* 302:316, 1991.

127. Linde K, Clausius N, Ramirez G, et al: Are the clinical effects of homeopathy placebo effects? A meta-analysis of placebo-controlled trials. *Lancet* 350:834, 1997.

128. Linde K, Melchart D: Randomized controlled trials of individualized homeopathy: A state of the art review. *J Alt Comp Med* 4:371, 1998.

129. NIH Consensus Conference on Acupuncture. *JAMA* 280:1518, 1998.

130. Avants SK, Margolin A, Holford TR, et al: A randomized, controlled trial of auricular acupuncture for cocaine dependence. *Arch Intern Med* 160:2305, 2000.

131. Melzack R: Myofacial trigger points: Relation to acupuncture and mechanisms of pain. *Arch Phys Med Rehabil* 62:114, 1981.

132. Bishop B: Pain: Its physiology and rationale for management. Part III. Consequences of current concepts of pain mechanism related to pain management. *Phys Ther* 60:24, 1980.

133. Chen GS: Enkephalin, drug addiction and acupuncture. *Am J Clin Med* 5:25, 1977.

134. Saler G, Iob I, Mingrino S: Cortical evoked responses and transcutaneous electrotherapy. *Neurology* 30:663, 1980.

135. Bjorntorp P: Effects of physical training on blood pressure in hypertension. *Eur Heart J* 8(Suppl B):71, 1987.

135a. Bueno EA, Mamtani R, Frishman WH: Alternative approaches to the management of angina pectoris: Acupuncture, electrical nerve stimulation and spinal cord stimulation. *Heart Dis* 3:236, 2001.

135b. Longhurst JC: Alternative approaches to the management of angina pectoris: acupuncture, electrical nerve stimulation and spinal cord stimulation (editorial). *Heart Dis* 3:215, 2001.

136. Blumenthal M, Busse WR, Goldberg J, et al: *The Complete German Commission E Monographs*. Austin, TX: American Botanical Council, 1998.

136a. Goldman P: Herbal medicines today and the roots of modern pharmacology. *Ann Intern Med* 135:594, 2001.

136b. Stein CM: Are herbal products dietary supplements or drugs? An important question for public safety. *Clin Pharmacol Therap* 71:411, 2002.

137. Tyler VE: Herbs of choice, in *The Therapeutic Use of Phytomedicinals*. New York: Pharmaceutical Product Press, 1994.

137a. Slifman NR, Obermeyer WR, Musser SM, et al: Contamination of botanical dietary supplements by *Digitalis lanata*. *N Engl J Med* 339:806, 1998.

138. Dickstein ES, Kunkel FW: Foxglove tea poisoning. *Am J Med* 69:167, 1980.

139. Radford DJ, Gillies AD, Hinds JA, et al: Naturally occurring cardiac glycosides. *Med J Aust* 144:540, 1986.

140. Cheung K, Hinds JA, Duffy P: Detection of poisoning by plant-origin cardiac glycoside with the Abbott TDx analyzer. *Clin Chem* 35:295, 1989.

141. Moxley RA, Schneider NR, Steinegger DH, et al: Apparent toxicosis associated with lily-of-the-valley (*Convallaria majalis*) ingestion in a dog. *J Am Vet Med Assoc* 195:485, 1989.

142. Bossi M, Brambilla G, Cavalli A, et al: Threatening arrhythmia by uncommon digitalic toxicosis (Italian). *G Ital Cardiol* 11:2254, 1981.

143. Haynes BE, Bessen HA, Wightman WD: Oleander tea: Herbal draught of death. *Ann Emerg Med* 14:350, 1985.

144. Ansford AJ, Morris H: Fatal oleander poisoning. *Med J Aust* 1:360, 1981.

145. Shaw D, Pearn J: Oleander poisoning. *Med J Aust* 2:267, 1979.

146. Tuncok Y, Kozan O, Cavdar C, et al: Urginea maritime (squill) toxicity. *J Toxicol Clin Toxicol* 33:83, 1995.

147. Oates JA: Antihypertensive agents and the drug therapy of hypertension. In: Hardman JG, Limbird LE, eds. Goodman & Gilman's *The Pharmacological Basis of Therapeutics,* 10th ed. New York: McGraw-Hill, 2001:871.

148. Rauwolfia alkaloids, in USP DI – Vol I: *Drug Information for the Health Care Professional,* 16th ed. Rockville, MD: United States Pharmacopeial Convention, 1996.

149. Raudixin, in *Physicians Desk Reference,* 43rd ed. Oradell, NJ: Medical Economics Company, 1989.

150. Brunton LL: Agents affecting gastrointestinal water flux; emesis and anti-emetics; bile acids and pancreatic enzymes. In: Hardman JG, Limbird LE, Molinoff PB, et al, eds. *Goodman & Gilman's The Pharmacological Basis of Therapeutics,* 9th ed. New York: McGraw-Hill, 1996.

151. Sutter MC, Wang YX: Recent cardiovascular drugs from Chinese medicinal plants. *Cardiovasc Res* 27:1891, 1993.

152. Rossier MF, Python CP, Capponi AM, et al: Blocking T-type calcium channels with tetrandrine inhibits steroidogenesis in bovine adrenal glomerulosa cells. *Endocrinology* 132:1035, 1993.

153. Kawashima K, Hayakawa T, Miwa Y, et al: Structure and hypotensive activity relationships of tetrandrine derivatives in stroke-prone spontaneously hyper-tensive rats. *Gen Pharmacol* 21:343, 1990.

154. Ody P: *The Complete Medicinal Herbal*. New York: Dorling Kindersley, 1993.

155. Kuramochi T, Chu J, Suga T: Gou-teng (from *Uncaria rhynchophylla* Miquel) induced endothelium-dependent and independent relaxations in the isolated rat aorta. *Life Sci* 54:2061, 1994.

156. Jaffe AM, Gephardt D, Courtemanche L: Poisoning due to ingestion of *Veratrum viride* (false hellebore). *J Emerg Med* 8:161, 1990.

157. Bahorun T, Trotin F, Pommery J, et al: Antioxidant activities of Crataegus monogyna extracts. *Planta Med* 60:323, 1994.

158. Vibes J, Lasserre B, Gleye J, et al: Inhibition of thromboxane A2 biosynthesis in vitro by the main components of *Crataegus oxyacantha* (hawthorn) flower heads. *Prostaglandins Leukot Essent Fatty Acids* 50:173, 1994.

159. Shanthi S, Parasakthy K, Deepalakshmi PD, et al: Hypolipidemic activity of tincture of *Crataegus* in rats. *Indian J Biochem Biophys* 31:143, 1994.

160. Nasa Y, Hashizume H, Hoque AN, et al: Protective effect of *Crataegus* extract on the cardiac mechanical dysfunction in isolated perfused working rat heart. *Arzneimittelforschung* 43:945, 1993.

161. Roddewig C, Hensel H: Reaction of local myocardial blood flow in non-anesthetized dogs and anesthetized cats to the oral and parenteral administration of a *Crataegus* fraction (oligomere procyanidines) [German] *Arzneimittelforschung* 27:1407, 1977.

162. Taskov M: On the coronary and cardiotonic action of crataemon. *Acta Physiol Pharmacol Bulg* 3:53, 1977.

163. Blesken R: *Crataegus* in cardiology (German). *Fortschr Med* 110:290, 1992.

164. Petkov V: Plants and hypotensive, antiatheromatous and coronarodilatating action. *Am J Chin Med* 7:197, 1979.

165. Zapfe jun G: Clinical efficacy of *Crataegus* extract WS® 1442 in congestive heart failure NYHA class II. *Phytomedicine* 8:262, 2001.

166. Schussler M, Holzl J, Fricke U: Myocardial effects of flavonoids from *Crataegus* species. *Arzneim Forsch* 45(8):842, 1995.

167. Mawrey DB: *Herbal Tonic Therapies*. New Canaan, CT: Keats Publishing, 1993.

168. Zhang W, Wojta J, Binder BR: Effect of notoginsenoside R1 on the synthesis of tissue-type plasminogen activator and plasminogen activator inhibitor-1 in cultured human umbilical vein endothelial cells. *Arterioscler Thromb* 14:1040, 1994.

169. Lin SG, Zheng XL, Chen QY, et al: Effect of *Panax notoginseng* saponins on increased proliferation of cultured aortic smooth muscle cells stimulated by hypercholesterolemic serum. *Chung Kuo Yao Li Hsueh Pao* 14:314, 1993.

170. Lei XL, Chiou GC: Cardiovascular pharmacology of *Panax notoginseng* Burk FH Chen and *Salvia miltiorrhiza*. *Am J Chin Med* 14:145, 1986.

171. Wang Z, Roberts JM, Grant PG, et al: The effect of a medicinal Chinese herb on platelet function. *Thromb Haemost* 48:301, 1982.

172. Yagi A, Fujimoto K, Tanonaka K, et al: Possible active components of tan-shen (Salvia miltiorrhiza) for protection of the myocardium against ischemia-induced derangements. *Planta Med* 55:51, 1989.

173. Mohamadi A, Jarrell ST, Shi SJ, et al: Effects of wild versus cultivated garlic on blood pressure and other parameters in hypertensive rats. *Heart Dis* 2:3, 2000.

173a. Ackermann RT, Mulrow CD, Ramirez G, et al: Garlic shows promise for improving some cardiovascular risk factors. *Arch Intern Med* 161:813, 2001.

173b. Ojewole JAO, Adewunmi CO: Possible mechanisms of antihypertensive effect of garlic: Evidence from mammalian experimental models (abstr). *Am J Hypertens* 14(4 Part 2):29A, 2001.

174. Silagy CA, Neil HA: A meta-analysis of the effect of garlic on blood pressure. *J Hypertens* 12:463, 1994.

175. Silagy C, Neil A: Garlic as a lipid lowering agent—a meta-analysis. *J R Coll Physicians Lond* 28:39, 1994.

176. Kendler BS: Garlic (*Allium sativum*) and onion (*Allium cepa*): A review of their relationship to cardiovascular disease. *Prev Med* 16:670, 1987.

177. Ernst E: Cardiovascular effects of garlic (*Allium sativum*): A review. *Pharmatherapeutica* 5:83, 1987.

178. Kleijnen J, Knipschild P, ter Riet G: Garlic, onions and cardiovascular risk factors: A review of the evidence from human experiments with emphasis on commercially available preparations. *Br J Clin Pharmacol* 28:535, 1989.

179. Ackermann RT, Mulrow CD, Ramirez G, et al: Garlic shows promise for improving some cardiovascular risk factors. *Arch Intern Med* 161:813, 2001.

180. Koch HP, Lawson LD: *Garlic: The Science and Application of Allium sativum L. and Related Species,* 2nd ed. Baltimore: Williams & Wilkins, 1996.

181. Mader FH: Treatment of hyperlipidaemia with garlic-powder tablets: Evidence from the German Association of General Practitioners multicentric placebo-controlled, double-blind study. *Arzneimittelforschung* 40:1111, 1990.

182. Warshafsky S, Kamer R, Sivak S: Effect of garlic on total serum cholesterol. *Ann Intern Med* 119:599, 1993.

183. Rose KD, Croissant PD, Parliament CF, et al: Spontaneous spinal epidural hematoma with associated platelet dysfunction from excessive garlic ingestion: A case report. *Neuroscurgery* 26:880, 1990.

184. Huxtable RJ: The pharmacology of extinction. *J Ethnopharmacol* 37:1, 1992.

185. Zbrun A: Ginkgo—myth and reality (German). *Schweiz Rundsch Med Prax* 84:1, 1995.

186. Kleijnen J, Knipschild P: Ginkgo biloba for cerebral insufficiency. *Br J Clin Pharmacol* 34:352, 1992.

187. Stevermer JJ, Lindbloom EJ: Ginkgo biloba for dementia. *J Fam Pract* 46(1):20, 1998.

187a. Solomon PR, Adams F, Silver A, et al: Ginkgo for memory enhancement. A randomized controlled trial. *JAMA* 288:835, 2002.

188. Ernst E: The risk-benefit profile of commonly used herbal therapies: Ginkgo, St. John's wort, ginseng, echinacea, saw palmetto, and kava. *Ann Intern Med* 136:42, 2002.

189. Warburton DM: Clinical psychopharmacology of Ginkgo biloba extract (French). *Presse Med* 15:1595, 1986.

190. Doly M, Droy-Lefaix MT, Braquet P: Oxidative stress in diabetic retina. *EXS* 62:299, 1992.

191. Vale S: Subarachnoid haemorrhage associated with Ginkgo biloba. *Lancet* 352:36, 1998.

192. Matthews MK: Association of Ginkgo biloba with intracerebral hemorrhage. *Neurology* 50:1933, 1998.

193. Rowin J, Lewis SL: Spontaneous bilateral subdural hematomas associated with chronic Ginkgo biloba ingestion. *Neurology* 46:1775, 1996.

194. Gianni L, Dreitlein WB: Some popular OTC herbals can interact with anti-coagulant therapy. *US Pharm* 23(5):80, 1998.

195. Offord EA, Mace K, Ruffieux C, et al: Rosemary components inhibit benzo(a)pyrene-induced genotoxicity in human bronchial cells. *Carcinogenesis* 16:2057, 1995.

196. Haraguchi H, Saito T, Okamura N, et al: Inhibition of lipid peroxidation and superoxide generation by diterpenoids from *Rosmarinus officinalis. Planta Med* 61:333, 1995.

197. Larrondo JV, Agut M, Calvo-Torras MA: Antimicrobial activity of essences from labiates. *Microbios* 82:171, 1995.

198. al-Hader AA, Hasan ZA, Aqel MB: Hyperglycemic and insulin release inhibiting effects of *Rosmarinus officinalis. J Ethnopharmacol* 43:217, 1994.

199. Swain AR, Dutton SP, Truswell AS: Salicylates in foods. *J Am Diet Assoc* 85:950, 1985.

200. Tyler VE: *The Honest Herbal: A Sensible Guide to the Use of Herbs and Related Remedies,* 3rd ed. New York: Pharmaceutical Product Press, 1993.

201. Zampieron ER: Horse chestnut for venous insufficiency. *Int J Integr Med* 3:41, 2000.

202. Guillaume M, Padioleau F: Veinotonic effect, vascular protection, antiinflammatory and free radical scavenging properties of horse chestnut extract. *Arzneimittelforschung* 44:25, 1994.

203. Rothkopf M, Vogel G: New findings on the efficacy and mode of action of the horse chestnut *Saponin escin* (German). *Arzneimittelforschung* 26:225, 1976.

204. Diehm C, Vollbrecht D, Amendt K, et al: Medical edema protection—clinical benefit in patients with chronic deep vein incompetence: A placebo controlled double blind study. *Vasa* 21:188, 1992.

205. Bisler H, Pfeifer R, Kluken N, et al: Effects of horse chestnut seed extract on transcapillary filtration in chronic venous insufficiency (German). *Dtsch Med Wochenschr* 111:3121, 1986.

206. Schorr DM, Gruber UF: Prophylaxis of thromboembolic complications in gynecological surgery (German). *Geburtshilfe Frauenheilkd* 38:291, 1977.

207. Lang W: Studies on the percutaneous absorption of 3H-aescin in pigs. *Res ExpMed* 169:175, 1977.

208. Takegoshi K, Tohyama T, Okuda K, et al: A case of venoplant-induced hepatic injury. *Gastroenterol Jpn* 21:62, 1986.

209. Voit E, Junger H: Acute posttraumatic renal failure following therapy with antibiotics and beta-aescin (German). *Anaesthesist* 27:81, 1978.

210. Hellberg K, Ruschewski W, de Vivie R: Drug induced acute renal failure after heart surgery (German). *Thoraxchir Vask Chir* 23:396, 1975.

211. Lang W: Dialysability of aescin (German). *Arzneimittelforschung* 34:221, 1984.

212. Bouskela E, Cyrino FZ, Marcelon G: Possible mechanisms for the inhibitory effect of *Ruscus* extract on increased microvascular permeability induced by histamine in hamster cheek pouch. *J Cardiovasc Pharmacol* 24:281, 1994.

213. Bouskela E, Cyrino FZ, Marcelon G: Possible mechanisms for the venular constriction elicited by *Ruscus* extract on hamster cheek pouch. *J Cardiovasc Pharmacol* 24:165, 1994.

214. Bouskela E, Cyrino FZ, Marcelon G: Effects of *Ruscus* extract on the internal diameter of arterioles and venules of the hamster cheek pouch microcirculation. *J Cardiovasc Pharmacol* 22:221, 1993.

215. Berg D: Venous constriction by local administration of ruscus extract (German). *Fortschr Med* 108:473, 1990.

216. Berg D: Venous tonicity in pregnancy varicose veins (German). *Fortschr Med* 110:67, 71, 1992.

217. Weindorf N, Schultz-Ehrenburg U: [Controlled study of increasing venous tone in primary varicose veins by oral administration of Ruscus aculeatus and trimethylhespiridinchalcone] [German]. *Z Hautkr* 62:28, 1987.

218. Li YP, Wang YM: Evaluation of tussilagone: A cardiovascular respiratory stimulant isolated from Chinese herbal medicine. *Gen Pharmacol* 19: 261, 1988.

219. Lambert B: Nassau to ban sale of herbal stimulant linked to a death. *New York Times,* April 17, 1996, pp E1, 4.

220. Haller CA, Benowitz NL: Adverse cardiovascular and central nervous system events associated with dietary supplements containing ephedra alkaloids. *N Engl J Med* 343:1833, 2000.

221. Hoffman BB: Adrenoceptor-activating drugs. In: Katzung BG, eds. *Basic and Clinical Pharmacology,* 6th ed. Norwalk, CT: Appleton & Lange, 1995.

222. Drugs used in bronchial disorders. In: Bennett DR, ed. *Drug Evaluations Annual 1991.* Milwaukee, WI: American Medical Association, 1990.

223. Chan TYK, Chan JCN, Tomlinson B, et al: Chinese herbal medicines revisited: a Hong Kong perspective. *Lancet* 342:1532, 1993.

224. Fatovich DM: Aconite: A lethal Chinese herb. *Ann Emerg Med* 21:309, 1992.

225. Tai YT, But PP, Young K, et al: Cardiotoxicity after accidental herb-induced aconite poisoning. *Lancet* 340:1254, 1992.

225a. Lin MC, Nahin R, Gershwin E, et al: State of complementary and alternative medicine in cardiovascular, lung, and blood research. Executive summary of a workshop. *Circulation* 103:2038, 2001.

225b. Knipschild P: Alternative treatments: Do they work? *Lancet* 356:S4, 2000.

Cardiovascular Drug Interactions

Lionel H. Opie

Cardiovascular drug interactions are numerous, sometimes unpredictable, and potentially serious to patient and physician. Fortunately, serious interactions are relatively uncommon and often avoidable by simple clinical precautions based on a prior knowledge of the properties of the drugs in question.[1,2] There are two types of drug interactions: pharmacokinetic and pharmacodynamic. *Pharmacokinetic interactions* concern all interactions at any stage of the pharmacokinetic steps that most drugs go through, that is, absorption, distribution in the blood and binding to plasma proteins, metabolism (often in the liver), and excretion, often in the urine. Active metabolites may have additional interactions. *Pharmacodynamic interactions,* on the other hand, result from additive cardiovascular hemodynamic or electrophysiologic effects. An example is added atrioventricular nodal block from the combination verapamil-β blocker (Fig. 48-1).[3] Although such an interaction could be predicted, its clinical relevance depends on specific unpredictable physiologic or pathologic variations found in the atrioventricular (AV) node of that particular individual.

The liver is the chief site of pharmacokinetic interactions (Fig. 48-2). An example is increased danger of myopathy with statins during the coadministration of erythromycin or ketoconazole, both inhibiting the cytochrome P450 3A4 system where most of the statins[4] and calcium-channel blockers are metabolized. A second example is the decreased rate of hepatic metabolism of lidocaine during cimetidine therapy, with possible risk of lidocaine toxicity. A third example of a pharmacokinetic interaction lies in those drugs that act on the P-glycoprotein that is the digoxin transmembrane transporter, showing how basic studies can help unravel well-known but poorly understood interactions such as that between quinidine and digoxin (Table 48-1). An example of a pharmacodynamic interaction arises when a calcium-channel blocker (CCB) is added to β-adrenergic blockade in the therapy of severe angina, sometimes with excess hypotension as a side effect.

This chapter analyzes cardiovascular drug interactions in two ways. First, the *major organ sites* of such interactions are considered, starting with the heart itself, followed by an evaluation of vascular smooth muscle as a site for drug interactions, after which come hepatic and renal interactions. There are only a few interactions at the level of plasma proteins. Second, the major classes of cardiovascular drug*s* are sequentially considered.

PERSPECTIVE ON DRUG INTERACTIONS: SIDE EFFECTS VERSUS BENEFITS OF COTHERAPY

The existence of a significant interaction does not necessarily mean that the apparently adverse combination must be avoided. Rather, the overall interests of the patient need to be considered. For example, in the case of the amiodarone-beta-blocker combination in postinfarct patients, the combination seems synergistically effective from the point of view of prolonging life.[5] In patients awaiting cardiac transplantation, a nonrandomized study suggested that the combination improves mortality, albeit at the cost of about 6% of patients requiring a permanent pacemaker.[6] Another example of the risk of the interaction having to be balanced against the expected benefits lies in combination lipid-modifying therapy with statins and fibrates.[7] In some patients with severe lipidemias, the combination brings about the risk of myopathy, albeit relatively low, with a consequent, but even lower, risk of renal failure. These risks must be balanced against the expected increase of life duration as a result of the combination achieving the dual aim of reducing the low-density lipoprotein (LDL)-cholesterol, for which statins are very effective, and increasing the high-density lipoprotein (HDL)-cholesterol for which the fibrates are very effective.[2] It is likely that computer-based decision making will become available to evaluate the exact probability of harm of a drug or drug class versus the expected therapeutic life-prolonging benefit, so that patient and doctor can make informed choices rather than relying on shrewd guesses.

THE HEART AS A SITE FOR DRUG INTERACTIONS

Sinoatrial and Atrioventricular Nodes

The SA node responds to at least three pacemaker currents, including the inward "funny" sodium current initially described in Purkinje's fibers, or I_f; long-acting calcium current, or $I_{Ca(L)}$; and the delayed rectifier, the outward potassium current, I_k.[1] Of these pacemaker currents, two are susceptible to beta-blockers and one to CCBs. There are several reasons why the combination of a beta-blocker with a CCB does not arrest the heart. First, neither type of drug affects the I_k pacemaker current. Second, the CCB effect is on the $I_{Ca(L)}$. The transient calcium current, $I_{Ca(T)}$, which probably accounts for the initial phases of depolarization in the SA and AV nodes, is not affected by standard CCBs. Third, only CCBs of the verapamil and diltiazem types are effective on the SA node in clinically used therapeutic levels.

Dihydropyridine CCBs (nifedipine, felodipine, isradipine, amlodipine, and others) have a much less marked effect on the SA node. In contrast, SA arrest has been reported when an intravenous bolus of verapamil or diltiazem is given to predisposed patients already receiving a beta-blocker. Thus, adverse drug reactions at the level

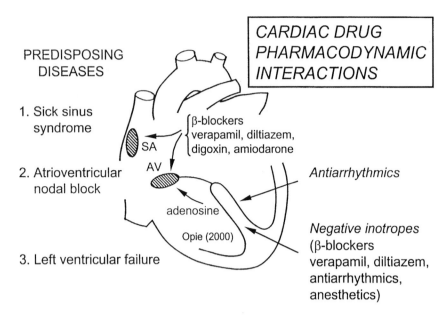

FIGURE 48-1. Cardiac pharmacodynamic interactions at the levels of the SA node, AV node, conduction system, and myocardium. The predisposing disease conditions are shown on the left. AV = atrioventricular; SA = sinoatrial. (*Reproduced with permission from Opie LH.* © *2000.*)

of the SA node causing excess bradycardia, excess tachycardia, or AV block often involve beta-blockers, CCBs, or digitalis.

Intraventricular Conduction System

There are a number of antiarrhythmics that inhibit the intraventricular (His-Purkinje) conduction system. When these are given as cotherapy, they may interact to produce serious additive intraventricular conduction defects.[1]

Proarrhythmic Drug Interactions

There are basically three possible proarrhythmic mechanisms.[1] First, prolongation of the QT interval may occur, especially in the presence of hypokalemia and/or bradycardia (Fig. 48-3). The type of arrhythmia produced by QT prolongation is highly specific, namely torsades de pointes. Second, agents increasing myocardial levels of cyclic adenosine monophosphate or cytosolic calcium levels cause arrhythmias through a different mechanism, namely the precipitation of ventricular tachycardia and/or fibrillation. Third, β-adrenergic stimulants decrease plasma potassium levels, which, in turn, promote automaticity.

Mood-altering drugs (thioridazine, chlorpromazine, amitriptyline, maprotiline, and nortriptyline) predispose to torsades de pointes, presumably by prolongation of the action potential duration.[7a,7b] The complex mechanism may include antimuscarinic, adrenergic, and quinidine-like effects.

Myocardial Contractile Mechanism

Drugs with negative inotropic effects include beta-blockers, CCBs, and certain arrhythmic agents. Often, a relatively well-functioning left ventricle is able to withstand cotherapy with these drugs, but when the left ventricle is diseased, then even one of these drugs may precipitate heart failure.

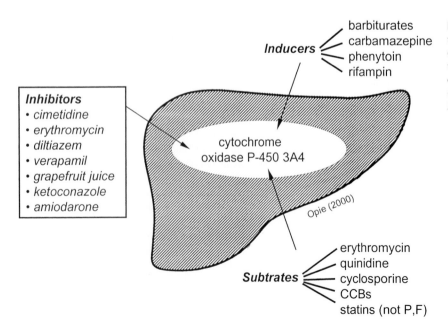

FIGURE 48-2. Potential hepatic pharmacokinetic interactions at the level of cytochrome oxidase P450 (isoform CYP 3A4). For details of cardiac drugs that might interact, see Table 48-1. CCB = calcium-channel blockers; F = fluvastatin; P = pravastatin. (*Reproduced with permission from Opie LH.* © *2000.*)

TABLE 48-1. Proposed P-Glycoprotein-Mediated Interactions of Cardiac Drugs: Comparison with Inhibition of Hepatic Cytochrome Isoforms

P-Glycoprotein Interaction	Cytochrome Inhibition
Antiarrhythmics	
Amiodarone	Inhibits several, including 3A4
Quinidine	Inhibits 2D6
Propafenone	None
Calcium-channel blockers	
Verapamil	Inhibits 3A4
Diltiazem (weak)	Inhibits 3A4
Other cardiac agents	
Digoxin	None
Reserpine	None
Spironolactone	None
Other agents	
Cyclosporine	None
Dipyridamole	None
Erythromycin	Inhibits 3A4
HIV protease inhibitors	Inhibit 2D6, 3A4
Ketoconazole	Inhibits 3A4
Phenothiazines	None

Source: Reproduced from Abernethy and Flockhart[32] and Opie.[1]

VASCULAR SMOOTH MUSCLE

In vascular smooth muscle, there can be interactions to cause excess vasoconstriction, for example, the combination of a drug inhibiting the reuptake of norepinephrine from the nerve terminals (such as cocaine) together with therapeutic administration of monoamine oxidase inhibitors, which also inhibit the reuptake of norepinephrine in the nerve terminals. The combination of cocaine with these inhibitors could, theoretically, promote powerful coronary vasoconstriction. When dopamine is infused into a patient receiving monoamine inhibitors, there is a risk of severe hypertension from excess sensitivity to dopamine.[8]

Conversely, there may be a number of drug interactions causing excess vasodilation and hypotension, for example, the combination of the α_1-blocker prazosin with the powerful calcium-antagonist vasodilator nifedipine.

Vascular smooth muscle can also be the site of drug interactions that lessen the effects of antihypertensive or heart failure therapy.

HEPATIC INTERACTIONS

Pharmacokinetic Interactions

Many cardiovascular drugs are metabolized in the liver, generally via the cytochrome oxidase system involving one of several isoforms (see Fig. 48-2). Of the various isoforms, the CYP 3A4 is the site of most hepatic interactions of cardiac drugs.[9,10] A number of interacting drugs, such as phenytoin, barbiturates, and rifampin, and the herbal remedy St. John's wort, can *induce the CYP 3A4 isoform.*[1] Accordingly, such drugs accelerate the breakdown of those cardiovascular drugs that are metabolized by this isoform, such as atorvastatin, cerivastatin, cyclosporine, disopyramide, felodipine, lidocaine, lovastatin, nifedipine, nisoldipine, propafenone, and simvastatin. Thus the inducers lessen the blood concentrations of these drugs and their therapeutic efficacy. On the other hand, blood levels of these same drugs are increased by those agents that act as *inhibitors of the CYP 3A4 isoform.* The prototype inhibitors are

FIGURE 48-3. Therapeutic agents, including antiarrhythmics, that may interact by QT prolongation to have proarrhythmic effects with risk of torsades de pointes. Class III antiarrhythmic agents (amiodarone and sotalol) act chiefly by prolonging the action potential duration. QT prolongation with quinidine may be dose-dependent with a greater effect at relatively low concentrations, whereas with sotalol there is a dose-dependent increase in QT. Diuretics may cause QTu prolongation to precipitate torsades de pointes during cotherapy, for example with sotalol. Less commonly, torsades de pointes may develop upon initiating antiarrhythmic drug therapy, when there is a preexisting QT prolongation. For further details see Opie and Gersh.[2] (*Reproduced with permission from Opie LH.* © 2001.)

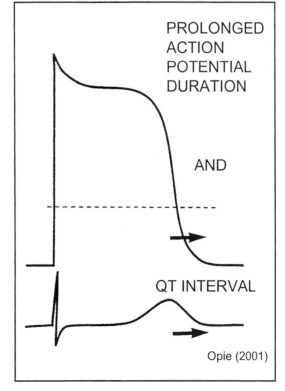

LONG QT WITH RISK OF TORSADES

PROLONGED ACTION POTENTIAL DURATION

AND

QT INTERVAL

- QUINIDINE DISOPYRAMIDE
- IBUTILIDE DOFETILIDE
- SOTALOL (AMIODARONE)
- BEPRIDIL
- TRICYCLICS HALOPERIDOL
- PHENOTHIAZINES
- IV ERYTHROMYCIN QUINOLONES (some)
- ANTIHISTAMINES
  - astemizole
  - terfenadine
- KETOCONAZOLE
- Prolonged QTU: Low K^+, Mg^{2+} (THIAZIDES)
- INDAPAMIDE

Opie (2001)

cimetidine and erythromycin, with grapefruit juice, the calcium blockers verapamil and diltiazem, and the antifungal agents such as ketoconazole all acting as inhibitors. Thus, in statin-treated patients, excess circulating levels may build up, with a greater risk of adverse effects, including greater risk of myopathy.

There may also be a greater therapeutic effect as result of such drug interactions. For example, the dose of the expensive immuno-suppressive cyclosporine can be reduced by cotherapy with verapamil or ketoconazole or high intake of grapefruit juice. Cimetidine inhibits a variety of other isoforms, so that it can increase blood levels of a host of drugs, including the antiarrhythmic drugs quinidine, lidocaine, and procainamide; the CCB verapamil; and the beta-blocker propranolol. Cimetidine, therefore, increases the blood levels of many of the cardiovascular drugs metabolized in the liver. Ranitidine inhibits fewer isoforms and is less likely to interact in this way.

Pharmacodynamic Interactions

These occur whenever altered hepatic blood flow changes the rate of first-pass liver metabolism. For example, when a beta-blocker and lidocaine are given together, as may occur during acute myocardial infarction, the beta-blocker reduces both the hepatic blood flow to the liver and the rate of hepatic metabolism of lidocaine.[11] The consequence is an increased blood lidocaine level, with the risk of lidocaine toxicity. Conversely, by increasing hepatic blood flow, nifedipine has the opposite effect, so that the breakdown of propranolol is increased, resulting in lower blood levels of propranolol.[12] The combination of nifedipine and atenolol, the latter not being metabolized in the liver at all, therefore seems theoretically better than that of nifedipine and propranolol.

P-GLYCOPROTEIN

This newly discovered digoxin transporter[13] operates whenever digoxin crosses the cell membrane (see Table 48-1), for example during renal excretion or when being taken up through the gut wall (Fig. 48-4). Inhibition of the transporter explains the major effects of quinidine and verapamil on blood digoxin levels, and lays aside the previous concept that erythromycin and tetracycline increased digoxin levels by inhibiting the gut flora that break down digoxin. Rather, these agents and especially erythromycin may act at least in part by inhibiting the P-glycoprotein.

RENAL PHARMACOKINETIC INTERACTIONS

A number of drugs interact with each other by competing for renal clearance mechanisms by altering the rate of renal clearance of the other drug.[1] For example, the renal clearance of digoxin is decreased by quinidine, by inhibition of the transporter P-glycoprotein, leading to an elevation of blood digoxin levels (see Fig. 48-4). This renal interaction attracted the attention of cardiologists because it explained certain strange aspects of the effects of these two drugs when given in combination. The knowledge of this interaction showed that apparently established properties of a drug could perhaps be explained more simply as drug interactions.[1] For example, "quinidine syncope" could be caused by digitalis-induced arrhythmias precipitated by cotherapy with quinidine. Other antiarrhythmics that inhibit the renal excretion of digoxin include verapamil,

amiodarone and propafenone, all acting on the same transporter (see Fig. 48-4).

PLASMA PROTEIN BINDING AS A SITE FOR DRUG INTERACTIONS

Sulfinpyrazone powerfully displaces warfarin from protein, so that the dose of warfarin required may be dramatically less.[14]

INTERACTIONS OF BETA-ADRENERGIC-BLOCKING DRUGS

Beta-adrenergic blockers, by their inhibitory effects on the SA and AV nodes can potentially interact negatively with several other cardioactive drugs, including some of the CCBs (verapamil and diltiazem) and amiodarone (see Fig. 48-1). Otherwise, they have relatively few serious drug interactions (Table 48-2). An example of a pharmacokinetic interaction is that with cimetidine,[15] which reduces hepatic blood flow and therefore increases blood levels of propranolol and metoprolol, which are both metabolized in the liver. However, there is no interaction of cimetidine with beta-blockers such as atenolol, sotalol, and nadolol, which are not metabolized in the liver. Another pharmacokinetic interaction is when verapamil raises blood levels of metoprolol through a hepatic interaction.[16] Presumably other beta-blockers metabolized by the liver may be subject to a similar interaction.

Now often used in the acute phase of myocardial infarction, beta-blockers may depress hepatic blood flow, thereby decreasing hepatic inactivation of lidocaine.[11] Thus beta-blockade increases lidocaine blood levels with enhanced risk of toxicity.

INTERACTIONS OF NITRATES

Pharmacodynamic

The major pharmacodynamic drug interaction of nitrates is with Viagra (sildenafil), both being powerful vasodilatory agents. Thus there is risk of life-threatening hypotension, so that the combination is absolutely contraindicated.[17] Other interactions of nitrates are also largely pharmacodynamic (Table 48-3). For example, during triple therapy of angina pectoris (nitrates, beta-blockers, calcium antagonists), the efficacy of the combination may be lessened, because each drug can predispose to excess hypotension. Even two components of triple therapy, such as diltiazem and nitrates, may interact adversely to cause significant hypotension.[1] Nonetheless, high doses of diltiazem can improve persistent effort angina when added to maximum doses of propranolol and isosorbide dinitrate, without any report of significant hypotension.[18] Therefore, individual patients vary greatly in their susceptibility to the hypotension of triple therapy.

Other Interactions

Unexpectedly, high doses of intravenous nitrates may induce heparin resistance by altering the activity of antithrombin III.[19] In dogs, nitroglycerin interferes with the therapeutic efficacy of the tissue plasminogen activator, alteplase.[20] There is a beneficial interaction between nitrates and hydralazine whereby the latter helps to lessen

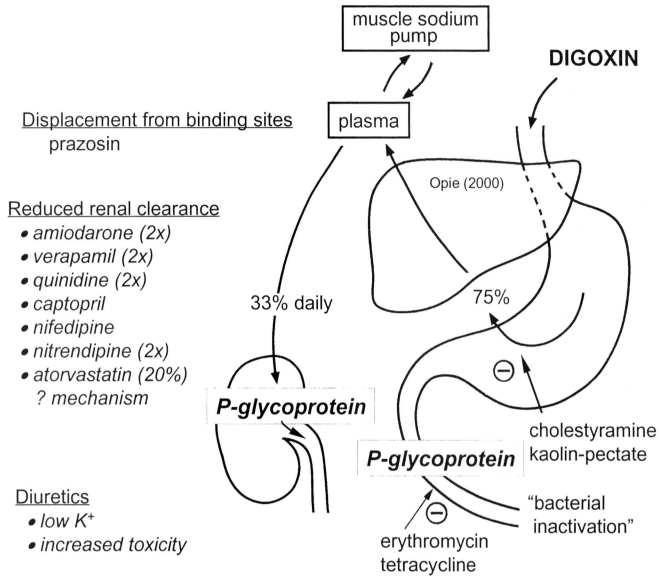

FIGURE 48-4. Potential sites of digoxin interactions. Note the importance of reduced renal clearance. Many of the inhibitory effect on digoxin excretion are probably mediated by inhibition of the digoxin transporter, P-glycoprotein (see Table 48-1). 2× indicates that an approximate doubling of digoxin blood levels has been reported. (*Reproduced with permission from Opie LH.* © *2000.*)

nitrate tolerance.[21] The proposed mechanisms are speculative, but may include vasodilation by a different mechanism to overcome the vasoconstriction of nitrate intolerance. Hydralazine is also a free-radical scavenger, whereas peroxynitrite triggers the vasoconstriction.

INTERACTIONS OF CALCIUM-CHANNEL BLOCKERS

Many of the interactions of CCBs are *pharmacokinetic.* Hepatic metabolic interactions are especially numerous (Table 48-4). Drugs metabolized by the cytochrome oxidase system, such as nifedipine and verapamil, have their breakdown inhibited by cimetidine but not by ranitidine.[1] Verapamil and diltiazem, both metabolized by the cytochrome oxidase system in the liver, can inhibit the hepatic oxidation of some other drugs whose blood levels therefore increase. For example, the blood level of cyclosporine may increase during diltiazem therapy, and during verapamil therapy the blood levels of prazosin, theophylline, and quinidine may all increase. Diltiazem can also interfere with hepatic nifedipine metabolism, potentiating dihydropyridine side effects when the drugs are used together.

In addition, many other interactions of CCBs are *pharmacodynamic,* such as added effects on the SA and AV nodes or on the systemic vascular resistance, with the risk of excess hypotension in predisposed subjects (Table 48-5). Specific examples are verapamil or diltiazem plus beta-blockers or excess digoxin (see Fig. 48-1). There may be two important properties of CCBs that distinguish the specific compounds from each other. First, accumulating evidence suggests that short-acting compounds with acute vasodilatory effects induce acute hypotension and repetitive neurohumoral activation and tachycardia. Thus, the long-acting

TABLE 48-2. Drug Interactions of Beta-Adrenergic-Blocking Agents

Cardiac Drug	Interacting Drugs	Mechanism	Consequence	Prophylaxis
Hemodynamic Interactions				
All beta-blockers	Calcium antagonists, especially nifedipine	Added hypotension	Risk of myocardial ischemia	Blood pressure control, adjust doses
	Verapamil or diltiazem; flecainide; most anesthetics	Added negative inotropic effect	Risk of myocardial failure; hypotension	Check for CHF, adjust doses; flecainide levels
Electrophysiologic Interactions				
Calcium blockers	Verapamil Diltiazem	Added inhibition of SA, AV nodes; added negative inotropic effect	Bradycardia, asystole, complete heart block, hypotension	Exclude "sick-sinus" syndrome, AV nodal disease, LV failure
	Amiodarone	Added nodal inhibition	Bradycardia, heart block	Exclude nodal disease
Hepatic Interactions				
All lipid-soluble beta-blockers: carvedilol, labetalol, metoprolol, propranolol (probably timolol)	Inhibitors of hepatic CYP2D6: cimetidine, ritonavir, quinidine	Decreased hepatic breakdown of the lipid-soluble beta-blocker	Excess beta-blocking effects	Avoid interaction or reduce beta-blocker dose
Antihypertensive Interactions				
All beta-blockers	Indomethacin (I), NSAIDs	I inhibits vasodilatory prostaglandins	Decreased antihypertensive effect	Omit indomethacin; use alternative drugs

Source: Adapted with permission from Opie LH, Frishman WH. Drug interactions. In: Fuster V, Alexander RW, O'Rourke RA, et al, eds. *Hurst's The Heart.* 10th ed. New York: McGraw-Hill, 2001:2251.

second-generation CCBs, such as amlodipine and nifedipine gastrointestinal therapeutic systems (GITS), are less likely to cause acute vasodilatory drug interactions than are shorter-acting compounds. Second, the dihydropyridine CCBs, such as nifedipine, amlodipine, and others, need to be distinguished from the nondihydropyridines, such as verapamil and diltiazem. The dihydropyridines have rather specific vascular dilatory effects, whereas the nondihydropyridines also inhibit the SA and AV nodes and are more negatively inotropic. Thus, the dihydropyridine CCBs have potentially fewer cardiac pharmacodynamic interactions, whereas the nondihydropyridine CCBs also interact with other nodal-inhibitor drugs such as beta-blockers and digoxin.

Another pharmacokinetic interaction, in this case at the level of the kidney, is that occurring between verapamil and digoxin, whereby digoxin clearance is decreased with consequent risk of digoxin toxicity.[1] In the case of nifedipine and diltiazem, such interactions with digoxin appear to be less prominent.

All CCBs are oxidized by the cytochrome P4503A4 system, so that inhibition of this isoenzyme by erythromycin or ketoconazole will increase blood levels of CCBs, with increased risks of adverse effects such as hypertension or heart block, depending on the variety of CCB. Amlodipine, weakly metabolized by CYP3A4, is an exception. Thus, amlodipine could be the CCB of choice in those taking known inhibitors of the CYP3A4 system, such as grapefruit juice, cimetidine, erythromycin, or ketoconazole (see Fig. 48-2). In each case, it could be anticipated that there would be a low, but not zero, probability of an interaction. Grapefruit juice is also an inhibitor of the cytochrome CYP4503A4 system,[9] leading to a doubling of the bioavailability of felodipine and lesser effects on most other dihydropyridine CCBs, with the exception of amlodipine.

TABLE 48-3. Drug Interactions of Nitrates

Cardiac Drug	Interacting Drugs	Mechanism	Consequence	Prophylaxis
All nitrates	CCBs	Excess vasodilation	Syncope, dizziness	Monitor BP, caution
	Prazosin; other α-blockers	Excess vasodilation	Syncope, dizziness	Check BP, low initial doses
	Sildenafil (Viagra)	Excess hypotension*	Excess hypotension, syncope, myocardial infarction	Before giving nitrates for acute coronary syndrome, question for Viagra use in preceding 24 h
	Alteplase (t-PA)	Decreased tPA effect	Thrombolytic benefit less	Avoid or reduce nitrate dose, policy not clear

*Viagra is metabolized by the 3A4 isoform so that inhibitors (see Table 48-4) predispose to excess Viagra levels and to nitrate interaction.

TABLE 48-4. Calcium-Channel Blockers: Hepatic Interactions

Hepatic and Other Interactions of CCBs	Interacting Drugs
Inhibitors of CYP3A4: tend to increase blood levels of CCBs	Cimetidine, erythromycin, grapefruit juice, ketoconazole and related antifungals, amiodarone; St John's wort, a herbal remedy.
Inducers of CYP3A4: tend to decrease blood levels of CCB, especially documented for verapamil	Barbiturates, carbamazepine, phenytoin, rifampin.
CCBs as inhibitors of CYP3A4: Verapamil (V), diltiazem (D), which should have similar effects	1. V increases blood levels of: carbamazepine, prazosin, theophylline, quinidine, cilostazol (expected). 2. D increases blood levels of: cyclosporine, some HIV protease inhibitors, some statins (lovastatin, atorvastatin, simvastatin), cilostazol.
Inhibition of digoxin transport P-glycoprotein	Digoxin blood levels increased by verapamil, nitrendipine.

CCBs = calcium-channel blockers.

TABLE 48-5. Nonhepatic Drug Interactions of Calcium-Channel Blockers

Cardiac Drug	Interacting Drugs	Mechanism	Consequence	Prophylaxis
Verapamil (V)	Beta-blockers	SA and AV nodal inhibition Myocardial failure	Added nodal and negative inotropic effects	Care during cotherapy; check ECG, BP, heart size
	Digitalis poisoning	Added SA and AV nodal inhibition	Asystole; complete heart block after IV verapamil	Avoid IV verapamil in digitalis poisoning
	Digoxin (D)	Decreased D clearance; inhibition of P-glycoprotein	Risk of D toxicity	Halve D dose; blood D level
	Disopyramide	Pharmacodynamic	Hypotension, constipation	Check BP, LV, and gut
	Flecainide (F)	Added negative inotropic effect	Hypotension	Check LV; F levels
	Prazosin, other α-blockers	Hepatic interaction	Excess hypotension	Check BP during cotherapy
	Quinidine (Q)	Added α-receptor inhibition; V decreased Q clearance	Hypotension; increased Q levels	Check Q levels and BP
Diltiazem	Beta-blockers	Added SA nodal inhibition; negative inotropism	Bradycardia, hypotension	Check ECG and LV function
	Digoxin (D)	Some fall in D clearance	Only in renal failure	Check D levels
	Flecainide (F)	Added negative inotropic effect	Hypotension	Check LV; F levels
Nicardipine (see also nifedipine)	Digoxin (D)	Decreased D clearance	Blood D doubles	Decrease; check D levels
Nifedipine (N)	Beta-blockers	Added negative inotropism	Excess hypotension	Check BP, use low initial dose
	Digoxin (D)	Minor/modest changes in D	Increased D levels	Check D levels
	Prazosin (PZ), other α-blockers	PZ blocks α-reflex to N	Postural hypotension	Low initial dose of N or PZ or other α-blocker
	Propranolol (P)	N and P have opposite effects on blood liver flow	N decreases P levels; P increases N levels	Readjust P and N doses if needed
	Quinidine (Q)	N improves poor LV function; Q clearance faster	Decreased Q effect	Check Q levels

AV = atrioventricular node; BP = blood pressure; ECG = electrocardiogram; LV = left ventricle; SA = sinoatrial node.

Source: Adapted with permission from Opie LH, Frishman WH. Drug interactions. In: Fuster V, Alexander RW, O'Rourke RA, et al, eds. *Hurst's The Heart.* 10th ed. New York: McGraw-Hill, 2001:2251.

TABLE 48-6. Drug Interactions of Diuretics

Cardiac Drug	Interacting Drugs	Mechanism	Consequence	Prophylaxis
Diuretics: loop and thiazide	Indomethacin and other NSAIDs	Pharmacodynamic	Decreased antihypertensive effect	Adjust diuretic dose or add another agent
	Probenecid	Decreased intratubular secretion of diuretic	Decreased diuretic effect	Increased diuretic dose
	ACE inhibitors, ARBs	Excess diuretics, high renins	Excess hypotension; prerenal uremia	Lower diuretic dose; initial low dose ACE inhibitor or ARB
Loop	Captopril	Possible interference with tubular secretion	Loss of diuretic efficacy of furosemide	Change to another ACE inhibitor
	Aspirin*	Inhibition of acute vasodilator response	Presumed less efficacy in heart failure	Delay aspirin when initiating acute therapy for heart failure
Spironolactone and other K-retainers	ACE inhibitors	Both retain K	Hyperkalemia	Monitor K, reduce ACE inhibitor dose

ACE = angiotensin converting enzyme; ARBs = angiotensin receptor blockers.

* Data from Jhund PS, Davie AP, McMurray JJV. Aspirin inhibits the acute venodilator response to furosemide in patients with chronic heart failure. *J Am Coll Cardiol* 37:1234, 2001.

Source: Adapted with permission from Opie LH, Frishman WH. Drug interactions. In: Fuster V, Alexander RW, O'Rourke RA, et al, eds. *Hurst's The Heart.* 10th ed. New York: McGraw-Hill, 2001: 2251.

INTERACTIONS OF DIURETICS

Thiazide Diuretics

Steroids, estrogens, indomethacin, and other nonsteroidal anti-inflammatory drugs (NSAIDs) lessen the antihypertensive effect of thiazide diuretics and may worsen congestive heart failure (Table 48-6). Diuretic-induced hypokalemia and/or hypomagnesemia may predispose to ventricular arrhythmias, including torsades de pointes; when that happens, usually an antiarrhythmic agent, such as class III agents, including sotalol, dofetilide, ibutilide, and probably to a lesser extent amiodarone, as well as class 1a agents, such as quinidine or disopyramide, is administered.[1] The common mechanism of action is that all may prolong the QT interval, with risk of further drug interactions (see Fig. 48-3). There is also some suggestion that diuretics may promote torsades independent of hypokalemia.[22] Probenecid interferes with the urinary excretion of thiazide and loop diuretics, so that diuretic efficacy is reduced. Diuretics may impair the renal clearance of lithium, thereby increasing the risk of lithium toxicity.[23]

Loop Diuretics

Loop diuretics, given acutely and intravenously, may cause hypokalemia, precipitating digitalis toxicity.[1] Furosemide decreases renal clearance of lithium. Aspirin and certain NSAIDs may antagonize the action of furosemide and other diuretics, particularly in patients with advanced congestive heart failure and cirrhosis.[24] In normal subjects, concurrent captopril therapy lessens the diuretic effect of furosemide.

Spironolactone and Other Potassium-Retaining Diuretics

Angiotensin-converting enzyme (ACE) inhibitors tend to be potassium-retaining and may cause hyperkalemia if combined with other potassium retainers, especially when there is renal failure. In the RALES study, spironolactone was successfully combined with ACE inhibition in the treatment of severe heart failure.[25] However, the serum potassium level had to be between 3.5 and 5.0 mmol/L, and if hyperkalemia developed, the dose of the ACE inhibitor was down titrated. Furthermore, significant renal impairment, which predisposes to hyperkalemia, (initial serum creatinine >2.5 mg/dL) was an exclusion criterion and medication could be withheld if the value rose >4.0 mg/dL. With these caveats, serious hypokalemia occurred in 14% and 10% of spironolactone- and placebo-treated subjects, respectively. Less well-known is that cyclosporine plus potassium-sparing diuretics may cause hyperkalemia (cyclosporine package insert), presumably via nephrotoxicity of the cyclosporine.

ANGIOTENSIN-CONVERTING ENZYME INHIBITORS AND ANGIOTENSIN-RECEPTOR BLOCKERS

In general, ACE inhibitors have few high-dose interactions (Table 48-7). The most feared interaction is with high-dose diuretics, with risk of excess hypotension in overdiuresed patients. The potassium-retaining diuretics or potassium supplements together with an ACE inhibitor can cause hyperkalemia. Nonetheless in the RALES trial,[25] spironolactone was cautiously added in low doses to heart-failure patients already receiving an ACE inhibitor, with reduced mortality and no serious hyperkalemia (see previous section). Of note, though, in some patients the dose of the ACE inhibitor had to be reduced. Indomethacin and NSAIDs may decrease the antihypertensive effects of ACE inhibitors (and almost all antihypertensives except for the dihydropyridine CCBs such as nifedipine).[26] Thus, NSAIDs may diminish the benefits of ACE inhibitors in heart failure.[27] Aspirin may also interact negatively with ACE inhibitors in heart failure.[28,29] The extent of this interaction is still controversial, and low-dose aspirin may lessen it.[30] Although few clinicians would regard such cotherapy as contraindicated, for example, in a postinfarct patient with LV dysfunction, common sense would advise using the lowest dose of aspirin thought to be protective.

Captopril

Cotherapy of high-dose captopril with other drugs that alter or impair the immune status (such as hydralazine and procainamide)

TABLE 48-7. Drug Interactions of Angiotensin-Converting Enzyme Inhibitors and Angiotensin-Receptor Blockers

Cardiac Drug	Interacting Drugs	Mechanism	Consequence	Prophylaxis
ACEi (class effect)	Excess diuretics; rare in hypertension	High renin levels in overdiuresed patients; volume depletion	"First" dose hypotension: risk of renal failure	Reduce diuretic dose; correct volume depletion
ACEi (class effect)	Potassium-sparing diuretics; spironolactone	Added potassium retention	Hyperkalemia	Avoid combination, or combine with care
ACEi (class effect)	Indomethacin	Less vasodilation	Less BP ↓; less antifailure effects	Avoid if possible
ACEi (class effect)	Aspirin, NSAIDs	Less vasodilation	Less heart failure effects	Low-dose aspirin
Captopril	Loop diuretic	Possible interference with tubular secretion	Lessened diuretic effect of furosemide	Consider alternate ACE inhibitor drug
Captopril (C)	Immunosuppressive drugs, procainamide-hydralazine	Added immune effects	Increased risk of neutropenia	Avoid combination; check neutrophils
	Probenecid (P)	P inhibits tubular secretion of C	Small rise in C levels	Decrease dose of C
ARBs (class effect)	Excess diuretics; rare in hypertension	High renin levels in overdiuresed patients; volume depletion	First dose hypotension; risk of renal failure	Reduce diuretic dose; correct volume depletion

ACEi = angiotensin-converting enzyme inhibitor; ARB = angiotensin-receptor blocker; NSAIDs = nonsteroidal anti-inflammatory drugs.

Source: Adapted with permission from Opie LH, Frishman WH. Drug interactions. In: Fuster V, Alexander RW, O'Rourke RA, et al, eds. *Hurst's The Heart.* 10th ed. New York: McGraw-Hill, 2001:2251.

may predispose to neutropenia. Probenecid inhibits the renal tubular secretion of captopril, thereby potentially increasing blood captopril levels so that doses of captopril may need downward adjustment.[1] Captopril may decrease digoxin clearance by 20 to 30%.[1]

All Other ACE Inhibitors (Including Enalapril)

Drug interactions are similar to those of captopril, except that the immune system is not involved and the risk of neutropenia is much less. It must be considered that because all these agents (except captopril) have a longer duration of action, adverse hypotensive interactions in diuresed patients are potentially more serious. Perindopril may give relative protection from first-dose hypotension, although the mechanism behind this is poorly understood.

Angiotensin-Receptor Blockers (ARBs)

Losartan and irbesartan, but not candesartan, are metabolized by the hepatic 2C9 isoform. Losartan is also metabolized by the 3A4 isoform. The 2C9 isoform is inhibited by fluvastatin. Although sources such as the Georgetown University Web site suggest the potential for an interaction of fluvastatin with losartan, no such interaction was observed in a drug-drug interaction study with fluvastatin and losartan.[31] The hepatic enzymes responsible for candesartan and valsartan breakdown have not been identified, but appear not to be part of the P450 isoform superfamily. Regarding pharmacodynamic interactions, blood pressure may drop significantly when these drugs are given to individuals who have been excessively diuresed and/or have a high renin form of hypertension. Hyperkalemia can occur both with ACE inhibitor and ARB therapy, particularly if a patient is predisposed to hyperkalemia. Hyperkalemia risk is highest in renal and/or heart failure patients, though the risk of hyperkalemia is less with ARBs than for ACE inhibitors.[31a] When ACE inhibitors and ARBs are used in the management of hypertension, the risk of hyperkalemia is substantially less.[31b] Drug interactions are rare for the ARBs with the possible exception of the ARB telmisartan,

wherein its coadministration with digoxin leads to increases in the serum digoxin level.[31c]

INTERACTIONS OF POSITIVE INOTROPIC AGENTS

Digoxin

The best known interaction is *quinidine-digoxin* (Table 48-8). Quinidine approximately doubles the blood digoxin levels, decreasing both renal and extrarenal clearance.[1] The mechanism is by the inhibition of the digoxin transmembrane transporter, P-glycoprotein.[13] Quinine given for muscle cramps acts likewise. The *verapamil-digoxin* interaction is equally significant; digoxin levels increase by 60 to 90%.[1] Again, the mechanism is by inhibition of the digoxin transporter.[32] Nitrendipine, not available in the U.S. but used in Europe, resembles verapamil in approximately doubling the digoxin levels.[1] In the case of addition of quinidine, verapamil, or nitrendipine to a patient already receiving digoxin, the previous dose of digoxin should be halved and the plasma digoxin rechecked. The other CCBs, nifedipine and diltiazem, increase digoxin levels much less than verapamil.[1] Adjustment of the digoxin dose with these agents is usually not necessary, except in the presence of renal failure (which decreases digoxin excretion). Amlodipine does not increase digoxin levels. Thus, there are no simple rules to explain which class of CCBs or which specific agent is likely to increase digoxin levels significantly.

Among antiarrhythmics other than quinidine or verapamil, amiodarone and propafenone[33] also elevate serum digoxin levels. Both inhibit the digoxin P-glycoprotein transporter.[32] Other antiarrhythmics, including procainamide and mexiletine, have no interaction with digoxin except for a relatively small rise of digoxin levels with flecainide.[1] When cotherapy elevates digoxin levels, the features of digitalis toxicity may depend on the agent added. With quinidine, tachyarrhythmias become more likely; whereas

TABLE 48-8. Interactions of Digoxin and Other Positive Inotropes

Cardiac Drug	Interacting Drugs	Mechanism	Consequence	Prophylaxis
Digoxin (D)	Amiodarone	Reduced renal clearance of D; P-glycoprotein (see Table 48-1)	D level may double	Check D level; halve dose
	Atorvastatin	Not known	D level may rise 20%	Check D level
	Captopril	Reduced D clearance	Blood D increases	Check D dose
	Diltiazem	Variable decrease of D clearance; P-glycoprotein (see Table 48-1)	Variable blood D increases	Check D level
	Diuretics: potassium-sparing amiloride or triamterene; spironolactone (S)	Reduced extrarenal D clearance; S reduces D clearance, inhibits P-glycoprotein (see Table 48-1)	D levels vary, may rise by 20% D levels increase, threat of toxicity	Check D level
	Erythromycin	Inhibits P-glycoprotein (see Table 48-1)	Decreased D loss into bowel; increased D levels, threat of toxicity	Check D levels, reduce dose if needed
	Nifedipine	Variable effect on D clearance	Variable blood D rises	Check D levels
	Nitrendipine	Reduced D clearance; mechanism not clear	Blood D Doubles	Check D levels, halve dose
	Prazosin (PZ)	PZ displaces D from binding sites	Blood D rises	(Needs confirmation in humans)
	Propafenone	P-glycoprotein (see Table 48-1)	D level increases	Check D level
	Quinidine, quinine	P-glycoprotein (see Table 48-1)	Blood D doubles	Check D levels, halve dose
	Verapamil	P-glycoprotein (see Table 48-1)	Blood D doubles or more	Check D levels; halve dose
Sympathomimetic Inotropes				
Dobutamine, inamrinone, milrinone	Diuretics, high doses	Additive hypokalemic effects	Arrhythmias	Check blood potassium

Source: Adapted with permission from Opie LH, Frishman WH. Drug interactions. In: Fuster V, Alexander RW, O'Rourke RA, et al, eds. *Hurst's The Heart.* 10th ed. New York: McGraw-Hill, 2001:2251.

amiodarone and verapamil seem to repress the ventricular arrhythmias of digitalis toxicity, so that bradycardia and AV block are more likely.

Diuretics may indirectly precipitate digitalis toxicity by causing hypokalemia, which, when really severe (plasma potassium <2 to 3 mEq/L), may limit the tubular secretion of digoxin. Potassium-sparing diuretics (amiloride, triamterene, and spironolactone), as well as captopril, decrease digoxin clearance by about 20 to 30% and may also elevate serum potassium levels. When these combinations with digoxin are used in the therapy of congestive heart failure, the blood digoxin level must be watched. Unexpectedly, spironolactone and its metabolite canrenone may decrease features of digitalis toxicity,[1] probably through increased potassium levels resulting from aldosterone inhibition. Nonetheless, the combination digoxin-quinidine-spironolactone markedly elevates digoxin levels.[1]

Cholestyramine may cause decreased gastrointestinal absorption of digoxin, probably because of the binding of digoxin to the resin; digoxin should therefore be given several hours before the resin or else digoxin capsules may be used. Digoxin capsules also decrease interaction with kaolin-pectate, which reduces digoxin absorption, and with erythromycin and tetracycline. Cancer chemotherapeutic agents may damage intestinal mucosa to depress digoxin absorption.

Increased digoxin bioavailability with erythromycin and tetracycline[1] was previously ascribed to changes in the gut flora caused by the antibiotics. An alternative and current explanation is that erythromycin inhibits the P-glycoprotein transporter.[32]

INTERACTION OF SYMPATHOMIMETIC AGENTS

Dopamine

Dopamine is contraindicated during the use of cyclopropane or halogenated hydrocarbon anesthetics (enhanced risk of arrhythmias). Monoamine-oxidase inhibitors decrease the rate of dopamine metabolism by the tissues; the dose of dopamine should therefore be cut to one-tenth of the usual dose.

Dobutamine

Dobutamine decreases plasma potassium and should be given with care together with diuretics, especially intravenous furosemide (see Table 48-8).

Inamrinone and Milrinone

Inamrinone and milrinone are phosphodiesterase inhibitors that can also provoke arrhythmias. During diuretic therapy, plasma K^+ needs monitoring. When these drugs are combined with digitalis, the digoxin level does not change, but digoxin toxicity should be

TABLE 48-9. Drug Interactions of Vasodilators

Cardiac Drug	Interacting Drugs	Mechanism	Consequence	Prophylaxis
Hydralazine	Beta-blockers (BB) (hepatic metabolized)	Hepatic shunting	BB metabolism ↓; blood levels ↑	Propranolol, metoprolol dose ↓
	Nitrates (N)	Renal blood flow ↑; added vasodilation; free radicals scavenged	Less N tolerance (benefit); risk of excess hypotension	Could be serious interaction with Viagra
Hydralazine/nitroprusside	Digoxin (D)	Increased renal D excretion	Decreased D levels	Check D levels
Prazosin (P), other α-blockers	Nifedipine; other dihydropyridine calcium blockers	Pharmacodynamic	Excess hypotension	Start with low dose of α-blocker or dihydropyridine calcium blocker
	Nitrates	Pharmacodynamic	Syncope, hypotension	Decrease P dose
	Verapamil	Hepatic metabolism	Synergistic antihypertensive effect	Adjust doses
Cilostazol (C)	Inhibitors of P450 3A4: diltiazem, verapamil, erythromycin, ketoconazole, cyclosporine	↓ Hepatic interaction	Increased C levels, risk of increased mortality in hear failure	Lessen C dose or avoid

Source: Adapted with permission from Opie LH, Frishman WH. Drug interactions. In: Fuster V, Alexander RW, O'Rourke RA, et al, eds. *Hurst's The Heart.* 10th ed. New York: McGraw-Hill, 2001:2251.

guarded against because of multiple mechanisms for arrhythmia development.

INTERACTIONS OF VASODILATORS

Nitroprusside and Hydralazine

Nitroprusside and hydralazine (Table 48-9) may decrease digoxin levels, possibly as a result of increased tubular secretion, by improving congestive heart failure and related renal hemodynamics.[1] Hydralazine, by creating hepatic shunts, may substantially increase the blood levels of those beta-blockers that undergo hepatic metabolism, such as propranolol and metoprolol.[34] Hydralazine interacts beneficially with nitrates, helping to lessen nitrate tolerance.[21]

Prazosin, Doxazosin, and Terazosin

There is an interaction between prazosin and the CCBs verapamil and nifedipine, resulting in excessive hypotension. In the case of verapamil, part of the effect may be explained by a pharmacokinetic hepatic interaction. Both nitrates and prazosin may cause syncope, and these agents should be combined with care. Similar interactions may hold for the other agents in this group. The package insert for terazosin warns of a specific hypotensive interaction with verapamil.

Cilostazol

This is a newly licensed peripheral vasodilator indicated for intermittent claudication. It acts by phosphodiesterase inhibition, and other similarly acting agents have increased mortality in heart failure. It is metabolized by the hepatic cytochrome P4503A4 system, so that there is a potential interaction with inhibitors of this system, such as verapamil, diltiazem, erythromycin, and ketoconazole, all of which could elevate cilostazol levels with increased risk of adverse effects in heart failure.

INTERACTIONS OF ANTIHYPERTENSIVE DRUGS

Interactions for diuretics, β-adrenergic blockers, CCBs, ACE inhibitors, and vasodilators have already been considered. Note that all vasodilators lower blood pressure except for cilostazol, are licensed for peripheral vascular disease. In general, NSAIDs interfere severely with the antihypertensive efficacy of all antihypertensives. An exception is nifedipine (and, presumably other dihydropyridines).[35] Unlike other NSAIDs, aspirin[1] and sulindac may give relative protection from this negative interaction.[1] When dihydropyridine CCBs are used as antihypertensives, part of their effect is by natriuresis, so that adding a diuretic is often relatively ineffective.[1]

INTERACTIONS OF ANTIARRHYTHMIC AGENTS

The emphasis of antiarrhythmic therapy has moved away from agents that do not save lives, such as the class 1a agents quinidine and disopyramide, and the class 1c agents flecainide or propafenone. All these compounds have potentially proarrhythmic drug interactions (Table 48-10). The new emphasis is on drugs that are known to save lives, such as the beta-blockers and amiodarone. Another trend is to intervene in those with serious recurrent supraventricular reentrant tachycardias of the Wolff-Parkinson-White and related syndromes rather than to face prolonged drug therapy. In ventricular tachycardia, the highest risk patients are now ideally treated by an implantable cardioverter defibrillator (ICD). Thus, lesser importance is attached to some of the numerous drug interactions of these agents, which, nevertheless, must be understood.[1]

The most frequent antiarrhythmic drug interactions are with digoxin (the levels of which increase with quinidine and verapamil due to inhibition of the P-glycoprotein transmembrane transporter for digoxin), with diuretics (there is a risk of QT prolongation with antiarrhythmics, such as quinidine, disopyramide, amiodarone, sotalol, dofetilide, and ibutilide, which all prolong duration of the action potential), and at the level of hepatic enzyme inhibition. The mechanism whereby quinidine increases blood digoxin levels has only recently been elucidated (see Table 48-1). There is also the

TABLE 48-10. Drug Interactions of Antiarrhythmic Drugs

Cardiac Drug	Interacting Drugs	Mechanism	Consequence	Prophylaxis
CLASS 1A				
Quinidine (Q)	Amiodarone	Added QT effects; blood Q rises	Torsades de pointes	Check QT, potassium
	Antibiotics (some)	Quinidine inhibits muscarinic receptors	Increased antibiotic-induced muscular weakness	Clinical care, drug levels
	Anticholinesterases	Quinidine inhibits muscarinic receptors	Decreased ACh efficacy in myasthenia gravis	Avoid Q if possible
	Antihypertensive agents; beta-blockers	Added hypotensive and added SA nodal effects	Hypotension, excess bradycardia	Regulate BP Check BP, ECG
	Cimetidine (C)	C inhibits oxidative metabolism of Q	Increased Q levels, risk of toxicity	Q levels, consider ranitidine
	Warfarin, other coumarin anticoagulants	Hepatic interaction with Q	Bleeding	Check prothrombin time
	Digoxin (D)	Decreased D clearance; inhibition of P-glycoprotein	Risk of D toxicity	Check D dose levels
	Diltiazem	Added inhibition of SA node	Excess bradycardia	Check ECG, heart rate
	Disopyramide	Added QT prolongation	Torsades de pointes	Check QT potassium
	Diuretic, potassium losing	Hypokalemia and QT prolongation	Torsades de pointes	Check QT, potassium
	Hepatic enzyme inducers (phenytoin, barbiturates, rifampin)	Increased Q hepatic metabolism by CYP 3A4	Decreased	Q levels, doses
	Nifedipine	Increased Q clearance	Decreased Q levels	Q levels, doses
	Class III agents: Sotalol, amiodarone, dofetilide, ibutilide	Added QT prolongation	Torsades de pointes	Check QT, potassium
	Verapamil	Decreased Q clearance	Excess bradycardia	Check ECG, Q levels
	Warfarin	Hepatic interaction with Q	Bleeding	Check prothrombin time
Procainamide (P)	Cimetidine	Decreased renal P clearance	Prolonged P halflife, excess P effect	Reduce P dose; consider ranitidine
Disopyramide (Dp)	Agents prolonging APD (quinidine, amiodarone, sotalol)	Added QT prolongation especially if hypokalemia	Torsades de pointes	Check TQ, potassium
CLASS 1A (ALL AGENTS)				
	Drugs inhibiting SA or AV nodes/conduction system (quinidine, beta-blockers, methyldopa, digoxin)	Pharmacodynamic additive effects	SA, AV block; conduction block	Check ECG; decrease doses
	Pyridostigmine	Inhibition of cholinesterase activity	Beneficial effect of P on D; harmful effect of D on P	In myasthenia gravis, avoid D
CLASS 1B				
Lidocaine (lignocaine)	Verapamil (V), diltiazem (Di)	Combined negative inotropism	Hypotension	Avoid IV Di or V cotherapy
	Cimetidine (C)	Decreased hepatic metabolism	Increased L levels	Decrease L infusion rate
	Halothane	Decreased hepatic blood flow	Increased L levels	Decrease L infusion rate
	Propranolol	Decreased hepatic blood flow	Increased L levels	Decrease L infusion rate
	Other beta-blockers	Decreased hepatic blood flow	Increased L levels	Decrease L infusion rate
Mexiletine	Hepatic enzyme inducers (Table 48-4)	Increased hepatic metabolism	Decreased plasma M levels	Increase M dose
CLASS 1C				
Flecainide (F)	Amiodarone	Unknown	Blood F rises; added effect on nodes, myocardium	Decrease F dose
	Digoxin (D)	Decreased D clearance	Blood D rises slightly	Check D level
	Drugs inhibiting SA or AV nodes, IV conduction or myocardial function	Pharmacodynamic additive	SA, AV block; conduction block, cardiogenic shock	Avoid combinations, decrease doses
	Cimetidine	Decreased hepatic F loss	Blood F rises	Check F dose
Propafenone	Digoxin (D)	Inhibition of P-glycoprotein	Increased D level	Decrease D dose

(continued)

TABLE 48-10. (*Continued*) Drug Interactions of Antiarrhythmic Drugs

Cardiac Drug	Interacting Drugs	Mechanism	Consequence	Prophylaxis
CLASS III				
Amiodarone (A) (see Table 48–11)	Drugs prolonging QT interval (see Fig. 48-2)	Additive effects on repolarization and QT interval	Torsades de pointes	Avoid low K^+; avoid combinations
	Beta-blockers	Added nodal depression	Bradycardia; heart block	Cotherapy can be very effective; may need pacemaker
	Quinidine (Q)	CYP 2D6 Inhibition	Blood Q rises	Check Q levels
	Procainamide (P)	Pharmacokinetic	Blood P rises	Check P dose
Sotalol, Dofetilide, Ibutilide	As for amiodarone and including amiodarone	Hypokalemia plus class III action, as for amiodarone	Torsades de pointes	Exclude low K^+; use K^+-retaining diuretic
CLASS IV				
Adenosine (Ad)	Dipyridamole (Dp)	Dp inhibits breakdown of Ad	Excess nodal inhibition	Reduce Ad dose to 25% or less
	Theophylline (T)	T blocks Ad receptor	Decrease Ad effect	Carefully adjust Ad dose upwards

ACh = acetylcholine; APD = action potential duration; IV = intravenous.

Source: Adapted with permission from Opie LH, Frishman WH. Drug interactions. In: Fuster V, Alexander RW, O'Rourke RA, et al, eds. *Hurst's The Heart.* 10th ed. New York: McGraw-Hill, 2001:2251.

risk of antiarrhythmic drug-drug interactions. Thus, amiodarone, when added to quinidine, enhances the risk of QT prolongation (see Fig. 48-3), while quinidine levels increase, so that quinidine toxicity is also more likely.[1] The combination of antiarrhythmic drugs that depress the sinus node, like amiodarone and beta-blockers, or CCBs, can occasionally lead to life-threatening bradycardia, requiring a pacemaker (see under amiodarone). Hepatic enzyme inducers can alter the metabolism of agents such as quinidine and other antiarrhythmics that are metabolized in the liver. Cimetidine decreases the hepatic metabolism of these agents, whereas phenytoin, barbiturates, and rifampin have opposite effects (see Fig. 48-2).

Adenosine is increasingly used to terminate supraventricular reentrant tachycardias. Dipyridamole inhibits its breakdown, so that the adenosine dose must be markedly reduced, perhaps to about one-eighth, in those receiving dipyridamole.[36] Rarely, in the presence of digoxin or verapamil, adenosine may precipitate ventricular fibrillation (package insert). As an AV nodal inhibitor (see Fig. 48-1), it may have additive inhibitory effects in the presence of digoxin, verapamil, diltiazem, amiodarone or beta-blockade.

INTERACTIONS OF ANTITHROMBOTIC AND THROMBOLYTIC AGENTS

Aspirin

Blood levels of uric acid may be increased by both low-dose aspirin and thiazide diuretics, so that special care is required in patients with a history of gout. Conversely, aspirin may decrease the uricosuric effects of sulfinpyrazone and probenecid (Table 48-11). Aspirin also reduces the natriuretic effect of spironolactone. Aspirin-induced gastrointestinal bleeding may be a greater hazard in patients receiving other NSAIDs or corticosteroid therapy. Antacids, by altering the pH of the stomach, may decrease the efficacy of enteric-coated preparations.

Hepatic enzyme inducers of cytochrome P450 (barbiturates, phenytoin, rifampin) increase aspirin breakdown. Aspirin tends to cause hypoglycemia in patients receiving oral hypoglycemics or insulin. Aspirin, especially in high doses, may exaggerate a bleeding tendency and worsen anticoagulant-induced bleeding.[37]

Clopidogrel

The use of this agent will increase following a large, recent, positive trial in unstable angina in which it was given together with aspirin. As expected, the incidence of bleeding, major and minor, was increased without more life-threatening bleeds. The package insert also indicates more gastrointestinal bleeding with NSAIDs and, by analogy with aspirin, there may be excess bleeding with warfarin. No heparin interaction as been found. In general there are few other documented drug interactions, but at high concentrations clopidogrel does inhibit the hepatic CYP2C9 that metabolizes carvedilol, cerivastatin, fluvastatin, irbesartan, losartan, torsemide, warfarin, and many NSAIDs. There are, therefore, potential drug interactions that merit caution during coadministration.

Ticlopidine

This drug inhibits platelet aggregation at the same site as clopidogrel, but may cause more serious adverse reactions, such as neutropenia. It similarly interacts with aspirin and NSAIDs, and increased bleeding with warfarin is also a risk. It is metabolized by the hepatic CYP2C9, with the same potential interactions as clopidogrel, and also by the CYP1A2, the latter explaining why cimetidine, an inducer of this isoenzyme, decreases the clearance of a single dose of ticlopidine by 50%.

Sulfinpyrazone

Sulfinpyrazone is highly bound to plasma proteins (98 to 99%) and may displace warfarin to precipitate bleeding. Like aspirin, sulfinpyrazone may sensitize patients who are given sulfonylureas and insulin to hypoglycemia.

TABLE 48-11. Drug Interactions of Antithrombotic Agents

Cardiac Drug	Interacting Drugs	Mechanism	Consequence	Prophylaxis
Aspirin (A)	ACE inhibitors	Vasodilation ↓	Antifailure effect ↓	Low A dose
	Hepatic enzyme inducers	Increased A metabolism	Decreased A effect	Adjust A dose; check A side effects
	Sulfinpyrazone (S), Probenecid (P)	A decreases urate excretion	Decreased uricosuric effect of S or P	Increase dose of S or P
	Thiazides	A decreases urate excretion	Hyperuricemia	Check blood urate
	Warfarin (W)	A is antithrombotic	Excess bleeding	Check INR or PT
Clopidogrel	Aspirin	Added platelet inhibition	Excess bleeding	Awareness of risk
	Warfarin (W)	A is antithrombotic	Excess bleeding	Check INR or PT
	Drugs metabolized by CYP 2C9	Isozyme inhibition	Excess effects of the other drug	Awareness of risk
Ticlopidine	Aspirin, warfarin	As for clopidogrel	As for clopidogrel	As for clopidogrel
	Cimetidine	Hepatic CYP 1A2	Increased levels of ticlopidine	Avoid use of cimetidine
Sulfinpyrazone (S)	Warfarin	S displaces W from plasma proteins	Excess bleeding	Check INR or PT
Warfarin (W)	*Potentiating drugs*			
	Allopurinol	Mechanism unknown	Excess bleeding	Check INR or PT
	Amiodarone	Mechanism unknown	Sensitizes to W for months	Avoid combination
	Aspirin	Added bleeding tendency	Excess bleeding	Check INR or PT
	Cimetidine	Decreased W degradation	Excess bleeding	Check INR or PT
	Quinidine	Hepatic interaction	Excess bleeding	Check INR or PT
	Statins	Hepatic interaction ?	Excess bleeding	Check INR or PT
	Sulfinpyrazone	Displaces W from plasma proteins	Excess bleeding	Check INR or PT
	Inhibitory drugs			
	Cholestyramine, colestipol	Decrease absorption of W	Decreased W effect	Check INR or PT
Alteplase, t-PA	Nitrates	Decreased t-PA effect	Less thrombolytic benefit	Avoid or reduce nitrate dose; policy not clear

INR = International Normalized Ratio; PT = prothrombin time.

Source: Adapted with permission from Opie LH, Frishman WH. Drug interactions. In: Fuster V, Alexander RW, O'Rourke RA, et al, eds. *Hurst's The Heart.* 10th ed. New York: McGraw-Hill, 2001:2251.

Dipyridamole

Dipyridamole is a potent vasodilator, so that care is required when it is used in combination with other vasodilators. Dipyridamole inhibits the breakdown of adenosine (see antiarrhythmics, Class IV).

Warfarin

Numerous Drug and Diet-Drug Interactions

Warfarin may be subject to many (up to 80) drug interactions.[38] Furthermore, there is a *diet-drug interaction*. Warfarin's effects are lessened by a diet rich in the precursor of prothrombin, vitamin K, as found in dark, green vegetables and certain plant oils, including those used in margarines and salad dressings.[39] Therefore, to avoid undue fluctuations in the International Normalized Ratio (INR), a measure of prothrombin time, the dietary intake of these should be constant. Overall, the safest rule is to persuade patients receiving oral anticoagulation to stay on a constant diet, and not to use any new or over-the-counter drugs without consultation, while the physician carefully checks out any planned added compounds. More frequent measurements of the INR and dose adjustments are required when potentially interfering drugs, including herbal agents, are added.

Mechanisms

The major known sites of interaction are, first, the plasma proteins where warfarin is bound while circulating and, second, the hepatic cytochrome P450 system, where warfarin is broken down by the CYP2C9 isoform. For example, with amiodarone a given dose of warfarin has a greater inhibition of prothrombin with increased risk of bleeding, resulting from the inhibition by amiodarone of the CYP2C9 isoform.[32] It should be recalled that coagulation is a complex process, and any drug impairing platelet function, such as aspirin, ticlopidine, or clopidogrel, may indirectly promote bleeding by warfarin. Very high doses of aspirin (six to eight tablets per day) may act differently by impairing synthesis of clotting factors. Heparin also potentiates the risk of bleeding; there are large individual variations.[1]

Interfering drugs include those that reduce absorption of vitamin K, warfarin (cholestyramine), or sulfinpyrazone (that displaces warfarin from the plasma protein binding sites) and those that induce hepatic enzymes (barbiturates, phenytoin, rifampin). The latter drugs, and also the herbal agent St. John's wort,[40] increase the rate of warfarin metabolism in the liver.

Potentiating drugs include those that decrease warfarin degradation by inhibiting the CYP2C9 isoform.[32] These include a variety of antibiotics such as metronidazole (Flagyl) and cotrimoxazole (Bactrim). Other antifungals, such as fluconazole and vaginal suppository miconazole, also potentiate warfarin.[41] Cimetidine likewise inhibits hepatic degradation; ranitidine does not. Other potentiating drugs include the cardiovascular agents allopurinol, propafenone, quinidine, and amiodarone.[1] Amiodarone is especially dangerous because of its excessively long half-life, so that this interaction can occur even after withdrawal of amiodarone.[41a] Grapefruit juice does not act on the CYP2C9 but on the CYP3A4; it has no interaction with warfarin.[1] It must be restressed that sulfinpyrazone powerfully displaces warfarin from blood proteins, so that the dose of warfarin may have to be reduced to only 1 mg in some patients.

Lipid-Lowering Drugs

Fibrates may markedly potentiate warfarin, while the statins in general have little or no effect. The latter is not too surprising because most of them (exceptions: pravastatin and fluvastatin) are metabolized by the CYP3A4 isoform and not through the isoform that metabolizes warfarin. In the case of fluvastatin, the absence of interaction noted in the package insert is surprising because this statin, unlike the others, inhibits the hepatic CYP2C9 according to the Georgetown University Web site data (see reference 1). Nonetheless, caution is advised. In one case, when warfarin was added to simvastatin, precipitating rhabdomyolysis with acute renal failure.[42] On first principles, the simplest statin to combine with warfarin would be pravastatin, because it is metabolized by a route quite different from the cytochrome P450 system.

Heparin

Physically, heparin is incompatible in a water solution with certain substances, including antibiotics, antihistamines, phenothiazines, and hydrocortisone. It is also incompatible with reteplase. However, direct pharmacokinetic or pharmacodynamic interactions have not been described except for a controversial interaction with nitrates.[43]

Tissue-Type Plasminogen Activator

Concurrent use of intravenous nitroglycerin diminishes the efficacy of recombinant tissue-type plasminogen activator (rt-PA or alteplase) possibly because of increased hepatic blood flow and enhanced catabolism of t-PA.[44]

INTERACTIONS OF STATINS AND OTHER LIPID-LOWERING AGENTS

Lipid-Lowering Drugs and Warfarin

A number of lipid-lowering agents may interact with warfarin (Table 48-12), either by decreased absorption (cholestyramine) or by hepatic interference (bezafibrate, fenofibrate, gemfibrozil).

No interaction occurs with niacin. The package inserts for gemfibrozil and fenofibrate, the only two *fibrates* licensed in the U.S., both give prominent warnings that the warfarin dose should be reduced and the prothrombin determined more frequently. The exact mechanism is not clear, but inhibition of the hepatic CYP2C9 that breaks down warfarin is possible. There has been a case report of profound hypoprothrombinemia and bleeding 4 weeks after starting gemfibrozil.[45] With fenofibrate, the INR increased after 5 to 10 days.[46]

In general, there appear to be less-severe interactions between statins and warfarin than with the fibrates. The package inserts indicate that there have been no interactions detected with fluvastatin, pravastatin or atorvastatin. There may be a modest increase of the INR with lovastatin and simvastatin. These effects cannot directly be related to the hepatic P450 isoform known to be concerned with the specific statin. For example, fluvastatin is the only statin that is an inhibitor of the CYP2C9 that breaks down warfarin,[32] but no interaction has been noted (package insert).

Other Interactions of the Statins

The HMG-COA reductase inhibitors such as lovastatin (Mevacor), simvastatin (Zocor), pravastatin (Pravachol), fluvastatin (Lescol), and atorvastatin (Lipitor) should ideally not be combined with the fibrates because of the higher risk of myositis with rhabdomyolysis and possible renal failure. Likewise, concurrent therapy with niacin or cyclosporine or erythromycin may also carry an increased risk of myopathy with further risk of rhabdomyolysis. Adding an antifungal azole (a group that includes ketoconazole, which is used in transplantation) has precipitated myolysis in a patient already receiving a statin and niacin.[47] Serum creatine kinase levels should be checked periodically, especially after increasing doses or after starting combination therapy. Yet, sometimes in clinical practice, the advantages of better lipid control with cautiously combined and monitored therapy seems to outweigh these risks, which may have been overestimated. In the case of cerivastatin, the drug had to be withdrawn after more than 50 fatalities, most ascribed to an interaction with gemfibrozil. Pravastatin is not metabolized by the cytochrome P450 system, as are all the other statins. Theoretically this may avoid many of the interactions leading to myopathy. Fluvastatin (Lescol) is metabolized by a different hepatic P450 enzyme system (2C9) from the others, except for pravastatin (see above), which may explain why it has not been associated with an increased

TABLE 48-12. Drug Interactions of Lipid-Lowering Agents

Lipid-Lowering Drug	Interacting Drugs	Mechanism	Consequence	Prophylaxis
Fibric acids (gemifibrozil, clofibrate, bezafibrate, fenofibrate)	Warfarin; statins (see below)	Hepatic interference	Risk of bleeding	Check PT
Bile acid sequestrants (cholestyramine, colestipol)	Warfarin; many other drugs	Decreased absorption; decreased absorption	Decreased warfarin effect; decreased drug effect	Check PT; space doses
HMG-CoA reductase inhibitors (statins: lovastatin, simvastatin)	Fibrates, inhibitors of CYP 3A4 (erythromycin, antifungal azoles others; see Fig. 48-1), nicotinic acid, cyclosporine	Added damage to muscle with myositis	Rhabdomyolysis and risk of renal failure; increased cyclosporine levels	Check creatine phosphokinase levels; avoid if possible
Statins	Warfarin	Hepatic interaction	Increased risk of bleeding	Check INR or PT
Pravastatin	Cyclosporine	Hepatic interaction; cyclosporine hepatotoxicity	Rhabdomyolysis and risk of renal failure; increased cyclosporine levels	Check creatine phosphokinase levels; avoid if possible

Source: Adapted with permission from Opie LH, Frishman WH. Drug interactions. In: Fuster V, Alexander RW, O'Rourke RA, et al, eds. *Hurst's The Heart.* 10th ed. New York: McGraw-Hill, 2001:2251.

incidence of myopathy during cotherapy with nicotinic acid (package insert).

Regarding statins and digoxin, there is no interaction with lovastatin or pravastatin, a small increase in blood digoxin levels occurs with simvastatin and fluvastatin, and a 20% increase with atorvastatin.

INTERACTIONS OF NONCARDIOVASCULAR DRUGS USED IN CARDIAC TRANSPLANTATION

Cyclosporine

Cyclosporine is metabolized by the hepatic 3A4 isoform cytochrome system, without inhibiting it. Thus, the potential interactions are with the inhibitors of this system (see Fig. 48-2). For example, grapefruit juice increases the area-under-the-curve (AUC) of cyclosporine by approximately 45%.[48] Both verapamil and diltiazem increase levels of cyclosporine, and may permit a lower dose to be used with cost-savings.[32] High levels of cyclosporine increase the risk of renal toxicity and hypertension. It is not clear why cyclosporine predisposes to myopathy with some statins; it does not inhibit the CYP3A4 that breaks down the statins. Presumably cyclosporine hepatotoxicity damages the statin breakdown system. In addition, cyclosporine nephropathy could inhibit that low percentage of the statin that is lost by renal secretion. Cyclosporine may predispose to digoxin toxicity, reducing the renal clearance and decreasing its volume of distribution. The mechanism may be by inhibition of the transmembrane digoxin transporter P-glycoprotein.[32]

Ketoconazole

This is an antifungal agent that increases blood cyclosporine levels by inhibition of the 3A4 isoform, so that the dose of the more expensive agent, cyclosporine, can be reduced. Its interactions are therefore both direct, via inhibition of the breakdown of those many drugs metabolized by this isoform (see Fig. 48-2), and indirect by increasing blood levels of cyclosporine.

INTERACTIONS OF HERBAL DRUGS

Herbal drugs are now commonly used (see Chap. 47). Often the physician is ignorant of the fact that the patient is taking an herbal drug, and, in addition, does not know that such drugs may have harmful interactions.[49] Garlic and ginkgo promote the action of warfarin, perhaps by causing platelet dysfunction.[49] Danshen increases the INR, probably by decreasing the elimination of warfarin.[50] Dong quai increases the INR because it contains coumarin.[50] St. John's wort, a supposed antidepressant, lowers serum warfarin, perhaps by its capacity to stimulate hepatic cytochrome P450.[40] It also decreases the blood digoxin concentration by about one-third.[51]

REFERENCES

1. Opie LH: Adverse cardiovascular drug reactions. *Curr Probl Cardiol* 25:621, 2000.
2. Opie LH, Gersh BJ: *Drugs for the Heart*. 5th ed. Philadelphia: WB Saunders, 2001.
3. Edoute Y, Nagachandran P, Svirski B, Ben-Ami H: Cardiovascular adverse drug reaction associated with combined β-adrenergic and calcium entry-blocking agents. *J Cardiovasc Pharmacol* 35:556, 2000.
4. White CM: An evaluation of CYP3A4 drug interactions with HMG-CoA reductase inhibitors. *Formulary* 35:343, 2000.
5. Boutitie F, Boissel JP, Connolly SJ, et al: Amiodarone interactions with beta-blockers. Analysis of the merged EMIAT (European Myocardial Infarct Trial) and CAMIAT (Canadian Amiodarone Myocardial Infarct Trial) databases. *Circulation* 99:2268, 1999.
6. Nägele H, Bohlmann M, Eck U, et al: Combination therapy with carvedilol and amiodarone in patients with severe heart failure. *Eur J Heart Fail* 2:71, 2000.
7. Backman JT, Kyrklund C, Kivisto KT, et al: Plasma concentrations of active simvastatin acid are increased by gemfibrozil. *Clin Pharmacol Ther* 68:122, 2000.
7a. Feinstein RE, Khawaja IS, Nurenberg JR, Frishman WH: Cardiovascular effects of psychotropic drugs. *Curr Probl Cardiol* 27:188, 2002.
7b. Haddad PM, Anderson IM: Antipsychotic-related QTC prolongation, torsade de pointes, and sudden death. *Drugs* 62:1649, 2002.
8. Horwitz D, Goldberg LI, Sjoerdsma A: Increased blood pressure responses to dopamine and norepinephrine produced by monoamine oxidase inhibitors in man. *J Lab Clin Med* 56:745, 1960.
9. Kane GC, Lipsky JJ: Drug-grapefruit juice interactions. *Mayo Clin Proc* 75:933, 2000.
10. Cheng JWM: Cytochrome P450-mediated cardiovascular drug interactions. *Heart Dis* 2:254, 2000.
11. Ochs HR, Carstens G, Greenblatt DJ: Reduction in lidocaine clearance during continuous infusion and by coadministration of propranolol. *N Eng J Med* 303:373, 1980.
12. Kleinbloesem CH, van Brummelen P, Sandberg TH, et al: Kinetic and haemodynamic interactions between nifedipine and propranolol in healthy subjects utilizing controlled rates of drug input. In: Kleinbloesem CH, ed. *Nifedipine: Clinical Pharmacokinetics and Haemodynamic Effects*. 's-Gravenhage: Drukkerij J H Pasmans BV, 1985: 151.
13. Fromm MF, Kim RB, Stein M, et al: Inhibition of P-glycoprotein-mediated drug transport. A unifying mechanism to explain the interaction between digoxin and quinidine. *Circulation* 99:552, 1999.
14. Bailey RR, Reddy J: Potentiation of warfarin action by sulphinpyrazone (letter). *Lancet* 1:254, 1980.
15. Kirch W, Spahn H, Kohler H, Mutschler E: Influence of β-receptor antagonists on pharmacokinetics of cimetidine. *Drugs* 25(Suppl 2):127, 1983.
16. McLean A, Knight R, Harrison P, Harper R: Clearance-based oral drug interaction between verapamil and metoprolol and comparison with atenolol. *Am J Cardiol* 55:1628, 1985.
17. ACC-AHA. Summary statement of the American College of Cardiology and the American Heart Association on the use of sildenafil (Viagra) in patients at clinical risk from cardiovascular effects. *Clin Rev* 8:91, 1998.
18. Boden WE, Bough EW, Reichman MJ, et al: Beneficial effects of high-dose diltiazem in patients with persistent effort angina on β-blockers and nitrates: A randomized, double-blind, placebo-controlled, crossover study. *Circulation* 71:1197, 1985.
19. Becker RC, Corrao JM, Bovill EG, et al: Intravenous nitroglycerin-induced heparin resistance: A qualitative antithrombin III abnormality. *Am Heart J* 119:1254, 1990.
20. Mehta S, Charbonneau F, Fitchett DH: The clinical consequences of a stiff left atrium. *Am Heart J* 122:1184, 1991.
21. Gogia H, Mehra A, Parikh S, et al: Prevention of tolerance to hemodynamic effects of nitrates with concomitant use of hydralazine in patients with chronic heart failure. *J Am Cardiol* 26:1575, 1995.
22. Roden D: Taking the "idio" out of "idiosyncratic": Predicting torsades de pointes. *PACE* 21:1029, 1998.
23. Jefferson JW, Kalin NH: Serum lithium levels and long-term diuretic use. *JAMA* 241:1134, 1979.
24. Jhund PS, Davie AP, McMurray JJV: Aspirin inhibits the acute venodilator response to furosemide in patients with chronic heart failure. *J Am Coll Cardiol* 37:1234, 2001.
25. Pitt B, Zannad F, Remme WJ, et al: for the Randomized Aldactone Evaluation Study Investigators. The effect of spironolactone on morbidity

and mortality in patients with severe heart failure. *N Engl J Med* 341:709, 1999.

26. Conlin PR, More TJ, Swartz SL, et al: Effect of indomethacin on blood pressure lowering by captopril and losartan in hypertensive patients. *Hypertension* 36:461, 2000.

27. Townend JN, Doran J, Lote CJ, Davies MK: Peripheral haemodynamic effects of inhibition of prostaglandin synthesis in congestive heart failure and interactions with captopril. *Br Heart J* 73:434, 1995.

28. Massie BM, Teerlink JR: Interaction between aspirin and angiotensin-converting enzyme inhibitors: Real or imagined. *Am J Med* 109:431, 2000.

29. Leor J, Reicher-Reiss H, Goldbourt U, et al: Aspirin and mortality in patients treated with angiotensin-converting enzyme inhibitors: A cohort study of 11,575 patients with coronary artery disease. *J Am Coll Cardiol* 33:1920, 1999.

30. Opie LH, Frishman WH, Thadani U: Angiotensin-converting enzyme inhibitors and conventional vasodilators. In: Opie LH, ed. *Drugs for the Heart.* 4th ed. Philadelphia: WB Saunders, 1994:105.

31. Meadowcroft AM, Williamson KM, Patterson JH, et al: The effects of fluvastatin, a CYP2C9 inhibitor, on losartan pharmacokinetics in healthy volunteers. *J Clin Pharmacol* 39:418, 1999.

31a. Bakris GL, Siomos M, Richardson D, et al: ACE inhibition or angiotensin receptor blockade: Impact on potassium in renal failure: VAL-K Study Group. *Kidney Intl* 58:2084, 2000.

31b. Reardon LC, MacPherson DS: Hyperkalemia in outpatients using angiotensin-converting enzyme inhibitors. How much should we worry? *Arch Intern Med* 158:26, 1998.

31c. Stangier J, Su CA, Hendriks MG, et al: The effect of telmisartan on the steady-state pharmacokinetics of digoxin in healthy male volunteers. *J Clin Pharmacol* 40:1373, 2000.

32. Abernethy DR, Flockhart DA: Molecular basis of cardiovascular drug metabolism. Implications for predicting clinically important drug interactions. *Circulation* 101:1749, 2000.

33. Hodges M, Salerno D, Granrud G: Double-blind placebo-controlled evaluation of propafenone in suppressing ventricular ectopic activity. *Am J Cardiol* 54:45D, 1984.

34. Schneck DW, Vary JE: Mechanism by which hydralazine increases propranolol bioavailability. *Clin Pharmacol Ther* 35:447, 1984.

35. Salvetti A, Magagna A, Abdel-Haq B, et al: Nifedipine interactions in hypertensive patients. *Cardiovasc Drugs Ther* 4:963, 1990.

36. Watt AH, Bernard MS, Webster J, et al: Intravenous adenosine in the treatment of supraventricular tachycardia: a dose-ranging study and interaction with dipyridamole. *Br J Clin Pharmacol* 21:227, 1986.

37. Moroz L: Increased blood fibrinolytic activity after aspirin ingestion. *N Engl J Med* 296:525, 1977.

38. Stratton F, Chalmers DG, Flute PT, et al: Drug interaction with coumarin derivative anticoagulants. *Br Med J* 285:274, 1982.

39. Booth SL, Centurelli MA. Vitamin K: a practical guide to the dietary management of patients on warfarin. *Nutr Rev* 57:288, 1999.

40. Ernst E: Second thoughts about safety of St. John's wort. *Lancet* 354:2014, 1999.

41. Thirion DJ, Zanetti LA: Potentiation of warfarin's hypoproteinemic effect with miconazole vaginal suppositories. *Pharmacotherapy* 20:98, 2000.

41a. Sanoski CA, Bauman JL: Clinical observations with the amiodarone/warfarin interaction. Dosing relationships with long-term therapy. *Chest* 121:19, 2002.

42. Mogyorosi A, Bradley B, Showalter A, Schubert ML: Rhabdomyolysis and acute renal failure due to combination therapy with simvastatin and warfarin. *J Intern Med* 246:599, 1999.

43. Koh KK, Park GS, Song JH, et al: Interaction of intravenous heparin and organic nitrates in acute ischemic syndromes. *Am J Cardiol* 76:706, 1995.

44. Romeo F, Rosano GM, Martuscelli E, et al: Concurrent nitroglycerin administration reduces the efficacy of recombinant tissue-type plasminogen activator in patients with acute anterior wall myocardial infarction. *Am Heart J* 130:692, 1995.

45. Rindone JP, Keng HC: Gemfibrozil-warfarin drug interaction resulting in profound hypoprothaminemia. *Chest* 114:641, 1998.

46. Ascah KJ, Rock GA, Wells PS: Interaction between fenofibrate and warfarin. *Ann Pharmacother* 32:765, 1998.

47. Lees RS, Lees AM: Rhabdomyolysis from the coadministration of lovastatin and the antifungal agent itraconazole. *N Engl J Med* 333:664, 1995.

48. Yee GC, Stanley DL, Pessa LJ, et al: Effect of grapefruit juice on blood cyclosporin concentration. *Lancet* 345:955, 1995.

49. Clinicians must remain alert for interactions between herbal medicines and prescribed drugs. *Drug Therap Perspect* 18:17, 2002.

50. Fugh-Berman A: Herb-drug interactions. *Lancet* 355:134, 2000.

51. Johne A, Brockmoller J, Bauer S, et al: Interaction of St. John's wort extract with digoxin (abstr.). *Eur J Clin Pharmacol* 55:A22, 1999.

CHAPTER 49

Pediatric Cardiovascular Pharmacology

Michael Gewitz

Paul Woolf

William H. Frishman

Joyce Wu

Increasingly, infants and children with cardiovascular disorders, even those with severe illnesses, are living through childhood into their adult years. The quality of life, with growth, development, and successful psychologic maturation as markers, continues to steadily improve as well for these patients. Much of this success is related to better refinement of pharmacologic supports, which has developed through increased understanding of the interplay of developing biologic systems and pharmacotherapeutics. This chapter reviews several important issues relating to the treatment of cardiovascular problems in infants and children with the broadening spectrum of agents available to the clinician. In many instances, pharmacologic treatments reflect modification of approaches learned from practice in the adult population. In others, novel approaches have been developed specifically for the unique problems encountered in children, either as a result of their primary disorder or as a result of its partial palliation. In all circumstances, however, documented differences in gastrointestinal physiology, in volumes of distribution, in receptor physiology, and in other key elements of metabolic and circulatory dynamics exist, which impact on cardiovascular pharmacotherapeutics. Many of these important differences are reviewed in this chapter as well. Recognition of the fact that, with regard to pharmacotherapeutics, important differences exist between infants and children as compared to adults, has led to an important initiative on the part of the FDA and the pharmaceutical industry to understand how these differences impact on the use of specific pharmaceuticals.[1] However, given the large amount of information still to be developed, the overall view should be one of a work in progress, as each day more and more agents become officially approved for use in children with attendant modification and alteration. Finally, this chapter builds upon the information developed in the pediatric chapter in the first edition of this text, reiterating important points made in that original effort, amplifying them where appropriate, and updating them as new information has developed.

There are many conditions that do have overlap between the adult and pediatric populations, and we will start with a review of the pharmacotherapeutics of these problems.

CONGESTIVE HEART FAILURE

Table 49-1 reviews the causes of congestive heart failure (CHF) in childhood. Most of these problems are amenable to surgical correction or to substantial palliation of the underlying anatomic disorder. An important proportion, however, are related to either inherited or acquired problems of cardiac muscle mechanics. Survival in this population is generally increasing, although recovery can require an extended period, even as long as 2 years.[2,2a] Thus, medical therapy has become increasingly important in the childhood management of CHF for several reasons: (a) to allow underlying reparative mechanisms to develop after acquired or iatrogenic acute insults to cardiac muscle; (b) to enable chronic survival while awaiting extreme interventions, such as orthotopic transplantation or longer-term mechanical supports; (c) to improve lifestyle quality after surgical intervention for complete repair or for palliation.

Inotropes and Vasopressors

Digoxin

In the pediatric population, digoxin is the most extensively used digitalis glycoside and, essentially, the only inotropic agent available for oral administration. The desired effects of digoxin are mechanical and electrical, that is, to improve contractility of the failing heart and prolong the refractory period of the atrioventricular (AV) node, respectively (also see Chap. 13). Inhibition of the sarcolemmal Na^+/K^+-ATPase pump and an associated increase in available intracellular calcium, result in digoxin's positive inotropic effect. It slows conduction velocity and increases refractoriness at the AV node, mediated mostly through its vagal effect. In canine studies, the electrophysiologic effects of digoxin are less pronounced in neonatal Purkinje fibers than they are in human adult myocardium.[3] This difference may be related, in part, to the increased concentrations of Na^+/K^+-ATPase (the enzyme inhibited by digoxin) in the neonatal myocardium.

Digoxin is used in a variety of circumstances causing CHF. In infants with large left-to-right shunts or with severe valvular regurgitation, surgical correction is preferred, but when not feasible, digoxin may help with the accommodation to large-volume loads. This has been a controversial indication because in many of these situations, normal or even increased myocardial contractility is present. In this circumstance, the effect of digoxin on sympathetic tone is probably key as it helps to counter the catabolic effects of increased catecholamine output in these babies. The classic indication

TABLE 49-1. Etiologic Considerations for Congestive Heart Failure

Congenital Heart Disease	Acquired Heart Disease	Endocrine/Metabolic	Other
Pressure Overload	Myocarditis	Electrolyte Disturbances	Ingestions/Toxins
Left ventricular outflow obstruction (e.g., aortic stenosis, severe coarctation)	Viral infections	Hypoglycemia	Cardiac toxins (e.g., digitalis)
Left ventricular inflow obstruction (e.g., cor triatriatum)	Kawasaki disease	Hypothyroidism	Arrhythmogenics (e.g., tricyclic antidepressants)
Volume Overload	Collagen-vascular disease	Calcium or magnesium disorders	Chemotherapy agents (e.g., adriamycin)
Left-to-right shunts (e.g., ventricular septal defect)	Cardiomyopathy	Lipid Disorders	
Anomalous pulmonary Venous return	Chronic anemia (e.g., thalassemia major)	Camitine deficiency	
Valvar regurgitation (e.g., aortic insufficiency)	Nutritional disorders	Carbolic acid disorders	
Arteriovenous fistulae	AIDS	Fatty acid disorders	
Other Structural Disease	Pericardial Disease	Storage Diseases	
Anomalous coronary artery	Rheumatic Heart Disease		
Traumatic injury	Cor Pulmonale		
Rhythm Disturbance	Acute (e.g., upper airway obstruction)		
Supraventricular tachycardia	Cystic fibrosis		
Complete heart block	Neuropathies		
Postoperative Heart Disease	Endocarditis		
Malfunctioning prosthetic valve			

AIDS = acquired immunodeficiency syndrome.

Source: Reprinted with permission from Gewitz MH, and Vetter VL.[13]

for digoxin involves diminished myocardial performance, when it is used in conjunction with diuretics and afterload reduction agents.

Digoxin toxicity is relatively common because of the drug's narrow therapeutic window. As in adults, digoxin toxicity in children includes sinus bradycardia, sinus arrest, complete AV block, and ventricular arrhythmias.[4] Other effects include anorexia in older children and vomiting in infants, as well as CNS disturbances. A variety of drugs may predispose to digoxin toxicity, especially antiarrhythmic medications such as quinidine, verapamil, and amiodarone, although the effects of quinidine on digoxin in childhood may differ from those seen in adults. It is well established that quinidine increases serum digoxin levels in adult patients on a stable dose of digoxin.[5] However, quinidine has no effect on the serum digoxin level of neonatal dogs. Yet, quinidine does result in higher levels of digoxin in the brain.[6] In one pediatric study, no relationship was observed between quinidine and digoxin levels. In fact, infants younger than 2 months of age did not show an increase in digoxin levels at all.[7] In adult patients taking maintenance digoxin, amiodarone is also reported to cause significant elevation of serum digoxin levels.[8] After the initiation of amiodarone therapy, significant increases of digoxin levels, associated with prolongation of the digoxin half-life, have been observed in children as well.[9] Verapamil, like quinidine, inhibits the renal elimination of digoxin without changing the glomerular filtration rate (GFR),[10] and thereby increases plasma digoxin concentrations. Hence, in settings where it is accepted practice to use verapamil and digoxin simultaneously, such as therapy for a variety of arrhythmias in children, frequent measurements of serum digoxin levels should be done.[11] It is recommended that when starting either quinidine or amiodarone in children on maintenance digoxin, the serum digoxin level should be measured and the digoxin dose reduced by 40 to 50%. Serial digoxin levels should then be measured and the digoxin dose titrated upward.

Because digoxin is primarily eliminated by the kidneys, any drug given simultaneously that causes renal impairment may change the pharmacokinetics of digoxin. This is particularly true when digoxin is used in combination with vasodilators (see below) such as enalapril and diuretics. Potassium loss can also potentiate toxicity and potassium monitoring is required whenever these drugs are used together. There is no specific correlation of higher serum levels and enhanced digoxin effect. Therefore, current recommendations[12] suggest a serum level of 1 to 2 ng/mL as an appropriate target for maintenance therapy. In neonates, endogenous "digoxin-like" substances can interfere with digoxin level interpretation.

Newborns, particularly premature, present a problem with regard to loading dosages, the commonly prescribed method of initiating treatment with digoxin because of the large volume of distribution. Thus, reductions in loading dose regimens have been devised, taking into account gestational age and weight, in order to decrease the risk for toxicity, as noted in Table 49-2.[13]

Dopamine

Dopamine is an endogenous catecholamine and the precursor of norepinephrine. In adults, it is particularly useful for the treatment of heart failure associated with hypotension and poor renal perfusion because of the unusual, dose-dependent combination of actions that it exerts (see also Chaps. 13 and 26). At low doses (0.5 to 2 μg/kg/min), it interacts primarily with D_1 dopaminergic receptors, which are distributed in the renal and mesenteric vascular beds. Their stimulation causes local vasodilation and augments renal blood and GFR, facilitating diuresis. Moderate doses of dopamine (2 to 5 μg/kg/min) directly increase contractility by stimulation of cardiac β_1 receptors and indirectly by causing the release of norepinephrine from sympathetic nerve terminals. At high doses (5 to 10 μg/kg/min), dopamine stimulates the systemic α-adrenergic receptors, thereby causing potent vasoconstriction and an elevation in systemic vascular resistance (SVR).

It is often stated that infants display reduced sensitivity to dopamine; however, the evidence is far from conclusive. In

TABLE 49-2. Digitalization with Digoxin

	Weight (g)	Dose (TDD)
Usual doses (IM or oral)		
Premature infants	500–1000	20 μg/kg or 0.02 mg/kg
	1000–1500	20–30 μg/kg or 0.02–0.03 mg/kg
	1500–2000	30 μg/kg or 0.03 mg/kg
	2000–2500	30–40 μg/kg or 0.03–0.04 mg/kg
Term to 12 yr		40–60 μg/kg or 0.04–0.06 mg/kg
		(no dose >1.5 mg TDD)
Alterations in usual doses		
Lower if renal function is impaired		
Lower in presence of poor myocardial function (cardiomyopathy, myocarditis)		
Lower in presence of metabolic imbalance (electrolyte abnormalities, hypoxia, acidosis)		
IV dose is 75% of oral or IM dose		

TDD = total digitalizing doses; Digitalizing regimen usually given as initial dose = one-half of TDD; second dose = one-fourth of TDD at 8 to 12 h; third dose = final one-fourth TDD at 8 to 12 h after second dose. Maintenance is then started as one-eighth TDD every 12 h. (Note: Parenteral preparation contains 100 μg/mL and oral preparation contains 50 μg/mL).

Source: Reprinted with permission from Gewitz MH and Vetter VL.[13]

support of reduced sensitivity, it has been found that in critically ill neonates, infusion rates of 50 μg/kg/min did not cause evidence of impairment of cutaneous or renal perfusion.[14] There is also some experimental evidence for diminished sensitivity to dopamine in infants; however, this is limited to studies in immature animals.[15,16] A contrary observation was made by Padbury and coworkers[17] who measured cardiac output in a group of infants and found that mean blood pressure increased at doses of 0.5 to 1 μg/kg/min, whereas heart rate increased with doses beyond 2 to 3 μg/kg/min. Cardiac output (and stroke volume) increased before heart rate, and SVR did not change within the range of dopamine infusion rates (0.5 to 8 μg/kg/min). The dose-response relationship is best described by a *threshold model;* that is, below a threshold level of drug concentration, no clinical response is seen, and beyond that level, a log-linear dose-response relationship is seen. The threshold values obtained were 14 ± 3.5 ng/mL for increase in mean blood pressure, 18 ± 4.5 ng/mL for increase in systolic blood pressure, and 35 ± 5 ng/mL for increase in heart rate. Steady-state concentration reached at infusion rates between 1 and 2 μg/kg/min was 16.5 ± 3.4 ng/mL. Thus, newborns may exhibit clinical response using doses as low as 0.5 to 1 μg/kg/min. This is good evidence against the concept that newborns are relatively insensitive to dopamine.

Low infusion rates of dopamine are frequently employed to augment renal function during critical illness.[18,19] Although there is evidence that this may promote salt excretion and urine flow rate, there are no adequate data to conclude that the chances of renal failure are thereby made lower.

Plasma dopamine clearance ranges from 60 to 80 mL/kg/min in normal adults.[20] The half-life has not been reliably determined but probably is in the range of 2 to 4 min. Clearance is lower in patients with renal or hepatic disease.[20] Age has a striking effect upon clearance of dopamine, and clearance in children younger than 2 years of age is approximately twice as rapid as it is in older children (82 vs 46 mL/kg/min).[21] This observation has been confirmed in a study by Allen et al[22] demonstrating that during the first 20 months of age, the clearance of infused dopamine decreases by almost 50% with an additional 50% decrease from ages 1 to 12 years. This pharmacokinetic difference, rather than a difference in receptors or myocardial sensitivity, may account for the observation that infants require tolerate higher infusion rates.

In clinical practice, dopamine is an effective inotropic and vasopressor agent in neonates and infants with a variety of conditions associated with circulatory failure, including hyaline membrane disease, asphyxia, sepsis syndrome, and cyanotic congenital heart disease.[23–25] Although there is surprisingly little formal data concerning use of dopamine in critically ill children, clinicians employ dopamine in order to enhance renal function and to exploit its inotropic and vasopressor properties. Dopamine is less likely to produce severe tachycardia or dysrhythmias than either epinephrine or isoproterenol.

Following volume depletion, dopamine is indicated in the context of moderately severe degrees of distributive shock (sepsis, hypoxia-ischemia) and cardiogenic shock. It is also indicated in the absence of hypotension, when clinical signs or hemodynamic measurements suggest a state of compensated shock or inadequate peripheral perfusion. Dopamine is not the agent of choice when hemodynamic measurements reveal an elevated cardiac output in the context of a markedly reduced SVR and profound hypotension. This pattern is commonly observed in septic shock, and suggests judicious use of a vasopressor such as norepinephrine (see below). Dopamine is also not the drug of choice to treat hypotension associated with major reductions in cardiac index (e.g., <2 to 2.5 L/min/M^2). Epinephrine is more appropriate. Children with primary myocardial disease not complicated by frank hypotension will benefit from a more selective inotropic agent such as dobutamine. Infusion rates of dopamine needed to improve signs of severe myocardial dysfunction may be associated with troublesome tachycardia or dysrhythmia, and may increase myocardial oxygen consumption disproportionately to myocardial perfusion. Although dopamine is extensively employed following cardiac surgery, there are reports that dopamine is less effective following cardiac surgery in infants than it is in older children or adults. Lang et al[26] treated five children with dopamine following cardiac surgery. For the group as a whole, hemodynamic improvement did not occur at infusion rates <15 μg/kg/min. When cardiac output did increase, it was attributed to an increase in heart rate, rather than to improved stroke volume. More recently, one study indicated that following cardiac surgery, dopamine and dobutamine have similar inotropic efficacy, but that dopamine was associated with pulmonary vasoconstriction at doses >7 μg/kg/min.[27]

To treat shock associated with hypotension, therapy is initiated with an infusion rate of 5 to 10 μg/kg/min. The rate of infusion is increased in steps of 2 to 6 μg/kg/min, guided by evidence of improved blood flow (skin temperature, capillary refill, sensorium, urine output) and by restoration of a blood pressure appropriate for age. Infusion rates >25 to 30 μg/kg/min of dopamine are not customary, even if they maintain a "normal" blood pressure. At infusion rates at this dose, the effect upon blood pressure is likely to represent an increase in SVR (α-adrenergic activation) rather than cardiac output. Although infusion rates of this magnitude or higher have been proposed, a requirement for a dopamine infusion at this high dose suggests that the physician reexamine the physiologic diagnosis or select a different agent, such as epinephrine or norepinephrine.

Dopamine can produce cardiovascular toxicity, including tachycardia, hypertension, and dysrhythmia. With the possible exception of the bipyridines, all inotropes increase myocardial oxygen consumption because they increase myocardial work. If the resulting increase in oxygen consumption is balanced by improved coronary blood flow, the net effect upon oxygen balance is beneficial. When shock is caused by or complicated by myocardial disease, then improved myocardial contractility may reduce preload and afterload (decrease oxygen consumption), improve coronary perfusion pressure (increase oxygen supply), and prolong diastolic coronary perfusion by reducing heart rate. If the same drug is administered to a patient with normal myocardial contractility, then the result may be an increase in cardiac oxygen consumption without an increase in oxygen delivery to the myocardium. Tachycardia, by both increasing oxygen consumption and shortening diastole, is a particular burden. Thus, the effect of dopamine upon myocardial oxygen balance is better than it is for isoproterenol, but not as good as for dobutamine, inamrinone, and milrinone.[28–30]

Dopamine depresses the ventilatory response to both hypoxemia and hypercarbia by as much as 60%.[31] Dopamine (and other β-agonists) can decrease P_aO_2 by interfering with hypoxic vasoconstriction. In one study, dopamine increased intrapulmonary shunting in patients with adult respiratory distress syndrome from 27 to 40%.[32] Dopamine can cause or worsen limb ischemia, gangrene of distal parts, and entire extremities, and result in extensive loss of skin.[33] Infusion rates as low as 1.5 μg/kg/min have been associated with limb loss.[34–36] The presence of an arterial catheter also increases the possibility of limb ischemia. Because dopamine promotes release of norepinephrine from synaptic terminals (and is also converted to norepinephrine in vivo), it is more often associated with limb ischemia than other adrenergic compounds. Extravasation of dopamine should be treated immediately by local infiltration with a solution of phentolamine (5 to 10 mg in 15 mL normal saline) administered with a fine hypodermic needle. Dopamine should not be administered by mixing with sodium bicarbonate because alkaline solutions inactivate this agent.

Dobutamine

Dobutamine is a synthetic analogue of dopamine that stimulates β_1-, β_2-, and α-adrenergic receptors (see Chap. 13). It increases cardiac contractility via its β_1 effect, and may not significantly alter SVR because of the balance between α_1-mediated vasoconstriction and β_2-mediated vasodilation. Unlike dopamine, dobutamine does not stimulate dopaminergic receptors (it is not a renal vasodilator), nor does it facilitate the release of norepinephrine from peripheral nerve endings.[37]

In adults with CHF, dobutamine produces a 50 to 80% increase in cardiac output, which is almost entirely due to improvement in stroke volume. Left atrial pressure falls, and SVR either decreases or remains the same. Heart rate increases little, if at all. Although renal function is not directly affected by dobutamine, renal function and urine output may improve as the increase in cardiac output fosters relaxation of sympathetic tone and improved perfusion. Dobutamine is a dilator of the pulmonary vasculature.[38]

A threshold model with a log-linear dose-response relationship above the threshold has been demonstrated in critically ill term and preterm neonates,[39] and in children between 2 and 168 months of age.[40] In one small study, dobutamine infusion (10 μ/kg/min) was associated with increase in cardiac output (30%), blood pressure (17%), and heart rate (7%). The thresholds for these increases were 13, 23, and 65 ng/mL, respectively, demonstrating that dobutamine is a relatively selective inotrope with little effect on heart rate at customary infusion rates.[41] Somewhat greater thresholds for improved cardiac output were observed in a second group of children[40] and in infants,[39] but in all studies, dobutamine improved cardiac contractility without substantially altering heart rate unless high infusion rates were employed.

The half-life is about 2 min in adults and the volume of distribution is 0.2 L/kg. Congestive heart failure increases the volume of distribution. In adults, clearance is about 2 L/M^2/min. Typical clearance values in children are 70 to 100 mL/kg/min. Infusions in the range used clinically yield plasma dobutamine concentrations from approximately 50 ng/mL to 160 to 190 ng/mL in both children[41] and in adults.[42] The principal route of elimination is methylation by catechol methyltransferase (COMT), followed by hepatic glucuronidation and excretion into urine and bile. Dobutamine is also cleared from the plasma by nonneuronal uptake. Some investigators report nonlinear elimination kinetics, but other data suggest that dobutamine's kinetics can be adequately described by a simple first-order (linear) model.[43]

Several studies in infants and children[39–41,44,45] demonstrate that dobutamine improves myocardial function in a variety of settings. Stroke volume and cardiac index improve without a substantial increase in cardiac rate. SVR and pulmonary vascular resistance (PVR) may decrease toward normal.

Dobutamine has been evaluated in children following cardiac surgery with cardiopulmonary bypass. In a study by Bohn et al,[46] dobutamine enhanced cardiac output by increasing heart rate. Indeed, tachycardia prompted discontinuation of the infusion in several patients. The expected fall in SVR was not observed in children receiving the drug after cardiopulmonary bypass. The authors found no benefit over isoproterenol or dopamine. These differences between adults and children may be due to the fact that myocardial dysfunction and congestive heart failure are not characteristic of the circulatory status of many children undergoing repair of congenital heart disease. Unlike adults, indication for operation involves abnormalities in ventricular architecture or abnormal circulatory anatomy. Berner and associates[47] found that children undergoing operations for mitral valve disease responded to dobutamine with an increase in stroke volume; children having repair of tetralogy of Fallot did not, and their cardiac output increased only through higher heart rate. A more recent report by the same group indicated that following repair of tetralogy of Fallot, dobutamine did enhance cardiac output when it was combined with atrial pacing to increase heart rate.[48] Isoproterenol without pacing provided a higher cardiac output than either dobutamine alone or dobutamine in combination with pacing.[48]

Specific indications for prescribing dobutamine in the pediatric age group include those conditions associated with a low cardiac output and normal to moderately decreased blood pressure. Typical examples include viral myocarditis, cardiomyopathy associated with use of anthracyclines, cyclophosphamide or hemochromatosis (related to hypertransfusion therapy), or myocardial infarction (Kawasaki disease). Patients with congestive heart failure who have a normal or slightly low blood pressure may benefit by combining dobutamine with a left ventricular afterload-reducing agent. For rapid titration in the unstable patient, nitroprusside is available. When rapid adjustment is not necessary, angiotensin-converting enzyme inhibitors such as captopril or enalapril (see below) can be employed for this purpose.[49] A decrease in afterload improves stroke volume and may enhance cardiac output at a lower cost of oxygen consumption than use of an inotropic agent alone.

Dobutamine is not a first-line agent to treat low output states caused by intracardiac shunt. Dobutamine is employed following corrective or palliative cardiovascular surgery in the child; however, in this context, its use should also be limited to occasions in which demonstrated or suspected myocardial dysfunction exists.

Dobutamine may be of adjunctive value in treating myocardial dysfunction that complicates a primary condition such as adult respiratory distress syndrome (ARDS) or septic shock. Rarely, however, is it appropriate to employ dobutamine as the sole agent to treat hemodynamic compromise associated with sepsis, ARDS, or shock following an episode of severe hypoxia-ischemia.

Dobutamine can be useful when combined with other adrenergic agonists such as norepinephrine to treat myocardial dysfunction associated with so-called "hyperdynamic" shock. For example, the child with anthracycline cardiotoxicity who develops septic shock may be candidate for this type of combined therapy.

Dobutamine usually increases myocardial oxygen demand. In subjects with myocardial dysfunction, coronary blood flow and oxygen supply improve with the increase in demand.[50] However, if dobutamine is employed when myocardial contractility is normal, oxygen balance will be adversely affected. Tachycardia greatly increases oxygen use by the heart, and should prompt a reduction in the dose of dobutamine (or an alternate agent).

Although less likely than other catecholamines to induce serious atrial and ventricular dysrhythmias, these do occur in patients receiving dobutamine, particularly in the context of myocarditis, electrolyte imbalance, or high infusion rates. Dobutamine and other inotropes should be administered cautiously, if at all, to patients with dynamic left ventricular outflow obstruction (hypertrophic subaortic stenosis).

Isoproterenol

Isoproterenol is an intravenously administered, synthetic catecholamine. As a nonselective β-agonist, it augments myocardial contractility, increases heart rate, reduces afterload, and dilates the bronchial tree. It is useful for the treatment of bradycardia in all age groups and for life-threatening reactive airway disease in young children. The dosage varies with clinical indication. Lower dosages are required for the treatment of bradyarrhythmias than those needed for bronchial hyperreactivity.[51–53] In the neonate, isoproterenol produces a greater increase in heart rate than either dopamine or dobutamine.[54]

In the past, isoproterenol was used for a variety of indications, including septic shock and cardiogenic shock associated with myocardial infarction. Newer agents, such as dopamine and dobutamine, together with a more subtle understanding of the pathophysiology of shock, have limited the use of isoproterenol to very few specific indications.

Isoproterenol may be employed to treat hemodynamically significant bradycardia. However, an epinephrine infusion is probably preferable.[55] When bradycardia results from heart block, then atropine is the initial urgent form of drug therapy, and placement of a pacemaker is definitive treatment. Bradycardia due to anoxia is treated by administering oxygen and improving gas exchange but isoproterenol may be a useful adjunct in this setting.

Some clinicians prefer isoproterenol as a first-time agent for infants following cardiac surgery with cardiopulmonary bypass. Although this indication is not well explored in the literature, the agent may be effective in improving cardiac output by combining inotropic and chronotropic activity with a capacity for both pulmonary and systemic vasodilation. Isoproterenol may provide greater improvement in cardiac output than either atrial pacing or atrial pacing combined with dobutamine.

The main concerns regarding the use of isoproterenol include sinus tachycardia, which can be counterproductive to ventricular filling and to myocardial oxygen debt burden, and induction of arrhythmias, especially ventricular extrasystoles. Patients must be monitored closely for this latter complication when receiving isoproterenol.

Epinephrine

Epinephrine is an endogenous catecholamine that acts on both α- and β-adrenergic receptors resulting in an increase in heart rate, contractility, and SVR. These actions make it especially useful under circumstances of severe myocardial dysfunction associated with hypotension.[56]

A wide interindividual variation in epinephrine clearance is observed in healthy adults. In critically ill children receiving epinephrine at doses from 0.03 to 0.2 μg/kg/min, plasma concentrations at steady state ranged from 0.67 to 8.5 ng/mL and were linearly related to dose.[56]

Epinephrine is employed to treat shock associated with myocardial dysfunction. Thus, it may be an appropriate drug for treatment of cardiogenic shock unresponsive to dopamine or following open cardiac surgery.[57]

The septic patient who does not improve adequately after intravascular volume repletion and treatment with dopamine or dobutamine may benefit from infusion of epinephrine. Epinephrine is most likely to be useful when hypotension exists in the context of a low cardiac index and stroke index. At modest infusion rates (0.05 to 0.1 μg/kg/min), SVR decreases slightly; heart rate, cardiac output, and systolic blood pressure increase somewhat. At intermediate infusion rates, α_1-adrenergic activation becomes important, but is balanced by the improved cardiac output and activation of vascular β_2 receptors. Even though epinephrine constricts renal and cutaneous arterioles, renal function and skin perfusion may improve. Very high infusion rates (>1 to 2 μg/kg/min) are associated with significant α_1-adrenergic-mediated vasoconstriction; blood flow to individual organs will be compromised and the associated increase in afterload may further impair myocardial function. Epinephrine by infusion is also the agent of choice for hypotension or shock following successful treatment of cardiac arrest. Shock following an episode of hypoxemia or ischemia is usually cardiogenic[58] and may respond to epinephrine infusion.

Bolus injections of epinephrine are used to treat asystole and other nonperfusing rhythms. The recommended initial dose (American Heart Association) is 0.01 mg/kg (10 μg/kg or 0.1 mL/kg of the 1:10,000 solution). Subsequent doses are tenfold greater ("high-dose epinephrine"): 0.1 mg/kg (100 μ/kg or 0.1 mL/kg of a 1:1000 solution). Although initial studies using high-dose epinephrine were encouraging, published reports indicate no improvement in return of spontaneous circulation or survival after high-dose epinephrine following out-of-hospital cardiac arrest in children.[59]

Epinephrine may also be given by endotracheal tube (dose is 100 μg/kg). Intraosseous administration is appropriate for both bolus and continuous administration of epinephrine. The dose is the same as for intravenous injection. The intraosseous route is effective in briskly achieving high plasma levels of epinephrine and other catecholamines when direct vascular access is difficult.[60]

Epinephrine has the potential to cause multiple adverse reactions. The drug produces CNS excitation manifested as anxiety, dread, nausea, and dyspnea. Enhanced automaticity and increased oxygen consumption are the main serious toxicities of epinephrine. Extreme tachycardia carries a substantial oxygen penalty, as does hypertension. A severe imbalance of myocardial oxygen delivery and oxygen consumption produces characteristic ECG changes of ischemia. A subischemic, but persistently unfavorable, ratio of oxygen delivery to consumption may also be harmful to the myocardium.

Epinephrine produces tachycardia and increases in infusion rate lead to successively more serious events, including atrial and ventricular extrasystoles, atrial and ventricular tachycardia and ultimately, ventricular fibrillation. Ventricular dysrhythmias in children are not frequent, but may occur in the presence of myocarditis, hypokalemia or hypoxemia.

Epinephrine overdose is serious. Several neonates have died when inadvertently subjected to oral administration of huge amounts of epinephrine. The syndrome mimicked an epidemic of neonatal sepsis with shock and metabolic acidosis.[61] Intra-aortic injection in infants (per umbilical artery) produces tachycardia, hypertension, and renal failure.[62] Intravenous overdosage of epinephrine is immediately life-threatening. Manifestations include myocardial infarction, ventricular tachycardia, extreme hypertension, cerebral hemorrhage, seizures, renal failure, and pulmonary edema. Paradoxically, bradycardia has also been observed.[63]

Manifestations of acute overdosage are treated symptomatically. β-Receptor antagonists, such as propranolol, are contraindicated. Hypertension is treated with short-acting antihypertensives (i.e., nitroprusside).

Hypokalemia can be produced during epinephrine infusion due to stimulation of β_2-adrenergic receptors, which are linked to sodium-potassium-ATPase located in skeletal muscle. Hyperglycemia results from α-adrenergic-mediated suppression of insulin release. Other metabolic abnormalities include hyperlactemia and hypophosphatemia.

Epinephrine is an α_1-adrenergic agonist and infiltration into local tissues or intra-arterial injection can produce severe vasospasm and tissue injury. Concurrent activation of β_2 receptors by epinephrine limits vasospasm, and local injury to tissue is less frequent than with either norepinephrine or dopamine.

Norepinephrine

Norepinephrine is an endogenous catecholamine that stimulates β_1- and α-adrenergic receptors, thereby increasing contractility and SVR. Its ultimate effect on heart rate is variable and is the net result of opposing forces. Some of its inotropic activity may result from α_1-receptor stimulation as well as β-receptor agonism.[64] Whereas its direct cardiac β1 effect favors an increase in heart rate, its peripheral α-adrenergic effect, which leads to activation of the baroreceptor reflex, favors a decrease in heart rate. Published pediatric data in infants and children are quite limited, but the observed hemodynamic response to norepinephrine seems to resemble that seen in adults. Its use, for the most part, is reserved for the persistently hypotensive patient, such as the child in whom hypotension persists in spite of being given doses as high as 20 μg/kg per minute of dopamine.[53] It should not be used as a positive inotrope in the context of depressed myocardial contractile function unaccompanied by hypotension, because its marked vasoconstrictive effects may result in an extremely high SVR with reduced renal blood flow. Its adverse effects profile is similar to epinephrine.

Norepinephrine improves perfusion in children with low blood pressure and a normal or elevated cardiac index as occurs in septic shock. Norepinephrine is administered only after intravascular volume repletion and is best guided by knowledge of cardiac output and SVR. There is very little published experience on the use of norepinephrine to treat distributive shock in children; however, a randomized study (in adults) indicates that norepinephrine is superior to dopamine for treating hypotension and other hemodynamic abnormalities associated with hyperdynamic septic shock.[65] In this study, the average infusion rate for norepinephrine was 1.5 μg/kg/min, although others have reported that somewhat lower average doses (0.4 μg/kg/min) were effective in adults with sepsis.[66] Thus, titration is important, and may entail fairly rapid escalation of dosage.

Norepinephrine produces increases in SVR, arterial blood pressure, and urine flow. It is most valuable in the context of tachycardia because infusion of the drug does not produce significant elevation of heart rate, and may even lower heart rate through reflex mechanisms.

The usual starting dose is an infusion of 0.1 μg/kg/min. The goal is to elevate perfusion pressure so that the flow to vital organs is above the threshold needed to meet metabolic requirements. The lowest infusion rate should be employed that improves perfusion as judged by skin color and temperature, mental status, urine flow, and reduction in plasma lactate level. Other causes of distributive shock (e.g., vasodilator ingestion, intoxication with CNS depressants) should also respond to norepinephrine infusion when the predominant hemodynamic problem is low SVR and blood pressure.

The net effect of norepinephrine infusion upon oxygen balance varies. The increase in afterload which it produces should increase myocardial oxygen consumption, but norepinephrine also decreases heart rate, which should reduce oxygen consumption and improve diastolic coronary perfusion. Injudicious use of norepinephrine will lead to compromised organ blood flow. Norepinephrine infusion may elevate blood pressure yet not improve clinical indices of perfusion.

Phosphodiesterase Inhibitors

Inamrinone and milrinone are intravenously administered nondigitalis, noncatecholamine, bipyridine derivatives that exert their positive inotropic effects by inhibiting cyclic adenosine monophosphate (AMP) phosphodiesterase (PDE) in cardiac myocytes (see Chap. 13). Increased levels of cyclic AMP, by inhibition of its breakdown, promote Ca^{2+} entry into the cell, thereby increasing contractility. These drugs may cause adverse effects, including ventricular arrhythmias.

Inamrinone, a PDE inhibitor, thereby prevents the degradation of cyclic AMP. It is used as an adjunct to dopamine or dobutamine in the intensive care unit. In adults, inamrinone acts as both a positive inotropic agent and as a vasodilator.[67] The cardiovascular effects of both inamrinone and milrinone appear to be markedly age dependent. Studies have shown a lack of responsiveness to either inamrinone or milrinone in the newborn dog [68–70] and rabbit.[71] Yet, by 2 weeks of age, the response of rabbit myocardium to milrinone exceeds that of an adult.[72] In the treatment of children with cor pulmonale using inamrinone, beneficial effects on the pulmonary vasculature have been reported.[73]

Compared to dobutamine, milrinone produces a greater reduction in SVR for a given degree of improvement in inotropic status.[74] Blood pressure is well maintained, even in the face of reduced SVR, because of the associated improvement in contractility and stroke volume. However, when inamrinone is administered to patients who are intravascularly volume depleted or in whom the expected improvement in cardiac output does not occur hypotension may result. In patients with CHF, amelioration in global hemodynamic function is associated with an improvement in the ratio of myocardial oxygen delivery to consumption. Inamrinone may improve contractility in patients who have failed to respond to catecholamines, and may further increase cardiac index even in patients who have responded to dobutamine.[75]

Inamrinone reduces pulmonary artery pressure and resistance in children with intracardiac left-to-right shunts. In one study, children with elevated PVR enjoyed a 47% reduction in PVR upon infusion of inamrinone.[76] The PVR/SVR ratio decreased by 45%. In these children, both pulmonary blood flow and left-to-right shunt increased. In children with normal pulmonary pressure, inamrinone infusion was associated with a decrease in SVR but not PVR. Inamrinone may be undesirable in children with an elevated pulmonary artery pressure associated with a high-flow left-to-right shunt but normal PVR. Conversely, inamrinone (and probably milrinone) may be effective adjunctive therapy in the child with elevated pulmonary vascular resistance and reduced pulmonary blood flow.[76]

Milrinone was licensed for use in the U.S. in 1992. A derivative of inamrinone, it shares the same mechanism of action and pharmacodynamic profile. The major advantage of milrinone is that, unlike inamrinone, it does not appear to evoke thrombocytopenia.[77] It is eliminated through the kidneys. In adults, milrinone acts both as an inotrope and vasodilator. In adults with CHF, milrinone causes a much greater change in left and right filling pressures and SVR than does dobutamine, even at equivalent increases in contractility.[78] It has been extensively employed following cardiac surgery and in adults with CHF where it increases cardiac index and reduces SVR, filling pressure, and, often, systemic blood pressure.[79,80] Although anecdotal reports indicate that use of milrinone is increasing in pediatric intensive care units, there is little data with which to evaluate this practice. One study evaluated treatment of neonates following congenital heart disease repair.[81] In this study, a loading dose of 50 μg/kg followed by a continuous infusion of 0.5 μg/kg/min was associated with mild tachycardia and a slight decrease in systemic blood pressure. Cardiac index increased from 2.1 to approximately 3.1 L/min/M^2, while SVR index decreased from approximately 2100 to 1300 dyne-sec/cm^{5}m^2. PVR index also decreased from approximately 488 to 360 dyne-sec/cm^{5}m^2, as did right and left atrial mean pressures. Thus, in children, the pharmacodynamic properties of milrinone are similar to those observed in the case of inamrinone, at least in this limited group of patients. Unfortunately, this study did not examine the pharmacokinetic properties of milrinone.

Inamrinone is metabolized by N-acetyl transferase. In addition, up to 40% is eliminated unchanged in the urine.[82] In healthy adults, the half-life of inamrinone in slow acetylators is 4.4 h and in fast

acetylators is 2 h.[83] It is not known whether this difference is clinically important. Protein binding is not extensive. The rate of elimination of inamrinone appears to be reduced in CHF.[84] There is little pharmacokinetic information available regarding the use of inamrinone in children, and virtually no information derived from children with organ system failure. One study of children younger than 1 year of age following cardiopulmonary bypass found that the half-life was prolonged in those younger than 4 weeks of age, and that volume of distribution (1.7 to 1.8 L/kg) was threefold greater than others have reported in adults.[85,86] A second study found wide interpatient variability in pharmacokinetic measurements. Beyond 1 month of age, there was no relation between age and any measured pharmacokinetic parameter. The average clearance was approximately 2 mL/kg/min, which is similar to that recorded in adults, and was associated with a mean half-life of about 5.5 h.[82] There are no published pharmacokinetic data for milrinone in infants or children. In adults, the volume of distribution of milrinone is 0.5 L/kg and the clearance is 0.11 to 0.1 L/kg/h. The half-life is approximately 2 h in adults with CHF.[87,88] Typically, the plasma level during therapy is in the range of 80 to 120 ng/mL.

In adults with CHF, inamrinone and milrinone are safe and effective and their clinical place in short-term management of patients with refractory heart failure is clearly established.[74] The bipyridines are most useful in management of children and adolescents with isolated cardiac dysfunction, particularly when it is due to myocardial failure. They provide both inotropic and afterload reduction and may be an alternative to coadministration of dobutamine and an afterload-reducing agent.

Inamrinone should not have a major role in management of critically ill children in whom the primary disturbance is other than myocardial failure. The relatively long half-life and the observation that clearance is depressed in patients with cardiac or hepatic dysfunction[89] are important limitations in the patient with multiple organ system failure. It is likely that these precautions should be applied to milrinone as well. In patients with septic shock or ARDS, for example, inamrinone or milrinone should be reserved for the individual with impaired myocardial performance who has not responded adequately to aggressive support with other agents, such as dobutamine, dopamine, or epinephrine.

Inamrinone produces reversible dose-dependent thrombocytopenia (incidence 2.4%),[89] which is more common during prolonged therapy. This was not seen in the largest published pediatric study[86] but anecdotal reports suggest that it occurs in children as well. Supraventricular and ventricular dysrhythmias have occurred during infusion of inamrinone, but may have been related to the underlying condition of the patient. Overdosage has been fatal in a child.[90] Progressive hypotension developed and peritoneal dialysis was not effective. This case involved excessive administration due to a computing error.

A rapid infusion of inamrinone or milrinone during the loading dose can produce hypotension. This problem is exacerbated in volume-depleted patients.

Diuretics

These drugs, which reduce central congestion and pulmonary edema directly, remain key to anticongestive therapy (see Chap. 11). In pediatrics, diuretics are a more common treatment for CHF than for hypertension. Traditionally, these agents are classified by principal site of action in the kidney.[91,92]

Loop Diuretics

Loop diuretics, which act by inhibiting the Na-K-2Cl transporter in the thick ascending limb of the nephron's loop of Henle, are widely used in pediatric patients.

Furosemide is the most commonly used agent of this type. This drug also has effects mediated through renal prostaglandin agonism. It increases renal blood flow, reduces renal vascular resistance, and stimulates renin release. There may also be beneficial pulmonary nondiuretic effects from furosemide making it a useful agent in children with combined cardiopulmonary disorders, such as bronchopulmonary dysplasia. In general it is used for both acute and chronic management of congestive circulatory states and for causing a diuresis after cardiac surgery. In the treatment of infants with CHF, the existing hyperaldosteronism may decrease the patient's response to furosemide.[93,94] The addition of an aldosterone antagonist such as spironolactone is then indicated to combat aldosterone's influence,[91] as well as to help reduce potassium loss.

Furosemide may be administered either orally or parenterally. With intravenous use in a newborn, 55% of the dose is excreted unchanged into the tubular lumen. For a given plasma level of furosemide, neonates exhibit higher urinary drug excretion due to lower protein-binding of the drug,[94] and plasma clearance has also been shown to increase with age. In the neonate, more of the unchanged drug appears in the urine because less biotransformation via glucuronidation occurs in its undeveloped renal epithelial cell.[94] Hence, in infants with immature renal function and in patients with renal failure the dosage must be adjusted accordingly.[95]

Adverse effects at all ages include hypovolemia and electrolyte disturbances. Hypokalemia is a relatively common side effect that is usually not of clinical significance in children during chronic therapy unless they also are taking digoxin. However, at high doses of furosemide, potassium supplementation may be necessary. Hypochloremic metabolic alkalosis is also a well-documented side effect with chronic therapy and, if severe, may necessitate chloride supplementation. In infants with bronchopulmonary dysplasia, chloride depletion has been implicated as a cause of increased mortality.[96] Hyponatremia may occur and, in the setting of CHF, furosemide may worsen existing hyponatremia.

Ototoxicity may also occur. There is an increased prevalence of ototoxicity in premature infants which may be due to an immature barrier to the inner ear.[97] Whereas in patients with normal renal function the risk of ototoxicity is minimal with standard dosages, in patients with renal dysfunction the risk of ototoxicity is higher. Additionally, the risk increases in those patients receiving other ototoxic drugs.

Ethacrynic acid is used in patients refractory to furosemide therapy, and the drug is sometimes used in the acute management of volume overload. While the pharmacokinetics in adults are similar to those observed with furosemide, in newborns and children this has yet to be determined.

Limited data are available for *bumetanide,* a newer loop diuretic, in the pediatric age group. Hence, its use is generally reserved for those patients in whom conventional diuretic therapy has failed. Bumetanide differs from furosemide in that it is partially metabolized in the liver and about 50% is excreted unchanged in the urine. Furthermore, in neonates and children, it is many times more potent than furosemide and must be monitored carefully.[98]

Bumetanide and metolazone (see below) may be particularly valuable in children with right heart failure, such as those post repair of tetralogy of Fallot or in children who have undergone the Fontan operation or its variants. Data definitively establishing this utility, however, need to be amplified.

Thiazide Diuretics

Hydrochlorothiazide (HCTZ) and chlorothiazide, structural analogues, are the primary thiazide diuretics used in pediatric patients with cardiovascular disease.[99] Their diuretic effect is primarily mediated by inhibition of sodium and chloride transport in the nephron's distal convoluted tubule.[100] Thiazides are effective until the GFR drops below 50% of normal, at which point a loop diuretic should be started instead. Thiazides are used in the chronic, outpatient management of congestive circulatory states. In addition, they are employed in the treatment of hypertension in older children and adolescents.[101] Whereas the mechanism of action, diuretic efficacy, and adverse effects of HCTZ and chlorothiazide are similar, their pharmacokinetics differ. HCTZ is more potent. Among its adverse effects are electrolyte imbalance, including hypokalemia and hypercalcemia, and hyperuricemia. Additionally, it may negatively alter the lipid profile and may cause carbohydrate intolerance.

Metolazone

Metolazone is a sulfonamide derivative whose site and mechanism of action is similar to that of thiazides. It is used in the short-term treatment of edematous states refractory to loop and thiazide diuretic therapy. Metolazone is commonly administered along with a more distally acting diuretic, since, which given by itself, the unaffected distal tubule compensates for the disabled proximal tubule.[102] It is administered once a day or every other day. The major adverse effects are severe electrolyte disturbances (hypokalemia) and significant volume depletion.

Potassium-Sparing Diuretics

Spironolactone, the most commonly used potassium-sparing diuretic,[103] is reserved for long-term therapy, because it is administered only orally. It exerts its diuretic effect by competitively inhibiting aldosterone at the distal tubule. It is weaker than either loop or thiazide diuretics, and thus is mostly used in combination with either. Its major adverse effects are hyperkalemia and renal dysfunction and patients with existing renal and/or hepatic dysfunction are at greatest risk. Concomitant potassium supplementation, as well as angiotensin-converting enzyme (ACE) inhibitor coadministration, should be done with extreme care. Gynecomastia and menstrual abnormalities have been reported in adults. Data regarding the use of other potassium-sparing diuretics, such as triamterene, eplerenone and amiloride, in pediatrics are limited, and recommendations cannot be made currently.

Spironolactone also has other, nondiuretic benefits for the patient with CHF. Recently, the findings of direct myocardial function enhancement, of inhibition of the collagen production and fibrosis stimulated by aldosterone, and of additive effects when combined with angiotensin converting enzyme inhibition (see below) have focused new attention on the use of spironolactone.[104] The Randomized Aldactone Evaluation Study (RALES) was interrupted early, in fact, because the findings of the value of spironolactone were impressive.[105,106]

Osmotic Diuretics

Mannitol is the most commonly used drug in this class used in pediatrics. Mannitol's cardiovascular use is reserved for the acute treatment of severe circulatory congestion in the face of limited renal output, that is, prerenal failure and azotemia. The primary site of action is the proximal tubule, and mannitol will maintain high rates of tubular flow to prevent obstruction. More of the total salt and water reabsorption occurs in the distal tubule in neonates than in older patients. Hence, mannitol as a proximally acting agent, is less effective than more distally acting agents in neonates.[92] Adverse effects are hemodynamic: immediately following its administration, mannitol may temporarily increase intravascular volume and the risk of electrolyte disturbances.

Vasodilators

Vasodilator therapy has become central to the management of impaired circulatory status in infants and children. With the tremendous development of the basic science knowledge base in microcirculatory function, particularly the factors involved with control of vasomotor tone, an increasing armamentarium of agents have become available. When vasodilators are combined with other agents, such as the inotropes reviewed above, efficacy is enhanced beyond the use of either class of agents alone.[107]

For acute usage, particularly in the intensive care unit, the nitrovasodilators have become agents of choice. These drugs have rapid onset of action and exceedingly short duration of action, making them specially suitable for the acutely ill patient. Principally, but not entirely, these are venoactive agents that work through nitric oxide activation and consequent cyclic guanosine monophosphate (GMP) mediation of regulatory proteins involved with smooth muscle contraction. In pediatric usage, nitroprusside is used most frequently, although nitroglycerin is used in the postoperative cardiac surgery patient.

Nitroprusside

This drug has both venous and arteriolar activity, and is the most widely used acute intravenous vasodilator in the pediatric population. Similar to nitroglycerin, it was used originally for pediatric patients following cardiac surgery during the immediate postoperative period.[108,109] With doses ranging from 1.5 to 12 μg/kg per minute, there is a decline in filling pressures, an increase in cardiac output (CO), and no change in heart rate. Nitroprusside is effective in pediatric patients with left ventricular dysfunction or mitral regurgitation.[110] Pulmonary and systemic vascular resistances and atrial pressures are reduced causing a net increase in CO. Heart rate may be unaffected or increase slightly. Its effects in neonates are comparable to those in older children. One neonatal study showed that 40% had improved systemic perfusion, and almost all the infants had improved urine output after initiation of therapy.[111] Nitroprusside must be administered parenterally by continuous infusion because it is metabolized so rapidly.

Nitroprusside's safety and efficacy have been demonstrated in neonates.[111] In hypoxemic neonatal and juvenile lambs, however, nitroprusside decreased PVR in the juvenile but not in the neonatal group. Moreover, the newborn lambs were not able to hemodynamically tolerate the nitroprusside-induced decrease in preload.[112] These age-related differences in vascular response suggest that nitroprusside should be used with extra caution in neonates.

Nitroprusside's metabolite, cyanide, is toxic. Symptoms of toxicity include headache, disorientation, fatigue, vomiting, anorexia, tachypnea, and tachycardia. In patients being given long-term or high-dose therapy, the meaningfulness of periodic red blood cell cyanide and plasma thiocyanate measurements are uncertain;

clinical evidence of toxicity has not been shown to correlate well with specific cyanide and thiocyanate concentrations.[113]

Nitroglycerin

In pediatrics, nitroglycerin is most commonly employed following cardiac surgery in the immediate postoperative period, with several studies demonstrating its beneficial effect in this setting.[114,115] It is most commonly used in patients with increased preload and symptoms of systemic and/or pulmonary venous congestion. Nitroglycerin has been demonstrated to be beneficial in newborns with low CO due to congenital heart disease, asphyxia, and sepsis. Although nitroglycerin can affect all smooth-muscle sites, its predominant action is to relax *venous* vascular smooth muscle, and therefore to reduce left ventricular preload. Nitroglycerin reduces pulmonary venous and arterial pressures.

The hemodynamic actions of nitroglycerin appear to be dose-related. At doses <2 μg/kg/min, a venodilation effect predominates. Doses from 3 to 5 μg/kg/min result in progressive arteriolar dilatation with a decrease in SVR and a resultant rise in CO. Higher than conventional doses may cause hypotension and reflex tachycardia. Conventional pediatric doses, such as a mean nitroglycerin dose of 20 μg/kg/min used in one study, may not significantly alter the mean arterial pressure (MAP) in children, but similar doses produce hypotension in adults. In children with pulmonary hypertension, a decrease in PVR is noted.[115a]

Nitroglycerin can be administered sublingually, intradermally, or intravenously, but *not* orally, because it undergoes extensive first-pass hepatic metabolism. When given intravenously, it must be given by continuous infusion because of its short serum half-life. Recommendations for chronic management in pediatric patients cannot be made because of insufficient data. Patients must be monitored for (a) the possibility of further reduction of CO secondary to even lower filling pressures than desired, and (b) hypotension accompanied by tachycardia and hypoxemia secondary to overdosage.

Nitric Oxide

Much recent attention has focused on nitric oxide and its role in modulating vascular smooth muscle vasomotor tone as noted above in the discussion of therapeutic infused nitrovasodilators. Use of nitric oxide itself as a pharmaceutical has relatively recently been widely accepted, in its inhaled form, to effect pulmonary vasodilation.[116,117,117a] As an inhaled agent with little systemic action, nitric oxide causes selective and prolonged reduction in pulmonary artery pressure in a variety of clinical settings with consequent beneficial effects on right ventricular mechanics and relief of cor pulmonale.[118] The most use for this therapy has been found for modulating pulmonary vasomotor tone in the newborn with congenital heart or lung disease or a combination of both.[119] Use in other forms of pulmonary hypertension and right heart failure has been more limited, but some studies do suggest a possible role in problems such as adult respiratory distress syndrome as well.[120]

Peripheral α_1-Adrenergic Receptor Blockers

Prazosin

Prazosin is an α_1 selective blocker that can cause a reduction in SVR and MAP. Its selectivity for the α_1 receptor explains its ability to produce less reflex tachycardia than can nonselective agents. It exerts an effect both on arteriolar and venous capacitance vessels. Prazosin has been used in pediatric patients with CHF due to systolic dysfunction.[121] The drug is administered orally, and its peak effect occurs within 2 to 3 h. Although its serum half-life is 2.5 to 4 h, prazosin's duration of action lasts for about 12 h. Prazosin is generally tolerated well with only minor side effects. However, the "first-dose phenomenon," characterized by dizziness, hypotension, and syncope, may occur within approximately 0.5 to 1.5 h after initiation of therapy. It may also occur after an increase in dosage. This effect can be avoided by giving the patient the drug at bedtime. It is unclear whether the tendency in adults having CHF to develop drug tachyphylaxis will apply to children as well.[122] There is little pediatric experience with other similar drugs, terazosin or doxazosin, two newer congeners with long-acting potential.

Phentolamine

Phentolamine is a nonselective α blocker. Unlike the selective α_1 blockers such as prazosin, phentolamine is more likely to cause tachycardia and arrhythmias by virtue of its α_2-blocking effect. It has been used in children who have CHF, following cardiac surgery, to reduce ventricular afterload and augment CO.[47] The published pediatric experience to date is limited to short-term parenteral therapy.

Angiotensin-Converting Enzyme Inhibitors

In the past several years, use of ACE inhibition therapy has become integral to the management of chronic left ventricular dysfunction in children as well as adults. These agents act as vasodilators through inhibition of the potent vasoconstrictor, angiotensin-II (see Chap. 10). In addition, they enhance the vasodilator action of bradykinin by decreasing its degradation and may inhibit norepinephrine release from sympathetic nerve endings. These actions result in reduced SVR and blood pressure resulting in decreased afterload and increased CO.

In the pediatric population, most of the published experience is with captopril and enalapril. A number of other ACE inhibitors are now available (fosinopril, lisinopril, ramipril, trandolapril, benazepril, quinipril, perindopril, moexipril),[122a] but captopril and enalapril continue to be used most frequently in children.[12] Clinical trials with fosinopril and ramipril are now underway at pediatric centers.

Captopril

The use of captopril has been studied in children of all ages and has proved to be an effective antihypertensive agent.[123] Initial pediatric experience with captopril was for the treatment of systemic hypertension in infants and children.[123–125] Dose-response studies in older children have shown similar responses to 0.5, 1.0, and 2.0 mg/kg per dose; hence the lowest dose of 0.5 mg/kg is recommended when therapy is initiated in children older than 6 months.[126] If the desired effect is not achieved with that low dose, then the dose should be increased to 1.0 mg/kg; further increase would most likely *not* result in better control, and another agent should be used. Captopril is given orally. Although twice-daily dosing has been successful, captopril is generally administered three times daily. In premature infants, as high as 60% reductions in blood pressure levels were achieved with doses of 0.3 mg/kg; oliguria was also reported.[127] Normotensive blood pressures have been achieved in premature and full-term infants with doses as low as 0.01 mg/kg.[128] Captopril's absorption is inhibited by food in the stomach, and therefore the drug should be given on an empty stomach. Peak plasma concentrations are reached within 1 to 2 h after an oral dose, and effects generally last for 6 to 8 h.[129] In young infants and newborns, captopril is more potent and its duration of action is longer as compared with older children.[128] Approximately half of the drug is excreted in the urine unchanged. Drug clearance is positively correlated with renal function, and therefore dosage should be reduced in renal disease. Side effects of captopril described in adults, including hypotension, hyperkalemia, renal insufficiency, and dry cough, are less common in children. However, in neonates, idiosyncratic side effects including significant hypotension, oliguria, and neurologic complications have occurred. Hence, it is obligatory to monitor blood pressure closely during the use of captopril. Increases in BUN and creatinine also must be monitored when using this drug.

Captopril has been used successfully in children with large left-to-right shunts and elevated SVR to reduce the magnitude of the left-to-right shunting.[130] Additionally, in patients with dilated cardiomyopathies or paradoxical hypertension following coarctation surgery, captopril appears to be beneficial.[131]

Patients with ventricular volume loading associated with chronic aortic or mitral regurgitation have also derived benefit from captopril. Recently, clinical practice has focused on the use of captopril and other agents of this group as prophylactic therapies in those at risk for declining ventricular function, such as postcancer chemotherapy patients, or patients with single ventricle conditions, such as those who have undergone Fontan's operation or its variations.[132,133] Multicenter clinical trials are needed to objectively verify the value of such prophylaxis.

Enalapril

Enalapril, the second commercially available ACE inhibitor in the U.S., is also effective in the treatment of children with systemic hypertension[134,134a] and CHF.[135,136] It is a prodrug that must be deesterified in the liver to the active form. (Enalaprilat is the only ACE inhibitor available for intravenous administration.) Enalapril differs from captopril in two significant ways: (a) its molecular structure contains no sulfhydryl group, postulated to be an etiologic factor in the development of some side effects, and (b) its half-life is longer. In general, enalapril's side effects are similar to captopril but may occur somewhat less frequently.

Lisinopril

Lisinopril, another long-acting ACE inhibitor, was evaluated in 115 hypertensive children (aged 6–16 years) and found to lower blood pressure in a dose-dependent manner. A starting dose of 0.07 mg/kg was appropriate, and the drug was well tolerated.[136a]

Beta-Adrenergic Blockers

While much experience in pediatric patients has been accumulated for beta-blockers in the treatment of hypertension and arrhythmias, only recently were these drugs found to be useful in heart failure as well. First- and second-generation drugs of this group are reviewed under arrhythmia treatment. In several important trials and reports on adult CHF patients, carvedilol, bisoprolol, and metoprolol appear to have important clinical benefit.[137–139] Their efficacy relates to interference with the deleterious effects of excess sympathetic activity in chronic heart failure, and, in pediatric patients, particularly to those with nonischemic cardiomyopathy.

Bisoprolol and metoprolol are both β_1-selective blockers. Carvedilol, a nonselective beta-blocker, is an α-adrenergic antagonist as well, with antioxidant capability.[137]

In pediatrics, a few favorable original studies with small numbers of patients have been supported by the recently published multicenter carvedilol trial,[140] demonstrating the value of this agent in patients deemed severe enough to warrant heart transplantation. As more information is developed,[140a] it seems likely that these drugs will secure as important a place in the management of pediatric patients with CHF as they currently have in adults.

ANTIHYPERTENSIVE AGENTS

In pediatrics, antihypertensive pharmacotherapy is primarily used to treat secondary forms of hypertension.[141] In more than 80% of children younger than 10 years of age, the cause of hypertension is likely to be a disease of the kidney, the cardiovascular system, or the endocrine system.[142] The prevalence of essential hypertension in the first decade of life is significantly less than 1% of this age group. During the second decade of life, the prevalence increases, but the percentage of teenagers with essential hypertension continues to be extremely low.[143] An aggressive approach to therapy with multidrug regimens is often necessary for adequate control of secondary hypertension, as it is generally more resistant to therapy than essential hypertension.[101] Repeated measurements exceeding the 95th percentile for age and gender, as defined by the Second Task Force on Blood Pressure Control in Children,[144] necessitates the initiation of drug therapy.

Hypertensive Emergencies

Hypertension accompanied by clinical evidence of end-organ injury is an emergency and requires immediate pharmacotherapy. Signs and symptoms such as retinal hemorrhages or papilledema, seventh nerve palsy, diplopia, symptoms of encephalopathy (headache, vomiting, altered mental status, or seizures), CHF, or renal insufficiency all reflect end-organ injury due to malignant hypertension. The patient's blood pressure must not be reduced too rapidly, because it may lead to hypotension, obtundation, or other disabling adverse effects.[145]

Nifedipine

Nifedipine, the most potent vasodilator of the calcium channel blockers, has been used to treat hypertension in children with hypertensive emergencies. Its rapid onset of action and relatively short duration of action make it ideal for this purpose. It has also been used to treat infants with hypertrophic cardiomyopathy,[146] primary pulmonary hypertension,[147] and ventricular septal defect with pulmonary hypertension.[148] It is supplied as an encapsulated liquid that must be swallowed and not taken sublingually, because very little absorption occurs via the latter route.[149] Uchiyama and Sakai[150] suggest that rectal administration of perforated nifedipine capsules may be a reliable way to acutely treat young children with severe hypertension. Pediatric patients appear to tolerate nifedipine better than do adult patients, with infrequent and mild side effects.[151] However, cardiovascular collapse and cardiac arrest after ingesting an extraordinary large dose of nifedipine can reflect nifedipine poisoning[152] in which the antihypertensive effect is not maintained.

Diazoxide

Diazoxide, a nondiuretic thiazide derivative, is a potent arteriolar dilator. Its antihypertensive effect is rapid in onset, and it has been used safely in children.[153] One may avoid an abrupt decrease in blood pressure and its associated complications (see above) by administering diazoxide as a slow, rather than as a rapid, infusion, as was done in one adult study,[154] which demonstrated the efficacy of the slower infusion. Adverse effects of diazoxide include fluid retention and hypertrichosis, especially with frequent administration.

Labetalol

Labetalol acts as a nonselective beta-blocker. It also has α-adrenergic blocking properties and direct vasodilating activity.[153] Its β-blocking properties, however, are about eight times as potent as its α-blocking ability.[155] It is well absorbed after an oral dose and undergoes extensive first-pass hepatic metabolism. The intravenous use of labetalol was recently reported in children. Bunchman et al[156] noted that the intravenous infusion of labetalol in children with severe hypertension or in those with uncontrollable hypertension was effective in controlling blood pressure when oral medication could not be tolerated. Labetalol's antihypertensive effect was observed within an hour after a starting dose of 0.2 to 1.0 mg/kg. Its effect was sustained with a continuous parenteral infusion of 0.25 to 1.5 mg/kg/h. Side effects were rare, and the response to labetalol was independent of kidney function. Labetalol is particularly useful in treating the hypertensive crisis of chronic renal failure.[142]

Hydralazine

Hydralazine's primary action is to relax precapillary arteriolar vascular smooth muscle. It reduces SVR and therefore afterload, which permits increased ventricular muscle fiber shortening during systole. This results in an enhanced stroke volume at any given end-diastolic volume. In infants and children, hydralazine has been shown to be effective in the treatment of ventricular systolic dysfunction.[157,158] It may also decrease shunt magnitude and increase systemic output by decreasing SVR to a greater degree than PVR in infants with left-to-right shunts.[159,160]

Hydralazine can be given both orally and parenterally. After an oral dose, the drug undergoes extensive first-pass metabolism by acetylation, which limits its bioavailability. Hemodynamic effects occur within 30 to 60 min and last for as long as 8 h. Unlike adults to whom hydralazine has been given by continuous infusion, infants and children should be given hydralazine by bolus infusions. Following intravenous administration, hemodynamic responses are apparent after approximately 5 to 10 min, peak by approximately 30 min, and last for 2 to 4 h.[161] Its rapid onset of action makes intravenous hydralazine useful for treating hypertensive urgencies.

Presently, the incidence of adverse effects in infants and children are not well delineated. The most common adverse effects seen in adults include headache, dizziness, nausea, and vomiting, postural hypotension, and tachycardia. About 10% of adult patients on long-term hydralazine therapy develop a generally reversible lupus-like syndrome. Without clinical suspicion of a lupus-like syndrome, routine monitoring of antinuclear antibody is not justified, because only some of the patients in whom antinuclear antibodies are present will subsequently develop clinical features of lupus. For a given dose, slow acetylators achieve higher plasma concentrations and are at increased risk for adverse effects. It is unclear whether tolerance to long-term hydralazine therapy, as demonstrated in adults, will occur in pediatric patients as well.

Chronic Hypertension Management

Calcium-Channel Blockers

Chronic drug therapy in hypertensive children is predicated on the expectation that reduction of high pressure will result in decreased long-term morbidity and mortality, which has been proved with at least some antihypertensive agents in adults.[162] In fact, there is mounting evidence, as the Bogalusa Heart Study[163] suggests, that hypertension in children may herald the development of essential hypertension later in life. Chronic antihypertensive drug therapy in children has been modified in recent years to include initially either an ACE inhibitor or a calcium-channel blocker.[101] Their once-a-day dosages and favorable side effect profile have tended to improve compliance, a major issue in childhood and adolescence.

Calcium-channel blockers reduce the influx of calcium responsible for cardiac and vascular smooth-muscle contraction. These agents are divided into two groups based on their molecular structure and clinical application. Type I agents are characterized by a tertiary amine structure similar to verapamil. They are used primarily to treat cardiac arrhythmias and are discussed in the section entitled "Antiarrhythmic Therapy." Type II agents have a dihydropyridine nucleus, similar to nifedipine. These agents exhibit less antiarrhythmic activity but are more potent vasodilators and are used in pediatrics to treat hypertension.

The effects of nitrendipine, a dihydropyridine compound, were studied in 25 hypertensive children (6 months to 16 years of age) who had systolic and diastolic blood pressure consistently exceeding the 95th percentile for age and gender.[164] Significant reductions in blood pressures (mean decrease 148/99 to 128/77 mm Hg after 1 day and to 121/75 mm Hg after 2 weeks) were observed within 24 h, and the effects were sustained through 3 months of treatment with a dose of 0.25 to 0.50 mg/kg given every 6 to 12 h. It was apparently safe. The duration of action and the long-term clinical response to nitrendipine was believed to be substantially better than that of nifedipine.

Amlodipine, another long-acting dihydropyridine calcium-channel blocker, was evaluated in an international, placebo-controlled study of 268 hypertensive children aged 1–17, and found to be both safe and effective. Headache was the most common adverse effect.[164a]

Beta-Blockers

Beta-blockers act at the β-adrenergic receptor. Although they share this common characteristic, they differ from each other with regard to the presence or absence of β_1 selectivity, lipid solubility, intrinsic sympathomimetic activity, membrane stabilization, and potency (also see Chap. 7). These drugs' high therapeutic index has been confirmed by reports in children.[165] The antihypertensive effect is poorly correlated with plasma concentrations and surpasses the anticipated duration of action based on plasma half-life. Hence, even preparations with short half-lives generally can be given on a twice-daily basis, and possibly even once a day. The reported incidence of side effects to beta-blockers in children is exceptionally low. Administration of any of the β-blocking agents, which can inhibit β_2-receptor bronchodilation, to children with obstructive forms of lung disease such as asthma, should be strongly discouraged. CNS side effects in children are more likely to present in the form of sleep disturbances as opposed to the depression, dreams, confusion, and agitation seen in adults. Glucose and lipid profile can be adversely affected.

The most extensive published clinical pediatric experience with beta-blockers has been with propranolol. Berenson et al[166] randomized 95 patients with persistent hypertension, defined as greater than the 90th percentile for blood pressure over a 4-month interval, to either a drug-treatment group consisting of low-dose propranolol and chlorthalidone therapy or to a control group. Both groups were exposed to an education program oriented toward the treatment of hypertension by diet and exercise. Those in the drug-treatment group, after 30 months of follow-up, had significantly lower mean systolic and diastolic blood pressures, with minimal side effects. Griswold et al[167] treated nine children with hypertension secondary to renal disease associated with high plasma renin levels who had failed pharmacotherapy with diuretics, hydralazine, and methyldopa. One patient developed resting bradycardia. Ruley and Magalnick[168] successfully treated hypertension in a 1-year-old male with Wilm's tumor and elevated plasma renin activity with doses as high as 24 mg/kg/d of propranolol. Boerth[169] reported a need for higher plasma propranolol levels to achieve therapeutic results in those patients with secondary hypertension due to renal parenchymal disease or hypoplastic abdominal aorta than in those patients with essential hypertension (140 vs 111 ng/mL). Mongeau et al[170] conducted a single-blind, 8-month, crossover trial that compared propranolol to placebo in 10 patients (14 to 17 years of age) with essential hypertension. Both systolic and diastolic pressures were significantly reduced with propranolol. None of the patients developed adverse effects severe enough to require cessation of propranolol therapy. Three of 10 patients did, however, experience fatigue after exercise, bradycardia, and transient Raynaud's phenomenon. Potter et al[171] conducted a prospective study on the effect of propranolol (1.0 to 9.0 mg/kg/d) in 13 postkidney transplant, high-renin, hypertensive children. Some of the patients were concomitantly administered diuretics, methyldopa, and hydralazine. There was a mean reduction of blood pressure from 139/94 to 127/84 mm Hg. Two of the 13 patients did not improve with propranolol therapy, and there was no correlation between change in renin levels and change in blood pressure. Propranolol has also been shown to be effective preoperatively in children with coarctation of the aorta. Gidding et al[172] addressed the question of whether preoperative administration of propranolol could prevent paradoxical hypertension noted in children following surgery for coarctation of the aorta. They found that propanolol effectively decreased postoperative rises in both blood pressure and plasma renin activity. Leenen et al[173] have also confirmed the effective use of propranolol in this regard in a randomized, controlled, double-blind trial.

In previously noted pediatric studies,[170,171] β blockade caused a fall in serum renin activity, but there was no relationship between that reduction and an antihypertensive response. Falkner et al[174] reported adequate blood pressure control with metoprolol and a blunted change in the systolic pressure and heart rate response to aerobic exercise and mental stress. At maximum exercise, patients were able to increase their heart rate to expected maximal levels, without limitation in endurance capacity (measured by exercise stress testing), suggesting that metoprolol may be useful in diabetics who fail propranolol therapy. In addition, metoprolol had no adverse effect on glucose levels and insulin requirements.

Central α_2-Adrenergic Agonists

These agents, including clonidine and guanabenz, act centrally by stimulating α_2-mediated inhibition of sympathetic outflow, which results in decreased SVR (also see Chap. 15). These drugs are primarily used in the treatment of hypertension. Abrupt discontinuation of therapy may result in rebound hypertension. Other side effects are sedation and dry mouth. Published pediatric experience with these agents is limited.

Minoxidil

Minoxidil results in arteriolar vasodilation without significant venous vasodilation, similar to hydralazine. Its use is primarily reserved for children with severe drug-resistant hypertension. Side effects of minoxidil include hypotension, tachycardia, hypertrichosis, and fluid retention.[175]

TREATMENT OF LIPID DISORDERS

Increasingly, evidence is accumulating that links atherosclerosis in adults with a juvenile onset.[176] In addition, there are primary lipid disorders with marked elevation of cholesterol and its congeners, which exist in childhood in their own right. As a result, over the past decade increasing attention has been focused on developing strategies of pharmacologic management of lipoprotein metabolism in childhood.

There is considerable experience with antilipid pharmacotherapy in children with familial hypercholesterolemia (FH), the most commonly recognized and best understood disorder of lipoprotein metabolism in childhood.[177] In FH heterozygotes (1 of 500), the plasma cholesterol [total and low-density lipoproteins (LDL)] are elevated approximately two- to threefold; FH homozygotes (1 of 1,000,000) have cholesterol levels that are elevated five- to sixfold.[178] The published studies have been small in size, making it difficult to thoroughly assess the potential adverse side effects of antilipid drug therapy. Furthermore, therapeutic approaches studied in FH may not have broad-based applicability to other types of childhood dyslipidemias. Additionally, in these studies, therapy for the most part has been oriented toward the reduction of serum total cholesterol and LDL-cholesterol without addressing other constituents of the serum lipid profile which may have both prognostic and therapeutic significance.[179]

In children with dyslipidemias, it may be reasonably assumed that atherosclerosis is developing at an accelerated rate.[180] The treatment of dyslipidemic children hinges on the assumption that modifying the serum lipoprotein concentrations will reduce the rate of atherogenesis. The use of combined diet-drug intervention has been shown to arrest the progression of arteriographically defined coronary atherosclerosis and to reduce cardiovascular disease risk in middle-aged men, although such data are not available in children.

As in adults, initial medical intervention for dyslipidemias in childhood is generally nonpharmacologic. On average, the LDL-cholesterol will decrease approximately 10 to 15% with diet therapy.[181] In some children, however, diet therapy alone will not suffice. The National Cholesterol Education Program (NCEP) Expert Panel on Blood Cholesterol Levels in Children and Adolescents[181] selected cut points for initiation of pharmacotherapy. According to those guidelines, in children 10 years of age and older, drug therapy should be initiated after a 6- to 12-month trial of diet if (a) serum LDL-cholesterol is greater than 190 mg/dL or (b) serum LDL-cholesterol is greater than 160 mg/dL along with either a positive family history of premature coronary artery disease or two or more other risk factors that remain present after vigor-

ous attempts have been made to control them. In children younger than 10 years of age, clinical judgment of the physician must dictate treatment.

Another set of recommendations has been issued by the American Academy of Pediatrics Committee on Nutrition.[182] While specific levels for screening algorithms differ to a limited extent, there is consensus agreement that indications for pharmacotherapy include a 190 mg/dL LDL-cholesterol value in children 10 years of age or older who have attempted diet modification or an LDL of >160 mg/DL if there is a family history of premature cardiovascular disease or if there are other risk factors present assuming a strong attempt at dietary control.[183] In addition, there are advocates for beginning treatment at even younger ages, although the value of this approach remains to be tested in large population samples.[184]

Approved medication options for use in the pediatric population are limited. The most widespread experience is with the bile acid sequestrants colestipol and cholestyramine. However, other drugs, including various statins, niacin, and fenofibrate, also reduce the total cholesterol.

Bile-Acid Binding Resins

Cholestyramine and Colestipol

The NCEP recommends only the use of the bile acid sequestrants. These agents have been used successfully to lower LDL-cholesterol in children over long intervals, apparently with relatively few side effects. Doses are not related to the body weight of the child, but to the postdietary LDL-cholesterol levels.[185] These drugs are the safest to use because they are not absorbed systemically. Both cholestyramine and colestipol have been used for up to 8 years in children,[179] without evidence of fat-soluble vitamin deficiencies, steatorrhea, calcium or vitamin D metabolic disturbances, or erythrocyte folic deficiency. However, no placebo-controlled, double-blind, prospective study of the safety and efficacy of these agents, particularly regarding long-term growth and development, has been done.

The dose range frequently recommended is 2 to 16 g/d. Most common side effects include flatulence, nausea, and constipation. Approximately a 15 to 20% reduction in LDL-cholesterol values can be achieved, on average, over the long-term, although greater reductions have been reported in selected circumstances.

HMG-CoA Reductase Inhibitors (Statins)

HMG-CoA reductase inhibitors have not been approved by the FDA for use in patients younger than 18 years of age. Nevertheless, many studies have recently been carried out that indicate a promising role for these agents, based upon the encouraging work that has been amassed in adults.[186,186a] In the last several years, placebo-controlled double-blind clinical trials have demonstrated reductions in LDL-cholesterol in children using statins and diet, both with and without concomitant bile acid sequestrant therapy.[187–190] Only limited side effects have been reported in these studies, involving pravastatin, lovastatin, or simvastatin in doses ranging from 5 to 40 mg/d, depending on the particular study. Some children were treated for as long as 12 months. Reductions in mean LDL-cholesterol ranged from as high as 21 to 36% in one study[188] to 17 to 27% in another,[189] with similar reductions found in other trials as well. As with adults, monitoring of cholecystokinin (CK) and liver function studies is required, as well as accurate reporting of muscle cramping, rash, and fatigue. Importantly, statin use in these trials has not had adverse effects on growth or on maturation in males. The caveat against their use in the pubertal female remains in place, however, as there are no data proving safety in this group for either the patient or a prospective fetus. Long-term studies are still needed, perhaps spanning decades, for obtaining secure data concerning the impact of such treatment in children on the development of cardiovascular complications in adults with lipid disorders.

Niacin

Niacin functions by suppressing hepatic production and secretion of LDL and very-low-density lipoproteins (VLDL). There are descriptions of the use of niacin in childhood, but its clinical utility use is limited because of well-documented adverse effects. The most worrisome is its potential hepatotoxicity at therapeutic doses, as suggested by elevation of liver enzymes. Common adverse effects include "niacin flush," which can be prevented by taking aspirin (dose is age-dependent) 20 to 30 min prior to the niacin dose. Less commonly, itching, dry skin, headaches, nausea, vomiting, diarrhea, and increased liver function tests may occur. Usually, niacin is recommended to be used in combination with diet therapy plus bile acid sequestrants in doses of 1 to 1.5 g/d.

ANTIARRHYTHMIC DRUGS

Arrhythmias are encountered much less frequently in children than in adults, but remain important reasons for pharmacotherapy in childhood. Arrhythmia therapy differs from that in adults because of the spectrum of arrhythmias most frequently encountered in children and the differences in pharmacokinetics and specific effects of antiarrhythmic drugs between children and adults. In addition, the strategy for fetal arrhythmia drug therapy given via the mother and the cardiac electrophysiologic effects of commonly used psychotropic medications in childhood also make discussion of this topic in childhood unique.

Children without congenital structural heart disease most frequently have supraventricular tachycardia and, rarely, ventricular tachycardia. After corrective surgery for congenital heart defects, supraventricular tachycardia, atrial flutter, atrial fibrillation, and ventricular tachycardia can all occur. Children with complex congenital heart disease are living longer postoperatively with an increasing incidence of arrhythmias with increasing age. Atkins et al recently extensively reviewed evidence-based drug therapy of arrhythmias in children and adults.[191]

Overview of Diagnoses in Children

Supraventricular Arrhythmias

Supraventricular tachycardia is the most frequent significant arrhythmia in children, with an estimated incidence of 1 in 250 to 1 in 1000.[192] The most common electrophysiologic mechanisms are atrioventricular and atrioventricular nodal reentry. In the hemodynamically unstable patient, electrical cardioversion is indicated. If the patient with SVT is hemodynamically stable, after a trial of vagal maneuvers, intravenous adenosine is the drug of choice for acute conversion to sinus rhythm. Intravenous procainamide or amiodarone have also been shown in children to be effective and may be used if adenosine is unsuccessful or unavailable. Intravenous

verapamil may be used, but not in patients younger than 1 year of age, because of reported cardiovascular collapse. For prevention of subsequent episodes, digoxin, propranolol, atenolol, verapamil, flecainide and amiodarone may all have a role. In the presence of preexcitation (Wolff-Parkinson-White syndrome), digoxin should be avoided because it can accelerate conduction along the bypass tract. Transcatheter radiofrequency ablation, however, has become an increasingly popular alternative to chronic pharmacologic therapy.

Atrial flutter and atrial fibrillation occur infrequently in infants without structural heart disease, as well as in children with surgical repairs involving extensive atrial suturing (Mustard, Senning, Fontan, or TAPVR repair). Electrical cardioversion is the definitive therapy and indicated for hemodynamic instability, although care must be taken to follow anticoagulation guidelines[193] in order to prevent thromboembolic complications. For pharmacologic rate control or conversion to sinus rhythm, beta-blockers, calcium-channel blockers, digoxin, amiodarone, procainamide, flecainide, and sotalol may all be effective. Therapy is determined by the presence or absence of preexcitation and the hemodynamic status. Junctional tachycardia may be encountered after open-heart surgery and may be treated by intravenous amiodarone, procainamide or propafenone.

Ventricular Tachycardia

In children, ventricular tachycardia is encountered much less frequently than supraventricular arrhythmias, but does occur in certain settings, including the long QT syndrome and after cardiac surgery involving ventricular suturing (e.g., tetralogy of Fallot repair). Hemodynamically unstable ventricular tachycardia warrants electrical cardioversion. In the hemodynamically stable child, effective acute drug therapy for monomorphic ventricular tachycardia includes intravenous amiodarone, procainamide, or lidocaine. Polymorphic ventricular tachycardia, that is torsades de pointes, may be treated by intravenous magnesium, pacing, beta-blockers, or isoproterenol. Other polymorphic ventricular tachycardia may be treated by intravenous lidocaine, amiodarone, procainamide, sotalol, beta-blockers, or phenytoin. Pulseless ventricular tachycardia and ventricular fibrillation are electrically cardioverted, but if refractory to electroshock, the arrhythmias can be treated with epinephrine, intravenous amiodarone, lidocaine, procainamide, or magnesium.

Chronic therapy for ventricular tachycardia may include beta-blockers, mexiletine, amiodarone, or phenytoin. In the presence of long QT syndrome, β blockade is the mainstay of therapy.

Prolonged QT Syndrome

It has been suggested that 10% of the 7000 annual crib deaths are the result of unrecognized cardiac causes—notably, concealed cardiac arrhythmias, including those related to a prolonged QT interval.[194] In 80% of untreated patients with prolonged QT syndrome, ventricular tachycardia occurs, especially torsade de pointes.[195,196] Although many cases are sporadic, there is a clear genetic pattern in the Romano-Ward (autosomal dominant) and Jervell-Lange-Nielsen (autosomal recessive) syndromes. The dominant disorder has no clinical marker aside from the arrhythmia, whereas the recessive syndrome is associated with hereditary neurosensory deafness. The congenital long QT syndrome is familial in 60% of cases.[197] The current understanding of the pathogenetic mechanism of the long QT syndrome involves the sympathetic nervous system either as the primary defect (sympathetic imbalance hypothesis) or as an intracardiac abnormality probably related to the control of potassium currents.[198] Recent findings of specific mutations on specific genes that determine specific abnormalities in cardiac ion channels leading to different forms of long QT syndrome will determine specific therapies for each type of ion channel disorder, allowing for more effective pharmacologic therapy.[199]

Whereas the length of QT intervals in infants deemed to be at high risk for crib death do not strictly correlate with the likelihood of sudden death,[200] corrected QT intervals lasting for longer than 500 milliseconds appear to confer upon patients the greatest risk.[197]

Therapy is oriented toward the prevention of sudden death by acutely terminating torsade de pointes and its immediate reinitiation, and chronically preventing its recurrence. Since (bradycardia or long pauses may potentiate the tachycardia and are important risk factors),[201] ventricular pacing and isoproterenol infusion have been studied. Lidocaine infusion has variable results.[202] In vitro, magnesium inhibits early after depolarizations and may play a role in suppressing reinitiation of torsade de pointes.[203,204] Experimental data suggest that calcium-channel blockers may be of some acute benefit.[200,205,206]

β Blockade with propranolol has been the mainstay for chronic therapy of long QT syndrome as it has proven effective in 75 to 80% of patients.[201,207] In some patients, antiarrhythmic agents, such as tocainide and mexiletine, have been used effectively.[208] However, despite full-dose beta-blockers, 20 to 25% of patients continue to have syncopal episodes and remain at a high risk for sudden cardiac death. For those unresponsive patients, high thoracic left sympathectomy has been used. Recently, an international prospective study provided evidence that left cardiac sympathetic denervation is a very effective therapy.[209]

The treatment of asymptomatic children with long QT syndrome remains controversial. Garson et al recommend that asymptomatic children with a corrected QT interval >0.44 and a positive family history of the long QT syndrome should be treated,[210] as a cardiac arrest may be the first symptom (9% presented with a cardiac arrest). This differs from adults where the majority of patients have syncopal episodes before a cardiac arrest.[211] The authors noted that ineffective treatment, particularly for symptoms, was a predictor for late symptoms and sudden death. Also, it has been noted that ineffective treatment with one agent likely predicted ineffective therapy with other pharmacologic agents. Hence, lack of clinical response to even one drug should prompt the clinician to consider alternative therapies, including pacing or left-cardiac sympathetic denervation.[212,213]

Propranolol is equal to other beta-blockers in providing effective treatment for symptoms and ventricular arrhythmias and is similar in terms of incidence of late sudden death. The sudden death risk was not related to the type of other beta-blocker used.

Specific Antiarrhythmic Drugs

When the pediatric cardiologist is challenged with the task of selecting an appropriate antiarrhythmic drug and finding pediatric drug-dosing guidelines for antiarrhythmics, one discovers the relative lack of information available. Antiarrhythmic medications can have different pharmacokinetics and effects in children than they do in adults. Use of antiarrhythmia medications in children are mostly based upon studies in adults, although pediatric data will hopefully be collected in the near future.[214] In fact, digoxin is the only agent that is officially approved by the U.S. Food and Drug administration for use in children with cardiac arrhythmias. In the following discussion, the Vaughan Williams classification of antiarrhythmics will be

used. The electrophysiologic actions of the drugs are summarized in Chap. 17.

Class IA Agents

Quinidine

Quinidine can be used for the treatment of supraventricular and ventricular tachycardias in children. Animal studies suggest that the effects of quinidine are less pronounced in the immature than in the mature heart.[215] Whereas quinidine's direct electrophysiologic effect tends to be antiarrhythmic, its indirect anticholinergic effect tends to be proarrhythmic. Quinidine will increase the SA node's rate of discharge and, at the AV node, indirectly augment conduction through its anticholinergic action. Quinidine can also act as an α-adrenergic blocker.

The clinician must attempt to ensure that the resulting in vivo effect of quinidine is the desired one. For example, in patients with atrial fibrillation or flutter, enhanced AV nodal conduction due to the anticholinergic effect may translate into an inappropriately accelerated ventricular rate. This can be avoided by combining quinidine with an agent that will combat quinidine's effect at the AV node such as digoxin which slows AV nodal conduction.

Quinidine is usually prescribed orally but may be slowly given parenterally, in either the gluconate or sulfate form. Quinidine gluconate is absorbed more slowly and takes longer to reach its peak concentration than quinidine sulfate, allowing for the less frequent dosing of every 8 hours. Significant age-related differences in protein binding have been shown—63% in newborns versus 86% in older children, approximating the 90% protein binding seen in adults.[115a] Similarly, in the presence of cyanotic heart disease, changes in protein binding have been demonstrated.[216] Quinidine is primarily metabolized by the liver; 20% is excreted unmetabolized in the urine along with its metabolites.[217] The elimination half-life of quinidine is shorter in children (about 4 h) than in adults (about 6 h).[217] The dose of quinidine in children is correspondingly higher than that for adults. Dosage for quinidine gluconate is generally 20% higher.[218]

The dreaded cardiovascular complication of quinidine therapy is excessive prolongation of the QT interval associated with a potentially fatal ventricular arrhythmia, torsade de pointes. In children, an association between "quinidine syncope" and the presence of structural heart disease and/or hypokalemia has been noted.[219] In adults, syncope usually occurs within 5 days of initiation of therapy.[220] In children, however, syncope may occur as late as 2 weeks after treatment initiation. Furthermore, the likelihood of syncope to occur does not appear to correlate with serum quinidine levels.[219] Hence, in such patients, it is advisable to initiate quinidine therapy only in the hospital. Hypotension, especially with parenteral administration, may also occur due to α-adrenergic blockade. Other adverse effects are GI (diarrhea, nausea, vomiting) and hematologic (antibody-mediated thrombocytopenia). Importantly, quinidine can raise serum digoxin levels, as is discussed earlier in this chapter.

Procainamide

Procainamide has similar indications to quinidine. It does not prolong the action potential and QT interval as much as quinidine. Also, it has weaker autonomic effects, which include less anticholinergic activity and no α-adrenergic blocking action. Procainamide does act as a mild ganglionic blocker and thereby may cause peripheral vasodilation and a negative chronotropic effect. Animal studies show that like quinidine, in neonates, higher concentrations of procainamide are necessary to produce effects similar to those on adult myocardium.[221]

Procainamide may be used intravenously. It is rapidly absorbed following oral administration, with peak plasma concentrations achieved in about 75 min. Unlike quinidine, only 20% of procainamide is protein bound.[115a] Conventional and sustained-release forms are available. More than 50% of the drug is excreted unmetabolized in the urine. The rest undergoes N-acetylation to form N-acetyl procainamide (NAPA), which is then excreted in the urine. The rate of metabolism corresponds to a genetically determined acetylator phenotype. NAPA itself displays class III antiarrhythmic properties. Whereas NAPA's parent drug exerts its effect on both the duration and the upstroke of the action potential, NAPA's electrophysiologic effect is limited to its ability to prolong the action potential.[115a]

Procainamide has a significantly shorter elimination half-life in children (1.7 h) than in adults.[222] Its cardiovascular adverse effects in children are similar to quinidine. However, torsade de pointes is less frequent and appears to be dose-related. GI effects occur less often than with quinidine. Approximately one-third of patients can develop a lupus-like syndrome with fever, rash, and thrombocytopenia after 6 months of therapy, and up to 70% of patients will develop antinuclear antibodies, conditions which are reversible with cessation of therapy. Slow acetylators carry an increased risk for developing adverse effects from treatment. Amiodarone may increase plasma levels of procainamide.[223]

Disopyramide

Not only does disopyramide exert class IA antiarrhythmic effects, but it also exhibits a pronounced negative inotropic effect. In fact, it has recently been used successfully in children with hypertrophic obstructive cardiomyopathy to reduce outflow tract gradients.[224] In addition, it exhibits much greater anticholinergic activity than the other class IA agents. It is administered orally, is well absorbed, and subject to first-pass hepatic metabolism. Apparent age-related differences in the ability of pediatric patients to maintain therapeutic disopyramide serum levels have been noted. Whereas older children may achieve satisfactory levels after being given 5 to 15 mg/kg/d, children younger than 2 years of age may require as much as 30 mg/kg/d to obtain the same levels.[225]

The cardiovascular adverse effects are similar to quinidine. It also may precipitate CHF due to its negative inotropic actions. Gastrointestinal side effects occur less frequently than with the other class IA agents. Anticholinergic side effects do occur and the drug does not increase serum digoxin levels.

Class IB Agents

Lidocaine

Lidocaine is useful in suppressing delayed after depolarizations and has little benefit for supraventricular tachycardias. Canine studies reveal that neonatal fibers require greater lidocaine concentrations to achieve the same effects on the action potential as that seen in adult dogs.[226] Lidocaine is less effective in reducing conduction velocity in young, as compared to adult, Purkinje fibers,[227] and the time constant of recovery from rate-dependent conduction delay in intact newborn canine heart is notably shorter than in the adult.[228] Lidocaine is not administered orally as it undergoes extensive first-pass hepatic metabolism. Its half-life, which is related to

hepatic blood flow, is approximately 3.2 h in neonate versus 1.8 in adults.[229] Adverse effects appear to be dose related and may occur at plasma levels as low as 5 μg/mL. Most commonly, CNS symptoms (confusion, dizziness, and seizures) occur, which can be avoided by reducing the infusion rate and by monitoring drug serum levels.[230] With serum levels exceeding 9 μg/mL, even more serious reactions have been seen, including, hypotension, low cardiac output, muscle twitching, and respiratory arrest.[231] Lidocaine may exacerbate preexisting electrophysiologic abnormalities (AV block, sinus node dysfunction).

Other IB Agents

In children, phenytoin is used as an antiarrhythmic agent for chronic therapy of ventricular arrhythmias after cardiac surgery and for treating digoxin-induced arrhythmias. Mexiletine and tocainide are used for chronic oral treatment of ventricular tachycardia which had previously responded to intravenous lidocaine.[100]

Class IC Agents

Flecainide

Some of flecainide's electrophysiologic effects appear to be less pronounced in the neonatal as compared to the adult myocardium.[232] Flecainide has been used in children to treat supraventricular tachycardias, atrial flutter, and ventricular arrhythmias. The adult CAST trial,[233] however, raised concern about the safety of flecainide and prompted the review of the use of flecainide in children. The pediatric patient with ventricular arrhythmias and structural heart disease most closely parallels the profile implicated in the CAST trial, namely the adult with ventricular arrhythmias after myocardial infarction. In their comprehensive review of the use of flecainide in children, Perry and Garson[234] concluded that in pediatric patients with supraventricular tachycardia (excluding atrial flutter) and normal hearts, flecainide appeared to be both effective and safe (no deaths with usual oral dosing and less than 1% serious proarrhythmia). In patients with atrial flutter or ventricular arrhythmias[235] with structurally abnormal hearts, flecainide may not be safe. However, for those patients with ventricular arrhythmias and structurally normal hearts, the safety of flecainide has yet to be established.[236]

The elimination half-life of flecainide manifests agedependence. Although children between 1 and 12 years of age have a mean elimination half-life of 8 h, pediatric patients outside of that age range have a longer elimination half-life of 11 to 12 h. The therapeutic flecainide dose is 100 to 200 mg/m²/d or 1 to 8 mg/kg/d.[235,236] The risk of toxicity is increased in patients who require high doses of flecainide because of persistently low plasma trough levels,[235] and in those patients whose diet changes to include less milk products, which can result in increased flecainide absorption.[236]

Propafenone

In addition to its possessing the electrophysiologic properties of flecainide, propafenone exerts a mild beta-blocking and calcium channel blocking effects. In children, intravenous propafenone has been used to treat postoperative junctional ectopic tachycardia[237] and congenital junctional ectopic tachycardia.[238] It appears to be effective for treating children with supraventricular tachycardias, particularly those arising from an ectopic site.[239] It can be given orally or intravenously. In a report by Janousek et al,[240] the use of oral propafenone (mean dose 353 mg/m²/d divided three times daily) effectively controlled supraventricular tachyarrhythmias in 41 of 47 (87%) patients studied, most of whom were infants. This report helps give dosing guidelines (200 to 600 mg/m^2/d divided into three doses) for oral propafenone use. Furthermore, the authors suggest that for monitoring drug effect, measuring QRS duration is preferred over measuring drug plasma levels. Because of propafenone's interaction with digoxin, it has been recommended that the digoxin maintenance dosage should be halved when initiating propafenone therapy in a child already taking digoxin.[241,242]

Class II Agents

Beta-Adrenergic Blockers

Beta-blockers have been used for years in children to treat supraventricular arrhythmias and ventricular arrhythmias. Propranolol can significantly inhibit SA node automaticity in children with normal SA node function and has had little effect, if any, on sinoatrial conduction.[243] The usefulness of β blockade in the treatment of children with supraventricular tachycardias has been elucidated in several studies reviewed by Kornbluth and Frishman[244] and are briefly summarized here. In one study,[245] in three of six children with supraventricular tachycardia in whom digoxin treatment failed, propranolol (1 to 3 mg/kg/d) restored normal sinus rhythm. Another report[246] again demonstrated the usefulness of digoxin plus propranolol in suppressing supraventricular tachycardia in a 4-month-old girl, but also illustrated propranolol's adverse effects of bronchospasm and sleep disturbances which necessitated its discontinuation. The substitution of propranolol with metoprolol (2 mg/kg/d) yielded effective arrhythmia suppression, which was devoid of side effects over the next 7 months. Pickoff et al[247] described five of five patients studied, who had supraventricular tachycardia inadequately controlled by digitalis, who were free of arrhythmias for up to 2 years with propranolol dosed at 7 to 14 mg/kg/d, maintaining peak serum drug levels between 118 and 250 ng/mL. Dworkin et al[248] reported beneficial effect in seven of nine children who failed to respond to other therapy (digoxin and/or quinidine and/or cardioversion), but who did respond to propranolol in doses of 0.5 to 4.0 mg/kg/d. The side effects that led to dosage reduction were sinus bradycardia, feeding difficulties, and worsening of ketotic hypoglycemia. Finally, Walters et al[249] described five patients with chronic supraventricular tachycardia, who were refractory to digitalis alone, who were successfully treated, without adverse effects, using the combination of digitalis and propranolol doses of 20 to 120 mg/d.

The efficacy of β blockade for the treatment of ventricular tachycardia has also been documented. Propranolol has been used for the acute termination of ventricular tachycardia[250] and chronically for the prevention of its recurrence. For chronic management, for the most part, β-blocking agents have not been effective when given alone, but have been effective when combined with either another drug such as procainamide[251] or another therapeutic modality, such as electrical pacing.[252] Ayabe and Chemmongkoltis,[253] however, reported both successful acute treatment and chronic suppression of ventricular tachycardia after 1.5 years follow-up, in an infant born to a heroin addict, with continued doses of 1 mg/kg propranolol used alone.

Because of its once-a-day and twice-a-day dosing, atenolol, a β-selective blocker, has gained popularity for the treatment of older children and adolescents with arrhythmias, but a high incidence of side effects limits its usefulness. Esmolol, an ultrashort-acting beta-blocker, is helpful in slowing an incessant supraventricular tachycardia in children while other long-term agents are being titrated. Hypotension is a serious limitation with esmolol, especially if ventricular dysfunction already exists as a result of an incessant arrhythmia. The pharmacokinetics of esmolol in children have recently been reviewed and the authors suggest using pediatric dosing guidelines.[254]

Class III Agents

Amiodarone

As in adults, amiodarone exhibits a broad spectrum of antiarrhythmic efficacy that includes the termination of supraventricular and ventricular tachycardias. Its use, however, is limited due to its multiple, serious adverse effects, including a tendency to be proarrhythmic. Chen et al[255] recently reported the successful treatment of SVT-induced cardiomyopathy in a neonate with amiodarone. Shuler et al[256] reported on oral amiodarone's safety and efficacy in 17 infants. Oral amiodarone was successful in relieving arrhythmias in 10 of 17 patients (59%). In three infants with primary atrial tachycardias, the combination of amiodarone with a class IC antiarrhythmic agent was effective. In two infants, amiodarone was found to be proarrhythmic as they developed "incessant episodes" of reentrant supraventricular tachycardia soon after the initiation of treatment. Those who "failed" amiodarone therapy were considered to have reentrant supraventricular tachycardias and were sent for ablative therapy. Perry et al[257] reported on the use of intravenous bolus amiodarone for life-threatening tachyarrhythmias in 10 pediatric patients. The drug was well-tolerated, devoid of significant adverse effects, and was effective in terminating rapid tachyarrhythmias in 6 of 10 patients. Among those who responded was one patient with postoperative junctional ectopic tachycardia.[242] Recently, Etheridge et al reported on 50 infants treated with amiodarone for supraventricular arrhythmias.[258] Amiodarone was felt to be highly effective, with a low incidence of adverse effects. The QTc interval increased during drug loading, but no ventricular arrhythmias were encountered. There were increases in alanine and aspartate aminotransferases and in thyroid-stimulating hormone, but no clinical abnormalities in liver or thyroid function.

Other Class III Agents

Ibutilide is a class III antiarrhythmic drug with an FDA indication for the rapid conversion of atrial fibrillation and atrial flutter to sinus rhythm. The dosage is 0.01 mg/kg intravenously over 10 min. The safety and efficacy of ibutilide in children has not been established.[193]

Dofetilide is a similar agent that can be used orally, but there is no published experience with the drug in children.

Intravenous bretylium use is reserved for patients with recurrent or refractory ventricular fibrillation. Significant hypotension may follow its administration because of the drug's antiadrenergic properties. Sotalol, similar to ibutilide, is a beta-blocker that possesses class III rather than class II antiarrhythmic properties. It appears to be effective in the treatment of supraventricular tachycardia.[259]

Class IV Agents

Class IV antiarrhythmic drugs exert their electrophysiologic effects by blockade of the slow calcium channels.

Verapamil

Verapamil has been used in the initial treatment of supraventricular tachycardia in older children. While the drug lengthens the action potential of mature Purkinje fibers, it shortens it in the neonatal myocardium.[260] Furthermore, verapamil's negative inotropic effect is greater on neonatal than on adult ventricular myocardium,[261,262] and the drug should not be used in conjunction with beta-blockers.[263] Pediatric pharmacokinetic studies have shown that verapamil can have slower and faster elimination half-lives than in adults.[264,265] Although as many as 44% of children develop adverse effects while on chronic oral verapamil therapy, less than 10% of those reactions are severe enough to necessitate discontinuation of the drug.[266] Verapamil is contraindicated in infants younger than 1 year of age, however, because it may reduce cardiac output and produce hypotension and cardiac arrest.[267,268]

Miscellaneous Antiarrhythmics

Adenosine

Adenosine has emerged as the drug of choice for the acute termination of supraventricular tachycardia in the hemodynamically stable infant or child in whom the use of nonpharmacologic vagal maneuvers have failed.[269–271] It is an endogenous nucleoside with a very short half-life (10 sec). Its net electrophysiologic effect is to slow the sinoatrial node firing rate and to decrease AV nodal conduction. It has a rapid onset of action and minimal effects on cardiac contractility. In a recent report, Ralston et al[272] used intravenous adenosine in 24 patients and achieved the desired AV block in 21 (88%). The investigators demonstrated both the diagnostic and therapeutic utilities of causing AV block with intravenous adenosine. In 11 patients, AV block terminated the reentrant tachycardia; in the remaining 10 patients, AV block allowed for proper diagnosis of the enduring atrial arrhythmias.[246] In a recent review of use of adenosine in children in the emergency room, the most effective dose was found to be between 0.1 and 0.3 mg/kg (max = 12 mg) by rapid intravenous push. No major adverse effects, including bronchospasm and sinus arrest, were reported. Minor adverse effects, including nausea, vomiting, headache, flushing, and chest pain, were found to occur with an incidence of 22%.[273]

Digoxin

Digoxin is described earlier in this chapter. It is commonly used for the long-term therapy of supraventricular tachycardia. In atrial flutter and fibrillation, it is used to lessen the ventricular response.

Fetal Arrhythmias

Currently, the most common indication for cardiovascular drug therapy for the fetus is for intrauterine supraventricular tachycardia.[12,12a] In 1969, supraventricular tachycardia was first implicated as a cause of fetal heart failure.[274] In 1980, first report of in utero treatment of supraventricular tachycardia appeared.[275] Soon after, in the mid-1980s, with the advent of new fetal echocardiographic techniques which facilitated the detection and diagnosis of fetal arrhythmias, the treatment of fetal arrhythmias became more common.[276,277]

The mother will be affected by any therapy of the fetus and maternal drug toxicity often limits the effective employment of commonly used antiarrhythmic agents for treating fetal arrhythmias.

Correspondingly, difficulties in controlling fetal arrhythmias stem from difficulties in maintaining adequately high drug concentrations in the mother to provide an effective concentration in the fetus. Some newer, technically more demanding approaches for fetal drug delivery, which bypass the placenta, have been used but may confer greater risk to the fetus.

The majority of those fetuses found to have an arrhythmia have unsustained, isolated ectopy, and this rhythm constitutes about 80% of all fetal arrhythmias detected by echocardiography, most of these being premature atrial contractions (PACs), isolated ventricular ectopy, and variable atrioventricular block. These arrhythmias are of little clinical significance because only 1% of fetuses will have underlying structural congenital heart disease and only 0.5% will go on to develop sustained supraventricular tachycardia. In the absence of structural heart disease, the arrhythmias are generally benign and do not necessitate drug therapy.

As mentioned above, supraventricular tachycardia, usually generated by a reentrant mechanism, is by far the most commonly treated fetal arrhythmia. Recently, Toro et al[278] postulated that atrial septal aneurysms, found in 78% of those fetuses with persistent arrhythmia, may serve as a nidus for PACs and subsequent supraventricular tachycardias. For the viable, near-term, nonhydropic fetus developing a sustained tachyarrhythmia, delivery is the treatment. For the immature fetus, however, who exhibits pulmonary immaturity or who displays signs of CHF, pharmacotherapy should be initiated. Atrial flutter or fibrillation with variable AV block and ventricular response is less commonly treated.[279] Digoxin is the drug of choice for the treatment of fetal supraventricular tachycardia. It may be more effective to load the mother with digoxin intravenously rather than orally.[280] In the hydropic fetus, who may display increased resistance to drug therapy, it may be necessary to administer digoxin directly, that is, either intraperitoneally or via the umbilical vein.[281,282] For the fetal supraventricular tachycardia patient refractory to digoxin alone, a class IA antiarrhythmic agent such as quinidine[283] or procainamide[284] may be added to the maternally administered regimen. Although verapamil has been used,[285,286] Klitzner and Friedman advocate against this[263] in view of Klitzner et al's more recent findings, which demonstrate the fetus' greater dependence on calcium influx to support myocardial contractility than later in life.[287]

Bradyarrhythmias account for about only 5% of all fetal arrhythmias. Etiologies include sinus bradycardia, nonconducted PACs, and complete heart block. In and of itself, sustained fetal bradycardia is not an indication for therapeutic intervention and the fetus should be monitored for fetal distress. In combination with fetal distress, such as hydrops fetalis, however, sustained bradycardia may herald demise. Sustained bradycardia in a fetus with structural heart disease renders the fetus a dismal prognosis.[288] The fetus should be delivered early and paced. Unfortunately, in utero pacing is not yet a widely available therapeutic option.

Arrhythmias and Psychotropic Drugs in Children

Psychotropic drugs are used with increasing frequency in children with a variety of disorders, including attention deficit disorder, hyperactivity, depression, and a number of other psychiatric disorders. There are reports of arrhythmias and sudden death related to the cardiac and, specifically, the cardiac electrophysiologic effects of these medications. In 1999, the American Heart Association issued recommendations for cardiac monitoring of children being treated with certain drugs of this type, based upon knowledge of their cardiac electrophysiologic effects.[289] Tricyclic antidepressants can cause prolonged QTc, QRS, and PR intervals. Phenothiazines, butyrophenones, and diphenylbutylpiperidines have all been reported to prolong the QTc. Phenothiazines and tricyclic antidepressants have also been reported to cause sinus tachycardia. Clinical and electrocardiographic monitoring have been recommended for these medications.

SPECIAL PHARMACOLOGIC APPROACHES

Patent Ductus Arteriosus

Pharmacologic manipulation of the ductus arteriosus has become central to the treatment of neonates with congenital heart disease and to the management of premature newborns, even those with structurally normal hearts.

The ductus arteriosus is a physiologically vital channel required for normal development of fetal circulation. It is found normally in all mammalian fetuses. As lung blood flow in the fetus only amounts to less than 10% of the right ventricular output, and the right ventricle ejects approximately 65% of the combined ventricular output, the ductus arteriosus carries 55 to 60% of the combined ventricular output of the fetus. After birth, as the transition from fetal to normal postnatal circulation develops, the ductus arteriosus closes, first functionally then anatomically. Functional closure occurs by 24, 48, and 96 h in 10%, 82%, and 100%, respectively, of term infants. Anatomic closure is usually finished by 2 to 3 weeks of age. In about 0.04% of term infants, however, the ductus fails to close and remains patent.[290–292]

A variety of factors are contributory to the initial closure process. These include oxygen, calcium, endogenous catecholamines, and other vasoactive compounds. The most important substances involved, however, are the prostaglandins: prostacyclin (PGI_2) produced by the ductus arteriosus and prostaglandin E_2 (PGE_2). While PGI_2 is produced more vigorously, PGE_2 is much more potent as a ductus relaxer.[292] Because PGE_2 metabolism by the lung is limited in the fetus, and the placenta also is a source of this hormone, relatively high circulating levels are maintained. After birth, PGE_2 levels decline substantially and ductal relaxation is less-well maintained allowing oxygen and other vasoconstrictors to become dominant. The effects and counter effects of these substances differ at different postnatal gestational ages, another factor relevant for clinical pharmacotherapeutics. In less-mature infants, the ductus is more sensitive to dilating prostaglandins. In as many as 40% of infants born weighing less than 2000 g, and as many as 80% of infants weighing less than 1200 g, the ductus remains patent after birth.[293] In addition, even in term infants, any lowering of arterial PO_2, such as with pulmonary disease or asphyxia, can result in delayed normal closure.[294]

These physiologic relationships underlie the development of pharmacologic strategies to modulate tone of the ductus. There are two distinct strategies necessitated by either the importance to augment or to reduce pulmonary blood flow in the newborn infant.

Indomethacin, as an example of a cyclooxygenase inhibitor, is currently the most widely used medication to effect closure of the ductus.[295] Indomethacin is most useful in the preterm infant in whom a PDA may complicate other problems of prematurity by causing circulatory overload and even congestive heart failure. Dosage varies based on weight and age and regimens vary from center to center. Table 49-3 outlines a typical regimen.[295]

TABLE 49-3. Indomethacin Dosing Regimen (mg)

Age and Weight	Time		
	0 h	12 h	24–36 h
<48 h, all weights	0.2	0.1	0.1
2–7 d, <1250 g	0.2	0.1	0.1
2–7 d, >1250 g	0.2	0.2	0.2
>7 d, all weights	0.2	0.2	0.2

Most infants should receive the third dose 24 h after the first dose; infants with poor renal function, most commonly those weighing <1000 g, should be given the third dose 36 h after the first dose. Use the same schedule for the second course unless it is begun within 24 h of the last dose, in which case 0.1 mg/kg × 3 is used. An alternate schedule for infants <1000 g, especially if treatment is initiated after 3 to 4 days of life, is to give 0.1 mg/kg q24h × 7 d.

Source: Reprinted with permission from Gewitz MH.[295]

Indomethacin also has vasoconstrictive action in other vascular beds. In humans, these include renal and cerebral artery vasoconstriction. Gut perfusion may also be affected. In view of this activity, the preferred route of administration is by slow intravenous infusion. In particular, this approach reduces cerebral blood flow alteration.[296] A similar salutary effect on renal blood flow also results from continuous infusion. While control of fluid volume including the use of diuretics, had been advocated in the past, currently vigorous diuresis, such as with furosemide, is no longer thought to be useful because furosemide may enhance release of PGE_1, helping to promote ductal dilation. The patent ductus arteriosus, even when treated with cyclooxygenase inhibition, can redilate, and this reopening has been linked to increasing dilator prostaglandin levels.[297]

Complications from indomethacin not only affect renal, cerebral, and mesenteric blood flow as noted above, but also affect platelet and neutrophil function. In addition, bilirubin metabolism must be monitored, as indomethacin can displace bilirubin from albumin-binding sites and may influence serum bilirubin levels. Some interest has been shown in the use of other prostaglandin synthesis inhibitors, such as ibuprofen, mefenamic acid, and others,[291] but use of these agents is not widespread in the U.S.

Pharmacologic manipulation of the ductus to maintain patency, instead of promoting closure, has become a mainstay of the management of the newborn with certain forms of congenital heart disease. In this circumstance, the aim of therapy is to overcome the physiologic cascade that normally results in a decline in circulating dilating prostaglandins shortly after term birth. PGE_1 has become the agent of choice for this purpose. Dosages of 0.05 to 0.1 mg/kg/min are usual, and the drug must be given by continuous intravenous infusion because more than 80% is metabolized on transhepatic and transpulmonary passage. Side effects include apnea, bradycardia, rash, seizures, hypotension, and hyperthermia. Maintenance intravenous infusion can be extended for a prolonged period until surgery is possible for more permanent palliation. However, oral PGE_1 administration is not efficacious for long-term treatment, because the drug has a very short half-life and absorption from the gastrointestinal tract can be unpredictable. If prolonged IV therapy is required (usually in the preterm or low-birth-weight infant), electrolyte depletion, metabolic alkalosis, and delayed wound healing can complicate management. In addition, during prolonged PGE_1 usage, the unique x-ray finding of periosteal calcification and cortical hyperostosis involving long bones, ribs, and clavicles can develop. Fortunately, this appears to be a reversible phenomenon once PGE_1 is discontinued.

Cyanotic Spells

In certain types of physiologic abnormalities, infants and young children can be predisposed to the rapid onset of extreme arterial desaturation, the so called "hypoxemic attack" or "cyanotic spell." These circumstances involve dynamic right ventricular outflow obstruction in the setting of baseline, pre-existing pulmonary or subpulmonary stenosis. An associated intracardiac shunt also is present, which allows egress of desaturated blood into the systemic circulation. The typical condition with this anatomic and physiologic arrangement is tetralogy of Fallot. Components of the tetrad include (a) right ventricular outflow obstruction, usually at the pulmonary valve and subvalve levels; (b) "malalignment" ventricular septal defect, which allows right ventricular blood access to the aorta; (c) dextroposition of the aortic root, which accepts blood flow from both right and left ventricles; and (d) right ventricular hypertrophy.

While definitive therapy for tetralogy of Fallot is surgical repair, pharmacologic management of the acute hypercyanotic episode can be critically important to allow the child to reach surgery in the first place.

The initial trigger for an episode of sudden extreme cyanosis has not been conclusively defined, but probably involves decreased systemic vascular resistance or excess endogenous catecholamine release, or both. Changes in cardiac rhythm, such as tachyarrhythmias, and peripheral vascular pooling, such as occurs with prolonged recumbent position can precipitate an event. Similarly, sudden or sharp pain, or prolonged agitation, can also lead to a hypercyanotic episode. Medications, such as isoproterenol, can also induce an episode.[298]

If an acute intervention is required to ameliorate a cyanotic "spell," morphine sulfate (0.1 mg/kg) has been demonstrated over many years to be an effective remedy. Morphine has primary sedating effects to interfere with catecholamine production and secondary effects to slow heart rate and respiratory rate, thus favorably effecting right ventricular filling. This drug, when used in combination with positional changes to augment systemic vascular resistance, is often singularly effective to improve oxygenation. Administration of oxygen, by raising the pulmonary-to-systemic vascular resistance ratio, also can be helpful, as long as the net right-to-left intracardiac shunt is reduced. On occasion, more direct pharmacologic manipulation of systemic vascular resistance is required. For this purpose, infusion of phenylephrine, an α-agonist, at 2 to 10 mg/kg/min is of value.[299] When a hypercyanotic spell is persistent despite these maneuvers, general anesthesia may be required and surgical augmentation of pulmonary blood should follow quickly.

Long-term pharmacologic palliation of tetralogy of Fallot and its variations is decreasingly used, coincident with advances in surgical techniques and perioperative management. Combined surgical and interventional cardiology approaches have made treatable available to many more children with even-marked pulmonary arterial bed anomalies.[300] However, there still is an occasional indication for extended medical management. Because positive inotropy may result in a hypercontractile right ventricular outflow tract ("infundibular") and promote intracardiac right-to-left shunting with resultant systemic cyanosis, agents that decrease contractility can be beneficial. Beta-blockers, specifically propranolol, are particularly useful in this context. In the 1980s, several major studies documented the usefulness of propranolol for long-term palliation (several months' duration),[301–303] confirming suggestions first raised 15 years earlier.[304] Potential complications, including bronchospasm, hypoglycemia, and bradycardia, must be monitored for once this therapy is initiated. Most clinicians continue beta-blocker therapy until shortly before surgery, but there is controversy in this regard because beta-blockers may adversely affect myocardial recovery postcardiopulmonary bypass.

CONCLUSION

Cardiovascular drugs evaluated in adults for clinical approval are frequently used to treat disorders in children with few therapeutic guidelines. Although most of the experiences with pediatric drug use are favorable, carefully done clinical trials need to be conducted to help guide physicians in the future drug management of cardiovascular disorders in children.

REFERENCES

1. Blumer JL: Labeling antihypertensive agents for children. *Curr Ther Res Clin Exp* 62:281, 2001.
2. Clark BJ: Treatment of heart failure in infants and children. *Heart Dis* 2:354, 2000.
2a. Kay JD, Colan SD, Graham, TP Jr: Congestive heart failure in pediatric patients. *Am Heart J* 142:923. 2001.
3. Hoffman BF, Bigger JT: Digitalis and allied cardiac glycosides. In: Gilman AG, Goodman LS, Gilman A, eds. *The Pharmacological Basis for Therapeutics.* 6th ed. New York: Macmillan, 1980:729.
4. Roberts RJ: *Drug Therapy in Infants: Pharmacologic Principles and Clinical Experience.* Philadelphia: WB Saunders, 1984.
5. Doering W: Quinidine-digoxin interaction, pharmacokinetics, underlying mechanism and clinical implications. *N Engl J Med* 301:400, 1979.
6. Pickoff AS, Stolfi A, Gelband H: Digoxin-quinidine interaction in the neonatal dog. *J Am Coll Cardiol* 8:669, 1986.
7. Koren G, Soldin SJ: Cardiac glycosides. *Clin Lab Med* 7:587, 1987.
8. Moysey JO, Jaggaro NSV, Grundy EN, et al: Amiodarone increases plasma digoxin concentrations. *Br Med J* 282:272, 1981.
9. Koren G, Hesslein P, MacLeod SM, et al: Digoxin toxicity associated with amiodarone therapy in children. *J Pediatr* 104:467, 1984.
10. Pederson KE, Dorph Pederson A, Huidt S, et al: Digoxin verapamil interaction, a single-dose pharmacokinetic study. *Clin Pharmacol Ther* 30:311, 1981.
11. Klein HO, Langer R, Weiss E, et al: The influence of verapamil on serum digoxin concentration, *Circulation* 65:998, 1982.
12. Artman M: Pharmacologic therapy. In: Emmanouilides GC, Riemenschneider TA, Allen HD, Gutgesell HP, eds. *Moss and Adams' Heart Disease in Infants, Children and Adolescents.* 6th ed. Baltimore: Lippincott Williams & Wilkins, 2001:333–349.
13. Gewitz MH, Vetter VL: Cardiac emergencies. In: Fleisher G, Ludwig S, eds. *Textbook of Pediatric Emergency Medicine.* 4th ed. Philadelphia: Lippincott Williams & Wilkins, 2000:665.
14. Perez CA, Reimer JM, Schreiber MD, et al: Effect of high-dose dopamine on urine output in newborn infants. *Crit Care Med* 14:1045, 1986.
15. Driscoll DJ, Gillette PC , Ezrailson EG, Schwartz A: Inotropic response of the neonatal canine myocardium to dopamine. *Pediatr Res* 12:42, 1978.
16. Rockson SG, Homcy CJ, Quinn P, et al: Cellular mechanisms of impaired adrenergic responsiveness in neonatal dogs. *J Clin Invest* 67:319, 1981.
17. Padbury JF, Agata Y, Baylen BG, et al: Dopamine pharmacokinetics in critically ill newborn infants. *J Pediatr* 110:2, 1987.
18. Girardin E, Berner M, Rouge JC, et al: Effect of low-dose dopamine on hemodynamic and renal function in children. *Pediatr Res* 26:200, 1989.
19. Tulassay T, Rascher W, Scharer K: Effect of low dose dopamine on kidney function and vasoactive hormones in pediatric patients with advanced renal failure. *Clin Nephrol* 28:22, 1987.
20. Gundert-Remy U, Penzien J, Hildebrandt R, et al: Correlation between the pharmacokinetics and pharmacodynamics of dopamine in healthy subjects. *Eur J Clin Pharmacol* 26:163, 1984.

21. Notterman DA, Greenwald BM, Moran F, et al: Dopamine clearance in critically ill infants and children: Effect of age and organ system dysfunction. *Clin Pharmacol Ther* 48:138, 1990.

22. Allen E: Alterations in dopamine clearance and catechol-o-methyltransferase activity by dopamine infusions in children. *Crit Care Med* (*in press*).

23. Driscoll DJ, Gillette PC, McNamara DG: The use of dopamine in children. *J Pediatr* 92:309, 1978.

24. Seri I, Tulassay T, Kiszel J, et al: Cardiovascular response to dopamine in hypotensive preterm neonates with severe hyaline membrane disease. *Eur J Pediatr* 142:3, 1984.

25. Zaritsky A, Chernow B: Use of catecholamines in pediatrics. *J Pediatr* 105:341, 1984.

26. Lang P, Williams RG, Norwood WI, et al: The hemodynamic effects of dopamine in infants after corrective cardiac surgery. *J Pediatr* 96:630, 1980.

27. Booker PD, Evans C: Franks R: Comparison of the hemodynamic effects of dopamine and dobutamine in young children undergoing cardiac surgery. *Br J Anaesth* 74:419, 1995.

28. Benotti JR, Grossman W, Braunwald E, Carabellow BA: Effects of amrinone on myocardial energy metabolism and hemodynamics in patients with severe congestive heart failure due to coronary artery disease. *Circulation* 62:28, 1980.

29. Fowler MB, Alderman EL, Oesterle SN, et al: Dobutamine and dopamine after cardiac surgery: Greater augmentation of myocardial blood flow with dobutamine. *Circulation* 70(Suppl I):103, 1981.

30. Mueller H, Ayres S, Gregory J: Hemodynamics, coronary blood flow, and myocardial metabolism in coronary shock: Response to 1–epinephrine and isoproterenol. *J Clin Invest* 49:1885, 1970.

31. Ward D, Bellville J: Reduction of hypoxic ventilatory drive by dopamine. *Anesth Analg* 61:333, 1982.

32. Lemaire F: Effect of catecholamines on pulmonary right-to-left shunt. *Int Anesthesiol Clin* 21:43, 1983.

33. Notterman D: Inotropic agents. *Crit Care Clin* 7:583, 1991.

34. Alexander CS, Sako Y, Mikulic E: Pedal gangrene associated with use of dopamine. *N Engl J Med* 293:591, 1975.

35. Golbranson FL, Lurie L, Vance RM, Vandell RF: Multiple extremity amputations in hypotensive patients treated with dopamine. *JAMA* 243:1145, 1980.

36. Greene SI, Smith JW: Dopamine gangrene. *N Engl J Med* 294:114, 1976.

37. Sonnenblick EH, Frishman WH, Le Jemtel TH: Dobutamine: A new synthetic cardioactive sympathetic amine. *N Engl J Med* 300:17, 1979.

38. Leier CV, Unverferth DV: Dobutamine. *Ann Intern Med* 99:4, 1983.

39. Martinez AM, Padbury F, Thio S: Dobutamine pharmacokinetics and cardiovascular responses in critically ill neonates. *Pediatrics* 89:47, 1992.

40. Berg RA, Padbury JF, Donnerstein RL, et al: Dobutamine pharmacokinetics and pharmacodynamics in normal children and adolescents. *J Pharmacol Exp Ther* 265:1232, 1993.

41. Habib DM, Padbury JF, Anas NG, et al: Dobutamine pharmacokinetics and pharmacodynamics in pediatrics intensive care patients. *Crit Care Med* 20:601, 1992.

42. Leier CV, Unverferth DV, Kates RE: The relationship between plasma dobutamine concentrations and cardiovascular responses in cardiac failure. *Am J Med* 66:238, 1979.

43. Steinberg C, Notterman D: Pharmacokinetics of cardiovascular drugs in children. *Clin Pharmacokinet* 27:345, 1994.

44. Perkin RM, Levin DL, Webb R, et al: Dobutamine: A hemodynamic evaluation of in children with shock. *J Pediatr* 100:977, 1982.

45. Schranz D, Stopfkuchen H, Jungst BK, et al: Hemodynamic effects of dobutamine in children with cardiovascular failure. *Eur J Pediatr* 139:4, 1982.

46. Bohn DJ, Poirier CS, Edmonds JF, et al: Haemodynamic effects of dobutamine after cardiopulmonary bypass in children. *Crit Care Med* 16:340, 1980.

47. Berner M, Rouge JC, Friedli B: The hemodynamic effect of phentolamine and dobutamine after open-heart operations in children: Influence of the underlying heart defect. *Ann Thorac Surg* 35:643, 1983.

48. Berner M, Oberhansli I, Rouge JC, et al: Chronotropic and inotropic supports are both required to increase cardiac output early after corrective operations for tetralogy of Fallot. *J Thorac Cardiovasc Surg* 97:297, 1989.

49. Lewis BS, Halon DA, Rodeanu ME, et al: Synergistic effect of captopril and dobutamine on left ventricular pressure volume and pressure shortening relations in severe cardiac failure. *Inl J Cardiol* 21:157, 1988.

50. Magorien R, Unverferth D, Brown G: Dobutamine and hydralazine: Comparative influences of positive inotropy and vasodilation on coronary blood flow and energetics in nonischemic congestive heart failure. *J Am Coll Cardiol* 1:499, 1983.

51. Steinberg C, Notterman DA: Pharmacokinetics of cardiovascular drugs in children: Inotropes and vasopressors. *Clin Pharmacokinet* 27:345, 1994.

52. Notterman D, Metakis L, Steinberg C, et al: Isoproterenol pharmacokinetics in children with status asthmaticus: Pronounced beta-adrenergic receptor desensitization (abstr. 185). *Pediatr Res* 31 (4 pt 22):33A, 1992.

53. Reyes G, Schwartz PH, Newth CJL, et al: The pharmacokinetics of isoproterenol in critically ill pediatric patients. *J Clin Pharmacol* 33:29, 1993.

54. Driscoll DJ, Gillette PC, Duff DF, et al: The hemodynamic effect of dopamine in children. *J Thorac Cardiovasc Surg* 78:765, 1979.

55. Notterman D: Cardiovascular disorders, in Joint Task Force on Advanced Pediatric Life Support. In: Notterman D, ed. *APLS. The Pediatric Emergency Medicine Course.* 2d ed. Elk Grove Village, IL: American Academy of Pediatrics, 1993:48.

56. Fisher DG, Schwartz PH, Davis AL: Pharmacokinetics of exogenous epinephrine in critically ill children. *Crit Care Med* 21:111, 1993.

57. Benzing G III, Helmsworth JA, Schreiber JT, et al: Nitroprusside and epinephrine for treatment of low output in children after open heart surgery. *Ann Thorac Surg* 27:523, 1979.

58. Lucking SE, Pollack MM, Fields AI: Shock following generalized hypoxic ischemic injury in previously healthy infants and children. *J Pediatr* 108:359, 1986.

59. Dieckmann R, Vardis R: High-dose epinephrine in pediatric out-of-hospital cardiopulmonary arrest. *Pediatrics* 95:901, 1995.

60. Orlowski JP, Porembka DT, Gallagher JM: Comparison study of intraosseous, central intravenous and peripheral intravenous infusion of emergency drugs. *Am J Dis Child* 144:112, 1990.

61. Solomon SL, Wallace EM, Fort-Jones EL, et al: Medication errors with inhalant epinephrine mimicking an epidemic of neonatal sepsis. *N Engl J Med* 310:166, 1984.

62. Levine DH, Levkoff AH, Pappu LD, et al: Renal failure and other serious sequelae of epinephrine toxicity in neonates. *South Med J* 78:874, 1985.

63. Kurachek SC, Rockoff MA: Inadvertent intravenous administration of racemic epinephrine. *JAMA* 253:1441, 1985.

64. Borthne K, Haga P, Langslet A, et al: Endogenous norepinephrine stimulates both alpha-1 and beta adrenoceptors in myocardium from children with congenital heart defects. *J Mol Cell Cardiol* 27:693, 1995.

65. Martin C, Papazian L, Perrin G, et al: Norepinephrine or dopamine for the treatment of hyperdynamic septic shock? *Chest* 103:1826, 1993.

66. Redl-Wenzl EM, Armbruster C, Edelman G, et al: The effects of norepinephrine on hemodynamics and renal function in severe septic shock states. *Intensive Care Med* 19:151, 1993.

67. Benotti RG, Grossman W, Braunwald E, et al: Effects of amrinone on myocardial energy metabolism and hemodynamics in patients with severe congestive heart failure due to coronary artery disease. *Circulation* 72:28, 1980.

68. Binah O, Legato MJ, Danilo P Jr, et al: Developmental changes in the cardiac effect of amrinone in the dog. *Circ Res* 52:747, 1983.

69. Binah O, Sodowick B, Vulliemoz Y, et al: The inotropic effect of amrinone and milrinone on neonatal and young canine cardiac muscle. *Circulation* 73:III-46, 1986.

70. Driscott DJ, Gillette PC, Fukushige J, et al: Comparison of the cardiovascular action of isoproterenol, dopamine, and dobutamine in the neonatal and mature dog. *Pediatr Cardiol* 1:307:1980.

71. Klitzner TS, Shapir Y, Ravin R, et al: The biphasic effect of amrinone on tension development in newborn mammalian myocardium. *Pediatr Res* 27:144, 1990.

72. Artman M, Kithas PA, Wike JS, et al: Inotropic responses to cyclic nucleotide phosphodiesterase inhibitors in immature and adult rabbit myocardium. *J Cardiovasc Pharmacol* 13:146, 1989.

73. Kulik TJ, Lock JE: Amrinone for pulmonary hypertension in infants and children (abstr.). *Pediatr Res* 18:125, 1984.

74. Colucci W, Wright R, Braunwald E: New positive inotropic agents in the treatment of congestive heart failure. *N Engl J Med* 314:291(pt 1), 349 (pt 2), 1986.

75. Gage J, Rutman H, Lucido D, et al: Additive effects of dobutamine and amrinone on myocardial contractility and ventricular performance in patients with severe heart failure. *Circulation* 74:367, 1986.

76. Robinson BW, Gelband H, Mas MS: Selective pulmonary and systemic vasodilator effects of amrinone in children: New therapeutic implication. *J Am Coll Cardiol* 21:1461, 1993.

77. Simonton C, Chatterjee K, Cody R: Milrinone in congestive heart failure: acute and chronic hemodynamic and clinical evaluation. *J Am Coll Cardiol* 6:453, 1985.

78. Colucci WS, Wright RF, Jaski BE, et al: Milrinone and dobutamine in severe heart failure: Differing hemodynamic effects and individual patient responsiveness. *Circulation* 73(3 pt 2):III-175, 1986.

79. De Hert SG, Moens MM, Jorens PG, et al: Comparison of two loading doses of milrinone for weaning from cardiopulmonary bypass. *J Cardiothoracic Vasc Anesth* 9:264, 1995.

80. Jaski B, Fifer M, Wright R: Positive inotropic and vasodilator actions of milrinone in patients with severe congestive heart failure: Dose-response relations and comparison to nitroprusside. *J Clin Invest* 75:643, 1985.

81. Chang AC, Atz AM, Wernovsky G, et al: Milrinone, systemic and pulmonary hemodynamic effects in neonates after cardiac surgery. *Crit Care Med* 23:1907, 1995.

82. Allen-Webb EM, Ross MP, Pappas JB, et al: Age-related amrinone pharmacokinetics in a pediatric population. *Crit Care Med* 22:1016, 1994.

83. Hamilton RA, Kowalsky Sf, Wright EM, et al: Effect of the acetylator phenotype on amrinone pharmacokinetics. *Clin Pharmacol Ther* 40:615, 1986.

84. Rocci ML Jr, Wilson H: The pharmacokinetics and pharmacodynamics of newer inotropic agents. *Clin Pharmacokinet* 13:91, 1987.

85. Edelson J, Stroshane R, Benziger DP, et al: Pharmacokinetics of the bipyridines amrinone and milrinone. *Circulation* 73(Suppl III):145, 1986.

86. Lawless S, Burckart G, Diven W, et al: Amrinone in neonates and infants after cardiac surgery. *Crit Care Med* 17:751, 1989.

87. Benotti JR, Lesko LJ, McCue JE, et al: Pharmacokinetics and pharmacodynamics of milrinone in chronic congestive heart failure. *Am J Cardiol* 56:685, 1985.

88. Stroshane R: Oral and intravenous pharmacokinetics of milrinone in healthy volunteers. *J Pharm Sci* 73:1438, 1984.

89. Bottoroff MB, Rutledge DR, Pieper A: Evaluation of intravenous amrinone: The first of a new class of positive inotropic agents with vasodilator properties. *Pharmcotherapy* 5:227, 1985.

90. Leibovitz D, Lawless S, Weise K: Fatal amrinone overdose in a pediatric patient. *Crit Care Med* 23:977, 1995.

91. Young JB, Robert R: Heart failure. In: Dirks JH, Sutton RAL, eds. *Diuretics: Physiology, Pharmacology, and Clinical Use.* Philadelphia: WB Saunders, 1986.

92. Radde IC: Renal Function and elimination of drugs during development. In: Radde IC, MacLeod SM, eds. *Pediatric Pharmacology and Therapeutics.* 2d ed. St. Louis: Mosby-Year Book, 1993:87–110.

93. Nau H, Luck W, Kuhnz W, et al: Serum protein binding of diazepam, desmethyl-diazepam, furosemide, indomethacin, warfarin, and phenobarbital in human fetus, mother and newborn infant. *Pediatr Pharmacol* 3:219, 1983.

94. Vert P, Broquaire M, Legagneur M, et al: Pharmacokinetics of furosemide in neonates. *Eur J Clin Pharmacol* 22:39, 1982.

95. Mirochnick MH, Micelli JJ, Kramer PA, et al: Furosemide pharmacokinetics in very low birthweight infants. *J Pediatr* 112:653, 1988.

96. Perlman JM, Moore V, Siegel MJ, et al: Is chloride depletion an important contributing cause of death in infants with bronchopulmonary dysplasia? *Pediatrics* 77:212, 1986.

97. Ryback LP, Green TP, John SK, et al: Probenecid reduces cochlear effects and perilymph penetration of furosemide in chinchilla. *J Pharmacol Exp Ther* 2230:706, 1984.

98. Davies DL, Lant AF, Millard NR, et al: Renal action, therapeutic use and pharmacokinetics of the diuretic bumetanide. *Clin Pharmacol Ther* 15:141, 1974.

99. Witte MK, Stork JE, Blumer JL: Diuretic therapeutics in the pediatric patients. *Am J Cardiol* 57:44A, 1986.

100. Kunau RT, Weller DR, Webb HL: Clarification of the site of action of chlorothiazide in the rat nephron. *J Clin Invest* 56;401, 1975.

101. Sinaiko AR: Pharmacologic management of childhood hypertension. *Pediatr Clin North Am* 40:195, 1993.

102. Arnold WC: Efficacy of metolazone and furosemide in children with furosemide resistant edema. *Pediatrics* 74:872, 1984.

103. Hobbins SM, Fowler RS, Rowe RD, Korey AG: Spironolactone therapy in infants with congestive heart failure secondary to congenital heart disease. *Arch Dis Child* 56:934, 1981.

104. Klug D, Robert V, Swynghedauw D: Role of mechanical and hormonal factors in cardiac remodeling and the biologic limits of myocardial adaptation. *Am J Cardiol* 71(Suppl):45A, 1993.

105. The Rales Investigators. Effectiveness of spironolactone added to an angiotensin converting enzyme inhibitor and a loop diuretic for severe chronic congestive heart failure. *Am J Cardiol* 91:457, 1996.

106. Pitt B, Zannad F, Remme WJ et al: The effect of spironolactone on morbidity and mortality in patients with severe heart failure. Randomized Aldactone Evaluation Study. *N Engl J Med* 341:709, 1999.

107. Beekman RH, Rochinni AP, Dick M, et al: Vasodilator therapy in children: acute and chronic effects in children with left ventricular dysfunction or mitral regurgitation. *Pediatrics* 73:43, 1984.

108. Benzing GIII, Helmsworth JS, Schriber JT, et al: Nitroprusside after open heart surgery. *Circulation* 54:467, 1976.

109. Applebaum A, Blackstone EH, Kouchoukos NT, et al: Afterload reduction and cardiac output in infants early after intracardiac surgery. *Am J Cardiol* 39:445, 1977.

110. Nakano H, Ueda K, Saito KR: Acute hemodynamic effects of nitroprusside in children with isolated mitral regurgitation. *Am J Cardiol* 56:351, 1985.

111. Benitz WE, Malachowski N, Cohen RS, et al: Use of sodium nitroprusside in neonates: Efficacy and safety. *J Pediatr* 106:102, 1985.

112. Getman CE, Goetzman BW, Bennet S: Age-dependent effects of sodium nitroprusside and dopamine in lambs. *Pediatr Res* 29:329, 1991.

113. Linakis JG, Lacouture PG, Woolf A: Monitoring cyanide and thiocyanate concentrations during infusion of sodium nitroprusside in children. *Pediatr Cardiol* 12:214, 1991.

114. Ilbawi MN, Idriss FS, DeLeon SY, et al: Hemodynamic effects of intravenous nitroglycerin in pediatric patients after open-heart surgery. *Circulation* 72(Suppl II):II, 101, 1985.

115. Benson LN, Bohn DJ, Edmonds JF, et al: Nitroglycerin therapy in children with low cardiac index after heart surgery. *Cardiovasc Med* 4:207, 1979.

115a. Gow RM, Bohn D, Koren G, et al: Cardiovascular pharmacology. In: Radde IC, MacLeod SM, eds. *Pediatric Pharmacology and Therapeutics.* 2d ed. St. Louis: Mosby-Year Book 1993:197–219.

116. Frostelli C, Frattaci MD, Wain JC, et al: Inhaled nitric oxide. A selective pulmonary vasodilator reversing hypoxic pulmonary vasoconstruction. *Circulation* 83:2038, 1991.

117. Hurford WE: Conference summary: is inhaled nitric oxide therapeutic? *Respir Care* 44:360, 1999.

117a. Ivy D: Diagnosis and treatment of severe pediatric pulmonary hypertension. *Cardiol in Rev* 9:227, 2001.

118. Golombek SG: The use of inhaled nitric oxide in newborn medicine. *Heart Dis* 2:342, 2000.

119. Roberts JD, Lang P, Bigatello LM, et al: Inhaled NO in congenital heart disease. *Circulation* 87:447, 1993.

120. Nelin LD, Hoffman GM: The use of inhaled nitric oxide in a wide variety of clinical problems. *Pediatr Clin North Am* 45:531, 1998.

121. Friedman WF and George BL: New concepts and drugs in the treatment of congestive heart failure. *Pediatr Clin North Am* 31:1197, 1984.

122. Kaplan NM: Systemic hypertension therapy: Mechanisms and diagnosis. In: Braunwald E, ed. *Heart Disease.* 5th ed. Philadelphia: WB Saunders, 1997:807.

122a. Hazama K, Nakazawa M, Momma K: Effective dose and cardiovascular effects of cilazapril in children with heart failure. *Am J Cardiol* 88:801, 2001.

123. Friedman A, Chesney RW, Ball D, et al: Effective use of captopril (angiotensin I-converting enzyme inhibitor) in severe childhood hypertension. *J Pediatr* 97:664, 1980.

124. Hymes LC, Warshaw BL: Captopril: long-term treatment of hypertension in a preterm infant and in older children. *Am J Dis Child* 137:263, 1983.

125. Bifano E, Post EM, Springer J, et al: Treatment of neonatal hypertension with captopril. *J Pediatr* 100:143, 1982.

126. Sinaiko AR, Mirkin BL, Hendrick DA, et al: Antihypertensive effect elimination kinetics of captopril in hypertensive children with renal disease. *J Pediatr* 103:799, 1983.

127. Tack ED, Perlman JM: Renal failure in sick hypertensive premature infants receiving captopril therapy. *J Pediatr* 112:805, 1988.

128. O'Dea RF, Mirkin BL, Alward CT, et al: Treatment of neonatal hypertension with captopril *J Pediatr* 113:403, 1988.

129. Pereira CM, Tam YK, Collins-Nakai RL: The pharmacokinetics of captopril in infants with congestive heart failure. *Ther Drug Monit* 13:209, 1991.

130. Shaddy RE, Teitel D, Brett C: Short-term hemodynamic effects of captopril in infants with congestive heart failure. *Am J Dis Child* 142:100, 1988.

131. Stern H, Weil J, Genz T, et al: Captopril in children with dilated cardiomyopathy: Acute and long-term effects in a prospective study of hemodynamic and hormonal effects. *Pediatr Cardiol* 11:22, 1990.

132. Alehan D, Ozkutlu S: Beneficial effects of 1 year captopril therapy in children with chronic aortic regurgitation who have no symptoms. *Am Heart J* 135:598, 1998.

133. Lipshultz SE, Colan SD, More SM, et al: Afterload reduction therapy in long-term survivors of childhood cancer treated with doxorubicin. *Circulation* 84:659, 1991.

134. Miller K, Atkin B, Rodel PV Jr, et al: Enalapril: A well-tolerated and efficacious agent for the pediatric hypertensive patient. *J Cardiovasc Pharmacol* 10(Suppl 7):S154, 1987.

134a. Wells T, Frame V, Soffer B, et al: A double-blind, placebo-controlled, dose-response study of the effectiveness and safety of enalapril for children with hypertension. *J Clin Pharmacol* 42:870, 2002.

135. Webster MWI, Neutz JM, Calder AL: Acute hemodynamic effects of converting enzyme inhibition in children with intracardiac shunts. *Pediatr Cardiol* 13:129, 1992.

136. Sluysmans T, Styns-Cailteaux M, Tremouroux-Wattiez M, et al: Intravenous enalaprilat and oral enalapril in congestive heart failure secondary to ventricular septal defect in infancy. *Am J Cardiol* 70:959, 1992.

136a. Herrera P, Soffer B, Zhang Z, et al: Effects of the ACE inhibitor, lisinopril, in children age 6–16 years with hypertension (abst). *Am J Hypertens* 15(Part 2):32A, 2002.

137. Frishman WH: Carvedilol. *N Engl J Med* 339:1759, 1998.

138. Effect of metoprolol CR/XL in chronic heart failure: Metoprolol CR/XL Randomised Intervention Trial in Congestive Heart Failure (MERIT-HF). *Lancet* 353:2001, 1999.

139. Dargie H: Recent clinical data regarding the use of beta blockers in heart failure: Focus on CIBIS II. *Heart* 83(Suppl 4):IV2, 1999.

140. Bruns LA, Chrisant MK, Lamour JM, et al: Carvedilol as therapy in pediatric heart failure: An initial multicenter experience. *J Pediatr* 138:457, 2001.

140a. Shaddy RE, Curtin L, Sower B, et al: The pediatric randomized carvedilol trial in children with chronic heart failure: Rationale and design. *Am Heart J* 144:383, 2002.

141. Friedman AL: Approach to the treatment of hypertension in children. *Heart Dis* 4:47, 2002.

142. Hanna JD, Chan JCM, Gill JR: Medical progress: Hypertension and the kidney. *J Pediatr* 118(3):327, 1991.

143. Sinaiko AR, Gomez-Marin O, Prineas RJ: Prevalence of significant hypertension in junior high school-aged children. The Children and Adolescent Blood Pressure Program. *J Pediatr* 114:664, 1989.

144. Task Force on Blood Pressure Control in Children. Report of the Second Task Force on Blood Pressure Control in Children. *Pediatrics* 79:1, 1987.

145. Hulse JA, Taylor DSI, Dillon MJ, et al: Blindness and paraplegia in severe childhood hypertension. *Lancet* 2:553, 1979.

146. Dickinson DF, Wilson N, Curry P: Use of nifedipine in hypertrophic cardiomyopathy in infants: A report of two cases. *Int J Cardiol* 7:159, 1985.

147. Rozkovec A, Stradling JR, Sheperd G, et al: Prediction of favorable responses to long-term vasodilator treatment of pulmonary hypertension by short-term administration of epoprostenol (prostacyclin) and nifedipine. *Br Heart J* 59:696, 1988.

148. Berisha S, Goda A, Kastratt A, et al: Acute hemodynamic effects of nifedipine in patients with ventricular septal defect. *Br Heart J* 60:149, 1988.

149. Van Harten J, Burggraaf K, Danhof M, et al: Negligible sublingual absorption of nifedipine. *Lancet* 2:1363, 1987.

150. Uchiyama M, Sakai K: Rectal administration of perforated nifedipine capsules in acute severe hypertension in children. *Br J Clin Pract* 46:100, 1992.

151. Siegler RL, Brewer ED: Effects of sublingual or oral nifedipine in the treatment of hypertension. *J Pediatr* 112:811, 1988.

152. Wells TG, Graham CJ, Moss M, et al: Nifedipine poisoning in a child. *Pediatrics* 86:91, 1990.

153. Frishman WH, Halprin S: Clinical pharmacology of the new beta-adrenergic blocking drugs. Part 7. New horizons in beta-adrenoceptor blockade therapy. *Am Heart J* 98:660, 1979.

154. Huysmans FTM, Thien T, Koene RA: Acute treatment of hypertension with slow infusion of diazoxide. *Arch Intern Med* 143:882, 1983.

155. Proceedings of the symposium on labetalol. *Br J Clin Pharmacol* 3(Suppl 3):627, 1976.

156. Bunchman TE, Lynch RE, Wood EG: Intravenously administered labetalol for treatment of hypertension in children. *J Pediatr* 120:140, 1992.

157. Beekman RH, Rocchini AP, Dick M, et al: Vasodilator therapy in children: Acute and chronic effects in children with left ventricular dysfunction or mitral regurgitation. *Pediatrics* 73:43, 1984.

158. Artman M, Parrish MD, Appleton S, et al: Hemodynamic effects of hydralazine in infants with idiopathic dilated cardiomyopathy and congestive heart failure. *Am Heart J* 113:144, 1987.

159. Nakazawa M, Takao A, Chen Y, et al: Significance of systemic vascular resistance in determining the hemodynamic effects of hydralazine on large ventricular septal defects. *Circulation* 68:420, 1983.

160. Artman M, Parrish MD, Boerth RC, et al: Short-term hemodynamic effects of hydralazine in infants with complete atrioventricular canal defects. *Circulation* 69:949, 1984.

161. Artman M, Graham TP: Guidelines for vasodilator therapy of congestive heart failure in infants and children. *Am Heart J* 113:994, 1987.

162. Joint National Committee. The Sixth report of the Joint National Committee on Prevention, Detection, Evaluation and Treatment of High Blood Pressure (JNC-VI). *Arch Intern Med* 157:2413, 1997.

163. Shear CL, Burke GL, Freedman DS, et al: Value of childhood blood pressure measurements and family history in predicting future blood pressure status: Results from 8 years of follow-up in the Bogalusa Heart Study. *Pediatrics* 77:862, 1986.

164. Wells TG, Sinaiko AR: Antihypertensive effect and pharmacokinetics of nitrendipine in children. *J Pediatr* 118:638, 1991.

164a. Flynn JT, Hogg RL, Portman RJ, et al: A randomized, placebo-controlled trial of amlodipine in the treatment of children with hypertension (abst). *Am J Hypertens* 15(Part 2):31A, 2002.

165. Mirkin BL, Sinaiko AR: Clinical pharmacology and therapeutic utilization of antihypertensives in children. In: New MI, Levine LS, eds. *Juvenile Hypertension.* New York: Raven Press, 1977.

166. Berenson GS, Shear CL, Chiang YK, et al: Combined low-dose medication and primary intervention over a 30-month period for sustained high blood pressure in childhood. *Am J Med Sci* 299:70, 1990.

167. Griswold WR, McNeal R, Mendoza SA, et al: Propranolol as an antihypertensive agent in children. *Arch Dis Child* 53:594, 1978.

168. Ruley EJ, Magalnick H: Control of hypertension in Wilm's tumor by the use of propranolol. *Pediatr Res* 8:460, 1974.

169. Boerth RC: Effect of propranolol in the treatment of hypertension in children. *Pediatr Res* 10:328, 1976.

170. Mongeau JG, Biron P, Pichardo ML: Propranolol efficacy in essential hypertension in adolescents. *Can Med Assoc J* 116:589, 1977.

171. Potter DE, Schambelan M, Salvatierra O, et al: Treatment of high-renin hypertension with propranolol in children after renal transplantation. *J Pediatr* 90:307, 1977.

172. Gidding SS, Rocchini AP, Beekman R, et al: Therapeutic effect of propranolol on paradoxical hypertension after repair of coarctation of the aorta. *N Engl J Med* 312:1224, 1985.

173. Leenen FH, Balfe JA, Pelech AN, et al: Postoperative hypertension after repair of coarctation of aorta in children: Protective effect of propranolol? *Am Heart J* 113:1164, 1987.

174. Falkner B, Lowenthal DT, Affrime MB: The pharmacodynamic effectiveness of metoprolol in adolescent hypertension. *Pediatr Pharmacol* 2:49, 1982.

175. Sinaiko AR, Mirkin BL: Management of severe childhood hypertension with minoxidil: A controlled clinical study. *J Pediatr* 91:138, 1977.

176. Gidding, SS: Preventive pediatric cardiology. Tobacco, cholesterol, obesity, and physical activity. *Pediatr Clin North Am* 46:253, 1999.

177. Kwiterovich PO Jr: Pediatric implication of heterozygous familial hyper-cholesterolemia: Screening and dietary treatment. *Arteriosclerosis* 9(Suppl I):I111, 1989.

178. Sprecher DL, Schaeffer EJ, Kent KM, et al: Cardiovascular features of homozygous familial hypercholesterolemia: Analysis of 16 patients. *Am J Cardiol* 54:20, 1984.

179. Hoeg JM: Pharmacological and surgical treatment of dyslipidemic children and adolescents. *Ann N Y Acad Sci* 623:275, 1991.

180. Goldstein JL, Brown MS: Familial hypercholesterolemia. In: Scriver CR, Beaudet AL, eds. *The Metabolic Basis of Inherited Disease*. New York: McGraw-Hill, 1215–1250, 2001.

181. National Cholesterol Education Program (NCEP). Highlights of the report of the Expert Panel on Blood Cholesterol Levels in Children and Adolescents. *Pediatrics* 89:495, 1992.

182. American Academy of Pediatrics. National Cholesterol Education Program: Report of the Expert Panel on Blood Cholesterol Levels in Children. *Pediatrics* 89:525, 1992.

183. Kronn, DF, Sapru, A, Satou, GM: Management of hypercholesterolemia in childhood and adolescence. *Heart Dis* 2:348, 2000.

184. Tonstad SA: A rational approach to treating hypercholesterolemia in children. Weighing the risks and benefits. *Drug Saf* 16:330, 1997.

185. Farah R, Kwiterovich PO Jr, Neill CA: A study of the dose effect of cholestyramine in children and young adults with familial hypercholesterolemia. *Lancet* i:59, 1977.

186. Shepherd J, Cobbe SM, Ford I, et al: Prevention of coronary heart disease with pravastatin in men with hypercholesterolemia. *N Engl J Med* 333:1301, 1995.

186a. Heart Protection Study Collaborative Group: MRC/BHF heart protection study of cholesterol lowering with simvastatin in 20, 536 high-risk individual: A randomised, placebo-controlled trial. *Lancet* 360: 7, 2002.

187. Knipscheer HC, Boelen CC, Kastelein JJ, et al: Short-term efficacy and safety of pravastatin in 72 children with familial hypercholesterolemia. *Pediatr Res* 39:867, 1996.

188. Lambert M, Lupien PJ, Gagne C: Treatment of familial hypercholesterolemia in children and adolescents: effect of lovastatin. Canadian Lovastatin in Children Study Group. *Pediatrics* 97:619, 1996.

189. Stein EH, Illingworth DR, Kwiterovich PO Jr, et al: Efficacy and safety of lovastatin in adolescent males with heterozygous familial hypercholesterolemia: A randomized controlled trial *JAMA* 281:37, 1999.

190. Stefanutti C, Vivenzio A, Colombo C et al: Treatment of homozygous and double heterozygous familial hypercholesterolemic children with LDL-apheresis. *Int J Artif Organs* 18:103, 1995.

191. Atkins DL, Durian P et al: Treatment of tachyarrhythmias. *Ann Emerg Med* 39:S91–S109, 2001.

192. Gillette PC, Garson A, eds. *Pediatric Arrhythmias: Electrophysiology and Pacing*. Philadelphia: WB Saunders, 1990:380.

193. Applegate TE: Atrial arrhythmias. *Primary Care* 27:677–708, 2000.

194. Valdes-Dapena M: Are some crib deaths sudden cardiac deaths? *J Am Coll Cardiol* 5(Suppl):113B, 1985.

195. Schwartz PJ, Locati EH, Moss AJ, et al: Left cardiac sympathetic denervation in the therapy of congenital long-QT syndrome: A worldwide report. *Circulation* 84:503, 1991.

196. Ben-David J, Zipes DP: Torsades de pointes and proarrhythmia. *Lancet* 341:1578, 1993.

197. Liberthson RR: Current concepts: Sudden death from cardiac causes in children and young adults. *N Engl J Med* 334:1039, 1996.

198. Fish F, Benson DW Jr: Disorders of cardiac rhythm and conduction. In: Emmanouilides GC, Riemenschneider TA, Allen HD, Gutgesell HP, eds. *Moss and Adams' Heart Disease in Infants, Children and Adolescents*. 5th ed. Baltimore: Williams & Wilkins, 1995:1555–1603.

199. Roden DM, Lazzara R, Rosen M, et al: Multiple mechanisms in the long QT syndrome. *Circulation* 94:1996, 1996.

200. Kelly DH, Shannon DC, Liberthson RR: The role of QT interval in the sudden infant death syndrome. *Circulation* 56:633, 1977.

201. Moss AJ, Schwartz PJ, Crampton RS, et al: The long QT syndrome: Prospective longitudinal study of 328 families. *Circulation* 84:1136, 1991.

202. Bansal AM, Jugler JD, Pinsky WW, et al: Torsades de pointes: Successful acute control by lidocaine and chronic control by tocainide in two patients one each with the acquired long QT syndrome and the congenital long QT syndrome. *Am Heart J* 112:618, 1986.

203. Perticone F, Adinolfi L, Bonaduce D, et al: Efficacy of magnesium sulfate in the treatment of torsades de pointes. *Am Heart J* 112:618, 1986.

204. Tzivoni D, Banai S, Shugar C, et al: Treatment of torsades de pointes with magnesium sulfate. *Circulation* 77:392, 1988.

205. Aloot E, Szabo B, Sweiden R, et al: Prevention of torsades de pointes with calcium channel blockade in an animal model. *J Am Coll Cardiol* 5:492, 1985.

206. January CT, Riddle JM: Early after depolarizations: Mechanism of induction and block: a role for L-type Ca^{2+} current. *Circ Res* 64:977, 1989.

207. Schwartz PJ, Locati E: The idiopathic long QT syndrome: Pathogenetic mechanisms and therapy. *Eur Heart J* 6:103,1985.

208. Shah A, Schwartz H: Mexiletine for treatment of torsades de pointes. *Am Heart J* 107:589, 1984.

209. Schwartz PJ, Locati E, Moss AJ, et al: Left cardiac sympathetic denervation in the therapy of congenital long QT syndrome: A worldwide report. *Circulation* 84:503, 1991.

210. Garson A Jr, Dick M, Fournier A, et al: The long QT syndrome in children: An international study of 287 patients. *Circulation* 87:1866, 1993.

211. Moss AJ, Schwartz PJ, Crampton RS, et al: Hereditable malignant arrhythmias: A prospective study of the long QT syndrome. *Circulation* 71:17, 1985.

212. Eldar M, Griffin JY, Abbott JA, et al: Permanent cardiac pacing inpatients with the long QT syndrome (LQTS). *J Am Coll Cardiol* 10:600, 1987.

213. Moss AJ, Liu JE, Gottlieb S, et al: Efficacy of permanent pacing in the management of the long QT syndrome (LQTS). *Circulation* 82(Suppl III):111–181, 1990.

214. Schreiner MS, Greeley WJ: Safe and effective for children (editorial)? *Am Heart J* 141:3–5, 2001.

215. Goldberg P, Caboto F, Roberts J: Alterations in reactivity to anti-arrhythmic agents produced by age. *Clin Res* 23:185, 1975.

216. Pickoff AS, Kessler KM, Singh S, et al: Age-related differences in the protein binding of quinidine. *Dev Pharmacol Ther* 3:108, 1981.

217. Szefler SJ, Shen D, Gingell RL: Quinidine elimination in pediatric patients. *Pediatr Res* 14:473, 1980.

218. Burckart GJ, Marin-Garcia J: Quinidine dosage in children using population estimates. *Pediatr Cardiol* 6:269, 1986.

219. Webb CL, Dick M, Rocchini AP, et al: Quinidine syncope in children. *J Am Coll Cardiol* 9:1031, 1987.

220. Roden DM, Woolsley RL, Primm RK: Incidence and clinical features of the quinidine associated long QT syndrome: Implications for patient care. *Am Heart J* 111:1088, 1986.

221. Ezrin AM, Epstein K, Bassett AL et al: Effects of procainamide on cellular electrophysiology of neonatal and adult dog myocardium. *Dev Pharmacol Ther* 1:352, 1980.

222. Singh S, Gelband H, Mehta A, et al: Procainamide elimination kinetics in pediatric patients. *Pediatr Res* 15:471, 1981.

223. Saal AK, Werner JA, Greene HL, et al: Effect of amiodarone on serum quinidine and procainamide levels. *Am J Cardiol* 53:1264, 1984.

224. Duncan WJ, Tyrrell MJ, Bharadwaj BB: Disopyramide as a negative inotrope in obstructive cardiomyopathy in children. *Can J Cardiol* 7:81, 1991.

225. Holt DW, Walsh AC, Curry PV et al: Pediatric use of mexiletine and disopyramide. *Br Med J* 2:1476, 1979.

226. Mary-Rabine L, Rosen MR: Lidocaine effects on action potentials of Purkinje fibers from neonatal and adult dogs. *J Pharmacol Exp Ther* 205:204, 1978.

227. Morikawa Y, Rosen MR: Developmental changes in the effects of lidocaine on the electrophysiological properties of canine Purkinje fibers. *Circ Res* 55:633, 1984.

228. Dise TL, Stolfi A, Clarkson CW, et al: Rate-dependent effects of lidocaine on His-Purkinje conduction in the intact neonatal heart-characterization and amplification of *N*-acetyl procainamide. *J Pharmacol Exp Ther* 259:535, 1991.

229. Mihaly GW, Moore G, Thomas J, et al: The pharmacokinetics and metabolism of the anilide local anesthetics in neonates. *Eur J Clin Pharmacol* 13:143, 1978.

230. Mofenson HC, Caraccio TR, Schauben J: Poisoning by antiarrhythmic drugs. *Pediatr Clin North Am* 33:723, 1986.

231. Pickoff AS, Singh S, Gelband H: The medical management of cardiac arrhythmias. In: Roberts N, Gelband H, eds. *Cardiac Arrhythmias in the Neonate, Infant and Child.* 2d ed. Norwalk, CT: Appleton-Century-Crofts, 1983:297.

232. Yabek SM, Kato R, Ideka N, et al: Effects of flecainide on the cellular electrophysiology of neonatal and adult myocardium. *Am Heart J* 113:70, 1987.

233. The Cardiac Arrhythmia Suppression Trial (CAST) Investigators. Preliminary report: Effect of encainide and flecainide on mortality in a randomized trial of arrhythmia suppression after myocardial infarction. *N Engl J Med* 321:406, 1989.

234. Perry JC, Garson A Jr: Flecainide acetate for treatment of tachyarrhythmias in children: Review of world literature on efficacy, safety and dosing. *Am Heart J* 124(6):1614, 1992.

235. Till JA, Shinebourne EA, Rowland E, et al: Pediatric use of flecainide in supraventricular arrhythmia: Clinical efficacy and pharmacokinetics. *Br Heart J* 62:133, 1989.

236. Russell GAB, Martin RP: Flecainide toxicity. *Arch Dis Child* 64:860, 1989.

237. Garson A Jr, Moak JP, Smith RT Jr, et al: Usefulness of intravenous and oral propafenone for control of postoperative junctional ectopic tachycardia. *Am J Cardiol* 59:1422, 1987.

238. Paul T, Reimer A, Janousek J, et al: Efficacy and safety of propafenone in congenital junctional ectopic tachycardia. *J Am Coll Cardiol* 20:911, 1992.

239. Reimer A, Paul T, Kallfelz HC, et al: Efficacy and safety of intravenous and oral propafenone in pediatric cardiac dysrhythmias. *Am J Cardiol* 68:741, 1991.

240. Janousek T, Paul T, Reimer A, et al: Usefulness of propafenone for supraventricular arrhythmias in infants and children. *Am J Cardiol* 72:294, 1993.

241. Zalztein E, Koren G, Bryson SM, et al: Interaction between digoxin and propafenone in children. *J Pediatr* 116:310, 1990.

242. Perry JC: Fetal arrhythmias, pediatric arrhythmias, and pediatric electrophysiology. *Curr Opinion Cardiol* 10:52, 1995.

243. Yabek SM, Berman W, Dillon T: Electrophysiologic effects of propranolol on sinus node function in children. *Am Heart J* 104:612, 1982.

244. Kornbluth A, Frishman WH, Ackerman M: Beta-adrenergic blockade in children. *Cardiol Clin* 5:629, 1987.

245. Gillette PC, Garson A: Electrophysiologic and pharmacologic characteristics of automatic ectopic atrial tachycardia. *Circulation* 56:571, 1977.

246. Hepner SI, Davoli E: Successful treatment of supraventricular tachycardia with metoprolol, a cardioselective beta-blocker. *Clin Pediatr* 7:523, 1983.

247. Pickoff AS, Zies L, Ferrer PL, et al: High-dose propranolol therapy in the management of supraventricular tachycardia. *J Pediatr* 94:144, 1979.

248. Dworkin PH, Bell BB, Mirowski M: Propranolol in supraventricular tachycardias of childhood. *Arch Dis Child* 48:382, 1973.

249. Walters L, Gepies LS, Noonan JA, et al: Long-term management of chronic tachycardias of childhood with orally administered propranolol. *Am J Cardiol* 21:119, 1968.

250. Roberts RJ, Mueller S, Lauer RM: Propranolol in the treatment of cardiac arrhythmias associated with amitriptyline intoxication. *J Pediatr* 82:65, 1973.

251. Dimich I, Steinfeld L, Richman R, et al: Treatment of recurrent paroxysmal ventricular tachycardia. *Am Heart J* 79:811, 1970.

252. Crawford MH, Karliner JS, O'Rourke RY, et al: Prolonged QT interval syndrome. Successful treatment with combined ventricular pacing and propranolol. *Chest* 68:369, 1975.

253. Ayabe T, Chemmongkoltis P: Persistent ventricular tachycardia in a newborn infant. *Clin Pediatr* 17:93, 1978.

254. Wiest DB, Trippel DL, Gillette PC, et al: Pharmacokinetics of esmolol in children. *Clin Pharmacol Ther* 49(6):618, 1991.

255. Chen RP, Ignaszewski AP, Robertson MA: Successful treatment of supraventricular tachycardia-induced cardiomyopathy with amiodarone: Case report and review of literature. *Can J Cardiol* 11:918, 1995.

256. Shuler CO, Case CL, Gillette PC: Efficacy and safety of amiodarone in infants. *Am Heart J* 125:1430, 1993.

257. Perry JC, Knilans TK, Marlow D, et al: Intravenous amiodarone for life-threatening tachyarrhythmias in children and young adults. *J Am Coll Cardiol* 22:95, 1993.

258. Ethridge SP, Craig JE and Compton SJ: Amiodarone is safe and highly effective therapy for supraventricular tachycardia in infants. *Am Heart J* 141:105–110, 2001.

259. Maragnes P, Tipple M: Fournier A: Effectiveness of oral sotalol for treatment of pediatric arrhythmias. *Am J Cardiol* 69:751, 1992.

260. Ezrin AM, Bassett AL, Gelband H: Cellular electrophysiology in developing mammalian heart: Modification by antiarrhythmic agents. In: Roberts NK, Gelband H, eds. *Cardiac Arrhythmias in the Neonatal Infant and Child.* 2d ed. Norwalk, CT: Appleton-Century-Crofts, 1983:37.

261. Boucek RJ, Shelton M, Artman M, et al: Comparative effects of verapamil, nifedipine and diltiazem on contractile function in the isolated immature and adult rabbit heart. *Pediatr Res* 18:948, 1984.

262. Seguchi M, Jarmakani JM, George BL, et al: Effects of CA^{2+} antagonists on mechanical function in the neonatal heart. *Pediatr Res* 20:839, 1986.

263. Klitzner TS, Friedman WF: Pharmacology and therapeutics in pediatric cardiology. In: Singh BN, LeJemtel TH, Sonnenblick EH, Yuen JL, eds. *Cardiovascular Pharmacology and Therapeutics.* New York: Churchill-Livingstone, 1994:1099–1125.

264. DeVonderweid U, Benettoni A, Piovan D, et al: Use of oral verapamil in long term treatment of neonatal, paroxysmal supraventricular tachycardia: A pharmacokinetic study. *Int J Cardiol* 6:581, 1984.

265. Wagner JG, Rocchini AP, Vasiliades J: Prediction of steady-state verapamil plasma concentrations in children and adults. *Clin Pharmacol Ther* 32:172, 1982.

266. Hesslein PS, Finlay CD, Garson A, et al: Chronic oral verapamil: Pediatric experience. *Circulation* 74(Suppl 2):176, 1986.

267. Epstein ML, Keil EA, Victorica BE: Cardiac decomposition following verapamil therapy in infants with supraventricular tachycardia. *Pediatrics* 75:737, 1985.

268. Bernstein D: Disturbances of rate and rhythm of the heart. In: Behrman RE, Kliegman RM, Arvin AM, Nelson WE, eds. *Nelson Textbook of Pediatrics.* 15th ed. Philadelphia: WB Saunders, 1996:1335–1343.

269. Overholt ED, Rheuban KS, Gutgessel HP et al: Usefulness of adenosine for arrhythmias in infants and children. *Am J Cardiol* 61:336, 1988.

270. Till J, Shinebourne EA, Rigby ML, et al: Efficacy and safety of adenosine in the treatment of supraventricular tachycardia in infants and children. *Br Heart J* 62:204, 1989.

271. Rossi AF, Burton DA: Use of adenosine in the management of perioperative arrhythmias in the pediatric cardiac intensive care unit. *Crit Care Med* 20:1107, 1992.

272. Ralston MA, Knilans TK, Hannon DW: Use of adenosine for diagnosis and treatment of tachyarrhythmias in pediatric patients. *J Pediatr* 124:139, 1994.

273. Losek JD, Endom E, et al: Adenosine and pediatric supraventricular tachycardia in the emergency department: Multicenter study and review. *Ann Emerg Med* 33:185–191, 1999.

274. Silber DL, Durnin RE: Intrauterine atrial tachycardia associated with massive edema in a newborn. *Am J Dis Child* 117:722, 1969.

275. Kerenyi TD, Gleicher N, Meller J, et al: Transplacental cardioversion of intrauterine supraventricular tachycardia with digitalis. *Lancet* 2:393, 1980.

276. Wladimiroff JW, Stewart PA: Fetal therapy: Treatment of fetal cardiac arrhythmias. *Br J Hosp Med* 34:134, 1985.

277. Bergmans MGM, Jonker GJ, Kock HCLV: Fetal supraventricular tachycardia. Review of the literature. *Obstet Gynecol Surv* 40:61, 1985.

278. Toro L, Weintraub RG, Shiota T, et al: Relation between persistent atrial arrhythmias and redundant septum primum flap (atrial septal aneurysm) in fetuses. *Am J Cardiol* 73:711, 1994.

279. Wheller JJ: Diagnosis of arrhythmias and congenital heart disease. In: Emmanouilides GC, Riemenschneider TA, Allen HD, Gutgesell HP, eds. *Moss and Adams' Heart Disease in Infants and Children and Adolescents.* 5th ed. Baltimore: Williams & Wilkins, 1995:554–568.

280. Schlebusch H, et al: Determination of digoxin in the blood of pregnant women, fetuses and neonates before and during antiarrhythmic therapy, using four immunochemical methods. *Eur J Clin Chem Clin Biochem* 29:57, 1991.

281. Gembruch U, Hansmann M, Bald R: Direct intrauterine fetal treatment of fetal tachyarrhythmia with severe hydrops fetalis by antiarrhythmic drugs. *Fetal Ther* 3:210, 1988.

282. Gembruch U, Hansmann M, Redel DA, Bald R: Intrauterine therapy of fetal tachyarrhythmias: Intraperitoneal administration of antiarrhythmic drugs to the fetus in fetal tachyarrhythmias with severe hydrops fetalis. *J Perinat Med* 16:39, 1988.

283. Spinnato JA, Shaver DC, Flinn GS, et al: Fetal supraventricular tachycardia: In utero therapy with digoxin and quinidine. *Obstet Gynecol* 64:730, 1984.

284. Given BD, Phillippe M, Sanders SP, et al: Procainamide cardioversion of fetal supraventricular tachyarrhythmia. *Am J Cardiol* 53:1460, 1982.

285. Lilja H, Karlsonn K, Lindecrantz K, et al: Treatment of intrauterine supraventricular tachycardia with digoxin and verapamil. *J Perinatol Med* 12:151, 1984.

286. Maxwell DJ, Crawford DC, Curry PVM, et al: Obstetric importance, diagnosis, and management of fetal tachycardia. *Br Med J* 297:107, 1988.

287. Klitzner TS: Maturational changes in excitation-contraction coupling in mammalian myocardium. *J Am Coll Cardiol* 17:218, 1991.

288. Wladimiroff JW, Stewart PA, Tongue HM: Fetal bradyarrhythmia: Diagnosis and outcome. *Prenat Diagn* 8:53, 1988.

289. Gutgesell H, Atkins D, et al: Cardiovascular monitoring of children and adolescents receiving psychotropic drugs. *Circulation* 99:979–982, 1999.

290. Lim MK, Hanretty K, Houston AB, et al: Intermittent ductal patency in healthy newborn infants: Demonstration by colour Doppler flow imaging. *Arch Dis Child* 67:1218, 1992.

291. Hammerman C: Patent ductus arteriosus: clinical relevance of prostaglandins and prostaglandin inhibitors in PDA pathophysiology and treatment. *Clin Perinatol* 22:457, 1995.

292. Clyman RI, Heymann RA: Pharmacology of the ductus arteriosus. *Pediatr Clin North Am* 28:77, 1981.

293. Ellison R, Peckham G, Lang P, et al: Evaluation of the preterm infant for patent ductus arteriosus. *Pediatrics* 71:364, 1983.

294. Heymann MA, Rudolph AM: Control of the ductus arteriosus. *Physiol Rev* 55:62, 1975.

295. Gewitz M: Patent ductus arteriosus. In: Burg FD, Ingelfinger JR, Wald ER et al, eds. *Gellis and Kagans' Current Pediatric Therapy.* 16th ed. Philadelphia: WB Saunders, 1999:354.

296. Hammerman C, Glaser J, Schimmel MS, et al: Continuous vs. multiple rapid infusions of indomethacin: Effects on cerebral blood flow velocity. *Pediatrics* 95:244, 1995.

297. Mellander M, Jeheup B, Lindsterom D, et al: Recurrence of symptomatic patent ductus arteriosus in extremely premature infants treated with indomethacin. *J Pediatr* 105:138, 1985.

298. Kothari SS: Mechanism of cyanotic spells in tetralogy of Fallot—the missing link? *Int J Cardiol* 37:1, 1992.

299. Shaddy RE, Viney J, Judd VE, et al: Continuous intravenous phenylephrine infusion for treatment of hypercyanotic spells in tetralogy of Fallot. *J Pediatr* 114:468, 1989.

300. Bridges ND, O'Laughlin MP, Mullins CE, Freed M: Cardiac catheterization, angiography and intervention. In: Allen HD, Gutgesell HP, Clark EB, et al, eds. *Moss and Adams' Heart Disease in Infants, Children, and Adolescents.* 6th ed., Chap. 16. Philadelphia: Lippincott Williams & Wilkins, 2001.

301. Garson A, Gillette PC, McNamara DG: Propranolol, the preferred palliation for tetralogy of Fallot. *Am J Cardiol* 47:1098, 1981.

302. Pickoff AS, Zies L, Ferrer PL, et al: High dose propranolol therapy in the management of supraventricular tachycardia. *J Pediatr* 94:144, 1979.

303. Garson A, Gorry GA, McNamara DG, et al: The surgical decision in tetralogy of Fallot: weighing risks and benefits with decision analysis. *Am J Cardiol* 45:108, 1980.

304. Honey MB, Chamberlain DA, Howard J: The effect of beta-sympathetic blockade on arterial oxygen saturation in Fallot's tetralogy. *Circulation* 30:501, 1964.

CHAPTER 50

Drug Treatment of Peripheral Vascular Disease

Robert T. Eberhardt

Jay D. Coffman

Despite intensive investigation over the past several decades, there remain a limited number of clinically useful agents available in the treatment of peripheral vascular disease. In particular, it has been most difficult to find effective drugs for the symptomatic relief of peripheral arterial obstructive disease (PAD). The treatment of PAD has focused on exercise training, modification of risk factors for atherosclerosis, and revascularization for critical limb ischemia. In contrast, treatment of Raynaud's phenomenon has primarily focused on symptomatic relief, with no therapy aimed at altering the underlying problem. The prevention and treatment of deep vein thrombosis has evolved with the development and refinement of antithrombotic and thrombolytic therapy. The treatment of vasculitides, particularly those affecting the large vessels, involves suppression of the inflammatory response.

This chapter reviews of the pharmacotherapeutic armamentarium available in the treatment of these peripheral vascular disorders. Emphasis is placed on agents used clinically, but investigational agents and emerging therapies are also covered.

ARTERIOSCLEROSIS OBLITERANS

The manifestations of PAD, typically due to arteriosclerosis obliterans, vary from asymptomatic to critical limb ischemia. However, the most common symptomatic manifestation of PAD is intermittent claudication (IC).[1,1a] Treatment for patients with PAD should focus on relieving symptoms, delaying or preventing disease progression, and reducing morbidity and mortality. There are few agents available for the management of symptomatic PAD (Table 50-1). There are a far greater number of agents useful in the treatment of risk factors for atherosclerosis.[1b] In addition, recent findings provide evidence that an angiotensin-converting–enzyme (ACE) inhibitor, ramipril, reduced cardiovascular events in a high-risk group of patients, many with PAD.[2] This cardioprotective benefit was beyond that anticipated simply from a blood pressure–lowering effect. Despite considerable interest in developing new and effective agents for the symptomatic treatment of claudication, few agents have demonstrated a clear benefit. In contrast, the effectiveness of exercise training in the treatment of IC is well established. A recent meta-analysis found that exercise training improved treadmill walking distances with an increase in initial claudicant distance (ICD) of 139 m and absolute claudicant distance (ACD) of 179 m compared with control.[3] Furthermore, exercise has been shown to improve cardiopulmonary function and functional status during daily activities, with enhanced community-based ambulation.[4,5]

Pentoxifylline

Pentoxifylline was the first agent approved—and is one of only two agents currently approved—by the U.S. Food and Drug Administration (FDA) for the symptomatic treatment of IC. It is a xanthine derivative that inhibits 3,5-monophosphate diesterase, leading to increased cyclic adenosine monophosphate (cAMP). The proposed mechanism of action involves decreased whole-blood viscosity, in part due to increased erythrocyte deformability; decreased platelet activity; and decreased fibrinogen levels.

Over the past several decades, numerous small studies have evaluated the effect of pentoxifylline for the treatment of IC, with conflicting results. Initial attempts to analyze the aggregate data concluded that a reliable conclusion regarding the drug's efficacy could not be reached due to inadequate data.[6] Two more recent meta-analysis concluded that pentoxifylline had a modest effect on treadmill walking distance with increases of approximately 20 to 30 m in ICD and 45 to 48 m in ACD compared with placebo.[3,7] The clinical relevance of an effect of this magnitude on walking distance has been questioned, but others conclude that it is highly relevant. This treadmill distance is equivalent to walking 90 m (or greater than one city block) on level ground, which may minimize the disability in these patients, enabling engagement in personal and social activities as well as employment.[7] There is limited (or discouraging) information regarding the impact of pentoxifylline on functional status or quality of life, however.

Perhaps the most benefit of pentoxifylline may be found in those with moderate disease and long duration.[8] It has been suggested that pentoxifylline may alter the natural history of PAD. Continuous use of pentoxifylline for 4 months reduced the number of diagnostic and therapeutic procedures within the first year in a small group of patients with IC.[9] The use of pentoxifylline was not associated with a greater cost of PAD-related care and, in fact, was possibly associated with a reduction in hospital costs.[10] The drug has also been used with mechanical compression in the management of venous ulcers and may be effective for patients not receiving compression for this indication.[10a]

The dose of pentoxifylline is 400 mg given three times daily, preferably with meals. The most common side effects are gastrointestinal in origin, including dyspepsia, nausea, and vomiting. Pentoxifylline is well tolerated despite these potential side effects, as only 3% of patients are unable to tolerate it. Although there is still uncertainty (and considerable skepticism) regarding the clinical uti- lity of this agent, many vascular clinicians will give a 6- to 12-week trial of pentoxifylline to assess its efficacy

TABLE 50-1. Drug Therapy for Intermittent Claudication

Agent	Dose	Increase in ICD (m)	Increase in ACD (m)
Pentoxifylline	400 mg tid	20–30	45–48
Cilostazol	100 mg bid	28–34	65–90
PLC	2 g qd	31	59
PGE$_1$	40 μg/bid	NS	35
Naftidrofuryl	400–800 mg qd	59	71
Defibrotide	200–400 mg bid	(?)	72
Buflomedil	600 mg qd	75	81
Exercise		139	179

ICD = initial claudicant distance; ACD = absolute claudicant distance; PLC = propionyl L-carnitine; PGE$_1$ = prostaglandin E$_1$; NS = not significant.

Source: Reproduced with permission from Eberhardt RT, Coffman JD: Drug treatment of peripheral vascular disease. *Heart Dis* 2:62, 2000.

after other measures (including exercise) have failed to diminish symptoms.

Cilostazol

Cilostazol is the second agent approved by the FDA for the symptomatic treatment of IC. Cilostazol is a type III phosphodiesterase inhibitor that blocks proteolysis and leads to an increase in intracellular cAMP levels. The proposed mechanisms of therapeutic action are vasodilation, due to direct smooth muscle relaxation and perhaps enhanced effect of prostacyclin, and inhibition of platelet function.[10b] Additionally, cilostazol appears to favorably influence serum lipids, and to have smooth muscle antiproliferative properties.[11,12]

An extensive clinical development program, with a number of randomized controlled trials, has been performed to evaluate the efficacy of cilostazol in the treatment of IC of varying severity. A randomized, double-blind, placebo-controlled trial involving 239 subjects with mild-moderate IC found that cilostazol, at a dose of 100 mg twice daily for 16 weeks, improved walking distance.[13] Cilostazol increased ACD by 62 m (32%) and ICD by 28 m (27%) compared with placebo ($P < .05$) on a variable-grade treadmill protocol. Another trial of cilostazol involving 81 subjects with moderately severe IC found significant improvements in ICD (35%) and ACD (41%) on a fixed-incline treadmill protocol.[14] Several other studies have reported a beneficial effect of cilostazol on walking distance, including a recent trial involving 698 subjects that compared the effectiveness of cilostazol to that of placebo and pentoxifylline.[15–17] Cilostazol increased ACD significantly more than pentoxifylline or placebo after 24 weeks of therapy (107 m with cilostazol versus 64 m with pentoxifylline and 65 m with placebo).[16] The withdrawal of treatment with cilostazol, by crossing over to placebo, worsened the walking distance in subjects with IC who benefited from therapy.[17]

Concomitant with the improved treadmill performance was a subjective improvement in walking performance and functional status. There was significant improvement in the physical component scale score of the Medical Outcome Scale Health Survey (SF-36) and walking speed and specific measures of walking difficulty on the Walking Impairment Questionnaire, although there was no change in the perceived walking distance.[13] Using a global therapeutic assessment, more subjects and investigators subjectively judged the claudication symptoms to be improved with cilostazol. More subjects receiving cilostazol rated their outcome as "better" or "much better" compared with pretreatment.[15] Several trials demonstrated an approximate 9% increase in ankle brachial index (ABI) with cilostazol; however, the clinical significance of this finding remains uncertain.[11,13]

The recommended dose of cilostazol is 50 to 150 mg twice daily, with 100 mg twice daily being used most commonly. One study found that 50 mg of cilostazol given twice daily also improved walking distance; however, a dose response was observed, as the standard dose of 100 mg twice daily seemed to provide greater efficacy.[15] Cilostazol is metabolized by cytochrome P450 isoenzymes, especially CYP3A4 and CYP2C19, but does not inhibit their action. It is excreted primarily (~75%) by the kidney; thus plasma levels are increased in renal insufficiency. The plasma levels of cilostazol are also increased by other drugs that utilize or inhibit the P450 isoenzymes, including erythromycin, omprazole, diltiazem, and ketoconazole as well as grapefruit juice.

Most vascular clinicians have found cilostazol to be useful in the treatment of patients with IC.[17a–17c] Despite these clear benefits, the use of cilostazol requires some consideration, careful instructions, and close monitoring. Side effects are reported frequently, including gastrointestinal complaints, headaches, and palpitations (in over 25% of patients). Patients need to be carefully instructed to anticipate side effects, which are often transient and will dissipate with continued use. The use of analgesics is often helpful to palliate symptoms such as headache. Despite the high rate of side effects, the rates of withdrawal among patients taking cilostazol were similar to those among patients receiving placebo or pentoxifylline.[14–17]

Since cilostazol is a phosphodiesterase inhibitor, it is contraindicated in patients with congestive heart failure of any severity, as a result of detrimental effect observed with other agents in this category in patients with NYHA class III to IV heart failure. It is recommended that patients be screened for a history and for signs or symptoms of congestive heart failure prior to initiating therapy. Such concerns have led some to recommend regular reassessment of the risk-benefit ratio based upon interval ischemic events and close monitoring for tachycardia during initiation of therapy.[18] There are no long-term data available regarding safety; however, experience in the eight U.S./U.K. phase III trials involving over 2000 subjects found no increased risk of death or ischemic cardiovascular events during the study period.

Antiplatelet Drugs

Platelets are well known to participate in the development and progression of atherosclerosis and its complications. Activated platelets release a number of vasoactive mediators that may also participate in the pathogenesis of limb ischemia. Inhibition of platelet function

TABLE 50-2. Antithrombotic Therapy in Peripheral Arterial Disease

Problem	Agent	Clinical Effect
Chronic arterial ischemia	Aspirin	Reduce cardiovascular morbidity and mortality
	Aspirin plus dipyridamole	? Modify the natural history of limb disease
	Clopidogrel	? Superiority to aspirin
Acute arterial occlusion	Heparin	Prevents thrombus propagation
	Thrombolysis	Facilitates recanalization and minimize need for surgery
Revascularization surgery	Aspirin	Reduce cardiovascular events
Infrainguinal with prosthetic	Aspirin plus dipyridamole	May provide additional benefit
Infrainguinal with high-risk thrombosis	Warfarin ± aspirin	Protect against graft thrombosis

Source: Modified from recommendation of the 6th American College of Chest Physicians Guideline for Antithrombotic Therapy for the Prevention and Treatment of Thrombosis. *Chest* 119:283S, 2001.

provides a potential site for the treatment of claudication. Furthermore, the increase in cardiovascular events among individuals with PAD warrants some form of antiplatelet therapy, given the well-established benefit of these agents in prevention of coronary events (Table 50-2).[19]

Aspirin, the traditional antiplatelet agent, inhibits cyclooxygenase, thereby preventing the formation of thromboxane A2 and thromboxane-dependent platelet activation. The benefit of antiplatelet therapy (primarily aspirin) in the prevention of cardiovascular events in patients with atherosclerotic vascular disease has been demonstrated in the meta-analysis of studies conducted by the Antiplatelet Trialists' Collaboration.[20] Analysis of the subgroup of patients with IC demonstrated an 18% reduction in cardiovascular events; however, this failed to reach statistical significance. This has led to various recommendations regarding the use of antiplatelet therapy in patients with PAD. The American College of Chest Physicians' recommended dose of aspirin is 81 to 325 mg daily as life-long therapy in those with PAD in the absence of contraindications.[19] The FDA expert panel found insufficient evidence to approve the labeling of aspirin as indicated for patients with PAD.[21]

There is no evidence to support the use of aspirin for the symptomatic treatment of claudication, but some suggestion that it may alter the natural history. The Antiplatelet Trialists' Collaboration found that antiplatelet therapy containing aspirin reduced the risk of graft or vessel occlusion by 43% in those with PAD undergoing revascularization.[22] In the U.S. Physician Health Study, aspirin (325 mg every other day) failed to prevent the development of claudication but decreased the need for peripheral artery surgery.[23]

Aspirin plus dipyridamole may have a modest effect in the treatment of IC. One study involving 54 subjects with IC found that the combination of these two drugs improved both resting limb blood flow and ICD compared with aspirin alone.[24] Two other studies involving 296 and 240 subjects with IC found that aspirin plus dipyridamole improved ABI and delayed progression of disease, as assessed by serial angiograms.[25,26] Neither study reported the effect on walking distance or functional status. Thus aspirin, particularly in combination with dipyridamole, may alter the natural history of lower extremity arterial insufficiency, although larger-scale trials supporting this are still lacking.

Ticlopidine is an adenosine diphosphate (ADP)–receptor antagonist that prevents ADP-mediated platelet activation and aggregation by inhibiting glycoprotein IIb/IIIa expression on the platelet surface. In 151 subjects with IC, ticlopidine was reported to significantly improve walking distance with an increase in both ICD and

ACD compared with placebo.[27] In contrast, another randomized trial involving 169 patients failed to find an effect of ticlopidine on treadmill walking distance.[28] Perhaps a more important finding has been a significant reduction in the combined cardiovascular end points in patients with IC who were treated with ticlopidine.[29] Ticlopidine is dosed at 250 mg twice daily; side effects include bleeding, dyspepsia, diarrhea, nausea, anorexia, rash, and dizziness. The potential for developing severe leukopenia and thrombocytopenia requires regular monitoring of the cell count for at least several months.

Clopidogrel is in the same class of agents as ticlopidine, but the frequency of side effects—including leukopenia and thrombocytopenia—is low. Clopidogrel is given at a dose of 75 mg once daily. The Clopidogrel vs Aspirin in Patients at Risk of Ischemic Events (CAPRIE) study demonstrated a benefit of clopidogrel over aspirin in preventing "vascular" events in 19,185 patients with atherosclerotic vascular disease, with a relative risk reduction of 8.7%.[30] The overall incidence of the composite endpoint of ischemic stroke, myocardial infarction (MI), or vascular death was 5.32% per year in the clopidogrel group compared to 5.83% per year in the aspirin group. Subgroup analysis demonstrated that this effect of clopidogrel was most pronounced among the subset of patients with established PAD, with a 23.8% relative risk reduction. Despite the possibility that this may have been due to chance, this finding has led many to consider clopidogrel as the preferred antiplatelet agent in patients with PAD.[18]

The aggregate data on the use of antiplatelet agents for the symptomatic treatment of IC indicates that they result in, at best, minimal improvement. However, due to the cardioprotective benefit of these drugs, antiplatelet therapy should be part of the medical regimen of nearly every patient with PAD provided that there are no absolute contraindications.[19]

Carnitine

Carnitine is an important cofactor for skeletal muscle metabolism during exercise (see Chap. 37). An impairment in muscle energetics and abnormalities in carnitine metabolism, with a deficiency of carnitine, is seen in skeletal muscle in severe PAD.[31–33] L-carnitine and its analogues are believed to act by replenishing the deficient carnitine and normalizing energy metabolism in ischemic muscle.[31]

Propionyl-L-carnitine (PLC) is a naturally occurring analogue of carnitine that has been evaluated in the treatment of IC. A double-blind, placebo-controlled trial involving 245 subjects with IC found a modest increase in ACD of 139 m (73%) in patients receiving PLC compared with 90 m (46%) in those receiving placebo.[34] There was a doubling in the ICD compared with placebo, which failed to reach significance. A follow-up report to this trial noted a subjective improvement in functional status and quality of life among individuals with the most severely impaired walking capacity.[35] A more recent study involving 485 patients with IC identified a potential target population, those with an ACD of less than 250 m, that may benefit from PLC therapy.[36] In this group, there was an improvement in walking distances with PLC with an increase in ACD of 98% (155 m) compared with 54% (95 m) in the placebo group ($P < .05$).[36]

The optimal dose of PLC is still under investigation, but the maximal benefit appears to occur at 2 g per day. Side effects reported with the use of PLC include occasional headache and gastrointestinal symptoms. PLC may improve exercise performance and functional status; however, further clarification is required. This agent is not approved for the treatment of IC in the United States.

Prostaglandins

Because of their potent vasodilator and antiplatelet properties, prostaglandins—including prostaglandin I_2 (PGI_2), iloprost, and prostaglandin E_1 (PGE_1)—have been evaluated primarily for the management of critical limb ischemia but also for IC (see Chap. 25). In the largest of the randomized, placebo-controlled trials, 1560 patients with chronic critical leg ischemia were treated with daily intravenous infusions of PGE_1 for up to 28 days.[37] This regimen resulted in improved tissue perfusion with diminished ongoing ischemia and reduced need for amputation at hospital discharge.[37] There was a significant reduction in the combined end point (including death, major amputation, persistent critical limb ischemia, myocardial infarction, and stroke) at hospital discharge, although this difference was no longer signi- ficant at 6 months.[37]

Several small studies have suggested a benefit of PGE_1 in the treatment of IC, with a moderate improvement in treadmill walking distance and an improvement in the quality of life.[38] A surprising finding in one study was a marked beneficial effect when PGE_1 infusion was added to an exercise program.[39] A more recent trial evaluated the effect of an oral PGI_2 analogue beraprost sodium (40 μg three time daily for 6 months) on treadmill walking distance in 549 patients with severe IC.[40] There was an improvement in ICD of 81.5% and ACD of 60.1% in the beraprost sodium group compared with respective increase of 52.5 and 35.0% in the placebo group.[40] The difference between the beraprost sodium and placebo groups was 36 m for the increase in ICD and 70 m for the increase in ACD at 6 months compared with baseline.[40]

These agents have been administered daily by intravenous infusion for up to 28 days in the management of critical limb ischemia. Therapy with prostaglandins is often complicated by the development of hypotension, flushing, nausea, diarrhea, abdominal pain, and vomiting. Prostaglandins, particularly PGE_1, may play a limited role in the treatment of critical limb ischemia to allow healing of ulcers or limb salvage attempts in patients who are not candidates for surgery. Newer oral prostaglandin analogues are still being tested for the treatment of symptomatic PAD.

Vasodilators

In theory, vasodilators may be beneficial in the treatment of IC by improving blood flow in muscle and decreasing tissue ischemia.

However, there have been no adequate controlled studies to demonstrate the efficacy of vasodilators in the treatment of IC. The lack of benefit may be explained by failure of these agents to dilate a fixed lesion in the peripheral vessels that limit blood flow in PAD and near maximal dilation of resistance vessels in ischemic limbs. As a result, most vascular specialists agree there is no role for vasodilators in the treatment of PAD.[41] A single trial suggested a benefit of verapamil in the treatment of IC, with an improvement in ICD and ACD of 29 and 49%, respectively, although this represented a small increase in walking distance and testing was performed on level ground.[42]

L-Arginine

Nitric oxide is a critical vasoregulatory mediator released from the endothelium; it participates in control of vascular tone and regulation of blood flow (see Chap. 33). Nitric oxide is generated during the conversion of L-arginine to L-citrulline by the action of nitric oxide synthase. Nitric oxide has multiple actions that may be beneficial in the treatment of limb ischemia including vasodilation, antiplatelet actions, and antiproliferative actions.

L-arginine and nutritional supplements that enhance nitric oxide generation have been gaining interest as a potential therapy for PAD. Experimentally, L-arginine administered intravenously increased limb perfusion and nutritive capillary flow, as determined by positron emission tomography, in ischemic limbs.[43] A trial involving 39 patients with IC found that both L-arginine and PGE_1 improved walking distance compared with placebo.[44] In this study, 8 g of L-arginine administered by daily infusion for 3 weeks increased ICD by 147 m (230%) and ACD by 216 m (155%).[44] These effects lasted for 6 weeks after the discontinuation of therapy and were associated with improved endothelium-dependent vasodilation, supporting enhanced nitric oxide generation.[44] Similar improvements in walking distance have been reported with a nutritional supplement designed to enhance nitric oxide metabolism.[45] These initial studies with L-arginine are promising and provide support for further investigations.

Growth Factors

The use of growth factors to stimulate the growth of new blood vessels, in an approach known as therapeutic angiogenesis, is an area of research that has gained widespread attention for the treatment of vascular disease (see Chap. 38). The two main agents being evaluated are vascular endothelial growth factor (VEGF) and basic fibroblast growth factor (bFGF) in both the coronary and peripheral circulations.[46,46a]

VEGF has been found to augment collateral development and improve tissue perfusion in experimental models of hind-limb ischemia.[47] In patients with critical limb ischemia, VEGF was found to stimulate the development of new vessels associated with ulcer healing and limb salvage.[48] In this uncontrolled study, intramuscular gene transfer of naked DNA encoding human VEGF was performed in 10 limbs of 9 patients with nonhealing ulcers or ischemic leg rest pain.[48] New visible collateral vessels were documented by computed tomographic angiography in 7 limbs, improved distal flow was seen by magnetic resonance angiography in 8 limbs, and marked improvement was observed by clinical assessment in 4 of 7 limbs with ulcers.[48] The only reported complication was transient peripheral edema, attributed to enhanced vascular permeability by the growth factor.[49] This typically responded to a brief course of oral diuretic therapy.

Similarly, bFGF has been shown to improve limb blood flow in experimental models and more recently in humans with IC.[50] In a phase I trial, 19 patients with IC were randomized to receive by intraarterial infusion one of three doses of bFGF or placebo. Intraarterial bFGF was safe and well tolerated without any detected retinal neovascularization during the 1-year follow-up. There was an improvement in resting calf blood flow measured by plethysmography in the two higher doses of bFGF at 1 month by 66% and 6 months by 153%.[50] The use of recombinant FGF-2 has been evaluated in a phase II trial, the Therapeutic Angiogenesis with FGF-2 for Intermittent Claudication (TRAFFIC) study, in patients with PAD and IC. Preliminary findings reported an improvement in the ACD at 90 days with a single infusion of recombinant FGF-2 compared with placebo.[51] However this benefit was no longer seen at 180 days, and there was no additional benefit of repeat infusions.[51] Although intriguing as potential therapeutic targets, these agents are in the early stages of development.

Other approaches to therapeutic angiogenesis include autologous transplantation of bone marrow cells.[51a]

Thrombolytics

Thrombolytic agents—including streptokinase, urokinase, and tissue plasminogen activator (t-PA)have been evaluated in the management of acute arterial occlusion of the limbs (see Chap. 19). As a group, these agents have been shown to be effective in dissolving thrombus and improving recanalization on angiography. They appear to reduce the need for surgical procedures and improve amputation-free survival.

Randomized trials have compared surgical thrombectomy and thrombolytic therapy in patients with acute arterial occlusion. For example, in a randomized multicenter trial, catheter-guided intraarterial recombinant urokinase was compared with vascular surgery for the management of acute arterial occlusion of the legs.[52] The amputation-free survival rates among patient treated with urokinase was similar to that observed among those treated with surgery at both 6 months and 1 year (71.8 versus 74.8% at 6 months and 65.0 versus 69.9% at 1 year).[52]

A comparison of agents is limited and primarily involves open trials. In one such trial, intraarterial recombinant t-PA (rt-PA) was superior to either intravenous rt-PA or intraarterial streptokinase, resulting in a rate of thrombolysis of 100%, compared to 45 and 80% for intravenous rt-PA or intraarterial streptokinase, respectively.[53] In another trial, rt-PA achieved more rapid thrombolysis than urokinase; however, there was no significant difference between treatments in success at 30 days.[54]

It is not possible, based upon the available data, to make an absolute recommendation on the selection of a specific agent or dose; however, the current clinical practice has favored the use of rt-PA.[55,56] The preferred route of administration is catheter-guided intraarterial or intrathrombus infusion rather than the intravenous administration. Although variable dosing schemes are available, a commonly used regimen for rt-PA is 1 mg/h or 0.05 mg/kg/h.[55,56] The common side effects are related to hemorrhagic complications.

Surgical revascularization is still indicated for profound limb-threatening ischemia, with emergent thromboembolectomy for proximal emboli. However, thrombolysis should be considered for acute limb ischemia due to thrombosis or embolus presenting within 24 to 48 h of onset. It is now an acceptable part of a treatment strategy designed to gradually restore blood flow to minimize reperfusion injury.[55] However, successful thrombolysis will often reveal an underlying lesion that requires correction by either a percutaneous or surgical approach. Furthermore, emboli, which may consist of old thrombus and atherosclerotic plaque, may be less amenable to thrombolysis.

Others Agents

Alpha tocopherol, the most active form of vitamin E, is a lipid-soluble antioxidant that participates in the defense against oxygen-derived free radicals. Vitamin E has been advocated for the treatment of claudication since the 1950s, when several small studies suggested some improvement.[57,58] Since that time, the data supporting the use of vitamin E have been limited. In a large cancer prevention study, alpha tocopherol (50 mg daily) did not prevent the development of claudication in male smokers, as assessed by the Rose questionnaire.[59] The results of the Heart Outcome Prevention Evaluation trial regarding the effect of vitamin E use on cardiovascular events in a high risk group of patients, many with established PAD, were disappointing.[60]

Ketanserin is a selective S_2-serotonin receptor antagonist with actions including vasodilation, decreased blood viscosity, and perhaps dilation of collateral vessels (see Chap. 29). Clinical trials evaluating the effect of ketanserin in the treatment of IC have been controversial. Although a small placebo-controlled study found an improvement in walking distance, ketanserin failed to improve treadmill walking distance compared to placebo in a multicenter trial involving 179 patients with IC.[61,62]

In this study, a serendipitous discovery of a higher incidence of cardiovascular complications in the placebo group was made, which was subsequently confirmed in a pooled analysis, suggesting that ketanserin may possess a protective effect against thrombovascular complications.[63] This led to the PACK trial (Prevention of Atherosclerotic Complications with Ketanserin), which was designed to determine the effect of ketanserin on cardiovascular events during 1 year of treatment.[64] In the PACK trial, 3899 patients with IC were randomized to receive ketanserin or placebo; however, many patients were withdrawn prematurely due to excessive mortality in the ketanserin group. This has since been attributed to QT-interval prolongation in association with hypokalemia caused by potassium-wasting diuretic agents. Ketanserin is not available in the U.S. and its role in the treatment of IC remains undefined.

Naftidrofuryl is a serotonin-receptor antagonist that inhibits platelet aggregation and enhances oxidative metabolism in ischemic tissue. A moderate beneficial effect of naftidrofuryl in the treatment of IC has been suggested in a number of randomized trials. A recent meta-analysis of four randomized trials found that naftidrofuryl increased ICD by 59 m and ACD by 71 m compared with placebo.[3] Another randomized trial involving 188 patients with severe IC found an improvement in ICD but no effect on ACD or ABI.[65] Subjectively there was a delay in the deterioration of symptoms with naftidrofuryl. The recommended dose of naftidrofuryl is 400 to 800 mg daily; the most common side effects being mild, tolerable gastrointestinal symptoms. This agent is not available in the U.S. but has been used in Europe for the symptomatic treatment of IC for over 20 years.

Defibrotide is a polydeoxyribonucleotide that modulates endothelial function, enhancing the release of t-PA, decreasing the release of tissue plasminogen inhibitor, stimulating the release of prostacyclin and other prostanoids, and perhaps inhibiting platelet aggregation. In a double-blind, placebo-controlled trial involving 227 patients with IC, defibrotide increased ACD by about 50%, compared with 17% in the placebo group.[66] A trend toward improvement in ABI was reported, although this may be explained by a reduction in systolic blood pressure. In another small open study, defibrotide improved walking distance and rest pain.[67] Defibrotide is dosed 200 to 400 mg twice daily. This agent deserves further investigation but is presently unavailable for use.

Buflomedil acts through several mechanisms to promote vasodilation and improve rheology, promoting platelet disaggregation and improving erythrocyte deformability. The results of clinical investigations evaluating its efficacy in the treatment of IC have been conflicting. In a randomized trial involving 93 patients with IC, treatment with buflomedil for 12 weeks improved both ICD and ACD (by 100 and 97%, respectively) compared with placebo (38 and 42%, respectively).[68] A small study comparing buflomedil to pentoxifylline failed to show an improvement in treadmill walking distance, although some subjective improvement was noted.[69] Another small study comparing buflomedil to pentoxifylline or nifedipine found that the improvement in ICD with buflomedil was less than that noted with pentoxifylline.[70] The dose of buflomedil is 600 mg daily; side effects include gastrointestinal symptoms, headache, dizziness, erythema, and pruritus. This agent has been used in selected countries for over 10 years, although it has been inadequately studied and no trials are under way in the U.S.

Hemodilution involves the removal of blood and its replacement with a colloid solution such as hydroxyethyl starch (HES) or a low-molecular-weight dextran. Hemodilution may decrease plasma viscosity and erythrocyte aggregation and increase resting limb blood flow. This approach may have a modest effect on walking distance in patients with IC. In one study of 75 patients, HES was superior to Ringer's lactate plus exercise or exercise alone in increasing the ICD (44 versus 20 and 14%, respectively).[71] Another study found a 50% improvement in walking distance with both 10% HES and dextran 40 infusions.[72] Current data do not support the routine use of this therapy, which is likely to be unacceptable to most patients.

Chelation therapy has been advocated for the treatment of IC as well as other atherosclerotic disorders. Chelation therapy involves the administration of agents such as ethylenediamine tetraacetic acid (EDTA), which are theorized to mobilize calcium within atherosclerotic lesions and to promote the regression of existing lesions. There are limited controlled data to suggest a benefit from this type of therapy. A randomized, double-blind, placebo-controlled trial of 153 patients with IC found that chelation therapy did not improve walking distance, angiographic findings, tissue oxygen tension, ankle/brachial indices, or subjective assessments of symptoms.[73,74] Despite its supporters, this type of treatment is of dubious benefit and has significant potential side effects, such as hypocalcemia and renal failure.[74a]

Other approaches under investigation include the use of drug-eluting stents using sirolimus for treatment of obstructive superficial femoral artery disease.[74b]

RAYNAUD'S PHENOMENON

Raynaud's phenomenon, described by Maurice Raynaud in 1888, is characterized by paroxysmal episodes of digital ischemia resulting from vasospasm of the digital arteries, with subsequent dilation and reperfusion. Clinically it is manifest by episodes of sharply demarcated "color changes" of the skin of the digits, often precipitated by cold exposure or emotional stress. Raynaud's phenomenon is considered primary (or idiopathic) if the symptoms occur in the absence of an associated systemic disorder and secondary if the they occur in association with a disorder such as systemic lupus erythematosus or scleroderma.

Primary Raynaud's phenomenon usually does not require drug therapy; typically, it responds well to conservative measures such as behavior modification and reassurance to the patient that loss of digits will not ensue. This would include advice on minimizing cold exposure through the use of mittens (rather than gloves), the use of hand and foot warmers, and—importantly—keeping the entire body warm (to avoid reflex sympathetic vasoconstriction).

Drug therapy becomes necessary if the frequency and severity of vasospastic episodes interfere with daily functioning or quality of life and is often required in patients with secondary Raynaud's phenomenon. A variety of agents have been evaluated for the treatment of Raynaud's phenomenon; most have potent direct or indirect vasodilator properties (Table 50-3).

TABLE 50-3. Drug Therapy for Raynaud's Phenomenon

Agent	Daily Dosage	Side Effects
Calcium-channel blocker		
Nifedipine	30–90 mg	Headache, leg edema, flushing, palpitations
Felodipine	5–10 mg	Same as above
Isradipine	5–20 mg	Same as above
Diltiazem	120–360 mg	Constipation, nausea, headache, flushing
Sympathetic blocking agents		
Prazosin	2–8 mg	Nausea, headache, dizziness, dyspnea, edema, diarrhea
Reserpine	0.25–1 mg	Postural hypotension, bradycardia, lethargy, depression
*Angiotensin-enzyme inhibitor**		
Captopril	75–150 mg	Cough, rash, renal, insufficiency, hyperkalemia, angioedema
Angiotensin-blocking agent[†]		
Losartan	50–100 mg	Same as above

*Comparable dose ranges of any of the available ACE inhibitors can be considered for use.

[†]Comparable dose ranges of any of the available angiotensin-receptor blockers can be considered for use.

Calcium-Channel Blockers

Calcium channel blockers are the pharmacologic agents most commonly used for the treatment of Raynaud's phenomenon. As a group, these agents have been shown to reduce the frequency, duration, and severity of attacks. However, calcium-channel blockers differ in their vasodilator potency, with the dihydropyridine class seeming to be the most potent and effective agents.

Nifedipine has been the most intensively investigated of the calcium-channel blockers. Several double-blind, placebo-controlled trials have shown it to decrease the frequency and severity of attacks. One such study used a crossover design and found that 60% of patients with Raynaud's phenomenon reported moderate to marked improvement in clinical symptoms, with a decreased attack rate while receiving nifedipine, compared with 13% of patients receiving placebo.[75] The largest trial, involving 313 patients with primary Raynaud's phenomenon, found a 66% reduction in vasospastic attacks in the nifedipine-treated subjects compared with placebo-treated subjects.[76] Although nifedipine is beneficial in patients with both primary and secondary Raynaud's phenomenon, it is less efficacious in secondary Raynaud's phenomenon, especially in patients with scleroderma.

Despite convincing subjective benefits, confirmation of objective improvement in digital blood flow with nifedipine and other calcium-channel blockers have been difficult to substantiate. Early studies reported that nifedipine had variable effects on the peripheral circulation in patients with Raynaud's phenomenon. The drug failed to attenuate cold-induced reduction in digital artery pressure in one study of patients with Raynaud's phenomenon.[75] In contrast, although nifedipine did not significantly increase finger blood flow following acute sublingual administration, it did decrease vascular resistance, indicating that vasodilation of digital vessels has occurred.[77] The largest of these trials, involving 158 patients with primary Raynaud's phenomenon, demonstrated higher digital pressure during cooling in nifedipine-treated patients.[78]

The recommended dose of nifedipine is 10 to 30 mg three times daily for the short-acting preparation or 30 to 90 mg once daily for the long-acting preparations. The long-acting, sustained-release preparations appear to be better tolerated and are probably as effective as the short-acting, immediate-release form.[75,76] Only 15% of participants discontinued therapy due to adverse effects. Nifedipine may be used intermittently for cold exposure if it is tolerated. The most common side effects are headache, dizziness, nausea, heartburn, pruritus, palpitations, and peripheral edema. The headache is often mild and transient, lasting for the first several days of use.

Numerous other dihydropyridine calcium-channel blockers—including amlodipine, felodipine, isradipine, nicardipine, and nisoldipine—have been shown to have favorable effects in patients with Raynaud's phenomenon.[79–84] Other types of calcium-channel blockers have played a limited role in the treatment of this condition. There is controversy regarding the effect of diltiazem. A reduction in the frequency and severity of attacks was shown with diltiazem, with the most benefit seen among patients with primary Raynaud's.[85] Another study found that diltiazem was ineffective in the treatment of Raynaud's phenomenon associated with connective tissue disease.[86] One trial reported that verapamil was ineffective in a group of patients with severe Raynaud's phenomenon.[87]

Sympathetic Blocking Agents

Sympathetic adrenergic stimulation, especially involving α-adrenergic receptors, of digital arteries plays an important role in the regulation of digital blood flow. A variety of sympatholytic drugs have been used in the treatment of Raynaud's phenomenon, but few controlled trials have been conducted to evaluate their efficacy.

Prazosin is the α_1-adrenoceptor antagonist that has been the best studied of this class of agents for the treatment of patients with Raynaud's phenomenon, particularly Raynaud's phenomenon in progressive systemic sclerosis.[88] Several placebo-controlled studies have found a decrease in the frequency, duration, and severity of vasospastic attacks in approximately two-thirds of patients with Raynaud's after 2 weeks of treatment with prazosin.[89–91] Its effectiveness, however, appears to decrease with prolonged use, despite titration to the maximally tolerated dose.[91] The recommended dose range is from 2 to 8 mg daily. Side effects—including palpitations, dizziness, fatigue, headache, dyspnea, edema, rash, and diarrhea—may limit its use.

Thymoxamine, another α_1-adrenoceptor antagonist, has also been evaluated in the treatment of Raynaud's phenomenon. In an uncontrolled study, thymoxamine at a dose of 40 mg four times daily resulted in clinical improvement, with a decrease in the frequency of attacks and an improvement in digital perfusion during cold challenge.[92] Side effects are reported to be less frequent than with prazosin; however, experience with this agent is limited and it is not available in the U.S.

Although popular two or three decades ago, reserpine and guanethidine are used infrequently in the treatment of Raynaud's phenomenon today. These agents are nonselective adrenoceptor antagonists that have been shown to increase capillary blood flow in patients with primary and secondary Raynaud's phenomenon.[93] However, adequate controlled studies have not been performed. In a small study, intraarterial reserpine did not provide benefit over placebo in patients with primary Raynaud's phenomenon.[94] The experience with several other sympatholytic agents—including methyldopa, phenoxybenzamine, and tolazoline—is also limited.

There are limited controlled data to support the routine use of sympatholytic agents in the treatment of Raynaud's phenomenon. In addition, these agents have not been shown to be more effective than calcium-channel blockers. They may be considered for patients who do not tolerate calcium-channel blockers well or for those with refractory symptoms that do not respond to other measures.

Prostaglandins

The potent vasoactive properties of prostaglandins, including PGI_2 and PGE_1, have led to interest in their potential use for the treatment of patients with refractory Raynaud's phenomenon with ischemic digital ulcerations. Early reports of studies with prostaglandin E_1 in patients with severe Raynaud's phenomenon suggested clinical improvement.[95] In 26 patients, PGE_1 infusion at 10 ng/kg/min for 72 h improved digital blood flow and temperature, lessened the frequency and severity of attacks, and promoted ulcer healing.[95] However, a multicenter placebo-controlled trial failed to show a benefit of PGE_1 over placebo in the treatment of Raynaud's phenomenon.[96]

Studies evaluating prostacyclin (PGI_2) and iloprost (a prostacylin analog) have shown a clinical benefit of these agents in patients with intractable Raynaud's phenomenon. Infusion of PGI_2 (7.5 to 10 ng/kg/min) decreased the frequency and severity of vasospastic attacks compared to placebo.[97,98] It is unclear whether this subjective improvement is associated with objective improvement in digital flow or finger temperature. Similarly, in a placebo-controlled, double-blind study involving 131 patients with Raynaud's phenomenon associated with scleroderma, iloprost decreased the frequency and severity of Raynaud's attacks.[99] Another study found that infusion of 0.5 to 2.0 ng/kg/min of iloprost for 8 h on 3 days was equivalent to nifedipine at decreasing the frequency, duration, and severity of vasospastic attacks and in promoting the healing of digital lesions.[100] A review of five trials found that intravenous iloprost was effective in the treatment of secondary Raynaud's phenomenon.[101] Iloprost decreased the frequency and severity of attacks and prevented digital ulceration or promoted healing in secondary Raynaud's phenomenon in progressive systemic sclerosis.[101]

Side effects of such treatment occur primarily during the infusion and include hypotension and flushing. Oral prostaglandins have been under intensive investigation over the past several years; however, the results have been mixed and often disappointing.[102,103] In the U.S., these agents have gained approval for select indications but not in the management of Raynaud's phenomenon. The exact role that prostaglandins play in the management of Raynaud's phenomenon awaits further clarification, but these agents may provide short-term palliation in patients with severe Raynaud's phenomenon who have ischemic digital ulcerations.

Ketanserin

Ketanserin has several actions on vascular reactivity that may be useful in the treatment of Raynaud's phenomenon. In addition to preventing vasoconstriction and inhibiting platelet aggregation caused by serotonin, ketanserin increases finger blood flow during reflex sympathetic vasoconstriction. In a double-blind, placebo-controlled trial involving 222 patients with Raynaud's phenomenon, ketanserin at a dose of 40 mg three times daily significantly reduced the frequency of vasospastic episodes (34% with ketanserin compared with 18% in placebo).[104] A subjective global evaluation of symptoms completed by both patients and physicians favored ketanserin; however, the severity and duration of attacks was not affected. There was no change in finger blood flow at rest or in response to cold challenge. A review of three trials found that ketaserin is not significantly different from placebo for the treatment of secondary Raynaud's phenomenon in progressive systemic sclerosis except for some decrease in the duration of attacks.[105] Ketanserin is available in several countries but not in the U.S.

Another serotonin receptor antagonist has been evaluated in Raynaud's phenomenon. Sarpogrelate hydrochloride, a 5-HT$_2$-receptor antagonist, was given for 1 year to 72 patients with secondary Raynaud's phenomenon.[106] There was a subjective improvement of symptoms in 59.3% of patients, with a significant increase in the acceleration plethysmograms compared with baseline, suggesting an improvement in peripheral hemodynamics. These studies have been inadequately controlled and further investigation is required.

Angiotensin-Blocking Agents

Both angiotensin-converting enzyme (ACE) inhibitors and angiotensin-receptor antagonists may have a role in the treatment of Raynaud's phenomenon. These agents may improve local blood flow by blocking the vasoconstrictive action of angiotensin II and, in the case of ACE inhibitors, potentiate the action of bradykinin.

Interest in the use of these agents developed following the report of remarkable improvement in the vasospastic-induced ischemic digital ulceration in a small number of subjects being treated with captopril for scleroderma-associated hypertensive renal crisis.[107] In uncontrolled studies, captopril at a dose of 25 mg three times daily has been reported to decrease the frequency and

severity of attacks in patients with primary Raynaud's phenomenon but not in those with Raynaud's phenomenon associated with scleroderma.[108] These subjective benefits were supported by attenuation in the cold-induced vasoconstriction. Similar findings were observed with the angiotensin-receptor antagonist losartan, which decreased the frequency and severity of attacks in primary Raynaud's phenomenon.[109] However, most vascular clinicians have not found ACE inhibitors to be useful clinically in the prevention or treatment of vasospastic attacks.

Others Agents

A large number of alternative vasodilators have been used in the treatment of severe Raynaud's phenomenon, including minoxidil, hydralazine, and sodium nitroprusside. The use of these agents is not recommended, however, because controlled trials have not been performed and alternative agents are readily available.

Nitroglycerin preparations have been recommended for the treatment of Raynaud's phenomenon for many years, but results of studies evaluating transdermal nitroglycerin have been varied. In one study, nitroglycerin ointment (1%) was beneficial in reducing the frequency and severity of attacks while promoting ulcer healing in patients with secondary Raynaud's phenomenon who were receiving maximally tolerated doses of sympatholytic drugs.[110] There has been limited clinical enthusiasm for using topical nitrates for the treatment of patients with Raynaud's phenomenon.

Pentoxifylline is reported to have some beneficial effects on the peripheral circulation, resulting in an increase in resting digital blood flow and an attenuation of cold-induced vasoconstriction in patients with Raynaud's phenomenon.[111] Despite a suggestion of clinical improvement, double-blind, placebo-controlled studies have not demonstrated convincing beneficial effects of pentoxifylline compared with placebo.

Thyroid preparations have been recommended for the treatment of Raynaud's phenomenon since the 1960s.[112] In a more recent double-blind, placebo-controlled, crossover trial of 18 patients with Raynaud's phenomenon, a daily dose of 80 μg of triiodothyronine significantly reduced the frequency, duration, and severity of attacks.[113] However, there was an increase in heart rate and one-third of patients reported episodic palpitations. The authors suggested that lower ("physiologic") doses of triiodothyronine should be evaluated.

Selective thromboxane synthetase inhibitors have also been evaluated in the treatment of Raynaud's phenomenon. This class of agents may have useful effects by inhibiting production of thromboxane A$_2$ and preserving production of endogenous prostacyclin, thus promoting vasodilation and inhibiting platelet aggregation. In a double-blind, placebo-controlled trial, administration of dazoxiben 400 mg daily for 6 weeks improved the clinical manifestations of primary Raynaud's phenomenon.[114] These results are controversial, however, as other studies have found dazoxiben to be ineffective in the treatment of Raynaud's phenomenon.[115,116]

L-arginine supplementation, which enhances the endogenous production of nitric oxide, is an intriguing potential agent in the treatment of Raynaud's phenomenon. In patients with primary Raynaud's phenomenon, L-arginine at a dose of 8 g/day for 28 days had no significant effect on the cutaneous vascular response to acetylcholine or sodium nitroprusside.[117] However, there was no description of the effect on the frequency or severity of vasospastic episodes. In contrast, topical application of a nitric oxide–generating gel in patient with primary Raynaud's phenomenon increased microcirculatory volume and flux.[118] Intraarterial infusion of L-arginine at

8.5 mg/min reduced cold-induced vasocontrictive response in subjects with Raynaud's phenomenon.[119] This line of therapy requires further investigation.

DEEP VEIN THROMBOSIS

Deep venous thrombosis (DVT) and pulmonary embolus are expressions of venous thromboembolism. DVT, especially involving the proximal lower extremity veins, is the principal source of pulmonary emboli and is a common cause of hospital morbidity and mortality. The goal of therapy for established DVT is to prevent thrombus propagation, recurrent thrombosis, pulmonary embolus, and mortality as well as the development of late complications.[120] The benefit of anticoagulation in the management of thromboembolic disease is undisputed.[121] Furthermore, prophylactic anticoagulant strategies are an effective means to prevent the development and complications of DVT, particularly in higher-risk patients.[122] Recently a clinical report described a reduced frequency of venous thrombosis in patients receiving statin therapy.[122a] The American College of Chest Physicians has specific recommendations, based upon risk, regarding prevention of thromboembolic complication in various medical and surgical patients (see Table 50-4). The evaluation of patients with "idiopathic" or recurrent DVT continues to evolve as knowledge mounts regarding inherited thrombophilias.[123,124]

Heparin

Unfractionated heparin has been the mainstay of treatment and prevention for DVT. Heparin complexes with antithrombin III, leading to the inactivation of factors IIa, Xa, and IXa and inhibition of factor V and VIII activation by thrombin. The beneficial effects of heparin in the treatment of venous thromboembolism have been known since 1960.[125] For the treatment of established DVT, heparin is usually administered by constant infusion and requires frequent monitoring with dose adjustment. In a randomized trial, patients with proximal DVT treated with continuous intravenous heparin had a lower rate of recurrent thromboembolism compared with those treated with subcutaneous heparin (5.2 versus 19.3% over 6 weeks).[126] The efficacy of heparin was found to be highly dependent upon achieving a therapeutic level within the first 24 h of therapy.[127] The use of weight-based nomograms has facilitated the time required to achieve a therapeutic activated partial thromboplastin time (APTT).[128] A therapeutic level of anticoagulation is an APTT of 1.5 to 2.5 times control and corresponds to a heparin blood level of 0.2 to 0.4 IU/mL by protamine sulfate titration assay. Complications of heparin therapy include bleeding, thrombocytopenia (often with paradoxical thrombosis), and osteoporosis.

Unfractionated heparin has also been shown to be effective in the prevention of DVT formation in many higher-risk patient populations. Fixed-dose subcutaneous heparin (5000 U given 2 h before and every 8 to 12 h after surgery) reduced the incidence of

TABLE 50-4. Recommendations for the Prophylaxis of Venous Thromboembolism

Clinical Situation	Suggested Prophylaxis
General surgery	
Low risk	Early ambulation
Moderate risk	UH, LMWH, ES, or IPC
Higher risk	UH, LMWM, or IPC
Very high risk	UH or LMWH combined with ES or IPC
Gynecologic surgery	
Brief procedure	Early ambulation
Major procedure	
Benign disease	UH twice daily, alternative daily LMWH or IPC
Malignant disease	UH thrice daily, alternative UH plus EC or IPC, or high-dose LMWH
Urologic surgery	
Low risk	Early ambulation
Major procedure	UH, ES, IPC, or LMWH
Highest risk	UH or LMWH plus ES ± IPC
Major orthopedic surgery	
Elective hip replacement	LMWH, fondaparinux or adjusted-dose warfarin
	Alternative adjusted-dose UH
Elective knee replacement	LMWH, fondaparinux or adjusted-dose warfarin
	Alternative IPC, UH not recommended
Hip fracture	LMWH, fondaparinux or adjusted-dose warfarin
	Alternative UH
Neurologic surgery	IPC ± ES, alternative UH or LMWH
Trauma	LMWH if no contraindications
	EC ± IPC if delay in starting LMWH
Acute spinal cord injury	LMWH; not UH, ES, or IPC alone
Medical conditions	
Myocardial infarction	SC or IV UH; LMWH*
Ischemic stroke	UH, LMWH, or danaparoid
Others with increased risk	UH or LMWH

UH = unfractionated heparin; LMWH = low-molecular-weight heparin; ES = elastic compression stockings; IPC = intermittent pneumatic compression; SC = subcutaneous; IV = intravenous.

*Not mentioned in the ACCP guidelines but generally accepted in being used for acute coronary syndrome.

Source: Modified from recommendation of the 6th American College of Chest Physicians Guideline for Antithrombotic Therapy for the Prevention and Treatment of Thrombosis. *Chest* 119:132S, 2001.

TABLE 50-5. Drug Therapy for Deep Venous Thrombosis

Agent	Indication	Typical Dose
Unfractionated heparin	Prophylaxis	5000 U bid or adjusted for PTT
	Treatment	per weight-based nomogram
LMWH		
Enoxaparin	Prophylaxis	30–40 mg once or twice daily*
	Treatment	1 mg/kg twice daily (?1.5 mg/kg once daily)
Dalteparin	Prophylaxis	2500–5000 U once or twice daily*
	Treatment	100 U/kg twice daily
Nadroparin	Prophylaxis	3100 U or 40 U/kg daily
	Treatment	90 U/kg twice daily
Tinzaparin	Prophylaxis	3500 U or 50 U/kg daily
	Treatment	175 U/kg daily
Hirudin	Prophylaxis	1250–2500 U twice daily
Danaparoid	Prophylaxis	10–20 mg twice daily
Warfarin	Prophylaxis	Start on day of surgery; adjust dose for INR
	"Treatment"	Adjust for INR 2.0–3.0
Fondaparinux	Prophylaxis	2.5 mg SC daily
Thrombolytic agents	Treatment	
SK		250,000 IU load; 100,000 IU/h for 48–72 h
UK		4400 IU/kg load; 2200 IU/kg/h for 48–72 h
t-PA		0.05 mg/kg/h for 8–24 h

LMWH = low-molecular weight heparin; SK = streptokinase; UK = urokinase; t-PA = tissue plasminogen activator; PTT = prothrombin time; INR = international normalized ratio.

*Dose varies according to the risk.

Source: Reproduced with permission from Eberhardt RT, Coffman JD: Drug treatment of peripheral vascular disease. *Heart Disease* 2:62, 2000.

venous thromboembolism by 70% and fatal pulmonary embolus by 50% following general surgical procedures.[129] Benefits have also been reported in neurosurgical, general medical, ischemic stroke, and trauma patients as well as those with acute spinal cord injuries and possibly also orthopedic patients.[122,129,130] However, the effect in orthopedic patients undergoing knee or hip surgery was relatively slight and less than that of alternative strategies.[122] Use of dose-adjusted subcutaneous heparin to keep the APTT in the high normal range may be more effective but has not been widely tried. One study found that following hip arthroplasty, only 5 of 38 patients on adjusted-dose heparin developed a DVT, compared to 16 of 41 patients on fixed-dose heparin.[131] The use of heparin prophylaxis appears to be safe, as the incidence of major bleeding is not increased, although minor wound hematomas may ensue.

Low-Molecular-Weight Heparins

Low-molecular-weight heparins (LMWHs) are currently replacing unfractionated heparin for the prevention and treatment of DVT. The constituents of unfractionated heparin have a molecular weight ranging from 3000 to 30,000 Da, while LMWHs have fragments of unfractionated heparin with a mean molecular weight of about 5000 Da.[132] Their mechanism of action is similar to that of unfractionated heparin, although they possess greater relative inhibitory activity against factor Xa compared with factor IIa. LMWH is used in both fixed and weight-adjusted dosing regimens and is administered subcutaneously once or twice daily. Compared to unfractionated heparin, LMWH has a more predictable anticoagulant response (with no need for routine monitoring), reflecting its better bioavailability, longer half-life, and non-dose-dependent clearance.[132] Additional potential advantages of LMWH include fewer bleeding complications and a lower risk of thrombocytopenia.[132] LMWH may be used in heparin-induced thrombocytopenia; however, there is a significant risk of cross-reactivity.

The use of LMWH in both the prophylaxis and treatment of DVT has been evaluated in numerous randomized, controlled trials and the subject of recent meta-analysis. LMWH was more effective than fixed-dose heparin and equivalent (or superior) to adjusted-dose unfractionated heparin in preventing DVT.[133] It has been shown to be effective in many patient populations, including acutely ill medical, general surgical, neurosurgical, and orthopedic surgical patients.[133,134] Similarly, LMWH appears to be at least as effective and safe as unfractionated heparin for the treatment of DVT, even DVT involving the proximal veins.[133] Several recent meta-analysis found that LMWH was more effective than unfractionated heparin in preventing thrombus propagation, reducing recurrent thromboembolism, and reducing mortality, with a similar or lower rate of major bleeding.[135-137] An open-label study found that a LMWH was more effective than unfractionated heparin in promoting thrombus regression as assessed by venography.[138] Furthermore, recent studies have supported the feasibility and safety of outpatient treatment of DVT with LWMH in 50 to 75% of patients, which would significantly lower the cost of therapy.[139-142] This has led to suggestions regarding the need for vigilance with the use of home therapy, including the need for appropriate patient selection, adequate resources for clinical services, and documentation of effectiveness of individual centers.[143] In the U.S., several agents in this class are currently approved for the prevention and treatment of DVT as well as for unstable coronary syndromes (see Table 50-5).

Warfarin

After the acute phase of DVT treatment with heparin or LMWH, anticoagulation with warfarin is usually continued for 3 to 6 months to prevent recurrent disease and late complications. Warfarin interferes with the action of vitamin K by inhibiting vitamin K epoxide reductase, which leads to impaired function of prothrombin, factor VII, factor IX, and factor X. In patients with proximal DVT, long-term administration of warfarin reduced the recurrence of venous thromboembolism from about 47 to about 2%.[144,145] Warfarin is dose-adjusted according to the international normalized ratio (INR), typically to maintain a therapeutic value in the range of 2.0 to 3.0. The INR standardizes the prothrombin time to an international reference thromboplastin to allow for comparison between different laboratories.

Recommendations regarding the duration of treatment with warfarin have been the subject of debate. One study found a marked reduction in the recurrence rate with prolonged therapy for idiopathic DVT compared to a standard 6 months of therapy (1.3 versus 27%).[146] Another study found that after a second DVT, 4 years of therapy with warfarin reduced the reduced the recurrence of venous thromboembolism (2.6 versus 20.7%), although the risk of bleeding significantly increased (8.6 versus 2.7%).[147] Despite its delayed onset of action, warfarin was also found to be effective in the prevention of DVT following orthopedic surgery,[148] but it has been replaced by LMWH for reasons of efficacy and convenience.

Warfarin remains an effective agent for preventing recurrent venous thromboembolism after initial anticoagulation with heparin or LMWH. The duration of therapy is typically 3 to 6 months, although more prolonged or indefinite therapy with warfarin has been advocated for idiopathic and recurrent DVT, respectively. Except for bleeding, side effects with warfarin are infrequent.

Hirudin

Hirudin is a direct thrombin inhibitor that directly binds to the fibrinogen recognition and catalytic site of thrombin. In addition to the management of acute coronary syndrome, this agent has been evaluated in the prevention of DVT following surgery. In a multicenter, randomized, controlled trial involving 1119 patients undergoing hip surgery, recombinant hirudin was found to be more effective than fixed-dose subcutaneous heparin at preventing DVT formation.[149] In another study involving 2070 patients, subcutaneous recombinant hirudin (desirubin) was compared with enoxaparin in the prevention of DVT following total hip replacement.[150] The rate of all DVT (18.4 versus 25.5%) and proximal DVT (4.5 versus 7.5%) was significantly lower among those receiving hirudin than among those receiving enoxaparin, as assessed by follow-up venography. Recombinant hirudin warrants further investigation and may be useful in heparin-induced thrombocytopenia.

Danaparoid

Danaparoid, a derivative of the intestinal mucosa of the pig after removal of heparin, is a mixture of heparan, dermatan, and chondroitin sulfates. It is an even more selective inhibitor of factor Xa than LMWH. It is reported to be safe and effective in the prophylaxis of DVT in patients after cancer surgery, hip fracture surgery, or hip replacements, and in patients with nonhemorrhagic stroke.[151] In an open-label, randomized, multicenter study, subcutaneous danaparoid was compared with continuous intravenous infusion of unfractionated heparin for the treatment of venous thromboembolism.[151] Danaparoid was more effective in the prevention of thrombus extension or recurrent thromboembolism, with a similar risk of bleeding. Danaparoid has all the advantages of LMWH and has minimal cross-reactivity with antibodies generated in heparin-induced thrombocytopenia. Danaparoid is approved for the prevention of DVT in patients undergoing elective hip replace-

ment surgery. The dose of danaparoid is 750 anti–factor Xa units twice per day; side effects include hemorrhage and fever.

Fondaparinux

Fondaparinux, a synthetic pentasaccharide that selectively inhibits factor Xa, is the latest heparin analogue to reach the market in the U.S. The drug is an entirely synthetic agent that is structually related to the antithrombin-binding site of heparin. The drug has been shown to prevent asymptomatic DVT somewhat more effectively than does enoxaparin after hip or knee surgery.[151a–151d] However, a reduction in symptomatic events has not been demonstrated, and the bleeding risk may be greater with fondaparinux.

The drug is approved for use in the prophylaxis of DVT that could lead to PE in patients undergoing hip fracture surgery, hip replacement surgery, and knee replacement surgery. The recommended dose is 2.5 mg SC daily for 5 to 9 days.

Thrombolytic Agents

Thrombolytic agents—including streptokinase, urokinase and t-PA—have been studied in the treatment of DVT.[152–154] Thrombolytics have been shown to enhance the rate of lysis in peripheral veins, with a greater likelihood of having complete or near complete resolution of the thrombus. In contrast, standard treatment with heparin reduces the extension and embolization of a thrombus but does not appear to effect the rate of lysis.

There remains controversy regarding the benefit of thrombolysis in the treatment of proximal DVT. These agents have not been shown to reduce the subsequent development of pulmonary embolus or to reduce mortality. It appears that their early use may decrease subsequent pain, limb swelling, and loss of venous valves; however, the benefit in reducing the late complications, such as postphlebitic syndrome, remains poorly defined.[121] Furthermore, delayed use of thrombolytics has been less successful, especially if thrombus has been present for more than 7 days. A recent review of randomized trials using rt-PA in the treatment of lower extremity DVT did not support the routine use of rt-PA.[155]

Thrombosis within other venous systems, primarily the subclavian veins, has been treated by direct infusion of thrombolytic agent into the distal vein, which has been successful in preventing surgical thrombectomy. However, this often discloses an anatomic abnormality that led to the development of the thrombus, such a thoracic outlet syndrome, which then requires surgical correction.

The present recommendations are to consider thrombolysis for massive iliofemoral DVT, typically with marked limb swelling and threatened foot ischemia, if there is a low risk of bleeding.[121] Many have also considered thrombolysis for subclavian vein thrombosis with occlusion. Commonly used dosing regimen of streptokinase is 250,000 IU load followed by an infusion of 100,000 IU/h for 48 h and t-PA 0.05 mg/kg/h for 8 to 24 h. Successful thrombolytic administration must be followed by systemic antithrombotic therapy and long-term anticoagulation.

VASCULITIS

The vasculitides are a heterogeneous group of disorders characterized by leukocyte infiltration into the vessel wall with reactive damage, leading to tissue ischemia and necrosis. The pattern of vessel involvement, in terms of size and location, varies with the specific disorders. Those involving the large vessels, such as Takayasu arteritis and giant-cell arteritis, are frequently encountered by the cardiovascular clinician. Takayasu arteritis primarily affects the aorta and its major branches. The presenting symptoms early in the course of the disease are those of systemic inflammation; whereas the later clinical syndrome is typified by vascular insufficiency. Giant-cell or temporal arteritis most prominently involves the cranial branches of the arteries originating from the aortic arch. The most common presenting symptom is headache but visual problems, scalp tenderness, mailase, fever, and weight loss are common.

Corticosteroids and immunosuppressive agents are useful in the treatment of most forms of vasculitis, particularly in the acute phase.[156] Systemic vasculitides usually require at least corticosteroid therapy to induce a remission. Rapidly progressive and steroid-refractory vasculitides require combination therapy with corticosteroids and cytotoxic drugs such as cyclophosphamide, azathioprine, or methotrexate.

Glucocorticoids

Glucocorticoids are the mainstay of therapy for many vasculitides including both giant-cell arteritis and Takayasu arteritis.[156a] These agents decrease inflammation by suppressing the migration of polymorphonuclear leukocytes and decreasing capillary permeability. There is suppression of the immune system by reducing the activity and volume of the lymphatic system.

Blindness occurred in up to 80 percent of patients with giant-cell arteritis prior to the use of steroids.[157] However, remission is induced in nearly all cases with an initial dose of 40 to 60 mg of prednisone in a single or divided daily dose.[158] Therapy with intravenous pulse methyprednisilone should be initiated in those with recent visual loss. Once a clinical remission has been induced, the dose of steroids are gradually reduced to a minimally suppressive dose. Laboratory evaluations, such as the sedimentation rate or C-reactive protein, are usually monitored to confirm the persistence of the remission. Steroids are often discontinued within a couple of years as giant-cell arteritis usually runs a self-limited course. However, approximately half of all patients will experience a relapse during corticosteroid tapering and the need for long-term corticosteroid therapy leads to adverse events from the steroids in a majority of patients.[159,160]

Glucocorticoids are effective to suppress systemic symptoms and arrest progression of arterial lesions in Takayasu arteritis. Early in the course of the disease, treatment with corticosteroids may reverse arterial stenoses, even with a restoration of pulses, and can improve ischemic symptoms.[161] The response is diminished once fibrosis or thrombosis has developed within the affected vessels. A commonly accepted initial dose of prednisone for Takayasu arteritis is 40 to 60 mg per day to induce a remission but then gradually tapered to sustain remission. Laboratory markers of systemic inflammation are monitored to confirm the persistence of a remission. As with giant-cell arteritis, many patients with Takayasu arteritis will experience a relapse during corticosteroid tapering and complications of long-term corticosteroid therapy are common.

Cytotoxic Drugs

Various cytotoxic agents are used for steroid-resistant disease that has failed to enter remission with corticosteroids. Cytotoxic agents have also been used for their steroid-sparing effects in an attempt to reduce the corticosteroid requirement to keep the disease quiesent. These agents, including cyclophosphamide, azathioprine, and methotrexate, should only be handled by physicians well versed in their use. With the large-vessel vasculitides, the use of methotrexate has been evaluated. The experience with the other agents is very limited.

There is controversy regarding the steroid-sparing effect of methotrexate in giant-cell arteritis. In a recent double-blind, placebo-controlled trial, 42 subjects with new-onset giant-cell arteritis were randomized to weekly methotrexate (at a dose of 10 mg) for 24 months plus prednisone, or placebo plus prednisone.[162] Treatment with methotrexate significantly reduced the proportion of patients who experienced a relapse (45 vs. 84%, $P = .02$), reduced the duration of use of prednisone (median time of 29 and 94 weeks, $P < .01$), and reduced the mean cumulative dose of prednisone (4.2 vs. 5.5, $P < .01$).[162] The rate and severity of side effects was similar in the two groups. In contrast, a preliminary report in another placebo-controlled trial found that weekly methotrexate failed to lower the dose of corticosteroids.[163]

The use of methotrexate has been evaluated in the treatment of persistent or recurrent Takayasu arteritis that is refractory to glucocorticoids. An open-label study evaluated the effect of low-dose methotrexate with glucocorticoids in 18 patients with refractory Takayasu arteritis; 16 were followed for a mean period of 2.8 years.[164] Weekly administration of methotrexate (mean dose of 17.1 mg) and glucocorticoids induced remission in 81% of patients (13 of 16). However, when the dose of glucocortcoid was tapered, relapse occurred in 44% of patients (7 of 13) requiring retreatment again leading to a remission. There was a sustained remission (with a mean of 18 months) in half of patients treated with low-dose weekly methotrexate.

CONCLUSION

Despite years of intense investigation, effective drug therapy for the symptomatic treatment of manifestations of arteriosclerosis obliterans remains elusive. The current focus is on the treatment of modifiable risk factors for atherosclerosis (including smoking cessation) and an exercise regimen. Only two agents, pentoxifylline and cilostazol, are available in the U.S. for the symptomatic treatment of IC. Antiplatelet agents hold promise in reducing cardiovascular morbidity and mortality among individuals with PAD. Investigational agents involving nitric oxide and carnitine metabolism remain viable therapeutic targets in the management of IC. There was minimal long-term benefit to the use of prostaglandins in the treatment of critical limb ischemia, and angiogenesis is still in the early stages of development. There is a role for catheter-guided thrombolytic therapy in the treatment of acute arterial occlusion of the extremities.

When Raynaud's phenomenon requires drug therapy, dihydropyridine-type calcium-channel blockers are effective at decreasing the frequency, duration, and severity of attacks but do not provide complete relief. Alternative vasodilators, such as prazosin, may be tried if calcium-channel blockers are ineffective or intolerable. Other agents, including prostaglandins, continue to be evaluated in the treatment of refractory Raynaud's phenomenon to allow wound healing.

Heparin has been the standard agent in the prevention and short-term management of DVT, followed by administration of warfarin for long-term management. The use of weight-based nomograms has facilitated achieving therapeutic anticoagulation with heparin more safely than with the prior regimens. LMWHs are becoming the preferred agents for the prevention and possibly for the treatment of DVT. The ease of administration and fewer side effects with equivalent (or better) efficacy are key to the recent flourishing in the use of LMWH. Heparinoids and direct antithrombin agents, such as danaparoid and hirudin, are emerging as alternative agents in the prevention and perhaps management of DVT. Warfarin should be continued for at least 3 to 6 months to maintain an INR of 2.0 to 3.0 for treatment of DVT, although more prolonged therapy should be considered for idiopathic and recurrent DVT. Thrombolysis may be used selectively for the treatment of proximal DVT, particularly if evidence for limb ischemia is present. Although great strides have been made in the prevention of DVT in high-risk patients, there is still a higher than acceptable incidence.

Glucocorticoids and cytoxic agents remain the treatments of choice for managing patients with vasculitis.

REFERENCES

1. Quriel K: Peripheral arterial disease. *Lancet* 358:1257, 2001.
1a. Hirsch AT, Criqui MH, Treat-Jacobson D, et al: Peripheral arterial disease detection, awareness, and treatment in primary care. *JAMA* 286:1317, 2001.
1b. Hiatt WR: Medical treatment of peripheral arterial disease and claudication. *N Engl J Med* 344:1608, 2001.
2. The Heart Outcome Prevention Evaluation Study Investigators: Effects of an angiotensin-converting-enzyme inhibitor, ramipril, on cardiovascular events in high-risk patients. *N Engl J Med* 342:145, 2000.
3. Girolami B, Bernardi E, Prins MH, et al: Treatment of intermittent claudication with physical training, smoking cessation, pentoxifylline, or nafronyl: A meta-analysis. *Arch Intern Med* 159:337, 1999.
4. Gardner AW, Katzel LI, Sorkin JD, et al: Improved functional outcomes following exercise rehabilitation in patients with intermittent claudication. *J Gerontol* 55:M570, 2000.
5. Regensteiner JG, Steiner JF, Hiatt WR: Exercise training improves functional status in patients with peripheral arterial disease. *J Vasc Surg* 23:104, 1996.
6. Radack K, Wyderski RJ: Conservative management of intermittent claudication. *Ann Intern Med* 113:135, 1999.
7. Hood SC, Moher D, Barber GG: Management of intermittent claudication with pentoxifylline: Meta-analysis of randomized controlled trials. *Can Med Assoc J* 155:1053, 1996.
8. Lindgarde F, Jelnes R, Bjorkman H, et al: Conservative drug treatment in patients with moderately severe chronic occlusive peripheral arterial disease. Scandinavian Study Group. *Circulation* 80:1549, 1989.
9. Stergachis A, Sheingold S, Luce BR, et al: Medical care and cost outcomes after pentoxifylline treatment for peripheral arterial disease. *Arch Intern Med* 152:1220, 1992.
10. Gillings DB: Pentoxifylline and intermittent claudication: Review of clinical trials and cost-effectiveness analyses. *J Cardiovasc Pharmacol* 25(Suppl 2):S44, 1995.
10a. Jull A, Waters J, Arroll B: Pentoxifylline for treatment of venous leg ulcers: A systematic review. *Lancet* 359:1550, 2002.
10b. Woo Sk, Kang Wk, Kwon K-i: Pharmacokinetic and pharmacodynamic modeling of the antiplatelet and cardiovascular effects of cilostazol in healthy humans. *Clin Pharmacol Ther* 71:246, 2002.
11. Elam MB, Heckman J, Crouse JR, et al: Effect of the novel antiplatelet agent cilostazol on plasma lipoproteins in patients with intermittent claudication. *Arterioscler Thromb Vasc Biol* 18:1942, 1998.
12. Ishizaka N, Taguchi J, Kimura Y, et al: Effects of a single local administration of cilostazol on neointimal formation in balloon-injured rat carotid artery. *Atherosclerosis* 142:41, 1999.
13. Money SR, Herd JA, Isaacsohn JL, et al: Effect of cilostazol on walking distances in patients with intermittent claudication caused by peripheral vascular disease. *J Vasc Surg* 27:267, 1998.
14. Dawson DL, Cutler BS, Meissner MH, Strandness DE: Cilostazol has beneficial effects in treatment of intermittent claudication: Results from a multicenter, randomized, prospective, double-blind trial. *Circulation* 98:678, 1998.
15. Beebe HG, Dawson DL, Cutler BS, et al: A new pharmacological treatment for intermittent claudication: Results of a randomized, multicenter trial. *Arch Intern Med* 159:2041, 1999.
16. Dawson DL, Cutler BS, Hiatt WR, et al: A comparision of cilostazol and pentoxifylline for treating intermittent claudication. *Am J Med* 109:523, 2000.
17. Dawson DL, DeMaioribus CA, Hagino RT, et al: The effect of withdrawal of drugs treating intermittent claudication. *Am J Surg* 178:141, 1999.
17a. Regensteiner JG, Hiatt WR: Current medical therapies for patients with peripheral arterial disease: A critical review. *Am J Med* 112:49, 2002.
17b. Creager MA: Medical management of peripheral arterial disease. *Cardiol in Rev* 9:238, 2002.
17c. Various interventions have potentially major economic impact in intermittent claudication. *Drugs Ther Perspect* 18:23, 2002.
18. Hiatt WR: Medical treatment of claudication. IV. Morbidity of PAD: medical approaches to claudication. In: Hirsh AT, Hiatt WR, eds. *An Office-Based Approach to the Diagnosis and Treatment of Peripheral Arterial Disease.* Continuing education monograph series from the American Journal of Medicine. Bellemead, NJ: Excerpta Medica, 1999:6.
19. Jackson MR, Clagett GP: Antithrombotic therapy in peripheral arterial occlusive disease. *Chest* 119:283S, 2001.
20. Collaborative overview of randomised trials of antiplatelet therapy: I. Prevention of death, myocardial infarction, and stroke by prolonged therapy in various categories of patients. *BMJ* 308:81, 1994.
21. Food and Drug Administration: Internal analgesic, antipyretic, and antirheumatic drug products for over-the-counter human use: Final rule for professional labeling of aspirin, buffered aspirin, and aspirin in combination with antacid products. *Fed Reg* 63:56802, 1998.
22. Collaborative overview of randomised trials of antiplatelet therapy. II. Maintenance of vascular graft or arterial patency by antiplatelet therapy. *BMJ* 308:159, 1994.
23. Goldhaber SZ, Manson JE, Stampfer MJ, et al: Low-dose aspirin and subsequent peripheral arterial surgery in the Physicians' Health Study. *Lancet* 340:143, 1992.
24. Libretti A, Catalano M: Treatment of claudication with dipyridamole and aspirin. *Int J Clin Pharm Res* 6:59, 1986.
25. Giansante C, Calabrese S, Fisicaro M, et al: Treatment of intermittent claudication with antiplatelet agents. *J Intern Med Res* 18:400, 1990.
26. Hess H, Mietaschk A, Deichsel G: Drug-induced inhibition of platelet function delays progression of peripheral occlusive arterial disease: A prospective double-blind arteriographically controlled trial. *Lancet* 1:415, 1985.
27. Balsano F, Coccheri S, Libretti A, et al: Ticlopidine in the treatment of intermittent claudication: A 21-month double-blind trial. *J Lab Clin Med* 114:84, 1989.
28. Arcan JC, Panak E: Ticlopidine in the treatment of peripheral occlusive arterial disease. *Semin Thromb Hemost* 15:167, 1989.
29. Janzon L, Bergqvist D, Boberg J, et al: Prevention of myocardial infarction and stroke in patients with intermittent claudication: Effects of ticlopidine. Results from STIMS, the Swedish Ticlopidine Multicentre Study. *J Intern Med* 227:301, 1990.
30. The Clopidogrel versus Aspirin in Patients at Risk of Ischemic Events (CAPRIE) Steering Committee: A randomised, blinded, trial of clopidogrel versus aspirin in patients at risk of ischaemic events (CAPRIE). *Lancet* 348:1329, 1996.
31. Brevetti G, Angelini C, Rosa M, et al: Muscle carnitine deficiency in patients with severe peripheral vascular disease. *Circulation* 84:1490, 1991.
32. Hiatt WR, Wolfel EE, Regensteiner JG, Brass EP: Skeletal muscle carnitine metabolism in patients with unilateral peripheral arterial disease. *J Appl Physiol* 73:346, 1992.
33. Brass EP, Hiatt WR: Acquired skeletal muscle metabolic myopathy in atherosclerotic peripheral arterial disease. *Vasc Med* 5:55, 2000.
34. Brevetti G, Perna S, Sabba C, et al: Propionyl-L-carnitine in intermittent claudication: Double-blind, placebo-controlled, dose titration, multicenter study. *J Am Coll Cardiol* 26:1411, 1995.
35. Brevetti G, Perna S, Sabba C, et al: Effect of propionyl-L-carnitine on quality of life in intermittent claudication. *Am J Cardiol* 79:777, 1997.

36. Brevetti G, Diehm C, Lambert D: European multicenter study on propionyl-L-carnitine in intermittent claudication. *J Am Coll Cardiol* 34:1618, 1999.

37. The ICAI study group: Prostanoids for chronic critical leg ischemia: A randomized, controlled, open-label trial with prostaglandin E1. *Ann Intern Med* 130:412, 1999.

38. Belch JJ, Bell PR, Creissen D, et al: Randomized, double-blind, placebo-controlled study evaluating the efficacy and safety of AS-013, a prostaglandin E_1 prodrug, in patients with intermittent claudication. *Circulation* 95:2298, 1997.

39. Scheffler P, de la Hamette D, Gross J, et al: Intensive vascular training in stage IIb of peripheral arterial occlusive disease: The additive effects of intravenous prostaglandin E1 or intravenous pentoxifylline during training. *Circulation* 90:818, 1994.

40. Lièvre M, Morand S, Besse Bi, et al: Oral beraprost sodium, a prostaglandin in I_2 analogue, for intermittent claudication: A double-blind, randomized multicenter controlled trial. *Circulation* 102:426, 2000.

41. Coffman JD: Drug therapy: Vasodilator drugs in peripheral vascular disease. *N Engl J Med* 300:713, 1979.

42. Bagger JP, Helligsoe P, Randsbaek F, et al: Effect of verapamil in intermittent claudication: A randomized, double-blind, placebo-controlled, cross-over study after individual dose-response assessment. *Circulation* 95:411, 1997.

43. Schellong SM, Boger RH, Burchert W, et al: Dose-related effect of intravenous L-arginine on muscular blood flow of the calf in patients with peripheral vascular disease: A H215O positron emission tomography study. *Clin Sci* 93:159, 1997.

44. Boger RH, Bode-Boger SM, Thiele W, et al: Restoring vascular nitric oxide formation by L-arginine improves the symptoms of intermittent claudication in patients with peripheral arterial occlusive disease. *J Am Coll Cardiol* 32:1336, 1998.

45. Maxwell AJ, Anderson B, Cooke JP: Nutritional therapy for peripheral arterial disease: A double-blind, placebo-controlled, randomized trial of HeartBar®. *Vasc Med* 5:11, 2000.

46. Pantely GA, Porter JM: Therapeutic angiogenesis: Time for the next phase. *J Am Coll Cardiol* 36:1245, 2000.

46a. Rajagopalan S, Trachtenberg J, Mohler E, et al: Phase 1 study of direct administration of a replication deficient adenovirus vector containing the vascular endothelial growth factor cDNA (CI-1023) to patients with claudication. *Am J Cardiol* 90:512, 2002.

47. Tsurumi Y, Takeshita S, Chen D, et al: Direct intramuscular gene transfer of naked DNA encoding vascular endothelial growth factor augments collateral development and tissue perfusion. *Circulation* 94:3281, 1996.

48. Baumgartner I, Pieczek A, Manor O, et al: Constitutive expression of phVEGF165 after intramuscular gene transfer promotes collateral vessel development in patients with critical limb ischemia. *Circulation* 97:1114, 1996.

49. Baumgartner I, Guenter R, Pieczek A, et al: Lower extremity edema associated with gene transfer of naked DNA encoding vascular endothelial growth factor. *Ann Intern Med* 132:880, 2000.

50. Lazarous DF, Unger EF, Epstein SE, et al: Basic fibroblast growth factor in patients with intermittent claudication: Results of a phase I trial. *J Am Coll Cardiol* 36:1239, 2000.

51. Lederman RT: TRAFFIC (Therapeutic Angiogenesis with rFGF-2 for Intermittent Claudication). Presentation at the American College of Cardiology 50th Scientific Session. Progress in Clinical Trials. *Clin Cardiol* 24:481, 2001.

51a. Tateishi-Yuyama E, Matsubara H, Murohara T, et al: Therapeutic angiogenesis for patients with limb ischaemia by autologous transplantation of bone-marrow cells: A pilot study and a randomised controlled trial. *Lancet* 360:427, 2002.

52. Ouriel K, Veith FJ, Sasahara AA: A comparison of recombinant urokinase with vascular surgery as initial treatment for acute arterial occlusion of the legs. Thrombolysis or Peripheral Arterial Surgery (TOPAS) Investigators. *N Engl J Med* 338:1105, 1998.

53. Berridge DC, Gregson RH, Hopkinson BR, Makin GS: Randomized trial of intra-arterial recombinant tissue plasminogen activator, intravenous recombinant tissue plasminogen activator and intra-arterial streptokinase in peripheral arterial thrombolysis. *Br J Surg* 78:988, 1991.

54. Lonsdale RJ, Berridge DC, Earnshaw JJ, et al: Recombinant tissue-type plasminogen activator is superior to streptokinase for local intra-arterial thrombolysis. *Br J Surg* 79:272, 1992.

55. Working Party on Thrombolysis in the Management of Limb Ischemia: Thrombolysis in the management of lower limb peripheral arterial occlusion: A consensus document. *Am J Cardiol* 81:207, 1998.

56. The Advisory Panel: Thrombolytic therapy with the use of altaplase (rt-PA) in peripheral arterial occlusive disease: Review of the clinical literature. *J Vasc Intervent Radiol* 11:149, 2000.

57. Hamilton M, Wilson GM, Armitage P, Boyd JT: The treatment of intermittent claudication with vitamin E. *Lancet* 1:367, 1953.

58. Livingstone PD, Jones C: Treatment of intermittent claudication with vitamin E. *Lancet* 2:602, 1958.

59. Tornwall M, Virtamo J, Haukka JK, et al: Effect of alpha-tocopherol (vitamin E) and beta-carotene supplementation on the incidence of intermittent claudication in male smokers. *Arterioscler Thromb Vasc Biol* 17:3475, 1997.

60. The Heart Outcome Prevention Evaluation Study Investigators: Vitamin E supplementation and cardiovascular events in high-risk patients. *N Engl J Med* 342:154, 2000.

61. De Cree J, Leempoels J, Geukens H, Verhaegen H: Placebo-controlled double-blind trial of ketanserin in treatment of intermittent claudication. *Lancet* 2:775, 1984.

62. Thulesius O, Lundvall J, Kroese A, et al: Ketanserin in intermittent claudication: Effect on walking distance, blood pressure, and cardiovascular complications. *J Cardiovasc Pharmacol* 9:728, 1987.

63. Clement DL, Duprez D: Effect of ketanserin in the treatment of patients with intermittent claudication: Results from 13 placebo-controlled parallel group studies. *J Cardiovasc Pharmacol* 10(Suppl 3): S89, 1987.

64. Prevention of Atherosclerotic Complications with Ketanserin Trial Group: Prevention of atherosclerotic complications: Controlled trial of ketanserin. *BMJ* 298:424, 1989.

65. Moody AP, al-Khaffaf HS, Lehert P, et al: An evaluation of patients with severe intermittent claudication and the effect of treatment with naftidrofuryl. *J Cardiovasc Pharmacol* 23(Suppl 3):S44, 1994.

66. Strano A, Fareed J, Sabba C, et al: A double-blind, multicenter, placebo-controlled, dose comparison study of orally administered defibrotide: Preliminary results in patients with peripheral arterial disease. *Semin Thromb Hemost* 17(Suppl 2):228, 1991.

67. Sabba C, Zupo V, Dina F, et al: A pilot evaluation of the effect of defibrotide in patients affected by peripheral arterial occlusive disease. *Int J Clin Pharmacol Ther Toxicol* 26:249, 1988.

68. Trubestein G, Balzer K, Bisler H, et al: Buflomedil in arterial occlusive disease: Results of a controlled multicenter study. *Angiology* 35:500, 1984.

69. Pignoli P, Ciccolo F, Villa V, Longo T: Comparative evaluation of bluflomedil and pentoxifylline in patients with peripheral arterial occlusive disease. *Curr Ther Res* 37:596, 1985.

70. Chacon-Quevedo A, Eguaras MG, Calleja F, et al: Comparative evaluation of pentoxifylline, buflomedil, and nifedipine in the treatment of intermittent claudication of the lower limbs. *Angiology* 45:647, 1994.

71. Kiesewetter H, Blume J, Jung F, et al: Haemodilution with medium molecular weight hydroxyethyl starch in patients with peripheral arterial occlusive disease stage IIb. *J Intern Med* 227:107, 1990.

72. Ernst E, Kollar L, Matrai A: A double-blind trial of dextran-haemodilution vs. placebo in claudicants. *J Intern Med* 227:19, 1990.

73. Sloth-Nielsen J, Guldager B, Mouritzen C, et al: Arteriographic findings in EDTA chelation therapy on peripheral arteriosclerosis. *Am J Surg* 162:122, 1991.

74. Guldager B, Jelnes R, Jorgensen SJ, et al: EDTA treatment of intermittent claudication: A double-blind, placebo-controlled study. *J Intern Med* 231:261, 1992.

74a. Frishman WH: Chelation therapy for coronary artery disease: Panacea or quackery? (editorial) *Am J Med* 111:729, 2001.

74b. Duda SH, Pusich B, Richter G, et al: Sirolimus-eluting stents for the treatment of obstructive superficial femoral artery disease. Six months results. *Circulation* 106:1505, 2002.

75. Rodeheffer RJ, Rommer JA, Wigley F, Smith CR: Controlled double-blind trial of nifedipine in the treatment of Raynaud's phenomenon. *N Engl J Med* 308:880, 1983.

76. Raynaud's Treatment Study Investigators: Comparison of sustained-release nifedipine and temperature biofeedback for treatment of primary Raynaud phenomenon: Results from a randomized clinical trial with 1-year follow-up. *Arch Int Med* 160:1101, 2000.

77. Creager MA, Pariser KM, Winston EM, et al: Nifedipine-induced fingertip vasodilation in patients with Raynaud's phenomenon. *Am Heart J* 108:370, 1984.

78. Maricq HR, Jennings JR, Valter I, et al: Evaluation of treatment efficacy of Raynaud phenomenon by digital blood pressure response to cooling. *Vasc Med* 5:135, 2000.

79. La Civita L, Pitaro N, Rossi M, et al: Amlodipine in the treatment of Raynaud's phenomenon. *Br J Rheumatol* 32:524, 1993.

80. Kallenberg CG, Wouda AA, Meems L, Wesseling H: Once daily felodipine in patients with primary Raynaud's phenomenon. *Eu J Clin Pharmacol* 40:313, 1991.

81. Schmidt JF, Valentin N, Nielsen SL: The clinical effect of felodipine and nifedipine in Raynaud's phenomenon. *Eu J Clin Pharmacol* 37:191, 1989.

82. Leppert J, Jonasson T, Nilsson H, Ringqvist I: The effect of isradipine, a new calcium-channel antagonist, in patients with primary Raynaud's phenomenon: A single-blind dose-response study. *Cardiovasc Drugs Ther* 3:397, 1989.

83. French Cooperative Multicenter Group for Raynaud's Phenomenon: Controlled multicenter double-blind trial of nicardipine in the treatment of primary Raynaud phenomenon. *Am Heart J* 122:352, 1991.

84. Gjorup T, Hartling OJ, Kelbaek H, Nielsen SL: Controlled double blind trial of nisoldipine in the treatment of idiopathic Raynaud's phenomenon. *Eu J Clin Pharmacol* 31:387, 1986.

85. Kahan A, Amor B, Menkes CJ: A randomised double-blind trial of diltiazem in the treatment of Raynaud's phenomenon. *Ann Rheum Dis* 44:30, 1985.

86. Da Costa JT, Gomes JAM, Santo JE, Queiros MV: Inefficacy of diltiazem in the treatment of raynaud's phenomenom with associated connective tissue disease: A double blind placebo controlled study. *J Rheumatol* 14:858, 1987.

87. Kinney EL, Nicholas GG, Gallo J, et al: The treatment of severe Raynaud's phenomenon with verapamil. *J Clin Pharmacol* 22:74, 1982.

88. Pope J, Fenlon D, Thompson A, et al: Prazosin for Raynaud's phenomenon in progressive systemic sclerosis. *Cochrane Database Syst Rev* [computer file] 2:CD000956, 2000.

89. Wollersheim H, Thien T, Fennis J, et al: Double-blind, placebo-controlled study of prazosin in Raynaud's phenomenon. *Clin Pharmocol Ther* 40:219, 1986.

90. Russell IJ, Lessard JA: Prazosin treatment of Raynaud's phenomenon: A double blind single crossover study. *J Rheumatol* 12:94, 1985.

91. Nielsen SL, Vitting K, Rasmussen K: Prazosin treatment of primary Raynaud's phenomenon. *Eu J Clin Pharmacol* 24:421, 1983.

92. Aylward M, Bater PA, Davies DE, et al: Long-term monitoring of the effects of thymoxamine hydrochloride tablets in the management of patients with Raynaud's disease. *Curr Med Res Opin* 8:158, 1982.

93. Coffman JD, Cohen AS: Total and capillary fingertip blood flow in Raynaud's phenomenon. *N Engl J Med* 285:259, 1971.

94. McFadyen IJ, Housley E, MacPherson AI: Intraarterial reserpine administration in Raynaud syndrome. *Arch Intern Med* 132:526, 1973.

95. Clifford PC, Martin MF, Sheddon EJ, et al: Treatment of vasospastic disease with prostaglandin E1. *BMJ* 281:1031, 1980.

96. Mohrland JS, Porter JM, Smith EA, et al: A multiclinic, placebo-controlled, double-blind study of prostaglandin E$_1$ in Raynaud's syndrome. *Ann Rheum Dis* 44:754–760, 1985.

97. Belch JJ, McKay A, McArdle B, et al: Epoprostenol (prostacyclin) and severe arterial disease: A double-blind trial. *Lancet* 1:315, 1983.

98. Dowd PM, Martin MF, Cooke ED, et al: Treatment of Raynaud's phenomenon by intravenous infusion of prostacyclin (PGI2). *Br J Dermatol* 106:81, 1982.

99. Wigley FM, Wise RA, Seibold JR, et al: Intravenous iloprost infusion in patients with Raynaud phenomenon secondary to systemic sclerosis: A multicenter, placebo-controlled, double-blind study. *Ann Intern Med* 120:199, 1994.

100. Rademaker M, Cooke ED, Almond NE, et al: Comparison of intravenous infusions of iloprost and oral nifedipine in treatment of Raynaud's phenomenon in patients with systemic sclerosis: A double blind randomised study. *BMJ* 298:561, 1989.

101. Pope J, Fenlon D, Thompson A, et al: Iloprost and cisaprost for Raynaud's phenomenon in progressive systemic sclerosis. *Cochrane Database Syst Rev* [computer file] 2:CD000953, 2000.

102. Wigley FM, Korn JH, Csuka ME, et al: Oral iloprost treatment in patients with Raynaud's phenomenon secondary to systemic sclero-

sis: A multicenter, placebo-controlled, double-blind study. *Arthritis Rheum* 41:670, 1998.

103. Belch JJ, Capell HA, Cooke ED, et al: Oral iloprost as a treatment for Raynaud's syndrome: A double blind multicentre placebo controlled study. *Ann Rheum Dis* 54:197, 1995.

104. Coffman JD, Clement DL, Creager MA, et al: International study of ketanserin in Raynaud's phenomenon. *Am J Med* 87:264, 1989.

105. Pope J, Fenlon D, Thompson A, et al: Ketanserin for Raynaud's phenomenon in progressive systemic sclerosis. *Cochrane Database Sys Rev* [computer file] 2:CD000954, 2000.

106. Igarashi M, Okuda T Oh-I T, Koga M: Changes in plasma serotonin concentration and acceleration plethysmograms in patients with Raynaud's phenomenon after long-term treatment with a 5–HT$_2$ receptor antagonist. *J Dermatol* 27:643, 2000.

107. Lopez-Ovejero JA, Saal SD, D'Angelo WA, et al: Reversal of vascular and renal crises of scleroderma by oral angiotensin-converting-enzyme blockade. *N Engl J Med* 300:1417, 1979.

108. Tosi S, Marchesoni A, Messina K, et al: Treatment of Raynaud's phenomenon with captopril. *Drugs Exp Clin Res* 13:37, 1987.

109. Pancera P, Sansone S, Secchi S, et al: The effects of thromboxane A2 inhibition (picotamide) and angiotensin II receptor blockade (losartan) in primary Raynaud's phenomenon. *J Intern Med* 242:373, 1997.

110. Franks AG: Topical glyceryl trinitrate as adjunctive treatment in Raynaud's disease. *Lancet* 1:76. 1982.

111. Neirotti M, Longo F, Molaschi M, et al: Functional vascular disorders: Treatment with pentoxifylline. *Angiology* 38:575, 1987.

112. Peacock JH: The treatment of primary Raynaud's disease of the upper limb. *Lancet* 2:65, 1960.

113. Dessein PH, Morrison RC, Lamparelli RD, van der Merwe CA: Triiodothyronine treatment for Raynaud's phenomenon: A controlled trial. *J Rheumatol* 17:1025, 1990.

114. Belch JJ, Cormie J, Newman P, et al: Dazoxiben, a thromboxane synthetase inhibitor, in the treatment of Raynaud's syndrome: A double-blind trial. *Br J Clin Pharmacol* 15(Suppl 1):113S, 1983.

115. Ettinger WH, Wise RA, Schaffhauser D, Wigley FM: Controlled double-blind trial of dazoxiben and nifedipine in the treatment of Raynaud's phenomenon. *Am J Med* 77:451, 1984.

116. Coffman JD, Rasmussen HM: Effect of thromboxane synthetase inhibition in Raynaud's phenomenon. *Clin Pharmacol Ther* 36:369, 1984.

117. Khan F, Litchfield SJ, McLaren M, et al: Oral L-arginine supplementation and cutaneous vascular responses in patients with primary Raynaud's phenomenon. *Arthritis Rheum* 40:352, 1997.

118. Tucker AT, Pearson RM, Cooke ED, Benjamin N: Effect of nitric oxide-generating system on microcirculatory blood flow in skin of patients with severe Raynaud's syndrome: A randomised trial. *Lancet* 354:1670, 1999.

119. Freedman RR, Girgis R, Mayes MD: Acute effect of nitric oxide on Raynaud's phenomenon in scleroderma. *Lancet* 354:73, 1999.

120. Ginsberg JS: Management of venous thromboembolism. *N Engl J Med* 335:1816, 1996.

121. Hyers TM, Agnelli G, Hull Rd, et al: Antithrombotic therapy for venous thromboembolic disease. *Chest* 119:176S, 2001.

122. Geerts WH, Heit JA, Clagett P, et al: Prevention of venous thromboembolism. *Chest* 119:132S, 2001.

122a. Ray JG, Mamdani M, Tsuyuki RG, et al: Use of statins and the subsequent development of deep vein thrombosis. *Arch Intern Med* 161:1405, 2001.

123. Seligsohn U, Lubetsky A: Genetic susceptibility to venous thrombosis. *N Engl J Med* 344:1222, 2001.

124. Federman DG, Kirsner RS: An update on hypercoagulable disorders. *Arch Intern Med* 161:1051, 2001.

125. Barritt DW, Jordan SC: Anticoagulant drugs in the treatment of pulmonary embolism: A controlled trial. *Lancet* 1:1309, 1960.

126. Hull RD, Raskob GE, Hirsh J, et al: Continuous intravenous heparin compared with intermittent subcutaneous heparin in the initial treatment of proximal-vein thrombosis. *N Engl J Med* 315:1109, 1986.

127. Hull RD, Raskob GE, Brant RF, et al: Relation between the time to achieve the lower limit of the APTT therapeutic range and recurrent venous thromboembolism during heparin treatment for deep vein thrombosis. *Arch Intern Med* 157:2562, 1997.

128. Raschke RA, Reilly BM, Guidry JR, et aL: The weight-based heparin dosing nomogram compared with a "standard care" nomogram: A randomized controlled trial. *Ann Intern Med* 119:874, 1993.

129. Collins R, Scrimgeour A, Yusuf S, Peto R: Reduction in fatal pulmonary embolism and venous thrombosis by perioperative administration of subcutaneous heparin: Overview of results of randomized trials in general, orthopedic, and urologic surgery. *N Engl J Med* 318:1162, 1988.

130. Halkin H, Goldberg J, Modan M, Modan B: Reduction of mortality in general medical in-patients by low-dose heparin prophylaxis. *Ann Intern Med* 96:561, 1982.

131. Leyvraz PF, Richard J, Bachmann F, et al: Adjusted versus fixed-dose subcutaneous heparin in the prevention of deep-vein thrombosis after total hip replacement. *N Engl J Med* 309:954, 1983.

132. Weitz JI: Low-molecular-weight heparins. *N Engl J Med* 337:688, 1997.

133. Nurmohamed MT, Rosendaal FR, Buller HR, et al: Low-molecular-weight heparin versus standard heparin in general and orthopaedic surgery: A meta-analysis. *Lancet* 340:152, 1992.

134. Samama MM, Cohen AT, Darmon J-Y, et al: A comparison of enoxaparin with placebo for the prevention of venous thromboembolism in acutely ill medical patients. *N Engl J Med* 341:793, 1999.

135. Gould MK, Dembitzer AD, Doyle RL, et al: Low-molecular-weight heparins compared with unfractionated heparin for treatment of acute deep venous thrombosis: A meta-analysis of randomized, controlled trials. *Ann Intern Med* 130:800, 1999.

136. Lensing AW, Prins MH, Davidson BL, Hirsh J: Treatment of deep venous thrombosis with low-molecular-weight heparins: A meta-analysis. *Arch Intern Med* 155:601, 1995.

137. Leizorovicz A, Simonneau G, Decousus H, Boissel JP: Comparison of efficacy and safety of low molecular weight heparins and unfractionated heparin in initial treatment of deep venous thrombosis: A meta-analysis. *BMJ* 309:299, 1994.

138. Breddin HK, Hach-Wunderle V, Nakov R, et al: Effects of low-molecular-weight heparin on thrombus regression and recurrent thromboembolism in patients with deep-vein thrombosis. *N Engl J Med* 344:626, 2001.

139. Levine M, Gent M, Hirsh J, et al: A comparison of low-molecular-weight heparin administered primarily at home with unfractionated heparin administered in the hospital for proximal deep-vein thrombosis. *N Engl J Med* 334:677, 1996.

140. Koopman MM, Prandoni P, Piovella F, et al: Treatment of venous thrombosis with intravenous unfractionated heparin administered in the hospital as compared with subcutaneous low-molecular-weight heparin administered at home. The Tasman Study Group. *N Engl J Med* 334:682, 1996.

141. Hull RD, Raskob GE, Rosenbloom D, et al: Treatment of proximal vein thrombosis with subcutaneous low-molecular-weight heparin vs intravenous heparin: An economic perspective. *Arch Intern Med* 157:289, 1997.

142. Schwarz T, Schmidt B, Hohlein U, et al: Eligibility for home treatment of deep vein thrombosis: Prospective study. *BMJ* 322:1212, 2001.

143. Eikelboom J, Baket R: Routine home treatment of deep vein thrombosis: Is now a reality. *BMJ* 322:1192, 2001.

144. Hull R, Delmore T, Genton E, et al: Warfarin sodium versus low-dose heparin in the long-term treatment of venous thrombosis. *N Engl J Med* 301:855, 1979.

145. Hull R, Hirsh J, Jay R, et al: Different intensities of oral anticoagulant therapy in the treatment of proximal-vein thrombosis. *N Engl J Med* 307:1676, 1982.

146. Kearon C, Gent M, Hirsh J, et al: A comparison of three months of anticoagulation with extended anticoagulation for a first episode of idiopathic venous thromboembolism. *N Engl J Med* 340:901, 1999.

147. Schulman S, Granqvist S, Holmstrom M, et al: The duration of oral anticoagulant therapy after a second episode of venous thromboembolism. The Duration of Anticoagulation Trial Study Group. *N Engl J Med* 336:393, 1997.

148. Francis CW, Pellegrini VDJ, Marder VJ, et al: Comparison of warfarin and external pneumatic compression in prevention of venous thrombosis after total hip replacement. *JAMA* 267:2911, 1992.

149. Eriksson BI, Ekman S, Kalebo P, et al: Prevention of deep-vein thrombosis after total hip replacement: Direct thrombin inhibition with recombinant hirudin, CGP 39393. *Lancet* 1996 347:635.

150. Eriksson BI, Wille-Jorgensen P, Kalebo P, et al: A comparison of recombinant hirudin with a low-molecular-weight heparin to prevent thromboembolic complications after total hip replacement. *N Engl J Med* 337:1329, 1997.

151. de Valk HW, Banga JD, Wester JW, et al: Comparing subcutaneous danaparoid with intravenous unfractionated heparin for the treatment of venous thromboembolism: A randomized controlled trial. *Ann Intern Med* 123:1, 1995.

151a. Bauer KA, Eriksson BI, Lassen MR, et al: Fondaparinux compared with enoxiparin for the prevention of venous thrombo embolism after elective major knee surgery. *N Engl J Med* 345:1305, 2001.

151b. Lassen MR, Bauer KA, Eriksson BI, et al: Postoperative fondaparinux versus preoperative enoxiparin for prevention of venous thromboembolism in elective hip-replacement surgery. A randomised, double-blind comparison *Lancet* 359:1715, 2002.

151c. Turpie AGG, Bauer KA, Eriksson BI, Lassen MR: Postoperative fondaparinux venous postoperative enoxiparin for prevention of venous thromboembolism after elective hip-replacement surgery. A randomised, double-blind trial. *Lancet* 359:1721, 2002.

151d. Ansani NT: Fondaparinux: The first pentasaccharide anticoagulant. *Pharm Therap* 27:310, 2002.

152. Goldhaber SZ, Meyerovitz MF, Green D, et al: Randomized controlled trial of tissue plasminogen activator in proximal deep venous thrombosis. *Am J Med* 88:235, 1990.

153. Goldhaber SZ, Polak JF, Feldstein ML, et al: Efficacy and safety of repeated boluses of urokinase in the treatment of deep venous thrombosis. *Am J Cardiol* 73:75, 1994.

154. Turpie AG, Levine MN, Hirsh J, et al: Tissue plasminogen activator (rt-PA) vs heparin in deep vein thrombosis: Results of a randomized trial. *Chest* 97:172S, 1990.

155. Forster A, Wells P: Tissue plasminogen activator for the treatment of deep venous thrombosis of the lower extremity: A systemic review. *Chest* 119:572, 2001.

156. Langford CA: Chronic immunosuppressive therapy for systemic vasculitis. *Curr Opin Rheumotol* 9:416, 1997.

156a. Salvarani C, Cantini F, Boiardi L, Hunder GG: Polymyalgia rheumatica and giant-cell arteritis. *N Engl J Med* 347:261, 2002.

157. Myles AB, Perera TE, Ridley MG: Prevention of blindness in giant cell arteritis by corticosteroid treatment. *Br J Rheumatol* 31:103, 1992.

158. Hunder GG, Sheps SG, Allen GC, et al: Daily and alternate-day corticosteroid regimens in treatment of giant cell arteritis: Comparison in a prospective study. *Ann Intern Med* 82:613, 1975.

159. Lundberg I, Hedfors E: Restricted dose and duration of corticosteroid treatment in patients with polymyalgia rheumatica and temporal arteritis. *J Rheumatol* 17:1340, 1990.

160. Gabriel SE, Sunku J, Savarani C, O'Fallon WM, Hunder CC: Adverse outcomes of antiinflammatory therapy among patients with polymyalgia rheumatica. *Arthritis Rheum* 40:1873, 1997.

161. Kerr G: Takayasu's arteritis. *Rheum Dis Clin North Am* 21:1041, 1995.

162. Jover JA, Hernandez-Garcia C, Morado I, et al: Combined treatment of giant-cell arteritis with methotrexate and prednisone: A randomized, double-blind, placebo-controlled trial. *Ann Intern Med* 134:106, 2001.

163. Rojo-Leyva F, Ratliff NB, Cosgrove DM, Hoffman GS: Study of 52 patients with idiopathic aortitis from a cohort of 1,204 surgical cases. *Arthritis Rheum* 43:901, 2000.

164. Hoffman GS, Leavitt RY, Kerr GS, et al: Treatment of glucocorticoid-resistant or relapsing Takayasu arteritis with methotrexate. *Arthritis Rheum* 37:578, 1994.

Quality-of-Life Issues with Cardiovascular Drug Therapy

Domenic A. Sica

James A. Schoenberger

Modern drug treatment has had a profound influence on cardiovascular (CV) disease. The natural history of asymptomatic diseases, such as hypertension and hypercholesterolemia, has been appreciably altered and morbidity and mortality significantly delayed. In clinical CV disease, life has also been prolonged following myocardial infarction (MI), congestive heart failure (CHF), and after surgical procedures such as angioplasty and coronary artery bypass surgery.

The prolongation of life achieved by these interventions does not come without cost. Although the short-term adverse side effects of drugs can be accepted in acute disease if symptoms are relieved, or long-term cure is achieved, use of CV drugs, often for the life of the patient, requires more careful consideration. The benefits must be clearly weighed against the disadvantages. It is not enough just to list the most frequently experienced side effects. A more global assessment of the impact of these side effects on the overall quality of life of the patient must be undertaken. If the effect of CV drug therapy on quality of life (QOL) is ignored, the consequences, at the very least, may be a lack of adherence to the regimen. At the very worst, the compliant patient may lead a life of resigned desperation. The purpose of ongoing research on QOL issues is to determine the impact of therapeutic regimens on the QOL in order to avoid these pitfalls. The implications for the clinician are obvious and an appreciation of the impact of any regimen on the QOL should always be present.

This chapter describes measurement of QOL and discusses methodologic issues. The results of key studies using these methods are reviewed. Finally, how these concepts can be put to use by the practicing clinician is discussed.

METHODOLOGIC ISSUES

Optimal pharmacologic management cannot simply be limited to objective findings from a patient's physiologic and metabolic profile. Care of the hypertensive patient should also incorporate an assessment of QOL, a concept that transcends documentation of side effects and appreciates a patients perception of functional capacity, productivity, and sense of well-being. In addition, clinically meaningful information may be obtained from individuals closest to the patient.[1,2] Unfortunately, there is no single, universally accepted, definition of QOL. The term refers to "the physical, psychological, and social domains of health, seen as distinct areas that are influenced by a person's experience, beliefs, expectations, and percep-

tions." The definition of a "good QOL" varies with one of two broad mechanisms. One mechanism involves a direct influence on the central nervous system, with agents such as reserpine, α-methyldopa, and beta-blockers.[3] For example, beta-blockers can influence affect by decreasing anxiety and/or by increasing depressive symptoms.[1,2] As a second mechanism, the distress induced by physical symptoms can also influence QOL, which can modify mood. This appears to be the case with calcium-channel blockers (CCBs), a drug class widely held to be free of direct central nervous system effects. To quantify changes in QOL as reported by the patient, it has been necessary to develop questionnaires (instruments), which have been thoroughly tested and validated. Instruments should be available to evaluate both psychological well-being and physical symptom distress.[4] The areas (domains) for such evaluations are shown in Table 51-1.[5]

Many questionnaires have been developed. Because most clinical studies arbitrarily pick and choose from these questionnaires, it is difficult to make direct comparisons between studies that have not used identical instruments.[6,7] An additional methodologic issue in QOL assessments relates to the clinical significance of changes in measurement scores. Most instruments use a five- to seven-point scale from least to most affected. In large studies, there may be only a fraction of a point change in the score, statistically significant, but of uncertain clinical importance. In a recent report, changes in QOL scores were plotted against scores for stressful life events (Fig. 51-1).[8] The observed correlation confirms, at least for a large population, that QOL measures do have clinical relevance.

A number of specific methodologic considerations should enter into the analysis of a QOL,[9] such as (a) QOL studies are generally underpowered because power analyses focus on primary efficacy outcomes; small sample sizes dramatically reduce the power and validity of the trial and have a tremendous impact on the statistical and clinical interpretations made from a trial. Small sample size generally means underrepresentation of important target groups; thus, age, gender, and ethnicity are often neglected considerations. The importance of this cannot be overstated because, for example, women have been observed to report more symptoms and have been shown to repeatedly report lower health-related QOL scores.[10,11] (b) Even in the case of a large sample size, the sensitivity to change of the QOL measure must be known because small differences in QOL may have important effects on the conclusions of pharmacoeconomic studies. (c) If the meaning of differences in QOL scores is to be understood, calibration in terms of commonly experienced life events is mandatory. (d) The common practice of reporting QOL change as overall mean differences may well wash out important treatment effect differences. (e) QOL reports not uncommonly fail

TABLE 51-1. Domains of Quality of Life

Physical status
    Symptoms
    Sleep and rest
    Sexual functioning
Functional status
    Physical activity
Emotional status
    Anxiety
    Depression
    Irritability and anger
    Stress
    Spiritual well-being
Cognitive functioning
    Attention and concentration
    Clarity of thinking
    Psychomotor functioning
Performance of social roles
    Work performance
    Household management
    Community activities
General well-being
    Life satisfaction
    Energy and vitality

Source: Modified with permission from Croog.[5]

to deal with issues of patient drop-out or missing data; if patients' having dropped out are excluded from data analysis, results are biased in favor of those having completed the trial and who had better QOL scores. Moreover, the issue of missing data, although ubiquitous as an issue in clinical trials, is rarely addressed in QOL studies. (f) QOL analyses will gain an order of magnitude in sensitivity if changes are indexed by the length of time that individuals spend in different health states. Currently, there is an appalling lack of long-term QOL change with therapeutic interventions. It has been suggested that the maximum effect of antihypertensive therapy on QOL requires at least 16 to 18 weeks of therapy.[1,3,12] (g) In this regard, it is claimed that patients who experience medication-related side effects do so shortly after drug initiation; thereafter, those who continue to receive medication "develop a tolerance or diminution

of effect over time" allowing short-term duration trials to detect all relevant differences in a short period.[3]

With these seven interpretive precautions in mind, publications on QOL have geometrically increased in the last two decades.[8] It has now become standard practice in many clinical studies to include information on the effect of the regimen or a specific treatment on QOL.

CLINICAL STUDIES

Clinical studies on QOL associated with the use of CV drug therapy can be divided into two categories. In the first category are those studies carried out in CV conditions either associated with no or minimal symptoms, the main examples being hypertension and hypercholesterolemia. Life-long treatment is the usual rule, and the effect of the drug on QOL becomes especially important if an asymptomatic patient believes that his or her QOL is worsened by the drug. In this regard, well-designed cognitive-behavioral interventions may be employed as adjunctive treatment in reducing or eliminating drug requirements in hypertensive subjects, a finding quite pertinent to QOL in treated hypertensives.[13] Nonadherence is a likely outcome, which is regrettable, because interventions against hypertension and hypercholesterolemia have proven quite effective in diminishing the morbidity and mortality of these illnesses. Adherence to drug therapy can be improved by low-dose fixed combination antihypertensive therapy, but few, if any, QOL studies have been conducted with combination drug therapy.[14] In the second group of CV diseases are those with obvious clinical symptoms; for example, angina, MI, and CHF. Far fewer QOL studies have been carried out on these conditions, but in ongoing and future research assessment of QOL will undoubtedly be included.

Hypertension

Interest in QOL studies in patients receiving antihypertensive drugs was greatly stimulated by the report of Croog et al.[3] This multicenter, randomized, double-blind study of 626 males with mild to moderate hypertension set the standard for studies using

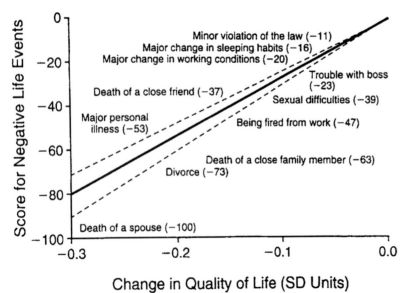

FIGURE 51-1. Calibration of changes in overall scores for quality of life with the corresponding scores for stressful life events. A total of 2938 pairs of change scores were obtained for 824 male patients with hypertension who participated in two randomized clinical trials of antihypertensive therapy. The changes in quality of life shown are computed from statistical summary scores of 11 components from the social, psychological, and physical domains. Examples of life events (followed in parentheses by their associated scores) are shown in the body of the figure, with lower negative numbers indicating greater stress and worse quality of life. The thick line is the regression slope, and the upper and lower dashed lines are the standard error. (*Modified with permission from Testa MA et al.*[8])

state-of-the-art measures for assessment of QOL. This study compared captopril, propranolol, and α-methyldopa and showed that these three drugs differed in their effects on QOL. Favorable effects correlated with withdrawal rates, varying from 8% for captopril, to 13% for propranolol, to 20% for α-methyldopa. Patients taking captopril scored significantly higher on measures of general well-being and life satisfaction, and they had fewer side effects and less sexual dysfunction. This report has been followed by a large number of other studies of antihypertensive drugs, some of which are summarized in Table 51-2.[1,3,10,12,15–28] In general, these studies suggest that use of angiotensin converting enzyme (ACE) inhibitors or angiotensin-receptor blockers (ARBs) is not associated with a decrease in general well-being and may even result in an improvement in mood, affect, or cognitive function.

There is an inherent risk in making cross-study comparisons because different survey instruments are generally used, duration of treatment typically lacks uniformity, and protocols vary widely. To avoid these confounding variables, a meta-analysis of 13 trials involving 2516 patients was carried out using strict criteria, which eliminated 41 other published studies.[29] The statistical technique employed in this meta-analysis allowed studies with different measurement scales to be combined. A χ^2 test for homogeneity was calculated for each drug and QOL domain, revealing nonsignificance and permitting individual studies to be merged. It should be considered that the published studies incorporated into a meta-analysis might present the best-case situation for an observation because negative results are less commonly published. Table 51-3 summarizes these findings. Of the 2516 patients included in this meta-analysis, 81% were male, 19% female, 72% white, and 28% black. The QOL constructs (domains) were sexual function, sleep, psychomotor function, general well-being, and mood. The authors concluded that only a small effect (0.2 scale units) or no effect was seen for all pharmacologic classes and all constructs.[29] No negative effect was seen with any treatment, and none of the drugs had a clearly superior effect. The ACE inhibitors, CCBs, and beta-blockers all had greater or more positive effects. ARBs were not yet available at the time of this meta-analysis, therefore they were not included. This meta-analysis fails to identify any drug groups that are clearly superior in lowering blood pressure while maintaining or improving QOL.

In a similar type analysis, QOL studies of antihypertensive therapy were questioned in a systematic review of 25 randomized, controlled trials that met specific criteria for selection.[30] Particular criticisms were levied at inconsistent definitions of the QOL, problems with validity and reliability of measures used, failures of standardization in the administration of questionnaires, inappropriate handling of data, and inadequate interpretation of results. Many of these same points are reinforced in a review by Testa and Lenderking.[9] QOL studies in patients receiving beta-blockers have also been reviewed.[31,32] Central nervous system side effects of beta-blockers can be minimized by low doses and by use of β_1-selective blockers. Although there are few QOL studies of diuretics, depression of sexual function, even in low doses, is a well-recognized thiazide diuretic side effect and can be a reason for significant impairment of quality of life.[33] As regards CCBs, QOL effect may be a function of duration of medication effect and/or differences in delivery systems. For example, nifedipine GITS produces a better pattern of QOL improvement than does amlodipine, a difference presumably related to the very long half-life of amlodipine.[34] Moreover, in studying treatment effects on QOL with CCBs, both the distress of physical symptoms and the change in psychosocial factors should

be assessed.[4] Thus, an important consideration in the treatment of hypertension is that the impact of therapy on QOL may not be uniform within a pharmacologic class of drugs. Optimal pharmacologic management cannot simply be limited to objective findings from a patient's physiologic and metabolic profile. Care of the hypertensive patient should also incorporate an assessment of QOL, a concept that transcends documentation of side effects and appreciates a patient's perception of functional capacity, productivity, and sense of well-being. In addition, clinically meaningful information may be obtained from individuals closest to the patient.[12]

Two additional QOL issues are of clinical importance. First, there has been concern over potential adverse effects of hypertension treatment in the elderly. In the elderly, concerns over the effects of blood pressure reduction have centered on cognition, depression, and mood. The Systolic Hypertension in the Elderly Program (SHEP), a trial in patients 60 years of age or older, compared the diuretic chlorthalidone with or without a beta-blocker or reserpine to placebo. The SHEP trial involved a range of psychometric testing, including global QOL, recording of troublesome symptoms that developed, and measurements of activities of daily living (ADL). The results of this testing were noteworthy, reassuring, and the first to point out that in the course of hypertension treatment, patients can "feel better."[35,36] In the SHEP trial, scores on tests of cognition, mood, and depression favored the active treatment group, although results were only statistically significant for mood. ADL and social leisure activities were also slightly better in the active treatment group. Alternatively, symptoms described as "minor adverse effects" were slightly more common in the active treatment group; these included fatigue, sexual dysfunction, muscle weakness, and self-reported memory problems.[35] Second, the effect of a change in diet and/or lifestyle, which represent noninvasive therapeutic changes, on QOL was speculated upon.[37,38] A substudy in the Dietary Approaches to Stop Hypertension (DASH) examined the effects on blood pressure and QOL of three diets: a typical U.S. diet; a diet that emphasized intake of fruits and vegetables; and a combination diet, which stressed fruit and vegetable intake as well as low-fat dairy products. In this substudy of 83 study participants, changes in health-related QOL as measured by the Medical Outcomes Short Form-36 favored both experimental groups over the control diet group, although results were only statistically significant for the subscale measuring perceived change in health.[37] The positive effects on QOL in this substudy are not surprising in that the DASH study mandated considerable social interaction and no restriction on caloric intake, even though dietary choices were restricted. Unfortunately, the small sample size in this substudy, and the limited sensitivity of the Medical Outcomes Short Form[38] subscales in detecting change, limit the strength of the findings.

Hypercholesterolemia

Elevated serum cholesterol is an asymptomatic condition and efforts to reduce cholesterol levels by diet and/or drugs must take this into account. If the patient perceives that his or her QOL is worsened by the prescribed regimen, failure to adhere is likely. Treatment of elevated cholesterol is rapidly increasing in clinical practice, for both persons free of clinical coronary heart disease (CHD) and those with clinical manifestations of CHF, such as angina and MI. Because diet and drugs are usually prescribed together, it will be difficult to avoid the confounding of the effects of the two regimens on QOL. It is strange that there are so few studies on the QOL in patients

TABLE 51-2. Recent Double-Blind, Randomized, Parallel-Design Quality-of-Life Studies in Hypertensive Subjects

Lead Author (y)	Treatment Groups	Number of Patients	Treatment Duration	QOL Results	Comments
Karlberg (1999)[27]	Telmisartan	139	3–5-wk placebo lead-in		
	Enalapril	139	16-wk titration	No difference between E and	Cough present in 16% of
	± HCTZ		10-wk maintenance	Tel in quality-of-life scores	E-treated subjects
Dahlof (1997)[28]	Losartan	300	4-wk placebo lead-in	Lo > Am for psychologic	30.6% of Am group reported
	Los + HCTZ	298	6-wk titration	well-being; (60% of Lo,	"swollen ankles"
	Amlodipine	298	6-wk maintenance	54% of Lo + HCTZ, and	
				50% of Am improved)	
Testa (1993)[12]	Captopril	192	4-wk placebo lead-in	C > E for vitality, general	BP lowering and side-effect
	Enalapril	187	10-wk titration	health status, behavioral/	profiles similar; baseline
	± HCTZ		14-wk maintenance	emotional control	QOL significant covariate
Omvik (1993)[15]	Amlodipine	231	4-wk placebo lead-in	No significant differences	BP reduction similar;
	Enalapril	230	12-wk titration		Enalapril—cough (13%)
	± HCTZ		38-wk maintenance		Amlod—edema (22%)
Fletcher (1992)[16]	Pinacidil	127	3–6 washout phase	P > N for psychological	Significant edema in both
	Nifedipine	130	6-wk titration	general well-being and	groups
	± thiazide diuretic		20-wk maintenance	cognitive function subscale	
Fletcher (1992)[10]	Cilazapril	179	4-wk placebo lead-in	CZ = A > N for physical	N > discontinued rate due to
	Nifedipine	179	12-wk titration	complaint score; N > CZ =	adverse events (17%) vs
	Atenolol	182	12-wk maintenance	A for fatigue subscale	A (8%) or CZ (5%);
	± HCTZ				multilingual QOL study
Testa (1991)[1]	Atenolol	193	4-wk placebo lead-in	N > A for completers for	More N patients discontinued
	Nifedipine	201	8-wk titration	psychological and physical	due to adverse events (16%)
			12-wk maintenance	well-being; no difference	vs 4% (A); GITS
				for all randomized patients	formulation
Frimodt-Moeller (1991)[17]	Lisinopril	175	2-wk placebo lead-in	L > M for work activity	More M patients discontinued
	Metoprolol	185	4-wk titration	visual analogue scale	due to adverse events
	± HCTZ		4-wk maintenance		
Dahlof (1991)[18]	Diltiazem	xx	2-wk placebo lead-in	No significant differences	Trend contentment, vitality
	Metoprolol	xx	8-wk titration	with high-dose M	
			4-wk maintenance		
Applegate (1991)[19]	Diltiazem	79	4–6-wk placebo lead-in	No significant differences	Females ≥ 65 years of age,
	Atenolol	79	4-wk titration		D > BP lowering, adequate
	Enalapril	84	8-wk maintenance		sample size?
Steiner (1990)[20]	Atenolol	90	3–5-wk placebo lead-in	A = C = E > PR for	Treatment duration short,
	Captopril	91	1–4-wk titration	psychological general	depressed mood improved
	Enalapril	90	4-wk maintenance	well-being	with C vs baseline
	Propranolol	89			
Palmer (1990)[21]	Verapamil	41	3-wk placebo lead-in	V > N for cognitive	Psychological well-being
	Nifedipine	40	16-wk treatment	performance	tended to improve with V
					and deteriorate with N
Fletcher (1990)[22]	Atenolol	62	3-wk lead-in phase	No significant differences	Trend toward decreased
	Captopril	63	8-wk maintenance		depression (C) &
					anxiety/hostility (A);
					adequate sample size?
Croog (1990)[23]	Atenolol	128	2–4-wk placebo lead-in	No significant differences	Black males and black
	Captopril	123	4-wk initial therapy		females; maintenance phase
	Verapamil	117	4-wk forced titration		short
Blumenthal (1990)[24]	Atenolol	15	4-wk placebo lead-in	No significant differences	Small sample size
	Enalapril	15	4-wk titration		
	± HCTZ		8-wk maintenance		
Herrick (1989)[25]	Atenolol	76	4-wk placebo lead-in	No significant differences	E produced greater
	Enalapril	86	16-wk treatment		BP-lowering effect
Fletcher (1989)[26]	Propranolol	47	3-wk placebo lead-in		
	Verapamil	47	6-wk titration	V > PR for health status index	
			10-wk maintenance	(activity, perceived health)	
Croog (1986)[3]	Captopril	213	4-wk placebo lead-in	C > M-D = PR for general	More M-D patients
	Methyldopa	201	10-wk titration	well-being; PR > M-D for	discontinued due to adverse
	Propranolol	212	14-wk maintenance	work performance; C > PR	events (20%) than PR
	± HCTZ			for less sexual dysfunction	(13%) or C (8%)

A = atenolol; Am = amlodipine; C = captopril; CZ = cilazapril; D = diltiazem; E = enalapril; HCTZ = hydrochlorothiazide; L = lisinopril; Lo = losartan; M = metoprolol; M-D = methyldopa; P = pinacidil; PR = propranolol; Tel = telmisartan; V = verapamil.

TABLE 51-3. Summary of Quality-of-Life Effect

Construct	ACEI	β-blocker	CAAA	CCB	Diuretic	Vaso	All drugs
Sexual function	0	0	0	0	nd	nd	0
Sleep	0	0	0	0	nd	nd	+
Psychomotor function	+	+	+	+	+	0	+
General well-being	0	0	0	+	w	nd	+
Mood	0	+	0	0	+	0	+
All constructs	+	+	0	+	+	0	

+ = positive; 0 = no difference; nd = no data available for analysis; ACEI = angiotensin-converting enzyme inhibitor; CAAA = centrally acting α_2-agonist; CCB = calcium-channel blocker; Vaso = direct vasodilator.

Source: Reproduced with permission from Bansal VK et al.[29]

on weight-reduction or fat-restricted diets, and a limited number of studies assessing the effect of lipid-lowering drugs on QOL. Studies in this area are necessary because cross-sectional studies suggest that serum lipid concentrations may influence cognitive function, mood, and behavior. To date, dose-ranging studies, head-to-head comparisons of different agents, different modes of dietary cholesterol reduction, and age have not identified substantive consequences to be associated with cholesterol reduction.[39–43]

That weight-reduction diets are usually ineffective because of nonadherence or recidivism is well known. Also, dietary restriction of fat and cholesterol usually, in practice, produces far less in cholesterol reduction than the maximum attainable (15%). Yet, some studies show that weight loss is associated with an improvement in QOL.[33,44] In view of these facts, physicians and patients have placed increasing reliance on lipid-lowering drugs. Those lipid-lowering drugs with obvious side effects (nicotinic acid) or unpleasant taste (resins) have been supplemented by the HMG-CoA reductase inhibitors (statins). Although there are extensive studies on the benefits of cholesterol reduction with the statin drugs, emphasis so far has been on mechanisms, pathogenesis, and end results.[45] In patients with symptomatic CHD, the relief of symptoms or the prevention of death outweighs, perhaps, any side effects of the drug regimen. Yet, as increased emphasis is placed on primary prevention, the issue of QOL in patients treated with the statin drugs will assume added importance and demand appropriate studies beyond the known side effects of lipid-lowering drug regimens.

Coronary Heart Disease

Drugs used in the acute syndromes of CHD, such as unstable angina and acute MI do not require QOL studies because the short-term nature of the illness requires immediate symptom relief or prevention of end points. In chronic CHD and/or intermittent claudication, quality-of-life becomes a more relevant issue.[6,46] Chronic CHD is a condition particularly well-suited to the use of QOL measures because many interventions are directed toward improving QOL rather than specifically extending survival.[47] Because the operating characteristics of the various QOL instruments for coronary artery disease differ in their psychometric properties, such as their internal reliability, test-retest reliability, and their responsiveness to change, the instrument selected can be as important as the reported findings.[6,48] In particular, the physical distress symptom index is a sensitive technique for assessing the influence of CV treatment on QOL. In studying treatment effects on QOL, both the distress specifically associated with physical symptoms and the change in psychosocial factors should be evaluated.[48]

Digitalis was compared with captopril in a 2-year study of post-MI patients with regional wall motion abnormalities and mild CHF [New York Heart Association (NYHA) Classes II and III].[49] Digitalis significantly improved general well-being, symptom score, as well as vitality, and improved the NYHA class in 45% of patients. Although early in the course of treatment with captopril angina worsened, by the completion of the study its use was accompanied by a marked improvement in QOL indices. Alternatively, in elderly patients, use of CV drugs, such as digitalis and diuretics, was associated with impaired QOL as well as increased feelings of loneliness.[50] Because this was a cross-sectional study, the use of digitalis, diuretics, and other CV drugs only served to identify sick people and did not technically answer the question as to whether QOL was, in fact, better before these medications were started. Finally, use of β_1-selective blockers has been reported to improve the QOL to the same degree as ACE inhibitors in patients with angina and following MI.[51]

Congestive Heart Failure

The use of agents that interrupt the renin-angiotensin-aldosterone axis are standard in the management of CHF, with ACE inhibitors being the first choice of most physicians.[52] Relief of symptoms and prevention of morbid and mortal events are the main criteria for successful treatment with ACE inhibitors. In other clinical settings, such as hypertension, use of ACE inhibitors is associated with an improvement in QOL, and it is reasonable to assume that they would be equally well tolerated by patients with CHF, although women with CHF who are treated with ACE inhibitors have worse quality-of-life ratings than do men for a range of intermediate activities, including daily living and social activity.[53] More recently, the ARB valsartan was shown to have a positive effect on QOL in CHF. Among the 1504 patients in the valsartan treatment group in the Valsartan Heart Failure Trial (VAL-HEFT) to whom the Minnesota Living with Heart Failure questionnaire was administered, there was little change in scores from baseline to the end-point, but among the 1506 patients in the placebo group, the mean score worsened by an average of 1.9.[54] Finally, recent studies in Class II to IV CHF patients stabilized with optimum standard therapy, employing a controlled-release form of the β_1-selective blocker metoprolol, showed a beneficial effect on patient well-being when compared to placebo.[55]

As the above suggests health-related QOL, representing a patient-driven end point, is increasingly emphasized in randomized clinical trials of new CHF therapies (Table 51-4).[56–64] Measurement of health-related QOL depends on the use of validated instruments,

TABLE 51-4. Sampling of Quality-of-Life Trials in Congestive Heart Failure

Study Name	Medication	N	EF/NYHA	QOL Results
SOLVD (treatment arm)[56]	Enalapril	2465	LVEF 0.35	Customized QOL scale; consistent superiority in QOL (social functioning and dyspnea) at 6 weeks and 1 year; an average of 40% of QOL responses were missing at 2 years of follow-up because of death or failure to complete the questionnaire
V-HEFT II[57]	Enalapril vs hydralazine + isosorbide dinitrate	804	LVEF 0.45	No significant differences amongst either treatment group; decline in QOL score despite treatment in both groups
ELITE II[58]	Losartan vs captopril	203	NYHA II-IV	Significant improvements in both treatment limbs, trend favoring losartan in drug tolerability/QOL; fewer study withdrawals for unfavorable reasons (10.9% for losartan and 19.6% for captopril)
RESOLVD[59]	Candesartan vs enalapril vs both	768	NYHA II-IV	Minnesota Living with Heart Failure Questionnaire: no significant difference in QOL or NYHA functional class at 18 or 43 weeks
V-HeFT III[60]	Felodipine vs placebo	450	LVEF 0.45	Minnesota Living with Heart Failure Questionnaire: trend for less worsening with felodipine treatment at 27 months (n = 112)
BEST[61]	Bucindolol	2708	NYHA III-IV	Not reported: health-related quality of life reported as secondary end point
CIBIS-II[62]	Bisoprolol	2647	NYHA III-IV	Not assessed
COPERNICUS[63]	Carvedilol	2289	LVEF < 0.29	More patients self-reported as improved
MERIT-HF[55]	Metoprolol	3991 (741 QOL)	NYHA II-IV	Improvement in treatment group ($P = .009$) using McMaster Overall Treatment Evaluation; $P = .2$ with Minnesota Living with Heart Failure Questionnaire
US Carvedilol Heart Failure Study Group[64]	Carvedilol	1094	NYHA II-IV	QOL questionnaire; unpublished

with attention paid to the timing of administration and analysis of data in the context of conventional morbidity and mortality endpoints. In a recent review of health-related QOL measurement in CHF drug trials published from 1966 to 1999, important data, such as the number of participating subjects, was often found lacking. Improvements in trial methodology are warranted if QOL data are to be meaningful in the determination of drug efficacy in CHF.[65]

Postmenopausal States

The use of estrogens in postmenopausal women for the prevention of osteoporosis and CHD is increasing, but is far from being universally accepted by women.[66] Because many of the distressing symptoms associated with menopause are relieved with estrogen therapy, QOL is improved and adherence to long-term treatment can be anticipated.

CLINICAL IMPLICATIONS OF QUALITY-OF-LIFE STUDIES

Quality-of-life studies can be of great value to clinicians by revealing the effects of a class of drugs or a particular drug, which might bear importantly on compliance.[67] However, a critical review of 75 articles in the current literature revealed that a conceptual definition of QOL was given in only 15%, the targeted domains were identified in only 47%, the reason for choosing the QOL instrument was given in only 36%, and aggregated results in a QOL score provided in only 36%.[68] In only 12% of articles were patients invited to

make their own appraisal of QOL. Therefore, published articles on QOL must be viewed critically before the clinician makes therapeutic decisions. Despite these caveats, QOL studies have a tremendous potential for improving medical care and reducing noncompliance.

Studies of large populations might not necessarily apply to the individual patient and, therefore, the clinician must be alert and mindful of the effect of treatment on the QOL of each person. This can be accomplished in a variety of ways. A questionnaire can be administered to individuals before and periodically during treatment, or the same done in small group sessions.[69] Such questionnaires, although widely available, may not necessarily provide a comprehensive view of all "side-effects." For example, sexual dysfunction is poorly established as a side-effect in women, due to the lack of established methodology.[70] How widely this or any other available questionnaire will be used by the time-pressured practitioner is uncertain. At the very least, clinicians must always be aware that their judgment of the effects of treatment might not be shared by the patient or immediate family members.[1,2] A more detailed interview going beyond the mere elicitation of side effects known to be associated with the drug or drugs used should attempt to make a global assessment of how the patient really feels. QOL studies in hypertension have focused primarily on drug side effects because of the strong correlation between side affects and adherence. The patient's short-term and long-term QOL depends on the physicians understanding of the complex relationship among human behavior, QOL, adherence, efficacy, and outcome, and the ability of the physician to use that knowledge to identify optimal therapies for the individual patient. This effort will be amply rewarded by greater adherence and patient satisfaction.[71]

REFERENCES

1. Testa MA, Hollenberg NK, Anderson RB, Williams GH: Assessment of quality of life by patient and spouse during antihypertensive therapy with atenolol and nifedipine gastrointestinal therapeutic system. *Am J Hypertens* 4:363, 1991.

2. Jachuck SJ, Brierly H, Jachuck S, Willcox PM: The effect of hypotensive drugs on the quality of life. *J R Coll Gen Pract* 32:103, 1982.

3. Croog SH, Levine S, Testa MA, et al: The effects of antihypertensive therapy on the quality of life. *N Engl J Med* 314:1657, 1986.

4. Anderson RB, Hollenberg NK, Williams GH: Physical symptoms distress index: A sensitive tool to evaluate the impact of pharmacological agents on quality of life. *Arch Intern Med* 159:693, 1999.

5. Croog SH: Quality of life and the hypertensive patient: Clinical aspects. In: Puzi H, Flamenbaum W, eds. *Clinical Cardiovascular Therapeutics.* Vol 1. Mt. Kisco, NY: Futura Publishing, 1989.

6. Dougherty C, Dewhurst T, Nichol WP, Spertus J: Comparison of three quality-of-life instruments in stable angina pectoris: Seattle Angina Questionnaire, Short Form Health Survey (SF-36) and Quality of Life Index-Cardiac Version III. *J Clin Epidemiol* 51:569, 1998.

7. Cote I, Gregoire JP, Moisan J: Health-related quality-of-life measurement in hypertension. A review of randomized controlled drug trials. *Pharmacoeconomics* 18:435, 2000.

8. Testa MA, Simonson DC: Assessment of quality-of-life outcomes. *N Engl J Med* 334:835, 1996.

9. Testa MA, Lenderking WR: Interpreting pharmacoeconomic and quality of life clinical trials for use in therapeutics. *Pharmacoeconomics* 2:107, 1992.

10. Fletcher AE, Bulpitt CJ, Chase DM, et al: Quality of life with three antihypertensive treatments: cilazapril, atenolol, nifedipine. *Hypertension* 19:499, 1992.

11. Ware JE, Snow KK, Kosinki M, et al: *SF-36 Health Survey Manual and Interpretation Guide.* Boston: Nimrod Press, 1993.

12. Testa MA, Anderson RB, Nackley JF, Hollenberg NK, and the Quality-of-Life Hypertension Study Group: Quality of life and antihypertensive therapy in men: a comparison of captopril and enalapril. *N Engl J Med* 328:907, 1993.

13. Shapiro D, Hui KK, Oakley ME, et al: Reduction in drug requirements for hypertension by means of a cognitive-behavioral intervention. *Am J Hypertens* 10:9, 1997.

14. Ambrosioni E: Pharmacoeconomics of hypertension management: The place of combination therapy. *Pharmacoeconomics* 19:337, 2001.

15. Omvik P, Thaulow E, Herland OB, et al: Double-blind, parallel, comparative study on quality of life during treatment with amlodipine or enalapril in mild to moderate hypertensive patients: A multicentre study. *J Hypertens* 1:103, 1993.

16. Fletcher AE, Battersby C, Adnitt P, et al: Quality of life on antihypertensive therapy: A double-blind trial comparing quality of life on pinacidil and nifedipine in combination with a thiazide diuretic. *J Cardiovasc Pharmacol* 20:108, 1992.

17. Frimodt-Moeller J, Loldrup Poulsen D, Bech P: Quality of life, side effects and efficacy of lisinopril compared with metoprolol in patients with mild to moderate essential hypertension. *J Hum Hypertens* 5:215, 1991.

18. Dahlof C, Hedner T, Thulin T, et al: The effects of diltiazem and metoprolol on blood pressure, adverse symptoms and general well-being. *Eur J Clin Pharmacol* 40:453, 1991.

19. Applegate WB, Phillips HL, Schnaper H, et al: A randomized controlled trial of the effects of three antihypertensive agents on blood pressure control and quality of life in older women. *Arch Intern Med* 151:1817, 1991.

20. Steiner SS, Friedhoff AJ, Wilson BL, et al: Antihypertensive therapy and quality of life: A comparison of atenolol, captopril, enalapril and propranolol. *J Hum Hypertens* 4:217, 1990.

21. Palmer A, Fletcher A, Hamilton G, et al: A comparison of verapamil and nifedipine on quality of life. *Br J Clin Pharmacol* 30:365, 1990.

22. Fletcher AE, Bulpitt CJ, Hawkins CM, et al: Quality of life on antihypertensive therapy: A randomized double-blind controlled trial of captopril and atenolol. *J Hypertens* 8:463, 1990.

23. Croog SH, Kong BW, Levine S, et al: Hypertensive black men and women; quality of life and effects of antihypertensive medications. Black Hypertension Quality of Life Multicenter Trial Group. *Arch Intern Med* 150:1733, 1990.

24. Blumenthal JA, Ekelund LG, Emery CF: Quality of life among hypertensive patients with a diuretic background who are taking atenolol and enalapril. *Clin Pharmacol Ther* 48:447, 1990.

25. Herrick AL, Waller PC, Berkin KE, et al: Comparison of enalapril and atenolol in mild to moderate hypertension. *Am J Med* 86:421, 1989.

26. Fletcher AE, Chester PC, Hawkins CM, et al: The effects of verapamil and propranolol on quality of life in hypertension. *J Hum Hypertens* 3:125, 1989.

27. Karlberg BE, Lins LE, Hermansson K for the TEES Study Group: Efficacy and safety of telmisartan, a selective AT_1-receptor antagonist, compared with enalapril in elderly patients with primary hypertension. *J Hypertens* 17:293, 1999.

28. Dahlof B, Lindholm LH, Carney S, et al: Main results of the losartan versus amlodipine study on drug tolerability and psychological general well-being. *J Hypertens* 15:1327, 1997.

29. Bansal VK, Beto JA: Antihypertensive therapy: Quality of life assessment. *Cardiovasc Rev Rep* Dec:21, 1994.

30. Hunt SM: Quality of life claims of anti-hypertensive therapy. *Qual Life Res* 6:185, 1997.

31. Dahlof C, Dimenas E, Kendall M, Wiklund I: Quality of life in cardiovascular diseases: Emphasis on beta-blocker treatment. *Circulation* 84(Suppl 6):VI108, 1991.

32. Wiklund I: Quality of life and cost-effectiveness in the treatment of hypertension. *J Clin Pharm Ther* 19:81, 1994.

33. Neaton JD, Grimm RH Jr, Prineas RP, et al: The Treatment of Mild Hypertension Study: Final results. Treatment of Mild Hypertension Study Research Group. *JAMA* 270:713, 1993.

34. Testa MA, Turner RR, Simonson DC, et al: Quality of life and calcium channel blockade with nifedipine GITS versus amlodipine in hypertensive patients in Spain. *J Hypertens* 16:1839, 1998.

35. Applegate WB: Quality of life during antihypertensive treatment: Lessons from the Systolic Hypertension in the Elderly Program. *Am J Hypertens* 11:57S, 1998.

36. Wiklund I, Halling K, Ryden-Bergsten T, et al: Does lowering the blood pressure improve the mood? Quality of life results from the Hypertension Optimal Treatment (HOT) study. *Blood Press* 6:357, 1997.

37. Plaisted CS, Lin PH, Ard JD, et al: The effects of dietary patterns on quality of life: A substudy of the Dietary Approaches to Stop Hypertension trial. *J Am Diet Assoc* 99(Suppl 8):S84,1999.

38. Grimm RH, Grandits GA, Cutler JA, et al: Relationship of quality-of-life measures to long-term lifestyle and drug treatment in the treatment of mild hypertension study. *Arch Intern Med* 157:638, 1997.

39. Weir MR, Berger ML, Weeks ML, et al: Comparison of the effects on quality of life and of the efficacy and tolerability of lovastatin versus pravastatin. The Quality of Life Multicenter Group. *Am J Cardiol* 77:475, 1996.

40. Santanello NC, Barber BL, Applegate WB, et al: Effect of pharmacological lipid lowering on health-related quality of life in older persons: Results from the Cholesterol Reduction in Senior Program Pilot Study. *J Am Geriatr Soc* 45:8, 1997.

41. Seed M, Weir MR: Double-masked comparison of the quality of life of hypercholesterolemic men treated with simvastatin or pravastatin. International Quality of Life Multicenter Group. *Clin Ther* 21:1758, 1999.

42. Wardle J, Rogers P, Judd P, et al: Randomized trial of the effects of cholesterol-lowering dietary treatment on psychological function. *Am J Med* 108:547, 2000.

43. Muldoon MF, Barger SD, Ryan CM, et al: Effects of lovastatin on cognitive function and psychological well-being. *Am J Med* 108:538, 2000.

44. Wassertheil-Smoller S, Oberman A, Blaufox MD, et al: The Trial of Antihypertensives Interventions and Management (TAIM): Final results with regard to blood pressure, cardiovascular risk and quality of life. *Am J Hypertens* 5:37, 1992.

45. Sacks JM, Pfeffer MA, Braunwald E, eds. A symposium: Cholesterol-lowering trials: New results and emerging issues. *Am J Cardiol* 76:1c, 1995.

46. Schmieder FA, Comerota AJ: Intermittent claudication: Magnitude of the problem, patient evaluation, and therapeutic strategies. *Am J Cardiol* 87(Suppl 1):3, 2001.

47. Toobert DJ, Glasgow RE, Radcliffe JL: Physiologic and related behavioral outcomes from the Women's Lifestyle Heart Trial. *Ann Behav Med* 22:1, 2000.

48. Hollenberg NK, Williams GH, Anderson R: Medical therapy, symptoms, and the distress they cause: Relation to quality of life in patients with angina pectoris and/or hypertension. *Arch Intern Med* 160:1477, 2000.

49. Just H, Drexler H, Taylor SH, et al: Captopril versus digoxin in patients with coronary artery disease and mild heart failure: A prospective, double-blind, placebo controlled multicentre study. The CADS Study Group. *Herz* 18(Suppl 1):436, 1993.

50. Jensen E, Dehlin O, Hagberg B, et al: Medical, psychological, and sociological aspects of drug treatment in 80-year-olds. *Z Gerontol* 27:140, 1994.

51. Cruickshank JM: The beta-1 hyperselectivity in beta-blocker treatment. *J Cardiovasc Pharmacol* 25(Suppl 1):S35, 1995.

52. Just H, Drexler H, Hasenfuss G: Pathophysiology and treatment of congestive heart failure. *Cardiology* 84(Suppl 2):99, 1994.

53. Riedinger MS, Dracup KA, Brecht ML, et al: Quality of life in patients with heart failure: do gender differences exist? *Heart Lung* 30:105, 2001.

54. Cohn JN, Tognoni G: A randomized trial of the angiotensin-receptor blocker valsartan in chronic heart failure. *N Engl J Med* 345:1667, 2001.

55. Hjalmarson A, Goldstein S, Fagerberg B, et al: Effects of controlled-release metoprolol on total mortality, hospitalizations, and well-being in patients with heart failure: The Metoprolol CR/XL Randomized Intervention Trial in congestive heart failure (MERIT-HF). MERIT-HF Study Group. *JAMA* 283:1295, 2000.

56. Rogers WJ, Johnstone DE, Yusuf S, et al: Quality of life among 5,025 patients with left ventricular dysfunction randomized between placebo and enalapril: The Studies of Left Ventricular Dysfunction. The SOLVD Investigators. *J Am Coll Cardiol* 23:393, 1994.

57. Rector TS, Johnson G, Dunkman WB, et al: Evaluation by patients with heart failure of the effects of enalapril compared with hydralazine plus isosorbide dinitrate on quality of life. V-HeFT II. The V-HeFT VA Cooperative Studies Group. *Circulation* 87(Suppl 6):VI71, 1993.

58. Cowley AJ, Wiens BL, Segal R, et al: Randomised comparison of losartan vs. captopril on quality of life in elderly patients with symptomatic heart failure: The losartan heart failure ELITE quality of life substudy. *Qual Life Res* 9:377, 2000.

59. McKelvie RS, Yusuf S, Pericak D, et al: Comparison of candesartan, enalapril, and their combination in congestive heart failure: Randomized evaluation of strategies for left ventricular dysfunction (RESOLVD) pilot study. The RESOLVD Pilot Study Investigators. *Circulation* 100:1056, 1999.

60. Cohn JN, Ziesche S, Smith R, et al: Effect of the calcium antagonist felodipine as supplementary vasodilator therapy in patients with chronic heart failure treated with enalapril: V-HeFT III. Vasodilator-Heart Failure Trial (V-HeFT) Study Group. *Circulation* 96:856, 1997.

61. Design of the Beta-Blocker Evaluation Survival Trial (BEST). The BEST Steering Committee. *Am J Cardiol* 75:1220, 1995.

62. The Cardiac Insufficiency Bisoprolol Study II (CIBIS-II): A randomised trial *Lancet* 353:9, 1999.

63. Louis A, Cleland JG, Crabbe S, et al: Clinical Trials Update: CAPRICORN, COPERNICUS, MIRACLE, STAF, RITZ-2, RECOVER and RENAISSANCE and cachexia and cholesterol in heart failure. Highlights of the scientific sessions of the American College of Cardiology, 2001. *Eur J Heart Fail* 3:381, 2001.

64. Packer M, Bristow MR, Cohn JN, et al: The effect of carvedilol on morbidity and mortality in patients with chronic heart failure. US Carvedilol Heart Failure Study Group. *N Engl J Med* 334:1349, 1996.

65. al-Kaade S, Hauptman PJ: Health-related quality of life measurement in heart failure: Challenges for the new millennium. *J Card Fail* 7:194, 2001.

66. Sinclair HK, Bond CM, Taylor RJ: Hormone replacement therapy: A study of women's knowledge and attitudes. *Br J Gen Pract* 43:365, 1993.

67. Turner RR: Role of quality of life in hypertension therapy: Implication for patient compliance. *Cardiology* 80(Suppl 1):11, 1992.

68. Gill TM, Feinstein AR: A cultural appraisal of the quality of quality-of-life measurements. *JAMA* 272:619, 1994.

69. Duquette RL, Dupuis G, Perrault J: A new approach for quality-of-life assessment in cardiac patients: Rationale and validation of the Quality of Life Systemic Inventory. *Can J Cardiol* 10:106, 1994.

70. Duncan LE, Lewis C, Smith CE, et al: Sex, drugs, and hypertension: A methodological approach for studying a sensitive subject. *Int J Impot Res* 13:31, 2001.

71. Testa MA: Methods and applications of quality-of-life measurement during antihypertensive therapy. *Curr Hypertens Rep* 2:530, 2000.

PART V

Appendices

Angela Cheng-Lai
William H. Frishman
Adam Spiegel
Pamela Charney

Pharmacokinetic Properties of Approved Cardiovascular Drugs

Generic Name	Bioavailability (%)	Protein Binding (%)	Volume of Distribution (liters/kg)	Half-Life (hours)	Urinary Excretion (% unchanged)	Clearance (mL·min⁻¹·kg⁻¹)	Therapeutic Range	References
Abciximab	NA	—	—	0.5	—	—	—	Faulds D, Sorkin EM: Abciximab (c7E Fab): A review of its pharmacology and therapeutic potential in ischemic heart disease. *Drugs* 48:583–598, 1994.
Acebutolol	37 ± 12	26 ± 3	1.2 ± 0.3	2.7 ± 0.4	40 ± 11	6.8 ± 0.8	—	Singh BN, Thoden WR, Wahl J: Acebutolol: A review of its pharmacology, pharmacokinetics, clinical uses, and adverse effects. *Pharmacotherapy* 6:45–63, 1986.
Adenosine	—	—	0.11–0.19	<10 sec.	—	59–152	—	Blardi P, Laghi-Pasini F, Urso R, et al: Pharmacokinetics of exogenous adenosine in man after infusion. *Eur J Clin Pharmacol* 44:505–507, 1993.
Alteplase	—	—	0.10–0.17	3–5 min $t_{1/2}$ is ↑ in HI	—	9.8–10.4 Cl is ↓ in HI	0.45 μg/mL	Seifried E, Tanswell P, Rijken DC, et al: Pharmacokinetics of antigen and activity of recombinant tissue-type plasminogen activator after infusion in healthy volunteers. *Arzneimittelforschung* 38:418–422, 1988.
Amiloride	15–25	23	17 ± 4	6–9 $t_{1/2}$ is ↑ in RF	49 ± 10 Cl is ↓ in eld and RI	9.7 ± 1.9	38–48 ng/mL	Vidt DG: Mechanism of action, pharmacokinetics, adverse effects, and therapeutic uses of amiloride hydrochloride, a new potassium-sparing diuretic. *Pharmacotherapy* 1:179–187, 1981.

(continued)

Generic Name	Bioavailability (%)	Protein Binding (%)	Volume of Distribution (liters/kg)	Half-Life (hours)	Urinary Excretion (% unchanged)	Clearance (mL·min⁻¹·kg⁻¹)	Therapeutic Range	References
Amiodarone	46 ± 22	99.98 ± 0.01	66 ± 44	25 ± 12 days	0	1.9 ± 0.4	1.0–2.5 μg/mL	Freeman MD, Somberg JC: Pharmacology and pharmacokinetics of amiodarone. *J Clin Pharmacol* 31:1061–1069, 1991.
Amlodipine	74 ± 17	93 ± 1	16 ± 4	39 ± 8 $t_{1/2}$ is ↑ in eld and HI	10	5.9 ± 1.5 Cl is ↓ in eld and HI	—	Abernethy DR: The pharmacokinetic profile of amlodipine. *Am Heart J* 118:1100–1103, 1989.
Amrinone (Inamrinone)	93 ± 12	35–49	1.3 ± 0.3	4.4 ± 1.4[1] 2.0 ± 0.6[2] $t_{1/2}$ is ↑ in CHF and neo	25 ± 10	4.0 ± 1.6[1] 8.9 ± 2.7[2] Cl is ↓ in CHF and neo	3.7 μg/mL	Steinberg C, Notterman DA: Pharmacokinetics of cardiovascular drugs in children; inotropes and vasopressors. *Clin Pharmacokinet* 27:345–367, 1994. [1]Slow acetylators. [2]Fast acetylators.
Anagrelide	—	—	12	1.3 h[1] 3 days[2]	<1	2.1	—	Spencer, CM, Brogden RN: Anagrelide: A review of its pharmacodynamic and pharmacokinetic properties, and therapeutic potential in the treatment of thrombocythaemia. *Drugs* 47:809–822, 1994. [1]Plasma half-life. [2]Terminal elimination half-life.
Anisindione	Variable	97–99	—	3–5 days	—	—	—	—
Anistreplase	—	—	0.084 ± 0.027	1.2 ± 0.4	—	0.92 ± 0.36 Cl is ↓ in HI	—	Gemmill JD, Hogg KJ, Burns JMA, et al: A comparison of the pharmacokinetic properties of streptokinase and anistreplase in acute myocardial infarction. *Br J Clin Pharmacol* 31:143–147, 1991.
Argatroban	NA	54	0.2	39–51 min	16	5	—	McKeage K, Plosker GL: Argatroban. *Drugs* 61(4):515–522, 2001.
Aspirin	50–100[1]	76–90	0.15–0.2	2.4–19[2] $t_{1/2}$ is ↑ in HI	2–30[3]	0.18–0.88 Cl is ↓ in HI and neo	150–300 μg/mL	Furst DE, Tozer TN, Melmon KL: Salicylate clearance, the resultant of protein binding and metabolism. *Clin Pharmacol Ther* 26:380–389, 1979. [1]Dependent on formulation. [2]Dependent on dose. [3]Dependent on urinary pH.
Atenolol	50–60	5–15	0.95 ± 0.15	6.1 ± 2.0 $t_{1/2}$ is ↑ in RI and eld	94 ± 8	2.0 ± 0.2 Cl is ↓ in eld and RI	0.1–1 μg/mL	Wadworth AN, Murdoch D, Brogden RN: Atenolol: A reappraisal of its pharmacological properties and therapeutic use in cardiovascular disorders. *Drugs* 42:468–510, 1991.
Atorvastatin	12	≥98	8	14 (11–24) ↑ in elderly	<2	—	—	Lea AP, McTavish D: Atorvastatin: A review of its pharmacology and therapeutic potential in the management of hyperlipidaemias. *Drugs* 53:828–847, 1997.

(continued)

Generic Name	Bioavailability (%)	Protein Binding (%)	Volume of Distribution (liters/kg)	Half-Life (hours)	Urinary Excretion (% unchanged)	Clearance (mL·min⁻¹·kg⁻¹)	Therapeutic Range	References
Atropine	50	14–22	2.0 ± 1.1 V_d is ↑ in child	3.5 ± 1.5 $t_{1/2}$ is ↑ in eld and child	57 ± 8	8 ± 4 Cl is ↓ in eld	—	Kentala E, Kaila T, Lisalo E, et al: Intramuscular atropine in healthy volunteers: A pharmacokinetic and pharmacodynamic study. *Int J Clin Pharmacol Ther Toxicol* 28:399–404, 1990.
Benazepril	37	95–97	0.12	0.6 10–11[1]	<1 18[1]	0.3–0.4	—	Kaiser G, Ackermann R, Brechbukler S, et al: Pharmacokinetics of the angiotensin converting enzyme inhibitor benazepril HCl (CGS 14 824 A) in healthy volunteers after single and repeated administration. *Biopharm Drug Dispos* 10:365–376, 1989. [1]Active metabolite.
Bendroflumethiazide	100	94	1.48	3–3.9	30	5.3 ± 1.4	—	Beermann B, Groschinsky-Grind M, Lindstrom B: Pharmacokinetics of bendroflumethiazide. *Clin Pharmacol Ther* 22:385–388, 1977.
Bepridil	60	>99	8 ± 5	12–24	<1	5.3 ± 2.5	—	Benet LZ: Pharmacokinetics and metabolism of bepridil. *Am J Cardiol* 55:8C–13C, 1985.
Betaxolol	76–89	50–55	4.9–9.8	14–22 $t_{1/2}$ is ↑ in eld	15	4.7 Cl is ↓ in eld	20–50 ng/mL	Frishman WH, Tepper D, Lazar EJ, et al: Betaxolol: A new long-acting beta₁-selective adrenergic blocker. *J Clin Pharmacol* 30:686–692, 1990.
Bisoprolol	85–91	30–35	3.2 ± 0.5	8.2–12 $t_{1/2}$ is ↑ in RI	50–60	3.7 ± 0.7 Cl is ↓ in RI	—	Lancaster SG, Sorkin EM: Bisoprolol: A preliminary review of its pharmacodynamic and pharmacokinetic properties, and therapeutic efficacy in hypertension and angina pectoris. *Drugs* 36:256–285, 1988.
Bivalirudin	40[1]	0	ID	25–36 min	≈20	3.4	—	Fox I, Dawson A, Loynds P, et al: Anticoagulant activity of Hirulog, a direct thrombin inhibitor, in humans. *Thromb Haemost* 69:157–163, 1993.
Bosentan	50	>98	~0.26	5	<3	1.9	—	[1]Bioavailability of subcutaneous injection. Actelion: Tracleer package insert: S. San Francisco, CA, 2002.
Bretylium	23 ± 9	0–8	5.9 ± 0.8	5–10 $t_{1/2}$ is ↑ in RI	70–80	10.2 ± 1.9 Cl is ↓ in RI	—	Rapaport WG: Clinical pharmacokinetics of bretylium. *Clin Pharmacokinet* 10:248–256, 1985.
Bumetanide	55–89	99 ± 0.3	0.13 ± 0.03 V_d is ↑ in RI and HI	0.3–1.5 $t_{1/2}$ is ↑ in RI, HI, and CHF	62 ± 20	2.6 ± 0.5 Cl is ↓ in RI, HI, and CHF	—	Cook JA, Smith DE, Cornish LA, et al: Kinetics, dynamics, and bioavailability of bumetanide in healthy subjects and patients with congestive heart failure. *Clin Pharmacol Ther* 44:487–500, 1988.

(continued)

Generic Name	Bioavailability (%)	Protein Binding (%)	Volume of Distribution (liters/kg)	Half-Life (hours)	Urinary Excretion (% unchanged)	Clearance (mL·min⁻¹·kg⁻¹)	Therapeutic Range	References
Candesartan	15	>99	0.13	9–13	26	0.37	—	McClellan KJ, Goa KL: Candesartan cilexetil: A review of its use in essential hypertension. *Drugs* 56(5):847–869, 1998.
Captopril	65–75	30 ± 6	0.81 ± 0.18	2.2 ± 0.5 $t_{1/2}$ is ↑ in RI and CHF	40–50	12.0 ± 1.4 Cl is ↓ in RI	0.05–0.5 µg/mL	Duchin KL, McKinstry DN, Cohen AI, et al: Pharmacokinetics of captopril in healthy subjects and in patients with cardiovascular diseases. *Clin Pharmacokinet* 14:241–259, 1988.
Carteolol	85	23–30	—	5–7 $t_{1/2}$ is ↑ in RI	50–70	—	—	Chrisp P, Sorkin EM: Ocular carteolol: A review of its pharmacological properties, and therapeutic use in glaucoma and ocular hypertension. *Drugs Aging* 2:58–77, 1992.
Carvedilol	25	95	1.5 ± 0.3	7–10[1] $t_{1/2}$ is ↑ in HI	<2	8.7 ± 1.7 Cl is ↓ in HI	—	Dunn CJ, Lea AP, Wagstaff AJ: Carvedilol: A reappraisal of its pharmacological properties and therapeutic use in cardiovascular disorders. *Drugs* 54:161–185, 1997. [1]Apparent mean terminal elimination half-life.
Chlorothiazide	10–21	20–80	0.20 ± 0.08	1.5 ± 0.2 $t_{1/2}$ is ↑ in RI and CHF	92 ± 5	4.5 ± 1.7 Cl is ↓ in RI	—	Osmon MA, Patel RB, Irwin DS, et al: Bioavailability of chlorothiazide from 50, 100, and 250 mg solution doses. *Biopharm Drug Dispos* 3:89–94, 1982.
Chlorthalidone	64 ± 10	75 ± 1	0.10 ± 0.04	47 ± 22 $t_{1/2}$ is ↑ in eld	65 ± 9	0.04 ± 0.01 Cl is ↓ in eld	—	Williams RL, Blume CD, Lin ET, et al: Relative bioavailability of chlorthalidone in humans: Adverse influence of polyethylene glycol. *J Pharm Sci* 71:533–535, 1982.
Cilostazol	ID	95–98	ID	11–13	0	ID	—	Reilly MP, Mohler ER 3rd: Cilostazol: Treatment of intermittent claudication. *Ann Pharmacother* 35(1):48–56, 2001.
Clofibrate	95 ± 10	95–98	0.11 ± 0.02	12–22 $t_{1/2}$ is ↑ in RI	5.7 ± 2.1	0.12 ± 0.01 Cl is ↓ in RI	162–200 µg/mL	Gugler R, Kurten JW, Jensen CJ, et al: Clofibrate disposition in renal failure and acute and chronic liver disease. *Eur J Clin Pharmacol* 15:341–347, 1979.
Clonidine	95	20	2.1 ± 0.4	12–16 $t_{1/2}$ is ↑ in RI	40–60	3.1 ± 1.2 Cl is ↓ in RI	0.2–2 ng/mL	Lowenthal DT, Matzek KM, McGregor TR: Clinical pharmacokinetics of clonidine. *Clin Pharmacokinet* 14:287–310, 1988.
Clopidogrel	—	98	—	8[1]	ID	—	—	Sanof: Plavix package insert, New York:1997. [1]Half-life of primary metabolite (inactive carboxylic-acid derivative).
Colesevelam	NA[1]	NA	NA	NA	0.05	ID	—	Wong N: Colesevelam: A new bile acid sequestrant. *Heart Dis* 3:63–70, 2001. [1]Colesevelam is not hydrolyzed by digestive enzymes and is not absorbed.
Dalteparin	87	—	0.04–0.06	3–5 $t_{1/2}$ is ↓ in RI	—	0.27–0.41	0.1–0.6 anti-Xa Units/mL	Simoneau G, Bergmann JF, Kher A, et al: Pharmacokinetics of a low molecular weight heparin (Fragmin) in young and elderly subjects. *Thromb Res* 66:603–607, 1992.

(continued)

Generic Name	Bioavailability (%)	Protein Binding (%)	Volume of Distribution (liters/kg)	Half-Life (hours)	Urinary Excretion (% unchanged)	Clearance (mL · min⁻¹ · kg⁻¹)	Therapeutic Range	References
Danaparoid	100[1]	—	0.11–0.13[1]	24[1] ↑ in RI	—	0.086–0.190[2]	0.15–0.40 units/mL[3]	Skoutakis VA: Danaparoid in the prevention of thromboembolic complications. *Ann Pharmacother* 31:876–887, 1997. [1]Based on plasma antifactor Xa activity. [2]Total plasma clearance of plasma antifactor Xa activity. [3]Plasma antifactor Xa level at 6 hours postdose; further studies are needed to determine whether a therapeutic window exists for danaparoid.
Diazoxide	NA[1]	94	0.21	48	ID	0.06	—	Kirsten R, Nelson K, Kirsten D, et al: Clinical pharmacokinetics of vasodilators. Part I. *Clin Pharmacokinet* 34(6):457–82, 1998. [1]Intravenous formulation.
Dicoumarol	Variable	99	—	1–2 days	—	—	—	
Digitoxin	>90	97 ± 0.5	0.54 ± 0.14 V_d is ↑ in child	6.7 ± 1.7 days	32 ± 15	0.055 ± 0.018 Cl is ↑ in child	14–26 ng/mL	Mooradian AD: Digitalis: An update of clinical pharmacokinetics, therapeutic monitoring techniques and treatment recommendations. *Clin Pharmacokinet* 15:165–179, 1988.
Digoxin	70 ± 1.3	20–25	—	39 ± 13 $t_{1/2}$ ↑ in RI, CHF, eld	60 ± 11	[(0.8 mL/min/kg) (wt in kg) + Cl_{cr}][1]; ↑ in neo, child	0.5–2 ng/mL	Mooradian AD: Digitalis: An update of clinical pharmacokinetics, therapeutic monitoring techniques and treatment recommendations. *Clin Pharmacokinet* 15:165–179, 1988. [1]Total digoxin clearance in patients without CHF (mL/min).
Diltiazem	40–67	70–80	3.1 ± 1.2 V_d ↓ in RI	3.7–6	2–4	12 ± 4 Cl is ↓ in RI	50–200 ng/mL	Echizen H, Eichelbaum M: Clinical pharmacokinetics of verapamil, nifedipine and diltiazem. *Clin Pharmacokinet* 11:425–449, 1986.
Dipyridamole	37–66	91–99	—	10–12	<5	—	—	Gregov D, Jenkins A, Duncan E, et al: Dipyridamole: Pharmacokinetics and effects on aspects of platelet function in man. *Br J Clin Pharmacol* 24:425–434, 1987.
Disopyramide	83 ± 11	68–89	0.59 ± 0.15	4–10 $t_{1/2}$ ↑ in RI, CHF	55 ± 6	1.2 ± 0.4, Cl ↓ in MI, CHF, RI, HI	2–4 μg/mL	Siddoway LA, Woosley RL: Clinical pharmacokinetics of disopyramide. *Clin Pharmacokinet* 11:214–222, 1986.
Dobutamine	NA	ID	0.20 ± 0.08	2.4 ± 0.7 min	0	59 ± 22 Cl ↑ in child	40–190 ng/mL	Steinberg C, Notterman DA: Pharmacokinetics of cardiovascular drugs in children: Inotropes and vasopressors. *Clin Pharmacokinet* 27:345–367, 1994.

(continued)

Generic Name	Bioavailability (%)	Protein Binding (%)	Volume of Distribution (liters/kg)	Half-Life (hours)	Urinary Excretion (% unchanged)	Clearance (mL · min⁻¹ · kg⁻¹)	Therapeutic Range	References
Dofetilide	>90	60–70	3–4	5–13	≈64	5.2	—	Lenz TL, Hilleman DE: Dofetilide, a new class III antiarrhythmic agent. *Pharmacotherapy* 20(7):776–86, 2000.
Dopamine	NA	0	—	2 min	<5	—	—	Kulka PJ, Tryba M: Inotropic support of the critically ill patient. *Drugs* 45:654–667, 1993.
Doxazosin	63 ± 14	98.9 ± 0.5	1.5 ± 0.3	19–22	—	1.7 ± 0.4	—	Donelly R, Meredith PA, Elliott HL: Pharmacokinetic-pharmacodynamic relationships of α-adrenoceptor antagonists. *Clin Pharmacokinet* 17:264–274, 1989.
Enalapril	41 ± 15	<50	1.7 ± 0.7	1.3 11[1] $t_{1/2}$ is ↑ in RI and HI	54 40[1]	4.9 ± 1.5 Cl is ↓ in RI, eld, CHF, neo and ↑ in child	5–20 ng/mL	Louis WJ, Conway EL, Krum H, et al: Comparison of the pharmacokinetics and pharmacodynamics of perindopril, cilazapril and enalapril. *Clin Exp Pharmacol Physiol* 19 (Suppl 19):55–60, 1992. [1]Enalaprilat.
Encainide	25–90[1]	75–85	3.6–3.9	1–2[2] 6–11[3]	5[2] 40–45[3]	30[2] 2.5[3]	250 ng/mL	Brogden RN, Todd PA: Encainide: A review of its pharmacological properties and therapeutic efficacy. *Drugs* 34:519–538, 1987. [1]Depends on metabolic phenotype. [2]Fast oxidizer. [3]Slow oxidizer.
Enoxaparin	92	—	0.08	4.5 $t_{1/2}$ is ↑ in RI	8–20	0.3 ± 0.1 Cl is ↓ in RI	—	Bendetowicz AV, Beguin S, Caplain H, et al: Pharmacokinetics and pharmacodynamics of a low molecular weight heparin (enoxaparin) after subcutaneous injection, comparison with unfractionated heparin—a three-way crossover study in healthy volunteers. *Thromb Haemost* 71:305–313, 1994.
Eprosartan	13	98	≈4.4[1]	5–9	≈6	11.5	—	Bottorff MB, Tenero DM: Pharmacokinetics of eprosartan in healthy subjects, patients with hypertension, and special populations. *Pharmacotherapy* 19(4 pt 2):73S–78S, 1999. [1]This value is the population mean steady-state volume of distribution (V_{ss}/F).
Eptifibatide	NA	25	0.23	2.5–2.8	ID	0.92–0.97	—	Goa KL, Noble S: Eptifibatide: A review of its use in patients with acute coronary syndromes and/or undergoing percutaneous coronary intervention. *Drugs* 57(3):439–462, 1999.
Esmolol	NA	55	1.9 ± 1.3	0.13 ± 0.07 $t_{1/2}$ is ↓ in child	<1	170 ± 70 Cl is ↓ in CAD and ↑ in child	—	Weist D: Esmolol: A review of its therapeutic efficacy and pharmacokinetic characteristics. *Clin Pharmacokinet* 28:190–202, 1995.

(continued)

Generic Name	Bioavailability (%)	Protein Binding (%)	Volume of Distribution (liters/kg)	Half-Life (hours)	Urinary Excretion (% unchanged)	Clearance (mL · min^{-1} · kg^{-1})	Therapeutic Range	References
Ethacrynic acid	100	90	—	0.5–1	65	—	—	
Felodipine	20	99.6 ± 0.2	10 ± 3	10–17 $t_{1/2}$ is ↑ in eld, CHF	<1	12 ± 5 Cl is ↓ in eld, HI, CHF	—	Edgar B, Lundborg P, Regardh CG: Clinical pharmacokinetics of felodipine: A summary. *Drugs* 34(Suppl 3):16–27, 1987.
Fenofibrate	60–90	>99[1]	0.89[1]	19.6–26.6[1]	ID	0.45[2]	—	Balfour JA, McTavish D, Heel RC: Fenofibrate. A review of its pharmacodynamic and pharmacokinetic properties and therapeutic use in dyslipidaemia. *Drugs* 40(2):260–90, 1990. [1]Properties of major active metabolite fenofibric acid. [2]Plasma clearance of fenofibric acid.
Fenoldopam	5.7	88	0.23–0.66	0.16	1	24.8–38.2	3.5–14.25 μg/L	Brogden RN and Markham A: Fenoldopam: A review of its pharmacodynamic and pharmacokinetic properties and intravenous clinical potential in the management of hypertensive urgencies and emergencies. *Drugs* 54(4):634–650, 1997.
Flecainide	85–90	40–50	4.9 ± 0.4	12–30 $t_{1/2}$ is ↑ in RI, HI, CHF and ↓ in child	10–50	5.6 ± 1.3 Cl is ↓ in RI, HI, CHF	0.4–0.8 μg/mL	Funck-Bretano C, Becquemont L, Kroemer HK, et al: Variable disposition kinetics and electrocardiographic effects of flecainide during repeated dosing in humans: Contribution of genetic factors, dose-dependent clearance and interaction with amiodarone. *Clin Pharmacol Ther* 55:256–269, 1994.
Fluvastatin	9–50	98	—	1.2 $t_{1/2}$ is ↑ in HI	<5	—	—	Tse FLS, Jaffe JM, Troendle A: Pharmacokinetics of fluvastatin after single and multiple doses in normal volunteers. *J Clin Pharmacol* 32:630–638, 1992.
Fondaparinux	≈100[1]	—	0.10–0.12[1]	13–15 $t_{1/2}$ ↑ in eld with reduced Cl$_{cr}$	≤77%	0.10–0.13[2] Cl is ↓ in eld with reduced Cl$_{cr}$	—	Boneu B, Necciari J, Cariou R, et al: Pharmacokinetics and tolerance of the natural pentasaccharide (SR90107/ORG31540) with high affinity to antithrombin III in man. *Thromb Haemost* 74:1468–1473, 1995. [1]After subcutaneous injection. [2]Plasma clearance.

(continued)

Generic Name	Bioavailability (%)	Protein Binding (%)	Volume of Distribution (liters/kg)	Half-Life (hours)	Urinary Excretion (% unchanged)	Clearance (mL·min⁻¹·kg⁻¹)	Therapeutic Range	References
Fosinopril	36 ± 7	≥ 95	0.13 ± 0.03	11.3 ± 0.7[1] $t_{1/2}$ is ↑ in RI	<2	0.51 ± 0.10 Cl is ↓ in HI, RI	—	Hui KK, Duchin KL, Kripalani KJ, et al: Pharmacokinetics of fosinopril in patients with various degrees of renal function. *Clin Pharmacol Ther* 49:457–467, 1991. [1]Fosinoprilat.
Furosemide	61 ± 17	98.8 ± 0.2	0.11 ± 0.02	0.5–1.0 $t_{1/2}$ ↑ in RI, CHF, neo, HI, eld	66 ± 7	2.0 ± 0.4 Cl is ↓ in RI, CHF, neo, eld	ID	Hammarlund-Udenaes M, Benet LZ: Furosemide pharmacokinetics and pharmacodynamics in health and disease—an update. *J Pharmacokinet Biopharm* 17:1–46, 1989.
Gemfibrozil	98 ± 1	>97	0.14 ± 0.03	1.1 ± 0.2	<1	1.7 ± 0.4	—	Todd PA, Ward A: Gemfibrozil, a review of its pharmacodynamic and pharmacokinetic properties and therapeutic use in dyslipidaemia. *Drugs* 36:314–339, 1988.
Guanabenz	ID	95	93–147	4–14	<1	—	—	Holmes B, Brogden RN, Heel RC, et al: Guanabenz: A review of its pharmacodynamic properties and therapeutic efficacy in hypertension. *Drugs* 26:212–229, 1983.
Guanadrel	85	<20	—	10–12 $t_{1/2}$ ↑ in RI	40	—	—	Finnerty FA Jr, Brogden RN: Guanadrel: A review of its pharmacodynamic and pharmacokinetic properties and therapeutic use in hypertension. *Drugs* 30:22–31, 1985.
Guanethidine	3–30	—	—	4–8 days	50	0.8	8–17 ng/mL	Woosley RL, Nies AS: Guanethidine. *N Engl J Med* 295:1053–1057, 1976.
Guanfacine	80	70	6.3	10–30	40–75	—	5–10 ng/mL	Sorkin EM, Heel RC: Guanfacine: A review of its pharmacodynamic and pharmacokinetic properties and therapeutic efficacy in the treatment of hypertension. *Drugs* 31:301–336, 1986.
Heparin	NA	—	0.058 ± 0.01	1–2[1]	≤50	0.5–0.6[2]	—	Estes JW: Clinical pharmacokinetics of heparin. *Clin Pharmacokinet* 5:204–220, 1980. [1]Increase with dose. [2]Plasma clearance.
Hydralazine	16 ± 15[1] 35 ± 4[2]	87	1.5 ± 1.0	2–4 $t_{1/2}$ is ↑ in CHF	1–15	56 ± 13 Cl is ↓ in CHF	—	Mulrow JP, Crawford MH: Clinical pharmacokinetics and therapeutic use of hydralazine in congestive heart failure. *Clin Pharmacokinet* 16:86–89, 1989. [1]Rapid acetylator. [2]Slow acetylator.

(continued)

Generic Name	Bioavailability (%)	Protein Binding (%)	Volume of Distribution (liters/kg)	Half-Life (hours)	Urinary Excretion (% unchanged)	Clearance (mL · min^{-1} · kg^{-1})	Therapeutic Range	References
Hydrochlorothiazide	65–75	58 ± 17	0.83 ± 0.31	2–15 $t_{1/2}$ is ↑ in RI, CHF and eld	>95	4.9 ± 1.1 Cl is ↓ in RI, CHF and eld	—	Beerman B, Groschinsky Grind M: Pharmacokinetics of hydrochlorothiazide in man. *Eur J Clin Pharmacol* 12:297–303, 1977.
Hydroflumethiazide	50	74	—	12–27	40–80	—	—	Brors O, Jacobsen S: Pharmacokinetics of hydroflumethiazide during repeated oral administration to healthy subjects. *Eur J Pharmacol* 15:281–286, 1979.
Ibutilide	—	40	11	6 ± 4	7	29	—	Jungbluth GL, et al: Evaluation of the pharmacokinetics and pharmacodynamics of ibutilide fumarate and its enantiomers in healthy male volunteers (abstr.). *Pharm Res* 8:S249, 1991.
Indapamide	93	71–79	0.86–1.57	14–18	7	—	—	Caruso FS, Szabadi RR, Vukovich RA: Pharmacokinetics and clinical pharmacology of indapamide. *Am Heart J* 106:212–220, 1983.
Irbesartan	60–80	~90	0.76–1.33	11–15	1	2.3–2.6	—	Gillis JC, Markham A: Irbesartan: A review of its pharmacodynamic and pharmacokinetic properties and therapeutic use in the management of hypertension. *Drugs* 54(6):885–902, 1997.
Isosorbide dinitrate	22 ± 14[1] 45 ± 16[2]	28 ± 12	3.9 ± 1.5	1.0 ± 0.5	<1	45 ± 20 Cl is ↓ in HI	—	Fung HL: Pharmacokinetics and pharmacodynamics of organic nitrates. *Am J Cardiol* 60:4H–9H, 1987. [1]Oral. [2]Sublingual.
Isosorbide mononitrate	93 ± 13	<4	0.73 ± 0.09	4.9 ± 0.8	<5	1.80 ± 0.24	100 ng/mL	Abshagen UWP: Pharmacokinetics of isosorbide mononitrate. *Am J Cardiol* 70:61G–66G, 1992.
Isoxsuprine	100	ID	—	1.25	—	—	—	
Isradipine	17 F ↑ in eld and HI	97	2.9	6.1–10.7	0	10	—	Fitton A, Benfield P: Isradipine. A review of its pharmacodynamic and pharmacokinetic properties, and therapeutic use in cardiovascular disease. *Drugs* 40(1):31–74, 1990.
Labetalol	18 ± 5 F ↑ in eld and HI	50	9.4 ± 3.4	4.9 ± 2.0 $t_{1/2}$ ↑ in eld	<5	25 ± 10 Cl ↓ in eld	—	Donnelly R, Macphee GJA: Clinical pharmacokinetics and kinetic-dynamic relationships of dilevalol and labetalol. *Clin Pharmacokinet* 21:95–109, 1991.

(continued)

Generic Name	Bioavailability (%)	Protein Binding (%)	Volume of Distribution (liters/kg)	Half-Life (hours)	Urinary Excretion (% unchanged)	Clearance (mL · min⁻¹ · kg⁻¹)	Therapeutic Range	References
Lepirudin	75–80[1]	ID	0.13–0.46	1.3	≈17	2.3–3.3	—	Cheng-Lai A: Hirudin. *Heart Dis* 1:41–49, 1999. [1]Bioavailability of lepirudin following subcutaneous administration.
Lidocaine	NA	50–70	1.1 ± 0.4	1.8 ± 0.4 $t_{1/2}$ is ↑ in HI, neo	<10	9.2 ± 2.4 Cl is ↓ in CHF, HI	1.5–6 µg/mL	Thompson PD, Melmon KL, Richardson JA, et al: Lidocaine pharmacokinetics in advanced heart failure, liver disease and renal disease in humans. *Ann Intern Med* 78:499–508, 1973.
Lisinopril	25 ± 20 F ↓ in CHF	0	2.4 ± 1.4	12 $t_{1/2}$ is ↑ in eld, RI	88–100	4.2 ± 2.2 Cl is ↓ in CHF, RI, eld	—	Sica DA, Cutler RE, Parmer RJ, et al: Comparison of the steady-state pharmacokinetics of fosinopril, lisinopril and enalapril in patients with chronic renal insufficiency. *Clin Pharmacokinet* 20:420–427, 1991.
Losartan	33 F is ↑ in HI	98	0.49	1.5–2.5 6–9[1]	4	8.6 Cl is ↓ in HI	—	Ohtawa M, Takayama F, Saitoh K, et al: Pharmacokinetics and biochemical efficacy after single and multiple oral administration of losartan, an orally active non-peptide angiotensin II receptor antagonist, in humans. *Br J Clin Pharmacol* 35:290–297, 1993. [1]Active metabolite.
Lovastatin	<5	>95	—	3–4	<5	4–18 Cl is ↓ in RI	—	McKenney JM: Lovastatin: A new cholesterol-lowering agent. *Clin Pharmacol* 7:21–36, 1988.
Mecamylamine	ID	—	—	ID	50[1]	—	—	[1]Depends on urinary pH.
Methyldopa	42 ± 16	1–16	0.46 ± 0.15	1.8 ± 0.6 $t_{1/2}$ is ↑ in RI, neo	40 ± 13	3.7 ± 1.0 Cl is ↓ in RI	—	Skerjanee A, Campbell NRC, Robertson S, et al: Pharmacokinetics and presystemic gut metabolism of methyldopa in healthy human subjects. *J Clin Pharmacol* 35:275–280, 1995.
Metolazone	40–65	95[1]	1.6	14	70–95	—	—	Tilstone WJ, Dargle H, Dargle EN, et al: Pharmacokinetics of metolazone in normal subjects and in patients with cardiac or renal failure. *Clin Pharmacol Ther* 16:322–329, 1974. [1]50% to 78% is bound to erythrocytes.
Metoprolol	38 ± 14 F is ↑ in HI	11 ± 1	4.2 ± 0.7	3–4 $t_{1/2}$ is ↑ in HI, neo	10 ± 3	15 ± 3	50–100 ng/mL	Dayer P, Leemann T, Marmy A, et al: Interindividual variation of beta-adrenoreceptor blocking drugs, plasma concentration and effect: Influence of genetic status on behavior of atenolol, bopindolol and metoprolol. *Eur J Clin Pharmacol* 28:149–153, 1985.

(continued)

Generic Name	Bioavailability (%)	Protein Binding (%)	Volume of Distribution (liters/kg)	Half-Life (hours)	Urinary Excretion (% unchanged)	Clearance (mL · min^{-1} · kg^{-1})	Therapeutic Range	References
Mexiletine	87 ± 13	50–60	4.9 ± 0.5	9.2 ± 2.1 $t_{1/2}$ is ↑ in MI, CHF, RI, and HI	10	6.3 ± 2.7 Cl is ↓ in MI, RI (Cl$_{cr}$ <10 mL/min), HI	0.5–2.0 µg/mL	Monk JP, Brogden RN: Mexiletine: A review of its pharmacodynamic and pharmacokinetic properties, and therapeutic use in the treatment of arrhythmias. *Drugs* 40:374–411, 1990.
Midodrine	90–93[1]	—	4–4.6[1]	0.5 3[1]	2–4	19.7–24.3[2]	—	McTavish D, Goa KL: Midodrine: A review of its pharmacological properties and therapeutic use in orthostatic hypotension and secondary hypotensive disorders. *Drugs* 38:757–777, 1989. [1]Based on desglymidodrine, active metabolite of midodrine. [2]Total-body plasma clearance of desglymidodrine.
Milrinone	≥80	70	0.32 ± 0.08	0.80 ± 0.22 $t_{1/2}$ is ↑ in CHF, RI	85 ± 10	6.1 ± 1.3 Cl is ↓ in CHF, RI	150–250 ng/mL	Young RA, Ward A, Milrinone: A preliminary review of its pharmacological properties and therapeutic use. *Drugs* 36:158–192, 1988.
Minoxidil	ID	0	2.7 ± 0.7	3.1 ± 0.6[1]	20 ± 6	24 ± 6	—	Fleishaker JC, Andreadis NA, Welshman IR, et al: The pharmacokinetics of 2.5 to 10 mg oral doses of minoxidil in healthy volunteers. *J Clin Pharmacol* 29:162–167, 1989. [1]Hypertensives.
Moexipril	13	90	—	1.3 2–9[1]	<10	—	—	Van Hecken A, Verbesselt R, Depre M, et al: Moexipril does not alter the pharmacokinetics or pharmacodynamics of warfarin. *Eur J Clin Pharmacol* 45:291–293, 1993. [1]Moexiprilat.
Moricizine	38	95	4.4	1.5–3.5 $t_{1/2}$ is ↑ in HI	<1	—	—	Fitton A, Buckley MM: Moricizine: A review of its pharmacological properties, and therapeutic efficacy in cardiac arrhythmias. *Drugs* 40:138–167, 1990.
Nadolol	34 ± 5	20 ± 4	1.9 ± 0.2	16 ± 2 $t_{1/2}$ is ↑ in RI and child	73 ± 4	2.9 ± 0.6 Cl is ↓ in RI	—	Morrison RA, Singhvi SM, Creasey WA, et al: Dose proportionality of nadolol pharmacokinetics after intravenous administration to healthy subjects. *Eur J Clin Pharmacol* 33:625–628, 1988.
Nesiritide	NA	—	0.19	18 min	—	9.2	—	Cheng JWM: Nesiritide: Review of clinical pharmacology and role in heart failure management. *Heart Dis* 4:199–203, 2002.
Nicardipine	18 ± 11	98–99.5	1.1 ± 0.3	2–4 $t_{1/2}$ is ↑ in HI	<1	10.4 ± 3.1 Cl is ↓ in HI	0.1 µg/mL	Singh BN, Josephson MA: Clinical pharmacology, pharmacokinetics and hemodynamic effects of nicardipine. *Am Heart J* 119:427–434, 1990.

(continued)

Generic Name	Bioavailability (%)	Protein Binding (%)	Volume of Distribution (liters/kg)	Half-Life (hours)	Urinary Excretion (% unchanged)	Clearance (mL · min^{-1} · kg^{-1})	Therapeutic Range	References
Nicotinic acid	88	<20	—	0.75–1	1	—	—	[1]Increases with ↑ dose.
Nifedipine	50 ± 13 F is ↑ in HI	96 ± 1	0.78 ± 0.22	2.5 ± 1.3	<1	7.0 ± 1.8	47 ± 20 ng/mL	Soons PA, Schoemaker HC, Cohen AF, et al: Intraindividual variability in nifedipine pharmacokinetics and effects in healthy subjects. *J Clin Pharmacol* 32:324–331, 1992.
Nimodipine	10 ± 4 F is ↑ in HI	98	1.7 ± 0.6	1.1 ± 0.3 $t_{1/2}$ is ↑ in HI and RI	<1	19 ± 6 Cl is ↓ in HI and RI	—	Langley MS, Sorkin EM: Nimodipine: A review of its pharmacodynamic and pharmacokinetic properties, and therapeutic potential in cerebrovascular disease. *Drugs* 37:669–699, 1989.
Nisoldipine	3.7 F is ↑ in HI	99	4–5	8–9 $t_{1/2}$ is ↑ in HI	—	—	—	Baksi AK, Edwards JS, Ahr G: A comparison of the pharmacokinetics of nisoldipine in elderly and young subjects. *Br J Clin Pharmacol* 31:367–370, 1991.
Nitroglycerin	Oral:<1 SL: 38 ± 26 TOP: 72 ± 20	60	2.9	1–4 min	—	—	—	Thadani U, Whitsett T: Relationship of pharmacokinetic and pharmacodynamic properties of the organic nitrates. *Clin Pharmacokinet* 15:32–43, 1988.
Olmesartan	28.6[1]	99	≈0.5	10–15	—	0.3	—	Brunner HR: The new oral angiotensin II antagonist olmesartan medoxomil: A concise overview. *J Hum Hypertens* 16(Suppl 2): S13–S16, 2002. [1]After oral administration.
Penbutolol	100	80–98	—	5 $t_{1/2}$ is ↑ in RI	<10	—	—	Brockmeier D, Hajdu P, Henke W, et al: Penbutolol: Pharmacokinetics, effect on exercise tachycardia, and in vitro inhibition of radioligand binding. *Eur J Clin Pharmacol* 35:613–623, 1988.
Pentoxifylline	33 ± 13 F is ↑ in HI	0	4.2 ± 0.9	0.9 ± 0.3 $t_{1/2}$ is ↑ in eld and HI	0	60 ± 13 Cl is ↓ in eld and HI	—	Ward A, Clissold SP: Pentoxifylline: A review of its pharmacodynamic and pharmacokinetic properties, and its therapeutic efficacy. *Drugs* 34:50–97, 1987.
Perindopril	≈75[1] ≈25[2]	60[1] 10–20[2]	0.22[1] 0.16[2]	0.8–1[1] 3–10[2] 30–120[3]	3–10	3.1–5.2	—	Todd PA, Fitton A: Perindopril: A review of its pharmacological properties and therapeutic use in cardiovascular disorders. *Drugs* 42:90–114, 1991. [1]Properties of perindopril. [2]Properties of perindoprilat. [3]Prolonged terminal elimination half-life of perindoprilat.
Pindolol	75 ± 9 F is ↓ in RI	40–60	2.3 ± 0.9	3.6 ± 0.6 $t_{1/2}$ is ↑ in RI and HI	35–50	8.3 ± 1.8 Cl is ↓ in RI and HI	—	Guerret M, Cheymol G, Aubry JP, et al: Estimation of the absolute oral bioavailability of pindolol by two analytical methods. *Eur J Clin Pharmacol* 25:357–359, 1983.

(continued)

Generic Name	Bioavailability (%)	Protein Binding (%)	Volume of Distribution (liters/kg)	Half-Life (hours)	Urinary Excretion (% unchanged)	Clearance (mL · min⁻¹ · kg⁻¹)	Therapeutic Range	References
Polythiazide	ID	84	—	25.7	25	—	—	
Pravastatin	18 ± 8	43–48	0.46 ± 0.04	1.8 ± 0.8	20	13.5[1] Cl is ↓ in HI	—	Quion JAV, Jones PH: Clinical pharmacokinetics of pravastatin. *Clin Pharmacokinet* 27:94–103, 1994. [1]Clearance after intravenous dose.
Prazosin	48–68	95 ± 1	0.60 ± 0.13	2.9 ± 0.8 $t_{1/2}$ is ↑ in CHF, eld	<1	3.0 ± 0.3 Cl is ↓ in CHF	—	Vincent J, Meredith PA, Reid JL, et al: Clinical pharmacokinetics of prazosin—1985. *Clin Pharmacokinet* 10:144–154, 1985.
Probucol	2–8	95	—	12–500	0	—	23.6 ± 17.2 μg/mL	
Procainamide	83 ± 16	16 ± 5	1.9 ± 0.3	3.0 ± 0.6 $t_{1/2}$ is ↑ in RI and MI, and ↓ in child and neo	67 ± 8	3.2[1] & 1.1[2] Cl is ↑ in child and ↓ in MI	3–10 μg/mL	Karlson E: Clinical pharmacokinetics of procainamide. *Clin Pharmacokinet* 3:97–107, 1978. [1]Fast acetylator. [2]Slow acetylator.
Propafenone	5–50[1]	85–95	3.6 ± 2.1	2–10[2] 10–32[3]	<1	17 ± 8 Cl is ↓ in HI	0.2–1.5 μg/mL	Bryson HM, Palmer KJ, Langtry HD, et al: Propafenone: A reappraisal of its pharmacology, pharmacokinetics and therapeutic use in cardiac arrhythmias. *Drugs* 45:85–130, 1993. [1]Dose dependent. [2]Fast metabolizers. [3]Slow metabolizers.
Propranolol	26 ± 10	87 ± 6	4.3 ± 0.6	3–5 $t_{1/2}$ is ↑ in HI	<0.5	11.4–17.1 Cl is ↓ in HI	20 ng/mL	McDevitt DG: Comparison of pharmacokinetic properties of beta-adrenoreceptor blocking drugs. *Eur Heart J* 8(Suppl. M):9–14, 1987.
Quinapril	60	97	0.4	2.2 ± 0.2[1] $t_{1/2}$ is ↑ in eld and RI	Trace	2.0 ± 0.6 Cl is ↓ in eld and RI	—	Wadworth AN, Brogden RN: Quinapril: A review of its pharmacological properties and therapeutic efficacy in cardiovascular disorders. *Drugs* 41:378–399, 1991. [1]Quinaprilat.
Quinidine	70–80 71 ± 17	87 ± 3	2.7 ± 1.2	6.2 ± 1.8 $t_{1/2}$ is ↑ in RI and eld	18 ± 5	4.7 ± 1.8 Cl is ↓ in RI, eld and severe CHF	2–6 μg/mL	Verme CN, Ludden TM, Clementi WA, et al: Pharmacokinetics of quinidine in male patients: A population analysis. *Clin Pharmacokinet* 22:468–480, 1992.
Ramipril	50–60	56	—	14 ± 7[1] $t_{1/2}$ is ↑ in RI	<2%	1.1 ± 0.4 Cl is ↓ in RI	—	Meisel S, Shamiss A, Rosenthal T: Clinical pharmacokinetics of ramipril. *Clin Pharmacokinet* 26:7–15, 1994. [1]Ramiprilat.

(continued)

Generic Name	Bioavailability (%)	Protein Binding (%)	Volume of Distribution (liters/kg)	Half-Life (hours)	Urinary Excretion (% unchanged)	Clearance (mL · min⁻¹ · kg⁻¹)	Therapeutic Range	References
Reserpine	50	—	—	33	<1	—	—	—
Reteplase	—	—	0.086[1]	13–16 min[2]	—	3.6–6.4[3]	2000 IU/mL (activity) 4200 µg/L (antigen)	Noble S, McTavish D: Reteplase: A review of its pharmacological properties and clinical efficacy in the management of acute myocardial infarction. *Drugs* 52:589–605, 1996. [1]Apparent volume of distribution during the terminal elimination phase. [2]Effective half-life. [3]Plasma clearance.
Simvastatin	<5	94	—	1.9	<0.5	7.6	—	Mauro VF, MacDonald JL: Simvastatin: A review of its pharmacology and clinical use. *DICP* 25:257–264, 1991.
Sodium nitroprusside	NA	ID	—	3–4 min 3–4 days[1] $t_{1/2}$ ↑ in RI	—	—	—	Schulz V: Clinical pharmacokinetics of nitroprusside, cyanide, thiosulphate and thiocyanate. *Clin Pharmacokinet* 9:239–251, 1984. [1]Thiocyanate.
Sotalol	90–100	0	2.0 ± 0.4	7–15 $t_{1/2}$ is ↑ in RI and eld	80.1	2.6 ± 0.5 Cl is ↓ in RI and eld	—	Antonaccio MJ, Gomoll A: Pharmacology, pharmacodynamics and pharmacokinetics of sotalol. *Am J Cardiol* 65:12A–21A, 1990.
Spironolactone	60–70	>90	—	1.3–1.4 13–24[1] $t_{1/2}$ is ↑ in eld	<1	— Cl is ↓ in eld	—	Overdiek HW, Merkus FW: The metabolism and biopharmaceutics of spironolactone in man. *Rev Drug Metab Drug Interact* 5:273–302, 1987. [1]Half-life of canrenone.
Streptokinase	NA	—	0.08 ± 0.04	0.61 ± 0.04	0	1.7 ± 0.7	—	Gemmill JD, Hogg KJ, Burns JMA, et al: A comparison of the pharmacokinetic properties of streptokinase and anistreplase in acute myocardial infarction. *Br J Clin Pharmacol* 31:143–147, 1991.
Telmisartan	43	>99	7.1	≈24	<1	>11	—	McClellan KJ, Markham A: Telmisartan. *Drugs* 56(6):1039–1044, 1998.
Tenecteplase	NA	ID	0.09–0.21	11–20 min[1] 41–138 min[2]	ID	2.2	—	Tsikouris JP, Tsikouris AP: A review of available fibrin-specific thrombolytic agents used in acute myocardial infarction. *Pharmacotherapy* 21(2):207–17, 2001. [1]$t_{1/2}\alpha$. [2]$t_{1/2}\beta$.
Terazosin	90	90–94	0.80 ± 0.18	9–12	12 ± 3	1.1 ± 0.2	—	Titmarsh S, Monk JP: Terazosin: A review of its pharmacodynamic and pharmacokinetic properties and therapeutic efficacy in essential hypertension. *Drugs* 33:461–477, 1987.

(continued)

Generic Name	Bioavailability (%)	Protein Binding (%)	Volume of Distribution (liters/kg)	Half-Life (hours)	Urinary Excretion (% unchanged)	Clearance (mL · min⁻¹ · kg⁻¹)	Therapeutic Range	References
Ticlopidine	80–90	98	—	4–5 days $t_{1/2}$ is ↑ in RI	trace	8–21 Cl is ↓ in RI	1–2 μg/mL	Saltiel E, Ward A: Ticlopidine: A review of its pharmacodynamic and pharmacokinetic properties and therapeutic efficacy in platelet-dependent disease states. *Drugs* 34:222–262, 1987.
Timolol	50	< 10[1] 60[2]	2.1 ± 0.8	3–5	15	7.3 ± 3.3	—	McGourty JC, Silas JH, Fleming JJ, et al: Pharmacokinetics and beta-blocking effects of timolol in poor and extensive metabolizers of debrisoquin. *Clin Pharmacol Ther* 38:409–413, 1985. [1]By equilibrium dialysis. [2]By ultrafiltration.
Tinzaparin	90[1]	ID	0.06[1]	3–4[1]	ID	0.4[2]	—[3]	Friedel HA, Balfour JA: Tinzaparin. A review of its pharmacology and clinical potential in the prevention and treatment of thromboembolic disorders. *Drugs* 48(4):638–660, 1994. [1]Based on anti-factor Xa activity. [2]Clearance following intravenous administration of 4500 IU of tinzaparin. [3]Monitoring based on anti-Xa activity is generally not advised.
Tirofiban	NA	ID[1]	0.3–0.6	≈2	<65[2]	3.0–4.5	—	McClellan KJ, Goa KL: Tirofiban. A review of its use in acute coronary syndromes. *Drugs* 56(6):1067–1080, 1998. [1]Tirofiban is not highly bound to plasma proteins. [2]Tirofiban is cleared from the plasma largely by renal excretion, with about 65% of an administered dose appearing in the urine, largely as unchanged drug.
Tocainide	89 ± 5	10–15	3.0 ± 0.2	13.5 ± 2.3 $t_{1/2}$ is ↑ in RI	38 ± 7	2.6 ± 0.5 Cl is ↓ in CHF and RI	3–9 μg/mL	Roden DM. Woosley RL: Drug therapy: Tocainide. *N Engl J Med* 315:41–45, 1986.
Tolazoline	NA	—	1.61 ± 0.21	3–10[1]	—	—	—	Ward RM, Daniel CH, Kendig JW, et al: Oliguria and tolazoline pharmacokinetics in the newborn. *Pediatrics* 77:307–315, 1986. [1]In neonates.
Torsemide	80–90	97–99	0.16	3–4	27	—	—	Knauf H, Spahn H, Mutschler P: The loop diuretic torsemide in chronic renal failure: Pharmacokinetic and pharmacodynamics. *Drugs* 41(Suppl 3):23–34, 1991.

(*continued*)

Generic Name	Bioavailability (%)	Protein Binding (%)	Volume of Distribution (liters/kg)	Half-Life (hours)	Urinary Excretion (% unchanged)	Clearance (mL·min⁻¹·kg⁻¹)	Therapeutic Range	References
Trandolapril	40–60[1]	80	—	0.7–1.3 16–24[1] $t_{1/2}$ is ↑ in RI	—	—	—	Wiseman LR, McTavish D: Trandolapril: A review of its pharmacodynamic and pharmacokinetic properties, and therapeutic use in essential hypertension. *Drugs* 48:71–90, 1994. [1]Trandolaprilat.
Triamterene	54 ± 12	61 ± 2	13.4 ± 4.9	4.2 ± 0.7 $t_{1/2}$ is ↑ in RI and eld	21	63 ± 20 Cl is ↓ in HI, RI, and eld	—	Gilfrich HJ, Kremer G, Möhrke W, et al: Pharmacokinetics of triamterene after IV administration to man: Determination of bioavailability. *Eur J Clin Pharmacol* 25:237–241, 1983.
Trichlormethiazide	ID	—	—	2.3–7.3	ID	—	—	Sketris IS, Skoutakis VA, Acchiardo SR, et al: The pharmacokinetics of trichlormethiazide in hypertensive patients with normal and compromised renal function. *Eur J Clin Pharmacol* 20:453–457, 1981.
Urokinase	NA	—	—	10–20 min $t_{1/2}$ ↑ in HI	—	—	—	Maizel AS, Bookstein JJ: Streptokinase, urokinase, and tissue plasminogen activator: Pharmacokinetics, relative advantages, and methods for maximizing rates and consistency of lysis. *Cardiovasc Intervent Radiol* 9:236–244, 1986.
Valsartan	25 (10–35)	95 (94–97)	0.24	6	<13	0.48	—	Criscione L, et al: Valsartan: Preclinical and clinical profile of an antihypertensive angiotensin-II antagonist. *Cardiovasc Drug Rev* 13:230–250, 1995.
Verapamil	22 ± 8	90 ± 2	5.0 ± 2.1	4.0 ± 1.5 $t_{1/2}$ is ↑ in HI and eld	<3	15 ± 6 Cl is ↓ in HI and eld	80–300 ng/mL	McTavish D, Sorkin EM: Verapamil: An updated review of its pharmacodynamic and pharmacokinetic properties and therapeutic use in hypertension. *Drugs* 38:19–76, 1989.
Warfarin	93 ± 8	99 ± 1	0.14 ± 0.06	37 ± 15	<2	0.045 ± 0.024	—[1]	Chan E, McLachlan AJ, Pegg M, et al: Disposition of warfarin enantiomers and metabolites in patients during multiple dosing with *rac*-warfarin. *Br J Clin Pharmacol* 37:563–569, 1994. [1]Dose of warfarin should be adjusted based on desired INR range.

↑ = increased; ↓ = decreased; CAD = coronary artery disease; CHF = congestive heart failure; Cl = clearance; Cl_{cr} = creatinine clearance; eld = elderly; F = bioavailability; HI = hepatic impairment; ID = insufficient data; MI = myocardial infarction; NA = not applicable; neo = neonate; RI = renal impairment; SL = sublingual; $t_{1/2}$ = half-life; TOP = topical; V_d = volume of distribution.

Therapeutic Use of Available Cardiovascular Drugs

ALPHA-ADRENERGIC BLOCKERS

1. Doxazosin (Doxazosin, Cardura®)

Indications
Hypertension
Benign prostatic hyperplasia (BPH)

Dosage

Adults

As an antihypertensive, initiate at 1 mg/d. Dosage may be increased gradually according to blood pressure response. May increase every 1 to 2 weeks to 2, 4, 8, and 16 mg/d as needed.

Elderly

Initiate at lowest dose and titrate to response.

Children

Safety and efficacy have not been established.

Preparations
Doxazosin (generic); Cardura (Pfizer): 1 mg, 2 mg, 4 mg, and 8 mg tablets

2. Prazosin (Prazosin, Minipress®)

Indication
Hypertension

Dosage

Adults

As an antihypertensive, initiate therapy at 1 mg two to three times daily and slowly increase to the usual maintenance dose of 6 to 15 mg/d in divided doses. Most patients can be maintained on a twice-daily regimen after initial titration. Doses above 20 mg usually do not have increased effect. Some patients may respond to up to 40 mg/d.

Elderly

Initiate at lowest dose and titrate to response.

Children

Safety and efficacy have not been established. However, there has been some experience with the use of this drug in children and the following dosage regimen has been suggested: for children younger than 7 years of age, initiate at 250 μg (0.25 mg) two to three times daily and adjust to response. For children 7 to 12 years of age, initiate at 500 μg (0.5 mg) two to three times daily and adjust to response.

Preparations
Prazosin (generic); Minipress (Pfizer): 1 mg, 2 mg, 5 mg capsules.

Fixed dose combinations for treatment of hypertension:
Minizide-prazosin/polythiazide combination tablet: 1 mg/0.5 mg, 2 mg/0.5 mg, 5 mg/0.5 mg

3. Terazosin (Terazosin, Hytrin®)

Indications
Hypertension
Benign prostatic hyperplasia (BPH)

Dosage

Adults

As an antihypertensive, initiate therapy with 1 mg at bedtime. Dosage may be increased slowly to achieve desired response. There seems to be little benefit in exceeding a dose of 20 mg/d. Usual maintenance dose is 1 to 5 mg/d.

Elderly

Initiate at lowest dose and titrate to response.

Children

Safety and efficacy have not been established.

Preparations
Terazosin (generic); Hytrin (Abbott Laboratories): 1 mg, 2 mg, 5 mg, 10 mg capsules

4. Phenoxybenzamine (Dibenzyline®)

Indication
Symptomatic management of pheochromocytoma

Dosage

Adults

Initiate with 10 mg twice daily. Dose may be increased every other day by 10 mg until the desired response is obtained. Usual dose range is 20 to 40 mg two to three times per day. Phenoxybenzamine may be used concurrently with a beta-blocker if troublesome tachycardia coexists.

Elderly

Initiate at lowest dose and titrate to response.

Children

Safety and efficacy have not been established. However, there has been some experience with the use of this drug in children and the following dosage regimen has been suggested: initiate at

0.2 mg/kg once daily (maximum dose of 10 mg/d). Dosage may be increased gradually by 0.2 mg/kg increments until an adequate response is achieved. The usual pediatric maintenance dosage is 0.4 to 1.2 mg/kg/d given every 6 to 8 h; higher doses may be needed in some cases.

Preparation
Dibenzyline (Wellspring): 10 mg capsules

5. Phentolamine (Regitine®)

Indications
Diagnosis of pheochromocytoma

Prevention/control of hypertensive episodes that may occur in a patient with pheochromocytoma as a result of stress or manipulation during preoperative preparation and surgical excision

Prevention/treatment of dermal necrosis and sloughing following intravenous administration or extravasation of norepinephrine

Dosage

Prevention/control of hypertensive episodes associated with pheochromocytoma

Adults
Preoperative—5 mg (1 mg for children) administered intravenously (IV) or intramuscularly (IM) 1 to 2 h before surgery and repeat if indicated.

Intraoperative—5 mg IV (1 mg for children) and repeat as indicated to prevent or control paroxysms of hypertension, tachycardia, respiratory depression, convulsions, or other effects related to epinephrine intoxication.

Elderly
No dosage adjustment is required.

Children
Use lower dose in children as described above.

Prevention/treatment of dermal necrosis and sloughing associated with IV norepinephrine

Adults
Prevention—10 mg of phentolamine is added to each liter of norepinephrine solution.

Treatment—Initiate within 12 h (as soon as possible) of extravasation; 5 to 10 mg of phentolamine in 10 mL of 0.9% sodium chloride is infiltrated into the area using a small needle syringe.

Diagnosis of pheochromocytoma (not the first test of choice; all nonessential medications should be withheld for at least 24 h prior to the test)

Adults
5 mg IV or IM (1 mg IV or 3 mg IM for children) is administered. Five milligrams of phentolamine should be dissolved in 1 mL of sterile water for injection before administration. Following the IV dose, blood pressure should be monitored immediately, every 30 sec for the first 3 min, and every minute for the next 7 min. Following IM dose, blood pressure should be monitored every 5 min for 30 to 45 min. A blood pressure decrease of at least 35 mm Hg systolic and 25 mm Hg diastolic within 2 min after IV or 20 min after

IM administration of phentolamine is considered a positive test for pheochromocytoma.

Elderly
No dosage adjustment is required.

Children
Use lower dose in children as described above.

Preparation
Phentolamine mesylate for injection (Bedford); Regitine (Ciba): 5 mg vials

ALPHA₂-ADRENERGIC AGONISTS

1. Clonidine (Clonidine, Catapres,® Catapres-TTS,® Duraclon®)

Indications
Hypertension (oral and transdermal formulations)
Severe cancer pain not adequately relieved by opioid analgesics alone (continuous epidural infusion)

Dosage

Adults

Oral Initiate therapy at 0.05 to 0.1 mg twice daily. The dose may be increased by 0.1 to 0.2 mg daily every few days until the desired response is achieved. For rapid blood pressure reduction in patients with severe hypertension, clonidine 0.1 to 0.2 mg may be given, followed by 0.05 to 0.2 mg every hour until a total dose of 0.5 to 0.7 mg or adequate blood pressure control is achieved. The usual dose range of clonidine is 0.2 to 2.4 mg/d given in two to three divided doses.

Transdermal Initiate with one TTS-1 (2.5 mg) patch; increase to the next largest dose every 1 to 2 weeks for additional control or use a combination of patches. The maximum dosage is two TTS-3 patches. Note: For patients who are already on oral clonidine, it is recommended that the oral dose be continued for 1 to 2 days after the first transdermal system is applied.

Intravenous Initial dose of clonidine for continuous epidural infusion is 30 μg/h. Dosage may be titrated up or down depending on pain relief and occurrence of adverse events. Experience with dosage rate >40 μg/h is limited.

Elderly
Initiate at lowest dose and titrate to response.

Children
Safety and efficacy have not been established.

Preparations
Clonidine (generic); Catapres (Boehringer Ingelheim): 0.1, 0.2, 0.3 mg tablets

Transdermal System—Catapres-TTS-1, TTS-2, TTS-3 (Boehringer Ingelheim): delivering 0.1 mg, 0.2 mg, and 0.3 mg/d, respectively

Injection, as hydrochloride; Duraclon: 100 μg/mL (10 mL vials)

Fixed-Dose Combinations for the Treatment of Hypertension:
Combipres—clonidine/chlorthalidone combination tablets: 0.1 mg/15 mg; 0.2 mg/15 mg; 0.3 mg/15 mg

2. Guanabenz (Guanabenz, Wytensin®)

Indication
Hypertension

Dosage

Adults
Initiate therapy at 4 mg twice daily; dose may be adjusted every 1 to 2 weeks in increments of 4 to 8 mg/d until adequate blood pressure control is achieved. The maximum daily dose is 32 mg given in two divided doses.

Elderly
Initiate at lowest dose and titrate to response.

Children
Safety and efficacy have not been established.

Preparations
Guanabenz (generic); Wytensin (Wyeth-Ayerst): 4, 8 mg tablets

3. Guanfacine (Guanfacine, Tenex®)

Indication
Hypertension

Dosage

Adults
Initiate with 1 mg at bedtime to minimize somnolence. The dose may be increased in 1-mg increments every 3 to 4 weeks until adequate blood pressure control is achieved. The maximum daily dose is 3 mg once daily.

Elderly
Initiate at lowest dose and titrate to response.

Children
Safety and efficacy have not been established.

Preparations
Guanfacine (generic); Tenex (A.H. Robins): 1 mg, 2 mg tablets

4. Methyldopa (Methyldopa, Aldomet®)

Indication
Hypertension

Dosage

Adults

Oral   Initiate therapy at 250 mg two to three times daily for 2 days. The dose is then increased at intervals of at least 2 days until adequate blood pressure control is achieved. The maximum oral dose is 3 g/d.

Note: In patients who are receiving concomitant antihypertensive therapy other than thiazides, limit the initial dosage to 500 mg/d.

Intravenous (methyldopate)   Add the dose, 250 to 500 mg, to 100 mL of 5% dextrose or give in 5% dextrose in water in a concentration of 10 mg/mL. Administer intravenously over 30 to 60 min every 6 h if necessary. Maximum dose is 1 g every 6 h.

Elderly
Initiate at lowest dose and titrate to response.

Children
Safety and efficacy have not been established. However, there has been some experience with the use of this drug in children and the following dosage regimen has been suggested:

Oral   Dose should be based on body weight. Initially, give 10 mg/kg/d in two to four divided doses. Dosage should be adjusted in daily increments of 10 mg/kg until adequate blood pressure control is achieved. The maximum daily dose is 65 mg/kg or 3 g, whichever is less.

Intravenous   Dose should be based on body weight: 20 to 40 mg/kg/d in divided doses every 6 h. The maximum daily dose is 65 mg/kg or 3 g, whichever is less.

Preparations
Methyldopa (generic); Aldomet (Merck): 125 mg, 250 mg, 500 mg tablets

Methyldopate HCl injection (generic); Aldomet injection (Merck): 50 mg/mL, 250 mg/5 mL

Aldomet oral Suspension (Merck): 250 mg/5 mL

Fixed-Dose Combinations for the Treatment of Hypertension:
Aldoclor (Merck)—methyldopa/chlorothiazide combination tablets: 250 mg/150 mg; 250 mg/250 mg

Aldoril (Merck)—methyldopa/hydrochlorothiazide combination tablets: 250 mg/15 mg; 250 mg/25 mg

Aldoril D (Merck)—methyldopa/hydrochlorothiazide combination tablets: 500 mg/30 mg; 500 mg/50 mg

ANGIOTENSIN-CONVERTING ENZYME INHIBITORS

1. Benazepril (Lotensin®)

Indication
Hypertension

Dosage

Adults
The usual initial dose is 10 mg once daily. Dose can be titrated up to 40 mg/d (in one or two divided doses.) The maximum dose is 80 mg/d. In renovascular hypertension, renal failure, or in patients in whom diuretics have not been discontinued, the starting dose should be 5 mg.

Elderly
Dose reduction generally not required.

Children
Safety and efficacy have not been established.

Preparations

Lotensin (Novartis Pharmaceuticals): 5, 10, 20, 40 mg tablets

Fixed-Dose Combinations for the Treatment of Hypertension:
Lotensin HCT—benazepril hydrochloride/hydrochlorothiazide combination tablets: 5 mg/6.25 mg; 10 mg/12.5 mg; 20 mg/12.5 mg; 20 mg/25 mg

Lotrel—amlodipine/benazepril hydrochloride combination capsules: 2.5 mg/10 mg; 5 mg/10 mg; 5 mg/20 mg; 10 mg/20 mg

2. Captopril (captopril, Capoten®)

Indications

Hypertension
Heart failure
Left ventricular dysfunction after myocardial infarction
Diabetic nephropathy

Dosage

Hypertension

Adults

Initiate therapy at 12.5 to 25 mg two to three times per day. Dosage may be increased according to response to 150 mg/d given in three divided doses. In renovascular hypertension, when diuretics have not been discontinued or in renal impairment, initial dose should be 6.25 mg, titrated cautiously according to response.

Elderly

Initiate at lowest dose and titrate to response.

Children

Safety and efficacy have not been established. However, the following regimen has been suggested: initiate with 0.3 mg/kg three times daily. Dosage may be increased in increments of 0.3 mg/kg at intervals of 8 to 24 h until adequate blood pressure control is achieved.

Heart failure

Adults

Initiate at 6.25 to 12.5 mg 3 times daily and increase dosage according to clinical response. The target dose is 150 mg/d given in three divided doses.

Diabetic nephropathy

Adults

25 mg 3 times daily in Type I diabetes

Left ventricular dysfunction after myocardial infarction

Adults

Initiate with 6.25 mg, followed by 12.5 mg 3 times daily. Then increase dose to 25 mg three times per day during the next several days. A target dose of 50 mg three times per day may be achieved over the next several weeks.

Preparations

Captopril (generic); Capoten (Bristol-Myers-Squibb): 12.5 mg, 25 mg, 50 mg, 100 mg tablets

Fixed-Dose Combinations for the Treatment of Hypertension:
Capozide (generic)—captopril/hydrochlorothiazide combination tablets: 25 mg/15 mg; 25 mg/25 mg; 50 mg/15 mg; 50 mg/25 mg

3. Enalapril (Enalapril, Vasotec®) and Enalaprilat (Enalaprilat, Vasotec® I.V.)

Indications

Hypertension
Heart failure
Left ventricular dysfunction-asymptomatic

Dosage

Hypertension

Adults

Oral Initiate therapy at 5 mg/d, dosage may be increased to the usual effective maintenance dose of 10 to 20 mg/d (maximum, 40 mg daily given in two divided doses). In renovascular hypertension or in patients in whom diuretics have not been discontinued 2 to 3 days previously, the starting dose should be 2.5 mg.

Intravenous The usual IV dose in hypertension is 1.25 mg every 6 h administered intravenously over a 5-minute period. An initial dose of 0.625 mg over 5 min should be used in patients who are sodium and volume depleted or who have renal impairment (CrCl <30 mL/min). Patients should be observed 1 h after dose to watch for hypotension. If response is inadequate after 1 h, the 0.625 mg dose may be repeated and therapy continued at a dose of 1.25 mg every 6 h.

Elderly

Initiate at lowest dose and titrate to response.

Children

Safety and efficacy have not been established.

Heart failure

Adults

Initiate therapy at 2.5 mg by mouth once or twice per day; dosage may be titrated according to clinical response. The usual maintenance dose is 5 to 40 mg/d given in two divided doses.

Asymptomatic left ventricular dysfunction

Adults

Initiate therapy at 2.5 mg by mouth once or twice per day, dosage may be titrated according to clinical response. The target daily dose is 20 mg/d given in two divided doses.

Preparations

Enalapril (generic); Vasotec (Merck): 2.5 mg, 5 mg, 10 mg, 20 mg tablets

Enalaprilat (generic); Vasotec I.V. (Merck): 1.25 mg/mL intravenous solution

Fixed-Dose Combinations for the Treatment of Hypertension:
Vaseretic—enalapril maleate/hydrochlorothiazide combination tablets: 5 mg/12.5 mg; 10 mg/25 mg

Teczem (Aventis) —enalapril maleate/diltiazem malate extended-release combination tablets: 5 mg/180 mg

Lexxel (Astra Zeneca) —enalapril maleate/felodipine extended-release combination tablets: 5 mg/2.5 mg, 5 mg/5 mg

4. Fosinopril (Monopril®)

Indications
Hypertension
Heart failure

Dosage

Hypertension

Adults
Initiate with 10 mg/d; dosage may be increased to the usual effective dose of 20 to 40 mg/d. Some patients may have a further response to 80 mg/d. The total daily dose may be divided into two if trough effect is inadequate. In renovascular hypertension or in patients in whom diuretics have not been discontinued, the starting dose should be 5 mg/d.

Elderly
Dose reduction generally not required.

Children
Safety and efficacy have not been established.

Heart failure

Adults
The usual initial dose is 10 mg/d. The patient should be observed under medical supervision for at least 2 h for the presence of hypotension or orthostasis following the initial dose of fosinopril. An initial dose of 5 mg may be used in patients with moderate to severe renal impairment or in those who have been vigorously diuresed. Dosage should be increased over a period of several weeks to a dose that is maximal and tolerated. The usual effective dosage range is 20 to 40 mg once daily.

Preparations
Monopril (Bristol-Myers-Squibb): 10 mg, 20 mg, 40 mg tablets

Fixed-Dose Combinations for Treatment of Hypertension:
Monopril HCT—fosinopril/hydrochlorothiazide combination tablets: 10 mg/12.5 mg; 20 mg/12.5 mg

5. Lisinopril (Prinivil®, Zestril®)

Indications
Hypertension
Heart failure
Acute myocardial infarction

Dosage

Hypertension

Adults
Initiate with 10 mg/d; dosage may be adjusted to the usual effective dose of 10 to 40 mg/d according to response. In patients with hyponatremia, patients with renal impairment (CrCl $\leq$30 mL/min),

or in patients in whom diuretics have not been discontinued, the starting dose should be 2.5 mg/d.

Elderly
Initiate at lowest dose and titrate to response.

Children
Safety and efficacy have not been established.

Heart failure

Adults
The usual initial dose is 5 mg/d administered under close medical observation, especially in patients with low blood pressure. The usual effective dosage range is 5 to 20 mg once daily.

Acute myocardial infarction

Adults
In hemodynamically stable patients, give 5 mg of lisinopril within 24 h of the onset of acute MI. Another dose of 5 mg may be given 24 h later, followed by 10 mg at 48 h, then 10 mg once daily thereafter for 6 weeks. Patients should receive, as appropriate, the standard recommended treatments, such as thrombolytics, aspirin, and beta-blockers. Patients with a low systolic blood pressure ($\leq$120 mm Hg) when treatment is initiated or during the first 3 days after the infarct should be given a lower dose of 2.5 mg. If hypotension occurs (systolic blood pressure $\leq$100 mm Hg), a daily maintenance dose of 5 mg may be given with temporary reductions to 2.5 mg if necessary.

Preparations
Lisinopril (generic); Prinivil (Merck): 2.5, 5, 10, 20, 40 mg tablets

Lisinopril (generic); Zestril (Astra Zeneca): 2.5, 5, 10, 20, 30, 40 mg tablets

Fixed-Dose Combinations for the Treatment of Hypertension:
Prinzide—lisinopril/hydrochlorothiazide combination tablets: 10 mg/12.5 mg; 20 mg/12.5 mg; 20 mg/25mg

Zestoretic—lisinopril/hydrochlorothiazide combination tablets: 10 mg/12.5 mg; 20 mg/12.5 mg; 20 mg/25mg

6. Moexipril (Univasc®)

Indication
Hypertension

Dosage

Adults
The usual initial dose is 7.5 mg once daily in patients not receiving diuretics. Dosage may be increased gradually to a maximum of 30 mg/d (given in one or two divided doses) according to response. In renovascular hypertension, or in patients in whom diuretics have not been discontinued, the recommended starting dose is 3.75 mg once daily given with close medical supervision. Similarly, for patients whose creatinine clearance is $\leq$40 mL/min/1.73^2, the recommended initial dose is 3.75 mg once daily given with caution. Note: moexipril should be taken on an empty stomach, preferably 1 h prior to a meal.

Elderly
Initiate at lowest dose and titrate to response.

Children
Safety and efficacy have not been established.

Preparations
Univasc (Schwarz Pharma): 7.5, 15 mg tablets

Fixed-Dose Combinations for the Treatment of Hypertension:
Uniretic—moexipril hydrochloride/hydrochlorothiazide combination tablets: 7.5 mg/12.5 mg; 15 mg/25 mg

7. Perindopril (Aceon®)
Indication
Hypertension

Dosage

Adults
The usual initial dose is 4 mg once daily in patients not receiving other antihypertensives. This dose may be titrated up to a maximum of 16 mg/d based on clinical response. The usual maintenance dose is 4 to 8 mg once daily. For patients older than 70 years of age and for patients with CrCl of 30 to 60 mL/min, initiate with 2 mg once daily and titrate according to response to a maximum of 8 mg/d. The safety and efficacy of perindopril have not been established for patients with CrCl of <30 mL/min.

Elderly
Initiate at lowest dose and titrate to response.

Children
Safety and efficacy have not been established.

Preparations
Aceon (Solvay): 2, 4, 8 mg tablets

8. Quinapril (Accupril®)
Indications
Hypertension
Heart failure

Dosage

Hypertension

Adults
The usual initial dose is 10 or 20 mg once daily in patients not receiving diuretics. This dose may be increased, at intervals of at least 2 weeks, to a maximum of 80 mg/d (given as a single dose or in two divided doses) according to response. In renovascular hypertension, or in patients in whom diuretics have not been discontinued, the starting dose should be 2.5 to 5 mg/d. For patients with creatinine clearance of 31 to 60 mL/min, the initial dose should be 5 mg daily. For patients with creatinine clearance of 10 to 30 mL/min, the initial dose should be 2.5 mg/d.

Elderly
Initiate at lowest dose and titrate to response.

Children
Safety and efficacy have not been established.

Heart failure

Adults
The usual initial dose is 5 mg twice daily titrated according to clinical response. The usual maintenance dose is 20 to 40 mg/d in two divided doses.

Preparations
Accupril (Parke-Davis/Pfizer): 5 mg, 10 mg, 20 mg, 40 mg tablets

Fixed-Dose Combinations for the Treatment of Hypertension:
Accuretic—quinapril/hydrochlorothiazide combination tablets: 10 mg/12.5 mg; 20 mg/12.5 mg; 20 mg/25 mg

9. Ramipril (Altace®)
Indications
Hypertension
Heart failure postmyocardial infarction
Reduction in risk of myocardial infarction, stroke, and death from cardiovascular causes

Dosage

Hypertension

Adults
The usual initial dose is 2.5 mg/d, this dose may be increased gradually to a maximum of 20 mg/d (given as a single daily dose or in two equally divided doses) according to response. In renovascular hypertension or in patients in whom diuretics have not been discontinued, the starting dose should be 1.25 mg/d. For patients with creatinine clearance of <40 mL/min/1.73 m^2, the initial dose should be 1.25 mg/d. Dosage may be titrated upward until blood pressure is controlled or to a maximum of 5 mg/d.

Elderly
Initiate at lowest dose and titrate to response.

Children
Safety and efficacy have not been established.

Heart failure post myocardial infarction

Adults
The usual initial dose is 2.5 mg twice daily. Patients who become hypotensive at this dose may be switched to 1.25 mg twice daily, but all patients should then be titrated toward a target dose of 5 mg twice daily if tolerated. For patients with creatinine clearance of <40 mL/min/1.73 m^2, the initial dose should be 1.25 mg daily. Dosage may then be increased to 1.25 mg twice daily up to a maximum dose of 2.5 mg twice daily, depending on clinical response and tolerance.

Reduction in risk of MI, stroke, and death from cardiovascular causes

Adults
Initiate at 2.5 mg once daily for one week, then increase dose to 5 mg once daily for the next 3 weeks, then increase dose as tolerated to 10 mg once daily (may be given as divided dose).

Preparations
Altace (Monarch): 1.25 mg, 2.5 mg, 5 mg, 10 mg capsules

10. Trandolapril (Mavik®)

Indications
Hypertension
Heart failure postmyocardial infarction
Left ventricular dysfunction postmyocardial infarction

Dosage

Hypertension

Adults
The usual initial dose is 1 mg/d in non-black patients and 2 mg/d in black patients. Dosage may be increased, according to response, at intervals of ≥1 week to a maximum of 8 mg/d. Most patients have required dosages of 2 to 4 mg/d. There is little experience with doses more than 8 mg/d. Patients inadequately treated with once-daily dosing at 4 mg may be treated with twice-daily dosing. In renovascular hypertension or in patients in whom diuretics have not been discontinued, the starting dose should be 0.5 mg/d. Similarly, for patients with a creatinine clearance <30 mL/min or with hepatic cirrhosis, the recommended initial dose is 0.5 mg/d.

Elderly
Initiate at lowest dose and titrate to response.

Children
Safety and efficacy have not been established.

Heart failure or left ventricular dysfunction postmyocardial infarction

Adults
The usual initial dose is 1 mg/d. This dose may be increased as tolerated to a target dose of 4 mg/d. If the 4-mg dose is not tolerated, patients can continue therapy with the greatest tolerated dose. For patients with a creatinine clearance <30 mL/min or with hepatic cirrhosis, the recommended initial dose is 0.5 mg/d.

Preparations
Mavik (Abbott): 1 mg, 2 mg, 4 mg tablets

Fixed-Dose Combinations for the Treatment of Hypertension:
Tarka—trandolapril/verapamil hydrochloride extended release tablets: 2 mg/180 mg; 1 mg/240 mg; 2 mg/240 mg; 4 mg/240 mg

ANGIOTENSIN-II RECEPTOR BLOCKERS

1. Candesartan (Atacand®)

Indication
Hypertension

Dosage

Adults
The usual initial dose is 16 mg once daily. Dosage may be titrated within the range of 8 to 32 mg/d according to response. Hydrochlorothiazide has an additive effect.

Elderly
No initial dosage adjustment is required.

Children
Safety and efficacy have not been established.

Preparations
Atacand (AstraZeneca): 4 mg, 8 mg, 16 mg, 32 mg tablets

Fixed-Dose Combinations for the Treatment of Hypertension:
Atacand HCT—candesartan cilexetil/hydrochlorothiazide combination tablets: 16 mg/12.5 mg; 32 mg/12.5 mg

2. Eprosartan (Teveten®)

Indication
Hypertension

Dosage

Adults
The usual initial dose is 600 mg once daily. Dosage may be titrated within the range of 400 to 800 mg/d given in one or two divided doses.

Elderly
No initial dosage adjustment is required.

Children
Safety and efficacy have not been established.

Preparations
Teveten (Unimed): 400 mg, 600 mg tablets

3. Irbesartan (Avapro®)

Indications
Hypertension
Type II diabetes with nephropathy to prevent end-stage renal disease

Dosage

Adults
The usual initial dose is 150 mg once daily. Dosage may be titrated to 300 mg once daily according to response. Hydrochlorothiazide has an additive effect.

Elderly
No initial dosage adjustment is required.

Children
Safety and efficacy have not been established.

Preparations
Avapro (Bristol-Myers Squibb/Sanofi): 75 mg, 150 mg, 300 mg tablets

Fixed-Dose Combinations for the Treatment of Hypertension:
Avalide—irbesartan/hydrochlorothiazide: 150mg/12.5 mg, 300 mg/12.5 mg

4. Losartan (Cozaar®)

Indications
Hypertension
Type II diabetes with nephropathy to prevent end-stage renal disease

Dosage

Adults

The usual initial dose is 50 mg once daily. Dosage may be titrated up to 100 mg/d (in one or two divided doses). Lower initial dose of 25 mg once daily should be given to patients at high risk for hypotension, volume depletion, and those with hepatic dysfunction.

For nephropathy in type 2 diabetic patients the usual starting dose is 50 mg once daily. The dose should be increased to 100 mg once daily based on blood pressure response.

Elderly

No initial dosage adjustment is required.

Children

Safety and efficacy have not been established.

Preparations

Cozaar (Merck): 25 mg, 50 mg, 100 mg tablets

Fixed-Dose Combinations for the Treatment of Hypertension: Hyzaar—losartan/hydrochlorothiazide: 50 mg/12.5 mg, 100 mg/25 mg

5. Olmesartan (Benicar®)

Indication

Hypertension

Dosage

Adults

The usual recommended initial dose is 20 mg once daily when used as monotherapy in patients who are not volume-contracted. If further reduction in blood pressure is required after 2 weeks of therapy, the dose may be increased to 40 mg. Doses above 40 mg do not appear to have greater effect. Twice-daily dosing offers no advantage over the same total dose given once daily.

Elderly

No initial dosage adjustment is required.

Children

Safety and efficacy have not been established.

Preparations

Benicar (Sankyo): 5 mg, 20 mg, and 40 mg tablets

6. Telmisartan (Micardis®)

Indication

Hypertension

Dosage

Adults

The usual initial dose is 40 mg once daily. Dosage may be titrated within the range of 20 to 80 mg/d according to response. Initiate treatment under close medical supervision for patients with hepatic impairment or biliary obstructive disorders. If intravascular volume depletion is present, correct this condition prior to initiation of telmisartan and monitor closely.

Elderly

No initial dosage adjustment is required.

Children

Safety and efficacy have not been established.

Preparations

Micardis (Boehringer Ingelheim): 40 mg, 80 mg tablets

Fixed-Dose Combinations for the Treatment of Hypertension: Micardis HCT—telmisartan/hydrochlorothiazide: 40 mg/12.5 mg; 80 mg/12.5 mg

7. Valsartan (Diovan®)

Indication

Hypertension

Dosage

Adults

The usual initial dose is 80 mg once daily. Dosage may be increased to 160 to 320 mg once daily according to response.

Elderly

No initial dosage adjustment is required.

Children

Safety and efficacy have not been established.

Preparations

Diovan (Novartis): 40 mg, 80 mg, 160 mg, 320 mg tablets

Fixed-Dose Combinations for the Treatment of Hypertension: Diovan HCT: valsartan/hydrochlorothiazide: 80 mg/12.5 mg; 160 mg/12.5 mg

ANTIARRHYTHMIC AGENTS

CLASS IA

1. Disopyramide (Disopyramide phosphate, Norpace®)

Indications

Life-threatening ventricular arrhythmias
Supraventricular arrhythmias (unlabeled use)

Dosage

Adults

The usual dosage in adults weighing more than 50 kg is 150 mg q 6 h as conventional capsules or 300 mg q 12 h as extended-release capsules. In adults weighing less than 50 kg, the usual dosage is 100 mg q 6 h as conventional capsules or 200 mg q 12 h as extended-release capsules. When rapid control of ventricular arrhythmias is required, 300 mg of disopyramide (200 mg for patients weighing <50 kg) may be given initially and followed by the usual maintenance dose in conventional capsules. The extended-release capsules should not be used initially when rapid control of ventricular arrhythmias is needed.

In patients with cardiomyopathy or possible cardiac decompensation, the initial loading dose should not be given and an initial dosage of 100 mg q 6 h should not be exceeded. Dosage should be carefully adjusted while the patient is closely monitored for hypotension and/or congestive heart failure.

In patients with moderately impaired renal function (CrCl >40 mL/min) or hepatic insufficiency, the usual dosage is 100 mg q 6 h as conventional capsules or 200 mg q 12 h as extended-release capsules. For rapid control of a ventricular arrhythmia, an initial dose of 200 mg may be given. In patients with severely impaired renal function (CrCl ≤40 mL/min), the usual dosages of disopyramide (with or without an initial 150-mg dose) given as conventional capsules are as follows:

CrCl	Maintenance Dose
30 to 40 mL/min	100 mg q 8 h
15 to 30 mL/min	100 mg q 12 h
<15 mL/min	100 mg q 24 h

Elderly

May be more sensitive to adult dose. Dose reduction is required.

Children

Dosing is age-specific. The total daily dose should be given in equally divided doses q 6 h or at intervals according to individual requirements. Pediatric patients should be hospitalized during initial period of therapy to allow close monitoring until maintenance dose is established.

Age	Maintenance Dose
<1 y	10 to 30 mg/kg/d
1 to 4 y	10 to 20 mg/kg/d
4 to 12 y	10 to 15 mg/kg/d
12 to 18 y	6 to 15 mg/kg/d

Preparations

Disopyramide phosphate (generic); Norpace (Pharmacia & Upjohn): 100 mg, 150 mg capsules

Disopyramide phosphate extended release (generic); Norpace CR (Pharmacia & Upjohn): 100 mg, 150 mg extended-release capsules

2. Procainamide (Procainamide HCl, Pronestyl®, Pronestyl^SR®, Procanbid®)

Indications

Ventricular arrhythmias
Supraventricular arrhythmias (unlabeled use)
Atrial fibrillation/atrial flutter (unlabeled use)

Dosage

Adults

For initial management of arrhythmias in adults, a loading dose intravenous infusion of 500 to 600 mg may be administered at a constant rate over a period of 25 to 30 min. Although it is unusual to require more than 600 mg to initially control an arrhythmia, the maximum recommended total dose is 1 g. A continuous intravenous infusion of 1 to 6 mg/min may be administered to maintain therapeutic plasma concentrations subsequently. Alternatively, a loading dose infusion of 12 to 17 mg/kg (at a rate of 20 to 30 mg/min) may be given followed by a continuous infusion of 1 to 4 mg/min.

Infusion rate should be lower in patients with renal impairment or hemodynamic instability. Consult procainamide package literature for information on proper dilution of procainamide prior to intravenous administration.

Extended-release tablets are intended for maintenance dosing regimen. Usual maintenance dose for ventricular arrhythmias is 50 mg/kg/d in divided doses q 6 h for extended-release tablets and q 12 h for Procanbid. Usual maintenance dose for supraventricular arrhythmias in adults is 1 g q 6 h using extended-release tablets.

For the treatment of arrhythmias that occur during surgery and anesthesia, an IM or IV (preferably IM) dose of 100 to 500 mg can be given.

Elderly

Dosage adjustment is required for reduced renal function and other comorbid conditions (e.g., CHF).

Children

Safety and efficacy have not been established. IM injection is not recommended.

Preparations

Pronestyl (Princeton Pharm): 250 mg, 375 mg, 500 mg tablets
Procainamide hydrochloride tablets (generic): 375 mg, 500 mg tablets
Procanbid (Monarch): 500 mg, 1000 mg extended-release tablets
Procainamide hydrochloride extended-release tablets (generic): 250 mg, 500 mg, 750 mg tablets
Procainamide hydrochloride capsules (generic); Pronestyl (Princeton Pharm): 250 mg, 375 mg, 500 mg capsules
Procainamide hydrochloride injection (generic): 100 mg/mL, 500 mg/mL

3. Quinidine (Quinidine gluconate, Quinaglute® Dura-Tabs®, Quinidine sulfate, Quinidex Extentabs®)

Indications

Maintenance of sinus rhythm after conversion of atrial fibrillation/flutter
Atrial or ventricular premature complexes
Conversion of atrial fibrillation/flutter
Paroxysmal supraventricular tachycardia
Paroxysmal ventricular tachycardia that is not associated with complete heart block
Life-threatening *Plasmodium falciparum* malaria (IV quinidine gluconate)

Dosage

Adults

Quinidine is expressed in molar basis   267 mg of quinidine gluconate or 275 mg of quinidine polygalacturonate is equivalent to 200 mg of quinidine sulfate. The following dosages are expressed in terms of the respective salts.

Quinidine sulfate   For the conversion of atrial fibrillation: 200 mg po q 2 to 3 h for 5 to 8 doses. Usually, clinicians used 300 to 400 mg po q 6 h. If pharmacologic conversion back to sinus rhythm does not occur with plasma concentrations of 9 μg/mL, increase in dose would increase the risk of toxicity. For paroxysmal supraventricular tachycardia and paroxysmal ventricular tachycardia: 400 to 600 mg po q 2 to 3 h until paroxysm is terminated. For the maintenance of sinus rhythm after conversion: 200 to 400 mg po tid or qid or 300 to 600 mg extended release tablets q 8 to 12 h.

Quinidine gluconate   For the suppression and prevention of atrial, AV junctional, and ventricular premature complexes, administer 324 to 648 mg po as extended release tablets q 8 to 12 h. Maintenance dose for sinus rhythm after conversion is 324 mg q 8 to 12 h as extended release tablets, increase to 648 mg q 8 to 12 h if necessary and tolerated.

Quinidine gluconate injections   For atrial fibrillation/flutter (can be used for ventricular arrhythmias), administer 5 to 10 mg/kg at an initial rate of up to 0.25 mg/kg/min. If conversion does not occur at 10 mg/kg, attempt another mean for conversion. There is a high risk for hypotension. Monitor ECG for widening of QRS and prolongation of QT intervals, disappearance of the P wave, symptomatic bradycardia, or tachycardia. Consult quinidine package literature for proper dilution of intravenous injection prior to administration.

Elderly
Initiate with lowest dose and titrate to response.

Children
Safety and efficacy have not been established. However, quinidine gluconate used to treat malaria in children has shown an efficacy and safety profile comparable to adults.

Preparations
Quinidine gluconate extended-release tablets (generic); Quinaglute Dura-Tabs (Berlex): 324 mg extended-release tablets
Quinidine sulfate extended-release tablets (generic); Quinidex Extentabs (A.H. Robins): 300 mg extended-release tablets
Quinidine sulfate tablets USP (generic): 200 mg, 300 mg tablets
Quinidine gluconate injection: 80 mg/mL (50 mg/mL quinidine)

CLASS IB

1. Lidocaine (Lidocaine HCl, Xylocaine®)

Indication
Acute treatment of ventricular tachyarrhythmias (intravenous formulation)

Dosage

Adults

Initial IV bolus dose   1 to 1.5 mg/kg at 25 to 50 mg/min, may repeat 0.5 to 0.75 mg/kg in 5 to 10 min if initial response is inadequate up to a total dose of 3 mg/kg. No more than 200 to 300 mg should be administered during a 1-h period. Patients with CHF or cardiogenic shock may require a smaller dose.

Maintenance infusion   1 to 4 mg/min (20 to 50 μg/kg/min). A slower rate of 1 to 2 mg/min may be sufficient for patients with CHF, liver disease, who are older than 70 years old, or who weigh less than 70 kg.

Elderly
Dose reduction is required due to reduction in patients' capacity to metabolize the drug.

Children
Safety and effectiveness have not been established; reduce dosage when used in children.

Preparations
Lidocaine for IV admixtures (generic): 40, 100, 200 mg/mL
Xylocaine (Astra Zeneca) for IV admixtures: 40, 200 mg/mL
Lidocaine direct intravenous injection (generic); Xylocaine (Astra Zeneca): 10, 20 mg/mL.
Lidocaine hydrochloride and dextrose injection (generic): 1, 2, 4, 8 mg/mL

2. Mexiletine (Mexiletine HCl, Mexitil®)

Indication
Life-threatening ventricular arrhythmias

Dosage

Adults
Initiate at 200 mg po q 8 h, increase or decrease dosage in increments or decrements of 50 to 100 mg/dose every 2 to 3 days as needed. For rapid control of ventricular arrhythmias, loading dose of 400 mg may be administered followed by a 200 mg dose 8 h later. Limit to 1200 mg/d when given q 8 h (i.e., 400 mg/dose) or 900 mg/d when given q 12 h (i.e., 450 mg/dose).

Patients with CHF or hepatic impairment may require dose reduction. Dosage adjustments should be made no more frequently than every 2 to 3 days. Some patients may tolerate twice-daily dosing. For patients adequately maintained on a dose of 300 mg or less q 8 h, total daily dose may be given divided q 12 h. Patients not adequately controlled by dosing q 8 h may respond to dosing q 6 h.

Elderly
Dosage adjustment is required due to reduction in patients' capacity to metabolize the drug.

Children
Safety and effectiveness have not been established.

Preparations
Mexilitine (generic); Mexitil (Boehringer Ingelheim): 150 mg, 200 mg, 250 mg capsules

3. Tocainide (Tonocard®)

Indication
Life-threatening ventricular arrhythmias

Dosage

Adults

Loading dose   600 mg then 400 mg after 4 to 6 h.

Maintenance dose   400 mg po q 8 h. Usual maintenance dose is 1.2 to 1.8 g daily. Maximum dose is 2.4 g/d in divided doses. Reduce initial maintenance dose by 50% in patients with hepatic dysfunction and in patients with CrCl <10 mL/min. Reduce initial maintenance dose by 25% in patients with CrCl of 10 to 30 mL/min.

Elderly

Dosage adjustment is required due to reduction in patients' capacity to eliminate the drug.

Children

Safety and effectiveness have not been established.

Preparations

Tonocard (Astra Zeneca): 400 mg, 600 mg tablets

CLASS IC

1. Flecainide (Tambocor®)

Indications

Life-threatening ventricular arrhythmias
Supraventricular tachyarrhythmias

Dosage

Adults

For sustained ventricular tachycardia, initiate at 100 mg q 12 h; increase dosage in increments of 50 mg twice daily every 4 days as needed. The usual maintenance dose is 150 mg q 12 h; limit to 400 mg/d. For patients with paroxysmal supraventricular tachycardia and patients with paroxysmal atrial fibrillation, initiate at 50 mg q 12 h. Increase dosage in increments of 50 mg twice daily every 4 days as needed; limit to 300 mg/d in patients with paroxysmal supraventricular tachycardia.

For patients with severe renal impairment (CrCl <35 mL/min), reduce initial dose to 50 mg q 12 h; increase doses at intervals of >4 days if needed and monitor plasma levels frequently to guide dosage adjustment.

Elderly

Lower doses are recommended due to age-related decline in clearance.

Children

Safety and effectiveness have not been established.

Preparations

Tambocor (3M Pharmaceuticals): 50 mg, 100 mg, 150 mg tablets

2. Propafenone (Propafenone, Rythmol®)

Indications

Life-threatening ventricular arrhythmias
Supraventricular tachyarrhythmias (unlabeled use)

Dosage

Adults

Initiate at 150 mg q 8 h. Increase dosage after 3 to 4 days to 225 mg q 8 h if needed. Dosage may be further increased to 300 mg q 8 h after an additional 3 to 4 days if needed and tolerated.

Elderly

Lower doses may be required due to reduction in patients' capacity to metabolize the drug.

Children

Safety and effectiveness have not been established.

Preparations

Propafenone (generic); Rythmol (Abbott): 150 mg, 225 mg, 300 mg tablets

3. Moricizine (Ethmozine®)

Indication

Life-threatening ventricular arrhythmias

Dosage

Adults

The usual dosage is 600 to 900 mg/d in three divided doses q 8 h. Dosage may be increased at 150 mg/d at 3-day intervals. Limit to 900 mg/d.

In patients with hepatic function impairment or significant renal impairment, an initial dose of 600 mg/d or less is recommended. In patients whose arrhythmias are well controlled, dosing q 12 h may aid compliance.

Elderly

Lower doses may be required due to reduction in patients' capacity to metabolize the drug.

Children

Safety and effectiveness have not been established.

Preparations

Ethmozine (Roberts): 200 mg, 250 mg, 300 mg tablets

CLASS II

BETA-ADRENERGIC BLOCKERS

CLASS III

1. Amiodarone (Amiodarone, Cordarone®, Pacerone®)

Indications

Life-threatening ventricular arrhythmias (ventricular fibrillation or hemodynamically unstable ventricular tachycardia)
Supraventricular arrhythmias (not FDA approved)

Dosage

Adults

Oral

Life-threatening ventricular arrhythmias   Loading dose is 800 to 1600 mg/d in divided doses for 1 to 3 weeks (occasionally longer). Dosage should then be reduced to 600 to 800 mg/d in one to two divided doses for 4 weeks. Maintenance dose is usually 400 mg/d. Some patients may require larger maintenance doses of 600 mg/d, others may be controlled on lower doses. Amiodarone may be administered as a single daily dose, or as a twice daily dose in patients with severe GI intolerance.

Supraventricular arrhythmias (not FDA approved)   Oral loading dose of 600 to 800 mg/d for 7 to 10 days, then 200 to 400 mg/d as maintenance dose.

Intravenous

Life-threatening ventricular arrhythmias   Load 150 mg over 10 min (15 mg/min), then 360 mg over the next 6 h (1 mg/min). A maintenance infusion of 540 mg is then given over the next 18 h (0.5 mg/min). Intravenous amiodarone should be used for acute treatment until the patient's ventricular arrhythmias are stabilized. Most patients require intravenous therapy for 48 to 96 h; however, the maintenance infusion of 0.5 mg/min (or less) can be administered up to 2 to 3 weeks. A supplemental dose of 150 mg over 10 min can be given for breakthrough arrhythmias. Consult amiodarone package literature for proper dilution of drug prior to administration. Intravenous amiodarone concentration should not exceed 2 mg/mL unless a central venous catheter is used.

Elderly

Dosage adjustment should be made based on comorbid conditions and concurrent therapy.

Children

Safety and effectiveness have not been established. Limited data suggest that amiodarone may be useful in the management of refractory supraventricular or ventricular arrhythmias in selected cases.

Preparations

Amiodarone (generic); Cordarone (Wyeth-Ayerst); Pacerone (Upsher Smith): 200 mg tablets

Cordarone IV (Wyeth-Ayerst): 3 mL ampule, 50 mg/mL

2. Bretylium (Bretylium tosylate)

Indications

Life-threatening ventricular arrhythmias (ventricular fibrillation or hemodynamically unstable ventricular tachycardia that are unresponsive to conventional antiarrhythmic drugs)

Dosage

Adults

Immediately life-threatening ventricular arrhythmias (ventricular fibrillation or hemodynamically unstable ventricular tachycardia that are unresponsive to conventional antiarrhythmic drugs)   Initiate with a 5 mg/kg undiluted intravenous injection over approximately 1 minute. CPR measures including cardioversion should be undertaken before and following bretylium administration as needed. If ventricular fibrillation persists, supplemental doses of 10 mg/kg may be given by rapid intravenous injection (over approximately 1 minute) and repeated as needed, usually at 5- to 30-minute intervals up to a total dose of 30 to 35 mg/kg.

Treatment of sustained ventricular tachycardia   A dosage of 5 to 10 mg/kg of bretylium diluted in 50 mL of 5% dextrose injection and given intravenously over 8 to 10 min is recommended. For continued suppression of persistently recurrent ventricular tachycardia, a continuous intravenous infusion of bretylium at a rate of

1 to 2 mg/min can be given following the initial 5- to 10-mg/kg loading dose. Alternatively, 5 to 10 mg/kg can be given by intermittent intravenous infusion over 8 min or longer q 6 h for continued suppression of ventricular tachycardia.

Treatment of other life-threatening ventricular arrhythmias   Administer diluted intravenous infusion in a dose of 5 to 10 mg/kg over a 8 to 10 min period and repeat this dose every 1 to 2 h if needed. Maintenance infusion can be given every 6 to 8 h as described above. Alternatively, bretylium can be administered as a constant infusion (diluted) at a rate of 1 to 2 mg/min. With intramuscular (IM) administration, give 5 to 10 mg/kg undiluted and repeated every 1 to 2 h as needed. Maintenance dose is 5 to 10 mg/kg every 6 to 8 h. Do not exceed 5 mL volume in any one site for IM injection. IM injections should not be made directly into or near a major nerve, and injection sites should be rotated.

Elderly

Dosage adjustment may be required based on renal function.

Children

Safety and effectiveness have not been established.

Preparations

Bretylium tosylate injection (generic): 50 mg/mL, 10 mL ampules, vials, and syringes

Bretylium tosylate in 5% dextrose injection (generic): 2 mg/mL (500 mg/vial), 4 mg/mL (1000 mg/vial).

3. Dofetilide (Tikosyn®)

Indications

Maintenance of normal sinus rhythm (delay in atrial fibrillation/atrial flutter recurrence)

Conversion of atrial fibrillation/flutter

Dosage

Adults

The usual recommended dose of dofetilide is 500 μg twice daily. The dose of dofetilide must be individualized according to creatinine clearance and QTc. Prior to administration of the first dose, the QTc must be determined using an average of 5 to 10 beats. If the QTc is greater than 440 msec (500 msec in patients with ventricular conduction abnormalities), dofetilide is contraindicated. If heart rate is <60 beats per minute, QT interval should be used. There are no data on use of dofetilide when the heart rate is <50 beats per minute.

The initial dose of dofetilide is determined as follows:

Creatinine Clearance	Dofetilide Dose
>60 mL/min	500 μg twice daily
40 to 60 mL/min	250 μg twice daily
20 to <40 mL/min	125 μg twice daily
<20 mL/min	Dofetilide is contraindicated in these patients

At 2 to 3 h after administering the *first* dose of dofetilide, determine the QTc. If the QTc has increased by more than 15% when compared to the baseline, or if the QTc is greater than 500 msec (550 msec in patients with ventricular conduction abnormalities), subsequent dosing should be adjusted as follows:

If the Starting Dose Based on Creatinine Clearance is:	Then the Adjusted Dose (for QTc Prolongation) is:
500 μg twice daily	250 μg twice daily
250 μg twice daily	125 μg twice daily
125 μg twice daily	125 μg once a day

At 2 to 3 h after each subsequent dose of dofetilide, determine the QTc (for in-hospital doses 2nd to 5th). No further down titration of dofetilide based on QTc is recommended. If at any time after the second dose of dofetilide is given, the QTc is greater than 500 msec (550 msec in patients with ventricular conduction abnormalities) dofetilide should be discontinued. Please consult dofetilide package insert for complete prescribing information.

Elderly
Dosage adjustment may be required based on renal function.

Children
Safety and effectiveness have not been established.

Preparations
Tikosyn (Pfizer): 125 μg, 250 μg, 500 μg capsules

4. Ibutilide (Corvert®)

Indications
Conversion of atrial fibrillation or atrial flutter of recent onset to sinus rhythm

Dosage

Adults
For patients who weigh ≥60 kg, give 1 mg intravenously over 10 min. For patients who weigh <60 kg, give 0.01 mg/kg intravenously over 10 min. If the arrhythmia does not terminate within 10 min after the end of the initial infusion, a second 10-min infusion of equal strength may be administered 10 min after completion of the first infusion.

Ibutilide may be administered undiluted or diluted in 50 mL of 0.9% sodium chloride injection or 5% dextrose injection.

Elderly
No dosage adjustment is required.

Children
Safety and effectiveness have not been established.

Preparation
Corvert (Pharmacia and Upjohn): 0.1 mg/mL, 10 mL vials

5. Sotalol (Betapace®, Betapace AF®)

Indications
Documented life-threatening ventricular arrhythmias (Betapace)

Maintenance of normal sinus rhythm in patients with symptomatic atrial fibrillation or atrial flutter who are currently in sinus rhythm (Betapace AF)

Dosage

Adults

Documented life-threatening ventricular arrhythmias   Initiate with low doses and titrate up slowly. Usual starting dose is 80 mg twice daily. Dosage may be titrated up every 3 days up to 240 mg or 320 mg daily given in two to three divided doses. The usual maintenance dose is 160 to 320 mg/d, but some patients may require doses as high as 480 to 640 mg/d. However, the higher doses should only be prescribed when the potential benefit outweighs the increased risk of adverse events. Because sotalol is excreted predominantly in urine and its elimination half-life is prolonged in patients with renal impairment, the dosing interval of sotalol should be modified according to creatinine clearance as follows:

Creatinine Clearance (mL/min)	Dosing Interval
>60	12
30 to 59	24
10 to 29	36 to 48
<10	Dose should be individualized

In addition, dose increments in patients with renal impairment should be made after administration of at least 5 to 6 doses.

Maintenance of normal sinus rhythm in patients with symptomatic atrial fibrillation or atrial flutter who are currently in sinus rhythm   Initiate with 80 mg twice daily if the creatinine clearance is >60 mL/min, and 80 mg once daily if the creatinine clearance is 40 to 60 mL/min. If the creatinine clearance is <40 mL/min, sotalol (Betapace AF) is contraindicated. If the 80-mg dose level is tolerated and the QT interval remains <500 msec after at least 3 days (after 5 or 6 doses if patient receiving once-daily dosing), the patient can be discharged. Patients should not be discharged within 12 h of electrical or pharmacologic conversion to normal sinus rhythm. Alternatively, during hospitalization, the dose can be increased to 120 mg twice daily or once daily depending upon the creatinine clearance and the patient followed for 3 days on this dose (followed for 5 or 6 doses if patient receiving once daily doses). If the 120 mg dose level does not reduce the frequency of early relapse of AFIB/AFL and is tolerated without excessive QT interval prolongation (≥520 msec), an increase to 160 mg (twice daily or once daily depending upon the creatinine clearance) can be considered.

Note   The QT interval is used to determine patient eligibility for sotalol (Betapace AF) treatment and for monitoring safety during treatment. The baseline QT interval must be ≤450 msec in order for a patient to be started on this medication. During initiation and titration, the QT interval should be monitored 2 to 4 h after each dose. If the QT interval prolongs to 500 msec or greater, the dose must be reduced or the drug discontinued. During maintenance of sotalol (Betapace AF) therapy, renal function and QT should be reevaluated regularly if medically warranted. If QT is 520 msec or greater (JT 430 msec or greater if QRS is >100 msec), the dose of sotalol (Betapace AF) therapy should be reduced and patients should be carefully monitored until QT returns to <520 msec. If the QT interval is ≥520 msec while on the lowest maintenance dose level (80 mg), the drug should be discontinued.

Elderly
Dosage adjustment may be required based on renal function.

Children
Safety and effectiveness have not been established.

Preparations
Betapace (Berlex): 80 mg, 120 mg, 160 mg, 240 mg tablets
Betapace AF (Berlex): 80 mg, 120 mg, 160 mg tablets

OTHER

1. Adenosine (Adenocard®)

Indications
Conversion to sinus rhythm of paroxysmal supraventricular tachyarrhythmias, including that associated with Wolff-Parkinson-White syndrome

Dosage

Adults

Initiate with 6 mg as a rapid intravenous bolus (administered over 1 to 2 seconds). If the first dose does not result in elimination of the supraventricular tachycardia within 1 to 2 min, give 12 mg as a rapid intravenous bolus. Repeat the 12-mg dose a second time if necessary.

Note   Adenosine injection should be given as a rapid bolus by the peripheral intravenous route. To assure the medication reaches the systemic circulation, adenosine should be administered either directly into a vein or, if given into an intravenous line, it should be given as close to the patient as possible and followed by a rapid saline flush.

Elderly
Dosage adjustment is not required.

Children
Safety and effectiveness have not been established.

Preparations
Adenocard (Fujisawa): 3 mg/mL, 2 and 5 mL vials

2. Atropine (Atropine sulfate)

Indications
Symptomatic sinus bradycardia (intravenous formulation)
Treatment of ventricular asystole during CPR (intravenous formulation)

Dosage

Adults

Treatment of bradycardia in advanced cardiac life support during CPR   usual adult dose is 0.5 to 1 mg given intravenously; this dose may be repeated every 3 to 5 min until the desired heart rate is achieved.

Treatment of ventricular asystole during CPR   1 mg intravenously; this dose may be repeated in 3 to 5 min if needed. The total dose usually should not exceed 2.5 mg (0.04 mg/kg) in patients with severe bradycardia or ventricular asystole because a 2.5-mg dose generally results in complete vagal blockade.

Note   Atropine sulfate may be administered orally or by intramuscular, subcutaneous, or direct intravenous administration. When atropine sulfate cannot be administered intravenously for advanced cardiac life support during CPR, the drug may be administered via an endotracheal tube or by intraosseous injection in adults and children. Some experts recommend that doses administered via endotracheal tube should be 2 to 2.5 times those administered intravenously and generally should be diluted in 10 mL of 0.9% sodium chloride or sterile water for adults, and in 1 to 2 mL of 0.45 or 0.9% sodium chloride for children. Such dilution may enhance tracheobronchial distribution and absorption of atropine. When atropine sulfate is given intravenously, it should generally be given rapidly because slow injection of the drug may cause a paradoxical slowing of the heart rate.

Elderly
Use usual dose with caution.

Children

Advanced cardiac life support during CPR   0.02 mg/kg intravenously, with a minimum pediatric dose of 0.1 mg and a maximum single dose of 0.5 and 1 mg in children and adolescents, respectively. The dose may be repeated at 5-minute intervals to a maximum total dose of 1 mg in children and 2 mg in adolescents.

Preparations
Atropine sulfate injection (generic): 0.05, 0.1, 0.3, 0.4, 0.5, 0.8, 1 mg/mL

ANTITHROMBOTICS

ANTICOAGULANTS

1. Argatroban

Indications
As an anticoagulant for prophylaxis or treatment of thrombosis in patients with heparin-induced thrombocytopenia (HIT)
As an anticoagulant in patients with or at risk for HIT undergoing percutaneous coronary intervention (PCI)

Dosage

Adults
Heparin-Induced Thrombocytopenia (HIT/HITTS)

The usual initial dose is 2 μg/kg/min administered as a continuous infusion (the concentrated drug, 100 mg/mL, must be diluted 100-fold prior to infusion). The dose can be adjusted as clinically indicated and according to steady-state aPTT (1.5 to 3 times the initial baseline value, not to exceed 100 seconds) up to 10 μg/kg/min. A lower initial dose of 0.5 μg/kg/min is recommended for patients with moderate hepatic impairment. aPTT should be monitored closely and dosage adjusted as clinically indicated.

PCI in HIT/HITTS (heparin-induced thrombocytopenia and thrombosis syndrome) patients

An infusion of argatroban should be started at 25 μg/kg/min and a bolus of 350 μg/kg administered via a large bore intravenous line over 3–5 min. Activated clotting time (ACT) should be obtained before dosing and 5–10 min after the bolus dose is completed. The procedure may proceed if the ACT is > 300 sec.

If the ACT is less than 300 sec, an additional IV bolus dose of 150 μg/kg should be administered, the infusion dose increased to 30 μg/kg/min, and the ACT checked 5–10 min later. If the ACT is greater than 450 sec, the infusion rate should be decreased to 15 μg/kg/min, and the ACT checked 5–10 min later. Once a therapeutic ACT (between 300–450 sec) has been achieved, this infusion dose should be continued for the duration of the procedure.

In case of dissection, impending abrupt closure, thrombus formation during the procedure, or inability to achieve or maintain an ACT over 300 sec, additional bolus doses of 150 μg/kg may be administered and the infusion dose increased to 40 μg/kg/min. The ACT should be checked after each additional bolus or change in the rate of infusion.

If a patient requires anticoagulation after the procedure, argatroban may be continued, but as a lower infusion dose. Use of high doses of argatroban in PCI patients with clinically significant hepatic disease or AST/ALT levels ≥ 3 times the upper limit of normal should be avoided. Such patients were not studied in PCI trials.

Conversion to oral anticoagulant therapy

Because coadministration of argatroban and warfarin may cause combined effects on INR, a loading dose of warfarin should not be used. Initiate therapy using the expected daily dose of warfarin. With doses of argatroban ≤2 μg/kg/min, argatroban can be discontinued when the INR is >4 on combined therapy. INR measurement should be repeated 4 to 6 h after discontinuation of argatroban infusion. If the repeated INR is below the desired therapeutic range, restart argatroban infusion and repeat the procedure daily until the desired therapeutic range on warfarin alone is achieved. For doses of argatroban >2 μg/kg/min, temporarily reduce the dose of argatroban to 2 μg/kg/min to get a more accurate INR measurement on warfarin alone. Obtain the INR measurement on argatroban and warfarin 4 to 6 hours after reduction of the argatroban dose and follow the process described above for administering argatroban at doses ≤2 μg/kg/min.

Elderly
Dosage adjustment is not required.

Children
Safety and effectiveness have not been established.

Preparation
Argatroban injection (Glaxo SmithKline): 100 mg/mL, 2.5 mL single-use vials

2. Bivalirudin (Angiomax®)
Indications

Unstable angina For use as an anticoagulant in patients with unstable angina undergoing percutaneous transluminal coronary angioplasty (PTCA). Bivalirudin is intended for use in patients receiving concomitant aspirin (300 to 325 mg daily).

Dosage

Adults
Treatment with bivalirudin should be initiated just prior to PTCA. Administer an intravenous bolus of 1 mg/kg followed by

a 4-h intravenous infusion at a rate of 2.5 mg/kg/h. If necessary, an additional intravenous bivalirudin infusion may be initiated at a rate of 0.2 mg/kg/h for ≤20 h after completion of the initial 4-h infusion. The dose may need to be reduced, and anticoagulation status monitored, in patients with renal impairment. Consult package insert for instructions on dilution of drug prior to administration.

Elderly
Dosage adjustment is not required.

Children
Safety and effectiveness have not been established.

Preparation
Angiomax (Medicines Company): 250 mg injection, lyophilized.

3. Dalteparin sodium (Fragmin®)
Indications

Prophylaxis of deep vein thrombosis which may lead to pulmonary embolism in patients undergoing hip replacement surgery, and in patients undergoing abdominal surgery who are at risk for thromboembolic complications.

Prevention of ischemic complications in patients with unstable angina or non-Q-wave myocardial infarction (use with concurrent aspirin therapy).

Dosage

Adults

Abdominal surgery

Patients with a low to moderate risk of thromboembolic complications 2500 IU subcutaneously once daily for 5 to 10 days starting 1 to 2 h prior to surgery.

Patients with a high risk of thromboembolic complications 5000 IU subcutaneously once daily for 5 to 10 days starting the evening before surgery. Alternatively, in patients with malignancy, 2500 IU of dalteparin can be administered subcutaneously 1 to 2 h prior to surgery followed by 2500 IU subcutaneously 12 h later, and then 5000 IU once daily for 5 to 10 days postoperatively.

Hip replacement surgery

Administer the first dose, 2500 IU, subcutaneously within 2 h before surgery and the second dose of 2500 IU subcutaneously in the evening of the day of surgery (at least 6 h after the first dose). If surgery is performed in the evening, omit the second dose on the day of surgery. Dalteparin 5000 IU is then administered subcutaneously once daily from first postoperative day and continued for 5 to 10 days. Alternatively, dalteparin 5000 IU can be administered the evening before the surgery, followed by 5000 IU once daily, starting in the evening of the day of surgery and continued for 5 to 10 days. Up to 14 days of treatment have been well tolerated in controlled clinical trials.

Unstable angina/non-Q-wave myocardial infarction

120 IU/kg (maximum single dose of 10,000 IU) subcutaneously every 12 h with concurrent aspirin therapy for 5 to 8 days or until the patient is clinically stable.

Elderly

No data; dosage adjustment is probably not required.

Children

Safety and effectiveness have not been established.

Preparations

Fragmin (Pharmacia and Upjohn): 2500 anti-Factor Xa IU/ 0.2 mL, 5000 anti-Factor Xa IU/0.2 mL syringes; 10,000 anti-Factor Xa IU/mL, 9.5 mL multiple-dose vials.

4. Danaparoid sodium (Orgaran®)

Indications

Prophylaxis of postoperative deep-venous thrombosis, which may lead to pulmonary embolism in patients undergoing elective hip replacement surgery

Dosage

Adults

750 anti-Xa units (0.6 mL) twice daily administered subcutaneously starting 1 to 4 h before surgery, and then not sooner than 2 h after surgery. Treatment should be continued until the patient is fully ambulatory (up to 14 days).

Monitor patients with serum creatinine ≥ 2 mg/dL carefully. In patients with renal failure undergoing hemodialysis, reduce maintenance dosages and titrate according to predialysis plasma antifactor Xa activity.

Elderly

Dosage adjustment is not required.

Children

Safety and effectiveness have not been established.

Preparations

Orgaran (Organon): 750 anti-Xa U/0.6 mL syringes; 750 anti-Xa U/0.6 mL ampules.

5. Enoxaparin sodium (Lovenox®)

Indications

Prophylaxis of deep-vein thrombosis, which may lead to pulmonary embolism in patients undergoing hip or knee replacement surgery and in high-risk patients undergoing abdominal surgery

Treatment of acute deep-vein thrombosis with or without pulmonary embolism when used in conjunction with warfarin

Prevention of ischemic complications in patients with unstable angina or non-Q-wave myocardial infarction with concurrent aspirin

Dosage

Adults

Knee replacement surgery

30 mg q 12 h subcutaneously for 7 to 10 days starting 12 to 24 h after the surgery. Up to 14 days administration has been well tolerated in clinical trials.

Hip replacement surgery

Administer 30 mg q 12 h or 40 mg once daily by subcutaneous injection. An initial dose of 40 mg once a day subcutaneously may be given approximately 12 h prior to surgery. Following the initial phase of thromboprophylaxis, continued prophylaxis with enoxaparin injection 40 mg once daily for 3 weeks is recommended.

Abdominal surgery

40 mg daily by subcutaneously injection for 7 to 10 days starting 2 h prior to surgery. Up to 12 days administration has been well tolerated in clinical trials.

Treatment of deep-vein thrombosis and pulmonary embolism

In patients with acute deep-vein thrombosis without pulmonary embolism who can be treated at home, the recommended dose is 1 mg/kg q 12 h by subcutaneous injection. In hospitalized patients with acute deep-vein thrombosis with pulmonary embolism, or patients with acute deep-vein thrombosis without pulmonary embolism (who are not candidates for outpatient treatment), the recommended dose is 1 mg/kg q 12 h or 1.5 mg/kg once daily by subcutaneous injection. Therapy with warfarin should be initiated when appropriate and enoxaparin should be continued for a minimum of 5 days and until the INR is therapeutic. The average duration of treatment is 7 days; up to 17 days administration has been well tolerated in clinical trials.

Unstable angina and non-Q-wave myocardial infarction

1 mg/kg administered subcutaneously q 12 h in conjunction with oral aspirin therapy (100 to 325 mg once daily) for a minimum of 2 days and continued until clinical stabilization. The usual duration of treatment is 2 to 8 days.

Elderly

Dosage adjustment is not required. However, dosage adjustment should be considered in patients with a creatinine clearance of <30 mL/min.

Children

Safety and effectiveness have not been established.

Preparations

Lovenox (Aventis): 30 mg/0.3 mL, 40 mg/0.4 mL, 60 mg/0.6 mL, 80 mg/0.8 mL, 100 mg/1 mL, 90 mg/0.6 mL, 120 mg/0.8 mL, 150 mg/1 mL injections.

6. Fondaparinux sodium (Arixtra®)

Indication

Prophylaxis of deep vein thrombosis which may lead to pulmonary embolism in patients undergoing hip fracture surgery, hip replacement surgery, or knee replacement surgery.

Dosage

Adults

The recommended dose of fondaparinux is 2.5 mg administered by subcutaneous injection once daily in patients undergoing hip fracture surgery, hip replacement surgery, or knee replacement surgery. After hemostasis has been established, the initial dose is given 6 to 8 h following surgery. Administration before 6 h following surgery has been associated with an increased risk of major bleeding. The usual duration of administration is 5 to 9 days, and up to 11 days of administration has been tolerated.

Elderly

The risk of fondaparinux-associated major bleeding increased with age, with an incidence of 1.8% in patients less than 65 years of age, 2.2% in those 65 to 74 years of age, and 2.7% in those 75 years of age or older. The kidney substantially eliminates fondaparinux, and the risk of toxic reactions to fondaparinux may be greater in patients with impaired renal function. Because elderly patients are more likely to have decreased renal function, it may be useful to monitor renal function.

Children

Safety and effectiveness have not been established.

Preparations

Arixtra (Organon/Sanofi-Synthelabo): 2.5 mg injection, in 0.5 mL single-dose prefilled syringes with needle

7. Heparin (Heparin Sodium)

Indications

Prophylaxis and treatment of: venous thrombosis, pulmonary embolism, atrial fibrillation with thromboembolism, and peripheral arterial embolism

Prophylaxis and treatment of unstable angina, evolving stroke, acute myocardial infarction (not FDA-approved)

Prevention of clotting in cardiac/arterial surgery, blood transfusion, dialysis and other extracorporeal interventions, and disseminated intravascular coagulation

Dosage

Adults

Prophylaxis for deep-venous thrombosis

5000 units subcutaneously q 8 to 12 h until the patient is fully ambulatory.

Treatment guidelines for thromboembolic events

Continuous intravenous administration   60 to 100 U/kg loading dose by intravenous injection, followed by an intravenous infusion of 15 to 25 U/kg/h and adjusted based on coagulation test results.

Intermittent intravenous administration   the usual initial dose for a 68-kg adult is 10,000 units, followed by 5,000 to 10,000 units q 4 to 6 h.

Deep subcutaneous injections   10,000 to 20,000 units loading dose, followed by 8,000 to 10,000 units q 8 h or 15,000 to 20,000 units q 12 h. Dose should be adjusted based on coagulation test results.

Open heart and vascular surgery

The minimum initial dose is 150 U/kg for patients undergoing total body perfusion for open heart surgery. For procedures <60 min, the usual dose used is 300 U/kg. For procedures >60 min, the usual dose used is 400 U/kg.

Heparin lock

To avoid clot formation in a heparin lock set, inject diluted heparin solution (Heparin Lock Flush Solution, USP; or a 10 to 100 U/mL heparin solution) via the injection hub to fill the entire set to the needle tip. Replace this solution each time the heparin lock is used. Consult the set manufacturer's instructions.

Elderly

Dosage adjustment is not required.

Children

Dosage adjustment should be made based on weight, age, and coagulation test results.

Preparations

Available in either bovine or porcine origin

Heparin sodium: 10, 100, 1000, 2500, 5000, 7500, 10,000, 20,000, 40,000 U/mL in various volumes as single use or multiple-dose packages.

8. Lepirudin (Refludan®)

Indications

Prevention of further thromboembolic complications in patients with heparin-induced thrombocytopenia and associated thromboembolic disease

Dosage

Adults

Bolus dose   0.4 mg/kg (up to 44 mg) intravenously over 15 to 20 seconds.

Maintenance dose   0.15 mg/kg/h (up to 16.5 mg/h) as a continuous intravenous infusion for 2 to 10 days or longer if indicated. Dosage should be adjusted based on aPTT measurements. The first aPTT determination should be made 4 h after initiation of the lepirudin infusion. Follow-up aPTT determinations should be made at least once a day. Adjustments of bolus dose and maintenance dose should be made in patients who are receiving thrombolytic therapy concurrently and in patients with renal impairment. Consult lepirudin package insert for full prescribing information.

Concurrent warfarin therapy   Reduce lepirudin dose to reach an aPTT ratio just above 1.5 before administering the first dose of warfarin. Lepirudin infusion should be discontinued once an INR of 2 is achieved.

Elderly

Dosage adjustment should be made based on creatinine clearance.

Children

Safety and effectiveness have not been established.

Preparation

Refludan (Hoechst-Marion Roussel): 50 mg/vial, powder for injection.

9. Tinzaparin Sodium (Innohep®)

Indications

Treatment of acute symptomatic deep vein thrombosis with or without pulmonary embolism when administered in conjunction with warfarin

Dosage

Adults

175 anti-Xa IU/kg, administered subcutaneously once daily for at least 6 days and until the patient is adequately anticoagulated with warfarin (INR ≥2 for 2 consecutive days). Use with caution in patients with renal impairment.

Elderly

Dosage adjustment is not required.

Children

Safety and effectiveness have not been established.

Preparation

Innohep (DuPont Pharma): 20,000 IU/mL, 2 mL vials.

10. Warfarin (Warfarin Sodium, Coumadin®)

Indications

Prophylaxis and treatment of venous thrombosis, pulmonary embolism, atrial fibrillation with embolization, thromboembolism associated with prosthetic heart valves.

Dosage

Adults

Initiate with 5 to 10 mg/d for 2 to 4 days; adjust dose to maintain desired therapeutic INRs according to recommendations by the American College of Chest Physicians (ACCP) and the National Heart, Lung and Blood Institute (NHLBI). Warfarin injection provides an alternative administration route for patients who cannot receive oral drugs. The dose of warfarin injection is the same as the oral dose and should only be administered intravenously. The dose should be given as a slow bolus injection over 1 to 2 min into a peripheral vein.

Elderly

Initiate therapy with a lower dose. Dosing is based on coagulation test results.

Children

Safety and effectiveness have not been established.

Preparations

Warfarin (generic); Coumadin (DuPont): 1 mg, 2 mg, 2.5 mg, 3 mg, 4 mg, 5 mg, 6 mg, 7.5 mg, 10 mg tablets.
Coumadin Injection (DuPont): 5 mg per vial

ANTIPLATELET AGENTS

1. Abciximab (ReoPro®)

Indications

Prevention of cardiac ischemic complications in patients undergoing percutaneous coronary intervention (PCI) or in patients with unstable angina not responding to conventional medical therapy when PCI is planned within 24 h.

Dosage

Adults

Percutaneous coronary intervention (PCI)

0.25 mg/kg intravenous bolus administered 10 to 60 min prior to the start of PCI, followed by a continuous intravenous infusion of 0.125 μg/kg/min (to a maximum of 10 μg/min) for 12 h.

Unstable angina with planned PCI within 24 h

0.25 mg/kg intravenous bolus followed by an 18- to 24-h intravenous infusion of 10 μg/min, concluding 1 h after the PCI.

Note   The safety and efficacy of abciximab have only been studied with concomitant administration of heparin and aspirin. The continuous infusion of abciximab should be stopped in cases of failed PCI because there is no evidence for the efficacy of abciximab in that setting. A filter must be used during the administration of abciximab; see package insert for detailed instructions on administration.

Elderly

No dosage adjustment is required. However, there may be an increased risk of major bleeding in patients over 65 years of age. Caution is recommended.

Children

Safety and effectiveness have not been established.

Preparation

ReoPro (Lilly): 2 mg/mL, 5 mL vials

2. Anagrelide Hydrochloride (Agrylin®)

Indication

Treatment of essential thrombocythemia to reduce the elevated platelet count and the risk of thrombosis

Dosage

Adults

Initiate treatment with anagrelide under close medical supervision. Initial dose is 0.5 mg four times daily or 1 mg twice daily, which should be maintained for at least 1 week. Dosage should then be adjusted to the lowest effective level required to reduce and maintain platelet count below 600,000/μL and ideally to the normal range. Dosage should be increased by not more than 0.5 mg/d in any 1 week. Dosage should not exceed 10 mg/d or 2.5 mg in a single dose. Most patients will experience an adequate response at a dose of 1.5 to 3.0 mg/d. Monitor patients with known or suspected heart disease, renal insufficiency, or hepatic dysfunction closely.

Elderly

No data; dosage adjustment is probably not required.

Children

Safety and effectiveness are not established in patients under 16 years of age. However, anagrelide has been used successfully in eight pediatric patients (age range, 8 to 17 years), including three patients with essential thrombocythemia, who were treated at a dose of 1 to 4 mg/d.

Preparations

Agrylin (Roberts): 0.5 mg, 1 mg capsules

3. Aspirin

Indications

Listed below are cardiovascular indications only (not all indications are FDA approved)

Prevention of arterial and venous thrombosis in:

Arteriovenous shunt for hemodialysis

Atrial fibrillation

Coronary bypass

Intracoronary stent placement (in combination with clopidogrel, ticlopidine, or warfarin)

Myocardial Infarction (primary/secondary prophylaxis)

Prosthetic heart valves (with an oral anticoagulant and with or without dipyridamole)

Transient ischemic attacks

Transluminal angioplasty of coronary, iliac, femoral, popliteal, or tibial artery (with or without dipyridamole)

Unstable angina

Dosage

Adults

Transient ischemic attacks in men

1300 mg/d in two to four divided doses; doses as low as 300 mg/d may be effective if tolerance is a problem with high doses.

Myocardial infarction/unstable angina

80 to 325 mg once daily; the first dose in patients experiencing chest pain should be plain aspirin (not enteric coated) and the dose should be chewed or crushed or dispersed in solution and administered as soon as possible for more rapid antiplatelet effect.

Elderly

Dosage adjustment is not required.

Children

Dosage recommendations are based on age and weight for the analgesic indication. Aspirin is not recommended in children with influenza or chickenpox due to the risk for Reye's syndrome.

Preparations

Available in various strengths and formulations

4. Cilostazol (Pletal®)

Indication

Intermittent claudication

Dosage

Adults

100 mg twice daily, taken ≥30 min before or 2 h after breakfast and dinner. A lower dose of 50 mg twice daily should be considered during coadministration of CYP3A4 inhibitors (i.e., ketoconazole, itraconazole, erythromycin, diltiazem) and CYP2C19 inhibitors (i.e., omeprazole). Because CYP3A4 is also inhibited by grapefruit juice, patients receiving cilostazol should avoid this beverage.

Elderly

Dosage adjustment is not required.

Children

Safety and effectiveness have not been established.

Preparations

Pletal (Otsuka America Pharmaceuticals/Pharmacia & Upjohn): 50 mg, 100 mg tablets

5. Clopidogrel (Plavix®)

Indications

Reduction of thrombotic events in patients with a history of recent myocardial infarction, recent stroke, or established peripheral arterial disease

Reduction of thrombotic events in patients with acute coronary syndrome

Dosage

Adults

Recent myocardial infarction, recent stroke or established peripheral arterial disease

75 mg once daily

Acute coronary syndrome   For patients with acute coronary syndrome (unstable angina/non-Q-wave MI), clopidogrel should be initiated with a single 300 mg loading dose and then continued at 75 mg once daily. Aspirin (75 mg to 325 mg once daily) should be initiated and continued in combination with clopidogrel. In the CURE trial, most patients with acute coronary syndrome also received heparin acutely.

Elderly

Dosage adjustment is not required.

Children

Safety and effectiveness have not been established.

Preparation

Plavix (Bristol Myers Squibb/Sanofi): 75 mg tablets

6. Dipyridamole (Dipyridamole, Persantine®)

Indications

Prophylaxis of thromboembolism after cardiac valve replacement (use as an adjunct to warfarin therapy)

An alternative to exercise during Thallium myocardial perfusion imaging for the evaluation of coronary artery disease in patients who cannot exercise adequately

Dosage

Adults

Adjunctive use in prophylaxis of thromboembolism after cardiac valve replacement

75 to 100 mg four times daily (as an adjunct to warfarin therapy).

Evaluation of coronary artery disease

Intravenous infusion: 0.14 mg/kg/min for 4 min; not to exceed 60 mg over 4 min). The radiopharmaceutical is injected within 3 to 5 min after completion of the dipyridamole infusion.

Elderly

Dosage adjustment is not required.

Children

Safety and effectiveness have not been established in children under 12 years of age.

Preparations

Dipyridamole (generic); Persantine (Boehringer Ingelheim): 25 mg, 50 mg, 75 mg tablets

Persantine Injection (Boehringer Ingelheim): 5 mg/mL (10 mg/2 mL ampule)

7. Dipyridamole and Aspirin (Aggrenox®)

Indication

Stroke To reduce the risk of stroke in patients who have had transient ischemia of the brain or complete ischemic stroke due to thrombosis

Dosage

Adults

Administer 1 capsule twice daily (one in the morning and one in the evening). Capsules should be swallowed whole; do not crush or chew capsule.

Elderly

Dosage adjustment is not required.

Children

Safety and effectiveness have not been established.

Preparation

Aggrenox (Boehringer Ingelheim): 200 mg extended-release dipyridamole/25 mg aspirin capsules

8. Eptifibatide (Integrilin®)

Indications

Treatment of patients with acute coronary syndrome (unstable angina or non-Q-wave myocardial infarction), including patients who are to be managed medically and those undergoing percutaneous coronary intervention (PCI).

Dosage

Adults

Acute coronary syndrome

180 μg/kg intravenous bolus (over 1 to 2 min) administered as soon as possible following diagnosis, followed by a continuous infusion of 2 μg/kg/min until hospital discharge or initiation of CABG surgery, up to 72 h. If PCI is performed during treatment with eptifibatide, consideration can be given to reducing the infusion rate to 0.5 μg/kg/min at the time of the procedure. Infusion should be continued for an additional 20 to 24 h after the PCI, allowing for up to 96 h of therapy. Patients weighing >121 kg have received a maximum bolus of 22.6 mg followed by a maximum infusion rate of 15 mg/h.

PCI in patients not presenting with an acute coronary syndrome

135 μg/kg intravenous bolus (over 1 to 2 min) administered immediately before the initiation of PCI followed by a continuous infusion of 0.5 μg/kg/min for 20 to 24 h. There has been little experience in patients weighing >143 kg.

Note The safety and efficacy of eptifibatide have only been established with concomitant administration of heparin and aspirin. Dosage adjustment is not required for patients with serum creatinine <2 mg/dL for the 180 μg/kg bolus and the 2.0 μg/kg/min infusion and <4 mg/dL for the 135 μg/kg bolus and the 0.5 μg/kg/min infusion. Plasma eptifibatide levels are expected to be higher in patients with more severe renal impairment and data are not available for this patient population.

Elderly

Dosage adjustment is not required.

Children

Safety and effectiveness have not been established.

Preparations

Integrilin (COR Therapeutics, Key): 0.75 mg/mL, 100 mL vials; 2 mg/mL, 10 mL vials.

9. Ticlopidine (Ticlopidine Hydrochloride, Ticlid®)

Indication

Stroke To reduce the risk of thrombotic stroke in patients who have experienced stroke precursors, and in patients who have had a completed thrombotic stroke.

Dosage

Adults

250 mg twice daily with food.

Elderly

Dosage adjustment is not required.

Children

Safety and effectiveness have not been established.

Preparation
Ticlopidine (generic); Ticlid (Roche): 250 mg tablets

10. Tirofiban Hydrochloride (Aggrastat®)

Indications
Treatment of acute coronary syndrome (in combination with heparin), including patients who are to be managed medically and those undergoing percutaneous transluminal coronary angioplasty (PTCA), or atherectomy

Dosage

Adults

Administer intravenously, at an initial rate of 0.4 μg/kg/min for 30 min and then continued at 0.1 μg/kg/min. In a clinical trial, PRISM-PLUS, tirofiban was administered in combination with heparin for 48 to 108 h. The infusion should be continued through angiography and for 12 to 24 h after angioplasty or atherectomy. Patients with severe renal impairment (creatinine clearance <30 mL/min) should receive half the usual rate of loading and maintenance infusion.

Note Tirofiban has been studied in a setting that included aspirin and heparin. The 250 μg/mL injection must be diluted to 50 μg/mL prior to administration.

Elderly

Dosage adjustment is not required.

Children

Safety and effectiveness have not been established.

Preparations
Aggrastat (Merck): 250 μg/mL, 50 mL vial; 50 μg/mL, 500 mL single-dose IntraVia containers

THROMBOLYTIC AGENTS

1. Alteplase, Recombinant (Activase®)

Indications
Acute myocardial infarction
Acute ischemic stroke
Pulmonary embolism

Dosage

Adults

Acute myocardial infarction
Treatment should be initiated as soon as possible after the onset of chest pain.

1. Accelerated Infusion—15 mg intravenous bolus, followed by 0.75 mg/kg (up to 50 mg) infused over the next 30 min, and then 0.5 mg/kg (up to 35 mg) infused over the next 60 min. The maximum total dose is 100 mg for patients who weigh more than 67 kg. The safety and efficacy of this accelerated infusion regimen has only been investigated with concomitant administration of heparin and aspirin.

2. Three-hour infusion—60 mg infused over 60 min (with 6 to 10 mg administered as a bolus over the first 1 to 2 min), followed by 20 mg/h infusion for the next 2 h to deliver a total dose of 100 mg. For patients weighing less than 65 kg, a total dose of 1.25 mg/kg given over 3 h is recommended. Although the use of anticoagulants during and following alteplase infusion has been shown to be of unclear benefit, heparin has been given concomitantly for ≥24 h in >90% of patients. Aspirin or dipyridamole has been administered either during or following heparin treatment.

Acute ischemic stroke

0.9 mg/kg (up to 90 mg) administered intravenously over 60 min with 10% of the total dose administered as a bolus over the first minute. Treatment should be initiated within 3 h after the onset of stroke symptoms. Avoid concurrent aspirin and heparin use during the first 24 h after symptom onset.

Pulmonary embolism

Administered 100 mg intravenously over 2 h. Heparin therapy should be instituted or reinstituted near the end of or immediately following the alteplase infusion when partial thromboplastin time or thrombin time returns to twice of normal or less.

Note Alteplase must be reconstituted before administration, consult package insert for detailed instructions.

Elderly

Generally, the adult dose can be used, but body weight should be considered. Patients older than 75 years of age, especially those with suspected arterial degeneration are at an increased risk for unwanted bleeding; monitor closely.

Children

Safety and effectiveness have not been established.

Preparations
Activase (Genentech): 50 mg (29 million IU)/vial, 100 mg (58 million IU)/vial

2. Anistreplase (Eminase®)

Indication
Acute myocardial infarction

Dosage

Adults

Thrombolytic therapy should be initiated as soon as possible after the onset of symptoms. The dose of anistreplase is 30 units administered intravenously over 2 to 5 min.

Reconstitution Slowly add 5 mL of sterile water for injection into the vial containing anistreplase, directing the stream of water against the side of the vial. Gently roll (do not shake) the vial to mix the powder with the liquid. The reconstituted solution should not be further diluted before administration. No other medication should be added to the vial containing anistreplase.

Elderly

Dosage adjustment is not required. Patients older than 75 years of age, especially those with suspected arterial degeneration, may be at risk for unwanted bleeding; monitor closely.

Children

Safety and effectiveness have not been established.

Preparation

Eminase (Roberts): 30 U/single-dose vial

3. Reteplase, Recombinant (Retavase®)

Indication

Acute myocardial infarction

Dosage

Adults

Treatment should be initiated as soon as possible, preferably within 12 h after the onset of chest pain. Reteplase should be administered as two 10-unit bolus injections each administered over 2 min, the second dose given 30 min after the initiation of the first injection. Patients should also receive adjunctive therapy with heparin and aspirin.

Note   Reteplase should be given through an intravenous line in which no other medications (e.g., heparin) are being injected or infused. If reteplase is to be administered through an intravenous line containing heparin, the line should be flushed before and after reteplase administration with either 0.9% sodium chloride or 5% dextrose solution. Reteplase should be reconstituted with 10 mL of sterile water for injection (without preservatives) to yield a solution of 1 U/mL. The vial should be swirled gently to dissolve the drug, taking precaution to avoid shaking. Once dissolved, 10 mL should be withdrawn from the vial into a syringe for administration to the patient. Approximately 0.7 mL will remain in the vial due to overfill.

Elderly

Dosage adjustment is not required.

Children

Safety and effectiveness have not been established.

Preparation

Retavase (Centocor): 10.8 units (18.8 mg)/single-use vial.

4. Streptokinase (Streptase®)

Indications

Acute myocardial infarction
Arterial thrombosis or embolism
Cannula, arteriovenous clearance
Deep-vein thrombosis
Pulmonary embolism

Dosage

Adults

Acute myocardial infarction

Treatment should be initiated as soon as possible, preferably within 4 h after the onset of chest pain.

Intravenous infusion—Administer a total dose of 1,500,000 IU within 60 min.

Intracoronary infusion—Administer 20,000 IU by bolus followed by 2000 IU/min for 60 min (a total dose of 140,000 IU).

Pulmonary embolism, deep-vein thrombosis, arterial thrombosis, or embolism

250,000 IU bolus infused intravenously over 30 min, followed by 100,000 IU/h continuous infusion for 24 h for pulmonary embolism, 72 h for deep-vein thrombosis, and 24 to 72 h for arterial thrombosis or embolism. Treatment should be initiated as soon as possible, preferably within 7 days after onset of the symptoms.

Arteriovenous cannula occlusion

Slowly instill 250,000 IU streptokinase in 2 mL solution into each occluded limb of the cannula. Clamp off cannula limb(s) for 2 h and observe closely for adverse effects. After treatment, aspirate contents of infused cannula limb(s), flush with saline, and reconnect cannula.

Note   Consult package insert for detailed instructions on reconstitution of streptokinase prior to administration.

Elderly

Dosage adjustment is not required. Patients older than 75 years of age may be more susceptible to unwanted bleeding events.

Children

Safety and effectiveness have not been established.

Preparations

Streptase (Astra Zeneca): 250,000, 750,000, 1,500,000 IU/vial

5. Tenecteplase (TNKase®)

Indication

Acute myocardial infarction

Dosage

Adults

Acute myocardial infarction

Treatment should be initiated as soon as possible after the onset of symptoms. Dosage of tenecteplase is based on patient weight as follows:

Patient Weight (kg)	Tenecteplase (mg)	Tenecteplase (mL)*
<60	30	6
≥60 to <70	35	7
≥70 to <80	40	8
≥80 to <90	45	9
≥ 90	50	10

*This is the volume of tenecteplase to be administered as a single bolus dose over 5 seconds after one vial of tenecteplase (50 mg) is reconstituted with 10 mL of sterile water for injection. Consult tenecteplase package insert for detailed instructions on reconstitution.

Elderly

Dosage determination is based on weight. Elderly patients may be more susceptible to unwanted bleeding events.

Children

Safety and effectiveness have not been established.

Preparation

TNKase (Genentech): 50 mg/vial; sterile water for injection, 10 mL

6. Urokinase (Abbokinase®)

Indications

Coronary artery thrombosis
Intravenous catheter clearance
Pulmonary Embolism

Dosage

Adults

Coronary artery thrombosis

For the treatment of coronary artery thrombi, urokinase is administered selectively into the thrombosed coronary artery via a coronary catheter. Treatment should be initiated within 6 h of the onset of symptoms. A bolus dose of heparin 2500 to 10,000 units should be administered by rapid intravenous injection, followed by intracoronary administration of urokinase at a rate of 6,000 IU/min (1500 IU/mL) for up to 2 h. The duration of treatment is guided by angiography performed every 15 min. The average urokinase dose used was 500,000 IU with a 60% response rate. Heparin should be continued after clot lysis.

Note Consult urokinase package insert for detailed instructions on reconstitution of medication prior to administration.

Pulmonary embolism

Treatment should be initiated as soon as possible after onset of pulmonary embolism, preferably within 7 days. Administered urokinase 4400 IU/kg intravenously over 10 min, followed by continuous infusion of 4400 IU/kg/h for 12 h. Thrombin time (TT) should be determined 3 to 4 h after initiation of therapy and maintained greater than twice the normal control. Appropriate anticoagulant therapy should be initiated about 3 to 4 h after discontinuance of urokinase infusion (until the TT has decreased to less than twice the normal control value).

Note Consult urokinase package insert for recommendations regarding rate of infusion, which is based on dilution volume of the drug.

Occluded catheter

Urokinase 5,000 IU/mL is used and only the amount that equals to the internal volume of the catheter should be injected slowly into the catheter. Specific instructions provided by the manufacturer should be followed to ensure aseptic application and proper urokinase indwelling time before each aspiration attempt, and to avoid the risk for air emboli.

Elderly

Dosage adjustment is not required. Elderly patients may be more susceptible to unwanted bleeding events.

Children

Safety and effectiveness have not been established.

Preparations

Abbokinase Open-Cath (Abbott): 5000, 9000 IU/mL vials (urokinase for catheter clearance)

Abbokinase (Abbott): 250,000 IU/5 mL vial (urokinase for injection)

BETA-ADRENERGIC BLOCKERS

NONSELECTIVE BETA-ADRENERGIC BLOCKERS WITHOUT ISA

1. Nadolol (Nadolol, Corgard®)

Indications

Angina pectoris
Hypertension

Dosage

Adults

Hypertension

Initiate with 20 to 40 mg once daily, dosage may be increased gradually in increments of 40 to 80 mg to a maximum of 240 to 320 mg/d. Usual maintenance dose is 40 to 80 mg once daily.

Angina pectoris

Initiate with 40 mg once daily, dosage may be increased by 40 to 80 mg/d every 3 to 7 days until adequate control of angina is achieved. The usual dose is 40 to 80 mg/d. Up to 160 to 240 mg/d may be needed.

Note Because of the long half-life of nadolol, once-daily dosing is sufficient to provide stable plasma concentrations. Adjustments in dosing intervals must be made for patients with renal impairment as follows:

CrCl (mL/min/1.73 m^2)	Dosing Interval
>50	q 24 h
31 to 50	q 24 to 36 h
10 to 30	q 24 to 48 h
<10	q 48 h or longer

Elderly

Initiate at lowest dose and titrate to response.

Children

Safety and efficacy have not been established.

Preparations

Corgard (Monarch): 20 mg, 40 mg, 80 mg, 120 mg, 160 mg tablets

Fixed-Dose Combinations for the Treatment of Hypertension:
Corizide 40/5 tablets—40 mg nadolol and 5 mg bendroflumethiazide

Corizide 80/5 tablets—80 mg nadolol and 5 mg bendroflumethiazide

2. Propranolol (Propranolol, Inderal®, Inderal® LA)

Indications

Angina pectoris
Cardiac arrhythmias
Essential tremor
Hypertension
Hypertrophic subaortic stenosis
Myocardial infarction
Migraine prophylaxis
Pheochromocytoma

Dosage

Adults

Angina pectoris

Regular formulation: Initiate with 10 to 20 mg three to four times per day, dosage may be increased gradually every 3 to 7 days according to response to a maximum dose of 320 mg/d.

Extended-Release formulation: Initiate with 80 mg once daily; increase dosage gradually every 3 to 7 days as needed up to a maximum of 320 mg/d.

Cardiac arrhythmias

Regular formulation: 10 to 30 mg three to four times per day given before meals and at bedtime.

Essential tremor

Regular formulation: Initiate with 40 mg twice daily, dosage may be titrated according to response to a maximum of 320 mg/d. The usual maintenance dose is 120 mg/d in divided doses.

Hypertension

Regular formulation: Initiate with 40 mg twice daily; dosage may be increased gradually according to response to a maximum of 640 mg/d. The usual maintenance dose is 120 to 240 mg/d given in two to three divided doses.

Extended-Release formulation: Initiate with 80 mg once daily, dosage may be increased gradually according to response to a maximum of 640 mg/d. The usual maintenance dose is 120 to 160 mg once daily.

Hypertrophic subaortic stenosis

Regular formulation: The usual dose range is 20 to 40 mg three to four times per day given before meals and at bedtime.

Extended-Release formulation: The usual dose range is 80 to 160 mg once daily.

Myocardial infarction

Regular formulation: The usual dose range is 180 to 240 mg/d given in three to four divided doses.

Migraine prophylaxis

Regular formulation: Initiate with 80 mg/d in divided doses, dosage may be increased gradually to the usual range of 160 to 240 mg/d in divided doses.

Extended-Release formulation: Initiate with 80 mg once daily. Dosage may be increased gradually to a maximum of 240 mg/d.

Pheochromocytoma (adjunct therapy to α-adrenergic blocker)

Regular formulation: 60 mg/d in divided doses for 3 days prior to surgery. To prevent severe hypertension caused by unopposed α-adrenergic stimulation, treatment with an α-adrenergic blocking agent must always be started prior to the use of propranolol and continued during propranolol therapy. As an adjunct to prolonged treatment of inoperable pheochromocytoma, 30 mg of propranolol daily in divided doses along with an α-adrenergic blocker is usually sufficient.

Intravenous administration for life-threatening arrhythmias

The usual dose is 1 to 3 mg given under careful monitoring. Rate of injection should not exceed 1 mg/min. A second dose may be given after 2 min if indicated. Thereafter, do not give additional dose in <4 h.

Elderly

Initiate at lowest dose and titrate to response.

Children

Initiate with oral dosage of 0.5 mg/kg twice daily for the treatment of hypertension. Dosage may be increased at 3- to 5-day intervals to usual range of 2 to 4 mg/kg/d given in divided doses. Intravenous use is not recommended; however, a dose of 0.01 to 0.1 mg/kg/dose to a maximum of 1 mg/dose by slow push has been used for the management of arrhythmias.

Preparations

Propranolol (generic); Inderal (Wyeth-Ayerst): 10 mg, 20 mg, 40 mg, 60 mg, 80 mg tablets

Propranolol extended-release capsules (generic); Inderal LA (Wyeth-Ayerst): 60 mg, 80 mg, 120 mg, 160 mg extended-release capsules

Propranolol injection (generic); Inderal injection (Wyeth-Ayerst): 1 mg/mL

Fixed-Dose Combinations for the Treatment of Hypertension:
Inderide LA 80/50: propranolol 80 mg/hydrochlorothiazide 50 mg capsules

Inderide LA 120/50: propranolol 120 mg/hydrochlorothiazide 50 mg capsules

Inderide LA 160/50: propranolol 160 mg/hydrochlorothiazide 50 mg capsules

Inderide 80/25: propranolol 80 mg/hydrochlorothiazide 25 mg tablets

Inderide 40/25: propranolol 40 mg/hydrochlorothiazide 25 mg tablets

Propranolol 80 mg/hydrochlorothiazide 25 mg tablets
Propranolol 40 mg/hydrochlorothiazide 25 mg tablets

3. Sotalol (Betapace®, Betapace AF®)

Please refer to the section on antiarrhythmic agents.

4. Timolol (Timolol, Blocadren®)

Indications

Hypertension
Myocardial infarction

Migraine prophylaxis
Open-angle glaucoma (ophthalmic preparation)

Dosage

Adults

Hypertension
Initiate with 10 mg twice daily, dosage may be increased gradually (at intervals of at least 7 days) to a maximum of 60 mg/d given in two divided doses. The usual maintenance dose is 20 to 40 mg/d.

Myocardial Infarction
Administer 10 mg twice daily for long-term prophylactic use in patients who have survived a myocardial infarction.

Migraine prophylaxis
Initiate with 10 mg twice daily. The dose should be adjusted based on clinical response to a maximum of 30 mg/d given in divided doses. Therapy should be tapered and discontinued if a satisfactory response is not achieved after 6 to 8 weeks of the maximum daily dosage.

Elderly
Initiate at lowest dose and titrate to response.

Children
Safety and effectiveness have not been established.

Preparations
Timolol (generic); Blocadren (Merck): 5 mg, 10 mg, 20 mg tablets

Timolol (generic): 0.25 and 0.50% ophthalmic solution
Timoptic (Merck): 0.25 and 0.50% ophthalmic solution
Timoptic XE (Merck): 0.25 and 0.50% ophthalmic gel

Fixed-Dose Combinations for the Treatment of Hypertension:
Timolide 10–25: 10 mg timolol/25 mg hydrochlorothiazide tablets

BETA₁ SELECTIVE β-ADRENERGIC BLOCKERS WITHOUT ISA

1. Atenolol (Atenolol, Tenormin®)

Indications
Angina pectoris
Hypertension
Myocardial infarction

Dosage

Adults

Angina pectoris
Initiate with 50 mg once daily, dosage may be increased to 100 mg/d according to response. Some patients may require 200 mg/d.

Hypertension
Initiate with 50 mg once daily, dosage may be increased (at 1 to 2 week intervals) to 100 mg/d according to response.

Myocardial infarction
Treatment should be initiated with intravenous atenolol 5 mg administered over 5 min, followed by a second intravenous dose of 5 mg 10 min later. If the patient tolerates the full intravenous therapy, 50 mg of atenolol should be administered orally 10 min after the last intravenous dose, followed by a second 50 mg oral dose 12 h later. Then the patient can receive atenolol orally either 100 mg once daily or 50 mg twice daily for 6 to 9 days or until discharge from the hospital.

Note   Because atenolol is eliminated mainly in the kidneys as unchanged drug, dosage adjustment should be made in patients with renal impairment.

CrCl (mL/min/1.73 m²)	Maximum Dose
15 to 35	50 mg/d
<15	25 mg/d
Hemodialysis	25 or 50 mg post hemodialysis

Elderly
Initiate at lowest dose and titrate to response.

Children
Safety and effectiveness have not been established.

Preparations
Atenolol (generic); Tenormin (Astra Zeneca): 25 mg, 50 mg, 100 mg tablets
Tenormin injection (Astra Zeneca): 5 mg/10 mL, 10 mL ampules

Fixed-Dose Combinations for the Treatment of Hypertension:
Generic; Tenoretic 50: 50 mg atenolol/25 mg chlorthalidone tablets
Generic; Tenoretic 100: 100 mg atenolol/25 mg chlorthalidone tablets

2. Betaxolol (Betaxolol, Kerlone®)

Indications
Hypertension
Ocular hypertension (ophthalmic preparation)
Open-angle glaucoma (ophthalmic preparation)

Dosage

Adults

Hypertension
Initiate with 10 mg once daily (5 mg for elderly patients or patients with renal impairment). Dosage may be doubled every 2 weeks to a maximum dose of 20 to 40 mg/d.

Elderly
Initiate at lowest dose and titrate to response.

Children
Safety and effectiveness have not been established.

Preparations
Betaxolol (generic); Kerlone: 10 mg, 20 mg tablets

3. Bisoprolol (Bisoprolol, Zebeta®)

Indications
Hypertension

Dosage

Adults

Hypertension
Initiate with 2.5 to 5 mg once daily, dosage may be increased according to response to a maximum of 20 mg once daily.

Elderly
Dosage adjustment is not necessary. However, a lower initial dose of 2.5 mg should be used in patients with CrCl <40 mL/min or in patients with hepatic impairment.

Children
Safety and effectiveness have not been established.

Preparations
Bisoprolol (generic); Zebeta (Lederle): 5 mg, 10 mg tablets

Fixed-Dose Combinations for the Treatment of Hypertension:
Generic; Ziac (Lederle) bisoprolol/hydrochlorothiazide combination tablets: 2.5 mg/6.25 mg; 5 mg/6.25 mg; 10 mg/6.25 mg

4. Esmolol (Brevibloc®)

Indications
Supraventricular tachycardia
Intraoperative and postoperative tachycardia and/or hypertension

Dosage

Adults

Supraventricular tachycardia
The dosage is established by means of a series of loading and maintenance doses. Administer a loading intravenous infusion of 500 μg/kg/min for 1 minute followed by a maintenance intravenous infusion of 50 μg/kg/min for 4 min. If adequate response is not observed at the end of 5 min, repeat sequence with loading intravenous infusion (as above) followed by an increased maintenance infusion rate of 100 μg/kg/min. The sequence is repeated until an adequate response is obtained, with an increment of 50 μg/kg/min in the maintenance dose at each step. As desired end-point (defined as desired heart rate/undesirable decrease in blood pressure) is approached, loading dose may be omitted and increments in maintenance dose reduced to 25 μg/kg/min or less. Intervals between titration steps may also be increased from 5 to 10 min. Established maintenance dose usually does not exceed 200 μg/kg/min (due to the risk of hypotension) and can be given for up to 24 h (up to 48 h of therapy have been given in limited studies). Maintenance doses as low as 25 μg/kg/min and as high as 300 μg/kg/min have been used.

Intraoperative and postoperative tachycardia and/or hypertension
Rapid intraoperative control—Administer an 80-mg (1 mg/kg) intravenous bolus dose over 30 sec, followed by a 150 μg/kg/min infusion and titrate the dose to maintain desired heart rate or blood pressure (up to 300 μg/kg/min)

Gradual postoperative control—Dose titration schedule is the same as the treatment in supraventricular tachycardia; however, higher dosages of up to 250 to 300 μg/kg/min may be needed for adequate blood pressure control.

Note   The 250 mg/mL strength of esmolol hydrochloride injection must be diluted before administration by intravenous infusion. The 10 mg/mL strength may be given by direct infusion. Concentrations >10 mg/mL may produce irritation. If a reaction occurs at the infusion site, the infusion should be stopped and resumed at another site. Avoid the use of butterfly needles and very small veins for infusion of esmolol.

Elderly
Initiate with a low dose and titrate according to response.

Children
Safety and effectiveness have not been established.

Preparations
Brevibloc (Baxter Healthcare): 10 mg/mL, 250 mg/mL

5. Metoprolol (Metoprolol tartrate, Lopressor®, Toprol XL®)

Indications
Angina pectoris
Hypertension
Myocardial infarction
Congestive heart failure (Toprol XL®)

Dosage

Adults

Hypertension
Initiate with 100 mg/d in single or divided doses. Dosage may be adjusted at weekly intervals (or longer) until desired blood pressure control is achieved. Effective maintenance dose ranged from 100 to 450 mg/d.

Note   The extended-release tablets are for once-a-day administration. The same total daily dose should be used when switching from immediate-release metoprolol tablets to extended-release tablets.

Angina pectoris
Initiate with 100 mg/d in two divided doses. Dosage may be increased at weekly intervals until optimum clinical response is achieved. Effective maintenance dose ranged from 100 to 400 mg/d.

Myocardial infarction
Treatment should be initiated as soon as the patient's hemodynamic status has stabilized. Three 5-mg intravenous bolus injections of metoprolol should be administered at 2-minute intervals. If the full 15-mg intravenous dose is tolerated by the patient, 50 mg of oral metoprolol (or 25 mg for those who cannot tolerate the full dose) every 6 h should be initiated 15 min after the last intravenous

dose and continued for 48 h. Thereafter, the dose may be adjusted to 100 mg twice daily.

Congestive heart failure

For NYHA Class II patients start with 25 mg once daily. For severe heart failure start with 12.5 mg once daily. Titrate by doubling dose every 2 weeks as tolerated; reduce dose if symptomatic bradycardia occurs. Maximal dose is 200 mg daily.

Elderly

Initiate with a low dose and titrate according to response.

Children

Safety and effectiveness have not been established.

Preparations

Metoprolol tartrate (generic); Lopressor (Novartis): 50 mg, 100 mg tablets

Toprol XL (Astra Zeneca): 25 mg, 50 mg, 100 mg, 200 mg extended-release tablets

Metoprolol tartrate injection (generic); Lopressor injection (Novartis): 1 mg/mL

Fixed-Dose Combinations for the Treatment of Hypertension:
Lopressor HCT tablets (Novartis):
50/25—50 mg metoprolol/25 mg hydrochlorothiazide
100/25—100 mg metoprolol/25 mg hydrochlorothiazide
100/50—100 mg metoprolol/50 mg hydrochlorothiazide

β-ADRENERGIC BLOCKERS WITH ISA

1. Acebutolol (Acebutolol, Sectral®)

Indications
Hypertension
Ventricular arrhythmia

Dosage

Adults

Hypertension

Initiate with 200 to 400 mg/d administered in one or two divided doses. Dosage may be increased gradually based on clinical response up to 600 mg twice daily. Most patients require 400 to 800 mg/d.

Ventricular arrhythmia

Initiate with 400 mg once daily or 200 mg twice daily. Dosage may be increased until optimal response is achieved. The usual maintenance dose is 600 to 1200 mg/d given in two divided doses.

Note The daily dose of acebutolol should be reduced by 50% when CrCl is <50 mL/min/1.73m². Reduce dose by 75% when CrCl is <25 mL/min/1.73 m². Use acebutolol with caution in patients with hepatic impairment.

Elderly
Initiate at lowest dose and titrate to response. Avoid doses >800 mg/d.

Children
Safety and effectiveness have not been established.

Preparations
Acebutolol (generic); Sectral (Wyeth-Ayerst): 200 mg, 400 mg capsules

2. Carteolol (Cartrol®)

Indication
Hypertension

Dosage

Adults

Hypertension

Initiate with 2.5 mg once daily. Dosage may be increased gradually according to response to a maximum of 10 mg once daily. The usual maintenance dose is 2.5 or 5 mg once daily.

Note Guidelines for dosing intervals in patients with renal impairment are as follows:

CrCl (mL/min/1.73 m²)	Dosage Interval (h)
>60	24
20 to 60	48
<20	72

Elderly
Initiate at lowest dose and titrate to response.

Children
Safety and effectiveness have not been established.

Preparations
Cartrol (Abbott): 2.5 mg, 5 mg tablets

3. Penbutolol (Levatol®)

Indication
Hypertension

Dosage

Adults

Hypertension

The usual starting and maintenance dose is 20 mg once daily. Doses of 40 to 80 mg/d have been well tolerated but have not shown greater effect.

Elderly
Initiate at lowest dose and titrate to response.

Children
Safety and effectiveness have not been established.

Preparation
Levatol (Schwarz Pharma): 20 mg tablets

4. Pindolol (Pindolol, Visken®)

Indication
Hypertension

Dosage

Adults

Hypertension
Initiate with 5 mg twice daily. Dosage may be increased by 10 mg/d at 3- to 4-week intervals to a maximum of 60 mg/d if necessary.

Elderly
Initiate at lowest dose and titrate to response.

Children
Safety and effectiveness have not been established

Preparations
Pindolol, Visken (Novartis): 5 mg, 10 mg tablets

DUAL-ACTING BETA-BLOCKERS

1. Carvedilol (Coreg®)

Indications
Congestive heart failure (mild-to-severe)
Hypertension

Dosage

Adults

Congestive heart failure
Dosage of carvedilol must be individualized and closely monitored during the up-titration period. Dosing of digitalis, diuretics, and ACE inhibitors (if used) must be stabilized prior to initiation of carvedilol. Initiate carvedilol with 3.125 mg twice daily for 2 weeks. If this dose is tolerated, it can then be increased to 6.25 mg twice daily. Dosing should then be doubled every 2 weeks to the highest level tolerated by the patient. The maximum recommended dose is 25 mg twice daily in patients weighing <85 kg and 50 mg twice daily in patients weighing >85 kg. If bradycardia occurs (pulse rate <55 beats/min), the dose of carvedilol should be reduced.

Hypertension
Initiate with 6.25 mg twice daily. Dosage may be increased to 12.5 mg twice daily after 7 to 14 days if tolerated and needed. A further increase to 25 mg twice daily may be made after an additional 7 to 14 days if necessary. The total daily dose should not exceed 50 mg.

Note Carvedilol should be taken with food to slow the rate of absorption and reduce the incidence of orthostatic hypotension. Because carvedilol is primarily metabolized in the liver, it should not be given to patients with severe hepatic impairment. In patients with heart failure, slower titration with temporary dose reduction or withdrawal may be required based on clinical assessment; however, this should not preclude later attempts to reintroduce or increase the dose of carvedilol.

Elderly
Although plasma levels of carvedilol average about 50% higher in the elderly compared with young subjects, the manufacturer has not suggested dosage adjustment.

Children
Safety and effectiveness have not been established.

Preparations
Coreg (Glaxo SmithKline): 3.125 mg, 6.25 mg, 12.5 mg, 25 mg tablets

2. Labetalol (Labetalol, Normodyne®, Trandate®)

Indications
Hypertension
Severe hypertension (intravenous formulation)

Dosage

Adults
Initiate with 100 mg orally twice daily, dosage may be adjusted in increments of 100 mg two times daily every 2 to 3 days until desired response is reached. The usual maintenance dose is 200 to 400 mg twice daily. For severe hypertension, oral doses of 1.2 to 2.4 g daily in two to three divided doses may be needed.

Labetalol may also be administered by repeated intravenous injections. Inject 20 mg (0.25 mg/kg for an 80-kg patient) slowly over 2 min. Additional injections of 40 and 80 mg may be given at 10-minute intervals until the desired blood pressure is reached or a total of 300 mg has been given. Alternatively, an intravenous infusion at a rate of 2 mg/min may be given (labetalol injection must be diluted properly for intravenous infusion); infusion rate should be adjusted according to response. The infusion should be continued until an adequate response is achieved or a total dose of 300 mg is infused. The infusion is then discontinued and oral therapy is initiated when supine blood pressure begins to increase. Initial oral dose should be 200 mg, followed by an additional oral dose of 200 or 400 mg in 6 to 12 h based on blood pressure response.

Elderly
Dosage adjustment based on age is not necessary.

Children
Safety and efficacy have not been established.

Preparations
Labetalol HCl (generic); Normodyne (Schering); Trandate (Prometheus): 100 mg, 200 mg, 300 mg tablets
Generic; Normodyne injection (Schering); Trandate injection (Prometheus): 5 mg/mL

CALCIUM ANTAGONISTS

1. Amlodipine (Norvasc®)

Indications
Hypertension
Chronic stable angina
Vasospastic (Prinzmetal's or variant) angina

Dosage

Adults

Hypertension

Initiate with 5 mg once daily; dosage may be increased to a maximum of 10 mg once daily based on response. A lower initial dose of 2.5 mg once daily is recommended for elderly patients and patients with hepatic insufficiency.

Angina

The usual dose is 5 to 10 mg once daily. Use lower dose for elderly patients and patients with hepatic impairment.

Elderly

Initiate at lowest dose and titrate to response.

Children

Safety and effectiveness have not been established.

Preparations

Norvasc (Pfizer): 2.5 mg, 5 mg, 10 mg tablets

2. Bepridil (Vascor®)

Indication

Chronic stable angina

Dosage

Adults

Dosage should be individualized according to clinical judgment and patient's response. The usual initial dose is 200 mg once daily. Upward adjustment may be made after 10 days depending on patient's response. The usual maintenance dose is 300 mg once daily. Maximum daily dose is 400 mg.

Note If nausea occurs, administer the drug with meals or at bedtime.

Elderly

Same initial dose as in adult patients may be used. However, elderly patients may require close monitoring due to underlying cardiac and organ system insufficiencies.

Children

Safety and effectiveness have not been established.

Preparations

Vascor (Ortho-McNeil): 200 mg, 300 mg tablets

3. Diltiazem (Diltiazem, Cardizem®, Cardizem® SR, Cardizem® CD, Dilacor® XR, Tiazac®)

Indications

Angina pectoris
Atrial fibrillation or flutter (Cardizem injectable)
Hypertension
Paroxysmal supraventricular tachycardia (Cardizem injectable)

Dosage

Adults

Short-acting (diltiazem, Cardizem)

As an antianginal agent, the usual initial dose is 30 mg four times daily (before meals and at bedtime). Dosage should be increased gradually at 1- to 2-day intervals. Maximum daily dose is 360 mg.

Sustained-release (Cardizem SR)

As monotherapy for hypertension, start with 60 to 120 mg twice daily, although some patients may respond well to lower doses. The usual dosage range is 240 to 360 mg/d.

Sustained-release (Cardizem CD)

As monotherapy for hypertension, initiate at 180 to 240 mg once daily. The usual dose range in clinical trials was 240 to 360 mg/d. Some patients may respond to higher doses of up to 480 mg once daily. For angina, start with 120 or 180 mg once daily. Dosage may be titrated upward every 7 to 14 days to a maximum of 480 mg once daily if necessary.

Sustained-release (Dilacor XR)

For hypertension, initiate at 180 to 240 mg once daily. Adjust dose as needed depending on antihypertensive response. In clinical trials, the therapeutic dose range is 180 to 540 mg once daily. For angina, initiate at 120 mg once daily. Dosage may be titrated upward every 7 to 14 days up to a maximum of 480 mg once daily if needed.

Sustained-release (Tiazac)

The usual initial dose is 120 to 240 mg once daily. Maximum effect is observed after 14 days. Doses up to 540 mg daily were shown to be effective in clinical trials.

Injection (diltiazem IV, Cardizem IV)

Direct intravenous single injections (bolus): Administer 0.25 mg/kg as a bolus over 2 min (20 mg is a reasonable dose for a patient with an average weight). If response is inadequate, a second dose may be administered after 15 min (25 mg or 0.35 mg/kg is a reasonable dose).

Intravenous infusion

An intravenous infusion may be administered for continued reduction of the heart rate (up to 24 h) in patients with atrial fibrillation or atrial flutter. Start an infusion at a rate of 10 mg/h immediately after bolus administration of 0.25 or 0.35 mg/kg. Some patients may maintain response to an initial rate of 5 mg/h. The infusion rate may be increased in 5 mg/h increments up to 15 mg/h as needed. Infusion duration longer than 24 h and infusion rate > 15 mg/h are not recommended (refer to manufacturer's package insert for proper dilution of diltiazem injection for continuous infusion).

Elderly

Initiate at lowest dose and titrate to response.

Children

Safety and effectiveness have not been established.

Preparations

Tablets (Diltiazem, Cardizem): 30 mg, 60 mg, 90 mg, 120 mg
Capsules (Cardizem SR): 60 mg, 90 mg, 120 mg

Capsules (Cardizem CD): 120 mg, 180 mg, 240 mg, 300 mg, 360 mg

Capsules (Dilacor XR): 120 mg, 180 mg, 240 mg

Capsules (Tiazac): 120 mg, 180 mg, 240 mg, 300 mg, 360 mg, 420 mg

Injection (as hydrochloride): 5 mg/mL (5 mL, 10 mL)

Fixed-Dose Combinations for the Treatment of Hypertension:
Teczem—5 mg of enalapril maleate/180 mg of diltiazem malate ER (extended-release) combination tablets

4. Felodipine (Plendil®)

Indication
Hypertension

Dosage

Adults

The usual initial dose is 5 mg once daily. Dosage may be increased by 5 mg at 2-week intervals according to response. Maintenance dose range from 2.5 to 10 mg once daily.

Elderly

A lower initial dose of 2.5 mg once daily is recommended.

Children

Safety and effectiveness have not been established.

Preparations

Plendil (Astra Zeneca): 2.5 mg, 5 mg, 10 mg extended-release tablets.

Fixed-Dose Combinations for the Treatment of Hypertension:
Lexxel—5 mg of enalapril maleate/5 mg of felodipine ER (extended-release) combination tablets

5. Isradipine (DynaCirc®, DynaCirc CR®)

Indication
Hypertension

Dosage

Adults

Immediate-release (DynaCirc)

Initiate at 2.5 mg twice daily alone or in combination with a thiazide diuretic. Dosage may be adjusted in increments of 2.5 to 5 mg/d at 2- to 4-week intervals if needed. The maximum daily dose is 20 mg.

Note Most patients show no further improvement with doses >10 mg/d; adverse reactions are increased in frequency with doses >10 mg/d.

Controlled-release (DynaCirc CR)

Initiate at 5 mg once daily alone or in combination with a thiazide diuretic.

Dosage may be adjusted in increments of 5 mg/d at 2- to 4-week intervals if needed. The maximum daily dose is 20 mg.

Elderly

Initiate at lowest dose and titrate to response.

Children

Safety and effectiveness have not been established.

Preparations

DynaCirc (Reliant): 2.5 mg, 5 mg capsules
DynaCirc CR (Reliant): 5 mg, 10 mg controlled-release tablets

6. Nicardipine (Nicardipine, Cardene®, Cardene SR®)

Indications

Hypertension (Cardene, Cardene SR)
Short-term treatment of hypertension when oral therapy cannot be given (Cardene I.V.)
Angina (Cardene)

Dosage

Adults

Immediate-release (Cardene)

As an antianginal or antihypertensive agent, administer 20 mg in capsule form three times daily. The usual maintenance dose is 20 to 40 mg three times daily. Allow at least 3 days between dose increases. For patients with renal impairment, titrate dose beginning with 20 mg three times daily. For patients with hepatic impairment, titrate dose starting with 20 mg twice daily.

Sustained-release (Cardene SR)

Initiate treatment with 30 mg twice daily. The effective dose ranges from 30 to 60 mg twice daily. For patients with renal impairment, carefully titrate dose beginning with 30 mg twice daily. The total daily dose of immediate-release product may not automatically be equivalent to the daily sustained-release dose; use caution in converting.

Injection (Cardene I.V.)

Intravenously administered nicardipine injection must be diluted before infusion. Administer (concentration of 0.1 mg/mL) by slow, continuous infusion. Blood pressure lowering effect is seen within minutes. For gradual blood pressure lowering, initiate at 50 mL/h (5 mg/h). Infusion rate may be increased by 25 mL/h (2.5 mg/h) every 15 min to a maximum of 150 mL/h (15 mg/h). For rapid blood pressure reduction, initiate at 50 mL/h. Increase infusion rate by 25 mL/h every 5 min to a maximum of 150 mL/h until desirable blood pressure lowering is reached. Infusion rate must be decreased to 30 mL/h (3 mg/h) when desirable blood pressure is achieved. Conditions requiring infusion adjustment include hypotension and tachycardia. The intravenous infusion rate required to produce an average plasma concentration equivalent to a given oral dose at steady state is as follows:

Oral Dose (Immediate-Release)	Equivalent IV Infusion Rate
20 mg q 8 h	0.5 mg/h
30 mg q 8 h	1.2 mg/h
40 mg q 8 h	2.2 mg/h

Intravenous nicardipine should be transferred to oral medication for prolonged control of blood pressure as soon as the clinical condition permits. If treatment includes transfer to an oral antihypertensive agent other than nicardipine, generally initiate therapy upon discontinuation of the infusion. If oral nicardipine is to be used, administer the first dose of a three times daily regimen 1 h before discontinuation of the infusion.

Elderly
Dosage adjustment is not necessary.

Children
Safety and effectiveness have not been established.

Preparations
Nicardipine HCl (generic); Cardene (Roche): 20 mg, 30 mg capsules

Cardene SR (Roche): 30 mg, 45 mg, 60 mg sustained-release capsules

Cardene I.V. (Wyeth-Ayerst): 2.5 mg/mL injection, 10 mL ampules

7. Nifedipine (Nifedipine, Adalat®, Adalat® CC, Procardia®, Procardia XL®)

Indications
Chronic stable angina (Nifedipine, Adalat, Procardia, Procardia XL)

Hypertension (Adalat CC, Procardia XL)

Vasospastic angina (Nifedipine, Adalat, Procardia, Procardia XL)

Dosage

Adults

Short-acting (Nifedipine, Adalat, Procardia)
As an antianginal, initiate nifedipine in the capsule form at 10 mg three times daily, dosage may be increased gradually over 7 to 14 days as needed. For hospitalized patients under close supervision, dosage may be increased by 10-mg increments over 4 to 6 h periods until symptoms are controlled. For elderly patients and patients with hepatic impairment, initiate treatment at 10 mg twice daily and monitor carefully.

Note   Current labeling states that the short-acting product should not be used for hypertension, hypertensive crisis, acute MI, and some forms of unstable angina and chronic stable angina.

Extended-release (Adalat CC)
Initiate with 30 mg once daily and titrate over a 7 to 14 day period according to response. The usual maintenance dose is 30 to 60 mg once daily. Titration to doses >90 mg daily is not recommended.

Extended-release (Procardia XL)
Initiate with 30 or 60 mg once daily and titrate over a period of 7 to 14 days according to response. Titration may proceed more rapidly if the patient is frequently assessed. Titration to doses >120 mg daily is not recommended. Angina patients maintained on the short-acting formulation (nifedipine capsule) may be switched to the extended-release tablet at the nearest equivalent total daily dose. Experience with doses >90 mg daily in patients with angina is limited.

Elderly
Initiate at lowest dose and titrate to response.

Children
Safety and effectiveness have not been established.

Preparations
Nifedipine (generic); Adalat (Bayer); Procardia (Pfizer): 10 mg, 20 mg liquid-filled capsules

Adalat CC (Bayer): 30 mg, 60 mg, 90 mg sustained-release tablets

Procardia XL (Pfizer): 30 mg, 60 mg, 90 mg sustained-release tablets

Generic SR tablets: 30 mg, 60 mg, 90 mg

8. Nimodipine (Nimotop®)

Indication
Subarachnoid hemorrhage

Dosage

Adults
The usual dose is 60 mg q 4 h beginning within 96 h of subarachnoid hemorrhage and continuing for 21 days. Dosage should be reduced to 30 mg q 4 h with close monitoring of blood pressure and heart rate in patients with hepatic cirrhosis.

Note   This medication is given preferably not less than 1 h before or 2 h after meals. If the capsule cannot be swallowed (e.g., time of surgery, unconscious patient), make a hole in both ends of the capsule with an 18-gauge needle and extract the contents into a syringe. Empty the contents into the patient's in situ nasogastric tube and wash down the tube with 30 mL of normal saline.

Elderly
Use usual dose with caution.

Children
Safety and effectiveness have not been established.

Preparation
Nimotop (Bayer): 30 mg liquid-filled capsules

9. Nisoldipine (Sular®)

Indication
Hypertension

Dosage

Adults
Initiate at 20 mg orally once daily; dosage may be increased by 10 mg per week (or at longer intervals) to attain adequate response. The usual maintenance dose is 20 to 40 mg once daily. Doses greater than 60 mg daily are not recommended. For elderly patients and patients with hepatic function impairment, initiate with a dose not exceeding 10 mg daily. Monitor blood pressure closely during any dosage adjustment.

Note Nisoldipine has been used safely with diuretics, ACE inhibitors, and beta-blockers. Administration of this medication with a high fat meal can lead to excessive peak drug concentration and should be avoided. In addition, grapefruit products should be avoided before and after dosing.

Elderly

Initiate at lower dose and titrate to response.

Children

Safety and effectiveness have not been established.

Preparations

Sular Astra (Zeneca): 10 mg, 20 mg, 30 mg, 40 mg extended-release tablets

10. Verapamil (Verapamil, Sustained-Release Verapamil, Calan®, Calan® SR, Isoptin®, Isoptin® SR, Verelan®, Verelan® PM, Covera-HS®, Verapamil IV, Isoptin® IV)

Indications

Angina (all oral immediate-release formulations and Covera-HS)
Arrhythmias (all oral immediate-release formulations)
Hypertension (all oral formulation)
Supraventricular tachyarrhythmias (intravenous formulations)

Dosage

Adults

Immediate-release tablets (verapamil, Calan, Isoptin)

As an antianginal, antiarrhythmic, and antihypertensive, initiate at 80 to 120 mg three times daily. Dosage may be increased at daily or weekly intervals as needed and tolerated. Limit to 480 mg daily in divided doses.

Sustained-release capsules (Verelan)

As an antihypertensive, initiate at 120 to 240 mg once daily. Dosage may be adjusted in increments of 60 to 120 mg/d at daily or weekly intervals as needed and tolerated. The usual daily dose range is 240 to 480 mg.

Sustained-release tablets (verapamil SR, Calan SR, Isoptin SR)

As an antihypertensive, initiate at 120 to 240 mg once daily with food. Dosage may be adjusted in increments of 60 to 120 mg/d at daily or weekly intervals as needed and as tolerated. The usual total daily dose range is 240 to 480 mg.

Extended-release tablets, controlled onset (Covera-HS)

Initiate with 180 mg at bedtime for both hypertension and angina. If response is inadequate, the dose may be titrated upward to 540 mg/d given at bedtime.

Extended-release capsules, controlled onset (Verelan PM)

Initiate with 200 mg dose at bedtime for hypertension; if response is inadequate, the dose may be titrated upward to 300 or 400 mg/d given at bedtime.

Injection (verapamil IV, Isoptin IV)

Initiate at 5 to 10 mg (or 0.075 to 0.15 mg/kg) slowly over at least 2 min with continuous electrocardiographic and blood pressure monitoring. If response is inadequate, 10 mg (or 0.15 mg/kg) may be administered 30 min after completion of the initial dose.

Note Less than 1% of patients may have life-threatening adverse responses (rapid ventricular rate in atrial flutter/fibrillation, marked hypotension or extreme bradycardia/asystole) to verapamil injections. Monitor the initial use of intravenous verapamil and have resuscitation facilities available. An intravenous infusion (5 mg/h) has also been used; precede the infusion with an intravenous loading dose.

Elderly

Initiate the oral formulation of verapamil at lower dose and titrate to response. Intravenous injections should be given slowly over a longer period of time (at least 3 min) to minimize undesired effects.

Children

Safety and effectiveness have not been established. However, there has been experience with the use of verapamil in the pediatric population.

Preparations

Tablets, immediate release (verapamil, Calan, Isoptin): 40 mg, 80 mg, 120 mg
Capsules, sustained-release (Verelan): 120 mg, 180 mg, 240 mg, 360 mg
Capsules, sustained-release (verapamil): 120 mg, 180 mg, 240 mg
Tablets, extended-release and controlled onset (Covera-HS): 180 mg, 240 mg
Capsules, extended-release and controlled onset (Verelan PM): 100 mg, 200 mg, 300 mg
Tablets, sustained-release (verapamil): 120 mg, 180 mg, 240 mg
Tablets, sustained-release (Calan SR, Isoptin SR): 120 mg, 180 mg, 240 mg
Injection (verapamil IV, Isoptin IV): 5 mg/2 mL (2- and 4-mL ampules and vials; syringes)

Fixed-Dose Combinations for the Treatment of Hypertension:
Tarka—trandolapril/verapamil hydrochloride ER combination tablets: 2 mg/180 mg, 1 mg/240 mg, 2 mg/ 240 mg, 4 mg/240 mg

DIURETICS

LOOP DIURETICS

1. Bumetanide (Bumetanide, Bumex®)

Indications

Edema associated with CHF, hepatic cirrhosis or renal disease, including the nephrotic syndrome

Dosage

Adults

Oral formulation

The usual dose range is 0.5 to 2 mg/d as a single dose. Higher dosage (>1 to 2 mg/d) may be required to achieve the desired therapeutic response in patients with renal insufficiency. If the initial diuresis is inadequate, repeated doses may be administered q 4 to 6 h until the desired diuretic response is achieved or until a maximum daily dosage of 10 mg is administered. An intermittent dose schedule, given on alternate days or daily for 3 to 4 days with rest periods of 1 to 2 days in between, may be used for the continued control of edema. Dosage should be kept to a minimum with careful adjustments in dosage for patients with hepatic impairment.

Intravenous or intramuscular formulations

Parenteral administration of bumetanide should be reserved for patients in whom GI absorption may be impaired or in whom oral administration is not feasible. Initiate at 0.5 to 1 mg intravenously or intramuscularly. Intravenous injection should be given over a period of 1 to 2 min. If the initial diuresis is inadequate, repeated doses may be administered q 2 to 3 h until the desired diuretic response is achieved or until a maximum daily dosage of 10 mg is administered.

Elderly

Initiate at lowest dose and titrate to response.

Children

Safety and effectiveness have not been established.

Preparations

Bumetanide (generic); Bumex (Roche): 0.5 mg, 1 mg, 2 mg tablets

Bumetanide injection (generic); Bumex injection (Roche): 0.25 mg/mL

2. Ethacrynic Acid (Edecrin®, Edecrin® Sodium Intravenous)

Indications

Ascites associated with malignancy, idiopathic edema, and lymphedema

Edema associated with CHF, hepatic cirrhosis, or renal disease, including the nephrotic syndrome

Hospitalized pediatric patients with congenital heart disease or the nephrotic syndrome (not indicated for infants)

Dosage

Adults

Oral formulation

Initiate at 25 to 50 mg (lower doses should be used in patients who are receiving other diuretics concurrently) once daily after a meal. Dosage may be adjusted at 25 to 50 mg increments daily until the desired response is achieved or until a maximum dose of 100 mg twice daily is given. A dose of 200 mg twice daily may be required to maintain adequate diuresis in patients with severe, refractory edema. An intermittent dose schedule, given on alternate days or daily for 3 to 4 days with rest periods of 1 to 2 days in between, may be used for the continued control of edema after an effective diuresis is obtained.

Intravenous formulations

Intravenous administration of ethacrynate sodium should be reserved for patients in whom a rapid onset of diuresis is desired such as in acute pulmonary edema, or when oral administration is not feasible. The usual adult intravenous dose is 0.5 to 1 mg/kg (up to 100 mg in a single intravenous dose) or 50 mg for an adult of average size. After reconstitution, ethacrynate sodium solution may be infused slowly (over 20 to 30 min) through the tubing of a running intravenous infusion or by direct intravenous injection over several minutes. If the desired diuresis is not achieved with the first dose of ethacrynate sodium, a second dose may be given after 2 to 3 h at a new injection site.

Elderly

Initiate at lowest dose and titrate to response.

Children

Safety and effectiveness have not been established in children for intravenous administration and in infants for oral as well as intravenous administration.

Preparations

Edecrin (Merck): 25 mg, 50 mg tablets
Edecrin Sodium (Merck): 50 mg/vial, powder for injection

3. Furosemide (Furosemide, Lasix®)

Indications

Edema associated with CHF, hepatic cirrhosis or renal disease, including the nephrotic syndrome

Hypertension (oral formulation)

Dosage

Adults

Edema (oral formulation)

The usual oral dose is 20 to 80 mg given as a single dose. The same dose may be repeated, or adjusted in increments of 20 to 40 mg q 6 to 8 h until the desired diuresis is achieved. The effective dose may then be given once or twice daily to maintain adequate fluid balance. For chronic maintenance therapy, furosemide given on alternate days or intermittently on 2 to 4 consecutive days each week is preferred. A maximum oral dose of 600 mg/d has been used in patients with severe fluid overload.

Edema (intravenous formulation)

The usual dose is 20 to 40 mg given as a single injection. The intravenous route is preferred when rapid diuresis is indicated. The same dose may be repeated, or adjusted in 20 to 40 mg increment q 1 to 2 h until the desired response is achieved. Each intravenous dose should be administered over a few minutes. Furosemide has also been administered as a continuous intravenous infusion in some patients to maintain adequate urine flow. A bolus of 20 to 40 mg should be given first, followed by an infusion with an initial rate of 0.25 to 0.5 mg/min. The infusion rate may be titrated up to a maximum of 4 mg/min according to clinical response.

Hypertension

The usual initial dose is 40 mg orally twice daily; dosage should then be adjusted according to clinical response. The maximum dose is 240 mg/d in two to three divided doses. Higher doses may be required for the management of edema or hypertension in patients with renal insufficiency or CHF. These patients should be monitored closely to ensure efficacy and avoid undesired toxicity.

Elderly

Initiate at lowest dose and titrate to response.

Children

Safety and effectiveness have been established in children for the management of edema, but not for hypertension.

Preparations

Furosemide (generic); Lasix (Aventis): 20 mg, 40 mg, 80 mg tablets

Furosemide (generic); Lasix (Aventis): 10 mg/mL, 40 mg/5 mL oral solution

Furosemide (generic); Lasix (Aventis): 10 mg/mL injection, in 2, 4, and 10 mL single-dose vials

4. Torsemide (Demadex®)

Indications

Edema associated with CHF, hepatic cirrhosis or renal disease, including the nephrotic syndrome

Hypertension (oral formulation)

Dosage

Adults

CHF/chronic renal failure

The usual initial dose is 10 to 20 mg once daily via oral or intravenous administration. If the diuretic response is inadequate, the dose may be doubled until the desired response is achieved or until a maximum single dose of 200 mg is given.

Hepatic cirrhosis

The usual initial dose is 5 to 10 mg once daily administered orally or intravenously along with an aldosterone antagonist or a potassium-sparing diuretic. If the diuretic response is inadequate, the dose may be doubled until the desired response is achieved or until a maximum single dose of 40 mg is given.

Note Because of high bioavailability, oral and intravenous doses are therapeutically equivalent. Therefore, patients may be switched to and from the intravenous form with no change in dose. The intravenous injection should be administered slowly over a period of 2 min.

Hypertension

The usual initial dose is 5 mg orally once daily. If adequate reduction in blood pressure is not achieved in 4 to 6 weeks, the dose may be increased up to 10 mg once daily. If the blood pressure response is still inadequate, an additional antihypertensive agent should be added.

Elderly

Initiate at lowest dose and titrate to response

Children

Safety and effectiveness have not been established.

Preparations

Demadex (Roche): 5 mg, 10 mg, 20 mg, 100 mg tablets
Demadex injection (Roche): 10 mg/mL

THIAZIDE DIURETICS

1. Bendroflumethiazide (Bendroflumethiazide, Naturetin®)

Indications

Edema
Hypertension

Dosage

Adults

Edema

Initiate at 5 to 20 mg/d given once daily in the morning or in two divided doses. The usual maintenance dose is 2.5 to 5 mg once daily in the morning. Electrolyte imbalance may occur less frequently by administering bendroflumethiazide every other day or on a 3 to 5 days per week schedule during maintenance therapy.

Hypertension

Initiate at 5 to 20 mg/d once daily in the morning or in two divided doses. The usual maintenance dose is 2.5 to 15 mg once daily given in the morning.

Elderly

Initiate at lowest dose and titrate to response.

Children

Safety and effectiveness have not been established.

Preparations

Naturetin (Apothecon): 2.5 mg, 5 mg, 10 mg tablets
Fixed-Dose Combinations for the Treatment of Hypertension:
Bendroflumethiazide 4 mg/Rauwolfia Serpentina 50 mg
Corzide 80/5—Bendroflumethiazide 5 mg/Nadolol 80 mg
Corzide 40/5—Bendroflumethiazide 5 mg/Nadolol 40 mg

2. Benzthiazide (Exna®)

Indications

Edema
Hypertension

Dosage

Adults

Edema

Initiate at 50 to 200 mg/d given in one to two doses for a few days until the desired diuresis is achieved (dosages above 100 mg/d should be divided and administered in two daily doses). The usual maintenance dose is 50 to 150 mg/d. Electrolyte imbalance may occur less frequently by administering benzthiazide every other day or on a 3 to 5 days per week schedule during maintenance therapy.

Hypertension

Initiate at 25 to 50 mg twice daily after breakfast and lunch; dosage may be titrated up to a maximum of 100 mg twice daily if necessary.

Elderly

Initiate at lowest dose and titrate to response.

Fixed-Dose Combinations for the Treatment of Hypertension:
Salutensin Tablets:
Hydroflumethiazide 50 mg/Reserpine 0.125 mg

7. Indapamide (Indapamide, Lozol®)

Indications
Edema
Hypertension

Dosage

Adults

Edema
Initiate at 2.5 mg once daily in the morning. Dosage may be increased to 5 mg once daily according to response. Electrolyte imbalance may occur less frequently by administering indapamide every other day or on a 3- to 5-days-per-week schedule during maintenance therapy.

Hypertension
Initiate at 1.25 mg once daily in the morning. Dosage may be increased gradually to 5 mg once daily according to response.

Elderly
Initiate at lowest dose and titrate to response.

Children
Safety and effectiveness have not been established.

Preparations
Indapamide (generic): 2.5 mg tablets
Lozol (Aventis): 1.25 mg, 2.5 mg tablets

8. Methyclothiazide (Methyclothiazide, Enduron®)

Indications
Edema
Hypertension

Dosage

Adults

Edema
Initiate at 2.5 to 10 mg once daily in the morning. The usual maintenance dose is 2.5 to 5 mg once daily. Electrolyte imbalance may occur less frequently by administering methyclothiazide every other day or on a 3- to 5-days-per-week schedule during maintenance therapy.

Hypertension
Administer 2.5 to 5 mg once daily in the morning.

Elderly
Initiate at lowest dose and titrate to response.

Children
Safety and effectiveness have not been established.

Preparations
Methyclothiazide (generic): 2.5 mg, 5 mg tablets
Aquatensen (Wallace); Enduron (Abbott): 5 mg tablets

Fixed-Dose Combinations for the Treatment of Hypertension:
Diutensen-R Tablets (Wallace): methyclothiazide 2.5 mg/ reserpine 0.1 mg

9. Metolazone (Mykrox®, Zaroxolyn®)

Indications
Edema (Zaroxolyn only)
Hypertension (Mykrox and Zaroxolyn)

Dosage

Adults

Edema
Administer Zaroxolyn at 5 to 10 mg/d given once daily in the morning. Dosage up to 20 mg once daily may be used in patients with renal insufficiency. The usual maintenance dose for Zaroxolyn is 2.5 to 10 mg given once daily in the morning. Electrolyte imbalance may occur less frequently by administering metolazone every other day or on a 3- to 5-days-per-week schedule during maintenance therapy.

Hypertension
Administer 2.5 to 5 mg of Zaroxolyn or 0.5 to 1 mg of Mykrox once daily in the morning.

Note   The metolazone formulations are not bioequivalent or therapeutically equivalent at the same doses. When switching from Zaroxolyn to Mykrox, determine the dose by titration starting at 0.5 mg once daily and increasing to 1 mg once daily according to response.

Elderly
Initiate at lowest dose and titrate to response.

Children
Safety and effectiveness have not been established.

Preparations
Mykrox (Celltech): 0.5 mg tablets
Zaroxolyn (Celltech): 2.5 mg, 5 mg, 10 mg

10. Polythiazide (Renese®)

Indications
Edema
Hypertension

Dosage

Adults

Edema
Administer 1 to 4 mg once daily in the morning. Electrolyte imbalance may occur less frequently by administering polythiazide every other day or on a 3- to 5-days-per-week schedule during maintenance therapy.

Hypertension
Administer 2 to 4 mg once daily in the morning.

Elderly

Initiate at lowest dose and titrate to response.

Children

Safety and effectiveness have not been established.

Preparations

Renese (Pfizer): 1 mg, 2 mg, 4 mg tablets

Fixed-Dose Combinations for the Treatment of Hypertension:
Minizide Capsules:
Polythiazide 0.5 mg/prazosin 1 mg
Polythiazide 0.5 mg/prazosin 2 mg
Polythiazide 0.5 mg/prazosin 5 mg

11. Quinethazone (Hydromox®)

Indications
Edema
Hypertension

Dosage

Adults

Edema

Administer 25 to 200 mg/d as a single dose in the morning or in two divided doses. Electrolyte imbalance may occur less frequently by administering quinethazone every other day or on a 3- to 5-days-per-week schedule during maintenance therapy.

Hypertension

Administer 25 to 100 mg/d as a single dose in the morning or in two divided doses.

Elderly

Initiate at lowest dose and titrate to response.

Children

Safety and effectiveness have not been established.

Preparation

Hydromox (Lederle): 50 mg tablets

12. Trichlormethiazide (Trichlormethiazide, Diurese®, Metahydrin®, Naqua®)

Indications
Edema
Hypertension

Dosage

Adults

Edema

Administer 2 to 4 mg once daily in the morning. Electrolyte imbalance may occur less frequently by administering trichlormethiazide every other day or on a 3- to 5-days-per-week schedule during maintenance therapy.

Hypertension

Administer 2 to 4 mg/d as a single dose in the morning or in two divided doses.

Elderly

Initiate at lowest dose and titrate to response.

Children

Safety and effectiveness have not been established.

Preparations

Trichlormethiazide (generic); Diurese (American Urologicals): 4 mg tablets
Metahydrin (Aventis); Naqua (Schering): 2 mg, 4 mg tablets

Fixed-Dose Combinations for the Treatment of Hypertension:
Metatensin #4 Tablets (Aventis): Trichlormethiazide 4 mg/reserpine 0.1 mg
Metatensin #2 Tablets (Aventis): Trichlormethiazide 2 mg/reserpine 0.1 mg

POTASSIUM-SPARING DIURETICS

1. Amiloride (Amiloride, Midamor®)

Indications
As adjunctive therapy with thiazide or other kaliuretic diuretics in CHF or hypertension to prevent excessive potassium loss

Dosage

Adults

Administer 5 to 10 mg once daily. Although dosages >10 mg/d are usually not necessary, higher doses (up to 20 mg/d) have been used occasionally in some patients with persistent hypokalemia.

Elderly

Initiate at lowest dose and titrate to response.

Children

Safety and effectiveness have not been established.

Preparations

Amiloride (generic); Midamor (Merck): 5 mg tablets

Fixed-Dose Combinations for the Treatment of Hypertension:
Moduretic Tablets and various generic products:
Amiloride 5 mg/hydrochlorothiazide 50 mg

2. Spironolactone (Spironolactone, Aldactone®)

Indications
Edema associated with CHF, liver cirrhosis, or nephrotic syndrome
Hypokalemia
Hypertension (usually used in conjunction with other agents such as a thiazide diuretic)
Primary hyperaldosteronism

Dosage

Adults

Edema

Initiate at 100 mg/d (range, 25 to 200 mg/d) administered as a singe dose or in divided doses. If spironolactone is used as a sole agent, the treatment should be continued for at least 5 days. Thereafter, the dose may be adjusted based on response or a more potent diuretic may be added.

Diuretic-induced hypokalemia

The usual dose ranged from 25 to 100 mg/d.

Hypertension

Initiate at 50 to 100 mg/d in single or divided doses. The usual dose ranged from 25 to 100 mg/d.

Primary hyperaldosteronism (diagnostic test)

Long test—Spironolactone 400 mg is administered daily for 3 to 4 weeks. Correction of hypokalemia and hypertension provides presumptive evidence for the diagnosis.

Short test—Spironolactone 400 mg is administered daily for 4 days. If serum potassium level increases during the therapy but declines after discontinuation of the drug, a presumptive diagnosis should be considered.

Hyperaldosteronism (maintenance therapy)

Administer 100 to 400 mg daily in preparation for surgery. For patients who are not suitable for surgery, long-term therapy with spironolactone may be used. Dosage should be titrated individually (maintain at the lowest possible dose).

Elderly

Initiate at lowest dose and titrate to response.

Children

Safety and effectiveness have been established for the management of edema only.

Preparations

Spironolactone (generic): 25 mg tablets
Aldactone (Pharmacia & Upjohn): 25 mg, 50 mg, 100 mg tablets

Fixed-Dose Combinations for the Treatment of Hypertension:
Aldactazide tablets and various generic products:
Spironolactone 25 mg/hydrochlorothiazide 25 mg
Spironolactone 50 mg/hydrochlorothiazide 50 mg

3. Triamterene (Dyrenium®)

Indications

Edema associated with CHF, hepatic cirrhosis, nephrotic syndrome, steroid use, or secondary hyperaldosteronism.

Dosage

Adults

When used as a single agent, the usual initial dose is 100 mg twice daily after meals. Dosage should not exceed 300 mg/d. Once edema is controlled, most patients can be maintained on 100 mg/d or every other day. When used in combination with a kaliuretic diuretic, the initial dose is 50 mg once daily. The dose should be titrated based on response to a maximum of 100 mg/d.

Elderly

Initiate at lowest dose and titrate to response.

Children

Safety and effectiveness have not been established.

Preparations

Dyrenium (Wellspring): 50 mg, 100 mg capsules

Fixed-Dose Combinations for Treatment of Hypertension:
Diazide capsules: triamterene 37.5 mg/hydrochlorothiazide 25 mg
Maxzide capsules: triamterene 37.5 mg/hydrochlorothiazide 25 mg
Maxzide capsules: triamterene 75 mg/hydrochlorothiazide 50 mg
Various generic triamterene/hydrochlorothiazide tablets and capsule.

ENDOTHELIN RECEPTOR ANTAGONIST

1. Bosentan (Tracleer®)

Indication

Treatment of pulmonary arterial hypertension in patients with WHO Class III or IV symptoms, to improve exercise ability and decrease the rate of clinical worsening

Dosage

Adults

Initiate at 62.5 mg twice daily for 4 weeks and then increased to the maintenance dose of 125 mg twice daily. Doses above 125 mg twice daily did not appear to confer additional benefit sufficient to offset the increased risk of liver injury. Refer to Tracleer package insert for recommendations on dosage adjustment and monitoring in patients developing aminotransferase abnormalities during therapy.

Note Because of potential liver injury and in an effort to make the chance of fetal exposure to bosentan as small as possible, bosentan may be prescribed only through the TRACLEER Access Program.

Elderly

Clinical experience has not identified differences in responses between elderly and younger patients.

Children

Safety and efficacy in pediatric patients have not been established. In patients with a body weight below 40 kg but who are over 12 years of age the recommended initial and maintenance dose is 62.5 mg twice daily.

Preparations

Tracleer (Actelion): 62.5 mg, 125 mg tablets

HUMAN B-TYPE NATRIURETIC PEPTIDE

1. Nesiritide (Natrecor®)

Indication

Treatment of patients with acutely decompensated congestive heart failure who have dyspnea at rest or with minimal activity.

Dosage

Adults

The recommended dose of nesiritide is an intravenous bolus of 2 μg/kg followed by a continuous infusion of 0.01 μg/kg/min. Nesiritide should not be initiated at a dose that is above the recommended dose. The dose-limiting side effect of nesiritide is hypotension. Blood pressure should be monitored closely during administration. If hypotension occurs during the administration of nesiritide, the dose should be reduced or discontinued and other measures to support blood pressure should be started (IV fluids, changes in body position). In the vasodilation in the management of acute congestive heart failure (VMAC) trial, when symptomatic hypotension occurred, nesiritide was discontinued and subsequently could be restarted at a dose that was reduced by 30% (with no bolus administration) once the patient was stabilized.

In the VMAC trial there was limited experience with increasing the dose of nesiritide above the recommended dose. In those patients, the infusion dose of nesiritide was increased by 0.005 μg/kg/min (preceded by a bolus of 1 μg/kg), no more frequently than every 3 hours up to a maximum dose of 0.03 μg/kg/min. Experience with administering nesiritide for longer than 48 hours is limited. Refer to Natrecor package insert for complete prescribing information.

Elderly

Use usual dose with caution.

Children

Safety and effectiveness have not been established.

Preparations

Natrecor (Scios): powder for injection, lyophilized: 1.5 mg single-use vials.

INOTROPIC AND VASOPRESSOR AGENTS

PHOSPHODIESTERASE INHIBITORS

1. Inamrinone Lactate (Inamrinone Lactate Inocor®)

Indications

Congestive heart failure, short-term management

Dosage

Adults

Initiate with an intravenous bolus dose of 0.75 mg/kg administered slowly over 2 to 3 min, followed by a continuous infusion of 5 to 10 μg/kg/min. A second bolus of 0.75 mg/kg may be given 30 min after the initial bolus dose. The total dose should not exceed 10 mg/kg/d. Rate of administration and duration of therapy should be determined by the responsiveness of the patient.

Elderly

Initiate at lowest dose and titrate to response.

Children

Safety and effectiveness have not been established.

Preparation

Inamrinone Lactate (Abbott Hospital): 5 mg/mL, 20 mL ampules

Inocor (Sanofi Winthrop): 5 mg/mL, 20 mL ampules

2. Milrinone Lactate (Primacor®)

Indication

Congestive heart failure, short-term management

Dosage

Adults

Initiate with an intravenous loading dose of 50 μg/kg administered slowly over 10 min, followed by a continuous infusion of 0.375 μg/kg/min. Rate of administration and duration of therapy should be determined by the responsiveness of the patient. The total dose should not exceed 1.13 mg/kg/d (or, 0.75 μg/kg/min).

The following infusion rates are recommended for patients with renal impairment:

CrCl (mL/min/1.73 m²)	Infusion rate (μg/kg/min)
50	0.43
40	0.38
30	0.33
20	0.28
10	0.23
5	0.20

Elderly

Dosage should be adjusted based on renal function.

Children

Safety and effectiveness have not been established.

Preparations

Primacor Injections (Sanofi/Synthelabo): 1 mg/mL, 10 mL, 20 mL single-dose vials; 200 μg/mL in 100 mL of 5% dextrose injection; 200 μg/mL in 200 mL of 5% dextrose injection.

ADRENERGIC RECEPTOR AGONISTS

1. Dobutamine (Dobutamine, Dobutrex®)

Indication

Short-term inotropic support in patients with cardiac decompensation due to depressed contractility

Dosage

Adults

The rate of infusion required to increase cardiac output usually ranges from 2.5 to 15 μg/kg/min. The infusion rate and the duration of therapy should be determined based on clinical response.

Note   Consult manufacturer's package insert for instructions on proper dilution of dobutamine injection prior to infusion.

Elderly

Initiate at lowest dose and titrate to response.

Children

Safety and effectiveness have not been established.

Preparations

Dobutamine(generic); Dobutrex (Lilly): 12.5 mg/mL injection, 20 mL vials

2. Dopamine (Dopamine, Intropin®)

Indication

Hemodynamic imbalances, after adequate fluid resuscitation

Dosage

Adults

Initially give dopamine intravenously at an infusion rate of 1 to 5 μg/kg/min. Adjust by increments of 1 to 4 μg/kg/min at intervals of 10 to 30 min according to clinical response. Lower initial doses are recommended for patients with chronic heart failure (0.5 to 2 μg/kg/min) and for patients with occlusive vascular disease ($\leq$1 μg/kg/min). Most patients respond to a dose of <20 μg/kg/min. Severely ill patients should be given a higher initial dose of 5 μg/kg/min. Dosage may be increased gradually according to response using 5 to 10 μg/kg/min increments, up to a maximum rate of 20 to 50 μg/kg/min.

Note   Consult manufacturer's package insert for instructions on proper dilution of dopamine injection prior to infusion.

Elderly

Initiate at lowest dose and titrate to response.

Children

Safety and effectiveness have not been established.

Preparations

Dopamine (generic); Intropin (Faulding): 40 mg/mL, 80 mg/mL, 160 mg/mL injections

Dopamine in 5% dextrose (Abbott): 80 mg/100 mL, 160 mg/100 mL, 320 mg/100 mL

3. Isoproterenol (Isoproterenol, Isuprel®)

Indications

Emergency Treatment of cardiac arrhythmias
Shock
Bronchospasm

Dosage

Adults

Emergency treatment of cardiac arrhythmias

The usual initial adult intravenous bolus dose is 0.02 to 0.06 mg (1 to 3 mL of a 1:50,000 dilution); subsequent doses range from 0.01 to 0.2 mg (0.5 to 10 mL of a 1:50,000 dilution). For intravenous infusion, the initial rate of administration is 5 μg/min (1.25 mL of

a 1:250,000 dilution per minute or 2.5 mL of a 1:500,000 dilution per minute); subsequent dosage is adjusted based on the patient's response and generally ranges from 2 to 20 μg/min.

Shock

As an adjunct therapy for the management of shock, isoproterenol is administered by intravenous infusion. Intravenous infusion rates of 0.5 to 5 μg (0.25 to 2.5 mL of a 1:500,000 dilution) per minute have been recommended; the rate of infusion should be adjusted based on the patient's response. Rates greater than 30 μg/min have been used in advanced stages of shock. Some clinicians have recommended that isoproterenol be administered only for a short time ($\leq$1 h) to patients with septic shock.

Bronchospasm

For the control of bronchospasm occurring during anesthesia, administer 0.01 to 0.02 mg (0.5 to 1 mL of a 1:50,000 dilution) of isoproterenol intravenously. This dose may be repeated if necessary.

Elderly

Initiate at lowest dose and titrate to response.

Children

Safety and effectiveness have not been established. However, intravenous isoproterenol has been used in children with asthma or in postoperative cardiac patients with bradycardia.

Preparations

Isoproterenol injection (generic); Isuprel injection (Sanofi): 1:5000 solution (0.2 mg/mL)

Isuprel injection (Sanofi): 1:50,000 (0.02 mg/mL)

4. Epinephrine (Epinephrine, Adrenalin®, Various Sources)

Indications

Cardiac arrest
Symptomatic bradycardia
Anaphylaxis, severe allergic reactions

Dosage

Adults

Cardiac arrest, ventricular fibrillation and pulseless ventricular tachycardia, pulseless electrical activity, or asystole in advanced cardiac life support

The usual intravenous dose is 0.5 to 1 mg (usually as 5 to 10 mL of a 1:10,000 injection) repeated every 3 to 5 min if needed. Each dose of epinephrine given by peripheral injection should be followed by a 20-mL flush of intravenous fluid in order to ensure delivery of the drug into the central compartment. The extremity where the drug is injected should be elevated for 10 to 20 sec.

Higher doses of 3 to 5 mg (about 0.1 mg/kg) repeated every 3 to 5 min as necessary may be considered if the 1-mg dose has failed. Doses as high as 0.2 mg/kg have been given, but caution with potentially severe adverse effects should be taken when high doses are used. Alternatively, initial intravenous administration may be followed by a continuous infusion, at an initial rate of 1 μg/min and titrated up to 3 to 4 μg/min as needed. Intravenous infusions of epinephrine should be administered via central venous access whenever possible in order to reduce the risk of extravasation and to ensure good bioavailability. If intravenous access is not available, epinephrine may be administered via the endotracheal tube. A dose of 2 to 2.5 mg diluted in 10 mL of 0.9% sodium chloride has been recommended.

Symptomatic bradycardia

The usual initial dose is 1 μg/min [infusion solution of 2 μg/mL may be prepared by adding 1 mg (1 mL of a 1:1000 injection) of epinephrine to 500 mL of a compatible intravenous solution] by continuous infusion. The rate of infusion is titrated based on clinical response and usually ranges from 2 to 10 μg/min.

Elderly

Initiate at lowest dose and titrate to response.

Children

Administer with caution to infants and children. Dosage should be adjusted based on weight.

Preparations

Syringes: 1 mg/mL (1:1,000) in 0.3 mL, 1 mL, 2 mL; 0.5 mg/mL (1:2,000) in 0.3 mL; 0.1 mg/mL (1:10,000) in 10 mL
Ampules: 5 mg/mL (1:200) in 0.3 mL; 1 mg/mL (1:1000) in 1 mL
Vials: 5 mg/mL (1:200) in 5 mL; 1 mg/mL (1:1000) in 30 mL

5. Metaraminol (Aramine®)

Indications

Hypotension associated with spinal anesthesia
Hypotension due to hemorrhage, reactions to medications, surgical complications; shock associated with brain damage due to trauma or tumor.

Dosage

Adults

Prevention of hypotension

The usual intramuscular dose ranges from 2 to 10 mg. The lowest effective dose for the shortest possible time should be used. At least 10 min should elapse before additional doses are administered.

Note Subcutaneous administration of metaraminol has also been used. However, this mode of administration is not recommended because of increased risk of local tissue injury. When given intravenously, metaraminol is preferably given in the large veins of the antecubital fossa or the thigh.

Severe hypotension or shock

The usual dose for a single direct intravenous injection ranges from 0.5 to 5 mg. If necessary, the direct intravenous injection may be followed by a continuous infusion (15 to 100 mg in 500 mL of compatible diluent) with the rate adjusted according to blood pressure response.

Elderly

Initiate at lowest dose and titrate to response.

Children

Safety and effectiveness have not been established.

Preparation

Aramine (Merck): 10 mg/mL (1% as bitartrate), 10 mL vials

6. Methoxamine (Vasoxyl)

Indications

Hypotension associated with anesthesia
Paroxysmal supraventricular tachycardia associated with hypotension or shock

Dosage

Adults

Hypotension

Intramuscular dose ranges from 5 to 20 mg. A dose of 5 to 10 mg may be adequate when only moderate hypotension is present. In an emergency, 3 to 5 mg of methoxamine may be administered slowly by direct intravenous injection. Intravenous administration may be supplemented with an intramuscular dose of 10 to 15 mg to provide more prolonged effects.

Prevention of hypotension during anesthesia

The usual dose is 10 to 15 mg (up to 20 mg may be required at high levels of anesthesia) given intramuscularly shortly before or at the time of administration of the spinal anesthetic. This dose may be repeated at intervals of at least 15 min if needed.

Paroxysmal supraventricular tachycardia

Administer 10 mg (range: 5 to 15 mg) intravenously over 3 to 5 min. Alternatively, 10 to 20 mg may be injected intramuscularly. Systolic blood pressure should not be raised above 160 mm Hg.

Elderly

Initiate at lowest dose and titrate to response.

Children

Safety and effectiveness have not been established.

Preparation

Vasoxyl (Glaxo SmithKline): 20 mg/mL injection

7. Midodrine (ProAmatine®)

Indication

Orthostatic hypotension

Dosage

Adults

The recommended dose is 10 mg three times daily (doses may be given at 3- to 4-h intervals). Dosing should take place during the daytime hours when the patient is upright and pursuing daily activities. Do not give midodrine after the evening meal or <4 h before bedtime due to the risk of supine hypertension.

Elderly

Dosage adjustment based on age is not necessary. However, lower initial doses of 2.5 mg should be administered to patients with renal impairment.

Children

Safety and effectiveness have not been established.

Preparations

ProAmatine (Shire): 2.5 mg, 5 mg tablets

8. Norepinephrine (Norepinephrine, Levophed®)

Indications

Hypotensive state
Cardiac arrest (as an adjunct for severe hypotension)

Dosage

Adults

Norepinephrine is administered by continuous intravenous infusion. The infusion solution is usually prepared by adding 4 mg of norepinephrine bitartrate (4 mL of the commercially available injection) to 1 L of 5% dextrose injection to yield a solution that contains 4 μg of base/mL. The usual initial dosage of norepinephrine is 8 to 12 μg of base per minute and the usual maintenance dosage is 2 to 4 μg of base per minute. Dosage should be titrated according to the patient's response. Alternatively, norepinephrine may be initiated at a rate of 0.5 to 1 μg of base per minute and titrated to maintain a desired blood pressure response. A few hypotensive patients have required as much as 68 mg of norepinephrine bitartrate daily. In patients requiring very large dosages of norepinephrine, occult blood volume depletion should be suspected and corrected if present; central venous pressure monitoring may be helpful in detecting and managing this situation.

Elderly

Dosage should be adjusted based on clinical response.

Children

Safety and effectiveness have not been established. However, there has been experience with the use of norepinephrine in the pediatric population.

Preparation

Norepinephrine injection (generic); Levophed (Sanofi): 1 mg (as bitartrate) per mL, 4 mL ampules

9. Phenylephrine (Phenylephrine, Neo-Synephrine®)

Indications

Management of vascular failure in shock, shock-like states, drug-induced hypotension, or hypersensitivity
Termination of paroxysmal supraventricular tachycardia attacks
Maintenance of adequate blood pressure during spinal and inhalation anesthesia

Dosage

Adults

Mild or moderate hypotension

The usual dose is 2 to 5 mg (range: 1 to 10 mg) administered subcutaneously or intramuscularly. The initial dose should not exceed 5 mg. Additional intramuscular or subcutaneous doses may be given in 1 to 2 h if needed. Alternatively, phenylephrine may be administered by slow intravenous injection in a dose ranging from 0.1 to 0.5 mg (0.2 mg is the usual dose). The intravenous dose may be repeated after 10 to 15 min if necessary. For convenience in administration by intravenous injection, 1 mL of phenylephrine injection containing 10 mg/mL may be diluted with 9 mL of sterile water for injection to yield a solution containing 1 mg/mL.

Severe hypotension

A continuous intravenous infusion at a rate of 100 to 180 μg/min should be initiated and titrated based on clinical response. Once the blood pressure is stabilized, a maintenance infusion rate of 40 to 60 μg/min is usually sufficient. Infusion solutions may be prepared by adding 10 mg of phenylephrine to 500 mL of diluent.

Hypotension associated with spinal anesthesia

For the prevention of hypotension during spinal anesthesia, a dose of 2 or 3 mg should be administered intramuscularly or subcutaneously 3 to 4 min before administration of the anesthetic agent.

For the management of hypotensive emergencies during spinal anesthesia, an initial dose of 0.2 mg may be given intravenously. Any subsequent dose should not exceed the previous dose by 0.1 to 0.2 mg and a single dose should not exceed 0.5 mg.

Paroxysmal supraventricular tachycardia

Up to 0.5 mg of phenylephrine may be given by rapid intravenous injection (over 20 to 30 sec). Subsequent doses may be given in increments of 0.1 to 0.2 mg if indicated and should not exceed 1 mg in a single dose.

Elderly

Dosage should be adjusted based on clinical response.

Children

Dosage should be adjusted based on weight and clinical response.

Preparations

Phenylephrine HCl (generic): Neo-Synephrine (Sanofi): 1% (10 mg/mL) injection

OTHER INOTROPIC AGENTS

1. Digoxin (Digoxin, Lanoxicaps®, Lanoxin®)

Indications

Congestive heart failure
Atrial fibrillation

Dosage

Rapid digitalization

A full digitalizing dosage of digoxin may be given if other cardiac glycosides have not been administered within the previous 2 weeks. The total dosages for rapid digitalization are listed in the table below. Peak body digoxin stores of 8 to 12 μg/kg are generally required for therapeutic effect with minimum risk of toxicity in most patients with heart failure and normal sinus rhythm. Higher body digoxin stores of 10 to 15 μg/kg are often required for control of ventricular rate in patients with atrial flutter or fibrillation. Lower loading doses (i.e., 6 to 10 μg/kg) should be considered in patients with severe renal impairment.

Usual Digitalizing Dosages Based on Lean Body Weight in patients with Normal Renal Function

Age	Capsules*	Elixir†	Injection*	Tablets†
Premature neonates	—	20 to 30 μg/kg	15 to 25 μg/kg	20 to 30 μg/kg
Full-term neonates	—	25 to 35 μg/kg	20 to 30 μg/kg	25 to 35 μg/kg
1 to 24 months	—	35 to 60 μg/kg	30 to 50 μg/kg	35 to 60 μg/kg
2 to 5 years old	25 to 35 μg/kg	30 to 40 μg/kg	25 to 35 μg/kg	30 to 40 μg/kg
5 to 10 years old	15 to 30 μg/kg	20 to 35 μg/kg	15 to 30 μg/kg	20 to 35 μg/kg
>10 years old	8 to 12 μg/kg	10 to 15 μg/kg	8 to 12 μg/kg	10 to 15 μg/kg

∗ This loading dose is usually given in three divided doses, with 50% of the total dose given as the first dose and two additional doses (25% each) given at 4- to 8-h intervals after assessing clinical response. For intravenous administration, digoxin injection is given either undiluted over a period of at least 5 min or diluted with a fourfold or greater volume of sterile water for injection, 5% dextrose injection, or 0.9% sodium chloride injection and given over a period of at least 5 min.

† This loading dose is usually given in three divided doses, with 50% of the total dose given as the first dose and two additional doses (25% each) given at 6- to 8-h intervals after assessing clinical response.

Slow digitalization or maintenance therapy

The usual maintenance dosage in adults is 100 to 375 μg daily. For slow digitalization in children <10 years of age, 25 to 35% of the total dose of digoxin for rapid digitalization is administered daily. Slow digitalization is the preferred regimen in patients with heart failure and the dose should be administered orally whenever possible. Dosage requirement for each individual should be adjusted based on clinical response and renal function. It may take 1 to 3 weeks for a patient to reach steady state serum digoxin concentrations depending on the renal function. In patients with severe renal impairment, a maintenance dose given every 2 to 3 days may be adequate to maintain desired serum digoxin concentrations.

Elderly

Dosage should be adjusted based on renal function, clinical response, and serum concentration.

Children

Dosage should be adjusted based on age, weight, renal function, clinical response, and serum concentration.

Preparations

Digoxin (generic): 0.125, 0.25 mg tablets
Lanoxin (Glaxo SmithKline): 0.125, 0.25 mg tablets
Digitek (Bertek): 0.125 mg, 0.25 mg tablets
Lanoxicaps (Glaxo SmithKline) 0.05, 0.1, 0.2 mg capsules
Digoxin elixir (generic); Lanoxin (Glaxo SmithKline): 50 μg/mL
Digoxin injection (generic): 250 μg/mL
Lanoxin injection (Glaxo SmithKline): 100 μg/mL, 250 μg/mL

LIPID-LOWERING AGENTS

BILE-ACID SEQUESTRANTS

1. Cholestyramine (Cholestyramine, Questran®, Questran Light®, Prevalite®)

Indications

As adjunctive therapy to diet in patients with elevated LDL-cholesterol (type II hyperlipidemia)
Relief of pruritus associated with partial biliary obstruction

Dosage

Adults

Initiate at 4 g (anhydrous cholestyramine resin) one to two times daily at mealtime. The contents of 1 powder packet or 1 level scoop must be mixed with 60 to 180 mL water or noncarbonated beverage before administration. Maintenance dose is up to 4 g (anhydrous cholestyramine resin) six times daily at mealtime and at bedtime. The maximum recommended daily dose is 24 g (anhydrous cholestyramine resin).

Note The administration time for cholestyramine should be modified to avoid interference with the absorption of other medications. Because cholestyramine may worsen constipation, patients who are constipated should be started on dosages of one packet or scoop once daily for 5 to 7 days, increasing by one dose per day every month up to a maximum of six doses per day.

Elderly

Dosage adjustment is not necessary.

Children

Optimal dosing has not been established; long-term effects are not known in this population.

Preparations

Cholestyramine (generic); Questran (Apothecon): 4 g anhydrous cholestyramine resin/9 g powder
Cholestyramine Light (generic): 4 g anhydrous cholestyramine resin/dose
Questran Light (Apothecon): 4 g (as anhydrous cholestyramine resin)/5 g powder
Prevalite (Upsher Smith): 4 g (as anhydrous cholestyramine resin)/5.5 g powder

2. Colestipol (Colestid®)

Indications

As adjunctive therapy to diet in patients with elevated LDL-cholesterol (type II hyperlipidemia)

Dosage

Adults

Granules Initiate at 5 g once or twice daily; dosage may be increased by 5 g daily at 1 to 2 month intervals. The usual daily dose is 5 to 30 g given once or in divided doses. The prescribed amount of granules must be mixed with a glassful of liquid before administration; do not take dry.

Tablets   Initiate at 2 g once or twice daily; dosage may be increased by 2 g once or twice daily at 1 to 2 month intervals. The usual daily dose is 2 to 16 g given once or in divided doses. Tablets should be swallowed whole, one at a time, with plenty of water or other appropriate fluids.

Note   The administration time for colestipol should be modified to avoid interference with the absorption of other medications. Because colestipol may worsen constipation, patients who are constipated should be started on a once daily dose for 5 to 7 days, increasing by one dose per day every month up to a maximum of six doses per day.

Elderly
Dosage adjustment is not necessary.

Children
Safety and effectiveness have not been established.

Preparations
Colestid Granules (Pharmacia and Upjohn): 5 g colestipol HCL/dose, 5 g colestipol HCl/7.5 g powder
Colestid Tablets (Pharmacia and Upjohn): 1 g

3. Colesevelam (Welchol®)

Indications
As adjunctive therapy to diet and exercise used alone or in combination with an HMG-CoA reductase inhibitor to reduce elevated LDL-cholesterol in patients with primary hypercholesterolemia (Type IIa hyperlipidemia)

Dosage

Adults

Monotherapy   The recommended initial dose is 3 tablets taken twice daily with meals (and water or other appropriate fluids) or 6 tablets once daily with a meal. The dose may be increased to 7 tablets daily as needed.

Combination therapy   When colesevelam is administered with an HMG-CoA reductase inhibitor concurrently, the recommended dose is 3 tablets taken twice daily with meals (and water or other appropriate fluids) or 6 tablets taken once daily with a meal. Doses of 4 to 6 tablets per day are safe and effective when coadministered with an HMG-CoA reductase inhibitor or when the two drugs are dosed apart.

Elderly
Dosage adjustment is not necessary.

Children
Safety and effectiveness have not been established.

Preparation
Welchol (Sankyo Parke Davis): 625 mg tablets

FIBRIC ACID DERIVATIVES

1. Clofibrate (Atromid-S®)

Indications
As adjunctive therapy to diet in patients with type III hyperlipidemia

As adjunctive therapy to diet in patients with elevated triglyceride concentrations (types IV and V hyperlipidemias) who are at risk for pancreatitis

Dosage

Adults
The usual dosage is 1 g twice daily. Some patients may respond to lower dosages.

Elderly
Dosage adjustment is not necessary.

Children
Safety and effectiveness have not been established.

Preparation
Atromid-S (Wyeth-Ayerst): 500 mg capsules

2. Fenofibrate (Tricor®)

Indications
As adjunctive therapy to diet for the reduction of LDL-cholesterol, total cholesterol, triglycerides, and apolipoprotein B, and to increase HDL cholesterol in patients with primary hypercholesterolemia or mixed dyslipidemia (types IIa and IIb hyperlipidemias)

As adjunctive therapy to diet for the reduction of elevated triglyceride concentrations (types IV and V hyperlipidemias)

Dosage

Adults

Primary hypercholesterolemia/Mixed hyperlipidemia
The initial dose is 160 mg/d.

Hypertriglyceridemia
The initial dose ranges from 54 to 160 mg/d. Dosage should be individualized according to patient response and adjust if necessary following repeat lipid determinations at 4 to 8 week intervals. The maximum dose is 160 mg/d.

Note   A dose of 54 mg/d should be initiate in patients with impaired renal function.

Elderly
Initiate with a dose of 54 mg/d.

Children
Safety and effectiveness have not been established.

Preparations
Tricor (Abbott): 54 mg, 160 mg tablets

3. Gemfibrozil (Gemfibrozil, Lopid®)

Indications

As adjunctive therapy to diet in patients with elevated triglyceride concentrations (types IV and V hyperlipidemias) who are at risk for pancreatitis

Reducing the risk of developing coronary heart disease (CHD) in patients with type IIb hypercholesterolemia with low HDL cholesterol and no history or symptoms of CHD after other treatments have failed

Dosage

Adults

The usual dosage is 600 mg twice daily 30 min before the morning and evening meal.

Note Gemfibrozil may worsen renal impairment in patients with serum creatinine concentrations >2.0 mg/dL and should therefore be used cautiously in this group.

Elderly

Dosage adjustment is not required.

Children

Safety and effectiveness have not been established.

Preparations

Gemfibrozil (generic); Lopid (Parke-Davis): 600 mg tablets

NICOTINIC ACID

1. Nicotinic Acid (Niacor®, Niaspan®, Slo-Niacin®)

Indications

As adjunctive therapy to diet for reduction of elevated total cholesterol, LDL-cholesterol, apolipoprotein B, and triglyceride concentrations, and to increase HDL cholesterol in patients with primary hypercholesterolemia (heterozygous familial and nonfamilial) and mixed dyslipidemia (types IIa and IIb)

As adjunctive therapy in the management of elevated triglyceride concentrations (types IV and V hyperlipidemias) who are at risk for pancreatitis

As adjunctive therapy to diet to reduce the risk of recurrent nonfatal myocardial infarction in patients with a history of myocardial infarction and hypercholesterolemia (extended-release niacin, Niaspan)

As combination therapy with a bile acid sequestrant to slow the progression or promote regression of atherosclerosis in patients with clinical evidence of coronary heart disease who have elevated cholesterol concentrations (extended-release niacin, Niaspan)

Dosage

Adults

Immediate-release preparations

The usual dose of immediate-release niacin (Niacor) is 1 to 2 g two to three times daily with meals. Initiate with 250 mg as a single daily dose after the evening meal and increase the frequency of dosing and total daily dose at 4- to 7-day intervals until the desired LDL or triglyceride level is reached or the first-level therapeutic dose of 1.5 to 2 g/d is reached. If hyperlipidemia is not adequately controlled after 2 months at this level, dosage may be further increased at 2- to 4-week intervals to 3 g/d (1 g three times per day). The maximum dose is 6 g/d.

Extended-release preparations

The usual initial dosage of extended-release niacin preparation (Niaspan) is 500 mg daily at bedtime. Dosage may be increased by no more than 500 mg daily at 4-week intervals as needed until the desired response is achieved. The maximum daily dose is 2 g.

Note Immediate and extended-release preparations are not interchangeable. For patients switching from immediate-release to extended-release preparations, therapy should be instituted with the recommended initial dose and gradually titrated upward.

Elderly

Dosage adjustment is not necessary.

Children

Safety and effectiveness have not been established.

Preparations

Niacor (Upsher-Smith): 500 mg tablets (scored)

Niaspan (Kos Pharmaceuticals): 500 mg, 750 mg, 1000 mg extended-release tablets

Niacin SR (generic): 125 mg, 250 mg extended-release tablets

Slo-Niacin (Upsher-Smith): 250 mg, 500 mg, 750 mg extended-release tablets

Fixed-Dose Combinations for the Treatment of Primary Hypercholesterolemia and Mixed Dyslipidemia:

Advicor (Kos Pharmaceuticals): niacin extended-release/lovastatin combination tablets: 500 mg/20 mg; 750 mg/20 mg; 1000 mg/20 mg

HMG-CoA REDUCTASE INHIBITORS

1. Atorvastatin (Lipitor®)

Indications

As adjunctive therapy to diet for reduction of elevated total cholesterol, LDL-cholesterol, apolipoprotein B, and triglyceride concentrations, and to increase HDL cholesterol in patients with primary hypercholesterolemia (heterozygous familial and nonfamilial) and mixed dyslipidemia (types IIa and IIb)

As adjunctive therapy to diet for the management of elevated triglyceride concentrations (type IV hyperlipidemia)

For the treatment of patients with primary dysbetalipoproteinemia (type III hyperlipidemia) who do not respond adequately to diet

To reduce total cholesterol and LDL-cholesterol in patients with homozygous familial hypercholesterolemia as an adjunct to other lipid-lowering treatments (e.g., LDL apheresis) or if such treatments are unavailable

Dosage

Adults

The usual initial dosage is 10 mg once daily. Dosage may be titrated every 2 to 4 weeks up to 80 mg once daily.

Elderly

Dosage adjustment is not necessary.

Children

Safety and effectiveness have not been established.

Preparations

Lipitor (Pfizer): 10 mg, 20 mg, 40 mg, 80 mg tablets

2. Fluvastatin (Lescol®)

Indications

As adjunctive therapy to diet for reduction of elevated total cholesterol, LDL-cholesterol, apolipoprotein B, and triglyceride concentrations in patients with primary hypercholesterolemia and mixed dyslipidemia (types IIa and IIb) whose response to dietary restriction of saturated fat and cholesterol and other nonpharmacologic measures alone has not been adequate

To slow the progression of coronary atherosclerosis in patients with coronary heart disease as part of a treatment strategy to lower total and LDL-cholesterol to target levels

Dosage

Adults

Initiate therapy at 20 to 40 mg once daily at bedtime. Dosage may be titrated every 4 weeks based on response up to a maximum dose of 80 mg/d. If 80 mg/d is required, the dose may be given as a single daily dose using the extended-release preparation or in divided doses as a 40-mg capsule twice daily.

Elderly

Dosage adjustment is not necessary.

Children

Safety and effectiveness have not been established.

Preparations

Lescol (Novartis/Reliant): 20 mg, 40 mg capsules
Lescol XL (Novartis/Reliant): 80 mg extended-release tablets

3. Lovastatin (Lovastatin, Mevacor®)

Indications

As adjunctive therapy to diet for reduction of elevated total cholesterol, LDL-cholesterol in patients with primary hypercholesterolemia (types IIa and IIb) whose response to dietary restriction of saturated fat and cholesterol and to other nonpharmacological measures alone has not been adequate

To slow the progression of coronary atherosclerosis in patients with coronary heart disease as part of a treatment strategy to lower total and LDL-cholesterol to target levels

To reduce the risk of myocardial infarction, unstable angina and coronary revascularization procedures in individuals without symptomatic cardiovascular disease who have average to moderately elevated total cholesterol and LDL-cholesterol, and below average HDL cholesterol concentrations

Dosage

Adults

The usual initial dosage is 20 mg once daily for patients requiring ≥20% reductions in LDL-cholesterol and 10 mg once daily for patients requiring LDL reductions of <20%, administered with the evening meal. Dosage may be titrated every 4 weeks or more up to a maximum of 80 mg given once daily or in two divided doses. If used in combination with cyclosporine, therapy should begin with 10 mg of lovastatin and should not exceed 20 mg/d. If used in combination with fibrates or niacin, the dose of lovastatin should not exceed 20 mg.

Elderly

Dosage adjustment is not necessary.

Children

Safety and effectiveness have not been established.

Preparations

Lovastatin (generic); Mevacor (Merck): 10 mg, 20 mg, 40 mg tablets

Altocor (Andrx Pharmaceuticals) 10 mg, 20 mg, 40 mg, 60 mg extended-release tablets

Fixed-Dose Combinations for the Treatment of Primary Hypercholesterolemia and Mixed Dyslipidemia:

Advicor (Kos Pharmaceuticals)—niacin extended-release/lovastatin combination tablets: 500 mg/20 mg; 750 mg/20 mg; 1000 mg/20 mg

4. Pravastatin (Pravachol®)

Indications

As adjunctive therapy to diet for reduction of elevated total cholesterol, LDL-cholesterol, apolipoprotein B, and triglyceride concentrations, and to increase HDL cholesterol in patients with primary hypercholesterolemia and mixed dyslipidemia (types IIa and IIb)

As adjunctive therapy to diet in the management of elevated triglyceride concentrations (type IV hyperlipidemia)

For the treatment of patients with primary dysbetalipoproteinemia (type III hyperlipidemia) who do not respond adequately to diet

To reduce the risk of myocardial infarction, to reduce the risk of undergoing myocardial revascularization procedures, and to reduce the risk of cardiovascular mortality with no increase in death from noncardiovascular causes in hypercholesterolemic patients without clinically evident coronary heart disease (primary prevention of coronary events)

To slow the progression of coronary atherosclerosis and reduce the risk of acute coronary events in hypercholesterolemic patients with clinically evident coronary heart disease (secondary prevention of cardiovascular events)

Dosage

Adults

Initiate therapy at 10, 20, or 40 mg once daily. Dosage may be titrated based on response at 4-week intervals. A lower starting dose of 10 mg is recommended for patients with significant renal or hepatic impairment. If used in combination with cyclosporine, therapy should begin with 10 mg of pravastatin once daily at bedtime and should generally not exceed 20 mg/d (dosage must be titrated with caution).

Elderly
Dosage adjustment is not necessary.

Children
Safety and effectiveness have not been established.

Preparations
Pravachol (Bristol-Myers Squibb): 10 mg, 20 mg, 40 mg, 80 mg tablets

5. Simvastatin (Zocor®)

Indications
As adjunctive therapy to diet for reduction of elevated total cholesterol, LDL-cholesterol, apolipoprotein B, and triglyceride concentrations, and to increase HDL cholesterol in patients with primary hypercholesterolemia (heterozygous familial and nonfamilial) and mixed dyslipidemia (types IIa and IIb)

As adjunctive therapy to diet in the management of elevated triglyceride concentrations (type IV hyperlipidemia)

For the treatment of patients with primary dysbetalipoproteinemia (type III hyperlipidemia)

To reduce total cholesterol and LDL-cholesterol in patients with homozygous familial hypercholesterolemia as an adjunct to other lipid-lowering treatments (e.g., LDL apheresis) or if such treatments are unavailable

To reduce the risk of death, nonfatal myocardial infarction, stroke, or transient ischemic attack, and to reduce the risk for undergoing myocardial revascularization procedures in patients with coronary heart disease and hypercholesterolemia

Dosage

Adults
The usual initial dosage is 20 mg once daily in the evening, 40 mg once daily for patients requiring a large reduction in LDL-cholesterol (>45%). Dosage may be titrated every 4 weeks or more up to a maximum dosage of 80 mg every evening. Patients taking cyclosporine or who have severe renal insufficiency should be started on 5 mg daily. The recommended dosage for patients with homozygous familial hypercholesterolemia is 40 mg every evening or 80 mg daily in three divided doses (20 mg, 20 mg, and an evening dose of 40 mg). If used in combination with cyclosporine, fibrates or niacin, the daily dosage of simvastatin should not exceed 10 mg.

Elderly
Dosages of ≤20 mg daily are generally sufficient for maximum LDL reduction in the elderly.

Children
Safety and effectiveness have not been established.

Preparations
Zocor (Merck): 5 mg, 10 mg, 20 mg, 40 mg, 80 mg tablets

NEURONAL AND GANGLIONIC BLOCKERS

1. Mecamylamine (Inversine®)

Indication
Severe hypertension

Dosage

Adults
Initiate at 2.5 mg twice daily. Dosage may be adjusted in increments of 2.5 mg at intervals of at least every 2 days according to response. The smallest dose should be taken in the mornings to limit the orthostatic adverse effects of the drug. The usual maintenance dose is 25 mg/d in three divided doses.

Note   It is recommended that mecamylamine be administered at consistent times in relation to meals because hypotension may occur after a meal. Ingestion of mecamylamine with meals may slow the drug's absorption and thereby produce desired gradual correction of severe hypertension. Therapy with mecamylamine should not be discontinued abruptly.

Elderly
Initiate at lowest dose and titrate to response.

Children
Safety and effectiveness have not been established.

Preparation
Inversine (Layton): 2.5 mg tablets

2. Reserpine (Reserpine)

Indications
Hypertension
Psychotic disorders

Dosage

Adults
The usual maintenance dose for hypertension is 0.1 to 0.25 mg/d, taken with meals to avoid gastric irritation.

Elderly
Initiate at lowest dose and titrate to response.

Children
Safety and effectiveness have not been established.

Preparations
Reserpine (generic): 0.1 mg, 0.25 mg tablets

Fixed-Dose Combinations for the Treatment of Hypertension:
Diutensen-R (Wallace)—Reserpine/methyclothiazide combination tablets: 0.1 mg/2.5 mg

3. Trimethaphan (Arfonad®)

Indications
Production of controlled hypotension during surgery
Short-term acute control of blood pressure in hypertensive emergencies

Emergency treatment of pulmonary edema in patients with pulmonary hypertension associated with systemic hypertension

Dosage

Adults

For controlled hypotension during surgery, initiate therapy as an intravenous infusion at 3 to 4 mg/min. Infusion rate should be adjusted according to response to a maintenance dose ranging from 0.2 to 6 mg/min. Trimethaphan should be administered after the patient is anesthetized and this drug should be discontinued prior to wound closure to allow blood pressure to return toward normal. For hypertensive emergency, initiate trimethaphan at 0.5 to 1 mg/min and adjust the infusion rate according to response. The usual maintenance infusion rate is 1 to 5 mg/min.

Note Trimethaphan should be diluted in the proper amount of compatible fluid prior to intravenous infusion (500 mg, 10 mL, of trimethaphan may be diluted in 500 mL of 5% dextrose injection to yield to final solution containing 1 mg/mL of trimethaphan).

Elderly
Initiate at lowest dose and titrate to response.

Children
Dosage is based on body weight; use with caution.

Preparation
Arfonad (Roche): 50 mg/mL injection

VASODILATORS

1. Cilostazol (Pletal®)

Please refer to the section on Antiplatelet Agents for the summary of this agent.

2. Diazoxide (Hyperstat® IV)

Indications
Hypertensive emergencies (intravenous formulation)

Dosage

Adults

Hypertensive emergencies
Administer 1 to 3 mg/kg (up to 150 mg in a single injection) by rapid intravenous injection every 5 to 15 min as needed to obtain the desired blood pressure response. Further doses may be given every 4 to 24 h as needed to maintain desired blood pressure until oral antihypertensive medication can be instituted. Continued treatment for >4 to 5 days is usually not necessary; do not use for >10 days.

Note Intravenous injection should be administered only into a peripheral vein. Treatment is most effective when intravenous administration is completed in ≤30 sec. The solution's alkalinity is irritating to tissue; avoid extravasation. Patient should remain recumbent during and for 15 to 30 min after medication administration.

Elderly
Initiate at lowest dose and titrate to response.

Children
Dosing is based on weight.

Preparations
Hyperstat IV (Schering): 15 mg/mL injection, 20 mL ampules

3. Epoprostenol (Flolan®)

Indication
Primary pulmonary hypertension (epoprostenol is indicated for the long-term intravenous treatment of primary pulmonary hypertension in NYHA Class III and Class IV patients)

Dosage

Adults

Acute dose-ranging
The infusion rate is initiated at 2 ng/kg/min and adjusted in increments of 2 ng/kg/min every 15 min or longer until dose-limiting pharmacologic effects occur. The most common dose-limiting pharmacologic effects are nausea, vomiting, headache, hypotension, and flushing. During acute dose-ranging in clinical trials, the mean maximum dose which did not result in dose-limiting pharmacologic effects was 8.6 ± 0.3 ng/kg/min.

Note Epoprostenol must be reconstituted only with sterile diluent for epoprostenol. Reconstituted solutions of epoprostenol must not be diluted or administered with other parenteral solutions or medications.

Continuous chronic infusion
Chronic infusions of epoprostenol should be initiated at 4 ng/kg/min less than the maximum-tolerated infusion rate determined during acute dose-ranging. If the maximum-tolerated infusion rate is <5 ng/kg/min, the chronic infusion should be initiated at one-half the maximum-tolerated infusion rate. During clinical trials, the mean initial chronic infusion rate was 5 ng/kg/min.

Note Chronic continuous infusion of epoprostenol should be administered through a central venous catheter. Temporary peripheral intravenous infusions may be used until central access is established.

Dosage adjustments
Adjustments in the chronic infusion rate should be based on persistence, recurrence, or worsening of the patient's symptoms of primary pulmonary hypertension and the occurrence of adverse events due to excessive doses of epoprostenol. In general, increases in dose from the initial chronic dose should be expected. Increments in dose should be considered if symptoms of primary pulmonary hypertension persist or recur after improving. The infusion should be adjusted by 1 to 2 ng/kg/min increments at intervals sufficient to allow assessment of clinical response; these intervals should be at least 15 min. In contrast, reduced dosage of epoprostenol should be considered when dose-related pharmacologic events occur. Dosage reductions should be made gradually in decrements of 2 ng/kg/min every 15 min or longer until the dose-limiting adverse effects resolve.

Note Abrupt withdrawal of epoprostenol or sudden large reductions in infusion rates should be avoided with the exception of life-threatening situations such as unconsciousness or collapse. Consult manufacturer's package insert for detailed information on administration and reconstitution of epoprostenol.

Elderly

Use usual dose with caution.

Children

Safety and effectiveness have not been established.

Preparations

Flolan (Glaxo SmithKline): 0.5 mg, 1.5 mg powder for reconstitution and 50 mL vials of sterile diluent for Flolan

4. Fenoldopam (Corlopam®)

Indications

In hospital, short-term (up to 48 h) management of severe hypertension when rapid, but quickly reversible, emergency reduction of blood pressure is indicated, including malignant hypertension with deteriorating end-organ function.

Dosage

Adults

The initial dose of fenoldopam is chosen according to the desired magnitude and rate of blood pressure reduction in a given clinical situation. In general, there is a greater and more rapid blood pressure reduction as the initial dose is increased. Lower initial doses (0.03 to 0.1 μg/kg/min) titrated slowly have been associated with less reflex tachycardia than have higher initial doses ($\geq$0.3 μg/kg/min). The recommended increments for titration are 0.05 to 0.1 μg/kg/min at intervals of $\geq$15 min. Doses of <0.1 μg/kg/min have very modest effects and appear only marginally useful in patients with severe hypertension. Doses from 0.01 to 1.6 μg/kg/min have been studied in clinical trials. Most of the effect of a given infusion rate is attained within 15 min. Fenoldopam infusion can be abruptly discontinued or gradually tapered prior to discontinuation. Oral antihypertensive agents can be added during fenoldopam infusion (after blood pressure is stable) or following its discontinuation.

Note Fenoldopam should be administered by continuous intravenous infusion only. A bolus dose should not be used. The fenoldopam injection ampule concentrate must be diluted with the appropriate amount of compatible fluid prior to infusion. Consult manufacturer's package insert for instructions on proper dilution of fenoldopam.

Elderly

Dosage adjustment is not necessary.

Children

Safety and effectiveness have not been established.

Preparation

Corlopam (Abbott): 10 mg/mL injection, concentrate

5. Hydralazine (Hydralazine, Apresoline®)

Indications

Essential hypertension (oral formulation)

Severe essential hypertension when the drug cannot be given orally or when the need to lower blood pressure is urgent (parenteral formulation)

Dosage

Adults

Oral formulation

Initiate therapy at 10 mg four times per day for the first 2 to 4 days; increase to 25 mg four times per day for the rest of the first week. Thereafter, the dosage may be increased to 50 mg four times per day during the second and subsequent weeks. Dosage should be maintained at the lowest effective level. The maximum dose is 300 mg/d. Higher doses have been used in the treatment of CHF.

Parenteral administration

The usual dose is 10 to 20 mg administered intravenously or 10 to 50 mg administered intramuscularly; low doses in these ranges should be used initially. Parenteral doses may be repeated as necessary and may be increased within the above ranges based on blood pressure response.

Note Because hydralazine interacts with stainless steel resulting in a pink discoloration, the injections should be used as quickly as possible after being drawn through a needle or syringe; stainless steel filters should also be avoided. In addition, hydralazine should not be diluted with solutions containing dextrose or other sugars.

Elderly

Initiate at lowest dose and titrate to response.

Children

Safety and effectiveness have not been established; however, there is experience with the use of hydralazine in children.

Preparations

Hydralazine (generic), Apresoline (Novartis): 10 mg, 25 mg, 50 mg, 100 mg tablets

Hydralazine (generic): 20 mg/mL injection, 1 mL vials

Fixed-Dose Combinations for the Treatment of Hypertension:
Hydra-Zide—Hydralazine hydrochloride/hydrochlorothiazide combination capsules: 25 mg/25 mg; 50 mg/50 mg; 100 mg/50 mg

6. Isosorbide dinitrate (Isosorbide dinitrate, Isordil®, Isordil Titradose®, Isordil Tembids®, Sorbitrate®, Dilatrate®-SR)

Indications

Angina pectoris (treatment and prevention)

Dosage

Adults

Short-acting oral tablets (isosorbide dinitrate, Isordil Titradose)
Administer 5 to 20 mg three times daily; dosage may be adjusted as needed and tolerated. The usual dose ranges form 10 to 40 mg three times daily. Use with caution in patients with hepatic or renal impairment.

Note A daily nitrate-free interval of at least 14 h has been recommended to minimize tolerance. The optimal nitrate-free interval may vary among different patients, doses, and regimens.

Sustained-release oral tablets and capsules (isosorbide dinitrate, Isordil Tembids, Dilatrate-SR) Administer sustained-release preparations once daily or twice daily in doses given 6 h apart (i.e., 8 a.m. and 2 p.m.). Do not exceed 160 mg/d.

Sublingual and chewable tablets (isosorbide dinitrate, Isordil, Sorbitrate) The usual initial dose is 2.5 to 5 mg for sublingual tablets and 5 mg for chewable tablets. Dosage may be titrated upward until angina is relieved or until dose-related adverse effects occur. For acute prophylaxis, 5 to 10 mg of sublingual or chewable tablets may be administered q 2 to 3 h. The use of sublingual or chewable isosorbide dinitrate for the termination of acute anginal attacks should be reserved for patients who are intolerant of or unresponsive to sublingual nitroglycerin.

Elderly
Initiate at lowest dose and titrate to response.

Children
Safety and effectiveness have not been established.

Preparations
Tablets, short-acting (isosorbide dinitrate): 5 mg, 10 mg, 20 mg, 30 mg
Tablets, short-acting (Isordil Titradose, Sorbitrate): 5 mg, 10 mg, 20 mg, 30 mg, 40 mg
Tablets, sublingual (isosorbide dinitrate, Isordil): 2.5 mg, 5 mg, 10 mg
Tablets, sublingual (Sorbitrate): 2.5 mg, 5 mg
Tablets, chewable (Sorbitrate): 5 mg, 10 mg
Tablets, sustained-release (isosorbide dinitrate, Isordil Tembids: 40 mg
Capsules, sustained-release (Dilatrate-SR, Isordil Tembids): 40 mg

7. Isosorbide mononitrate (Isosorbide mononitrate, ISMO®, Monoket®, Imdur®)

Indication
Angina pectoris (prevention)

Dosage

Adults

Tablets (isosorbide mononitrate, Monoket, ISMO)
Administer 20 mg twice daily with doses given 7 h apart. An initial dose of 5 mg twice daily may be appropriate for persons of small stature; dosage should be increased to at least 10 mg by the second or third day of therapy.

Extended-release tablets (isosorbide mononitrate, Imdur)
Initiate at 30 or 60 mg once daily. Dosage may be increased to 120 mg once daily after several days if necessary. Rarely, 240 mg may be required in some patients.

Elderly
Dosage adjustment is not necessary.

Children
Safety and effectiveness have not been established.

Preparations
Tablets (isosorbide mononitrate, ISMO): 20 mg
Tablets (Monoket): 10 mg, 20 mg
Tablets, extended-release (isosorbide mononitrate): 60 mg
Tablets, extended-release (Imdur): 30 mg, 60 mg, 120 mg

8. Minoxidil (Minoxidil, Loniten®)

Indications
Severe hypertension (oral formulation)

Dosage

Adults

Oral formulation
Initiate therapy at 5 mg once daily; dosage may be increased by 10 mg at intervals of ≥ 3 days as needed. The usual maintenance dose is 10 to 40 mg/d in one to two divided doses. The maximum dose is 100 mg/d.

Elderly
Initiate at lowest dose and titrate to response.

Children
Safety and effectiveness have not been established; however, there is experience with the use of minoxidil in children.

Preparations
Minoxidil (generic); Loniten (Pharmacia and Upjohn): 2.5 mg, 10 mg tablets

9. Nitroglycerin (Various sources)

Indications
Prevention of angina pectoris (oral sustained-release tablets and capsules, transdermal system)
Prevention and treatment of angina pectoris (sublingual tablets, translingual spray, transmucosal tablets, topical ointment)
Control of blood pressure in perioperative hypertension (intravenous formulation)
Congestive heart failure associated with acute myocardial infarction (intravenous formulation)
Angina pectoris unresponsive to recommended doses of organic nitrates or beta-blockers (intravenous formulation)

Controlled hypotension during surgical procedures (intravenous formulation)

Dosage

Adults

Sublingual tablets (Nitrostat)

Dissolve one tablet under the tongue or in the buccal pouch at first sign of an acute anginal attack. Repeat approximately every 5 min until relief is obtained. No more than three tablets should be taken in 15 min. If pain persists, notify physician or get to the emergency room immediately. Sublingual tablets may also be used prophylactically 5 to 10 min prior to activities that might trigger an acute attack.

Translingual spray (Nitrolingual PumpSpray)

At the onset of an attack, spray one to two metered doses onto or under the tongue. No more than three metered doses should be administered within 15 min. If chest pain continues, seek immediate medical attention. Translingual spray may also be used prophylactically 5 to 10 min prior to activities that might trigger an acute attack. Do not inhale spray.

Transmucosal, buccal tablets (Nitrogard)

Administer 1 mg q 3 to 5 h during waking hours. Place tablet between lip and gum above incisors, or between cheek and gum. Do not chew or swallow tablet.

Sustained-release capsules (nitroglycerin, Nitro-Bid Plateau Caps)

Initiate therapy at 2.5 mg three times daily. Dosage may be titrated upward to an effective dose or until dose-related adverse effects occur. Tolerance may develop when nitroglycerin is administered without a nitrate-free interval. Consider administering on a reduced schedule (one or twice daily).

Sustained-release tablets (Nitrong)

Initiate therapy at 2.6 mg three times daily. Dosage may be titrated upward to an effective dose or until dose-related adverse effects occur. Tolerance may develop when nitroglycerin is administered without a nitrate-free interval. Consider administering on a reduced schedule (once or twice daily).

Topical ointment (nitroglycerin, Nitro-Bid)

Initiate therapy at 15 to 30 mg (1 to 2 inches) q 8 h; dosage may be increased by one-half inch per application q 6 h to a maximum of 75 mg (5 inches) per application q 4 h.

Note Any regimen of nitroglycerin ointment administration should include a daily nitrate-free interval of about 10 to 12 h to avoid tolerance. To apply the ointment using the dose-measuring paper applicator, place the applicator on a flat surface, printed side down. Squeeze the necessary amount of ointment from the tube onto the applicator, place the applicator (ointment side down) on the desired area of skin (usually on nonhairy skin of chest or back), and tape the applicator into place. Do not rub in.

Transdermal Systems (Nitroglycerin Transdermal, Minitran, Nitro-Dur)

Initiate therapy with a 0.1 or 0.2 mg/h patch. Apply patch for 12 to 14 h; remove for 10 to 12 h before applying a new patch. Patch should be applied on to clean, dry, hairless skin of chest, inner upper arm, or shoulder. Avoid placing below knee or elbow. Vary site of placement to decrease skin irritation. Apply a new patch if the first patch loosens or falls off.

Intravenous formulations (nitroglycerin IV, Tridil IV, Nitro-Bid IV, nitroglycerin in 5% dextrose)

Initiate intravenous infusion at 5 μg/min; increase by increments of 5 μg/min at 3- to 5-minute intervals until desired effect is obtained or to 20 μg/min. Dosage may be increased beyond 20 μg/min by 10 μg/min increments at 3- to 5-minute intervals, then by 20 μg/min increments until desired effect is achieved. Reduce dosage increments and frequency of dosage increments as partial effects are noted. There is no fixed optimum dose. Continuously monitor physiologic parameters such as blood pressure and heart rate and other measurements, such as pulmonary capillary wedge pressure, to achieve accurate dose. Maintain adequate blood and coronary perfusion pressures.

Note Intravenous infusion must be given through a special non-polyvinylchloride (non-PVC) intravenous infusion set or infusion pump. Consult manufacturer's package insert for instructions on dilution and administration of intravenous nitroglycerin.

Elderly

Initiate at lowest dose and titrate to response.

Children

Safety and effectiveness have not been established.

Preparations

Sublingual tablets (Nitrostat): 0.3 mg, 0.4 mg, 0.6 mg

Translingual spray (Nitrolingual pump spray): 0.4 mg per metered dose

Transmucosal tablets, controlled-release: 1 mg, 2 mg, 3 mg

Capsules, sustained-release (nitroglycerin, Nitro-Bid Plateau Caps: 2.5 mg, 6.5 mg, 9 mg

Capsules, sustained-release (Nitroglyn): 13 mg

Tablets, sustained-release (Nitrong): 2.6 mg, 6.5 mg, 9 mg

Topical ointment (nitroglycerin, Nitro-Bid): 2% in a lanolin petrolatum base

Transdermal systems (nitroglycerin): 0.1 mg/h, 0.2 mg/h, 0.4 mg/h, 0.6 mg/h

Transdermal systems (Minitran, Nitro-Dur): 0.1 mg/h, 0.2 mg/h, 0.3 mg/h, 0.4 mg/h, 0.6 mg/h

Intravenous (nitroglycerin IV, Nitro-Bid IV, Tridil IV): 5 mg/mL (1, 5, 10 mL vials)

Intravenous (Tridil IV): 0.5 mg/mL, 10 mL ampules

Intravenous (nitroglycerin in 5% dextrose): 25 mg in 250 mL, 50 mg in 250 and 500 mL, 100 mg in 250 mL, 200 mg in 500 mL

10. Papaverine (Papaverine, SR)

Indications

Relief of cerebral and peripheral ischemia associated with arterial spasm and myocardial ischemia complicated by arrhythmias

Dosage

Adults

Oral formulation

Administer 150 mg in an extended-release formulation q 8 to 12 h or 300 mg q 12 h.

Note   It is uncertain if effective plasma concentrations are maintained for 12 h with extended-release preparations. In the past, the Food and Drug Administration has recommended that papaverine products be withdrawn from the market.

Elderly

Initiate at lowest dose and titrate to response.

Children

Safety and effectiveness have not been established.

Preparations

Papaverine HCl (generic); 150 mg extended-release capsules

11. Pentoxifylline (Pentoxifylline, Trental®)

Indications

Intermittent claudication

Dosage

Adults

Initiate therapy at 400 mg three times daily with meals; dosage may be reduced to 400 mg twice daily if GI or CNS adverse effects occur. Although therapeutic effects may be observed within 2 to 4 weeks, continue treatment for ≥ 8 weeks.

Elderly

Use usual dose with caution.

Children

Safety and effectiveness have not been established.

Preparations

Pentoxifylline (generic): 400 mg tablets
Pentoxifylline (generic): 400 mg extended-release tablets
Trental (Aventis): 400 mg extended-release tablets

12. Nitroprusside (Sodium Nitroprusside Nitropress®)

Indications

Hypertensive crises
Production of controlled hypotension in order to reduce bleeding during surgery
Acute congestive heart failure

Dosage

Adults

The usual initial dose is 0.3 μg/kg/min (range, 0.1 to 0.5 μg/kg/min) as an intravenous infusion. Dosage may be adjusted slowly in increments of 0.5 μg/kg/min according to response. The usual infusion rate is 3 μg/kg/min. The maximum recommended infusion rate is 10 μg/kg/min; infusion at the maximum dose rate should never last for > 10 min. To keep the steady-state thiocyanate concentration below 1 mmol/L, the rate of a prolonged infusion should not exceed 3 μg/kg/min (1 μg/kg/min in anuric patients). When > 500 μg/kg of nitroprusside is administered faster than 2 μg/kg/min, cyanide is generated faster than the unaided patient can eliminate it.

Note   After reconstitution with the appropriate diluent, sodium nitroprusside injection is not suitable for direct injection. The reconstituted solution must be further diluted in the appropriate amount of sterile 5% dextrose injection before infusion. The diluted solution should be protected from light by promptly wrapping the medication container with the supplied opaque sleeve. Sodium nitroprusside should be administered through an infusion pump, preferably a volumetric pump. Consult manufacturer's package insert for complete prescribing information.

Elderly

Use usual dose with caution.

Children

Appropriate studies have not been performed; however, pediatrics-specific problems that would limit the usefulness of this agent in children are not expected.

Preparations

Sodium nitroprusside (generic); Nitropress (Abbott): 50 mg per vial, powder for injection

13. Treprostinil (Remodulin®)

Indications

For the treatment of pulmonary arterial hypertension in patients with NYHA class II-IV symptoms, to diminish symptoms associated with exercise.

Dosage

Adults

The infusion rate is initiated at 1.25 ng/kg/min SQ continuous infusion. The infusion rate is reduced to 0.625 ng/kg/min if not tolerated. The dose can then be titrated by no more than 1.25 ng/kg/min per week for the first 4 weeks, then no more than 2.5 ng/kg/min per week thereafter, depending on the clinical response. The dose should be decreased with excessive pharmacologic effects or with unacceptable infusion site reactions (pain).

Elderly

Use usual dose with caution.

Children

Safety and effectiveness have not been established.

Preparations

Remodulin (United Therapeutics): injection 1 mg/mL, 2.5 mg/mL, 5 mg/mL, 10 mg/mL (20 mL).

Guide to Cardiovascular Drugs Use in Pregnancy and with Nursing

Drugs	Pregnancy	Lactation	Pregnancy Category
α-Adrenergic Antagonists			
Doxazosin	Weigh benefits vs risk	Breastfeeding not recommended; excretion in milk unknown	C
Phenoxybenzamine	Weigh benefits vs risk	Breastfeeding not recommended; excretion in milk unknown	C
Phentolamine	Weigh benefits vs risk	Breastfeeding not recommended; excretion in milk unknown	C
Prazosin	Weigh benefits vs risk	Breastfeed with caution; drug excreted in breast milk	C
Terazosin	Weigh benefits vs risk	Breastfeeding not recommended; excretion in milk unknown	C
α₂-Adrenergic Agonists			
Clonidine	Weigh benefits vs risk	Breastfeed with caution; drug excreted in breast milk	C
Guanabenz	Weigh benefits vs risk	Breastfeeding not recommended; excretion in milk unknown	C
Guanfacine	Use only if clearly indicated	Breastfeeding not recommended; excretion in milk unknown	C
Methyldopa	Weigh benefits vs risk	Breastfeed with caution; drug excreted in breast milk	B(PO), C(IV)
ACE Inhibitors			
Benazepril	The use of ACE inhibitors during the	Breastfeeding not recommended; excretion in milk unknown	C (1st trimester)
Captopril	second and third trimesters of	Breastfeeding not recommended; drug excreted in breast milk	D (2nd, 3rd Trimesters)
Enalapril	pregnancy has been associated with	Breastfeeding not recommended; drug excreted in breast milk	
Fosinopril	fetal and neonatal injury, including	Breastfeeding not recommended; drug excreted in breast milk	
Lisinopril	hypotension, neonatal skull	Breastfeeding not recommended; excretion in milk unknown	
Moexipril	hypoplasia, anuria, reversible or	Breastfeeding not recommended; excretion in milk unknown	
Perindopril	irreversible renal failure and death	Breastfeeding not recommended; excretion in milk unknown	
Quinapril		Breastfeeding not recommended; drug excreted in breast milk	
Ramipril		Breastfeeding not recommended; excretion in milk unknown	
Trandolapril		Breastfeeding not recommended; excretion in milk unknown	
Angiotensin-II-Receptor Blockers			
Candesartan	The use of medications that act	Breastfeeding not recommended; excretion in milk unknown	C (1st trimester)
Eprosartan	directly on the RAS during the	Breastfeeding not recommended; excretion in milk unknown	D (2nd, 3rd trimesters)
Irbesartan	second and third trimesters of	Breastfeeding not recommended; excretion in milk unknown	
Losartan	pregnancy has been associated with	Breastfeeding not recommended; excretion in milk unknown	
Olmesartan	fetal and neonatal injury including	Breastfeeding not recommended; excretion in milk unknown	
Telmisartan	hypotension, neonatal skull	Breastfeeding not recommended; excretion in milk unknown	
Valsartan	hypoplasia, anuria, reversible or	Breastfeeding not recommended; excretion in milk unknown	
	irreversible renal failure, and death.		

(continued)

Drugs	Pregnancy	Lactation	Pregnancy Category
Antiarrhythmic Agents			
Class IA			
Disopyramide	Weigh benefits vs risk	Breastfeeding not recommended; drug excreted in breast milk	C
Procainamide	Weigh benefits vs risk	Breastfeeding not recommended; drug excreted in breast milk	C
Quinidine	Weigh benefits vs risk	Breastfeeding not recommended; drug excreted in breast milk	C
Class IB			
Lidocaine	Use only if clearly indicated	Breastfeed with caution; drug excreted in breast milk	B
Mexiletine	Weigh benefits vs risk	Breastfeeding not recommended; drug excreted in breast milk	C
Tocainide	Weigh benefits vs risk	Breastfeeding not recommended; drug excreted in breast milk	C
Class IC			
Flecainide	Weigh benefits vs risk	Breastfeeding not recommended; drug excreted in breast milk	C
Moricizine	Use only if clearly indicated	Breastfeeding not recommended; drug excreted in breast milk	B
Propafenone	Weigh benefits vs risk	Breastfeeding not recommended; excretion in breast milk unknown	C
Class II (Beta-Blockers)			
Acebutolol	Use only if clearly indicated	Breastfeeding not recommended; drug excreted in breast milk	B
Atenolol	Weigh benefits vs risk	Breastfeeding not recommended; drug excreted in breast milk	C
Betaxolol	Weigh benefits vs risk	Breastfeed with caution; drug excreted in breast milk	C
Bisoprolol	Weigh benefits vs risk	Breastfeeding not recommended; excretion in milk unknown	C
Carteolol	Weigh benefits vs risk	Breastfeeding not recommended; excretion in milk unknown	C
Carvedilol	Weigh benefits vs risk	Breastfeeding not recommended; excretion in milk unknown	C
Esmolol	Weigh benefits vs risk	Breastfeeding not recommended; excretion in milk unknown	C
Labetalol	Weigh benefits vs risk	Breastfeed with caution; drug excreted in breast milk	C
Metoprolol	Weigh benefits vs risk	Breastfeeding not recommended; drug excreted in breast milk	C
Nadolol	Weigh benefits vs risk	Breastfeed with caution; drug excreted in breast milk	C
Penbutolol	Weigh benefits vs risk	Breastfeeding not recommended; excretion in milk unknown	C
Pindolol	Use only if clearly indicated	Breastfeed with caution; drug excreted in breast milk	B
Propranolol	Weigh benefits vs risk	Breastfeed with caution; drug excreted in breast milk	C
Timolol	Weigh benefits vs risk	Breastfeed with caution; drug excreted in breast milk	C
Class III			
Amiodarone	Not recommended	Breastfeeding not recommended; drug excreted in breast milk	D
Bretylium	Weigh benefits vs risk	Breastfeeding not recommended; excretion in milk unknown	C
Dofetilide	Weigh benefits vs risk	Breastfeeding not recommended; drug excreted in breast milk	C
Ibutilide	Weigh benefits vs risk	Breastfeeding not recommended; excretion in milk unknown	C
Sotalol	Use only if clearly indicated	Breastfeeding not recommended; drug excreted in breast milk	B
Class IV (Calcium Antagonists)*			
Amlodipine	Weigh benefits vs risk	Breastfeeding not recommended; excretion in milk unknown	C
Bepridil	Weigh benefits vs risk	Breastfeeding not recommended; drug excreted in breast milk	C
Diltiazem	Weigh benefits vs risk	Breastfeeding not recommended; drug excreted in breast milk	C
Felodipine	Weigh benefits vs risk	Breastfeeding not recommended; excretion in milk unknown	C
Isradipine	Weigh benefits vs risk	Breastfeeding not recommended; excretion in milk unknown	C
Nicardipine	Weigh benefits vs risk	Breastfeeding not recommended; excretion in milk unknown	C
Nifedipine	Weigh benefits vs risk	Breastfeeding not recommended; drug excreted in breast milk	C
Nimodipine	Weigh benefits vs risk	Breastfeeding not recommended; excretion in milk unknown	C
Nisoldipine	Weigh benefits vs risk	Breastfeeding not recommended; excretion in milk unknown	C
Verapamil	Weigh benefits vs risk	Breastfeeding not recommended; drug excreted in breast milk	C

(continued)

Drugs	Pregnancy	Lactation	Pregnancy Category
Antithrombotic Agents			
Anticoagulants			
Argatroban	Use only if clearly needed	Breastfeeding not recommended; excretion in milk unknown	B
Bivalirudin	Use only if clearly needed	Breastfeeding not recommended; excretion in milk unknown	B
Dalteparin	Use only if clearly needed	Breastfeeding not recommended; excretion in milk unknown	B
Danaparoid	Use only if clearly needed	Breastfeeding not recommended; excretion in milk unknown	B
Enoxaparin	Use only if clearly needed	Breastfeeding not recommended; excretion in milk unknown	B
Fondaparinux	Use only if clearly needed	Breastfeeding not recommended; excretion in milk unknown	B
Heparin	Weigh benefits vs risk	Not excreted in breast milk	C
Lepirudin	Use only if clearly needed	Breastfeeding not recommended; excretion in milk unknown	B
Tinzaparin	Use only if clearly needed	Breastfeeding not recommended; excretion in milk unknown	B
Warfarin	Contraindicated	Breastfeeding not recommended; drug excreted in breast milk	X
Antiplatelets			
Anagrelide	Weigh benefits vs risk	Breastfeeding not recommended; excretion in milk unknown	C
Aspirin	Contraindicated in third trimester	Breastfeed with caution; drug excreted in breast milk	D
Abciximab	Weigh benefits vs risk	Breastfeeding not recommended; excretion in milk unknown	C
Clopidogrel	Use only if clearly needed	Breastfeeding not recommended; excretion in milk unknown	B
Dipyridamole	Use only if clearly needed	Breastfeed with caution; drug excreted in breast milk	B
Eptifibatide	Use only if clearly needed	Breastfeeding not recommended; excretion in milk unknown	B
Ticlopidine	Use only if clearly needed	Breastfeeding not recommended; excretion in milk unknown	B
Tirofiban	Use only if clearly needed	Breastfeeding not recommended; excretion in milk unknown	B
Thrombolytics			
Alteplase (t-PA)	Weigh benefits vs risk	Breastfeeding not recommended; excretion in milk unknown	C
Anistreplase	Weigh benefits vs risk	Breastfeeding not recommended; excretion in milk unknown	C
Reteplase	Weigh benefits vs risk	Breastfeeding not recommended; excretion in milk unknown	C
Streptokinase	Weigh benefits vs risk	Breastfeeding not recommended; excretion in milk unknown	C
Tenecteplase	Weigh benefits vs risk	Breastfeeding not recommended; excretion in milk unknown	C
Urokinase	Use only if clearly needed	Breastfeeding not recommended; excretion in milk unknown	B
Diuretics			
Loop			
Bumetanide	Weigh benefits vs risk	Breastfeeding not recommended; excretion in milk unknown	C
Ethacrynic acid	Use only if clearly needed	Breastfeeding not recommended; excretion in milk unknown	B
Furosemide	Weigh benefits vs risk	Breastfeeding not recommended; drug excreted in breast milk	C
Torsemide	Use only if clearly needed	Breastfeeding not recommended; excretion in milk unknown	B
Thiazides			
Bendroflumethiazide	Weigh benefits vs risk	Breastfeed with caution; drug excreted in breast milk	C
Benzthiazide	Weigh benefits vs risk	Breastfeed with caution; drug excreted in breast milk	C
Chlorothiazide	Use only if clearly needed	Breastfeed with caution; drug excreted in breast milk	B
Chlorthalidone	Use only if clearly needed	Breastfeeding not recommended; drug excreted in breast milk	B
Hydrochlorothiazide	Use only if clearly needed	Breastfeed with caution; drug excreted in breast milk	B
Hydroflumethiazide	Weigh benefits vs risk	Breastfeeding not recommended; drug excreted in breast milk	C
Indapamide	Use only if clearly needed	Breastfeeding not recommended; drug excreted in breast milk	B
Methyclothiazide†	Use only if clearly needed	Breastfeeding not recommended; drug excreted in breast milk	B
Metolazone	Use only if clearly needed	Breastfeeding not recommended; drug excreted in breast milk	B

(continued)

Drugs	Pregnancy	Lactation	Pregnancy Category
Polythiazide	Weigh benefits vs risk	Breastfeed with caution; drug excreted in breast milk	D
Quinethazone	Weigh benefits vs risk	Breastfeed with caution; drug excreted in breast milk	D
Trichlormethiazide	Weigh benefits vs risk	Breastfeed with caution; drug excreted in breast milk	C
Potassium-Sparing			
Amiloride	Use only if clearly needed	Breastfeeding not recommended; excretion in milk unknown	B
Spironolactone	Weigh benefits vs risk	Breastfeeding not recommended; drug excreted in breast milk	D
Triamterene	Use only if clearly needed	Breastfeeding not recommended; excretion in milk unknown	B
Endothelin Receptor Antagonist			
Bosentan	Contraindicated	Breastfeeding not recommended; excretion in milk unknown	X
Human B-Type Natriuretic Peptide			
Nesiritide	Weigh benefits vs risk	Breastfeeding not recommended; excretion in milk unknown	C
Inotropic and Vasopressor Agents			
Digoxin	Weigh benefits vs risk	Breastfeed with caution; drug excreted in breast milk	C
Amrinone (Inamrinone)	Weigh benefits vs risks	Breastfeeding not recommended; excretion in milk unknown	C
Milrinone	Weigh benefits vs risk	Breastfeeding not recommended; excretion in milk unknown	C
Dobutamine	Use only if clearly needed	Breastfeeding not recommended; excretion in milk unknown	B
Dopamine	Weigh benefits vs risk	Breastfeeding not recommended; excretion in milk unknown	C
Isoproterenol	Weigh benefits vs risk	Breastfeeding not recommended; excretion in milk unknown	C
Epinephrine	Weigh benefits vs risk	Breastfeed with caution; drug excreted in breast milk	C
Metaraminol	Weigh benefits vs risk	Breastfeeding not recommended; excretion in milk unknown	C
Methoxamine	Weigh benefits vs risk	Breastfeeding not recommended; excretion in milk unknown	C
Midodrine	Weigh benefits vs risk	Breastfeeding not recommended; excretion in milk unknown	C
Norepinephrine	Weigh benefits vs risk	Breastfeeding not recommended; excretion in milk unknown	C
Phenylephrine	Weigh benefits vs risk	Limited absorption in GI tract; excretion in milk unknown	C
Lipid-Lowering Agents			
BAS			
Cholestyramine	Weigh benefits vs risk	Breastfeed with caution; excretion in breast milk unknown	C
Colestipol	Weigh benefits vs risk	Breastfeed with caution; excretion in breast milk unknown	Not evaluated
Colesevelam	Use only if clearly needed	Breastfeed with caution; excretion in breast milk unknown	B
FADS			
Clofibrate	Weigh benefits vs risk	Breastfeeding not recommended; excretion in milk unknown	C
Fenofibrate	Weigh benefits vs risk	Breastfeeding not recommended; excretion in milk unknown	C
Gemfibrozil	Weigh benefits vs risk	Breastfeeding not recommended; excretion in milk unknown	C
Nicotinic Acid	Weigh benefits vs risk	Breastfeed with caution; excretion in milk unknown	C
HMG-CoA Reductase Inhibitors			
Atorvastatin	Contraindicated	Breastfeeding not recommended; excretion in milk unknown	X
Fluvastatin	Contraindicated	Breastfeeding not recommended; drug excreted in breast milk	X
Lovastatin	Contraindicated	Breastfeeding not recommended; excretion in milk unknown	X
Pravastatin	Contraindicated	Breastfeeding not recommended; drug excreted in breast milk	X
Simvastatin	Contraindicated	Breastfeeding not recommended; excretion in milk unknown	X
Neuronal and Ganglionic Blockers			
Guanadrel	Use only if clearly needed	Breastfeeding not recommended; excretion in milk unknown	B
Guanethidine	Weigh benefits vs risk	Breastfeeding not recommended; drug excreted in breast milk	C
Mecamylamine	Weigh benefits vs risk	Breastfeeding not recommended; excretion in milk unknown	C
Reserpine	Weigh benefits vs risk	Breastfeeding not recommended; drug excreted in breast milk	C
Trimethaphan	Not recommended	Breastfeeding not recommended; excretion in milk unknown	D

(continued)

Drugs	Pregnancy	Lactation	Pregnancy Category
Vasodilators			
Cilostazol	Weigh benefits vs risk	Breastfeeding not recommended; excretion in milk unknown	C
Diazoxide	Weigh benefits vs risk	Breastfeeding not recommended; excretion in milk unknown	C
Epoprostenol	Use only if clearly needed	Breastfeeding not recommended; excretion in milk unknown	B
Fenoldopam	Use only if clearly needed	Breastfeeding not recommended; excretion in milk unknown	B
Hydralazine	Weigh benefits vs risk	Breastfeeding not recommended; drug excreted in breast milk	C
Isosorbide Dinitrate	Weigh benefits vs risk	Breastfeeding not recommended; excretion in milk unknown	C
Isosorbide Mononitrate	Weigh benefits vs risk	Breastfeeding not recommended; excretion in milk unknown	C
Isoxsuprine	Weigh benefits vs risk	Breastfeeding not recommended; excretion in milk unknown	C
Minoxidil	Weigh benefits vs risk	Breastfeeding not recommended; drug excreted in breast milk	C
Nitroglycerin	Weigh benefits vs risk	Breastfeeding not recommended; excretion in milk unknown	C
Nitroprusside	Weigh benefits vs risk	Breastfeeding not recommended; excretion in milk unknown	C
Papaverine	Weigh benefits vs risk	Breastfeeding not recommended; excretion in milk unknown	C
Pentoxifylline	Weigh benefits vs risk	Breastfeeding not recommended; drug excreted in breast milk	C
Tolazoline	Weigh benefits vs risk	Breastfeeding not recommended; excretion in milk unknown	C

Pregnancy Categories/US Food and Drug Administration Pregnancy Risk Classification:

B = Either animal reproduction studies have not demonstrated fetal risk or else they have not shown an adverse effect (other than a decrease in fertility). However, there are no controlled studies of pregnant women in the first trimester to confirm these findings and no evidence of risk in the later trimesters.

C = Either animal studies have revealed adverse effects (teratogenic or embryocidal), but there are no confirmatory studies in women, or studies in both animals and women are not available. Because of the potential risk to the fetus, drugs should be given only if justified by potentially greater benefits.

D = Evidence of human fetal risk is available. Despite the risk, benefits from use in pregnant women may be justifiable in select circumstances (e.g., if the drug is needed in a life-threatening situation and/or no other safer acceptable drugs are effective). An appropriate "warning" statement will appear on the labeling.

X = Studies in animals and humans have demonstrated fetal abnormalities and/or evidence of fetal risk based on human experience. Thus, the risk of drug use and consequent fetal harm outweighs any potential benefit, and the drug is contraindicated in pregnant women. An appropriate "contraindicated" statement will appear on the labeling.

*Only diltiazem and verapamil are indicated for arrhythmias.

†The pregnancy category of methyclothiazide has ranged from B to D.

ACE = angiotensin converting enzyme; BAS = bile acid sequestrants; FADS = fibric acid derivatives; HMG-CoA = hydroxymethylglutaryl coenzyme A.

Source: Adapted from Ngo A, Frishman WH, Elkayam E. Cardiovascular pharmacotherapeutic considerations during pregnancy and lactation. In: Frishman WH, Sonnenblick EH, eds. *Cardiovascular Pharmacotherapeutics.* New York: McGraw-Hill, 1997:1309.

Dosing Recommendations of Cardiovascular Drugs in Patients with Hepatic Disease and/or Congestive Heart Failure

Drug	Cirrhosis	CHF
α-Adrenergic Antagonists		
Doxazosin	Usual dose with frequent monitoring	Usual dose with frequent monitoring
Phenoxybenzamine	Usual dose with frequent monitoring	Usual dose with frequent monitoring
Phentolamine	Usual dose with frequent monitoring	Usual dose with frequent monitoring
Prazosin	Usual dose with frequent monitoring	Usual dose with frequent monitoring
Terazosin	Usual dose with frequent monitoring	Usual dose with frequent monitoring
α₂-Adrenergic Agonists		
Clonidine	Usual dose with frequent monitoring	Usual dose with frequent monitoring
Guanabenz	Initiate with lower dose	Usual dose with frequent monitoring
Guanfacine	Initiate with lower dose	Usual dose with frequent monitoring
Methyldopa	Initiate with lower dose	Usual dose with frequent monitoring
ACE Inhibitors		
Benazepril	Usual dose with frequent monitoring	Usual dose with frequent monitoring
Captopril	Usual dose with frequent monitoring	Usual dose with frequent monitoring
Enalapril	Usual dose with frequent monitoring	Usual dose with frequent monitoring
Fosinopril	Usual dose with frequent monitoring	Usual dose with frequent monitoring
Lisinopril	Usual dose with frequent monitoring	Usual dose with frequent monitoring
Moexipril	Dose reduction may be necessary	Usual dose with frequent monitoring
Perindopril	Usual dose with frequent monitoring	Usual dose with frequent monitoring
Quinapril	Usual dose with frequent monitoring	Usual dose with frequent monitoring
Ramipril	Usual dose with frequent monitoring	Usual dose with frequent monitoring
Trandolapril	Initiate with lower dose	Usual dose with frequent monitoring
Angiotensin-II-Receptor Antagonists		
Candesartan	Usual dose with frequent monitoring	Usual dose with frequent monitoring
Eprosartan	Usual dose with frequent monitoring	Usual dose with frequent monitoring
Irbesartan	Usual dose with frequent monitoring	Usual dose with frequent monitoring
Losartan	Initiate with lower dose	Usual dose with frequent monitoring
Olmesartan	Usual dose with frequent monitoring	Usual dose with frequent monitoring
Telmisartan	Dose reduction may be necessary; consider alternative treatment	Dose reduction may be necessary
Valsartan	Usual dose with frequent monitoring	Usual dose with frequent monitoring
Antiarrhythmics		
Adenosine	Usual dose with frequent monitoring	Usual dose with frequent monitoring
Amiodarone	Usual dose with frequent monitoring	Usual dose with frequent monitoring
Atropine	Usual dose with frequent monitoring	Usual dose with frequent monitoring
Bretylium	Usual dose with frequent monitoring	Usual dose with frequent monitoring
Disopyramide	Initiate with lower dose	Dose reduction may be necessary
Dofetilide	Usual dose with frequent monitoring	Usual dose with frequent monitoring
Flecainide	Use lower dose or alternative treatment	Dose reduction may be necessary
Ibutilide	Usual dose with frequent monitoring	Usual dose with frequent monitoring
Lidocaine	Initiate with lower dose	Initiate with lower dose
Mexiletine	Initiate with lower dose	Initiate with lower dose
Moricizine	Use lower dose or alternative treatment	Dose reduction may be necessary
Procainamide	Dose reduction may be necessary	Dose reduction may be necessary
Propafenone	Initiate with lower dose	Contraindicated in uncontrolled CHF

(continued)

Drug	Cirrhosis	CHF
Quinidine	Reduce maintenance dose and monitor serum concentration*	Contraindicated in uncontrolled CHF
Sotalol	Usual dose with frequent monitoring	Contraindicated in uncontrolled CHF
Tocainide	Avoid loading dose; limit dose to 1200 mg/d	Dose reduction may be necessary
Antithrombotics		
Anticoagulants		
Argatroban	Initiate with lower dose	Usual dose with frequent monitoring
Bivalirudin	Usual dose with frequent monitoring	Usual dose with frequent monitoring
Dalteparin	Usual dose with frequent monitoring	Usual dose with frequent monitoring
Danaparoid	Usual dose with frequent monitoring	Usual dose with frequent monitoring
Enoxaparin	Usual dose with frequent monitoring	Usual dose with frequent monitoring
Fondaparinux	Usual dose with frequent monitoring	Usual dose with frequent monitoring
Heparin	Dose reduction may be necessary; titrate dose based on coagulation test results	Usual dose with frequent monitoring
Lepirudin	Usual dose with frequent monitoring	Usual dose with frequent monitoring
Tinzaparin	Usual dose with frequent monitoring	Usual dose with frequent monitoring
Warfarin	Initiate at lower dose	Dose reduction may be necessary
Antiplatelets		
Anagrelide	Dose reduction may be necessary; weigh benefits vs risk when LFT >1.5 times the upper limit of normal	Weigh benefits vs risk; use of anagrelide may cause CHF
Aspirin	Usual dose with frequent monitoring	Usual dose with frequent monitoring
Dipyridamole	Reduce dose with biliary obstruction	Usual dose with frequent monitoring
Ticlopidine	Contraindicated	Usual dose with frequent monitoring
Clopidogrel	Usual dose with frequent monitoring	Usual dose with frequent monitoring
Abciximab	Usual dose with frequent monitoring	Usual dose with frequent monitoring
Eptifibatide	Usual dose with frequent monitoring	Usual dose with frequent monitoring
Tirofiban	Initiate at lower dose	Usual dose with frequent monitoring
Thrombolytics		
Alteplase	Usual dose with frequent monitoring	Usual dose with frequent monitoring
Anistreplase	Dose reduction may be necessary	Usual dose with frequent monitoring
Streptokinase	Dose reduction may be necessary	Usual dose with frequent monitoring
Urokinase	Dose reduction may be necessary	Usual dose with frequent monitoring
Reteplase	Usual dose with frequent monitoring	Usual dose with frequent monitoring
Tenecteplase	Use usual dose with caution; risk of bleeding may increase	Usual dose with frequent monitoring
β-Adrenergic Blockers		
Nonselective		
Nadolol	Usual dose with frequent monitoring	Usual dose with frequent monitoring
Propranolol	Initiate with lower dose	Usual dose with frequent monitoring
Sotalol	Usual dose with frequent monitoring	Usual dose with frequent monitoring
Timolol	Initiate with lower dose	Usual dose with frequent monitoring
β1-Selective		
Atenolol	Usual dose with frequent monitoring	Usual dose with frequent monitoring
Betaxolol	Usual dose with frequent monitoring	Usual dose with frequent monitoring
Bisoprolol	Initiate with lower dose	Usual dose with frequent monitoring
Esmolol	Usual dose with frequent monitoring	Usual dose with frequent monitoring
Metoprolol	Dose reduction may be necessary	Usual dose with frequent monitoring
With ISA: Nonselective		
Carteolol	Usual dose with frequent monitoring	Usual dose with frequent monitoring
Penbutolol	Dose reduction may be necessary	Usual dose with frequent monitoring
Pindolol	Dose reduction may be necessary	Usual dose with frequent monitoring
With ISA: β1-Selective		
Acebutolol	Usual dose with frequent monitoring	Usual dose with frequent monitoring
Dual-Acting		
Carvedilol	Initiate with lower dose	Initiate at lower dose; contraindicated in severely decompensated CHF
Labetalol	Dose reduction may be necessary	Usual dose with frequent monitoring
Calcium-Channel Blockers		
Amlodipine	Initiate with lower dose	Usual dose with frequent monitoring
Bepridil	Dose reduction may be necessary	Contraindicated in uncompensated cardiac insufficiency
Diltiazem	Dose reduction may be necessary	Usual dose with frequent monitoring
Felodipine	Dose reduction may be necessary	Usual dose with frequent monitoring
Isradipine	Dose reduction may be necessary	Usual dose with frequent monitoring

(continued)

Drug	Cirrhosis	CHF
Nicardipine	Initiate with lower dose	Usual dose with frequent monitoring
Nifedipine	Dose reduction may be necessary	Usual dose with frequent monitoring
Nimodipine	Initiate with lower dose	Usual dose with frequent monitoring
Nisoldipine	Initiate with lower dose	Usual dose with frequent monitoring
Verapamil	Initiate with lower dose	Avoid in patients with severe left ventricular dysfunction
Diuretics		
Loop		
Bumetanide, Ethacrynic Acid, Furosemide, Torsemide	May precipitate hepatic coma. Dose reduction is probably not necessary; titrate dosage based on clinical response	Usual dose with frequent monitoring
Thiazide		
Bendroflumethiazide, Benzthiazide, Chlorothiazide, Hydrochlorothiazide, Hydroflumethiazide, Methyclothiazide, Polythiazide, Quinethazone, Trichlormethiazide	May precipitate hepatic coma; diuretic effect is decreased in patients with renal insufficiency (CrCl <30 mL/min). Dosage adjustment is probably not required in hepatic impairment; titrate dosage based on clinical response	Usual dose with frequent monitoring
Indapamide	Dose reduction may be necessary	Usual dose with frequent monitoring
Metolazone	May precipitate hepatic coma; diuretic effect is preserved in patients with renal insufficiency. Dosage adjustment is probably not required in hepatic impairment	Usual dose with frequent monitoring
Potassium-Sparing		
Amiloride	Dose reduction may be necessary	Usual dose with frequent monitoring
Spironolactone	Usual dose with frequent monitoring	Usual dose with frequent monitoring
Triamterene	Usual dose with frequent monitoring	Usual dose with frequent monitoring
Endothelin Receptor Antagonist		
Bosentan	Caution should be exercised during the use of bosentan in patients with mildly impaired liver function. Bosentan should generally be avoided in patients with moderate or severe liver impairment	Usual dose with frequent monitoring
Human B-Type Natriuretic Peptide		
Nesiritide	Cirrhotic patients with ascites and avid sodium retention were shown to have blunted natriuretic response to low-dose brain natriuretic peptide	Usual dose with frequent monitoring
Inotropic Agents and Vasopressors		
Amrinone (inamrinone)	Dose reduction may be necessary	Usual dose with frequent monitoring
Digoxin, dobutamine,	Usual dose with frequent monitoring	Usual dose with frequent monitoring
Dopamine, milrinone	Usual dose with frequent monitoring	Usual dose with frequent monitoring; initiate dopamine at lower dose in patients with chronic heart failure
Midodrine	Usual dose with frequent monitoring	Usual dose with frequent monitoring
Norepinephrine, epinephrine,	Usual dose with frequent monitoring	Usual dose with frequent monitoring
Isoproterenol, metaraminol	Usual dose with frequent monitoring	Usual dose with frequent monitoring
Methoxamine, phenylephrine	Usual dose with frequent monitoring	Usual dose with frequent monitoring
Lipid-Lowering		
BAS		
Cholestyramine	Contraindicated in total biliary obstruction	Usual dose with frequent monitoring
Colestipol	Contraindicated in total biliary obstruction	Usual dose with frequent monitoring
Colesevelam	Contraindicated in total biliary obstruction	Usual dose with frequent monitoring
FADs		
Clofibrate	Contraindicated in clinically significant hepatic dysfunction	Usual dose with frequent monitoring
Fenofibrate	Contraindicated in clinically significant hepatic dysfunction, including primary biliary cirrhosis and in patients with unexplained persistent transaminase elevation.	Unknown
Gemfibrozil	Contraindicated in clinically significant hepatic dysfunction, including primary biliary cirrhosis	Unknown
HMG-CoA Reductase		
Inhibitors		
Atorvastatin, Fluvastatin, lovastatin, Pravastatin, simvastatin	Start at lowest dose and titrate cautiously; contraindicated in patients with active liver disease or unexplained persistent transaminase elevation	Usual dose with frequent monitoring

(continued)

Drug	Cirrhosis	CHF
Nicotinic acid	Use with caution; contraindicated in patients with active liver disease or unexplained persistant transaminase elevation	Usual dose with frequent monitoring
Neuronal and Ganglionic Blockers		
Guanadrel	Usual dose with frequent monitoring	Contraindicated in frank CHF
Guanethidine	Dose reduction may be necessary	Contraindicated in frank CHF
Mecamylamine	Usual dose with frequent monitoring	Usual dose with frequent monitoring
Reserpine	Dose reduction may be necessary	Usual dose with frequent monitoring
Trimethaphan	Dose reduction may be necessary	Contraindicated in severe cardiac disease
Vasodilators		
Alprostadil	Usual dose with frequent monitoring	Usual dose with frequent monitoring
Cilostazol	Usual dose with frequent monitoring	Contraindicated
Diazoxide	Dose reduction may be necessary	Contraindicated in uncompensated CHF
Epoprostenol	Usual dose with frequent monitoring	Contraindicated in severe left ventricular systolic dysfunction
Fenoldopam	Usual dose with frequent monitoring	Usual dose with frequent monitoring
Hydralazine	Dose reduction may be necessary	Higher doses have been used
Isosorbide dinitrate	Use lower dose; avoid in severe hepatic impairment	Used in combination with hydralazine
Isosorbide mononitrate	Caution in severe hepatic impairment	Avoid in acute CHF
Isoxsuprine	Dose reduction may be necessary	Usual dose with frequent monitoring
Minoxidil	Usual dose with frequent monitoring	Usual dose with frequent monitoring
Nitroglycerin	Dose reduction may be necessary; avoid in severe hepatic impairment	Usual dose with frequent monitoring
Sodium nitroprusside	Initiate with lower dose	Usual dose with frequent monitoring
Papaverine	Dose reduction may be necessary	Usual dose with frequent monitoring
Pentoxifylline	Usual dose with frequent monitoring	Unknown
Sildenafil	Initiate with lower dose	Usual dose with frequent monitoring
Tolazoline	Unknown	Unknown

ACE = angiotensin-converting enzyme; BAS = bile acid sequestrants; CHF = congestive heart failure; FADS = fibric acid derivatives; HMG-CoA = hydroxymethylglutaryl coenzyme A; ISA = intrinsic sympathomimetic activity.

*Due to an increased volume of distribution, a larger loading dose of quinidine may be indicated.

Source: Adapted from Frishman WH, Sokol SI. Cardiovascular drug therapy in patients with intrinsic hepatic disease and impaired hepatic function secondary to congestive heart failure. In: Frishman WH, Sonnenblick EH, eds. *Cardiovascular Pharmacotherapeutics.* New York: McGraw-Hill, 1997:1561–1576.

Dose Adjustment in Patients with Renal Insufficiency

Drug	CrCl: 30 to 60 mL/min	CrCl <30 mL/min	Dialyzability (Hemodialysis)
α-Adrenergic Antagonists			
Doxazosin	Use usual dose	Use usual dose	No
Phenoxybenzamine	Use usual dose	Use usual dose	No
Phentolamine	Use usual dose	Use usual dose	No
Prazosin	Use usual dose	Start with low dose and titrate based on response	No
Terazosin	Use usual dose	Use usual dose	No
α₂-Adrenergic Agonists			
Clonidine	Use usual dose	Start with low dose and titrate based on response	No
Guanabenz	Use usual dose	Use usual dose	Unknown
Guanfacine	Use usual dose	Start with low dose and titrate based on response	No
Methyldopa	Use usual dose	Start with low dose and titrate based on response	Yes
Angiotensin-Converting Enzyme Inhibitors			
Benazepril	Use usual dose	Start with low dose and titrate based on response	No*
Captopril	Start with low dose and titrate based on response	Start with low dose and titrate based on response	Yes
Enalapril	Use usual dose	Start with low dose and titrate based on response	Yes
Fosinopril	Use usual dose	Start with low dose and titrate based on response	No
Lisinopril	Use usual dose	Start with low dose and titrate based on response	Yes
Moexipril	For patients with CrCl ≤40 mL/min, start with low dose and titrate based on response	Start with low dose and titrate based on response	Unknown
Perindopril	Start with low dose and titrate based on response	The use of this drug is not recommended because of significant perindoprilat accumulation	Yes
Quinapril	Start with low dose and titrate based on response	Start with low dose and titrate based on response	No
Ramipril	For patients with CrCl <40 mL/min, start with low dose and titrate based on response	Start with low dose and titrate based on response; up to a max of 5 mg/d	Unknown
Trandolapril	Use usual dose	Start with low dose and titrate based on response	Yes (trandolaprilat)
Angiotensin-II-Receptor Blockers			
Candesartan	Use usual dose	Start with low dose and titrate based on response	No
Eprosartan	Use usual dose	Start with low dose and titrate based on response	No
Irbesartan	Use usual dose	Use usual dose	No
Losartan	Use usual dose	Use usual dose	No
Olmesartan	Use usual dose	Start with low dose and titrate based on response; maximum dose should not exceed 20 mg	Unknown
Telmisartan	Use usual dose	Use usual dose with caution	No
Valsartan	Use usual dose	Use usual dose with caution	Unknown (probably no)

(continued)

Drug	CrCl: 30 to 60 mL/min	CrCl <30 mL/min	Dialyzability (Hemodialysis)
Antiarrhythmic Agents			
Adenosine	Use usual dose	Use usual dose	No
Atropine	Use usual dose with caution	Use usual dose with caution	No
Class IA			
Disopyramide	↓ loading dose by 25% to 50% ↓ maintenance dose by 25% or give 100 mg (nonsustained release) q 6 to 8 h	↓ loading dose by 50% to 75% ↓ maintenance dose by 50% to 75% or give 100 mg (nonsustained release) q 12 to 24 h	No*
Procainamide	↑ dosing interval to q 4 to 6 h	↑ dosing interval to q 8 to 24 h	Yes (give maintenance dose after dialysis or supplement with 250 mg post hemodialysis)
Quinidine	Use usual dose	Use usual dose with caution; ↓ maintenance dose by 25% if CrCl <10 mL/min	Yes (give maintenance dose after dialysis or supplement with 200 mg post hemodialysis)
Class IB			
Lidocaine	Use usual dose	Use usual dose with caution	No
Mexiletine	Use usual dose	Reduce dose if CrCl <10 mL/min	No
Tocainide	Use usual dose	↓ 25% to 50% or ↑ dosing interval to q 24 h	Yes (give maintenance dose after dialysis or supplement with 25% of maintenance dose post hemodialysis)
Class IC			
Flecainide	Use usual dose	Initiate with 100 mg q 24 h or 50 mg q 12 h; titrate based on response	No
Moricizine	Use usual dose	Start with low dose and titrate based on response	Unknown
Propafenone	Use usual dose	Use usual dose with caution	No
Class II (β-Adrenergic Antagonists)			
Acebutolol	↓ 50%	↓ 75%	Yes—both acebutolol and diacetolol
Atenolol	Use usual dose with caution	Up to a max of 50 mg q 24 to 48 h	No
Betaxolol	Use usual dose with caution	Up to a max of 20 mg q 24 h	No
Bisoprolol	Use usual dose with caution	Start with low dose and titrate based on response	No
Carteolol	↑ dosing interval to q 48 h	↑ dosing interval to q 48 to 72 h	Unknown
Carvedilol	Use usual dose with caution	Start with low dose and titrate based on response	No
Esmolol	Use usual dose	Use usual dose	No
Labetalol	Use usual dose	Use usual dose	No
Metoprolol	Use usual dose	Use usual dose	No
Nadolol	Use usual dose with caution	↑ dosing interval to q 48 to 72 h	Yes
Penbutolol	Use usual dose	Use usual dose	No
Pindolol	Use usual dose	Use usual dose	Unknown
Propranolol	Use usual dose	Use usual dose	No
Timolol	Use usual dose	Use usual dose	No
Class III			
Amiodarone	Use usual dose	Use usual dose	No
Bretylium	↓ 50%	↓ 50% to 75%	No
Dofetilide	Start with lower dose and titrate based on response	Start with lower dose and titrate based on response; dofetilide is contraindicated in patients with CrCl of <20 mL/min	Unknown
Ibutilide	Use usual dose	Use usual dose with caution	Unknown (probably no)
Sotalol	↑ dosing interval to q 24 h	↑ dosing interval to q 36 to 48 h; individualize dosage for patients with CrCl of <10 mL/min	Yes (give maintenance dose after dialysis or supplement with 80 mg post hemodialysis)
Class IV (Calcium Antagonists†)			
Amlodipine	Use usual dose	Use usual dose with caution	No
Bepridil	Use usual dose	Use usual dose with caution	No
Diltiazem	Use usual dose	Use usual dose with caution	No
Felodipine	Use usual dose	Use usual dose	No

(continued)

Drug	CrCl: 30 to 60 mL/min	CrCl <30 mL/min	Dialyzability (Hemodialysis)
Isradipine	Use usual dose	Use usual dose with caution	No
Nicardipine	Use usual dose	Use usual dose; titrate dose carefully	No
Nifedipine	Use usual dose	Use usual dose	No
Nimodipine	Use usual dose	Use usual dose	No
Nisoldipine	Use usual dose	Use usual dose	No
Verapamil	Use usual dose	Use usual dose with caution	No
Antithrombotic Agents			
Antiplatelet Agents			
Abciximab	Use usual dose	Use usual dose with caution	No
Anagrelide	Weigh benefit vs risk when SCr ≥2 mg/dL	Weigh benefit vs risk when SCr ≥2 mg/dL	Unknown
Aspirin	Use usual dose	Use usual dose with caution	Yes
Clopidogrel	Use usual dose	Use usual dose	No
Dipyridamole	Use usual dose	Use usual dose	No
Eptifibatide	Use lower dose if SCr >2 mg/dL	Contraindicated if SCr >4 mg/dL	Yes
Ticlopidine	Use usual dose	Use with caution; dose reduction may be required	No
Tirofiban	Use usual dose with caution	↓ 50%	Yes
Anticoagulants			
Argatroban	Use usual dose	Use usual dose	Unknown
Bivalirudin	Reduce infusion dose by ≈20%	Reduce infusion dose by ≈60% to 90%	Yes (≈25% removed)
Dalteparin	Use usual dose	Use usual dose with caution; specific recommendations on dosage adjustments are not available	No
Danaparoid	Use usual dose	Use usual dose with caution if SCr ≥2 mg/dL	No
Enoxaparin	Use usual dose	Use with caution; dose reduction may be required (↓ 20% to 30%)	No
Fondaparinux	Use usual dose with caution	Contraindicated	Yes
Heparin	Use usual dose	Use usual dose with caution	No
Lepirudin	Bolus dose: 0.2 mg/kg; Infusion rate: 30% to 50% of usual dose	Bolus dose: 0.2 mg/kg; Infusion rate: 15% of usual dose; Contraindicated if SCr >6 mg/dL	Yes
Tinzaparin	Use usual dose	Use usual dose with caution; specific recommendations on dosage adjustments are not available	No
Warfarin	Use usual dose	Use usual dose with caution	No
Thrombolytic Agents			
Alteplase	Use usual dose with caution	Use usual dose with caution	No
Anistreplase	Use usual dose with caution	Use usual dose with caution	No
Reteplase	Use usual dose with caution	Use usual dose with caution	No
Streptokinase	Use usual dose with caution	Use usual dose with caution	No
Tenecteplase	Use usual dose with caution	Use usual dose with caution	No
Urokinase	Use usual dose with caution	Use usual dose with caution	No
Diuretics (Contraindicated in anuric patients)			
Loop Diuretics			
Bumetanide	Use usual dose	Use usual dose with caution	No
Ethacrynic Acid	Use usual dose	Use usual dose with caution	No
Furosemide	Use usual dose	Use usual dose with caution	No
Torsemide	Use usual dose	Use usual dose with caution	No
Thiazide Diuretics			
Chlorthalidone	Use usual dose with caution	Ineffective	No
Hydrochlorothiazide and similar agents	Use usual dose with caution	Ineffective	No
Indapamide	Use usual dose with caution	Ineffective if CrCl <15 mL/min	No
Metolazone	Use usual dose with caution	Use usual dose with caution	No
Potassium-Sparing Diuretics			
Amiloride	Use usual dose with caution	Contraindicated	Unknown
Spironolactone	Use usual dose with caution	Contraindicated	No
Triamterene	Use usual dose with caution	Contraindicated	Unknown

(continued)

Drug	CrCl: 30 to 60 mL/min	CrCl <30 mL/min	Dialyzability (Hemodialysis)
Endothelin Receptor Antagonist			
Bosentan	Use usual dose	Use usual dose	Unknown (probably no)
Human B-Type Natriuretic Peptide			
Nesiritide	Use usual dose	Use usual dose with caution	Unknown (probably no)
Inotropic Agents and Vasopressors			
Amrinone (Inamrinone)	Start with low dose and titrate based on response	Start with low dose and titrate based on response	No
Digoxin	Use usual dose and titrate based on response	Start with low dose, many patients only need a dose q 48 to 72 h; if loading dose is indicated, ↓ 25%	No
Dobutamine	Use usual dose and titrate based on response	Use usual dose and titrate based on response	Unknown
Dopamine	Use usual dose and titrate based on response	Use usual dose and titrate based on response	No
Epinephrine	Use usual dose with caution	Use usual dose with caution	Unknown
Isoproterenol	Use usual dose with caution	Use usual dose with caution	Unknown
Metaraminol	Start with low dose and titrate to response	Start with low dose and titrate to response	Unknown
Methoxamine	Use usual dose with caution	Use usual dose with caution	Unknown
Midodrine	Start with low dose and titrate based on response	Start with low dose and titrate based on response	Yes—both midodrine and desglymidodrine
Milrinone	↓ 25% to 50%; start with low dose and titrate based on response	↓ 50% to 75%; start with low dose and titrate based on response	Unknown
Norepinephrine	Use usual dose with caution	Use usual dose with caution	Yes
Phenylephrine	Use usual dose with caution	Use usual dose with caution	Unknown
Lipid-Lowering Agents			
BAS			
Cholestyramine	The possibility of hyperchloremic acidosis is increased in patients with renal insufficiency; use usual dose with caution		
Colestipol	The possibility of hyperchloremic acidosis is increased in patients with renal insufficiency; use usual dose with caution		
Colesevelam	The possibility of hyperchloremic acidosis is increased in patients with renal insufficiency; use usual dose with caution		
FADS			
Clofibrate	↑ dosing interval to q 6 to 12 h	↑ dosing interval to q 12 to 24 h; avoid use if CrCl is <10 mL/min	No
Fenofibrate	Start with low dose and titrate based on response	Start with low dose and titrate based on response	No
Gemfibrozil	Use usual dose with caution	Use usual dose with caution	No
HMG-CoA Reductase Inhibitors			
Atorvastatin	Use usual dose	Use usual dose	No
Fluvastatin	Use usual dose	Use usual dose with caution	No
Lovastatin	Use usual dose	Use usual dose with caution	No
Pravastatin	Use usual dose	Use usual dose with caution	No
Simvastatin	Use usual dose	Start with low dose and titrate based on response	No
Nicotinic Acid	Start with low dose and titrate based on response; use with caution	Start with low dose and titrate based on response; use with caution	Unknown
Neuronal and Ganglionic Blockers			
Guanadrel	↑ dosing interval to q 24 h; dosage increments should be made cautiously at intervals ≥7 days	↑ dosing interval to q 48 h; dosage increments should be made cautiously at intervals ≥14 days	Unknown (probably no)
Guanethidine	Start with low dose and titrate based on response	Start with low dose and titrate based on response; use with caution	Unknown
Mecamylamine	Start with low dose and titrate based on response	Start with low dose and titrate based on response; use with caution, if at all	Unknown
Reserpine	Use usual dose	Use usual dose with caution; avoid use if CrCl is <10 mL/min	No

(*continued*)

Drug	CrCl: 30 to 60 mL/min	CrCl <30 mL/min	Dialyzability (Hemodialysis)
Trimethaphan	Start with low dose and titrate based on response	Start with low dose and titrate based on response; use with caution	Unknown
Vasodilators			
Alprostadil	Individualize dose	Individualize dose	Unknown
Cilostazol	Use usual dose	Use usual dose with caution. Patients on hemodialysis have not been studied.	No
Diazoxide	Start with low dose and titrate based on response	Start with low dose and titrate based on response; use with caution	No
Epoprostenol	Individualize dose	Individualize dose	Unknown
Fenoldopam	Individualize dose	Individualize dose	Unknown
Hydralazine	↑ dosing interval to q 6 to 8 h	↑ dosing interval to q 8 to 24 h	No
Isosorbide dinitrate	Use usual dose	Start with low dose and titrate based on response; use with caution	Unknown
Isosorbide mononitrate	Use usual dose	Use usual dose with caution	No
Isoxsuprine	Start with low dose and titrate based on response	Start with low dose and titrate based on response; use with caution	Unknown
Minoxidil	Use usual dose	Start with low dose and titrate based on response	No
Nitroglycerin	Use usual dose	Use usual dose with caution	No
Nitroprusside	Start with low dose and titrate based on response; use with caution	Start with low dose and titrate based on response; use with caution	Yes
Papaverine	Use usual dose	Use usual dose with caution	Unknown
Pentoxifylline	Use usual dose	Use usual dose with caution	Unknown
Sildenafil	Use usual dose	Start with low dose and titrate based on response	No
Tolazoline	Start with low dose and titrate based on response; use with caution. Specific dosing guidelines are lacking	Start with low dose and titrate based on response; use with caution. Specific dosing guidelines are lacking	Unknown

BAS = bile acid sequestrants; CrCl = creatinine clearance; FAD = fibric acid derivatives; HMG-CoA = hydroxymethylglutaryl coenzyme A; SCr = serum creatinine.

*Hemodialysis does not remove appreciable amounts of this drug. However, dialysis may be considered in overdosed patients with severe renal impairment.

†Only diltiazem and verapamil are indicated for arrhythmias.

Selected Cardiovascular Medications and Gender Issues

Drug	Evidence for Efficacy in Women	Considerations when Treating Women
Antiplatelet Drugs		
Aspirin	Primary Prevention: US Nurses' Cohort shows decreased MI*	Women have higher rate of hemorrhagic stroke than men; Physician's Health Study showed an increased risk of bleeding when on aspirin; increased risk of bleeding at term in pregnancy; present in breast milk
	Secondary CAD Prevention: Decreases reinfarction[†]	
Glycoprotein IIb/IIIa antagonists	Effective in women undergoing PTCA	Women have higher risk than men with PTCA, but benefit as much from treatment
Agents that Affect Blood Pressure		
ACE Inhibitors	Post-MI: decreased mortality[†]	Cough is two to three times greater in women; increased fetal abnormalities possible; present in breast milk
	CHF: decreased mortality[†]	
Angiotensin-II-Receptor Blockers		Increased fetal abnormalities possible
Beta-Blockers	Antihypertension: effective in preventing MI, CVA, and death in women[†]	Present in breast milk; blood levels of propranolol may be higher in men
	Post-MI: decreases mortality[†]	
Calcium Blockers	Increased risk of MI in women[†]	Edema may be more common in women; verapamil clearance may be greater in women than in men; present in breast milk
	Increased effect of amlodipine in women in reducing blood pressure[†]	
Clonidine	No data about efficacy in women	Inability to achieve orgasm; possible decreased craving for tobacco more common in women[†]
Thiazide Diuretics	Decreased CVA, MI, death[†]	Decreased urinary calcium excretion; women have greater increase in risk of gout; acute pulmonary edema and allergic interstitial pneumonitis is more common in women; excreted in breast milk
Guanethidine		Orthostatic hypotension more common in women
Hydralazine	Effective in hypertension in pregnancy and peripartum	SLE more common in women than men; present in breast milk
Methyldopa	Often preferred in pregnancy for treating hypertension	Painful breast enlargement; decreased libido
Nitrates	Decreased mortality after MI[†]	Potential for difference in metabolism in women
Antiarrhythmic Agents		
Disopyramide	No data looking at efficacy in women	Complication of torsade de pointes more frequent in women[†]
Procainamide	No gender-specific data available	Drug-induced SLE more common in women
Quinidine	No gender-specific data available	Torsade de pointes more common in women; clearance may be faster in women; present in breast milk
Conjugated Estrogens		
	Increased HDL-cholesterol decreases total cholesterol and lipoprotein*	Need for progestin in women with intact uterus to prevent endometrial abnormalities
	Post-MI: not effective*	
	Primary prevention: ineffective	
Hypolipidemic Agents		
Colestipol	No effect on primary prevention[†]	
Clofibrate	Effective in secondary prevention in women[†]	
HMG-CoA	Primary and secondary prevention:	Gastrointestinal side effects more common in women
Reductase	Possible efficacy in women[†]	
Inhibitors	Decreases cholesterol and slows plaque progression without respect to gender	
Nicotine Preparations	Gum equally effective in women[†]	Gum may suppress weight gain; not recommended in pregnancy
	Patch effective in women[†]	

CAD = coronary artery disease; CVA = cerebrovascular accident; HDL = high-density lipoprotein; HMG-CoA = hydroxymethylglutaryl coenzyme A; MI = myocardial infarction; PTCA = percutaneous transluminal coronary angioplasty; SLE = systemic lupus erythematosus; US = United States.

*Studies of efficacy in women.

[†]Studies of efficacy in both men and women, with analysis by gender.

Source: Adapted from Charney P, Meyer BR, Frishman WH, Ginsberg A, Eastwood B: Gender, race and genetic issues in cardiovascular pharmacotherapy. In: Frishman WH, Sonnenblick EH, eds. *Cardiovascular Pharmacotherapeutics.* New York: McGraw-Hill, 1997:1350–1351.

Pharmacokinetic Changes, Route of Elimination, and Dosage Adjustment of Selected Cardiovascular Drugs in the Elderly

Drug	$T_{1/2}$	V_D	Cl	Primary Route(s) of Elimination	Dosage Adjustment
α-Adrenergic Antagonists					
Doxazosin	↑	↑	↑*	Hepatic	Initiate at lowest dose; titrate to response
Prazosin	↑	—	—	Hepatic	Initiate at lowest dose; titrate to response
Terazosin	↑	—	—	Hepatic	Initiate at lowest dose; titrate to response
α₂-Adrenergic Agonists					
Clonidine	—	—	—	Hepatic/renal	Initiate at lowest dose; titrate to response
Guanabenz	—	—	—	Hepatic	Initiate at lowest dose; titrate to response
Guanfacine	↑	—	↓	Hepatic/renal	Initiate at lowest dose; titrate to response
Methyldopa	—	—	—	Hepatic	Initiate at lowest dose; titrate to response
Angiotensin-Converting Enzyme Inhibitors					
Benazepril	↑	—	↓	Renal	No initial dosage adjustment is needed
Captopril	NS	—	↓	Renal	Initiate at lowest dose; titrate to response
Enalapril	—	—	—	Renal	Initiate at lowest dose; titrate to response
Fosinopril	—	—	—	Hepatic/renal	No initial dosage adjustment is needed
Lisinopril	↑	NS	↓	Renal	Initiate at lowest dose; titrate to response
Moexipril	—	—	—	Hepatic/renal	Initiate at lowest dose; titrate to response
Perindopril	—	—	↓	Renal	Initiate at lowest dose; titrate to response
Quinapril	—	—	—	Renal	Initiate at lowest dose; titrate to response
Ramipril	—	—	—	Renal	Initiate at lowest dose; titrate to response
Trandolapril	—	—	—	Hepatic/renal	Initiate at lowest dose; titrate to response
Angiotensin-II- Receptor Blockers					
Candesartan	—	—	—	Hepatic/renal	No initial dosage adjustment is needed
Eprosartan	—	—	—	Hepatic/biliary/renal	No initial dosage adjustment is needed
Irbesartan	NS	—	—	Hepatic	No initial dosage adjustment is needed
Losartan	—	—	—	Hepatic	No initial dosage adjustment is needed
Olmesartan	—	—	—	Renal/biliary	No initial dosage adjustment is needed
Telmisartan	—	—	—	Hepatic/biliary	No initial dosage adjustment is needed
Valsartan	↑	—	—	Hepatic	No initial dosage adjustment is needed
Antiarrhythmic Agents					
Class I					
Disopyramide	↑	—	↓	Renal	Initiate at lowest dose; titrate to response
Flecainide	↑	↑	↓	Hepatic/renal	Initiate at lowest dose; titrate to response
Lidocaine	↑	↑	NS	Hepatic	Initiate at lowest dose; titrate to response
Mexiletine	—	—	—	Hepatic	Initiate at lowest dose; titrate to response
Moricizine	—	—	—	Hepatic	Initiate at lowest dose; titrate to response
Procainamide	—	—	↓	Renal	Initiate at lowest dose; titrate to response
Propafenone	—	—	—	Hepatic	Initiate at lowest dose; titrate to response
Quinidine	↑	NS	↓	Hepatic	Initiate at lowest dose; titrate to response
Tocainide	↑	—	↓	Hepatic/renal	Initiate at lowest dose; titrate to response
Class II (see Beta-Blockers)					
Class III					
Amiodarone	—	—	—	Hepatic/biliary	Initiate at lowest dose; titrate to response
Bretylium	—	—	—	Renal	Initiate at lowest dose; titrate to response
Dofetilide	—	—	—	Renal	Adjust dose based on renal function

(continued)

Drug	T$_{1/2}$	V$_D$	Cl	Primary Route(s) of Elimination	Dosage Adjustment
Ibutilide	—	—	—	Hepatic	No adjustment needed
Sotalol	—	—	—	Renal	Adjust dose based on renal function
Class IV (see Calcium Channel Blockers)					
Other Antiarrhythmics					
Adenosine	—	—	—	Erythrocytes/vascular endothelial cells	No adjustment needed
Atropine	—	—	—	Hepatic/renal	Use usual dose with caution
Antithrombotics					
Anticoagulants					
Argatroban	—	—	—	Hepatic/biliary	Use usual dose with caution
Bivalirudin	—	—	—	Renal/proteolytic cleavage	Adjust dose based on renal function
Dalteparin	—	—	—	Renal	Use usual dose with caution
Danaparoid	NS	NS	NS	Renal	Use usual dose with caution
Enoxaparin	—	—	—	Renal	Use usual dose with caution
Fondaparinux	↑	—	↓	Renal	Use usual dose with caution
Heparin	—	—	—	Hepatic/reticuloendothelial system	Use usual dose with caution
Lepirudin	↑	—	↓	Renal	Adjust dose based on renal function
Tinzaparin	—	—	—	Renal	Use usual dose with caution
Warfarin	NS	NS	NS	Hepatic	Initiate at lowest dose; titrate to response
Antiplatelets					
Abciximab	—	—	—	Unknown	Use usual dose with caution
Anagrelide	—	—	—	Hepatic/renal	Use usual dose with caution
Aspirin	—	—	↓	Hepatic/renal	Use usual dose with caution
Clopidogrel	NS	—	—	Hepatic	Use usual dose with caution
Dipyridamole	—	—	—	Hepatic/biliary	Use usual dose with caution
Eptifibatide	—	—	—	Renal/plasma	Use usual dose with caution
Ticlopidine	—	—	↓	Hepatic	Use usual dose with caution
Tirofiban	↑	—	↓	Hepatic	Use usual dose with caution
Thrombolytics					
Alteplase	—	—	—	Hepatic	Use usual dose with caution
Anistreplase	—	—	—	Unknown	Use usual dose with caution
Reteplase	—	—	—	Hepatic	Use usual dose with caution
Streptokinase	—	—	—	Circulating antibodies/ reticuloendothelial system	Use usual dose with caution
Tenecteplase	—	—	—	Hepatic	Use usual dose with caution
Urokinase	—	—	—	Hepatic	Use usual dose with caution
β-Adrenergic Blockers					
Nonselective without ISA					
Nadolol	NS	—	—	Renal	Initiate at lowest dose; titrate to response
Propranolol	↑	NS	↓	Hepatic	Initiate at lowest dose; titrate to response
Timolol	—	—	—	Hepatic	Initiate at lowest dose; titrate to response
β$_1$-Selective Without ISA					
Atenolol	↑	NS	↓	Renal	Initiate at lowest dose; titrate to response
Betaxolol	—	—	—	Hepatic	Initiate at lowest dose; titrate to response
Bisoprolol	—	—	—	Hepatic/renal	Initiate at lowest dose; titrate to response
Esmolol	—	—	—	Erythrocytes	Use usual dose with caution
Metoprolol	NS	NS	NS	Hepatic	Initiate at lowest dose; titrate to response
Nonselective with ISA					
Carteolol	—	—	—	Renal	Initiate at lowest dose; titrate to response
Penbutolol	—	—	—	Hepatic	Use usual dose with caution
Pindolol	—	—	—	Hepatic/renal	Initiate at lowest dose; titrate to response
β$_1$-Selective with ISA					
Acebutolol	↑	↓	—	Hepatic/biliary	Initiate at lowest dose; titrate to response
Dual-Acting					
Carvedilol	—	—	—	Hepatic/biliary	Initiate at lowest dose; titrate to response
Labetalol	—	—	NS	Hepatic	No initial dosage adjustment is needed
Calcium-Channel Blockers					
Amlodipine	↑	—	↓	Hepatic	Initiate at lowest dose; titrate to response
Bepridil	—	—	—	Hepatic	Use usual dose with caution
Diltiazem	↑	NS	↓	Hepatic	Initiate at lowest dose; titrate to response
Felodipine	—	NS	↓	Hepatic	Initiate at lowest dose; titrate to response

(continued)

Drug	$T_{1/2}$	V_D	Cl	Primary Route(s) of Elimination	Dosage Adjustment
Isradipine	—	—	—	Hepatic	Initiate at lowest dose; titrate to response
Nicardipine	NS	—	—	Hepatic	No initial dosage adjustment is needed
Nifedipine	↑	NS	↓	Hepatic	Initiate at lowest dose; titrate to response
Nimodipine	—	—	—	Hepatic	Use usual dose with caution
Nisoldipine	—	—	—	Hepatic	Initiate at lowest dose; titrate to response
Verapamil	↑	NS	↓	Hepatic	Initiate at lowest dose; titrate to response
Diuretics					
Loop					
Bumetanide	—	NS	—	Renal/hepatic	Initiate at lowest dose; titrate to response
Ethacrynic Acid	—	—	—	Hepatic	Initiate at lowest dose; titrate to response
Furosemide	↑	NS	↓	Renal	Initiate at lowest dose; titrate to response
Torsemide	—	—	—	Hepatic	Initiate at lowest dose; titrate to response
Thiazides					
Bendroflumethiazide	—	—	—	Renal	Initiate at lowest dose; titrate to response
Benzthiazide	—	—	—	Unknown	Initiate at lowest dose; titrate to response
Chlorothiazide	—	—	—	Renal	Initiate at lowest dose; titrate to response
Chlorthalidone	—	—	—	Renal	Initiate at lowest dose; titrate to response
Hydrochlorothiazide	—	—	↓	Renal	Initiate at lowest dose; titrate to response
Hydroflumethiazide	—	—	—	Unknown	Initiate at lowest dose; titrate to response
Indapamide	—	—	—	Hepatic	Initiate at lowest dose; titrate to response
Methyclothiazide	—	—	—	Renal	Initiate at lowest dose; titrate to response
Metolazone	—	—	—	Renal	Initiate at lowest dose; titrate to response
Polythiazide	—	—	—	Unknown	Initiate at lowest dose; titrate to response
Quinethazone	—	—	—	Unknown	Initiate at lowest dose; titrate to response
Trichlormethiazide	—	—	—	Unknown	Initiate at lowest dose; titrate to response
Potassium-Sparing					
Amiloride	—	—	↓	Renal	Initiate at lowest dose; titrate to response
Spironolactone	—	—	—	Hepatic/biliary/renal	Initiate at lowest dose; titrate to response
Triamterene	↑	—	—	Hepatic/renal	Initiate at lowest dose; titrate to response
Endothelin Receptor Antagonist					
Bosentan	—	—	—	Hepatic/biliary	Use usual dose with caution
Human B-Type Natriuretic Peptide					
Nesiritide	—	—	—	Cellular internalization and lysosomal proteolysis/proteolytic cleavage/renal filtration	Use usual dose with caution
Inotropic and Vasopressor Agents					
Amrinone (Inamrinone)	—	—	—	Hepatic/renal	Initiate at lowest dose; titrate to response
Digoxin	↑	↓	↓	Renal	Initiate at lowest dose; titrate to response
Dobutamine	—	—	—	Hepatic/tissue	Initiate at lowest dose; titrate to response
Dopamine	—	—	—	Renal/hepatic/plasma	Initiate at lowest dose; titrate to response
Epinephrine	—	—	—	Sympathetic nerve endings/ hepatic/plasma	Initiate at lowest dose; titrate to response
Isoproterenol	—	—	—	Renal	Initiate at lowest dose; titrate to response
Metaraminol	—	—	—	Hepatic/biliary/renal	Initiate at lowest dose; titrate to response
Methoxamine	—	NS	—	Unknown	Initiate at lowest dose; titrate to response
Midodrine	—	—	—	Tissue/hepatic/renal	No initial dosage adjustment is needed
Milrinone	—	—	—	Renal	Adjust based on renal function
Norepinephrine	—	—	—	Sympathetic nerve endings/ hepatic/plasma	Initiate at lowest dose; titrate to response
Phenylephrine	—	—	—	Hepatic/intestinal	Initiate at lowest dose; titrate to response
Lipid-Lowering Drugs					
BAS					
Cholestyramine	—	—	—	Not absorbed from GI tract	No adjustment needed
Colestipol	—	—	—	Not absorbed from GI tract	No adjustment needed
Colesevelam	—	—	—	Not absorbed from GI tract	No adjustment needed
FADS					
Clofibrate	—	—	—	Hepatic/renal	Adjust based on renal function
Fenofibrate	—	—	—	Renal	No adjustment necessary
Gemfibrozil	—	—	—	Hepatic/renal	No adjustment necessary
Nicotinic Acid	—	—	—	Hepatic/renal	No initial dosage adjustment is needed

(continued)

Drug	$T_{1/2}$	V_D	Cl	Primary Route(s) of Elimination	Dosage Adjustment
HMG-CoA Reductase					
Inhibitors					
Atorvastatin	↑	—	—	Hepatic/biliary	No initial dosage adjustment is needed
Fluvastatin	—	—	—	Hepatic	No initial dosage adjustment is needed
Lovastatin	—	—	—	Hepatic/fecal	No initial dosage adjustment is needed
Pravastatin	—	—	—	Hepatic	Initiate at lowest dose; titrate to response
Simvastatin	—	—	—	Hepatic/fecal	Initiate at lowest dose; titrate to response
Neuronal and Ganglionic					
Blockers					
Guanadrel	—	—	—	Hepatic/renal	Initiate at lowest dose; titrate to response
Guanethidine	—	—	—	Hepatic/renal	Initiate at lowest dose; titrate to response
Mecamylamine	—	—	—	Renal	Initiate at lowest dose; titrate to response
Reserpine	—	—	—	Hepatic/fecal	Initiate at lowest dose; titrate to response
Trimethaphan	—	—	—	Hepatic/renal	Initiate at lowest dose; titrate to response
Vasodilators					
Alprostadil	—	—	—	Pulmonary/renal	Initiate at lowest dose; titrate to response
Cilostazol	—	—	—	Hepatic	No adjustment necessary
Diazoxide	—	—	—	Hepatic/renal	Initiate at lowest dose; titrate to response
Epoprostenol	—	—	—	Hepatic/renal	Initiate at usual dose with caution
Fenoldopam	—	—	—	Hepatic	No adjustment necessary
Hydralazine	—	—	—	Hepatic	Initiate at lowest dose; titrate to response
ISDN	—	—	—	Hepatic	Initiate at lowest dose; titrate to response
ISMN	NS	—	NS	Hepatic	No adjustment necessary
Isoxsuprine	—	—	—	Renal	Initiate at lowest dose; titrate to response
Minoxidil	—	—	—	Hepatic	Initiate at lowest dose; titrate to response
Nitroglycerin	—	—	—	Hepatic	Initiate at lowest dose; titrate to response
Nitroprusside	—	—	—	Hepatic/renal/erythrocytes	Use usual dose with caution
Papaverine	—	—	—	Hepatic	Initiate at lowest dose; titrate to response
Pentoxifylline	—	—	↓	Hepatic/renal	Use usual dose with caution
Sildenafil	—	—	—	Hepatic/fecal	Initiate at lowest dose; titrate to response

*Increase in Cl is small when compared to increase in V_D; $T_{1/2}$ = half-life; V_D = volume of distribution; Cl = clearance; ↑ = increase; ↓ = decrease; — = no information or not relevant; BAS = bile acid sequestrants; FADS = fibric acid derivatives; GI = gastrointestinal; HMG-CoA = hydroxymethylglutaryl coenzyme A; ISA = intrinsic sympathomimetic activity; ISDN = isosorbide dinitrate; ISMN = isosorbide mononitrate; LMWH = low-molecular-weight heparin; NS = no significant change.

Selected Cardiovascular Medications and Ethnic Issues

Drug or Drug Class	Evidence of Efficacy in Various Ethnic Groups	Consideration in Treatment
α-Adrenergic Antagonists	Prazosin is less effective in blacks.	Blacks may need higher doses, generally a second-line agent.
Beta-Blockers		
Propranolol	No difference in plasma concentrations of propranolol between Malays, Indians, and Chinese.	Blacks may need higher doses of propranolol to achieve same effects as whites.
	Compared to white patients, black patients have lower plasma concentration of propranolol when this drug is taken orally.	
	S-isomer clears more slowly than R-isomer. All metabolic pathways have higher metabolic rates in blacks as compared to whites.	
	Chinese have lower plasma concentrations and higher clearance of propranolol, mainly secondary to increased ring oxidation and conjugation.	
Metoprolol	No differences in metabolism of metoprolol between whites and blacks in the United States. Chinese have a higher incidence of slow metabolizers (with one or two copies of CYP2D6*10) and have significantly higher plasma concentrations of R- and S-metoprolol.	Lower doses of metoprolol required in Chinese.
	The S-isomer (which confers beta-blocking activity) reaches higher concentrations than the R-isomer. In poor metabolizers, there is a lasting effect after 24 hours, which correlates with reduced clearance of the S-isomer.	
Others	Response of blacks to other beta-blockers is similar to the response of whites.	Carvedilol can be used in blacks for heart failure.
	Labetalol seems to be effective in blacks.	Bucindolol should be avoided in blacks with advanced heart failure.
	Carvedilol was effective in CHF treatment in all subgroups.	
	In blacks, bucindolol was worse than placebo in advanced heart failure.	
	Unusually high plasma concentrations of alprenolol and timolol have been found in subjects with CYP2D6-poor metabolizer phenotype.	
	The plasma concentrations and the degree of beta-blockade were greater in subjects with the CYP2D6-PM-phenotype taking timolol.	
Calcium-Channel Blockers	Nifedipine clearance is faster in whites than in blacks.	Nifedipine might be a good initial treatment for hypertension in Asians, Hispanics, and blacks.
	South Asians, Mexicans, and Nigerians have higher drug exposure and longer half-life, when compared with whites.	Diltiazem may not be a good choice in young white patients.
	Diltiazem is less effective in younger white men when compared to blacks.	
Diuretics	Blacks respond better to thiazide diuretics than do whites.	Good initial choice for antihypertensive therapy in blacks.
Antiarrhythmics	Propafenone concentrations elevated in poor metabolizers of dextromorphan in a Chinese population and CNS side effects were more frequent.	Close observation of side effects may be warranted in CYP2D6-intermediate metabolizers, such as many Asians, and in CYP2D6-poor metabolizers.
	Poor metabolizers of propafenone have a higher incidence of side effects.	

(continued)

Drug or Drug Class	Evidence of Efficacy in Various Ethnic Groups	Consideration in Treatment
	Encainide extensive metabolizers accumulate active metabolites that lead to more QRS-widening.	
	Poor metabolizers of flecainide have higher drug exposure and longer half-lives.	
Warfarin	Mean maintenance dose of warfarin in Chinese subjects is around 3.1 mg vs 6.1 mg in whites.	Use lower warfarin doses in Chinese.
Aspirin	In Nigerians, overall excretion (particularly the glucuronide conjugate) is higher in males than in females.	Some populations may have increased side effects or decreased effectiveness.
ACE-Inhibitors and Angiotensin-Receptor Blockers (ARB)	Fosinoprilat has lower clearance and distribution volume in Chinese as compared to whites.	Chinese may need lower doses.
	Less antihypertensive effect in blacks at lower doses. However, the antihypertensive effect of ACE inhibitors is increased when a diuretic is given concurrently.	Blacks may need additional drug (such as a diuretic) to achieve blood pressure control.
	ACE-inhibitors may not be as effective in blacks as in whites for heart failure, which might partially explain worse outcome of left ventricular dysfunction in blacks.	Alternative or additional therapy in blacks with left ventricular dysfunction may be needed.

Index

Index

Note: Page numbers followed by *f* indicate figures; page numbers followed by *t* indicate tables.

ISBN 0-07-136981-3

90000

9 780071 369817

FRISHMAN/CARDIOVASCULAR PHARM 2/E